Medical-Surgical Nursing

Volume 2

Assessment and Management
of Clinical Problems

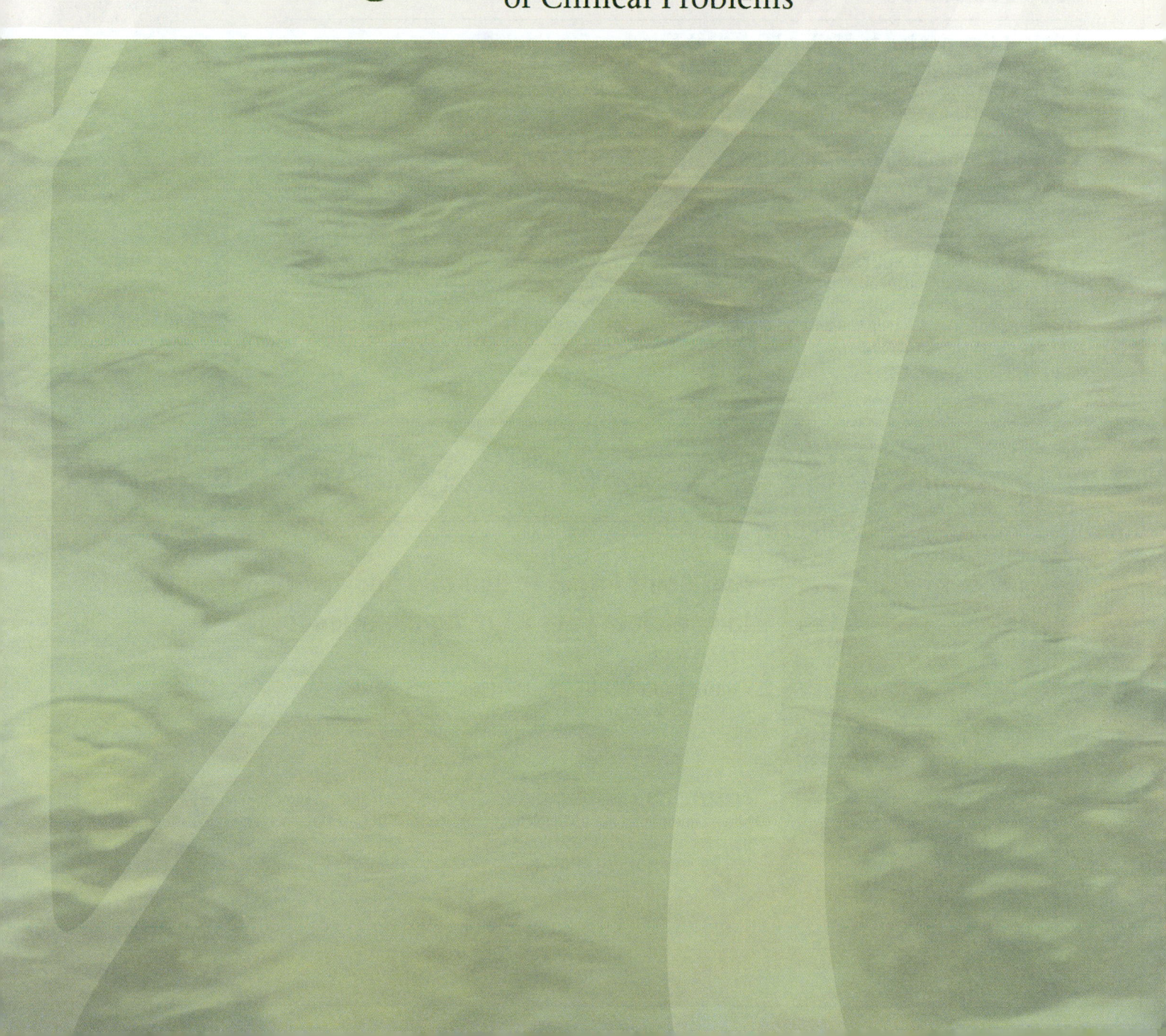

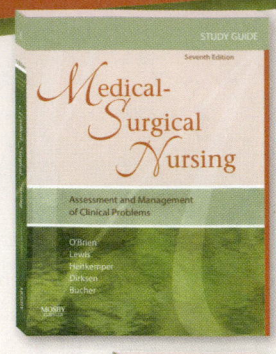
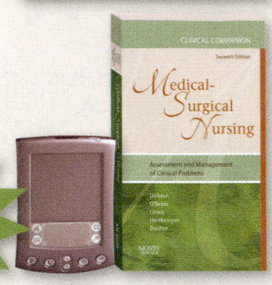
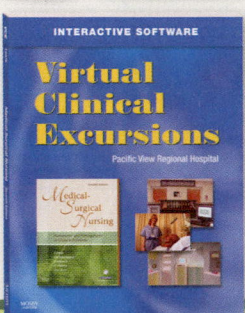
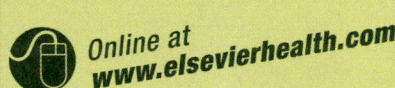
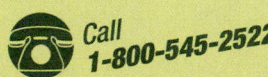
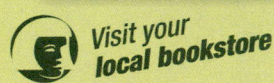
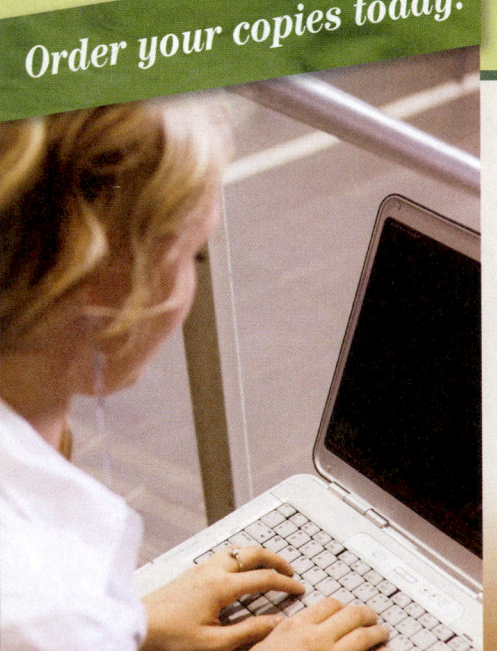
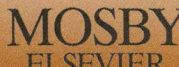

Seventh Edition

Medical-Surgical Nursing

Volume **2**

Assessment and Management of Clinical Problems

Sharon L. Lewis, RN, PhD, FAAN

Professor, Schools of Nursing and Medicine
Castella Distinguished Professor in Nursing
University of Texas Health Science Center at San Antonio;
Clinical Nurse Scientist
Geriatric Research, Education, and Clinical Center
South Texas Veterans Health Care System
San Antonio, Texas

Margaret McLean Heitkemper, RN, PhD, FAAN

Professor and Chairperson, Biobehavioral Nursing and Health Systems
Elizabeth Sterling Soule Endowed Chair in Nursing
School of Nursing;
Adjunct Professor, Division of Gastroenterology
School of Medicine
University of Washington
Seattle, Washington

Shannon Ruff Dirksen, RN, PhD

Associate Professor, College of Nursing and Health Care Innovation
Arizona State University
Phoenix, Arizona

Patricia Graber O'Brien, APRN-BC, MA, MSN

Instructor, College of Nursing
University of New Mexico;
Clinical Research Coordinator
Lovelace Scientific Resources
Albuquerque, New Mexico

Linda Bucher, RN, DNSc

Associate Professor
School of Nursing
University of Delaware;
Nursing Research Facilitator
Christiana Care Health System
Newark, Delaware

MOSBY
ELSEVIER

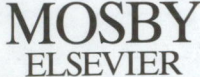

11830 Westline Industrial Drive
St. Louis, Missouri 63146

MEDICAL-SURGICAL NURSING: ASSESSMENT AND
MANAGEMENT OF CLINICAL PROBLEMS
**Copyright © 2007, 2004, 2000, 1996, 1992, 1987, 1983 by Mosby, Inc., an affiliate
of Elsevier Inc.**

ISBN: 978-0-323-03688-7

Notice

Knowledge and best practice in this field are constantly changing. As new research and experience broaden
our knowledge, changes in practice, treatment and drug therapy may become necessary or appropriate.
Readers are advised to check the most current information provided (i) on procedures featured or (ii) by the
manufacturer of each product to be administered, to verify the recommended dose or formula, the method
and duration of administration, and contraindications. It is the responsibility of the practitioner, relying on
their own experience and knowledge of the patient, to make diagnoses, to determine dosages and the best
treatment for each individual patient, and to take all appropriate safety precautions. To the fullest extent of
the law, neither the Publisher nor the Authors assume any liability for any injury and/or damage to persons
or property arising out or related to any use of the material contained in this book.

The Publisher

ISBN: 978-0-323-03688-7

Executive Publisher: Robin Carter
Acquisitions Editor: Kristin Geen
Senior Developmental Editor: Lauren Lake
Publishing Services Manager: Jeffrey Patterson
Senior Project Manager: Mary Stueck
Cover Design Director: Mark Oberkrom
Text Designer: Paula Ruckenbrod

Printed in China

Last digit is the print number: 9 8 7 6 5 4 3 2

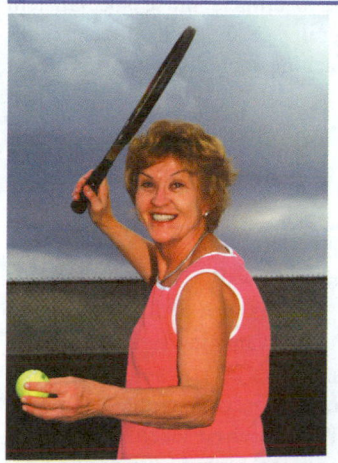

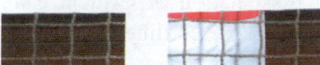

SHARON L. LEWIS, RN, PhD, FAAN

Sharon Lewis is Professor, Schools of Nursing and Medicine and Castella Distinguished Professor at the University of Texas Health Science Center–San Antonio and Clinical Nurse Scientist at the Geriatric Research, Education, and Clinical Center at the South Texas Veterans Health Care System. She received her Bachelor of Science in nursing from the University of Wisconsin-Madison, Master of Science in nursing with a minor in biological sciences from the University of Colorado-Denver, and PhD in immunology from the Department of Pathology at the University of New Mexico School of Medicine. She had a 2-year postdoctoral fellowship from the National Kidney Foundation. Her more than 35 years of teaching experience include inservice education and teaching in associate degree, baccalaureate, master's degree, and doctoral programs in Maryland, Illinois, Wisconsin, New Mexico, and Texas. Favorite teaching areas are pathophysiology, immunology, renal disease, and caregiving. She has been actively involved in clinical research for the past 25 years, investigating altered immune responses in various disorders. Her current research focus is on the newly emerging field of psychoneuroimmunology. At this time she is using biofeedback and immune parameters to study the effects of relaxation therapy and stress management for caregivers of patients with Alzheimer's and Parkinson's disease. Her free time is spent playing tennis, landscaping, and gardening.

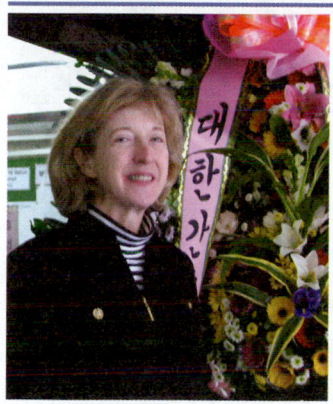

MARGARET McLEAN HEITKEMPER, RN, PhD, FAAN

Margaret Heitkemper is Professor and Chairperson, Department of Biobehavioral Nursing and Health Systems at the School of Nursing, and Adjunct Professor, Division of Gastroenterology at the School of Medicine at the University of Washington. She is also Director of the National Institutes of Health–National Institute for Nursing Research–funded Center for Women's Health and Gender Research at the University of Washington. In the fall of 2006, Dr. Heitkemper was appointed the Elizabeth Sterling Soule Endowed Chair in Nursing. Dr. Heitkemper received her Bachelor of Science in nursing from Seattle University, a Master of Science in gerontologic nursing from the University of Washington, and a doctorate in Physiology and Biophysics from the University of Illinois at the Medical Center, Chicago. She has been on faculty at the University of Washington since 1981 and has been the recipient of three School of Nursing Excellence in Teaching awards and the University of Washington Distinguished Teaching Award. In addition, in 2002 she received the Distinguished Nutrition Support Nurse Award from the American Society for Parenteral and Enteral Nutrition (ASPEN), in 2003 the American Gastroenterological Association and Janssen Award for Clinical Research in Gastroenterology, and in 2005 she was the first recipient of the Pfizer and Friends of the National Institutes for Nursing Research Award for Research in Women's Health.

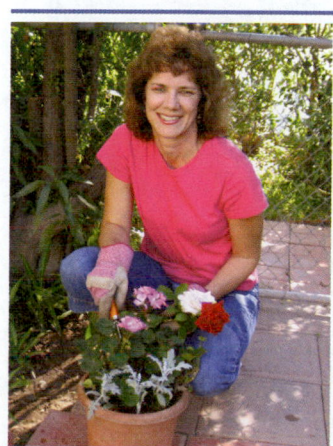

SHANNON RUFF DIRKSEN, RN, PhD

Shannon Dirksen is Associate Professor at the College of Nursing and Health Care Innovation, Arizona State University. She received her Bachelor of Science in nursing from Arizona State University, Master of Science in nursing from the University of Arizona, and doctorate in nursing with a minor in psychology from the University of Arizona. She has over 20 years of undergraduate and graduate teaching experience at the University of Arizona, Edith Cowan University (Western Australia), Intercollegiate College of Nursing–Washington State University, and University of New Mexico. She has been on the faculty at Arizona State University since 1996. She currently teaches management and leadership, and nursing research, including evidence-based practice. Her research focuses on cancer survivorship, with current studies examining behavioral interventions that positively impact insomnia, fatigue, mood, and quality of life in persons diagnosed with breast and prostate cancer. In her free time, she enjoys gardening, reading, and bicycling.

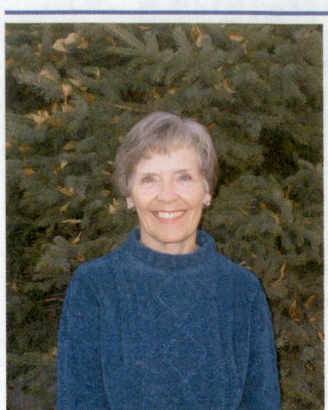

PATRICIA GRABER O'BRIEN, APRN-BC, MA, MSN

Patricia O'Brien retired from Albuquerque Technical-Vocational Institute, a community college, in 1993, and continues to teach part-time at the College of Nursing at the University of New Mexico. She is also employed part-time as a clinical research coordinator at Lovelace Scientific Resources in Albuquerque. She received her Bachelor of Science in nursing from the University of Kansas, Master of Arts in adult education from the University of New Mexico, and Master of Science in nursing with majors in medical-surgical nursing and nursing administration from the University of Texas at El Paso. During her nursing career, she has worked in medical-surgical nursing and home health care, but most of her experience is in nursing education. She is a certified clinical nurse specialist in medical-surgical nursing. She has directed and taught in nursing programs of all levels of basic nursing preparation for more than 30 years. Her primary interests in teaching include nursing process, pharmacology, and metabolic problems.

LINDA BUCHER, RN, DNSc

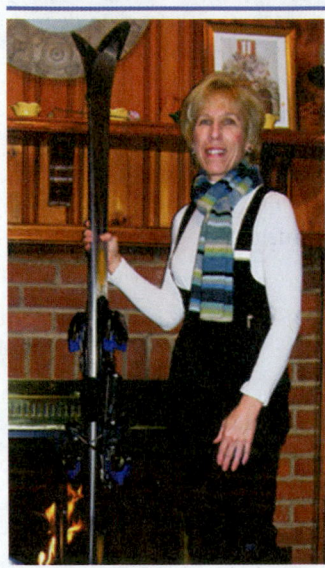

Linda Bucher has a joint appointment as an Associate Professor at the University of Delaware and a Nursing Research Facilitator at Christiana Care Health Services, both in Newark, Delaware. She received her Bachelor of Science in nursing from Thomas Jefferson University in Philadelphia, her Master of Science in adult health and illness from the University of Pennsylvania in Philadelphia, and her DNSc in nursing from Widener University in Chester, Pennsylvania. Her 26 years of nursing experience has spanned staff and patient education, and teaching in associate, baccalaureate, and graduate nursing programs in New Jersey, Pennsylvania, and Delaware. Her preferred teaching areas include cardiac and emergency nursing and research. She maintains her clinical practice by working per diem as an emergency nurse, is an active member of the American Association of Critical Care Nurses, and enjoys working as a volunteer nurse for Operation Smile. In her free time, she enjoys traveling and skiing with her family.

Margaret M. Andrews, RN, PhD, CTN, FAAN
Professor of Nursing and Director, Department of Nursing
School of Health Professions and Studies
The University of Michigan
Flint, Michigan

Richard B. Arbour, RN, MSN, CCRN, CNRN
Staff Nurse/Clinical Researcher
Albert Einstein Healthcare Network
Philadelphia, Pennsylvania

Margaret Wooding Baker, RN, PhD
Assistant Professor, School of Nursing
Biobehavioral Nursing and Health Systems Department
University of Washington
Seattle, Washington

Bobbie Berkowitz, RN, PhD, FAAN
Alumni Endowed Professor of Nursing, School of Nursing
University of Washington
Seattle, Washington

Paula Blackwell, BS, MBA, MT(ASCP)
Senior Research Assistant
University of Texas Health Science Center at San Antonio
San Antonio, Texas

Audrey J. Bopp, RN, MSN, CNS
Assistant Professor of Nursing
University of Northern Colorado
Greeley, Colorado

Elisabeth G. Bradley, APRN-BC, MS, CCRN
Clinical Nurse Specialist, Cardiology/Critical Care
Christiana Care Health System
Newark, Delaware

Lucy Bradley-Springer, RN, PhD, ACRN, FAAN
Associate Professor of Medicine
University of Colorado Health Sciences Center;
Principal Investigator
Mountain Plains AIDS Education and Training Center
Denver, Colorado

Linda Bucher, RN, DNSc
Associate Professor
School of Nursing
University of Delaware
Nursing Research Facilitator
Christiana Care Health System
Newark, Delaware

Elizabeth Burkhart, RN, MPH, PhD
Assistant Professor
Marcella Niehoff School of Nursing
Loyola University–Chicago
Chicago, Illinois

Jormain Cady, ARNP, MS, AOCN
Nurse Practitioner
Department of Radiation Oncology
Virginia Mason Medical Center
Seattle, Washington

Sharon G. Childs, APRN-BC, MS, NP/CS, ONC
Adult, Acute Care Nurse Practitioner
The Sports Center
Baltimore, Maryland

Janet T. Crimlisk, RN, MS, NP-C, APRN-BC
Clinical Nurse Specialist
Boston Medical Center
Boston, Massachusetts

Paula Cox-North, RN, MN, NP-C
Advanced Registered Nurse Practitioner
Pacific Medical Centers
Seattle, Washington

Anne Croghan, ARNP, MN
Nurse Practitioner
Seattle Gastroenterology Associates
Seattle, Washington

Shannon Ruff Dirksen, RN, PhD
Associate Professor, College of Nursing and
    Health Care Innovation
Arizona State University
Phoenix, Arizona

Angela J. DiSabatino, RN, MS
Manager, Cardiovascular Research and Database
Christiana Care Health System
Newark, Delaware

Laura Dulski, RNC, MSN
Instructor
West Suburban College of Nursing
Oak Park, Illinois

Stephanie A. Elms, RN, MSN
Clinical Instructor, School of Nursing
Acute Care Department
University of Texas Health Science Center
San Antonio, Texas

Connie Engelking, RN, MS, OCN
President
The CHE Group, Inc
Mt. Kisco, New York

Mary Ersek, RN, PhD
Director of Research, Center for Nursing Excellence
Swedish Medical Center
Seattle, Washington

Ellen Fineout-Overholt, RN, PhD
Associate Professor of Clinical Nursing, College of Nursing and
    Health Care Innovation
Director, Center for the Advancement of Evidence-Based
    Practice
Arizona State University
Phoenix, Arizona

Hatice Y. Foell, ARNP-C, MSN
Nurse Practitioner
Diagnostic and Interventional Cardiology
Melbourne, Florida

Kathleen M. Geib, RN, DNSc
Associate Professor
Palm Beach Atlantic University
West Palm Beach, Florida

Shari Goldberg, RN, MS
Women's Health Nurse Practitioner;
Assistant Professor, Department of Nursing
Colby-Sawyer College
New London, New Hampshire

Peggi Guenter, RN, PhD, CNSN
Managing Editor for Special Projects
American Society for Parenteral and Enteral Nutrition
Silver Spring, Maryland

Elise F. Hazzard, ARNP-C, MS, ONC
Dermatology ARNP
Bloomingdale Medical Associates
Riverview, Florida

Margaret McLean Heitkemper, RN, PhD, FAAN
Professor and Chairperson, Biobehavioral Nursing and
    Health Systems
Elizabeth Sterling Soule Endowed Chair in Nursing
School of Nursing;
Adjunct Professor, Division of Gastroenterology
School of Medicine
University of Washington
Seattle, Washington

Sherry Garrett Hendrickson, APRN-BC, PhD
Assistant Professor of Clinical Nursing, School of Nursing
University of Texas at Austin
Austin, Texas

Mary Ann House-Fancher, ACNP, MSN, CCRN-CSC
Adult Acute Care Nurse Practitioner
Division of Cardio-Thoracic Surgery
University of Florida
Gainesville, Florida

Valerie Bender Howard, RN, MSN
Clinical Assistant Professor, Nursing
Robert Morris University
Moon Township, Pennsylvania

**Gordon A. Irving, MD, MB, BS, FFA(SA), MMed, MSc,
Diplomate ABA, ABPM, ABA Certificate in Pain
Management**
Clinical Associate Professor, Department of Anesthesiology
University of Washington School of Medicine;
Medial Director, Swedish Pain and Headache Center
Swedish Medical Center
Seattle, Washington

Vicki Y. Johnson, RN, PhD, CUCNS
Assistant Professor
University of Alabama School of Nursing at Birmingham
Birmingham, Alabama

Jane Steinman Kaufman, RN, MS, CS, ANP
Clinical Associate Professor, School of Nursing
University of North Carolina
Chapel Hill, North Carolina

Jack R. Kless, CRNA, MA, MSN
Instructor/Program Director
Frances Payne Bolton School of Nursing
Case Western Reserve University
Cleveland, Ohio

Judy A. Knighton, RegN, MScN
Clinical Nurse Specialist–Burns
Ross Tilley Burn Centre
Sunnybrook and Women's College
Health Sciences Centre
Toronto, Ontario, Canada

JoAnne Konick-McMahan, RN, MSN, CCRN
Staff Nurse–Respiratory Unit
Harrisburg Hospital, Pinnacle Health System
Harrisburg, Pennsylvania

Jennifer Kretzschmar, BBA
Senior Research Data Management Coordinator
University of Texas Health Science Center at San Antonio
San Antonio, Texas

Nancy Stoetzner Kupper, RN, MSN
Associate Professor of Nursing
Tarrant Community College
Fort Worth, Texas

Linda Laskowski-Jones, RN, MS, APRN-BC, CCRN, CEN
Vice President, Emergency, Trauma, and Aeromedical Services
Christiana Care Health System
Newark, Delaware

Sharon L. Lewis, RN, PhD, FAAN
Professor, Schools of Nursing and Medicine
Castella Distinguished Professor in Nursing
University of Texas Health Science Center at San Antonio;
Clinical Nurse Scientist
Geriatric Research, Education, and Clinical Center
South Texas Veterans Health Care System
San Antonio, Texas

Kathy Lucke, RN, PhD
Associate Dean for Academic Programs and Administration,
    School of Nursing
University of Texas Medical Branch
Galveston, Texas

Nancy J. MacMullen, RN, APN, CNS, PhD
Assistant Professor
Governors State University
University Park, Illinois

Linda Griego Martinez, RN, MSN, CCRN, APRN-BC
Clinical Nurse Specialist
Presbyterian Heart Group
Albuquerque, New Mexico

Terran R. Mathers, RN, DNS
Associate Professor, Division of Nursing
Spring Hill College
Mobile, Alabama

Cynthia Matthews WHNP, MSN
Nurse Practitioner
The Breast Center
Marietta, Georgia

De Ann Mitchell, RN, PhD
Professor of Nursing
Tarrant Community College
Fort Worth, Texas

Teri A. Murray, RN, PhD
Associate Director, School of Nursing
Doisy College of Health Sciences
Saint Louis University
St. Louis, Missouri

Sherry Neely, RN, MSN, CRNP
Assistant Professor
Butler County Community College
Butler, Pennsylvania

Janice A. Neil, RN, PhD
Associate Professor
East Carolina University
Greenville, North Carolina

Diane K. Newman, RNC, MSN, CRNP, FAAN
Co-Director
Penn Center for Continence and Pelvic Health, Division of
    Urology
University of Pennsylvania Medical Center
Philadelphia, Pennsylvania

Patricia Graber O'Brien, APRN-BC, MA, MSN
Instructor, College of Nursing
University of New Mexico;
Clinical Research Coordinator
Lovelace Scientific Resources
Albuquerque, New Mexico

Maureen Reilly, RN, PhD, MHS, CRNA
Associate Professor, United States Army Graduate Program in
    Anesthesia Nursing
University of Texas Health Science Center at Houston
Houston, Texas

Kathleen A. Rich, RN, DNSc, CCNS, CCRN, CEN, CNN
Cardiovascular Clinical Nurse Specialist
LaPorte Regional Health System
LaPorte, Indiana

Nancy C. Robbins, RN, MSN, CFNP, CDE
Family Nurse Practitioner
Virginia Beach Family Practice
Virginia Beach, Virginia

Dottie Roberts, MSN, MACI, RN, CMSRN, OCNS-C
Clinical Nurse Specialist
Rehabilitative and Medical Services
Palmetto Health Baptist Medical Center
Columbia, South Carolina

Sandra Irene Rome, RN, MN, AOCN
Clinical Nurse Specialist, Hematology/Oncology
Cedars-Sinai Medical Center
Los Angeles, California

Julie T. Sanford, RN, DNS
Associate Professor
College of Nursing
University of South Alabama
Mobile, Alabama

Marilee Schmelzer, RN, PhD
Associate Professor, School of Nursing
The University of Texas at Arlington
Arlington, Texas

Alyce Schultz, RN, PhD, FAAN
Clinical Professor, College of Nursing and Health Care
    Innovation
Associate Director, Center for the Advancement of
    Evidence-Based Practice
Arizona State University
Phoenix, Arizona

Maureen A. Seckel, RN, MSN, APRN-BC, CCNS, CCRN
Clinical Nurse Specialist, Medical Critical Care/Pulmonary
Christiana Care Health System
Newark, Delaware

Cory A. Shaw, MSTOM, L.Ac.
Laboratory Technical Assistant, Acute Nursing
University of Texas Health Science Center
Traditional Chinese Medicine Practitioner, Licensed
    Acupuncturist
San Antonio, Texas

Virginia Shaw, RN, MSN
Assistant Professor, School of Nursing
University of Texas Health Science Center
San Antonio, Texas

Brenda K. Shelton, RN, MS, AOCN, CCRN
Clinical Nurse Specialist
The Sidney Kimmel Comprehensive Cancer Center at
    Johns Hopkins
Baltimore, Maryland

Anita J. Shoup, RN, MSN, CNOR
Clinical Nurse Consultant
Regent Medical
Edmonds, Washington

Barbara Sinni-McKeehen, ARNP, MSN, DNC
Dermatology Nurse Practitioner/Clinical Administrator
Bay Pines VAMC
Bay Pines, Florida

Debra J. Smith, RN, MSN, CCRN
Instructor, College of Nursing
University of New Mexico
Albuquerque, New Mexico

Sarah C. Smith, RN, MA, CRNO
Advanced Practice Nurse/Educational Associate
Department of Ophthalmology
University of Iowa Healthcare
Iowa City, Iowa

Cheryl Ross Staats, RN, MSN, APRN-BC
Associate Professor/Clinical
Department of Acute Nursing Care
University of Texas Health Science Center at San Antonio
San Antonio, Texas

Colleen R. Walsh RN, MSN, ONC, CS, ACNP-BC
Faculty, Graduate Nursing, School of Nursing and
    Health Professions
University of Southern Indiana
Evansville, Indiana

Deirdre D. Wipke-Tevis, RN, PhD, BC
Associate Professor, Sinclair School of Nursing
University of Missouri-Columbia
Columbia, Missouri

Reviewers

Kathryn C. Anderson, RN, CEN, BA, AD, ACLS
Vernon, New Jersey

Lisa Anderson-Shaw, RN, DrPh
Chicago, Illinois

Margaret M. Andrews, RN, PhD, CTN
Flint, Michigan

Helen Wash Asbury, RN, ASN, BSHA, MSN, LNC
Albuquerque, New Mexico

Robert B. Babiak, RN, BSN, CWOCN
San Antonio, Texas

Martha C. Beeker, RN, PhD, CCRN, APRN
Springfield, Missouri

Marietta Bell-Scriber, MSN, APRN-BC, PhD
Big Rapids, Michigan

Nancy Mansueto Berg, RN, MSN, ANCC
Williston, Vermont

Mary-Liz Bilodeau, RN, MS, CCRN, CCNS, CS, BC
Boston, Massachusetts

Audrey J. Bopp, RN, MSN, CNS
Greeley, Colorado

Alexandra Bowen, RN, CGRN
Charleston, South Carolina

Josie M. Bowman, RN, DSN
Greenville, North Carolina

Caralee Brommé, RN, MSN, CCRN
Oakland, California

Janet Witucki Brown, RN, PhD
Knoxville, Tennessee

Karen R. Bruni, RN, MSN, NP, CVN
Albany, New York

Quincealea Brunk, RN, PhD
Valdosta, Georgia

Kathryn Bucks, RN, PhD
Columbia, Missouri

Teresa S. Burckhalter, RN, MSN, C
Beaufort, South Carolina

Barbara J. Burgel, RN, MS, COHNS, FAAN
San Francisco, California

Elizabeth Burkhart, RN, MPH, PhD
Chicago, Illinois

Jormain Cady, ARNP, MS, AOCN
Seattle, Washington

Susan Gallagher Camden, RN, PhD
Houston, Texas

Carolyn Carty, RN, MSN, CEN
Marlton, New Jersey

Sheila M. Choppala, RN, PhD
Vancouver, Washington

Phyllis L. Christianson, MN, ANCC, ARNP
Seattle, Washington

Maureen Chrzanowski, RN, MSN, CNM, FNP
Grand Rapids, Michigan

Mary Ciechanowski, RN, MSN, APRN-BC, CCRN
Newark, Delaware

Katherine M. Crawford, RN, MSN
Newark, Delaware

Virginia Crocker, RN, MS, CEN
Winchester, Massachusetts

Nancy Curry, RN, MSN
Shreveport, Louisiana

Judi Daniels, PhD, ARNP-BC
Lexington, Kentucky

Gayle H. Dasher, RN, PhD, CCRN, CNRN
San Antonio, Texas

Angele H. Davis, RN, MSN, CCRN
Thibodaux, Louisiana

Rhonda S. Davis, RN, MSN
Decatur, Alabama

David Derrico, RN, MSN
Gainesville, Florida

Louise Diehl-Oplinger, RN, MSN, CCRN, APRN-BC
Easton, Pennsylvania

Rose Ann DiMaria, RN, PhD, CNSN
Charleston, West Virginia

Angela J. DiSabatino, RN, MS
Newark, Delaware

Kelly Dodds, RN, MSN, APRN-BC
St Louis, Missouri

Cynthia L. Donell, RN, MSN
Reading, Pennsylvania

Penny Downer, APRN-BC, MSN,
Sidney, Michigan

MaryAnne Dudley, RN, MSN
Cheyenne, Wyoming

Sharon Dudley-Brown, APRN-BC, PhD, FNP
Washington, DC

Patti Eisenberg, APRN-BC, MSN
Indianapolis, Indiana

Marsha L. Ellett, RN, DNS, CGRN
Indiana Pohls, Indiana

Peggy Ellis, RN, PhD, FNP, ANP
St. Louis, Missouri

Coleen R. Elmers, RN, MSN
San Antonio, Texas

Stephanie A. Elms, RN, MSN
San Antonio, Texas

Christy H. Erickson, RN, MSN, NP, AOCN
Burlington, Vermont

Susan A. Ezzone, RN, MS, CNP
Columbus, Ohio

Kathryn Feigenbaum, CGRN, MSN
Bethesda, Maryland

Eleanor R. Fitzpatrick, RN, MSN, CRNP, CCRN
Philadelphia, Pennsylvania

Jan Foecke, RN, MS, ONC
Kansas City, Kansas

Karen Lee Fontaine, RN, MSN, ASSECT
Hammond, Indiana

Rebecca A. Fountain, RN, MSN
Tyler, Texas

John J. Gallagher, RN, MSN, CCNS, CCRN, RRT
Philadelphia, Pennsylvania

Cathy Garcia, RN-BC, CNA BC
Tyler, Texas

Beverly George-Gay, RN, MSN, CCRN
Richmond, Virginia

Eileen P. Geraci, MA, ANP-C, PhD(c)
Danbury, Connecticut

Shari Goldberg, RN, MS
New London, New Hampshire

Karen E. Greco, RN, MN, PhD, ANP
Portland, Oregon

Mary Ellen Grohar-Murray, RN, PhD
St. Louis, Missouri

Shelia Grossman, PhD, APRN-BC
Fairfield, Connecticut

Kathleen Halcomb, APRN-BC, MSN
Richmond, Kentucky

Margaret T. Haynes, RN, BSN, MN
Jackson, Mississippi

Judy Hendricks, MS, ANP, CDE
Newark, Delaware

Sherry Garrett Hendrickson, APRN-BC, PhD
Austin, Texas

Frank D. Hicks, RN, PhD
Chicago, Illinois

Doris Leal Hill, RN, PhD, CNOR
Bloomington, Minnesota

Janice J. Hoffman, RN, PhD
Baltimore, Maryland

Sandra Hoffman, APRN-BC, MSN
Chapel Hill, North Carolina

Linda M. Hoke, RN, PhD, CCRN
Philadelphia, Pennsylvania

M. Catherine Hough, RN, PhD
Jacksonville, Florida

Robert M. Hovis, CRNA
St. Louis, Missouri

Valerie M. Howard, RN, MSN
Pittsburgh, Pennsylvania

Sarah M. Howell, RN, MSN
Columbus, Mississippi

Donna Walker Hubbard, RN, MSN, CNN
Belton, Texas

Beth Hurley, BSN, CRNO, COE
Phoenix, Arizona

Patricia Jansen, APRN, CS, MS, BC
San Jose, California

Suzanne L. Jed, APRN-BC, MSN, FNP
Denver, Colorado

Ann-Marie John, RN, MS
Rochester, New York

Jane Steinman Kaufman, RN, MS, CS, ANP
Chapel Hill, North Carolina

Colleen Keller, RN, PhD, ANCC
Phoenix, Arizona

Mary Ellen Kern, RN, MSN, CCRN, APRN
Philadelphia, Pennsylvania

Jack R. Kless, CRNA, MA, MSN
Cleveland, Ohio

Paula Scharf Kohn, RN, PhD
Pleasantville, New Jersey

JoAnne Konick-McMahan, RN, MSN, CCRN
Harrisburg, Pennsylvania

Caroline Kuhlman, APRN-BC, MS, AOCN
Boston, Massachusetts

Kristine L. Kwekkeboom, RN, PhD
Iowa City, Iowa

Judy M. LaBonte, APRN-BC, MSN, FNP
Memphis, Tennessee

Linda LaCasse, RN, MSN
New Britain, Connecticut

Ann Marie Lagonegro, RN-C, MS, FNP
Rochester, New York

Linda Laskowski-Jones, RN, MS, APRN-BC, CCRN, CEN
Newark, Delaware

Canelia Layton, RN, MSN, PNP
Texas City, Texas

Kathleen Lopez-Bushnell, RNC (FNP), MPH, COHN-S, EdD
Albuquerque, New Mexico

Carolyn M. Lowe, RN, BSN, CDE
San Antonio, Texas

Joyce A. Marrs, APRN-BC, MS, AOCNP
Dayton, Ohio

Jeanne M. Martinez, RN, MPH, CHPN
Chicago, Illinois

Dorothy Mathers, RN, MSN
Williamsport, Pennsylvania

Terran R. Mathers, RN, DNS
Mobile, Alabama

Cynthia Matthews RN, MSN, NP
Kennesaw, Georgia

Barbara Maxwell, RNC, CNS, MSN
Stone Ridge, New York

Anthony W. McGuire, RN, MSN, CCRN, ACNP
Orange, California

Margaret A. Medvedev, RN, MSN
Carthage, Texas

Brenda Michel, RN, EdD
Springfield, Illinois

Douglas W. Mitchell, RN, MSN
Phoenix, Arizona

Diana King Mixon, RN, MSN
Boise, Idaho

Leigh W. Moore, RN, MSN, CNOR
Alberta, Virginia

Debra A. Morgan, RN, EdD
Wichita Falls, Texas

Mary L. Moser-Gautreauz, RN, EdD, CEN, CNS
Albuquerque, New Mexico

Anne C. Muller, RN, MSN, CRNP, CNS
Philadelphia, Pennsylvania

Claire Murphy-Marshall, (BScHons) RN
Perth, Western Australia

Teri A. Murray, RN, PhD
St. Louis, Missouri

Sherry Neely, RN, MSN, CRNP
Butler, Pennsylvania

Janice A. Neil, RN, PhD
Greenville, North Carolina

Geri B. Neuberger, RN, EdD
Kansas City, Kansas

Diane Newman, RNC, MSN, CRNP, FAAN
Philadelphia, Pennsylvania

Marian O'Rourke, RN, CCTC
New Orleans, Louisiana

Barbara Owens, RN, PhD, OCN
San Antonio, Texas

Judith A. Paice, RN, PhD, FAAN
Chicago, Illinois

Elizabeth A. Palmer, RN, PhD
Indiana, Pennsylvania

Barbara Pope, RN, MSN, CCRN, CCNS
Philadelphia, Pennsylvania

Renee Pozza, RN, PhD, CNS, CFNP
Azusa, California

Barbara D. Powe, RN, PhD
Atlanta, Georgia

Lola M. Prince, APRN-BC, PhD(c), FNP
Chicago, Illinois

Virginia E. Printz-Feddersen, RN, MSN, CNS
Albuquerque, New Mexico

Cynthia Zackrison Pritchett, RN, MSN
Mobile, Alabama

Dana Reeves, RN, MSN
Fort Smith, Arkansas

Darryl E. Reid, Sr., RN, MSN
San Antonio, Texas

Diane Reynolds, RN, MS, OCN
Brooklyn, New York

Donna Ricketts, RN, MSN
Richmond, Kentucky

Janet Riggs, RN, MSN, CCRN, CCNS
Philadelphia, Pennsylvania

Nancy C. Robbins, RN, MSN, CFNP, CDE
Virginia Beach, Virginia

Dana Rosdahl, RN, PhD, APRN-BC
Phoenix, Arizona

Kathleen Rourke, RN, BSN, ANP, ONC
Boston, Massachusetts

Judith L. Roy, RN, BSN, BC
Scarborough, Maine

Kathleen K. Salati, MSN, CCRN, NP-C
Newark, Delaware

Julie T. Sanford, RN, DNS
Mobile, Alabama

Bette A. Schans, PhD, RT(R)
Grand Junction, Colorado

Teri W. Scott, RN, MSN, FNP-C, COHN-S
Kansas City, Missouri

Lucinda Seidl, RN, MSN
Lincoln, Nebraska

Camille A. Servodidio, RN, MPH, CRNO, OCN
Hartford, Connecticut

Virginia Shaw, RN, MSN
San Antonio, Texas

Mary Shelkey, ARNP, PhD
Seattle, Washington

Brenda K. Shelton, RN, MS, CCRN, AOCN
Baltimore, Maryland

Tamara Shields, RN, MSN, CFNP
Lafayette, Indiana

Deborah Shows-Rushing, RN, MSN
Troy, Alabama

Barbara Sinni-McKeehen, ARNP, MSN, DNC
Bay Pines, Florida

Susan E. Sitter, RN, MSN
Edinboro, Pennsylvania

Diana Kristin Smith, RN, MSN, CDE, APRN-BC
Wilmington, Delaware

Julie S. Snyder, RN, MSN, BC
Norfolk, Virginia

Sheryl Sommer, RN, PhD
Chicago, Illinois

Debra Gartman Spring, RN, MS
Jackson, Mississippi

Darrell Spurlock, RN, MSN, CCRN, CEN
Columbus, Ohio

Susan K. Steele, RN, DNS, AOCN
New Orleans, Louisiana

Mary M. Sullivan-Whalen, RN, MSN, FNP
New York, New York

Suzanne Sutherland, RN, PhD, CCRN
Sacramento, California

Cheryl Swallow, RN, MSN
St. Louis, Missouri

Karen K. Swenson, RN, PhD(c), AOCN
St. Louis Park, Minnesota

Joanne Thanauaro, RN, MSN, CS, ANP
St. Louis, Missouri

Georgianna M. Thomas, RN, EdD
Oak Park, Illinois

Tamekia L. Thomas, RN, BSN
Newark, Delaware

Rosie Thompson, RN, MS, CS
Kansas City, Kansas

Cheryl L. Touhy, RN, MSN, FNP-C
Newark, Delaware

Sarah Reidunn Tvedt-Pool, RN, MS
Rochester, Minnesota

Pamela A. Van Bevern, MPAS
St. Louis, Missouri

Donna F. Wallner, RN, MS
St. Louis, Missouri

Colleen R. Walsh, RN, MSN, ONC, CS, ACNP-BC
Evansville, Indiana

Brian A. Weber, ARNP, PhD
Gainesville, Florida

Mary Ann Wehmer, RN, MSN, CNOR
Evansville, Indiana

Joyce E. Wenger, RN, MSN, CCRN
Lancaster, Pennsylvania

Elizabeth Wheeler, RN, DNS, WHNP
Staten Island, New York

Erlinda C. Wheeler, RN, DNS
Newark, Delaware

Christine L. Willis, RN, MSN, ANP-C
Durham, North Carolina

Anita K. Witzke, RN, CCRN
Newark, Delaware

Juvann M. Wolff, RN, MSN, ARNP
Seattle, Washington

Patricia Worthington, RN, MSN, CNSN
Philadelphia, Pennsylvania

Thomas Worms, RN, MSN
Chicago, Illinois

Kathleen R. Wren, CRNA, PhD
New Orleans, Louisiana

Nancy H. Wright, RN, BS, CNOR
Birmingham, Alabama

Julie A. Wubs, RN, MSN, CNP, CCRN
Chicago, Illinois

Mary Zaccagnini, RN, MS, AOCN
Minneapolis, Minnesota

Polly Gerber Zimmerman, RN, MS, MBA, CEN
Chicago, Illinois

To the
Profession of Nursing
and to the
Important People in Our Lives

Sharon: My husband, Peter, our sons and their wives, Marc and Heidi, Aaron and Roberta, Michael and Brianna, and Jeremy and Monica, and our grandchildren Malia Belle and Halle Gisele

Margaret: My husband, David, and our daughters Elizabeth and Ellen

Shannon: My husband, John, our children Marshall and Meaghan, and my mother, Marilyn

Pat: My husband, Lawrence, our daughter, Lisa, and the more than a thousand students who taught me so well

Linda: My mother, Charlotte, my siblings Millie, Janet, Barb, Rich, and Joanne, and my very good friend and hypnotherapist, Beth

The seventh edition of *Medical-Surgical Nursing: Assessment and Management of Clinical Problems* has been thoroughly revised to incorporate the most current medical-surgical nursing information in an easy-to-use format. More than just a textbook, this is a comprehensive resource containing essential information that students need to prepare for lectures, classroom activities, examinations, clinical assignments, and comprehensive care of patients. In addition to the readable writing style and full-color illustrations, the text includes many special features to help students learn medical-surgical nursing content, including patient and family teaching, gerontology, collaborative care, cultural and ethnic considerations, nutrition and drug therapy, home care, evidence-based practice, and much more.

The comprehensive and timely content, special features, attractive layout, and student-friendly writing style combine to make this the number one medical-surgical nursing textbook used in more nursing schools than any other medical-surgical nursing textbook.

The strengths of the first six editions have been retained, including the use of the nursing process as an organizational theme for nursing management. Numerous new features have been added to address some of the rapid changes in practice. Contributors have been selected for their acknowledged expertise in specific content areas; one or more specialists in the subject area have thoroughly reviewed each chapter to increase accuracy. The editors have undertaken final rewriting and editing to achieve internal consistency. All efforts have been directed toward building on the strengths of the previous edition while preparing an even more effective new edition.

ORGANIZATION

Content is organized into two major divisions. The first division, Section One (Chapters 1 through 12), discusses general concepts related to adult patients. The second division, Sections Two through Twelve (Chapters 13 through 69), presents nursing assessment and nursing management of medical-surgical problems.

The various body systems are grouped to reflect their interrelated functions. Each section is organized around two central themes: assessment and management. Chapters dealing with assessment of a body system include a discussion of the following:

1. A brief review of anatomy and physiology, focusing on information that will promote understanding of nursing care
2. Health history and noninvasive physical assessment skills to expand the knowledge base on which treatment decisions are made
3. Common diagnostic studies, expected results, and related nursing responsibilities to provide easily accessible information

Management chapters focus on the pathophysiology, clinical manifestations, diagnostic studies, collaborative care, and nursing management of various diseases and disorders. The nursing management sections are organized into assessment, nursing diagnoses, planning, implementation, and evaluation. To emphasize the importance of patient care in various clinical settings, nursing implementation of all major health problems is organized by the following levels of care:

1. Health Promotion
2. Acute Intervention
3. Ambulatory and Home Care

CLASSIC FEATURES

- **Patient and family teaching** is an ongoing theme throughout the text. Coverage includes a separate chapter (Chapter 5: Patient and Family Teaching) and 87 Patient and Family Teaching Guides throughout the text.
- **Home care/community-based care** is also emphasized. Coverage includes a separate chapter (Chapter 7: Community-Based Nursing and Home Care) and special Ambulatory and Home Care headings in the Nursing Implementation sections of the management chapters.
- **Collaborative care** is highlighted in special Collaborative Care sections in all management chapters and 90 Collaborative Care tables throughout the text.
- **Gerontology** is discussed in Chapter 6: Older Adults, and included throughout the text under Gerontologic Considerations and Effects of Aging headings and in Gerontologic Differences in Assessment tables.
- **Nutrition** is highlighted throughout the book. Nutritional Therapy tables summarize nutritional interventions and promote healthy lifestyles in patients with various health problems.
- **Nursing management** is presented in a consistent and comprehensive format, with headings for Health Promotion, Acute Intervention, and Ambulatory and Home Care. In addition, **56 Nursing Care Plans** appear in management chapters.
- A separate chapter on **complementary and alternative therapies** (CAT) addresses timely issues in today's health care settings related to these therapies. In addition, **Complementary and Alternative Therapies boxes** located in disorders chapters expand upon the information presented in the chapter, and summarize what nurses need to know about therapies such as herbal remedies, acupuncture, and biofeedback.
- **Cultural and ethnic health disparities** information is integrated into the text and appears in special boxes highlighting risk factors and other important issues related to the nursing care of various ethnic groups. A special **Culturally Competent Care heading** highlights expanded cultural and ethnic content as it relates to specific diseases and disorders.
- **Genetics in Clinical Practice boxes** highlight the genetic basis, genetic testing, and clinical implications for genetic disorders that affect adults.
- **Ethical Dilemmas boxes** promote critical thinking for timely and sensitive issues that nursing students may deal with in clinical practice—topics such as informed consent, advance directives, and confidentiality.

- **Emergency Management tables** outline the emergency treatment of health problems most likely to require emergency intervention.
- **Common Assessment Abnormalities tables** in assessment chapters alert the nurse to frequently encountered abnormalities and their possible etiologies.
- **Nursing Assessment tables** summarize the key subjective and objective data related to common diseases. Subjective data are organized by functional health patterns.
- **Health History tables** in assessment chapters present key questions to ask patients related to a specific disease or disorder.
- Student-friendly pedagogy includes:
  - **Learning Objectives** and **Key Terms** at the beginning of each chapter help students identify the key content for that body system or disorder.
  - **Electronic Resources** boxes included in each chapter opener alert students to supplemental content and exercises on the companion CD and Evolve website, making it easier than ever for students to integrate the textbook with media supplements such as animations, video and audio clips, and much more.
  - **NCLEX® Examination Review Questions** at the end of each chapter, which are matched to the learning objectives, help students learn the important points in the chapter. Answers are provided in an appendix so that the review questions serve as a self-study tool.
  - **Critical Thinking Exercises** appearing at the end of nursing management chapters include Case Studies with Critical Thinking Questions for clinical application.
  - **Resources** at the end of each chapter contain information about nursing and health care organizations that provide patient teaching and disease and disorder information. Resources include Internet sites to help students find current information online.

NEW FEATURES

- *New* **Chapter 2: Health Disparities** discusses differences in health status between groups of people as they relate to access to care, economic aspects of health care, gender and cultural issues, and disease risk in the context of overall health promotion and the government's *Healthy People* initiative.
- *New* **Chapter 41: Nursing Management: Obesity** discusses this increasingly common condition with which so many health risks are associated. It discusses weight reduction strategies, commonly used diets (Atkins, South Beach, Zone, etc.), bariatric surgical procedures, and metabolic syndrome.
- *New* **Gender Differences boxes** summarize how women and men are affected differently by conditions such as pain, irritable bowel syndrome, headaches, addiction, osteoporosis, stroke, coronary artery disease, multiple sclerosis, hypertension, and more.
- *New* **All nursing care plans** now incorporate **Nursing Interventions Classification (NIC)** and **Nursing Outcomes Classification (NOC)** in a way that clearly shows the linkages among NIC, NOC, and nursing diagnoses, and applies them to nursing practice.
- *New* **Drug Alerts** highlight important safety considerations applicable to key drugs throughout the management chapters.

- Each chapter has been carefully revised to ensure a **lower reading level** throughout the book making the content more reader-friendly and understandable than ever.
- *New* **Glossary** of key terms and definitions has been added to the book. It was developed in response to feedback from students. An expanded version of the glossary with audio pronunciations is included on the companion CD and Evolve website.
- *New* **Healthy People boxes** summarize government health care goals as they relate to specific disorders such as diabetes, obesity, cancer, and heart disease.
- The **Companion CD** packaged with this text has been completely revamped to include the following learning tools:
  - A completely unique **Stress-Busting Kit for Nursing Students** provides students with practical strategies for managing their patients' stress as well as their own. This includes imagery, breathing, yoga, meditation, and other relaxation strategies.
  - More than 50 **in-depth case studies** include state-of-the-art animations and a variety of interactive learning activities, which provide students with immediate feedback.
  - A dynamic collection of **Multimedia Supplements** includes animations, video clips, and audio clips.
  - A bank of **375 NCLEX® Examination Review Questions** allow for test preparation.
  - An expanded **glossary** provides pronunciations and definitions for the key terms in the book, and is available as one comprehensive glossary and organized by chapter.
- NCLEX Examination Review Questions in each chapter now include a **focus on prioritization of patient care.**
- **Evidence-Based Practice boxes** have been completely revamped to include updated material that provides synthesis of evidence for application to clinical practice.
- **Enhanced case studies** feature photos that "bring patients to life" and incorporate multiple disorders so that students learn how to **prioritize care and manage patients** in the clinical setting.
- *New* **content on organ transplant** covers organ donation, histocompatibility, rejection, and immunosuppressive therapy with new visual aids.
- **Chapter 9: Stress and Stress Management** replaces the former more theoretical and research-focused stress chapter with more practical information on basic stress management techniques (e.g., breathing, imagery, and meditation) and even self-care strategies for nurses.
- **Chapter 15: Infection and Human Immunodeficiency Virus Infection** now covers emerging infections, multi-resistant drugs, and the nursing care of patients with HIV.
- **Chapter 16: Cancer** reflects a new "healthy" focus on cancer survivors and their long-term care needs.
- **Chapter 18: Nursing Management: Preoperative Care** has been expanded with a new focus on ambulatory and outpatient surgery.
- **Chapter 34: Nursing Management: Coronary Artery Disease and Acute Coronary Syndrome** features expanded information on cardiac surgery and postoperative considerations.
- **Chapter 49 Nursing Management: Diabetes Mellitus** includes extensively revised and updated material with new figures and teaching materials.

- **Chapter 67: Nursing Management: Shock, Systemic Inflammatory Response Syndrome, and Multiple Organ Dysfunction Syndrome** has been completely rewritten for increased readability and student comprehension of this complex topic.
- **Chapter 69: Nursing Management: Emergency and Disaster Nursing** features expanded content on agents of terrorisms, and emergency and mass casualty incidents preparedness.

LEARNING SUPPLEMENTS FOR STUDENTS

- **Clinical Companion to *Medical-Surgical Nursing*, Seventh Edition,** presents approximately 200 common medical-surgical conditions and procedures in a concise, alphabetical format for quick clinical reference. Designed for portability, this popular reference includes the essential, need-to-know information for medical-surgical nursing practice. An attractive and functional two-color design highlights key information for quick, easy reference. This edition features a strong focus on treatments and procedures in which the nurse plays a major role. **Also available on Skyscape PDA!**
- An exceptionally thorough **Study Guide** contains over 500 pages of review material that has been thoroughly updated to reflect the revision of the textbook. Written by textbook co-author Patricia O'Brien, it features a wide variety of clinically relevant exercises and activities, including fill-in-the-blank worksheets, anatomy identification review, true-false questions, critical thinking activities, crossword puzzles, case studies, matching exercises, word scrambles, and multiple-choice questions in NCLEX format. This edition features highlighted Alternate Item questions to better prepare students for the NCLEX exam. Answers to all questions are included in the back to provide students with immediate feedback as they study.
- **Evolve Student Resources** are available online at *http://evolve. elsevier.com/Lewis/medsurg/* and include the following valuable learning aids organized by chapter:
  - Content Updates
  - Audio Key Points summaries for each chapter that can be downloaded to a CD-ROM or iPod
  - Printable Key Points summaries for each chapter
  - Concept Map Creator
  - Key Term Flash Cards
  - Customizable Nursing Care Plans
  - 40 Patient and Family Instruction handouts in both English and Spanish that can be printed and distributed to patients
  - Physical Examination Video
  - Fluids and Electrolytes Tutorial
  - Electronic Calculators
  - WebLinks
  - Audio glossary of key terms, available as comprehensive alphabetical glossary and organized by chapter
- **Virtual Clinical Excursions 3.0** is an exciting learning tool that brings learning to life in a "virtual" hospital setting. Completely updated for easier use and more control, the VCE Pacific View workbook/CD-ROM package features textbook reading assignments that correspond with the CD-ROM and workbook activities. The workbook acts as a map, guiding students through the CD-ROM as they care for patients in the virtual hospital to help students make connections between what they experience through the CD-ROM and what they have

learned in their textbook. Each virtual hospital visit allows the student to access realistic information resources essential to patient care resulting in a true-to-life, hands-on learning experience. Instructors receive an Implementation Manual with directions for using VCE as a teaching tool.

TEACHING SUPPLEMENTS FOR INSTRUCTORS

- The **Instructor's Electronic Resource with Integrated Lesson Plans on CD** remains the most comprehensive set of instructor's materials available, containing:
  - **Integrated Lesson Plans** with electronic resources organized by chapter to help instructors develop and manage the course curriculum. This exciting new resource includes:
    - Four-column lesson plans listing chapter outlines, classroom strategies, collaborative/active learning activities with critical thinking questions, and a "putting it all together" section that lists specific teaching resources available for each content section
    - Quizzes with answer guidelines
    - Case studies with answer guidelines
    - Learning objectives
    - Key terms with audio pronunciations

  This unique teaching aid includes links and cross-references to additional instructor and student materials for each chapter to help faculty "put it all together" and truly make the best use of all of the teaching/learning supplements. Included are links to the relevant content in the image collection, PowerPoint presentations, i-Clicker Question Suite, test bank, animation collection, content updates—as well as the related components of the companion CD and student Evolve resources. Also provided are quick-access links to resources useful for all chapters, including the concept map creator, electronic calculators, and much more.
- The **ExamView® Test Bank** features approximately 1800 NCLEX® Examination test questions with text page references and answers coded for NCLEX Client Needs category, nursing process, and cognitive level. The 7th edition test bank has been revamped to include rationales, more application-based questions, additional questions in NCLEX alternate-item formats, and to incorporate prioritization and delegation content. The ExamView program allows instructors to create new tests; edit, add, and delete test questions; sort questions by NCLEX category, cognitive level, and nursing process step; and administer/grade online tests.
- The **Image Collection** contains more than 800 full-color images from the text for use in lectures.
- An extensive collection of **PowerPoint Presentations** is organized by chapter and includes over 8000 customizable slides for use in lectures. The presentations include applicable illustrations from the image collection and links to applicable animations.
- A new **i-Clicker Question Suite** for each chapter developed especially for use with audience response systems.
- **Evolve Instructor Resources** are available online at *http:// evolve.elsevier.com/Lewis/medsurg/* and feature the following valuable teaching aids:
  - Online access to the Integrated Lesson Plans, Test Bank, PowerPoint Presentations, Image Collection, and i-Clicker Question Suite

- A collection of additional "faculty only" state-of-the-art animations
- Course Management System
- Access to all student resources listed above

Evolve Select

This exciting new program is available to faculty who adopt a number of Elsevier texts, including *Medical-Surgical Nursing: Assessment and Management of Clinical Problems,* 7th edition. Evolve Select is an integrated electronic study center consisting of a collection of textbooks made available electronically in CD format. It is carefully designed to "extend" the textbook for an easier and more efficient teaching and learning experience. It includes study aids such as highlighting, e-note taking, and cut and paste capabilities. Even more importantly, it allows students and instructors to do a comprehensive search within the specific text or across a number of titles. Please check with your Elsevier sales representative for more information.

ACKNOWLEDGMENTS

The editors are especially grateful to many people at Elsevier who assisted with this major revision effort. In particular, we wish to thank the team of Kristin Geen, Lauren Lake, Mary Stueck, Jeff Patterson, and Paula Ruckenbrod. In addition, we want to thank the marketing team of Bob Boehringer and Tricia Schroeder.

A team of special persevering contributors put together our excellent ancillary package. These include Pat O'Brien (Study Guide and i-Clicker Question Suite), Barbara Bartz (Test Bank), Dorothy Mathers (Interactive Case Studies for Companion CD), and Jennie Shaw and Stephanie Elms (Instructor's Manual). Elizabeth Burkhart, Pat O'Brien, and Sara Doeberling revised the nursing care plans to incorporate NANDA nursing diagnoses, Nursing Interventions Classifications, and Nursing Outcomes Classifications.

Special thanks and appreciation go to Peter Bonner who assisted with many details of manuscript preparation. Our special assistants have earned our respect and thanks and include Cory Shaw, Alissa Calaway, Jennifer Kretzschmar, Brianna Chavez, Crystal Ninan, Bevin O'Connor, Kamilah Newland, Paula Blackwell, and Lisa Grabarec.

Ellen Fineout-Overholt and Alyce Schultz, Center for the Advancement of Evidence-Based Practice at the College of Nursing and Health Care Innovation, Arizona State University, Phoenix, Arizona, assisted with content on evidence-based practice.

Our exciting new Stress-Busting kit was a team effort of many people. Cory Shaw helped write and produce it. She and Allen Novian were our actors. Peter Bonner played guitar and contributed photos. Russ Keys played synthesizer. Our wonderful animations and illustrations were prepared by David Baker, Chris McKee, and Jeanne Robertson. The video, photography, and editing were done by Lester Rosebrock. Brian Luke Seaward was our narrator and contributed imagery scripts and photos. For additional information on stress management, see his website at *www. brianlukeseaward.net.*

We are particularly indebted to the faculty, nurses, and student nurses who have put their faith in our book to assist them on their path to excellence. The increasing use of this book throughout the United States, Canada, Australia, and other parts of the world has been gratifying. We appreciate the many users who have shared their comments and suggestions on the previous editions. All feedback is welcome.

We also wish to thank our contributors and reviewers for their assistance with the revision process. We sincerely hope that this book will assist both students and clinicians in practicing truly professional nursing.

Sharon Lewis
Margaret Heitkemper
Shannon Dirksen
Patricia O'Brien
Linda Bucher

Contents

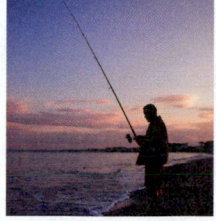

Section 1

CONCEPTS IN NURSING PRACTICE

1   Nursing Practice Today, 2

2   Health Disparities, 19

3   Culturally Competent Care, 26

4   Health History and Physical Examination, 39

5   Patient and Family Teaching, 53

6   Older Adults, 66

7   Community-Based Nursing and Home Care, 85

8   Complementary and Alternative Therapies, 94

9   Stress and Stress Management, 110

10 Pain, 125

11 End-of-Life and Palliative Care, 151

12 Addictive Behaviors, 165

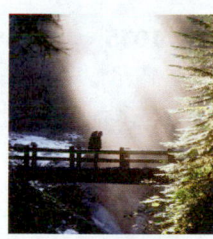

Section 2

PATHOPHYSIOLOGIC MECHANISMS OF DISEASE

13 Inflammation and Wound Healing, 193

14 Genetics, Altered Immune Responses, and Transplantation, 213

15 Infection and Human Immunodeficiency Virus Infection, 243

16 Cancer, 271

17 Fluid, Electrolyte, and Acid-Base Imbalances, 314

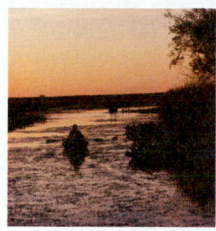

Section 3

PERIOPERATIVE CARE

18 Nursing Management
    Preoperative Care, 343

19 Nursing Management
    Intraoperative Care, 359

20 Nursing Management
    Postoperative Care, 376

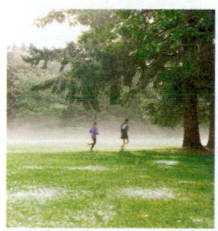

Section 4

PROBLEMS RELATED TO ALTERED SENSORY INPUT

21 Nursing Assessment
    Visual and Auditory Systems, 398

22 Nursing Management
    Visual and Auditory Problems, 416

23 Nursing Assessment
    Integumentary System, 449

24 Nursing Management
    Integumentary Problems, 460

25 Nursing Management
    Burns, 483

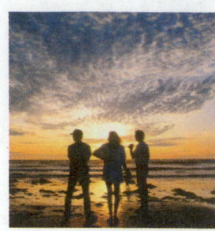

Section 5

PROBLEMS OF OXYGENATION: VENTILATION

26   Nursing Assessment
     Respiratory System, 509

27   Nursing Management
     Upper Respiratory Problems, 533

28   Nursing Management
     Lower Respiratory Problems, 560

29   Nursing Management
     Obstructive Pulmonary Diseases, 607

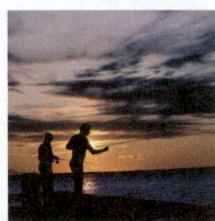

Section 6

PROBLEMS OF OXYGENATION: TRANSPORT

30   Nursing Assessment
     Hematologic System, 665

31   Nursing Management
     Hematologic Problems, 684

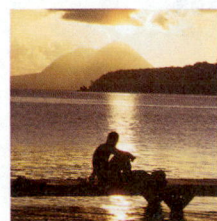

Section 7

PROBLEMS OF OXYGENATION: PERFUSION

32   Nursing Assessment
     Cardiovascular System, 739

33   Nursing Management
     Hypertension, 761

34   Nursing Management
     Coronary Artery Disease and Acute Coronary
     Syndrome, 784

35   Nursing Management
     Heart Failure, 821

36   Nursing Management
     Dysrhythmias, 842

37   Nursing Management
     Inflammatory and Structural Heart
     Disorders, 865

38   Nursing Management
     Vascular Disorders, 892

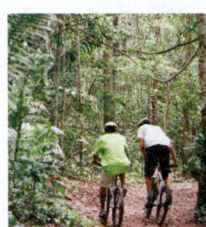

Section 8

PROBLEMS OF INGESTION, DIGESTION, ABSORPTION, AND ELIMINATION

39   Nursing Assessment
     Gastrointestinal System, 926

40   Nursing Management
     Nutritional Problems, 948

41   Nursing Management
     Obesity, 971

42   Nursing Management
     Upper Gastrointestinal Problems, 990

43   Nursing Management
     Lower Gastrointestinal Problems, 1035

44   Nursing Management
     Liver, Pancreas, and Biliary Tract
     Problems, 1087

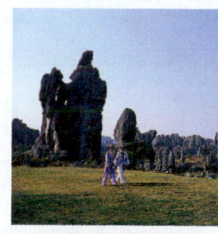

Section 9

PROBLEMS OF URINARY FUNCTION

45   Nursing Assessment
     Urinary System, 1136

46   Nursing Management
     Renal and Urologic Problems, 1154

47   Nursing Management
     Acute Renal Failure and Chronic Kidney
     Disease, 1197

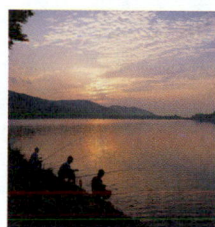

Section 10

PROBLEMS RELATED TO REGULATORY AND REPRODUCTIVE MECHANISMS

48   Nursing Assessment
     Endocrine System, 1234

49   Nursing Management
     Diabetes Mellitus, 1253

50   Nursing Management
     Endocrine Problems, 1290

51   Nursing Assessment
     Reproductive System, 1323

52   Nursing Management
     Breast Disorders, 1343

53   Nursing Management
     Sexually Transmitted Diseases, 1366

54   Nursing Management
     Female Reproductive Problems, 1381

55   Nursing Management
     Male Reproductive Problems, 1414

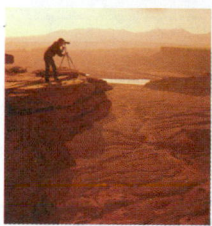

Section 11

PROBLEMS RELATED TO MOVEMENT AND COORDINATION

56   Nursing Assessment
     Nervous System, 1441

57   Nursing Management
     Acute Intracranial Problems, 1467

58   Nursing Management
     Stroke, 1502

59   Nursing Management
     Chronic Neurologic Problems, 1527

60   Nursing Management
     Alzheimer's Disease and Dementia, 1561

61   Nursing Management
     Peripheral Nerve and Spinal Cord
     Problems, 1580

62   Nursing Assessment
     Musculoskeletal System, 1614

63   Nursing Management
     Musculoskeletal Trauma and Orthopedic
     Surgery, 1629

64   Nursing Management
     Musculoskeletal Problems, 1668

65   Nursing Management
     Arthritis and Connective Tissue
     Diseases, 1693

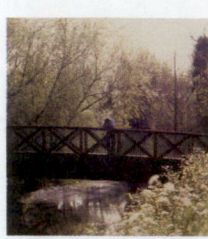

Section 12

NURSING CARE IN SPECIALIZED SETTINGS

66 Nursing Management
Critical Care, 1733

67 Nursing Management
Shock, Systemic Inflammatory Response
Syndrome, and Multiple Organ Dysfunction
Syndrome, 1772

68 Nursing Management
Respiratory Failure and Acute Respiratory
Distress Syndrome, 1799

69 Nursing Management
Emergency and Disaster Nursing, 1821

APPENDIXES

A Cardiopulmonary Resuscitation (CPR) and Basic
Life Support, 1845
B Nursing Diagnoses, 1850
C Laboratory Values, 1854
D Answer Key to Review Questions, 1865

GLOSSARY, G-1

ILLUSTRATION CREDITS, IL-1

INDEX, I-1

ELECTRONIC RESOURCES, ER-1

HEALTHY PEOPLE BOXES

Access to Health Care, 2, p. 20
Arthritis Prevention, 65, p. 1701
Avoiding Smoking and Environmental Tobacco Smoke, 12, p. 185
Avoiding Substance Abuse, 12, p. 185
Cancer, Prevention and Early Detection, 16, p. 282
Chronic Kidney Disease, Prevention and Detection, 47, p. 1205
Diabetes Mellitus, 49, p. 1275
Good Oral Hygiene, 42, p. 1003
Heart Disease, Prevention, 34, p. 791
HIV, Prevention and Early Detection, 15, p. 260
Hypertension, Prevention and Control, 33, p. 768
Immunization, 14, p. 219
Low Back Pain, Prevention, 64, p. 1677
Maintaining a Healthy Weight, 41, p. 973
Regular Physical Activity, 63, p. 1631
Respiratory Diseases, Prevention, 28, p. 569
Responsible Eye Care, 22, p. 420
Responsible Sexual Behavior, 53, p. 1377
Stroke, Prevention, 58, p. 1510
Wearing Ear Protection, 22, p. 444
Well-Balanced Diet, 40, p. 958

GENDER DIFFERENCES BOXES

Acute Coronary Syndrome (ACS), 34, p. 802
Addictive Behaviors, 12, p. 167
Alzheimer's Disease and Dementia, 60, p. 1565
Asthma, 29, p. 608
Cancer, 16, 272
Cardiac Assessment, 32, p. 747
Cholelithiasis, 44, p. 1127
Chronic Obstructive Pulmonary Disease, 29, p. 629
Coronary Artery Disease, 34, p. 785
Endocrine Problems, 50, p. 1299
Gout, 65, p. 1715
Headaches, 59, p. 1528
Heart Failure, 35, p. 823
Hernia, 43, p. 1079
Hip Fracture, 63, p. 1653
Hypertension, 33, p. 762
Irritable Bowel Syndrome, 43, 1046
Lung Cancer, 28, p. 579
Older Adults, 6, p. 70
Osteoarthritis, 65, p. 1694
Osteoporosis, 64, p. 1687
Pain, 10, p. 127
Stroke, 58, p. 1503
Urinary Incontinence, 46, p. 1180
Urinary Tract Calculi, 46, p. 1169
Vascular Disorders, 38, p. 893

CULTURAL AND ETHNIC HEALTH DISPARITIES BOXES

Anorexia and Bulimia, 40, p. 969
Arthritis and Connective Tissue Disorders, 65, p. 1702
Brain Tumors, 57, p. 1487
Breast Cancer, 52, p. 1348
Cancer, 16, p. 273
Cancers of the Female Reproductive System, 54, p. 1400
Cancers of the Male Reproductive System, 55, p. 1423
Chronic Kidney Disease, 47, p. 1204
Colon Disorders, 43, p. 1051
Coronary Artery Disease, 34, p. 787
Diabetes Mellitus, 49, p. 1254
Heart Failure, 35, p. 822
Hematologic Problems, 31, p. 685
Hypertension, 33, p. 762
Integumentary Problems, 24, p. 461
Liver, Pancreas, and Gallbladder Disorders, 44, p. 1089
Lung Cancer, 28, p. 579
Obesity, 41, p. 972
Obstructive Pulmonary Diseases, 29, p. 608
Oral, Pharyngeal, and Esophageal Problems, 42, p. 1001
Osteoporosis, 64, p. 1687
Stroke, 58, p. 1503
Tuberculosis, 28, p. 570
Urologic Disorders, 46, p. 1155
Visual and Auditory Problems, 22, p. 417

COMPLEMENTARY AND ALTERNATIVE THERAPIES BOXES

Acupuncture, 64, p. 1682
Assessment of Use of Herbal Products and Dietary
    Supplements, 4, p. 44
Bilberry, 22, p. 425
Biofeedback for Urinary Incontinence, 46, p. 1182
Clotting, Herbs that Affect, 38, p. 903
Complementary and Alternative Therapies Boxes, 8, p. 103
Echinacea, 27, p. 536
Fish Oil/Omega-3 Fatty Acids, 33, p. 771
Ginger, 42, p. 993
Ginkgo Biloba, 60, p. 1569
Ginseng, 9, p. 120
Glucosamine, 65, p. 1697
Glucose, Herbs That Affect, 49, p. 1276
Goldenseal, 27, p. 536
Hawthorn, 35, p. 831
Imagery, 52, p. 1361
Kava, 9, p. 121
Menopause, Herbs and Supplements for, 54, p. 1393
Milk Thistle, 44, p. 1131

Music Therapy, 19, p. 364
Natural Lipid-Lowering Agents, 34, p. 796
Perioperative Period, Effects of Herbs and Supplements during, 18, p. 347
Saw Palmetto, 55, p. 1417
St. John's Wort, 9, p. 121
Valerian, 54, p. 1393
Yoga, 9, p. 121
Zinc, 27, p. 539

EVIDENCE-BASED PRACTICE BOXES

Activity for Patients with Low-Back Pain, 64, p. 1681
Basal Cell Carcinoma Therapy, 24, p. 465
Cardiac Rehabilitation Programs, 34, p. 794
Ethnicity and Hepatitis C Patients, 44, p. 1095
Exercise to Improve Quality of Life in Multiple Sclerosis Patients, 59, p. 1547
Exercise Programs for Stroke Patients, 58, p. 1514
Group-Based Educational Programs for Diabetic Patients, 49, p. 1259
Increasing Breast Cancer Screenings, 52, p. 1359
Initiating Nutritional Support for Head Injury Patients, 57, p. 1475
Invasive Screening Methods for Early Diagnosis of Ovarian Cancer, 54, p. 1403
Localized Estrogen Preparations for Vaginal Atrophy, 54, p. 1391
Low-Molecular Weight Heparin Versus Compression Therapy in Deep Vein Thrombosis, 38, p. 912
Male Condom Breakage During Intercourse, 53, p. 1373
Managing Stable COPD, 29, p. 639
Nicotine-Replacement Therapy for Smoking Cessation, 12, p. 172
Noninvasive Interventions in Patients with Lung Cancer, 28, p. 583
Noninvasive Physical Treatments for Chronic Headaches, 59, p. 1531
Patient Discharge Education in Chronic Heart Failure, 35, p. 830
Physical Training to Improve Health in Patients with Asthma, 29, p. 609
Postoperative Analgesia and Pain Control, 20, p. 389
Prophylactic Antibiotics for Recurrent Urinary Tract Infection, 46, p. 1158
Psychologic Interventions for Weight Loss, 41, p. 981
Reducing Incidence of Falls, 63, p. 1646
Reducing Risk Factors for COPD, 29, p. 640
Reduction of Dietary Salt to Decrease Blood Pressure, 33, p. 780
Retin-A for Sun-Damaged Skin, 24, p. 463
Self-Management Programs for Irritable Bowel Syndrome, 43, p. 1047
Sexuality Following Spinal Cord Injury, 61, p. 1607
Stress Management for Crohn's Disease Symptoms, 43, p. 1054
Surgical Location for Cataract Surgery, 22, p. 428
Treating Osteoarthritis with Acetaminophen or NSAIDs, 65, p. 1697
Urinary Incontinence Therapy After Radical Prostatectomy, 55, p. 1425
Use of Music to Prevent Confusion and Delirium in Surgical Patients, 60, p. 1577
Weight-Bearing Exercises for Hip Fracture Patients, 63, p. 1655
Weight-Loss Interventions for Patients with Prediabetes, 49, p. 1257
Withholding Fluids Before Elective Surgery, 18, p. 353

GENETICS IN CLINICAL PRACTICE BOXES

a_1-Antitrypsin Deficiency, 29, p. 632
Alzheimer's Disease, 60, p. 1565
Ankylosing Spondylitis, 65, p. 1712
Breast Cancer, 52, p. 1349
Cystic Fibrosis, 29, p. 656
Diabetes Mellitus, Type 1 and 2, 49, p. 1256
Duchenne Muscular Dystrophy, 64, p. 1675
Familial Adenomatous Polyposis, 43, p. 1063
Familial Hypercholesterolemia, 34, p. 788
Genetics in Clinical Practice Boxes, 14, p. 216
Hemochromatosis, 31, p. 699
Hemophilia A and B, 31, p. 707
Hereditary Nonpolyposis Colorectal Cancer or Lynch Syndrome, 43, p. 1064
Human Genome Project, 14, p. 214
Huntington's Disease, 59, p. 1559
Ovarian Cancer, 54, p. 1402
Polycystic Kidney Disease, 46, p. 1176
Sickle Cell Disease, 31, p. 696

ETHICAL DILEMMAS BOXES

Abortion, 54, p. 1385
Advance Directives, 29, p. 637
Allocation of Resources, 47, p. 1226
Alternative Healers, 50, p. 1309
Brain Death, 57, p. 1485
Competence, 35, p. 830
Confidentiality, 53, p. 1378
Do Not Resuscitate, 37, p. 882
Durable Power of Attorney, 29, p. 655
End-of-Life Care, 11, p. 159
Entitlement to Treatment, 63, p. 1652
Genetic Testing, 14, p. 218
Guardianship, 42, p. 1009
Health Disparities, 2, p. 22
Impaired Health Care Providers, 12, p. 174
Individual vs. Public Health Protection, 15, p. 256
Informed Consent, 18, p. 353
Justice, 34, p. 809
Medical Futility, 16, p. 309
Pain Management, 31, p. 698
Patient Adherence, 28, p. 575
Payment for Organs, 47, p. 1225
Rationing, 44, p. 1115
Religious Interest, 31, p. 730
Sterilization, 55, p. 1433
Withdrawing Treatment, 47, p. 1230
Withholding Treatment, 57, p. 1492

COLLABORATIVE CARE TABLES

Acute Decompensated Heart Failure and Pulmonary Edema, Table 35-6, p. 827
Acute Glomerulonephritis, Table 46-9, p. 1166
Acute Pancreatitis, Table 44-20, p. 1120
Acute Pericarditis, Table 37-9, p. 874
Acute Pulmonary Embolism, Table 28-27, p. 599
Acute Pyelonephritis, Table 46-7, p. 1162

Acute Renal Failure, Table 47-4, p. 1202
Acute Respiratory Distress Syndrome, Table 68-10, p. 1817
Acute Respiratory Failure, Table 68-5, p. 1806
Addison's Disease, Table 50-16, p. 1317
Alzheimer's Disease, Table 60-7, p. 1568
Amputation, Table 63-13, p. 1658
Aortic Dissection, Table 38-1, p. 900
Asthma, Table 29-4, p. 614
Bacterial Meningitis, Table 57-17, p. 1495
Benign Prostatic Hyperplasia, Table 55-2, p. 1417
Bladder Cancer, Table 46-16, p. 1179
Breast Cancer, Table 52-5, p. 1351
Burns, Table 25-10, p. 493
Cardiomyopathy, Table 37-20, p. 886
Cataract, Table 22-4, p. 426
Cervical Cord Injury, Table 61-5, p. 1597
Chlamydial Infection, Table 53-7, p. 1372
Cholelithiasis and Acute Cholecystitis, Table 44-24, p. 1128
Chronic Heart Failure, Table 35-7, p. 827
Chronic Otitis Media, Table 22-14, p. 440
Cirrhosis of the Liver, Table 44-15, p. 1107
Colorectal Cancer, Table 43-26, p. 1065
Conservative Therapy of Chronic Kidney Disease,
    Table 47-7, p. 1209
COPD, Table 29-19, p. 638
Cor Pulmonale, Table 28-28, p. 603
Cushing Syndrome, Table 50-14, p. 1314
Diabetes Mellitus, Table 49-2, p. 1259
Diabetic Ketoacidosis and Hyperosmolor Hyperglycemic
    Syndrome, Table 49-18, p. 1280
Diverticulosis and Diverticulitis, Table 43-35, p. 1077
Endometriosis, Table 54-10, p. 1397
Erectile Dysfunction, Table 55-11, p. 1435
Esophageal Cancer, Table 42-15, p. 1010
External Otitis, Table 22-12, p. 438
Fractures, Table 63-6, p. 1638
Gastroesophageal Reflux Disease (GERD) and Hiatal Hernia,
    Table 42-12, p. 1005
Genital Herpes, Table 53-8, p. 1375
Glaucoma, Table 22-9, p. 434
Gonorrhea, Table 53-2, p. 1369
Gout, Table 65-13, p. 1716
Headaches, Table 59-3, p. 1530
Hypertension, Table 33-5, p. 768
Hyperthyroidism, Table 50-7, p. 1301
Hypoglycemia, Table 49-20, p. 1282
Hypothyroidism, Table 50-9, p. 1306
Increased Intracranial Pressure, Table 57-3, p. 1472
Infertility, Table 54-1, p. 1382
Inflammatory Bowel Disease, Table 43-19, p. 1053
Intervertebral Lumbar Disk Damage, Table 64-9, p. 1682
Iron-Deficiency Anemia, Table 31-7, p. 690
Lung Cancer, Table 28-15, p. 581
Ménière's Disease, Table 22-17, p. 442
Multiple Sclerosis, Table 59-14, p. 1543
Myasthenia Gravis, Table 59-20, p. 1556
Neurogenic Bladder, Table 61-9, p. 1605
Neutropenia, Table 31-22, p. 715
Obesity, Table 41-5, p. 978

Oral Cancer, Table 42-9, p. 1002
Osteoarthritis, Table 65-2, p. 1696
Osteoporosis, Table 64-14, p. 1688
Otosclerosis, Table 22-16, p. 441
Ovarian Cancer, Table 54-12, p. 1403
Parkinson's Disease, Table 59-17, p. 1551
Peptic Ulcer Disease, Table 42-19, p. 1019
Peripheral Arterial Disease, Table 38-3, p. 902
Peritonitis, Table 43-16, p. 1050
Pneumonia, Table 28-5, p. 566
Premenstrual Syndrome, Table 54-4, p. 1386
Prostate Cancer, Table 55-6, p. 1424
Retinal Detachment, Table 22-8, p. 430
Rheumatic Fever, Table 37-11, p. 877
Rheumatoid Arthritis, Table 65-8, p. 1706
Seizure Disorders and Epilepsy, Table 59-7, p. 1536
Specific Strategies for the Treatment of Shock,
    Table 67-10, p. 1789
Stomach Cancer, Table 42-26, p. 1029
Stroke, Table 58-4, p. 1510
Syphilis, Table 53-4, p. 1371
Systemic Lupus Erythematosus, Table 65-15, p. 1719
Systemic Sclerosis, Table 65-18, p. 1724
Thrombocytopenia, Table 31-13, p. 704
Trigeminal Neuralgia, Table 61-1, p. 1582
Pulmonary Tuberculosis, Table 28-8, p. 572
Urinary Tract Infection, Table 46-4, p. 1158
Valvular Heart Disease, Table 37-15, p. 881
Viral Hepatitis, Table 44-6, p. 1094

NUTRITIONAL THERAPY TABLES

Calcium Sources, Table 64-15, p. 1689
Calorie-Restricted Weight-Reduction Diet, Table 41-6, p. 978
Celiac Disease, Table 43-38, p. 1080
Daily Requirements for the Patient with Chronic Kidney Disease,
    Table 47-8, p. 1212
DASH Diet for Hypertension, Table 33-7, p. 770
Diabetes Mellitus, Table 49-9, p. 1268
Erythropoiesis and Nutrients Needed, Table 31-5, p. 689
Foods High in Iron, Table 40-4, p. 951
High-Calorie Foods, Table 16-21, p. 307
High-Calorie, High Protein Diet, Table 40-14, p. 958
High-Fiber Foods, Table 43-9, p. 1043
High-Potassium Foods, Table 47-9, p. 1213
Low-Sodium Diets, Table 35-11, p. 834
Postgastrectomy Dumping Syndrome, Table 42-25, p. 1027
Protein Foods with High Biologic Value, Table 16-20, p. 306
Sodium Content in Different Food Groups, Table 35-13, p. 834
Stoma Output and Effects of Food, Table 43-33, p. 1075
Therapeutic Lifestyle Changes Diet, Table 34-4, p. 793
Therapeutic Lifestyle Changes Diet Menu, Table 34-5, p. 793
Urinary Tract Calculi, Table 46-13, p. 1171

PATIENT AND FAMILY TEACHING GUIDE TABLES

Acute or Chronic Sinusitis, Table 27-4, p. 541
Acute Coronary Syndrome, Table 34-18, p. 815
Addison's Disease, Table 50-17, p. 1317
After Ear Surgery, Table 22-15, p. 440
After Eye Surgery, Table 22-6, p. 428

Alzheimer's Disease, Table 60-10, p. 1574

Alzheimer's Disease Warning Signs, Table 60-6, p. 1567

Amputation, Table 63-14, p. 1661

Anticoagulation Therapy, Table 38-14, p. 917

Antiretroviral Drugs, Table 15-23, p. 265

Asthma, Table 29-15, p. 630

Autonomic Dysreflexia, Table 61-7, p. 1604

Back Exercises, Table 64-7, p. 1677

Bowel Management after Spinal Cord Injury, Table 61-10, p. 1606

Cardiomyopathy, Table 37-21, p. 889

Cast Care, Table 63-9, p. 1646

Chronic Kidney Disease, Table 47-10, p. 1216

Chronic Obstructive Pulmonary Disease, Table 29-28, p. 654

Cirrhosis, Table 44-18, p. 1115

Colostomy Irrigation, Table 43-34, p. 1075

Constipation, Table 43-11, p. 1044

Corticosteroid Therapy, Table 50-20, p. 1319

Decrease Risk for Antibiotic-Resistant Infection, Table 15-7, p. 247

Decreasing Risk Factors for Coronary Artery Disease, Table 34-3, p. 792

Diabetes Mellitus Management, Table 49-15, p. 1277

Dry Powder Inhaler (DPI) Use, Table 29-9, p. 623

Effective Coughing Guidelines, Table 29-25, p. 646

Exercise for Patients with Diabetes Mellitus, Table 49-11, p. 1269

Femoral Head Prosthesis, Table 63-11, p. 1654

FITT Physical Activity Guidelines After Acute Coronary Syndrome, Table 34-20, p. 816

Foot Care, Table 49-22, p. 1287

Gastroesophageal Reflux Disease (GERD) Prevention, Table 42-14, p. 1007

Good Nutrition, Table 40-13, p. 958

Halo Vest Care, Table 61-12, p. 1606

Head Injury, Table 57-11, p. 1486

Headaches, Table 59-5, p. 1533

Heart Failure, Table 34-13, p. 838

Heat and Cold Therapy, Table 10-11, p. 144

Herbal Therapies, Table 8-9, p. 101

Home Oxygen Use, Table 29-24, p. 645

How to Reduce Symptoms of Allergic Rhinitis, Table 27-1, p. 536

Hypertension, Table 33-14, p. 779

Hypokalemia Prevention, Table 17-7, p. 329

Hypothyroidism, Table 50-10, p. 1309

Ileal Conduit, Changing Appliances, Table 46-24, p. 1193

Implantable Cardioverter-Defibrillator (ICD), Table 36-9, p. 858

Instructions for Patients with Diabetes Mellitus, Table 49-16, p. 1277

Insulin Therapy, Table 49-5, p. 1262

Joint Protection and Energy Conservation, Table 65-4, p. 1701

Low Back Problems, Table 64-6, p. 1677

Lyme Disease Prevention (Endemic Areas), Table 65-11, p. 1714

Menstruation Characteristics, Table 51-2, p. 1329

Mitral Valve Prolapse, Table 37-14, p. 880

Musculoskeletal Problem Prevention in the Older Adult, Table 63-1, p. 1630

Neck Exercises, Table 64-11, p. 1684

Neutropenia, Table 31-23, p. 715

Older Adults, Table 6-12, p. 79

Ostomy Self-Care, Table 43-32, p. 1072

Pacemaker, Table 36-12, p. 861

Pain Management, Table 10-13, p. 145

Peak Flow Meter Use, Table 29-14, p. 628

Pelvic Floor Muscle or Kegel Exercises, Table 46-20, p. 1184

Peptic Ulcer Disease, Table 42-24, p. 1025

Peripheral Artery Bypass Surgery, Table 38-5, p. 907

Postoperative Laparoscopic Cholecystectomy, Table 44-27, p. 1132

Preoperative Preparation, Table 18-7, p. 352

Pressure Ulcer, Table 13-15, p. 210

Preventing Food Poisoning, Table 42-28, p. 1032

Proper Use of Drug-Using Equipment, Table 15-21 p. 263

Proper Use of the Female Condom, Table 15-20, p. 263

Proper Use of the Male Condom, Table 15-19, p. 262

Protection of Small Joints, Table 65-10, p. 1710

Radiation Skin Reactions, Table 16-16, p. 300

Reducing Barriers to Pain Management, Table 10-15, p. 146

Seizure Disorders and Epilepsy, Table 59-12, p. 1541

Self-Monitoring of Blood Glucose (SMBG), Table 49-12, p. 1270

Sexual Activity After Acute Coronary Syndrome, Table 34-21, p. 817

Sexual Assault Prevention, Table 54-16, p. 1411

Sexually Transmitted Diseases, Table 53-10, p. 1377

Signs and Symptoms that HIV Patients Need to Report, Table 15-25, p. 266

Skin Care for Patient with Spinal Cord Injury, Table 61-11, p. 1606

Smoking and Tobacco Use Cessation, Table 12-6, p. 173

Stroke Warning Signs, Table 58-7, p. 1515

Supraglottic Swallow Steps, Table 27-8, p. 553

Systemic Lupus Erythematosus, Table 65-17, p. 1720

Testicular Self-Examination, Table 55-9, p. 1433

Thrombocytopenia, Table 31-15, p. 707

Urinary Tract Infection, Table 46-6, p. 1161

GERONTOLOGIC DIFFERENCES IN ASSESSMENT TABLES

Adaptations in Physical Assessment Techniques, Table 4-7, p. 50

Adult Mental Functioning, Table 6-4, p. 70

Auditory System, Table 21-7, p. 410

Cardiovascular System, Table 32-1, p. 744

Endocrine System, Table 48-5, p. 1242

Factors Affecting Nutritional Intake in Older Adults, Table 40-15, p. 959

Gastrointestinal System, Table 39-5, p. 933

Hematologic Studies, Table 30-4, p. 672

Immune System, Table 14-8, p. 224

Integumentary System, Table 23-1, p. 452

Musculoskeletal System, Table 62-1, p. 1619

Nervous System, Table 56-5, p. 1454

Reproductive Systems, Table 51-3, p. 1331

Respiratory System, Table 26-4, p. 517

Urinary System, Table 45-2, p. 1411

Visual System, Table 21-1, p. 401

EMERGENCY MANAGEMENT TABLES

Abdominal Trauma, Table 43-14, p. 1048

Acute Abdominal Pain, Table 43-13, p. 1045

Acute Soft Tissue Injury, Table 63-3, p. 1632
Anaphylactic Shock, Table 14-13, p. 230
Chemical Burns, Table 25-5, p. 489
Chest Pain, Table 34-13, p. 806
Chest Trauma, Table 28-19, p. 586
Cocaine and Amphetamine Toxicity, Table 12-7, p. 175
Depressant Drugs Overdose, Table 12-11, p. 179
Diabetic Ketoacidosis, Table 49-19, p. 1280
Dysrhythmias, Table 36-6, p. 848
Electrical Burns, Table 25-7, p. 490
Emergency Management Tables, Table 69-1, p. 1822
Eye Injury, Table 22-3, p. 421
Fractured Extremity, Table 63-7, p. 1642
Head Injury, Table 57-9, p. 1484
Hyperthermia, Table 69-8, p. 1830
Hypothermia, Table 69-9, p. 1832
Inhalation Injury, Table 25-6, p. 489
Sexual Assault, Table 54-14, p. 1410
Shock, Table 67-7, p. 1785
Spinal Cord Injury, Table 61-4, p. 1596
Stroke, Table 58-5, p. 1511
Submersion Injuries, Table 69-10, p. 1833
Thermal Burns, Table 25-8, p. 490
Thoracic Injuries, Table 28-20, p. 586
Tonic-Clonic Seizures, Table 59-8, p. 1537

NURSING CARE PLANS

Abdominal Hysterectomy, NCP 54-1, p. 1398
Acute Coronary Syndrome, NCP 34-1, p. 811
Acute Infectious Diarrhea, NCP 43-1, p. 1039
Acute Pancreatitis, NCP 44-3, p. 1122
Acute Renal Lithiasis, NCP 46-2, p. 1173
Acute Respiratory Failure, NCP 68-1, p. 1807
Acute Viral Hepatitis, NCP 44-1, p. 1097
Alcohol Withdrawal, NCP 12-1, p. 183
Alzheimer's Disease, NCP 60-1, p. 1571
Anemia, NCP 31-1, p. 688
Asthma, NCP 29-1, p. 625
Bacterial Meningitis, NCP 57-2, p. 1496
Burn Patient, NCP 25-1, p. 494
Chronic Kidney Disease, NCP 47-1, p. 1214
Cirrhosis, NCP 44-2, p. 1112
Colostomy/Ileostomy, NCP 43-3, p. 1073
COPD, NCP 29-2, p. 651
Diabetes Mellitus, NCP 49-1, p. 1273
Enteral Nutrition, NCP 40-1, p. 963
Fracture, NCP 63-1, p. 1644
Headache, NCP 59-1, p. 1533
Heart Failure, NCP 35-1, p. 836
Hyperthyroidism, NCP 50-1, p. 1303
Hypothyroidism, NCP 50-2, p. 1307
Ileal Conduit, NCP 46-3, p. 1191
Increased Intracranial Pressure, NCP 57-1, p. 1479
Infective Endocarditis, NCP 37-1, p. 870
Inflammatory Bowel Disease, NCP 43-2, p. 1058
Low Back Pain, NCP 64-2, p. 1678
Mastectomy or Lumpectomy, NCP 52-1, p. 1357
Mechanical Ventilation, NCP 66-1, p. 1754
Multiple Sclerosis, NCP 59-3, p. 1547
Nausea and Vomiting, NCP 42-1, p. 994
Neutropenia, NCP 31-3, p. 716
Orthopedic Surgery, NCP 63-2, p. 1647
Osteomyelitis, NCP 64-1, p. 1671
Parenteral Nutrition, NCP 40-2, p. 968
Parkinson's Disease, NCP 59-4, p. 1554
Peptic Ulcer Disease, NCP 42-2, p. 1023
Peripheral Arterial Disease of the Lower Extremities, NCP 38-1, p. 905
Pneumonia, NCP 28-1, p. 568
Postoperative Patient, NCP 20-1, p. 383
Pressure Ulcer, NCP 13-1, p. 210
Prostate Surgery, NCP 55-1, p. 1420
Rheumatoid Arthritis, NCP 65-1, p. 1708
Seizure Disorder or Epilepsy, NCP 59-2, p. 1540
Shock, NCP 67-1, p. 1791
Spinal Cord Injury, NCP 61-1, p. 1598
Stroke, NCP 58-1, p. 1516
Systemic Lupus Erythematosus, NCP 65-2, p. 1721
Thoracotomy, NCP 28-2, p. 594
Thrombocytopenia, NCP 31-2, p. 706
Total Laryngectomy and/or Radical Neck Surgery, NCP 27-2, p. 554
Tracheostomy, NCP 27-1, p. 548
Urinary Tract Infection, NCP 46-1, p. 1160
Valvular Heart Disease, NCP 37-2, p. 884

COMMON ASSESSMENT ABNORMALITIES TABLES

Auditory System, Table 21-10, p. 413
Breast, Table 51-9, p. 1336
Cardiovascular System, Table 32-5, p. 749
Endocrine System, Table 48-7, p. 1246
Female Reproductive System, Table 51-10, p. 1336
Fluid and Electrolyte Imbalances, Table 17-17, p. 338
Gastrointestinal System, Table 39-11, p. 939
Hematologic System, Table 30-7, p. 675
Integumentary System, Table 23-9, p. 457
Male Reproductive System, Table 51-11, p. 1337
Musculoskeletal System, Table 62-6, p. 1623
Nervous System, Table 56-8, p. 1460
Respiratory System, Table 26-8, p. 524
Urinary System, Table 45-7, p. 1145
Visual System, Table 21-5, p. 406

DRUG THERAPY TABLES

Acute and Chronic Glaucoma, Table 22-10, p. 434
Acute and Chronic Pancreatitis, Table 44-21, p. 1121
Adjuncts to General Anesthesia, Table 19-6, p. 370
Adjuvant Drugs Used for Pain Management, Table 10-9, p. 139
Agents Used to Treat Leukemia, Table 31-25, p. 720
α-Interferon and Ribavirin Side Effects, Table 44-7, p. 1094
Allergic Rhinitis and Sinusitis, Table 27-2, p. 537
Alzheimer's Disease, Table 60-8, p. 1569
Angina and Acute Coronary Syndrome, Table 34-12, p. 800
Antacid Preparations, Table 42-21, p. 1020
Antacid Therapy Side Effects, Table 42-22, p. 1020
Anticoagulant Therapy, Table 38-9, p. 913
Antidiarrheal Drugs, Table 43-3, p. 1037
Antidysrhythmic Drugs, Table 36-8, p. 856
Antiretroviral Agents Used in HIV Infection, Table 15-15, p. 258

Antiretroviral Therapy in the Chronically HIV-Infected Patient, Table 15-13, p. 257

Arthritis and Connective Tissue Disorders, Table 65-3, p. 1698

Asthma and COPD, Table 29-7, p. 618

Asthma Management, Stepwise Approach, Table 29-5, p. 616

Biologic and Targeted Therapy, Table 16-17, p. 303

Blood Glucose Level Effects, Table 49-8, p. 1267

Burn Treatment, Table 25-14, p. 499

Cirrhosis, Table 44-16, p. 1110

Classification of Chemotherapy Drugs, Table 16-9, p. 287

Combination Drug Therapy for Hypertension, Table 33-9, p. 777

Common Causes of Medication Errors by Older Adults, Table 6-14, p. 81

Commonly Used Preoperative Medications, Table 18-10, p. 355

Constipation, Table 43-8, p. 1042

Corticosteroids, Table 50-18, p. 1318

Corticosteroids, Side Effects, Table 50-19, p. 1318

Diabetes Mellitus, Table 49-7, p. 1266

Digitalis Toxicity Manifestations, Table 35-10, p. 833

Drugs Influencing Lower Urinary Tract Function, Table 46-17, p. 1180

Gastroesophageal Reflux Disease (GERD), Table 42-13, p. 1006

Gastrointestinal Bleeding, Table 42-5, p. 998

General Anesthesia, Table 19-5, p. 369

Heart Failure, Table 35-9, p. 831

Helicobacter pylori Infection, Table 42-17, p. 1014

Hematopoietic Growth Factors Used in Cancer Treatment, Table 16-18, p. 304

Hormonal Therapy for Breast Cancer, Table 52-8, p. 1355

Hormonal Therapy for Prostate Cancer, Table 55-7, p. 1426

Hyperlipidemia, Table 34-6, p. 795

Hypertension, Table 33-8, p. 773

Immunosuppressive Therapy, Table 14-18, p. 239

Infective Endocarditis Treatment with Antibiotic Therapy, Table 37-5, p. 869

Infertility, Table 54-2, p. 1383

Inflammation and Healing, Table 13-8, p. 202

Inflammatory Bowel Disease, Table 43-20, p. 1055

Insulin Regimens, Table 49-4, p. 1261

Insulin Types, Table 49-3, p. 1260

Leukemia Treatments, Table 31-26, p. 721

Long-Term Control Versus Quick Relief of Asthma, Table 29-6, p. 617

Mechanisms of Action of Drugs Used to Treat HIV Infection, Table 15-14, p. 257

Medication Use by Older Adults, Table 6-15, p. 81

Methods of Chemotherapy Administration, Table 16-10, p. 288

MOPP Chemotherapeutic Drug Schedule, Table 16-12, p. 291

Multiple Sclerosis, Table 59-15, p. 1544

Nausea and Vomiting, Table 42-1, p. 992

Nonopioid Analgesics, Table 10-7, p. 136

Opioid Analgesics, Table 10-8, p. 137

Pain Medications' Side Effects, Table 10-6, p. 135

Parkinson's Disease, Table 59-18, p. 1552

Patient Categories and Treatment for Community Acquired Pneumonia, Table 28-4, p. 563

Peptic Ulcer Disease, Table 42-20, p. 1019

Photosensitivity, Drugs that May Cause, Table 24-2, p. 461

Replacement Factors Used in Treating Hemophilia, Table 31-18, p. 709

Seizure Disorders and Epilepsy, Table 59-9, p. 1538

Shock, Table 67-9, p. 1787

Syphilis, Table 53-5, p. 1371

Topical Medications, Common Bases for, Table 24-11, p. 474

Topical Medications for Pupil Dilation, Table 22-5, p. 427

Tuberculosis, Table 28-9, p. 573

Tuberculosis, Regimen Options for the Initial Treatment, Table 28-10, p. 574

Voiding Dysfunction, Table 46-21, p. 1185

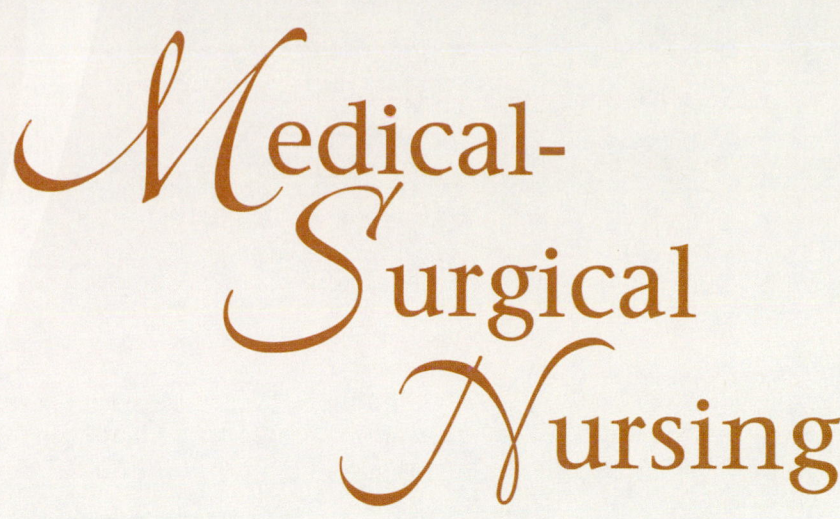

Medical-Surgical Nursing

Volume 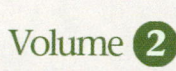 Assessment and Management
of Clinical Problems

Problems of Ingestion, Digestion, Absorption, and Elimination

Section Outline

39 **Nursing Assessment
Gastrointestinal System,** p. 926

40 **Nursing Management
Nutritional Problems,** p. 948

41 **Nursing Management
Obesity,** p. 971

42 **Nursing Management
Upper Gastrointestinal Problems,** p. 990

43 **Nursing Management
Lower Gastrointestinal Problems,** p. 1035

44 **Nursing Management
Liver, Pancreas, and
Biliary Tract Problems,** p. 1087

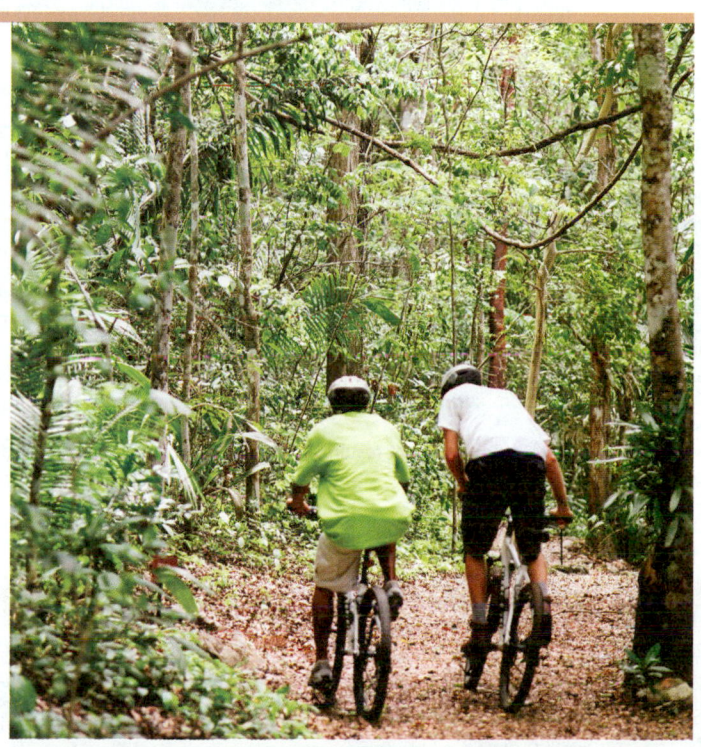

It's supposed to be a professional secret, but I'll tell you anyway. We doctors do nothing. We only help and encourage the doctor within.

Albert Schweitzer

39

Nursing Assessment
Gastrointestinal System

Anne Croghan

LEARNING OBJECTIVES

1. Describe the structures and functions of the organs of the gastrointestinal tract.
2. Describe the structures and functions of the liver, gallbladder, biliary tract, and pancreas.
3. Explain the processes of ingestion, digestion, absorption, and elimination.
4. Explain the processes of biliary metabolism, bile production, and bile excretion.
5. Describe age-related changes in the gastrointestinal system and differences in assessment findings.
6. Identify the significant subjective and objective data related to the gastrointestinal system that should be obtained from a patient.
7. Describe the appropriate techniques used in the physical assessment of the gastrointestinal system.
8. Differentiate normal from common abnormal findings of a physical assessment of the gastrointestinal system.
9. Describe the purpose, significance of results, and nursing responsibilities related to diagnostic studies of the gastrointestinal system.

KEY TERMS

borborygmi,* p. 940
cheilosis,* p. 939
endoscopy, p. 944
hematemesis,* p. 939
hepatocytes, p. 930
Kupffer cells, p. 931
melena,* p. 940
pyorrhea,* p. 939
pyrosis,* p. 939
steatorrhea,* p. 940
tenesmus,* p. 940
Valsalva maneuver, p. 930

*See Table 39-11 on pp. 939 to 940.

Electronic Resources

Supplemental content related to Chapter 39 can be found . . .

Companion CD
- Stress-Busting Kit for Nursing Students
- NCLEX Examination Review Questions
- Animation: Rectal Examination
- Video Clips:
  - Auscultation: Abdomen, Bowel Sounds
  - Percussion: Abdomen
  - Percussion: Liver
  - Percussion: Spleen
  - Palpation: Abdomen, Superficial and Deep
- Comprehensive Glossary

Evolve Website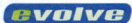
http://evolve.elsevier.com/Lewis/medsurg
- Content Updates
- Key Points (Printable and CD/MP3 Download)
- Concept Map Creator
- Expanded Audio Glossary
- Key Term Flash Cards
- Electronic Calculators

- Physical Examination Video Clips:
  - Abdomen: Inspection, Auscultation, and Percussion
  - Abdomen: Palpation
- WebLinks

The main function of the gastrointestinal (GI) system is to supply nutrients to body cells. This is accomplished through the processes of *ingestion* (taking in food), *digestion* (breakdown of food), and *absorption* (transfer of food products into circulation). *Elimination* is the process of excreting the waste products of digestion.

The GI system (also called the digestive system) consists of the GI tract and its associated organs and glands. Included in the GI tract are the mouth, esophagus, stomach, small intestine, large in-

testine, rectum, and anus. The associated organs are the liver, pancreas, and gallbladder (Fig. 39-1).

Factors outside the GI tract can influence its functioning. Both psychologic and emotional factors, such as stress and anxiety, influence GI functioning in many people. Stress may be manifested as anorexia, epigastric and abdominal pain, or diarrhea. However, GI problems should never be attributed solely to psychologic factors. Organic and psychologically based problems

Reviewed by Juvann M. Wolff, RN, MSN, ARNP, Lecturer, School of Nursing, University of Washington, Seattle, Wash.

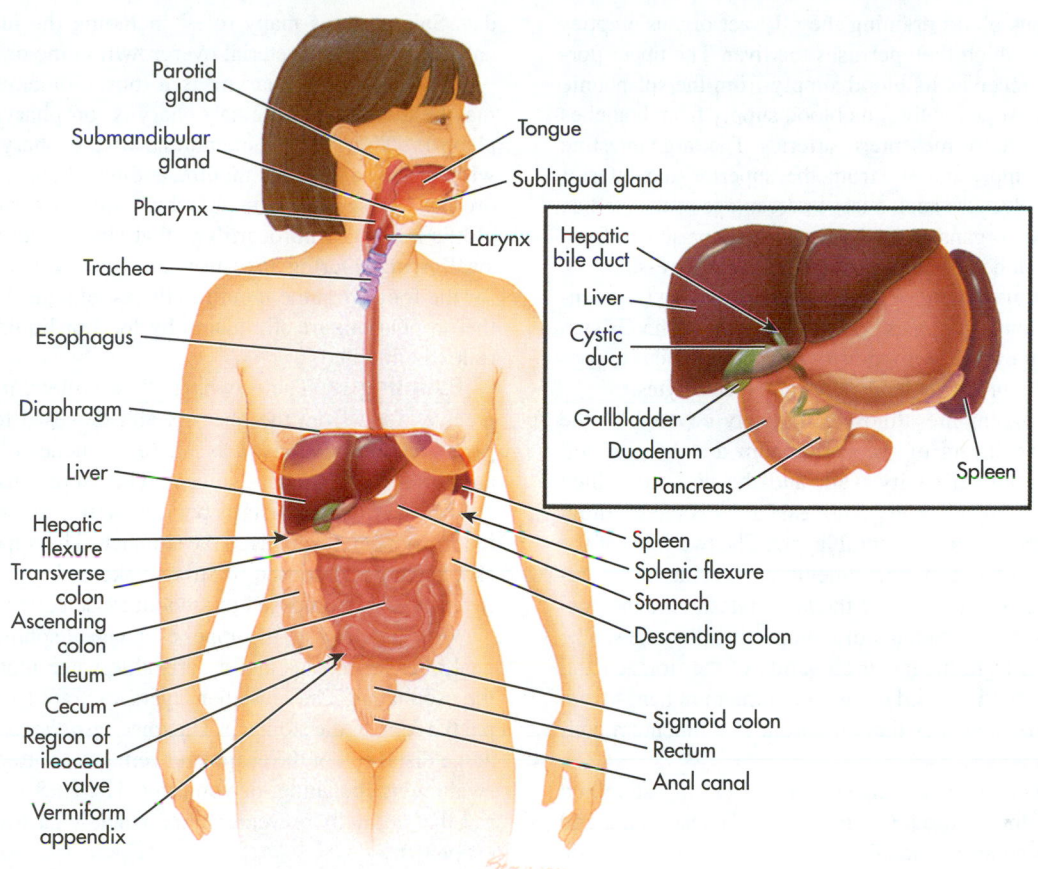

FIG. 39-1 Location of organs of the gastrointestinal system.

can exist independently or concurrently. Physical factors, such as dietary intake, ingestion of alcohol and caffeine-containing products, cigarette smoking, poor sleep, and fatigue, may also affect GI function. Some organic diseases of the GI system, such as peptic ulcer disease and ulcerative colitis, may be aggravated by stress.

STRUCTURES AND FUNCTIONS OF THE GASTROINTESTINAL SYSTEM

The GI tract is a tube approximately 30 feet (9 m) long extending from the mouth to the anus. The entire tract is composed of four common layers. From the inside to the outside, these layers are (1) mucosa, (2) submucosa, (3) muscle, and (4) serosa (Fig. 39-2). In the esophagus the outer coat is fibrous tissue rather than serosa. The muscular coat consists of two layers: the circular (inner) and the longitudinal (outer).

The GI tract is innervated by the parasympathetic and the sympathetic branches of the autonomic nervous system. The parasympathetic system is mainly excitatory, and the sympathetic system is mainly inhibitory. For example, peristalsis is increased by parasympathetic stimulation and decreased by sympathetic stimulation. Sensory information is relayed via both sympathetic and parasympathetic afferent fibers.

The GI tract also has its own nervous system: the enteric, or intrinsic, nervous system. The enteric nervous system is composed of two nerve layers that lie between the mucosa and the circular muscle layer and the circular and longitudinal muscle layers. These neurons contribute to the coordination of GI motor and secretory activities. The enteric nervous system is also known as the

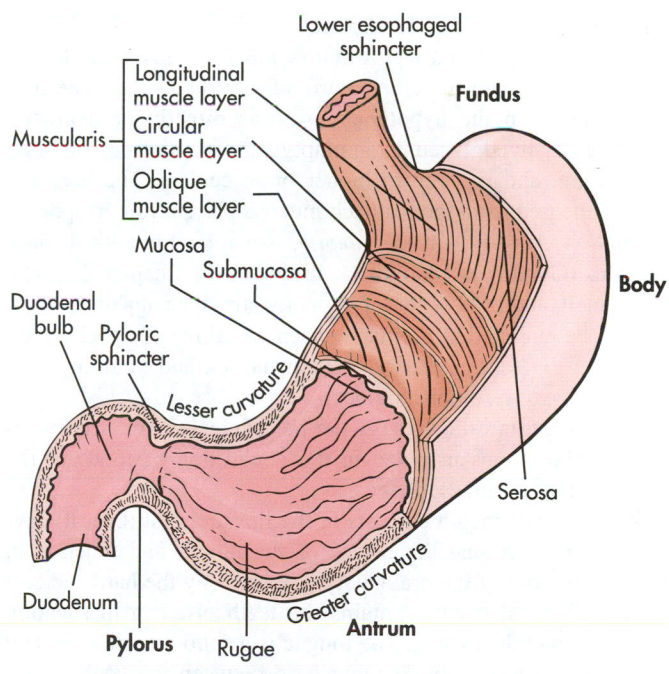

FIG. 39-2 Parts of the stomach.

"gut brain." It contains numerous neurons (about as many as the spinal cord) and has the ability to control movement and secretion of the GI tract.

The GI tract and accessory organs receive approximately 25% to 30% of the cardiac output. Circulation in the GI system is unique in that venous blood draining the GI tract organs empties into the portal vein, which then perfuses the liver. The upper portion of the GI tract receives its blood supply from the splanchnic artery. The small intestine receives its blood supply from branches of the hepatic and superior mesenteric arteries. The large intestine receives its blood supply mainly from the superior and inferior mesenteric arteries. Because such a large percentage of the cardiac output perfuses these organs, the GI tract is a major source from which blood flow can be diverted during exercise or stress.

The two types of movement of the GI tract are mixing (segmentation) and propulsion (peristalsis). The secretions of the GI system consist of enzymes and hormones for digestion, mucus to provide protection and lubrication, and water and electrolytes.

The abdominal organs are almost completely covered by the peritoneum. The two layers of the peritoneum are the *parietal,* which lines the abdominal cavity wall, and the *visceral,* which covers the abdominal organs. The peritoneal cavity is the potential space between the parietal and visceral layers. The two folds of the peritoneum are the mesentery and omentum. The mesentery attaches the small intestine and part of the large intestine to the posterior abdominal wall and contains blood and lymph vessels. The lesser omentum goes from the lesser curvature of the stomach and upper duodenum to the liver, and the greater omentum hangs from the stomach over the intestines like an apron. The omentum contains fat and lymph nodes.

The primary functions of the GI system are (1) ingestion and propulsion (movement) of food, (2) digestion, (3) absorption, and (4) elimination. Each part of the GI system performs different activities to accomplish these functions.

Ingestion and Propulsion of Food

Ingestion is the intake of food. A person's appetite or desire to ingest food is a significant factor in how much food is eaten. Multiple factors are involved in the control of appetite. An appetite center is located in the hypothalamus. It is directly or indirectly stimulated by hypoglycemia, an empty stomach, decrease in body temperature, and input from higher brain centers. The hormone *ghrelin* released from the stomach mucosa plays a role in appetite stimulation. Another hormone, *leptin,* is involved in appetite suppression. (Ghrelin and leptin are discussed in Chapter 41.) The sight, smell, and taste of food frequently stimulate appetite. Appetite may be inhibited by stomach distention, illness (especially accompanied by fever), hyperglycemia, nausea and vomiting, and certain drugs (e.g., amphetamines).

Deglutition (swallowing) is the mechanical component of ingestion. The organs involved in the deglutition of food are the mouth, pharynx, and esophagus.

Mouth. The mouth consists of the lips and oral (buccal) cavity. The lips surround the orifice of the mouth and function in speech. The roof of the oral cavity is formed by the hard and soft palates. The oral cavity contains the teeth, used in mastication (chewing), and the tongue. The tongue is a solid muscle mass and assists in mastication by keeping food between the teeth during chewing and moving the food to the back of the throat for swallowing (deglutition). Taste receptors are found on the sides and tip of the tongue. The tongue is also important in speech.

Within the oral cavity are three pairs of salivary glands: the parotid, submaxillary, and sublingual. These glands produce saliva, which consists of water, protein, mucin, inorganic salts, and salivary amylase. Approximately 1 L of saliva is produced each day. Saliva serves many roles, including the lubrication of food and prevention of bacterial overgrowth in the oral cavity.

Pharynx. The pharynx is a musculomembranous tube that may be divided into the nasopharynx, oropharynx, and laryngeal pharynx. The mucous membrane of the pharynx is continuous with the nasal cavity, mouth, auditory tubes, and larynx. The oropharynx secretes mucus, which aids in swallowing. The epiglottis is a lid of fibrocartilage that closes over the larynx during swallowing. During ingestion the oropharynx provides a route for the food from the mouth to the esophagus. When receptors in the oropharynx are stimulated by food or liquid, the swallowing reflex is initiated.

Esophagus. The esophagus is a hollow, muscular tube that receives food from the pharynx and moves it to the stomach by peristaltic contractions. It is 9.2 to 10 inches (23 to 25 cm) long and 0.8 inch (2 cm) in diameter. The esophagus is located in the thoracic cavity, and it starts behind the trachea at the lower end of the pharynx and extends to the stomach. The upper one third of the esophagus is composed of striated skeletal muscle, and the distal two thirds are composed of smooth muscle.

With swallowing, the upper esophageal sphincter (cricopharyngeal muscle) relaxes and a peristaltic wave moves the bolus into the esophagus. The muscular layers contract (peristalsis) and propel the food to the stomach. The *lower esophageal sphincter* (LES) at the distal end of the esophagus remains contracted except during swallowing, belching, or vomiting. The LES is an important barrier that normally prevents reflux of acidic gastric contents into the esophagus.

Digestion and Absorption

Mouth. Digestion begins in the mouth. **Digestion** involves both mechanical (mastication) and chemical digestion. Saliva is the first secretion involved in digestion, and its main function is to lubricate and soften the food mass, thus facilitating swallowing. Saliva contains amylase (ptyalin), which hydrolyzes starches to maltose. However, salivary amylase is not necessary for the digestion of carbohydrates.

Stomach. The functions of the stomach are to store food, mix the food with gastric secretions, and empty contents into the small intestine at a rate at which digestion can occur. The stomach absorbs only small amounts of water, alcohol, electrolytes, and certain drugs.

The stomach lies obliquely in the epigastric, umbilical, and left hypochondriac regions of the abdomen (see Fig. 39-7 later in the chapter). The shape and position of the stomach change based on the degree of gastric distention. It always contains gastric fluid and mucus. The three main parts of the stomach are the fundus, body, and antrum (see Fig. 39-2). The pylorus is a small portion of the antrum that lies proximal to the pyloric sphincter. Sphincter muscles (the LES and the pyloric sphincter) guard the entrance to and exit from the stomach.

The serous (outer) layer of the stomach is formed by the peritoneum. The muscular layer consists of the longitudinal (outer) layer, circular (middle) layer, and oblique (inner) layer. The mucosal layer forms folds called *rugae* that contain many small glands. In response to nutrient intake, these glands secrete most of the gastric juice. In the fundus the glands contain chief cells, which secrete pepsinogen, and parietal cells, which secrete hydrochloric (HCl) acid, water, and intrinsic factor. The secretion of HCl acid makes gastric juice acidic in comparison with other body fluids. This acidic pH aids in the protection against ingested organisms. Intrinsic factor promotes cobalamin (vitamin B_{12}) absorption in the small intestine. Mucus is secreted by glands in the fundus and pyloric areas.

Small Intestine. The two primary functions of the small intestine are digestion and **absorption** (uptake of nutrients from the gut lumen to the bloodstream). The small intestine is a coiled tube approximately 23 feet (7 m) in length and from 1 to 1.1 inches (2.5 to 2.8 cm) in diameter, diminishing in diameter at the lower end. It extends from the pylorus to the ileocecal valve. The small intestine is composed of the duodenum, jejunum, and ileum. The ileocecal valve, which separates the small intestine from the large intestine, prevents reflux of large intestine contents into the small intestine.

The serous coat of the small intestine is formed by the peritoneum. The mucosa is thick, vascular, and glandular. The circular folds in the mucous and submucous layers provide a greater surface area for digestion and absorption.

The functional units of the small intestine are villi. They are present in the entire small intestine. **Villi** are minute, fingerlike projections in the mucous membrane. They contain goblet cells that secrete mucus and epithelial cells that produce the intestinal digestive enzymes. The epithelial cells on the villi also have *microvilli,* which compose the brush border. Thus the presence of villi and microvilli greatly increases the surface area for absorption.

The digestive enzymes on the brush border of the microvilli chemically break down nutrients so that they can be absorbed. The villi are surrounded by the crypts of Lieberkühn, which contain the base columnar cells that are the stem cells for the other epithelial cell types. Brunner's glands in the submucosa of the duodenum secrete mucus.

Physiology of Digestion. *Digestion* is the physical and chemical breakdown of food into absorbable substances. Digestion in the GI tract is facilitated by the timely movement of food through the various organs and the secretion of specific enzymes. These enzymes break down foodstuffs to particles of appropriate size for absorption (Table 39-1).

The process of digestion begins in the mouth, where the food is chewed, mechanically broken down, and mixed with saliva. The saliva lubricates the food. In addition, salivary amylase begins the breakdown of starch. Salivary gland secretion is stimulated by chewing movements and the sight, smell, thought, and taste of food. The food is swallowed and passes into the esophagus, where peristaltic waves propel it to the stomach. No digestion or absorption occurs in the esophagus.

In the stomach the digestion of proteins begins with the release of pepsinogen from chief cells. The acidic environment of the stomach results in the conversion of pepsinogen to its active form, pepsin. Pepsin begins the initial breakdown of proteins. In the stomach there is minimal digestion of starches and fats. The food is mixed with gastric secretions, which are under neural and hormonal control (Tables 39-2 and 39-3). The stomach also serves as a reservoir for food, which is slowly expelled into the small intestine. The length of time that food remains in the stomach depends on the composition of the food, but average meals remain from 3 to 4 hours.

Digestion is completed in the small intestine, where carbohydrates are hydrolyzed to monosaccharides, fats to glycerol and fatty acids, and proteins to amino acids. The physical presence of *chyme* (food mixed with gastric secretions), along with its chemical nature in the small intestine, stimulates motility and secretion. Secretions involved in digestion include enzymes from the pancreas, bile from the liver (see Table 39-1), and intestinal secretions from glands in the small intestine. Both secretion and motility are under neural and hormonal control.

When food enters the stomach and small intestine, hormones are released into the bloodstream (see Table 39-3). The hormone secretin stimulates the pancreas to secrete fluid with a high concentration of bicarbonate. This alkaline secretion enters the duodenum and neutralizes acid in the chyme. The duodenal mucosa also secretes mucus to protect against the HCl acid. In response to the presence of chyme, the hormone cholecystokinin (CCK), produced by the duodenal mucosa, enters the bloodstream and stimulates contraction of the gallbladder and relaxation of the sphincter of Oddi. These actions permit bile to flow from the common bile duct into the duodenum. Bile is necessary for the digestion of fats. CCK also stimulates the pancreas to synthesize and secrete enzymes for enzymatic digestion of carbohydrates, fats, and proteins.

TABLE 39-1	Gastrointestinal Secretions Related to Digestion		
Location	**Daily Amount (ml)**	**Secretions/Enzymes**	**Action**
Salivary glands	1000-1500	Salivary amylase (ptyalin)	Initiation of starch digestion
Stomach	2500	Pepsinogen	Protein digestion
		HCl acid	Activation of pepsinogen to pepsin
		Lipase	Fat digestion
		Intrinsic factor	Essential for cobalamin absorption in ileum
Small intestine	3000	Enterokinase	Activation of trypsinogen to trypsin
		Amylase	Carbohydrate digestion
		Peptidases	Protein digestion
		Aminopeptidase	
		Maltase	Maltose to two glucose molecules
		Sucrase	Sucrose to glucose and fructose
		Lactase	Lactose to glucose and galactose
		Lipase	Fat digestion
Pancreas	700	Trypsinogen	Protein digestion
		Chymotrypsin	Protein digestion
		Amylase	Starch to disaccharides
		Lipase	Fat digestion
Liver and gallbladder	1000	Bile	Emulsification of fats and aid in absorption of fatty acids and fat-soluble vitamins (A, D, E, K)

Enzymes present on the brush border of the microvilli complete the digestion process. These enzymes hydrolyze disaccharides to monosaccharides and peptides to amino acids for absorption.

Absorption is the transfer of the end products of digestion across the intestinal wall to the circulation. Most absorption occurs in the small intestine. The surface area of the small intestine is greatly increased by its circular folds, villi, and microvilli. The movement of the villi enables the end products of digestion to come in contact with the absorbing membrane. Monosaccharides (from carbohydrates), fatty acids (from fats), amino acids (from proteins), water, electrolytes, and vitamins are absorbed.

Elimination

Large Intestine. The large intestine is a hollow, muscular tube approximately 5 to 6 feet (1.5 to 2 m) long and 2 inches (5 cm) in diameter. The four parts of the large intestine are (1) the cecum and appendix, a narrow tube at the end of the cecum; (2) the colon (ascending colon on the right side, transverse colon across the abdomen, descending colon on the left side, and the sigmoid colon); (3) the rectum; and (4) the anus, the terminal portion of the large intestine (Fig. 39-3).

The most important function of the large intestine is the absorption of water and electrolytes. It also forms feces and serves as a reservoir for the fecal mass until defecation occurs. Feces are composed of water (75%), bacteria, unabsorbed minerals, undigested foodstuffs, bile pigments, and desquamated epithelial cells. The large intestine secretes mucus, which acts as a lubricant and protects the mucosa.

Microorganisms in the colon are responsible for the breakdown of proteins not digested or absorbed in the small intestine. These amino acids are deaminated by the bacteria, leaving ammonia, which is carried to the liver and converted to urea. Bacteria in the colon also synthesize vitamin K and some of the B vitamins. Bacteria also play a part in the production of flatus.

The movements of the large intestine are usually slow. When the circular muscles contract, they produce a kneading action termed *haustral churning*. Propulsive (mass movements) peristalsis also occurs. When food enters the stomach and duodenum, the gastrocolic and duodenocolic reflexes are initiated, resulting in peristalsis in the colon. These reflexes are more active after the first daily meal and frequently result in bowel evacuation.

Defecation is a reflex action involving voluntary and involuntary control. Feces in the rectum stimulate sensory nerve endings that produce the desire to defecate. The reflex center for defecation is in the sacral portion of the spinal cord (parasympathetic nerve fibers). These fibers produce contraction of the rectum and relaxation of the internal anal sphincter. Defecation is controlled voluntarily by relaxing the external anal sphincter when the desire to defecate is felt. An acceptable environment for defecation is usually necessary or the urge to defecate will be ignored. If defecation is suppressed over long periods, problems can occur, such as constipation or stool impaction.

Defecation can be facilitated by the **Valsalva maneuver.** This maneuver involves contraction of the chest muscles on a closed glottis with simultaneous contraction of the abdominal muscles. These actions result in increased intraabdominal pressure. The Valsalva maneuver may be contraindicated in the patient with a head injury, eye surgery, cardiac problems, hemorrhoids, abdominal surgery, or liver cirrhosis with portal hypertension.

Constipation is common in the older adult and is due to many factors, including slower peristalsis, inactivity, decreased dietary fiber, decreased fluids, depression, constipating medications, and laxative abuse.[1] (Constipation is discussed in Chapter 43.)

Liver, Biliary Tract, and Pancreas

Liver. The liver is the largest internal organ in the body, weighing approximately 3 lb (1.37 kg) in the adult. It lies in the right epigastric region (see Fig. 39-7 later in the chapter). Most of the liver is enclosed in peritoneum. It has a fibrous capsule that divides it into right and left lobes (Fig. 39-4).

The functional units of the liver are lobules (Fig. 39-5). The lobule consists of rows of hepatic cells (**hepatocytes**) arranged around a central vein. The capillaries (sinusoids) are located be-

TABLE 39-2	Phases of Gastric Secretion	
Phase	**Stimulus to Secretion**	**Secretion**
Cephalic (nervous)	Sight, smell, taste of food (before food enters stomach); initiated in the CNS and mediated by the vagus nerve	HCl acid, pepsinogen, mucus
Gastric (hormonal and nervous)	Food in antrum of stomach, vagal stimulation	Release of gastrin from antrum into circulation to stimulate gastric secretions and motility
Intestinal (hormonal)	Presence of chyme in small intestine	Acidic chyme (pH <2): release of secretin, gastric inhibitory polypeptide, cholecystokinin into circulation to decrease HCl acid secretion Chyme (pH >3): release of duodenal gastrin to increase acid secretion

CNS, Central nervous system.

TABLE 39-3	Major Hormones Controlling Gastrointestinal Secretion and Motility		
Hormone	**Source**	**Activating Stimuli**	**Function**
Gastrin	Gastric and duodenal mucosa	Stomach distention, partially digested proteins in pylorus	Gastric acid secretion, increased motility, maintenance of lower esophageal sphincter tone
Secretin	Duodenal mucosa	Acid entering small intestine	Inhibition of gastric motility and acid secretion, stimulation of pancreatic bicarbonate secretion
Cholecystokinin	Duodenal mucosa	Fatty acids and amino acids in small intestine	Contraction of gallbladder and relaxation of sphincter of Oddi, allowing increased flow of bile into duodenum; release of pancreatic digestive enzymes
Gastric inhibitory peptide	Duodenal mucosa	Fatty acids and lipids in the small intestine	Inhibition of gastric acid secretion and gastric motility

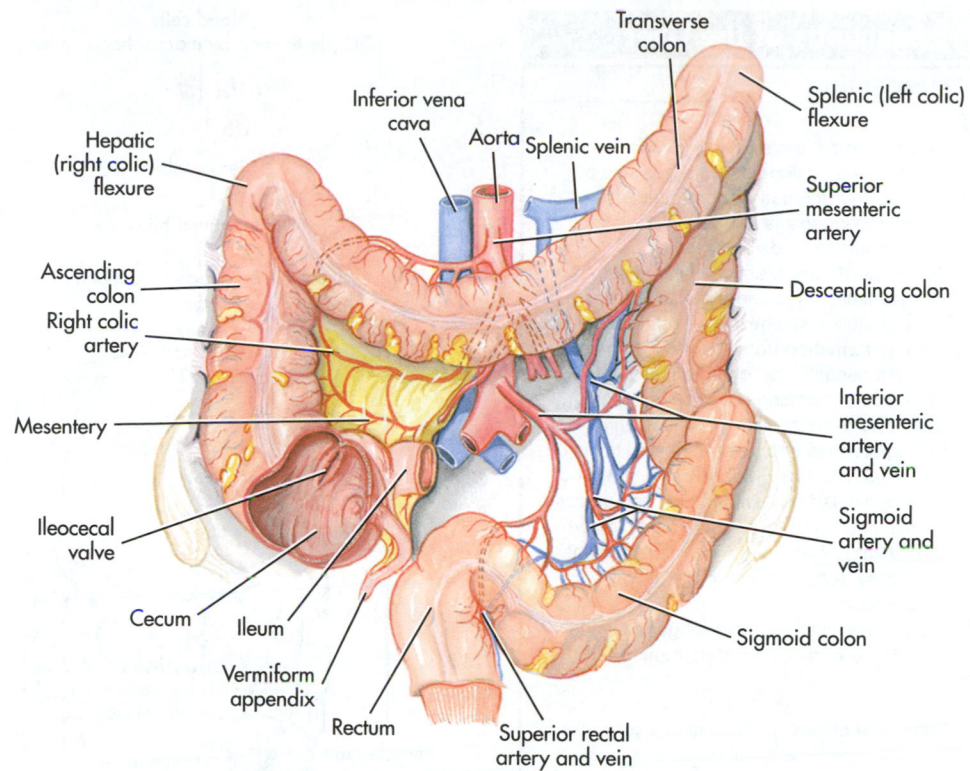

FIG. 39-3 Anatomic locations of the large intestine.

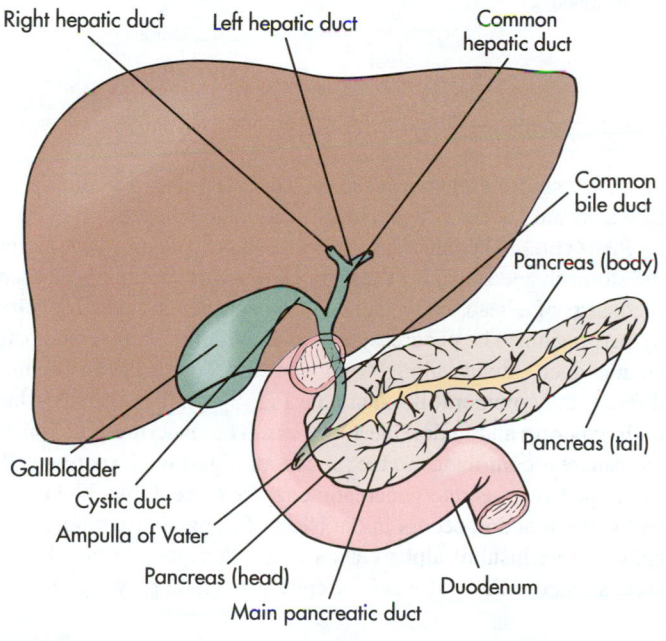

FIG. 39-4 Gross structure of the liver, gallbladder, pancreas, and duct system.

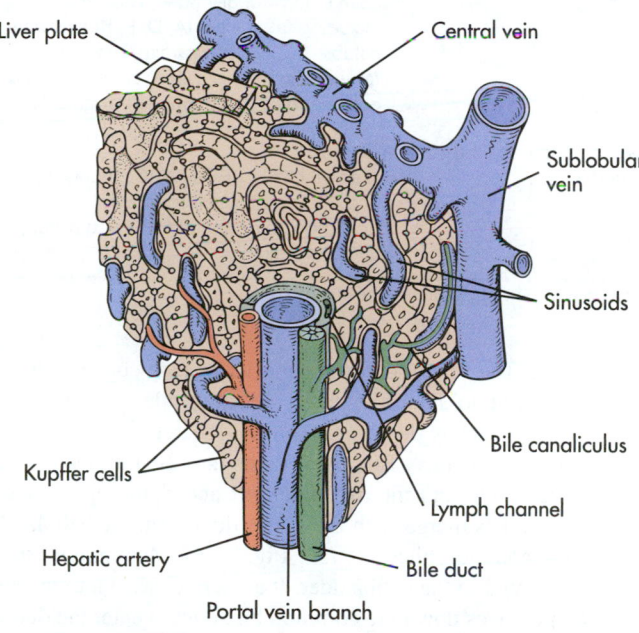

FIG. 39-5 Microscopic structure of liver lobule.

tween the rows of hepatocytes and are lined with **Kupffer cells,** which carry out phagocytic activity (removal of bacteria and toxins from the blood). Interlobular bile ducts form from bile capillaries (canaliculi). The hepatic cells secrete bile into the canaliculi.

The nerve supply to the liver is from the left vagus and sympathetic celiac plexus. About one third of the blood supply comes from the hepatic artery (branch of the celiac artery), and two thirds come from the portal vein.

The portal circulatory system (enterohepatic) brings blood to the liver from the stomach, intestines, spleen, and pancreas. This blood enters the liver through the portal vein. The portal vein carries absorbed products of digestion directly to the liver. In the liver the portal vein branches and comes in contact with each lobule. The blood in the sinusoids is a mixture of arterial and venous blood.

The liver is essential for life. It functions in the manufacture, storage, transformation, and excretion of a number of substances involved in metabolism. The functions of the liver are numerous but can be classified into four main areas, as identified in Table 39-4.

Biliary Tract. The biliary tract consists of the gallbladder and the duct system. The gallbladder is a pear-shaped sac located be-

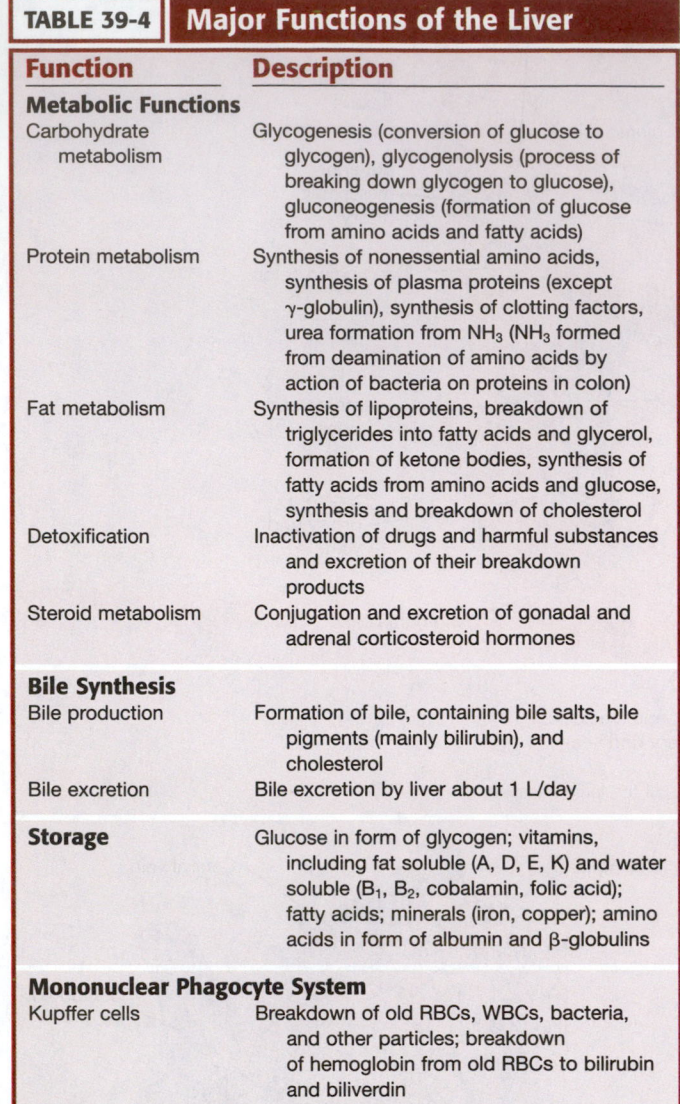

TABLE 39-4 | **Major Functions of the Liver**

Function	Description
Metabolic Functions	
Carbohydrate metabolism	Glycogenesis (conversion of glucose to glycogen), glycogenolysis (process of breaking down glycogen to glucose), gluconeogenesis (formation of glucose from amino acids and fatty acids)
Protein metabolism	Synthesis of nonessential amino acids, synthesis of plasma proteins (except γ-globulin), synthesis of clotting factors, urea formation from NH_3 (NH_3 formed from deamination of amino acids by action of bacteria on proteins in colon)
Fat metabolism	Synthesis of lipoproteins, breakdown of triglycerides into fatty acids and glycerol, formation of ketone bodies, synthesis of fatty acids from amino acids and glucose, synthesis and breakdown of cholesterol
Detoxification	Inactivation of drugs and harmful substances and excretion of their breakdown products
Steroid metabolism	Conjugation and excretion of gonadal and adrenal corticosteroid hormones
Bile Synthesis	
Bile production	Formation of bile, containing bile salts, bile pigments (mainly bilirubin), and cholesterol
Bile excretion	Bile excretion by liver about 1 L/day
Storage	
	Glucose in form of glycogen; vitamins, including fat soluble (A, D, E, K) and water soluble (B_1, B_2, cobalamin, folic acid); fatty acids; minerals (iron, copper); amino acids in form of albumin and β-globulins
Mononuclear Phagocyte System	
Kupffer cells	Breakdown of old RBCs, WBCs, bacteria, and other particles; breakdown of hemoglobin from old RBCs to bilirubin and biliverdin

RBCs, Red blood cells; *WBCs,* white blood cells.

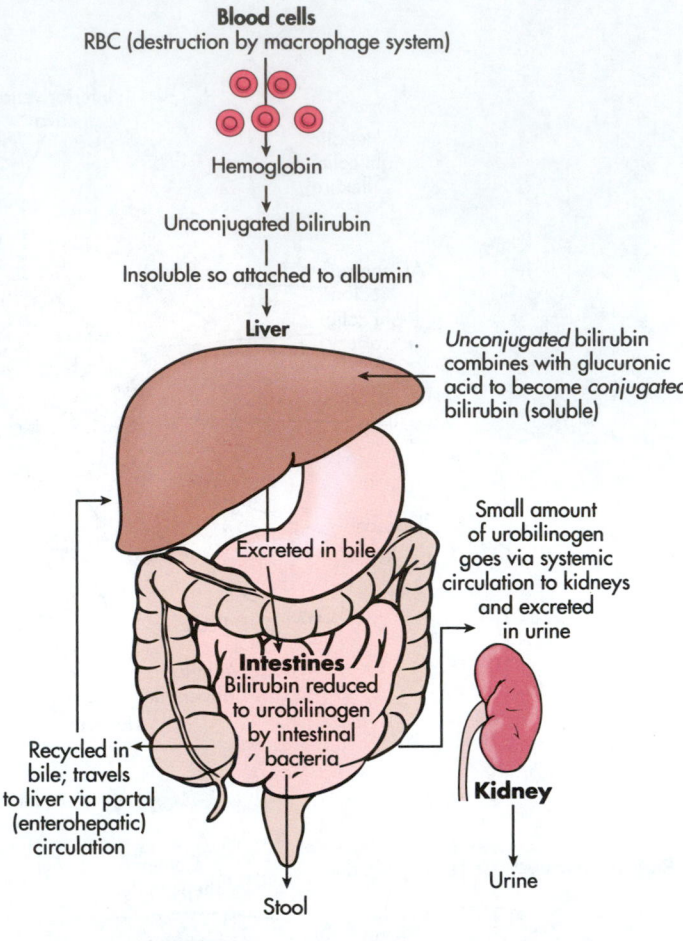

FIG. 39-6 Bilirubin metabolism and conjugation.

low the liver. The function of the gallbladder is to concentrate and store bile. It can hold approximately 45 ml of bile.

Bile is produced by the hepatic cells and secreted into the biliary canaliculi of the lobules. Bile then drains into the interlobular bile ducts, which unite into the two main left and right hepatic ducts. The hepatic ducts merge with the cystic duct from the gallbladder to form the common bile duct (see Fig. 39-4). Most bile is stored and concentrated in the gallbladder. It is then released into the cystic duct and moves down the common bile duct to enter the duodenum at the ampulla of Vater. In the intestines, bilirubin is reduced to stercobilinogen and urobilinogen by bacterial action. Stercobilinogen accounts for the brown color of stool. A small amount of conjugated bilirubin is reabsorbed by the blood. Some urobilinogen is reabsorbed by the blood and returned to the liver through the portal circulation (enterohepatic) and excreted in the bile. An insignificant amount of urobilinogen is excreted in the urine.[2]

Bilirubin Metabolism. Bilirubin, a pigment derived from the breakdown of hemoglobin, is constantly produced (Fig. 39-6). Because it is insoluble in water, it is bound to albumin for its transport to the liver. This form of bilirubin is referred to as unconjugated. In the liver bilirubin is conjugated with glucuronic acid. Conjugated bilirubin is soluble and is excreted in bile. Bile also consists of water, cholesterol, bile salts, electrolytes, and phospholipids. Bile salts are needed for fat emulsification and digestion.

Pancreas. The pancreas is a long, slender gland lying behind the stomach and in front of the first and second lumbar vertebrae. It consists of a head, body, and tail. The anterior surface is covered by peritoneum. The pancreas contains lobes and lobules. The pancreatic duct extends along the gland and enters the duodenum through the common bile duct (see Fig. 39-4). The pancreas has both exocrine and endocrine functions. The exocrine function of the pancreas contributes to the process of digestion. Exocrine cells in the pancreas secrete pancreatic enzymes (see Table 39-1). The endocrine function occurs in the islets of Langerhans, whose beta cells secrete insulin; alpha cells secrete glucagon; delta cells secrete somatostatin; and F cells secrete pancreatic polypeptide.

GERONTOLOGIC CONSIDERATIONS
EFFECTS OF AGING ON THE GASTROINTESTINAL SYSTEM

The process of aging causes changes in the functional ability of the GI system, although less than in other organ systems (Table 39-5). Tooth enamel and dentin wear down and make the teeth susceptible to cavities. Periodontal disease can lead to the loss of teeth. *Xerostomia* (decreased saliva production), or dry mouth, affects many older adults and may be associated with difficulty swallowing (dysphagia).[3] Taste buds decrease, the sense of smell diminishes, and salivary secretions diminish, all of which can lead to a decrease in appetite and make eating less pleasurable.

TABLE 39-5	*GERONTOLOGIC DIFFERENCES IN ASSESSMENT* Gastrointestinal System	

Expected Aging Changes	Differences in Assessment Findings
Mouth	
Gingival retraction	Loss of teeth, presence of dentures, difficulty chewing
Decreased taste buds, decreased sense of smell	Diminished sense of taste (especially salty and sweet)
Decreased volume of saliva	Dry oral mucosa
Atrophy of gingival tissue	Poor-fitting dentures
Esophagus	
Lower esophageal sphincter pressure decreased, motility decreased	Epigastric distress, dysphagia, potential for hiatal hernia and aspiration
Abdominal Wall	
Thinner and less taut	More visible peristalsis, easier palpation of organs
Decrease in number and sensitivity of sensory receptors	Less sensitivity to surface pain
Stomach	
Atrophy of gastric mucosa, decrease in blood flow	Food intolerances, signs of anemia as result of cobalamin malabsorption, decreased gastric emptying
Small Intestines	
Slight decreases in secretion of most digestive enzymes and motility	Complaints of indigestion, slowed intestinal transit, delayed absorption of fat-soluble vitamins
Liver	
Decreased size and lowered in position	Easier palpation due to lower border extending past costal margin
Decrease in protein synthesis, ability to regenerate decreased	Decrease in drug metabolism
Large Intestine, Anus, Rectum	
Decreased anal sphincter tone and nerve supply to rectal area	Fecal incontinence
Decreased muscular tone, decreased motility	Flatulence, abdominal distention, relaxed perineal musculature
Increase in transit time, sensation to defecation decreased	Constipation, fecal impaction
Pancreas	
Pancreatic ducts distended, lipase production decreased, pancreatic reserve impaired	Impaired fat absorption, decreased glucose tolerance

Age-related changes in the esophagus include delayed emptying resulting from smooth muscle weakness and an incompetent lower esophageal sphincter.[1] Decreased esophageal clearance of acid may put the older patient at risk for gastroesophageal reflux disease (GERD).[3] Motility of the GI system decreases with age, but secretion and absorption are affected to a lesser extent. The elderly patient often experiences a decrease in HCl acid secretion (hypochlorhydria), delayed gastric emptying, and constipation. With chronic atrophic gastritis there is a decrease in the number of

parietal cells and subsequent reduction in the amount of acid and intrinsic factor secreted. Although constipation is a common complaint of elderly patients, age-related changes in colonic secretion or motility have not been consistently shown.[3]

The liver size decreases after 50 years of age, but results of liver function tests remain within normal ranges. Enzyme changes in the liver that are age related decrease the ability of the liver to metabolize drugs and hormones. The size of the pancreas is unaffected by aging but does undergo structural changes such as fibrosis, fatty acid deposits, and atrophy. Aging does not cause changes in the structure and function of the gallbladder and bile ducts. There is an increase in the incidence of gallstones.[3]

Older adults, especially those over 85, are at risk for decreased food intake.[3] The economic inability to purchase food supplies may affect nutritional intake, especially in the older adult. Economic constraints may also reduce the number of fresh fruits and vegetables consumed and thus the amount of fiber. Immobility limits the ability to obtain and prepare meals. A reduction in dietary fiber, along with reduced fluid intake and decreased physical activity, contributes to constipation. Approximately 35% of individuals over 65 are obese.[3] Age-related changes in the GI system and differences in assessment findings are presented in Table 39-5.

ASSESSMENT OF THE GASTROINTESTINAL SYSTEM

Subjective Data

Important Health Information

Past Health History. Information should be gathered from the patient about the history or existence of the following problems related to GI functioning: abdominal pain, nausea and vomiting, diarrhea, constipation, abdominal distention, jaundice, anemia, heartburn, dyspepsia, changes in appetite, hematemesis, food intolerance or allergies, indigestion, excessive gas, bloating, melena, hemorrhoids, or rectal bleeding. In addition, the patient should be asked about the history or existence of diseases such as gastritis, hepatitis, colitis, gallbladder disease, peptic ulcer, cancer, or hernias, especially hiatal hernias.

The patient should be questioned about weight history. Any unexplained or unplanned weight loss or weight gain within the past 12 months should be explored in detail. A history of chronic dieting and repeated weight loss and gain should be documented.

Medications. The health history should include an assessment of the patient's past and current use of medications. The names of all drugs, their frequency of use, and their duration of use are important. This is a critical aspect of history taking because many medications may not only have an effect on the GI system but also may be affected by abnormalities of the GI system and surrounding organs. The medication assessment should include information about over-the-counter medications, prescription drugs, herbal products, and nutritional supplements (see the Complementary and Alternative Therapies box in Chapter 4 on p. 44). The use of prescription or over-the-counter appetite suppressants should be noted.

Many chemicals and drugs are potentially hepatotoxic (Table 39-6) and result in significant patient harm unless monitored closely. For example, chronic high doses of acetaminophen and nonsteroidal antiinflammatory drugs (NSAIDs) may be hepatotoxic. NSAIDs may also predispose to upper GI bleeding with increasing risk/frequency with age. Other medications such as antibiotics have the potential to change the normal bacterial composition in the GI tract,

TABLE 39-6	Potentially Hepatotoxic Chemicals and Drugs

acetaminophen	6-mercaptopurine (6-MP)
amiodarone	mercury
arsenic	methotrexate
azathioprine	nevirapine
carbamazepine	niacin
chloroform	statins
gold compounds	sulfonamides
halothane	thiazide diuretics
isoniazid (INH)	thiazolidinediones
ketoconazole	

TABLE 39-7	Surgeries of the Gastrointestinal System

Surgical Procedure	Description
Antrectomy	Removal of antrum portion of stomach
Appendectomy	Removal of the appendix
Cecostomy	Opening into cecum
Cholecystectomy	Removal of gallbladder
Cholecystostomy	Opening into gallbladder
Choledochojejunostomy	Opening between common bile duct and jejunum
Choledocholithotomy	Opening into common bile duct for removal of stones
Colectomy	Removal of the colon
Colostomy	Opening into colon
Esophagoenterostomy	Removal of portion of esophagus with segment of colon attached to remaining portion
Esophagogastrostomy	Removal of esophagus and anastomosis of remaining portion to stomach
Gastrectomy	Removal of stomach
Gastrostomy	Opening into stomach
Glossectomy	Removal of tongue
Hemiglossectomy	Removal of half of tongue
Herniorrhaphy	Removal of a hernia
Ileostomy	Opening into ileum
Mandibulectomy	Removal of mandible
Pyloroplasty	Enlargement and repair of pyloric sphincter area
Vagotomy	Resection of branch of vagus nerve

resulting in diarrhea. Antacids and laxatives may affect the absorption of certain medications. The nurse should ask the patient if laxatives or antacids are taken, including the kind and frequency.

Surgery or Other Treatments. Information should be obtained about hospitalizations for any problems related to the GI system. Data should also be obtained related to any abdominal or rectal surgery, including the year, reason for surgery, postoperative course, and possible blood transfusions. Terms related to surgery of the GI system are presented in Table 39-7.

Functional Health Patterns. Key questions to ask a patient with a GI problem are presented in Table 39-8.

Health Perception–Health Management Pattern. The nurse should ask about the patient's health practices related to the GI system, such as maintenance of normal body weight, attention to proper dental care, maintenance of adequate nutrition, and effective elimination habits.

The patient should be asked about recent foreign travel with possible exposure to hepatitis, parasitic infestation, or bacterial infestation. Past history of receiving hepatitis A and/or hepatitis B vaccination should be documented.

The patient should be assessed in relation to certain habits that directly affect GI functioning. The consumption of alcohol in large quantities has detrimental effects on the mucosa of the stomach and also increases the secretion of HCl acid and pepsinogen. Chronic alcohol exposure causes fatty infiltration of the liver and can cause damage leading to cirrhosis. The nurse should obtain a history of cigarette smoking. Nicotine is irritating to the entire GI tract mucosa. Cigarette smoking is related to various GI cancers (especially mouth and esophageal cancers), esophagitis, and ulcers. Smoking will also delay the healing of ulcers.

Nutritional-Metabolic Pattern. A thorough nutritional assessment is essential. A dietary history should be taken and compared with the food pyramid (see Fig. 40-1 and Table 40-1). Open-ended questions will allow the patient to express beliefs and feelings about the diet. For example, the nurse can say, "Please tell me about your food and beverage intake over the past 24 hours." A 24-hour dietary recall can be used to analyze the adequacy of the diet. The nurse should assist the patient in recalling the preceding day's food intake, including early morning and nighttime intake, as well as snacks, liquids, and vitamin supplements. The diet will then be evaluated by the nurse in terms of the recommended groups and servings on the food pyramid and try to determine whether the 24-hour recall is typical of the patient's usual eating habits. If weekend eating habits vary greatly, the nurse should obtain a separate weekend diet history and assess the patient's intake for both quality and quantity of food.

The nurse should ask the patient about the use of sugar and salt substitutes, use of caffeine, and amount of fluid and fiber intake.

Any changes in appetite, food tolerance, and weight should be noted. Anorexia and weight loss may indicate the presence of cancer. The nurse should ask the patient about food allergies and determine what GI symptoms such allergic responses cause. The patient should be asked about dietary intolerances, including lactose and gluten.

Elimination Pattern. A detailed account of the patient's bowel elimination pattern should be elicited. The frequency, time of day, and usual consistency of stool should be noted. The use of laxatives and enemas, including type, frequency, and results, should be documented. Any recent change in bowel patterns should be investigated.

The amount and type of fluid and fiber intake should be determined because they have an important effect on the frequency and consistency of stools. Inadequate intake of fiber can be associated with constipation. Analysis of fluid intake and output could indicate the presence of a urinary problem and the possibility of fluid retention.

Food allergies can cause lesions, pruritus, and edema. Diarrhea can result in redness, irritation, and pain in the perianal area. External drainage systems, such as an ileostomy or ileal conduit, can cause local skin irritation. The possible association between a skin problem and a GI problem should be investigated.

Activity-Exercise Pattern. The patient's ambulatory status should be assessed to determine if the patient is capable of securing and preparing food. If the patient is unable to do these tasks, it should be determined if family or an outside agency is meeting this need. Any limitation in the patient's ability to feed himself or herself independently should be noted. Any difficulty accessing a safe environment of elimination should be assessed. Use of and access to elimination supplies should be assessed, such as a commode or ostomy supplies. Activity and exercise may affect GI motility. Immobility is a risk factor for constipation.

Gastrointestinal System

TABLE 39-8	*HEALTH HISTORY* **Gastrointestinal System**

Health Perception–Health Management Pattern
- Describe any measures used to treat GI symptoms such as diarrhea or vomiting.
- Do you smoke?* Do you drink alcohol?*
- Are you exposed to any chemicals on a regular basis?* Have you been exposed in the past?*
- Have you recently traveled outside the United States?*

Nutritional-Metabolic Pattern
- Describe your usual daily food and fluid intake.
- Do you take any supplemental vitamins or minerals?*
- Have you experienced any changes in appetite or food tolerance?*
- Has there been a weight change in the past?*
- Are you allergic to any foods?*

Elimination Pattern
- Describe the frequency and time of day you have bowel movements. What is the consistency of the bowel movement?
- Do you use laxatives or enemas?* If so, how often?
- Have there been any recent change in your bowel pattern?*
- Describe any skin problems caused by GI problems.
- Do you need any assistive equipment, such as ostomy equipment, raised toilet seat, commode?

Activity-Exercise Pattern
- Do you have limitations in mobility that make it difficult for you to procure and prepare food?*
- Are you able to feed yourself?
- Do you have any GI symptoms, such as vomiting or diarrhea, that affect your activity?*
- Do you have any difficulty accessing a toilet when needed?*
- Is a safe and comfortable environment for elimination available?

Sleep-Rest Pattern
- Do you experience any difficulty sleeping because of a GI problem?*
- Are you awakened by symptoms such as gas or esophageal burning?*

Cognitive-Perceptual Pattern
- Have you experienced any change in taste or smell that has affected your appetite?*
- Do you have any heat or cold sensitivity that affects eating?*
- Does pain interfere with food preparation, appetite, or chewing?*
- Do pain medications cause constipation or appetite suppression?*

Self-Perception–Self-Concept Pattern
- Describe any changes in your weight that have affected how you feel about yourself.
- Have you had any changes in normal elimination that have affected how you feel about yourself?*
- Have any symptoms of GI disease caused physical changes that are a problem for you?*

Role-Relationship Pattern
- Describe the impact of any GI problem on your usual roles and relationships.
- Have any changes in elimination affected your relationships?*
- Do you live alone? Describe how your family or others assist you with your GI problems.

Sexuality-Reproductive Pattern
- Describe the effect of your GI problem on your sexual activity.

Coping–Stress Tolerance Pattern
- Do you experience GI symptoms in response to stressful or emotional situations?
- Describe how you deal with any GI symptoms that result.

Value-Belief Pattern
- Describe any culturally specific health beliefs regarding food and food preparation that may influence the treatment of this GI problem.

GI, Gastrointestinal.
*If yes, describe.

Sleep-Rest Pattern. Many food-related events can interrupt and interfere with the quality of sleep. Nausea, vomiting, diarrhea, indigestion, bloating, and hunger can produce sleep problems and should be investigated. The patient should be asked if GI symptoms affect sleep or rest. For example, a patient with a hiatal hernia may be awakened because of burning pain; sleep may be improved by elevating the head of the bed for this patient.

A patient often has a bedtime ritual that involves the use of a particular food or beverage. Milk is known to induce sleep through the effect of the serotonin precursor L-tryptophan. Herbal teas and melatonin are often sleep inducing. Individual routines should be noted and complied with whenever possible to avoid sleeplessness. Hunger can prevent sleep and should be relieved by a light, easily digested snack unless contraindicated.

Cognitive-Perceptual Pattern. Decreases in sensory adequacy can result in problems related to the acquisition, preparation, and ingestion of food. Changes in taste or smell can affect appetite and eating pleasure. Vertigo can make shopping and standing at a stove difficult and dangerous. Heat or cold sensitivity could make certain foods painful to eat. Problems in expressive communication could make it difficult and frustrating for the patient to make personal desires and preferences known. The nurse should assess the patient in this pattern to judge the effect

of deficiencies on adequate nutritional intake. If the patient has been diagnosed as having a GI disorder, the nurse should ask questions to determine the patient's understanding of the illness and its treatment.

Pain is another area that requires careful assessment related to its effect on the GI system and nutrition. Relevant behaviors associated with chronic pain include avoidance of activity, fatigue, and disruption of eating patterns. The possible effects of opioid pain medication related to constipation, nausea, sedation, and appetite suppression should be assessed.

Self-Perception–Self-Concept Pattern. Many GI and nutritional problems can have serious effects on the patient's self-perception. Overweight and underweight persons often have problems related to self-esteem and body image. Repeated attempts to achieve a personally acceptable weight can be discouraging and depressing for the patient. The manner in which a person recounts a weight history can alert the nurse to potential problems in this area.

Another potentially problematic area is the need for external devices to manage elimination, such as a colostomy or an ileostomy. The patient's willingness to engage in self-care and to discuss this situation should provide the nurse with valuable information related to body image and self-esteem.

The altered physical changes often associated with advanced liver disease can be problematic for the patient. Jaundice and ascites cause significant changes in external appearance. The patient's attitude toward these changes should be assessed.

Role-Relationship Pattern. Problems related to the GI system such as cirrhosis, alcoholism, hepatitis, ostomies, obesity, and carcinoma can have a major impact on the patient's ability to maintain usual roles and relationships. A chronic illness may necessitate leaving a job or reducing the number of hours worked. Changes in body image and self-esteem can affect relationships. The availability of and satisfaction with support should be determined. It is important that the nurse be aware of these possible consequences and assess for their presence.

Sexuality-Reproductive Pattern. Changes related to sexuality and reproductive status can result from problems of the GI system. For example, obesity, jaundice, anorexia, and ascites could decrease the acceptance of a potential sexual partner. The presence of an ostomy could affect the patient's confidence related to sexual activity. Chronic alcoholism could discourage a meaningful relationship that could develop into a sexual relationship. Sensitive questioning by the nurse could determine the presence of potential problems.

Anorexia can affect the reproductive status of a female patient. Alcoholism can affect the reproductive status of both men and women. A poor nutritional intake before and during pregnancy can result in a low-birth-weight infant.

Coping–Stress Tolerance Pattern. The nurse should try to determine what is a stressor for the patient and what coping mechanisms the patient uses to function with these stressors. GI symptoms such as epigastric pain, nausea, and diarrhea develop in many people in response to stressful or emotional situations. Some GI problems such as peptic ulcers and irritable bowel syndrome are aggravated by stress.

Value-Belief Pattern. The patient's spiritual and cultural beliefs regarding food and food preparation should be assessed. Whenever possible, these preferences should be respected by the health care provider. In addition, it should be determined if any value or belief could interfere with planned interventions. For example, if the patient with anemia is a vegetarian, the prescription of a high-meat diet would be met with patient resistance. Thoughtful assessment and consideration of the patient's beliefs and values will usually increase patient compliance and satisfaction.

Objective Data

In addition to collecting subjective data related to a diet history and functional health patterns, objective data related to a nutritional assessment should be collected. Anthropometric measurements (height, weight, skinfold thickness) and blood studies such as serum protein, albumin, and hemoglobin are examples of important objective data related to the GI system. A physical examination also adds valuable information.

Physical Examination

Mouth

Inspection. The lips should be inspected for symmetry, color, and size. They should be observed for abnormalities such as pallor or cyanosis, cracking, ulcers, or fissures. The dorsum (top) of the tongue should have a thin white coating; the undersurface should be smooth. The nurse should observe for any lesions. Using a tongue blade, the nurse should inspect the buccal mucosa and note the color, any areas of pigmentation, and any lesions. Dark-skinned

individuals normally have patchy areas of pigmentation. In assessing the teeth and gums, the nurse should look for caries; loose teeth; abnormal shape and position of teeth; and swelling, bleeding, discoloration, or inflammation of the gingivae. Any distinctive breath odor should be noted.

The pharynx is inspected by tilting the patient's head back and depressing the tongue with a tongue blade. The tonsils, uvula, soft palate, and anterior and posterior pillars should be observed. The nurse should have the patient say "ah." The uvula and soft palate should rise and remain in the midline.

Palpation. The nurse should palpate any suspicious areas in the mouth. Ulcers, nodules, indurations, and areas of tenderness should be noted.

The mouth of the older adult requires careful assessment. Particular attention should be given to dentures (e.g., fit, condition), ability to swallow, the tongue, and lesions. The patient who has dentures must remove the dentures during an oral examination to allow for good visualization and palpation of the area.

Abdomen. Two systems are used to anatomically describe the surface of the abdomen. One system divides the abdomen into four quadrants by a perpendicular line from the sternum to the pubic bone and a horizontal line across the abdomen at the umbilicus (Fig. 39-7, *A,* and Table 39-9). The other system divides the abdomen into nine regions (Fig. 39-7, *B*), but only the epigas-

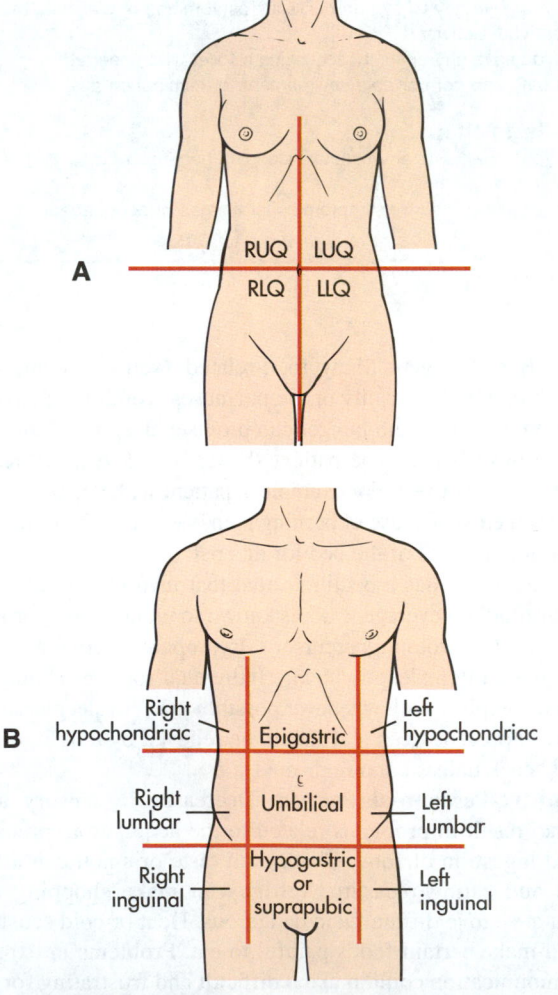

FIG. 39-7 **A,** Abdominal quadrants. **B,** Abdominal regions.

TABLE 39-9	Abdominal Structures in Regions of the Abdomen		
Right Upper Quadrant	**Left Upper Quadrant**	**Right Lower Quadrant**	**Left Lower Quadrant**
Liver and gallbladder	Left lobe of liver	Lower pole of right kidney	Lower pole of left kidney
Pylorus	Spleen	Cecum and appendix	Sigmoid flexure
Duodenum	Stomach	Portion of ascending colon	Portion of descending colon
Head of pancreas	Body of pancreas	Bladder (if distended)	Bladder (if distended)
Right adrenal gland	Left adrenal gland	Right ovary and salpinx	Left ovary and salpinx
Portion of right kidney	Portion of left kidney	Uterus (if enlarged)	Uterus (if enlarged)
Hepatic flexure of colon	Splenic flexure of colon	Right spermatic cord	Left spermatic cord
Portion of ascending and transverse colon	Portion of transverse and descending colon	Right ureter	Left ureter

tric, umbilical, and suprapubic or hypogastric regions are commonly addressed.

For the abdominal examination, good lighting should shine across the abdomen. The patient should be in the supine position and as relaxed as possible. To help relax the abdominal muscles, the patient should slightly flex the knees and the head of the bed should be raised slightly. The patient should have an empty bladder. The examiner should use warm hands when doing the abdominal examination to avoid eliciting muscle guarding. The patient should be asked to breathe slowly through the mouth.

Inspection. The nurse should assess the abdomen for skin changes (color, texture, scars, striae, dilated veins, rashes, and lesions), umbilicus (location and contour), symmetry, contour (flat, rounded [convex], concave, protuberant, distention), observable masses (hernias or other masses), and movement (pulsations and peristalsis). A normal aortic pulsation may be seen in the epigastric area. The nurse should look across the abdomen tangentially (across the abdomen in a line) for peristalsis. Peristalsis is not normally visible in an adult but may be visible in a thin person.

Auscultation. During examination of the abdomen, auscultation is done before percussion and palpation because these latter procedures may alter the bowel sounds. Auscultation of the abdomen includes listening for increased or decreased bowel sounds and vascular sounds. The diaphragm of the stethoscope is used to auscultate bowel sounds because they are relatively high pitched. The bell of the stethoscope is used to detect lower-pitched sounds. Normal bowel sounds occur 5 to 35 times per minute and sound like high-pitched clicks or gurgles.[4,5] Before auscultation, warming the stethoscope in the hands helps prevent abdominal muscle contraction. The nurse should listen in the epigastrium and in all four quadrants. The nurse should listen for bowel sounds for 2 to 5 minutes. Bowel sounds cannot be described as absent until no sound is heard for 5 minutes (in each quadrant).[5] The frequency and intensity of bowel sounds will vary, depending on the phase of digestion. Normally they will sound relatively high pitched and gurgling. Loud gurgles indicate hyperperistalsis and are termed *borborygmi* (stomach growling). The bowel sounds will be more high pitched (rushes and tinkling) when the intestines are under tension, such as in intestinal obstruction. The nurse should listen for decreased or absent bowel sounds. Terms used to describe bowel sounds include *present, absent, increased, decreased, high pitched, tinkling, gurgling,* and *rushing.* Normally no aortic bruits should be heard. A bruit, best heard with the bell of the stethoscope, is a swishing or buzzing sound and indicates turbulent blood flow.

Percussion. The purpose of percussion of the abdomen is to determine the presence of fluid, distention, and masses. Sound waves vary according to the density of underlying tissues; the presence of air produces a higher-pitched, hollow sound termed *tympany;* the presence of fluid or masses produces a short, high-pitched sound with little resonance termed *dullness.* The nurse should lightly percuss all four quadrants of the abdomen and assess the distribution of tympany and dullness. Tympany is the predominant percussion sound of the abdomen.

To percuss the liver, the nurse should start below the umbilicus in the right midclavicular line and percuss lightly upward until dullness is heard, thus determining the lower border of liver dullness. After the lower border of the liver has been determined, the nurse should start at the nipple line in the right midclavicular line and percuss downward between ribs to the area of dullness indicating the upper border of the liver. The height or vertical space between the two areas should be measured to determine the size of the liver. The normal range of liver height in the right midclavicular line is 2.4 to 5 inches (6 to 12 cm).

Palpation. Light palpation is used to detect tenderness or cutaneous hypersensitivity, muscular resistance, masses, and swelling. It also helps the patient to relax for deeper palpation. The nurse should keep fingers together and press gently with the pads of the fingertips, depressing the abdominal wall about 0.4 inch (1 cm). Smooth movements should be used and all quadrants palpated (Fig. 39-8, *A*).

Deep palpation is used to delineate abdominal organs and masses (Fig. 39-8, *B*). The palmar surfaces of the fingers should be used to press more deeply. Again, all quadrants should be palpated. When palpating masses, the nurse should note the location, size, shape, and presence of tenderness. The patient's facial expression should be observed during these maneuvers because it will provide nonverbal cues of discomfort or pain.

An alternative method for deep abdominal palpation is the two-hand method. One hand is placed on top of the other. The fingers of the top hand apply pressure to the bottom hand. The fingers of the bottom hand feel for organs and masses. The nurse should practice both methods of palpation to determine which one is most effective.[6]

A problem area on the abdomen can be checked for rebound tenderness by pressing in slowly and firmly over the painful site. The palpating fingers are withdrawn quickly. Pain on withdrawal of the fingers indicates peritoneal inflammation. Because assessing for rebound tenderness may produce pain and severe muscle spasm, it should be done at the end of the examination and only by an experienced practitioner.

To palpate the liver, the nurse's left hand is placed behind the patient to support the right eleventh and twelfth ribs (Fig. 39-9). The patient may relax on the nurse's hand. The nurse should press the left hand forward and place the right hand on the patient's right abdomen lateral to the rectus muscle. The fingertips should be be-

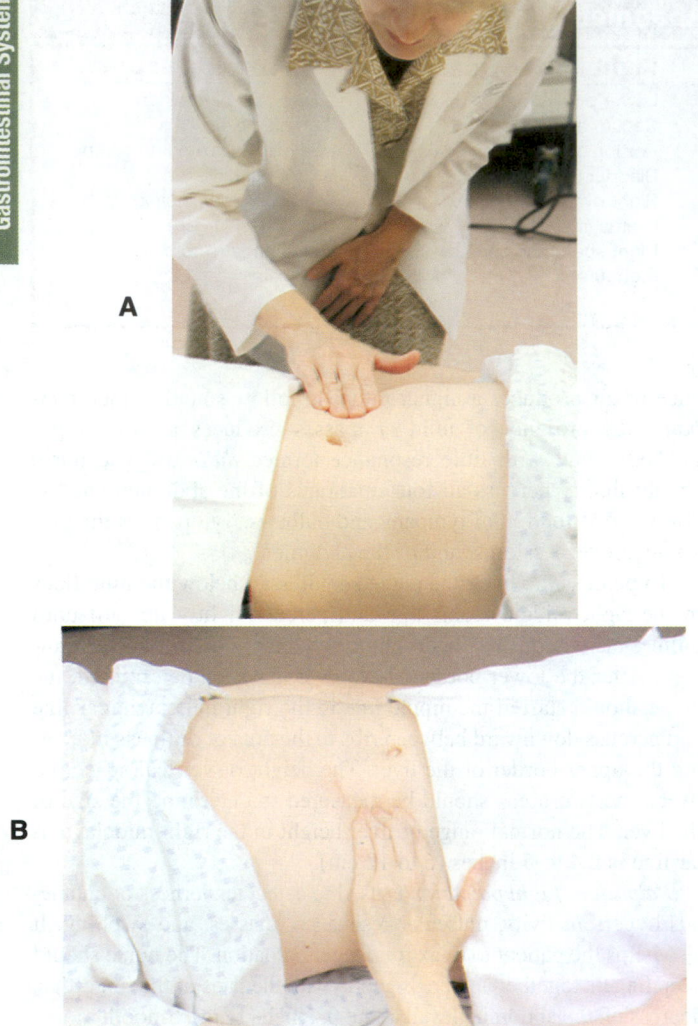

FIG. 39-8   **A,** Technique for light palpation of the abdomen. **B,** Technique for deep palpation.

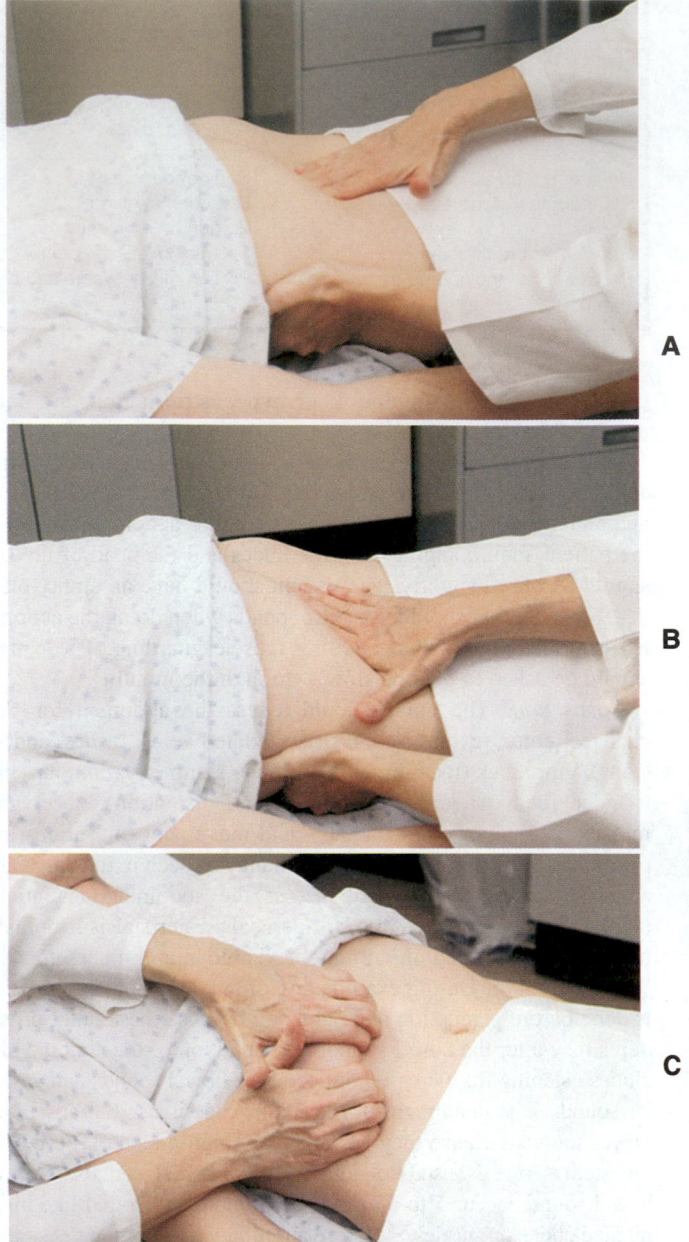

FIG. 39-9   **A,** Technique for liver palpation. **B,** Alternative technique. **C,** Palpation of liver with fingers hooked over the costal region.

low the lower border of liver dullness and pointed toward the right costal margin. The nurse should gently press in and up. The patient should take a deep breath with the abdomen so that the liver drops and is in a better position to be palpated. The nurse should try to feel the liver edge as it comes down to the fingertips. During inspiration the liver edge should feel firm, sharp, and smooth. The surface and contour and any tenderness should be described.

To palpate the spleen, the nurse moves to the left side of the patient. The nurse places the right hand under the patient and supports and presses the patient's left lower rib cage forward. The left hand is placed below the left costal margin and presses it in toward the spleen. The nurse should ask the patient to breathe deeply. The tip or edge of an enlarged spleen will be felt by the fingertips. The spleen is normally not palpable. If it is palpable, the nurse should not continue because manual compression of an enlarged spleen may cause it to rupture.

The standard approach for examining the abdomen can be used on the older adult.[7] Palpation is important because it may reveal a tumor. The abdomen may be thinner and more lax unless the patient is obese. If the patient has chronic obstructive pulmonary disease, large lungs, or a low diaphragm, the liver may be palpated 0.4 to 0.8 inch (1 to 2 cm) below the right costal margin.

Rectum and Anus. The perianal and anal areas should be inspected for color, texture, lumps, rashes, scars, erythema, fissures, and external hemorrhoids. Any lumps or unusual areas should be palpated with a gloved hand.

For the digital examination of the rectum, the gloved, lubricated index finger is placed against the anus while the patient strains (Valsalva maneuver). Then, as the sphincter relaxes, the finger is inserted. The finger is pointed toward the umbilicus. The nurse should try to get the patient to relax. The finger is inserted into the rectum as far as possible, and all surfaces are palpated. Nodules, tenderness, or any irregularities should be assessed. A sample of stool can be removed with the gloved finger and should be checked for occult blood.

Recording of the normal physical assessment of the GI system is found in Table 39-10. Gerontologic differences in the GI system

TABLE 39-10	Normal Physical Assessment of the Gastrointestinal System

Mouth
- Moist and pink lips
- Pink and moist buccal mucosa and gingivae without plaques or lesions
- Teeth in good repair
- Protrusion of tongue in midline without deviation or fasciculations
- Pink uvula in midline, soft palate, tonsils, and posterior pharynx
- Swallows smoothly without coughing or gagging

Abdomen
- Flat without masses or scars
- No abdominal tenderness
- No bruises
- Bowel sounds in all quadrants
- Nonpalpable liver and spleen
- Liver 10 cm in right midclavicular line
- Generalized tympany

Anus
- Absence of lesions, fissures, and hemorrhoids
- Good sphincter tone
- Rectal walls smooth/soft
- No masses
- Stool soft, brown, and heme negative

and differences in assessment findings are described in Table 39-5. Common assessment abnormalities are presented in Table 39-11.

DIAGNOSTIC STUDIES OF THE GASTROINTESTINAL SYSTEM

Diagnostic studies provide important information to the nurse in monitoring the patient's condition and planning appropriate interventions. These studies are considered to be objective data. Table 39-12 presents diagnostic studies common to the GI system. For most diagnostic studies, nurses should make sure a signed consent form for the procedure has been completed and is in the medical record. It is the responsibility of the health care provider doing the procedure to explain the procedure and obtain the written consent. However, nurses play an important role in educating patients regarding the procedures. When preparing the patient it is important to ask about any known allergies to drugs or contrast media.

Many of the diagnostic procedures of the GI system require measures to cleanse the GI tract, as well as the ingestion or injection of a contrast medium or a radiopaque tracer. Often the patient has a series of GI diagnostic tests done. The nurse must monitor the patient closely to ensure adequate hydration and nutrition during the testing period. Some diagnostic studies of the GI system are especially difficult and uncomfortable for the older adult. It

TABLE 39-11	COMMON ASSESSMENT ABNORMALITIES Gastrointestinal System

Finding	Description	Possible Etiology and Significance
Mouth		
Ulcer, plaque on lips or in mouth	Sore or lesion	Carcinoma, viral infections
Cheilosis	Softening, fissuring, and cracking of lips at angles of mouth	Riboflavin deficiency
Cheilitis	Inflammation of lips (usually lower) with fissuring, scaling, crusting	Often unknown
Geographic tongue	Scattered red, smooth (loss of papillae) areas on dorsum of tongue	Unknown
Smooth tongue	Red, slick appearance	Cobalamin deficiency
Leukoplakia	Thickened white patches	Premalignant lesion
Pyorrhea	Recessed gums, purulent pockets	Periodontitis
Herpes simplex	Benign vesicular lesion	Herpesvirus
Candidiasis	White, curd-like lesions surrounded by erythematous mucosa	*Candida albicans*
Glossitis	Reddened, ulcerated, swollen tongue	Exposure to streptococci, irritation, injury, vitamin B deficiencies, anemia
Acute marginal gingivitis	Friable, edematous, painful, bleeding gingivae	Irritation from ill-fitting dentures, calcium deposits on teeth, food impaction
Esophagus and Stomach		
Dysphagia	Difficulty in swallowing, sensation of food sticking in esophagus	Esophageal problems, cancer of esophagus
Hematemesis	Vomiting of blood	Esophageal varices, bleeding peptic ulcer
Pyrosis	Heartburn, burning in epigastric or substernal area	Hiatal hernia, esophagitis, incompetent lower esophageal sphincter
Dyspepsia	Burning or indigestion	Peptic ulcer disease, gallbladder disease
Odynophagia	Painful swallowing	Cancer of esophagus, esophagitis
Eructation	Belching	Gallbladder disease
Nausea and vomiting	Feeling of impending vomiting, expulsion of gastric contents through mouth	GI infections, common manifestation of many GI diseases; stress, fear, and pathologic conditions

GI, Gastrointestinal.

Continued

Gastrointestinal System

TABLE 39-11	**COMMON ASSESSMENT ABNORMALITIES** **Gastrointestinal System—cont'd**

Finding	Description	Possible Etiology and Significance
Abdomen		
Distention	Excessive gas accumulation, enlarged abdomen; generalized tympany	Obstruction, paralytic ileus
Ascites	Accumulated fluid within abdominal cavity; eversion of umbilicus (usually)	Peritoneal inflammation, heart failure, metastatic carcinoma, cirrhosis
Bruit	Humming or swishing sound heard through stethoscope over vessel	Partial arterial obstruction (narrowing of vessel), turbulent flow (aneurysm)
Hyperresonance	Loud, tinkling rushes	Intestinal obstruction
Borborygmi	Waves of loud, gurgling sounds	Hyperactive bowel as result of eating
Absent bowel sounds	No auscultation of bowel sounds	Peritonitis, paralytic ileus, obstruction
Absence of liver dullness	Tympany on percussion	Air from viscus (e.g., perforated ulcer)
Masses	Lump on palpation	Tumors, cysts
Rebound tenderness	Sudden pain when fingers withdrawn quickly	Peritoneal inflammation, appendicitis
Nodular liver	Enlarged, hard liver with irregular edge or surface	Cirrhosis, carcinoma
Hepatomegaly	Enlargement of liver, liver edge >1-2 cm below costal margin	Metastatic carcinoma, hepatitis, venous congestion
Splenomegaly	Enlargement of spleen	Chronic leukemia, hemolytic states, portal hypertension, some infections
Hernia	Bulge or nodule in abdomen, usually appearing on straining	Inguinal (in inguinal canal), femoral (in femoral canal), umbilical (herniation of umbilicus), or incisional (defect in muscles after surgery)
Rectum and Anus		
Hemorrhoids	Thrombosed veins in rectum and anus (internal or external)	Portal hypertension, chronic constipation, prolonged sitting or standing, pregnancy
Mass	Firm, nodular edge	Tumor, carcinoma
Pilonidal cyst	Opening of sinus tract, cyst in midline just above coccyx	Probably congenital
Fissure	Ulceration in anal canal	Straining, irritation
Melena	Abnormal, black, tarry stool containing digested blood	Cancer, bleeding in upper GI tract from ulcers, varices
Tenesmus	Painful and ineffective straining at stool	Ulcerative colitis, diarrhea secondary to GI infection such as food poisoning
Steatorrhea	Fatty, frothy, foul-smelling stool	Chronic pancreatitis, biliary obstruction, malabsorption problems

may be necessary to individualize and make adjustments. It is particularly important to prevent diarrhea from bowel-cleansing procedures and dehydration from prolonged fluid restriction.

Many radiologic studies use either barium sulfate or meglumine diatrizoate (Gastrografin) as a contrast medium. Barium sulfate is more effective for visualizing mucosal detail. Gastrografin is water soluble and rapidly absorbed, so it is preferred when a perforation is suspected. Spillage of barium into the peritoneal cavity can result in peritonitis. Under other circumstances in a person at high risk for aspiration, water-soluble media are contraindicated and barium is preferred.

Radiologic Studies

Upper Gastrointestinal Series. An upper GI x-ray allows examination of the esophagus after swallowing a thick barium solution. An upper GI series with small bowel follow-through provides visualization of the esophagus, stomach, and small intestine by means of fluoroscopy and x-ray examination. The procedure consists of the patient swallowing contrast medium (a thick barium solution) and then assuming different positions on the x-ray table. The movement of the contrast medium is observed with fluoroscopy, and several x-rays are taken (see Table 39-12). An upper GI is used to identify esophageal, stomach, and small intestine disorders such as esophageal strictures, varices, polyps, tumors, hiatal hernia, foreign bodies, and peptic ulcers in the stomach or duodenum.

Lower Gastrointestinal Series. The purpose of a lower GI series (barium enema) x-ray examination is to observe by means of fluoroscopy the filling of the colon with contrast medium and to observe by x-ray the filled colon. This procedure identifies polyps, tumors, and other lesions in the colon. It consists of administering an enema of contrast medium to the patient. The air-contrast barium enema provides better visualization of an inflammatory bowel disease, polyps, and tumors (Fig. 39-10). Because it requires the patient to retain the barium, it is not tolerated as well in an older or immobile patient.

Abdominal Ultrasound. Ultrasonography is used to show the size and configuration of organs. It is the diagnostic procedure of choice for detecting cholelithiasis (gallstones). Ultrasound is also used for detecting appendicitis, acute cholecystitis, and other changes in abdominal organs (Fig. 39-11; see Table 39-12).

Virtual Colonoscopy. *Virtual colonoscopy* combines computed tomography (CT) scanning or magnetic resonance imaging (MRI) with sophisticated computer software to produce images of the colon and rectum. The test is less invasive than a conventional colonoscopy. (The technique is described in Table 39-12.)

TABLE 39-12	*DIAGNOSTIC STUDIES* Gastrointestinal System

Study	Description and Purpose	Nursing Responsibility
Radiology		
Upper gastrointestinal (GI) or **Barium swallow**	X-ray study with fluoroscopy with contrast medium. Study is used to diagnose structural abnormalities of the esophagus, stomach, and duodenum.	Explain procedure to patient, the need to drink contrast medium, and the need to assume various positions on x-ray table. Keep patient NPO for 8-12 hr before procedure. Tell patient to avoid smoking after midnight the night before the study. After x-ray, take measures to prevent contrast medium impaction (fluids, laxatives). Tell patient that stool may be white up to 72 hr after test.
Small bowel series	Contrast medium is ingested and films taken every 30 min until medium reaches terminal ileum.	Same as for upper GI.
Lower GI or barium enema	Fluoroscopic x-ray examination of colon using contrast medium, which is administered rectally (enema) (see Fig. 39-10). Double-contrast or air-contrast barium enema is test of choice. Air is infused after thick barium flows through the transverse colon.	Before the procedure, administer laxatives and enemas until colon is clear of stool evening before procedure. Administer clear liquid diet evening before procedure. Keep patient NPO for 8 hr before test. Instruct patient about being given barium by enema. Explain that cramping and urge to defecate may occur during procedure and that patient may be placed in various positions on tilt table. After the procedure, give fluids, laxatives, or suppositories to assist in expelling barium. Observe stool for passage of contrast medium.
Ultrasound	Noninvasive procedure uses high-frequency sound waves (ultrasound waves), which are passed into body structures and recorded as they are reflected (bounded). A conductive gel (lubricant jelly) is applied to the skin and a transducer is placed on the area.	
• Abdominal ultrasound	Study detects abdominal masses (tumors and cysts) and is also used to assess ascites.	Instruct patient to be NPO 8-12 hr before ultrasound. Air or gas can reduce quality of images. Food intake can cause gallbladder contraction, resulting in suboptimal study.
• Hepatobiliary ultrasound	Study detects subphrenic abscesses, cysts, tumors, and cirrhosis and to visualize biliary ducts.	Same as abdominal ultrasound.
• Gallbladder (GB) ultrasound	Study detects gallstones (see Fig. 34-11).	Same as abdominal ultrasound.
• Esophageal endoscopic ultrasound	Study detects and stages esophageal tumors. Fine-needle aspiration can validate cancer or dysplasia.	Same as upper GI endoscopy.

NPO, Nothing by mouth.

Continued

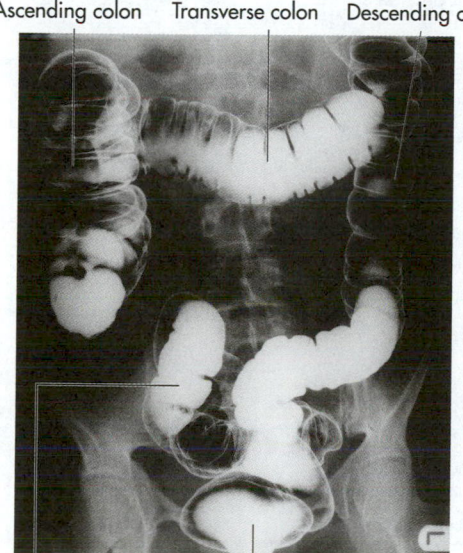

Ascending colon   Transverse colon   Descending colon

Sigmoid colon   Rectum

FIG. 39-10   Barium enema x-ray showing the large intestine.

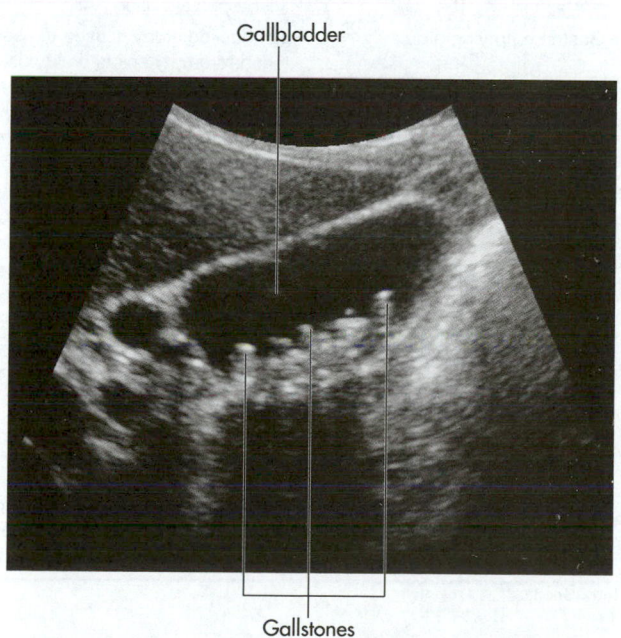

Gallbladder

Gallstones

FIG. 39-11   Ultrasound of gallbladder showing multiple gallstones.

Gastrointestinal System

TABLE 39-12	DIAGNOSTIC STUDIES Gastrointestinal System—cont'd

Study	Description and Purpose	Nursing Responsibility
Radiology—cont'd **Computed tomography (CT)**	Noninvasive radiologic examination combines special x-ray machine used for CT that allows for exposures at different depths. Study detects biliary tract, liver, and pancreatic disorders. Use of contrast medium accentuates density differences.	Explain procedure to patient. Determine sensitivity to iodine if contrast material is used.
Magnetic resonance imaging (MRI)	Noninvasive procedure using radiofrequency waves and a magnetic field. Procedure is used to detect hepatic metastases and sources of GI bleeding and to stage colorectal cancer.	Explain procedure to patient. Contraindicated in patient with metal implants (e.g., pacemaker) or who is pregnant.
Virtual colonoscopy	Technique combines CT scanning or MRI with computer virtual reality software to detect colon and bowel diseases, including polyps, colorectal cancer, diverticulosis, and lower GI bleeding. Air is introduced via a tube placed in rectum to enlarge colon to enhance visualization. Images are obtained while patient is on back and stomach. Computer combines images to form 2- and 3-D pictures, which are viewed on monitor.	Bowel prep similar to colonoscopy (see Colonoscopy below). Unlike conventional colonoscopy, no sedatives are needed and no scope is used. Procedure takes about 15-20 min.
Cholangiography		
• Percutaneous transhepatic Cholangiogram (PTC)	After local anesthesia, liver is entered with long needle (under fluoroscopy), bile duct is entered, bile withdrawn, and radiopaque contrast medium injected. Fluoroscopy is used to determine filling of hepatic and biliary ducts.	Observe patient for signs of hemorrhage or bile leakage. Assess patient's medication for possible contraindications, precautions, or complications with the use of contrast medium.
• Surgical cholangiogram	Study is performed during surgery on biliary structures, such as GB. Contrast medium is injected into common bile duct.	Explain to patient that anesthetic will be used. Assess patient's medication for possible contraindications, precautions, or complications with the use of contrast medium.
• Magnetic resonance cholangiopancreatography (MRCP)	Noninvasive study uses MRI technology to obtain images of biliary and pancreatic ducts.	Same as MRI.
Nuclear imaging scans (scintigraphy)	Purpose is to show size, shape, and position of organ. Functional disorders and structural defects may be identified. Radionuclide (radioactive isotope) is injected IV and a counter (scanning) device picks up radioactive emission, which is recorded on paper. Only tracer doses of radioactive isotopes are used.	Tell patient that substances contain only traces of radioactivity and pose little to no danger. Schedule no more than one radionuclide test on the same day. Explain to patient need to lie flat during scanning.
• Gastric emptying studies	Radionuclide study is used to assess ability of stomach to empty solids or liquids. In solid-emptying study, cooked egg white containing Tc-99m is eaten. In liquid-emptying study, orange juice with Tc-99m is drunk. Sequential images from gamma camera are recorded q2min for up to 60 min. Study is used in patients with emptying disorders from peptic ulcer, ulcer surgery, diabetes, or gastric malignancies.	Same as above.
• Hepatobiliary scintigraphy (HIDA)	Patient is given IV injection of Tc-99m and positioned under camera to record distribution of tracer in the liver, biliary tree, gallbladder, and proximal small bowel. Useful for identifying diffuse hepatic disease (such as cirrhosis or neoplasm), as well as to confirm acute cholecystitis.	Same as above.
• Scintigraphy of GI bleeding	Tc-99m–labeled sulfur colloid or Tc-99m labeling of the patient's own red blood cells (RBCs) can accurately determine the site of active GI blood loss. The sulfur colloid or the patient's RBCs are injected, and images of the abdomen are obtained at intermittent intervals.	Same as above.

IV, Intravenous.

TABLE 39-12	DIAGNOSTIC STUDIES Gastrointestinal System—cont'd

Study	Description and Purpose	Nursing Responsibility
Endoscopy **Esophagogastroduodenoscopy** (EGD)	Technique directly visualizes mucosal lining of esophagus, stomach, and duodenum with flexible, fiberoptic endoscope. Test may use video imaging to visualize stomach motility. Inflammations, ulcerations, tumors, varices, or Mallory-Weiss tear may be detected. Biopsies may be taken and varices can be treated with band ligation or sclerotherapy.	Before the procedure, keep patient NPO for 8 hr. Make sure signed consent is on chart. Give preoperative medication if ordered. Explain to patient that local anesthetic may be sprayed on throat before insertion of scope and that patient will be sedated during the procedure. After the procedure, keep patient NPO until gag reflex returns. Gently tickle back of throat to determine reflex. Use warm saline gargles for relief of sore throat. Check temperature q15-30min for 1-2 hr (sudden temperature spike is sign of perforation).
Colonoscopy	Study directly visualizes entire colon up to ileocecal valve with flexible fiberoptic scope. Patient's position is changed frequently during procedure to assist with advancement of scope to cecum. Test is used to diagnose inflammatory bowel disease, detect tumors, diagnose diverticulosis, and dilate strictures. Procedure allows for biopsy and removal of polyps without laparotomy.	Before the procedure, a bowel preparation is done. Type of preparation varies depending on physician. For example, patients may be kept on clear liquids 1-2 days before procedure. Cathartic and/or enema may be given the night before. An alternative is to give 1 gal of polyethylene glycol (GoLYTELY, Colyte) evening before (8 oz glass q10min). Explain to patient that flexible scope will be inserted while patient is in side-lying position. Explain to patient that sedation will be given. After the procedure, be aware that patient may experience abdominal cramps caused by stimulation of peristalsis because the bowel is constantly inflated with air during procedure. Observe for rectal bleeding and signs of perforation (e.g., malaise, abdominal distention, tenesmus). Check vital signs.
Capsule endoscopy	Patient swallows a capsule with camera (approximately the size of a large vitamin) that provides endoscopic evaluation of GI tract (see Fig. 39-13 on p. 945). Most commonly used to visualize small intestine and diagnose diseases such as Crohn's disease, celiac disease, and malabsorption syndrome and to identify sources of possible GI bleeding in areas not accessible by upper endoscopy or colonoscopy. Camera takes about 57,000 images during 8-hr examination. Capsule relays images to data recorder that patient wears on belt. After examination, images are downloaded to monitor.	Dietary preparation: similar to colonoscopy. The video capsule is swallowed, and the patient is usually kept NPO until 4–6 hr later. Procedure is comfortable for most patients. Eight hours after swallowing the capsule, the patient returns to have the monitoring device removed. Peristalsis causes passage of the disposable capsule with a bowel movement.
Sigmoidoscopy	Study directly visualizes rectum and sigmoid colon with lighted flexible endoscope. Sometimes special table is used to tilt patient into knee-chest position. Test may detect tumors, polyps, inflammatory and infectious diseases, fissures, and hemorrhoids.	Administer enemas evening before and morning of procedure. Patient may have clear liquids day before, or no dietary restrictions may be necessary. Explain to patient knee-chest position (unless patient is older or very ill), need to take deep breaths during insertion of scope, and possible urge to defecate as scope is passed. Encourage patient to relax and let abdomen go limp. Observe for rectal bleeding after polypectomy or biopsy.
Endoscopic retrograde cholangiopancreatography (ERCP)	Fiberoptic endoscope (using fluoroscopy) is inserted through the oral cavity into descending duodenum, then common bile and pancreatic ducts are cannulated. Contrast medium is injected into ducts and allows for direct visualization of structures. Technique can also be used to retrieve a gallstone from distal common bile duct, dilate strictures, obtain biopsy of tumors, and diagnose pseudocysts.	Before the procedure, explain procedure to patient, including patient role. Keep patient NPO 8 hr before procedure. Ensure that consent form is signed. Administer sedation immediately before and during procedure. Administer antibiotics if ordered. After the procedure, check vital signs. Check for signs of perforation or infection. Be aware that pancreatitis is most common complication. Check for return of gag reflex.
Endoscopic ultrasound	Combined use of endoscopy and ultrasound using an ultrasound transducer attached to an endoscope. Enables visualization of the esophagus, stomach, intestine, liver, pancreas, and gallstones.	Similar to upper GI endoscopy.

Continued

TABLE 39-12	*DIAGNOSTIC STUDIES* Gastrointestinal System—cont'd	

Study	Description and Purpose	Nursing Responsibility
Endoscopy—cont'd Laparoscopy (peritoneoscopy)	Peritoneal cavity and contents are visualized with laparoscope. Biopsy specimen may also be taken. Done under general anesthesia in operating room. Double-puncture peritoneoscopy permits better visualization of abdominal cavity, especially liver. Technique can eliminate need for exploratory laparotomy in many patients.	Make sure signed permit is on chart. Keep patient NPO 8 hr before study. Administer preoperative sedative medication. Ensure that bladder and bowel are emptied. Instruct patient that local anesthetic is used before scope insertion. Observe for possible complications of bleeding and bowel perforation after the procedure.
Blood Chemistries Serum amylase	Study measures secretion of amylase by pancreas and is important in diagnosing acute pancreatitis. Level of amylase peaks in 24 hr and then drops to normal in 48-72 hr. Depending on method, *normal finding* is 0-130 U/L (0-2.17 μkat/L).	Obtain blood sample in acute attack of pancreatitis. Explain procedure to patient.
Serum lipase	Study measures secretion of lipase by pancreas. Level stays elevated longer than serum amylase. *Normal finding* is 0-160 U/L (0-2.66 μkat/L)	Explain procedure to patient.
Liver Biopsy	Percutaneous procedure uses needle inserted between sixth and seventh or eighth and ninth intercostal spaces on the right side to obtain specimen of hepatic tissue. Often done using ultrasound or CT guidance.	Before the procedure, check patient's coagulation status (prothrombin time, clotting or bleeding time). Ensure that patient's blood is typed and crossmatched. Take vital signs as baseline data. Explain holding of breath after expiration when needle is inserted. Ensure that informed consent has been signed. After the procedure, check vital signs to detect internal bleeding q15min × 2, q30min × 4, q1hr × 4. Keep patient lying on right side for minimum of 2 hr to splint puncture site. Keep patient in bed in flat position for 12-14 hr. Assess patient for complications such as bile peritonitis, shock, and pneumothorax.

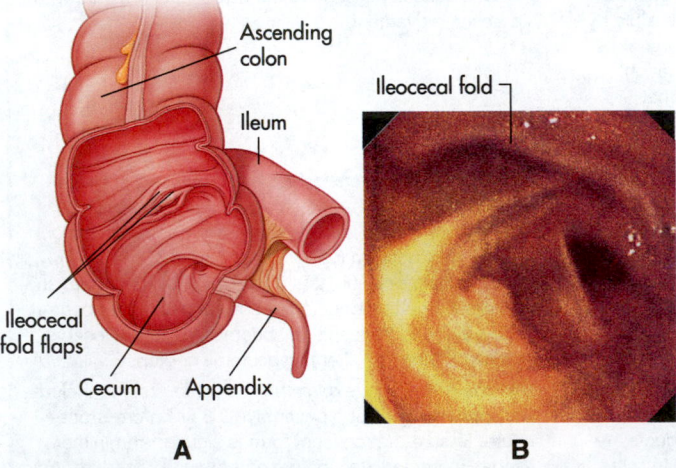

FIG. 39-12 Ileocecal junction. **A,** Illustration showing the ileocecal junction and the ileocecal fold. **B,** Endoscopic image of the ileocecal fold.

Virtual colonoscopy is better able to visualize the ascending colon than conventional colonoscopy and is as good as conventional colonoscopy at assessing polyps larger than 1 cm. However, if a polyp is discovered using virtual colonoscopy, a conventional colonoscopy will then be done to obtain a biopsy or remove it. Another advantage of virtual colonoscopy is its more acceptable use in older adults. It is this group of people who especially need to be screened for colorectal cancer. However, they may find the actual procedure of having a conventional colonoscopy very difficult.

A disadvantage of virtual colonoscopy is that it may be less sensitive to obtaining information on the details and color of the mucosa. In addition, it is less sensitive at detecting small polyps.

Endoscopy

Endoscopy refers to the direct visualization of a body structure through a lighted fiberoptic instrument. The GI structures that can be examined by endoscopy include the esophagus, stomach, duodenum, colon, and, with the aid of fluoroscopy and x-rays, the pancreas and biliary tree. The pancreatic, hepatic, and common bile ducts can be visualized with side-viewing flexible endoscopes. This procedure is called *endoscopic retrograde cholangiopancreatography* (ERCP).[8]

The endoscope is an instrument channel through which biopsy forceps and cytology brushes may be passed. Cameras may be attached and video and still pictures taken (Fig. 39-12). Endoscopy of the GI tract is often done in combination with biopsy and cytologic studies. The major complication of GI endoscopy is perforation through the structure being scoped. This complication is

TABLE 39-12	*DIAGNOSTIC STUDIES* Gastrointestinal System—cont'd		
Study	**Description and Purpose**		**Nursing Responsibility**
Miscellaneous Tests			
Gastric analysis	Purpose is to analyze gastric contents for acidity and volume. NG tube is inserted, and gastric contents are aspirated. Contents are analyzed mainly for HCl acid, but pH, pepsin, and electrolytes may be determined. Histalog and pentagastrin may be used to stimulate HCl acid secretion. Exfoliative cytology may be done to determine whether malignant cells are present. With fasting, *normal acidity* is 2.5 mEq/L (2.5 mmol/L) and *normal volume* is 62 ml/hr; 30 min after Histalog or pentagastrin administration, *normal acidity* is 1.5 mEq/L (1.5 mmol/L) and *normal volume* is 110 ml/hr.		Keep patient NPO for 8-12 hr. Explain insertion of NG tube. Withhold drugs affecting gastric secretions 24-48 hr before test. Ensure no smoking morning of test (nicotine increases gastric secretion).
Fecal analysis	Form, consistency, and color are noted. Specimen examined for mucus, blood, pus, parasites, and fat content. Tests for occult blood (guaiac test, Hemoccult, Hematest) are done.		Observe patient's stools. Collect stool specimens. Check stools for blood with Hemoccult or Hematest. Keep diet free of red meat for 24-48 hr before guaiac test.
Stool culture	Tests for the presence of bacteria, including *Clostridium difficile*.		Collect stool specimen.

NG, Nasogastric.

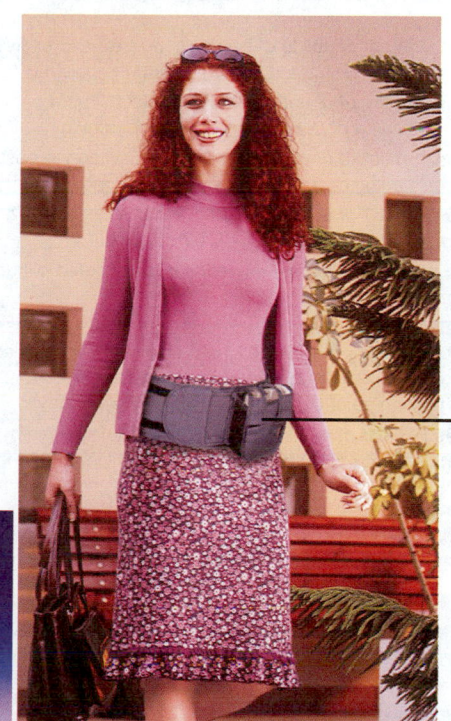
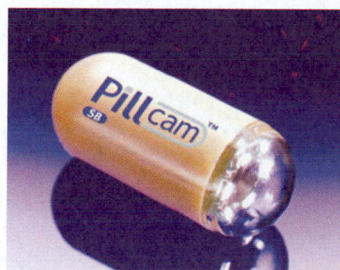

Data recorder

FIG. 39-13   Capsule endoscopy. **A,** The video capsule has its own camera and light source. After it is swallowed, it travels through the GI tract and allows visualization of the small intestine. It sends messages to a data recorder that is worn on a waist belt **(B).** During the 8-hour examination, the patient is free to move about. After the test, the images are viewed on a video monitor.

decreased with the use of the flexible fiberoptic scopes. All endoscopic procedures require informed, written consent. Specific endoscopy procedures are discussed in Table 39-12. In addition to diagnostic procedures, many invasive and therapeutic procedures may be done with endoscopes. These include procedures such as polypectomy, sclerosis of varices, laser treatment, cauterization of bleeding sites, papillotomy, common bile duct stone removal, and balloon dilations. Many endoscopic procedures require intravenous short-acting sedation.

Capsule endoscopy is a noninvasive approach to visualize the GI tract[9] (see Fig. 39-13 on p. 945). (See Table 39-12 for further discussion of this diagnostic technique.)

Liver Biopsy

The purpose of a liver biopsy is to obtain hepatic tissue to be used in establishing a diagnosis such as fibrosis, cirrhosis, and neoplasms. It may also be useful for following the progress of liver disease, such as chronic hepatitis.

The two types of liver biopsy are open and closed. The *open method* involves making an incision and removing a wedge of tissue. It is done in the operating room with the patient under general anesthesia, often concurrently with another surgical procedure. The *closed,* or *needle, biopsy* is a percutaneous procedure in which the site is infiltrated with a local anesthetic and a needle is inserted between the sixth and seventh or eighth and ninth intercostal spaces on the right side. The patient lies supine with the right arm over the head. The patient should be instructed to expire fully and not breathe while the needle is inserted (see Table 39-12). Nursing assessment before and after a liver biopsy is important.

Liver Function Studies

Liver function tests are usually described separately from other GI diagnostic studies. Liver function tests are laboratory (blood) studies that reflect hepatic disease. Table 39-13 describes some common liver function tests.

TABLE 39-13	*DIAGNOSTIC STUDIES* **Liver Function Tests**
Test	**Description and Purpose**
Bile Formation and Excretion	
Serum bilirubin	Measurement of ability of liver to conjugate and excrete bilirubin, allowing differentiation between unconjugated (indirect) and conjugated (direct) bilirubin in plasma
Total	Measurement of direct and indirect total bilirubin *Normal finding* of 0.2-1.3 mg/dl (3.4-22 μmol/L)
Direct	Measurement of conjugated bilirubin; elevation in obstructive jaundice *Normal finding* of 0.1-0.3 mg/dl (1.7-5.1 μmol/L)
Indirect	Measurement of unconjugated bilirubin; elevation in hepatocellular and hemolytic conditions *Normal finding* of 0.1-1 mg/dl (1.7-17 μmol/L)
Urinary bilirubin	Measurement of urinary excretion of conjugated bilirubin *Normal finding* of 0
Urinary urobilinogen	Measurement of urinary excretion of urobilinogen; maximum excretion midafternoon to early evening, collection of total urinary output for 2 hr in afternoon, sent to laboratory in dark container immediately because of oxidation of urobilinogen to urobilin on exposure to air *Normal finding* of 0.5-4 mg/day (0.8-6.8 μmol/day)
Fecal urobilinogen	Measurement of fecal urobilinogen in stool specimen *Normal finding* of 30-220 mg/100 g stool (55-372 μmol/100 g of stool)
Dye Excretion Tests (Detoxification)	
Indocyanine green	Determination of liver's ability to take up and excrete dye given IV; drawing of blood samples every 5 min for 20-30 min *Normal finding* of 500-800 ml/m² of body surface/min
Protein Metabolism	
Serum protein levels	Measurement of serum proteins that are manufactured by the liver; measurement of albumin, *normal finding* of 3.5-5 g/dl (35-50 g/L); measurement of globulin, *normal finding* of 2-3.5 g/dl (20-35 g/L) *Normal total protein* of 6-8 g/dl (60-80 g/L) *Normal A/G ratio* of 1.5:1-2.5:1
α-Fetoprotein	Indication of hepatic cancer *Normal finding* of <15 ng/ml (<15 mcg/L)
Blood ammonia levels	Conversion of ammonia to urea normally occurs in the liver; elevation can result in hepatic encephalopathy secondary to liver cirrhosis *Normal finding* of 30-70 mcg/dl (17.6-41.1 μmol/L)
Hemostatic Functions	
Prothrombin	Determination of prothrombin activity *Normal finding* of 10-14 sec
Vitamin K production	Determination of response of liver to vitamin K; checking of prothrombin time necessary 24 hr after injection of vitamin K

TABLE 39-13	*DIAGNOSTIC STUDIES* **Liver Function Tests—cont'd**

Test	Description and Purpose
Serum Enzyme Tests	
Alkaline phosphatase (ALP)	Originating in bone and liver; serum levels rise when excretion is impaired as a result of obstruction in the biliary tract *Normal finding* of 30-120 U/L (0.5-2 µkat/L), depending on method and age
Aspartate aminotransferase (AST)	Elevation in liver damage and inflammation *Normal finding* of 7-40 U/L (0.12-0.67 µkat/L)
Alanine aminotransferase (ALT)	Elevation in liver damage and inflammation *Normal finding* of 5-36 U/L (0.08-0.6 µkat/L)
γ-Glutamyl transpeptidase (GGT)	Present in biliary tract (not in skeletal or cardiac muscle), increase in hepatitis and alcoholic liver disease; more sensitive for liver dysfunction than ALP *Normal finding* of 0-30 U/L (0-0.5 µkat/L)
Lipid Metabolism	
Serum cholesterol	Synthesis and excretion by liver, increase in biliary obstruction, decrease in extensive liver disease and malnutrition *Normal finding* of 140-200 mg/dl (3.6-5.2 mmol/L), varying with age

NCLEX EXAMINATION REVIEW QUESTIONS

The number of the question corresponds to the same-numbered objective at the beginning of the chapter.

1. A patient is admitted to the hospital with a diagnosis of diarrhea with dehydration. The nurse recognizes that increased peristalsis resulting in diarrhea can be related to
   a. sympathetic inhibition.
   b. mixing and propulsion.
   c. sympathetic stimulation.
   d. parasympathetic stimulation.

2. A patient has an elevated blood level of indirect (unconjugated) bilirubin. One cause of this finding is that
   a. the gallbladder is unable to contract to release stored bile.
   b. bilirubin is not being conjugated and excreted into the bile by the liver.
   c. the Kupffer cells in the liver are unable to remove bilirubin from the blood.
   d. there is an obstruction in the biliary tract preventing flow of bile into the small intestine.

3. As gastric contents move into the small intestine, the bowel is normally protected from the acidity of gastric contents by the
   a. inhibition of secretin release.
   b. release of bicarbonate by the pancreas.
   c. release of pancreatic digestive enzymes.
   d. release of gastrin by the duodenal mucosa.

4. A patient is jaundiced and her stools are clay colored (gray). This is most likely related to
   a. decreased bile flow into the intestine.
   b. increased production of urobilinogen.
   c. increased production of cholecystokinin.
   d. increased bile and bilirubin in the blood.

5. An 80-year-old man states that although he adds a lot of salt to his food it still does not have much taste. The nurse's response is based on the knowledge that the older adult
   a. should not experience changes in taste.
   b. has a loss of taste buds, especially for sweet and salt.
   c. has some loss of taste but no difficulty chewing food.
   d. loses the sense of taste because the ability to smell is decreased.

6. When assessing the health promotion–health maintenance pattern as related to GI function, an appropriate question by the nurse is,
   a. "What is your usual bowel elimination pattern?"
   b. "What percentage of your income is spent on food?"
   c. "Have you traveled to a foreign country in the last year?"
   d. "Do you have diarrhea when you are under a lot of stress?"

7. During an examination of the abdomen the nurse should
   a. position the patient in the supine position with the bed flat and knees straight.
   b. listen in the epigastrium and all four quadrants for 2 to 5 minutes for bowel sounds.
   c. use the following order of techniques: inspection, palpation, percussion, auscultation.
   d. describe bowel sounds as absent if no sound is heard in the lower right quadrant after 2 minutes.

8. A normal physical assessment finding of the GI system is
   a. tympany on percussion of the abdomen.
   b. liver edge 2 to 4 cm below the costal margin.
   c. finding of a firm, nodular edge on the rectal examination.
   d. easy palpation of the spleen edges with moderate pressure.

9. In preparing a patient for a colonoscopy, the nurse explains that
   a. a signed permit is not necessary.
   b. sedation may be used during the procedure.
   c. only one cleansing enema is necessary for preparation.
   d. a light meal should be eaten the day before the procedure.

REFERENCES

1. Eliopoulos C: *Gerontological nursing*, ed 6, Philadelphia, 2005, Lippincott Williams & Wilkins.
2. Hall KE, Proctor DD, Fisher L, et al: American Gastroenterological Association Future Trends Committee report: effects of aging of the population on gastroenterology practice, education, and research, *Gastroenterology* 129:1305, 2005.
3. Porth CM: *Pathophysiology concepts of altered health states*, ed 7, Philadelphia, 2005, Lippincott Williams & Wilkins.
4. Wilson SF, Giddens JF: *Health assessment for nursing practice,* ed 3, St Louis, 2005, Elsevier Mosby.
5. Seidel HM, Ball J, Dains J, et al: *Mosby's guide to physical examination*, ed 6, St Louis, 2006, Mosby.
6. Jarvis C: *Physical examination and health assessment*, ed 4, St Louis, 2004, Elsevier Mosby.
7. Ebersole P, Hess P: *Toward healthy aging*, ed 6, St Louis, 2004, Mosby.
8. Wolfe MM, Davis GL, Farraye FA, et al: Therapy of digestive disorders, ed 2, Philadelphia, 2006, Saunders.
9. Carlo JT, DeMarco D, Smith BA, et al: The utility of capsule endoscopy and its role for diagnosing pathology in the gastrointestinal tract, *Am J Surg* 190(6):886, 2005.

RESOURCES

Resources for this chapter are listed in Chapter 40 on page 970, Chapter 42 on page 1034, Chapter 43 on page 1086, and Chapter 44 on page 1134.

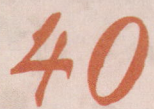

40

Nursing Management
Nutritional Problems

Peggi Guenter

LEARNING OBJECTIVES

1. Describe the essential components of a nutritionally good diet and their importance to health.
2. Describe possible adverse interactions between drugs and various foods.
3. Describe the common etiologic factors, clinical manifestations, and management of malnutrition.
4. Explain the indications for use, complications, and nursing management of tube feedings.
5. Describe the types of feeding tubes and related nursing management.
6. Define the indications, complications, and nursing management related to the use of parenteral nutrition.
7. Compare the etiologic factors, clinical manifestations, and nursing management of eating disorders.

KEY TERMS

anorexia nervosa, p. 968
bulimia nervosa, p. 969
enteral nutrition, p. 960
malabsorption syndrome, p. 953
malnutrition, p. 951
marasmus, p. 952
parenteral nutrition, p. 965
protein-calorie malnutrition, p. 951

Electronic Resources

Supplemental content related to Chapter 40 can be found . . .

Companion CD
- Stress-Busting Kit for Nursing Students
- NCLEX Examination Review Questions
- Comprehensive Glossary

Evolve Website *evolve*
http://evolve.elsevier.com/Lewis/medsurg
- Content Updates
- Key Points (Printable and CD/MP3 Download)
- Concept Map Creator
- Expanded Audio Glossary
- Key Term Flash Cards
- Table: Nutritional Therapy: High-Calorie, High-Protein Diet

- Customizable Nursing Care Plans:
  - Enteral Nutrition
  - Parenteral Nutrition
- Electronic Calculators
- WebLinks

This chapter focuses on problems related to nutrition. The primary nutritional problems discussed are malnutrition and eating disorders. Obesity is discussed in Chapter 41.

NUTRITIONAL PROBLEMS

Nutritional problems can occur in all age-groups, cultures, ethnic groups, and socioeconomic classes. Intelligence and wealth do not necessarily preclude the development of poor nutritional habits. The nurse in the roles of caregiver, teacher, and resource person can have a strong influence on the nutritional practices of patients and their families. Together with the physician, the dietitian, and the pharmacist, the nurse is in an excellent position to assess the dietary practices of the patient and provide important information, as well as provide nutritional resources within and outside the institutional setting.

The nutritional status of a person or a family may be influenced by many factors. Attitudes toward the importance of food and eating habits are established early. Cultural or religious preferences and requirements are frequently reflected in dietary intake. The financial status of a family or an individual can determine the type and amount of nutritionally sound food that can be purchased. Findings support that generally the lower the socioeconomic status, the poorer the nutritional state.[1] The availability of food sources also contributes to the individual's nutritional status.

NORMAL NUTRITION

Nutrition is the process by which the body uses food for energy, growth, and maintenance and repair of body tissues. Good nutrition in the absence of any underlying disease process results from the ingestion of a balanced diet. The United States Department of Agricul-

---

Reviewed by Rose Ann DiMaria, RN, PhD, CNSN, Associate Professor, West Virginia University School of Nursing—Charleston Division, Charleston, W.Va.

ture (USDA) has adopted the MyPyramid *(www.mypyramid.gov)*, which consists of food groups that are presented in proportions appropriate for a healthy diet. Fig. 40-1 and Table 40-1 show these food groups with the recommended daily requirements and examples of common sources. The essential components of the basic food groups are carbohydrates, fats, proteins, vitamins, and minerals.

Carbohydrates, the body's primary source of energy, yield approximately 4 kilocalories per gram. (Kilocalorie is the correct unit to designate caloric intake and expenditure. However, calorie is more commonly used.) Carbohydrates are either simple or complex. Simple carbohydrates come in two forms: *monosaccharides* (e.g., glucose and fructose), which are found in fruits and honey, and *disaccharides* (e.g., sucrose, maltose, and lactose), which are found in such substances as table sugar, malted cereal, and milk, respectively. Complex carbohydrates or polysaccharides commonly appear in the diet as starches, such as cereal grains, potatoes, and legumes. Carbohydrates are the chief protein-sparing ingredient in a nutritionally sound diet and compose approximately 47% of the daily caloric needs of the body. The National Research Council recommends that at least half of the body's energy needs should come from carbohydrates, especially complex carbohydrates.[2]

Approximately 36% of the daily caloric intake in current American diets is derived from fat.[2] This level is considerably higher than that found in many other societies and is a cause for concern. The Dietary Guidelines for Americans 2005 from *Healthy People 2010* recommends that people reduce their fat intake to 20% to 35% of their total daily caloric intake.[3] One gram of fat yields 9 calories. Fats are stored in adipose tissue and in the abdominal cavity. Besides being a major source of energy, fats act as insulation, which reduces loss of body heat in cold environments and provides padding and protection for vital organs. Fats also act as carriers of essential fatty acids and fat-soluble vitamins. Fats provide a feeling of satiety after eating, partly from the flavor added and partly from their slow rate of digestion, which delays hunger. The daily caloric requirements of a person are influenced by body build, age, gender, and physical activity. Adjustments in caloric intake are necessary depending on changes in health status and daily activity level. An average adult requires an estimated 20 to 35 calories per kilogram of body weight per day, leaning toward the higher end if the person is critically ill or very active and the lower end if the person is sedentary.[4]

Proteins, another essential component of a well-balanced diet, are obtained from both animal and plant sources. Ideally, proteins provide 15% to 20% of daily caloric needs. The recommended daily protein intake is 0.8 to 1 g/kg of body weight. One gram of protein yields 4 calories. Proteins are complex nitrogenous organic compounds, of which amino acids are the fundamental units of structure. The 22 amino acids can be classified as essential and nonessential. The body is capable of synthesizing nonessential amino acids if an adequate supply of protein is available. However, the nine essential amino acids cannot be synthesized, and their availability depends totally on dietary sources. Protein sources containing all the essential amino acids are called *complete proteins*. Proteins that lack one or more of the essential amino acids are called *incomplete proteins*. Table 40-2 lists good sources of protein. Proteins are essential for tissue growth, repair, and maintenance; body regulatory functions; and energy production.

Vitamins are organic compounds required in small amounts by the body for normal metabolism. Vitamins function primarily in enzyme reactions that facilitate the metabolism of amino acids, fats, and carbohydrates. The body must rely on a dietary source to meet requirements for some vitamins, such as cobalamin (vitamin B_{12}).

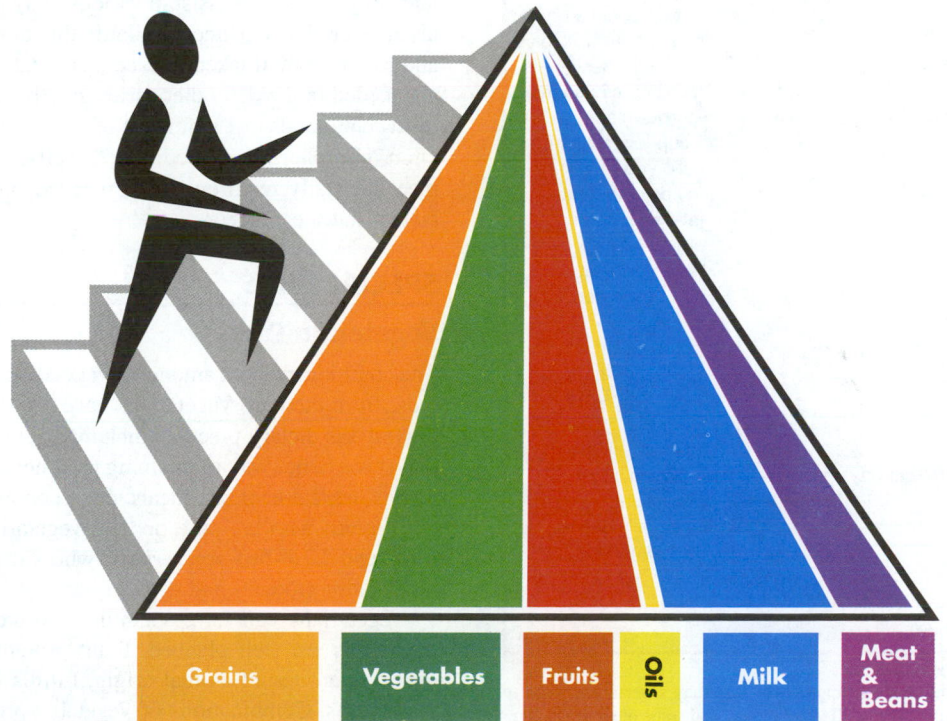

FIG. 40-1 In the MyPyramid, each food group is characterized by varying widths, representative of the proportion of each group that should be eaten. The person climbing the stairs on the side of the pyramid indicates the need to include daily physical activity in a healthy lifestyle. *(Modified from U.S. Department of Agriculture, Center for Nutrition Policy and Promotion, www.Mypyramid.gov.)*

TABLE 40-1	**Pyramid Food Groups and Recommended Number of Servings**

Amounts of various food groups that are recommended each day or week in the Food Guide and in the Eating Plan (amounts are daily unless otherwise specified) at the 2000-calorie level.

Food Groups and Subgroups	Food Guide Amount*	Equivalent Amounts
Fruit group	2 cups (4 servings)/day	1/2 cup equivalent: • 1/2 cup fresh, frozen, or canned fruit • 1 med fruit • 1/4 cup dried fruit • 1/2 cup fruit juice
Vegetable group	2 1/2 cups (5 servings)/day	1/2 cup equivalent: • 1/2 cup of cut-up raw or cooked vegetable • 1 cup raw leafy vegetable • 1/2 cup vegetable juice
• Dark green vegetables	3 cups/wk	
• Orange vegetables	2 cups/wk	
• Legumes (dry beans)	3 cups/wk	
• Starchy vegetables	3 cups/wk	
• Other vegetables	6 1/2 cups/wk	
Grain group	6 oz/day	1 oz equivalent: • 1 slice bread • 1 cup dry cereal • 1/2 cup cooked rice, pasta, cereal
• Whole grains	3 oz	
• Other grains	3 oz	
Meat and beans group	5 1/2 oz/day	1 oz equivalent: • 1 oz cooked lean meats, poultry, fish • 1 egg • 1/4 cup cooked dry beans or tofu, 1 tbs peanut butter, 1/2 oz nuts or seeds
Milk group	3 cups/day	1 cup equivalent: • 1 cup low-fat/fat-free milk, yogurt • 1 1/2 oz of low-fat or fat-free natural cheese • 2 oz of low-fat or fat-free processed cheese
Oils	27 g (6 tsp)/day	1 tsp equivalent: • 1 tbs low-fat mayo • 2 tbs light salad dressing • 1 tsp vegetable oil
Discretionary calorie allowance	267 cal/day	1 tbs added sugar equivalent: • 1/2 oz jelly beans • 8 oz lemonade
Example of distribution:		
• Solid fat†	18 g	
• Added sugars	8 tsp	

From *www.health.gov/dietaryguidelines.*
The 2000-calorie USDA Food Guide is appropriate for many sedentary men 51 to 70 years of age, sedentary women 19 to 30 years of age, and some other gender/age-groups who are more physically active.
*All servings are per day unless otherwise noted. Vegetable subgroup amounts and amounts of nuts, seeds, and dry beans are per week.
†The oils listed in this table are not considered to be part of discretionary calories because they are a major source of the vitamin E and polyunsaturated fatty acids, including the essential fatty acids, in the food pattern. In contrast, solid fats (i.e., saturated and *trans* fats) are listed separately as a source of discretionary calories.

TABLE 40-2	**Good Sources of Protein**

Complete Proteins	Incomplete Proteins
Milk and milk products (e.g., cheese)	Grains (e.g., corn)
Eggs	Legumes (e.g., navy beans, soybeans, peas)
Fish	Nuts (e.g., peanuts)
Meats	Seeds (e.g., sesame seeds, sunflower seeds)
Poultry	

TABLE 40-3	**Major Minerals and Trace Elements**

Major Minerals	Trace Elements
Calcium	Chromium
Chloride	Copper
Magnesium	Fluoride
Phosphorus	Iodine
Potassium	Iron
Sodium	Manganese
Sulfur	Molybdenum
	Selenium
	Zinc

Vitamins are divided into two categories: water-soluble vitamins (vitamin C and the B-complex vitamins) and fat-soluble vitamins (vitamins A, D, E, and K).

Mineral salts (e.g., magnesium, iron, calcium) make up approximately 4% of the total body weight. When minerals are present in minute amounts, they are referred to as trace elements. Minerals required in amounts greater than 100 mg per day are called major minerals. Table 40-3 lists the major minerals and trace elements. Minerals are necessary for the body to build tissues, regulate body fluids, and assist in various body functions. Some minerals are stored in a manner similar to that of the fat-soluble vitamins and can be toxic if taken in excess amounts. The amount of minerals needed in the daily diet varies greatly, from a few micrograms of trace minerals to 1 g or more of the major minerals, such as calcium, phosphorus, and sodium. A well-balanced diet can usually meet the daily requirements of needed minerals. However, deficiency states can occur.

SPECIAL DIETS

Vegetarian Diet

The common element among all vegetarians is the exclusion of red meat from the diet. Vegetarians have a variety of reasons for following this dietary practice, including religious or cultural beliefs that it is a better way of attaining total health, respect for all living beings, ethical-ecologic ideals, and economics. Many vegetarians are *vegans,* who are pure or total vegetarians and eat only plant food, and *lacto-ovo-vegetarians,* who eat plant foods and sometimes dairy products and eggs.

Vegetarians can have vitamin or protein deficiencies unless their diets are well planned. Plant protein, although of a lesser quality than that of animal origin, fulfills most of the protein requirements. Combinations of vegetable protein foods (e.g., cornmeal, kidney beans) can increase the nutritional value. Lacto-ovo-vegetarians obtain additional protein sources from dairy products and eggs. Milk made from soybeans is an excellent protein source, especially for the true vegan. The primary deficiency of a strict vegan is lack of cobalamin (vitamin B_{12}). This vitamin

TABLE 40-4	**NUTRITIONAL THERAPY** Foods High in Iron*

Food	Selected Serving Size
Breads, Cereals, and Grain Products	
Farina, regular or quick cooked (enriched)	2/3 cup
Oatmeal, instant, fortified, prepared (enriched)	2/3 cup
Ready-to-eat cereals, fortified (enriched)	1 oz
Meat, Poultry, Fish, and Alternatives	
Beef liver, braised	3 oz
Pork liver, braised	3 oz
Chicken or turkey liver, braised	1/2 cup diced
Clams: steamed, boiled, or canned (drained)	3 oz
Oysters: baked, broiled, steamed, or canned (undrained)	3 oz
Soybeans, cooked	1/2 cup

*These foods provide 25% to 39% of the recommended dietary allowance (RDA) of iron.

can be obtained only from animal protein, special supplements, or foods that have been fortified with the vitamin. Vegans not using cobalamin supplements are susceptible to the development of megaloblastic anemia and the neurologic signs of cobalamin deficiency. Strict vegetarians and lacto-ovo-vegetarians are also at risk for iron deficiency. Iron-enriched foods or iron supplements are prescribed during pregnancy, early childhood, and adolescence and after major blood loss. Table 40-4 lists examples of foods high in iron. Other deficiencies that may be present in a vegan diet include calcium, zinc, vitamins A and D, and protein.

CULTURALLY COMPETENT CARE
NUTRITION

People have unique cultural heritages that may affect eating customs and nutritional status. Culture, along with personal preferences, socioeconomic status, and religious preferences, can influence food choices. Each culture has its own beliefs and behaviors related to food and the role that food plays in the etiology and treatment of disease. In addition, culture can dictate what food is considered edible, as well as how it is prepared and when it is eaten. There are a wide array of cultural influences on diet ranging from what foods are selected to when meals are eaten and how and who prepares them. For example, some religions require periods of fasting.

The nurse should include cultural and ethnic considerations when assessing the patient's diet history and implementing interventions that require dietary changes. At the same time, the nurse needs to avoid *cultural stereotyping* by making assumptions or generalizations about diet based on the individual's cultural background. For example, not all Jewish patients eat only kosher foods.

It is important to know whether the patients eats "traditional foods" associated with the culture. If traditional foods are eaten, the nurse should assess for their impact on health. For example, "soul foods," which include traditional foods eaten by some African Americans, tend to be high in fat, cholesterol, and sodium. Traditional foods eaten by some Asian Americans may be high in fiber and low in fat and cholesterol but also low in calcium content because of the lack of milk products.

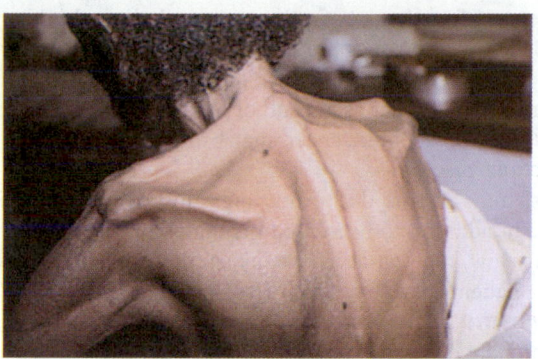

FIG. 40-2   Patient with malnutrition.

Consideration of cultural beliefs is very important when planning dietary changes and monitoring acceptance of dietary changes. For example, perception of body weight and size may also be influenced by culture. Thus the nurse needs to ask the patient or family about how culture affects dietary choices and weight maintenance. In some cultures an overweight person may be seen as a sign of success. Thus the nurse would have a challenging time trying to convince that person to lose weight. Another example is that a Jewish patient who eats only kosher food may be comforted in knowing that most enteral formulas are manufactured kosher and are labeled as such.

Teaching related to dietary restrictions and recommended dietary changes should involve the patient's family. In many situations it is a family member who does the grocery shopping and cooking.

MALNUTRITION

Malnutrition is a deficit, excess, or imbalance of the essential components of a balanced diet. Terms such as *undernutrition* and *overnutrition* are also used to describe malnutrition. **Undernutrition** describes a state of poor nourishment as a result of inadequate diet or diseases that interfere with normal appetite and assimilation of ingested food. **Overnutrition** refers to the ingestion of more food than is required for body needs, as in obesity. An example of nutrient imbalance is a vitamin deficiency state such as *rickets,* a bone disorder caused by inadequate vitamin D. *Scurvy* is a condition characterized by weakness, anemia, and oral ulcerations that is associated with inadequate vitamin C intake.

Undernutrition is most prevalent in developing countries in which adequate food sources do not exist, the inhabitants are not well educated about their nutritional needs, and economic conditions often preclude the purchase of a balanced diet. Undernutrition does exist in the United States, and it is usually found in individuals or groups from the lower socioeconomic class or in individuals who have chronic or acute illnesses. Malnutrition is common in hospitalized patients, with an incidence of 30% to 55%[5] (Fig. 40-2). The prevalence of elderly long-term care residents who can be found to have protein-calorie malnutrition ranges from 23% to 85%.[6]

Types of Malnutrition

Protein-Calorie Malnutrition. **Protein-calorie malnutrition** (PCM) is the most common form of undernutrition and can result from either primary or secondary factors. Primary PCM is present when nutritional needs are not met as a result of poor eating habits. Secondary PCM is the result of an alteration or defect in ingestion, digestion, absorption, or metabolism. In this type of malnutrition, tissue needs are not met even though the dietary intake would be satisfactory under normal conditions. Secondary malnutrition may occur as a result of gastrointestinal (GI) obstruction, surgical procedure, cancer, malabsorption syndromes, drugs, or infectious diseases.

PCM may also be due to the ingestion of foods deficient in protein. In addition to decreased quantities of protein, the diet is generally low in necessary vitamins and minerals. Most malnourished ill patients have this type of combined PCM.

Marasmus and Kwashiorkor. Marasmus is the result of a concomitant deficiency of both caloric and protein intake leading to generalized loss of body fat and muscle. Patients generally appear "wasted," or emaciated, but may have normal serum protein levels. **Kwashiorkor** is caused by a deficiency of protein intake that is superimposed on a catabolic stress event, such as a GI obstruction, a surgical procedure, cancer, a malabsorption syndrome, or an infectious disease. These patients may appear well nourished but have very low serum protein levels (hypoalbuminemic malnutrition).

Etiology and Pathophysiology

Starvation Process. Knowledge of the phases of the starvation process is essential to better understand the physiologic changes that occur in PCM. Initially, the body selectively uses carbohydrates (glycogen) rather than fat and protein to meet metabolic needs. These carbohydrate stores, found in the liver and muscles, are minimal and may be totally depleted within 18 hours. During this early phase of starvation, the only use of protein is in its obligatory participation in cellular metabolism. However, once carbohydrate stores are depleted, protein begins to be converted to glucose for energy. Alanine and glutamine are the first amino acids to be used by the liver for the formation of glucose in a process termed *gluconeogenesis*. The resulting available plasma glucose allows the metabolic processes to continue. With these amino acids being used as energy sources, the person may be in negative nitrogen balance (nitrogen excretion exceeds nitrogen intake). However, within 5 to 9 days, body fat is fully mobilized to supply much of the needed energy.

In prolonged starvation up to 97% of calories are provided by fat, and protein is conserved. Depletion of fat stores depends on the amount available, but fat stores are generally used up in 4 to 6 weeks. Once fat stores are used, body proteins, including those in internal organs and plasma, can no longer be spared and rapidly decrease because they are the only remaining body source of energy available.

If the malnourished patient has surgery, experiences physical trauma, or has an infection, the stress response with concomitant increase in energy expenditure is superimposed on the starvation response. These body insults cause an increase in the metabolic rate, with a subsequent increase in energy requirements. Protein stores are no longer spared and are used with increasing frequency for body energy because of the increased metabolic energy needs.

As the protein depletion continues, liver function is impaired, and synthesis of proteins is diminished. The plasma oncotic pressure is decreased because of decreased protein synthesis. A major function of plasma proteins, primarily of albumin, is the maintenance of the osmotic pressure of the blood. Because of this decreased pressure, a shift in body fluids occurs from the vascular space into the interstitial compartment. As protein ingestion de-

creases and body stores are depleted, albumin eventually leaks into the interstitial space along with the fluid. Edema becomes clinically observable. Often the edema present in the face and legs of the patient masks the muscle wasting that occurs.

As the total blood volume is reduced, the skin appears dry and wrinkled. Along with the shift of fluids to the interstitial space, ions also move. Sodium (a predominant extracellular ion) is found in increased amounts within the cell, and potassium (a predominant intracellular ion) and magnesium are shifted to the extracellular space. The sodium-potassium exchange pump has high energy needs, using 20% to 50% of all calories ingested. When the diet is extremely deficient in calories and essential proteins, the pump will fail, leaving sodium inside the cell (along with water), and the cell will expand.

The liver is the body organ that loses the most mass during protein deprivation. It gradually becomes infiltrated with fat secondary to decreased synthesis of lipoproteins. Immediate restoration to a diet of protein and other necessary constituents must be instituted, or death will rapidly ensue.

Causes of Malnutrition. Many factors contribute to the development of malnutrition, including socioeconomic status, cultural influences, psychologic disorders, medical conditions, and medical treatments. Table 40-5 lists conditions that increase the risk for malnutrition. Because individuals and families from lower socioeconomic classes spend a greater percentage of their income on food, there is a tendency to seek out cheaper foods as the cost of food increases. These foods may not provide adequate or balanced nutrition. In contrast, some lower-income persons may prefer to select foods that are more expensive but only marginally nutritious because of their prestige value. The nurse and the dietitian can assist patients in making food choices that meet nutritional requirements while staying within their limited resources.

Patients with Physical Illnesses. Regardless of the cause of the illness, most sick persons have increased nutritional needs. Pathologic conditions are frequently aggravated by undernutrition, and an existing deficiency state is likely to become more severe during illness. Malnutrition is not an uncommon consequence of illness, surgery, injury, or hospitalization. Anorexia, nausea, vomiting, diarrhea, abdominal distention, and abdominal cramping may accompany diseases of the GI system. Any combination of these symptoms interferes with normal food consumption and metabolism. In addition, a patient may restrict the dietary intake to a few foods or fluids that may not be nutritionally sound out of fear of aggravating the already disturbed GI function.

TABLE 40-5	**Conditions That Increase the Risk for Malnutrition**

- Dementia
- Depression
- Chronic alcoholism
- Excessive dieting to lose weight
- Swallowing disorders (e.g., head and neck cancer)
- Decreased mobility that limits access to food or its preparation
- Nutrient losses from malabsorption, dialysis, fistulas, or wounds
- Drugs with antinutrient or catabolic properties such as corticosteroids and oral antibiotics
- Extreme need for nutrients because of hypermetabolism or stresses such as infection, burns, trauma, or fever
- No oral intake and/or receiving standard intravenous solutions (5% dextrose) for 10 days (adults) or for 5 days (older adults)

Malabsorption syndrome is defined as the impaired absorption of nutrients from the GI tract. It may result from decreased amounts of necessary enzymes or a reduced bowel surface area and can quickly lead to a deficiency state. Many drugs may have undesirable GI side effects, as well as alter normal digestive and absorptive processes. For example, antibiotics change the normal flora of the intestines, decreasing the body's ability to synthesize biotin.

Fever accompanies many illnesses, injuries, and infections, with a concomitant increase in the body's basal metabolic rate (BMR). Each degree of temperature increase on the Fahrenheit scale raises the BMR by about 7%.[7] Without an increase in the amount of calories ingested in the diet, body protein stores will be used to supply calories, and protein depletion can become a problem.

The hospitalized patient, especially the older adult, is at risk of becoming malnourished. Prolonged illness, major surgery, sepsis, draining wounds, burns, hemorrhage, fractures, and immobilization can all contribute to malnutrition. The nurse must assume responsibility, along with the health care provider and the dietitian, for meeting the patient's nutritional needs. The nurse must also be knowledgeable of the requirements of a patient who is not overtly ill but who is undergoing diagnostic studies. This patient may be nutritionally fit on entering the hospital but can develop nutritional problems because of the dietary restrictions imposed by multiple diagnostic studies.

Incomplete Diets. Vitamin deficiencies are rare in most of the developed countries of the world. When vitamin deficiencies are present, several vitamins are usually involved rather than a single vitamin deficiency. The recommended dietary allowances or Dietary Reference Intakes (DRIs) for essential vitamins and minerals can be obtained by eating a diet consisting of foods from the five basic food groups. DRIs from the Food and Nutrition Board have a safety margin because the levels exceed minimum daily requirements for most people.[8] When vitamin imbalances do occur, they are usually found among persons with a pattern of alcohol and drug abuse, persons who are chronically ill, and individuals who follow poor dietary practices. Followers of fad diets or poorly planned vegetarian diets are also subject to a potential deficiency state. Clinical manifestations of vitamin imbalances are most commonly exhibited as neurologic manifestations (Table 40-6). In the growing child, the central nervous system (CNS) is primarily involved, whereas the peripheral nervous system is most affected in the adult.

Food-Drug Interactions. When health conditions require drug therapy, drug and food interactions may not be explored before starting a prescription. Adverse interactions can include incompatibilities, altered drug effectiveness, and impaired nutritional status. Table 40-7 outlines examples of common drug and food/nutrient interactions. As members of the health care team, nurses have a responsibility for monitoring and preventing these potential interactions for patients while in the hospital and at home.

Clinical Manifestations. The adult who is deprived of adequate protein and calories may have many of the clinical manifestations presented in Table 40-8. The most obvious clinical signs on physical examination are apparent in the skin, eyes, mouth, muscles, and CNS. The speed at which the malnutrition develops depends on the quantity and quality of the protein intake, caloric value, illness, and the age of the person.

TABLE 40-6	Recommended Dietary Reference Intakes and Manifestations of Imbalance		
Vitamin	**DRI**	**Manifestations of Overdose**	**Manifestations of Deficiencies**
Fat Soluble			
A	Men: 900 mcg/retinol equivalents* Women: 700 mcg/retinol equivalents	Hair loss, dry skin; headaches; dry mucous membranes; liver damage; bone and joint pain; blurred vision; nausea and vomiting	Dry, scaly skin; increased susceptibility to infection; night blindness; anorexia; eye irritation; xerosis (dry skin); keratinization of respiratory and GI mucosa; bladder stones; anemia; retarded growth
D	Adults: 5-10 mcg of cholecalciferol†	Deposits of calcium and phosphorus in soft tissue; kidney and heart damage; bone fragility; constipation; anorexia, nausea, vomiting; headache	Muscular weakness; excessive sweating; diarrhea and other GI disturbances; bone pain; active rickets; healed rickets; osteomalacia
E	Adults: 15 mg	Relatively nontoxic	Neurologic deficits
K	Men: 120 mcg Women: 90 mcg	Anemia	Defective blood coagulation
Water Soluble			
B$_1$	Men: 1.2 mg Women: 1.1 mg	Not stored in body, therefore overdose does not occur	Loss of appetite; fatigue; nervous irritability; constipation; paresthesias; insomnia
B$_6$	Men: 1.3-1.7 mg Women: 1.3-1.5 mg	Not stored in body, therefore overdose does not occur	Seizures; dermatitis; anemia; neuropathy with motor weakness; anorexia
Cobalamin (B$_{12}$)	Adults: 2-4 mcg	Not stored in body, therefore overdose does not occur	Megaloblastic anemia; inadequate myelin synthesis; anorexia; glossitis; sore mouth and tongue; pallor; neurologic problems such as depression and dizziness; weight loss; nausea; constipation
C	Adults: 75-90 mg	Not stored in body, therefore overdose does not occur	Bleeding gums; loose teeth; easy bruising; poor wound healing; scurvy; dry, itchy skin
Folate (folic acid)	Adults: 400 mcg	Not stored in body, therefore overdose does not occur	Impaired cell division and protein synthesis; megaloblastic anemia; anorexia; fatigue; sore tongue; diarrhea; forgetfulness

GI, Gastrointestinal; *DRI*, Dietary Reference Intake.
*1 retinol equivalent = 10 international units vitamin A activity from β-carotene or 3.33 international units vitamin A activity from retinol.
†1 mcg of cholecalciferol = 40 international units vitamin D.

TABLE 40-7	Common Drug and Food/Nutrient Interactions	
Drug Category/Drug	**Food/Nutrient**	**Drug-Food Effects or Cautions**
Anticoagulants	Dietary vitamin K (e.g., green leafy vegetables, green tea, dairy products/meats)	Decrease or loss of anticoagulant effect
Antiseizure agents • phenytoin (Dilantin)	Folate (folic acid)	Long-term drug use may increase folic acid requirement
Antidepressants • trazodone (Desyrel) • tricyclic antidepressants (e.g., amitriptyline [Elavil])	Food Riboflavin	Food slows drug absorption Riboflavin requirements may increase with amitriptyline (Elavil) or imipramine (Tofranil)
Antidiabetic agents • glyburide (Micronase, DiaBeta)	High-fat diet	Drug should not be taken with high-fat diet
Barbiturates • phenobarbital • mephobarbital (Mebaral)	Folate (folic acid)	Drugs may increase folic acid requirements; long-term therapy may require vitamin D supplements for osteomalacia
β-Adrenergic blockers • labetalol (Normodyne) • metaproterenol (Alupent) • carteolol (Cartrol) • sotalol (Betapace)	Food	Bioavailability of these drugs may be enhanced when taken with food
Bronchodilators • theophylline • oxtriphylline (Choledyl) • dyphylline (Lufyllin)	High-carbohydrate, low-protein diets Caffeine-containing foods and fluids	↓ Drug elimination Caffeine may increase CNS-stimulant effects of xanthine-derivative bronchodilators
• cholestyramine (Questran)	Fat-soluble vitamins	Drug may interfere with their absorption
Corticosteroids (prolonged therapy)	Salt seasonings	May require decreased sodium and/or potassium supplementation intake
• etidronate (Didronel)	Foods, fluids, or drugs high in calcium	May prevent drug absorption
• isoniazid (INH)	Cheese (e.g., Swiss) or fish (e.g., tuna, skipjack)	Concurrent ingestion may lead to redness or itching, HR changes, sweating, chills or clammy feeling, headache or light-headedness; thought to be related to altered metabolism of tyramine in foods
Phenothiazines	Riboflavin	Drugs may increase riboflavin requirements
• procarbazine (Matulane)	Food and fluids containing tyramine (e.g., aged cheese, smoked or pickled meats or poultry, fermented meat, beer, wine, liqueurs)	When used concurrently, may cause sudden and severe hypertensive reactions; dietary restrictions need to continue for at least 2 wk after MAO inhibitors discontinued
• selegiline (Eldepryl)	Food and fluids containing tyramine (e.g., see above)	Same as above
• ticlopidine (Ticlid)	Food	Drug absorption increased when taken after a meal
• zafirlukast (Accolate)	High-fat and high-protein meal	When taken concurrently, drug bioavailability reduced by about 40%
Zinc supplements	Foods	Many foods (e.g., fiber, milk casein) impair zinc absorption

CNS, Central nervous system; *HR,* heart rate; *MAO,* monoamine oxidase.

Clinical manifestations of malnutrition are the result of numerous interactions occurring at the cellular level. As protein intake is severely reduced, the muscles, which make up the largest reservoir of protein in the body, become wasted and flabby, leading to weakness, fatigability, and decreased endurance. There is decreased protein available for repair, and as a result, wound healing may be delayed. Malnutrition in the hospitalized patient may result in delayed recovery and prolonged hospitalization. The person is more susceptible to all types of infections. Both humoral and cell-mediated immunity are deficient in PCM. There is a decrease in leukocytes in the peripheral blood. Phagocytosis is altered as a result of the lack of energy (adenosine triphosphate [ATP]) necessary to drive the process. Many malnourished persons are anemic. Anemia resulting from PCM is usually caused by nutritional deficiencies in iron and folic acid, the necessary building blocks for red blood cells (RBCs).

The severity of complications from malnutrition ranges from mild to emaciation and death. Major complications center around delayed wound healing and increased susceptibility to infection from decreased immune function.

Diagnostic Studies

History and Physical Examination. A diet history of foods eaten over the past week will reveal a great deal about the patient's dietary habits and knowledge of good nutrition. In addition to the height, weight, and vital signs, the patient's physical state should be thoroughly assessed and documented. Each body system should be assessed. Table 40-9 summarizes the assessment and findings of the patient with malnutrition.

Laboratory Studies. The diagnosis of PCM can be determined by a variety of laboratory studies used in conjunction with the physical examination. Serum albumin is somewhat useful in the diagnosis of malnutrition. The degree of protein depletion can be identified with the use of the scale in Table 40-10. Serum albumin has a half-life of approximately 20 to 22 days. In the absence of marked fluid loss, such as from hemorrhage or burns, the serum albumin value lags behind actual protein changes by more than 2 weeks and there-

TABLE 40-8	Manifestations of Protein-Calorie Malnutrition

Body System	Subclinical Manifestations	Clinical Manifestations
Integumentary	Slowed tissue turnover rate, surface temperature 1°-2° F cooler	Brittle nails, ↓ tone and elasticity of skin, xeroderma (dry skin), pigment changes (brown-gray), erythematous seborrheic dermatitis, scrotal dermatitis
Visual	Night blindness	Hair: easy loss of hair, color changes, lack of luster
		Blood vessel growth in cornea, Bitot's spots (gray keratinized epithelium on conjunctiva), dryness of conjunctiva and cornea, pale to red conjunctiva
Gastrointestinal		
Mouth and lips	Reduction in saliva production	Cheilosis (crusting and ulceration at angle of mouth)
Tongue	Mucosa more permeable to bacteria	Raw and beefy red, edematous and smooth, atrophy or hypertrophy of papillae
Teeth	Improper development, delayed eruption	Cavities, loose teeth, discolored enamel
Gingivae		Periodontal disease, tendency to bleed easily, receding, pale, and soft
Stomach	↓ Gastric secretion, delayed gastric emptying	Constant hunger, ↑ incidence of ulcers
Intestines	↓ Motility and absorption, normal flora causing infection from ↑ permeability of mucosa	Diarrhea and flatulence, protruding abdomen, ↑ incidence of parasitic diseases
Liver-biliary	Fatty liver, ↓ absorption of fat-soluble vitamins	Hepatomegaly
Cardiovascular	↓ Cardiac output, ↓ hemoglobin, shift in heart position, ↑ risk of thrombophlebitis	↓ BP and pulse, slight cyanosis, anemia, body edema
Endocrine	↓ Insulin production	Thyroid enlargement, polydipsia, polyuria, ↓ ↓ sensitivity to cold
Immunologic	↓ Lymphocyte proliferation, ↓ albumin levels, ↓ acute-phase protein production, ↓ antibody production, diminished febrile response to infection	↑ Number of infections, ↓ response to delayed hypersensitivity skin tests
Musculoskeletal	↓ Growth rate, ↓ body stature with chronic PCM, ↓ muscle mass	Prominence of bony structures such as face, clavicle, scapula, ribs, iliac crests, and spinal vertebrae due to subcutaneous tissue loss; weak and spindly arms and legs, flat buttocks, weak and flabby muscles; ↓ physical activity and ability to work; severe weight loss
Neurologic	Loss of ambition, feeling of being tired	Depression, confusion, ↓ reflexes in legs and ankles, ↓ position sense, ↓ vibratory sense, paresthesias of hands and feet, syncope, motor weakness
Renal	Negative nitrogen balance, ↓ BUN and creatinine levels	Nocturia, ↓ urinary output
Reproductive	↓ Gonadotropin levels	Amenorrhea, impotence, atrophied breasts
Respiratory	Pulmonary edema, ↓ strength of respiratory muscles	↑ Susceptibility to respiratory infection, ↓ respiratory rate, ↓ vital capacity

BUN, Blood urea nitrogen; *PCM,* protein-calorie malnutrition.

fore is not a good indicator of acute changes in nutritional status. Prealbumin, a protein synthesized by the liver, has a half-life of 2 days and is a better indicator of recent or current nutritional status. Serum transferrin level is another indicator of protein status. Transferrin, a protein synthesized by the liver and used to transport iron, decreases during states of protein deficiency.

Serum electrolyte levels reflect changes taking place between the intracellular and the extracellular spaces. The serum potassium level is often elevated. The RBC count and the hemoglobin level indicate the presence and degree of anemia. The total lymphocyte count decreases during malnutrition states. The total lymphocyte count is calculated by multiplying the percent of lymphocytes times the total white blood cell (WBC) count. Liver enzyme levels, a reflection of liver function, may be elevated during malnutrition. Serum levels of both fat-soluble and water-soluble vitamins are usually diminished in malnutrition. The lowered levels of the fat-soluble vitamins correlate with the clinical signs of *steatorrhea* (fatty stools).

Anthropometric Measurements. Anthropometric measurements, which include gross measures of fat and muscle contents, may be ordered. These measurements tend to be most beneficial in evaluating long-term effects of malnutrition or responses to nutritional interventions. They consist of measures of skinfold thickness at various sites, which is an indicator of subcutaneous fat stores, and midarm muscle circumference, an indicator of protein stores. These measurements are then compared with standards for healthy persons of the same age and gender. Training and practice are required to perform these measurements accurately and reliably. To provide information on the patient's nutritional status in response to treatment, serial measurements are needed. Sites most reflective of body fat are those over the biceps and the triceps, below the scapula, above the iliac crest, and over the upper thigh. Both skinfold thickness and midarm muscle circumference measurements are decreased in chronic PCM and acute protein malnutrition. These measurements may also be influenced by shifts in hydration status. The exact relationship of the midarm circumference measure to body composition of functional protein, both muscle and nonmuscle, remains to be established.

NURSING MANAGEMENT
MALNUTRITION

▪ *Nursing Assessment*

In many institutions (acute and long-term care) and in home care, the nurse is responsible for nutritional screening. Nutritional screening identifies individuals who are malnourished or at risk for malnutrition. The purpose of the nutritional screening is to determine if a more detailed nutritional assessment is necessary.[9-12] Ta-

Gastrointestinal System

TABLE 40-9	*NURSING ASSESSMENT* **Malnutrition**

Subjective Data
Important Health Information
Past health history: Severe burns, major trauma, hemorrhage, draining wounds, bone fractures with prolonged immobility, chronic renal or liver disease, cancer, malabsorption syndrome, GI obstruction, infectious diseases (TB, AIDS)
Medications: Corticosteroids, chemotherapeutic agents, diet pills
Surgery or other treatments: Recent surgery, radiation

Functional Health Patterns
Health perception–health management: Alcohol or drug abuse; malaise, apathy
Nutritional-metabolic: Increase or decrease in weight, weight problems; increase or decrease in appetite, typical dietary intake; food preferences and aversions; food allergies or intolerance; ill-fitting or absent dentures; dry mouth, difficulty in chewing or swallowing; bloating or gas; ↑ sensitivity to cold; delayed wound healing
Elimination: Constipation, diarrhea, nocturia, decreased urinary output
Activity-exercise: Increase or decrease in activity patterns; weakness, fatigue, decreased endurance
Cognitive-perceptual: Pain in mouth; paresthesias; loss of position and vibratory sense
Role-relationship: Change in family (e.g., loss of a spouse); financial resources
Sexual-reproductive: Amenorrhea, impotence, decreased libido

Objective Data
General
Listless, cachectic; underweight for height

Integumentary
Dry, brittle, sparse hair with color changes and lack of luster, alopecia; dry, scaly lips, fever blisters, angular crusts and lesions at corners of mouth (cheilosis); brittle, ridged nails; decreased tone and elasticity of skin; cool, rough, dry, scaly skin with brown-gray pigment changes; reddened, scaly dermatitis, scrotal dermatitis; slight cyanosis; peripheral edema

Eyes
Pale or red conjunctivae, gray keratinized epithelium on conjunctiva (Bitot's spots); dryness and dull appearance of conjunctiva and cornea, soft cornea; blood vessel growth in cornea; redness and fissuring of eyelid corners

Respiratory
Decreased respiratory rate, ↓ vital capacity, crackles, weak cough

Cardiovascular
Increase or decrease in heart rate, ↓ BP, dysrhythmias

Gastrointestinal
Swollen, smooth, raw, beefy red tongue (glossitis), hypertrophic or atrophic papillae; dental cavities, absent or loose teeth, discolored tooth enamel; spongy, pale, receded gums with a tendency to bleed easily, periodontal disease; ulcerations, white patches or plaques, redness, swelling of oral mucosa; distended, tympanic abdomen; ascites, hepatomegaly, decreased bowel sounds; steatorrhea

Neurologic
Decreased or loss of reflexes, tremor; inattention, irritability, confusion, syncope

Musculoskeletal
Decreased muscle mass with poor tone, "wasted" appearance; bowlegs, knock-knees, beaded ribs, chest deformity, prominent bony structures

Possible Findings
↓ Hemoglobin and hematocrit; ↓ MCV, MCH, or MCHC (iron deficiency); ↓ MCV or MCH (folic acid or cobalamin deficiency); altered serum electrolyte levels, especially hyperkalemia; ↓ BUN and creatinine; ↓ serum albumin, transferrin, and prealbumin; ↓ lymphocytes; ↑ liver enzymes; ↓ serum vitamin levels

AIDS, Acquired immunodeficiency syndrome; *BUN,* blood urea nitrogen; *GI,* gastrointestinal; *MCH,* mean corpuscular hemoglobin; *MCHC,* mean corpuscular hemoglobin concentration; *MCV,* mean corpuscular volume; *TB,* tuberculosis.

TABLE 40-10	**Serum Albumin and Prealbumin Levels**

Albumin	
Normal value	3.8-4.5 g/dl (38-45 g/L)
Mild depletion	3.0-3.7 g/dl (30-37 g/L)
Moderate depletion	2.5-2.9 g/dl (25-29 g/L)
Severe depletion	<2.5 g/dl (<25 g/L)
Prealbumin	
Normal value	20 mg/dl (200 mg/L)
Mild depletion	10-15 mg/dl (100-150 mg/L)
Moderate depletion	5-10 mg/dl (50-100 mg/L)
Severe depletion	<5 mg/dl (<50 mg/L)

ble 40-11 provides an example of a nursing nutritional screening tool.[10] In long-term care, the Minimum Data Set (MDS) form is used to obtain information about a person's nutritional status.[11] In home care, the Outcome and Assessment Information Set (OASIS) prompts the nurse to collect information on diet, oral intake, dental health, swallowing difficulties, and any needs for meal assistance. If nutritional problems are identified, a referral to a dietitian is suggested.

If the nutritional screening identifies that an individual is at nutritional risk, a full nutritional assessment is most often warranted.

A nutritional assessment is a comprehensive approach to defining nutritional status that uses medical, nutritional, and medication histories; physical examination; anthropometric measurements; and laboratory data.

Across all settings of care delivery, the nurse must be aware of the nutritional status of the patient. Obtaining an accurate measure of body weight and height and recording this information are important components of this assessment. When possible, the patient's actual height should be measured rather than based on the patient's self-report. The patient's current weight relative to usual body weight and ideal body weight should be noted. An easy way to determine ideal body weight is to use the Hamwi "rule of thumb" method (Table 40-12). The percent change in body weight over time provides information on the degree of weight loss.

Body mass index (BMI) is a measure of weight for height (see Fig. 41-4). BMI is calculated as follows:

$$BMI = Weight\ (kg)/Height^2\ (m^2)$$

In adults a BMI of less than 15 kg/m^2 is associated with a significant increase in morbidity, and a BMI of less than 18.5 kg/m^2 is considered underweight. A healthy weight is considered a BMI between 18.5 and 24.9 kg/m^2. A BMI between 25 and 29.9 kg/m^2 is considered overweight, and a BMI of 30 kg/m^2 or greater is considered obese.[4]

TABLE 40-11 Admission Nutrition Screening Tool

A. Diagnosis

If the patient has at least *one* of the following diagnoses, circle and proceed to section E to consider the patient AT NUTRITIONAL RISK and stop here.

- Anorexia nervosa/bulimia nervosa
- Malabsorption (celiac sprue, ulcerative colitis, Crohn's disease, short bowel syndrome)
- Multiple trauma (closed head injury, penetrating trauma, multiple fractures)
- Pressure ulcers
- Major gastrointestinal surgery within the past year
- Cachexia (temporal wasting, muscle wasting, cancer, cardiac)
- Coma
- Diabetes
- End-stage liver disease
- End-stage renal disease
- Nonhealing wounds

B. Nutrition Intake History

If the patient has at least *one* of the following symptoms, circle and proceed to section E to consider the patient AT NUTRITIONAL RISK and stop here.

- Diarrhea (500 ml × 2 days)
- Vomiting (5 days)
- Reduced intake (<½ normal intake for 5 days)

C. Ideal Body Weight Standards

Compare the patient's current weight for height to the ideal body weight chart.

If at 80% of ideal body weight, proceed to section E to consider the patient AT NUTRITIONAL RISK and stop here.

D. Weight History

Any recent unplanned weight loss? No _____ Yes _____
    Amount (lb or kg) _____
    If yes, within the past _____ wk or _____ mo
    Current weight (lb or kg) _____
    Usual weight (lb or kg) _____
    Height (ft, in, or cm) _____
Find percentage of weight loss:

$$\frac{\text{Usual wt} - \text{Current wt}}{\text{Usual wt}} \times 100 = _____ \% \text{ wt loss}$$

Compare the % wt loss with the following chart and circle appropriate value:

Length of Time	Significant (%)	Severe (%)
1 wk	1-2	>2
2-3 wk	2-3	>3
1 mo	4-5	>5
3 mo	7-8	>8
5+ mo	10	>10

If the patient has experienced a significant or severe weight loss, proceed to section E and consider the patient AT NUTRITIONAL RISK.

E. Nurse Assessment

Using the above criteria, what is this patient's nutritional risk? (circle one)
LOW NUTRITIONAL RISK   AT NUTRITIONAL RISK

Adapted from Kovacevich DS, Boney AR, Braunschweig CL, et al: Nutrition risk classification: a valid and reproducible tool for nurses, *Nutr Clin Pract* 12:20, 1997. Reprinted with permission of the American Society for Parenteral and Enteral Nutrition (ASPEN).

TABLE 40-12 Desirable Body Weight—Hamwi Formula (Rule of Thumb)

Women: 100 lb for first 5 ft + 5 lb for every inch thereafter
Men: 106 lb for first 5 ft + 6 lb for every inch thereafter

Percent desirable body weight = (current wt./desirable wt.) × 100

Small frame: subtract 10%
Large frame: add 10%

Source: Hamwi GJ: Changing dietary concepts. In Danowski TS, editor: *Diabetes mellitus: diagnosis and treatment*, vol 1, New York, 1964, American Diabetes Association.

etitian, pharmacist, and physician should also be involved in the assessment and planning of care. However, the nurse, as the first-line health care professional dealing with the patient, should take the initiative in determining the severity of any nutritional problems.

■ Nursing Diagnoses

Nursing diagnoses for the patient with malnutrition include, but are not limited to, the following:

- Imbalanced nutrition: less than body requirements *related to* decreased access, ingestion, digestion, or absorption of food or *related to* anorexia
- Self-care deficit (feeding) *related to* decreased strength and endurance, fatigue, and apathy
- Constipation or diarrhea *related to* poor eating patterns, immobility, or medication effects
- Fluid volume deficit *related to* factors affecting access to or absorption of fluids
- Risk for impaired skin integrity *related to* poor nutritional state
- Noncompliance *related to* alteration in perception, lack of motivation, or incompatibility of regimen with lifestyle or resources
- Activity intolerance *related to* weakness, fatigue, and inadequate caloric intake or iron stores

■ Planning

The overall goals are that the patient with malnutrition will (1) achieve weight gain, (2) consume a specified number of calories per day (with a diet individualized for the patient), and (3) have no adverse consequences related to malnutrition or nutrition therapies.

■ Nursing Implementation

Health Promotion. The nurse is in a good position to teach and reinforce healthy eating habits with individuals and groups of persons throughout their life span. The gap between perceived importance of nutrition and care in selecting foods has widened. To assist in these efforts are the Food and Drug Administration (FDA)–mandated food labels that are now on all packaged foods. The Dietary Guidelines for Americans 2005 offers key recommendations for improving nutrition that are useful points for a teaching program[12] (Table 40-13).

Acute Intervention. The nurse must assess the patient's nutritional state, as well as focus on the other physical problems of the patient. The nurse must become more aware of who is at risk, why, and how to intervene appropriately. In states of increased stress, such as surgery, severe trauma, and sepsis, more calories and protein are needed. Wound healing requires increased protein synthe-

In addition, the nurse should get a record of the complete diet history from the patient or the family. The patient's nutritional state may not be the reason medical assistance was sought. However, it may be a contributing factor to the disease, and have an impact on management of and recovery from the disease. The di-

Gastrointestinal System

TABLE 40-13   PATIENT AND FAMILY TEACHING GUIDE
Good Nutrition

The following recommendations apply to most people:
- Eat a variety of foods.
- Modify diet habits slowly.
- Plan your meals ahead of time.
- Choose a diet moderate in sugars.
- Choose a diet moderate in salt and sodium.
- Avoid foods described as crispy, creamy, or fried.
- If you drink alcoholic beverages, do so in moderation.
- Choose a diet low in fat, unsaturated fat, and cholesterol.
- Learn to modify your favorite foods so they are healthier.
- Choose a diet with plenty of grain products, vegetables, and fruits.
- Set small goals for yourself and reward yourself when you achieve them.
- When eating out, look for foods described as baked, broiled, grilled, or steamed.
- Balance the food you eat with physical activity to maintain or improve your weight.
- Allow yourself healthy snacks so you will not feel deprived and you are less likely to binge on foods.
- Encourage family members to adopt healthy habits or enlist friends to make healthy eating a part of their lives.

TABLE 40-14   NUTRITIONAL THERAPY
High-Calorie, High-Protein Diet

General Principles
1. A normal diet is supplemented with larger portions to increase the protein and caloric content. It is used for patients with hypermetabolism, burns, excessive stress, and cancer.
2. It is important to eat regularly and not to skip meals or snacks.

Meal	Protein (g)	Menu Plan*
Fruit	2	Large orange juice
Starch, fat		1 toast with butter or jelly
Starch, protein supplement	4	Cream of wheat with 2 tbs skim milk powder
2 meat	14	Omelet with 2 eggs
Milk, protein supplement	10	High-protein milk shake (2 tbs skim milk powder added)
4 meat	28	2 burritos with extra cheese, meat
4 starches	8	
Vegetable	2	Lettuce and tomato salad with dressing
4 fats		Sugar cookies
Milk, protein supplement	10	High-protein milk shake
4 meat	28	Spaghetti with 4 oz meat sauce, Parmesan cheese
3 starches	6	
Vegetable	2	Green beans with 2 tbs margarine
7 fats		Bread with butter
		Tapioca pudding
Milk, protein supplement	10	High-protein milk shake
Snack		
Milk	8	$^1/_2$ sandwich with peanut butter
Fruit		
TOTAL	**132**	

*Additional menu plans are available on the website at *http://evolve.elsevier.com/Lewis/medsurg*.

sis. When fever is present, the metabolic rate is increased and nitrogen loss is accelerated. Despite the return of body temperature to normal, the rate of protein breakdown and resynthesis may be accelerated for several weeks. After major surgery, several weeks of increased protein and calorie intake are needed to promote healing and replenish body stores.

The nurse must have a thorough understanding of nutritional support and the rationale for recording the daily weight, intake, and output. Daily weights can give an ongoing record of body weight gain or loss. However, rapid gains and losses are usually the result of shifts in fluid balance. The body weight, in conjunction with accurate recording of food and fluid intake, provides a clearer picture of the patient's fluid and nutritional state. To obtain an accurate weight, the nurse should weigh the patient at the same time each day, on the same scale, with the same type or amount of clothing, and preferably with the bladder recently emptied.

The protein and calorie intake required in the malnourished patient depends on the cause of the malnutrition, the treatment being employed, and other stressors affecting the patient. If the patient is able to take food by mouth, a daily calorie count and diet diary can be obtained to give an accurate record of food intake. The nurse and the dietitian working with the patient and family can assist in the selection of high-calorie and high-protein foods (unless medically contraindicated). Preparation of foods preferred by the pa-

tient enhances the daily intake. Discussion with the patient and family about foods that should be eaten to provide high-protein, high-calorie content is important. The family can be encouraged to bring the patient's favorite foods from home while the patient is still hospitalized. Table 40-14 gives an example of a high-calorie, high-protein diet.

The undernourished patient usually needs to have between-meal supplements. These may consist of items prepared in the dietary department or commercially prepared products. Eating these items between meals increases the total daily intake and provides extra calories, proteins, fluids, and nutrients. In addition, multiple small feedings improve the tolerance for food intake by distributing the amount more evenly throughout the day. If the patient is unable to consume enough nutrition with a high-calorie, high-protein diet, oral liquid nutrition supplements can be added. Some patients may benefit from appetite stimulants such as megestrol acetate (Megace) or dronabinol (Marinol) to improve nutritional intake.

If the patient is still unable to take in enough calories, tube feedings may be considered. Parenteral nutrition (PN) may be initiated if enteral feedings are not feasible.

Ambulatory and Home Care. With shortened hospital stays, many patients are discharged on a therapeutic diet. Discharge preparation for both the patient and the family is important. They must be carefully instructed on the cause of the undernourished state and ways to avoid the problem in the future. The patient must be made aware that undernourishment, whatever the cause, can recur and that adhering to a diet high in protein and calories for a few weeks cannot fully restore a normal nutritional state. Many months may be needed to reach this goal. Diet instruction is usually carried out by the dietitian, but it is important for the nurse to assess the patient's understanding and reinforce the information whenever possible. The patient's ability to comply with the dietary instructions must be examined in light of past eating habits, religious and ethnic preferences, age, income, other resources, and state of health.

Unless the patient and the family can be convinced of the necessity for dietary change and have the resources to effect change, it is likely that no long-term benefits will be achieved. Ways should be found in which the patient can become actively involved in the recovery. The need for continuous follow-up care must be strongly emphasized if rehabilitation is to be accomplished and maintained.

The nurse is in an ideal position to determine the need for nutritious meals and snacks after discharge from the hospital. In addition, it is important to consider the availability and acceptability of community resources that provide meals. Such aspects can be integrated into discharge planning, and visits by the home health nurse can ensure follow-up.

Keeping a diet diary or a calorie count for 3 days at a time is one way to analyze and reinforce healthful eating patterns. These records are also helpful to the health care team in the follow-up care. Self-assessment of progress can be encouraged by having the patient weighed once or twice a week and keeping a weight record.

■ Evaluation

The expected outcomes are that the patient who is malnourished will

- achieve and maintain optimal body weight
- consume a well-balanced diet
- experience no adverse outcomes related to malnutrition

GERONTOLOGIC CONSIDERATIONS
MALNUTRITION

Older adults are at risk for malnutrition, with many factors influencing their nutritional intake[13] (Table 40-15). Many of these factors may occur at the same time, thus further increasing the risk of malnutrition. The unique nutritional requirements of an older adult are often overlooked. The older person frequently reduces the consumption of needed protein, vitamins, and minerals and may take in "empty calories," such as candy and pastries. As a group, older adults may be less well informed about what constitutes a well-balanced diet.

When these factors are added to already existing medical problems, it is easy to see why poor dietary practices develop. In addition, poor dentition, ill-fitting dentures, anorexia, multiple losses affecting the social setting of meals, low income, and medical conditions involving the GI tract contribute to the type and amount of foods that are eaten.

Some of the physiologic changes associated with aging affect the nutritional status of older adults. The following changes are of particular interest:

1. Changes in the oral cavity (e.g., change in bite surfaces of the teeth, periodontal disease, drying of the mucous membrane of the mouth and tongue, poorly fitting dentures, de-

| TABLE 40-15 | GERONTOLOGIC DIFFERENCES IN ASSESSMENT
Factors Affecting Nutritional Intake in Older Adults |

Physical Factors
- Age
- Anorexia
- Decreased number of taste buds
- Dental problems
- Food intolerances
- Health status
- Physical disability
- Prescribed diets
- Prescribed or over-the-counter drugs

Psychosocial Factors
- Importance of food in the past
- Loneliness or loss
- Mental awareness
- Social isolation

Socioeconomic Factors
- Available time for food preparation and eating
- Availability of desired foods
- Availability of transportation to food stores
- Education level and nutritional knowledge
- Food fads
- Income level
- Lack of food preparation equipment

creased muscle strength for chewing, decreased number of taste buds, decreased saliva production)
2. Changes in digestion and motility (e.g., decreased absorption of cobalamin, vitamin A, and folic acid, and decreased GI motility)
3. Changes in the endocrine system (e.g., decreased tolerance to glucose)
4. Changes in the musculoskeletal system (e.g., degenerative joint changes can decrease mobility and ability to prepare food)
5. Decrease in vision and hearing (e.g., procurement and preparation of food are more difficult)

Certain illnesses that are more prevalent in the older population are considered to be diet related. These include atherosclerosis, osteoporosis, diabetes mellitus, and diverticulosis. Multiple drugs are often required to treat these and other common chronic illnesses of the older patient. These drugs often have an adverse effect on the appetite of older adults, increasing the possibility of inadequate intake caused by anorexia.

To date, with the exception of calories, it has not been determined that older adults have different requirements for specific nutrients from those of middle-aged adults. Generally, caloric intake should decrease with age because of the progressive loss of lean body mass and a decrease in the basal metabolic rate. Therefore fewer calories are needed to meet metabolic needs. Unless caloric intake is decreased by careful attention to food intake, or energy expenditure is increased through greater physical activity and exercise, obesity will result.

Socioeconomic factors are important variables when assessing the nutritional status of an older adult. Because more than one third of older adults have incomes below the poverty level, obtaining adequate and nutritious food can be an ongoing problem. In many cases the older person cannot afford to purchase meat, fresh vegetables, and fruits that provide many necessary nutrients.

Lifestyle changes such as retirement or relocation to a nursing home can have a significant impact on the eating habits of the older

Gastrointestinal System

adult. Other important considerations that should be assessed include the ethnic background, previous dietary practices, food preferences, knowledge of proper diet, availability and accessibility of food stores, transportation, and health status. Problems related to any or all of these areas can alert the nurse to the possibility of a nutritional problem.

Malnutrition can occur in an older person even though the caloric requirements decrease with age. If malnutrition is present, it may be difficult to ingest enough food to correct the problem. Special strategies, such as adaptive devices (e.g., large-handled eating utensils), often are helpful in increasing dietary intake. Some older persons may require nutritional support therapies until their strength and general health are improved.

Many community nutritional programs are available to the older person to make mealtime a pleasant, social event. Improving the social setting of a meal often improves the dietary intake. Home-delivered meals and meal sites in a central location are popular meal alternatives for many older adults. The use of food stamps is another alternative that allows low-income households, regardless of age, to buy more food of a greater variety.

TYPES OF SPECIALIZED NUTRITION SUPPORT

Oral Feeding

High-calorie oral supplements may be used in the patient whose nutritional intake is deficient. This may include milk shakes, puddings, or commercially available products (e.g., Ensure, Sustacal). Research suggests that ingestion of these beverages may have a role in improving the nutritional status of elderly patients.[14] These supplements should not be used as meal substitutes but between meals as snacks. In some long-term care facilities, these beverages are used instead of water with oral medication administration to increase caloric intake. If patients are unable to maintain or achieve adequate nutritional status, nutrition support may be necessary. For a decision-making plan related to nutrition, see the algorithm in Fig. 40-3.

Tube Feeding

Tube feeding (also known as **enteral nutrition**) refers to the administration of a nutritionally balanced liquefied food or formula through a tube inserted into the stomach, duodenum, or jejunum.[15] Tube feedings may be ordered for the patient who has a functioning GI tract but

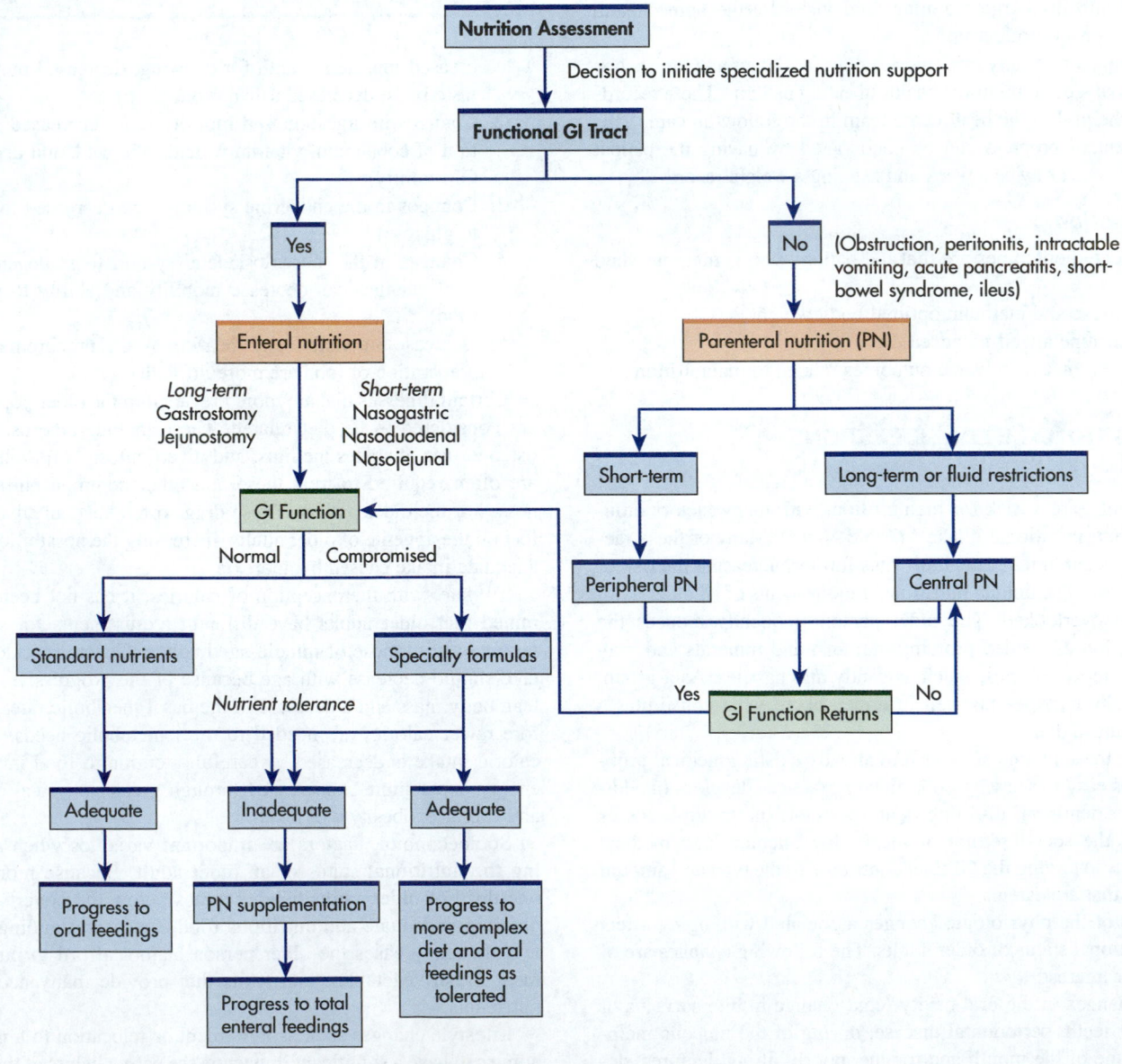

FIG. 40-3 Nutrition support algorithm.

is unable to take any or enough oral nourishment. Specific indications for tube feeding include those persons with anorexia, orofacial fractures, head and neck cancer, neurologic or psychiatric conditions that prevent oral intake, extensive burns, and those who are receiving chemotherapy or radiation therapy. Tube feedings are considered to be easily administered, safer, more physiologically efficient, and definitely less expensive than parenteral nutrition. Enteral nutrition is used to provide nutrients by way of the GI tract either alone or as a supplement to oral or parenteral nutrition.

Common delivery options are continuous infusion by pump, intermittent by gravity, intermittent bolus by syringe, and cyclic feedings by infusion pump. Continuous infusion is most often used with critically ill patients and feedings into the small intestine. Intermittent feeding may be preferred as the patient improves or is receiving such feedings at home.[16]

A nasogastric (NG) tube is most commonly used for short-term feeding problems. If the feedings are necessary for an extended time, other means of feeding may be used, such as an esophagostomy tube, a gastrostomy tube (placed surgically, endoscopically, or radiologically), or a jejunostomy tube that empties directly into the jejunum. Transpyloric (nasointestinal) tube placement or placement into the jejunum is used when physiologic conditions warrant feeding the patient below the pyloric sphincter. (Fig. 40-4 shows the locations of commonly used enteral feeding tubes.)

Nasogastric and Nasointestinal Tubes. Feeding tubes made of polyurethane or silicone materials have added to the comfort level of the patient over extended periods. These tubes are long, small in diameter, soft, and flexible, thereby decreasing the risk of mucosal damage from prolonged placement. The older tubes made of rubber or polyvinyl chloride tend to stiffen with time. Polyurethane and silicone tubes are radiopaque, making their position readily identified by x-ray. Placement into the intestine theoretically decreases the likelihood of regurgitation of contents into the esophagus and subsequent aspiration. With the use of a stylet, these tubes can be placed in a comatose patient because the ability to swallow is not essential during insertion.

Although the smaller feeding tubes have many advantages over wider-lumen tubes, such as the standard decompression NG tube, there are some disadvantages. Because of the small diameter, these tubes are more easily clogged when feedings are thick and are more difficult to use for checking residual volumes. They are particularly prone to obstruction when oral drugs have not been thoroughly crushed and dissolved in water before administration. They can become dislodged by vomiting or coughing and can also become knotted or kinked in the GI tract. Failure to flush the tubing after both drug administration and residual volume determinations can result in tube clogging. When the tube becomes clogged, it may necessitate removal and insertion of a new tube, adding to cost and patient discomfort.

Gastrostomy and Jejunostomy. A gastrostomy tube may be used for a patient who requires tube feedings over an extended time (Fig. 40-5). Gastrostomy tubes can be placed surgically, radiologically, or endoscopically. See Fig. 40-6 for the placement procedure of a percutaneous endoscopic gastrostomy (PEG). The patient must have an intact, unobstructed GI tract, and the esophageal lumen must be wide enough to pass the endoscope for this type of gastrostomy tube placement. A PEG and a radiologically placed gastrostomy have several advantages. These procedures have fewer risks than surgical placement. Because they require no

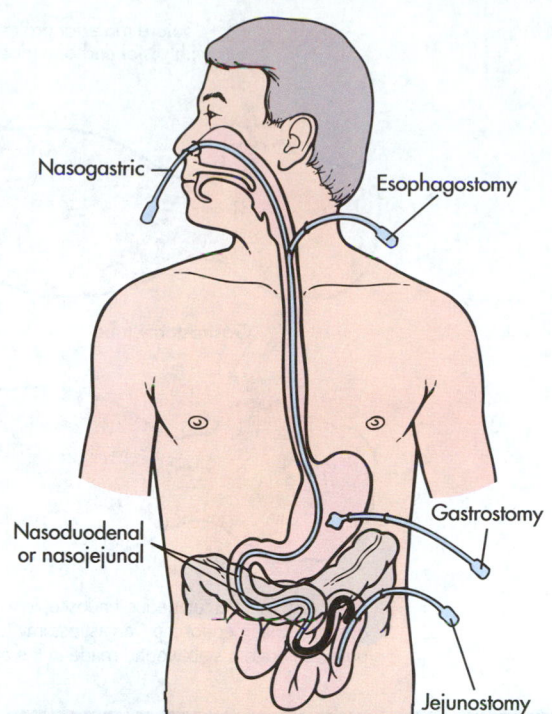

FIG. 40-4   Common enteral feeding tube placement locations.

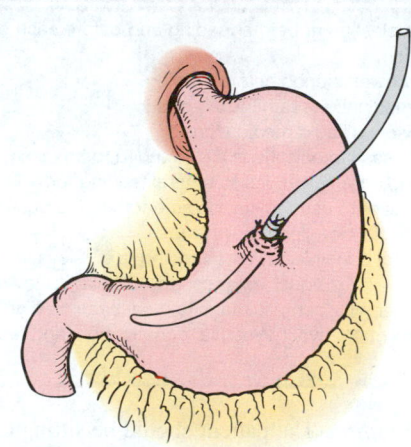

FIG. 40-5   Placement of a gastrostomy tube.

general anesthesia and only minimum or no sedation of the patient, these techniques can be done at a lower cost.

Gastrostomy tube feedings can usually be started when bowel sounds are present, usually within 24 hours after tube placement. Immediately after tube insertion, the tube length from the insertion site to the distal end should be measured and recorded. The tube is then marked at the skin insertion site, although many tubes are premarked. At regular intervals the tube insertion length should be rechecked. The tube is most often connected to a pump for continuous feeding. Water may be infused within 2 hours after placement.

For the patient with chronic reflux, a jejunostomy tube with continuous feedings may be necessary to reduce risk of aspiration.[17] Some important nursing implications for care and feeding of patients with tube feedings are listed in Table 40-16.

Procedures for Tube Feedings. The procedure for the administration of tube feeding through an enteral feeding tube should be outlined in a standard protocol. The following principles apply.

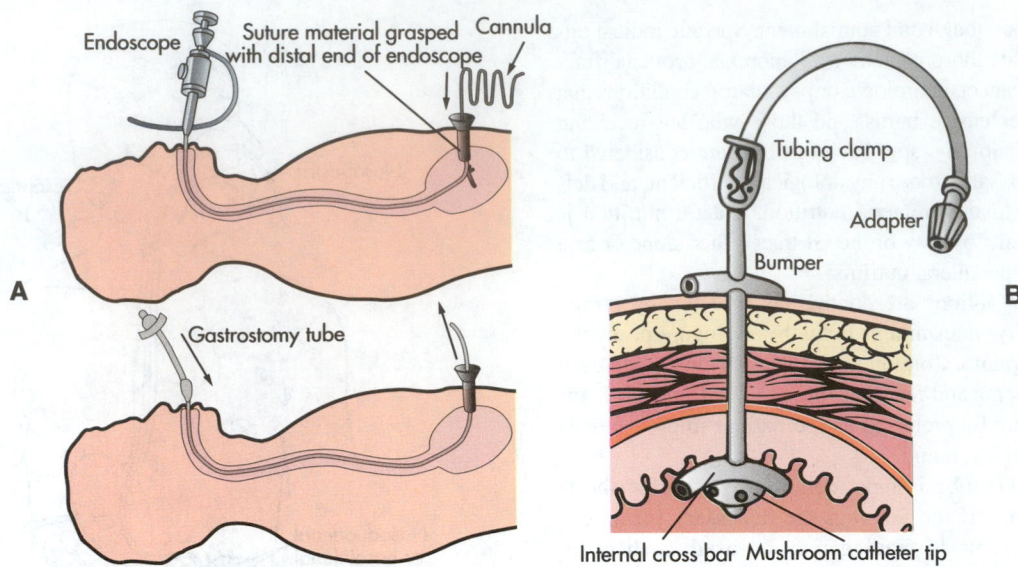

FIG. 40-6 Percutaneous endoscopic gastrostomy. **A,** Gastrostomy tube placement via percutaneous endoscopy. Using endoscopy, a gastrostomy tube is inserted through the esophagus into the stomach and then pulled through a stab wound made in the abdominal wall. **B,** A retention disk and bumper secure the tube.

TABLE 40-16	Nursing Management: Feeding Tubes

1. Check tube placement before feeding and before each drug administration.
2. Assess for bowel sounds before feeding.
3. Use liquid medications rather than pills.
   - Dilute viscous liquid medications.
   - Check to see if medications are intended to be taken with meals.
   - Avoid adding medications to enteral feeding formula.
4. If it is necessary to use tablets, be sure to crush drugs to a fine powder to avoid clogging feeding tubes.
5. Follow general principles of tube feeding (e.g., elevating head of bed, checking for residual volumes, and flushing tube with water).
6. Assess regularly for complications (e.g., aspiration, diarrhea, abdominal distention, hyperglycemia, constipation, and fecal impaction).

1. *Patient position.* The patient should be sitting or lying with the head of the bed elevated 30 to 45 degrees to prevent aspiration. If intermittent delivery is used, the head should remain elevated for 30 to 60 minutes after feeding.
2. *Patency of tube.* If feedings are intermittent, the tube should be irrigated with water before and after each feeding to ensure tube patency. If the feedings are continuous, they should be administered by a feeding pump with a built-in alarm that will sound if the tube becomes occluded. If no pump is available, the feedings require frequent monitoring of the drip rate so that blockage does not occur from the patient lying on the tubing inadvertently or from too slow a drip rate.
3. *Tube position.* Proper placement of the tube is checked before each feeding or every 8 hours with continuous feedings. Methods used to check for tube placement can include aspiration of stomach contents and checking the pH of contents using a pH meter or pH paper. The smaller feeding tubes may be passed directly into the bronchus on insertion or may become dislodged and slip into the bronchus without any obvious respiratory manifestations. This is more likely to occur in a patient with decreased cough or gag reflex. Because gastric contents are primarily acidic, as opposed to

the more alkaline environment of the small intestine and lungs, a pH value less than 5 on aspirated contents is indicative of the stomach. The most accurate assessment for correct tube placement is by x-ray visualization.

Checking gastric residual volumes is important when feedings are administered into the stomach. For example, when the infusion rate is 100 ml/hr, the total infused volume of 400 ml may accumulate when gastric emptying is delayed. In addition, gastric secretions can increase the volume beyond 400 ml. With increased residual volume there is increased risk for aspiration of formula into the pulmonary tract.

4. *Formula.* In the home setting, blenderized foods from a normal diet may be used as tube feedings, although this is rare. Commercial formulas are preferable over blenderized foods for small-lumen tubes because of the lower risk of tube clogging, completeness of nutrition, and decreased risk of formula contamination.

The feeding should be given at room or body temperature to decrease the likelihood of diarrhea and other GI complaints. The pleasurable aspects of eating, such as smelling, seeing, tasting, and chewing the food, are frequently denied the tube-fed patient. If the clinical condition permits, the patient may be allowed to smell, taste, and even chew small amounts of food before the feeding, and then the chewed food must be spit out. Before initiating the feeding, the nurse should aspirate gastric contents and measure the amount. If the volume is greater than 200 ml and there are clinical signs of intolerance, including nausea or increase in abdominal girth, the next feeding is held for 1 hour and then the residual volume is rechecked. The aspirate should be reinstilled.[17]

5. *Administration of feeding.* Feedings are administered either by gravity drip method or by feeding pump. Applying pressure to force the feeding can damage the tube. The feeding rate or volume is increased gradually for 24 to 48 hours to minimize side effects, such as nausea or diarrhea. If intermittent feedings are ordered, the volume is usually 200 to 500 ml/feeding. It is important to remember that the patient

still needs water, and this may be administered with flush water or as additional boluses of water as tolerated.

6. *General nursing considerations.* The patient should be weighed daily or several times a week, and accurate intake and output records should be maintained. Initially blood glucose checks to assess glucose tolerance are performed at the bedside. An older patient who has baseline glucose intolerance is particularly at risk for hyperglycemia. Feedings that have been opened and not refrigerated or feedings that have been infusing longer than 8 hours should be discarded to prevent the administration of possible contaminated feedings. Feedings should be labeled with the date and time they are initially used. If a pump is used, pump tubing should be changed every 24 hours or per manufacturer's guidelines. See NCP 40-1 for care of the patient receiving enteral nutrition.

Complications Related to Tubes and Feedings. The types of problems encountered in patients receiving tube feedings and corrective measures are presented in Table 40-17. When commercial products are used, the concentration, flavor, osmolarity, and amounts of protein, sodium, and fat vary according to the manufacturer. Most commercial formulas are lactose free. The concentrations range from 1 to 2 kcal/ml, with most between 1 and 1.5 kcal/ml.

The osmolality of the solution is determined by the number and size of particles in solution. With regard to feeding formulas, the more hydrolyzed or broken down the nutrients, the greater the osmolality. The more calorically dense the formula, the less water it contains. Protein content greater than 16% can lead to dehydration unless the patient is given supplemental fluids or is sufficiently alert to request additional fluids. The nurse must be aware of this potential problem and provide extra fluids through the feeding tube or, if permitted, by mouth. Tube feedings with high sodium content are contraindicated in the patient with cardiovascular problems, such as heart failure. High fat content is not advocated for a patient with short bowel syndrome or ileocecal resections because of impaired fat absorption.

With regard to enteral nutrition (and nutrition in general), the dietitian is an important health care team member. Some institutions have nutrition support teams composed of a physician, nurse, dietitian, and pharmacist whose function is to oversee the nutrition

NURSING CARE PLAN 40-1

Patient Receiving Enteral Nutrition

NURSING DIAGNOSIS **Imbalanced nutrition: less than body requirements** *related to* inability to ingest food due to physiologic or psychologic factors *as evidenced by* body weight at least 20% less than ideal, pale conjunctival and mucous membranes, poor muscle tone

PATIENT GOAL Achieves adequate nutritional status

OUTCOMES (NOC)	INTERVENTIONS (NIC) and *RATIONALES*
Nutritional Status	*Nutrition Therapy*
• Nutrient intake ____	• Determine—in collaboration with the dietitian—the number of calories and type of nutrients needed to meet nutrition requirements.
• Weight/height ratio ____	• Determine need for enteral tube feedings.
• Hematocrit ____	• Administer enteral feedings.
• Muscle tone ____	
• Food intake ____	*Enteral Tube Feeding*
• Hydration ____	• Monitor weight three times a week initially, decreasing to once a month, *to make adjustments as needed in calorie intake.*
Measurement Scale	• Monitor for presence of bowel sounds every 4-8 hr *to ensure presence of GI function.*
1 = Severe deviation from normal range	• Slow tube feeding rate and/or decrease strength *to control diarrhea.*
2 = Substantial deviation from normal range	• Keep open containers of enteral feeding refrigerated *to prevent bacterial growth.*
3 = Moderate deviation from normal range	• Discard enteral feeding containers and administration sets every 24 hr *because they can become contaminated over time.*
4 = Mild deviation from normal range	
5 = No deviation from normal range	

NURSING DIAGNOSIS **Risk for aspiration** *related to* enteral tube and tube feedings

PATIENT GOAL Experiences no aspiration

OUTCOMES (NOC)	INTERVENTIONS (NIC) and *RATIONALES*
Aspiration Prevention	*Enteral Tube Feeding*
• Positions self upright for eating/drinking ____	• Check for residual every 4 to 6 hours for the first 24 hr, then every 8 hr during continuous feedings, *to validate gastric emptying.*
• Identifies risk factors ____	• Hold tube feedings if residual is greater than 200 ml or more than 110% to 120% of the hourly rate.
• Avoids risk factors ____	• Elevate head of the bed 30 to 45 degrees during feedings *to prevent aspiration.*
Measurement Scale	• Monitor for sensation of fullness, nausea, and vomiting *because these are signs of gastric retention.*
1 = Never demonstrated	• Discontinue feedings 30 to 60 min before putting patient in a head-down position *to prevent aspiration.*
2 = Rarely demonstrated	
3 = Sometimes demonstrated	
4 = Often demonstrated	
5 = Consistently demonstrated	

Continued

NURSING CARE PLAN 40-1

Patient Receiving Enteral Nutrition—cont'd

NURSING DIAGNOSIS **Risk for deficient fluid volume** *related to* diarrhea or inadequate fluid intake

PATIENT GOAL Maintains adequate fluid volume

OUTCOMES (NOC)	INTERVENTIONS (NIC) and *RATIONALES*
Fluid Balance • Blood pressure ____ • Radial pulse rate ____ • 24-hr intake and output balance ____ • Skin turgor ____ • Moist mucous membranes ____ • Serum electrolytes ____ **Measurement Scale** 1 = Severely compromised 2 = Substantially compromised 3 = Moderately compromised 4 = Mildly compromised 5 = Not compromised	**Hypovolemia Management** • Observe for indications of dehydration (e.g., poor skin turgor, delayed capillary refill, weak/thready pulse, severe thirst, dry mucous membranes, decreased urine output, and hypotension) *to identify signs of fluid volume deficit.* **Diarrhea Management** • Identify factors (e.g., medications, bacteria, tube feedings) that may cause or contribute to diarrhea. **Enteral Tube Feeding** • Check gravity drip rate or pump rate every hour *to maintain adequate fluid intake.* • Slow tube feeding rate and/or decrease strength *to control diarrhea.* • Irrigate the tube every 4-6 hr as appropriate during continuous feedings and after every intermittent feeding *to provide free water.*

TABLE 40-17	Common Problems of Patients Receiving Tube Feedings

Problems and Possible Causes	Corrective Measures
Vomiting and/or Aspiration	
Improper placement of tube	Replace tube in proper position. Check tube position before beginning feeding and every 8 hr if continuous feedings.
Delayed gastric emptying, increased residual volume	Hold feeding 1 hr; then if residual volume is less than previous rate, resume feeding.
Potential for aspiration	Keep head of bed elevated to 30- to 45-degree angle. Have patient sit up on side of bed or in chair. Encourage ambulation unless contraindicated.
Contamination of formula	Refrigerate unused formula and record date opened. Discard outdated formula every 24 hr. Discard formula left standing for longer than manufacturer's guidelines: 8-12 hr for ready-to-feed formulas (cans) or 4 hr for reconstituted formula. Use closed system to prevent contamination.
Diarrhea	
Feeding too fast	Decrease rate of feeding. Change to continuous drip feedings.
Medications	Check for drugs that may cause diarrhea (e.g., antibiotics).
Contamination of formula or tubing	Change tubing every 24 hr. Hang 8 hr of formula at a time. Do not exceed manufacturer's guidelines.
Low-fiber formula	Change to formula with more fiber.
Tube moving distally	Properly secure tube before beginning feeding. Check before each feeding or at least every 24 hr if continuous feedings.
Constipation	
Formula components	Consult health care provider for change in formula to one with more fiber content. Obtain laxative order.
Poor fluid intake	Increase fluid intake if not contraindicated. Give free water, as well as formula. Give total fluid intake of 30 ml/kg body weight.
Drugs	Check for drugs that may be constipating.
Impaction	Perform rectal examinations to check and manually remove feces if present.
Dehydration	
Excessive diarrhea, vomiting	Decrease rate or change formula. Check drugs that patient is receiving, especially antibiotics. Take care to prevent bacterial contamination of formula and equipment.
Poor fluid intake	Increase intake and check amount and number of feedings. Increase amount of intake if appropriate.
High-protein formula	Change formula.
Hyperosmotic diuresis	Check blood glucose levels frequently. Change formula.

support of select inpatients and outpatients. The nutrition support nurse on that team is a key resource for issues regarding patients' nutrition.[18]

In patients receiving gastrostomy or jejunostomy feeding, the nurse should be alert to two possible problems: (1) skin irritation and (2) pulling out of the tube. Skin care around the tube site is important because the action of the digestive juices is irritating to the skin. The skin around the feeding tube should be assessed daily

for signs of redness and maceration. To keep the skin clean and dry, initially it should be rinsed with sterile water and dried. Once the site has healed, it can be washed with mild soap and water. A protective ointment (zinc oxide, petroleum gauze) or a skin barrier (Karaya, Stomahesive) may be used on the skin around the tube. A small dressing may be placed around the tube until the site is healed and must be changed promptly if it gets wet. Other types of drain or tube pouches may be used if there is a problem with skin irritation, and an enterostomal therapist can be of great assistance to the nurse if these issues arise. The patient and family members can be taught how to care for the feeding tube. Accidental tube removal by the patient or caregiver can result in delayed feedings, as well as potential discomfort with tube replacement. Teaching should include skin care, care of the tube, and complete information about feeding administration and potential complications.[19]

GERONTOLOGIC CONSIDERATIONS
ENTERAL NUTRITION

Enteral nutrition strategies, including NG, nasointestinal, and gastrostomy feedings, are often used in the older patient to improve nutritional status. Because of physiologic changes associated with aging, the older adult is more vulnerable to complications associated with these interventions, especially fluid and electrolyte imbalances. Complications such as diarrhea can leave the patient dehydrated. Decreased thirst perception or impaired cognitive function decreases the ability of the patient to seek additional fluids.

With aging there is decreased ability to handle glucose loads (glucose intolerance). As a result, the older patient may be more susceptible to problems of hyperglycemia in response to the high carbohydrate load of some enteral feeding formulas. If the older adult has compromised cardiovascular function (e.g., heart failure), there will be a decreased ability to handle large volumes of formula. In this situation the use of more concentrated formulas may be warranted. The older adult also is at increased risk for aspiration caused by gastroesophageal reflux disease (GERD), hiatal hernia, or diminished gag reflex. Physical mobility, fine motor movement, and visual system changes associated with aging may contribute to difficulties in managing enteral nutrition equipment at home. In addition, age-related changes such as a decrease in lean muscle mass influence the reliability of measures used for nutritional assessment.

Parenteral Nutrition

When the GI tract cannot be used for the ingestion, digestion, and absorption of essential nutrients, parenteral nutrition may be substituted. **Parenteral nutrition** (PN) refers to the administration of nutrients by a route other than the GI tract (e.g., the bloodstream). **Central parenteral nutrition** is the delivery of a nutritionally adequate hypertonic solution consisting of glucose, crystalline amino acids, fat emulsion, minerals, and vitamins using a central venous route. PN has become a relatively safe and practical method of delivering complete nutritional needs. The goal of using PN is to meet the patient's nutritional needs and to allow growth of new body tissue. Regular IV solutions of 5% dextrose (5 g dextrose/100 ml) in water (D_5W) or 5% dextrose in lactated Ringer's solution (D_5LR) contain no protein and have approximately 170 cal/L. The normal adult requires a minimum of 1200 to 1500 cal/day to carry out normal physiologic functions. Patients who sustain severe injury, surgery, or burns and those who are malnourished as a result of medical treatment or disease processes have greatly increased nutritional needs. The volume of regular dextrose solutions needed to meet these high caloric requirements could exceed the capacity of the cardiovascular system. Table 40-18 lists common indications for the use of PN.

Composition. Commercially prepared PN base solutions are available for both central and peripheral use. These base solutions contain dextrose and protein in the form of amino acids. The pharmacy adds the prescribed electrolytes (e.g., sodium, potassium, chloride, calcium, magnesium, and phosphate), vitamins, and trace

TABLE 40-18	Common Indications for Parenteral Nutrition

- Chronic severe diarrhea and vomiting
- Complicated surgery or trauma
- Gastrointestinal obstruction
- Gastrointestinal tract anomalies and fistulae
- Intractable diarrhea
- Severe anorexia nervosa
- Severe malabsorption
- Short bowel syndrome

elements (e.g., zinc, copper, chromium, and manganese) to customize the solution for the patient. A three-in-one or total nutrient admixture containing an IV fat emulsion, dextrose, and amino acids is widely used.

Calories. Calories in PN are supplied primarily by carbohydrates in the form of dextrose and by fat in the form of fat emulsion. The administration of between 100 and 150 g of dextrose (1 g provides approximately 3.4 calories, as opposed to oral carbohydrates, which provide 4 calories) daily has a protein-sparing effect. Adequate nonprotein calories in the form of glucose and fat must be provided to allow metabolism of amino acids for wound healing and not as energy. However, overfeeding can lead to metabolic complications. To minimize these problems, an energy intake of 25 to 30 cal/kg/day in a nonobese patient is often recommended. The FDA has approved the use of 10%, 20%, and 30% fat-emulsion solutions. Fat emulsions provide approximately 1 cal/ml (10% solution) or 2 cal/ml (20% solution). The contents of fat emulsion are primarily soybean or safflower triglycerides with egg phospholipids added as an emulsifier. The maximum fat-emulsion amount should not exceed a dose of 2.5 g/kg/day,[20] and it should be administered slowly over 12 to 24 hours. Critically ill patients may not tolerate this dose and close monitoring of triglyceride levels may be indicated. Nausea, vomiting, and elevated temperature have been reported, especially when lipids are infused quickly. The administration of fat emulsion is contraindicated in the patient with a disturbance in fat metabolism. It should also be used with caution in the patient who is in danger of fat embolism (e.g., fractured femur) and the patient with an allergy to eggs.

Protein. The normal healthy person of average body size needs approximately 45 to 65 g of protein daily. Protein should be provided at the rate of 1 to 1.5 g/kg/day depending on the patient's needs. In a nutritionally depleted patient under the stress of illness or surgery, requirements can exceed 150 g/day to ensure a positive nitrogen balance. In the most recent guidelines, protein intake levels of 1.5 to 2 g/kg/day are suggested for most patients with moderate to severe stress.[4]

Electrolytes. The assessment of individual requirements should take place daily at the beginning of therapy and then several times a week as the treatment progresses. The following are ranges for average daily electrolyte requirements for adult patients without renal or hepatic impairment:[20]

- Sodium: 1 to 2 mEq/kg
- Potassium: 1 to 2 mEq/kg
- Chloride: as needed to maintain acid-base balance
- Magnesium: 8 to 20 mEq
- Calcium: 10 to 15 mEq
- Phosphate: 20 to 40 mmol

The exact amount needed depends on the patient's health problem and on electrolyte levels as determined by blood testing.

Trace Elements. Zinc, copper, chromium, manganese, selenium, molybdenum, and iodine supplements may be added according to the patient's condition and needs. Levels of these elements are monitored in the patient receiving PN. The health care provider may order additional amounts of these elements to be added to the solutions according to the patient's requirements.

Vitamins. The daily addition of a multivitamin preparation to the PN generally meets the vitamin requirements. If multivitamin infusion is used, the cobalamin (vitamin B_{12}) requirement may be met without the need for supplemental preparations.

Methods of Administration.
PN may be administered by central or peripheral veins. Central parenteral nutrition is given through a catheter whose tip lies in the superior vena cava. The central venous catheter often originates at the subclavian or jugular vein. More recently, single- or double-lumen peripherally inserted central catheters (PICCs) are being placed, usually into the basilic or cephalic vein and then advanced into the central circulation. Such catheters are made of soft, flexible material (silicon, polymer) and are 20 to 24 inches long. Ease of placement, cost, and limited complications make this an attractive alternative to a subclavian vein catheter.[21] Central PN is indicated when long-term parenteral support is necessary or when the patient has high protein and caloric requirements.

Peripheral parenteral nutrition (PPN) is administered through a peripherally inserted catheter or vascular access device, which uses a large peripheral vein. PPN is used when (1) nutritional support is needed for only a short time, (2) protein and caloric requirements are not high, (3) the risk of a central catheter is too great, or (4) parenteral nutrition is used to supplement inadequate oral intake. Both central and peripheral parenteral nutrition are used in a patient who is not a candidate for enteral support.

Central and peripheral parenteral nutrition differ in tonicity, which is measured in milliosmoles (mOsm; the concentration of particles in a fluid). Blood is isotonic and measures approximately 280 mOsm/L. The standard IV solutions of D_5W and normal saline are essentially isotonic. Central PN solutions are hypertonic, measuring at least 1600 mOsm/L. The high glucose content ranges from 20% to 50%. Central PN must be infused in a large central vein so that rapid dilution can occur. The use of a peripheral vein for central PN would cause irritation and thrombophlebitis. Nutrients can be infused using smaller volumes than PPN. PPN is hypertonic (using as much as 20% glucose), but less so than central PN, and can be safely administered through a large peripheral vein, although phlebitis can occur. Another potential complication of PPN is fluid overload.

All PN solutions should be prepared by a pharmacist or a trained technician using strict aseptic techniques under a laminar flow hood. Nothing should be added to parenteral nutrition solutions after they are prepared in the pharmacy. The danger of drug incompatibilities and contamination is high.[22] The fewer the personnel involved in the preparation and administration of PN, the lower the risk of infection for the patient. In most hospitals the health care provider must order the PN solution daily. In this way the solution and additives can be adjusted to the patient's current needs. Each PN solution label indicates the nutrient content, all additives, the time mixed, and the date and time of expiration. In general, solutions are good for 24 hours and must be refrigerated until a half hour before use.

Catheter Placement.
The central placement of the catheter into a large main vein for PN is performed by the physician or a specially trained advanced practice nurse. The vein most commonly used is the subclavian, although the innominate or the jugu-

lar vein may be used. The procedure is the same as for the insertion of a central venous pressure line and should be done under strict aseptic conditions.

A standard isotonic IV solution is infused through the central line until x-ray confirms proper placement of the catheter tip in the superior vena cava and not in the jugular vein. The catheter insertion site is covered with a sterile dressing. The date is marked on the dressing.

Placement of a PICC is done under sterile conditions, often by a specially trained nurse. A baseline measurement of the upper arm circumference is recommended. A tourniquet is then placed around the upper arm near the axilla to allow examination of the antecubital fossa and selection of a vein. If possible, the patient should be supine with the arm straight and at a 90-degree angle. Preparation of the insertion site should be done according to institutional policy. The sterile catheter is cut to the predetermined length, depending on the vein selected.

A local anesthetic is usually used at the insertion site. This site should be cleaned, protected, and maintained according to institutional policy. As with the centrally placed line, a chest x-ray is needed to verify proper tip placement before administering any PN solution. Proper placement of a catheter for central PN is illustrated in Fig. 40-7. Complications frequently associated with catheter placement are hemorrhage, hydrothorax and pneumothorax, hemothorax, air embolus, and venous thrombosis. Once established for PN, a single-lumen central catheter should not be used for the administration of blood or antibiotics, the drawing of blood samples, or the monitoring of central venous pressure.

Administration of Solution.
Because PN solutions are excellent media for microbial growth, it is essential that proper aseptic techniques be followed. The FDA recommends that a 0.22-micron Millipore filter be placed on parenteral solutions not containing fat emulsion and a 1.2-micron filter be placed on solutions containing fat emulsion.[20] Filters and IV tubing are changed every 24 hours if PN with lipids is being administered and every 72 hours for PN with amino acids and dextrose. The tubing and the filter should be clearly labeled with the date and the time they are put into use. Complications of PN can be divided into three catego-

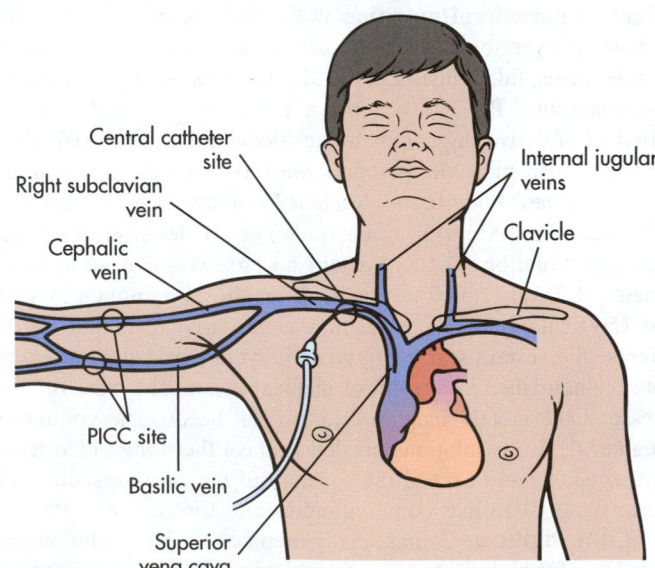

FIG. 40-7 Placement of a catheter for parenteral nutrition using subclavian vein. Peripherally inserted central catheters (PICCs) are inserted using the basilic or cephalic vein.

TABLE 40-19	Complications of Parenteral Nutrition

Infection
Fungus
Gram-positive bacteria
Gram-negative bacteria

Metabolic Problems
Hyperglycemia; hypoglycemia; and hyperosmolar, hyperglycemic state
Prerenal azotemia
Essential fatty acid deficiency
Electrolyte and vitamin excesses and deficiencies
Trace mineral deficiencies
Hyperlipidemia

Mechanical Problems
Insertion
- Air embolus
- Pneumothorax, hemothorax, chylothorax, and hydrothorax
- Hemorrhage
Dislodgement
Thrombosis of great vein
Phlebitis

ries: (1) infection, (2) metabolic, and (3) mechanical. The major complications of each category are presented in Table 40-19.

To control the rate of infusion, peripheral PN solutions should be administered with a volumetric controller while a pump is used for central PN solutions. If a PN formula bag should empty before the next solution is available, a 10% or 20% dextrose solution (based on the amount of dextrose in the central PN solution) or 5% dextrose solution (based on the amount of dextrose in the peripheral PN solution) may be administered to prevent hypoglycemia.

NURSING MANAGEMENT
PARENTERAL NUTRITION

Initially vital signs should be monitored every 4 to 8 hours in the patient receiving PN. Daily weights give an indication of the patient's hydration status as therapy progresses. Body weight is considered the sum of the changes in protein, fat, and water. On a daily basis, body water fluctuates more than protein or fat. Analysis must be made of whether gains or losses in weight are caused by fluid gained from edema, fluid lost through diuresis, or actual increase or decrease in tissue weight. Blood levels of glucose, electrolytes, and urea nitrogen; a complete blood count; and hepatic enzyme studies are followed a minimum of three times per week until stable and then weekly as the patient's condition warrants. Assessment of these important values assists the nurse in evaluating the patient's tolerance of PN. A nursing care plan for the patient receiving PN is presented on p. 968.

Dressings covering the catheter site are changed according to institutional protocol, ranging from every other day to once a week. The procedure for changing the dressing is similar to that followed after catheter insertion. The site is carefully observed for signs of inflammation and infection. Phlebitis can readily occur in the vein as a result of the hypertonic infusion, and the area can become infected. The patient receiving parenteral nutrition may be immunosuppressed and thus more susceptible to opportunistic infections. In this patient, signs of inflammation or infection can be subtle, if present at all. Some patients receiving PN may also be receiving chemotherapy, corticosteroids, or antibiotics, which can mask signs of infection.

If an infection is suspected during dressing change, a culture specimen of the site and drainage should be sent for analysis, and the health care provider should be notified immediately.

Hyperglycemia is a metabolic complication of parenteral nutrition. Initially blood glucose levels should be checked at the bedside every 4 to 6 hours with a glucose-testing meter (see Chapter 49). Some increase in the blood glucose level is expected during the first few days after PN is started. In general, the dextrose dose of PN should not be increased until the blood glucose concentrations are consistently less than 180 mg/dl. A sliding scale dose of insulin may be ordered to keep the glucose level in normal range.

Refeeding syndrome is characterized by fluid retention; electrolyte imbalances, including hypophosphatemia, hypokalemia, and hypomagnesemia; and hyperglycemia.[23] Conditions that predispose patients to refeeding syndrome include long-standing malnutrition states such as chronic alcoholism, vomiting and diarrhea, chemotherapy, and major surgery. Hypophosphatemia is the hallmark of refeeding syndrome and is associated with serious outcomes, including cardiac dysrhythmias, respiratory arrest, and neurologic disturbances (e.g., paresthesias).[23]

An infusion pump must be used during administration of PN so that the infusion rate can be maintained, and an alarm will sound if the tubing becomes obstructed. Even though an infusion pump is being used, the nurse should periodically check the volume infused because pump malfunctions can alter the rate.

Before setting up and administering PN, the nurse must check the label and ingredients in the solution to see that they are what the health care provider ordered. Solutions must also be examined for leaks, color changes, particulate matter, clarity, and fat emulsion cracking. If any of these abnormalities is suspected, the solution should be returned promptly to the pharmacy for replacement. It is the nurse's responsibility to ensure that the PN solution is discontinued and replaced with a new solution if the bag is not empty at the end of 24 hours. At room temperature, the solution, especially solutions containing fat emulsions, is a medium for microorganism growth.

Sometimes fat emulsions are infused separately from the parenteral nutrition solution. The preferred delivery method is a continuous low volume, such as 20% lipids delivered over 12 hours, depending on patient needs. Adverse reactions that can occur are allergic manifestations, dyspnea, cyanosis, fever, flushing, phlebitis, chest and back pain, and pain at the IV site. A major benefit derived from IV fat administration is that a large number of calories can be provided in a relatively small amount of fluid. This is especially beneficial when the patient is at risk for fluid overload.

Catheter-related infection and septicemia can occur in patients receiving PN through both peripherally and centrally placed lines. Local manifestations of infection include erythema, tenderness, and exudate at the catheter insertion site. Systemically the patient may have fever, chills, nausea, vomiting, and malaise. If no other causes can be identified, a catheter-related infection is suspected. Because of the risk of infection, catheters with antibiotic or antiseptic surfaces may be used. To diagnose the presence of infection and to determine the causative organism, cultures are performed of the catheter tip if the catheter has been removed or of the blood in the catheter if still in place. Blood cultures are drawn simultaneously from the catheter and a peripheral vein. A chest x-ray is taken to detect changes in pulmonary status. When the catheter tip of a short-term catheter is the source of infection, antibiotic therapy may not be necessary because removal of the catheter can eliminate the problem.[24] More permanent catheter-related infections may require anti-

NURSING CARE PLAN 40-2

Patient Receiving Parenteral Nutrition

NURSING DIAGNOSIS **Risk for infection** *related to* placement of a central venous catheter, administration of fluids that support rapid bacterial growth, and decreased defense mechanisms

PATIENT GOAL Experiences no manifestations of infection

OUTCOMES (NOC)	INTERVENTIONS (NIC) and *RATIONALES*
Infection Severity	***Infection Control***
• Fever _____	• Maintain an optimal aseptic environment during bedside insertion of central lines *to minimize the possibility of infection.*
• Malaise _____	• Maintain an aseptic environment while changing PN tubing and bags *to minimize the possibility of infection.*
• Blood culture colonization _____	• Change peripheral IV and central line sites and dressings according to current CDC guidelines *to prevent infection.*
• Wound site culture colonization _____	• Wash hands before and after each patient care activity *to minimize possibility of infection.*
• WBC count elevation _____	• Encourage rest *so that nutrition is used for healing purposes.*
Measurement Scale	***Infection Protection***
1 = Severe	• Monitor for systemic and localized signs and symptoms of infection *to ensure early detection of infection.*
2 = Substantial	• Monitor absolute granulocyte count, WBC count, and differential results *to ensure early detection of infection.*
3 = Moderate	
4 = Mild	
5 = None	

COLLABORATIVE PROBLEMS

NURSING GOALS	NURSING INTERVENTIONS and *RATIONALES*
Potential Complications	**Hyperglycemia, hypoglycemia, and electrolyte imbalances**
• Monitor blood glucose and serum electrolytes.	• Monitor for signs of hyperglycemia such as thirst, polyuria, confusion, elevated blood glucose, blurred vision, dizziness, nausea and vomiting, and dehydration *to plan appropriate treatment.*
• Report deviations from acceptable parameters.	• Monitor for signs of hypoglycemia such as sweating, hunger, weakness, and tremors *to ensure early intervention.*
• Carry out appropriate medical and nursing interventions.	• Monitor serum electrolyte levels daily *to identify and treat complications early.*
	• Check for symptoms of hyperkalemia (e.g., muscle weakness, flaccid paralysis, cardiac dysrhythmias, abdominal cramps, diarrhea) and hypokalemia (e.g., general weakness, decreased muscle tone, weak or irregular pulse, low BP, shallow respirations, abdominal distention, and ileus).*
	• Maintain accurate infusion rate to control the amount of glucose administered and prevent fluctuations in blood glucose levels.

CDC, Centers for Disease Control and Prevention; *IV,* intravenous; *PN,* parenteral nutrition; *WBC,* white blood cell.
*Other manifestations of electrolyte imbalances are discussed in Chapter 17.

biotics. A new central line may or may not be immediately placed depending on the clinical circumstances. When the PN therapy is completed and the catheter is removed, the dressing should be changed daily until the wound heals. Oral nourishment should be encouraged, and a careful record of intake should be maintained.

■ Home Nutrition Support

Home parenteral or enteral nutrition is an accepted mode of nutritional therapy for the person who does not require hospitalization but who requires continued nutrition support. Some patients have been successfully treated at home for many months and even years. It is important for the nurse to educate the patient or the family about catheter or tube care, proper technique in mixing and handling of the solutions and tubing, and side effects.

Home nutrition therapies are expensive. For patients to be reimbursed for expenses, there are specific criteria that must be met. The nurse should have the discharge planning personnel involved early in the admission to help plan for such issues. Home nutrition support

may also be a burden on the patient and caregivers and may affect quality of life. The nurse should make the family aware of support groups such as the OLEY Foundation (see Resources at end of chapter for information) who provide peer support and advocacy.[4]

EATING DISORDERS

Eating disorders are primarily psychiatric disorders. However, a number of nutritional problems associated with these disorders require the nurse to implement a nutritional plan of care. According to the American Dietetic Association, over 5 million Americans suffer from eating disorders. They primarily affect young women. It is estimated that 6% of those with severe eating disorders will die, and only 50% report being cured.[25]

Anorexia Nervosa

Anorexia nervosa is characterized by a self-imposed weight loss, endocrine dysfunction, and a distorted psychopathologic attitude toward weight and eating.[26] Anorexia nervosa clinically manifests

CULTURAL AND ETHNIC HEALTH DISPARITIES
Anorexia and Bulimia

- Anorexia nervosa is most common among women from middle and upper-middle classes.
- Anorexia nervosa and bulimia have a higher incidence among whites than African Americans and Asian Americans.

as abnormal weight loss, deliberate self-starvation, intense fear of gaining weight, *lanugo* (soft, downy hair covering the body except the palms and soles), refusal to eat, continuous dieting, hair loss, sensitivity to cold, compulsive exercise, absent or irregular menstruation, dry skin, and constipation. Diagnostic studies often show iron deficiency anemia and an elevated blood urea nitrogen level that is reflective of marked intravascular volume depletion and prerenal azotemia. Lack of potassium in the diet and loss of potassium in the urine lead to potassium deficiency. Manifestations of potassium deficiency include muscle weakness, cardiac dysrhythmias, and renal failure. If the eating pattern is permitted to continue for a prolonged time, body wasting and signs of severe malnutrition are evident.

Multidisciplinary treatment must involve a combination of nutritional support and psychiatric care.[27] Hospitalization may be necessary if there are severe physical complications that cannot be managed in an outpatient therapy program. Nutritional replenishment must be closely supervised to ensure consistent and ongoing weight gains. The use of tube or parenteral feedings may be necessary. Voluntary nasogastric tube feeding in inpatient settings has been shown to be effective for weight gain.[28] Improved nutrition, however, is not a cure for anorexia nervosa. The underlying psychiatric problem must be addressed by identification of the disturbed patterns of individual and family interactions, followed by individual and family counseling.

Bulimia Nervosa

Bulimia nervosa is a disorder characterized by frequent binge eating and self-induced vomiting associated with loss of control related to eating and a persistent concern with body image.[29] These individuals may have normal weight for height, or their weight may fluctuate with bingeing and purging. They may also abuse laxatives, diuretics, exercise, or diet drugs. They may have signs of frequent vomiting, such as macerated knuckles, swollen salivary glands, broken blood vessels in the eyes, and dental problems.

Bulimia is increasing in incidence and may be even more prevalent than anorexia nervosa. Female college students seem to be most susceptible to this syndrome. The cause remains unclear but is thought to be similar to that of anorexia nervosa. Substance abuse, anxiety, affective disorders, and personality disturbances have been reported among persons with bulimia.

The patient with bulimia, similar to the one with anorexia nervosa, goes to great lengths to conceal abnormal eating habits. As the behavior persists, many problems associated with the condition become increasingly hard to deal with effectively. As with anorexia, a treatment combination of psychologic counseling and diet therapy is essential. Education and emotional support for the patient and family are vital. Support groups such as the National Association of Anorexia Nervosa and Associated Disorders (see Resources for information) are extremely helpful to those affected by these disorders.

CRITICAL THINKING EXERCISE
CASE STUDY

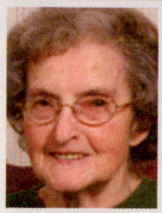

Case Study photo ©iStockphoto.com/ Stan Rohrer.

Undernutrition
Patient Profile. Mrs. Mary Smith is a 70-year-old white woman who is 5 feet 4 inches tall and weighs 100 pounds. She was recently admitted to the medical unit.
Subjective Data
- Reports 30-pound weight loss during past 2 months
- Has recently had a thrombotic stroke with hemiparesis and dysphagia
- Has had nothing by mouth for the past 24 hours and just started tube feedings
- Lives with her daughter, who is at her bedside

Objective Data
Physical Examination
- Has left-sided weakness
- BP is 150/90 mm Hg
- A PEG tube was recently placed

Laboratory Results
- Serum albumin 2.9 g/dl
- Prealbumin 11.0 mg/dl

Critical Thinking Questions

1. What are Mrs. Smith's risk factors for malnutrition?
2. What is her BMI?
3. What are contributing factors to her developing dysphagia and malnutrition?
4. What should the nurse include in a successful weight gain program for Mrs. Smith?
5. What possible complications of tube feeding could Mrs. Smith be at risk for?
6. What is the priority of the nursing care for Mrs. Smith?
7. Based on the assessment data presented, write one or more appropriate nursing diagnoses. Are there any collaborative problems?

NCLEX EXAMINATION REVIEW QUESTIONS

The number of the question corresponds to the same-numbered objective at the beginning of the chapter.

1. The nurse identifies a need for dietary teaching for the patient whose daily intake of food groups consists of
   a. 2 to 4 servings of the fruit group.
   b. 3 cups of the milk, yogurt, and cheese group.
   c. 4 ounces of the bread, cereal, rice, and pasta group.
   d. 5 ounces of the meat, poultry, fish, beans, egg, and nut group.
2. In general, nutrient or food interactions with drugs can result in all of the following except
   a. enhancing drug absorption.
   b. decreasing drug bioavailability.
   c. increasing a nutrient requirement.
   d. all of the above options can happen.
3. During the first 24 hours of starvation, the order in which the body obtains substrate for energy is
   a. glycogen, skeletal protein.
   b. visceral protein, fat stores, glycogen.
   c. fat stores, skeletal protein, visceral protein.
   d. liver protein, muscle protein, visceral protein.

Gastrointestinal System

4. An elderly patient with a recent stroke is exhibiting signs of severe dysphagia. The optimal form of nutrition support at this time would be
   a. regular diet.
   b. parenteral nutrition.
   c. nasoenteric tube feedings.
   d. nothing by mouth (NPO) until dysphagia resolves.

5. One advantage of a percutaneous endoscopic gastrostomy (PEG) tube placement relative to NG feedings for the patient receiving long-term enteral nutrition is that
   a. it increases patient comfort.
   b. it eliminates the risk of aspiration.
   c. feedings can be initiated before bowel sounds are present.
   d. more calories can be delivered compared with NG feeding.

6. A nutritionally stressed patient weighing 60 kg is NPO and receiving central PN. In evaluating the patient's nutritional intake, the nurse calculates that the daily central PN solution should provide
   a. 40 g fat.
   b. 80 g protein.
   c. 20 calories per kilogram.
   d. 2000 calories from carbohydrate.

7. The nurse recognizes that the major goal of treatment for a patient with anorexia nervosa is being met when the patient
   a. demonstrates a rapid weight gain.
   b. consumes the required daily intake of nutrients.
   c. commits to long-term individual and family counseling.
   d. verbalizes feelings regarding self-image and fears of becoming obese.

REFERENCES

1. Payette H, Shatenstein B: Determinants of healthy eating in community-dwelling elderly people, *Can J Public Health* 96:S27, 2005.
2. National Research Council: *Dietary Reference Intakes for energy, carbohydrate, fiber, fatty acids, cholesterol, protein, and amino acids,* Washington, DC, 2002, National Academy of Sciences.
3. Dietary guidelines for Americans 2005. In *Healthy people 2010.* Office of disease prevention and health promotion. US Department of Health and Human Services. Available at *www.healthypeople.gov* (accessed July 21, 2006).
4. ASPEN Board of Directors: Guidelines for the use of parenteral and enteral nutrition in adult and pediatric patients, *J Parenter Enteral Nutr* 26(suppl 1):1SA, 2002.
5. Sabol VK: Nutrition assessment of the critically ill adult, *AACN Clin Issues* 15:595, 2004.
6. Nutrition Screening Initiative: Nutrition statement of principle, 2002. Available at *www.eatright.org/Public/Files/nutrition(1).pdf* (accessed July 21, 2006).
7. Wilmore DW: *The metabolic management of the critically ill,* New York, 1977, Plenum Publishing.
8. Institute of Medicine, Food, and Nutrition Board: *Dietary Reference Intakes: vitamins and elements,* Washington, DC, 2004, National Academy Press. Available at *www.nap.edu.*
9. American Dietetic Association: ADA's definition for nutrition screening and assessment, *J Am Diet Assoc* 94:838, 1994.
10. Project of the American Academy of Family Physicians, the American Dietetic Association, and National Council on Aging: *Nutrition interventions manual for professional caring for older Americans,* Washington, DC, 1994, Nutrition Screening Initiative.
*11. Kovacevich DS, Boney AR, Braunschweig CL, et al: Nutrition risk classification: a reproducible and valid tool for nurses, *Nutr Clin Pract* 12:20, 1997.
*12. Salva A, Corman B, Andrieu S, et al: Minimum data set for nutritional intervention studies in elderly people, *J Gerontol A Biol Sci Med Sci* 59:722, 2004.
13. Hamwi GJ: Changing dietary concepts. In Danowski TS, editor: *Diabetes mellitus: diagnosis and treatment,* vol 1, New York, 1964, American Diabetes Association.
14. DiMaria-Ghalili RA, Amelia E: Nutrition in older adults, *Am J Nurs* 105:40, 2005.

*15. Arnaud-Battandier F, Malvy D, Jeandel C, et al: Use of oral supplements in malnourished elderly patients living in the community: a pharmacoeconomic study, *Clin Nutr* 23:1096, 2004.
16. Cottrell DB, Aturi E: Gastric intubation: assessment and intervention, *Crit Care Nurs Clin North Am* 16:480, 2004.
17. Guenter P: Tube feeding administration. In Guenter P, Silkroski M, editors: *Tube feeding: practical guidelines and nursing protocols,* Gaithersburg, Md, 2001, Aspen.
18. Metheny NA, Schallom ME, Edwards SJ: Effect of gastrointestinal motility and feeding tube site on aspiration risk in critically ill patients: a review, *Heart Lung* 33:131, 2004.
19. Guenter P, Curtas S, Murphy L, et al: The impact of nursing practice on the history and effectiveness of total parenteral nutrition, *J Parenter Enteral Nutr* 28:54, 2004.
20. Guenter P: Nursing care of patients with enteral feeding devices. In Guenter P, Silkroski M, editors: *Tube feeding: practical guidelines and nursing protocols,* Gaithersburg, Md, 2001, Aspen.
21. Task Force for the Revision of Safe Practices for Parenteral Nutrition: safe practices for parenteral nutrition, *J Parenter Enteral Nutr* 28:S38, 2004.
22. Penney-Timmons E, Sevedge S: Outcome data for peripherally inserted central catheters used in an acute care setting, *J Infus Nurs* 27:431, 2004.
23. Mirtallo JM: Complications associated with drug and nutrient interactions, *J Infus Nurs* 27:19, 2004.
24. Worthington P, Reyen L: Administration and management of parenteral nutrition. In Worthington P, editor: *Practical aspects of nutritional support: an advanced practice guide,* Philadelphia, 2004, Saunders.
25. Krzywda EA, Andris DA, Edmiston CE: Catheter infections: diagnosis, etiology, treatment, and prevention, *Nutr Clin Pract* 14:178, 1999.
26. American Dietetic Association: Position of the ADA: nutrition intervention in the treatment of anorexia nervosa, bulimia nervosa, and eating disorders not otherwise specified, *J Am Diet Assoc* 101:810, 2001.
27. Muse DM, Lucas AR: Behavioral disorders affecting food intake: anorexia nervosa, bulimia nervosa and other psychiatric conditions. In Shils ME, Ross CA, Caballero B, et al, editors: *Modern nutrition in health and disease,* ed 10, Baltimore, 2005, Lippincott Williams & Wilkins.
28. Cartwright MM: Eating disorder emergencies: understanding the medical complexities of the hospitalized eating disordered patient, *Crit Care Nurs North Am* 16:515, 2004.
29. Zuercher JN, Cumella EJ, Woods BK, et al: Efficacy of voluntary nasogastric tube feeding in female inpatients with anorexia nervosa, *J Parenter Enteral Nutr* 27:268, 2003.

RESOURCES

Academy for Eating Disorders
   847-498-4274
   www.aedweb.org
American Dietetic Association
   800-877-1600
   www.eatright.org
American Society for Parenteral and Enteral Nutrition
   301-587-6315
   www.nutritioncare.org
FDA Center for Food Safety and Applied Nutrition (CFSAN)
   888-463-6332
   www.cfsan.fda.gov
Institute of Medicine, Food and Nutrition Board
   888-624-8373
   www.nap.edu
National Association of Anorexia Nervosa and Associated Disorders (ANAD)
   847-831-3438
   www.anad.org
National Eating Disorder Information Centre
   866-NEDIC-20 or 416-340-4156
   www.nedic.ca
National Eating Disorders Association
   206-382-3587
   Helpline: 800-931-2237
   www.nationaleatingdisorders.org
OLEY Foundation
   800-776-OLEY or 518-262-5079
   www.oley.org
For additional Internet resources, see the website for this book at *http://evolve.elsevier.com/Lewis/medsurg.*

*Nursing research–based reference.

Yesterday is gone. Tomorrow has not yet come. We have only today. Let us begin.

Mother Teresa

Nursing Management
Obesity

41

Jennifer Kretzschmar, Paula Blackwell, Sharon L. Lewis

LEARNING OBJECTIVES

1. Discuss the etiologies and collaborative care of obesity.
2. Describe the classification systems for determining a person's body size.
3. Explain the health risks associated with obesity.
4. Discuss nutritional therapy and exercise plans for the obese patient.
5. Describe the different bariatric surgical procedures used to treat obesity.
6. Describe the nursing management related to conservative and surgical therapies for obesity.
7. Describe the etiology, clinical manifestations, and nursing and collaborative management of metabolic syndrome.

KEY TERMS

bariatric surgery, p. 982
body mass index, p. 974
lipectomy, p. 984
metabolic syndrome, p. 987
morbidly obese, p. 974
obese, p. 974
overweight, p. 974
waist-to-hip ratio, p. 974

Electronic Resources

Supplemental content related to Chapter 41 can be found . . .

Companion CD
- Stress-Busting Kit for Nursing Students
- Interactive Case Study: Obese Patient
- NCLEX Examination Review Questions
- Comprehensive Glossary

Evolve Website *evolve*
http://evolve.elsevier.com/Lewis/medsurg
- Content Updates
- Key Points (Printable and CD/MP3 Download)
- Concept Map Creator
- Expanded Audio Glossary
- Key Term Flash Cards

- Table: Nutritional Therapy: 1200-Calorie-Restricted Weight-Reduction Diet
- Electronic Calculators
- WebLinks

OBESITY

Obesity is an abnormal increase in the proportion of fat cells. Weight gain during adulthood is characterized predominantly by adipocyte hypertrophy, a process by which adipocytes can increase their volume several thousand–fold to accommodate large increases in lipid storage. This primarily occurs in the visceral (intraabdominal) and subcutaneous tissues of the body (Fig. 41-1).

Overweight and obesity result from a complex interaction between genes and the environment. An imbalance between energy expenditure and energy intake from a long-term sedentary lifestyle and/or excessive calorie intake causes an individual to become overweight or obese. In developed and developing countries, obesity has reached epidemic proportions. In the United States, obesity is the most common nutritional problem, affecting almost one third of the population. The Centers for Disease Control and Prevention (CDC) reports that 65% of Americans over age 20 are either overweight or obese. The percentage of young people who are overweight has tripled since 1980. Among children and teens ages 6 to 19 years, 16% are considered overweight and 31% are considered at risk for being overweight.[1] Obesity occurs at higher rates in certain racial/ethnic groups than in whites (Fig. 41-2 and Cultural and Ethnic Health Disparities box).

The U.S. Surgeon General has identified obesity as a major health problem with detrimental health care problems. The goal of *Healthy People 2010* is to reduce the prevalence of obesity to 15%. Obesity is the second leading cause of preventable deaths after smoking. Obesity is also the third leading reason for liver transplantation.[2] Obesity is a societal problem as much as a complex medical concern, due to adverse health conditions related to weight gain and the associated expenses for health care. It is esti-

Reviewed by Judi Daniels, PhD, ARNP-BC, Assistant Professor, College of Nursing, University of Kentucky, Lexington, Ky.; and Colleen Keller, RN, PhD, ANCC, Family Nurse Practitioner, Professor and Director, Center of Healthy Outcomes in Aging, Arizona State University, Phoenix, Ariz.

mated that costs related to obesity are greater than $75 billion to $78 billion dollars per year,[3] and obesity accounts for greater than 9% of all medical expenses nationally.[1]

Etiology and Pathophysiology

In one sense the etiology of obesity can be considered simplistically. It occurs because energy intake exceeds energy output. However, the processes leading to obesity are much more complex and still undergoing investigation. The cause of obesity involves significant genetic/biologic susceptibility factors that are highly influenced by environmental and psychosocial factors. Once obesity is present, caloric consumption (energy intake) must exceed the energy expended for the condition to continue.

Genetic/Biologic Basis. There is strong evidence that there is a genetic predisposition to obesity. Studies of twins, adoptees, and families all suggest the existence of genetic factors in obesity. The heritability of obesity estimated from twin studies is high, with only slightly lower values in twins raised apart than in those

raised together. Estimates of obesity as an inherited problem are over 50%.[4,5] Similarly, in adoptees the body mass index (BMI) of the children correlates with their biologic parents rather than that of their adoptive parents.[6]

The most common form of obesity is considered to be polygenic arising from the interaction of multiple genetic and environmental factors. Identifying these genes will contribute to a better understanding of the pathogenesis of obesity. This could potentially lead to the development of strategies for the prevention and management of obesity.

Regulation of eating behavior, energy metabolism, and body fat metabolism is controlled by signals from the periphery that act on the hypothalamus (Fig. 41-3). Appetite is influenced by many factors that are integrated by the brain, most importantly within the hypothalamus. Input to the hypothalamus is received from the periphery from many different hormones and peptides (Table 41-1). Obesity is associated with increased circulating plasma levels of leptin, insulin, and ghrelin, and decreased levels of peptide YY.[7,8] Interaction of these hormones and peptides at the level of the hypothalamus may be an important determinant in factors contributing to obesity.

Adipocytes secrete a number of hormones and cytokines known as *adipokines*. Visceral fat accumulation results in alterations of these adipokines, thus contributing to causes and complications of obesity.[9] Some of these adipokines include the following:

* *Adiponectin* regulates lipid and glucose levels. It is antiinflammatory, antidiabetic, and antiatherogenic. High levels

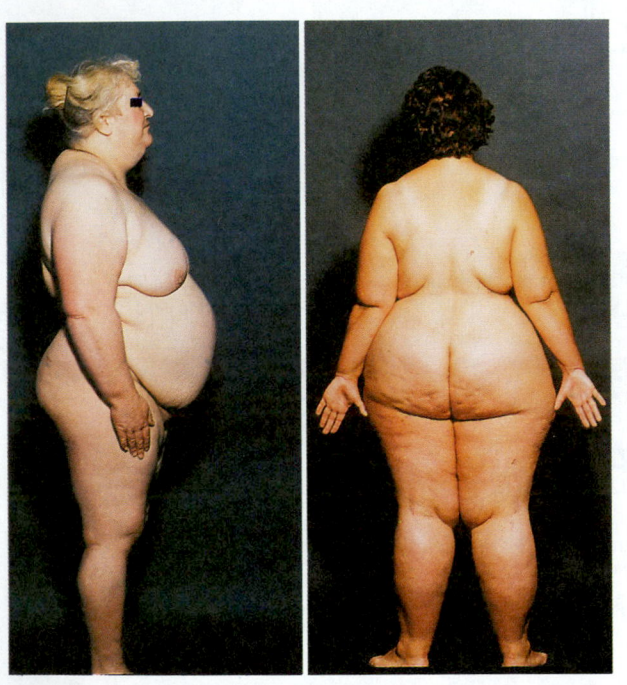

FIG. 41-1   Obese women. **A,** This woman has excessive fat deposits in her abdominal area, upper arms, and breasts. **B,** This woman has excessive fat deposits in her upper arms, buttocks, and thighs. The fat distribution in both of these women is common in obese people.

CULTURAL AND ETHNIC HEALTH DISPARITIES
Obesity

* Among women, African American women have the highest prevalence of being overweight and obese
* Among men, Mexican American men have the highest prevalence of being overweight and obese
* African American and Hispanic women with low incomes appear to have the greatest likelihood of being overweight when compared with other socioeconomic groups
* Native Americans have a higher prevalence of being overweight compared with the general population
* Among Native Americans ages 45 to 74, over 30% of women are overweight and over 40% are obese
* Asian Americans have the lowest prevalence of being overweight and obese compared with the general population

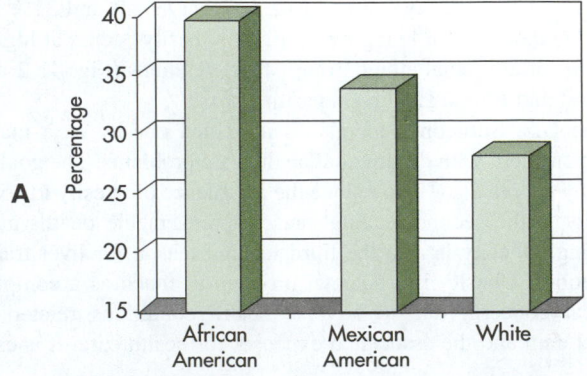

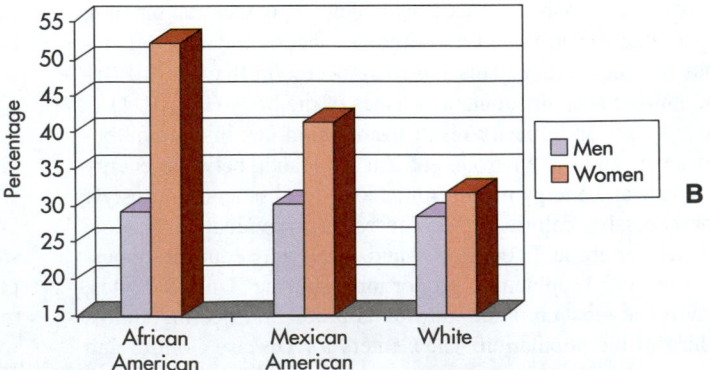

FIG. 41-2   Comparison of the percentage of obesity among different ethnic groups **(A)** and different ethnic groups based on gender **(B).**

prevent myocardial infarctions. Low levels are found in obese people.

- *Resistin* promotes insulin resistance and increases blood glucose. It is increased in obesity.

Environmental Factors. Environmental factors play an important role in obesity. In today's culture there is greater access to food, particularly prepackaged and fast foods, as well as soft drinks, which have poor nutritional quality. Portion size of meals has also increased (see Table 41-8 later in this chapter). Obese individuals tend to underestimate food and caloric intake. Eating outside of the home also restricts the ability to control the composition and quality of food.

Lack of physical exercise is another factor that contributes to weight gain and obesity. There is a reduction in physical activity,

HEALTHY PEOPLE

Health Impact of Maintaining a Healthy Weight

- Reduces the risk of developing type 2 diabetes
- Increases chance of longevity and better quality of life
- Lowers the risk of hypertension and elevated cholesterol
- Reduces the risk of heart disease, stroke, and gallbladder disease
- Reduces the likelihood of breathing problems, including sleep apnea and asthma
- Decreases the risk of developing osteoarthritis, low back pain, and certain types of cancers

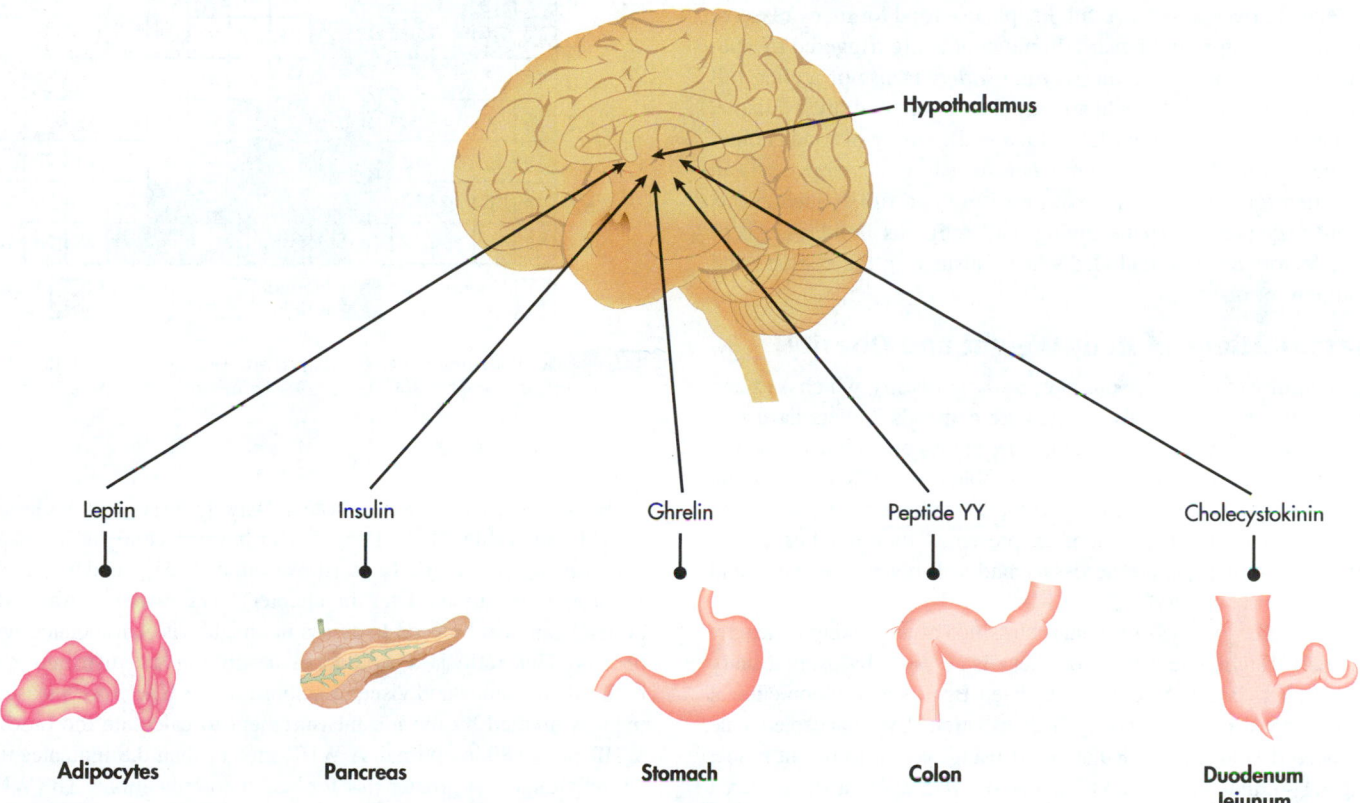

FIG. 41-3   Some of the common hormones and peptides that interact with the hypothalamus to control and influence eating patterns, metabolic activities, and digestion. Obesity causes a disruption in this balance (see Table 41-1).

TABLE 41-1   Hormones and Peptides in Obesity

Hormone/Peptide	Where Produced	Normal Function	Alteration in Obesity
Leptin	Adipocytes	Suppresses appetite and hunger Regulates eating behavior	Obesity is associated with high levels; leptin resistance develops, thus obese people may lose the effect of appetite suppression
Insulin	Pancreas	Decreases appetite	Frequently have high circulating levels
Ghrelin	Stomach (primarily)	Stimulates appetite ↑ After food deprivation ↓ In response to the presence of food in the stomach	Normal postprandial decline does not occur, which can lead to increased appetite and overeating
Peptide YY	Descending colon and rectum	Inhibits appetite by slowing GI motility and gastric emptying	Circulating levels are decreased; decreased release after eating
Cholecystokinin	Duodenum Jejunum	Inhibits gastric emptying and sends satiety signals to hypothalamus	Unknown role

GI, Gastrointestinal.

both in the workplace and at home. With increases in technology and labor-saving devices, Americans are expending less energy in their everyday lives. Elimination of physical education programs in elementary and secondary schools and increased time spent playing video games and watching TV have contributed to the increase in sedentary habits.

Socioeconomic status can affect obesity in a variety of indirect ways. People with low incomes may buy food that is less expensive, but the food may have poor nutritional quality and have greater caloric content. For example, people with low incomes are more likely to purchase pasta than fresh fish. Low-income residents may be more likely to live in environments that do not accommodate outdoor activities (e.g., tennis, swimming pools).[10] Gyms tend to be attended by more affluent individuals.

Psychosocial Factors. The emotional component of the tendency to overeat is powerful. People use food for many reasons, including comfort and reward. Some people are triggered by specific foods to continue eating beyond *satiety* (sense of feeling full after eating), especially when many flavors of food are available, such as in casseroles or buffets with a wide variety of food choices to select from. The social component of eating develops early in life when food is associated with pleasure and fun at such events as birthday parties, Thanksgiving, and religious holidays. All of these factors must be included when considering the etiology and treatment of obesity.

Classifications of Body Weight and Obesity

The majority of obese persons have *primary obesity,* which is excess calorie intake for the body's metabolic demands. Others have *secondary obesity,* which can result from various congenital anomalies, chromosomal anomalies, metabolic problems, or CNS lesions and disorders. The first step in the treatment of obesity is to determine whether any physical conditions are present. A thorough history and physical examination are necessary and will reveal the extent and duration of the obesity.

The degree to which a patient is classified as underweight, healthy (normal) weight, overweight, or obese is assessed by using a **body mass index** (BMI) chart. The calculated BMI is a common clinical index of obesity or altered body fat distribution. A well-accepted scale has been developed to calculate BMI using weight-to-height ratios[1] (Fig. 41-4). Individuals with a BMI below 18.5 kg/m² are considered underweight. Individuals with a BMI between 18.5 and 24.9 kg/m² are considered to be normal weight. Individuals with a BMI of 25 to 29.9 kg/m² are classified as being **overweight,** those with values of 30 kg/m² or more are classified as **obese**, and those with a BMI of more than 40 kg/m² are classified as **morbidly obese.**

Approximately 13% of Americans have a BMI greater than 35.[1] Table 41-2 shows the classification of overweight and obesity by BMI. Obesity is not the same as being overweight. Obesity carries many more risk factors and is a chronic condition with a strong familial element. For persons with a BMI of 30 kg/m² or greater, mortality rates from all causes, and especially from cardiovascular disease, are generally increased by 50% to 100% above those of persons with BMIs in the normal range. Over 4 million Americans are morbidly obese, with a BMI of at least 40 kg/m².[11] Men are more frequently overweight than women. However, current statistics provided by the National Health and Nutrition Examination Survey (NHANES) show that among obese individuals, women are more likely to have a BMI over 35 kg/m.[2] The 2004 NHANES reported that the prevalence of men over age 20 with a BMI $\geq$ 40 kg/m² was 3.3%; women were twice as likely to be morbidly obese at 6.4%.[1]

$$\text{BMI} = \left\{\frac{\text{WEIGHT (pounds)}}{\text{HEIGHT (inches)}^2}\right\} \times 703$$

Weight in Pounds

Height in Feet and Inches	120	130	140	150	160	170	180	190	200	210	220	230	240	250
4′6	29	31	34	36	39	41	43	46	48	51	53	56	58	60
4′8	27	29	31	34	36	38	40	43	45	47	49	52	54	56
4′10	25	27	29	31	34	36	38	40	42	44	46	48	50	52
5′0	23	25	27	29	31	33	35	37	39	41	43	45	47	49
5′2	22	24	26	27	29	31	33	35	37	38	40	42	44	46
5′4	21	22	24	26	28	29	31	33	34	36	38	40	41	43
5′6	19	21	23	24	26	27	29	31	32	34	36	37	39	40
5′8	18	20	21	23	24	26	27	29	30	32	34	35	37	38
5′10	17	19	20	22	23	24	26	27	29	30	32	33	35	36
6′0	16	18	19	20	22	23	24	26	27	28	30	31	33	34
6′2	15	17	18	19	21	22	23	24	26	27	28	30	31	32
6′4	15	16	17	18	20	21	22	23	24	26	27	28	29	30
6′6	14	15	16	17	19	20	21	22	23	24	25	27	28	29
6′8	13	14	15	17	18	19	20	21	22	23	24	25	26	28

Underweight · Normal weight · Overweight · Obese

FIG. 41-4 Body mass index (BMI) chart. Healthy weight: BMI 18 to 24.9 kg/m²; overweight: BMI 25 to 29.9 kg/m²; obesity: BMI $\geq$30 kg/m². BMI = weight (kg)/height (m²).

Waist circumference is another way to assess and classify weight (see Table 41-2). People who have visceral fat are especially at increased risk for cardiovascular disease and metabolic syndrome (discussed later in chapter). The **waist-to-hip ratio** (WHR) can also be used to assess the health risks associated with obesity. This ratio is a method of describing the distribution of both subcutaneous and visceral adipose tissue. The waist measurement is divided by the hip measurement to calculate the ratio. A WHR of $<$0.80 is optimal. A WHR greater than 0.8 indicates that an individual is at greater risk for health complications. The WHR is a preferred tool to measure for overweight and obesity when the patient is predominantly muscular.

Another way to classify obesity is by body shape or fat distribution. Individuals with fat located primarily in the abdominal area (apple-shaped body) are at a greater risk for obesity-related complications than those whose fat is primarily located in the upper legs (pear-shaped body) (Table 41-3 and Fig. 41-5). Individuals whose fat is distributed over the abdomen and upper body (neck, arms, and shoulders) are classified as having *android obesity. Gynoid obesity* is a term used to classify persons who are pear shaped. Genetics play an important role in determining body fat distribution patterns.

Gynoid obesity carries a better prognosis but is more difficult to treat. It is believed that abdominal fat is more readily available and can be mobilized to maintain elevated triglyceride and lipid levels. Individuals with abdominal fat carry more visceral fat than that of the person with a pear shape. Pear-shaped individuals carry more subcutaneous fat, which causes more cellulite to appear. Abdominal and visceral fat have been linked to metabolic syndrome, a major complication of obesity. Visceral fat is more active, causing the body harm by decreasing insulin sensitivity and levels of high-density li-

TABLE 41-2	**Classification of Overweight and Obesity by BMI, Waist Circumference, and Associated Disease Risk***			

			Disease Risk Based on Waist Circumference*	
	BMI (kg/m²)	**Obesity Class**	**Men ≤40 in (102 cm)** **Women ≤35 in (88 cm)**	**Men >40 in (102 cm)** **Women >35 in (88 cm)**
Underweight	<18.5		—	—
Normal†	18.5-24.9		—	—
Overweight	25.0-29.9		Increased	High
Obese	30.0-34.9	Class I	High	Very high
	35.0-39.9	Class II	Very high	Very high
Morbid obesity	≥40.0	Class III	Extremely high	Extremely high

Source: National Heart, Lung, and Blood Institute, North American Association for the Study of Obesity: *The practical guide: identification, evaluation, and treatment of overweight and obesity in adults,* Publication No. 00-4084, 2000, US Department of Health and Human Services.
BMI, Body mass index.
*Disease risk for type 2 diabetes, hypertension, and cardiovascular disease relative to person of normal weight.
†Increased waist circumference can also be a marker for increased risk in persons of normal weight.

TABLE 41-3	**Relationship Between Body Shape and Health Risks**

Gynoid (Pear)	**Android (Apple)**
Health risks	Health risks
• Osteoporosis	• Heart disease
• Varicose veins	• Diabetes mellitus
• Cellulite	• Breast cancer
• Subcutaneous fat traps and stores dietary fat	• Endometrial cancer
• Trapped fatty acids are stored as triglycerides	Visceral fat is more active, causing
	• ↓ insulin sensitivity
	• ↑ triglycerides
	• ↓ HDL cholesterol
	• ↑ BP
	• ↑ free fatty acid release into blood

HDL, High-density lipoprotein.

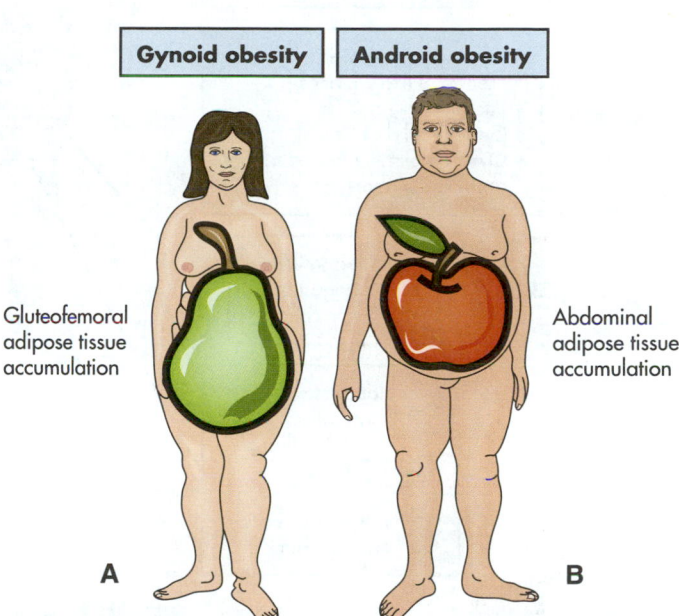

FIG. 41-5   Two general classifications used to classify people by body fat distribution are **(A)** pear shape and **(B)** apple shape. Health risks are associated with each classification (see Table 41-3).

poprotein (HDL) cholesterol and increasing BP. Visceral fat also releases more free fatty acids into the bloodstream.

Health Risks Associated with Obesity

Hippocrates wrote that "corpulence is not only a disease itself, but the harbinger of others," thus recognizing that obesity has major adverse effects on health. Many problems occur in obese people at higher rates than people of normal weight (Fig. 41-6). Mortality rate rises as obesity increases, especially when obesity is associated with visceral fat.[12] In addition to these problems, obese patients have a reduced quality of life.[13] Fortunately, most of these conditions can improve if an individual loses weight.

Cardiovascular Problems. Obesity is a significant risk factor for predicting cardiovascular disease in both men and women. The waist-to-hip ratio is the best predictor of these risks. Obesity, especially android obesity, is associated with increased low-density lipoproteins (LDLs) and triglycerides and decreased high-density lipoproteins (HDLs). Obesity is also associated with hypertension. Hypertension can occur because of increased circulating blood volume, abnormal vasoconstriction, decreased vascular relaxation, and increased cardiac output. Measurement of BP requires the use of a larger cuff size to avoid artifactual increases.

Respiratory Problems. Severe obesity may be associated with sleep apnea and obesity hypoventilation syndrome. Patients also have reduced chest wall compliance, increased work of breathing, and decreased total lung capacity and functional resid-

ual capacity. Weight loss can bring substantial improvement in lung function.

Diabetes Mellitus. Hyperinsulinemia and insulin resistance are common features of obesity. Insulin resistance is more strongly related to visceral fat than to fat in other locations. Obesity is a major risk factor for type 2 diabetes. As many as 80% of patients with type 2 diabetes are obese. Weight loss and exercise are associated with improved glucose control in diabetes.

Musculoskeletal Problems. Obesity is associated with an increased incidence of osteoarthritis, probably because of the trauma to the weight-bearing joints. Hyperuricemia and gout are often found in people who are obese and in those who have metabolic syndrome (discussed later in this chapter).

Gastrointestinal and Liver Problems. Gastroesophageal reflux disease (GERD) and gallstones are more prevalent in obese patients. Gallstones occur because of the supersaturation of the bile with cholesterol. Nonalcoholic steatohepatitis (NASH) is more common in obese patients. In NASH lipid is deposited in the liver, resulting in a fatty liver. It is associated with elevated hepatic

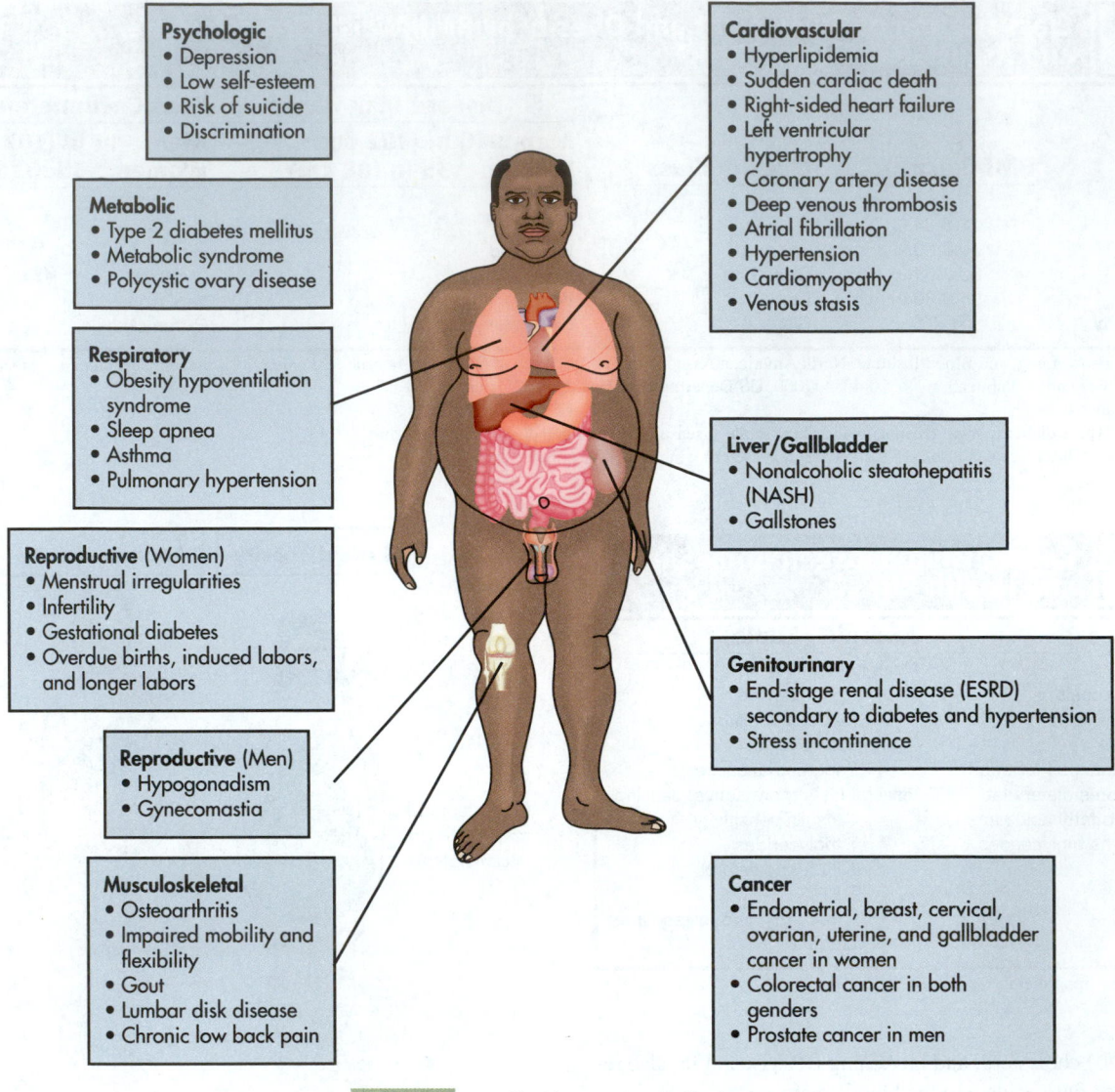

Psychologic
• Depression
• Low self-esteem
• Risk of suicide
• Discrimination

Metabolic
• Type 2 diabetes mellitus
• Metabolic syndrome
• Polycystic ovary disease

Respiratory
• Obesity hypoventilation
  syndrome
• Sleep apnea
• Asthma
• Pulmonary hypertension

Reproductive (Women)
• Menstrual irregularities
• Infertility
• Gestational diabetes
• Overdue births, induced labors,
  and longer labors

Reproductive (Men)
• Hypogonadism
• Gynecomastia

Musculoskeletal
• Osteoarthritis
• Impaired mobility and
  flexibility
• Gout
• Lumbar disk disease
• Chronic low back pain

Cardiovascular
• Hyperlipidemia
• Sudden cardiac death
• Right-sided heart failure
• Left ventricular
  hypertrophy
• Coronary artery disease
• Deep venous thrombosis
• Atrial fibrillation
• Hypertension
• Cardiomyopathy
• Venous stasis

Liver/Gallbladder
• Nonalcoholic steatohepatitis
  (NASH)
• Gallstones

Genitourinary
• End-stage renal disease (ESRD)
  secondary to diabetes and hypertension
• Stress incontinence

Cancer
• Endometrial, breast, cervical,
  ovarian, uterine, and gallbladder
  cancer in women
• Colorectal cancer in both
  genders
• Prostate cancer in men

FIG. 41-6   Health risks associated with obesity.

glucose production. NASH can eventually progress to cirrhosis and can be fatal. Weight loss can improve NASH.

Cancer. Obesity is one of the most important known preventable causes of cancer. The underlying mechanisms are difficult to determine. The risk of breast, endometrial, ovarian, and cervical cancer is increased in obese women. This may be due to the increased estrogen levels (estrogen is stored in fat cells) associated with obesity in postmenopausal women. Colorectal cancer has been linked to hyperinsulinemia. Waist circumference and WHR, indicators of abdominal obesity, are associated with colon cancer risk in both men and women. Obese men have higher mortality rates with cancer of the prostate.

NURSING *and* CONSERVATIVE COLLABORATIVE MANAGEMENT
OBESE PATIENT

■ *Nursing Assessment*

Information that can assist the nurse in understanding an obese patient and provide a basis for intervention is presented in Table 41-4. By being sensitive when asking specific and leading ques-

tions, the nurse can often obtain information that the patient may withhold out of embarrassment or shyness. The nurse must provide acceptable reasons for such personally intrusive questions, respond to the patient's concerns about diagnostic tests, and interpret test outcomes. The patient's answers to questions must be treated with respect, understanding, and a nonjudgmental attitude.

When assessing patients with obesity, the nurse should consider several different types of questions, such as the following:
• What is their history with weight gain and weight loss?
• Are they interested in losing weight or managing their weight differently?
• What do they think contributes to their weight?
• What sort of barriers do they feel impede their weight loss efforts?
• What does food mean to them? How do they use food (e.g., to relieve stress, provide comfort)?
• Are other family members overweight?
• Are there environmental or genetic factors influencing the weight gain?

The health care provider should explore genetic and endocrine factors such as hypothyroidism, hypothalamic tumors, Cushing

TABLE 41-4	*NURSING ASSESSMENT* **Obese Patient**

Subjective Data
Important Health Information
Past health history: Time of obesity onset; diseases related to metabolism and obesity, such as hypertension, cardiovascular problems, stroke, cancer, chronic joint pain, respiratory problems, diabetes mellitus, cholelithiasis, metabolic syndrome
Medications: Thyroid preparations, use of diet pills, use of herbal products
Surgery or other treatments: Prior weight-reduction procedures (bariatric surgery)

Functional Health Patterns
Health perception–health management: Family history of obesity; perception of problem; methods of weight loss attempted
Nutritional-metabolic: Amount and frequency of eating; overeating in response to boredom, stress, specific times, or activities; history of weight gain and loss
Elimination: Constipation
Activity-exercise: Typical physical activity; drowsiness, somnolence; dyspnea on exertion, orthopnea, paroxysmal nocturnal dyspnea
Sleep-rest: Sleep apnea
Cognitive-perceptual: Feelings of rejection, depression, isolation, guilt, or shame; meaning or value of food; compliance with prescribed reducing diets, degree of long-term commitment to a weight loss program
Role-relationship: Change in financial status or family relationships; personal, social, and financial resources to support a reducing diet
Sexuality-reproductive: Menstrual irregularity, heavy menstrual flow in women, infertility; effect of obesity on sexual activity and attractiveness to significant other

Objective Data
General
Body mass index ≥30 kg/m^2; waist circumference: woman >35 in (88 cm), man >40 in (102 cm)

Respiratory
Increased work of breathing; wheezing; rapid, shallow breathing

Cardiovascular
Hypertension, tachycardia, dysrhythmias

Musculoskeletal
Decreased joint mobility and flexibility; knee, hip, and low back pain

Reproductive
Menstrual irregularities and infertility in women; gynecomastia and hypogonadism in men

Possible Findings
Elevated serum glucose, cholesterol, triglycerides; chest x-ray demonstrating enlarged heart; electrocardiogram showing dysrhythmia; abnormal liver function tests

syndrome, hypogonadism in men, and polycystic ovary disease in women. Laboratory tests of liver function, fasting glucose level, triglyceride level, and LDL and HDL cholesterol levels assist in evaluating the cause and effects of obesity.

As part of the initial nursing history and physical examination, each body system should be examined with particular attention to the organ system in which the patient has expressed a problem or concern. Measurements used with the obese person may include skinfold thickness, height, weight, and BMI. Providing specific documentation on these areas assists the health care provider with a more in-depth history and physical examination.

■ Nursing Diagnoses

Nursing diagnoses for the patient with obesity include, but are not limited to, the following:

- Imbalanced nutrition: more than body requirements *related to* excessive intake in relationship to metabolic needs
- Impaired skin integrity *related to* alterations in nutritional state (obesity), immobility, excess moisture, and multiple skinfolds
- Ineffective breathing pattern *related to* decreased lung expansion from obesity
- Chronic low self-esteem *related to* body size, inability to lose weight, and perceived unattractiveness
- Health-seeking behaviors: practices that reduce the risk of obesity-related health problems

■ Planning

The overall goals are that the obese patient will (1) modify eating patterns, (2) participate in a regular physical activity program, (3) achieve weight loss to a specified level, (4) maintain weight loss at a specified level, and (5) minimize or prevent health problems related to obesity.

■ Nursing Implementation

The nurse, working closely with the other members of the health care team, plays a major role in the planning and management of the obese patient. To be effective, the nurse must be aware of perceptions of and beliefs about obesity. Clear and consistent stigmatization of obese people, and in some cases discrimination, can be documented in three important areas of living: employment, education, and health care.[14] In addition to the negative social impact experienced by many obese persons in the United States, many obese people suffer low self-esteem, withdraw from social interaction, and experience major depression.

In the workplace, obese women experience greater wage disparity from their normal-weight counterparts than men. For obese men and women, fewer are hired into higher-level positions. Although health care for obese people has inherently greater demands, health care providers regularly fail to address these needs, and obese people routinely underutilize health care opportunities available to them. Health care providers are often reluctant to counsel patients about obesity because of the time constraints during appointments, the fact that weight management is professionally unrewarding, and it is difficult to receive reimbursement for weight management services.

If a health care provider associates obesity with lack of willpower and with overindulgence, the patient can experience shame in a setting that claims to be a caring one. Nurses are in a pivotal position to help overweight and obese people deal with negative experiences and to educate other health care professionals to eliminate their bias against overweight patients.

Before selecting a weight loss strategy with the patient, the following questions should be asked:

- What is the patient's motivation for losing weight?
- Are there any major stresses that will make it difficult to focus on weight control?
- Does the patient have any psychiatric illnesses, such as severe depression, substance abuse, or a binge eating disorder, that will derail weight-loss efforts?
- Can the patient devote a minimal amount of time for exercise (e.g., at least 15 to 30 minutes per day for the next 6 months) that is needed for a serious weight-loss effort?

Motivation should be assessed because it is essential for a favorable outcome. Lack of motivation is a huge barrier to change. However, the reasons for wanting to lose weight should be focused on as the patient faces the challenges in dealing with obesity.

When no organic cause (e.g., hypothyroidism) can be found for obesity, it should be considered a chronic, complex illness. Any supervised plan of care should be directed at (1) successful weight loss, requiring a short-term energy deficit, and (2) successful weight control, requiring long-term behavior changes. These are two different processes. A multipronged approach ought to be used with attention to multiple factors, including dietary intake, physical activity, behavior modification, and perhaps drug therapy. Focusing on more than one aspect will likely give better balance to weight-loss and weight-control efforts. All opportunities for patient education should stress healthy eating habits and adequate physical activity as lifestyle patterns to develop and maintain (Table 41-5).

Even with a comprehensive action plan, there is a high rate of weight regain among people in all age-groups. This is discouraging when one considers the amount of time and effort expended in the process of attempting to lose weight. For successful management of obesity, it helps if obesity is viewed as a chronic condition that necessitates day-to-day attention to lose weight and maintain weight loss. It is essential that the nurse have a nonjudgmental approach in helping patients manage their problems related to obesity.

Nutritional Therapy. Restricted food intake is a cornerstone for any weight loss or maintenance program. A good weight loss plan should contain foods from the basic food groups (see Fig. 40-1 and Table 40-1). Diets may be classified as low calorie (800 to 1200 calories per day) or very low calorie (less than 800 calories per day) (Table 41-6).

Persons on low-calorie and very-low-calorie diets need frequent professional monitoring because the severe energy restriction places them at risk for multiple nutrient deficiencies. A diet that includes adequate amounts of fruits and vegetables provides enough bulk to prevent constipation and meets daily vitamin A and vitamin C requirements. Lean meat, fish, and eggs provide sufficient protein, as well as the B-complex vitamins. Restricting dietary intake so that it is below energy requirements is an effective way to reduce body weight. It is rare to find an overweight person who has not at some time attempted to lose weight. Some people

have met with limited and temporary success, and others have met only with failure. It is likely that the majority of these persons attempted weight loss by trying out at least one of the many fad diets that offer the enticement to eat and get slim. Weight reduction diets found in popular media that advocate the elimination of any one category of foods should be discouraged. For example, although eliminating all carbohydrates can lead to weight reduction, it is only because total calories are reduced, and the elimination of carbohydrates reduces the opportunity to get enough foods that provide fiber, vitamins, and minerals.

In general, fad diets claim weight loss quickly, easily, and inexpensively. Although it is true that initially weight is lost, it is not fat but body water that is lost. The normal fat cell is composed of approximately 80% fat, 18% water, and 2% protein. It is also a storage area for small amounts of glycogen. Glycogen is known to bind with water. When reducing diets severely restrict carbohydrates, the body's glycogen stores become depleted within a few days. It is only when the glycogen pool is almost depleted that protein and adipose tissues are burned to release energy for bodily functions. An obese patient must understand that following a well-balanced, low-calorie diet is an essential part of weight loss.

The degree of success of any reducing diet depends in part on the amount of weight to be lost. A moderately obese person will obviously attain the goal more easily than a morbidly obese person.

TABLE 41-5	**COLLABORATIVE CARE** **Obesity**

Diagnostic
History and physical examination
BMI
Waist-to-hip ratio

Collaborative Therapy
Nutritional therapy
Exercise
Behavior modification
Support groups
Drug therapy
- Appetite-suppressing drugs
  - Noradrenergic agents
  - Mixed noradrenergic-serotonergic agents
- Nutrient absorption–blocking drugs
Surgical therapy
- See Table 41-7

BMI, Body mass index.

TABLE 41-6	**NUTRITIONAL THERAPY** **1200-Calorie-Restricted Weight-Reduction Diet***

General Principles
1. Eat regularly. Do not skip meals.
2. Measure foods to determine the correct portion size.
3. Avoid concentrated sweets, such as sugar, candy, honey, pies, cakes, cookies, and regular sodas.
4. Reduce fat intake by baking, broiling, or steaming foods.
5. Maintain a regular exercise program for successful weight loss.

Meal	Exchanges	Menu Plan‡
Breakfast	1 meat	1 hard-boiled egg
	2 bread	1 slice toast
		¾ cup dry cereal (unsweetened)
	1 fruit	½ small banana
	1 fat	1 tsp margarine
	1 dairy†	1 cup low-fat milk
	Beverage	Coffee
Lunch	2 meat	Cheese enchiladas (made with 2 oz
	2 bread	cheese, 2 corn tortillas, lettuce,
	Vegetable	chili sauce)
	1 fruit	Fresh grapes (12)
	Beverage	Diet soda
Dinner	2 meat	2 oz baked chicken
	1 bread	Corn on the cob with 1 tsp margarine
	Vegetable	Tossed salad and 1 tbs salad dressing
	1 fruit	¾ cup strawberries
	1 milk	1 cup low-fat milk

*For 1000 calories, omit 1 fruit exchange and change low-fat milk to skim milk. For 1500 calories, add 1 meat exchange, 1 fruit exchange, and 2 fat exchanges; change low-fat milk to whole milk. For 1800 calories, add 2 bread exchanges, 3 meat exchanges, 3 fat exchanges, and 1 fruit exchange; change low-fat milk to whole milk.
†One extra fat exchange allowed for each cup of 2% low-fat milk; 2 extra fat exchanges allowed for each cup of skim milk.
‡Additional sample meal plans are available on the website at *http://evolve.elsevier.com/Lewis/medsurg*.

TABLE 41-7	Comparison of Fad Diets	
Diet	**Philosophy**	**Diet Composition**
Atkins	Obesity and other health problems caused by eating too many carbohydrates Ketosis leads to decreased hunger	Protein: 27% Carbohydrates: 5% Fat: 68% (saturated fat: 26%)
Zone	Eating the right combination of food makes body's metabolism perform at its best Ideally, every meal and snack would have a ratio of 40% carbohydrates, 30% protein, and 30% fat Once individuals determine the amount of protein they should have (size of palm) at each meal, they determine how much carbohydrates they need (size of fist) and how much fat they need	Protein: 34% Carbohydrates: 36% Fat: 29% (saturated fat: 9%) Alcohol: 1%
South Beach	Much of excess weight comes from highly processed carbohydrates To make up for the overall cut in carbohydrates, diet permits ample fats and animal proteins Diet is in two phases Phase one is the strictest part of the diet, lasting for 2 weeks, and allows protein, monounsaturated fats, and carbohydrates with the lowest glycemic index (GI)* (e.g., chocolate powder (no added sugar), hard candy, sugar substitute (all sugar-free unless otherwise specified) Phase two reintroduces the body to carbohydrates with low GI (e.g., apples, berries, grapefruit, high-fiber cereal, whole-grain breads)	*Phase one* Protein: 50% Carbohydrates: 10% Fat: 40%
Sugar Busters	Sugar is toxic to the body and causes the body to create more insulin Increases in insulin promote fat storage	Protein: 27% Carbohydrates: 5% Fat: 68% (saturated fat: 26%)

Glycemic index is the term used to describe the rise in blood glucose levels after a person has consumed a carbohydrate-containing food.

Perhaps because men have a higher percentage of lean body mass, men are able to lose weight more quickly than women. Women have a higher percentage of body fat, which is metabolically less active than muscle tissue. Postmenopausal women are particularly prone to weight gain, including increased abdominal fat.

Current fad diets include those that are either low in fat or low in carbohydrates (Table 41-7). They have been shown to have good effects on blood lipid concentrations, BP, and glucose control. However, these effects are generally short lived and not superior to standard approaches over the longer term. The degree of weight loss strongly depends on the ability of patients to adhere to their diets. The more restrictive the regimen, the greater the demand for intense discipline in the face of an intense desire to eat foods not allowed on the diet.[15]

Motivation is an essential ingredient for successful achievement of weight loss. The obese patient must see the need for weight loss and weight control and the advantages that will occur. The nurse can assist by helping the patient track eating patterns by keeping a diet diary. A frank discussion of eating habits helps the patient realize that often eating is the result of bad habits picked up with time and not of hunger. The bad habits must be changed, or weight loss will only be temporary.

Setting a realistic and healthy goal, such as losing 1 to 2 pounds per week, must be mutually agreed on at the outset. Trying to lose too much too fast usually results in a sense of frustration and failure for the patient. The nurse can help the patient understand that losing large amounts of weight in a short period causes skin and underlying tissue to lose elasticity and tone, which causes unsightly folds of flabby tissue. Slower weight loss offers better cosmetic results. Inevitably, the patient reaches plateau periods during which no weight is lost. These plateaus may last from several days to several weeks. It is especially important for the patient to realize that these are normal occurrences during weight reduction, so that discouragement, frustration, and giving up of the prescribed dietary plan are prevented. A weekly check of body weight is a good method of monitoring progress. Daily weighing is not recommended because of the frequent fluctuations resulting from retained water (including urine) and elimination of feces. The patient should be instructed to record the weight at the same time of the day, wearing the same type of clothing.

There is no firm agreement on the number of meals to be eaten when a person is on a diet. Some nutritionists advocate several small meals per day because the body's metabolic rate is temporarily increased immediately after eating. When several small meals a day are ingested, more calories are used. There seems to be general agreement that consumption of most of the daily caloric intake at a large evening meal results in less weight loss than when the calories are evenly distributed throughout the day.

When a person is first starting on a weight-reduction program, food portion sizes need to be carefully determined to stay within the dietary guidelines. Portion sizes over the past 20 years have increased considerably[16] (Table 41-8). Food portions can be weighed using a scale, or everyday objects can be used as a visual cue to determine portion sizes. The size of a woman's fist or a baseball is equivalent to a serving of vegetables or fruit. A serving of meat is about the size of a human's palm or a deck of cards. A serving of cheese is about the size of a thumb or six dice. A test on portion sizes is available at the following website: *http://hin.nhlbi.nih.gov/portion/index.htm.*

Another aspect of the American diet that needs to be considered is the proportion of calories from animal sources and calories from fruits, grains, and vegetables. The American Institute for Cancer Research advocates that two thirds or more of an individual's diet should be plant-source foods and the other one third or less from animal protein. Maintaining an awareness of personal consumption habits and striving for the two thirds to one third ratio is a simple goal that can be achieved without weighing and measuring foods at every meal. Once this ratio has been adopted into the pa-

TABLE 41-8	**Portion Sizes: Yesterday versus Today**	
	20 Years Ago	**Today**
Turkey sandwich	320 calories	820 calories
Bagel	3-in diameter 140 calories	6-in diameter 350 calories
Cheeseburger	333 calories	590 calories
Soda	6½ ounces 85 calories	20 ounces 250 calories

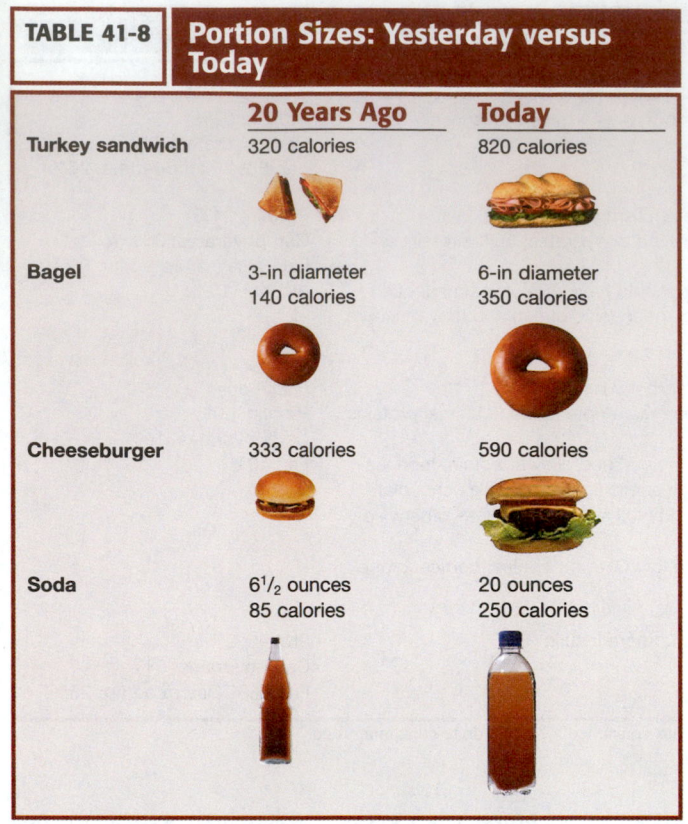

tient's meal planning, portions can gradually be reduced as activity levels are gradually increased to achieve healthy weight loss. The recommended portion size of animal protein is 3 ounces. The standard size for chopped vegetables is ½ cup according to MyPyramid guidelines (see Table 40-1).

A list of permitted foods serves as a good reference and permits an occasional meal to be eaten at a restaurant. The patient who carefully follows the prescribed diet may not need to take vitamin supplements. Appropriate fluid intake should be encouraged. Alcoholic beverages are usually not permitted on a reducing diet because they increase the caloric intake and are low in nutritional value.

Exercise. Exercise is an essential part of a weight control program. Exercise should be done daily, preferably 30 minutes to an hour a day. There is no evidence that increased activity promotes an increase in appetite or leads to dietary excess. In fact, exercise frequently has the opposite effect. The addition of exercise produces more weight loss than does dieting alone. Increasing exercise has a favorable effect on body fat distribution with a reduction in waist-to-hip ratio. Exercise is especially important in maintaining weight loss in overweight and obese persons.

The nurse should explore with the patient possible ways to increase exercise in daily routines. It may be as simple as parking farther from the place of employment or taking the stairs versus an elevator. Individuals should be encouraged to wear a pedometer to track their activity. The goal is 10,000 steps a day. However, success may be in walking a third of the recommended steps with incremental increases over time.

Joining a health club can be one mechanism of getting exercise. Walking, swimming, and cycling are sensible forms of exercise and have long-term benefits. Engaging in weekend exercise only or in spurts of strenuous activity is not advantageous and can actu-

ally be dangerous. When large muscles are involved in the exercise program, a primary benefit is cardiovascular conditioning. Overweight men and women who are active and fit have lower rates of morbidity and mortality than overweight persons who are sedentary and unfit. Therefore exercise is of benefit to overweight persons even if it does not make them lean.

Many psychologic benefits can be derived from an increased physical activity program. Reduction in tension and stress, better-quality sleep and rest, increased stamina and energy, improved self-concept and self-confidence, better attitudes toward work and play, and increased optimism about the future can be achieved.

Behavior Modification. The assumption behind behavior modification is that obesity is a learned disorder caused by overeating and that the critical difference between an obese person and a person of normal weight is in the cues that regulate eating behavior. Therefore most behavior-modification programs deemphasize the diet and focus on how and when the person eats. Participants often are taught to restrict their eating to designated meals and to increase the amount of physical activity in their lives. Persons who have undergone behavior therapy are more successful in maintaining their losses over an extended time than those who do not participate in such training.

Useful basic techniques include (1) self-monitoring, (2) stimulus control, and (3) rewards. Self-monitoring can focus on a record that shows what and when foods are eaten, as well as how the person was feeling when the foods were consumed. Stimulus control is aimed at separating events that trigger eating from the act of eating. Rewards may be used as incentive for weight loss. Short- and long-term goals are useful benchmarks for earning rewards. It is important that the reward for a specified weight loss not be associated with food, such as dinner out or a favorite treat. Reward items do not have to have a monetary component. For example, time for a hot bath or an hour of pleasure reading would be an enjoyable reward for many people. People may participate in group or individual sessions, or both, as they work toward their goals.

Support Groups. The person who is on any type of restrictive dietary program is often encouraged to join a group of other obese persons who are receiving professional counseling to help them modify their eating habits. Many self-help groups are available to the person who wants to learn more about successful dieting and who likes the support of others having the same problems and experiences. Take Off Pounds Sensibly (TOPS) is the oldest nonprofit organization of this type. Behavior modification is an integral part of the program, along with nutrition education. Weight Watchers International, Inc., is probably the most successful commercial weight-reduction enterprise. Weight Watchers offers a food plan that is nutritionally balanced and practical to follow, and it has used behavior-modification techniques since 1974.

There has been a proliferation of commercial weight-reduction centers across the nation. Many of these programs are staffed by nurses or dietitians, or both, and require an initial physical examination by a care provider before a candidate is accepted for weight reduction. These weight-reduction centers are costly and therefore are cost prohibitive for those with limited financial resources. Many of these programs also offer special prepackaged foods and supplements that must be purchased as part of the weight-reduction plan. Only these prescribed foods and drinks are to be consumed until an agreed-on amount of weight is lost. The patient is encouraged to buy the same type of foods for the maintenance phase of the pro-

EVIDENCE-BASED PRACTICE

Are Psychologic Interventions Effective in Helping Overweight Individuals Lose Weight?

Clinical Question

In overweight or obese persons (P), do psychologic interventions combined with diet and exercise (I) compared with diet and exercise alone (C) improve weight loss (O)?

Best Available Evidence

- Systematic review of randomized controlled trials (RCTs)

Critical Appraisal and Synthesis of the Evidence

Eight RCTs (*n* = 530) assessed success of behavior therapy (e.g., enhancing dietary restraint and motivation to increase physical activity) and cognitive-behavior therapy (CBT) (e.g., identify and modify aversive thinking patterns and mood states) in achieving sustained weight loss. Follow-up was 12 to 156 weeks.

- Behavior therapy combined with diet/exercise increased weight loss more than diet and exercise alone.
- CBT combined with diet and exercise also increased weight loss more than diet and exercise alone.

Conclusion

- Behavior and cognitive-behavior strategies can assist overweight and obese individuals to lose weight, especially when combined with diet and exercise.

Implications for Nursing

- Assist patients desiring to lose weight to access psychologic interventions when providing diet and exercise counseling.
- Other psychotherapies, including relaxation and hypnotherapy, need greater evaluation before being recommended as weight-loss treatments.

Reference for Evidence

Shaw K, O'Rourke P, Del Mar C, et al.: Psychological interventions for overweight or obesity, *Cochrane Database of Systematic Reviews* 2, 2005.

PICO: P, patient population of interest; *I,* intervention or area of interest; *C,* comparison of interest or comparison group; *O,* outcome(s) of interest (see p. 6).

gram, lasting from 6 months to 1 year. Behavior-modification training is incorporated within these programs as well.

Regardless of the commercial products used, successful weight loss and control are limited and require individualized programs consisting of restricted caloric intake, behavior modification, and exercise. Although persons who follow this type of program are likely to lose weight, once they leave the program the weight is usually regained because they tend to resume previous eating behaviors and return to the foods previously eaten.

A new concept of influencing health behavior and better employee health has occurred recently. Programs on health teaching and maintenance have been started at places of employment. The rationale for such programs is that better health repays the cost of the programs through improved work performance, decreased absenteeism, and eventually less hospitalization. Weight-reduction and hypertension-reduction programs have been instituted and are popular with employees.

Drug Therapy

Drugs have been used in the treatment of obesity but only as adjuncts to a good diet and exercise program. Drugs approved for weight loss can be classified into two categories: (1) those that decrease food intake by reducing appetite or increasing satiety and (2) those that decrease nutrient absorption. Drugs that increase energy expenditure (e.g., ephedrine) are not approved by the Food and Drug Administration (FDA) for weight loss in the United States at this time.

Appetite-Suppressing Drugs. Appetite suppressants reduce food intake through noradrenergic (drugs that mimic norepinephrine) or serotonergic mechanisms in the central nervous system (CNS). Noradrenergic agents include phentermine (Adipex-P, Fastin, Ionamin), diethylpropion (Tenuate, Tepanil), phendimetrazine (Bontril, Plegine), and benzphetamine (Didrex). Amphetamines are not recommended because of their abuse potential. Benzphetamine and phendimetrazine are classified as Schedule III drugs by the Drug Enforcement Administration because of their potential for abuse. These drugs are only recommended for short-term use (i.e., less than 12 weeks) in the management of obesity. Adverse effects of these drugs include palpitations, tachycardia, overstimulation, restlessness, dizziness, insomnia, weakness, and fatigue.[17,18]

Serotonergic drugs act to either increase the release of serotonin or decrease its uptake, thus reducing its metabolism. Fenfluramine (Pondimin) and dexfenfluramine (Redux) were the first drugs in this class. However, in 1997 these drugs were withdrawn from the market because of reported adverse effects (e.g., valvular heart disease, pulmonary hypertension). These drugs are mentioned to advise patients that their use is dangerous.[17]

Mixed noradrenergic-serotonergic agents are also used in weight management. Sibutramine (Meridia) inhibits both serotonin and norepinephrine uptake, thus increasing their levels in the CNS. Sibutramine, along with a reduced-calorie diet, has been shown to reduce body weight. Unlike fenfluramine it does not stimulate the release of serotonin, which is thought to be associated with adverse side effects.[18] Side effects include increased BP and heart rate, dry mouth, headache, insomnia, and constipation. Other selective serotonin reuptake inhibitors that are approved for the management of depression and other psychiatric conditions may have a short-term effect on weight loss, but the effect does not appear to last over time.

 Drug Alert - *Sibutramine (Meridia)*
- *Dose-related increases in BP and heart rate can occur.*

Nutrient Absorption–Blocking Drugs. Orlistat (Xenical), a drug that was developed for weight loss and maintenance, works by blocking fat breakdown and absorption in the intestine. It inhibits the action of intestinal lipases. The undigested fat is excreted in the feces. Although this drug has a high safety profile, some fat-soluble vitamin levels may decrease and may need to be supplemented. The FDA is considering making a low-dose form of orlistat available for over-the-counter use. Orlistat is associated with leakage of stool, flatulence, diarrhea, and abdominal bloating, which is accentuated if a high-fat diet is consumed. These side effects limit its acceptance as a weight-loss tool.

Because drugs will not cure obesity without substantial changes in food intake and increased physical activity, weight gain will occur when short-term drug therapy is stopped. Supervised long-term drug therapy with safe compounds can contribute to weight management, as well as weight loss. As with any pharmacologic treatment, there are side effects. Careful evaluation for the presence of other medical conditions can help determine which drugs, if any, would be advisable for a given patient.

The role of the nurse in relation to drug therapy should center on teaching the patient about proper administration and side effects and how the drugs fit into the larger weight-loss plan. The modification of dosage without consultation with the health care provider can have detrimental effects. The nurse should reemphasize that the diet and exercise regimens are the cornerstones of permanent weight loss. Drugs may be helpful, but they do not help the patient change eating behavior. The purchase of over-the-counter diet aids should be discouraged.

COLLABORATIVE SURGICAL THERAPY

Bariatric surgery is a surgical procedure that is used to treat morbid obesity. Bariatric surgery is currently the only treatment that has been found to have a successful and lasting impact for sustained weight loss for severely obese individuals.[2,19] The majority of patients who undergo bariatric surgery have successfully improved their overall quality of life. A great deal of excess weight is lost, and patients experience resolution of comorbidities and improve their appearance, social opportunities, and economic opportunities.[20]

An individual needs to meet all of the following criteria to be considered for bariatric surgery.

1. Has a BMI $\geq$40 kg/m^2 or a BMI $\geq$35 kg/m^2 with one or more severe obesity-related medical complications (e.g., hypertension, type 2 diabetes mellitus, heart failure, or sleep apnea)
2. Is 18 years old or older
3. Understands the risks and benefits of surgery
4. Has been obese for >5 years
5. Has tried and failed other methods to lose weight
6. Has no serious endocrine problem causing the obesity
7. Has psychiatric and social stability and willingness to cooperate with long-term follow-up
8. Availability of a team of health care providers (nurses, physicians, dietitians) to provide immediate and long-term care
9. Surgery would lessen or eradicate the high risks of a condition (e.g., degenerative joint disease)

Patients are not good candidates for bariatric surgery if they are obese from a treatable disorder (e.g., hypothyroidism), have a substance abuse problem, or have a major psychiatric disorder.

Bariatric surgeries fall into one of three broad categories: restrictive, malabsorptive, or a combination of malabsorptive and restrictive (Table 41-9 and Fig. 41-7). In restrictive procedures the

TABLE 41-9	**Surgical Interventions for Morbid Obesity***		
Procedure	**Anatomic Changes**	**Advantages**	**Complications**
Restrictive Surgery			
Vertical banded gastroplasty (VBG)	Small gastric pouch created	Easy to perform procedure (i.e., no anastomosis necessary) More normal anatomy and physiology maintained Lower risk of infection	Weight regain Staple line disruption Dilated pouch Dumping syndrome (nausea, light-headedness, upset stomach, vomiting, and/or diarrhea related to ingestion of sweets, high-calorie liquids, or dairy products)
Adjustable gastric banding (AGB)	Band encircles the stomach, creating a stoma and a gastric pouch	Food digestion occurs through normal process Band can be adjusted to $\uparrow$ or $\downarrow$ restriction Surgery can be reversed Absence of dumping syndrome Lack of malabsorption Short hospital stay	Gastric perforation Incisional hernia Stomal stenosis
Malabsorptive Surgery			
Biliopancreatic diversion (BPD) with or without duodenal switch	Anastomosis between the stomach and the intestine 70% of the stomach is removed horizontally Decreases the amount of small intestine available for nutrient absorption Duodenal switch cuts the stomach vertically and is shaped like a tube	Increased amount of food intake Less food intolerance Greater long-term weight loss Rapid weight loss	Abdominal bloating, diarrhea, and foul-smelling gas (steatorrhea) 3-4 loose bowel movements a day Malabsorption of fat-soluble vitamins Iron deficiency Protein-calorie malnutrition Ulcers Dumping syndrome (With duodenal switch, last two problems are less common)
Combination of Restrictive and Malabsorptive Surgery			
Roux-en-Y gastric bypass (RYGB)	Part of intestine connected to a very small stomach pouch Remaining stomach and first segment of small intestine are bypassed	Better weight loss results than gastric restrictive procedures Lower incidences of malnutrition and diarrhea Rapid improvement of weight-related comorbidities	Leak at site of anastomosis Pulmonary embolism GI hemorrhage Incisional hernia Bowel obstruction Stomal stenosis Marginal ulcer

*See Fig. 41-7.

stomach is reduced in size, and in malabsorptive procedures the length of the small intestine is decreased.

Restrictive Surgeries

Restrictive bariatric surgery reduces the size of a stomach to 30 ml or less, which causes the patient to feel full quicker.[21] The stomach and intestine digests and absorbs food normally when a restrictive gastrointestinal surgery is performed. Since digestion is not altered, the risk of anemia or cobalamin deficiency is low.

Vertical Banded Gastroplasty. *Vertical banded gastroplasty* (VBG) involves partitioning the stomach into a small pouch in the upper portion along the lesser curvature of the stomach. This small pouch drastically limits capacity. In addition, the stoma opening to the rest of the stomach is banded to delay emptying of solid food from the proximal pouch. This procedure has achieved considerable success in management of weight loss. Problems associated with this gastric restriction operation include intractable vomiting from too rapid intake of solids, distention of the wall of the proximal pouch, rupture of the staple line, and erosion of the band into the stomach.

Adjustable Gastric Banding. With *adjustable gastric banding* (AGB), the stomach size is limited by an inflatable band placed around the fundus of the stomach. This is the newest restrictive procedure and is often referred to as the *LapBand* ß(Inamed). The band is connected to a subcutaneous port and can be inflated or deflated (by fluid injection in the health care provider's office) to change the stoma size to meet the patient's needs as weight is lost.[18] The procedure can be done laparoscopically and can be modified or reversed after the initial procedure. AGB can be a better choice for patients who are surgical risks because it is a less invasive approach.

Weight loss is slower in patients who undergo AGB as compared with other procedures. Another disadvantage of this procedure is that the band may slip or erode into the stomach wall. Another operation would be needed to correct this problem.

Malabsorptive Surgeries

If a patient chooses to have malabsorptive surgery to reduce his or her weight, the surgeon will bypass various lengths of the small intestine so that less food is absorbed.

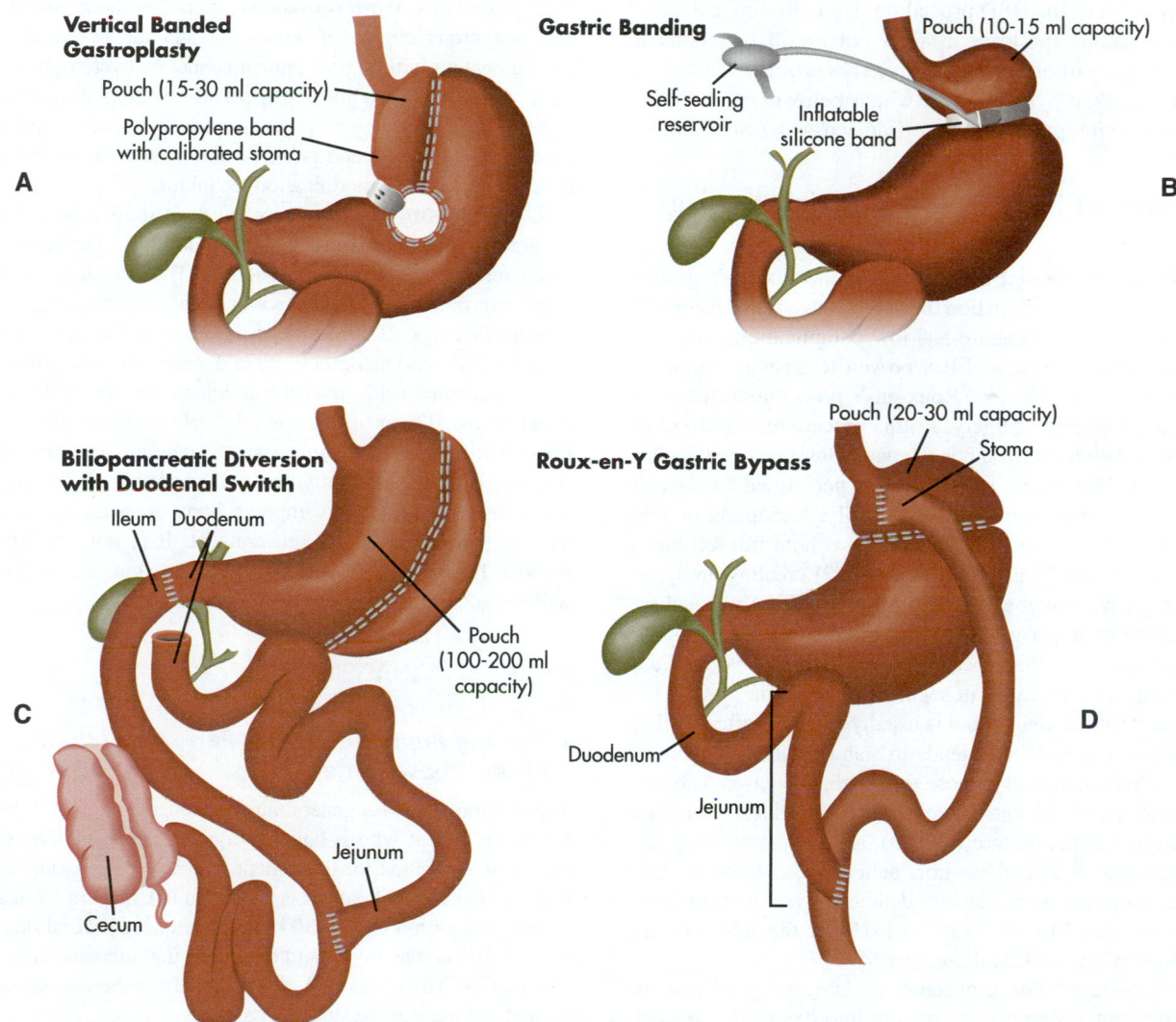

FIG. 41-7 Bariatric surgical procedures. **A,** Vertical banded gastroplasty involves creating a small gastric pouch. **B,** Adjustable gastric banding uses a band to create a gastric pouch. **C,** Biliopancreatic diversion with duodenal switch procedure creates an anastomosis between the stomach and intestine. **D,** Roux-en-Y gastric bypass procedure involves constructing a gastric pouch whose outlet is a Y-shaped limb of small intestine.

Gastrointestinal System

Biliopancreatic Diversion. Biliopancreatic diversion (BPD) involves removing approximately three fourths of the stomach to produce both restriction of food intake and reduction of acid output. The remaining portion of the stomach is connected to the lower portion of the small intestine. Pancreatic enzymes and bile enter the final segment of the small intestine. Nutrients pass without being digested. The patient loses weight because most of the calories and nutrients are routed into the colon where they are not absorbed.

This procedure can increase the risk of gallstones forming and may require the gallbladder to be removed. Patients should be aware of the possibilities of intestinal irritation and ulcers. Other risks from BPD include abdominal bloating and foul-smelling stool or gas. There is also a period when the intestines adjust and bowel movements can be very liquid and frequent. This condition may lessen over time, but may be a lifelong condition. Patients should also monitor their protein, iron, and cobalamin intake to ensure that they do not develop malnutrition or anemia. Supplements and vitamins should be taken to offset these risks.

Biliopancreatic Diversion with Duodenal Switch. This is a variation of the BPD procedure. By including a duodenal switch, surgeons can leave a larger portion of the stomach intact and a small part of the duodenum. This procedure also lets the surgeon keep the pyloric valve, which helps prevent dumping syndrome. (Dumping syndrome is discussed below and in Chapter 42.)

Combination of Restrictive and Malabsorptive Surgery

Roux-en-Y Surgical Procedure. The Roux-en-Y gastric bypass procedure is a combination of restrictive and malabsorptive surgery. This surgical procedure has low complication rates, has excellent patient tolerance, and has proven to sustain long-term weight loss. Because of this, the Roux-en-Y procedure is the most commonly used bariatric surgery. In this procedure, the stomach size is decreased with a gastric pouch anastomosis that empties directly into the jejunum. This surgery can be performed through an open abdominal incision or laparoscopically. Variations of this procedure include (1) stapling the stomach without transection to create a small, 20- to 30-ml gastric pouch; (2) creating an upper and a lower gastric pouch and totally disconnecting the pouches; and (3) creating an upper gastric pouch and completely removing the lower pouch. After the procedure, food bypasses 90% of the stomach, duodenum, and a small segment of jejunum.[22]

The greatest rate of weight loss is usually achieved after the first year following surgery. Weight tends to stabilize after 18 months. Outcomes include increased glucose tolerance, decreased diabetes, decreased BP, decreased cholesterol and triglycerides, decreased gastroesophageal reflux disease (GERD), and decreased sleep apnea. Adverse outcomes include iron deficiency, cobalamin deficiency, folic acid deficiency, calcium deficiency, and increased homocysteine levels.[23] Mortality rates are 2% in the first 30 days following surgery and 10% in those over 65.[24]

A complication of this procedure is *dumping syndrome*, in which gastric contents empty too rapidly into the small intestine, overwhelming its ability to digest nutrients. Symptoms can include vomiting, nausea, weakness, sweating, faintness, and, on occasion, diarrhea. Some patients are unable to eat sugary foods after surgery. Because sections of the small intestine are bypassed, poor absorption of iron and calcium can cause iron-deficiency anemia. Patients who experience chronic blood loss during excessive menstrual flow or bleeding hemorrhoids should be aware of the chance of iron-deficiency anemia. By taking a multivitamin and calcium supplements, patients can maintain a healthy level of minerals and vitamins. Chronic anemia caused by cobalamin deficiency may also occur. The problem usually can be managed with cobalamin pills, injections, or nasal spray.

Cosmetic Surgeries to Reduce Fatty Tissue and Skinfolds

Lipectomy. **Lipectomy** (adipectomy) is performed to remove unsightly flabby folds of adipose tissue. The patient who chooses lipectomy does so for cosmetic reasons. In some patients, up to 15% of the total fat cells can be removed from the breasts, abdomen, and lumbar and femoral areas. There is no evidence that a regeneration of adipose tissue occurs at the surgical sites. However, it must be emphasized to the patient that surgical removal does not prevent obesity from recurring, especially if lifetime eating habits remain the same. Although body image and self-esteem may be enhanced by such procedures, these operations are not without complications. The dangerous effects of anesthesia and the potential for poor wound healing in the obese patient cannot be overemphasized. It is more useful for the majority of patients contemplating a lipectomy to be instructed in preventive health measures, such as slow weight reduction to maintain and preserve tissue integrity, the value of exercise, and behavior-modification techniques.

Liposuction. Another surgical procedure is *liposuction,* or suction-assisted lipectomy. The current use is for cosmetic purposes and not for weight reduction. This surgical intervention helps improve facial appearance or body contours. A good candidate for this type of surgery is a person who has achieved weight reduction but who has excess fat under the chin, along the jawline, in the nasolabial folds, over the abdomen, or around the waist and upper thighs. The procedure is relatively free of major complications. A long, hollow, stainless steel cannula is inserted through a small incision over the fatty tissue to be suctioned. The purpose of this type of surgery is to improve body appearance, thereby enhancing body image and self-concept. It is not usually recommended for the older person because the skin is less elastic and will not accommodate the new underlying shape.

NURSING MANAGEMENT
OBESE PATIENT UNDERGOING SURGERY

■ *Nursing Implementation: Perioperative Care of the Obese Patient*

This section discusses general nursing considerations for the care of the obese patient who is having surgery. Special nursing considerations are described for the patient who is having bariatric surgery. (Care of the surgical patient is discussed in Chapters 18 to 20.)

Patients with a BMI >30 kg/m^2 often have several other medical conditions that are related to obesity that increase their surgical risk factors. These medical conditions affect the care of the obese patient before, during, and after surgery.

Preoperative Care. Special considerations are necessary in the care of the patient who is admitted to the hospital for surgical treatment, especially the morbidly obese. Before surgery, it is important that an interview with the patient is conducted. The primary reasons that a preoperative interview should be conducted are to obtain past and current patient health information and to ensure the patient understands the surgical procedure that he or she is scheduled to undergo. Patients who are obese are likely to suffer from other comorbidities, including diabetes, altered cardiorespiratory function, abnormal metabolic function, hemostasis, and atherosclerosis.[25] A team approach to treatment of the obese patient may be necessary. If the patient suffers from a disease other than obesity, it may be necessary to coordinate with the patient's cardiologist, pulmonologist, gynecologist, gastroenterologist, or other specialist to address concerns related to any other medical problems that the patient may have.

To ensure the patient's dignity and privacy, the nursing care team should have the room prepared and supplies ready before the patient arrives. Most nursing units are not prepared to meet the needs of a patient who is often too large for a typical hospital or recovery room bed or who has arms that even a large-size BP cuff will not fit. To eliminate embarrassment for the patient and frustration for the staff, plans for these special needs should be made before the patient's admission. Oversized BP cuffs should be ready for use when the patient arrives. A private room may be necessary for privacy of the patient and to accommodate the bed and sitting arrangements. A strongly reinforced trapeze bar should be placed over the bed to facilitate movement and positioning. In some cases a specially constructed chair may have to be built and beds joined together to allow the patient to sit and sleep in comfort.

Consideration should be given to questions such as how the patient will be weighed, how the patient will be transported throughout the hospital, and how simple physical assessment strategies may have to be adjusted to accommodate the morbidly obese patient. Another need is a wheelchair with removable arms that is large enough to safely accommodate the patient and pass easily through doorways.

Strategies for bathing, turning, and ambulating the patient, including the number of extra people needed to carry out these measures, are invaluable when the actual need arises. Special gowns are also needed for the patient. Routine physical assessment strategies do not work well with morbidly obese patients who have numerous layers of skinfolds covering areas that need to be assessed. Without identifying alternatives or unique methods of dealing with this problem, assessment of respiratory status and bowel sounds or even wound inspection could be awkward for the nurse and embarrassing for the patient.

Wound infection is one of the most common complications after surgery. Because of the many layers of flabby skinfolds, especially in the abdominal area, preoperative skin preparation is important. Frequently the patient is instructed to take several showers a day for a few days before admission to the hospital. Careful cleansing with soap and warm water of the abdominal area from the breasts to below the waist is emphasized.

Obesity can cause a patient's breathing to become shallow and rapid. The extra adipose tissue in the chest and abdomen compresses the diaphragmatic, thoracic, and abdominal structures. This compression restricts the chest's ability to expand, causing the lungs to not work as efficiently as they would otherwise. Thus the patient retains more carbon dioxide. In addition, there is less oxygen delivered to the lungs. This results in hypoxemia, pulmonary hypertension, and polycythemia. The patient must be in-

structed in the proper coughing technique, deep breathing, and methods of turning and positioning to prevent pulmonary complications after surgery. The use of a spirometer may be introduced before surgery. Use of the spirometer helps prevent and alleviate postoperative lung congestion. Practicing these strategies preoperatively can aid in performing them correctly postoperatively.

Obtaining venous access may also be complicated by excess adipose tissue. An assistant may be needed to help. If a patient has pitting edema, or excess fat, the nurse should hold a firm finger over the spot with pressure. The nurse may also want to mark the spot of injection with a sterile skin marker once a vein is found. Edema can become worse if the nurse chooses to anchor the catheter by taping the arm. This action can further impede venous return, causing venous stasis, pooling of intravenous fluids, extravasation, or infiltration. The nurse may also want to use multiple tourniquets to distend veins and hold back excess tissue. The tourniquet should be removed as soon as it is no longer needed to avoid aggravating the edema. The nurse may also need a longer catheter (longer than 1 inch) to transverse overlying tissue. It is important that the cannula is far enough into the vein to ensure that it is not dislodged or infiltrated.

If the patient is going to be undergoing anesthesia during the surgery, the nurse will want to encourage the anesthesia care provider to inform the patient about the increased risk of failure to wean from mechanical ventilation. This risk is important for the patient to know so that the patient is aware of what to expect when he or she wakes up from the anesthesia.

Special Considerations for Bariatric Surgery. All patients admitted for major gastric surgery procedures have a nasogastric (NG) tube inserted during surgery and attached to low suction after surgery. Allowing the patient to see a typical tube and explaining why it is necessary is a good method of involving the patient in the plan of care. The patient should know that oral nourishment will be impossible for a few days after the surgery and that intravenous fluids will be the main source of intake.

Postoperative Care. Trained staff members should assist the transfer of the unconscious patient. The transfer may require up to five trained staff members.[26] During the transfer, the patient's airway should remain stabilized and attention should be given to maintaining pain at a manageable level. The head of the patient should be maintained at a 35- to 40-degree angle to reduce abdominal pressure and increase tidal flow. If the patient is severely obese, the nursing team should closely monitor the patient for rapid oxygen desaturation. The body stores anesthetics in adipose tissue, placing patients with excess adipose tissue at risk for resedation. As adipose cells release anesthesic back into the bloodstream, the patient may become sedated after surgery. If this happens, the nursing care team should be prepared to perform a head-tilt or jaw-thrust maneuver and keep the patient's oral and nasal airways opened.[27]

Early ambulation is essential for the obese patient. It is important that the patient know that it is usually necessary to get out of bed soon after surgery and with increasing frequency thereafter, generally three to four times each day. The dangers of thrombophlebitis and measures to counteract its development are a routine part of preoperative teaching. The patient should know that elastic stockings, pneumatic compression devices, elastic compression stockings, or elastic wraps will be applied to the legs and that active and passive range-of-motion exercises will be a frequent part of daily care. Low-dose heparin often will be ordered. Depending on the size of the patient and the amount of pain he or she is experiencing, the patient may not be able to assist the nurse in turning. Extra nurses may be needed to turn the patient safely.

The nursing care team will also want to assess the patient's skin for delayed wound healing, the development of seromas, hematomas, wound dehiscence, wound evisceration, and wound infection. Skinfolds should be kept clean and dry to prevent dermatitis and secondary bacterial or fungal infections.[27]

Special Considerations for Bariatric Surgery. The patient experiences considerable abdominal pain after surgery. Administration of pain medications should be given as frequently as necessary during the immediate postoperative period. Encouraging and assisting the patient to turn, cough, and deep breathe at least every 1 to 2 hours minimizes the risk for atelectasis and pneumonia. Frequent mouth and nose care also helps breathing efforts because the NG tube is inserted through one nostril.

Position changes and range-of-motion exercises are instituted immediately after surgery and carried out every 1 to 2 hours. Ambulatory efforts generally are begun on the evening of surgery. For patient safety, the nurse should enlist the assistance of other staff members during these initial efforts, while encouraging the patient to help.

The abdominal wound requires frequent observation for the amount and type of drainage, condition of the sutures, and signs of infection. The incision must be protected against undue straining that accompanies turning and coughing. Wound dehiscence and wound healing are potential problems for all obese patients. Monitoring the vital signs assists in identifying problems such as infection.

It is important that the NG tube be kept patent and in the correct position. Vomiting is common following gastric procedures. If tube patency is blocked or the tube requires repositioning, the physician should be notified at once. The upper gastric pouch is small, and irrigating the tube with too much solution or manipulating tube position can lead to disruption of the anastomosis or staple line. In most cases the NG tube can be removed in approximately 48 hours, or when bowel sounds have resumed.

Skin care should be carried out several times each shift. Perspiration may be excessive at times. The many layers of skin should be kept clean and dry so that this source of irritation is eliminated. For the patient who has an indwelling catheter, perineal care is important so that a urinary tract infection can be prevented.

During the immediate postoperative period (first 24 hours) water and sugar-free clear liquids are given (30 ml every 2 hours while awake). At 1 day to 2 weeks postoperatively, a high-protein liquid diet (e.g., 30 to 60 ml of Boost HP, Ensure Plus, or Carnation Instant Breakfast) is offered every 2 hours while awake. During this time fluid intake should be carefully monitored. At 2 to 4 weeks postoperatively, a pureed diet is provided at frequent intervals. The patient is taught to eat slowly and to stop when feeling full and not to consume liquids with solid food. Vomiting is a common complication during this time. At 4 to 6 weeks the patient starts on a transition diet that includes solids, as well as pureed foods.

Ambulatory and Home Care

Special Considerations for Bariatric Surgery. The patient who has undergone major surgical treatment for obesity has not, in the past, been successful in following or maintaining a prescribed diet. Now the patient is forced to reduce the oral intake as a result of the anatomic changes brought about by the operation. This patient finds that adherence to a reduced intake is necessary because of the concern for abdominal distention, cramping abdominal pain, and perhaps diarrhea.

Weight loss is considerable during the first 6 to 12 months. It is during this time that the patient must learn to adjust intake sufficiently to maintain a stable weight. Although behavior modification was not an intended outcome when these surgical procedures were devised, it becomes an unexpected secondary gain. The diet generally prescribed should be high in protein and low in carbohydrates, fat, and roughage and consist of six small feedings daily. Fluids should not be ingested with the meal, and in some cases, fluids should be restricted to less than 1000 ml per day. Fluids and foods high in carbohydrate tend to promote diarrhea and symptoms of the dumping syndrome. Generally, calorically dense foods (foods high in fat) should be avoided to permit more nutritionally sound food to be consumed.

Proper diet must be clearly understood by the patient. Late complications can be anticipated after gastric bypass or gastroplasty, including anemia, vitamin deficiencies, diarrhea, and psychiatric problems. Failure to lose weight or loss of too much weight may be caused by the surgical formation of too large a stomach pouch or of an outlet that is much too small, respectively. Peptic ulcer formation, dumping syndrome, and small bowel obstruction may be seen late in the recovery and rehabilitative stage.

Long-term follow-up care must be stressed, in part because of complications late in the recovery period. The patient must be encouraged to adhere strictly to the prescribed diet and to keep the care provider informed of any changes in physical or emotional condition. Some patients have been known to overeat when they return home and gain rather than lose weight.

The nurse must anticipate and recognize several potential psychologic problems after surgery. Some patients express guilt feelings concerning the fact that the only way they could lose weight was by surgical means rather than by the "sheer willpower" of reduced dietary intake. The nurse should be ready to provide support so that this patient does not dwell on negative feelings.

Many morbidly obese patients who blamed their feelings of social inferiority or inadequacies on their appearance before bypass surgery may suffer from episodes of depression. By 6 to 8 months after surgery, considerable weight loss has occurred, and they are able to see clearly how much their appearance has changed. Massive weight loss often leaves the patient with large quantities of flabby skin that can result in problems related to altered body image. Reconstructive surgery at least 1 full year after the initial surgery may alleviate this situation. Reductions of the breasts, upper arms, thighs, and excess abdominal skinfolds are possible solutions. Discussion of this possible outcome with the patient before surgery and again during the rehabilitation phase of recovery helps facilitate the patient's adjustment to a new body image and social reintegration.

■ Evaluation

The expected outcomes are that the obese patient will
- experience long-term weight loss
- have improvement in obesity-related comorbidities
- integrate healthy practices into daily routines
- monitor for adverse side effects of surgical therapy
- have an improved self-image

GERONTOLOGIC CONSIDERATIONS
OBESITY IN OLDER ADULTS

The prevalence of obesity is increasing in all age-groups, including older people. The number of obese older persons has markedly risen because of both an increase in the total number of older persons and the percentage of the older adults who are obese. Obesity is more common in older women than in older men.[28] A decrease in energy expenditure is an important contributor to a gradual increase in body fat with increasing age.

Obesity in older adults can exacerbate age-related declines in physical function and lead to frailty and disability.[29] Obesity is associated with decreased survival. Individuals who are obese live 6 to 7 years less than people of normal weight.

Arthritis is a leading cause of physical disability in older adults. The age-related increase in the prevalence of osteoarthritis reflects body changes related to a lifetime of being overweight, which results in mechanical strain on weight-bearing joints.[29]

Pulmonary complications of obesity may occur. Hypoventilation syndrome and obstructive sleep apnea are major problems for older adults. Older obese men are especially predisposed to develop weight-related sleep apnea.

Obesity contributes to the increase in the prevalence of urinary incontinence in older persons. In addition, obesity is associated with an increased risk of several types of cancers that occur more commonly in older adults, including breast, colorectal, gallbladder, endometrial, and prostate cancers.[29]

Obesity affects quality of life for older adults. Weight loss can improve quality of life, physical function, and obesity-related health complications. The same therapeutic approaches for obesity as were discussed earlier also apply to the older adult.

METABOLIC SYNDROME

Metabolic syndrome, also known as *syndrome X, insulin resistance syndrome,* and *dysmetabolic syndrome,* is a collection of risk factors that increase an individual's chance of developing cardiovascular disease and diabetes mellitus. It is estimated that around 50 million, or one in five, Americans have metabolic syndrome.[30] Metabolic syndrome is diagnosed if an individual has three or more of the conditions listed in Table 41-10.

Etiology and Pathophysiology

The main underlying risk factors for metabolic syndrome are abdominal obesity and insulin resistance. Other conditions associated with the syndrome include physical inactivity, presence of inflammatory markers, prothrombotic tendencies, hormonal imbalance, aging, and genetic or ethnic predisposition. African Americans, Hispanics, American Indians, and Asians are at risk for development of metabolic syndrome, as well as women who had gestational diabetes.[31] Patients who have been diagnosed with metabolic syndrome typically are individuals who have diabetes that cannot maintain a proper level of glucose, have hypertension, and secrete a large amount of insulin, or who have survived a heart attack and have hyperinsulinemia.[32]

Although there are no symptoms of metabolic syndrome, medical problems will develop over time if the condition remains unaddressed. Patients with the syndrome are at a higher risk of developing heart disease, stroke, diabetes, and renal disease. Patients who have metabolic syndrome and smoke are at an even higher risk.

TABLE 41-10	Diagnostic Criteria for Metabolic Syndrome*
Measure	**Categorical Cut Point**
Waist circumference	≥40 in (102 cm) in men
	≥35 in (88 cm) in women
Triglycerides	>150 mg/dl (1.7 mmol/L)
	or
	Drug treatment for elevated triglycerides
High-density lipoprotein (HDL) cholesterol	<40 mg/dl (0.9 mmol/L) in men
	<50 mg/dl (1.1 mmol/L) in women
	or
	Drug treatment for reduced HDL cholesterol
BP	≥130 mm Hg systolic BP
	or
	≥85 mm Hg diastolic BP
	or
	Drug treatment for hypertension
Fasting glucose	≥100 mg/dl
	or
	Drug treatment for elevated glucose

Source: Grundy S, Cleeman JI, Daniels SR, et al: Diagnosis and management of the metabolic syndrome: an American Heart Association/National Heart, Lung, and Blood Institute scientific statement, *Circulation* 112:1, 2005.
BP, Blood pressure.
*Any three of the five measures are needed for a diagnosis of metabolic syndrome.

NURSING *and* COLLABORATIVE MANAGEMENT
METABOLIC SYNDROME

Lifestyle therapies are the first-line interventions to reduce the risk factors for metabolic syndrome. Management or reversal of metabolic syndrome can be achieved by reducing the major risk factors of cardiovascular disease: reducing LDL cholesterol, stopping smoking, lowering BP, and reducing glucose levels. For long-term reduction in risk, weight should be decreased to a desirable weight, physical activity should be increased, and healthy dietary habits should be established.[32]

There is only management of metabolic syndrome and no specific treatment is available, but nurses can assist patients by providing information on healthy diets, exercise, and positive lifestyle changes. To address metabolic syndrome, a diet should be low in saturated fats and promote weight loss. Although low-carbohydrate diets may offer short-term weight loss, there is no strong evidence to support long-term weight loss with such diets. Weight reduction and maintenance of a lower weight should be the first priority in those with abdominal obesity and metabolic syndrome.

Because sedentary lifestyles contribute to metabolic syndrome, increasing regular physical activity will lower a patient's risk factors. According to the U.S. Behavioral Risk Factor Surveillance System, a sedentary lifestyle is defined as "one in which demanding physical activity does not exceed 20 minute sessions or when such activity occurs fewer than three times per week." As well as assisting in weight reduction, regular exercise has been found to decrease the triglyceride level and increase the HDL cholesterol level in patients with metabolic syndrome.

Patients unable to lower risk factors with lifestyle therapies alone or those at high risk for a coronary event may be considered for drug therapy. Although there is no medication for metabolic syndrome specifically, medication can be prescribed to lower individual risk factors, such as metformin (Glucophage), which reduces glucose levels.

Gastrointestinal System

CRITICAL THINKING EXERCISE

CASE STUDY

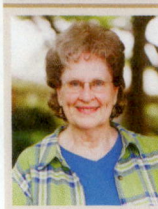

Obesity

Patient Profile. Mrs. Stella Roman is a 60-year-old white woman who is 5 feet 4 inches tall and weighs 210 pounds.

Subjective Data

- Reports gradual weight gain during past 40 years
- Spends most of her free time watching television
- Reports health problems related to type 2 diabetes mellitus, shortness of breath, hypertension, chest pressure, and osteoarthritis
- Had knee replacement surgery at age 56 for osteoarthritis

Objective Data

Physical Examination

- Has obese, nontender, soft abdomen
- BP 160/100 mm Hg

Laboratory Results

- Fasting blood glucose: 250 mg/dl (13.9 mmol/L)
- Total cholesterol: 205 mg/dl (5.3 mmol/L)
- Triglyceride: 298 mg/dl (3.36 mmol/L)
- HDL cholesterol: 31 mg/dl (0.8 mmol/L)

Critical Thinking Questions

1. What are Mrs. Roman's obesity risk factors?
2. What is her estimated BMI?
3. Of the possible complications of obesity, which ones does Mrs. Roman have? What are contributing factors to her developing type 2 diabetes mellitus, cardiovascular disease manifestations, and osteoarthritis?
4. What would you, as the nurse, include in a successful weight loss and weight management program for Mrs. Roman?
5. Is Mrs. Roman at risk for metabolic syndrome? Why or why not?
6. Is Mrs. Roman a candidate for surgical intervention for obesity? If so, why? If not, why not?
7. Based on the assessment data presented, write one or more appropriate nursing diagnoses. Are there any collaborative problems?

NCLEX EXAMINATION REVIEW QUESTIONS

The number of the question corresponds to the same-numbered objective at the beginning of the chapter.

1. Which of the following statements best describes the etiology of obesity?
   a. Obesity primarily results from a genetic predisposition.
   b. Psychosocial factors can override the effects of genetics in the etiology of obesity.
   c. Obesity is the result of complex interactions between genetic and environmental factors.
   d. Genetic factors are more important than environmental factors in the etiology of obesity.

2. The obesity classification that is most often associated with cardiovascular health problems is
   a. primary obesity.
   b. secondary obesity.

   c. gynoid fat distribution.
   d. android fat distribution.

3. Health risks associated with obesity include
   a. hypothyroidism and colorectal cancer.
   b. rheumatoid arthritis and diabetes mellitus.
   c. gynecomastia and systemic lupus arthritis.
   d. polycystic ovary disease and stress incontinence.

4. The best nutritional therapy plan for a person who is obese is
   a. the Zone diet.
   b. the Atkins diet.
   c. Sugar Busters.
   d. foods from the basic food groups.

5. This bariatric surgical procedure involves creating a stoma and gastric pouch that is reversible and no malabsorption occurs. What surgical procedure is this?
   a. Vertical gastric banding
   b. Biliopancreatic diversion
   c. Adjustable gastric banding
   d. Roux-en-Y gastric bypass

6. A morbidly obese patient has undergone Roux-en-Y gastric bypass surgery. In planning postoperative care, the nurse anticipates that the patient
   a. may have severe diarrhea early in the postoperative period.
   b. will not be allowed to ambulate for 1 to 2 days postoperatively.
   c. will require nasogastric suction until healing of the incision occurs.
   d. may have only liquids orally, and in very limited amounts, during the early postoperative period.

7. Which of the following criteria are needed for a diagnosis of a metabolic syndrome?
   a. Abdominal obesity and diabetes
   b. Elevated triglycerides and anemia
   c. Hypertension and elevated plasma glucose
   d. Gestational diabetes and increased waist circumference

REFERENCES

1. Centers for Disease Control and Prevention: Overweight and obesity. Available at *www.cdc.gov/nccdphp/dnpa/obesity* (accessed July 21, 2006).
2. National Heart, Lung, and Blood Institute, North American Association for the Study of Obesity: *The practical guide: identification, evaluation, and treatment of overweight and obesity in adults,* Publication No. 00-4084, 2000, US Department of Health and Human Services.
3. Bloch A: Low carbohydrate diets, pro: time to rethink our current strategies, *Nutr Clin Prac* 20(1):3, 2005.
4. Malis C, Rasmussen EL, Foulsen P, et al: Total and regional fat distribution is strongly influenced by genetic factors in young and elderly twins, *Obesity Research* 13:2139, 2005.
5. Allison DB, Matz PE, Pietrobelli A, et al: Genetic and environmental influences on obesity. In Bendich A, Deckelbaum RJ, editors: *Primary and secondary preventive nutrition,* Totowa, NJ, 2001, Humana Press.
6. Stunkard A, Sorensen TI, Hanis C, et al: An adoption study of human obesity, *N Engl J Med* 314(4):1483, 1986.
7. Broberger C: Brain regulation of food intake and appetite: molecules and networks, *J Intern Med* 258(4):307, 2005.
8. Vendrell J, Broch M, Vilarrasa N, et al: Resistin, adiponectin, ghrelin, leptin, and proinflammatory cytokines: relationships in obesity, *Obesity Research* 12:962, 2004.
9. McCance K, Huether SE: *Pathophysiology: the biologic basis for disease in adults and children,* ed 5, St Louis, 2005, Elsevier Mosby.
10. Oliver L, Hayes MV: Neighbourhood socioeconomic status and the prevalence of overweight Canadian children and youth, *Can J Public Health* 96(6):415, 2005.
11. National Institutes of Health: *Statistics related to overweight and obesity,* Publication No. 03-4158, 2003, US Department of Health and Human Services.
12. Kern P, Rasouli N: Pathogenesis and treatment of high-risk obesity. In Fonseca V, editor: *Clinical diabetes: translating research into practice,* St Louis, 2006, Saunders Elsevier.
13. Daniels J: Obesity: America's epidemic, *Am J Nurs* 106:40, 2006.

14. Latner J, Stunkard AJ, Wilson GT: Stigmatized students: age, sex, and ethnicity effects in the stigmatization of obesity, *Obesity Research* 13:226, 2005.

15. Dansinger ML, Gleason JA, Griffith JL, et al: Comparison of the Atkins, Ornish, Weight Watchers, and Zone diets for weight loss and heart disease risk reduction: a randomized trial, *JAMA* 293:43, 2005.

16. Ello-Martin JA, Ledikwe JH, Rolls BJ: The influence of food portion size and energy density on energy intake: implications for weight management, *Am J Clin Nutr* 82(suppl):236S, 2005.

17. Kaya A, Aydin N, Topsever P, et al: Efficacy of sibutramine, orlistat, and combination therapy on short-term weight management in obese patients, *Biomed Pharmacother* 58:582, 2004.

18. Snow V, Barry P, Fitterman N, et al: Pharmacologic and surgical management of obesity in primary care, *Ann Intern Med* 142(7):525, 2005.

19. Korenkov M, Sauerland S, Junginger T: Surgery for obesity, *Curr Opin Gastroenterol* 21:679, 2005.

20. Buchwald H, Avidor Y, Braunwald E, et al: Bariatric surgery. A systematic review and meta-analysis, *JAMA* 292(14):1724, 2004.

21. Gallagher S: Taking the weight off with bariatric surgery, *Nursing* 34(3):58, 2004.

22. Blackwood H: Help your patient downsize with bariatric surgery, *Med/Surg Insider* (suppl 4), Fall 2005.

23. Libeton M, Dixon JB, Laurie C, et al: Patient motivation for bariatric surgery: characteristics and impact on outcomes, *Obesity Surgery* 14(3):392, 2004.

24. Flum D, Salem L, Elrod JA, et al: Early mortality among Medicare beneficiaries undergoing bariatric surgical procedures, *JAMA* 294(15):1903, 2005.

25. Whittemore AD, Kelly J, Shirkora S, et al: Specialized staff and equipment for weight loss surgery patients: best practice guidelines, *Obesity Research* 13(2):283, 2005.

26. Davidson JE, Kruse MW, Cox DH, et al: Critical care of the morbidly obese, *Crit Care Nurs Q* 26:105, 2003.

27. Dunn D: Preventing perioperative complications in special population, *Nursing* 35(11):36, 2005.

28. Villareal D, Apovian C, Kushner R, et al: Obesity in older adults: technical review and position statement of the American Society for Nutrition and NAASO, the Obesity Society, *Am J Clin Nutr* 82:923, 2005.

29. Reynolds SL, Saito Y, Crimmins EM: The impact of obesity on active life expectancy in older American men and women, *Gerontologist* 45(4):438, 2005.

30. Kahn R, Buse J, Ferrannini E, et al: The metabolic syndrome: time for a critical appraisal, *Diabetes Care* 28:2289, 2005.

31. Appel S: Sizing up patients for metabolic syndrome, *Nursing* 35(12):20, 2005.

32. Grundy S, Cleeman JI, Daniels SR, et al: Diagnosis and management of the metabolic syndrome: an American Heart Association/National Heart, Lung, and Blood Institute scientific statement, *Circulation* 112:1, 2005.

RESOURCES

Academy for Eating Disorders
703-556-9222
www.aedweb.org

American Dietetic Association
800-877-1600
312-899-0040
www.eatright.org

American Institute for Cancer Research
800-843-8114
202-328-7744
www.aicr.org

American Obesity Association
202-776-7711
www.obesity.org

American Society for Bariatric Surgery
352-331-4900
www.asbs.org

National Eating Disorder Information Centre
866-NEDIC-20
416-340-4156
Email: nedic@uhn.on.ca
www.nedic.ca

National Eating Disorders Association
800-931-3327
206-382-3587
www.nationaleatingdisorders.org

North American Association for the Study of Obesity (NAASO)
301-563-6526
www.naaso.org

Overeaters Anonymous Headquarters
505-891-2664
www.overeatersanonymous.org

Take Off Pounds Sensibly (TOPS)
414.482.4620
www.tops.org

US Drug Enforcement Administration
800-DEA-4288
www.dea.gov

US Food and Drug Administration
888-INFO-FDA (888-463-6332)
www.fda.gov

Weight Control Information Network
National Institute of Diabetes and Digestive and Kidney Diseases
301-570-2177
800-WIN-8098
www.niddk.nih.gov/health/nutrit/nutrit.htm

Weight Watchers, Inc.
www.weightwatchers.com

For additional Internet resources, see the website for this book at *http://evolve.elsevier.com/Lewis/medsurg.*

42

Nursing Management
Upper Gastrointestinal Problems

Margaret McLean Heitkemper

LEARNING OBJECTIVES

1. Describe the etiology, complications, collaborative care, and nursing management of nausea and vomiting.
2. Explain the common etiology, clinical manifestations, collaborative care, and nursing management of upper gastrointestinal bleeding.
3. Describe the etiology, clinical manifestations, and treatment of common oral inflammations and infections.
4. Describe the etiology, clinical manifestations, complications, collaborative care, and nursing management of oral cancer.
5. Explain the types, pathophysiology, clinical manifestations, complications, and collaborative care, including surgical therapy and nursing management, of gastroesophageal reflux disease (GERD) and hiatal hernia.
6. Describe the pathophysiology, clinical manifestations, complications, and collaborative care of esophageal cancer, diverticula, achalasia, and esophageal strictures.
7. Differentiate between acute and chronic gastritis, including the etiology, pathophysiology, collaborative care, and nursing management.
8. Compare and contrast gastric and duodenal ulcers, including etiology and pathophysiology, clinical manifestations, complications, collaborative care, and nursing management.
9. Describe the clinical manifestations, collaborative care, and nursing management of gastric cancer.
10. Identify common types of food poisoning and nursing responsibilities related to food poisoning.

KEY TERMS

achalasia, p. 1012
Barrett's esophagus, p. 1004
dysphagia, p. 1001
esophageal cancer, p. 1009
esophageal diverticula, p. 1011
esophagitis, p. 1004
gastritis, p. 1013
gastroesophageal reflux disease, p. 1003
hiatal hernia, p. 1007
leukoplakia, p. 1001
Mallory-Weiss tear, p. 995
nausea, p. 990
peptic ulcer disease, p. 1014
physiologic stress ulcers, p. 1017
stomach cancer, p. 1028
stress-related mucosal disease, p. 1017
vomiting, p. 990

Electronic Resources

Supplemental content related to Chapter 42 can be found . . .

Companion CD
- Stress-Busting Kit for Nursing Students
- Interactive Case Studies:
  - Oral Cancer
  - Peptic Ulcer Disease
- NCLEX Examination Review Questions
- Comprehensive Glossary

Evolve Website **evolve**
http://evolve.elsevier.com/Lewis/medsurg
- Content Updates
- Key Points (Printable and CD/MP3 Download)
- Concept Map Creator
- Expanded Audio Glossary
- Key Term Flash Cards

- Customizable Nursing Care Plans:
  - Nausea and Vomiting
  - Peptic Ulcer Disease
- Electronic Calculators
- WebLinks

NAUSEA AND VOMITING

Nausea and vomiting are the most common manifestations of gastrointestinal (GI) diseases. Although nausea and vomiting can occur independently, they are usually closely related and treated as one problem. **Nausea** is a feeling of discomfort in the epigastrium with a conscious desire to vomit. **Vomiting** is the forceful ejection of partially digested food and secretions *(emesis)* from the upper GI tract. Vomiting is a complex act that requires the coordinated activities of several structures: closure of the glottis, deep inspiration with contraction of the diaphragm in the inspiratory position, closure of the pylorus, relaxation of the stomach and lower esophageal sphincter, and contraction of the abdominal muscles with in-

Reviewed by Alexandra Bowen, RN, CGRN, Clinical Nurse Leader, Digestive Disease Center, Medical University of South Carolina, Charleston, S.C.

creasing intraabdominal pressure. These simultaneous activities force the stomach contents up through the esophagus, into the pharynx, and out the mouth.

Etiology and Pathophysiology

Nausea and vomiting are found in a wide variety of GI disorders, as well as in conditions that are unrelated to GI disease. These include pregnancy, infectious diseases, central nervous system (CNS) disorders (e.g., meningitis, CNS tumor), cardiovascular problems (e.g., myocardial infarction, heart failure), metabolic disorders (e.g., diabetes mellitus, Addison's disease, uremia), side effects of drugs (e.g., chemotherapy, opioids, digitalis), and psychologic factors (e.g., stress, fear).

Generally, nausea occurs before vomiting and is physiologically related to slowing of gastric motility and emptying. A single episode of nausea accompanied by vomiting may not be significant. However, if vomiting occurs several times, it is important that the cause be identified.

A vomiting center in the brainstem coordinates the multiple components involved in vomiting. This center receives input from various stimuli. Neural impulses reach the vomiting center via afferent pathways through branches of the autonomic nervous system. Receptors for these afferent fibers are located in the GI tract, kidneys, heart, and uterus. When stimulated, these receptors relay information to the vomiting center, which then initiates the vomiting reflex (Fig. 42-1).

In addition, the chemoreceptor trigger zone (CTZ) located on the floor of the fourth ventricle in the brain responds to chemical stimuli of drugs and toxins. The CTZ also plays a role in vomiting due to labyrinthine stimulation (e.g., motion sickness) and is the site of action of drugs (e.g., ipecac) used to induce vomiting. Once stimulated, the CTZ transmits impulses directly to the vomiting center.

Vomiting also can occur when the GI tract becomes overly irritated, excited, or distended. It can be a protective mechanism to rid the body of spoiled or irritating foods and liquids. Irregular gastric

motor activity has also been associated with nausea and vomiting. Immediately before the act of vomiting, the person becomes aware of the need to vomit. The autonomic nervous system is activated, resulting in both parasympathetic and sympathetic nervous system stimulation immediately before vomiting. Sympathetic activation produces tachycardia, tachypnea, and diaphoresis. Parasympathetic stimulation causes relaxation of the lower esophageal sphincter, an increase in gastric motility, and a pronounced increase in salivation.

Clinical Manifestations

Nausea is a subjective complaint. *Anorexia* (lack of appetite) usually accompanies nausea. When nausea and vomiting are prolonged, dehydration can rapidly occur. Water plus essential electrolytes (e.g., potassium, sodium, chloride, hydrogen) are lost. As vomiting persists, there may be severe electrolyte imbalances, loss of extracellular fluid volume, decreased plasma volume, and eventually circulatory failure. Metabolic alkalosis can result from loss of gastric hydrochloric (HCl) acid. When contents of the small intestine are vomited, metabolic acidosis can occur. However, metabolic acidosis as a result of severe vomiting is less common than metabolic alkalosis. Weight loss resulting from fluid loss is evident in a short time when vomiting is severe.

The threat of pulmonary aspiration is a concern when vomiting occurs in the patient who is elderly, is unconscious, or has other conditions that impair the gag reflex. The patient who cannot adequately manage self-care should be put in a semi-Fowler's or side-lying position to prevent aspiration.

Collaborative Care

The goals of collaborative care are to determine and treat the underlying cause of the nausea and vomiting and to provide symptomatic relief. Determining the cause is often difficult because nausea and vomiting are manifestations of many conditions of the GI tract and other body systems.

A careful history must elicit important information regarding when the vomiting occurs, precipitating factors, and a description of the contents of the emesis. Women are more likely to suffer from nausea and vomiting associated with both surgical procedures and motion sickness.[1]

In all patients, differentiation must be made between vomiting, regurgitation, and projectile vomiting. *Regurgitation* is a process in which partially digested food is slowly brought up from the stomach. Retching or vomiting seldom precedes it. *Projectile vomiting* is a very forceful expulsion of stomach contents without nausea and is characteristic of CNS (brain and spinal cord) tumors.

The presence of fecal odor and bile after prolonged vomiting indicates intestinal obstruction below the level of the pylorus. The presence of bile in the emesis may suggest obstruction below the ampulla of Vater or bile reflux gastritis. The presence of partially digested food several hours after a meal is indicative of gastric outlet obstruction or delay in gastric emptying.

The color of the emesis aids in identifying the presence and source of bleeding. Vomitus with a "coffee ground" appearance is related to gastric bleeding, where blood changes to dark brown as a result of its interaction with HCl acid. Bright red blood indicates active bleeding. This could be due to tears in the mucosal lining of the esophagus (Mallory-Weiss), esophageal varices, gastric or duodenal ulcer, or neoplasm.

The time of day at which the vomiting occurs is often helpful in determining the cause. Early morning vomiting is a frequent

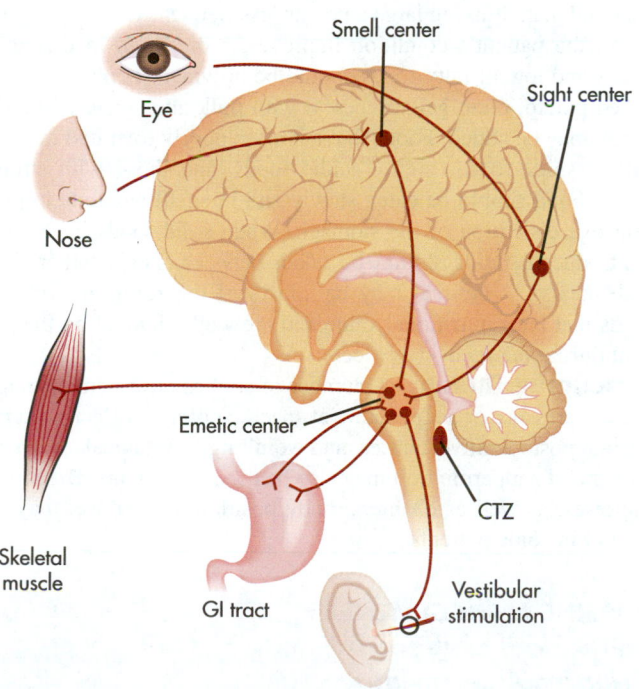

FIG. 42-1   Stimuli involved in the act of vomiting. *CTZ,* Chemoreceptor trigger zone; *GI,* gastrointestinal.

occurrence in pregnancy. Emotional stressors with no evident pathologic disorder may elicit vomiting during or immediately after the ingestion of a meal.

Drug Therapy. The use of drugs in the treatment of nausea and vomiting depends on the cause of the problem. Many different drugs can be used (Table 42-1). Because the cause cannot always be readily determined, drugs must be used with caution. The use of antiemetics before the cause of the vomiting is established can mask the underlying disease process and delay diagnosis and treatment. Many antiemetic drugs act in the CNS at the level of the CTZ. In general, they block the neurochemicals that appear to trigger nausea and vomiting.

Drugs that control nausea and vomiting include anticholinergics (e.g., scopolamine), antihistamines (e.g., promethazine [Phenergan]), phenothiazines (e.g., chlorpromazine [Thorazine], prochlorperazine [Compazine]), and butyrophenones (e.g., droperidol [Inapsine]). Because many of these drugs have anticholinergic actions, they are contraindicated for the patient with glaucoma, prostatic hyperplasia, pyloric or bladder neck obstruction, or biliary obstruction. They share many common side effects, which include dry mouth, hypotension, sedative effects, rashes, and GI disturbances such as constipation. Consultation with a pharmacist may be indicated before administering these drugs to the patient with multiple medical problems who is taking other medications.

Other drugs with antiemetic properties include benzamides such as metoclopramide (Reglan), which acts both centrally and peripherally on dopamine receptors. Peripherally it enhances the release of acetylcholine, resulting in increased gastric emptying. Because of this effect, metoclopramide is considered a *prokinetic* drug. However, about 10% to 20% of patients taking metoclo-

pramide experience CNS side effects ranging from anxiety to hallucinations. Extrapyramidal side effects including tremor and dyskinesias similar to Parkinson's disease may also occur.

Antagonists to specific serotonin (5-HT) receptors act centrally and peripherally to reduce nausea and vomiting. The 5-HT$_3$ receptor antagonists are effective in reducing cancer chemotherapy–induced vomiting, vomiting caused by total body radiation, GI motility disturbances, and nausea and vomiting related to migraine headache and anxiety. They are also used in prevention and treatment of postoperative nausea and vomiting. Examples of 5-HT$_3$ antagonists include ondansetron (Zofran), granisetron (Kytril), and dolasetron (Anzemet).

Dexamethasone (Decadron) is used in the management of cancer chemotherapy–induced emesis, usually in combination with other antiemetics. Dexamethasone alone or in combination with ondansetron reduces both acute and delayed chemotherapy-induced nausea and vomiting. Dronabinol (Marinol) is an orally active cannabinoid. It can be used alone or in combination with other antiemetics for the prevention of chemotherapy-induced emesis. Because of the potential for abuse, as well as CNS side effects including drowsiness and sedation, this drug is used when other therapies are ineffective.

Nutritional Therapy. The patient with severe vomiting requires intravenous (IV) fluid therapy with electrolyte and glucose replacement until able to tolerate oral intake. In some cases a nasogastric (NG) tube and suction are used to decompress the stomach. Once the symptoms have subsided, oral nutrition beginning with clear liquids is started. Extremely hot or cold liquids are not usually well tolerated. Carbonated beverages at room temperature and with the carbonation gone and warm tea are better tolerated. The addition of dry toast or crackers may alleviate the feeling of nausea and help prevent vomiting. Although broth and Gatorade have been used widely for the patient with severe vomiting, these substances are high in sodium and should be administered with caution. Water is the initial fluid of choice for rehydration by mouth. Sipping small amounts of fluid (5 to 15 ml) every 15 to 20 minutes is usually better tolerated than drinking large amounts less frequently.

As the patient's condition improves, a diet high in carbohydrates and low in fatty foods should be provided. Items such as a baked potato, plain gelatin, cereal with milk and sugar, and hard candy may be added. Foods that are often poorly tolerated include coffee, spicy foods, highly acidic foods, and those with strong odors. Food should be eaten slowly and in small amounts to prevent overdistention of the stomach. When solid foods have been reintroduced, fluids should be taken between meals rather than with meals. A dietitian may be consulted regarding appropriate foods that have nutritional value and are well tolerated by the patient during the recovery process.

Nondrug Therapy. A number of studies have demonstrated that acupressure or acupuncture at specific points is effective in reducing postoperative nausea and vomiting.[1] Botanicals such as ginger and peppermint oil may also be used by patients. Breathing exercises, as well as changing body position or exercise, may be helpful in some patients.

NURSING MANAGEMENT
NAUSEA AND VOMITING

■ *Nursing Assessment*

Each patient with a history of prolonged and persistent nausea or vomiting requires a thorough nursing assessment before a specific plan of care is developed. Although the conditions asso-

TABLE 42-1	*DRUG THERAPY* **Nausea and Vomiting**
Classification	**Drug**
Phenothiazine	chlorpromazine (Thorazine)
	perphenazine (Trilafon)
	prochlorperazine (Compazine)
	promazine (Sparine)
	trifluoperazine (Stelazine)
	triflupromazine (Vesprin)
Antihistamine	buclizine (Bucladin-S)
	cyclizine (Marezine)
	dimenhydrinate (Dramamine)
	hydroxyzine (Vistaril)
	meclizine (Antivert, Bonine)
	promethazine (Phenergan)
Prokinetic	domperidone (Motilium)
	metoclopramide (Reglan)
Serotonin antagonist	dolasetron (Anzemet)
	granisetron (Kytril)
	ondansetron (Zofran)
	palonosetron (Aloxi)
Anticholinergic	scopolamine transdermal (Transderm Scōp)
Butyrophenone	droperidol (Inapsine)
Others	benzquinamide (Emete-Con)
	dexamethasone (Decadron)
	diphenidol (Vontrol)
	dronabinol (Marinol)
	thiethylperazine (Torecan)
	trimethobenzamide (Tigan)
	aprepitant (Emend)
	nabilone (Cesamet)

ciated with nausea and vomiting are numerous, the nurse should have a basic understanding of the more common conditions and should be able to identify the patient who is at high risk. Knowledge of the physiologic mechanisms involved in nausea and vomiting is important to the assessment process. Table 42-2 presents subjective and objective data that is obtained from a patient with nausea and vomiting, regardless of the underlying cause.

■ Nursing Diagnoses

Nursing diagnoses for the patient with nausea and vomiting may include, but are not limited to, those presented in NCP 42-1.

■ Planning

The overall goals are that the patient with nausea and vomiting will (1) experience minimal or no nausea and vomiting, (2) have normal electrolyte levels and hydration status, and (3) return to a normal pattern of fluid balance and nutrient intake.

■ Nursing Implementation

Acute Intervention. The majority of individuals with nausea and vomiting can be managed at home. However, when nausea and vomiting persist regardless of home treatment strategies, hospitalization may be necessary for diagnosis of the underlying problem. Until a diagnosis is confirmed, the patient is kept on nothing-by-mouth (NPO) status and given IV fluids. An NG tube connected to suction may be necessary for the patient with persistent vomiting, as well as for the patient in whom the possible diagnosis may be

bowel obstruction or paralytic ileus. Keeping the stomach empty reduces the stimulus to vomit. The NG tube is secured to prevent its movement in the nose and back of the throat because this can stimulate nausea and vomiting.

With prolonged vomiting, there is a probability of dehydration and acid-base and electrolyte imbalances. The nurse records intake and output, monitors vital signs, assesses for signs of dehydration, positions the patient to prevent aspiration, and observes for changes in the patient's physical comfort and mentation. The nurse provides physical and emotional support; maintains a quiet, odor-free environment; and gives explanations regarding diagnostic tests or procedures performed.

Ambulatory and Home Care. The patient and family need instructions on (1) how to manage the unpleasant sensation of nausea, (2) methods of preventing nausea and vomiting, and (3) strategies to maintain fluid and nutritional intake. The occurrence of nausea or vomiting may be minimized if measures are taken to keep the immediate environment quiet, free of noxious odors, and well ventilated. The avoidance of sudden changes of position and unnecessary activity is also helpful. Use of relaxation techniques, frequent rest periods, and diversional tactics may help prevent nausea and vomiting or facilitate recovery from their effects. Cleansing the face and hands with a cool washcloth and mouth care between episodes increase the person's comfort level. When the symptoms occur, all foods and drugs should be stopped until the acute phase is past.

If a medication is suspected as the cause, the health care provider should be notified immediately so that either the dosage can be altered or a new drug prescribed. The patient is reminded that stopping the drug without consulting the health care provider may eliminate the immediate cause of the nausea and vomiting but that omission of the prescribed drug may have detrimental effects on health or the disease state.

When food is identified as the precipitating cause of nausea and vomiting, the nurse helps the patient identify the specific food. In addition, when it was eaten, prior history with that food, and whether anyone else in the family is sick are also important to identify.

Patients may be reluctant to resume fluid intake due to fear of nausea recurring and may need encouragement. When the patient

TABLE 42-2	**NURSING ASSESSMENT** **Nausea and Vomiting**

Subjective Data
Important Health Information
Past health history: GI disorders, chronic indigestion, food allergies, pregnancy, infection, CNS disorders, recent travel, bulimia, metabolic disorders, cancer, cardiovascular disease, renal disease
Medications: Use of antiemetics, digitalis, opioids, ferrous sulfate, aspirin, aminophylline, alcohol, antibiotics; general anesthesia; chemotherapy
Surgery or other treatments: Recent surgery

Functional Health Patterns
Nutritional-metabolic: Amount, frequency, character, and color of vomitus; dry heaves; anorexia; weight loss
Activity-exercise: Weakness, fatigue
Cognitive-perceptual: Abdominal tenderness or pain
Coping–stress tolerance: Stress, fear

Objective Data
General
Lethargy, sunken eyeballs

Integumentary
Pallor, dry mucous membranes, poor skin turgor

Gastrointestinal
Amount, frequency, character (e.g., projectile), content (undigested food, blood, bile, feces), and color of vomitus (red, "coffee ground," green-yellow)

Urinary
Decreased output, concentrated urine

Possible Findings
Altered serum electrolytes (especially hypokalemia), metabolic alkalosis, abnormal upper GI findings on endoscopy or abdominal x-rays

CNS, Central nervous system; *GI,* gastrointestinal.

COMPLEMENTARY AND ALTERNATIVE THERAPIES
Ginger

Clinical Uses
- Nausea and vomiting of pregnancy*
- Nausea and vomiting (postoperative or chemotherapy induced), motion sickness†

Effects
- Antiemetic and antiinflammatory. Has analgesic and sedative effects on gastrointestinal motility.

Nursing Implications
- Large doses may interfere with cardiac, antidiabetic, or anticoagulant therapy. Patients with gallstones should consult a health care practitioner before use.

Ulbricht CE, Basch EM: *Natural standard herb and supplement reference: evidence-based clinical reviews,* St Louis, 2005, Mosby.
www.naturalstandard.com.
*Good scientific evidence exists for its use.
†Unclear scientific evidence exists for its use.

NURSING CARE PLAN 42-1

Patient with Nausea and Vomiting

NURSING DIAGNOSIS   **Nausea** *related to* multiple etiologies *as evidenced by* episodes of nausea and vomiting

PATIENT GOAL   Reports minimal or no nausea and vomiting

OUTCOMES (NOC)	INTERVENTIONS (NIC) and *RATIONALES*
Nausea and Vomiting Control	**Nausea Management**
• Recognizes precipitating stimuli ____ • Uses preventive measures ____ • Uses antiemetic medications appropriately ____ • Reports nausea, retching, and vomiting controlled ____ **Measurement Scale** 1 = Never demonstrated 2 = Rarely demonstrated 3 = Sometimes demonstrated 4 = Often demonstrated 5 = Consistently demonstrated	• Perform complete assessment of nausea, including frequency, duration, severity, and precipitating factors, *to plan appropriate interventions.* • Reduce or eliminate personal factors that precipitate or increase the nausea (anxiety, fear, fatigue, and lack of knowledge) *to avoid precipitating factors of nausea/vomiting.* • Use frequent oral hygiene, unless it stimulates nausea, *to promote comfort.* • Ensure that effective antiemetic drugs are given when possible *to prevent nausea and vomiting.* • Teach the use of nonpharmacologic techniques (e.g., relaxation, guided imagery, music therapy, distraction, acupressure) *to manage nausea and vomiting.* • Promote adequate rest and sleep *to facilitate nausea relief.*

NURSING DIAGNOSIS   **Deficient fluid volume** *related to* prolonged vomiting and inability to ingest, digest, or absorb food and fluids *as evidenced by* decreased urine output and increased urine concentration, increased pulse rate, hypotension (postural), decreased intake, decreased skin turgor, dry skin and mucous membranes

PATIENT GOAL   Achieves normal fluid and electrolyte balance

OUTCOMES (NOC)	INTERVENTIONS (NIC) and *RATIONALES*
Fluid Balance	**Fluid/Electrolyte Management**
• Blood pressure ____ • Radial pulse rate ____ • Stable body weight ____ • Skin turgor ____ • Moist mucous membranes ____ • Serum electrolytes ____ **Measurement Scale** 1 = Severely compromised 2 = Substantially compromised 3 = Moderately compromised 4 = Mildly compromised 5 = Not compromised	• Assess the patient's buccal membranes, sclera, and skin for indications of altered fluid and electrolyte balance (e.g., dryness, cyanosis) *to plan appropriate interventions.* • Keep an accurate record of intake and output daily *to monitor trends and to accurately monitor fluid balance.* • Weigh patient daily *to monitor trends.* • Give fluids *to maintain fluid and electrolyte balance.* • Obtain laboratory specimens for monitoring of altered fluid or electrolyte levels (e.g., hematocrit, BUN, protein, sodium, and potassium levels) *to identify fluid and electrolyte imbalance.*

NURSING DIAGNOSIS   **Imbalanced nutrition: less than body requirements** *related to* nausea and vomiting *as evidenced by* lack of interest in or aversion to food, perceived or actual inability to ingest food, weight loss

PATIENT GOAL   Maintains body weight with adequate intake of nutrients

OUTCOMES (NOC)	INTERVENTIONS (NIC) and *RATIONALES*
Nutritional Status	**Nausea Management**
• Weight/height ratio ____ • Nutrient intake ____ • Food intake ____ • Fluid intake ____ • Hydration ____ **Measurement Scale** 1 = Severe deviation from normal range 2 = Substantial deviation from normal range 3 = Moderate deviation from normal range 4 = Slight deviation from normal range 5 = No deviation from normal range	• Provide information about the nausea, such as causes of the nausea and how long it will last. • Monitor recorded intake for nutritional content and calories *to evaluate nutritional status.* • Encourage eating small amounts of food that are appealing to the nauseated person. • Give cold, clear liquid and odorless and colorless food *to avoid irritating the stomach and initiating recurrence of nausea and vomiting.* **Nutrition Therapy** • Assist patient to select soft, bland, and nonacidic foods *to avoid irritating the stomach.*

believes some foods and fluids can be tolerated, the nurse might suggest that it would be helpful to begin with clear liquids or cola beverages, Gatorade, tea or broth, dry crackers or toast, and then plain gelatin. Bland foods, such as pasta, rice, and cooked chicken, are generally well tolerated in small amounts. An antiemetic drug is taken only if prescribed by the health care provider. Taking over-the-counter (OTC) drugs for relief of symptoms may make the problem worse.

Evaluation

The expected outcomes are that the patient with nausea and vomiting will

- be comfortable with minimal or no nausea and vomiting
- have electrolyte levels within normal range
- be able to maintain adequate intake of fluids and nutrients
- maintain body weight

GERONTOLOGIC CONSIDERATIONS
NAUSEA AND VOMITING

The older patient experiencing nausea and vomiting requires careful assessment and monitoring, particularly during periods of fluid loss and subsequent rehydration therapy. Older patients are more likely to have cardiac or renal insufficiency that places them at greater risk for life-threatening fluid and electrolyte imbalances. In addition, excessive replacement of fluid and electrolytes may result in adverse consequences for the elderly person who has heart failure or renal disease. Finally, the older adult with a decreased level of consciousness may be at high risk for aspiration of vomitus. Close monitoring of the patient's physical status and level of consciousness during episodes of vomiting is important.

In addition, the elderly are particularly susceptible to the CNS side effects of antiemetic drugs; these drugs may produce confusion. Dosages should be reduced and efficacy closely evaluated. Safety precautions also should be instituted for these patients.

UPPER GASTROINTESTINAL BLEEDING

In the United States there are approximately 150,000 to 200,000 hospital admissions each year for upper GI bleeding.[2] Despite advances in intensive care, hemodynamic monitoring, and endoscopy, there has been little change in the mortality rate for upper GI bleeding, which has remained at approximately 6% to 10% for the past 40 years. This is due in part to the greater incidence of upper GI bleeding in older adults, especially women, related to the use of nonsteroidal antiinflammatory drugs (NSAIDs).

Etiology and Pathophysiology

Although the most serious loss of blood from the upper GI tract is characterized by a sudden onset, insidious occult bleeding can also be a major problem. The severity of bleeding depends on whether the origin is venous, capillary, or arterial. (Types of upper GI bleeding are shown in Table 42-3.) Bleeding from an arterial source is profuse, and the blood is bright red. The bright red color indicates that the blood has not been in contact with the stomach's acid secretions. In contrast, "coffee ground" vomitus reveals that the blood and other contents have been in the stomach for some time and have been changed by contact with gastric secretions. A

TABLE 42-3	Types of Upper Gastrointestinal Bleeding	
Type	**Clinical Manifestations**	
Obvious Bleeding		
Hematemesis	Bloody vomitus appearing as fresh, bright red blood or "coffee ground" appearance (dark, grainy digested blood)	
Melena	Black, tarry stools (often foul smelling) caused by digestion of blood in the GI tract. The black appearance is from the presence of iron	
Occult Bleeding	Small amounts of blood in gastric secretions, vomitus, or stools not apparent by appearance; detectable by guaiac test	

TABLE 42-4	Common Causes of Upper Gastrointestinal Bleeding	
Drug Induced	**Stomach and Duodenum**	
Corticosteroids	Gastric cancer	
Nonsteroidal antiinflammatory drugs (NSAIDs)	Hemorrhagic gastritis	
Salicylates	Peptic ulcer disease	
	Polyps	
Esophagus	Stress-related mucosal disease	
Esophageal varices	**Systemic Diseases**	
Esophagitis	Blood dyscrasias (e.g., leukemia, aplastic anemia)	
Mallory-Weiss tear	Renal failure (uremia)	

massive upper GI hemorrhage is generally defined as a loss of more than 1500 ml of blood or a loss of 25% of intravascular blood volume. *Melena* (black, tarry stools) indicates slow bleeding from an upper GI source. The longer the passage of blood through the intestines, the darker the stool color, due to the breakdown of hemoglobin and the release of iron.

Discovering the cause of the bleeding is not always easy. A variety of areas in the GI tract may be involved. Table 42-4 lists the common causes of bleeding. Although systemic diseases (e.g., leukemia, blood dyscrasias) that interfere with normal blood clotting must be considered whenever upper GI bleeding occurs, the most common sites are the esophagus, stomach, and duodenum.

Esophageal Origin. Bleeding from the esophagus is most likely due to chronic esophagitis, **Mallory-Weiss tear** (a tear in the mucosa near the esophagogastric junction), or esophageal varices. Chronic esophagitis can be caused by gastroesophageal reflux disease (GERD), the ingestion of drugs irritating to the mucosa, alcohol, and smoking cigarettes. A Mallory-Weiss tear is most often related to severe retching and vomiting.

Esophageal varices usually occur secondary to cirrhosis of the liver. Branches of the vena cava and the azygos vein from the systemic circulation converge with the smaller vessels of the lower esophagus. These vessels are inelastic and become engorged and tortuous because of increased pressure exerted on them secondary to portal hypertension. Anything that may increase the pressure (e.g., coughing, sneezing, trauma) or cause mechanical irritation (e.g., vomiting, irritation, erosion) may re-

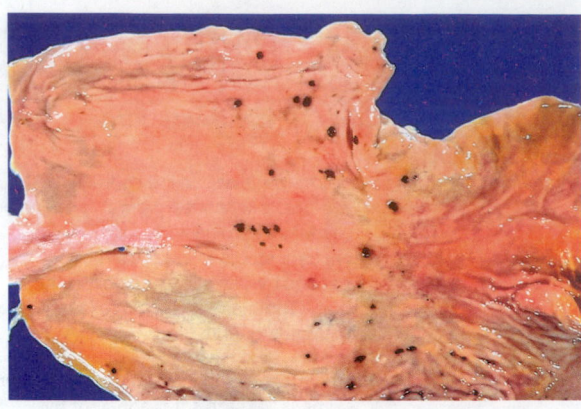

FIG. 42-2 Multiple stress ulcers of the stomach, highlighted by dark digested blood on their surfaces.

sult in sudden, massive bleeding. (Esophageal varices are discussed in Chapter 44.)

Stomach and Duodenal Origin. Bleeding ulcers account for 50% of the cases of upper GI bleeding.[2] Erosion of a blood vessel by a gastric or duodenal ulcer is always considered as a possible cause of upper GI bleeding. Most bleeding ulcers are related to the presence of *Helicobacter pylori* or drug use (NSAIDs).

Drugs, either prescribed by the health care provider or OTC, are a major cause of upper GI bleeding. For example, the patient who regularly takes aspirin or aspirin-containing compounds may be at risk for bleeding episodes. Aspirin, NSAIDs (e.g., ibuprofen), and corticosteroids can cause irritation and disruption of the gastric mucosal barrier. Many OTC preparations contain aspirin. It is not unusual for a patient to deny the use of aspirin yet be self-medicating with aspirin-containing drugs, such as Alka-Seltzer, Bufferin, and Excedrin. A careful history of all commonly used drugs is necessary whenever upper GI bleeding is suspected.

Stress-related mucosal disease (SRMD), also called *physiologic stress ulcers,* occurs in patients who have sustained severe burns or trauma or had major surgery. In SRMD there is erosion of more superficial blood vessels than with peptic ulcer disease (Fig. 42-2). Mucosal injury is found in approximately 70% to 90% of intensive care unit (ICU) patients.[3] Less common causes of upper GI bleeding include tumors and vascular lesions. Gastric cancer causes steady blood loss as it grows and ulcerates through the mucosa and blood vessels located in its path.

Emergency Assessment and Management

Although approximately 80% to 85% of patients who have massive hemorrhage spontaneously stop bleeding, the cause must be identified and treatment initiated immediately. A complete history of events leading to the bleeding episode is deferred until emergency care has been initiated. The immediate physical examination includes a systemic evaluation of the patient's condition with emphasis on blood pressure (BP), rate and character of pulse, peripheral perfusion with capillary refill, and observation for the presence or absence of neck vein distention. Vital signs are monitored every 15 to 30 minutes. Signs and symptoms of shock are evaluated, and treatment is started as soon as possible (see Chapter 67). The patient's respiratory status is carefully assessed, along with a thorough abdominal examination. The pres-

ence or absence of bowel sounds should be assessed and noted. A tense, rigid, boardlike abdomen may indicate a perforation and peritonitis.

Once the immediate interventions have begun, the patient or family should answer the following questions. Is there a history of previous bleeding episodes? Has weight loss been a recent problem? Has the patient received blood transfusions in the past, and were there any transfusion reactions? Are there any other illnesses (e.g., liver disease, cirrhosis) or medications that may contribute to bleeding or interfere with treatment? Is there a religious preference that prohibits the use of blood or blood products?

Laboratory studies are ordered, including a complete blood count (CBC), blood urea nitrogen (BUN), serum electrolytes, blood glucose, prothrombin time, liver enzymes, arterial blood gases (ABGs), and a type and crossmatch for possible blood transfusions. All vomitus and stools are tested for gross and occult blood. A urinalysis including specific gravity provides information on the patient's hydration status.

IV lines, preferably two, with a 16- or 18-gauge needle are placed for fluid and blood replacement. The type and amount of fluids infused are dictated by physical and laboratory findings. It is generally best to begin with an isotonic crystalloid solution (e.g., lactated Ringer's solution). Whole blood, packed red blood cells (RBCs), and fresh frozen plasma may be used for replacement of volume in massive hemorrhage. Because of the potential for fluid overload and immunologic reactions, packed RBCs are often preferred over whole blood. (The use of blood transfusions and volume expanders is discussed in Chapter 31.) The hemoglobin and hematocrit values are not of immediate help in estimating the degree of blood loss, but they provide a baseline for guiding further treatment. The initial hematocrit may be normal and may not reflect the loss until 4 to 6 hours after fluid replacement has taken place, since initially the loss of plasma and RBCs is equal. When upper GI bleeding is less profuse, infusion of isotonic saline solution followed by packed RBCs permits restoration of the hematocrit more quickly and does not create complications related to fluid volume overload. The use of supplemental oxygen delivered by face mask or nasal cannula may help increase blood oxygen saturation.

For most patients who are bleeding profusely, an indwelling urinary catheter is inserted so that urine volume can be accurately assessed hourly. A central venous pressure line may be inserted so that the patient's fluid volume status can be monitored easily. If the patient has a history of valvular heart disease, coronary artery disease, or heart failure, a pulmonary artery catheter may be necessary to monitor the patient.

Before performing endoscopy, some endoscopists prefer lavage to provide a clearer view, whereas others prefer to perform endoscopy immediately to avoid delays in treatment. For lavage, a nasogastric (NG) or an orogastric tube is placed and room temperature water or saline is used. Passage through the mouth is easier, but no tube should ever be advanced against resistance because of the likelihood of damaging the gastric mucosa or causing perforation. Aspiration of stomach contents through a large-bore tube such as an Ewald tube facilitates the removal of clots from the stomach and alleviates the patient's need to vomit. Lavage allows for better endoscopic visualization of the gastric mucosa.[4] Several techniques have been developed, including the two-syringe Easi-Lav Code Blue Kit (Ballard Medical).

Diagnostic Studies

Endoscopy is the primary tool for diagnosing the source of upper GI bleeding. When a skilled practitioner performs the procedure, bleeding from severe gastritis can be easily distinguished from that of a gastric or duodenal ulcer or esophageal and gastric varices.

Angiography is used in diagnosing upper GI bleeding only when endoscopy cannot be done. It is an invasive procedure requiring preparation and setup time and may not be appropriate for a high-risk, unstable patient. In this procedure a catheter is placed into the left gastric or superior mesenteric artery and advanced until the site of bleeding is discovered.

Barium contrast studies have limited use in the identification of major bleeding sites during the acute phase of treatment. After the acute bleeding phase, barium studies can document an actual lesion but cannot verify that it is the bleeding source.

Collaborative Care

Endoscopic Therapy. The goal of endoscopic hemostasis is to coagulate or thrombose the bleeding vessel. Endoscopic therapy can be useful to stop bleeding in patients with severe gastritis, Mallory-Weiss tear, esophageal and gastric varices, bleeding peptic ulcers, and polyps. Several techniques are used, including (1) thermal (heat) probe, (2) multipolar and bipolar electrocoagulation probe, (3) argon plasma coagulation (APC), and (4) neodymium:yttrium-aluminum-garnet (Nd:YAG) laser. Multipolar electrocoagulation and thermal probe are the two most commonly used procedures. The heat probe coagulates tissue by directly applying a heating element to the bleeding site. The APC is a noncontact coagulation that delivers monopolar current to tissue. For variceal bleeding, other strategies include variceal ligation, injection sclerotherapy, and balloon tamponade (see Chapter 44). Overall, endoscopic therapy is more effective than medical management alone in reducing bleeding episodes.

Surgical Therapy. Surgical intervention is indicated when bleeding continues regardless of the therapy provided and when the site of the bleeding has been identified. A high percentage of patients are known to have another massive hemorrhage within 5 years after the first bleeding episode. Some physicians regard surgical therapy as necessary when the patient continues to bleed after rapid transfusion of up to 2000 ml of whole blood or remains in shock after 24 hours. The site of the hemorrhage determines the choice of operation. In addition, the surgeon must consider the age of the patient because mortality rates increase considerably in those over 60 years of age.

Drug Therapy. During the acute phase, drugs are used to decrease bleeding, decrease HCl acid secretion, and neutralize the HCl acid that is present. Injection therapy with epinephrine (1:10,000 dilution) during endoscopy is effective for acute hemostasis. Epinephrine produces tissue edema and, ultimately, pressure on the source of bleeding. To prevent rebleeding, injection therapy is often combined with other therapies (e.g., thermocoagulation or laser treatment).

For variceal bleeding, vasopressin (Pitressin), which is posterior pituitary extract, is used to produce vasoconstriction. It is used to treat upper GI bleeding in those patients who do not respond to other therapies and are poor surgical risks. It is administered systemically through a vein or intraarterially at the local site of actual bleeding.

Side effects of IV vasopressin include decreased myocardial contractility and decreased coronary blood flow. The patient undergoing vasopressin therapy is closely monitored for its myocardial, visceral, and peripheral ischemic side effects. Vasopressin is used cautiously in the patient with a known history of vascular disease.

Efforts are made to reduce acid secretion because the acidic environment can alter platelet function, as well as interfere with clot stabilization. Histamine$_2$-receptor (H$_2$R) blockers (e.g., cimetidine [Tagamet]) or proton pump inhibitors (PPIs) (e.g., pantoprazole [Protonix]) are administered intravenously to decrease acid secretion. Table 42-5 reviews the mechanism of action of H$_2$R blockers and PPIs. Although these drugs have no proven ability to control active bleeding, they have become part of standard treatment protocols.

In patients with upper GI bleeding, early administration of the somatostatin analog octreotide (Sandostatin) may be used. The drug reduces splanchnic blood flow, as well as acid secretion. This drug is given in IV boluses up to 5 to 6 days after the initiation of bleeding.

Antacids neutralize HCl acid and continue to be used as an adjunct therapy for peptic ulcer disease and GERD. Because antacids neutralize HCl acid and increase the pH of gastric contents to above 5, there is inhibition of the conversion of pepsinogen to its active form pepsin. The most frequently used antacid preparations are magnesium hydroxide, magnesium trisilicate, aluminum hydroxide, calcium carbonate, and sodium bicarbonate (see Table 42-21 later in this chapter). Aluminum hydroxide and magnesium trisilicate are the most useful because they are nonabsorbable. Calcium carbonate and sodium bicarbonate are absorbable, and prolonged use can lead to systemic alkalosis.

Sedatives to control agitation and restlessness should be administered cautiously. They make accurate assessment of the patient's condition more difficult. Anticholinergic drugs are contraindicated in acute upper GI bleeding episodes.

NURSING MANAGEMENT
UPPER GASTROINTESTINAL BLEEDING

■ Nursing Assessment

As the nurse begins care of the patient admitted with upper GI bleeding, a thorough and accurate nursing assessment is an essential first step. Subjective and objective data that should be obtained from the patient or significant others are presented in Table 42-6.

The patient experiencing upper GI bleeding may not be able to provide specific information about the cause of the bleeding until the immediate physical needs are met. An immediate nursing assessment is performed while getting the patient ready for initial treatment. The assessment includes the patient's level of consciousness, vital signs, appearance of neck veins, skin color, and capillary refill. The abdomen is checked for distention, guarding, and peristalsis. Immediate determination of vital signs indicates whether the patient is in shock from blood loss and also provides a baseline BP and pulse by which to monitor the progress of treatment. Signs and symptoms of shock include low BP; rapid, weak pulse; increased thirst; cold, clammy skin; and restlessness. Vital signs are monitored every 15 to 30 minutes, and the health care provider is informed of any significant changes.

TABLE 42-5	DRUG THERAPY Gastrointestinal Bleeding	
Drug	**Source of GI Bleeding**	**Mechanism of Action**
Antacids*	Duodenal ulcer, gastric ulcer, acute gastritis (corrosive, erosive, and hemorrhagic)	Neutralizes acid and maintains gastric pH above 5.5; elevated pH inhibits activation of pepsinogen
H₂-receptor blockers cimetidine (Tagamet) famotidine (Pepcid) nizatidine (Axid) ranitidine (Zantac)	Duodenal ulcer, gastric ulcer, esophagitis, acute gastritis (especially hemorrhagic)	Inhibits action of histamine at H_2 receptors on parietal cells and decreases HCl acid secretion
Proton pump inhibitors esomeprazole (Nexium) lansoprazole (Prevacid) omeprazole (Prilosec) pantoprazole (Protonix) rabeprazole (Aciphex)	Duodenal ulcer, gastric ulcer, acute gastritis (corrosive, erosive, and hemorrhagic)	Suppresses gastric secretion by inhibiting H^+, K^+, ATPase enzyme system in gastric parietal cells; inhibits the gastric acid pump, which is necessary for secretion of HCl acid
vasopressin (Pitressin)	Esophageal varices	Causes vasoconstriction and increases smooth muscle activity of the GI tract; reduces pressure in the portal circulation and arrests bleeding
octreotide (Sandostatin)	Upper gastrointestinal bleeding, esophageal varices	Somatostatin analog that decreases splanchnic blood flow; decreases HCl acid secretion via decrease in release of gastrin
epinephrine	Bleeding due to ulceration	Injection during endoscopy produces hemostasis; causes tissue edema and pressure on the source of bleeding; injection therapy is often combined with other therapies (e.g., laser)

*See Table 42-21.

When obtaining vital signs, the nurse considers the patient's age and physical condition. Orthostatic vital signs should be obtained. The older the patient, the more changes in vital signs should be expected.

■ Nursing Diagnoses

Nursing diagnoses for the patient with upper GI bleeding include, but are not limited to, the following:

- Fluid volume deficit *related to* acute loss of blood, as well as gastric secretions
- Ineffective tissue perfusion *related to* loss of circulatory volume
- Anxiety *related to* upper GI bleeding, hospitalization, uncertain outcome, source of bleeding
- Ineffective coping *related to* situational crisis and personal vulnerability
- Risk for aspiration *related to* active bleeding and altered level of consciousness
- Decreased cardiac output *related to* loss of blood

■ Planning

The overall goals are that the patient with upper GI bleeding will (1) have no further GI bleeding, (2) have the cause of the bleeding identified and treated, (3) experience a return to a normal hemodynamic state, and (4) experience minimal or no symptoms of pain or anxiety.

■ Nursing Implementation

Health Promotion. Although not all cases of upper GI bleeding can be anticipated and prevented, the nurse shares responsibility with the health care provider in identifying patients at high risk. The patient with a history of chronic gastritis or peptic ulcer disease is always considered in the high-risk category because of the increased incidence of bleeding associated with chronic irritation or chronic ulcers. The patient who has had one major bleeding episode is more likely to have another bleed. Patients with cirrhosis and those with previous upper GI bleeding from varices are also at high risk. The at-risk patient is instructed to avoid gastric irritants such as alcohol and smoking, to prevent or decrease stress-inducing situations at home or at work, and to take only prescribed medications. OTC drugs can be harmful because they may contain ingredients (e.g., aspirin) that have potentially irritating effects on the mucosa. The patient is instructed in the methods of testing vomitus or stools for the presence of occult blood. Positive results should be promptly reported to the health care provider or the nurse.

The patient who requires regular administration of ulcerogenic drugs, such as aspirin, corticosteroids, or NSAIDs, needs instruction regarding the potential adverse effects related to GI bleeding. If possible, these drugs are avoided. However, if aspirin must be prescribed, enteric-coated tablets can be substituted for regular tablets. Taking the drugs with meals or snacks lessens the potential irritating effects. The coadministration of an NSAID with a PPI can reduce bleeding risk. For the patient at risk for gastric ulcers because of NSAID use, misoprostol (Cytotec) may also be prescribed. This prostaglandin analog inhibits acid secretion and reduces upper GI bleeding episodes associated with NSAID use. However, the drug has important side effects, including uterine cramping in women and diarrhea. Because of its effects on the uterus, it is contraindicated in women who are pregnant or of childbearing age and not using contraception.

When the nurse is working with the patient who has a history of liver cirrhosis with esophageal varices, the instructions must be specific regarding the importance of avoiding known irritants, such as alcohol and smoking. The prompt treatment of an upper respiratory tract infection should be stressed. Severe coughing or sneez-

TABLE 42-6	*NURSING ASSESSMENT* **Upper Gastrointestinal Bleeding**

Subjective Data
Important Health Information
Past health history: Precipitating events before bleeding episode, previous bleeding episodes and treatment, peptic ulcer disease, esophageal varices, esophagitis, acute and chronic gastritis, stress-related mucosal disease
Medications: Use of aspirin, nonsteroidal antiinflammatory drugs, corticosteroids, anticoagulants

Functional Health Patterns
Health perception–health management: Family history of bleeding, smoking, alcohol use
Nutritional-metabolic: Nausea, vomiting, weight loss; thirst
Elimination: Diarrhea; black, tarry stools; decreased urinary output; sweating
Activity-exercise: Weakness, dizziness, fainting
Cognitive-perceptual: Epigastric pain, abdominal cramps
Coping–stress tolerance: Acute or chronic stressors

Objective Data
General
Fever

Integumentary
Clammy, cool, pale skin; pale mucous membranes, nail beds, and conjunctivae; spider angiomas; jaundice; peripheral edema

Respiratory
Rapid, shallow respirations

Cardiovascular
Tachycardia, weak pulse, orthostatic hypotension, slow capillary refill

Gastrointestinal
Red or "coffee ground" vomitus; tense, rigid abdomen, ascites; hypoactive or hyperactive bowel sounds; black, tarry stools

Urinary
Decreased urinary output, concentrated urine

Neurologic
Agitation, restlessness; decreasing level of consciousness

Possible Findings
↓ Hematocrit and hemoglobin; hematuria; guaiac-positive stools, emesis, or gastric aspirate; ↓ levels of clotting factors; ↑ liver enzymes; abnormal upper GI studies or endoscopy results

per hour indicates adequate renal perfusion. Lesser amounts may indicate renal ischemia secondary to hypovolemia. Urine specific gravity is measured because it provides information about the patient's hydration status. Consistent readings greater than 1.025 (normal is 1.005 to 1.025) indicate that the urine is extremely concentrated and that there is probably a low blood volume. The health care provider must be kept informed of these important results so that the IV solutions can be increased or decreased accordingly. If the patient has a central venous pressure line or pulmonary artery catheter in place, readings should be recorded every 1 to 2 hours. Hemodynamic monitoring provides an accurate and quick assessment of blood flow and pressure within the cardiovascular system (see Chapter 66).

The older adult or the patient with a history of cardiovascular problems is observed closely for signs of fluid overload. However, volume overload and pulmonary edema are concerns in all patients who are receiving large amounts of IV fluids within a short time. Auscultation of breath sounds and close observation of respiratory effort are important. Electrocardiographic (ECG) monitoring is also used to evaluate cardiac function.

Foods such as beets or even swallowed mouthwash can give vomitus a bloody appearance. Unless the contents of the vomitus are checked for occult blood, false information may be recorded. Swallowed blood from a nosebleed must also be noted to avoid misdiagnosis of an upper GI bleeding episode. When an NG tube is inserted, the nurse must pay special attention to keeping it in proper position and observing the aspirate for blood.

The majority of upper GI bleeding episodes cease spontaneously, even without intervention. Although the use of room temperature, cool, or iced gastric lavage is used in some institutions, its effectiveness as a treatment for upper GI bleeding is questionable. When lavage is used, approximately 50 to 100 ml of fluid is instilled at a time into the stomach. The lavage fluid may be aspirated from the stomach or drained by gravity. When aspiration is the method used, it is important not to aspirate if resistance is felt. The tip of the NG tube may be up against the gastric mucosal lining. The pressure from attempts to aspirate may cause injury to the mucosa. When resistance is a factor, gravity is used as the method of drainage. Close monitoring of vital signs, especially in the patient with cardiovascular disease, is important because dysrhythmias may occur. Keeping the head of the bed elevated provides comfort and prevents possible aspiration.

The nurse caring for a patient with upper GI bleeding assesses the stools for blood. Black, tarry stools are not usually associated with a brisk hemorrhage but are indicative of the presence of bleeding of prolonged duration. Bright red blood (*hematochezia*) in the stool is usually from a source in the lower bowel. Menses and bleeding hemorrhoids should be ruled out as possible sources of blood in the stools. When vomitus contains blood but the stool contains no gross or occult blood, the hemorrhage is considered to have been of short duration.

Monitoring the patient's laboratory studies enables the nurse to estimate the effectiveness of therapy. The hemoglobin and hematocrit are usually evaluated about every 4 to 6 hours if the patient is actively bleeding. At first the hematocrit level may not accurately reflect the amount of blood lost or the amount of blood replaced and will appear falsely high or low. The patient's BUN level is assessed. During a significant hemorrhage blood proteins are broken down by GI tract bacteria, resulting in elevated BUN levels. However, hypoperfusion to the kidneys, as well as renal disease, may also result in elevated BUN levels. Many patients re-

ing can create increased pressure on the already fragile varices and may result in massive hemorrhage (see Chapter 44).

The patient who is known to have blood dyscrasias (e.g., aplastic anemia) or liver dysfunction or who is taking cancer chemotherapeutic drugs has a potential bleeding problem because of altered hemostasis caused by a decrease in clotting factors and platelets. When these patients also have a history of ulcer disease, gastritis, varices, or drug and alcohol abuse, they should be carefully instructed regarding their disease process and drugs, and they should be closely observed for bleeding.

Acute Intervention. The patient should be approached in a calm and assured manner to help decrease the level of anxiety. Caution should be used before administering sedatives for restlessness because it is one of the warning signs of shock and may be masked by the drugs.

Once an infusion has been started, the IV line must be maintained for fluid or blood replacement. An accurate intake and output record is essential so that the patient's hydration status can be assessed. Urine output should be measured hourly. A rate of at least 0.5 ml/kg

ceive oxygen by mask or nasally to ensure that the circulating blood has an adequate oxygen content.

When oral nourishment is begun, the patient is observed for symptoms of nausea and vomiting and a recurrence of bleeding. Feedings initially consist of clear fluids or milk and are given hourly until tolerance is determined. These feedings help neutralize the gastric secretions and assist in the mucosal repair. Gradual introduction of foods follows if the patient exhibits no signs of discomfort.

The patient in whom hemorrhage was the result of chronic alcohol abuse requires close observation for delirium tremens as withdrawal from alcohol takes place. Symptoms indicating the beginning of delirium tremens are agitation, uncontrolled shaking, sweating, and vivid hallucinations. (Alcohol withdrawal is discussed in Chapter 12.)

Ambulatory and Home Care. The patient and family are taught how to avoid future bleeding episodes. Ulcer disease, drug or alcohol abuse, and liver and respiratory diseases can all result in upper GI bleeding. The patient and family must be made aware of the consequences of noncompliance with diet and drug therapy. It must be emphasized that no drugs (especially aspirin, NSAIDs) other than those prescribed by the health care provider should be taken. Smoking and alcohol should be eliminated because they are sources of irritation and interfere with tissue repair. The need for long-term follow-up care may be necessary because of possible recurrence. The patient and family should be instructed on what to do if an acute hemorrhage occurs in the future.

■ **Evaluation**

The expected outcomes are that the patient with upper GI bleeding will

- have no upper GI bleeding
- maintain normal fluid volume
- experience a return to a normal hemodynamic state
- experience absence or tolerable levels of pain and be comfortable
- understand potential etiologic factors and make appropriate lifestyle modifications

ORAL INFLAMMATIONS AND INFECTIONS

Oral infections and inflammations may be specific mouth diseases, or they may occur in the presence of systemic disorders such as leukemia or vitamin deficiency. When oral inflammations and infections are present, they can severely impair the ingestion of food and fluids. Common inflammations and infections of the oral cavity are presented in Table 42-7. The patient who is immunosup-

TABLE 42-7	Infections and Inflammation of the Mouth		
Condition	**Etiology**	**Clinical Manifestations**	**Treatment**
Gingivitis	Neglected oral hygiene, malocclusion, missing or irregular teeth, faulty dentistry, eating of soft rather than fibrous foods	Inflamed gingivae and interdental papillae; bleeding during toothbrushing; development of pus; formation of abscess with loosening of teeth (periodontitis)	Prevention through health teaching, dental care, gingival massage, professional cleaning of teeth, fibrous foods, conscientious brushing habits with flossing
Vincent's infection (acute necrotizing ulcerative gingivitis, trench mouth)	Fusiform bacteria; Vincent spirochetes; predisposing factors of stress, excessive fatigue, poor oral hygiene, nutritional deficiencies (B and C vitamins)	Painful, bleeding gingivae; eroding necrotic lesions of interdental papillae; ulcerations that bleed; increased saliva with metallic taste; fetid mouth odor; anorexia, fever, and general malaise	Rest (physical and mental); avoidance of smoking and alcoholic beverages; soft, nutritious diet; correct oral hygiene habits; topical applications of antibiotics; mouth irrigations with hydrogen peroxide and saline solutions
Oral candidiasis (moniliasis or thrush)	*Candida albicans* (a yeastlike fungus), debilitation, prolonged high-dose antibiotic or corticosteroid therapy	Pearly, bluish white "milk-curd" membranous lesions on mucosa of mouth and larynx; sore mouth; yeasty halitosis	Nystatin or amphotericin B as oral suspension or buccal tablets, good oral hygiene
Herpes simplex (cold sore, fever blister)	Herpes simplex virus, type I or II; predisposing factors of upper respiratory infections, excessive exposure to sunlight, food allergies, emotional tension, onset of menstruation	Lip lesions, mouth lesions, vesicle formation (single or clustered); shallow, painful ulcers	Spirits of camphor, corticosteroid cream, mild antiseptic mouthwash, viscous lidocaine; removal or control of predisposing factors, antiviral agents (e.g., acyclovir [Zovirax]; penciclovir [Denavir])
Aphthous stomatitis (canker sore)	Recurrent and chronic form of infection secondary to systemic disease, trauma, stress, or unknown causes	Ulcers of mouth and lips, causing extreme pain; ulcers surrounded by erythematous base	Corticosteroids (topical or systemic), tetracycline oral suspension
Parotitis (inflammation of parotid gland, surgical mumps)	Usually *Staphylococcus* species, *Streptococcus* species occasionally, debilitation and dehydration with poor oral hygiene, NPO status for an extended time	Pain in area of gland and ear, absence of salivation, purulent exudate from gland, erythema, ulcers	Antibiotics, mouthwashes, warm compresses; preventive measures such as chewing gum, sucking on hard candy (lemon drops), adequate fluid intake
Stomatitis (inflammation of mouth)	Trauma; pathogens; irritants (tobacco, alcohol); renal, liver, and hematologic diseases; side effect of many cancer chemotherapy drugs and radiation	Excessive salivation, halitosis, sore mouth	Removal or treatment of cause, oral hygiene with soothing solutions, topical medications; soft, bland diet

pressed (e.g., patient with acquired immunodeficiency syndrome or receiving chemotherapy) is most susceptible to oral infections. Patients receiving corticosteroid inhalant treatment for asthma are at risk for oral infections (e.g., candidiasis).

Oral infections may predispose to infections in other body organs. For example, the oral cavity can be considered a potential reservoir for respiratory pathogens. In addition, oral pathogens have been associated with heart disease.[5]

An important element in reducing oral infections and inflammation is good oral and dental hygiene. Management of oral infections and inflammation is focused on identification of the cause, elimination of infection, provision of comfort measures, and maintenance of nutritional intake.

ORAL CANCER

Oral (or oropharyngeal) cancer may occur on the lips or anywhere within the mouth (e.g., tongue, floor of the mouth, buccal mucosa, hard palate, soft palate, pharyngeal walls, and tonsils). Head and neck squamous cell carcinoma (HNSCC) is an umbrella term for cancers of the oral cavity, pharynx, and larynx and accounts for 90% of malignant oral tumors. Oral cancer is diagnosed in 30,100 Americans annually, and it is estimated that 7800 persons a year die from the disease.[6] It is more common after 40 years of age, with 60 years being the average age at onset. Oral cancer occurs in all ethnic groups. It is more common in men (male-to-female ratio of 2:1). Mortality rates have been decreasing since the early 1980s.

The 5-year survival rate for all stages of cancer of the oral cavity and pharynx combined is 53%, and the 10-year rate is 43%.[6]

Most of the oral malignant lesions occur on the lower lip in men. Other common sites are the lateral border and undersurface of the tongue, the labial commissure, and the buccal mucosa. Carcinoma of the lip has the most favorable prognosis of any of the oral tumors. This is probably because lip lesions are more apparent to the patient than other oral lesions and are usually diagnosed earlier.

Etiology and Pathophysiology

Although the definitive cause of oral cancer is unknown, there are a number of predisposing factors (Table 42-8). Factors that influence the development of oral cancer include tobacco use (e.g., cigar, cigarette, pipe, snuff), excessive alcohol intake, and chronic irritation such as from a jagged tooth or poor dental care. Individuals who smoke have a 7 to 10 times higher risk of developing oral cancer than nonsmokers.[7] Constant overexposure to ultraviolet radiation from the sun is also a factor in the development of cancer of the lip. Irritation from the pipe stem resting on the lip is a factor in pipe smokers. Human papillomavirus (HPV) has also been postulated to have a role in HNSCC development, although further research is needed to confirm this.

Clinical Manifestations

The common manifestations of oral cancer are leukoplakia, erythroplakia, ulcerations, a sore that bleeds easily and does not heal, and a rough area (felt with the tongue). Patients may also report nonspecific symptoms such as chronic sore throat and voice changes. **Leukoplakia,** called "white patch" or "smoker's patch," is often considered a precancerous lesion, although less than 15% of these lesions actually transform into malignant cells. It is a whitish patch on the mouth or tongue mucosa.[8] The patch becomes *keratinized* (hard and leathery) and is sometimes described as hyperkeratosis. Leukoplakia is the result of chronic irritation, especially from smoking. *Erythroplasia* (erythroplakia), which is seen as a red velvety patch on the mouth or tongue, is also considered a precancerous lesion. Over 50% of cases of erythroplakia progress to squamous cell carcinoma. Later symptoms of oral cancer are pain, **dysphagia** (difficulty swallowing), and difficulty in moving the jaw (e.g., chewing and speaking).

Cancer of the lip usually appears as an indurated, painless ulcer on the lip. The first sign of carcinoma of the tongue is an ulcer or area of thickening. Soreness or pain of the tongue may occur, es-

TABLE 42-8	**Types and Characteristics of Oral Cancer**		
Location	**Predisposing Factors**	**Clinical Manifestations**	**Treatment**
Lip	Constant overexposure to sun, ruddy and fair complexion, recurrent herpetic lesions, irritation from pipe stem, syphilis, immunosuppression	Indurated, painless ulcer	Surgical excision, radiation
Tongue	Tobacco, alcohol, chronic irritation, syphilis	Ulcer or area of thickening; soreness or pain; increased salivation, slurred speech, dysphagia, toothache, earache (later signs)	Surgery (hemiglossectomy or glossectomy), radiation
Oral cavity	Poor oral hygiene, tobacco usage (pipe and cigar smoking, snuff, chewing tobacco), chronic alcohol intake, chronic irritation (jagged tooth, ill-fitting prosthesis, chemical or mechanical irritants)	Leukoplakia; erythroplakia; ulcerations; sore spot; rough area; pain, dysphagia, difficulty in chewing and speaking (later signs)	Surgery (mandibulectomy, radical neck dissection, resection of buccal mucosa), internal and external radiation

pecially when eating hot or highly seasoned foods. Cancerous lesions are most likely to develop in the proximal half of the tongue. Some patients experience limitation of movement of the tongue. Later symptoms of cancer of the tongue include increased salivation, slurred speech, dysphagia, toothache, and earache. Approximately 30% of patients with oral cancer have an asymptomatic neck mass.

Diagnostic Studies

Biopsy of the suspected lesion with cytologic examination is the definitive diagnostic study for oral cancer.[9] Oral exfoliative cytology involves scraping the suspicious lesion and spreading this scraping on a slide. Unlike biopsy, a negative cytologic smear does not reliably rule out the possibility of a malignant condition, but it may be used as an initial screening test. The toluidine blue test may also be used as a screening test for oral cancer. Toluidine blue is applied topically to stain an area, and cancer cells preferentially take up the dye.

Collaborative Care

Collaborative care of oral carcinoma usually consists of surgery, radiation, chemotherapy, or a combination of these (Table 42-9).

Surgical Therapy. Surgery remains the most effective treatment, especially for removing the central core of the tumor. Many of the operations are radical procedures involving extensive resections. Various surgical procedures may be performed, depending on the location and extent of the tumor. Some examples are partial *mandibulectomy* (removal of the mandible), *hemiglossectomy* (removal of half of the tongue), *glossectomy* (removal of the tongue), resections of the buccal mucosa and floor of the mouth, and radical neck dissection. Composite resections, which are combinations of the various surgical procedures, may be performed.

Because cancers of the oral cavity metastasize early to the cervical lymph nodes, a radical neck dissection is commonly performed. It includes wide excision of the involved primary lesion with removal of the regional lymph nodes, the deep cervical lymph nodes, and their lymphatic channels. In addition, the following structures may also be removed or transected (depending on the extent of the primary lesion): sternocleidomastoid muscle and other closely associated muscles, internal jugular vein, mandible, submaxillary gland, part of the thyroid and parathyroid glands, and

TABLE 42-9	COLLABORATIVE CARE Oral Cancer
Diagnostic	
History and physical examination	
Biopsy	
Oral exfoliative cytology	
Toluidine blue test	
CT, MRI	
Collaborative Therapy*	
Surgery	
• Surgical excision of the tumor	
• Radical neck dissection	
Radiation (internal or external)	
Combined surgical resection with radiation	
Chemotherapy	

CT, Computed tomography; *MRI*, magnetic resonance imaging.
*Any of these approaches may be used, depending on the primary lesion and the extent of metastasis.

spinal accessory nerve. A tracheostomy is commonly performed along with the radical neck dissection. Drainage tubes are inserted into the surgical area and connected to suction to remove fluid and blood.

Nonsurgical Therapy. Chemotherapy and radiation therapy are used together when the lesions are more advanced or involve several structures of the oral cavity. Chemotherapy may also be used when surgery and radiation therapy fail or as the initial therapy for smaller tumors. Chemotherapeutic agents used include 5-fluorouracil (5-FU), methotrexate, cisplatin (Platinol), carboplatin (Paraplatin), paclitaxel (Taxol), docetaxel (Taxotere), and bleomycin (Blenoxane). Combination drug therapies are also used. (Chemotherapy is discussed in Chapter 16.)

Palliative treatment may be the best management when the prognosis is poor, the cancer is inoperable, or the patient decides against surgery. Palliation aims to treat the symptoms and make the patient more comfortable. If it becomes difficult for the patient to swallow, a gastrostomy may be performed to allow for adequate nutritional intake. (Gastrostomy is discussed in Chapter 40.) Analgesic medication should be given freely to this patient. Frequent suctioning of the oral cavity becomes necessary when swallowing becomes difficult. (Other nursing measures for the terminally ill patient are discussed in Chapter 11.)

Nutritional Therapy. Because of depression, alcoholism, or presurgery radiation treatment, patients may be malnourished before surgery. A percutaneous endoscopic gastrostomy (PEG) placement may be considered before radiation treatment or surgery. After radical neck surgery, the patient may be unable to orally ingest nutrients because of swelling, location of sutures, or difficulty with swallowing. Parenteral fluids will be given for the first 24 to 48 hours. After this time, tube feedings are usually given via an NG, gastrostomy, or nasointestinal tube. (Enteral feedings are described in Chapter 40.) Cervical esophagostomy and pharyngostomy have also been used. The nurse observes for feeding tolerance and adjusts the amount, time, and formula if nausea, vomiting, diarrhea, or distention occurs. When the patient can swallow, small amounts of water are given. Close observation for choking is essential. Suctioning may be necessary to prevent aspiration.

NURSING MANAGEMENT
ORAL CANCER

■ *Nursing Assessment*

Subjective and objective data that should be obtained from a patient with oral cancer are presented in Table 42-10.

■ *Nursing Diagnoses*

Nursing diagnoses for the patient with oral cancer may include, but are not limited to, the following:

- Imbalanced nutrition: less than body requirements *related to* oral pain, difficulty chewing and swallowing, surgical resection, and radiation treatment
- Chronic pain *related to* the tumor, surgery, and/or radiation
- Anxiety *related to* diagnosis of cancer, uncertain future, potential for disfiguring surgery, potential for recurrence, and prognosis
- Ineffective coping *related to* body image change
- Ineffective health maintenance *related to* lack of knowledge of disease process and therapeutic regimen and unavailability of a support system

TABLE 42-10	*NURSING ASSESSMENT* Oral Cancer

Subjective Data
Important Health Information
Past health history: Recurrent oral herpetic lesions, syphilis, exposure to sunlight
Medications: Immunosuppressants
Surgery or other treatments: Removal of prior tumors or lesions

Functional Health Patterns
Health perception–health management: Use of alcohol and tobacco, pipe smoking; poor oral hygiene
Nutritional-metabolic: Reductions in oral intake, weight loss; difficulty in chewing food; increased salivation; intolerance to certain foods or temperatures of food
Cognitive-perceptual: Mouth or tongue soreness or pain, toothache, earache, neck stiffness, dysphagia, difficulty speaking

Objective Data
Integumentary
Indurated, painless ulcer on lip; painless neck mass

Gastrointestinal
Areas of thickening or roughness, ulcers, leukoplakia, or erythroplakia on the tongue or oral mucosa; limited movement of the tongue; increased salivation, drooling; slurred speech; foul breath odor

Possible Findings
Positive exfoliative smear cytology (microscopic examination of cells removed by scraping); positive biopsy

■ Planning

The overall goals are that the patient with carcinoma of the oral cavity will (1) have a patent airway, (2) be able to communicate, (3) have adequate nutritional intake to promote wound healing, and (4) have relief of pain and discomfort.

■ Nursing Implementation

Health Promotion. The nurse has a significant role in early detection and treatment of oral cancer. The nurse needs to provide the patient with information regarding predisposing factors, such as constant overexposure to the sun, tobacco, and other irritants. Smoking, long-term use of smokeless tobacco, and alcohol are the major risk factors for oral cancer. A patient identified as a smoker should be informed about smoking cessation programs available in the community. (Smoking cessation is discussed in Chapter 12 and Tables 12-4 and 12-6.)

It is important that adolescents and teenagers be informed about the danger of using snuff, or chewing tobacco. In addition, oral cancers have an increased chance of recurrence if risk factors are not reduced. The nurse should also teach correct oral hygiene and dental care and encourage the patient to seek preventive dental care. Because early detection of oral cancer is important, the patient is taught to report unexplained pain or soreness of the mouth, unusual bleeding, dysphagia, sore throat, voice changes, or swelling or lump in the neck. Any individual with an ulcerative lesion that does not heal within 2 to 3 weeks should be referred to a health care provider, and a biopsy of the lesion should probably be performed. The nurse also inspects the patient's oral cavity for suspicious lesions.

Acute Intervention. Preoperative care for the patient who is to have a radical neck dissection involves consideration of the patient's physical and psychosocial needs. Physical preparation is the

HEALTHY PEOPLE
Health Impact of Good Oral Hygiene

- Improves quality of life
- Lowers risk of teeth loss
- Decreases cost of care needed from dental professionals
- Assists in early detection of oral and pharyngeal cancers
- Decreases risk of developing periodontal disease, gingivitis, and dental caries

same as that for any major surgery, with special emphasis on oral hygiene. Thorough assessment of alcohol intake should be done, and measures to assess and treat withdrawal if it is a problem should be implemented early. Explanations and emotional support should include information on postoperative communication and feeding. The surgical procedure is explained to the patient, and the nurse ensures that the patient understands the information. Radical neck dissection and related nursing management are discussed in Chapter 27 and NCP 27-2.

■ Evaluation

The expected outcomes are that the patient with oral cancer will

- have no respiratory complications
- be able to communicate
- participate in regular follow-up examinations
- maintain an adequate nutritional intake to promote wound healing
- experience minimal pain and discomfort with eating, drinking, and talking

Esophageal Disorders

GASTROESOPHAGEAL REFLUX DISEASE

Gastroesophageal reflux disease (GERD) is not a disease but a syndrome. GERD is any clinically significant symptomatic condition or histopathologic alteration secondary to reflux of gastric contents into the lower esophagus. GERD is the most common upper GI problem seen in adults. Approximately 14% to 20% of the U.S. population experience GERD symptoms at least once a week.[10]

Etiology and Pathophysiology

There is no one single cause of GERD. Several factors or combinations of factors can be involved (Fig. 42-3). It results when the defenses of the lower esophagus are overwhelmed by the reflux of acidic gastric contents into the esophagus. The lower esophageal sphincter (LES) is the antireflux barrier. Predisposing conditions include hiatal hernia, incompetent LES, decreased esophageal clearance (ability to clear liquids or food from the esophagus into the stomach) resulting from impaired esophageal motility, and decreased gastric emptying. The acidic gastric secretions that reflux up into the lower esophagus can result in esophageal irritation and inflammation (esophagitis). The gastric enzyme pepsin and intestinal enzymes (e.g., trypsin) and bile salts are also corrosive to the esophageal mucosa. The degree of inflammation depends on the amount and composition of gastric reflux and on the ability of the esophagus to clear the acidic contents.

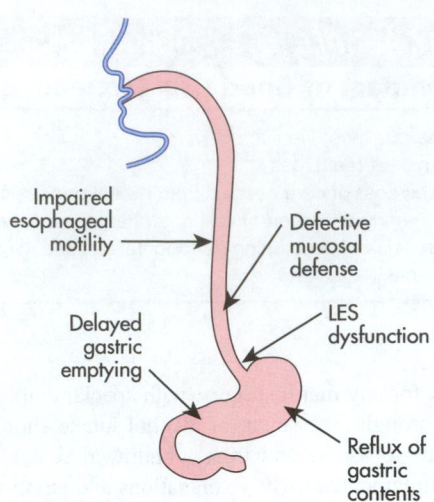

FIG. 42-3   Factors involved in the pathogenesis of gastroesophageal reflux disease (GERD). *LES,* Lower esophageal sphincter.

One of the primary factors in GERD is an incompetent LES. An incompetent LES results in a decrease in pressure in the distal portion of the esophagus. As a result, gastric contents are able to move from an area of higher pressure (stomach) to an area of lower pressure (esophagus) when the patient is in a supine position or has an increase in intraabdominal pressure. Decreased LES pressure can be due to certain foods (e.g., caffeine, chocolate) and drugs (e.g., anticholinergics). Obesity is a risk factor for GERD although the mechanism remains to be determined.[11] Pregnant women are also at greater risk for GERD. Cigarette and cigar smoking can also contribute to GERD. A common cause of GERD is a hiatal hernia, which is discussed in the next section.

Clinical Manifestations

The symptoms of GERD vary from individual to individual. Heartburn *(pyrosis)* from gastroesophageal reflux of acidic gastric secretions is the most common clinical manifestation. Heartburn is described as a burning, tight sensation that is felt intermittently beneath the lower sternum and spreads upward to the throat or jaw. Patients may also complain of dyspepsia. *Dyspepsia* is defined as pain or discomfort centered in the upper abdomen (mainly in or around the midline as opposed to the right or left hypochondrium). Episodes of hypersalivation (water brash) are another common complaint. Complaints of noncardiac chest pain are more common in older adults with GERD.

Most individuals have mild symptoms (e.g., heartburn after a meal that occurs about once a week with no evidence of mucosal damage). However, the persistence of mild symptoms for a period of 5 years or more or symptoms associated with difficulty swallowing should be evaluated. A health care provider should evaluate heartburn that occurs more than once a week, is rated as severe, or occurs at night and wakes a person from sleep. Older adults who complain of recent onset of heartburn should receive medical evaluation.

Heartburn may occur following ingestion of food or drugs that decrease the LES pressure or directly irritate the esophageal mucosa (Table 42-11). Heartburn may be relieved with milk, alkaline substances, or water. An individual with GERD may also report respiratory symptoms, including wheezing, coughing, and dyspnea. Nocturnal coughing can awaken the patient, resulting in disturbed sleep patterns. Otolaryngologic symptoms include hoarseness, sore throat, a *globus sensation* (sense of a lump in the throat), and choking. *Regurgitation* (effortless return of food or gastric contents from the stomach into esophagus or mouth) is a fairly common manifestation of GERD. It is often described as hot, bitter, or sour liquid coming into the throat or mouth. Gastric symptoms including early satiety, postmeal bloating, nausea, and vomiting are related to delayed gastric emptying.

Complications

Complications of GERD are related to the direct local effects of gastric acid on the esophageal mucosa. **Esophagitis** (inflammation of the esophagus) is a frequent complication of GERD. Other risk factors for esophagitis include hiatal hernia, chemical irritation from lye or physical irritants such as smoking, cold or hot liquids, and excessive alcohol intake. Trauma to the esophagus can produce inflammation. Esophagitis with esophageal ulcerations is shown in Fig. 42-4.

Repeated exposure may cause scar tissue formation and decreased distensibility *(esophageal stricture)* of the esophagus. This may result in dysphagia.

Another complication of GERD is **Barrett's esophagus** (esophageal metaplasia). Barrett's esophagus is considered a precancerous lesion that increases the patient's risk for esophageal cancer. Approximately 10% to 15% of patients with chronic reflux have Barrett's esophagus. In Barrett's esophagus there is replacement of the normal squamous epithelium with columnar epithelium. These cell changes are thought to be due to GERD. However,

TABLE 42-11	**Factors Affecting Lower Esophageal Sphincter Pressure**

Increase Pressure
bethanechol (Urecholine)
metoclopramide (Reglan)

Decrease Pressure

alcohol	β-adrenergic blockers
anticholinergics	calcium channel blockers
chocolate (theobromine)	diazepam (Valium)
fatty foods	morphine sulfate
nicotine	nitrates
peppermint, spearmint	progesterone
tea, coffee (caffeine)	theophylline

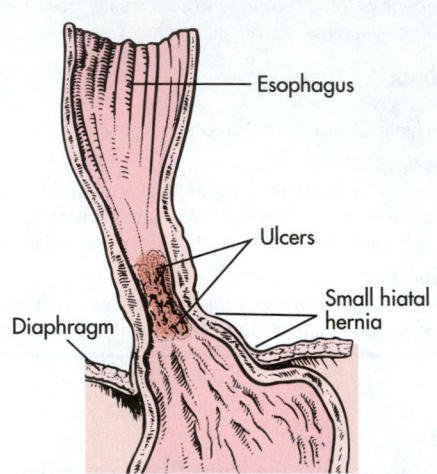

FIG. 42-4   Esophagitis with esophageal ulcerations.

TABLE 42-12	COLLABORATIVE CARE — Gastroesophageal Reflux Disease (GERD) and Hiatal Hernia

Diagnostic
History and physical examination
Upper GI endoscopy with biopsy and cytologic analysis
Barium swallow
Motility (manometry) studies
pH monitoring (laboratory or 24-hr ambulatory)
Radionuclide studies

Collaborative Therapy
Conservative
Elevation of head of bed on 4- to 6-in blocks
High-protein, low-fat diet with avoidance of foods that decrease LES
    pressure or irritate acid-sensitive esophagus
Antacids
Antisecretory agents
    H₂-receptor blockers*
    Proton pump inhibitors*
Prokinetic drug therapy*
Cholinergic drugs

Surgical
Nissen fundoplication
Toupet fundoplication
Hill gastropexy
Belsey fundoplication

Endoscopic
Intraluminal valvuloplasty
Radiofrequency therapy
Injection or implantation of foreign material

LES, Lower esophageal sphincter.
*See Table 42-13.

patients with no history of reflux can still develop Barrett's esophagus.[12] Signs and symptoms of Barrett's esophagus can range from none to mild to bleeding and perforation. Because patients with Barrett's esophagus are at higher risk for adenocarcinoma, they may need to be monitored on a regular basis (every 1 to 3 years) by endoscopy.

Respiratory complications of GERD include cough, bronchospasm, laryngospasm, and cricopharyngeal spasm. These complications are due to irritation of the upper airway by gastric secretions. With GERD there is also the potential for asthma, chronic bronchitis, and pneumonia as a result of aspiration of gastric contents into the respiratory system. Dental erosion, especially in the posterior teeth, may result from acid reflux into the mouth.

Diagnostic Studies

Diagnostic studies are performed to determine the cause of the GERD (Table 42-12). Barium swallow can detect if there is protrusion of the upper part of the stomach (*gastric fundus*). Endoscopy is useful in assessing the LES competence and the degree of inflammation (if present), potential scarring, and strictures. Biopsy and cytologic specimens can be taken to differentiate stomach or esophageal carcinoma from Barrett's esophagus. Manometric studies may be performed to measure pressure in the esophagus and LES. The determination of pH using specially designed probes can be used in the laboratory or as ambulatory monitoring systems to determine esophageal pH. With reflux there is acid in the normally alkaline esophagus. Radionuclide tests may also be performed to detect reflux of gastric contents and the rate of esophageal clearance.

Because of the cost and discomfort of diagnostic procedures, it has been suggested that high-dose proton pump inhibitor (PPI) treatment (explained under Drug Therapy) for a short period (2 weeks) can be used as a first step in the diagnosis of GERD.[13] In patients with GERD, PPI treatment should result in a marked reduction or elimination of symptoms.

Collaborative Care

Most patients with GERD can be successfully managed by lifestyle modifications and drug therapy. These are long-term approaches requiring patient teaching and compliance with therapies. When these therapies are ineffective, surgery is an option (see Table 42-12).

Lifestyle Modifications. The patient with GERD is taught to avoid factors that aggravate symptoms. Particular attention is given to diet and drugs that may affect the LES, acid secretion, or gastric emptying. Patients who smoke are encouraged to stop. Cigarette smoking has been associated with decreased acid clearance from the lower esophagus.

Nutritional Therapy. Diet does not cause GERD, but food can aggravate symptoms. No specific diet is necessary, but foods that cause reflux should be avoided. Fatty foods stimulate the release of cholecystokinin, a hormone from the duodenum that decreases LES pressure. High-fat foods also decrease the rate of gastric emptying. Foods that decrease LES pressure, such as chocolate, peppermint, coffee, and tea (see Table 42-11), should be avoided because they predispose to reflux. Milk products should be avoided, especially at bedtime, because milk increases gastric acid secretion. Small, frequent meals are advised to prevent overdistention of the stomach. The patient should avoid late evening meals and nocturnal snacking. Fluids should be taken between rather than with meals to reduce gastric distention. Certain foods (e.g., tomato-based products, orange juice) may irritate the acid-sensitive esophagus and may need to be avoided. To reduce intraabdominal pressure, weight reduction is recommended if the patient is overweight.

Drug Therapy. Drug therapy for GERD is focused on improving LES function, increasing esophageal clearance, decreasing volume and acidity of reflux, and protecting the esophageal mucosa (Table 42-13). There are two approaches to drug therapy. The first is the "step-up" approach, which means starting with antacids and OTC H₂R blockers and increasing to prescription H₂R blockers and, finally, PPIs. The "step-down" approach involves starting with a PPI and over time titrating down to prescription H₂R blockers and, finally, OTC H₂R blockers and antacids. More recently, "on-demand" (or prn) PPIs are being used with greater frequency.

Antacids produce quick but short-lived relief of heartburn. They act by neutralizing HCl acid. They should be taken 1 to 3 hours after meals and at bedtime. Antacids with or without alginic acid (e.g., Gaviscon) may be useful in patients with mild, intermittent heartburn. However, in patients with moderate to severe or frequent symptoms or patients with documented esophagitis, these regimens are not effective in relieving symptoms or healing lesions.

Antisecretory agents decrease the secretion of HCl acid by the stomach. H₂R blockers (e.g., cimetidine [Tagamet], ranitidine [Zantac], famotidine [Pepcid], nizatidine [Axid]) are available in OTC and prescription formulations. OTC preparations (e.g., Pepcid AC, Tagamet HB, Zantac 75, Axid AR) have lower drug dosages compared with prescription drugs. Some formulations include

TABLE 42-13	*DRUG THERAPY* **Gastroesophageal Reflux Disease (GERD)**	
Mechanism of Action	**Examples**	
Increase LES Pressure Cholinergic	bethanechol (Urecholine)	
Promotility Prokinetic	metoclopramide (Reglan)	
Acid Neutralizing Antacids	Gelusil, Maalox, Mylanta	
Antisecretory H₂-receptor blockers	cimetidine (Tagamet) famotidine (Pepcid) nizatidine (Axid) ranitidine (Zantac)	
Proton pump inhibitors (PPIs)	esomeprazole (Nexium) lansoprazole (Prevacid) omeprazole (Prilosec) pantoprazole (Protonix) rabeprazole (Aciphex)	
Cytoprotective Alginic acid-antacid Acid protective	Gaviscon sucralfate (Carafate)	

LES, Lower esophageal sphincter.

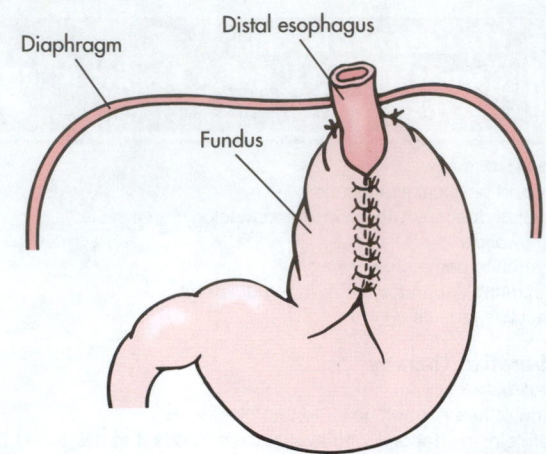

FIG. 42-5 Nissen fundoplication for repair of hiatal hernia. Fundus of stomach is wrapped around distal esophagus and sutured to itself.

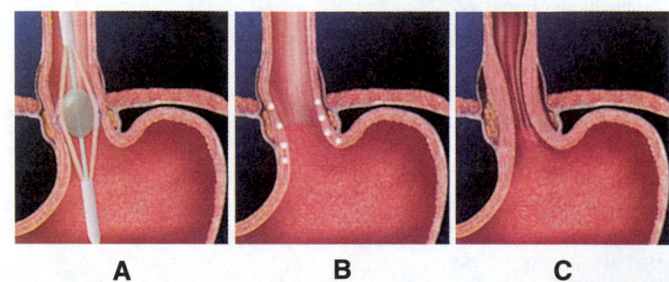

FIG. 42-6 Stretta procedure used to treat GERD. **A,** Catheter positioned. **B,** Multiple sites treated with radiofrequency energy. **C,** Remodeling occurs with collagen formation.

an H₂R plus antacid combination. For example, Pepcid Complete includes famotidine, calcium carbonate, and magnesium hydroxide. In prescription doses, H₂R blockers reduce symptoms and promote esophageal healing in approximately 50% of patients. Patients frequently relapse (i.e., symptoms return) with discontinuance of the drug.

PPIs such as omeprazole (Prilosec), esomeprazole (Nexium), pantoprazole (Protonix), lansoprazole (Prevacid), and rabeprazole (Aciphex) also decrease gastric HCl acid secretion. These agents act by inhibiting the proton pump mechanism responsible for the secretion of H⁺ ions. PPIs promote esophageal healing in approximately 80% to 90% of patients but are more expensive than H₂R blockers. PPIs may also be beneficial in decreasing the incidence of esophageal strictures, a complication of chronic GERD. Omeprazole is available as an OTC preparation and in an immediate-release form (Zegerid).

Sucralfate (Carafate), an antiulcer drug, may be used in patients with GERD for its cytoprotective properties. Cholinergic drugs, such as bethanechol (Urecholine), may be used to increase LES pressure, improve esophageal emptying in the supine position, and increase gastric emptying. However, the value of current cholinergic drugs is limited because they also stimulate HCl acid secretion. Prokinetic (motility-enhancing) drugs such as metoclopramide (Reglan) promote gastric emptying and reduce the risk of gastric acid reflux (see Table 42-13).

Surgical Therapy. Surgical therapy (antireflux surgery) may be necessary if conservative therapy fails; if a hiatal hernia is present; or if complications, such as esophageal stricture and stenosis (narrowing), chronic esophagitis, and bleeding, exist. Most surgical procedures are performed laparoscopically. The objective of surgical interventions for GERD (called *antireflux* procedures) is to reduce reflux of gastric contents by enhancing the integrity of the LES. In these procedures the fundus of the stomach is wrapped around the lower portion of the esophagus to reinforce and repair the defective barrier.

The Nissen fundoplication is shown in Fig. 42-5. Laparoscopically performed Nissen and Toupet fundoplications are common antireflux surgeries. The use of laparoscopic antireflux surgery has reduced complications, overall morbidity, and the cost of hospitalization compared with a thoracic or an open abdominal approach.

Endoscopic Therapy. Currently, three types of endoscopic procedures are used for GERD: endoscopic intraluminal valvuloplasty, endoscopic radiofrequency therapy, and endoscopic injection or implantation of foreign material. Endoscopic valvuloplasty or gastroplication utilizes gastric tissue to increase the integrity of the LES. Endoscopic radiofrequency procedure uses an instrument called the Stretta device, which is a balloon-tipped four-needle catheter that delivers radiofrequency energy to the smooth muscle of the LES[14] (Fig. 42-6). The radiofrequency energy induces collagen contraction, which helps to form a barrier against reflux. Endoscopic injection includes insertion of polymers, such as polymethyl-methylacrylaten and Gatekeeper hydrogel. These procedures are performed endoscopically under conscious sedation.

NURSING MANAGEMENT
GASTROESOPHAGEAL REFLUX DISEASE

Patients with GERD must avoid factors that cause reflux. A patient and family teaching guide is provided in Table 42-14. The patient who is a smoker should stop smoking. The patient may need to be

TABLE 42-14	**PATIENT AND FAMILY TEACHING GUIDE** Prevention of Gastroesophageal Reflux Disease (GERD)

The following are teaching guidelines for the patient and family:
1. Explain the rationale for a high-protein, low-fat diet.
2. Encourage the patient to eat small, frequent meals to prevent gastric distention.
3. Explain the rationale for avoiding alcohol, smoking (causes an almost immediate, marked decrease in LES pressure), and beverages that contain caffeine.
4. Teach the patient not to lie down for 2 to 3 hr after eating, wear tight clothing around the waist, or bend over (especially after eating).
5. Avoid eating within 3 hr of bedtime.
6. Encourage the patient to sleep with head of bed elevated on 4- to 6-in blocks (gravity fosters esophageal emptying).
7. Teach information regarding drugs, including rationale for their use and common side effects.
8. Discuss strategies for weight reduction if appropriate.
9. Encourage patient and family to share concerns about lifestyle changes and living with a chronic problem.

LES, Lower esophageal sphincter.

referred to community resources for assistance in stopping smoking. (See Chapter 12 for additional information related to smoking cessation.) Substances that decrease LES pressure and tone should be avoided (see Table 42-11). If stress seems to cause symptoms, measures to cope with stress should be discussed. (See Chapter 9 for stress management techniques.)

Nursing care for the patient with acute symptoms consists of encouraging the patient to follow the necessary regimen. The nurse should ensure that the head of the bed is elevated to approximately 30 degrees (usually on 4- to 6-inch blocks) and that the patient does not lie down for 2 to 3 hours after eating. Teaching the patient to avoid food and activities that cause reflux is important (e.g., late-night eating should be avoided). The patient may be taking drugs to treat heartburn, so the nurse must observe for side effects, as well as evaluate their effectiveness. Even when acute symptoms subside, the patient may need to continue drugs because the underlying problem is still present. Because of the link between GERD and Barrett's esophagus, patients are instructed to see their health care provider if symptoms persist.

The nurse instructs the patient about side effects of the drugs being taken. Side effects with H_2R blockers are uncommon. Headache is the most common complaint of patients taking a PPI. Antacids that contain aluminum can cause constipation, whereas those that contain magnesium can cause diarrhea. Several of the antacids are combinations of aluminum and magnesium designed to minimize these side effects. Side effects of cholinergic drugs (e.g., urinary frequency, abdominal cramping, diarrhea, hypotension) such as bethanechol limit their effectiveness in treating GERD. Side effects of metoclopramide include restlessness, anxiety, insomnia, and hallucinations. The most common side effect of sucralfate is constipation.

Postoperative care focuses on concerns related to prevention of respiratory complications, maintenance of fluid and electrolyte balance, and prevention of infection. If an open abdominal incision is used, respiratory complications can occur because of the high abdominal incision. Respiratory assessment includes respiratory rate and rhythm, pulse rate and rhythm, and signs of pneumothorax (e.g., dyspnea, chest pain, cyanosis). Deep breathing is essential to fully expand the lungs. Because most procedures are performed laparoscopically, the risk of respiratory complications is reduced. For some patients, the laparoscopic fundoplication is performed as an outpatient procedure. However, patients at risk for complications, including those with prior upper abdominal surgeries and those with comorbidities (e.g., cardiac disease, obesity), are hospitalized after the procedure. During the postoperative phase patients require medications to prevent postoperative nausea and vomiting and to control pain. A small percentage of patients experience complications, including pneumothorax, perforation, hemorrhage, and pneumonia.[15]

When peristalsis returns, only fluids are given initially. Solids are added gradually so that the stomach is not overdistended. The nurse must maintain an accurate recording of intake and output and observe for fluid and electrolyte imbalances (see Chapter 17). A normal diet is gradually resumed. The patient should avoid foods that are gas forming and should try to prevent gastric distention. Food should be chewed thoroughly.

After surgical therapy, there should be a decrease in reflux symptoms. However, the recurrence rate may range from 10% to 30% over a 20-year period following surgery. In the first month after surgery the patient may report mild dysphagia caused by edema, but it should resolve. The patient is instructed to report persistent symptoms such as heartburn and regurgitation.

Following endoscopic therapy (e.g., Stretta procedure) the patient is monitored for complaints of chest pain.[14] The patient is instructed to remain on clear liquids for 24 hours and then a soft diet for the next 2 weeks. Patients should take liquid medications to decrease irritation to the esophageal mucosa. If nausea and vomiting occur, the patient is instructed to contact his or her physician. The patient should not take NSAIDs for 10 days following the procedure.

HIATAL HERNIA

Hiatal hernia is herniation of a portion of the stomach into the esophagus through an opening, or hiatus, in the diaphragm. It is also referred to as diaphragmatic hernia and esophageal hernia. The incidence of hiatal hernia is difficult to determine. However, it is the most common abnormality found on x-ray examination of the upper GI tract. Hiatal hernias are common in older adults and occur more often in women than in men.

Types

Hiatal hernias are classified into the following two types (Fig. 42-7):
1. *Sliding:* The junction of the stomach and esophagus is above the hiatus of the diaphragm, and a part of the stomach slides through the hiatal opening in the diaphragm. The stomach "slides" into the thoracic cavity when the patient is supine and usually goes back into the abdominal cavity when the patient is standing upright. This is the most common type of hiatal hernia.
2. *Paraesophageal or rolling:* The esophagogastric junction remains in the normal position, but the fundus and the greater curvature of the stomach roll up through the diaphragm, forming a pocket alongside the esophagus.

Etiology and Pathophysiology

The actual cause of hiatal hernia is unknown. Many factors contribute to the development of hiatal hernia. Structural changes, such as weakening of the muscles in the diaphragm around the

Gastrointestinal System

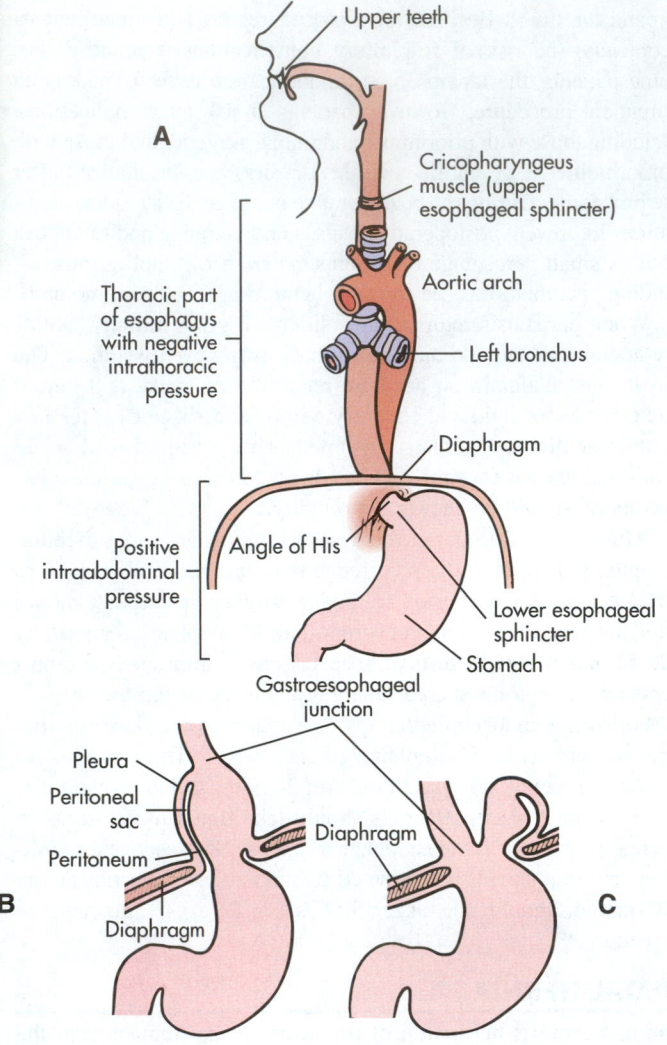

FIG. 42-7 **A,** Normal esophagus. **B,** Sliding hiatal hernia. **C,** Rolling or paraesophageal hernia.

esophagogastric opening, are usually contributing factors. Factors that increase intraabdominal pressure, including obesity, pregnancy, ascites, tumors, tight girdles, intense physical exertion, and heavy lifting on a continual basis, may also predispose to development of a hiatal hernia. Other predisposing factors are increased age, trauma, poor nutrition, and a forced recumbent position, as when a prolonged illness confines the person to bed. In some cases, congenital weakness is a contributing factor.

Clinical Manifestations

Persons with hiatal hernia may be asymptomatic. When present, the signs and symptoms of hiatal hernia are similar to those described for GERD. Heartburn, especially after a meal or after lying supine, is a common symptom. Bending over may cause a severe burning pain, which is usually relieved by sitting or standing. Other common precipitating factors of pain include large meals, alcohol, and smoking. Nocturnal symptoms of heartburn are common, especially if the person has eaten before lying down. Patients may complain of dysphagia. Frequently the symptoms of hiatal hernia mimic gallbladder disease, peptic ulcer disease, and angina.

Complications

Complications that may occur with hiatal hernia include GERD, esophagitis, hemorrhage from erosion, stenosis (narrowing of the esophagus), ulcerations of the herniated portion of the stomach, strangulation of the hernia, and regurgitation with tracheal aspiration. Patients with a history of hiatal hernia are more at risk for respiratory problems ranging from dyspnea to acute bronchoconstriction.[16]

Diagnostic Studies

A barium swallow may show the protrusion of gastric mucosa through the esophageal hiatus in the patient with hiatal hernia. Endoscopic visualization of the lower esophagus provides information on the degree of mucosal inflammation or other abnormalities. Other tests are described in Table 42-12.

NURSING *and* COLLABORATIVE MANAGEMENT
HIATAL HERNIA

▪ *Conservative Therapy*

Conservative therapy of hiatal hernia is similar to that described under GERD, including lifestyle modifications (e.g., reduction of intraabdominal pressure by eliminating constricting garments, avoiding lifting and straining, eliminating alcohol and smoking, elevating the head of the bed), and the use of antacids and antisecretory agents (PPIs, H2R blockers). Elevation of the bed on 4- to 6-inch blocks assists gravity in maintaining the stomach in the abdominal cavity and also helps prevent reflux and tracheal aspiration. If overweight, the patient should be encouraged to lose weight.

▪ *Surgical Therapy*

Surgical approaches to hiatal hernias can include reduction of the herniated stomach into the abdomen, *herniotomy* (excision of the hernia sac), *herniorraphy* (closure of the hiatal defect), an antireflux procedure, and *gastropexy* (attachment of the stomach subdiaphragmatically to prevent reherniation). The goals are to reduce the hernia, provide an acceptable LES pressure, and prevent movement of the gastroesophageal junction. Laparoscopically performed Nissen and Toupet techniques are the standard antireflux surgeries for hiatal hernia (see Fig. 42-5). A thoracic or an open abdominal approach is used in selected cases.

GERONTOLOGIC CONSIDERATIONS
HIATAL HERNIA AND GERD

The incidences of hiatal hernia and GERD increase with age. Hiatal hernia is associated with weakening of the diaphragm, obesity, kyphosis, or other factors (e.g., wearing girdles) that increase intraabdominal pressure. Medications commonly taken by older patients, including nitrates, calcium channel blockers, and antidepressants, decrease LES pressure. Others such as NSAIDs and potassium can irritate the esophageal mucosa. Some older adults with hiatal hernia and GERD are asymptomatic or have less severe symptoms.[17] The first indications may include esophageal bleeding secondary to esophagitis or respiratory complications (e.g., aspiration pneumonia) related to aspiration of gastric contents. The LES may become less competent with aging in some individuals.

The clinical course and management of GERD and hiatal hernia in the older adult are similar to that for the younger adult. With the increased use of laparoscopic procedures, surgical risks have

Situation

A 32-year-old man, institutionalized almost all of his life for profound developmental disabilities, is hospitalized for his fourth aspiration-related pneumonia in the last year. His health care provider believes that a feeding tube would solve the problem of aspiration and wants the family to agree to the procedure. The family believes his life span should not be extended by artificial means and refuses to give consent. The hospital is considering seeking a court-appointed guardian because the family is not acting in the best interest of the patient.

Important Points for Consideration

- Before making an ethical or legal decision, it is important that all contextual factors relating to the case be explored, such as possible reasons for the increase in aspiration pneumonia. These may include the technique used to feed the patient, how the patient is positioned during and after feedings, and how the patient might respond to the placement of a feeding tube.
- In most cases, families are considered in the best position to make treatment decisions for incompetent patients, unless there is some evidence they are not acting in the best interests of the patient. Courts are usually reserved as a last resort for treatment decisions in these situations.
- Two standards are used in decision making for incompetent patients: substituted judgment and best interest. *Substituted judgment* is basing the decision on what previously competent patients would have decided for themselves. The *best interest standard* involves making the best decision possible under the circumstances using experiences from the patient's life that are meaningful or bring satisfaction to the patient, if known.
- A consultation with an ethics committee may be helpful to clarify the issues or assist the health care team to understand quality of life from the perspective of the patient and family.
- Certain states require that specific criteria or qualifying conditions must be met to withhold or withdraw treatment from a patient.

Critical Thinking Questions

1. What are your thoughts and beliefs about the two opposing positions of preserving life in all circumstances versus maintaining an adequate quality of life?
2. In your opinion, who is in the best position to define quality of life for this patient?

been reduced. An older adult with cardiovascular and pulmonary problems may not be a good candidate for surgical intervention. In addition, changes in lifestyle, including elimination of dietary factors, such as caffeine-containing beverages and chocolate, and elevating the head of the bed on blocks, may be more difficult for the older adult.

ESOPHAGEAL CANCER

Esophageal cancer (malignant neoplasm of the esophagus) is a growing health concern. Compared with other cancers, esophageal cancer remains rare. However, during the last decade there has been a 200% increase in its rate in the United States.[6] In the United States an estimated 14,520 new cases of esophageal cancer (11,220 in men) and 13,570 deaths occur annually. Because esophageal cancer is rarely diagnosed in early stages, the 5-year survival rate is less than 20%.[6]

The percentage of esophageal cancers that are adenocarcinomas ranges from 30% to 70%, with the remainder being squamous cell. The incidence of squamous cell esophageal cancer is currently decreasing in the United States, whereas the incidence of adenocarcinoma of the distal esophagus is increasing.[6] Adenocarcinomas arise from the glands lining the esophagus and resemble cancers of the stomach and small intestine. The incidence of esophageal cancer increases with age. There is a higher incidence of esophageal cancer in African Americans and Alaska Natives than in whites.

One risk factor for esophageal adenocarcinoma is Barrett's esophagus. It is estimated that 1 of 200 cases of Barrett's esophagus will progress to esophageal cancer. (Barrett's esophagus is described earlier under GERD.)

Etiology and Pathophysiology

The cause of esophageal cancer is unknown. Two important risk factors are smoking and excessive alcohol intake. Diets that are low in fruits and vegetables and certain minerals and vitamins may increase the risk of this cancer. Lye that is found in strong cleaners such as drain cleaners can burn and destroy esophageal cells. As a result, a person who has swallowed lye has a higher risk of squamous cell cancer. A patient with a history of *achalasia,* a condition in which there is delayed emptying of the lower esophagus, is also at greater risk for squamous cell cancer. Other risk factors include exposure to asbestos and metal.[6]

The majority of esophageal tumors are located in the middle and lower portions of the esophagus. The malignant tumor usually appears as an ulcerated lesion and has often advanced by the time the patient experiences symptoms. The tumor may penetrate the muscular layer and even extend outside the wall of the esophagus. Obstruction of the esophagus occurs in the later stages.

Clinical Manifestations

The onset of symptoms is usually late relative to tumor growth. Progressive dysphagia is the most common symptom and may be described as a substernal feeling as if food is not passing (*globus sensation*). Initially the dysphagia occurs only with meat, then with soft foods, and eventually with liquids.

Pain develops late and is described as occurring in the substernal, epigastric, or back areas and usually increases with swallowing. The pain may radiate to the neck, jaw, ears, and shoulders. If the tumor is in the upper third of the esophagus, symptoms such as sore throat, choking, and hoarseness may occur. Weight loss is fairly common. When esophageal stenosis (narrowing) is severe, regurgitation of blood-flecked esophageal contents is common.

Complications

Hemorrhage occurs if the cancer erodes through the esophagus and into the aorta. Esophageal perforation with fistula formation into the lung or trachea sometimes develops. The tumor may enlarge enough to cause esophageal obstruction. The cancer spreads via the lymph system, with the liver and lung being common sites of metastasis.

Diagnostic Studies

Endoscopy with biopsy is necessary to make a definitive diagnosis of carcinoma by identification of malignant cells. Endoscopic ultrasonography (EUS) is an important tool used to stage esophageal cancer. Barium swallow with fluoroscopy may demonstrate a narrowing of the esophagus at the tumor site (Table 42-15). Some-

TABLE 42-15	COLLABORATIVE CARE — Esophageal Cancer

Diagnostic
History and physical examination
Endoscopy of esophagus with biopsy
Barium swallow
Endoscopic ultrasonography
Bronchoscopy
CT, MRI

Collaborative Therapy
Surgery
- Esophagectomy
- Esophagogastrostomy
- Esophagoenterostomy

Radiation therapy
Chemotherapy
Palliative treatment
- Dilation
- Stent or prosthesis
- Laser therapy
- Gastrostomy

CT, Computed tomography; *MRI,* magnetic resonance imaging.

times a crater is visible. A bronchoscopic examination may be performed to detect malignant involvement of the lung. Computed tomography (CT) scanning and magnetic resonance imaging (MRI) are also used to assess the extent of the disease.

Collaborative Care

The treatment of esophageal cancer depends on the location of the tumor and whether invasion or metastasis has occurred (see Table 42-11). Esophageal cancer has a poor prognosis, mainly because it is not usually diagnosed until the disease is advanced. The best results may be obtained with a combination of surgery, chemotherapy, and radiation. Cancer in the cervical esophagus is treated similar to oral carcinoma described earlier in this chapter.

Endoscopy. Endoscopic approaches utilizing photodynamic and/or laser therapy may be used to ablate mucosal adenocarcinoma or Barrett's esophagus (high-grade dysplasia). In photodynamic therapy, porfimer (Photofrin), which is a photosensitizer, is intravenously injected. The porfimer is absorbed by most tissues but selectively kept to a greater degree by neoplastic tissue. The light (activator) is transmitted via a fiber passed through the endoscope. Patients should be warned to avoid direct sunlight for up to 4 weeks after the procedure. Other endoscopic procedures include endoscopic mucosal resection (EMR). EMR is used to remove superficial lesions or submucosal neoplasms.

Surgery. The types of surgical procedures that can be performed are (1) removal of part or all of the esophagus *(esophagectomy)* with use of a Dacron graft to replace the resected part, (2) resection of a portion of the esophagus and anastomosis of the remaining portion to the stomach *(esophagogastrostomy),* and (3) resection of a portion of the esophagus and anastomosis of a segment of colon to the remaining portion *(esophagoenterostomy).* The surgical approaches may be open (thoracic, abdominal incision) or laparoscopic. Surgery may not be performed if the patient is an older adult or in poor physical health.

Concurrent radiation and chemotherapy are used to slow the progression of esophageal cancer. In some patients treatment is started before surgery.[18,19] Chemotherapy is used in advanced esophageal cancer to reduce symptoms, especially dysphagia, and

to increase survival. Currently, there is no standard single-agent or combination drug therapy recommended for esophageal cancer. Single-agent chemotherapeutic agents include bleomycin (Blenoxane), mitomycin (Mutamycin), methotrexate, paclitaxel (Taxol), docetaxel (Taxotere), and irinotecan (Camptosar). Combination therapies include cisplatin and 5-FU with other agents listed above. Vinorelbine (Navelbine) and vindesine are drugs under investigation for their effectiveness in treating esophageal cancer.

Palliative therapy consists of restoration of the swallowing function and maintenance of nutrition and hydration. Dilation, stent placement, or both can relieve obstruction. Self-expandable metal stents are available with features to prevent stent migration and tumor ingrowth. Dilation is done with various types of dilators (e.g., Celestin tube). Dilation often relieves dysphagia and allows for improved nutrition. Placement of a stent or prosthesis may help when dilation is no longer effective. The prostheses are composed of silicone rubber or nylon-reinforced latex tubes with distal and proximal collars. The prosthesis is placed in the esophagus so that food and fluids can pass through the stenotic segment of the esophagus. The prosthesis can be placed endoscopically.

Endoscopic laser therapy of the tumor may be used in combination with dilation. Obstruction recurs as the tumor grows, but laser therapy can be repeated. Sometimes these procedures are combined with radiation therapy. Other measures for palliation include gastrostomy or esophagostomy tube placements for nutrition support and pain management.

Nutritional Therapy. After esophageal surgery, parenteral fluids are given. A jejunostomy feeding tube may be used depending on the type of surgery (e.g., esophagogastrectomy) performed. A swallowing study may be given before the patient is allowed to have oral fluids. When fluids are permitted, water (30 to 60 ml) is given hourly, with gradual progression to small, frequent, bland meals. The patient should be in an upright position to prevent regurgitation of the fluid. The patient is observed for signs of intolerance to the feeding or leakage of the feeding into the mediastinum. Symptoms that indicate leakage are pain, increased temperature, and dyspnea. A gastrostomy may be performed for the purpose of feeding the patient. (Gastrostomy and tube feedings are discussed in Chapter 40.)

NURSING MANAGEMENT
ESOPHAGEAL CANCER

■ *Nursing Assessment*

The patient should be asked about any history of GERD, hiatal hernia, achalasia, or Barrett's esophagus. The patient is also questioned regarding tobacco and alcohol use. The patient should be assessed for progressive dysphagia and *odynophagia* (burning, squeezing pain while swallowing). The nurse asks the patient about the type of substances (e.g., meats, soft foods, liquids) that cause dysphagia. The patient is also assessed for pain (substernal, epigastric, or back areas), choking, heartburn, hoarseness, cough, anorexia, weight loss, and regurgitation.

■ *Nursing Diagnoses*

Nursing diagnoses for the patient with esophageal cancer include, but are not limited to, the following:
- Imbalanced nutrition: less than body requirements *related to* dysphagia, odynophagia, weakness, chemotherapy, and radiation therapy

- Chronic pain *related to* the compression of tumor on surrounding tissues, esophageal stenosis
- Deficient fluid volume *related to* inadequate intake
- Risk for aspiration *related to* impaired esophageal function
- Anxiety *related to* diagnosis of cancer, uncertain future, and poor prognosis
- Grieving *related to* diagnosis of life-threatening malignancy
- Ineffective health maintenance *related to* lack of knowledge of disease process and therapeutic regimen, unavailability of a support system, and chronic debilitating disease

■ Planning

The overall goals are that the patient with esophageal cancer will (1) have relief of symptoms, including pain and dysphagia; (2) achieve optimal nutritional intake; (3) understand the prognosis of the disease; and (4) experience a quality of life appropriate to disease progression.

■ Nursing Implementation

Health Promotion. Patients with diagnosed GERD, Barrett's esophagus, and hiatal hernia need to be counseled regarding regular follow-up evaluation. Health counseling should focus on elimination of smoking and excessive alcohol intake, as well as other risk factors for GERD. Maintenance of good oral hygiene and dietary habits (intake of fresh fruits and vegetables) may also be helpful.

Patients diagnosed with Barrett's esophagus need to be monitored because this is considered a premalignant condition. Early diagnosis and treatment of esophageal cancer is essential to increase survival. Patients are encouraged to seek medical attention for any esophageal problems, especially dysphagia. Patients who are at risk for esophageal adenocarcinoma, such as those with evidence of Barrett's esophagus and a diagnosis of achalasia (discussed under Other Esophageal Disorders later in this chapter), may need regular endoscopic screening with biopsy and cytologic study.

Acute Intervention

Preoperative Care. In addition to general preoperative teaching and preparation, particular attention is given to the patient's nutritional needs. Many patients are poorly nourished because of the inability to ingest adequate amounts of food and fluids before surgery. A high-calorie, high-protein diet is recommended. It may have to be in liquid form. Some patients may need IV fluid replacement or parenteral nutrition. The patient and/or a family member is instructed on how to keep an intake and output record and assess for signs of fluid and electrolyte imbalance. Some treatment protocols necessitate preoperative radiation and chemotherapy.

Meticulous oral care is essential. The mouth, including tongue, gingivae, and teeth or dentures, must be cleaned thoroughly. It may be necessary to use swabs or a gauze pad and to scrub the mouth, including the tongue. Milk of magnesia with mineral oil may be used to remove crust formation.

Teaching should include information about chest tubes (if an open thoracic approach is used), IV lines, NG tubes, gastrostomy feeding, turning, coughing, and deep breathing. (General preoperative care is discussed in Chapter 18.)

Postoperative Care. The patient usually has an NG tube in place, and there may be bloody drainage for 8 to 12 hours. The drainage gradually changes to greenish yellow. Assessment of the drainage, maintenance of the tube, and oral and nasal care are nursing responsibilities. The NG tube should not be repositioned or reinserted without consulting the surgeon.

Because of the location of the surgery and the general condition of the patient, emphasis is placed on prevention of respiratory complications. Turning and deep breathing should be done every 2 hours. Use of an incentive spirometer helps prevent respiratory complications.

The patient should be positioned in a semi-Fowler's or Fowler's position to prevent reflux and aspiration of gastric secretions. When the patient can drink fluids or eat, the upright position should be maintained for at least 2 hours after eating to assist with gastric emptying.

Ambulatory and Home Care. Many patients require long-term follow-up care after surgery for esophageal cancer. The patient may undergo chemotherapy and radiation treatment following surgery. The patient needs encouragement and assistance in maintaining adequate nutrition. A permanent feeding gastrostomy may be required. The patient usually has fears and anxieties about a diagnosis of cancer. The nurse should know what the health care provider has told the patient regarding the prognosis and then provide appropriate counseling.

Referral to a home health nurse may be necessary for continued care of the patient (e.g., gastrostomy teaching, follow-up wound care). (See Chapter 11 for a discussion of end-of-life and palliative care and Chapter 16 for care of the cancer patient.)

■ Evaluation

The expected outcomes are that the patient with esophageal cancer will

- maintain a patent airway
- have relief of pain
- be able to swallow comfortably
- consume adequate nutritional intake
- understand the prognosis of the disease
- experience quality of life appropriate to disease progression

OTHER ESOPHAGEAL DISORDERS

Esophageal Diverticula

Esophageal diverticula are saclike outpouchings of one or more layers of the esophagus. They occur in three main areas: (1) above the upper esophageal sphincter (*Zenker's diverticulum*), which is the most common location; (2) near the esophageal midpoint (traction diverticulum); and (3) above the LES (epiphrenic diverticulum) (Fig. 42-8). Pharyngeal pouches (Zenker's diverticula) occur most commonly in older adult patients (over 60 years), and typical symptoms include dysphagia, regurgitation, chronic cough, aspiration, and weight loss. Traction diverticulum may not cause signs and symptoms. The patient frequently complains of tasting sour food and smelling a foul odor caused by the stagnant food. Complications include malnutrition, aspiration, and perforation. A diagnosis is easily established by endoscopy or barium studies.

There is no specific treatment for diverticula. Some patients find they can empty the pocket of food that collects by applying pressure at a point on the neck. The diet may have to be limited to foods that pass more readily (e.g., blenderized foods). Treatment of the diverticulum may be necessary if nutrition becomes disrupted. Treatment is surgical via an endoscopic or external cervical approach and should include a cricopharyngeal myotomy. Open approaches have been associated with significant morbidity because the majority of patients are older and often have other medi-

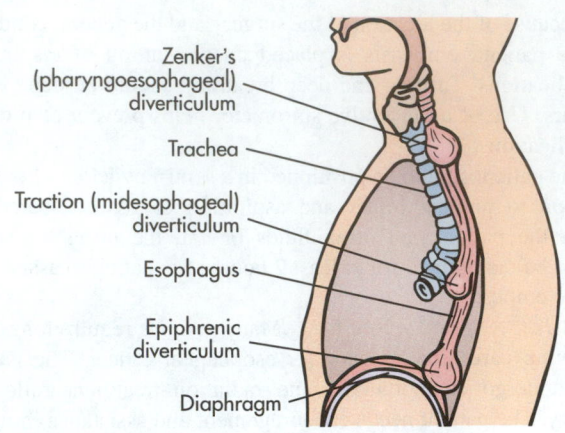

FIG. 42-8 Possible sites for the occurrence of esophageal diverticula. These hollow outpouchings may occur just above the upper esophageal sphincter (Zenker's, the most common type of pulsion diverticulum), near the midpoint of the esophagus (traction), and just above the lower esophageal sphincter (epiphrenic).

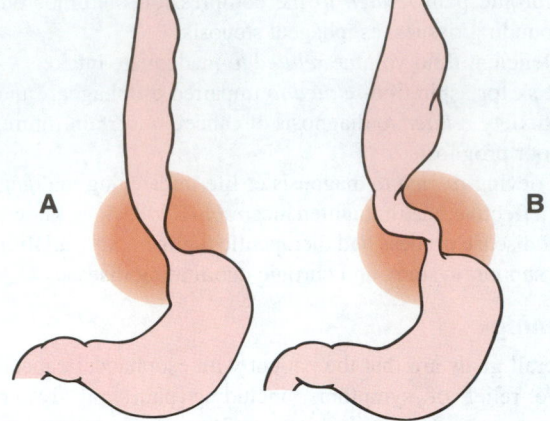

FIG. 42-9 Esophageal achalasia. **A,** Early stage, showing tapering of lower esophagus. **B,** Advanced stage, showing dilated, tortuous esophagus.

cal problems. Treatment by endoscopic stapling diverticulotomy or diverticulostomy has become increasingly popular with its distinct advantages related to decreased complications.[20]

Esophageal Strictures

Common causes of esophageal strictures include GERD and the ingestion of strong acids or alkalis. Trauma such as throat lacerations and gunshot wounds may also lead to strictures as a result of scar formation (collagen deposition). The strictures usually develop over a long time and can result in dysphagia, regurgitation, and ultimately weight loss. Strictures can be dilated endoscopically using *bougies* (dilating instruments). Strictures dilated with bougies, wire-guided dilators, or balloon dilation rarely use fluoroscopy. Surgical excision with anastomosis is sometimes necessary. The patient may have a temporary or permanent gastrostomy.

Achalasia

In **achalasia,** peristalsis of the lower two thirds (smooth muscle) of the esophagus is absent. Pressure in the LES is increased, along with incomplete relaxation of the LES. Obstruction of the esophagus at or near the diaphragm occurs. Food and fluid accumulate in the lower esophagus. The result of this condition is dilation of the lower esophagus (Fig. 42-9). The altered peristalsis is due to impairment of the neurons that innervate the lower esophagus. There is a selective loss of inhibitory neurons, resulting in unopposed contraction of the LES. Achalasia is a rare, chronic disorder affecting 1 in 100,000 Americans. It affects all ages and both genders.

Dysphagia is the most common symptom and occurs with both liquids and solids. Patients may report a globus sensation and/or substernal chest pain (similar to the angina pain) that occurs during or immediately after a meal. *Halitosis* (foul-smelling breath) and the inability to eructate (belch) are other symptoms. Patients with achalasia also report symptoms of GERD and regurgitation of sour-tasting food and liquids, especially when lying down. Weight loss is typical.

Diagnosis is made with radiologic studies, manometric studies of the lower esophagus, and/or endoscopy. The exact cause of achalasia is not known, so treatment is focused on symptom management. The goals of achalasia treatment are to relieve symptoms

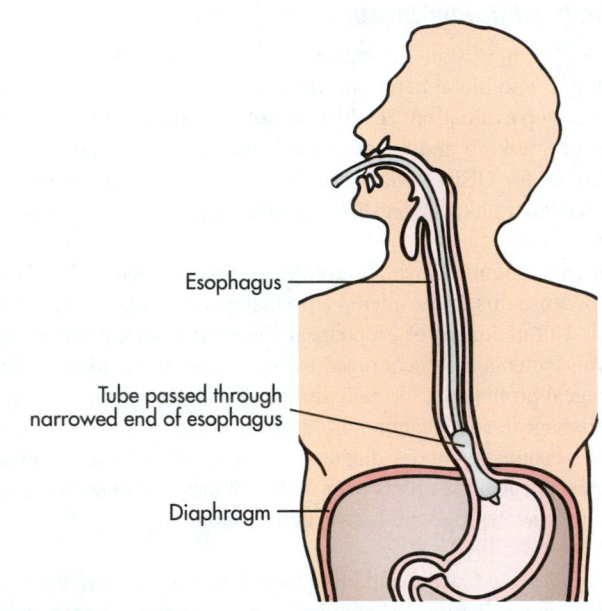

FIG. 42-10 Pneumatic dilation attempts to treat achalasia by maintaining an adequate lumen and decreasing lower esophageal sphincter (LES) tone.

(dysphagia and regurgitation), improve esophageal emptying by disrupting the LES, and prevent development of megaesophagus (enlargement of the lower esophagus).[21] Endoscopic pneumatic dilation is done as an outpatient procedure. The LES muscle is disrupted from within using balloons of progressively larger diameter (3.0, 3.5, and 4.0 cm) (Fig. 42-10). Repeat dilations are often required. A surgical procedure, Heller myotomy, is done laparoscopically. In this procedure the LES is surgically disrupted.[22] Because GERD with esophagitis and peptic stricture is a common complication, the patient often has antireflux surgery performed at the same time. The patient can usually return to work 1 to 2 weeks following this procedure.

Medical therapy is less effective than invasive procedures. Smooth muscle relaxants (nitrates and calcium channel blockers, e.g., nifedipine [Procardia]) taken immediately before meals improve dysphagia, but side effects and drug tolerance are common. The injection of botulinum toxin endoscopically into the LES gives short-term relief of symptoms and improves esophageal emptying. It works by inhibiting the release of acetylcholine from nerve endings, thereby promoting relaxation of the smooth muscle. This treatment is most effective in the elderly, because symptom relief can last up to 1 to 2 years with a single injection. Symptomatic treatment consists of a semisoft bland diet, eating slowly and drinking fluid with meals, and sleeping with the head elevated.

Esophageal Varices

Esophageal varices are dilated, tortuous veins occurring in the lower portion of the esophagus as a result of portal hypertension. Esophageal varices are a common complication of liver cirrhosis and are discussed in Chapter 44.

Disorders of the Stomach and Upper Small Intestine

GASTRITIS

Types

Gastritis, an inflammation of the gastric mucosa, is one of the most common problems affecting the stomach. Gastritis may be acute or chronic and may be diffuse or localized.

Etiology and Pathophysiology

Gastritis occurs as the result of a breakdown in the normal gastric mucosal barrier. This mucosal barrier normally protects the stomach tissue from autodigestion by HCl acid and the proteolytic enzyme pepsin. When the barrier is broken, HCl acid and pepsin can diffuse back into the mucosa. This back diffusion results in tissue edema, disruption of capillary walls with loss of plasma into the gastric lumen, and possible hemorrhage. Causes of gastritis are listed in Table 42-16.

Risk Factors

Drug-Related Gastritis. Drugs such as aspirin, nonsteroidal antiinflammatory drugs (NSAIDs), digitalis, and alendronate (Fosamax) have direct irritating effects on the gastric mucosa. For example, the ingestion of even small amounts of aspirin by a susceptible person is known to result in asymptomatic GI bleeding manifested by positive stool tests for occult blood. Corticosteroids and NSAIDs inhibit the synthesis of prostaglandins that are protective to the gastric mucosa. This leaves the gastric mucosa more susceptible to injury. NSAID-related gastritis is associated with many drugs, including piroxicam (Feldene), naproxen (Naprosyn), sulindac (Clinoril), indomethacin (Indocin), diclofenac (Voltaren), and ibuprofen (Motrin, Advil). The use of cyclooxygenase-2 (COX-2) inhibitors (e.g., celecoxib [Celebrex]) has been associated with fewer GI side effects as compared with nonselective NSAIDs. However, even these drugs are associated with an increased risk of upper GI inflammation and bleeding. Risk factors for NSAID-induced gastritis include being female, being over age 60, having a history of ulcer disease, and taking other ulcerogenic drugs, including corticosteroids and anticoagulants (warfarin [Coumadin]).

Dietary indiscretions can also result in acute gastritis. After an alcoholic drinking binge, acute damage to the gastric mucosa can range from localized injury of superficial epithelial cells to desquamation and destruction of the mucosa, with mucosal congestion, edema, and hemorrhage. Prolonged damage induced by repeated alcohol abuse can result in chronic gastritis. Eating large quantities

TABLE 42-16	Causes of Gastritis

Drugs
- Aspirin
- Corticosteroids
- Nonsteroidal antiinflammatory drugs (NSAIDs)

Diet
- Alcohol
- Spicy, irritating food

Microorganisms
- *Helicobacter pylori*
- *Salmonella*
- *Staphylococcus* organisms

Environmental Factors
- Radiation
- Smoking

Pathophysiologic Conditions
- Burns
- Large hiatal hernia
- Physiologic stress
- Reflux of bile and pancreatic secretions
- Renal failure (uremia)
- Sepsis
- Shock

Other Factors
- Endoscopic procedures
- Nasogastric tube
- Psychologic stress

of spicy, irritating foods and metabolic conditions such as uremia can also cause acute gastritis.

Helicobacter pylori. An important cause of chronic gastritis is *Helicobacter pylori (H. pylori)* infection. *H. pylori*–associated gastritis is a common problem in adults, many of whom are asymptomatic. For reasons not clearly understood, *H. pylori* is capable of promoting the breakdown of the gastric mucosal barrier, given certain "triggers" or conditions. Over time, *H. pylori* has a destructive effect on its host environment. This is consistent with the finding that the incidence of chronic gastritis increases with age. The role of *H. pylori* in ulcer development is discussed in greater detail on pp. 1016 to 1017.

Autoimmune. *Autoimmune atrophic gastritis* is a form of chronic gastritis that affects both the fundus and body of the stomach and is associated with an increased risk of gastric cancer. Approximately 30% of patients with *H. pylori* infection are also found to have antigastric antibodies. Thus there may be a link between the host's response to the presence of *H. pylori* and the development of autoimmune chronic gastritis.

Although not as common, other causes of chronic gastritis have been identified. Bacterial, viral, and fungal infections, including *Mycobacterium,* cytomegalovirus (CMV), and syphilis, are associated with chronic gastritis. Gastritis can occur from reflux of bile salts from the duodenum into the stomach as a result of anatomic changes following surgical procedures such as gastroduodenostomy and gastrojejunostomy. Prolonged vomiting may also cause reflux of bile salts. Intense emotional responses and CNS lesions may also produce inflammation of the mucosal lining as a result of hypersecretion of HCl acid or corticosteroids.

Clinical Manifestations

The symptoms of acute gastritis include anorexia, nausea and vomiting, epigastric tenderness, and a feeling of fullness. Hemorrhage is commonly associated with alcohol abuse and at times may be the only symptom. Acute gastritis is self-limiting, lasting from a few hours to a few days, with complete healing of the mucosa expected.

The manifestations of chronic gastritis are similar to those described for acute gastritis. Some patients have no symptoms directly associated with the gastric lesion. However, when the acid-secreting cells are lost or do not function as a result of atrophy, the source of intrinsic factor is also lost. The loss of *intrinsic factor,* a substance secreted by the gastric mucosa that is essential for the absorption of cobalamin (vitamin B_{12}) in the terminal ileum, ultimately results in cobalamin deficiency. With time, the body's storage of cobalamin in the liver is depleted, and a deficiency state exists. Lack of cobalamin, which is essential for the growth and maturation of RBCs, results in pernicious anemia and neurologic complications. (Cobalamin deficiency anemia is discussed in Chapter 31.)

Diagnostic Studies

Diagnosis of acute gastritis is most often based on a history of drug and alcohol use. The diagnosis of chronic gastritis may be delayed or completely missed because the symptoms are nonspecific. Endoscopic examination with biopsy is necessary to obtain a definitive diagnosis. Breath, urine, serum, stool, and gastric tissue biopsy tests are available for the determination of *H. pylori*. These tests are described under Peptic Ulcer Disease later in this chapter. Radiologic studies are not helpful because the superficial mucosa is generally involved, and changes will not show clearly on x-ray. A CBC may demonstrate the presence of anemia from blood loss or lack of intrinsic factor. Stools are tested for the presence of occult blood. A gastric analysis may be done to determine achlorhydria (lack of acid secretion), which is associated with severe atrophic gastritis. Serum tests for antibodies to parietal cells and intrinsic factor may be performed. Tissue biopsy with cytologic examination is necessary to rule out gastric carcinoma.

NURSING *and* COLLABORATIVE MANAGEMENT GASTRITIS

■ Acute Gastritis

Eliminating the cause and preventing or avoiding it in the future is generally all that is needed to treat acute gastritis. The plan of care is supportive and similar to that described for nausea and vomiting. If vomiting accompanies acute gastritis, rest, NPO status, and IV fluids may be prescribed. Dehydration can occur rapidly in acute gastritis with vomiting. Antiemetics are given for nausea and vomiting (see Table 42-1). In severe cases of acute gastritis, an NG tube may be used for several reasons: (1) to observe for bleeding; (2) for lavage of the precipitating agent from the stomach; or (3) to keep the stomach empty and free of noxious stimuli. Clear liquids are resumed when acute symptoms have subsided, with gradual reintroduction of solid, bland foods.

If hemorrhage is considered likely, frequent checking of vital signs and testing the vomitus for blood are indicated. All of the management strategies discussed in the section on upper GI bleeding also apply to the patient with severe gastritis.

Drug therapy is focused on reducing irritation of the gastric mucosa and providing symptomatic relief. Antacids are beneficial in the relief of abdominal discomfort by raising intragastric pH to

TABLE 42-17	*DRUG THERAPY* *Helicobacter pylori* Infection		
Treatment		**Duration**	**Eradication Rate**
Triple-drug therapy		7 days	>90%
proton pump inhibitor* or ranitidine bismuth citrate (Tritec) amoxicillin clarithromycin (Biaxin)			
Dual therapy		7 days	>90%
ranitidine bismuth citrate (Tritec) clarithromycin (Biaxin)			
Quadruple therapy		14 days	60%-80%
proton pump inhibitor* bismuth tetracycline metronidazole (Flagyl)			

*See Table 42-5.

above 6. H_2R blockers (e.g., ranitidine [Zantac], cimetidine [Tagamet]) or PPIs (e.g., omeprazole [Prilosec], lansoprazole [Prevacid]) may be used to reduce gastric HCl acid secretion. Combination of an H_2R blocker plus bismuth (ranitidine bismuth citrate [Tritec]) may also be used. It is important for the nurse to teach the patient about the therapeutic effects of PPIs and H_2R blockers and how to monitor for adverse effects.

■ Chronic Gastritis

The treatment of chronic gastritis focuses on evaluating and eliminating the specific cause (e.g., cessation of alcohol intake, abstinence from drugs, *H. pylori* eradication). Currently, antibiotic combinations are used to eradicate infection with *H. pylori* (Table 42-17). For the patient with pernicious anemia, oral cobalamin, nasal cobalamin, or injection of cobalamin is needed (see Chapter 31). Discussion of the lifelong need for cobalamin is provided.

The patient undergoing treatment for chronic gastritis may have to adapt to many lifestyle changes and adopt a strict adherence to a drug regimen. A nonirritating diet consisting of six small feedings a day and the use of an antacid after meals may help provide symptomatic relief. Smoking is contraindicated in all forms of gastritis. An interdisciplinary team approach in which the physician, nurse, dietitian, and pharmacist provide consistent information and support may increase the patient's success in making these alterations. Because the incidence of gastric cancer is higher in the patient who has a history of chronic gastritis, especially atrophic gastritis, close medical follow-up should be stressed.

PEPTIC ULCER DISEASE

Peptic ulcer disease (PUD) is a condition characterized by erosion of the GI mucosa resulting from the digestive action of HCl acid and pepsin. Any portion of the GI tract that comes into contact with gastric secretions is susceptible to ulcer development, including the lower esophagus, stomach, duodenum, and margin of gastrojejunal anastomosis after surgical procedures. There are approximately 500,000 new cases of ulcers diagnosed and over 4 million recurrences of PUD each year.[23]

Types

Peptic ulcers can be classified as acute or chronic, depending on the degree and duration of mucosal involvement (Fig. 42-11), and gastric or duodenal, according to the location. The *acute ulcer* (see Fig. 42-11) is associated with superficial erosion and minimal inflammation. It is of short duration and resolves quickly when the cause is identified and removed. A chronic ulcer (Fig. 42-12) is one of long duration, eroding through the muscular wall with the formation of fibrous tissue. It is present continuously for many months or intermittently throughout the person's lifetime. A chronic ulcer is at least four times as common as acute erosion.

Gastric and duodenal ulcers, although defined as PUD, are different in their etiology and incidence (Table 42-18). Generally, the treatment of all types of ulcers is similar.

Etiology and Pathophysiology

Peptic ulcers develop only in the presence of an acid environment. Patients with achlorhydria rarely have PUD. An excess of HCl acid may not be necessary for ulcer development. The typi-

cal person with a gastric ulcer has normal to less than normal gastric acidity compared with the person with a duodenal ulcer. However, some intraluminal acid does seem to be essential for an ulcer to occur.

Pepsinogen, the precursor of pepsin, is activated to pepsin in the presence of HCl acid and a pH of 2 to 3. The secretion of HCl acid by the parietal cells has a pH of 0.8. After mixing with the stomach contents, the pH reaches 2 to 3, a highly favorable range of acidity for pepsin activity. When the stomach acid level is neutralized by the presence of food or antacids or acid secretion is blocked by drugs, the pH is increased to 3.5 or more. At a pH of 3.5 or more, pepsin has little or no proteolytic activity.

The stomach is normally protected from autodigestion by the gastric mucosal barrier. The GI tract has a high cell turnover rate, and the surface mucosa of the stomach is renewed about every 3 days. As a result of this high turnover rate, the mucosa can continually repair itself except in extreme instances when the cell breakdown surpasses the cell renewal rate. Normally, water, electrolytes, and water-soluble substances (e.g., glucose) can easily pass through the barrier. However, the mucosal barrier prevents the back-diffusion of acid and pepsin from the gastric lumen through the mucosal layers to the underlying tissue. However, with certain conditions the mucosal barrier can be disrupted and back-diffusion

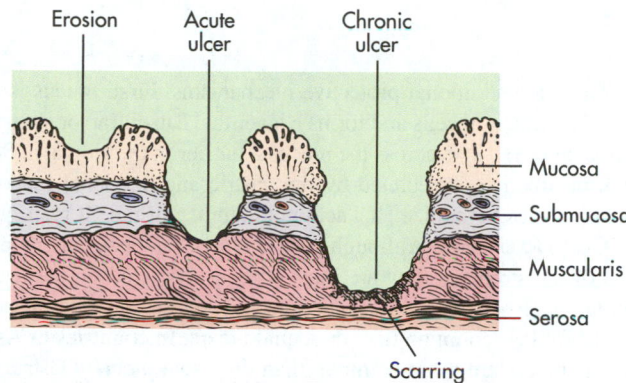

FIG. 42-11 Peptic ulcers, including an erosion, an acute ulcer, and a chronic ulcer. Both the acute ulcer and the chronic ulcer may penetrate the entire wall of the stomach.

Labels: Erosion, Acute ulcer, Chronic ulcer, Mucosa, Submucosa, Muscularis, Serosa, Scarring

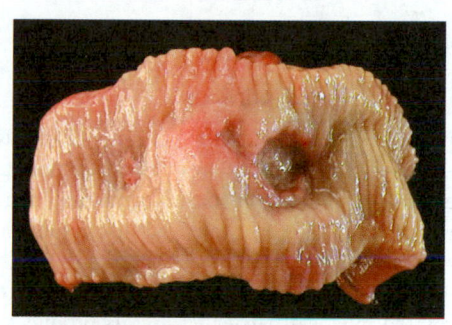

FIG. 42-12 Peptic ulcer of the duodenum.

TABLE 42-18	Comparison of Gastric and Duodenal Ulcers	
	Gastric Ulcers	**Duodenal Ulcers**
Lesion	Superficial; smooth margins; round, oval, or cone shaped	Penetrating (associated with deformity of duodenal bulb from healing of recurrent ulcers)
Location of lesion	Predominantly antrum, also in body and fundus of stomach	First 1–2 cm of duodenum
Gastric secretion	Normal to decreased	Increased
Incidence	Greater in women	Greater in men, but increasing in women, especially postmenopausal
	Peak age 50–60 yr	
	More common in persons of lower socioeconomic status	Peak age 35–45 yr
	Increased with smoking, drug use (aspirin, NSAID), and alcohol use	Associated with psychologic stress
	Increased with incompetent pyloric sphincter and bile reflux	Increased with smoking, drug use, and alcohol use
		Associated with other diseases (e.g., chronic obstructive pulmonary disease, pancreatic disease, hyperparathyroidism, Zollinger-Ellison syndrome, chronic renal failure)
Clinical manifestations	Burning or gaseous pressure in high left epigastrium and back and upper abdomen	Burning, cramping, pressurelike pain across midepigastrium and upper abdomen; back pain with posterior ulcers
	Pain 1–2 hr after meals; if penetrating ulcer, aggravation of discomfort with food	Pain 2–4 hr after meals and midmorning, midafternoon, middle of night, periodic and episodic
	Occasional nausea and vomiting, weight loss	Pain relief with antacids and food; occasional nausea and vomiting
Recurrence rate	High	High
Complications	Hemorrhage, perforation, gastric outlet obstruction, intractability	Hemorrhage, perforation, obstruction

NSAID, Nonsteroidal antiinflammatory drug.

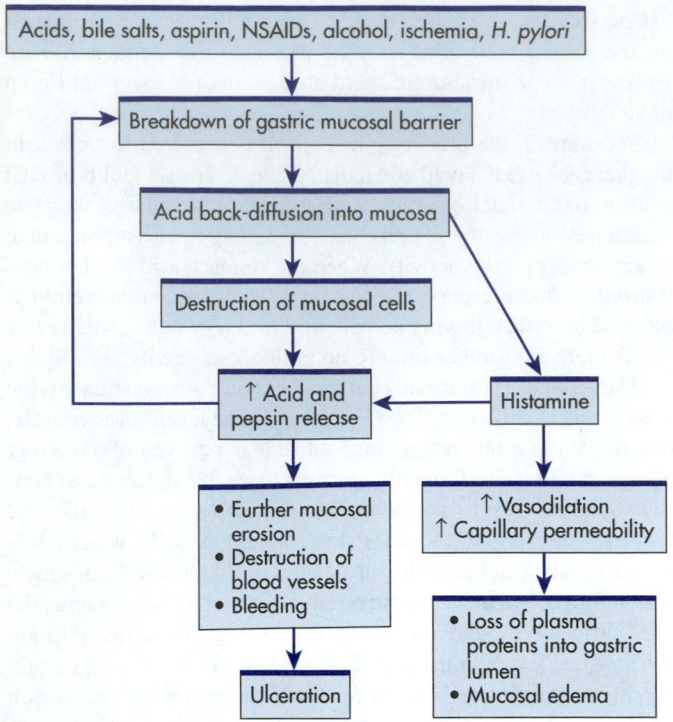

FIG. 42-13 Disruption of gastric mucosa and pathophysiologic consequences of back-diffusion of acids.

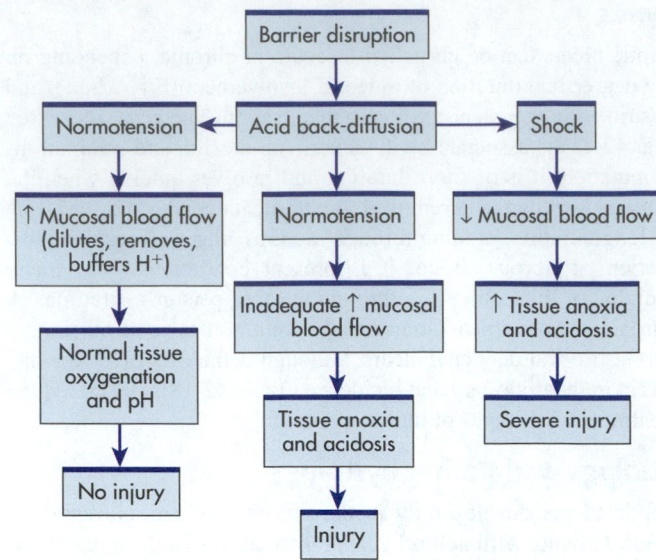

FIG. 42-14 Relationship between mucosal blood flow and disruption of the gastric mucosal barrier.

of acid and pepsin can occur (Fig. 42-13). This back-diffusion results in cellular destruction and inflammation. Histamine is released from the damaged mucosa, resulting in vasodilation and increased capillary permeability. The released histamine stimulates further secretion of acid and pepsin.

As described in the section on gastritis, a variety of agents are known to destroy the mucosal barrier. *H. pylori* produces the enzyme *urease,* which buffers the area around it through the production of ammonia, thus protecting itself from destruction. Urease also mediates inflammation, which makes the gastric mucosa more vulnerable to other noxious substances.[24] Ulcerogenic drugs, such as aspirin and NSAIDs, inhibit synthesis of prostaglandins and cause abnormal permeability. Corticosteroids have the ability to decrease the rate of mucosal cell renewal and thereby decrease its protective effects. Lipid-soluble cytotoxic drugs can pass through the barrier and destroy it. Increased vagus nerve stimulation from a variety of causes (e.g., emotions) results in hypersecretion of HCl acid and can alter the mucosal barrier. Duodenal ulcers are associated with high acid content.

When the mucosal barrier is disrupted, there is a compensatory increase in blood flow (Fig. 42-14). This occurs because of several factors, including the release of histamine, that increase capillary blood flow. As blood flow increases within the affected mucosa, hydrogen (H^+) ions are rapidly removed from the area, buffers are delivered to help neutralize the H^+ ions present, nutrients necessary for cell function arrive, and the rate of mucosal cell replication increases. When the increase is sufficient to dilute, buffer, and remove the excess H^+ ions, tissue damage may be minor or not occur at all. When blood flow is not sufficient, tissue injury results. Fig. 42-14 shows a representation of the interrelationship between the mucosal blood flow and disruption of the gastric mucosal barrier.

There are additional protective mechanisms. First, mucus is secreted by mucosal cells and forms a layer that can entrap or slow the diffusion of H^+ ions across the mucosal barrier in the stomach. Second, bicarbonate is secreted by the gastric and duodenal mucosa, and this helps neutralize HCl acid in the lumen of the GI tract.

Gastric Ulcers. Although gastric ulcers can occur in any portion of the stomach, they are most commonly found on the lesser curvature close to the antral junction. In Western countries, gastric ulcers are less common than duodenal ulcers. In countries of Asia, gastric ulcers are more common than duodenal ulcers. Gastric ulcers are more prevalent in women and in older adults. Because the peak incidence of gastric ulcers is in persons over 50 years of age, the mortality rate from gastric ulcers is greater than that from duodenal ulcers. Gastric ulcers are more likely than duodenal ulcers to result in hemorrhage, perforation, and obstruction.

Although gastric ulcers are characterized by a normal to low secretion of gastric acid, the back diffusion of acid is greater with chronic gastric ulcers than with duodenal ulcers or in the healthy person. *H. pylori* is present in 60% to 80% of patients with gastric ulcers.[25] The role of *H. pylori* in ulcer development is discussed in the section on duodenal ulcers. Injury to gastric mucosa by noxious agents such as drugs or smoking may be increased by the presence of *H. pylori.*

Drugs can cause acute and chronic gastric ulcers. The drugs most often implicated include aspirin, NSAIDs (e.g., ibuprofen), corticosteroids, and reserpine (Serpasil). It is estimated that 1% to 3% of patients taking NSAIDs for 1 year experience GI complications, including gastritis, gastric ulcer, upper GI hemorrhage, or perforation. Other known causative factors of gastric ulcer formation are chronic alcohol abuse, chronic gastritis, and bile reflux gastritis from an incompetent pyloric sphincter. Cigarette smoking is positively linked with gastric ulcers. Nicotine seems to enhance reflux of duodenal contents into the antrum of the stomach. The ingestion of hot, rough, or spicy foods has been suggested as a causative factor, but there is no evidence to substantiate this claim. Infection with herpes and CMV in immunocompromised patients may also lead to gastric ulcers.

Duodenal Ulcers. Duodenal ulcers account for about 80% of all peptic ulcers. Approximately 10% of men and 5% of women at some time in their lives will experience a duodenal ulcer.[23] Duodenal ulcers may occur at any age, but the incidence is especially high between 35 and 45 years of age. Duodenal ulcers can develop in anyone, regardless of occupation or socioeconomic group.

The development of duodenal ulcers is associated with a high HCl acid secretion. Several patient groups are at high risk of duodenal ulcer development, including those with chronic obstructive pulmonary disease, cirrhosis of the liver, chronic pancreatitis, hyperparathyroidism, chronic kidney disease, and the Zollinger-Ellison syndrome. (*Zollinger-Ellison syndrome* is a rare condition characterized by severe peptic ulceration, gastric acid hypersecretion, elevated serum gastrin levels, and gastrinoma of the pancreas or duodenum.) It is possible that the treatments used for these conditions may also promote ulcer development. Alcohol ingestion and smoking habits are also associated with duodenal ulcer formation because both are known stimulants of acid secretion.

Although many factors are associated with the development of duodenal ulcers, *H. pylori* has been identified as playing a key role. *H. pylori* is found in approximately 90% to 95% of patients with duodenal ulcers.[23] However, not all individuals with evidence of *H. pylori* go on to develop ulcers. Examination of different strains of *H. pylori* suggests differences in virulence across subtypes of the organism. *H. pylori* survives in the human upper GI tract for a long time as a result of its ability to move in mucus and attach to mucosal cells and the production of urease.

Infection with *H. pylori* is highest in underdeveloped countries and in persons of low socioeconomic status. Infection likely occurs during childhood with transmission from family members to the child, possibly through a fecal-oral and/or oral-oral route. In the United States and Canada, persons born before 1940 have a significantly higher risk of carrying *H. pylori* than persons in younger age-groups. This enhanced prevalence in older persons has been attributed to the presence of crowded living conditions and poor sanitation practices, which were more common in the first half of the last century. *H. pylori* has also been linked to gastric carcinoma and non-Hodgkin's lymphoma.[23]

Research into a genetic cause for PUD has shown that there is a familial tendency. Supporting a genetic etiology is the fact that persons with blood group O have an increased incidence of duodenal ulcers. This may be related to increased susceptibility to *H. pylori*. There is an increasing proportion of ulcers that are not due to NSAID use or *H. pylori*. In these patients it is important to rule out Zollinger-Ellison syndrome and gastric cancer.[25]

Stress-Related Mucosal Disease. Stress-related mucosal disease (SRMD) or **physiologic stress ulcers** refer to acute ulcers that develop following a major physiologic insult such as trauma or surgery (see Fig. 42-2). SRMD was described earlier in the section on acute upper GI bleeding. Because of their prevalence and high morbidity, patients at risk for SRMD receive prophylaxis with antisecretory agents, including H_2R blockers and proton pump inhibitors.

Clinical Manifestations

It is common for the person with PUD to have no pain or other symptoms. The gastric and duodenal mucosas are not rich in sensory pain fibers, which may account for this phenomenon. The pain associated with gastric ulcers is located high in the epigastrium and occurs about 1 to 2 hours after meals. The pain is described as "burning" or "gaseous." The pain can occur when the stomach is empty or when food has been ingested. If the ulcer has eroded through the gastric mucosa, food tends to aggravate rather than alleviate the pain. For some patients the earliest symptoms will be due to a serious complication such as perforation.

The patient with a duodenal ulcer may describe the pain as "burning" or "cramplike." It is most often located in the midepigastric region beneath the xiphoid process. Ulcers located on the posterior aspect of the duodenum can be manifested by back pain. The pain usually occurs 2 to 4 hours after meals. It is relieved by antacids alone or in combination with an H_2R blocker and sometimes by foods that neutralize and dilute the HCl acid. A characteristic of duodenal ulcer is its tendency to occur continuously for a few weeks or months and then disappear for a time, only to recur some months later. Some patients claim their symptoms worsen in the spring and fall of the year, suggesting a seasonal trend.

Complications

The three major complications of chronic PUD are hemorrhage, perforation, and gastric outlet obstruction. All are considered emergency situations and are initially treated conservatively. However, surgery may become necessary at any time during therapy.

Hemorrhage. Hemorrhage is the most common complication of PUD. It develops from erosion of the granulation tissue found at the base of the ulcer during healing or from erosion of the ulcer through a major blood vessel. Duodenal ulcers account for a greater percentage of upper GI bleeding episodes than gastric ulcers.

Perforation. Perforation is considered the most lethal complication of PUD. Perforation is commonly seen in large penetrating duodenal ulcers that have not healed and are located on the posterior mucosal wall (Fig. 42-15). Perforated gastric ulcers are most often located on the lesser curvature of the stomach. Even though duodenal ulcers are more prevalent and perforate more frequently, mortality rates associated with perforation of gastric ulcers are higher. The older age of the patient with gastric ulcers, who often has other concurrent medical problems, is thought to account for the higher mortality rates.

Perforation of a peptic ulcer occurs when the ulcer penetrates the serosal surface, with spillage of either gastric or duodenal contents into the peritoneal cavity. The size of the perforation is directly proportional to the length of time the patient has had the ul-

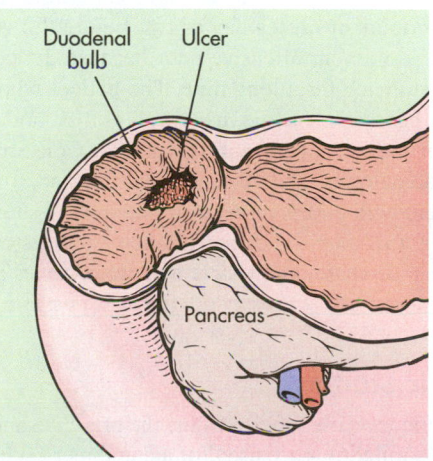

FIG. 42-15 Duodenal ulcer of the posterior wall penetrating into the head of the pancreas, resulting in walled-off perforation.

cer. The larger the perforation, the longer the history of the ulcer. Small perforations seal themselves and result in a cessation of symptoms; larger perforations require immediate surgical closure. Spontaneous sealing occurs as a result of large amounts of fibrin being produced in response to the perforation. This can lead to fibrinous fusion of the duodenum or gastric curvature to adjacent tissue, mainly the liver.

The clinical manifestations of perforation are characterized by their sudden and dramatic onset. The patient experiences sudden, severe upper abdominal pain that quickly spreads throughout the abdomen. The visceral and parietal layers of the peritoneum have an abundance of pain receptors. This contributes to the abrupt, intense pain experienced. There may be shoulder pain if the spillage causes irritation to the phrenic nerve. The abdominal muscles contract, appearing rigid and boardlike as they attempt to protect the abdomen from further injury. The patient's respirations become shallow and rapid. Bowel sounds are usually absent. Nausea and vomiting may occur. Many patients report a history of PUD or recent symptoms of indigestion.

The contents entering the peritoneal cavity from the stomach or duodenum may contain air, saliva, food particles, HCl acid, pepsin, bacteria, bile, and pancreatic fluid and enzymes. Bacterial peritonitis may occur within 6 to 12 hours. The intensity of the peritonitis is proportional to the amount and duration of the spillage through the perforation. It is difficult to determine from symptoms alone whether a gastric or duodenal ulcer has perforated because the clinical characteristics of intestinal perforation are the same (see Chapter 43).

Gastric Outlet Obstruction. Ulcers located in the antrum and the pyloric areas of the stomach and the duodenum can predispose to gastric outlet obstruction. The obstruction is due to edema, inflammation, pylorospasm, as well as fibrous scar tissue formation, all of which contribute to the narrowing of the pylorus. In the early phase of obstruction, gastric emptying is normal to near normal. Over time, increased contractile force needed to empty the stomach results in hypertrophy of the stomach wall. After longstanding obstruction, the stomach dilates and becomes atonic.

The patient with gastric outlet obstruction generally has a long history of ulcer pain. The pain progresses to a more generalized upper abdominal discomfort that becomes worse toward the end of the day as the stomach fills and dilates. Relief may be obtained by belching or by self-induced vomiting. Vomiting is common and often projectile. The vomitus contains food particles that were ingested many hours or even a day or two before the vomiting episode. There is often an offensive odor because the contents have been in the stomach for a long time. The patient who vomits frequently will become anorectic, have weight loss, and complain of thirst and an unpleasant taste in the mouth. Constipation occurs because of dehydration and decreased diet intake.

The patient with gastric outlet obstruction may show a swelling in the upper abdomen indicating dilation of the stomach. Loud peristalsis can be heard, and visible peristaltic waves are often observed. If the stomach is grossly dilated, it is possible to palpate it as well.

Diagnostic Studies

The diagnostic tests used to determine the presence and location of an ulcer are similar to those used for acute upper GI bleeding. Endoscopy is the procedure most often used because it allows for direct viewing of the gastric and duodenal mucosa. Endoscopy is also used to determine the degree of ulcer healing after treatment. During endoscopy, tissue specimens can be obtained for identification of *H. pylori* and to rule out gastric cancer.

Several diagnostic tests are available to confirm *H. pylori* infection. These are classified as noninvasive and invasive. Noninvasive tests include serum or whole blood antibody tests, in particular, immunoglobulin G (IgG). This test is approximately 90% to 95% sensitive for *H. pylori* infection. However, because of the length of time that IgG levels remain elevated in the blood after the infection, the serologic tests will not distinguish active from recently treated disease. The urea breath test can determine the presence of active infection. Urea is a by-product of the metabolism of *H. pylori* bacteria. Although not as accurate as the urea breath test, stool antigen tests can also be performed. Invasive tests involve biopsy of the stomach and include the rapid urease test, as well as other histologic markers of infection. These tests have greater sensitivity and specificity but involve an endoscopic procedure.

Barium contrast studies, although widely used, are not accurate in identifying shallow, superficial ulcers because of failure of the barium to properly fill the ulcer crater. X-ray studies are also ineffective in differentiating PUD from a malignant tumor. In addition, x-rays do not demonstrate the degree of healing that can be visually determined with the endoscope. Barium studies are of benefit in the diagnosis of gastric outlet obstruction.

Gastric analysis can help determine the presence of a possible gastrinoma (Zollinger-Ellison syndrome). Elevated serum gastrin levels combined with elevated gastric acid secretion levels are suggestive of a gastrinoma. Gastric analysis procedure is described in Table 39-12.

Laboratory tests, including a CBC, urinalysis, liver enzyme studies, serum amylase determination, and stool examination, should be performed. A CBC may indicate the presence of anemia secondary to ulcer bleeding. Liver enzyme studies help determine any liver problems, such as cirrhosis, that may complicate PUD treatment. Stools are routinely tested for the presence of blood. A serum amylase determination is done to determine pancreatic function when posterior duodenal ulcer penetration of the pancreas is suspected.

Collaborative Care: Conservative Therapy

When the patient's clinical manifestations and health history suggest the diagnosis of PUD and diagnostic studies confirm it, a medical regimen is instituted (Table 42-19). The regimen consists of adequate rest, dietary modifications, drug therapy, elimination of smoking, and long-term follow-up care. The aim of treatment is to decrease gastric acidity, enhance mucosal defense mechanisms, and minimize the harmful effects on the mucosa.

Patients are generally treated in ambulatory care clinics. The healing of a peptic ulcer requires many weeks of therapy. Pain disappears after 3 to 6 days, but ulcer healing is much slower. Complete healing may take 3 to 9 weeks, depending on ulcer size, treatment regimen, and patient compliance. Healing of the ulcer may be assessed by means of endoscopic examination or x-rays. Endoscopic examination is the most accurate method to monitor for ulcer healing.

Adequate rest, both physical and emotional, is important for ulcer healing. A quiet, calm environment at home or on the job is not easy to achieve and may require some modifications in the patient's daily routine. The benefits derived from the elimination or reduction of stressors may help decrease HCl acid secretion.

TABLE 42-19	*COLLABORATIVE CARE* **Peptic Ulcer Disease**

Diagnostic
History and physical examination
Upper GI endoscopy with biopsy
H. pylori testing of breath, urine, blood, tissue
Upper GI barium contrast study
Complete blood count
Urinalysis
Liver enzymes
Serum electrolytes

Collaborative Therapy
Conservative Therapy
Adequate rest
Dietary modifications
Cessation of smoking
Drug therapy
- H₂-receptor blockers (see Table 42-20)
- Proton pump inhibitors (see Table 42-20)
- Antibiotics for *H. pylori* (see Table 42-17)
- Antacids (see Table 42-21)
- Anticholinergics
- Cytoprotective drugs (see Table 42-20)
Stress management

Acute Exacerbation without Complications
NPO
NG suction
Adequate rest
Cessation of smoking
IV fluid replacement
Drug therapy
- H₂-receptor blockers
- Proton pump inhibitors
- Antacids
- Anticholinergics
- Sedatives

Acute Exacerbation with Complications (Hemorrhage, Perforation, Obstruction)
NPO
NG suction
Bed rest
IV fluid replacement (lactated Ringer's solution)
Blood transfusions
Stomach lavage (possible)

Surgical Therapy
Perforation—simple closure with omentum graft
Gastric outlet obstruction—pyloroplasty and vagotomy
Ulcer removal/reduction
- Billroth I and II
- Vagotomy and pyloroplasty

GI, Gastrointestinal; *IV*, intravenous; *NG*, nasogastric; *NPO*, nothing by mouth.

TABLE 42-20	*DRUG THERAPY* **Peptic Ulcer Disease**

Antisecretory
H₂-receptor blockers
- cimetidine (Tagamet)
- famotidine (Pepcid)
- nizatidine (Axid)
- ranitidine (Zantac)
Proton pump inhibitors
- esomeprazole (Nexium)
- lansoprazole (Prevacid)
- omeprazole (Prilosec)
- pantoprazole (Protonix)
- rabeprazole (Aciphex)
Anticholinergics

Antisecretory and Cytoprotective
misoprostol (Cytotec)

Cytoprotective
sucralfate (Carafate)
bismuth subsalicylate (Pepto-Bismol)

Neutralizing
Antacids (see Table 42-21)

Antibiotics for *H. pylori*
amoxicillin
metronidazole (Flagyl)
tetracycline
clarithromycin (Biaxin)

Others
Tricyclic antidepressants
- imipramine (Tofranil)
- doxepin (Sinequan)

pected benefits. Strict adherence to the prescribed regimen of drugs is important. Drug therapy is outlined in Tables 42-19 through 42-22.

Because recurrence of ulcers is frequent, interruption or discontinuation of therapy can have detrimental results. The patient is encouraged to comply with therapy and continue with follow-up care as prescribed. Antacids, H₂R blockers, and PPIs may be stopped after the ulcer has healed or may be prescribed in the form of low-dose maintenance therapy. No other drugs, unless prescribed by the health care provider, should be taken because they may have an ulcerogenic effect. Finally, the patient and family are told what to do in the event that pain and discomfort recur or blood is noted in the vomitus or stools.

Histamine (H₂)-Receptor Blockers. H₂R blockers, cimetidine (Tagamet), ranitidine (Zantac), famotidine (Pepcid), and nizatidine (Axid), are frequently used in PUD treatment. These drugs block the action of histamine on the H₂ receptors and thus reduce HCl acid secretion. This decreases the conversion of pepsinogen to pepsin, and accelerates ulcer healing. (Antihistamine drugs used to treat allergies are H₁R blockers and have no effect on HCl acid secretion.)

H₂R blocker drugs may be administered orally or intravenously. Depending on the specific drug, therapeutic effects last up to 12 hours. However, the onset of action (i.e., symptom relief) is longer than antacids. Famotidine, ranitidine, and nizatidine have longer half-lives than cimetidine, thus requiring fewer doses and providing nocturnal HCl acid suppression. More side effects are

Aspirin and nonselective NSAIDs may be discontinued. Patients requiring NSAIDs may be prescribed a COX-2 inhibitor. When aspirin or nonselective NSAIDs must be continued, enteric-coated preparations or coadministration with a PPI or misoprostol (Cytotec) should be considered.

Smoking has an irritating effect on the mucosa, increases gastric motility, and delays mucosal healing. It should be eliminated completely or severely reduced. Avoidance or restriction of alcohol intake will also enhance healing. The combination of adequate rest and abstinence from smoking accelerates ulcer healing.

Drug Therapy. Drugs are a vital part of therapy. The patient is taught about each drug prescribed, why it is ordered, and the ex-

TABLE 42-21

DRUG THERAPY
Antacid Preparations

Ingredient	Trade Name
Single Substance	
Aluminum carbonate	Basaljel
Aluminum hydroxide gel tablets	Amphojel, Alu-Cap
Aluminum phosphate	Phosphajel
Calcium carbonate	Alka-2, Tums
Dihydroxyaluminum aminoacetate	Robalate
Dihydroxyaluminum sodium carbonate	Rolaids
Magaldrate	Riopan
Magnesium oxide	Mag-Ox
Sodium bicarbonate	Alka-Seltzer
Mixtures of Aluminum Hydroxide and Magnesium Salts	
	Aludrox
	Delcid
	Gaviscon
	Gelusil and Gelusil M
	Maalox
	Mylanta
	WinGel
Mixtures of Calcium Carbonate and Aluminum and Magnesium Hydroxides	
	Camalox
Mixtures of Calcium Carbonate, Magnesium Carbonate, and Magnesium Oxide	
	Alkets

TABLE 42-22

DRUG THERAPY
Side Effects of Antacid Therapy

Antacid	Reactions
Aluminum hydroxide gels	Constipation, phosphorus depletion with chronic use
Calcium carbonate	Constipation or diarrhea, hypercalcemia, milk-alkali syndrome, renal calculi
Magnesium preparations	Diarrhea, hypermagnesemia
Sodium preparations	Milk-alkali syndrome if used with large amounts of calcium; used with caution in patients on sodium restrictions

associated with cimetidine. These include granulocytopenia, gynecomastia, diarrhea, fatigue, dizziness, rash, and mental confusion in the older adult. However, the rate of these side effects is low. Famotidine and nizatidine are considered more potent at reduced dosage levels as compared with cimetidine, and side effects are minimal. There are OTC forms of H$_2$R blockers currently available at a lower dose than drugs that are prescribed. H$_2$R blockers are used in combination with antibiotics to treat ulcers related to *H. pylori* and are used prophylactically to reduce SRMD.

Proton Pump Inhibitors. PPIs, such as omeprazole (Prilosec), lansoprazole (Prevacid), pantoprazole (Protonix), rabeprazole (Aciphex), and esomeprazole (Nexium), block the ATPase enzyme that is important for the secretion of HCl acid. PPIs are more effective than H$_2$R blockers in reducing gastric acid secretion and promoting ulcer healing. PPIs are also used in combination with antibiotics to treat ulcers caused by *H. pylori*.

Antibiotic Therapy. Antibiotics to eradicate *H. pylori* infection are prescribed. The treatment of *H. pylori* is the most important element of treating PUD in patients positive for *H. pylori*. When *H. pylori* is present, ulcer recurrence rates with H$_2$R blockers alone can be as high as 75% to 90%, whereas with antibiotic treatment the recurrence rate may be less than 10%. Antibiotic therapy for *H. pylori* is shown in Table 42-17. A growing percentage of patients will not have the *H. pylori* eradicated with a single round of therapy because of the development of antibiotic-resistant organisms. Thus second-line therapies for those who relapse are being tested.[26]

Once the presence of *H. pylori* has been determined, antibiotic treatment is instituted. The regimen of choice is based on the antibiotic susceptibility of the *H. pylori* organism, patient compliance, side effects, and costs. Most drug regimens involve treatment for 7 to 14 days. No single agents have been effective in eliminating *H. pylori* (see Table 42-17).

Antacids. Antacids are used as adjunct therapy for PUD. They increase gastric pH by neutralizing the HCl acid. As a result, the acid content of chyme reaching the duodenum is reduced. In addition, some antacids, such as aluminum hydroxide, can bind to bile salts, thus decreasing the detrimental effects of bile on the gastric mucosa. Patients who are at risk for SRMD may be treated prophylactically with antacids along with an antisecretory agent.

Antacids consist of systemic and nonsystemic types. Systemic antacids, such as sodium bicarbonate, are extremely soluble and are absorbed into the circulation. Their long-term use can lead to systemic alkalosis; therefore they are rarely used in PUD treatment. The nonsystemic antacids are insoluble and poorly absorbed. The common commercial nonsystemic antacids consist of magnesium hydroxide or aluminum hydroxide as single preparations or in various combinations (see Table 42-21).

The antacid preparation may be in liquid or tablet form. A large number of tablets may be required to equal the same dose of a liquid preparation. Because the tablets are chewable, some of the drug is left coating the teeth and gingivae instead of the stomach.

The neutralizing effects of antacids taken on an empty stomach last only 20 to 30 minutes because they are quickly evacuated. When antacids are taken after meals, the effects may last as long as 3 to 4 hours. Therapy recommending frequent dosing (e.g., hourly) often results in poor compliance.

After the acute phase of bleeding has diminished, antacids are generally administered hourly, either orally or through the NG tube. If the tube is in place, the stomach contents should be aspirated and tested periodically for pH level. If pH is less than 5, intermittent suction may be used, or the frequency or dosage of the antacid or antisecretory agent may be increased.

The type and dosage of antacid prescribed depends on side effects (see Table 42-22), as well as potential drug interactions. Preparations high in sodium (e.g., Titralac) should be used with caution in older adults and in the patient with liver cirrhosis, hypertension, heart failure, and renal disease. Magnesium preparations should not be prescribed for the patient with renal failure because of the risk of magnesium toxicity. The most frequent side effect experienced with magnesium antacids is diarrhea. Aluminum hydroxide causes constipation. An antacid combination of aluminum and magnesium salts seems to lessen the side effects of both.

Antacids have the capacity to interact unfavorably with some drugs. They can enhance the absorption of drugs such as dicumarol and amphetamines. The action of digitalis preparations can be potentiated when taken in combination with calcium or magnesium antacids. In some instances, antacids may decrease the absorption rates of prescribed drugs, such as tetracycline. Therefore it is important to inform the health care provider of any drugs that are being taken before antacid therapy is begun.

Cytoprotective Drug Therapy. Sucralfate (Carafate) is used for the short-term treatment of ulcers. It provides cytoprotection for the esophagus, stomach, and duodenum. Its ability to accelerate ulcer healing is thought to be due to the formation of an ulcer-adherent complex covering the ulcer and thereby protecting it from erosion caused by pepsin, acid, and bile salts. Sucralfate does not have acid-neutralizing capabilities. Its action is most effective at a low pH, and it should be given at least 30 minutes before or after an antacid. Adverse side effects are minimal. However, it does bind with cimetidine, digoxin, warfarin (Coumadin), phenytoin (Dilantin), and tetracycline, causing reduced bioavailability of these drugs.

Misoprostol (Cytotec) is a synthetic prostaglandin analog. It has protective and some antisecretory effects on gastric mucosa. Misoprostol is the only drug approved in the United States for the prevention of gastric ulcers induced by NSAIDs and aspirin. Misoprostol does not interfere with the therapeutic effects of aspirin and NSAIDs. Persons who require chronic NSAID therapy, such as those with osteoarthritis, may benefit from the use of misoprostol. Misoprostol should not be used in women of reproductive age who are pregnant or not using contraception.

Anticholinergic Drugs. Anticholinergic drugs are only occasionally used for PUD treatment. These drugs decrease cholinergic (vagal) stimulation of HCl acid. Because they decrease gastric motility, they are not used when gastric outlet obstruction is a concern. Anticholinergics are associated with a number of side effects, such as dry mouth and skin, flushing, thirst, tachycardia, dilated pupils, blurred vision, and urine retention. Anticholinergics must be prescribed with caution in the patient with narrow-angle glaucoma and benign prostatic hyperplasia.

Other Drugs. Tricyclic antidepressants (e.g., imipramine [Tofranil], doxepin [Sinequan]) and serotonin reuptake inhibitors may be prescribed for patients with PUD. Antidepressants may contribute to overall pain relief through their effects on afferent pain fiber transmission. In addition, tricyclic antidepressants have, to varying degrees, some anticholinergic properties, which results in reduced acid secretion.

Nutritional Therapy. Dietary modifications may be necessary so that foods and beverages irritating to the patient can be avoided or eliminated. A nonirritating or bland diet consisting of six small meals a day may be recommended during the symptomatic phase. However, there is controversy over the benefits of bland diets because there is little scientific evidence for their use. Each patient should be instructed to eat and drink foods and fluids that do not cause any distressing symptoms. Alcohol and caffeine-containing products should be eliminated because of their irritating effects.

Dietary instructions should include a sample diet with a list of foods that usually cause distress and should therefore be eliminated from the diet. Foods known to irritate the gastric mucosa include hot, spicy foods and pepper, alcohol, carbonated beverages, tea, coffee, and broth (meat extract). These foods also have limited buffering ability in addition to stimulating gastric acid secretion. Foods high in roughage, such as raw fruit, salads, and vegetables, may irritate an inflamed mucosa. If these foods are well chewed, this seems to be less of a problem.

Protein is considered the best neutralizing food, but it also stimulates HCl acid secretion. Carbohydrates and fats are the least stimulating to HCl acid secretion, but they do not neutralize well. The patient must determine a suitable combination of nutrients without causing undue distress.

Therapy Related to Complications of Peptic Ulcer Disease

Acute Exacerbation. The patient with an acute exacerbation of PUD can usually be treated with the same regimen used for conservative therapy. However, the situation is considered more serious because of the possible complications of perforation, hemorrhage, and gastric outlet obstruction.

An acute exacerbation is frequently accompanied by bleeding, increased pain and discomfort, and nausea and vomiting. If the patient experiences recurrent vomiting or gastric outlet obstruction, an NG tube is placed into the stomach with intermittent suction for about 24 to 48 hours. If there is a history of an incompetent pyloric sphincter allowing reflux of duodenal contents into the stomach, an NG tube will remove intestinal contents from the stomach. This period of stomach rest eliminates any causative factors that may have precipitated the acute exacerbation and permits the resolution of edema and inflammation of the mucosa. Fluids and electrolytes are replaced by IV infusion until the patient is able to tolerate oral feedings. Management is similar to that described for upper GI bleeding (see pp. 997 to 1000).

Endoscopic evaluation is performed to reveal the degree of inflammation or bleeding, as well as the ulcer location. It is important to ascertain the presence of a prepyloric or pyloric ulcer that can cause gastric outlet obstruction. When endoscopic examination reveals no major problems and the patient's physical condition stabilizes, the plan of care for the patient should follow the same regimen of diet, activity, and drugs used in conservative therapy. A 5-year follow-up program is recommended after acute exacerbation. Although conservative treatment may enhance ulcer healing, it may not prevent scar formation and gastric outlet obstruction.

Perforation. The immediate focus of management of a patient with a perforation is to stop the spillage of gastric or duodenal contents into the peritoneal cavity and restore blood volume. An NG tube is inserted into the stomach to provide continuous aspiration and gastric decompression to halt spillage through the perforation. Although duodenal aspiration is not achieved as promptly, placement of the tube as near to the perforation site as possible facilitates decompression.

Circulating blood volume must be replaced with lactated Ringer's and albumin solutions. These solutions substitute for the fluids lost from the vascular and interstitial space as the peritonitis develops. Blood replacement in the form of packed RBCs may be necessary. A central venous pressure line and an indwelling urinary catheter may be inserted and monitored hourly. The patient with a history of cardiac disease requires ECG monitoring or placement of a pulmonary artery catheter for more accurate assessment of left ventricular function. Broad-spectrum antibiotic therapy should be started immediately to treat bacterial peritonitis. Administration of pain medications provides comfort.

Either open or laparoscopic procedures are used for perforation repair depending on the location of the ulcer and the surgeon's preference. The procedure involving the least risk to the patient is simple oversewing of the perforation and reinforcement of the area with a graft of omentum. The excess gastric contents are suctioned from the peritoneal cavity during the surgical procedure. There is controversy regarding the need for more definitive surgical treatment of a perforated ulcer than can be achieved with simple closure.

Gastric Outlet Obstruction. The aim of therapy for obstruction is to decompress the stomach, correct any existing fluid and electrolyte imbalances, and improve the patient's general state of health. An NG tube is used as described previously. With continuous decompression for several days, the stomach has the opportunity to regain its normal muscle tone, the ulcer can begin healing, and the inflammation and edema will subside.

After several days of suction, the NG tube is clamped and gastric residual volume is measured periodically. The frequency and amount of time the tube remains clamped are proportional to the amount of aspirate obtained and the comfort level of the patient. A method commonly followed is to clamp the tube overnight for approximately 8 to 12 hours and to measure the gastric residue in the morning. When the aspirate falls below 200 ml, it is considered to be within a normal range and the patient can begin oral intake of clear liquids. Initially, oral fluids are begun at 30 ml per hour and then gradually increased in amount. The patient is assessed for signs of distress or vomiting. As the amount of gastric residue decreases, solid foods are added and the tube is removed.

IV fluids and electrolytes are administered according to the degree of dehydration, vomiting, and electrolyte imbalance indicated by laboratory studies. Pain relief results from the decompression and analgesics are usually not necessary. Antacids and antisecretory drug therapy (i.e., H_2R blockers, PPIs) are used if the obstruction is due to an active ulcer as determined by endoscopy. Pyloric obstruction may be treated endoscopically by balloon dilations. Surgical intervention may be necessary to remove scar tissue.

NURSING MANAGEMENT
PEPTIC ULCER DISEASE

▪ *Nursing Assessment*

Subjective and objective data that should be obtained from a patient with PUD are presented in Table 42-23.

▪ *Nursing Diagnoses*

Nursing diagnoses related to PUD may include, but are not limited to, those presented in NCP 42-2.

▪ *Planning*

Overall goals are that the patient with PUD will (1) comply with the prescribed therapeutic regimen, (2) experience a reduction or absence of discomfort, (3) exhibit no signs of GI complications, (4) have complete healing of the peptic ulcer, and (5) make appropriate lifestyle changes to prevent recurrence.

▪ *Nursing Implementation*

Health Promotion. Nurses need to be involved in identifying patients at risk for PUD. Early detection and treatment of ulcers are important aspects of reducing morbidity associated with PUD. Patients who are taking ulcerogenic drugs (e.g., aspirin, NSAIDs) are at risk for PUD. Patients are encouraged to take these drugs with food or milk. Patients need to be taught to report symptoms related to gastric irritation, including epigastric pain, to their health care provider.

TABLE 42-23	*NURSING ASSESSMENT* **Peptic Ulcer Disease**

Subjective Data
Important Health Information
Past health history: Chronic kidney disease, pancreatic disease, chronic obstructive pulmonary disease, serious illness or trauma, hyperparathyroidism, cirrhosis of the liver, Zollinger-Ellison syndrome
Medications: Use of aspirin, corticosteroids, nonsteroidal antiinflammatory drugs
Surgery or other treatments: Complicated or prolonged surgery

Functional Health Patterns
Health perception–health management: Chronic alcohol abuse, smoking, caffeine use; family history of peptic ulcer disease
Nutritional-metabolic: Weight loss, anorexia; nausea and vomiting, hematemesis; dyspepsia, heartburn, belching
Elimination: Black, tarry stools
Cognitive-perceptual: Duodenal ulcers—burning, midepigastric or back pain occurring 2 to 4 hours after meals and relieved by food; nocturnal pain common; gastric ulcers—high epigastric pain occurring 1 to 2 hours after meals; pain may be precipitated or aggravated by food
Coping–stress tolerance: Acute or chronic stress

Objective Data
General
Anxiety, irritability

Gastrointestinal
Epigastric tenderness

Possible Findings
Anemia; guaiac-positive stools; gastric analysis indicating high gastric acid secretion; positive blood, urine, breath, or stool tests for *H. pylori*; abnormal upper gastrointestinal endoscopic and barium studies

---

Acute Intervention. During the acute exacerbation of an ulcer, the patient often complains of increased pain and nausea and vomiting, and some may have evidence of bleeding. Initially many patients attempt to cope with the symptoms at home before seeking medical assistance.

During this acute phase the patient may be NPO for a few days, have an NG tube inserted and connected to intermittent suction, and have IV fluid replacement. The rationale for this therapy must be conveyed to the anxious patient and family. They must understand that the advantages far outweigh any temporary discomfort imposed by the presence of the NG tube. Regular mouth care alleviates the dry mouth. Cleansing and lubrication of the nares facilitate breathing and decrease soreness. Gastric contents may be analyzed for pH, blood, bile, or other substances. When the stomach is kept empty of gastric secretions, the ulcer pain diminishes and ulcer healing begins.

The volume of fluid lost, signs and symptoms of the patient, and laboratory test results (hemoglobin, hematocrit, and electrolytes) determine the type and amount of IV fluids administered. The nurse should be aware of any other current health problem (e.g., heart failure) that could be adversely affected by the type or amount of fluid used. Vital signs are initially taken at least hourly so that shock can be detected and treated.

Physical and emotional rest is conducive to ulcer healing. The patient's immediate environment should be quiet and restful. The

NURSING CARE PLAN 42-2

Patient with Peptic Ulcer Disease

NURSING DIAGNOSIS   **Acute pain** *related to* increased gastric secretions, decreased mucosal protection, and ingestion of gastric irritants *as evidenced by* burning cramplike pain in epigastrium and abdomen; pain onset 1 to 2 hr after meals with gastric ulcer; pain onset 2 to 4 hr after meals (midmorning, midafternoon) and middle of night with duodenal ulcer

PATIENT GOAL   Reports pain controlled without the use of analgesics

OUTCOMES (NOC)	INTERVENTIONS (NIC) and *RATIONALES*
Pain Control	**Pain Management**
• Describes causal factors ____	• Perform a comprehensive assessment of pain to include location, characteristics, onset/duration, frequency, quality, intensity or severity of pain, and precipitating factors *to determine appropriate intervention*.
• Uses preventive measures ____	• Provide the person optimal pain relief with prescribed analgesics *to provide comfort*.
• Uses nonanalgesic relief measures ____	
• Uses analgesics appropriately ____	• Select and implement a variety of measures (e.g., pharmacologic, nonpharmacologic, interpersonal) *to facilitate pain relief*.
• Reports change in pain symptoms or sites to health care professional ____	• Teach the use of nonpharmacologic techniques (e.g., relaxation, guided imagery, music therapy, distraction, acupressure, massage) before, after, and, if possible, during painful activities; before pain occurs or increases; and along with other pain-relief measures *because relaxation results in decreased acid production and reduction in pain*.
• Reports pain controlled ____	
Measurement Scale	
1 = Never demonstrated	
2 = Rarely demonstrated	
3 = Sometimes demonstrated	
4 = Often demonstrated	
5 = Consistently demonstrated	

NURSING DIAGNOSIS   **Ineffective therapeutic regimen management** *related to* lack of knowledge of long-term management of peptic ulcer disease and consequences of not following treatment plan and unwillingness to modify lifestyle *as evidenced by* frequent questions about home care, incorrect responses to questions about peptic ulcer disease, noncompliance with medical regimen

PATIENT GOALS   1. Verbalizes understanding of the therapeutic regimen, including knowledge of disease, rationale for treatment plan, and benefits of disease management
2. Verbalizes a commitment to self-care and management of the disease

OUTCOMES (NOC)	INTERVENTIONS (NIC) and *RATIONALES*
Knowledge: Treatment Regimen	**Teaching: Disease Process**
• Description of specific disease process ____	• Explain the pathophysiology of the disease and how it relates to anatomy and physiology *to foster understanding*.
• Description of self-care responsibilities for ongoing treatment ____	• Discuss lifestyle changes that may be required to prevent future complications and/or control the disease process.
• Description of prescribed diet ____	• Instruct patient on which signs and symptoms to report to health care provider *to ensure early initiation of treatment*.
• Description of prescribed medication(s) ____	
Measurement Scale	• Discuss therapy/treatment options.
1 = None	• Describe rationale behind management/therapy/treatment recommendations.
2 = Limited	
3 = Moderate	
4 = Substantial	
5 = Extensive	

Continued

use of a mild sedative or tranquilizer has beneficial effects when the patient is anxious and apprehensive. The nurse must use good judgment before sedating a person who is becoming increasingly restless. There is danger that the drug will mask the signs of shock secondary to upper GI bleeding.

If the patient's condition improves without progression of symptoms (e.g., increased pain, vomiting, hemorrhage), the regimen outlined for conservative therapy is followed. However, complications such as hemorrhage, perforation, and obstruction can occur.

Hemorrhage. Changes in the vital signs and an increase in the amount and redness of the aspirate often signal massive upper GI bleeding. When there is bleeding, the patient's pain is often decreased because the blood helps neutralize the acidic gastric contents. It is important to maintain the patency of the NG tube so that blood clots do not obstruct the tube. If the tube becomes blocked, the patient can develop abdominal distention. Similar interventions to those described for upper GI bleeding on pp. 999 to 1000 are used.

Perforation. When there is sudden, severe abdominal pain unrelated in intensity and location to the pain that brought the patient to the hospital, the nurse must recognize the possibility of ulcer perforation. Perforation is indicated by a rigid, boardlike

NURSING CARE PLAN 42-2

Patient with Peptic Ulcer Disease—cont'd

NURSING DIAGNOSIS   **Nausea** *related to* acute exacerbation of disease process *as evidenced by* episodes of nausea and/or vomiting (see NCP 42-1)

COLLABORATIVE PROBLEMS

POTENTIAL COMPLICATION   **Hemorrhage** secondary to eroded mucosal tissue

NURSING GOALS	NURSING INTERVENTIONS and *RATIONALES*
• Monitor for signs of hemorrhage. • Carry out appropriate medical and nursing interventions if hemorrhage occurs.	• Assess for evidence of hematemesis, bright red or melena stool, abdominal pain or discomfort, symptoms of shock (e.g., decreased BP; cool, clammy skin; dyspnea; tachycardia; decreased urine output) *to plan appropriate interventions.* • If ulcer is actively bleeding, observe NG tube aspirate or emesis for amount and color *to assess degree of bleeding.* • Take vital signs every 15-30 min *to determine patient's hemodynamic status and as indicators of shock.* • Maintain IV infusion line *to provide ready access for blood and fluid replacement.* • If RBC transfusion is given, observe for transfusion reaction *so appropriate actions can be taken immediately.* • Monitor hematocrit and hemoglobin *as indicators of severity of hemorrhage and need for fluid and blood replacement.* • Record intake and output *to monitor fluid balance.* • Reassure patient and family *to decrease their anxiety.* • Remain calm and confident in plan of care *to foster calm and confidence in patient and family.* • Prepare patient for possible endoscopy or surgery.

POTENTIAL COMPLICATION   **Perforation of GI mucosa** secondary to impaired mucosal tissue integrity

NURSING GOALS	NURSING INTERVENTIONS and *RATIONALES*
• Monitor for signs of perforation. • Carry out appropriate medical and nursing interventions.	• Observe for manifestations of perforation (e.g., sudden, severe abdominal pain; rigid, boardlike abdomen; radiating pain to shoulders; increasing distention; decreasing bowel sounds) *to ensure early recognition and intervention.* • Take vital signs every 15-30 min *to determine patient's hemodynamic status and as indicators of shock.* • Maintain NG tube to suction *to provide continuous aspiration and gastric decompression to prevent further leakage of gastric fluid through the perforation.* • Administer pain medication *to promote comfort and reduce anxiety.* • Prepare patient for emergency diagnostic tests and possible surgery *to foster timely intervention.*

abdomen; severe generalized abdominal and shoulder pain; drawing up of the knees; and shallow, grunting respirations. The bowel sounds that may have been previously normal or hyperactive may diminish and become absent. When the patient with an ulcer demonstrates these changes, perforation should be suspected and the health care provider notified immediately.

Vital signs are promptly taken and recorded every 15 to 30 minutes. The nurse should temporarily stop all oral or NG drugs and feedings until the health care provider can be notified and a definitive diagnosis made. If perforation does exist, anything taken orally can add to the spillage into the peritoneal cavity and increase discomfort. If IV fluids are being administered at the time of the perforation, the rate should be maintained or increased to replace the depleted plasma volume.

When perforation is confirmed, antibiotic therapy is usually started. When the perforation fails to seal spontaneously, surgical or laparoscopic closure is necessary and is performed as soon as

possible. There is often little time to adequately prepare the patient and family thoroughly for the surgical intervention.

Gastric Outlet Obstruction. Gastric outlet obstruction can occur at any time. It is most likely to occur in the patient whose ulcer is located close to the pylorus. Because the onset of symptoms is usually gradual, the condition is not generally as emergent as hemorrhage or perforation. Relief of symptoms may be achieved by constant NG aspiration of stomach contents. This allows edema and inflammation to subside and then permits normal flow of gastric contents through the pylorus.

Obstruction can also occur during the treatment of an acute exacerbation. If these symptoms are experienced while the patient is still on NPO status, the patency of the NG tube should be suspected. Regular irrigation of the tube with a saline solution facilitates proper functioning. It may be helpful to reposition the patient from side to side so that the tube tip is not constantly lying against the mucosal surface.

When oral feedings have been resumed and symptoms of obstruction are observed, the health care provider should be promptly informed. Generally, all that is necessary to treat the problem is to resume gastric aspiration so that the edema and inflammation resulting from the acute episode have time to resolve. IV fluids with electrolyte replacement keep the patient hydrated during this period. The NG tube can be clamped and gastric fluids can be aspirated to check for retention. It is important to maintain accurate intake and output records, especially of the gastric aspirate. When conservative treatment is not successful, surgery may be performed after the acute phase has passed.

Ambulatory and Home Care. The patient in whom PUD has been diagnosed has specific needs that must be met to prevent and avoid recurrence or complications. General instructions should cover aspects of the disease process itself, drugs, possible changes in lifestyle (including diet), and regular follow-up care. Table 42-24 provides a patient and family teaching guide for the patient with PUD.

Knowing the etiology and pathophysiology of PUD may motivate the patient to become involved in care and increase compliance with therapy. The patient must understand the dietary modifications and why they are important for recovery and health maintenance. The nurse and the dietitian should elicit a dietary history from the patient and plan for ways that dietary modifications can be easily incorporated into the patient's home and work setting. The patient who is following a diet prescribed for another illness needs to know how to balance the two so that neither condition is harmed by dietary interventions.

The patient does not always give the health care provider accurate information regarding habitual use of alcohol or cigarettes. The nurse should provide useful information about the detrimental effects of alcohol and cigarettes on PUD and ulcer healing.

The nurse should teach the patient about prescribed drugs, including their actions, side effects, and inherent dangers if omitted for any reason. The patient should know why OTC drugs (e.g., aspirin) should not be taken unless approved by the health care provider. Because antacids and some H_2R blockers and PPIs may be bought without a prescription, the patient needs to be informed that interchanging brands without checking with the health care provider or nurse can lead to harmful side effects.

Efforts should be made to obtain information about the patient's psychosocial status. Knowledge of lifestyle, occupation, and coping behaviors can be helpful in planning care. The patient may be reluctant to talk about personal subjects, the stress experienced at home or on the job, the usual methods of coping, or dependence on drugs or alcohol.

The need for long-term follow-up care must be stressed. Because successful treatment is often followed by a recurrence of the PUD, the patient is encouraged to seek immediate intervention if symptoms return. The patient who has recurrence following initial healing must learn to live with a chronic disease. The patient may be angry and frustrated, especially if the prescribed mode of therapy has been faithfully followed yet has failed to prevent the recurrence.

Some patients do not comply with the plan of care originally designed, and they experience repeated exacerbations. Patients quickly learn that they often experience no discomfort when they omit prescribed drugs or indulge in occasional dietary indiscretions. Consequently, they make no or little alteration in lifestyle. After an acute exacerbation the patient is often more amenable to following the plan of care and open to suggestions for changes in lifestyle. Changes, such as smoking cessation and alcohol abstinence, are difficult for many people. The patient may fare better from a reduction in his or her use of these substances rather than from total elimination. Although alcohol and smoking are known to interfere with ulcer healing, they frequently serve as coping mechanisms. From the patient's point of view, the distress caused by their total elimination may outweigh the benefits to be gained from abstention. The goal, however, should always be total cessation. A patient with chronic PUD must be aware of the complications, the clinical manifestations indicating their presence, and what to do until the health care provider can be seen.

■ **Evaluation**

Expected outcomes for the patient with peptic ulcer disease are addressed in NCP 42-2.

Collaborative Care: Surgical Therapy for Peptic Ulcer Disease

Because of antisecretory agents currently available, surgery for PUD is uncommon. Surgery is performed on those patients who are unresponsive to medical management, where there is a concern about gastric cancer, and in those patients whose ulcers are drug induced but the patients cannot be withdrawn from the drugs (e.g., patients with rheumatoid arthritis).

Surgical procedures include partial gastrectomy, vagotomy, and pyloroplasty. Partial gastrectomy with removal of the distal two thirds of the stomach and anastomosis of the gastric stump to the duodenum is called a *gastroduodenostomy* or *Billroth I* operation (Fig. 42-16). Partial gastrectomy with removal of the distal two thirds of the stomach and anastomosis of the gastric stump to the jejunum is called a *gastrojejunostomy* or *Billroth II* operation. To

TABLE 42-24	**PATIENT AND FAMILY TEACHING GUIDE** Peptic Ulcer Disease

The following are teaching guidelines for the patient and family:
1. Explain dietary modifications, including avoidance of foods that cause epigastric distress. This may include black pepper, spicy foods, and acidic foods. Small, frequent meals are better tolerated than large meals.
2. Explain the rationale for avoiding cigarettes. In addition to promoting ulcer development, smoking will delay ulcer healing.
3. Encourage the need to reduce or eliminate alcohol ingestion.
4. Explain the rationale for avoiding OTC drugs unless approved by the patient's care provider. Many preparations contain ingredients, such as aspirin, that should not be taken unless approved by the health care provider. Check with the care provider regarding the use of nonsteroidal antiinflammatory drugs.
5. Explain the rationale for not interchanging brands of antacids and H_2-receptor blockers that can be purchased OTC without checking with the health care provider. This can lead to harmful side effects.
6. Teach the need to take all medications as prescribed. This includes both antisecretory and antibiotic drugs. Failure to take medications as prescribed can result in relapse.
7. Explain the importance of reporting any of the following:
   • Increased nausea and/or vomiting
   • Increase in epigastric pain
   • Bloody emesis or tarry stools
8. Explain the relationship between symptoms and stress. Stress-reducing activities or relaxation strategies are encouraged.
9. Encourage patient and family to share concerns about lifestyle changes and living with a chronic illness.

OTC, Over-the-counter.

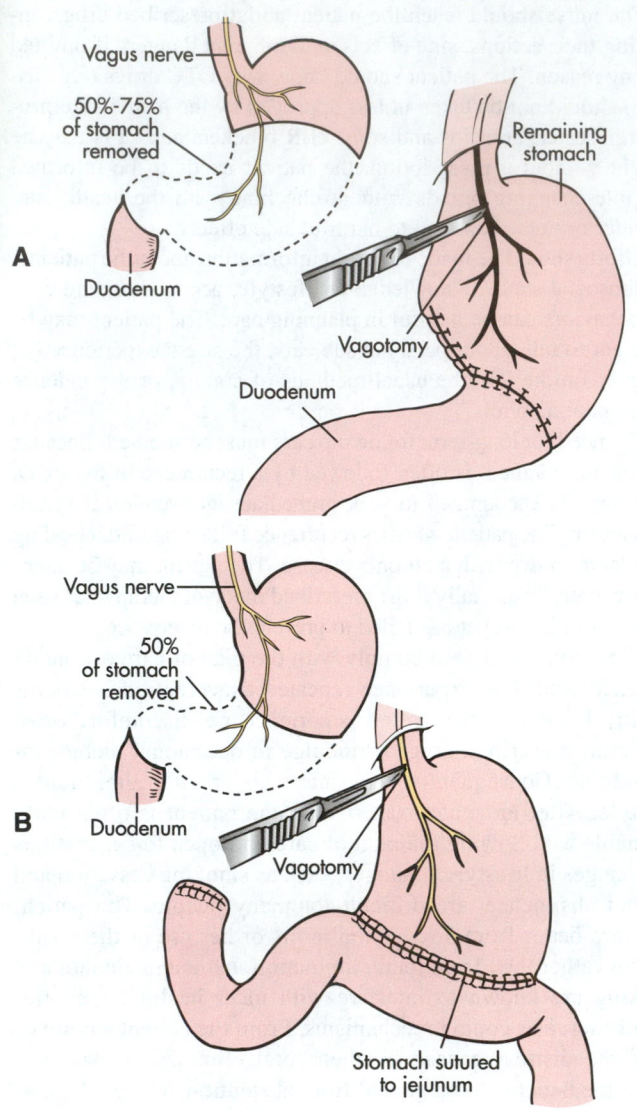

FIG. 42-16   **A,** Billroth I procedure (subtotal gastric resection with gastroduodenostomy anastomosis). **B,** Billroth II procedure (subtotal gastric resection with gastrojejunostomy anastomosis).

prevent recurrence of duodenal ulcers, the Billroth II operation is the preferred surgical procedure.

Vagotomy is the severing of the vagus nerve, either totally (truncal) or selectively at some point in its innervation to the stomach. *Selective vagotomy* consists of cutting the nerve at a particular branch of the vagus nerve, resulting in denervation of only a portion of the stomach, such as the antrum or the parietal cell mass. Vagotomy is done in conjunction with gastrectomy.

Pyloroplasty consists of surgical enlargement of the pyloric sphincter to facilitate the easy passage of contents from the stomach. It is commonly done after vagotomy or to enlarge an opening that has been constricted from scar tissue. A vagotomy decreases gastric motility and, subsequently, gastric emptying. A pyloroplasty accompanying vagotomy increases gastric emptying.

Postoperative Complications. The most common postoperative complications from PUD surgery are (1) dumping syndrome, (2) postprandial hypoglycemia, and (3) bile reflux gastritis.

Dumping Syndrome. *Dumping syndrome* is the direct result of surgical removal of a large portion of the stomach and the pyloric

sphincter. Approximately one third to one half of patients experience dumping syndrome after PUD surgery.

Dumping syndrome is associated with meals having a hyperosmolar composition. Normally, gastric chyme enters the small intestine in small amounts, and shifts in fluid from the extracellular space are minimal. After surgery, however, the stomach no longer has control over the amount of gastric chyme entering the small intestine. Consequently, a large bolus of hypertonic fluid enters the intestine and results in fluid being drawn into the bowel lumen. This creates a decrease in plasma volume along with distention of the bowel lumen and rapid intestinal transit.

The onset of symptoms occurs at the end of a meal or within 15 to 30 minutes after eating. The patient usually describes feelings of generalized weakness, sweating, palpitations, and dizziness. These symptoms are attributed to the sudden decrease in plasma volume. The patient complains of abdominal cramps, *borborygmi* (audible abdominal sounds produced by hyperactive intestinal peristalsis), and the urge to defecate. These manifestations usually last for no longer than an hour after meals.

Postprandial Hypoglycemia. *Postprandial hypoglycemia* is considered a variant of the dumping syndrome because it is the result of uncontrolled gastric emptying of a bolus of fluid high in carbohydrate into the small intestine. The bolus of concentrated carbohydrate results in hyperglycemia and the release of excessive amounts of insulin into the circulation. A secondary hypoglycemia then occurs, with symptoms appearing about 2 hours after meals. The symptoms experienced are the ones observed in any hypoglycemic reaction and include sweating, weakness, mental confusion, palpitations, tachycardia, and anxiety.

Bile Reflux Gastritis. Gastric surgery that involves the pylorus, either reconstruction or removal, can result in reflux alkaline gastritis. Prolonged contact of bile, especially bile salts, causes damage to the gastric mucosa. Chronic gastritis of this form may result in the back-diffusion of H^+ ions through the gastric mucosa. Paradoxically, PUD may recur after surgical treatment that was intended as a cure.

The symptoms associated with reflux alkaline gastritis are continuous epigastric distress that increases after meals. Vomiting relieves the distress, but only temporarily. The administration of cholestyramine (Questran), either before or with meals, has met with success. Cholestyramine binds with the bile salts that are the source of irritation in this condition. Aluminum hydroxide antacids have also been used in the treatment of this condition.

Nutritional Therapy. Discharge planning and instruction should be started as soon as the immediate postoperative period is successfully passed. Dietary instructions may be given by the dietitian and reinforced by the nursing staff. Because the stomach's reservoir is diminished after gastric resection, the meal size must be reduced accordingly. The patient should be advised to reduce drinking fluids (approximately 4 ounces) with meals. Dry foods with a low carbohydrate content and moderate protein and fat content are better tolerated initially. These dietary changes, along with a short rest period after each meal, reduce the likelihood of dumping syndrome. Reassurance that following these dietary measures will result in decreased symptoms within a few months is essential to long-term compliance.

Postprandial hypoglycemic reaction can be avoided if these dietary instructions are followed. The immediate ingestion of sugared fluids or candy relieves the hypoglycemic symptoms. The treatment of hypoglycemia is similar to that of dumping syndrome. To avoid similar occurrences the patient should be instructed to

TABLE 42-25	*NUTRITIONAL THERAPY* **Postgastrectomy Dumping Syndrome**

Purposes
- To slow the rapid passage of food into the intestine
- To control symptoms of the dumping syndrome (dizziness, sense of fullness, diarrhea, tachycardia), which sometimes occur following a partial or total gastrectomy

Diet Principles
- Meals are divided into six small feedings to avoid overloading intestines at mealtimes.
- Fluids should not be taken with meals but at least 30-45 min before or after meals; this helps prevent distention or a feeling of fullness.
- Concentrated sweets (e.g., honey, sugar, jelly, jam, candies, sweet pastries, sweetened fruit) are avoided because they sometimes cause dizziness, diarrhea, and a sense of fullness.
- Protein and fats are increased to promote rebuilding of body tissues and to meet energy needs. Meat, cheese, eggs, and milk products are specific foods to increase in the diet.
- Amount of time these restrictions should be followed varies. The health care provider decides the proper amount of time to remain on this prescribed diet according to the patient's clinical condition and progress.

limit the amount of sugar consumed with each meal and to eat small, frequent meals with moderate amounts of protein and fat. Although only a small percentage of patients experience bile reflux gastritis, the patient must be cautioned to notify the health care provider of any continuous epigastric distress after meals that is similar to that felt before surgery.

With regard to dumping syndrome, the symptoms are self-limiting and often disappear within several months to a year after surgery. The diet should consist of small dry feedings daily that are low in carbohydrate, are restricted in refined sugars, and contain moderate amounts of protein and fat (Table 42-25). Fluids should be taken between meals but not with the meal, and the patient should plan rest periods of at least 30 minutes after each meal. Reassuring the patient that the unpleasant symptoms are usually of short duration is helpful in gaining cooperation. A small percentage of patients experience long-term problems and may require further reconstructive surgery.

NURSING MANAGEMENT
SURGICAL THERAPY FOR PEPTIC ULCER DISEASE

■ *Preoperative Care*

Given the greater use of endoscopic procedures for the treatment of PUD, surgical procedures are used less frequently. Surgery can involve either laparoscopic or open surgery techniques. When surgery is planned, the surgeon should provide necessary information about the procedure and the expected outcome so that the patient can make an informed decision. The nurse can help the patient and family by clarifying and interpreting their questions. Instructions should be clear on what to expect after surgery, including comfort measures, pain relief, coughing and breathing exercises, use of an NG tube, and IV fluid administration (see Chapter 18).

■ *Postoperative Care*

Care of the patient after major abdominal surgery is similar to the postoperative care after abdominal laparotomy (see Chapter 43). An NG tube is used to decompress the remaining portion of the stomach to decrease pressure on the suture line and to allow for resolution of edema and inflammation resulting from surgical trauma.

The gastric aspirate is observed for color, amount, and odor during the immediate postoperative period. The color of the aspirate is expected to be bright red at first, with a gradual darkening within the first 24 hours after surgery. Normally the color changes to yellow-green within 36 to 48 hours. If the tube becomes clogged during this period, the health care provider may order periodic gentle irrigations with normal saline solution. It is essential that the NG suction is working and that the tube remains patent so that accumulated gastric secretions do not put a strain on the anastomosis. This can lead to distention of the remaining portion of the stomach and result in (1) rupture of the sutures, (2) leakage of gastric contents into the peritoneal cavity, (3) hemorrhage, and (4) possible abscess formation. If the tube must be replaced or repositioned, the health care provider must be called to perform this task because of the danger of perforating the gastric mucosa or disrupting the suture line.

The nurse observes the patient for signs of decreased peristalsis and lower abdominal discomfort that may indicate intestinal obstruction. Accurate intake and output records must be kept. Vital signs are monitored and recorded every 4 hours.

The patient is kept comfortable and free of pain by the administration of the prescribed drugs and by frequent changes in position. If open surgery was performed, the incision is relatively high in the epigastrium and may interfere with deep-breathing and coughing measures. Splinting the area with a pillow while gently and persistently encouraging the patient helps prevent pulmonary complications. Splinting also protects the abdominal suture line from rupturing during coughing. The dressing must be observed for signs of bleeding or odor and drainage indicative of an infection. Early ambulation is encouraged.

While the NG tube is connected to suction, IV therapy is maintained. Potassium and vitamin supplements are added to the infusion until oral feedings are resumed. Before the NG tube is removed, the patient is started on oral feedings of clear liquids to determine the tolerance level. The stomach may be aspirated within 1 or 2 hours to assess the amount remaining and its color and consistency. When fluids are well tolerated, the tube is removed and fluids are increased in frequency with a slow progression to regular foods. The regimen of six small meals a day is begun.

Pernicious anemia is a long-term complication of total gastrectomy and may occur after partial gastrectomy. Pernicious anemia is due to the loss of intrinsic factor, which is produced by the parietal cells. Depending on the amount of parietal cell mass removed in surgery, the patient may eventually require cobalamin replacement therapy (see Chapter 31).

PUD is a chronic problem, and ulcers can recur, especially at the site of the anastomosis. Adequate rest, adequate nutrition, and avoidance of known irritants and stressors are keys to recovery. Avoiding the use of drugs not prescribed by the health care provider is reemphasized, along with restrictions on smoking and alcohol use. If the patient is willing to make these kinds of adjustment in lifestyle, a successful rehabilitation is more likely.

GERONTOLOGIC CONSIDERATIONS
PEPTIC ULCER DISEASE

The incidence of PUD and, in particular, gastric ulcers in patients over 60 years of age is increasing. This is related to the increased use of NSAIDs. In the older patient, pain may not be the first symptom associated with an ulcer. For some patients the first manifestation may be frank gastric bleeding (e.g., hematemesis, melena) or a decrease in hematocrit. The morbidity and mortality rates associated with PUD in the elderly patient are higher than those for younger adults because of concomitant health problems (e.g., cardiovascular, pulmonary) and a decreased ability to withstand hypovolemia.

The treatment and management of PUD in older adults are similar to those in younger adults. An emphasis is placed on prevention of both gastritis and PUD. This includes teaching the patient to take NSAIDs and other gastric-irritating drugs with food, milk, or antacids. The patient may be treated with antisecretory agents (i.e., PPIs or H_2R blockers). The patient should be instructed to avoid irritating substances, such as alcohol and smoking, and to report abdominal pain or discomfort to his or her health care provider.

STOMACH CANCER

Stomach (gastric) **cancer** is an adenocarcinoma of the stomach wall (Fig. 42-17). The rate of stomach cancer has been steadily declining in the United States since the 1930s. However, it still accounts for more than 11,550 deaths and 21,860 new cancer cases annually.[1] Worldwide, gastric adenocarcinoma is the second most common cancer. Stomach cancer is more prevalent in men of the lower socioeconomic class, primarily those living in urban areas. Stomach cancer is more common in Hispanics, African Americans, and Asians/Pacific Islanders than in whites. The incidence of stomach cancer increases with age, with most individuals diagnosed in their 70s. Only 10% to 20% of patients have disease confined to the stomach, and over 50% have advanced metastatic disease at the time of diagnosis. The 5-year survival rate is 80% in patients with early stages (confined to the stomach) and less than 30% in those with advanced disease.

Etiology and Pathophysiology

Many factors have been implicated in the development of stomach cancer, yet no single causative agent has been identified. Stomach carcinogenesis probably begins with a nonspecific mucosal injury as a result of aging, autoimmunity, or repeated exposure to irritants such as bile, antiinflammatory agents, or smoking. Stomach cancer has been associated with diets containing smoked foods, salted fish and meat, and pickled vegetables. Whole grains and fresh fruits and vegetables are associated with reduced rates of stomach cancer. Infection with *H. pylori,* especially at an early age, is considered a risk factor for stomach cancer. It is possible that *H. pylori*

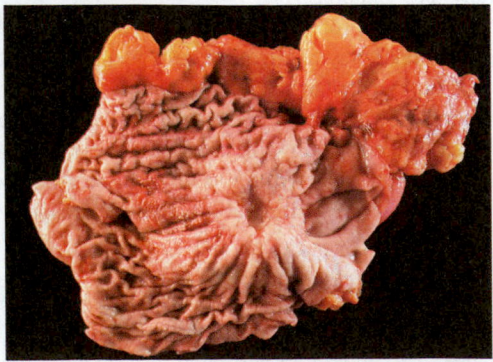

FIG. 42-17   Stomach carcinoma. Gross photograph showing an ill-defined, excavated central ulcer surrounded by irregular, heaped-up borders.

and resulting metabolic changes can induce a sequence of transitions from dysplasia to cancer.[27]

Other predisposing factors associated with stomach cancer include atrophic gastritis, pernicious anemia, adenomatous polyps, hyperplastic polyps, hypertrophic gastropathy (Ménétrier's disease), and achlorhydria. Smoking and obesity both increase the risk of stomach cancer. Stomach cancer is more likely to develop in the patient who has had a gastrectomy for PUD. Although first-degree relatives of patients with stomach cancer are at increased risk, only 8% to 10% of stomach cancers have an inherited familial component.[27] Additional genetic factors are being explored.

Adenocarcinomas account for more than 95% of the cancers, and sarcomas (comprising lymphomas and leiomyomas) make up the rest. Stomach cancer can occur in any portion of the stomach. Tumors located at the cardia and fundus are associated with a poor prognosis. These tumors spread by direct extension and typically infiltrate rapidly to the surrounding tissue and liver. The rich lymphatic plexuses in the stomach facilitate distant metastasis. Seeding of tumor cells into the peritoneal cavity may occur late in the course of the disease. Evidence of spread to the peritoneal cavity is manifested by ascites.

Clinical Manifestations

Stomach cancers often spread to adjacent organs before any distressing symptoms occur. The tumor may grow to large dimensions without obstructing the lumen of the stomach simply because the lumen itself is so large. The clinical manifestations include signs and symptoms of anemia, PUD, or indigestion. Anemia is common. It is caused by chronic blood loss as the lesion erodes through the mucosa or as a result of pernicious anemia (due to loss of intrinsic factor). The person appears pale and weak and complains of fatigue, weakness, dizziness, and, in extreme cases, shortness of breath. The stool may be positive for occult blood.

The pain and discomfort of stomach cancer may be alleviated by belching and by the use of antacids, antisecretory agents, and diet modifications similar to PUD. Manifestations related to indigestion include vague epigastric fullness with feelings of early satiety after meals *(dyspepsia).* Weight loss, dysphagia, and constipation frequently accompany epigastric distress. When nausea, vomiting, and hematemesis occur, they may indicate gastric outlet obstruction or may be a warning of impending hemorrhage.

With more advanced disease, the physical examination may reveal that the patient is pale and lethargic. When the appetite has been poor and weight loss has been considerable, the patient may appear cachectic. A mass can often be detected beneath the abdominal wall and is seen to move with each inspiration. On palpation the mass may be felt in the epigastrium. Tumors in the gastric antrum are generally found to the left of the midline. Masses located to the right of midline tend to be metastases to the liver or indicate involvement of the perigastric lymph nodes. Supraclavicular lymph nodes that are hard and enlarged and located on the left side are suggestive of metastasis via the thoracic duct. The presence of ascites is a poor prognostic sign.

Diagnostic Studies

The diagnostic studies for stomach cancer are presented in Table 42-26. Endoscopic examination of the stomach remains the best diagnostic tool. Lesions that go undetected on x-ray can be more easily viewed and a biopsy performed when endoscopy is used.

TABLE 42-26	COLLABORATIVE CARE Stomach Cancer

Diagnostic
History and physical examination
Endoscopy and biopsy
Upper GI barium study
Exfoliative cytology
Endoscopic ultrasonography
Complete blood count
Urinalysis
Stool examination
Liver enzymes
Serum amylase
Tumor markers
    Carcinoembryonic antigen (CEA)
    Carbohydrate antigen (CA) 19-9

Collaborative Therapy
Surgery
• Subtotal gastrectomy—Billroth I or II procedure
• Total gastrectomy with esophagojejunostomy
Adjuvant therapy
• Radiation therapy
• Chemotherapy
• Combination radiation therapy and chemotherapy

GI, Gastrointestinal.

The stomach can be distended with air during the procedure so that the mucosal folds can be stretched. Biopsy of the tissue and subsequent histologic examination are important for the diagnosis of stomach cancer. Endoscopic ultrasound and CT scanning can be used for the staging of the disease.

Upper GI barium studies may demonstrate alterations in gastric contractility and emptying. On x-ray examination the malignant ulcer crater is more irregular around the edges and more elevated than the craters found with benign PUD. Barium studies do not always detect small lesions of the cardia and fundus.

Blood chemistry studies detect anemia and its severity. Elevations in liver enzymes and serum amylase levels may indicate liver and pancreatic involvement. Stool examination provides evidence of occult or gross bleeding. Tumor markers, including CA 19-9 and CEA (see Table 42-26), are being examined for their potential roles as indicators of prognosis and tumor growth.[27]

Collaborative Care

When the diagnosis of stomach cancer has been confirmed, the treatment of choice is surgical removal of the tumor. The preoperative management of the patient with stomach cancer focuses on the correction of nutritional deficits and treatment of anemia.

Transfusions of packed RBCs correct the anemia. If a gastric lesion is located at or near the pylorus and is causing gastric outlet obstruction, gastric decompression may be necessary before surgery. When the tumor has extended into the transverse colon and partial colon resection is also required, special preparation of the bowel is necessary. This preparation may include a low-residue diet, enemas to cleanse the bowel, and the use of antibiotics to reduce the intestinal bacteria. Correction of malnutrition is important if surgery is planned. Malnutrition is associated with increased postoperative complications and mortality rates.

Surgical Therapy. The surgical intervention used in the treatment of stomach cancer may be the same surgical procedures

used for PUD. The location and extent of the lesion, the patient's physical condition, and preference of the surgeon determine the specific surgery employed (e.g., open versus laparoscopic). For patients with lymph node–negative stomach cancer, surgical treatment alone results in a 75% 5-year survival rate.[27] For patients with lymph node–positive cancer, the 5-year survival rate following surgery is 10% to 30%. The negative outcomes are due to the high incidence of local recurrence and distant metastases after surgery. Survival rates are less when organs adjacent to the stomach show evidence of invasion at the time of surgery.

The surgical aim is to remove as much of the stomach as necessary to remove the tumor and a margin of normal tissue. When the lesion is located in the fundus, a total gastrectomy with esophagojejunostomy is performed (Fig. 42-18). Lesions located in the antrum or the pyloric region are generally treated by either a Billroth I or II procedure. The omentum is often removed as well. When metastasis has occurred to adjacent organs, such as the spleen, ovaries, or bowel, the surgical procedure is modified and extended as necessary.

Adjuvant Therapy. Surgery is the only definitive means of achieving a cure. When the patient is a poor surgical candidate or when surgical cure is not feasible, radiation therapy or chemotherapy alone or in combination may be used. Neither radiation therapy nor chemotherapy alone has been successful when used as the primary mode of treatment. Because the radiosensitivity of stomach cancer is low, radiation therapy is of little value. However, radiation therapy may be used as a palliative measure to decrease tumor mass and provide temporary relief of obstruction.

The combination of chemotherapy and radiation therapy may be used for patients who are at high risk for disease recurrence following surgery. Chemotherapeutic agents identified as having some effect on stomach cancer are 5-FU, cisplatin, and either epirubicin (Ellence) or etoposide (Toposar). The combination of radiation therapy and chemotherapy involving 5-FU and leucovorin following surgical resection increases survival. Additional therapies, including intraperitoneal administration of chemotherapeutic

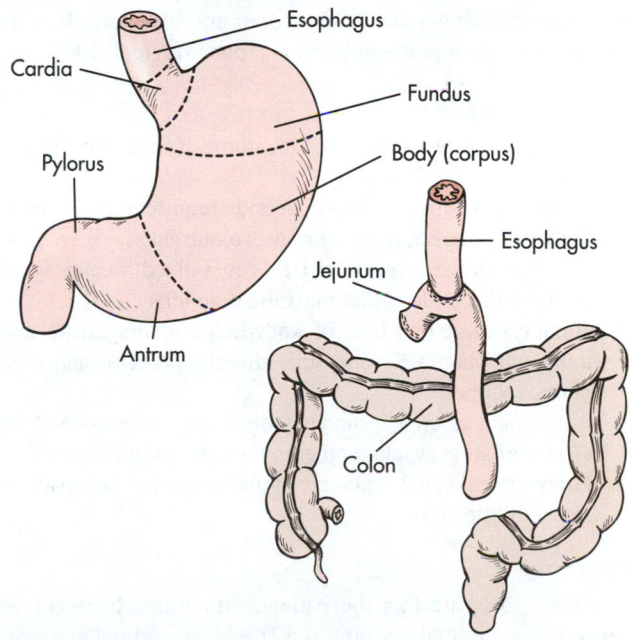

FIG. 42-18   Total gastrectomy for stomach cancer (total gastrectomy with esophagojejunostomy).

agents and immunotherapy, are undergoing evaluation. (These therapies are discussed in Chapter 16.)

NURSING MANAGEMENT
STOMACH CANCER

■ Nursing Assessment

The assessment of a person with possible stomach cancer is similar to that done for PUD (see Table 42-23). Important data to be obtained from the patient and the family should include a nutritional assessment, a psychosocial history, the patient's perceptions of the health problem and need for care, and the physical examination of the patient.

The nutritional assessment elicits information regarding appetite and changes in eating patterns over the previous 6 months. It is necessary to determine the patient's normal weight and any recent changes that may have occurred. Unexplained weight loss is common. A history of vague symptoms of dyspepsia, early satiety, feeling full after consuming even a small amount of food, or reporting symptoms of gas pain should help the nurse differentiate these typical stomach cancer symptoms from those of PUD. The nurse should determine whether pain is present, where and when it occurs, and how it is relieved.

It is important to determine the patient's personal perception of the health problem and method of coping with hospitalization, diagnostic tests, and procedures. The possibility of a diagnosis of cancer and a treatment regimen that may include surgery, chemotherapy, or radiation treatment is stressful. It is important for the nurse to support the patient and family if tests result in a cancer diagnosis and complex treatment interventions are planned. If surgery is probable, the nurse assesses the patient's expectations regarding surgery (cure or palliation) and how the patient has responded to previous surgical procedures.

A physical examination reveals the patient's current functional abilities, the presence of other health problems, and an estimate of how well the patient may respond to therapy. Cachexia may be evident if the nutritional intake has been reduced for an extended period of time. A malnourished patient does not respond well to chemotherapy or radiation therapy and is a poor surgical risk.

■ Nursing Diagnoses

Nursing diagnoses for the patient with stomach cancer include, but are not limited to, the following:

- Imbalanced nutrition: less than body requirements *related to* inability to ingest, digest, or absorb nutrients
- Activity intolerance *related to* generalized weakness, abdominal discomfort, and nutritional deficits
- Anxiety *related to* lack of knowledge of diagnostic tests, unknown diagnostic outcome, disease process, and therapeutic regimen
- Acute pain *related to* underlying disease process and side effects of surgery, chemotherapy, or radiation therapy
- Grieving *related to* perceived unfavorable diagnosis and impending death

■ Planning

The overall goals are that the patient with stomach cancer will (1) experience minimal discomfort, (2) achieve optimal nutritional status, and (3) maintain a degree of spiritual and psychologic well-being appropriate to the disease stage.

■ Nursing Implementation

Health Promotion. The nursing role in the early detection of stomach cancer is focused on identification of the patient at risk because of specific disorders such as pernicious anemia and achlorhydria. The nurse should be aware of symptoms associated with stomach cancer, method of spread, and the significant findings on physical examination. The nurse should understand that the cure rate is often low because symptoms arise late in the course of the disease process, are vague, and often mimic other conditions, such as PUD.

The nurse must be alert to early signs of stomach cancer, such as poor appetite, weight loss, fatigue, and persistent stomach distress. If any of these manifestations are present, medical attention should be obtained and the necessary diagnostic tests performed.

Patients with a positive family history of stomach cancer should be encouraged to undergo diagnostic evaluation if manifestations of anemia, PUD, or vague epigastric distress are present. It is important that the nurse recognize the possible existence of stomach cancer in a patient who is treated for PUD and who fails to have relief after 3 weeks of prescribed therapy. The ulcer, if it is benign, should show signs of healing on x-ray examination.

Acute Intervention

Preoperative Care. When the diagnostic tests confirm the presence of a malignancy, the patient and the family generally react with shock, disbelief, and depression. Throughout this period the nurse gives emotional and physical support, provides information, clarifies test results, and maintains a positive attitude with respect to the patient's immediate recovery and long-term survival.

On admission to the hospital, the patient may be in poor physical condition. Surgery may be delayed while the patient becomes more physically able to withstand surgery. A positive nutritional state enhances wound healing, as well as the ability to withstand infection and other possible postoperative complications. The patient may be better able to tolerate several small meals a day rather than three regular meals. The diet may be supplemented by a variety of commercial liquid supplements (see Chapter 40) and vitamins. The nurse is challenged to find innovative ways of persuading the patient to eat when lack of appetite and depression make eating difficult. Getting the patient's family to assist with meals and encourage intake may be beneficial. If the patient is unable to ingest oral feedings, it may be necessary to provide for nutritional needs with tube feedings or parenteral nutrition.

If needed, blood replacement and fluid volume restoration may be carried out in the preoperative period. Because anemia is usually present, packed RBCs may be administered. Close observation for reactions to the transfusions is important. Hemoglobin and hematocrit levels are monitored.

The preoperative teaching plan before gastric surgery for cancer is much the same as that for PUD (see the previous section, Surgical Therapy for Peptic Ulcer Disease).

Postoperative Care. Postoperative care of the patient with stomach cancer is similar to that following a Billroth I or II procedure (see the previous section, Surgical Therapy for Peptic Ulcer Disease). When the surgical intervention has involved a total gastrectomy, the plan of care is somewhat different. A total gastrectomy requires resecting of the lower esophagus along with the removal of the entire stomach and anastomosis of the esophagus to the jejunum. If the chest cavity is entered, postoperative drainage is accomplished by the insertion of chest tubes. (Chest surgery and drainage tubes are discussed in Chapter 28.) After total gastrectomy, the NG tube does not drain a large quantity of secretions because removal of the stomach has eliminated the reservoir capacity. The NG tube is removed when intestinal peristalsis has resumed. Small amounts of clear fluid may then be started. The patient requires close observation for signs of leakage of the fluids at the anastomosis as evidenced by an elevation in the temperature and increasing dyspnea. When fluids are well tolerated without distress, fluid intake is increased along with the addition of some solid foods.

As a consequence of a total gastrectomy, a patient experiences the symptoms of the dumping syndrome. Weight loss often occurs, and poor nutritional intake contributes. Postoperative wound healing may be impaired because of poor nutritional intake. This necessitates the IV or oral replacement of vitamins C, D, and K and the B-complex vitamins and replacement of cobalamin. Because these vitamins (with the exception of cobalamin) are normally absorbed in the duodenum, they must be replaced because the duodenum has been bypassed in the surgical procedure. For the patient who has had a Billroth I or II procedure, the postoperative care is similar to that of the patient having this procedure for PUD.

Most chemotherapeutic regimens include the use of 5-FU. When this drug or any of the combination drugs is prescribed, the nurse provides information regarding the action and side effects of the drugs (see Chapter 16). The patient with advanced malignant disease may be offered palliative treatment.

Radiation therapy can be used as an adjuvant to surgery or for palliation. The nurse provides detailed instruction, to reassure the patient and ensure completion of the designated number of treatments. The nurse should assess the patient's knowledge of radiation, care of the skin, the need for good nutrition and fluid intake during therapy, and the appropriate use of antiemetic drugs. (Specific care of the patient receiving radiation therapy is discussed in Chapter 16.)

Ambulatory and Home Care. Most dietary measures useful after PUD surgery are applicable after surgery for stomach cancer. Plans should be made for the relief of pain, including comfort measures and the judicious use of analgesics. Wound care, if needed, must be taught to the primary caregiver in the home situation. Dressings, special equipment, or special services may be required for the patient's care at home. A list of community agencies (e.g., American Cancer Society) that are available for assistance can be provided before the patient goes home.

When chemotherapy or radiation treatment is to be continued after discharge, a referral to the home health nurse may be beneficial. The home health nurse can assist with recovery, determine the degree of patient compliance, and provide consultation to the patient and family members. The patient is encouraged to comply with the prescribed therapies, to keep appointments for chemotherapy administration or radiation treatments, and to keep the health care provider informed of changes in physical condition. (Long-term management of the cancer patient is discussed in Chapter 16.)

■ **Evaluation**

Expected outcomes are that the patient with stomach cancer will
- experience no or minimal discomfort, pain, or nausea
- achieve optimal nutritional status
- maintain a degree of psychologic well-being appropriate to the disease stage

FOOD POISONING

Food poisoning is a nonspecific term that describes acute GI symptoms such as nausea, vomiting, diarrhea, and colicky abdominal pain caused by the intake of contaminated food or liquids. Food most commonly causes illness if it is contaminated with microorganisms or their products. The epidemiology of food-borne illness is changing. There are new organisms, and many have spread worldwide. The two main types of food poisoning are (1) acute gastroenteritis from bacteria and (2) neurologic symptoms from botulism. The most common bacterial food poisonings are presented in Table 42-27. Poisonous chemicals, such as mercury, arsenic, zinc, and potassium chlorate, may contaminate foods. Poisoning can also occur from ingestion of poisonous plants (e.g., certain mushroom species).

Prevention of occurrence is the focus of interventions. Teaching should include correct food preparation and cleanliness, adequate cooking, and refrigeration (Table 42-28). If the patient is hospitalized, care focuses on correction of fluid and electrolyte imbalance from diarrhea and vomiting. With botulism, additional assessment and care relative to neurologic symptoms are indicated (see Chapter 61).

Escherichia coli O157:H7 Poisoning

Escherichia coli O157:H7 causes hemorrhagic colitis. It is estimated that there are 73,000 cases of infection and 60 deaths in the United States each year.[28] Poisoning with *E. coli* O157:H7 can be life threatening, particularly in the very young and the elderly. *E. coli* O157:H7 is found primarily in undercooked meats, such as hamburger, roast beef, ham, and turkey. Most illnesses are due to eating undercooked, contaminated ground beef. Person-to-person contact in families, nursing homes, and child care centers is also an important mode of transmission. Infection can also occur after drinking raw milk or unpasteurized juice or from contaminated fruit juices and after swimming in or drinking sewage-contaminated water.

Most strains of *E. coli* are harmless and live in the intestines of healthy humans and animals. *E. coli* O157:H7 produces a powerful toxin and can cause severe illness. *E. coli* O157:H7 infection often results in severe bloody diarrhea and abdominal cramps; sometimes the infection causes nonbloody diarrhea or no symptoms. *E. coli* O157:H7 may be responsible for 0.6% to 2.4% of all nonbloody diarrhea and 15% to 36% of all cases of bloody diarrhea.[28] Usually little or no fever is present, and the illness resolves in 5 to 10 days. In approximately 2% to 7% of infections, particularly in young children, hemolytic uremic syndrome occurs, in which the RBCs are destroyed and the kidneys fail.

The clinical manifestations of *E. coli* O157:H7 vary from mild diarrhea to bloody diarrhea and systemic complications, including hemolytic uremia and thrombocytopenic purpura, and even death. The diarrhea may start out as watery but may progress to bloody. Infection with *E. coli* O157:H7 is diagnosed by detecting the bacterium in the stool. All persons who suddenly have diarrhea with blood should get their stool tested for *E. coli* O157:H7.

Treatment involves supportive care to maintain intravascular volume. The use of antibiotics remains controversial. Most persons recover without antibiotics or other specific treatment. There is no evidence that antibiotics improve the course of disease, and it is thought that treatment with some antibiotics may precipitate kidney complications. Antidiarrheal agents, such as loperamide

TABLE 42-27	**Bacterial Food Poisoning**					
Type	**Causative Agent**	**Sources**	**Onset of Symptoms**	**Manifestations**	**Treatment**	**Prevention**
Staphylococcal	Toxin from *Staphylococcus aureus*	Meat, bakery products, cream fillings, salad dressings, milk; skin and respiratory tract of food handlers	30 min-7 hr	Vomiting, nausea, abdominal cramping, diarrhea	Symptomatic, fluid and electrolyte replacement, antiemetics	Immediate refrigeration of foods, monitoring of food handlers
Clostridial	*Clostridium perfringens*	Meat or poultry dishes cooked at lower temperature (stew or pot pie), rewarmed meat dishes, gravies, improperly canned vegetables	8-24 hr	Diarrhea, nausea, abdominal cramps, vomiting (rare); midepigastrium pain	Symptomatic, fluid replacement	Correct preparation of meat dishes, serving of food immediately after cooking or rapid cooling of food
Salmonella	*Salmonella typhimurium* (grows in gut)	Improperly cooked poultry, pork, beef, lamb, and eggs	8 hr-several days	Nausea and vomiting, diarrhea, abdominal cramps, fever and chills	Symptomatic, fluid and electrolyte replacement	Correct preparation of food
Botulism	Toxin from *Clostridium botulinum,* ingested toxin absorbed from gut and blocks acetylcholine at neuromuscular junction	Improperly canned or preserved food, home-preserved vegetables (most common), preserved fruits and fish, canned commercial products	12-36 hr	GI symptoms of nausea, vomiting, abdominal pain, constipation, distention. Central nervous system symptoms of headache, dizziness, muscular incoordination, weakness, inability to talk or swallow, diplopia, breathing difficulties, paralysis, delirium, coma	Maintenance of ventilation, polyvalent antitoxin, guanidine hydrochloric acid (enhances acetylcholine release)	Correct processing of canned foods, boiling of suspected canned foods for 15 min before serving
Escherichia coli	*E. coli* serotype O157:H7	Contaminated beef, pork, milk, cheese, fish	Varies by strain: 8 hr-1 wk	Bloody stools, hemolytic uremic syndrome, abdominal cramping, profuse diarrhea	Symptomatic, fluid and electrolyte replacement	Correct preparation of food

TABLE 42-28	***PATIENT AND FAMILY TEACHING GUIDE*** **Preventing Food Poisoning**

1. Cook all ground beef and hamburger thoroughly.
   - Use a digital instant-read meat thermometer to ensure thorough cooking (ground beef can turn brown before disease-causing bacteria are killed).
   - Ground beef should be cooked until a thermometer inserted into several parts of the patty, including the thickest part, reads at least 160° F.
   - Persons who cook ground beef without using a thermometer can decrease their risk of illness by not eating ground beef patties that are still pink in the middle.
2. If you are served an undercooked hamburger or other ground beef product in a restaurant, send it back for further cooking. Also ask for a new bun and a clean plate.
3. Avoid spreading harmful bacteria. Keep raw meat separate from ready-to-eat foods. Wash hands, counters, and utensils with hot soapy water after they touch raw meat. Never place cooked hamburgers or ground beef on the unwashed plate that held raw patties. Wash meat thermometers in between tests of patties that require further cooking.
4. Drink only pasteurized milk, juice, or cider. Commercial juice with an extended shelf-life that is sold at room temperature (e.g., juice in cardboard boxes, vacuum-sealed juice in glass containers) has been pasteurized. Juice concentrates are also heated sufficiently to kill pathogens.
5. Wash fruits and vegetables thoroughly, especially those that will not be cooked.
6. Persons who are immunocompromised or elderly should avoid eating alfalfa sprouts until their safety can be ensured.

(Imodium), should also be avoided. Other therapies may include dialysis and plasmapheresis. Hemolytic uremic syndrome is a life-threatening condition usually treated in an ICU. Blood transfusions and kidney dialysis are often required. The death rate for hemolytic uremic syndrome is 3% to 5%. About one third of persons with hemolytic uremic syndrome have abnormal kidney function many years later, and a few require long-term dialysis. Less than 10% of persons with hemolytic uremic syndrome have other lifelong complications, such as high BP, seizures, blindness, and paralysis.

CRITICAL THINKING EXERCISE

CASE STUDY

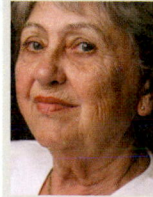

Hiatal Hernia

Patient Profile. Mary, a 63-year-old white elementary school teacher, has had a sliding hiatal hernia for 10 years. Mary is admitted to the hospital for a hiatal hernia repair.

Subjective Data
• Reports increasing heartburn, especially at night
• Is currently on a bland diet and taking antacids

Case Study photo ©iStockphoto.com/ Joseph Jean Rolland Dubé.

• Complains of substernal pain and heartburn
• Reports some problems with regurgitation

Objective Data
Physical Examination
• 5 feet 2 inches tall and weighs 195 pounds

Diagnostic Study
• Barium swallow and an endoscopy revealed a large sliding hiatal hernia.

Collaborative Care
• Mary had a Nissen fundoplication through a laparoscopic approach.

Critical Thinking Questions

1. Explain the pathophysiology of a hiatal hernia. What is the difference between a sliding and a paraesophageal hiatal hernia?
2. What are the characteristic symptoms of a hiatal hernia? Which of these did Mary have?
3. Describe a Nissen fundoplication procedure. What is the objective of this surgical procedure? Why was a laparoscopic approach used?
4. What are potential postoperative complications? What nursing measures prevent them?
5. What is the priority of care?
6. What should be included in a teaching plan for Mary?
7. Based on the assessment data presented, write one or more nursing diagnoses. Are there any collaborative problems?

NCLEX EXAMINATION REVIEW QUESTIONS

The number of the question corresponds to the same-numbered objective at the beginning of the chapter.

1. Mrs. Jones calls to tell you that her elderly mother, who is 85 years of age, has been nauseated all day and has vomited twice. Before you hang up and telephone the health care provider to communicate your assessment data, you instruct Mrs. Jones to
   a. administer antispasmodic drugs and observe skin turgor.
   b. give her mother sips of water and elevate the head of her bed to prevent aspiration.
   c. offer her mother a high-protein liquid supplement to drink to maintain her nutritional needs.
   d. offer her mother large quantities of Gatorade to drink because elderly people are at risk for sodium depletion.

2. Your teaching plan for the patient being discharged following an acute episode of GI bleeding will include information concerning the importance of
   a. taking only drugs prescribed by the health care provider.
   b. avoiding taking aspirin with acidic beverages such as orange juice.
   c. taking all drugs 1 hour before mealtime to prevent further bleeding.
   d. reading all OTC drug labels to avoid those containing stearic acid and calcium.

3. The nurse explains to the patient with Vincent's infection that treatment will include
   a. smallpox vaccinations.
   b. viscous lidocaine rinses.
   c. amphotericin B suspension.
   d. topical application of antibiotics.

4. The nurse is involved in health promotion related to oral cancer. Teaching of adolescents regarding behaviors that put them at risk for oral cancer includes
   a. discouraging use of chewing gum.
   b. avoiding use of perfumed lip gloss.
   c. avoiding use of smokeless tobacco.
   d. discouraging drinking of carbonated beverages.

5. The nurse explains to the patient with gastroesophageal reflux disease that this disorder
   a. results in acid erosion and ulceration of the esophagus caused by the frequent vomiting.
   b. will require surgical wrapping or repair of the pyloric sphincter to control the symptoms.
   c. is the protrusion of a portion of the stomach into the esophagus through an opening in the diaphragm.
   d. often involves relaxation of the lower esophageal sphincter, allowing stomach contents to back up into the esophagus.

6. A patient who has undergone an esophagectomy for esophageal cancer develops increasing pain, fever, and dyspnea when a full liquid diet is started postoperatively. The nurse recognizes that these symptoms are most indicative of
   a. an intolerance to the feedings.
   b. extension of the tumor into the aorta.
   c. leakage of fluid or foods into the mediastinum.
   d. esophageal perforation with fistula formation into the lung.

7. The pernicious anemia that may accompany gastritis is due to which of the following?
    a. Chronic autoimmune destruction of cobalamin stores in the body
    b. Progressive gastric atrophy from chronic breakage in the mucosal barrier and blood loss
    c. A lack of intrinsic factor normally produced by acid-secreting cells of the gastric mucosa
    d. Hyperchlorhydria resulting from an increase in acid-secreting parietal cells and degradation of RBCs

8. You are teaching your patient and her family about possible causative factors for peptic ulcers. You explain that ulcer formation is
    a. caused by a stressful lifestyle and other acid-producing factors such as *C. pylori*.
    b. inherited within families and reinforced by bacterial spread of *Staphylococcus aureus* in childhood.
    c. promoted by factors that tend to cause oversecretion of acid, such as excess dietary fats, smoking, and *B. pylori*.
    d. promoted by a combination of possible factors that may result in erosion of the gastric mucosa, including certain drugs and alcohol.

9. An optimal teaching plan for an outpatient with gastric cancer receiving radiation therapy should include information about
    a. cancer support groups, alopecia, and stomatitis.
    b. avitaminosis, ostomy care, and community resources.
    c. prosthetic devices, skin conductance, and grief counseling.
    d. wound and skin care, nutrition, drugs, and community resources.

10. Several patients are seen at an urgent care center with symptoms of nausea, vomiting, and diarrhea that began 2 hours ago while attending a large family reunion potluck dinner. The nurse questions the patients specifically about foods they ingested containing
    a. beef.
    b. meat and milk.
    c. poultry and eggs.
    d. home-preserved vegetables.

REFERENCES

1. Golembiewski J, Chernin E, Chopra T: Prevention and treatment of postoperative nausea and vomiting, *Am J Health Syst Pharm* 15:1247, 2005.
2. Rivkin K, Lyakhovetskiy A: Treatment of nonvariceal upper gastrointestinal bleeding, *Am J Health Syst Pharm* 62:1159, 2005.
3. Spirt MJ: Stress-related mucosal disease: risk factors and prophylactic therapy, *Clin Ther* 26:197, 2004.
4. Lee SD, Kearney DJ: A randomized controlled trial of gastric lavage prior to endoscopy for acute upper gastrointestinal bleeding, *J Clin Gastroenterol* 38:861, 2004.
5. Pussinen PJ, Nyyssonen K, Alfthan G, et al: Serum antibody levels to *Actinobacillus actinomycetemcomitans* predict the risk for coronary heart disease, *Arterioscler Thromb Vasc Biol* 25:833, 2005.
6. American Cancer Society: Cancer facts and figures 2005. Available at *www.cancer.org* (accessed December 31, 2005).
7. Warnakulasuriya S, Sutherland G, Scully C: Tobacco, oral cancer, and treatment of dependence, *Oral Oncol* 41:244, 2005.
8. Hunter KD, Parkinson EK, Harrison PR: Profiling early head and neck cancer, *Nat Rev Cancer* 5:127, 2005.
9. Kujan O, Glenny AM, Duxbury J, et al: Evaluation of screening strategies for improving oral cancer mortality: a Cochrane systematic review, *J Dent Educ* 69:255, 2005.
10. Camilleri M, Dubois D, Coulie B, et al: Prevalence and socioeconomic impact of upper gastrointestinal disorders in the United States: results of the US upper gastrointestinal study, *Clin Gastroenterol Hepatol* 3:543, 2005.
11. El-Serag HB, Graham DY, Satia JA, et al: Obesity is an independent risk factor for GERD symptoms and erosive esophagitis, *Am J Gastroenterol* 100:1243, 2005.
12. Shaheen NJ: Advances in Barrett's esophagus and esophageal adenocarcinoma, *Gastroenterology* 128:1554, 2005.
13. Lee TJ, Fennerty MB, Howden CW: Systematic review: is there excessive use of proton pump inhibitors in gastro-oesophageal reflux disease? *Aliment Pharmacol Ther* 20:1241, 2004.
14. McCormick DG: Stretta procedure for the treatment of gastroesophageal reflux disease, *Gastroenterol Nurs* 27:22, 2004.
15. Redmond MC: Perianesthesia care of the patient with gastroesophageal reflux disease, *J Perianesth Nurs* 18:335, 2003.
16. Greub G et al: Respiratory complications of gastroesophageal reflux associated with paraesophageal hiatal hernia, *J Clin Gastroenterol* 37:129, 2003.
17. Johnson DA: Gastroesophageal reflux disease in the elderly—a prevalent and severe disease, *Rev Gastroenterol Disord* 4:S16, 2004.
18. Rebecca W, Richard M: Combined chemotherapy and radiotherapy (without surgery) compared with radiotherapy alone in localized carcinoma of the esophagus, Cochrane Upper Gastrointestinal and Pancreatic Diseases Group, *Cochrane Database of Systematic Reviews* 4, 2005.
19. Malthaner R, Fenlon D: Preoperative chemotherapy for resectable thoracic esophageal cancer, Cochrane Upper Gastrointestinal and Pancreatic Diseases Group, *Cochrane Database of Systematic Reviews* 4, 2005.
20. Altman JI, Genden EM, Moche J: Fiberoptic endoscopic-assisted diverticulotomy: a novel technique for the management of Zenker's diverticulum, *Ann Otol Rhinol Laryngol* 114:347, 2005.
21. Richter JE: Modern management of achalasia, *Curr Treat Options Gastroenterol* 8:275, 2005.
22. Cacchione RN, Tran DN, Rhoden DH: Laparoscopic Heller myotomy for achalasia, *Am J Surg* 190:191, 2005.
23. Modlin IM, Sachs G: *Acid related diseases: biology and treatment*, Philadelphia, 2004, Lippincott Williams & Wilkins.
24. Peek RM: Events at the host-microbial interface of the gastrointestinal tract IV: the pathogenesis of *Helicobacter pylori* persistence, *Am J Physiol Gastrointest Liver Physiol* 289:G8, 2005.
25. Gastroenterology and hepatology for the primary care provider: principles, practices, and guidelines for referral. Available at *www.uwgi.org/guidelines/main.htm* (accessed August 1, 2005).
26. Fischbach LA, van Zanten S, Dickason J: Meta-analysis: the efficacy, adverse events, and adherence related to first-line anti–*Helicobacter pylori* quadruple therapies, *Aliment Pharmacol Ther* 15:1071, 2004.
27. Dicken BJ, Bigam DL, Cass C, et al: Gastric adenocarcinoma: review and considerations for future directions, *Ann Surg* 241:27, 2005.
28. Centers for Disease Control and Prevention: *Escherichia coli* O157:H7. Available at *www.cdc.gov/ncidod/dbmd/diseaseinfo/escherichiacoli_g.htm* (accessed December 31, 2005).

RESOURCES

American College of Gastroenterology
    301-263-9000
    www.acgi.gi.org
American Gastroenterological Association
    301-654-2055
    www.gastro.org
Digestive Disease National Coalition
    202-544-7497
    www.ddnc.org
National Digestive Diseases Information Clearinghouse
    800-891-5389
    http://digestive.niddk.nih.gov
National Heartburn Alliance
    877-471-2081
    www.heartburnalliance.org
National Institute of Diabetes and Digestive and Kidney Diseases (NIDDK)
    www.niddk.nih.gov/index.htm
Society of Gastroenterology Nurses and Associates (SGNA)
    800-245-7462 or 312-321-5165
    www.sgna.org
For additional Internet resources, see the website for this book at *http://evolve.elsevier.com/Lewis/medsurg*.

There are three ingredients to the good life: learning, earning, and yearning.

Christopher Morley

Nursing Management
Lower Gastrointestinal Problems

43

Marilee Schmelzer

LEARNING OBJECTIVES

1. Explain the common etiologies, collaborative care, and nursing management of diarrhea, fecal incontinence, and constipation.
2. Describe common causes of acute abdominal pain and nursing management of the patient following an exploratory laparotomy.
3. Describe the collaborative care and nursing management of acute appendicitis, peritonitis, and gastroenteritis.
4. Compare and contrast the inflammatory bowel diseases of ulcerative colitis and Crohn's disease, including pathophysiology, clinical manifestations, complications, collaborative care, and nursing management.
5. Differentiate among mechanical, neurogenic, and vascular bowel obstructions, including causes, collaborative care, and nursing management.
6. Describe the clinical manifestations and collaborative management of colorectal cancer.
7. Explain the anatomic and physiologic changes and nursing management of the patient with an ileostomy and a colostomy.
8. Differentiate between diverticulosis and diverticulitis, including clinical manifestations, collaborative care, and nursing management.
9. Compare and contrast the types of hernias, including etiology and surgical and nursing management.
10. Describe the types of malabsorption syndrome and collaborative care of celiac disease, lactase deficiency, and short bowel syndrome.
11. Describe the types, clinical manifestations, collaborative care, and nursing management of anorectal conditions.

KEY TERMS

appendicitis, p. 1048
celiac disease, p. 1079
colostomy, p. 1069
Crohn's disease, p. 1051
diverticulum, p. 1076
gastroenteritis, p. 1050
hemorrhoids, p. 1082
hernia, p. 1077
ileostomy, p. 1069
inflammatory bowel disease, p. 1051
irritable bowel syndrome, p. 1046
lactase deficiency, p. 1081
ostomy, p. 1069
paralytic (adynamic) ileus, p. 1060
peritonitis, p. 1049
short bowel syndrome, p. 1081
steatorrhea, p. 1079
ulcerative colitis, p. 1051

Electronic Resources

Supplemental content related to Chapter 43 can be found . . .

Companion CD
- Stress-Busting Kit for Nursing Students
- NCLEX Examination Review Questions
- Interactive Case Study: Ulcerative Colitis
- Comprehensive Glossary

Evolve Website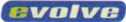
http://evolve.elsevier.com/Lewis/medsurg
- Content Updates
- Key Points (Printable and CD/MP3 Download)
- Concept Map Creator
- Expanded Audio Glossary
- Key Term Flash Cards
- Audio Lectures:
  - Inflammatory Bowel Disease
  - Irritable Bowel Syndrome
- Figure: Intestinal Tubes

- Customizable Nursing Care Plans:
  - Acute Infectious Diarrhea
  - Colostomy/Ileostomy
  - Inflammatory Bowel Disease
  - Laparotomy
- Patient and Family Instruction Guides in English and Spanish:
  - Colostomy Irrigation
  - Managing Constipation
- Electronic Calculators
- WebLinks

Reviewed by Sharon Dudley-Brown, APRN-BC, PhD, FNP, Assistant Professor, The Catholic University of America School of Nursing, Washington, D.C.

Gastrointestinal System

DIARRHEA

Diarrhea, the frequent passage of loose, liquid stools, is not a disease but a symptom. The term *diarrhea* may mean different things to different people. It is commonly used to denote an increase in stool frequency or volume and an increase in the looseness of stool.

Etiology and Pathophysiology

Causes of diarrhea can be divided into the general classifications of decreased fluid absorption, increased fluid secretion, motility disturbances, or a combination of these (Table 43-1). For example, large amounts of undigested carbohydrate in the bowel produce an osmotic diarrhea that promotes rapid transit through the bowel and prevents absorption of fluid and electrolytes. Lactose intolerance and certain laxatives (e.g., lactulose, sodium phosphate, and polyethylene glycol) produce an osmotic diarrhea. Infectious agents (e.g., *Escherichia coli, Salmonella*), bile salts, and undigested fats lead to excessive fluid secretion in the gut. The diarrhea from celiac disease and short bowel syndrome results from malabsorption in the small intestine. A combination of mechanisms leads to the diarrhea of Crohn's disease: decreased absorption because of inflammation and destruction of surface epithelium, increased secretion caused by excessive bile salts, and osmotic diarrhea from lactose intolerance.

Clinical Manifestations

Diarrhea may be acute or chronic. Acute diarrhea most commonly results from infection. Causes of acute infectious diarrhea are listed in Table 43-2. Bacterial or viral infection of the intestine may result in symptoms such as explosive watery diarrhea, tenesmus (spasmodic contraction of anal sphincter with pain and persistent desire to defecate), and abdominal cramping or pain. Liquid stools can also lead to perianal skin irritation. Systemic manifestations include fever, nausea, vomiting, and malaise. Leukocytes, blood, and mucus may be present in the stool, depending on the causative agent (see Table 43-2). Acute diarrhea is often self-limiting in the adult. Symptoms continue until the irritant or causative agent is excreted. The epithelial cells lining the lumen of the gastrointestinal (GI) tract regenerate after the inflammatory response resolves.

Diarrhea is considered chronic when it lasts for at least 4 weeks.[1] Severe diarrhea produces life-threatening dehydration, electrolyte disturbances (e.g., hypokalemia), and acid-base imbalances (metabolic acidosis). Infants and the elderly are particularly vulnerable to severe diarrhea. Malabsorption and malnutrition are also sequelae of chronic diarrhea.

Diagnostic Studies

Accurate diagnosis and management require a thorough history, physical examination, and laboratory testing. The patient should be asked about recent travel to foreign countries, medication use, diet, previous surgery, interpersonal contacts, and a family history of diarrhea. Deficiencies in iron and folate occur with long-standing diarrhea and can result in anemia. Increased hemoglobin, hematocrit, and blood urea nitrogen (BUN) levels suggest that fluid deficits and electrolyte levels may be abnormal. Infectious diarrhea may be associated with an elevated white blood cell (WBC) count. Stools are examined for the presence of blood, mucus, WBCs, and parasites, and cultures are performed to identify infectious organisms.

In a patient with chronic diarrhea, measurements of stool electrolytes, pH, and osmolality help determine whether the diarrhea is related to decreased fluid absorption or increased fluid secretion (secretory diarrhea). Measurement of stool fat and undigested muscle fibers may indicate fat and protein malabsorption conditions, including pancreatic insufficiency. Elevated serum levels of GI hormones such as vasoactive intestinal polypeptide and gastrin are present in some patients with secretory diarrhea. Colonoscopy is used to examine the mucosa and obtain biopsies for histologic examination. Upper and lower radiologic studies with barium contrast may be helpful in detecting mucosal disease or structural abnormalities.

Collaborative Care

Treatment depends on the cause. Foods and medications that cause diarrhea should be avoided. Acute diarrhea from infectious causes is usually self-limiting. The major concern is fluid and electrolyte replacement and resolution of the diarrhea. Oral solutions containing glucose and electrolytes (e.g., Gatorade, Pedialyte) may be sufficient to replace losses from mild diarrhea, but parenteral administration of fluids, electrolytes, vitamins, and nutrition is necessary if losses are severe.

Antidiarrheal agents are sometimes given to coat and protect mucous membranes, absorb irritating substances, inhibit GI motility, decrease intestinal secretions, and decrease central nervous system stimulation of the GI tract (Table 43-3). They are contraindicated in the treatment of infectious diarrhea because they potentially prolong exposure to the infectious organism, and are used cautiously in inflammatory bowel disease because of the danger of toxic megacolon (colonic dilation greater than 5 cm). Regardless of the cause of diarrhea, antidiarrheal drugs should only be given for a short period of time.

Antibiotics are rarely used to treat acute diarrhea, since the infection generally runs its course. Some antibiotics destroy the normal bowel flora, thereby allowing pathogenic organisms to flourish. For example, patients receiving antibiotics (e.g., clindamycin [Cleocin], ampicillin, amoxicillin, and cephalosporin) are suscep-

---

TABLE 43-1 | **Causes of Diarrhea**

Decreased Fluid Absorption
- Oral intake of poorly absorbable solutes (e.g., laxatives)
- Maldigestion and malabsorption (e.g., maldigestion of fat with pancreatitis, poorly absorbed bile salts in terminal ileum disease)
- Mucosal damage (e.g., tropical sprue, celiac disease, Crohn's disease, radiation injury, ulcerative colitis, ischemic bowel disease)
- Intestinal enzyme deficiencies (e.g., lactase)
- Decreased surface area (e.g., intestinal resection)
- Osmotic diarrhea (candy, gum, mints containing sorbitol, laxatives)

Increased Fluid Secretion
- Infectious: bacterial endotoxins (e.g., *Vibrio cholerae, Escherichia coli, Shigella, Salmonella, Staphylococcus, Clostridium difficile,* viral agents [rotavirus], and parasitic agents [*Giardia lamblia*])
- Hormonal: vasoactive intestinal polypeptide secretion from adenoma of the pancreas; gastrin secretion caused by Zollinger-Ellison syndrome; calcitonin secretion from carcinoma of the thyroid
- Tumor: Villous adenoma

Motility Disturbances
- Irritable bowel syndrome: ↑ visceral sensitivity and transit
- Diabetic enteropathy: ↓ transit secondary to peripheral neuropathy
- Gastrectomy: ↑ transit as a result of dumping syndrome

TABLE 43-2	Causes of Acute Infectious Diarrhea		
	Onset	**Duration**	**Symptoms and Signs**
Viral			
Rotavirus, Norwalk	18-24 hr	24-48 hr	Explosive, watery diarrhea; nausea; vomiting; abdominal cramps
Bacterial			
Escherichia coli	6-24 hr	3-4 days	Four or five loose stools per day, nausea, malaise, low-grade fever
Enterohemorrhagic *E. coli* (O157:H7)	8-24 hr	4-9 days	Bloody diarrhea, severe cramping, fever
Shigella	24 hr	7 days	Watery stools containing blood and mucus, tenesmus, urgency, severe cramping, fever
Salmonella	6-48 hr	2-5 days	Watery diarrhea, nausea, vomiting, abdominal cramps, fever
Staphylococcal (toxin from *S. aureus*)	30 min-7 hr	24-48 hr	Diarrhea, abdominal cramping, vomiting, nausea
Campylobacter species	24 hr	<7 days	Profuse, watery diarrhea; malaise, nausea, abdominal cramps, low-grade fever
Clostridium perfringens	8-24 hr	24 hr	Watery diarrhea, abdominal cramps, vomiting (rare)
Clostridium difficile	4-9 days after start of antibiotics	24 hr	Associated with antibiotic treatment; symptoms range from mild, watery diarrhea to severe abdominal pain, fever, leukocytosis, leukocytes in stool
Parasitic			
Giardia lamblia	1-3 wk	Few days to 3 mo	Sudden onset; malodorous, explosive, watery diarrhea; flatulence, epigastric pain and cramping, nausea
Entamoeba histolytica	4 days	Wk to mo	Frequent soft stools with blood and mucus (in severe cases, watery stools), flatulence, distention, abdominal cramps, fever, leukocytes in stool
Cryptosporidium	2-10 days	1-6 mo	Watery diarrhea, nausea, vomiting, abdominal cramps, weight loss in AIDS

AIDS, Acquired immunodeficiency syndrome.

TABLE 43-3	DRUG THERAPY Antidiarrheal Drugs		
Type	**Mechanism of Action**		**Examples**
Demulcent	Soothes, coats, and protects mucous membranes		bismuth subsalicylate* (Pepto-Bismol); calcium polycarbophil (Mitrolan-OTC); activated charcoal; kaolin,† pectin, hyoscyamine sulfate, and hyoscine hydrobromide (Donnagel)*†; Donnagel and opium (Donnagel-PG)*†
Anticholinergic	Inhibits GI motility		Donnagel,*† Donnagel-PG,*† diphenoxylate with atropine sulfate (Lomotil, Colonaid), loperamide (Imodium)†‡
Antisecretory	Decreases intestinal secretion		octreotide (Sandostatin), a synthetic analog of somatostatin
Opioid	Decreases CNS stimulation of GI tract motility and secretion; directly inhibits GI motility		camphorated tincture of opium (paregoric); Donnagel-PG†; paregoric, pectin, and kaolin (Parepectolin)†; tincture of opium, homatropine methylbromide, and pectin§

CNS, Central nervous system; *GI,* gastrointestinal.
*Also inhibits bacterial activity and is used prophylactically to prevent traveler's diarrhea.
†Also absorbent, which contributes to the adhesiveness of the stool.
‡Has cholinergic and noncholinergic actions.
§Also an anticholinergic.

tible to *Clostridium difficile (C. difficile),* which is a serious bacterial infection. *C. difficile* causes mild to severe diarrhea, abdominal cramping, and fever. *C. difficile* infection can also result in pseudomembranous enterocolitis and intestinal perforation. Immunosuppressed patients and the elderly are particularly susceptible. *C. difficile* is a particularly hazardous nosocomial infection because hospitalized patients are often immunosuppressed, antibiotic therapy is common, and *C. difficile* spores can survive for up to 70 days on inanimate objects. The spores have been found on commodes, telephones, thermometers, bedside tables, floors, and other objects in the room, as well as on the hands of health care workers. Health care workers who do not adhere to infection control precautions can transmit *C. difficile* from patient to patient. In many cases, the infection resolves when antibiotic therapy ceases. If not, metronidazole (Flagyl) is the first line of therapy. Vancomycin (Vancocin) is used if metronidazole is ineffective.[2]

NURSING MANAGEMENT
ACUTE INFECTIOUS DIARRHEA

■ Nursing Assessment

Nursing assessment begins with a thorough history and physical examination (Table 43-4). The patient is asked to describe the stool pattern and associated symptoms. Questions focus on the duration, frequency, character, and consistency of stool. A medication history includes use of antibiotics, laxatives, and other drugs known to cause diarrhea. Recent travel, stress, and health and family illnesses should be discussed. The patient is asked about eating habits, appetite, and food intolerances, especially milk and dairy products, and food preparation practices.

Physical examination includes vital signs and height and weight measurements. The patient's skin is inspected for signs of dehydration (poor turgor, dryness, and areas of breakdown). The abdo-

TABLE 43-4	*NURSING ASSESSMENT* Diarrhea

Subjective Data
Important Health Information
Past health history: Recent travel, infections, stress; diverticulitis or malabsorption; metabolic disorders; inflammatory bowel disease; irritable bowel syndrome
Medications: Use of laxatives or enemas, magnesium-containing antacids, sorbitol-containing suspensions or elixirs, antibiotics, methyldopa, digitalis, colchicine; OTC antidiarrheal medications
Surgery or other treatments: Stomach or bowel surgery, radiation

Functional Health Patterns
Health perception–health management: Chronic laxative abuse, malaise
Nutritional-metabolic: Ingestion of greasy and spicy foods, food intolerances; anorexia, nausea, vomiting; weight loss; thirst
Elimination: Increased stool frequency, volume, and looseness; change in color and character of stools; steatorrhea, abdominal bloating; decreased urinary output
Cognitive-perceptual: Abdominal tenderness, abdominal pain and cramping; tenesmus

Objective Data
General
Lethargy, sunken eyeballs, fever, malnutrition

Integumentary
Pallor, dry mucous membranes, poor skin turgor, perianal irritation

Gastrointestinal
Frequent soft to liquid stools that may alternate with constipation; altered stool color; abdominal distention, hyperactive bowel sounds; presence of pus, blood, mucus, or fat in stools; fecal impaction

Urinary
Decreased output, concentrated urine

Possible Findings
Abnormal serum electrolyte levels; anemia; leukocytosis; eosinophilia; hypoalbuminemia; positive stool cultures; presence of ova, parasites, leukocytes, blood, or fat in stool; abnormal sigmoidoscopic or colonoscopic findings; abnormal lower GI series

GI, Gastrointestinal; *OTC,* over-the-counter.

men is inspected for distention, auscultated for bowel sounds, and palpated for tenderness.

■ *Nursing Diagnoses*

Nursing diagnoses for the patient with acute infectious diarrhea may include, but are not limited to, those presented in NCP 43-1.

■ *Planning*

The overall goals are that the patient with diarrhea will (1) not transmit the microorganism causing the infectious diarrhea, (2) cease having diarrhea and resume normal bowel patterns, (3) have normal fluid and electrolyte and acid-base balance, (4) have normal nutritional status, and (5) have no perianal skin breakdown.

■ *Nursing Implementation*

All cases of acute diarrhea should be considered infectious until the cause is known. Strict infection control precautions are necessary (see Table 15-9) to prevent the infection from spreading to others. Hands should be washed before and after contact with each patient and when body fluids of any kind are handled. The patient

and family should be taught the principles of hygiene, infection control precautions, and the potential dangers of an illness that is infectious to themselves and others. Proper food handling, cooking, and storage are discussed with the patient suspected of having infectious diarrhea.

Patients with *C. difficile* should be placed in a private room and gloves and gowns should be worn for all care. A disposable stethoscope and individual patient thermometer are kept in the room. Objects in the room must be considered contaminated and can be disinfected with a 10% solution of household bleach. Strict hand washing is vital, and patients and their families should be taught ways to prevent the spread of infection.[2]

FECAL INCONTINENCE

Etiology and Pathophysiology

Fecal incontinence, the involuntary passage of stool, occurs when the normal structures that maintain continence are disrupted. Normally, fecal contents pass from the sigmoid colon into the rectum, causing rectal distention. Sensory (stretch) receptors in the muscles surrounding the rectum are stimulated. This causes a reflex relaxation of the internal anal sphincter and contraction of the external anal sphincter. Sensory receptors in the epithelium of the anal canal are able to distinguish between solid, liquid, and gas. The combination of contraction of the abdominal muscles, relaxation of the pelvic muscles, squatting (which straightens the anorectal angle), and voluntary relaxation of the external anal sphincter allows for elimination of feces. Problems with motor function (contraction of muscles) and/or sensory function (ability to perceive presence of stool or to experience the urge to defecate) can result in fecal incontinence. Weakness or disruption of the internal or external anal sphincter, damage to the pudendal nerve or other nerves that innervate the anorectum, damage to the anal tissue, and weakness of or trauma to the puborectalis muscle all contribute to incontinence.

For women, obstetric trauma is the most common cause of sphincter disruption. However, fecal incontinence usually develops years later when the woman is in her fifties or older.[3] Constipation and diarrhea are common risk factors for fecal incontinence[4] (Table 43-5). Fecal incontinence can occur secondary to **fecal impaction,** which is an accumulation of hardened feces in the rectum or sigmoid colon that cannot be expelled. Fecal incontinence caused by fecal impaction is a common problem in older adults with limited mobility.

Diagnostic Studies and Collaborative Care

The diagnosis and effective management of fecal incontinence require a thorough health history and physical examination with appropriate diagnostic studies. The patient is asked about the number of incontinent episodes weekly and stool consistency and volume. A rectal examination should be performed. Fecal impaction, internal prolapse, increased perineal descent, and rectocele can be detected during a rectal examination. If the impaction is higher in the colon, an abdominal x-ray or a computed tomography (CT) scan may be helpful. Sigmoidoscopy or colonoscopy may identify inflammation, tumors, fissures, and other sigmoid-rectum pathologic conditions. Anorectal manometry, electromyography, pudendal nerve latency testing, and ultrasound imaging of the anal sphincter may be used in the diagnosis. Defecography also provides useful information about difficulties with defecation and continence.[4]

NURSING CARE PLAN 43-1

Patient with Acute Infectious Diarrhea

NURSING DIAGNOSIS   **Diarrhea** *related to* acute infectious process *as evidenced by* frequent loose, liquid stools

PATIENT GOAL   Resumes normal bowel patterns

OUTCOMES (NOC)	INTERVENTIONS (NIC) and *RATIONALES*
Bowel Elimination	**Diarrhea Management**
• Diarrhea _____ • Pain with passage of stool _____ **Measurement Scale** 1 = Severe 2 = Substantial 3 = Moderate 4 = Mild 5 = None	• Obtain stool for culture and sensitivity if diarrhea continues to *provide appropriate treatment.* • Perform actions *to rest bowel* (e.g., NPO, liquid diet). • Instruct patient to notify staff of each episode of diarrhea *to monitor effectiveness of treatment.* • Instruct patient/family members to record color, volume, frequency, and consistency of stools *to monitor treatment.* • Teach patient appropriate use of antidiarrheal medication *to prevent patient's use of OTC antiperistaltic agents that prolong exposure to infectious organisms.*

NURSING DIAGNOSIS   **Deficient fluid volume** *related to* excessive fluid loss and decreased fluid intake secondary to diarrhea *as evidenced by* dry skin and mucous membranes, poor skin turgor, orthostatic hypotension, tachycardia, decreased urine output, electrolyte imbalance

PATIENT GOALS   1. Maintains fluid and electrolyte balance
2. Demonstrates no hypovolemia or hypervolemia

OUTCOMES (NOC)	INTERVENTIONS (NIC) and *RATIONALES*
Fluid Balance	**Hypovolemia Management**
• Blood pressure _____ • Radial pulse rate _____ • Stable body weight _____ • 24-hour intake and output balance _____ • Moist mucous membranes _____ • Serum electrolytes _____ • Skin turgor _____ **Measurement Scale** 1 = Severely compromised 2 = Substantially compromised 3 = Moderately compromised 4 = Mildly compromised 5 = Not compromised	• Observe for indications of dehydration (e.g., poor skin turgor, delayed capillary refill, weak/thready pulse, severe thirst, dry mucous membranes, decreased urine output, and hypotension) *as indicators of fluid volume deficit.* • Monitor fluid status, including intake and output, *to determine fluid balance.* • Monitor vital signs *because changes can indicate hypovolemia.* • Monitor weight *to monitor fluid loss.* • Encourage oral fluid intake *if intake does not stimulate intestinal hypermotility.* • Maintain a steady IV infusion flow rate *to replace fluids and electrolytes lost in stools.* **Fluid/Electrolyte Management** • Administer prescribed supplemental electrolytes *to replace electrolytes lost in stools.* • Monitor laboratory results relevant to fluid balance (e.g., hematocrit, BUN, albumin, total protein, serum osmolality, and urine specific gravity levels).

BUN, Blood urea nitrogen; *IV,* intravenous; *NPO,* nothing by mouth; *OTC,* over-the-counter.

Treatment of incontinence depends on the underlying cause. If fecal incontinence is related to noninfectious diarrhea, bulking agents are the first choice for treating diarrhea. If bulking agents are ineffective, antidiarrheal agents such as loperamide (Imodium) may be useful in reducing diarrhea and increasing sphincter tone.

Fecal incontinence from fecal impaction usually resolves after manual disimpaction of the hard feces and cleansing enemas. To prevent recurrence, a high-fiber diet (see Table 43-9 later in this chapter), along with increased fluid intake, should be given unless contraindicated.[4]

Dietary fiber supplements or bulk-forming laxatives (e.g., psyllium in Metamucil) can improve continence by increasing stool bulk, firming consistency, and promoting sensation of rectal filling. Perianal pouching or disposable pads or briefs provide containment of stool, protect skin, and promote comfort and dignity.

Biofeedback therapy is aimed at improving awareness of rectal sensation and coordination of the internal and external anal sphincters and increasing the strength of contraction of the external sphinc-

ter.[5] Biofeedback training requires adequate mental status and motivation to learn. Components of biofeedback include education, reinforcement, and concentration. It is a safe, painless, and relatively inexpensive treatment for fecal incontinence, but further investigation is needed to evaluate the effectiveness of various biofeedback programs.[5] (Biofeedback is discussed further in Chapter 8.)

Surgery (e.g., sphincter repair procedures) should be considered only when conservative treatment fails, in cases of full-thickness prolapse, and when the sphincter needs repair. A colostomy is sometimes necessary.

NURSING MANAGEMENT
FECAL INCONTINENCE

■ *Nursing Assessment*

Fecal incontinence is embarrassing, uncomfortable, and irritating to the skin. An assessment of the patient's general condition and mental alertness is necessary to identify the best alternative for

TABLE 43-5	Causes of Fecal Incontinence

Traumatic
- Anorectal surgery for hemorrhoids, fistula, and fissures
- Childbirth injury (episiotomy is believed to be a risk factor)
- Perineal trauma or pelvic fracture

Neurologic
- Brain tumor
- Cauda equina nerve injury
- Congenital abnormalities (e.g., spina bifida and myelomeningocele)
- Dementia
- Diabetes mellitus (secondary to neuropathy)
- Multiple sclerosis
- Rectal surgery
- Spinal cord injuries
- Stroke

Inflammatory
- Infection
- Inflammatory bowel disease
- Radiation

Other
- Chronic constipation
- Denervation of pelvic muscles from chronic excessive straining
- Fecal impaction
- Loss of rectal elasticity
- Rapid transit of large diarrheal stools

Pelvic Floor Dysfunction
- Medications
- Rectal prolapse

Functional
- Physical or mobility impairments affecting toileting ability (e.g., elderly person cannot get to the bathroom in time)

managing the patient with fecal incontinence. The nurse should ask about bowel patterns before the incontinence developed; usual bowel habits; stool consistency; and current symptoms, including pain during defecation, blood or mucus in the stool, and a feeling of incomplete evacuation. The nurse determines whether the patient has defecation urgency and is aware of leaking stool. Further assessment includes questions about the coexistence of urinary incontinence, a history of multiple or traumatic childbirths, previous anorectal surgery or injury, and any loss of sensation in the perineal region.

■ Nursing Diagnoses

Nursing diagnoses for the patient with fecal incontinence include, but are not limited to, the following:
- Bowel incontinence *related to* inability to control bowel function
- Self-care deficit (toileting) *related to* inability to manage bowel evacuation voluntarily
- Risk for situational low self-esteem *related to* inability to control bowel movements
- Risk for impaired skin integrity *related to* incontinence of stool
- Social isolation *related to* inability to control bowel functions

■ Planning

The overall goals are that the patient with fecal incontinence will (1) have normal bowel control, (2) maintain perianal skin integrity,

and (3) avoid self-esteem problems related to problems with bowel control.

■ Nursing Implementation

Prevention and treatment of fecal incontinence may be managed by implementing a bowel training program. Bowel training is effective in many patients because once the bowel is empty the rectum does not fill until the next day. If there is no stool, the person is continent. Bowel elimination occurs at regular intervals in most people, and the nurse uses knowledge of the patient's regular pattern to time elimination. The patient is put on a bedpan, assisted to a bedside commode, or walked to the bathroom at a regular time daily to promote bowel regularity. A good time to establish this pattern is within 30 minutes after breakfast. Most people experience an urge to defecate following the first meal of the day because of the gastrocolic reflex. If the usual bowel habits differ from this pattern, efforts should be made to adhere to the patient's individual timing.

If these techniques are ineffective in reestablishing bowel regularity, a bisacodyl (Dulcolax) glycerin suppository or a small phosphate enema may be administered 15 to 30 minutes before the usual evacuation time. These preparations stimulate the anorectal reflex and should be discontinued when a regular pattern is reestablished.

Maintenance of skin integrity is of utmost importance, especially in the bedridden and older adult patient. Nursing management may necessitate the use of drainage tubes or catheters, incontinence briefs, and meticulous skin care. Rectal tubes and catheters are avoided because they can decrease responsiveness of the rectal sphincter and cause ulceration of the rectal mucosa. Incontinence briefs may be helpful in maintaining skin integrity if changed frequently, but can be demeaning and humiliating to the patient. Meticulous cleaning after each stool is essential for skin integrity. The skin is cleaned with a mild soap and rinsed to remove feces, the area is dried, and a protective skin barrier cream is applied. Because the patient may have several stools each day, maintaining skin integrity is an important task for the nurse and the family.

CONSTIPATION

Normal bowel movement frequency varies from three bowel movements daily to one bowel movement every 3 days. **Constipation** can be defined as a decrease in frequency of bowel movements from what is "normal" for the individual; hard, difficult-to-pass stools; a decrease in stool volume; and/or retention of feces in the rectum. Since individuals vary, it is important to compare current symptoms with the patient's normal pattern of elimination. Changes in bowel habits may also indicate bowel obstruction produced by a tumor.

Etiology and Pathophysiology

Common causes of constipation include insufficient dietary fiber, inadequate fluid intake, decreased physical activity, and ignoring the defecation urge. Many medications, especially opioids, cause constipation. Constipation occurs with many diseases that slow GI transit and hamper neurologic function such as diabetes mellitus, Parkinson's disease, and multiple sclerosis. Emotions affect the GI tract, and both depression and stress can contribute to constipation (Table 43-6). For many patients with constipation, however, it is not possible to identify the underlying cause.

Some patients believe that they are constipated if they do not have a daily bowel movement. This can result in chronic laxative use and subsequent cathartic colon syndrome. In this condition, the colon becomes dilated and atonic (lacking muscle tone) and the person cannot defecate without the laxative.

TABLE 43-6	Causes of Constipation	
Colonic Disorders	**Systemic Disorders**	
Luminal or extraluminal obstructing lesions	**Metabolic/Endocrine**	
Inflammatory strictures	Diabetes mellitus	
Volvulus	Hypokalemia	
Intussusception	Hypothyroidism	
Irritable bowel syndrome	Pregnancy	
Diverticular disease	Hypercalcemia/	
Rectocele	hyperparathyroidism	
	Pheochromocytoma	
Drug Induced		
Antacids (calcium and aluminum)	**Collagen Vascular Disease**	
Antidepressants	Systemic sclerosis (scleroderma)	
Anticholinergics	Amyloidosis	
Antipsychotics		
Antihypertensives	**Neurologic Disorders**	
Barium sulfate	Hirschsprung's megacolon	
Bismuth	Neurofibromatosis	
Calcium supplements	Autonomic neuropathy (secondary to diabetes mellitus)	
Iron supplements	Multiple sclerosis	
Laxative abuse	Parkinson's disease	
Opioids	Spinal cord lesions or injury	
	Stroke	

TABLE 43-7	Clinical Manifestations of Constipation	
Abdominal distention/bloating	Increased rectal pressure	
Abdominal pain	Nausea	
Anorexia	Palpable mass	
Decreased frequency of bowel movements	Stone- or rock-shaped stool	
Hard, dry stool	Stool with blood	
Headache	Straining	
Increased flatulence	Tenesmus	

Ignoring the urge to defecate for a prolonged period can cause the muscles and mucosa of the rectum to become insensitive to the presence of feces. In addition, the prolonged retention of feces results in drying of stool due to water absorption. The harder and drier the feces, the more difficult it is to expel.

Clinical Manifestations

The clinical presentation of constipation may vary from a chronic discomfort to an acute event mimicking an "acute abdomen." Stools are absent or hard, dry, and difficult to pass. Other clinical manifestations are presented in Table 43-7. Hemorrhoids are the most common complication of chronic constipation. They result from venous engorgement caused by repeated Valsalva maneuvers (straining) and venous compression from hard impacted stool.

Valsalva maneuver, which occurs during straining to pass a hardened stool, may cause serious problems in patients with heart failure, cerebral edema, hypertension, and coronary artery disease. During straining, the patient inspires deeply and holds the breath while contracting abdominal muscles and bearing down. This increases both intraabdominal and intrathoracic pressures and reduces venous return to the heart. The heart slows temporarily (bradycardia), the cardiac output is decreased, and there is a transient drop in arterial pressure. When the patient relaxes, thoracic pressure falls, resulting in a sudden flow of blood into the heart, increased heart rate, and an immediate rise in arterial pressure. These changes may be fatal for the patient who cannot compensate for the sudden increased blood flow returning to the heart.

In the presence of obstipation, or fecal impaction secondary to constipation, colonic perforation may occur. Perforation, which is life threatening, causes abdominal pain, nausea, vomiting, fever, and an elevated WBC count. An abdominal x-ray shows the presence of free air, which is diagnostic of perforation. Rectal mucosal ulcers and fissures may also occur as a result of stool stasis or straining. Diverticulosis is another potential complication of chronic constipation and is described later in this chapter. These complications are most common in older patients.

Diagnostic Studies and Collaborative Care

A thorough history and physical examination should be performed so that the underlying cause of constipation can be identified and treatment started. Abdominal x-rays, barium enema, colonoscopy, sigmoidoscopy, and anorectal manometry may be helpful in the diagnosis. Many cases of constipation can be prevented by increasing dietary fiber, fluid intake, and exercise. Laxatives (Table 43-8) and enemas may be used to treat acute constipation, but are used cautiously because overuse leads to chronic constipation. People who continue to use laxatives and enemas eventually become unable to have a bowel movement without them.

The choice of laxative or enema depends on the severity of the constipation and the health of the individual. The health care provider may prescribe daily bulk-forming preparations to prevent constipation because they work like dietary fiber and do not cause dependence. Stool softeners are also used to prevent constipation. Bisacodyl tablets and suppositories, milk of magnesia, and lactulose are more potent and thus more likely to cause dependence and mucosal changes. Tegaserod (Zelnorm), a serotonergic drug, has been approved for the management of chronic constipation, as well as constipation associated with irritable bowel syndrome.[6] This drug acts by increasing GI transit time.

Enemas are fast acting and beneficial for immediate treatment of constipation, but must be used cautiously. Soapsuds enemas produce inflammation of colon mucosa, tap water enemas can lead to water intoxication, and sodium phosphate enemas may cause electrolyte imbalances in patients with cardiac and renal problems.

Biofeedback therapy may benefit patients who are constipated as a result of *anismus* (uncoordinated contraction of the anal sphincter during straining). For the patient in whom perceived constipation is related to rigid beliefs regarding bowel function, the nurse should initiate a discussion about these beliefs with the patient. Appropriate information on normal bowel function needs to be given and discussed along with the adverse consequences of excessive use of laxatives and enemas.

A patient with severe constipation related to bowel motility or mechanical disorders may require more intensive treatment. Diagnostic studies such as anorectal manometry, GI tract transit studies, and sigmoidoscopic rectal biopsies should be performed before treatment. In a patient with unrelenting constipation, a subtotal colectomy with ileorectal anastomosis is the procedure of choice.

Nutritional Therapy. Diet is an important factor in the prevention of constipation. Many patients experience an improvement in their symptoms when they increase their intake of dietary fiber and fluids. Dietary fiber is found in plant foods: fruits, vegetables, and grains (Table 43-9). Wheat bran and prunes are especially effective for preventing and treating constipation.

Insoluble fiber, which is found in higher concentrations in whole wheat and bran, remains essentially unchanged as it moves

TABLE 43-8

DRUG THERAPY
Constipation

Category	Mechanism of Action	Example	Onset of Action	Comments
Bulk forming	Absorbs water; increases bulk, thereby stimulating peristalsis	methylcellulose: Citrucel psyllium: Metamucil, Perdiem, Konsyl, Hydrocil, Fiberall	Usually within 24 hr	Contraindicated in patients with abdominal pain, nausea, and vomiting and in patients suspected of having appendicitis, biliary tract obstruction, or acute hepatitis; must be taken with fluids (at least 8 oz); best choice for initial treatment of constipation
Stool softeners and lubricants	Lubricate intestinal tract and soften feces, making hard stools easier to pass; do not affect peristalsis	Softeners: docusate (Colace, Surfak, Peri-Colace, Doxidan) Lubricants: mineral oil (Fleets Oil retention enema, Kondremul Plain)	Softeners up to 72 hr, lubricants up to 8 hr	Can block absorption of fat-soluble vitamins such as vitamin K, which may increase risk of bleeding in patients on anticoagulants
Saline and osmotic solutions	Cause retention of fluid in intestinal lumen caused by osmotic effect	Magnesium salts: magnesium citrate, Milk of Magnesia Sodium phosphates: Fleet enema, Phospho-Soda lactulose (Constulose) polyethylene glycol (MiraLax, GoLYTELY, Colyte)	15 min to 3 hr	Magnesium-containing products may cause hypermagnesemia in patients with renal insufficiency
Stimulants	Increase peristalsis by irritating colon wall and stimulating enteric nerves	cascara sagrada, senna (Senokot) phenolphthalein: Ex-Lax, Correctol, Feen-a-Mint, bisacodyl (Dulcolax)	Usually within 12 hr	Cause melanosis coli (brown or black pigmentation of colon); are most widely abused laxatives; should not be used in patients with impaction or obstipation
Selective chloride channel activator	Increases intestinal fluid secretion and motility	lubiprostone (Amitiza)	Usually within 24 hr	Used in the treatment of idiopathic constipation; contraindicated in patients with history of mechanical GI obstruction
Serotonin type 4 (5-HT$_4$) receptor partial agonist	Triggers peristaltic activity in gut, increasing bowel motility	tegaserod (Zelnorm)	Usually within 24 hr	Indicated for patients <65 yr old (male and female) with chronic idiopathic constipation

GI, Gastrointestinal.

through the GI tract, until it reaches the colon, where fermentation occurs. Dietary fiber adds to the stool bulk directly and by attracting water. Large, bulky stools decrease pressure within the lumen of the colon and move through the colon much more quickly than small stools. Therefore stool frequency increases and constipation is prevented. Fluid intake of approximately 3000 ml daily is important because much of the stool bulk and softening comes from the attraction of water to the stool. The person who eats large amounts of dietary fiber and does not drink enough fluids will have dry, hard stools that are difficult to pass. The recommended fluid intake may be contraindicated in the patient with cardiac disease or renal insufficiency or failure. The patient's understanding of the diet and the importance of dietary fiber is important to ensure compliance. Patients should be told that initially fiber may increase gas production because of fermentation in the colon, but that this effect decreases with use.

NURSING MANAGEMENT
CONSTIPATION

■ Nursing Assessment

Subjective and objective data that should be obtained from a patient with constipation are presented in Table 43-10.

■ Nursing Diagnosis

Nursing diagnosis for the patient with constipation includes, but is not limited to, the following:

- Constipation *related to* inadequate intake of dietary fiber and fluid and decreased physical activity

■ Planning

The overall goals are that the patient with constipation will (1) increase dietary intake of fiber and fluids; (2) increase physical activity; (3) have the passage of soft, formed stools; and (4) not have any complications, such as bleeding hemorrhoids.

■ Nursing Implementation

Nursing management should be based on the patient's symptoms (see Table 43-7) and the assessment of the patient (see Table 43-10). An important role of the nurse is teaching the patient the importance of dietary measures to prevent constipation. A patient and family teaching guide for constipation is presented in Table 43-11. Emphasis should be placed on maintenance of a high-fiber diet, increasing fluid intake, and a regular exercise program. The patient should be taught to establish a regular time to defecate and not to suppress the urge to defecate. The patient should be discouraged from using laxatives and enemas to achieve fecal elimination.

TABLE 43-9	**NUTRITIONAL THERAPY** **High-Fiber Foods**

High-fiber foods are especially recommended for patients with diverticulosis, irritable bowel syndrome, constipation, hemorrhoids, colorectal cancer, atherosclerosis, hyperlipidemia, and diabetes mellitus.

	Fiber per Serving (g)	Size of Serving	Calories per Serving
Vegetables			
Asparagus	3.5	½ cup	18
Beans			
Navy	8.4	½ cup	80
Kidney	9.7	½ cup	94
Lima	8.3	½ cup	63
Pinto	8.9	½ cup	78
String	2.1	½ cup	18
Broccoli	3.5	½ cup	18
Carrots, raw	1.8	½ cup	15
Corn	2.6	½ medium ear	72
Peas, canned	6.7	½ cup	63
Potatoes			
Baked	1.9	½ medium	72
Sweet	2.1	½ medium	79
Squash			
Acorn	7	1 cup	82
Tomato, raw	1.5	1 small	18
Fruits			
Apple	2.0	½ large	42
Blackberries	6.7	¾ cup	40
Orange	1.6	1 small	35
Peach	2.3	1 medium	38
Pear	2	½ medium	44
Raspberries	9.2	1 cup	42
Strawberries	3.1	1 cup	45
Grain Products			
Bread			
Whole wheat	1.3	1 slice	59
Cereal			
All Bran (100%)	8.4	⅓ cup	70
Corn Flakes	2.6	¾ cup	70
Shredded Wheat	2.8	1 biscuit	70
Popcorn	3	3 cups	62

TABLE 43-10	**NURSING ASSESSMENT** **Constipation**

Subjective Data
Important Health Information
Past health history: Colorectal disease, neurologic dysfunction, bowel obstruction, environmental changes, cancer, irritable bowel syndrome
Medications: Use of aluminum and calcium antacids, anticholinergics, antidepressants, antihistamines, antipsychotics, diuretics, opioids, iron, laxatives, enemas

Functional Health Patterns
Health perception–health management: Chronic laxative or enema abuse; rigid beliefs regarding bowel function; malaise
Nutritional-metabolic: Changes in diet or mealtime; inadequate fiber and fluid intake; anorexia, nausea
Elimination: Change in usual elimination patterns; hard, difficult-to-pass stool, decrease in frequency and amount of stools; flatus, abdominal distention; tenesmus, rectal pressure; fecal incontinence (if impacted)
Activity-exercise: Change in daily activity routines; immobility; sedentary lifestyle
Cognitive-perceptual: Dizziness, headache, anorectal pain; abdominal pain on defecation
Coping–stress tolerance: Acute or chronic stress

Objective Data
General
Lethargy

Integumentary
Anorectal fissures, hemorrhoids, abscesses

Gastrointestinal
Abdominal distention; hypoactive or absent bowel sounds; palpable abdominal mass; fecal impaction; small, hard, dry stool; stool with blood

Possible Findings
Guaiac-positive stools; abdominal x-ray demonstrating stool in lower colon

Proper position is important when defecating. Defecation is easiest when the person is sitting on a commode with the knees higher than the hips. It is extremely difficult to defecate while sitting on a bedpan. For a patient in bed, the bedpan should be placed, and the head of the bed should be elevated as high as the patient can tolerate. For the person who can sit on a toilet, a footstool may be placed in front of the toilet. Placing the feet on the footstool promotes flexion of the thighs, which assists in defecation.

Most people are embarrassed by the sights and sounds of defecation, and the nurse should ensure that patients have as much privacy as possible.

The patient with poor muscle tone should be encouraged to exercise the abdominal muscles and can be taught to contract the abdominal muscles several times a day. Sit-ups and straight leg raises can also be used to improve abdominal muscle tone.

Patients taking bulking products need to be taught to follow product recommendations in terms of fluid intake. Similar to increasing fiber intake, patients may initially experience an increase in flatus that will decrease with time.

ACUTE ABDOMINAL PAIN

Etiology and Pathophysiology

Acute abdominal pain is a symptom of many different types of tissue injury and can arise from damage to abdominal or pelvic organs and blood vessels. The most common causes of an acute onset of abdominal pain are listed in Table 43-12. Certain causes (e.g., hemorrhage, obstruction, and rupture) are life threatening because large fluid losses from the vascular space lead to shock. Other problems require only conservative medical treatment.

Clinical Manifestations

Pain is the most common symptom of an acute abdominal problem. The patient may also complain of nausea, vomiting, diarrhea, constipation, flatulence, fatigue, fever, and an increase in abdominal girth.

Diagnostic Studies and Collaborative Management

Many disorders must be ruled out before a diagnosis is confirmed. Diagnosis begins with a complete history and physical examination. A complete description of the pain (frequency, timing, dura-

TABLE 43-11	*PATIENT AND FAMILY TEACHING GUIDE* Constipation

The following are teaching guidelines for the patient and family:

1. Eat Dietary Fiber
Eat 20 to 30 g of fiber per day. Gradually increase the amount of fiber eaten over 1 to 2 weeks. Fiber softens hard stool and adds bulk to stool, promoting evacuation.
- Foods high in fiber: raw vegetables and fruits, beans, breakfast cereals (All Bran, oatmeal)
- Fiber supplements: Metamucil, Citrucel, FiberCon

2. Drink Fluids
Drink 3 quarts per day. Drink water or fruit juices; avoid caffeinated coffee, tea, and cola. Fluid softens hard stools; caffeine stimulates fluid loss through urination.

3. Exercise Regularly
Walk, swim, or bike at least three times per week. Contract and relax abdominal muscles when standing or by doing sit-ups to strengthen muscles and prevent straining. Exercise stimulates bowel motility and moves stool through the intestine.

4. Establish a Regular Time to Defecate
First thing in the morning or after the first meal of the day is a good time because people often have the urge to defecate at this time.

5. Do Not Delay Defecation
Respond to the urge to have a bowel movement as soon as possible. Delaying defecation results in hard stools and a decreased "urge" to defecate. Water is absorbed from stool by the intestine over time. The intestine becomes less sensitive to the presence of stool in the rectum.

6. Record your Bowel Elimination Pattern
Develop a habit of recording when you have a bowel movement on your calendar. Regular monitoring of bowel movement will assist in early identification of a problem.

7. Avoid Laxatives and Enemas
Do not overuse laxatives and enemas because they cause dependence. People who overuse them are unable to have a bowel movement without them.

TABLE 43-12	Common Causes of Acute Abdominal Pain

- Appendicitis
- Bowel obstruction
- Cholecystitis
- Diverticulitis
- Gastroenteritis
- Pelvic inflammatory disease
- Perforated gastric or duodenal ulcer
- Peritonitis
- Ruptured abdominal aneurysm
- Ruptured ectopic pregnancy

tion, location) and accompanying symptoms provides vital clues about the origin of the problem. Physical examination should include a rectal and pelvic examination in addition to the abdomen. A complete blood count (CBC), a urinalysis, an abdominal x-ray, and an electrocardiogram are done initially, along with an ultrasound or CT scan. Pregnancy tests should be done in women of childbearing age with acute abdominal pain to rule out ectopic pregnancy. The health care provider attempts to make a differential diagnosis because many causes of abdominal pain do not require surgery (see Table 43-12).

Emergency management of the patient with acute abdominal pain is presented in Table 43-13. The goal of management is to identify and treat the cause, and monitor and treat complications, especially shock. It was previously thought that pain medication should be withheld because analgesics might obscure progression of clinical manifestations and impede diagnosis. Appropriate pain management that does not result in altered consciousness (e.g., ketorolac [Toradol]) can decrease diffuse pain and abdominal rigidity and help localize the pain. This can lead to earlier diagnosis and treatment.

In the case of acute abdominal pain, surgery can be a diagnostic as well as therapeutic procedure. An exploratory laparotomy, in which an opening is made through the abdominal wall into the peritoneal cavity, is done after a careful examination of the patient. This procedure is done when "look and see" is better than "wait and see." If the cause of the acute abdomen can be surgically removed (e.g., inflamed appendix) or surgically repaired (e.g., ruptured abdominal aneurysm), surgery is considered definitive therapy.

NURSING MANAGEMENT
ACUTE ABDOMINAL PAIN

■ Nursing Assessment

Vital signs should be taken immediately. Increased pulse and decreasing blood pressure (BP) are indicative of hypovolemia. An elevated temperature may indicate an inflammatory or infectious process. Intake and output measurement provides essential information about the adequacy of vascular volume. The abdomen should be inspected for distention, masses, abnormal pulsation, rashes, scars, and pigmentation changes. Bowel sounds should be auscultated. Bowel sounds that are diminished or absent in a quadrant may indicate a complete bowel obstruction, acute peritonitis, or paralytic ileus. Palpation should be gentle.

A thorough assessment of the patient's symptoms should be made to determine the onset, location, intensity, duration, frequency, and character of pain. The nurse should determine whether the pain has spread or moved to new locations (quadrants), as well as what makes the pain worse or better. It should also be determined whether the pain is associated with other symptoms, such as nausea, vomiting, changes in bowel and bladder habits, or vaginal discharge in women. Assessment of vomiting should include the amount, color, consistency, and odor of the emesis. Bowel patterns and habits should also be carefully assessed.

■ Nursing Diagnoses

Nursing diagnoses for the patient with acute abdominal pain include, but are not limited to, the following:
- Acute pain *related to* inflammation of the peritoneum and abdominal distention
- Risk for deficient fluid volume *related to* collection of fluid in peritoneal cavity secondary to inflammation or infection
- Imbalanced nutrition: less than body requirements *related to* anorexia, nausea, and vomiting
- Anxiety *related to* pain and uncertainty of cause or outcome of condition

■ Planning

The overall goals are that the patient with acute abdominal pain will have (1) resolution of inflammation, (2) relief of abdominal pain, (3) freedom from complications (especially hypovolemic shock), and (4) normal nutritional status.

TABLE 43-13	*EMERGENCY MANAGEMENT* **Acute Abdominal Pain**

Etiology	Assessment Findings	Interventions
Inflammation Appendicitis Cholecystitis Crohn's disease Gastritis Pancreatitis Pyelonephritis Ulcerative colitis **Vascular Problems** Ruptured aortic aneurysm Mesenteric vascular occlusion **Gynecologic Problems** Pelvic inflammatory disease Ruptured ectopic pregnancy Ruptured ovarian cyst **Infectious Disease** *E. coli* O157:H7 *Giardia* *Salmonella* **Other** Obstruction or perforation of abdominal organ Gastrointestinal bleeding Trauma	**Abdominal/Gastrointestinal Findings** Diffuse, localized, dull, burning, or sharp abdominal pain or tenderness Rebound tenderness Abdominal distention Abdominal rigidity Nausea and vomiting Diarrhea Hematemesis Melena **Hypovolemic Shock** ↓ Blood pressure ↓ Pulse pressure Tachycardia Cool, clammy skin ↓ Level of consciousness ↓ Urine output (<0.5 ml/kg/hr)	**Initial** Ensure patent airway. Administer oxygen via nasal cannula or non-rebreather mask. Establish IV access with large-bore catheter and infuse warm normal saline or lactated Ringer's solution. Insert additional large-bore catheter if shock present. Obtain blood for CBC and electrolytes. Anticipate order for amylase level, pregnancy tests, clotting studies, and type and crossmatch as appropriate. Insert indwelling urinary catheter. Obtain urinalysis. Insert NG tube as needed. **Ongoing Monitoring** Monitor vital signs, level of consciousness, O₂ saturation, and intake/output. Assess quality and amount of pain. Assess amount and character of emesis. Anticipate surgical intervention. Keep NPO.

CBC, Complete blood count; *IV,* intravenous; *NG,* nasogastric; *NPO,* nothing by mouth.

■ *Nursing Implementation*

General care for the patient involves management of fluid and electrolyte imbalances, pain, and anxiety. The quality and intensity of pain are measured at regular intervals, and medication and other comfort measurements are administered. A calm environment, a confident attitude, and prompt provision of information help allay anxiety. The nurse continues to monitor vital signs, intake and output, and level of consciousness, which are key indicators of hypovolemic shock. If the patient has an exploratory laparotomy or other surgery, the nurse provides preoperative and postoperative care.

Acute Intervention

Preoperative Care. Preoperative care includes the emergency care of the patient described in Table 43-13 and general care of the preoperative patient (see Chapter 18).

Postoperative Care. Postoperative care depends on the type of surgical procedure performed. The increased use of laparoscopic procedures has reduced the risk of postoperative complications related to wound care, and postoperative paralytic ileus is rare. Early ambulation and advancement of diet result in shorter hospital stays. A general nursing care plan for the postoperative patient is presented in Chapter 20 on pp. 383 to 386.

A nasogastric (NG) tube with low suction may be used to empty the stomach of secretions and gas to prevent gastric dilation. However, the NG tube is used less frequently because of increased use of laparoscopic procedures. If the upper GI tract has been entered, drainage from the NG tube may be dark brown to dark red for the first 12 hours. Later it should be light yellowish brown, or it may have a greenish tinge because of the presence of bile. If a dark red color continues or if bright red blood is observed, the

health care provider should be notified at once of the possibility of hemorrhage. "Coffee ground" granules in the drainage are due to the presence of blood that has been chemically acted on by acidic gastric secretions.

The NG tube is checked frequently for patency. If the tube is obstructed with mucus, sediment, or blood clots, the nurse should request a physician's order to irrigate it with 20 to 30 ml of normal saline solution as necessary. Repositioning the tube may facilitate drainage. When bowel sounds are auscultated, the health care provider usually orders the removal of the NG tube. An accurate record of intake and output, including emesis and gastric drainage, is essential. The nurse assesses serum electrolyte values and acid-base balance because prolonged gastric suctioning can result in loss of sodium, chloride, potassium, water, and hydrochloric acid (HCl).

Routine mouth care and nasal care are essential. The patient tends to breathe through the mouth while the NG tube is in place, and mouth breathing dries the mucosal membranes of the mouth. The tube irritates nasal mucosa leading to increased secretions and crusting. Parenteral fluids are administered to provide the patient with fluids and electrolytes until bowel sounds return. Occasionally, ice chips may be ordered because they aid in the flow of saliva and prevent a dry mouth. When bowel sounds return, fluids and food are increased gradually.

Nausea and vomiting are not uncommon after abdominal surgery, and may be caused by the surgery, decreased peristalsis, or pain medications. Antiemetics such as prochlorperazine (Compazine), promethazine (Phenergan), ondansetron (Zofran), or trimethobenzamide (Tigan) may be ordered. Management of nausea and vomiting are discussed in Chapter 42. Swallowed air and decreased peristalsis from decreased mobility, manipulation of abdominal organs during surgery, and anesthesia can lead to abdominal distention and gas pains. Early ambulation helps restore peristalsis and eliminate flatus and gas pain. If gas pain is severe, the health care provider sometimes prescribes a medication (e.g., metoclopramide [Reglan]) to stimulate peristalsis. The health care provider should be informed of abdominal distention and rigidity. Gradually, as intestinal activity increases, distention and gas pain disappear.

Ambulatory and Home Care. Preparation for discharge begins soon after surgery. Instructions to the patient and the family should include any modifications in activity, care of the incision, diet, and drug therapy. Clear liquids are given initially after surgery and if tolerated, the patient progresses to a regular diet.

Early ambulation speeds recovery, but normal activities should be resumed gradually, with planned rest periods. After surgery the patient is generally instructed not to lift anything heavier than a few pounds. The patient should be aware of possible complications after surgery and should notify the health care provider immediately if vomiting, pain, weight loss, incisional drainage, or changes in bowel function occur.

■ Evaluation

The expected outcomes are that the patient with acute abdominal pain will have

- resolution of the cause of the acute abdominal pain
- relief of abdominal pain and discomfort
- freedom from complications (especially hypovolemic shock and septicemia)
- normal fluid, electrolyte, and nutritional status

Chronic Abdominal Pain

Chronic abdominal pain may originate from abdominal structures or may be referred from a site with the same or a similar nerve supply. Common causes include irritable bowel syndrome (IBS), diverticulitis, peptic ulcer disease, chronic pancreatitis, hepatitis, cholecystitis, pelvic inflammatory disease, and vascular insufficiency. (Some of these disorders are discussed in this chapter. The other diseases and disorders are discussed in other chapters.)

Diagnosis of the cause of chronic abdominal pain begins with a thorough history and description of specific pain characteristics. Character and severity of pain, location, duration, and onset should be determined. The assessment also includes the relationship of pain to meals, defecation, and activity and factors that increase or decrease the pain. Chronic abdominal pain is often described as dull, aching, or diffuse.

Endoscopy, CT scan, magnetic resonance imaging (MRI), laparoscopy, and barium studies may be used in the patient evaluation. Treatment for chronic abdominal pain is comprehensive and directed toward palliation of symptoms using nonopiate analgesics and antiemetics, as well as psychologic or behavioral therapies (e.g., relaxation therapies).

IRRITABLE BOWEL SYNDROME

Irritable bowel syndrome (IBS) is a symptom complex characterized by intermittent and recurrent abdominal pain and stool pattern irregularities. It is classified as IBS with diarrhea, IBS with constipation, and IBS with mixed diarrhea and constipation. Other common symptoms include abdominal distention, excessive flatu-

GENDER DIFFERENCES
Irritable Bowel Syndrome

Men
- More men report manifestations of diarrhea.
- Less likely to admit to symptoms or seek help for them than women.

Women
- More women report manifestations of constipation.
- Affects women 2-2.5 times as often as men.
- More women report extraintestinal manifestations (e.g., migraine headache, insomnia, fibromyalgia) than men.
- Alosetron (Lotronex) (antidiarrheal) and tegaserod (Zelnorm) (anticonstipation) are approved for treating IBS only in women.

lence, bloating, a continual defecation urge, urgency, and sensation of incomplete evacuation. IBS is a common problem, affecting approximately 10% to 15% of Western populations.[7] In the United States, approximately 2 to 2.5 times as many women as men seek health care services for IBS.[7] Stress, psychologic factors, prior gastroenteritis, and specific food intolerances have been identified as major factors that precipitate IBS symptoms.

The abdominal pain or discomfort associated with IBS is most likely due to increased visceral sensitivity. That is, the presence of stool or gas in the GI tract stimulates visceral afferent fibers, which results in perception of discomfort or pain. Several neurochemicals, including serotonin, are likely involved in bowel symptoms of diarrhea, constipation, and pain sensitivity.[8]

There are no specific physical findings with IBS. The diagnosis is made when the patient displays the characteristic symptoms and other conditions are ruled out. The key to accurate diagnosis is a thorough history and physical examination. Emphasis should be on symptoms, past health history (including psychosocial factors such as physical or sexual abuse), family history, and drug and diet history. Diagnostic tests should be selectively used to rule out more serious disorders with symptoms similar to those of IBS, such as colorectal cancer, peptic ulcer disease, inflammatory bowel disease, and malabsorption disorders (e.g., celiac disease). Symptom-based criteria for IBS have been standardized and are referred to as the Rome criteria. The Rome II criteria include the following: abdominal discomfort or pain for at least 12 weeks (not necessarily consecutive) within 12 months that has at least two of the following characteristics: (1) relieved with defecation; (2) onset associated with a change in stool frequency; and (3) onset associated with a change in stool appearance.[6,7]

The health care provider should establish a trusting relationship with the patient at the onset of treatment. The patient should be encouraged to verbalize concerns and anxiety. Since treatment is often focused on symptoms, patients are encouraged to keep a diary of symptoms, diet, and episodes of stress to help identify factors that seem to trigger the IBS symptoms.[7] Health care providers have traditionally prescribed a diet containing at least 20 g per day of dietary fiber (see Table 43-9), or a bulking agent such as Metamucil. Unfortunately, fermentation of large amounts of fiber can increase bloating and gas pain (at least initially), two symptoms that are already problematic for many patients with IBS.[6]

PICO: P, Patient population of interest; *I,* intervention or area of interest; *C,* comparison of interest or comparison group; *O,* outcome(s) of interest (see p. 6).

The patient whose primary symptoms are abdominal distention and increased flatulence should be advised to eliminate common gas-producing foods (e.g., broccoli, cabbage) from the diet and to substitute yogurt for milk products to help determine if there is lactose intolerance. Antispasmodic agents (e.g., dicyclomine [Bentyl]) may be tried before meals to alleviate the pain associated with ingestion of food, but their effectiveness has been questioned.[6,9] Loperamide (Imodium), a synthetic opioid that decreases intestinal transit and enhances intestinal water absorption and sphincter tone, has been found to be effective for IBS patients with diarrhea.[6,9] Two serotonergic agents have been approved by the Food and Drug Administration (FDA) for IBS: tegaserod (Zelnorm), for women whose primary bowel symptom is constipation, and alosetron (Lotronex), for women with severe IBS and diarrhea. Because of serious side effects (e.g., severe constipation, ischemic colitis), alosetron is available only in a restricted access program for women who have not responded to other IBS therapies, and in whom other anatomic and chemical abnormalities have been ruled out.[9] Other therapies include cognitive-behavioral therapy, relaxation and stress management techniques, acupuncture, hypnosis, and Chinese herbs.[10] No single therapy has been found to be effective for all patients with IBS.

> ### Drug Alert - Alosetron (Lotronex)
> - *Patients may experience severe constipation and ischemic colitis (reduced blood flow to intestines).*
> - *If constipation occurs, drug should be discontinued.*
> - *Symptoms of ischemic colitis include abdominal pain and blood in stool.*

ABDOMINAL TRAUMA

Etiology and Pathophysiology

Injuries to the abdominal area most often occur as a result of blunt trauma or penetration injuries. Blunt trauma commonly occurs with motor vehicle accidents and falls, and may not be obvious because it does not leave an open wound. Both compression injuries (e.g., direct blow to the abdomen) and shearing injuries (e.g., rapid deceleration in a motor vehicle crash allows some tissue to move forward while other tissues are held stationary) occur with blunt trauma. Penetrating injuries occur when a gunshot or stabbing produces an obvious, open wound into the abdomen. Regardless of whether it is a blunt or penetration injury, the abdominal organs are damaged. Solid organs (liver, spleen) bleed profusely when injured. Damage to hollow organs such as the bladder, stomach, and intestines causes peritonitis when the contents spill into the peritoneal cavity.[11]

Common injuries of the abdomen include lacerated liver, ruptured spleen, pancreatic trauma, mesenteric artery tears, diaphragm rupture, urinary bladder rupture, great vessel tears, renal injury, and stomach or intestine rupture. These injuries can result in massive blood loss and hypovolemic shock. Surgery is performed as early as possible to repair the damaged organs and to stop the bleeding. Common sequelae of intraabdominal trauma are peritonitis and sepsis, particularly when the bowel is perforated.

Clinical Manifestations

Careful assessment provides important clues to the type and severity of injury. Clinical manifestations of abdominal trauma are (1) guarding and splinting of the abdominal wall (indicating peritonitis); (2) a hard, distended abdomen (indicating intraabdominal bleeding); (3) decreased or absent bowel sounds; (4) contusions, abrasions, or bruising over the abdomen; (5) abdominal pain; (6) pain over the scapula caused by irritation of the phrenic nerve by free blood in the abdomen; (7) hematemesis or hematuria; and (8) signs of hypovolemic shock (Table 43-14). If the patient was in an automobile accident, a contusion or abrasion across the lower abdomen indicates that the seat belt probably did damage to the internal organs. Ecchymosis around the umbilicus (Cullen's sign) or flanks (Grey-Turner's sign) may indicate retroperitoneal hemorrhage. Loss of bowel sounds occurs with peritonitis. Bowel sounds are heard in the chest when the diaphragm ruptures. Auscultation of bruits signals arterial or aortic damage.[11] Intraabdominal injuries are often associated with low rib fractures, fractured femur, fractured pelvis, and thoracic injury. If any of these injuries are present, the patient should be observed for abdominal trauma.

TABLE 43-14	*EMERGENCY MANAGEMENT* Abdominal Trauma	
Etiology	**Assessment Findings**	**Interventions**
Blunt Falls Motor vehicle collisions Pedestrian event Assault with blunt object Crush injuries Explosions **Penetrating** Knife Gunshot wounds Other missiles	**Hypovolemic Shock** ↓ Level of consciousness Tachypnea Tachycardia ↓ Blood pressure ↓ Pulse pressure **Surface Findings** Abrasions or ecchymoses on abdominal wall, flank, or peritoneum Open wounds: lacerations, eviscerations, puncture wounds, gunshot wounds Impaled object Healed incisions or old scars **Abdominal/Gastrointestinal Findings** Nausea and vomiting Bloody urine Abdominal distention Abdominal rigidity Abdominal pain with palpation Rebound tenderness Pain radiation to shoulder and back	**Initial** Ensure patent airway. Administer O_2 via non-rebreather mask. Control external bleeding with direct pressure or sterile pressure dressing. Establish IV access with two large-bore catheters and infuse warm normal saline or lactated Ringer's solution. Obtain blood for type and crossmatch and CBC. Remove clothing. Stabilize impaled objects with bulky dressing—*do not remove.* Cover protruding organs or tissue with sterile, saline dressing. Insert indwelling urinary catheter if there is no blood at the meatus, pelvic fracture, or boggy prostate. Obtain urine for urinalysis. Insert NG tube if no evidence of facial trauma. Anticipate diagnostic peritoneal lavage. **Ongoing Monitoring** Monitor vital signs, level of consciousness, O_2 saturation, and urine output. Maintain patient warmth using blankets, warm IV fluids, or warm humidified oxygen.

CBC, Complete blood count; *IV,* intravenous; *NG,* nasogastric.

Diagnostic Studies

Laboratory tests include a baseline CBC and urinalysis. Even when bleeding, the patient's hemoglobin and hematocrit will remain normal because fluids are lost at the same rate as the red blood cells (RBCs). Deficiencies will be evident after fluid resuscitation begins. Blood in the urine may be a sign of damage to the kidney or bladder. Additional laboratory work includes arterial blood gases, prothrombin time, electrolytes, BUN and creatinine, and type and crossmatch (in anticipation of possible blood transfusions). Ultrasound is often used because it is portable and noninvasive. An abdominal CT scan can identify specific injury sites, but its use requires that the patient be stable enough to transport to radiology.

Diagnostic peritoneal lavage may also be used.[11] Peritoneal lavage is performed by inserting a large angiocatheter or peritoneal dialysis catheter into the abdomen after a local anesthetic has been injected. A syringe is attached to the catheter, and an attempt is made to gently aspirate any blood. If less than 10 ml of blood is aspirated, a liter of saline solution is then infused into the abdomen and drained. The fluid is observed for gross abnormalities, especially blood, and is sent to the laboratory for microscopic evaluation. Positive findings include (1) RBC count greater than 100,000/μl; (2) WBC count greater than 500/μl; (3) high amylase level; and (4) presence of bacteria, bile, or fecal material. If the results are positive, immediate surgery is indicated. If the results are negative, continued observation of the patient is warranted.

NURSING *and* COLLABORATIVE MANAGEMENT
ABDOMINAL TRAUMA

Emergency management of abdominal trauma focuses on establishing a patent airway and adequate breathing, fluid replacement, and prevention of hypovolemic shock (see Table 43-14). Intravenous (IV) lines are inserted, and volume expanders or blood is given if the patient is hypotensive. An NG tube is inserted to decompress the stomach and prevent the aspiration. Frequent ongoing assessment is necessary to detect deterioration in condition and the necessity of surgery. An impaled object should never be removed until skilled care is available. Removal may cause further injury and bleeding.

Regardless of the type of injury, physical evidence of abdominal trauma in a patient who is hemodynamically unstable mandates immediate laparotomy. Otherwise, the laparotomy may be delayed. If surgery is performed, the postoperative nursing care is similar to the care of the patient after laparotomy.

Inflammatory Disorders

APPENDICITIS

Appendicitis is an inflammation of the appendix, a narrow blind tube that extends from the inferior part of the cecum. Appendicitis occurs in 7% to 12% of the world's population. It can occur at any age but is most common in young adults.[12]

Etiology and Pathophysiology

The most common causes of appendicitis are obstruction of the lumen by a fecalith (accumulated feces) (Fig. 43-1), foreign bodies, tumor of the cecum or appendix, or intramural thickening caused by excessive growth of lymphoid tissue. Obstruction results in distention, venous engorgement, and the accumulation of mucus and bacteria, which can lead to gangrene and perforation.[12]

Clinical Manifestations

Symptoms vary and diagnosis can be difficult.[12] Appendicitis typically begins with periumbilical pain, followed by anorexia, nausea, and vomiting. The pain is persistent and continuous, eventually shifting to the right lower quadrant and localizing at McBurney's point (located halfway between the umbilicus and the right iliac crest). Further assessment of the patient reveals localized tenderness,

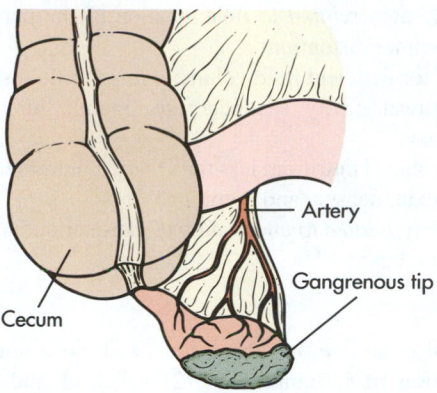

FIG. 43-1 In appendicitis the blood supply of the appendix is impaired by inflammation and bacterial infection in the wall of the appendix, which may result in gangrene.

Labels: Artery, Gangrenous tip, Cecum

TABLE 43-15	**Causes of Peritonitis**	
Primary	**Secondary**	
Blood-borne organisms	Appendicitis with rupture	
Genital tract organisms	Blunt or penetrating trauma to abdominal organs	
Cirrhosis with ascites	Diverticulitis with rupture	
	Ischemic bowel disorders	
	Obstruction in the gastrointestinal tract	
	Pancreatitis	
	Perforated peptic ulcer	
	Peritoneal dialysis	
	Postoperative (breakage of anastomosis)	

rebound tenderness, and muscle guarding. The patient usually prefers to lie still, often with the right leg flexed. Low-grade fever may or may not be present, and coughing aggravates pain. Rovsing's sign may be elicited by palpation of the left lower quadrant, causing pain to be felt in the right lower quadrant. Complications of acute appendicitis are perforation, peritonitis, and abscesses.

Diagnostic Studies and Collaborative Care

Examination of the patient includes a complete history and physical examination (particularly palpation of the abdomen) and a differential WBC count. The WBC count may be elevated with appendicitis. A urinalysis may be done to rule out genitourinary conditions that mimic the manifestations of appendicitis. The gold standard is either an ultrasound or a CT scan.

NeutroSpec imaging is a new technique to diagnose appendicitis. It uses a technetium-labeled anti-CD15 monoclonal antibody that selectively binds to neutrophils. When injected into the blood, NeutroSpec binds to neutrophils present at the infection site, labeling these cells with technetium. As a result, physicians can rapidly detect an infection using a gamma camera that records radioactivity. NeutroSpec's advantage over the current standard of care is in vivo labeling of WBCs and a diagnosis in less than 1 hour.

If diagnosis and treatment are delayed, the appendix can rupture, and the resulting peritonitis can be fatal. The treatment of appendicitis is immediate surgical removal (appendectomy) if the inflammation is localized. If the appendix has ruptured and there is evidence of peritonitis or an abscess, conservative treatment consisting of antibiotic therapy and parenteral fluids is given for 6 to 8 hours before the appendectomy in order to prevent sepsis and dehydration.

NURSING MANAGEMENT
APPENDICITIS

The patient with abdominal pain is encouraged to see a health care provider and to avoid self-treatment. Laxatives and enemas are especially dangerous because the resulting increased peristalsis may cause perforation of the appendix. Until a health care provider sees the patient, nothing should be taken by mouth (NPO) to ensure that the stomach is empty in the event that surgery is needed. An ice bag may be applied to the right lower quadrant to decrease the flow of blood to the area and impede the inflammatory process. Heat is never used because it may cause the appendix to rupture. Surgery, generally performed laparoscopically, is performed as soon as the diagnosis is made.

Postoperative nursing management is similar to postoperative care of the patient after laparotomy. In addition, the patient is observed for evidence of peritonitis. Ambulation begins the day of surgery or the first postoperative day. The diet is advanced as tolerated. The patient is usually discharged on the first or second postoperative day, and normal activities are resumed 2 to 3 weeks after surgery.

PERITONITIS
Etiology and Pathophysiology

Peritonitis results from a localized or generalized inflammatory process of the peritoneum. Causes of peritonitis are listed in Table 43-15. Primary peritonitis occurs when blood-borne organisms enter the peritoneal cavity. For example, the ascites that occurs with cirrhosis of the liver provides an excellent liquid environment for bacteria to flourish. Secondary peritonitis is much more common. It occurs when abdominal organs perforate or rupture and release their contents (bile, enzymes, and bacteria) into the peritoneal cavity. Common causes include a ruptured appendix, perforated gastric or duodenal ulcer, severely inflamed gallbladder, and trauma from gunshot or knife wounds.[13] Intestinal contents and bacteria irritate the normally sterile peritoneum and produce an immediate chemical peritonitis that is followed a few hours later by a bacterial peritonitis. Patients who use continuous ambulatory peritoneal dialysis are also at high risk.[14] (Peritoneal dialysis is described in Chapter 47.) No matter what the cause, the resulting inflammatory response leads to massive fluid shifts (peritoneal edema) and adhesions as the body attempts to wall off the infection.

Clinical Manifestations

Abdominal pain is the most common symptom of peritonitis. A universal sign of peritonitis is tenderness over the involved area. Rebound tenderness, muscular rigidity, and spasm are other major signs of irritation of the peritoneum. Patients may lie very still and take only shallow respirations because movement causes pain. Abdominal distention or ascites, fever, tachycardia, tachypnea, nausea, vomiting, and altered bowel habits may also be present. These manifestations vary depending on the severity and acuteness of the underlying cause. Complications of peritonitis include hypovolemic shock, sepsis, intraabdominal abscess formation, paralytic ileus, and acute respiratory distress syndrome. Peritonitis can be fatal if treatment is delayed.

Diagnostic Studies

A CBC is done to determine elevations in WBC count and hemoconcentration from fluid shifts (Table 43-16). Peritoneal aspiration may be performed and the fluid analyzed for blood, bile, pus, bac-

TABLE 43-16	COLLABORATIVE CARE Peritonitis

Diagnostic
History and physical examination
CBC
Serum electrolytes
Abdominal x-ray
Abdominal paracentesis and culture of fluid
CT scan or ultrasound
Peritoneoscopy

Collaborative Therapy
Preoperative or Nonoperative
NPO status
IV fluid replacement
Antibiotic therapy
NG suction
Analgesics (e.g., morphine)
Oxygen prn
Preparation for surgery to include the above and parenteral nutrition

Postoperative
NPO status
NG tube to low-intermittent suction
Semi-Fowler's position
IV fluids with electrolyte replacement
Parenteral nutrition as needed
Antibiotic therapy
Blood transfusions as needed
Sedatives and opioids

CBC, Complete blood count; *CT,* computed tomography; *IV,* intravenous; *NG,* nasogastric; *NPO,* nothing by mouth; *prn,* as required.

teria, fungus, and amylase content. An x-ray of the abdomen may show dilated loops of bowel consistent with paralytic ileus, free air if perforation has occurred, or air and fluid levels if an obstruction is present. Ultrasound and CT scans may be useful in identifying the presence of ascites and abscesses. Peritoneoscopy (placement of an endoscope through a stab wound in the abdomen to inspect the peritoneum) may be helpful in the patient without ascites. Direct examination of the peritoneum can be obtained, along with biopsy specimens for diagnosis.

Collaborative Care

Surgery is usually indicated to locate the cause, drain purulent fluid, and repair the damage. Appropriate antibiotics are given to treat the infection. Patients with milder cases of peritonitis or those who are poor surgical risks may be managed nonsurgically. Treatment consists of antibiotics, NG suction, analgesics, and IV fluid administration. Patients who require surgery need preoperative preparation as previously described.

NURSING MANAGEMENT
PERITONITIS

■ Nursing Assessment

Assessment of the patient's pain, including the location, is important and may help in determining the cause of peritonitis. The patient should be assessed for the presence and quality of bowel sounds, increasing abdominal distention, abdominal guarding, nausea, fever, and manifestations of hypovolemic shock.

■ Nursing Diagnoses

Nursing diagnoses for the patient with peritonitis include, but are not limited to, the following.

- Acute pain *related to* inflammation of the peritoneum and abdominal distention
- Risk for deficient fluid volume *related to* fluid shifts into the peritoneal cavity secondary to trauma, infection, or ischemia
- Imbalanced nutrition: less than body requirements *related to* anorexia, nausea, and vomiting
- Anxiety *related to* uncertainty of cause or outcome of condition and pain

■ Planning

The overall goals are that the patient with peritonitis will have (1) resolution of inflammation, (2) relief of abdominal pain, (3) freedom from complications (especially hypovolemic shock), and (4) normal nutritional status.

■ Nursing Implementation

The patient with peritonitis is extremely ill and needs skilled supportive care. An IV line is inserted to replace vascular fluids lost to the peritoneal cavity and as an access for antibiotic therapy. The patient is monitored for pain and response to analgesic therapy. The patient may be positioned with knees flexed to increase comfort. The nurse should provide rest and a quiet environment. Sedatives may be given to allay anxiety.

Accurate monitoring of fluid intake and output and electrolyte status is necessary to determine replacement therapy. Vital signs are monitored frequently. Antiemetics may be administered to decrease nausea and vomiting and prevent further fluid and electrolyte losses. The patient is placed on NPO status and may need an NG tube to decrease gastric distention and further leakage of bowel contents into the peritoneum. Low-flow oxygen may be needed.

If the patient has an open surgical procedure, drains are inserted to remove purulent drainage and excessive fluid. Postoperative care of the patient is similar to the care of the patient with an exploratory laparotomy.

GASTROENTERITIS

Gastroenteritis is an inflammation of the mucosa of the stomach and small intestine. Clinical manifestations include nausea, vomiting, diarrhea, abdominal cramping, and distention. Fever, increased WBC count, and blood or mucus in the stool may be present. Causative agents are varied (see Table 43-2). Most cases are self-limiting and do not require hospitalization. However, older adults and chronically ill patients may be unable to consume sufficient fluids orally to compensate for fluid loss. Until vomiting has ceased, the patient should be on NPO status. If dehydration occurs, IV fluid replacement may be necessary. As soon as tolerated, fluids containing glucose and electrolytes (e.g., Pedialyte) should be given. If the causative agent is identified, appropriate antibiotic and antimicrobial drugs are given.

NURSING MANAGEMENT
GASTROENTERITIS

Accurate monitoring of intake and output is important for successful replacement of lost fluid. Strict medical asepsis and infection control precautions should be instituted when indicated. The patient is instructed in the importance of proper food handling and preparation of food to prevent infections such as *Salmonella* and trichinosis (see Chapter 42, Table 42-28).

Symptomatic nursing care is given for nausea, vomiting, and diarrhea. The importance of rest and increased fluid intake should be stressed. The nurse should assess complaints of pain, vomiting, and diarrhea because gastroenteritis is often confused with appendicitis. To allay the patient's apprehension, the nurse should explain that gastroenteritis usually runs an acute course with no sequelae.

Inflammatory Bowel Disease

Crohn's disease and ulcerative colitis are immunologically related disorders that are referred to as **inflammatory bowel disease** (IBD) (Table 43-17). Both diseases are characterized by chronic inflammation of the intestine with periods of remission interspersed with periods of exacerbation. The cause is unknown and there is no cure. Therefore treatment relies on medications to treat the acute inflammation and maintain a remission. Surgery is reserved for patients who are unresponsive to medications or who develop life-threatening complications.

Etiology and Pathophysiology

IBD is an autoimmune disease. Although an antigen probably initiates the inflammation, the actual tissue damage is due to an overactive, inappropriate, and sustained inflammatory response. Both genetic and environmental factors seem to play a role in IBD. The prevalent theory is that an unidentified organism that is usually innocuous stimulates a poorly regulated immune response in genetically susceptible people.[15] According to this theory, a genetically susceptible person who is never exposed to the organism will not become ill, and a person who is not genetically susceptible will not develop IBD even if exposed to the organism.

Both ulcerative colitis and Crohn's disease commonly occur during the teenage years and early adulthood, but both have a second peak in the sixth decade. Both are more prevalent in whites and in industrialized regions of the world.

Studies of twins and family members provide support for a genetic influence in IBD. Not only are family members of patients with Crohn's disease at increased risk for Crohn's disease, but they also have an increased risk of ulcerative colitis and vice versa.[16] One susceptibility gene, CARD15 on chromosome 16, has been identified for Crohn's disease. However, this gene is only present in a minority of people with IBD. There is strong support for the existence of at least four additional susceptibility genes.[16] The antigen that initiates IBD remains to be found. Various bacteria have

---

CULTURAL AND ETHNIC HEALTH DISPARITIES

Colon Disorders

- African Americans are at the highest risk for colorectal cancer compared with other ethnic groups.
- The incidence of colorectal cancer is declining in the United States except among African American men.
- Among Asian Americans, colorectal cancer is the second most commonly diagnosed cancer, and it is the third most frequent cause of cancer-related death.
- The incidence of inflammatory bowel disease (IBD) is about four times higher among whites compared with other ethnic groups.
- IBD has the highest incidence among the Ashkenazi Jewish people and those of middle European origin.

TABLE 43-17	Comparison of Ulcerative Colitis and Crohn's Disease	
Characteristic	**Ulcerative Colitis**	**Crohn's Disease**
Clinical		
Usual age at onset	Teens to mid-30s	Teens to mid-30s
Diarrhea	Common	Common
Abdominal cramping pain	Common	Common
Fever (intermittent)	During acute attacks	Common
Weight loss	Rare	Common, may be severe
Rectal bleeding	Common	Infrequent
Tenesmus	Common	Rare
Malabsorption and nutritional deficiencies	Minimal incidence	Common
Pathologic		
Location	Usually starts in rectum and spreads in a continuous pattern up the colon	Occurs anywhere along GI tract in characteristic skip lesions; most frequent site is terminal ileum
Distribution	Continuous areas of inflammation	Healthy tissue is interspersed with areas of inflammation (skip lesions)
Depth of involvement	Mucosa and submucosa	Entire thickness of bowel wall (transmural)
Granulomas (noted on biopsy)	Occasional	Common
Cobblestoning of mucosa	Rare	Common
Pseudopolyps	Common	Rare
Small bowel involvement	Minimal, only backwash into ileum	Common
Complications		
Fistulas	Rare	Common
Strictures	Occasional	Common
Anal abscesses	Rare	Common
Perforation	Common (because of toxic megacolon)	Common (because inflammation involves entire bowel wall)
Toxic megacolon	Relatively more common	Rare
Carcinoma	Increased incidence after 10 yr of disease	Small intestine, increased; colon, increased but not as much as with ulcerative colitis
Recurrence after surgery	Cure with colectomy	Common at site of anastomosis

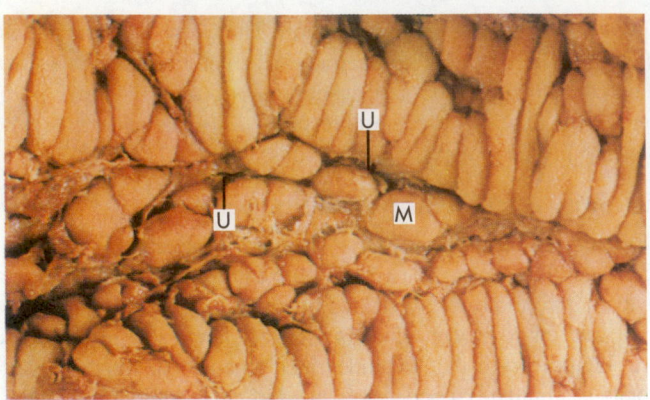

FIG. 43-2 Crohn's disease. The mucosa in Crohn's disease demonstrates a cobblestone pattern as a result of fissured ulcers (*U*) with intervening areas of edematous mucosa (*M*).

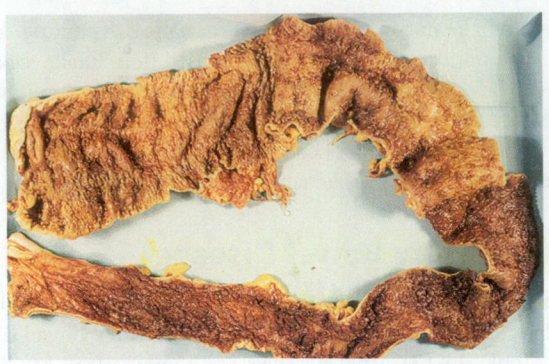

FIG. 43-3 Acute ulcerative colitis. Colitis with extensive mucosal ulceration involving the entire colon.

been proposed, and some patients respond favorably to antibiotic therapy. The normal inflammatory response is altered in patients with IBD.[17]

Certain criteria are used to differentiate ulcerative colitis from Crohn's disease, but the diseases have much in common, and a clear differentiation between the two cannot be made in about a third of the cases. The fact that people with ulcerative colitis commonly have a relative with Crohn's disease and vice versa supports the existence of a common gene.

Although symptoms are often the same (diarrhea, bloody stools, weight loss, abdominal pain, fever, and fatigue), the pattern of inflammation is different for the two diseases. In Crohn's disease the inflammation involves all layers of the bowel wall. Crohn's disease can occur anywhere in the GI tract from the mouth to the anus, but occurs most commonly in the terminal ileum and colon. Furthermore, segments of normal bowel can occur between diseased portions, the so-called skip lesions (see Table 43-17). Typically, ulcerations are deep and longitudinal and penetrate between islands of inflamed edematous mucosa, causing the classic cobblestone appearance (Fig. 43-2). Strictures at the areas of inflammation may cause bowel obstruction. Since the inflammation goes through the entire wall, microscopic leaks can allow bowel contents to enter the peritoneal cavity and form abscesses or peritonitis.

Sometimes the leaks form tracts or fistulas between adjacent organs. Fistulas develop between adjacent areas of bowel, between the bowel and the bladder, and between the bowel and the vagina, and can also form a tract through the skin to the outside of the body. Urinary tract infections are usually the first sign of a bowel/bladder fistula, and feces is sometimes seen in the urine. Fistulas between the bowel and vagina allow feces to leak out through the vagina, and feces leaks onto the skin if there is a cutaneous fistula.

Ulcerative colitis usually starts in the rectum and moves in a continual fashion toward the cecum. Although there is sometimes mild inflammation in the terminal ileum, ulcerative colitis is a disease of the colon and rectum (Fig. 43-3). Unlike Crohn's disease, in which healthy tissue is interspersed with inflamed tissue, ulcerative colitis spreads in a continuous pattern. The inflammation and ulcerations occur in the mucosal layer, the innermost layer of the bowel wall. Since it does not extend through all bowel wall layers, fistulas and abscesses are rare. Water and electrolytes are absorbed when the mucosal epithe-

lium is healthy, but cannot be absorbed through inflamed mucosa. Therefore diarrhea with large fluid and electrolyte losses is a characteristic feature of damage to the colonic mucosa epithelium. Breakdown of cells results in protein loss through the stool. Areas of inflamed mucosa form pseudopolyps, tongue-like projections into the bowel lumen.

Clinical Manifestations

Both forms of IBD are chronic disorders with mild to severe acute exacerbations that occur at unpredictable intervals over many years. With Crohn's disease, diarrhea and colicky abdominal pain are common symptoms. If the small intestine is involved, weight loss occurs from malabsorption. A mass is sometimes felt in the right iliac fossa. Rectal bleeding sometimes occurs with Crohn's disease although not as often as with ulcerative colitis. In addition, patients may have systemic symptoms such as fever.

About 90% of patients with ulcerative colitis have mild to moderately severe disease. The primary symptoms of ulcerative colitis are bloody diarrhea and abdominal pain. Pain may vary from the mild lower abdominal cramping associated with diarrhea to the severe, constant pain associated with acute perforations. With mild disease, diarrhea may consist of one to two semiformed stools daily that contain small amounts of blood. The patient may have no other systemic manifestations. In moderate ulcerative colitis there is increased stool output (four to five stools per day), increased bleeding, and systemic symptoms (fever, malaise, anorexia). In severe cases, diarrhea is bloody, contains mucus, and occurs 10 to 20 times a day. In addition, fever, weight loss greater than 10% of total body weight, anemia, tachycardia, and dehydration are present.

Complications

Patients with IBD experience both local (confined to the GI tract) and systemic (extraintestinal) complications. GI tract complications include hemorrhage, strictures, perforation (with possible peritonitis), fistulas, and colonic dilation. Colonic dilation greater than 5 cm is called *toxic megacolon*. Patients with toxic megacolon are at risk of perforation and may need an emergency colectomy.[17] Hemorrhage may lead to anemia and is corrected with blood transfusions and iron supplements. Perineal abscess and fistulas occur in up to a third of patients with Crohn's disease.[17] Some patients develop skin tags around the anus.

Nutritional problems are especially common with Crohn's disease when the terminal ileum is involved. Bile salts and cobalamin

TABLE 43-18	**Extraintestinal Complications of Inflammatory Bowel Disease**

Joints	Mouth
Peripheral arthritis (colitic)	Aphthous ulcers
Ankylosing spondylitis	Eye
Sacroiliitis	Conjunctivitis
Finger clubbing	Uveitis
Skin	Episcleritis
Erythema nodosum	Gallstones
Pyoderma gangrenosum	Kidney stones
Thromboembolism	Liver disease—primary
	sclerosing cholangitis
	Osteoporosis

TABLE 43-19	***COLLABORATIVE CARE*** *Inflammatory Bowel Disease*

Diagnostic
History and physical examination
CBC, erythrocyte sedimentation rate, genetic studies
Serum chemistries
Testing of stool for occult blood
Testing of stool for infection
Capsule endoscopy
Radiologic studies with barium contrast
Sigmoidoscopy and colonoscopy with biopsy

Collaborative Therapy
High-calorie, high-vitamin, high-protein, low-residue, lactose-free (if lactase deficiency) diet

Drug therapy
• Aminosalicylates*
• Antimicrobial agents*
• Corticosteroid drugs*
• Immunosuppressants*
• Biologic therapy (immunomodulator)*

Elemental diet or parenteral nutrition
Physical and emotional rest
Referral for counseling and/or support group
Surgery†

CBC, Complete blood count.
*See Table 43-20.
†See Table 43-21.

are exclusively absorbed in the terminal ileum. Thus disease at this location can result in fat malabsorption and anemia. Toxic megacolon is more common with ulcerative colitis, but strictures and fistulas occur most commonly with Crohn's disease. Patients with long-standing ulcerative colitis are at risk for colorectal cancer, and those with Crohn's disease are at risk for small bowel cancer.[18] Periodic colonoscopy is recommended for patients who developed IBD at a young age or have had it more than 10 years. Systemic complications of IBD, including fever, anorexia, and malaise, are due to the general inflammatory response.

Some people with IBD suffer from arthritis, ankylosing spondylitis, eye inflammation, and skin lesions (erythema nodosum and pyoderma gangrenosum) (Table 43-18). It is believed that circulating products of inflammation (e.g., cytokines) trigger inflammations in these areas.[17,19] An increased incidence of thromboembolism is seen in both Crohn's disease and ulcerative colitis. Kidney stones are also common, probably because of fluid deficits from chronic diarrhea. Primary sclerosing cholangitis and gallstones are also associated with IBD. Routine liver function tests are important because primary sclerosing cholangitis can lead to liver failure.[20]

Diagnostic Studies

The diagnosis of IBD includes ruling out other diseases with similar symptoms and then determining whether the patient has Crohn's disease or ulcerative colitis. Infectious causes of diarrhea are determined by stool cultures. Microperforation and peritonitis from Crohn's disease is sometimes confused with appendicitis, and is only discovered during surgery. Early Crohn's disease has symptoms that are similar to those of IBS. Diagnostic studies also provide information about disease severity and complications. Stool cultures should be obtained because treatable bacterial infections can trigger IBD.[17,21] A CBC typically shows iron deficiency anemia from blood loss. An elevated WBC count may indicate toxic megacolon or perforation. Decreases in serum sodium, potassium, chloride, bicarbonate, and magnesium levels are due to fluid and electrolyte losses from diarrhea and vomiting. Hypoalbuminemia is present with severe disease and is due to poor nutrition or protein loss from the bowel. An elevated erythrocyte sedimentation rate reflects chronic inflammation. The stool should be examined for blood, pus, and mucus.

Sigmoidoscopy and colonoscopy allow direct examination of the large intestine mucosa. Since ulcerative colitis usually begins in the rectum, rectal biopsies may be adequate for diagnosis. These samples can be obtained with a sigmoidoscope. Colonoscopy allows for examination of the entire large intestine and sometimes the most distal ileum. The extent of inflammation, ulcerations,

pseudopolyps, and strictures is determined, and biopsy specimens are taken for a definitive diagnosis.

A double-contrast barium enema may show areas of granular inflammation with ulcerations. The colon may appear narrow and shortened, and pseudopolyps may be present. A double-contrast study (in which air is introduced into the bowel after the expulsion of barium) is effective in detecting mucosal abnormalities in ulcerative colitis. Since an endoscope can enter very little of the small intestine, it has not been possible to get a direct view of the ileal inflammation of Crohn's disease. Capsule endoscopy (see Chapter 39) is used in the diagnosis of small intestine diseases. Thus far, capsule endoscopy has been shown to have greater sensitivity than radiography when diagnosing Crohn's disease.[22,23] Unfortunately, biopsies cannot be obtained with either capsule endoscopy or barium enema.

Collaborative Care

The goals of treatment are to (1) rest the bowel, (2) control the inflammation, (3) combat infection, (4) correct malnutrition, (5) alleviate stress, (6) provide symptomatic relief, and (7) improve quality of life. A variety of medications are available to treat IBD (Table 43-19). Hospitalization is indicated if the patient fails to respond to drug therapy, if the disease is severe, and when complications are suspected. Since there is a high recurrence rate following surgical treatment of Crohn's disease, medications are the preferred treatment.

Drug Therapy. The goals of drug treatment for IBD are to induce and then maintain a remission in order to improve the quality of life. Five major classes of medications are used to treat IBD: (1) aminosalicylates, (2) antimicrobials, (3) corticosteroids, (4) immunosuppressants, and (5) biologic therapy. All five classes of medication are used to treat Crohn's disease. Aminosalicylates and corticosteroids are the mainstays of treatment for ulcerative colitis (Table 43-20).

The first aminosalicylate was sulfasalazine (Azulfidine), a combination drug that was developed in the 1940s to treat rheumatoid arthritis.[24] Sulfasalazine contains sulfapyridine and 5-aminosalicylic acid (5-ASA). The 5-ASA accounts for its therapeutic benefits for IBD. Its exact mechanism of action is unknown, but topical application to the intestinal mucosa suppresses proinflammatory cytokines and other inflammatory mediators.[24] When given orally, 5-ASA alone is absorbed before it reaches the lower GI tract where it is needed. When combined with sulfapyridine, 5-ASA reaches the colon. However, many people are unable to tolerate sulfapyridine.[24] Newer preparations have been developed to deliver 5-ASA to the terminal ileum and colon (e.g., olsalazine [Dipentum], mesalamine [Pentasa], and balsalazide [Colazal]). These drugs are as effective as sulfasalazine and are better tolerated when administered orally.

Drug Alert - *Sulfasalazine (Azulfidine)*
- *May cause yellowish orange discoloration of skin and urine.*
- *Avoid exposure to sunlight and ultraviolet light until photosensitivity is determined.*

Preparations with 5-ASA can be administered rectally as suppositories, enemas, and foams. Topical treatment offers the advantage of delivering the 5-ASA directly to the tissue where it is needed and minimizes systemic effects. Aminosalicylates are also first-line therapies for mildly to moderately active Crohn's disease, especially when the colon is involved, but are more effective for ulcerative colitis. They are recommended for both achieving and maintaining a remission.[24]

Antimicrobials are used to treat IBD, although no specific infectious agent has been discovered. Metronidazole (Flagyl), ciprofloxacin (Cipro), and clarithromycin (Biaxin) have been used successfully with Crohn's disease, but have not been shown to be as effective for ulcerative colitis.[25]

Corticosteroids such as prednisone are used to achieve remission in IBD, but are not effective for maintaining the remission. They are helpful for acute flare-ups, but are given for the shortest possible time because of side effects associated with long-term use. Patients with disease in the left colon, sigmoid, and rectum can be given suppositories, enemas, and foams that deliver the corticosteroid directly to the inflamed tissue with minimal systemic effects.[26] Oral prednisone is given to patients with mild to moderate disease who do not respond to either 5-ASA or topical corticosteroids. IV corticosteroids are reserved for those with severe inflammation. Corticosteroids must be tapered to very low levels when surgery is planned to prevent postoperative complications (e.g., infection, delayed wound healing).

Two immunosuppressants, azathioprine (Imuran) and 6-mercaptopurine (Purinethol), are given orally and take 3 to 6 months to exhibit full effectiveness. They are most useful for patients with Crohn's disease who do not respond to aminosalicylates, antimicrobials, or corticosteroids. These drugs have lower long-term toxicity than corticosteroids, but require regular CBC monitoring because they can suppress the bone marrow and lead to inflammation of the pancreas or gallbladder.

Methotrexate has also been found to be effective for Crohn's disease, but patients may suffer flu-like symptoms, bone marrow depression, and liver dysfunction. CBCs and liver enzymes are monitored. Methotrexate should not be used in women who are pregnant because it causes birth defects and fetal death.

Infliximab (Remicade) is the first major biologic drug therapy (immunomodulator) to be approved for the treatment of IBD.[19,27] Infliximab is a monoclonal antibody to the cytokine tumor necrosis factor. It is given IV to induce and maintain remission in patients with active Crohn's disease and in patients with draining fistulas who do not respond to conventional drug therapy. Infliximab is immunogenic, meaning that patients receiving it frequently produce antibodies against it. Immunogenicity leads to an acute infusion reaction and delayed hypersensitivity–type reactions. Strategies that decrease the incidence of immunogenicity include coadministration of immunosuppressants (e.g., azathioprine, 6-mercaptopurine, and methotrexate) and pretreatment with IV hydrocortisone. Clinical trials are currently investigating infliximab's ability to decrease the inflammation of ulcerative colitis.[19,27]

Surgical Therapy. About 75% of patients with Crohn's disease will eventually require surgery.[21,22] Although surgery produces remission for patients with Crohn's disease, recurrence rates are high. Surgical removal of large segments of the small intestine

---

EVIDENCE-BASED PRACTICE

Do Stress Management Strategies Improve Symptoms of Crohn's Disease?

Clinical Question
In individuals with Crohn's disease (P), will the use of stress management skills (I) reduce the occurrence of symptoms associated with the disease (O) compared with a control group (C)?

Best Available Evidence
Randomized controlled trial (RCT)

Critical Appraisal and Synthesis of Evidence
- Patients with Crohn's disease ($n = 45$) were assigned to one of three groups.
  - Group 1 learned progressive muscle relaxation (PMR), group 2 was taught self-directed stress management, and group 3 received conventional medical treatment.
- The self-directed group was instructed in problem solving and repetition of autogenic phrases. They were also given an audio tape to assist in relaxation.
- Gastrointestinal symptoms were monitored with a daily diary of symptoms and interviews. Follow-ups were conducted at 6 and 12 months.
- Subjects who were trained in PMR experienced a reduction in tiredness, constipation, abdominal pain, and abdominal distention. Those in the self-directed group saw a reduction in tiredness and abdominal pain. No change was seen in the control group.

Conclusions
- Stress management strategies are an effective method for reducing the occurrence of Crohn's disease symptoms.
- Individuals who were instructed in PMR techniques observed the most improvement in symptoms during instruction and at all follow-up sessions.

Implications for Nursing Practice
- Nurses need to learn PMR and other stress management strategies (see Chapter 9) so they can use them for personal use and then teach their patients about their benefits.
- Teach patients with Crohn's disease about the stress components of the disease.

Reference for Evidence
Garcia-Vega E, Fernandez-Rodriguez C: A stress management programme for Crohn's disease, *Behavior Research and Therapy* 42:367, 2004.

PICO: P, Patient population of interest; I, intervention or area of interest; C, comparison of interest or comparison group; O, outcome(s) of interest (see p. 6).

TABLE 43-20	*DRUG THERAPY* Inflammatory Bowel Disease

Category	Action	Examples
5-Aminosalicylates (5-ASA)	Decrease GI inflammation through direct contact with bowel mucosa	*Systemic* sulfasalazine (Azulfidine) mesalamine (Asacol, Pentasa) olsalazine (Dipentum) *Topical* 5-ASA enema (Rowasa) mesalamine suppositories (Canasa)
Antimicrobials	Prevent or treat secondary infection	metronidazole (Flagyl) ciprofloxacin (Cipro) clarithromycin (Biaxin)
Corticosteroids	Decrease inflammation	*Systemic:* corticosteroids (prednisone, budesonide [Entocort]) (oral); hydrocortisone or methylprednisolone (IV for severe IBD) *Topical:* hydrocortisone suppository or foam (Cortifoam) or enema (Cortenema)
Immunosuppressants	Suppress immune response	azathioprine (Imuran), 6-mercaptopurine (6-MP), cyclosporine
Biologic therapy (immunomodulator)	Inhibits the cytokine tumor necrosis factor (TNF)	infliximab (Remicade)
Antidiarrheals	Decrease GI motility*	diphenoxylate with atropine (Lomotil) loperamide (Imodium)
Hematinics and vitamins	Correct iron deficiency anemia and promote healing	oral ferrous sulfate, ferrous gluconate; iron dextran injection (Imferon) cobalamin, zinc, folate

GI, Gastrointestinal; *IBD*, inflammatory bowel disease; *IV*, intravenous.
*Used with caution during severe disease because of potential to produce toxic megacolon.

can lead to short bowel syndrome, a condition in which inadequate absorption surface is available to maintain life unless parenteral nutrition is used. Surgery is reserved for emergency situations (excessive bleeding, obstruction, peritonitis) or when medical treatment has failed (Table 43-21). The principle surgical technique for Crohn's disease is strictureplasty to widen areas of narrowed bowel. It is sometimes necessary to resect the diseased bowel and anastomose the ends together. Unfortunately, the disease commonly recurs at the area of anastomosis. Emergency surgery is necessary when perforation allows bowel contents to drain into the abdominal cavity. In this situation, the pus is drained, the abdomen is washed out, and the person has a temporary ostomy. An abscess that is walled off may be surgically drained.

Approximately 25% to 40% of patients with ulcerative colitis will need surgery at some time during their illness.[21,22] Surgery is indicated if (1) the patient fails to respond to treatment; (2) exacerbations are frequent and debilitating; (3) massive bleeding, perforation, strictures, and/or obstruction occur; (4) tissue changes suggest that dysplasia is occurring; or (5) carcinoma develops. Since ulcerative colitis affects only the colon, a total proctocolectomy is curative.

Surgical procedures used to treat chronic ulcerative colitis include (1) total colectomy with rectal mucosal stripping and ileoanal reservoir; (2) total proctocolectomy with permanent ileostomy; and (3) total proctocolectomy with continent ileostomy (Kock pouch).

Total Colectomy with Ileoanal Reservoir. The most commonly used procedure involves total colectomy and ileoanal anastomosis with the formation of an ileoanal reservoir (Fig. 43-4). This combination of two procedures is performed approximately 8 to 12 weeks apart. The initial procedure includes colectomy, rectal mucosectomy, ileal reservoir construction, ileoanal anastomosis, and temporary ileostomy. The second surgery involves closure of the ileostomy

TABLE 43-21	Indications for Surgical Therapy for Inflammatory Bowel Disease

- Drainage of abdominal abscess
- Failure to respond to conservative therapy
- Fistulas
- Inability to decrease corticosteroids
- Intestinal obstruction
- Massive hemorrhage
- Perforation
- Severe anorectal disease
- Suspicion of carcinoma

to direct stool toward the new reservoir. Adaptation of the reservoir occurs over the next 3 to 6 months, which usually results in a decreased number of bowel movements over a 24-hour period. The patient is able to control defecation at the anal sphincter.

Patient selection criteria include absence of colorectal cancer, small intestine free of disease (e.g., Crohn's disease), competent anorectal sphincter, and physical status adequate to permit lengthy surgery. In addition, the patient needs to be motivated and capable of understanding self-care instructions.

Total Proctocolectomy with Permanent Ileostomy. Total proctocolectomy with a permanent ileostomy is a one-stage operation involving the removal of the colon, rectum, and anus with closure of the anus. The end of the terminal ileum is brought out through the abdominal wall and forms a stoma, or **ostomy.** The stoma is usually placed in the right lower quadrant below the belt line. With a permanent ileostomy, continence is not possible.

Total Proctocolectomy with Continent Ileostomy. Total proctocolectomy with continent ileostomy (Kock pouch) (Fig. 43-5) is rarely used today. When forming the Kock pouch, the distal segment of the ileum is surgically split, a fold is made, and a one-

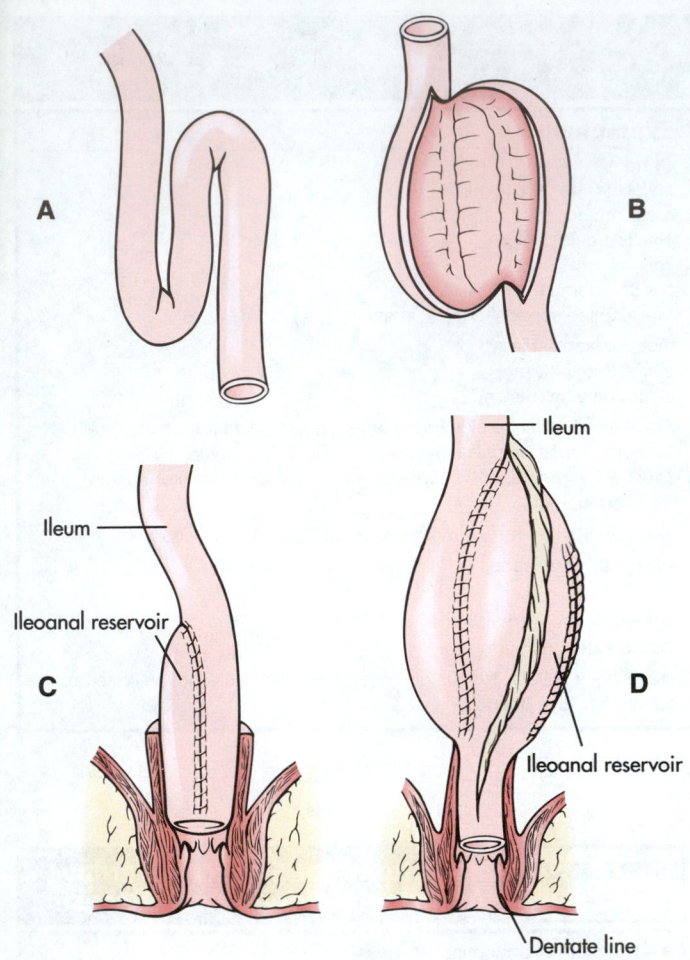

FIG. 43-4 Ileoanal reservoir. **A,** Formation of a reservoir. **B,** Posterior suture lines completed. **C,** J-shaped configuration for ileoanal reservoir. **D,** S-shaped configuration for ileoanal reservoir.

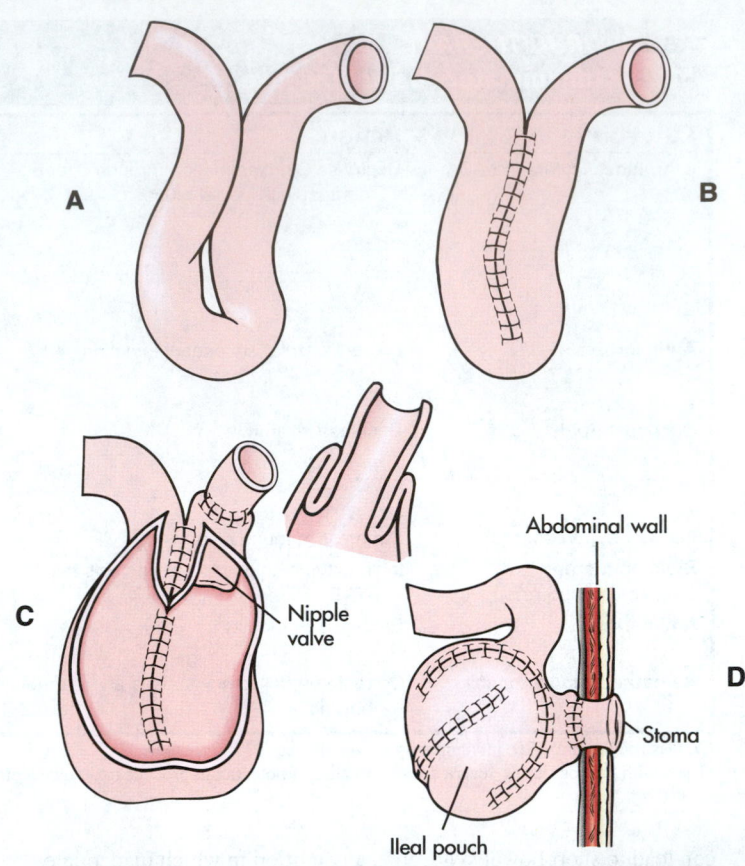

FIG. 43-5 Surgical formation of continent ileostomy (Kock pouch). **A,** Loop of terminal ileum. **B,** Both limbs sutured together and incised in a U shape. **C,** Pouch created with nipple valve. **D,** Pouch sutured to abdominal wall.

way nipple valve is created and sutured into place on the abdomen. The pouch acts as a reservoir and is drained at regular intervals by insertion of a catheter. Valve failure, leakage, and pouchitis are common problems with the Kock pouch.

Postoperative Care. Postoperative care following surgical procedures for IBD is similar to that described in the general nursing care plan for the postoperative patient presented in NCP 20-1. If an ileostomy is formed, stoma viability, the mucocutaneous juncture (the area where the mucous membrane of the bowel interfaces with the skin), and peristomal skin integrity must be monitored. An end ileostomy will be used if the ileostomy is permanent. A loop ileostomy may be used when a temporary ileostomy is constructed to allow the ileoanal reservoir to heal. The loop ostomy presents a pouching challenge because it retracts or drains inferiorly, resulting in effluent contact with the skin and predisposing to a denuded epidermis. An enterostomal therapy (ET) nurse should help with these challenging problems. Self-care instructions should be reviewed and written information provided before discharge. Stoma care is presented later in this chapter.

Ileostomy output initially may be as high as 1500 to 2000 ml per 24 hours. The patient must be observed for signs of hemorrhage, abdominal abscess, small bowel obstruction, dehydration, and other related complications. If an NG tube is used, it will be removed when bowel function returns.

Transient incontinence of mucus is a result of intraoperative manipulation of the anal canal. Initial drainage through the ileoanal anastomosis will be liquid. Kegel exercises are recommended to strengthen the pelvic floor and sphincter muscles (see Table 46-20). However, they are not recommended in the immediate postoperative period. Perianal skin care is important to protect the epidermis from mucous drainage and maceration. The patient should be instructed to gently clean the skin with a mild cleanser, rinse well, and dry thoroughly. A moisture barrier ointment may be used, and a perineal pad may be required.

Nutritional Therapy. Diet is an important component in the treatment of IBD. The dietitian is an important member of the team and should be consulted regarding dietary recommendations. The goals of diet management are to provide adequate nutrition without exacerbating symptoms, to correct and prevent malnutrition, to replace fluid and electrolyte losses, and to prevent weight loss. Overall, it is essential that people with IBD eat a balanced, healthy diet with sufficient calories, protein, and nutrients. Patients can use MyPyramid guidelines to ensure that they get adequate portions from all of the food groups (see Fig. 40-1 and Table 40-1). The diet for each patient must be individualized. Promoting good nutrition is essential for patients with ulcerative colitis and Crohn's disease.

Patients with diarrhea often decrease their oral intake to reduce diarrhea. The anorexia that accompanies inflammation also results in decreases in food intake. Blood loss leads to iron deficiency anemia. When the terminal ileum is involved in Crohn's disease there is reduced absorption of cobalamin, contributing to anemia.

Cobalamin is available in injection form, given monthly, or as a daily oral or nasal spray. Bile salts are also absorbed in the terminal ileum and disease here can lead to fat malabsorption. The presence of bile salts in the feces contributes to diarrhea. Cholestyramine, an ion-exchange resin that binds unabsorbed bile salts, helps control the diarrhea. Patients receiving sulfasalazine should receive 1 mg of folate (folic acid) daily, and those receiving corticosteroids need calcium supplements.

Patients with Crohn's disease are more likely to have a bowel obstruction, fistulas, fissures, and abscesses. All contribute to nutritional problems since patients cannot eat when they have a bowel obstruction, and hypermetabolism occurs with fistulas, fissures, and abscesses. Surgical resection of the diseased ileum removes surface area necessary for absorption and may cause severe nutritional problems.

There are no universal food triggers for IBD, but individuals may find that certain foods initiate diarrhea. A food diary helps them identify problem foods to avoid. Many patients with IBD are often lactose intolerant and improve when milk products are avoided. High-fat foods also tend to trigger diarrhea. Cold foods and high-fiber foods (cereal with bran, nuts, raw fruit) may increase GI transit. Smoking stimulates the GI tract (increases motility and secretion) and should be avoided. Patients with significant fluid and electrolyte losses or malabsorption may need parenteral nutrition or enteral feedings, such as elemental diets. Elemental diets are high in calories and nutrients, lactose free, and absorbed in the proximal small intestine, which allows the more distal bowel to rest.

Parenteral nutrition allows for a positive nitrogen balance while resting the bowel. Vitamins, minerals, electrolytes, and other important nutrients (e.g., glucose, amino acids) can be administered to promote healing and correct nutritional deficiencies. A number of potential side effects are associated with parenteral nutrition, as described in Chapter 40.

Supplemental iron (ferrous sulfate or ferrous gluconate) may be necessary to prevent or treat iron deficiency anemia resulting from chronic blood loss. Parenteral iron may be needed for patients who cannot tolerate oral iron. Iron dextran (Imferon) intramuscularly by Z-track or IV injection may be necessary if anemia is severe. In patients receiving long-term sulfasalazine therapy, folic acid deficiency may develop, and supplementation may be necessary. Potassium supplements may be necessary if corticosteroid therapy is used because retention of sodium and loss of potassium can result in hypokalemia and subsequent toxic megacolon. Zinc deficiency can result from severe or chronic diarrhea, and supplementation may be necessary.

NURSING MANAGEMENT
INFLAMMATORY BOWEL DISEASE

■ Nursing Assessment

Subjective and objective data that should be obtained from a patient with IBD are presented in Table 43-22.

■ Nursing Diagnoses

Nursing diagnoses for the patient with IBD include, but are not limited to, those presented in NCP 43-2.

■ Planning

The overall goals are that the patient with IBD will (1) experience a decrease in number and severity of acute exacerbations, (2) maintain normal fluid and electrolyte balance, (3) be free from pain or

TABLE 43-22	*NURSING ASSESSMENT* **Inflammatory Bowel Disease**

Subjective Data
Important Health Information
Past health history: Infection, autoimmune disorders
Medications: Use of antidiarrheal medications

Functional Health Patterns
Health perception–health management: Family history of ulcerative colitis; fatigue, malaise
Nutritional-metabolic: Nausea, vomiting; anorexia; weight loss
Elimination: Diarrhea, blood, mucus or pus in stools
Cognitive-perceptual: Lower abdominal pain (worse before defecation), cramping, tenesmus

Objective Data
General
Intermittent fever; emaciated appearance, fatigue

Integumentary
Pale skin with poor turgor, dry mucous membranes; skin lesions; anorectal irritation, skin tags, cutaneous fistulas

Gastrointestinal
Abdominal distention, hyperactive bowel sounds, abdominal cramps

Cardiovascular
Tachycardia, hypotension

Possible Findings
Anemia; leukocytosis; electrolyte imbalance; hypoalbuminemia; vitamin and trace metal deficiencies; guaiac-positive stool; abnormal sigmoidoscopic, colonoscopic, and/or barium enema findings

discomfort, (4) comply with medical regimens, (5) maintain nutritional balance, and (6) have improved quality of life.

■ Nursing Implementation

During the acute phase, attention is focused on hemodynamic stability, pain control, fluid and electrolyte balance, and nutritional support. Accurate intake and output records must be maintained. The number and appearance of stools are monitored. Nursing care is directed toward an intensive therapeutic and supportive program (see NCP 43-2). It is important that the nurse establishes rapport and encourages the patient to talk about self-care strategies. Honesty, patience, and understanding are essential in the relationship with the patient. An explanation of all procedures and treatment will build trust and may allay some apprehension. Teaching the patient strategies for managing stress may be helpful because there is a well-recognized association between the emotions and the gut. Smokers should be encouraged to quit because smoking exacerbates Crohn's disease.

Psychotherapy may be indicated if the patient is experiencing emotional problems, but the nurse must recognize that the patient's behavior may result from factors other than emotional ones. Any person who has 10 to 20 bowel movements a day, rectal discomfort, and an unpredictable disease may be anxious, frustrated, discouraged, and depressed. It is essential that nurses communicate clearly and fulfill promises to establish trust. Nurses and other team members can assist patients to accept the chronicity of IBD and learn strategies to cope with its recurrent, unpredictable nature. Inadequate coping mechanisms are sometimes due to early onset of the disease (often at 10 to 15 years of age or earlier) before the person has the emotional development and maturity needed to cope.

Patients suffer severe fatigue, which limits energy for physical activity. Rest is important. Patients may lose sleep because of fre-

Gastrointestinal System

NURSING CARE PLAN 43-2

Patient with Inflammatory Bowel Disease

NURSING DIAGNOSIS   **Diarrhea** *related to* bowel inflammation and intestinal hyperactivity *as evidenced by* frequent loose, liquid stools (>10 per day)

PATIENT GOALS   1. Experiences a decrease in the number of diarrhea stools
2. Stools are soft and formed

OUTCOMES (NOC)

Bowel Elimination

- Elimination pattern _____
- Comfort of stool passage _____
- Stool soft and formed _____

Measurement Scale

1 = Severely compromised
2 = Substantially compromised
3 = Moderately compromised
4 = Mildly compromised
5 = Not compromised

INTERVENTIONS (NIC) and RATIONALES

Diarrhea Management

- Instruct patient/significant other to record color, volume, frequency, and consistency of stools *to evaluate effectiveness of therapy and dietary restrictions.*
- Perform actions to rest the bowel (e.g., NPO, liquid diet).
- Teach patient stress-reduction techniques *to reduce the incidence of exacerbations.*
- Encourage frequent, small feedings, adding bulk gradually, *to prevent bowel irritation.*
- Teach patient/significant other to eliminate gas-forming and spicy foods from diet.
- Instruct in low-fiber, high-protein, high-calorie diet *to meet nutritional needs with minimum bowel irritation.*

NURSING DIAGNOSIS   **Anxiety** *related to* possible social embarrassment, unfamiliar environment, diagnostic tests, and treatment *as evidenced by* expression of concerns about effect of disease on social relationships, questions about disease and treatment

PATIENT GOALS   1. Reports decrease in anxiety
2. Uses effective coping strategies

OUTCOMES (NOC)

Anxiety Self-Control

- Plans coping strategies for stressful situations _____
- Uses effective coping strategies _____
- Maintains social relationships _____
- Controls anxiety response _____

Measurement Scale

1 = Never demonstrated
2 = Rarely demonstrated
3 = Sometimes demonstrated
4 = Often demonstrated
5 = Consistently demonstrated

INTERVENTIONS (NIC) and RATIONALES

Anxiety Reduction

- Observe for verbal and nonverbal signs of anxiety *to plan appropriate interventions.*
- Encourage verbalization of feelings, perceptions, and fears *to demonstrate acceptance and concern for the patient and allow verbalization of concerns.*
- Provide factual information concerning diagnosis, treatment, and prognosis *because understanding may reduce anxiety.*
- Stay with patient *to promote safety and reduce fear.*

NURSING DIAGNOSIS   **Ineffective coping** *related to* chronic disease, lifestyle changes, stress, and pain *as evidenced by* inability to express feelings and concerns; display of dependent, attention-getting behavior

PATIENT GOALS   1. Demonstrates the use of effective coping strategies
2. Expresses a sense of self-control and reduced stress

OUTCOMES (NOC)

Coping

- Identifies ineffective coping patterns _____
- Uses behaviors to reduce stress _____
- Uses effective coping strategies _____

Measurement Scale

1 = Never demonstrated
2 = Rarely demonstrated
3 = Sometimes demonstrated
4 = Often demonstrated
5 = Consistently demonstrated

INTERVENTIONS (NIC) and RATIONALES

Coping Enhancement

- Confront patient's ambivalent (angry or depressed) feelings.
- Foster constructive outlets for anger and hostility.
- Encourage verbalization of feelings, perceptions, and fears.
- Provide an atmosphere of acceptance.
- Assist the patient to identify available support systems.
- Assist patient to solve problems in a constructive manner.
- Appraise and discuss alternative responses to situation.
- Encourage patient to evaluate own behavior *to assist patient in recognizing effective and ineffective behaviors.*

NPO, Nothing by mouth.

NURSING CARE PLAN 43-2

Patient with Inflammatory Bowel Disease—cont'd

NURSING DIAGNOSIS   **Imbalanced nutrition: less than body requirements** *related to* decreased intake, decreased absorption, and increased nutrient loss through diarrhea *as evidenced by* anorexia, weight loss, weakness, lethargy, anemia

PATIENT GOALS
1. Consumes calories and nutrients adequate to meet nutritional needs
2. Maintains body weight within a normal range
3. Demonstrates increased muscle tone and strength

OUTCOMES (NOC)	INTERVENTIONS (NIC) and *RATIONALES*
Nutritional Status	***Nutritional Monitoring***
• Nutrient intake _____	• Weigh patient at specified intervals *to evaluate nutritional status and response to treatment.*
• Food intake _____	• Monitor albumin, total protein, hemoglobin, and hematocrit levels *to determine nutritional status.*
• Energy _____	• Note significant changes in nutritional status and initiate treatments *to prevent worsening malnutrition.*
• Weight/height ratio _____	• Monitor energy level, malaise, fatigue, and weakness *as signs of inadequate nutrition.*
• Hematocrit _____	
• Muscle tone _____	***Nutrition Therapy***
	• Monitor food/fluid ingested and calculate daily caloric intake *to determine adequacy of caloric intake.*
Measurement Scale	• Select nutritional supplements *to provide additional calories, iron, protein, and fluid.*
1 = Severe deviation from normal range	• Instruct patient and family about prescribed diet that will maintain nutrition without irritation of the bowel.
2 = Substantial deviation from normal range	• Refer for diet teaching and planning as needed.
3 = Moderate deviation from normal range	
4 = Mild deviation from normal range	
5 = No deviation from normal range	

NURSING DIAGNOSIS   **Ineffective therapeutic regimen management** *related to* lack of knowledge of course of disease, appropriate lifestyle adjustments, and nutritional and drug therapy *as evidenced by* questioning about the disease and treatment, poor decisions about activities of daily living

PATIENT GOALS
1. Describes the disease process and treatment regimen
2. Expresses confidence in ability to care for self with regard to medication administration and diet therapy

OUTCOMES (NOC)	INTERVENTIONS (NIC) and *RATIONALES*
Knowledge: Treatment Regimen	***Teaching: Disease Process***
• Description of specific disease process _____	• Appraise the patient's current level of knowledge related to specific disease process *to establish knowledge basis for teaching.*
• Description of rationale for treatment regimen _____	• Describe disease process *to ensure patient has adequate knowledge about the disease and treatment.*
• Description of self-care responsibilities for ongoing treatment _____	• Describe the rationale behind management/therapy/treatment recommendations *to enhance compliance with treatment.*
• Description of prescribed medication(s) _____	• Reinforce information provided by other health care professionals.
• Description of prescribed diet _____	• Discuss lifestyle changes that may need to be required to prevent future complications and/or control the disease process.
Measurement Scale	• Instruct the patient on which signs and symptoms to report to health care provider *to prevent complications.*
1 = None	
2 = Limited	
3 = Moderate	
4 = Substantial	
5 = Extensive	

quent episodes of diarrhea and abdominal pain. Nutritional deficiencies and anemia leave the patient feeling weak and listless. Activities should be scheduled around rest periods.

Until diarrhea is controlled, the patient must be kept clean, dry, and free of odor. A deodorizer should be placed in the room, and patients must have ready access to a toilet. Meticulous perianal skin care using plain water (no harsh soap) is necessary to treat and prevent skin breakdown. Dibucaine (Nupercainal), witch hazel, or other soothing compresses or prescribed ointment and sitz baths may reduce irritation and relieve discomfort of the anus.

In the majority of patients with IBD the course is chronic and intermittent, and is characterized by exacerbations and remissions of symptoms. The patient and significant others may need help in setting realistic short- and long-term goals. Teaching is important and should include (1) the importance of rest and diet management, (2) perianal care, (3) action and side effects of drugs, (4) symptoms of recurrence of disease, (5) when to seek medical care, and (6) use of diversional activities to reduce stress. Excellent teaching resources written in easily comprehensible language are available from the Crohn's and Colitis Foundation of America (see Resources at the end of the chapter.)

■ **Evaluation**

The expected outcomes for the patient with IBD are presented in NCP 43-2.

GERONTOLOGIC CONSIDERATIONS
INFLAMMATORY BOWEL DISEASE

Although IBD is considered a disease of teenagers and young adults, a second peak in occurrence is in the sixth decade. The etiology, natural history, and clinical course of ulcerative colitis and Crohn's disease in older adults are similar to those observed in younger patients. However, in the older patient with ulcerative colitis, the distal colon (proctitis) is usually involved.[28] In the older patient with Crohn's disease, the colon rather than the small intestine tends to be involved. There is less recurrence of Crohn's disease in older patients treated with surgical resection. The degree of inflammation associated with both conditions is less in the older adult than in the younger patient.

Collaborative care of the older patient with one of these conditions is similar to care of the younger patient. However, because of increased risk of cardiovascular and pulmonary complications, older adults tend to have increased morbidity associated with surgical procedures.

In addition to Crohn's disease and ulcerative colitis, older adults are also vulnerable to inflammation of the colon (colitis) from medication use and systemic vascular disease. Drugs such as nonsteroidal antiinflammatory drugs (NSAIDs), digitalis, vasopressin, estrogen, and allopurinol (Zyloprim) have been associated with colitis development in the elderly patient. Colitis may also be secondary to ischemic bowel disease related to atherosclerosis and heart failure.

Older adults are more vulnerable to the volume depletion consequences of diarrhea, which may be bloody. Volume depletion is particularly problematic in the patient with diminished renal and cardiovascular function. Nursing management is focused on careful assessment of fluid and electrolyte status and evaluation of the replacement therapies.

INTESTINAL OBSTRUCTION

Intestinal obstruction occurs when intestinal contents cannot pass through the GI tract. The obstruction may occur in the small intestine or colon and can be partial or complete. The causes of intestinal obstruction can be classified as mechanical or nonmechanical. Intestinal obstruction requires prompt treatment.

Types of Intestinal Obstruction

Mechanical. Mechanical obstruction is a detectable occlusion of the intestinal lumen. Most intestinal obstructions occur in the small intestine. Surgical adhesion is the most common cause of small bowel obstructions and can occur within days of surgery or several years later[29] (Fig. 43-6). Hernias and tumors are the next most common causes. Carcinoma is the most common cause of large bowel obstruction, followed by volvulus and diverticular disease.

Nonmechanical. A nonmechanical obstruction may result from a neuromuscular or vascular disorder. **Paralytic (adynamic) ileus** (lack of intestinal peristalsis and the presence of no bowel sounds) is the most common form of nonmechanical obstruction. It occurs to some degree after any abdominal surgery. It can be difficult to know whether postoperative obstruction is due to paralytic ileus or adhesions. One clue is that bowel sounds usually return before postoperative adhesions develop. Other causes of para-

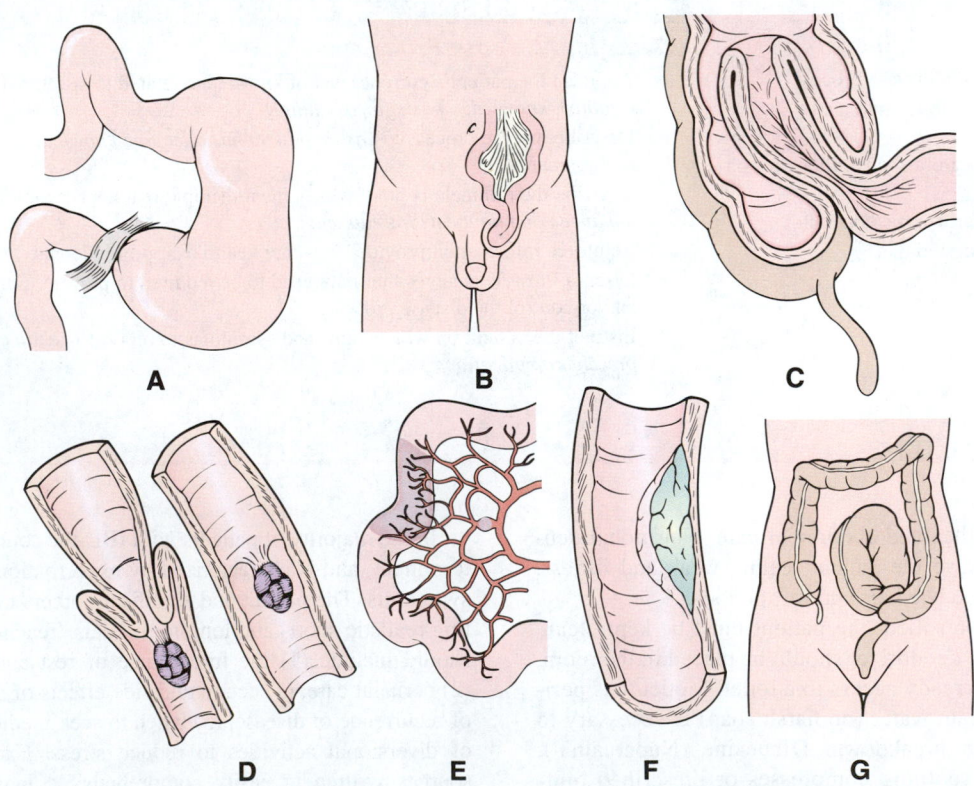

FIG. 43-6 Bowel obstructions. **A,** Adhesions. **B,** Strangulated inguinal hernia. **C,** Ileocecal intussusception. **D,** Intussusception from polyps. **E,** Mesenteric occlusion. **F,** Neoplasm. **G,** Volvulus of the sigmoid colon.

lytic ileus include peritonitis, inflammatory responses (e.g., acute pancreatitis, acute appendicitis), electrolyte abnormalities (especially hypokalemia), and thoracic or lumbar spinal fractures.

Pseudo-obstruction is an apparent mechanical obstruction of the intestine without demonstration of obstruction by radiologic methods. Collagen vascular diseases and neurologic and endocrine disorders may cause pseudo-obstruction, but many times the cause is unknown.

Vascular obstructions are rare and are due to an interference with the blood supply to a portion of the intestines. The most common causes are emboli and atherosclerosis of the mesenteric arteries. The celiac, inferior, and superior mesenteric arteries supply blood to the bowel. Emboli may originate from thrombi in patients with chronic atrial fibrillation, diseased heart valves, and prosthetic valves. Venous thrombosis may be seen in low-blood-flow states, such as heart failure and shock.

Etiology and Pathophysiology

About 6 to 8 L of fluid enters the small bowel daily. Most of the fluid is absorbed before it reaches the colon. Approximately 75% of intestinal gas is swallowed air. Normally, gastric HCl acid secretion and rapid movement of chyme through the small intestine inhibit bacterial growth in the small intestine, but bacteria flourish when the small bowel is obstructed. Fluid, gas, and intestinal contents accumulate proximal to the obstruction. The distal bowel collapses. The distention reduces the absorption of fluids and stimulates intestinal secretions. Bacteria flourish proximal to the obstruction and stimulate additional secretion of fluids into the bowel. The proximal bowel becomes increasingly distended, and intraluminal bowel pressure rises. The increased pressure leads to an increase in capillary permeability and extravasation of fluids and electrolytes into the peritoneal cavity. The retention of fluid in the intestine and peritoneal cavity can lead to a severe reduction in circulating blood volume and result in hypotension and hypovolemic shock. If blood flow is inadequate, bowel tissue becomes ischemic, then necrotic, and the bowel may rupture. The most dangerous obstruction is when the bowel becomes strangulated and the blood supply is cut off. If not corrected quickly, the bowel will become necrotic and rupture, leading to massive infection and death.

When the bowel is obstructed, electrolyte-rich fluids cannot be absorbed from the bowel, and are subsequently lost into the peritoneal cavity. The location of the obstruction determines the extent of fluid, electrolyte, and acid-base imbalances. If the obstruction is high, as in the pylorus, metabolic alkalosis may result from the loss of gastric HCl acid through vomiting or NG intubation. When the obstruction is located in the small bowel, dehydration occurs rapidly. Dehydration and electrolyte imbalances do not occur early in large bowel obstruction. If the obstruction is below the proximal colon, most GI fluids have been absorbed before reaching the point of the obstruction. Solid fecal material accumulates until symptoms of discomfort appear.

Obstructions may be partial or complete. Some obstructions, especially those due to surgical adhesions, may resolve without surgery. Others, such as strangulated obstructions, require emergency surgery for survival. Simple obstructions of the intestine involve blockage of the lumen in one spot. A closed-loop obstruction occurs when the lumen is blocked in two different spots (e.g., volvulus). This results in an isolated segment of bowel and obstruction proximal to that segment. Strangulation and gangrene are likely to develop if treatment is not immediate.

TABLE 43-23	Clinical Manifestations of Small and Large Intestinal Obstructions	
Clinical Manifestation	**Small Intestine**	**Large Intestine**
Onset	Rapid	Gradual
Vomiting	Frequent and copious	Rare
Pain	Colicky, cramplike, intermittent	Low-grade, cramping abdominal pain
Bowel movement	Feces for a short time	Absolute constipation
Abdominal distention	Greatly increased	Increased

Clinical Manifestations

The clinical manifestations of intestinal obstruction vary, depending on the location of the obstruction, and include nausea, vomiting, abdominal pain, distention, inability to pass flatus, and obstipation (Table 43-23). Patients with obstructions located high in the small intestine rapidly develop nausea and vomiting, which is sometimes projectile in nature and contains bile. Vomiting from more distal obstructions of the small intestine is more gradual in onset. The vomitus may be orange-brown and foul smelling like feces because of bacterial overgrowth.

Vomiting usually relieves abdominal pain in high intestinal obstructions. Persistent, colicky abdominal pain is seen with lower intestinal obstruction. A characteristic sign of mechanical obstruction is pain that comes and goes in waves. This is due to intestinal peristalsis trying to move bowel contents past the obstructed area. In contrast, paralytic ileus produces a more constant generalized discomfort. Strangulation causes severe, constant pain that is rapid in onset. Abdominal distention is a common manifestation of intestinal obstructions. It is usually absent or minimally noticeable in high obstructions of the small intestine and greatly increased in lower intestinal obstructions. Abdominal tenderness and rigidity are usually absent unless strangulation or peritonitis has occurred.

Auscultation of bowel sounds reveals high-pitched sounds above the area of obstruction. Bowel sounds may also be absent. The patient often notes *borborygmi* (audible abdominal sounds produced by hyperactive intestinal motility). The patient's temperature rarely rises above 100° F (37.8° C) unless strangulation or peritonitis has occurred.

Diagnostic Studies

A thorough history and physical examination should be performed. Abdominal x-rays are the most useful diagnostic aids. Upright and lateral abdominal x-rays show the presence of gas and fluid in the intestines. The presence of intraperitoneal air indicates perforation. Barium enemas are helpful in locating large intestinal obstructions. However, barium is not used if perforation is suspected. If the location is unknown, a lower GI tract study is done before an upper GI series. Sigmoidoscopy or colonoscopy may provide direct visualization of an obstruction in the colon. CT scans may also be used in diagnosis.

Laboratory tests are important and provide essential information. A CBC and serum electrolyte, amylase, and BUN determinations should be performed. An elevated WBC count may indicate strangulation or perforation; elevated hematocrit values may reflect hemoconcentration. Decreased hemoglobin and hematocrit values may indicate bleeding from a neoplasm or strangulation with necrosis. Serum electrolytes should be monitored frequently to provide essential information about the patient's fluid and electrolyte balance. Serum sodium, potassium, and chloride concentrations are decreased in small bowel obstruction. The BUN and serum creatinine should be monitored to determine if fluid resuscitation is adequate to prevent acute renal failure. The stool should be checked for occult blood.

Collaborative Care

Emergency surgery is performed if the bowel is strangulated, but many bowel obstructions resolve with conservative treatment. Initial medical treatment of bowel obstruction caused by adhesions includes placing the patient on NPO status, insertion of an NG tube, IV fluid resuscitation with either normal saline or lactated Ringer's, addition of potassium to IV fluids after renal function is verified, and analgesics for pain control. Long intestinal tubes (10 feet [300 cm]) (e.g., Cantor, Miller-Abbott) may be used instead of NG tubes to decompress the bowel. Their use is controversial and limited because they are more difficult and time consuming to insert, and they may not be any more effective than NG tubes.

If the situation does not improve within 24 to 48 hours or if the patient's condition deteriorates, surgery is performed to relieve the obstruction. The goals of treatment are relief of the obstruction and correction and maintenance of fluid and electrolyte balance. Parenteral nutrition may be necessary in some cases to correct nutritional deficits, improve the patient's nutritional status before surgery, and promote postoperative healing.

Surgery may involve simply resecting the obstructed segment of bowel and anastomosing the remaining healthy bowel back together. Partial or total colectomy, colostomy, or ileostomy may be required when extensive obstruction or necrosis is present. Occasionally obstructions can be removed nonsurgically. A colonoscope can be used to remove polyps, dilate strictures, and remove and destroy tumors with a laser.

NURSING MANAGEMENT
INTESTINAL OBSTRUCTION

■ Nursing Assessment

Intestinal obstruction is a potentially life-threatening condition. Major concerns are preventing fluid and electrolyte deficiencies and early recognition of deteriorations in the patient's condition. Nursing assessment must begin with a detailed patient history and physical examination. The type and location of obstruction usually cause characteristic symptoms. The nurse should determine the location, duration, intensity, and frequency of abdominal pain and whether abdominal tenderness or rigidity is present. Onset, frequency, color, odor, and amount of vomitus should be recorded. Bowel function, including passage of flatus, should be determined. The nurse auscultates for bowel sounds and documents their character and location; inspects the abdomen for scars, visible masses, and distention; and palpates for muscle guarding and tenderness. If the surgeon decides to wait and see if the obstruction resolves on its own, regular abdominal assessments are vital to detect deteriorations that would demand emergency surgery.

Nursing assessment of fluid and electrolyte balance is also essential. Intake and output is accurately measured. A urinary catheter is usually ordered to monitor hourly urine outputs. Urine output less than 0.5 ml/kg of body weight per hour must be reported immediately because it signals inadequate vascular volume and the potential for acute renal failure. Rising serum creatinine and BUN levels are additional indicators of acute renal failure.

■ Nursing Diagnoses

Nursing diagnoses for the patient with intestinal obstructions include, but are not limited to, the following:
- Acute pain *related to* abdominal distention and increased peristalsis
- Deficient fluid volume *related to* decrease in intestinal fluid absorption, third space fluid shifts into the bowel lumen and peritoneal cavity, NG suction, and vomiting
- Imbalanced nutrition: less than body requirements *related to* intestinal obstruction and vomiting

■ Planning

The overall goals are that the patient with an intestinal obstruction will have (1) relief of the obstruction and return to normal bowel function, (2) minimal to no discomfort, and (3) normal fluid and electrolyte status.

■ Nursing Implementation

The patient should be monitored closely for signs of dehydration and electrolyte imbalance. A strict intake and output record should be maintained and include all emesis and tube drainage. IV fluids should be administered as ordered. Serum electrolyte levels are monitored closely. A patient with a high intestinal obstruction is more likely to have metabolic alkalosis; a patient with a low obstruction is at greater risk of metabolic acidosis. The patient is often restless and constantly changes position to relieve the pain. The nurse should provide comfort measures, promote a restful environment, and keep distractions and visitors to a minimum. Nursing care of the patient after surgery for an intestinal obstruction is similar to care of the patient after a laparotomy (see pp. 1045 to 1046).

Care of Nasogastric Tubes. Once the NG tube is in place, mouth care is extremely important. Vomiting leaves a terrible taste in the patient's mouth, and fecal odor may be present. When an NG tube is in place, the patient breathes through the mouth, drying the mouth and lips. The nurse should encourage and assist the patient to brush the teeth frequently. Mouthwash and water for rinsing the mouth and petroleum jelly or water-soluble lubricant for the lips should be readily available to the patient.

The patient's nose should be checked for signs of irritation from the NG tube. This area should be cleaned and dried daily with application of a water-soluble lubricant and retaping of the tube. NG tubes should be checked every 4 hours for patency.

POLYPS OF THE LARGE INTESTINE

Colonic polyps arise from the mucosal surface of the colon and project into the lumen. They may be sessile (flat, broad based, and attached directly to the intestinal wall) or pedunculated (attached to the intestinal wall by a thin stalk). Polyps tend to be sessile when small and become pedunculated as they enlarge, especially if they are in the left or descending colon (Fig. 43-7). They may be found anywhere in the large intestine but are most commonly found in the rectosigmoid area. Rectal bleeding and occult blood in the stool are the most common symptoms, but most polyps are asymptomatic.

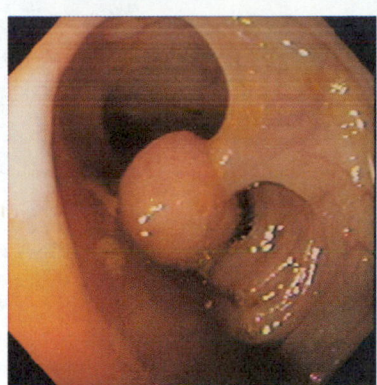 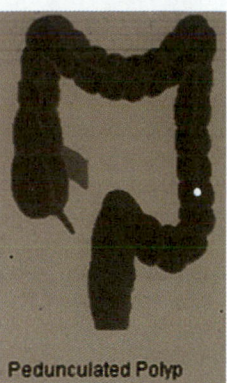

Pedunculated Polyp

FIG. 43-7 Endoscopic image of pedunculated polyp in descending colon.

Types of Polyps

The most common types of polyps are hyperplastic and adenomatous. Hyperplastic polyps originate from the epithelium and are nonneoplastic growths. They rarely grow larger than 5 mm in size and never cause clinical symptoms. Other benign (nonneoplastic) polyps include inflammatory polyps, lipomas, and juvenile polyps (Table 43-24). Adenomatous polyps are characterized by neoplastic changes in the epithelium. They are closely linked to colorectal adenocarcinoma. Structurally, there are three types, with tubular adenomas being the most prevalent. The risk of cancer in the polyp increases with polyp size and villous structure. Villous adenomas have a higher risk of turning cancerous than tubular adenomas. Removing adenomatous polyps has been reported to substantially decrease the occurrence of subsequent colorectal cancer.[30,31]

Although there are several polyposis syndromes, they are relatively rare. Of these, familial adenomatous polyposis (FAP) is the most common (see the Genetics in Clinical Practice box). This disorder is characterized by multiple polyps that at times number in the thousands and that are located in the large intestine and sometimes in other areas of the GI tract. Patients with a history of FAP have a lifetime risk of developing colorectal cancer of approximately 80%.[31] They also develop cancer at an earlier age (i.e., 40 years of age) than patients with non-FAP colorectal cancer. For children of patients with FAP, screening must be initiated at puberty and then conducted annually. There is a 50% risk for these children to develop FAP. When there is indication of disease, total colectomy with ileostomy is the treatment of choice.

Diagnostic Studies and Collaborative Care

Barium enema, sigmoidoscopy, colonoscopy, and virtual colonoscopy are used to diagnose polyps.[32] All polyps are considered abnormal and should be removed. In patients whose polyps are identified through barium enema or capsule endoscopy, removal (polypectomy) must be done through a colonoscope. If the polyp is not removable, a biopsy specimen should be taken for tissue examination. Surgery is not indicated unless carcinoma is present or certain cases of polyposis syndromes warrant it. The patient should be observed for rectal bleeding, fever, severe abdominal pain, and abdominal distention, which may indicate hemorrhage or perforation.

COLORECTAL CANCER

Colorectal cancer is the third most common form of cancer and the second leading cause of cancer-related deaths in the United States. Colorectal cancer has an insidious onset, and symptoms do

TABLE 43-24	**Types of Polyps of the Large Intestine**

Neoplastic
Epithelial polyps (adenomatous)
 Tubular adenoma
 Tubular villous adenoma
 Villous adenoma
Hereditary polyposis syndromes (adenomatous polyposis syndrome)
 Familial adenomatous polyposis (FAP)

Nonneoplastic
Epithelial polyps (hyperplastic)
Hereditary polyposis syndromes
 Familial juvenile polyposis
Inflammatory polyps
 Pseudopolyps
 Benign lymphoid polyp
Submucosal
 Lipomas
 Leiomyomas
 Fibromas

GENETICS IN CLINICAL PRACTICE
Familial Adenomatous Polyposis (FAP)

Genetic Basis
- Autosomal dominant disorder—classic form of disease
  - Mutations in the FAP gene located on chromosome 5
- Autosomal recessive disorder—mild form of disease
  - Mutations in the mutY homolog (MUTYH) *(E. coli)* gene

Incidence
- 1 in 6800 to 30,000 people
- Men and women affected equally

Genetic Testing
- DNA testing available

Clinical Implications
- Accounts for at least 1% of all colorectal cancers.
- Classical FAP is characterized by the presence of colorectal polyps (usually hundreds to thousands).
- Polyps are not present at birth but appear during adolescence and early adulthood.
- Autosomal recessive FAP is characterized by fewer polyps, typically fewer than 100.
- If untreated, FAP almost always results in the development of colorectal cancer before age 40.
- With classic FAP, other benign and malignant tumors are sometimes found, especially in the duodenum, stomach, bones, skin, and other tissues.
- Many deaths related to FAP could be prevented with early and aggressive monitoring and treatment, including frequent colonoscopies and total colectomy.
- Individuals with a family history of FAP could benefit from genetic counseling.

not appear until the disease is quite advanced. Therefore regular screening is necessary to detect precancerous lesions. About one half of all colorectal cancers occur in the rectosigmoid area (Fig. 43-8). Fortunately, about 85% of colorectal cancers arise from adenomatous polyps, which can be detected and removed from the rectum and sigmoid colon by sigmoidoscopy or colonoscopy. Since half of all cases are found in areas of the colon that are inaccessible by sigmoidoscopy, colonoscopy is considered the gold

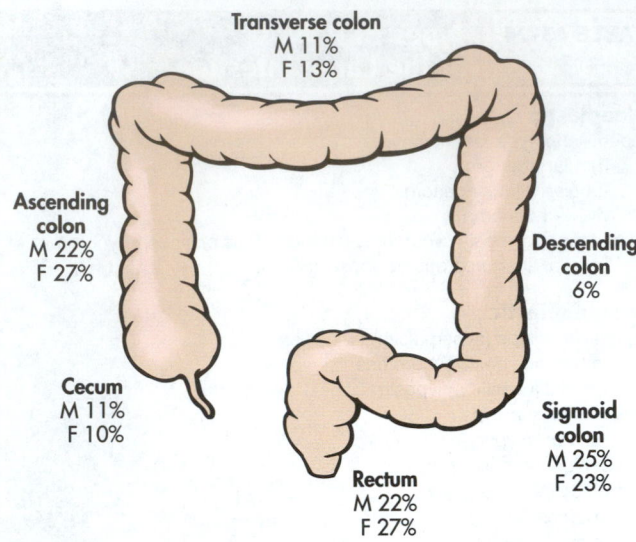

FIG. 43-8 Incidence of cancer. Approximately one half of all colon cancers occur in the rectosigmoid area. Percentages are listed for males *(M)* and females *(F)*.

standard for colorectal cancer screening and the detection and removal of precancerous polyps.[31]

Etiology and Pathophysiology

Colorectal cancer is more common in men than women, and mortality rates are highest among African American men and women. Major risk factors include increasing age, family or personal history of colorectal cancer, colorectal polyps, and IBD. About 90% of new colorectal cancer cases are detected in people older than 50, and about 25% occur in patients with a family history of colorectal cancer. Hereditary diseases (e.g., FAP) account for about 5% to 10% of colorectal cancer cases. Hereditary nonpolyposis colorectal cancer (HNPCC) syndrome, also called Lynch syndrome, is the most common inherited form of hereditary colorectal cancer[33] (see Genetics in Clinical Practice Box).

Certain lifestyle factors are also associated with colorectal cancer. Obesity, smoking, alcohol, and a large intake of red meat increase the risk. Physical exercise and a diet with large amounts of fruits, vegetables, and grains may decrease the risk. NSAIDs (e.g., aspirin) and hormone replacement therapy in women also seem to decrease the risk.[34] (See Table 43-25 for a list of risk factors.)

Adenocarcinoma is the most common type of colorectal cancer. Most colorectal cancers begin as adenomatous polyps that arise from the mucosa lining the lumen of the colon and rectum. As it grows, the cancer progresses down from the tip of the polyp through the body and stalk. It becomes invasive and penetrates the muscularis mucosae. Once through the muscularis mucosae, tumor cells gain access to the regional lymph nodes and vascular system, and can spread to distant sites. (Carcinomas of the cecum and colon are shown in Fig. 43-9.) The most common sites of metastasis are the regional lymph nodes, liver, lungs, and peritoneum. Since venous blood leaving the colon and rectum flows through the portal vein and the inferior rectal vein, the liver and lung are common sites of metastasis. The cancer spreads from the liver to other sites, including the lungs, bones, and brain. The cancer can also spread directly into adjacent structures. The growing tumor can obstruct

---

GENETICS IN CLINICAL PRACTICE

Hereditary Nonpolyposis Colorectal Cancer (HNPCC) or Lynch Syndrome

Genetic Basis
- Autosomal dominant disorder
- Mutations in repair genes
- Repair genes are involved in repair of mistakes when DNA is replicated
- Genes include MLH1, MSH2, MSH6, PMS2

Incidence
- 1 in 500 to 2000 people

Genetic Testing
- DNA testing available

Clinical Implications
- Accounts for 5% of all colorectal cancers.
- Individual with gene mutation has 80%-90% lifetime risk of developing colorectal cancer.
- Average age of diagnosis is in the mid-40s.
- Cancers tend to occur on right side of colon.
- HNPCC is less aggressive and survival rates are longer than colorectal cancer that develops without known risk factors.
- People with HNPCC have an increased risk of cancers of the stomach, small intestine, liver, gallbladder ducts, upper urinary tract, brain, skin, and prostate.
- Women with HNPCC also have a greatly increased risk of endometrial and ovarian cancer.
- Occasionally, people with HNPCC also have colon polyps, which occur at an earlier age than do colon polyps in the general population and are more prone to become malignant.
- Individuals with known gene mutations need to be monitored with colonoscopy every year. Examination by pelvic ultrasound and endometrial biopsy should also be considered to screen for endometrial cancer.

TABLE 43-25	**Risk Factors for Colorectal Cancer**

- Family history of colorectal cancer (first-degree relative)
- Inflammatory bowel disease for 10 yr or more
- Personal history of colorectal cancer
- Familial adenomatous polyposis (FAP)
- Hereditary nonpolyposis colorectal cancer (HNPCC) syndrome
- Obesity (body mass index $\geq$30 kg/m²)
- Red meat ($\geq$7 servings/wk)
- Cigarette use
- Alcohol ($\geq$4 drinks/wk)

the bowel. Other complications include bleeding, perforation, peritonitis, and fistula formation.

Clinical Manifestations

Most people with colorectal cancer have hematochezia (passage of blood through rectum) or melena (black, tarry stools), abdominal pain, and/or changes in bowel habits. Other symptoms include weakness, anemia, and weight loss. Clinical manifestations are usually nonspecific or do not appear until the disease is advanced. Cancer on the right side of the colon gives rise to clinical manifestations that are different from those on the left side of the colon (Fig. 43-10). Rectal bleeding, the most common symptom of

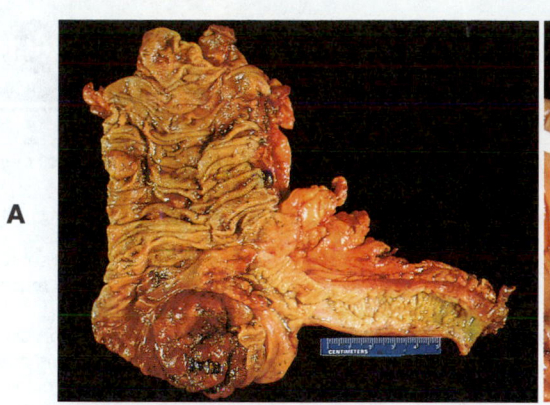
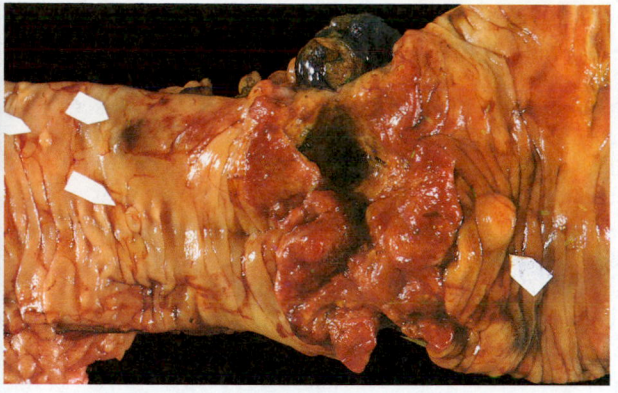

FIG. 43-9   **A,** Carcinoma of the cecum. The fungating carcinoma projects into the lumen but has not caused obstruction. **B,** Carcinoma of the descending colon. This circumferential tumor has heaped-up edges and an ulcerated central portion. The *arrows* identify separate mucosal polyps.

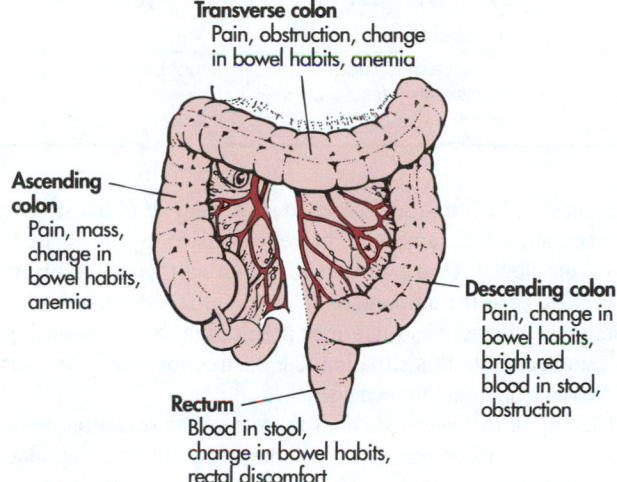

Transverse colon
Pain, obstruction, change in bowel habits, anemia

Ascending colon
Pain, mass, change in bowel habits, anemia

Descending colon
Pain, change in bowel habits, bright red blood in stool, obstruction

Rectum
Blood in stool, change in bowel habits, rectal discomfort

FIG. 43-10   Signs and symptoms of colorectal cancer by location of primary lesion.

TABLE 43-26	*COLLABORATIVE CARE* Colorectal Cancer

Diagnostic
History and physical examination
Digital rectal examination
Testing of stool for occult blood
Barium enema
Sigmoidoscopy
Colonoscopy
CBC
Liver function tests
CT scan of abdomen
MRI
Ultrasound
Carcinoembryonic antigen (CEA) test

Collaborative Therapy
Surgery
- Right hemicolectomy
- Left hemicolectomy
- Abdominal-perineal resection
- Laparoscopic colectomy
Radiation
Chemotherapy
Biologic and targeted therapy

CBC, Complete blood count; *CT,* computed tomography; *MRI,* magnetic resonance imaging.

colorectal cancer, is most often seen with left-sided lesions. Other manifestations of left-sided lesions include alternating constipation and diarrhea, change in stool caliber (narrow, ribbonlike), and sensation of incomplete evacuation. Obstruction symptoms appear earlier with left-sided lesions because lesions in the descending colon and rectum tend to progressively constrict the lumen and those in the more proximal lumen do not (see Fig. 43-10).

Cancers of the right side of the colon are usually asymptomatic. Vague abdominal discomfort or cramping, colicky abdominal pain may be present. Iron deficiency anemia and occult bleeding lead to weakness and fatigue.

Diagnostic Studies

A thorough history with close attention to family history should be obtained (Table 43-26). Since symptoms of colorectal cancer do not become evident until the disease is advanced, regular screening is advocated to detect and remove polyps before they become cancerous. Routine physical examinations should include a digital rectal examination because rectal polyps and cancer can be reached with a finger. The American Cancer Society recommends that a person who has no established risk factors should have a fecal occult blood test

(FOBT) or a fecal immunochemical test (FIT) yearly, a double-contrast enema every 5 years, a sigmoidoscopy every 5 years, or a colonoscopy every 10 years starting at age 50.[30] All positive tests are followed up with colonoscopy. (Screening recommendations for colorectal cancer are presented in Table 16-7.)

Persons with a history of colorectal cancer or adenomatous polyps, a strong family history of colorectal cancer or polyps in a first-degree relative younger than 60 or in two first-degree relatives of any age, a history of IBD, or a history of a hereditary colorectal cancer syndrome (e.g., FAP, HNPCC) should begin screening earlier and have screening done more often. If polyps are detected or colorectal cancer is suspected, the person should have a colonoscopy.

Colonoscopy is the gold standard for colorectal cancer screening because the entire colon is examined (only 50% of colorectal cancers are detected by sigmoidoscopy), biopsies can be obtained, and polyps can be immediately removed and sent to the laboratory for histologic examination.[35,36] Virtual colonoscopy can also detect colorectal lesions. However, biopsies cannot be obtained with this technique. (The difference between conventional and virtual colonoscopies is discussed in Chapter 39.)

Since cancerous tumors bleed intermittently into the colon, fecal occult blood tests are used to detect very small quantities of blood. Two tests are available. The guaiac-based tests (FOBT) require that the person avoid NSAIDs, vitamin C, citrus juices, and red meat for 3 days before the test. Six samples from three consecutive bowel movements are collected and smeared onto a special card. The FIT does not require special dietary restrictions and often needs only two stool specimens. Neither detects nonbleeding tumors.

Ongoing studies are evaluating the sensitivity and specificity of a stool DNA test. DNA markers are shed from premalignant adenomas and cancer cells into the stool and are not degraded. Stools are collected and sent to the laboratory for DNA analysis. Although promising, the DNA test is not yet sensitive enough to replace the other screening methods.[35,36]

Once colonoscopy and tissue biopsies confirm the diagnosis of colorectal cancer, additional laboratory studies are done, including a CBC to check for anemia, coagulation studies, and liver function tests. Carcinoembryonic antigen (CEA) is a complex glycoprotein produced by 90% of colorectal cancers. It is helpful in monitoring disease recurrence following surgery or chemotherapy. A CT scan or MRI of the abdomen may be helpful in detecting liver metastases, retroperitoneal and pelvic disease, and depth of penetration of tumor into the bowel wall. However, liver function tests may be normal even when metastasis has occurred.

Collaborative Care

Colorectal cancer prognosis and treatment correlate with pathologic staging of the disease. Two staging systems are used: the tumor, node, metastasis (TNM) staging system of the American Joint Committee on Cancer (Table 43-27) and the Dukes' classification system[37,38] (Table 43-28). The TNM system is currently the preferred classification system. As with other cancers, prognosis worsens with greater size and depth of tumor, lymph node involvement, and metastasis.[38]

Surgical Therapy. Polypectomy during colonoscopy can be used to resect colorectal cancer in situ and is considered successful when the resected margin of the polyp is free of cancer, the cancer is well differentiated, and there is no apparent lymphatic or blood vessel involvement. If the cancer is localized, it can be resected together with a margin of healthy tissue on either side and the remaining cancer-free ends sewn back together. Nearby lymph nodes are also removed. Chemotherapy or radiation therapy is used if the cancer has spread to lymph nodes or into nearby tissue. Once the cancer has spread to distant sites (e.g., liver, lungs, peritoneum, ovaries), surgery is palliative.

Surgical goals include complete resection of the tumor together with adequate margins of healthy tissue, a thorough exploration of the abdomen to determine if the cancer has spread, removal of all lymph nodes that drain the area where the cancer is located, restoration of bowel continuity so that normal bowel function will return, and prevention of surgical complications.[39,40] The optimal procedure is bowel resection with reanastomosis of the remaining segments. Reduction of colonic bacteria is necessary to decrease

TABLE 43-27	TNM Classification of Colorectal Cancer
T	**Primary Tumor**
T_x	Primary tumor cannot be assessed because of incomplete information.
T_{is}	Carcinoma in situ. Cancer is in earliest stage and has not grown beyond mucosa layer.
T_1	Tumor has grown beyond mucosa into the submucosa.
T_2	Tumor has grown through submucosa into muscularis propria.
T_3	Tumor has grown through the muscularis propria into the subserosa but not to neighboring organs or tissues.
T_4	Tumor has spread completely through the colon or rectal wall and into nearby tissues or organs.
N	**Lymph Node Involvement**
N_x	Lymph nodes cannot be assessed.
N_0	No regional lymph node involvement is found.
N_1	Cancer is found in one to three nearby lymph nodes.
N_2	Cancer is found in four or more nearby lymph nodes.
M	**Metastasis**
M_x	Presence of distant metastasis cannot be assessed.
M_0	No distant metastasis is seen.
M_1	Distant metastasis is present.

postoperative infection and breakdown at the site of anastomosis. In preparation for surgery, a bowel cleansing agent is used to empty the bowel. Oral erythromycin and neomycin are given to further decrease the amount of colonic and rectal bacteria. If the patient has a bowel obstruction or perforation, bowel cleansing is contraindicated. In this situation, the obstruction is relieved and a temporary colostomy is formed.

The site of the cancer dictates the site of the resection. For example, cecal cancer resection includes removal of a segment of terminal ileum and its mesentery and the right colon. The transverse colon is removed if the cancer is in the middle of the transverse colon. Right hemicolectomy is performed when the cancer is located in the cecum, ascending colon, hepatic flexure, or transverse colon to the right of the middle colic artery. A left hemicolectomy involves resection of the left transverse colon, the splenic flexure, the descending colon, the sigmoid colon, and the upper portion of the rectum. When the tumor is not resectable or if metastasis is present, palliative surgery is done to control hemorrhage or relieve an obstruction.

Clear margins are most difficult to obtain with rectal carcinoma. Location of the rectal lesion determines the surgical procedure to be performed. Unless sufficient rectum remains to ensure a secure anastomosis, an abdominal-perineal resection is indicated. Abdominal-perineal resection is most often performed when the cancer is located within 5 cm of the anus.

In the abdominal-perineal resection, an abdominal incision is made, and the proximal sigmoid is brought through the abdominal wall to form a permanent colostomy. The distal sigmoid, rectum, and anus are removed through a perineal incision. The perineal wound may be closed around a drain or left open with packing to allow healing by granulation. Complications that can occur are delayed wound healing, hemorrhage, persistent perineal sinus tracts, infections, and urinary tract and sexual dysfunctions.

Low anterior resection may be indicated for tumors of the rectosigmoid and the mid to upper rectum. The use of end-to-end

TABLE 43-28	Classification Systems Used to Stage Colon Cancer			
Dukes'	**Pathology**	**Stage***	**TNM†**	**Prognosis‡**
A	No invasion beyond submucosa	I	$T_1 N_0 M_0$	>90%
B_1	Extension into muscularis	I	$T_2 N_0 M_0$	85%
B_2	Extension into or through serosa	II	$T_3 N_0 M_0$	70%-80%
C	Involvement of lymph nodes	III	Any T, $N_1 M_0$	35%-65%
D	Distant metastases present	IV	Any T, any N, M_1	5%

Adapted from DuBois RN: Neoplasms of the large and small intestine. In Goldman L, Ausielo D, editors: *Cecil textbook of medicine*, ed 22, Philadelphia, 2005, Saunders Elsevier.
*Staging system is based on TNM classification.
†See Table 43-27.
‡Estimated 5-year survival rates.

anastomosis (EEA) staplers has allowed lower and more secure anastomoses. The stapler is passed through the anus, where the colon is stapled to the rectum. This technique has made it possible to resect lesions as close as 5 cm to the anus.

Sphincter-sparing procedures are being performed for the patient with early disease. In these procedures a local resection is performed, and the anal sphincters are left intact. The number of these procedures may increase with continued early detection and surveillance. Laparoscopic colectomy is being used with greater frequency. Benefits are faster return of bowel function, decreased incisional infections, shortened hospital stay, and improved cosmetic appearance.

Chemotherapy. Chemotherapy is recommended when a patient has positive lymph nodes at the time of surgery or has metastatic disease. Chemotherapy is used both as an adjuvant therapy following colon resection and as primary treatment for nonresectable colorectal cancer. At present, the combination of 5-fluorouracil (5-FU) plus leucovorin and irinotecan (Camptosar) is approved as first-line chemotherapy for patients with metastatic colorectal cancer. Additional treatment protocols include the use of 5-FU and levamisole (Ergamisol) with or without leucovorin (Wellcovorin). For patients who are not considered appropriate candidates for this triple therapy, either leucovorin-modulated 5-FU (Orzel) or capecitabine (Xeloda) is used as an acceptable alternative first-line treatment.[41] Additional agents include oxaliplatin (Eloxatin) and raltitrexed (Tomudex). (Chemotherapy drugs are discussed in Chapter 16.)

Drug Alert - *Capecitabine (Xeloda)*
• *Instruct patient not to get immunizations without physician's approval.*
• *Report temperature >100.5° F immediately.*

Biologic and Targeted Therapy. Targeted therapies used to treat colon cancer include three monoclonal antibodies. Two drugs target epidermal growth factor receptor (cetuximab [Erbitux], panitumumab [Vectibix]), and the other drug targets vascular endothelial growth factor (bevacizumab [Avastin]) (see Table 16-17 and Fig. 16-21). Bevacizumab works by preventing the formation of new blood vessels, a process known as *angiogenesis*. These drugs can be used alone or in conjunction with other chemotherapeutic agents.[41] One combination drug regimen for colorectal cancer is FOLFOX (see Table 16-12). (Biologic and targeted therapy is discussed in Chapter 16.)

Radiation Therapy. Radiation therapy may be used postoperatively as an adjuvant to surgery and chemotherapy or as a palliative measure for patients with metastatic cancer. As a palliative measure, its primary objective is to reduce tumor size and

TABLE 43-29	*NURSING ASSESSMENT* **Colorectal Cancer**

Subjective Data
Important Health Information
Past health history: Previous breast or ovarian cancer, familial polyposis, villous adenoma, adenomatous polyps, inflammatory bowel disease
Medications: Use of any medications affecting bowel function (e.g., cathartics, antidiarrheal drugs)

Functional Health Patterns
Health perception–health management: Family history of colorectal, breast, or ovarian cancer; weakness, fatigue
Nutritional-metabolic: High-calorie, high-fat, low-fiber diet; anorexia, weight loss; nausea and vomiting
Elimination: Change in bowel habits; alternating diarrhea and constipation, defecation urgency; rectal bleeding; mucoid stools; black, tarry stools; increased flatus, decrease in stool caliber; feelings of incomplete evacuation
Cognitive-perceptual: Abdominal and low back pain, tenesmus

Objective Data
General
Pallor, cachexia, lymphadenopathy (later signs)

Gastrointestinal
Palpable abdominal mass, distention, ascites, and hepatomegaly (liver metastasis)

Possible Findings
Anemia; guaiac-positive stools, palpable mass on digital rectal examination; positive sigmoidoscopy, colonoscopy, barium enema, or CT scan; positive biopsy

provide symptomatic relief. (Radiation therapy is described in Chapter 16.)

NURSING MANAGEMENT
COLORECTAL CANCER

■ **Nursing Assessment**

Subjective and objective data that should be obtained from a patient with colorectal cancer are presented in Table 43-29.

■ **Nursing Diagnoses**

Nursing diagnoses for the patient with colorectal cancer include, but are not limited to, the following:
• Diarrhea or constipation *related to* altered bowel elimination patterns

- Acute pain *related to* difficulty in passing stools because of partial or complete obstruction from tumor
- Fear *related to* diagnosis of colorectal cancer, surgical or therapeutic interventions, and possible terminal illness
- Ineffective coping *related to* diagnosis of cancer and side effects of treatment

■ Planning

The overall goals are that the patient with colorectal cancer will have (1) normal bowel elimination patterns, (2) quality of life appropriate to disease progression, (3) relief of pain, and (4) feelings of comfort and well-being.

■ Nursing Implementation

Health Promotion. The nurse can encourage all patients over 50 to have regular colorectal cancer screening. Screening for high-risk patients should begin before age 50, usually beginning with colonoscopy and continuing at more frequent intervals that vary according to risk factors. Participation in early cancer screening is effective in decreasing mortality rates, but barriers exist, including lack of information and fear of diagnosis.

Colonoscopy only detects polyps when the bowel has been adequately prepared to eliminate stool. When screening is done in the outpatient setting, the nurse must teach the patient how to take the bowel preparation. In the hospitalized patient, nurses have a more direct role in ensuring that the bowel cleansing preparation is followed. The American Society of Gastrointestinal Endoscopy (ASGE) recommends emptying the bowel by ingesting clear liquids for 24 hours before the colonoscopy and using one of the following oral preparations: a large-volume polyethylene glycol (PEG) lavage solution (e.g., GoLYTELY), sodium phosphate liquid, or sodium phosphate pills.[42] Many people find the large-volume PEG lavage solution difficult to drink, and side effects include nausea and bloating. The sodium phosphate liquid and tablets are easier to swallow, but can cause fluid and electrolyte imbalance in patients with heart, kidney, and/or liver disease.

Acute Intervention

Preoperative Care. Acute nursing care for the patient with a colon resection is similar to care of the patient having a laparotomy (see p. 1046). If the cancer was resected and the ends were reanastomosed, bowel function is maintained and routine postoperative care is appropriate. Patients will need information about prognosis and future screening, and will need support dealing with the diagnosis of cancer. If formation of an ostomy is necessary, patients must be prepared as described below.

An abdominal-perineal resection results in closure of the anus and a permanent ostomy. These patients will likely need intense emotional support to cope with their prognosis and the radical change in body appearance and function. The patient should be taught side-to-side positioning. The nurse should teach and assist the patient in proper positioning for taking a sitz bath.

Postoperative Care. After an abdominal-perineal resection, there are two wounds, and a stoma. There is an abdominal incision through which the colon is resected, and an incision is made in the perineum. The management of a perineal incision differs depending on the type of wound. Three techniques are used: (1) packing of the entire open wound, (2) partial closure with Penrose drains for open drainage, and (3) primary closure of the perineal wound with closed-suction drainage of the pelvic cavity. The type of management of the perineal wound is individualized. The open and packed method is used in patients with extensive surgery or uncontrollable bleeding in the pelvic wound. When infection or contamination is minimal, a partial closure with drains is used. Low intermittent wall suction, a Jackson-Pratt drain, and Hemovac suction are commonly used to drain the operative site during the early postoperative period. Drains remain in place until drainage is less than 50 ml/24 hr, which usually occurs after 3 to 5 days.

A patient who has open and packed wounds requires meticulous postoperative care. The perineal dressing is reinforced and changed frequently during the first several hours postoperatively when drainage is likely to be most profuse. All drainage is carefully assessed for amount, color, and consistency. The drainage is usually serosanguineous.

The packing is usually left in place for 2 to 3 days because packing the pelvic cavity for prolonged periods may result in sepsis and rigidity of the cavity wall and thus impede the healing process. The nurse should examine the wound regularly and record bleeding, excessive drainage, and unusual odor. The perineal wound is usually irrigated with a normal saline solution when the dressings are changed. Dressings are changed several times a day, and aseptic technique is always used.

If the wound is partially closed and drains are in place, the nurse assesses the incision for suture integrity and signs and symptoms of wound inflammation and infection. The drainage is examined for amount, color, and characteristics. The area around the drain is observed for signs of inflammation and kept clean and dry. The nurse monitors for edema, erythema, and drainage around the suture line, fever, and elevated WBC count. If the perineal wound was not closed, warm sitz baths at 100.4° to 106° F (38° to 41° C) for 10 to 20 minutes three to four times a day assist in tissue debridement, provide comfort, and increase circulation to the area. Moist heat causes vasodilation, which allows more oxygen to flow to the affected area. Sitz baths of more than 20 minutes may result in too much vasodilation, causing congestion and discomfort.

The patient may complain of pain and itching in and around the wound, which are treated with antipruritic agents and sitz baths. Use of a pressure-reducing chair cushion provides comfort when sitting. Sitting on a toilet for prolonged periods is discouraged until the perineal wound is well healed.

The patient may experience phantom rectal sensation because the sympathetic nerves responsible for rectal control are not severed during the surgery. The nurse must be astute in distinguishing phantom sensations from perineal abscess pain.

Sexual dysfunction is a possible complication of an abdominal-perineal resection. Although the likelihood of sexual dysfunction depends on the surgical technique used, the surgeon should discuss the possibility with the patient. Members of the health care team should be available to address the patient's questions and concerns. Erection, ejaculation, and orgasm involve different nerve pathways, and a dysfunction of one does not mean complete sexual dysfunction. The ET nurse is an important source of information concerning sexual dysfunction resulting from an abdominal-perineal resection.

Ambulatory and Home Care. Psychologic support for the patient and family is important. The recovery period is long, and the cancer could return. The overall 5-year survival rate for all patients undergoing resection for colorectal cancer is greater than 55%.[43] Recurrent cancer is painful, debilitating, and demoralizing, and patients need much emotional support. (The special needs of the cancer patient are discussed in Chapter 16.) Issues surrounding end-of-life preparation and hospice need to be addressed (see Chapter 11).

The perineal wound may not be completely healed before discharge. After discharge the health care provider, the home health nurse, and the ET nurse in an outpatient clinic may be involved in wound management. The wound is usually irrigated and debrided. The skin around the wound should be assessed for loose hair. Shaving may be necessary to prevent the development of a chronic draining sinus. Continual drainage may indicate the presence of a foreign body, a fistula, or rectal tissue not removed during surgery. The patient and significant others are taught management of the wound and the procedure to take a sitz bath at home. The patient and the family should be aware of all community services available for assistance.

■ Evaluation

The expected outcomes for the patient with colorectal cancer are that the patient will have
- minimal alterations in bowel elimination patterns
- relief of pain
- balanced nutritional intake
- quality of life appropriate to disease progression
- feelings of comfort and well-being

OSTOMY SURGERY

Types

An **ostomy** is a surgical procedure that allows intestinal contents to pass from the bowel through an opening in the skin on the abdomen. The opening is called a **stoma.** The stoma is created when the intestine is brought through the abdominal wall and sutured to the skin. The intestinal contents then empty through the hole on the surface of the abdomen rather than being eliminated through the anus.

An ostomy is used when the normal elimination route is no longer possible. For example, if the person has colorectal cancer, the diseased portion must be removed together with a certain margin of healthy tissue. Sometimes the tumor can be resected, leaving enough healthy tissue to immediately *anastomose* (reconnect) the two remaining ends of healthy bowel, and no ostomy is necessary. If the tumor involves the rectum and is large enough to necessitate the removal of the anal sphincters, the anus is sutured shut and a permanent ostomy is created.

Patients with high risk for colorectal cancer, such as those with FAP, may have a total colectomy. As discussed earlier, patients with ulcerative colitis may also need to have a total proctocolectomy. In both situations, the surgeon will form an ileal pouch anal anastomosis if the anal sphincters are not diseased and can be left intact. If not, the person will need to have a permanent ileostomy.

Ostomies are described according to location and type (Fig. 43-11). An ostomy in the ileum is called an **ileostomy.** An ostomy in the sigmoid colon is called a **sigmoid colostomy.** An ostomy in the transverse colon is called a **transverse colostomy,** and so on. The more distal the ostomy, the more the intestinal contents resemble feces that is eliminated from an intact colon and rectum. Normally, water and electrolytes are reabsorbed from the feces as they pass through the colon. Since output from an ileostomy has never entered the colon, it will be liquid and the ileostomy will drain continually. A bag must be worn constantly over the ileostomy to collect the drainage. In contrast, output from a sigmoid colostomy will resemble normal formed stool and some patients are able to regulate emptying time so they do not need to wear a collection bag. (See Colostomy Irrigations later in this chapter.) A comparison of colostomies and ileostomies is shown in Table 43-30.

The major types of ostomies are end stoma, double-barreled, and loop ostomy.

End Stoma. An end stoma is surgically constructed by dividing the bowel and bringing out the proximal end as a single stoma. The distal portion of the GI tract is surgically removed, or the distal segment is oversewn and left in the abdominal cavity with its mesentery intact. An end colostomy or ileostomy is then constructed. When the distal bowel is oversewn rather than removed, the procedure is known as a Hartmann's pouch (Fig. 43-12). If the distal bowel is removed, the stoma is permanent. If the distal bowel remains intact and oversewn, the potential exists for the bowel to be reanastomosed and the stoma to be closed (referred to as a *takedown*).

Loop Stoma. A loop stoma is constructed by bringing a loop of bowel to the abdominal surface and then opening the anterior wall of the bowel to provide fecal diversion. This results in one stoma with a proximal and distal opening and an intact posterior wall that separates the two openings. The loop of bowel is frequently held in place with a plastic rod for 7 to 10 days after surgery to prevent it from slipping back into the abdominal cavity (Fig. 43-13). A loop stoma is usually temporary.

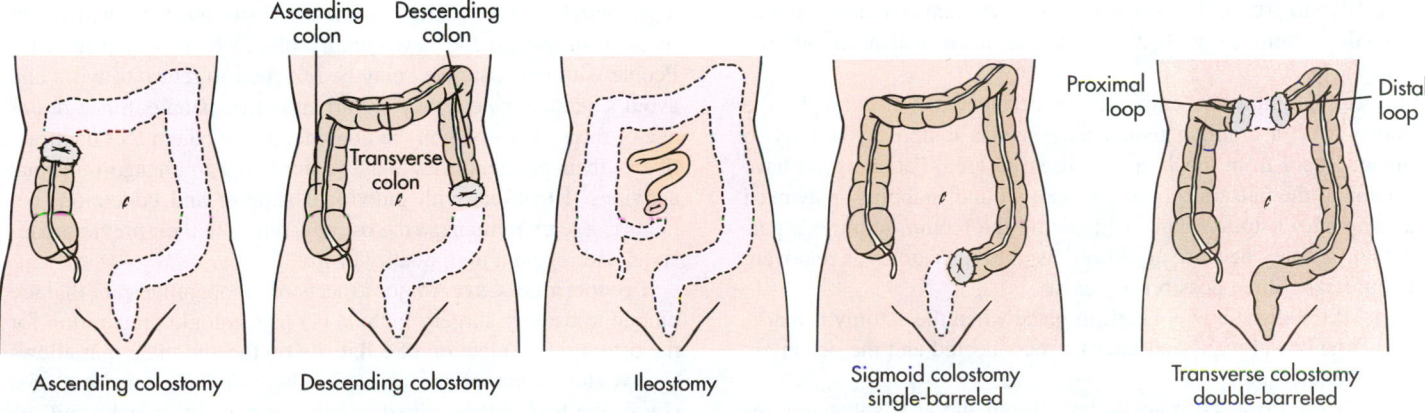

Ascending colon   Descending colon

Transverse colon

Proximal loop   Distal loop

Ascending colostomy   Descending colostomy   Ileostomy   Sigmoid colostomy single-barreled   Transverse colostomy double-barreled

FIG. 43-11   Types of ostomies.

TABLE 43-30	Comparison of Ileostomy and Colostomy			
		Colostomy		
	Ileostomy	**Ascending**	**Transverse**	**Sigmoid**
Stool consistency	Liquid to semiliquid	Semiliquid	Semiliquid to semiformed	Formed
Fluid requirement	Increased	Increased	Possibly increased	No change
Bowel regulation	No	No	No	Yes (if there is a history of a regular bowel pattern)
Pouch and skin barriers	Yes	Yes	Yes	Dependent on regulation
Irrigation	No	No	No	Possibly every 24-48 hr (if patient meets criteria)
Indications for surgery	Ulcerative colitis, Crohn's disease, diseased or injured colon, birth defect, familial polyposis, trauma, cancer	Perforating diverticulitis in lower colon; trauma; inoperable tumors of colon, rectum, or pelvis; rectovaginal fistula	Same as for ascending; birth defect	Cancer of the rectum or rectosigmoidal area; perforating diverticulum; trauma

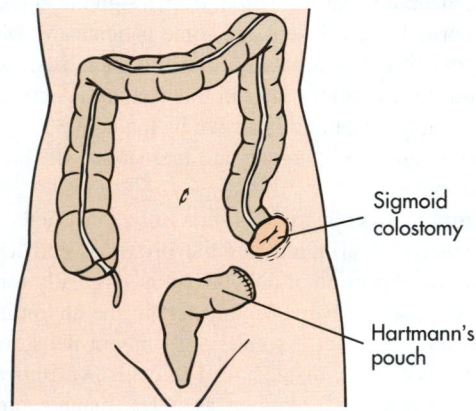

FIG. 43-12 Sigmoid colostomy. Distal bowel is oversewn and left in place to create Hartmann's pouch.

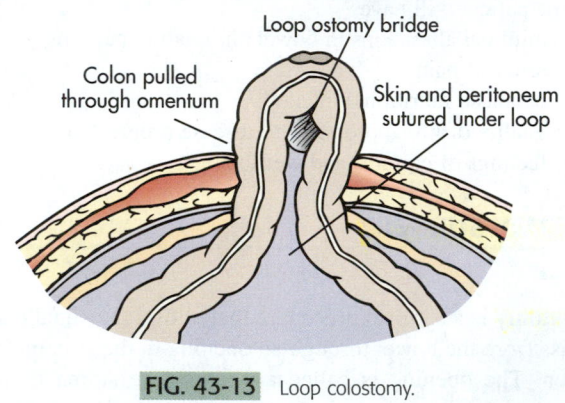

FIG. 43-13 Loop colostomy.

Double-Barreled Stoma. When the bowel is divided, both the proximal and distal ends are brought through the abdominal wall as two separate stomas (see Fig. 43-11). The proximal one is the functioning stoma; the distal, nonfunctioning stoma is referred to as the mucus fistula. The double-barreled stoma is usually temporary.

Kock Pouch. As described previously in this chapter (see p. 1056), the Kock pouch is a continent ileostomy, which is a variation from the traditional ileostomy (see Fig. 43-5).

Ileoanal Reservoir. As previously described in this chapter (pp. 1055 to 1056), this procedure involves total colectomy and ileoanal anastomosis with the formation of an ileal reservoir (see Fig. 43-4).

Ostomies may be temporary or permanent. For example, the person with a draining fistula may need a temporary ostomy to prevent stool from reaching the diseased area. Patients who have trauma to the intestines (e.g., gunshot wound, stabbing) may need a temporary ostomy. Cancer involving the rectum requires a permanent ostomy because all bowel distal to the ostomy is removed. In summary, three possibilities exist:

1. If the distal bowel is left in place when the ostomy is made, the bowel walls can later be reconnected and the ostomy is temporary.
2. If the distal bowel is removed, but the anal sphincters remain, an ileal pouch anal anastomosis is possible and the ostomy is temporary.
3. If the distal bowel and sphincters are removed, the anus will be sewn shut and the ostomy is permanent.

NURSING MANAGEMENT
OSTOMY SURGERY

Two major aspects of nursing care are (1) emotional support as the patient copes with a radical change in body image and (2) patient teaching about the many aspects of stoma care and the ostomy. Control of bowel elimination occurs by about age 2, and most people consider bowel elimination a private matter and the accompanying sounds and smells embarrassing. People with ostomies lose control over defecation and worry about odor and leakage of feces from around the bag. Quality of life is usually affected.[44] People with new ostomies may be reluctant to return to work and avoid situations where they are around other people. Since drainage of feces into a bag on the abdomen makes them feel unattractive to their partners, they may be unwilling to engage in sexual activities. However, with emotional support and education, patients can learn to manage the ostomy, return to their previous lifestyle, and regain a high quality of life.

Preoperative Care. Major aspects of preoperative care that are unique to ostomy surgery include (1) psychologic preparation for the ostomy; (2) selection of a flat site on the abdomen that allows secure attachment of the collection bag; and (3) selection of a stoma site that will be clearly visible to the patient who will be taking care of it. Psychologic preparation and emotional support are particularly important as the person copes with the change in body image, the loss of control over elimination, and the odors. Providing opportunities for patients to state their concerns and have questions answered in understandable terms enhances the patients' feelings of control and thus their ability to cope.

The Wound, Ostomy and Continence Nurses Society (WOCN) recommends that wound, ostomy, and continence (WOC) nurses (also called enterostomal therapy [ET] nurses) select the site where the ostomy should be positioned and mark the abdomen preoperatively. The surgeon uses these markings as a guideline, but may need to make adjustments based on the individual's internal anatomy. Criteria for site selection include that it lies "within the rectus muscle, is a flat, crease-free surface, and is in the patient's visual field."[45] Stomas placed outside the rectus muscle increase the chance of developing a hernia. A flat site makes it much easier to create a good seal and avoid leakage from the bag. Patients who cannot see the stoma are unable to care for it.

The family and the patient usually have many questions concerning the procedures. If available, an ET nurse should visit with the patient and the family. The ET nurse determines the patient's ability to perform self-care, identifies support systems, and determines potential adverse factors that could be modified to facilitate learning during rehabilitation. Preoperative assessment must be comprehensive and include physical, psychologic, social, cultural, and educational components. The patient and the family should understand the extent of surgery, the type of stoma, and its care.

If the patient desires a referral and the health care provider agrees, a trained ostomy visitor from the United Ostomy Association can provide psychologic support. The patient and family have an opportunity to see a person who has adjusted well to an ostomy and who has experienced some of the same feelings and concerns that they have.

Bowel preparations are used to empty the intestines before surgery to decrease the chance of a postoperative infection caused by bacteria in the feces. Nonabsorbable neomycin and erythromycin are given orally to decrease the number of intracolonic bacteria.

Postoperative Care. Postoperative nursing care includes assessment of the stoma and provision of an appropriate pouching system that protects the skin and contains drainage and odor. The nurse helps patients cope with the stoma and with the underlying disease that led to stoma formation; provides information; teaches practical stoma care techniques; and helps patients address issues surrounding social interactions, employment, body image, and sexuality.[44] The ET nurse is especially prepared to help the patient in these areas, but all nurses working with patients who have had ostomies should develop the knowledge and skills to help them.

The stoma should be pink. A dusky blue stoma indicates ischemia, and a brown-black stoma indicates necrosis. The nurse should assess and document stoma color every 8 hours. There is mild to moderate swelling of the stoma the first 2 to 3 weeks after surgery (Table 43-31). An appropriate pouching system is vital for protecting the skin and providing dependable drainage collection. The pouching system consists of a skin barrier and a bag or pouch to collect the feces. The skin barrier is a piece of pectin-based or karaya wafer that has a measurable thickness and hydrocolloid adhesive properties. The adhesion occurs in two phases. First, the wafer's backing has adhesive material that forms an immediate bond with the skin. Later, the hydrocolloids interface with the moisture on the skin to form a tighter seal. The skin barrier remains in place for about 5 to 7 days.[46] The length of adhesion depends on such factors as the strength of the seal and the

TABLE 43-31	Characteristics of Stoma
Characteristic	**Description or Cause**
Color*	
Rose to brick-red	Viable stoma mucosa
Pale	May indicate anemia
Blanching, dark red to purple	Indicates inadequate blood supply to the stoma or bowel from adhesions, low-flow state, or excessive tension on the bowel at the time of construction
Edema†	
Mild to moderate edema	Normal in the initial postoperative period
	Trauma to the stoma
	Any medical condition that results in edema
Moderate to severe edema	Obstruction of the stoma
	Allergic reaction to food
	Gastroenteritis
Bleeding	
Small amount	Oozing from the stoma mucosa when touched is normal because of its high vascularity
Moderate to large amount‡	Moderate to large amount‡ of bleeding from the stoma mucosa could indicate coagulation factor deficiency; stomal varices secondary to portal hypertension
	Moderate to large amount‡ of bleeding from intestinal stoma opening could indicate lower gastrointestinal bleeding

*Sustained color changes must be reported to surgeon.
†Closely observe and report to the surgeon and adjust the stoma opening size in the pouch.
‡Report moderate to large amounts of bleeding to surgeon.

amount of drainage from the stoma. If the abdominal stoma site has bends or creases, it is difficult to get a good seal and the skin barrier will pull away faster. Also, the weight of drainage from the stoma pulls the wafer away from the skin. For this reason, ostomy bags should be emptied when one third full.

The pouch must be compatible with the patient's abdominal contours. A flat pouch is used for a flat abdominal surface, and a convex pouching system is used when the stoma is located in a concave plane.[47] Pouches come as one- or two-piece systems. The one-piece system has the skin barrier attached, and the two-piece system allows removal of the pouch without removing the skin barrier. The skin should be washed with mild soap, rinsed with warm water, and dried thoroughly before the barrier is applied. Vigorous cleaning with strong soaps will damage the skin. A plasticizing skin sealant (e.g., Skin Prep) can be applied to the skin before the skin barrier to further protect the skin and improve adherence by increasing the skin's tackiness.[47]

With an open-ended, transparent, plastic, odor-proof pouch, it is easy to protect the skin and to observe and collect the drainage. The pouch must fit snugly to prevent leakage around the stoma. The size of the stoma is determined with a stoma-measuring card. Although the pouch is applied after surgery, the colostomy functions when peristalsis has been adequately restored. When a temporary colostomy is performed and the stoma is opened in the operating room with no bowel preparation being done previously, the stoma functions immediately.

The volume, color, and consistency of the drainage are recorded. Each time the pouch is changed, the condition of the skin is observed for irritation. A pouch should never be placed directly on irritated skin without the use of a skin barrier.

The patient should be able to perform a pouch change, provide appropriate skin care, control odor, care for the stoma, and identify signs and symptoms of complications. The patient should know the importance of fluids and a healthy diet, have names and addresses of the United Ostomy Association, and know when to seek health care. Home care and outpatient follow-up by an ET nurse is highly recommended. Patients should be discharged with written information about their particular ostomy, instructions for pouch changes, a list of supplies and where to purchase them (including names and phone numbers of retailers), outpatient follow-up appointments with the surgeon and ET nurse, and the phone numbers of the surgeon and nurse. The patient and family teaching guidelines are included in Table 43-32.

Teaching is often complicated by the emotional responses to the stoma. Emotional support, interventions from skillful ET nurses, and visits from people who have successfully learned to manage their ostomies will help patients learn to cope with and manage the new stoma.[48]

■ Colostomy Care

Nursing care for the patient with a colostomy is presented in NCP 43-3.

A colostomy in the ascending and transverse colon has semiliquid stools. The patient needs to be instructed to use a drainable pouch. A colostomy in the sigmoid or descending colon has semiformed or formed stools and can sometimes be regulated by the irrigation method. The patient may or may not wear a drainage pouch. A nondrainable pouch should have a gas filter.

A well-balanced diet and adequate fluid intake are important, and most patients with colostomies can eat anything they choose. However, dietary modifications are helpful for decreasing gas production and odor. Colonic bacteria act on certain poorly digested carbohydrates to form gas. Major gas-producing foods include beans, cabbage, cauliflower, brussels sprouts, broccoli, and asparagus. Potatoes, corn, noodles, and wheat also produce gas, but rice does not. The time between ingestion of gas-producing food and actual flatulence is 6 to 8 hours for the patient with a distal colostomy.[47] Table 43-33 lists foods and their effects on stoma output.

Colostomy Irrigations. Colostomy irrigations are used to stimulate emptying of the colon in order to achieve a regular bowel pattern. If control is achieved, there should be little or no spillage between irrigations. The patient who establishes regularity may need to wear only a pad or small pouch over the stoma. The patient who cannot or chooses not to establish regularity by irrigations must wear a pouch at all times. Regularity is only possible when the stoma is in the distal colon or rectum. Irrigations are not used for more proximal ostomies. The procedure for colostomy irrigation is presented in Table 43-34.

All equipment should be assembled before the irrigation. A commercially obtained irrigation set usually has all the equipment needed. The nurse should encourage the patient to watch the procedure and should explain each step to the patient. The cone tip on the tubing controls the depth of insertion and prevents the water from coming out from the stoma and not going into the colon. If resistance is met, force should not be used because perforation of the intestine can result. However, this is unlikely

TABLE 43-32	**PATIENT AND FAMILY TEACHING GUIDE** Ostomy Self-Care

Patients and their families must be able to do the following:
1. Explain what an ostomy is and how it functions.
2. Describe the underlying condition that resulted in the need for an ostomy.
3. Perform the following activities:
   - Remove the old skin barrier, cleanse the skin, and correctly apply new skin barriers.
   - Apply, empty, clean, and remove the pouch.
   - Empty the pouch before it is one third full to prevent leakage.
   - Irrigate the colostomy to regulate bowel elimination (optional).
4. Explain how to contact the enterostomal therapy nurse with questions.
5. Describe how to obtain additional ostomy supplies.
6. Explain dietary and fluid management.
   - Identify a well-balanced diet and dietary supplements to prevent nutritional deficiencies.
   - Identify foods to avoid to reduce diarrhea, gas, or obstruction (with ileostomy).
   - Drink at least 3000 ml/day of fluid to prevent dehydration (unless contraindicated).
   - Increase fluid intake during hot weather, excessive perspiration, and diarrhea to replace losses and prevent dehydration.
   - Describe symptoms of fluid and electrolyte imbalance.
   - Explain how to contact the registered dietitian with questions.
   - Explain how to recognize problems (fluid and electrolyte deficits, fever, diarrhea, skin irritation, stomal problems) and how to contact the appropriate health care provider.
7. Describe community resources to assist with emotional and psychologic adjustment to the ostomy.
8. Explain the importance of follow-up care.
9. Describe the ostomy's potential effects on sexual activity, social life, work, and recreation and strategies to manage these influences.

when using a stoma cone. A hard plastic catheter is not recommended because of the risk of intestinal perforation. The procedure should not be rushed; the patient should feel relaxed. The patient or family member must be instructed in the procedure and must be able to demonstrate how to do it. This can be done in the outpatient setting.

■ Ileostomy Care

Care of the ileostomy is presented in NCP 43-3. An ileostomy stoma protrusion of at least 1 to 1.5 cm makes care easier. When the stoma is flat, seepage occurs, resulting in altered skin integrity. Drainage is frequent and extremely irritating to the skin. Since regularity cannot be established, a pouch must be worn at all times. An open-ended, drainable pouch is preferable because drainage can be easily emptied. The drainable pouch is usually worn for 4 to 7 days before being changed unless leakage occurs. In that case, the pouch should be promptly removed, the skin cleansed, and a new pouch applied. A solid skin barrier should always be used. A transparent pouch should be used in the initial postoperative period to facilitate assessment of stoma viability and ease of pouch application by the patient.

The patient should be observed for signs and symptoms of fluid and electrolyte imbalance, particularly potassium, sodium, and fluid deficits. In the first 24 to 48 hours after surgery the amount of drainage from the stoma may be negligible. People with new ileostomies lose the absorptive functions provided by the colon and the delay provided by the ileocecal valve. As a result, they may experi-

NURSING CARE PLAN 43-3

Patient with a Colostomy/Ileostomy

NURSING DIAGNOSIS **Risk for impaired skin integrity** *related to* irritation from fecal drainage around peristomal area, irritation of appliance, and lack of knowledge of skin care

PATIENT GOAL Maintains intact, healthy skin around stoma

OUTCOMES (NOC)

Tissue Integrity: Skin and Mucous Membranes
- Tissue perfusion (stoma) _____
- Skin intactness _____
- Sensation _____

Measurement Scale
1 = Severely compromised
2 = Substantially compromised
3 = Moderately compromised
4 = Mildly compromised
5 = Not compromised

INTERVENTIONS (NIC) and *RATIONALES*

Ostomy Care
- Monitor stoma/surrounding tissue healing and adaptation to ostomy equipment *to initiate treatment if indicated.*
- Apply appropriately fitting ostomy appliance *to prevent drainage contact with skin.*
- Change/empty ostomy bag *to prevent drainage leakage onto the skin.*

Skin Care: Topical Treatments
- Use mild soap on the skin *to prevent irritation from intestinal contents or pouch adhesive.*
- Initiate consultation services of the enterostomal therapy nurse *to provide specialized care.*

NURSING DIAGNOSIS **Disturbed body image** *related to* presence of ostomy and malodor *as evidenced by* verbalization of embarrassment or shame due to malodor and presence of stoma and refusal to participate in care or look at or touch stoma

PATIENT GOALS   1. Verbalizes acceptance of changes in body appearance and function
2. Touches affected body part and participates in care of ostomy
3. Identifies methods to control ostomy odor

OUTCOMES (NOC)

Body Image
- Internal picture of self _____
- Congruence between body reality, body ideal, and body presentation _____
- Description of affected body part _____
- Willingness to touch affected body part _____
- Adjustment to changes in physical appearance _____
- Adjustment to changes in body function _____

Measurement Scale
1 = Never positive
2 = Rarely positive
3 = Sometimes positive
4 = Often positive
5 = Consistently positive

INTERVENTIONS (NIC) and *RATIONALES*

Body Image Enhancement
- Help patient determine the extent of actual changes in the body or its level of functioning *to assist with issues and misconceptions and plan appropriate interventions.*
- Monitor whether patient can look at the changed body part *to assess readiness to participate in self-care.*
- Assist patient to separate physical appearance from feelings of personal worth *to provide support and convey a sense of worth.*
- Facilitate contact with individuals with similar changes in body image *to provide realistic experiences of having an ostomy.*

Ostomy Care
- Instruct patient on mechanisms to reduce odor *to minimize embarrassing odors from drainage.*
- Instruct patient how to monitor for complications (e.g., mechanical breakdown, chemical breakdown, rash, leaks, dehydration, infection) *to prevent odors and functional problems of ostomy.*

Continued

---

ence a period of high-volume output of 1000 to 1800 ml per day when peristalsis returns. Later on, the average amount can be 500 ml daily because the proximal small bowel adapts. If the small bowel has been shortened as a result of surgical resections, the drainage from the ileostomy may be greater. The patient needs to increase fluid intake to 2 to 3 L of fluid daily, and pay particular attention to excessive fluid losses from heat and sweating. Patients must learn signs and symptoms of fluid and electrolyte imbalance so that they can take appropriate action. Because ileostomy output contains significant amounts of sodium and potassium, fluid intake should include sports drinks, not just water.

A low-fiber diet is ordered initially, and fiber-containing foods are reintroduced gradually. The ileostomy patient is susceptible to obstruction because the lumen is less than an inch in diameter and may narrow further at the point where the bowel passes through

the fascia/muscle layer of the abdomen. Foods such as popcorn, coconut, mushrooms, olives, stringy vegetables, foods with skins, dried fruits, and meats with casings must be chewed extremely well so that they are very small when swallowed.[47] The goal for the patient is a return to a normal, presurgical diet.

The stoma may bleed easily when it is touched because it has a high vascular supply. The patient should be told that minimal oozing of blood is normal. If the terminal ileum has been removed, the patient may need cobalamin treatment.

■ Adaptation to an Ostomy

Adaptation to the ostomy is a gradual process. The patient experiences a grief reaction from the loss of a body part and an alteration in body image. The adjustment period is unique to each individual. Psychologic support is needed during the grieving process. Pa-

NURSING CARE PLAN 43-3

Patient with a Colostomy/Ileostomy—cont'd

NURSING DIAGNOSIS   **Risk for deficient fluid volume** *related to* excess fluid loss from ileostomy or diarrhea with a colostomy and inadequate oral intake

PATIENT GOALS   1. Demonstrates no signs of hypovolemia
2. Maintains fluid and electrolyte balance

OUTCOMES (NOC)	INTERVENTIONS (NIC) and *RATIONALES*
Fluid Balance	**Hypovolemia Management**
• Blood pressure ____	• Observe for indications of dehydration (e.g., poor skin turgor, delayed capillary refill, weak/thready pulse, severe thirst, dry mucous membranes, decreased urine output, and hypotension) *to determine presence of fluid volume deficit and, if present, plan appropriate interventions.*
• Radial pulse rate ____	
• Peripheral pulses ____	
• Skin turgor ____	
• Moist mucous membranes ____	• Monitor fluid status including intake and output *to have an accurate record of fluid balance.*
• Serum electrolytes ____	
• 24-hour intake and output balance ____	• Encourage oral fluid intake (e.g., distribute fluids over 24 hr and give fluids with meals).
• Stable body weight ____	• Maintain steady IV infusion flow rate *to prevent dehydration.*
Measurement Scale	**Fluid/Electrolyte Management**
1 = Severely compromised	• Monitor for abnormal serum electrolyte levels *to detect any imbalances.*
2 = Substantially compromised	
3 = Moderately compromised	
4 = Mildly compromised	
5 = Not compromised	

NURSING DIAGNOSIS   **Ineffective sexuality patterns** *related to* perceived loss of sexual appeal and possibility of accidental seepage of fecal material during sexual activity *as evidenced by* verbalization of concern about intimate relations with spouse or significant other

PATIENT GOAL   Reports comfort with body in sexual activities

OUTCOMES (NOC)	INTERVENTIONS (NIC) and *RATIONALES*
Sexual Functioning	**Sexual Counseling**
• Expresses comfort with sexual expression ____	• Discuss the effect of the illness/health situation on sexuality *to determine if a problem exists and if there is a need to plan interventions.*
• Expresses self-esteem ____	
• Expresses comfort with body ____	• Encourage patient to verbalize fears and to ask questions to allow patient opportunity *to discuss sensitive topic in a nonthreatening situation.*
• Expresses ability to be intimate ____	
Measurement Scale	• Introduce patient to positive role models who have successfully conquered a similar problem *to discuss sexual concerns and share potential solutions, to provide an opportunity to ask questions, and to get practical, realistic answers from a supportive, understanding other.*
1 = Never demonstrated	
2 = Rarely demonstrated	
3 = Sometimes demonstrated	
4 = Often demonstrated	
5 = Consistently demonstrated	

tients have concerns about body image, sexual activity, family responsibilities, and changes in lifestyle. The patient may become resentful and have fears of odor or soiling. Supportive measures include encouraging patients to share their concerns and ask questions, providing information in a manner that is easily understood by patients, recommending support services, and helping patients develop confidence and competence in managing the stoma. The nurse provides support by responding to the physiologic needs of stoma care and the psychosocial need for self-esteem.

Activities of daily living are resumed within 6 to 8 weeks. Heavy lifting should be avoided. The patient's physical condition determines when sports may be resumed. Patients must know that they cannot participate in sports where direct trauma to the stoma is likely. Bathing and swimming may be done with or without the pouching system in place because water does not harm the stoma.

■ Sexual Dysfunction After Ostomy Surgery

Discussion of sexuality and sexual function must be incorporated in the plan of care. The nurse can help the patient understand that sexual function or sexual activity may be affected, but sexuality does not have to be altered.

Pelvic surgery can disrupt nerve and vascular supply to the genitals. Radiation therapy, chemotherapy, and medications can also alter sexual function. The overall physical health of the patient influences sexual desire. Generalized fatigue caused by illness can also influence desire. By communicating this information to patients, they can plan sexual activity around a drug schedule and energy levels. Any pelvic surgery that removes the rectum has the potential of damaging the parasympathetic nerve plexus. Erection in men depends on the parasympathetic nerves that control blood flow and vascular supply to the pelvis and the pudendal nerves that transmit sensory responses from the genital area. Nerve-sparing

NURSING CARE PLAN 43-3

Patient with a Colostomy/Ileostomy—cont'd

NURSING DIAGNOSIS   **Deficient knowledge of ostomy care** *related to* lack of exposure and unfamiliarity with information resources *as evidenced by* verbalization of lack of knowledge and inaccurate performance of care

PATIENT GOALS   1.   Describes the function of the ostomy and factors involved in the care and maintenance of the ostomy
2.   Demonstrates use of equipment and removal and application of ostomy appliance

OUTCOMES (NOC)

Knowledge: Ostomy Care
- Description of functioning of ostomy _____
- Description of skin care around ostomy _____
- Description of procedure to change/empty ostomy pouch _____
- Description of complications related to stoma/skin _____
- Description of diet modifications _____

Measurement Scale
1 = None
2 = Limited
3 = Moderate
4 = Substantial
5 = Extensive

INTERVENTIONS (NIC) and *RATIONALES*

Ostomy Care
- Instruct patient/significant other in the use of ostomy equipment and care.
- Have patient/significant other demonstrate use of equipment *to ensure proper technique for long-term care.*
- Instruct patient how to monitor for complications (e.g., mechanical breakdown, chemical breakdown, rash, leaks, dehydration, infection) *to obtain early treatment of complications.*
- Instruct patient/significant other in appropriate diet and expected changes in elimination function.
- Teach patient to chew thoroughly, avoid foods that caused digestive upset in the past, add new foods one at a time, and drink plenty of fluids *to help establish normal bowel patterns.*
- Encourage participation in ostomy support groups after discharge *to help patient learn to live with an ostomy.*

TABLE 43-33	*NUTRITIONAL THERAPY* Effects of Food on Stoma Output

Odor Producing*	Diarrhea Causing*
Eggs	Alcohol
Garlic	Beer
Onions	Cabbage family
Fish	Spinach
Asparagus	Green beans
Cabbage	Coffee
Broccoli	Spicy foods
Alcohol	Fruits (raw)
Gas Forming*	**Potential Obstruction in Ileostomy†**
Beans	Nuts
Cabbage family	Raisins
Onions	Popcorn
Beer	Seeds
Carbonated beverages	Vegetables (raw)
Cheeses (strong)	Celery
Sprouts	Corn

*The effect of food on stoma output is individual. Patients are not discouraged from eating the above-listed foods and beverages.
†Patients are encouraged to chew high-roughage food well and initially limit the amount, and to drink increased amounts of fluids.

TABLE 43-34	*PATIENT AND FAMILY TEACHING GUIDE* Colostomy Irrigation

Equipment
Lubricant
Irrigation set (1000- to 2000-ml container, tubing with irrigating stoma cone, clamp)
Irrigating sleeve with adhesive or belt
Toilet tissue to clean around the stoma
Disposal sack for soiled dressing

Procedure
1.   Place 500 to 1000 ml of lukewarm water (not to exceed 105° F [40.5° C]) in container. The volume is titrated for the individual; use enough irrigant to distend the bowel but not enough to cause cramping pain. Most adults use 500 to 1000 ml of water.
2.   Ensure comfortable position. Patient may sit in chair in front of toilet or on the toilet if the perineal wound is healed.
3.   Clear tubing of all air by flushing it with fluid.
4.   Hang container on hook or IV pole (18 to 24 inches) above stoma (about shoulder height).
5.   Apply irrigating sleeve and place bottom end in toilet bowl.
6.   Lubricate stoma cone, insert cone tip gently into the stoma, and hold tip securely in place.
7.   Allow irrigation solution to flow in steadily for 5 to 10 minutes.
8.   If cramping occurs, stop the flow of solution for a few seconds, leaving the cone in place.
9.   Clamp the tubing and remove irrigating cone when the desired amount of irrigant has been delivered or when the patient senses colonic distention.
10. Allow 30 to 45 minutes for the solution and feces to be expelled. Initial evacuation is usually complete in 10 to 15 minutes. Close off the irrigating sleeve at the bottom to allow ambulation.
11. Clean, rinse, and dry peristomal skin well.
12. Replace the colostomy drainage pouch or desired stoma covering.
13. Wash and rinse all equipment and hang to dry.

surgical techniques are used when possible to preserve sexual function. Radiation therapy to the pelvis can reduce blood flow to the pelvis by causing scarring in the small blood vessels. A woman's sexual functioning after healing includes expansion and lubrication of the vagina. Radiation therapy can affect vaginal expansion and lubrication. Pelvic surgery usually does not affect a woman's arousal unless part of or the entire vagina is removed. Muscle contraction and genital pleasure that occur during orgasm are not disrupted by pelvic surgery. If the sympathetic nerves in the male's presacral area are damaged, ejaculation may be disrupted. This can occur with an abdominal-perineal resection. Orgasms can occur in both men and women who have had stoma surgery, although other aspects of the sexual response may be affected.

The psychologic impact of the stoma and how it affects the patient's body image and self-esteem must be discussed. Emotional factors can contribute to sexual problems. A life-threatening illness can override concerns about sexual function. The nurse assists patients to identify ways of coping with depression and anxiety resulting from illness, surgery, or postoperative problems.

The social impact of the stoma is interrelated with the psychologic, physical, and sexual aspects. Concerns of people with stomas include the ability to resume sexual activity, as well as altering clothing styles, the effect on daily activities, sleeping while wearing a pouch, passing gas, the presence of odor, cleanliness, and deciding when or if to tell others about the stoma. The fear of rejection from a partner or the fear that others will not find him or her desirable as a sexual partner can be a concern. The nurse should encourage open communication about feelings and should realize that the patient needs time to adjust to the pouch and to body changes before feeling secure in his or her sexual functioning.

Although pregnancy is possible, the health care provider may recommend a limited number of pregnancies on the basis of the patient's physical condition. The person with an ostomy who becomes pregnant should have regular medical care.

DIVERTICULOSIS AND DIVERTICULITIS

A **diverticulum** is a saccular dilation or outpouching of the mucosa through the circular smooth muscle of the intestinal wall (Figs. 43-14 and 43-15). Clinically, diverticular disease covers a spectrum from asymptomatic, uncomplicated diverticulosis to diverticulitis with complications such as perforation, abscess, fistula, and bleeding.[49] Multiple noninflamed diverticula are present in diverticulosis. Diverticulitis is an infection of the diverticular sacs that is thought to be caused by obstruction with fecal matter.[50] In diverticulitis, inflammation of the diverticula occurs, which can result in perforation of one or more diverticula. Diverticula may occur at any point within the GI tract but are most commonly found in the sigmoid colon.

Etiology and Pathophysiology

Diverticular disease is a common disorder that affects 5% of the U.S. population by age 40 years and 50% by age 80 years.[50] Since most cases of diverticulosis are asymptomatic, it is difficult to calculate the true prevalence of the disease.[51]

Diverticula in the left (descending, sigmoid) colon are prevalent in Western populations, whereas diverticula in the right (ascending) colon occur more commonly in Asian populations and younger patients.[49] The etiology of diverticulosis of the ascending colon is unknown, but diverticula in the sigmoid colon are thought to be associated with high luminal pressures from a deficiency in dietary fiber intake and perhaps combined with a loss of muscle mass and collagen with the aging process. The disease is more prevalent in Western, industrialized populations that consume diets low in fiber and high in refined carbohydrates, and it is virtually unknown in areas of the world, such as rural Africa, where high-fiber diets are consumed. The incidence of diverticulosis rises with increasing age and is associated with obesity in people under age 40.[50]

When diverticula form, the smooth muscle of the colon wall becomes thickened. Lack of dietary fiber slows transit time, and

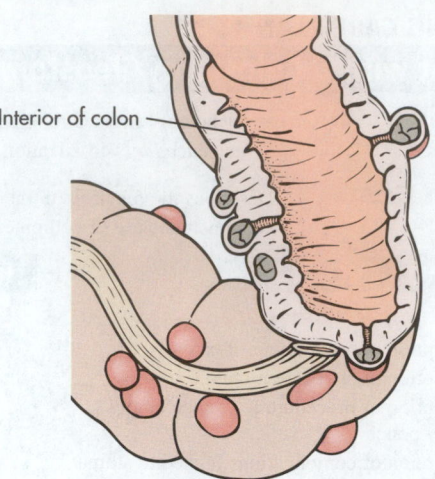

FIG. 43-14   Diverticula are outpouchings of the colon. When they become inflamed, the condition is diverticulitis. The inflammatory process can spread to the surrounding area in the intestine.

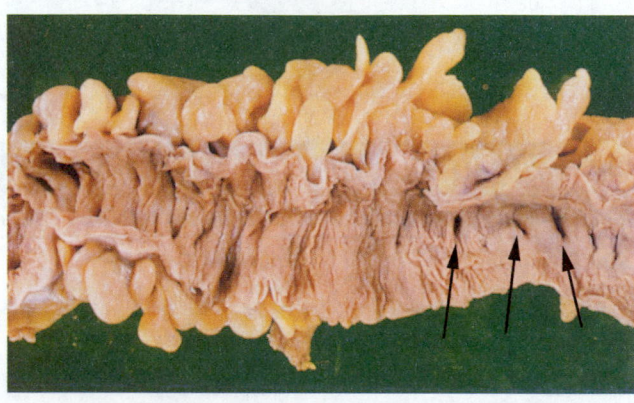

FIG. 43-15   In diverticular disease, the outpouches (*arrows*) of mucosa appear as slitlike openings from the mucosal surface of the open bowel.

more water is absorbed from the stool, making it more difficult to pass through the lumen. Decreased stool size raises intraluminal pressure, thus promoting diverticula formation. Diverticulitis results from retention of stool and bacteria in the diverticulum, forming a hardened mass called a *fecalith*. This causes inflammation and usually small perforations. Inflammation of the diverticulum spreads to the surrounding area in the intestines (Fig. 43-16), causing the tissue to become edematous.

Asymptomatic diverticular disease is typically diagnosed on routine sigmoidoscopy or colonoscopy. Symptomatic diverticular disease can be further broken down into painful diverticular disease and diverticulitis.

Clinical Manifestations

The majority of patients with diverticulosis have no symptoms. Those with symptoms typically have abdominal pain and/or changes in bowel habits, but no symptoms of inflammation.[49] Approximately 15% of patients with diverticulosis progress at some point to acute diverticulitis. In patients with diverticulitis, abdominal pain is localized over the involved area of the colon. The most common symptoms of diverticulitis in the sigmoid colon include left lower quadrant abdominal pain, fever, leukocytosis, and sometimes a palpable ab-

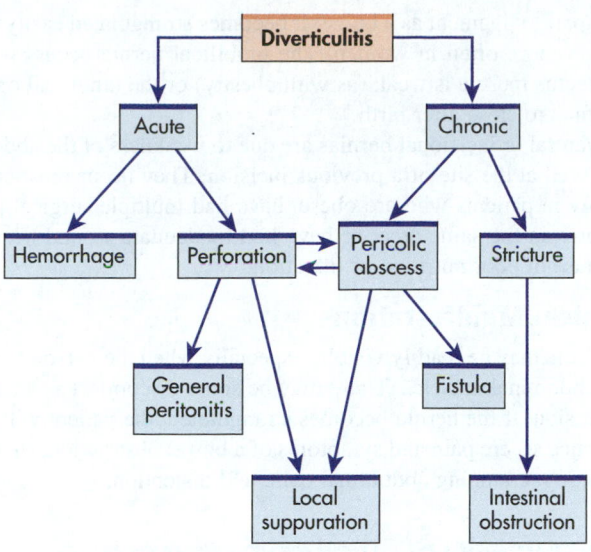

FIG. 43-16 Complications of diverticulitis.

TABLE 43-35	***COLLABORATIVE CARE*** **Diverticulosis and Diverticulitis**

Diagnostic
History and physical examination
Testing of stool for occult blood
Barium enema
Sigmoidoscopy
Colonoscopy
CBC
Urinalysis
Blood culture

Collaborative Therapy
Conservative Therapy
High-residue diet
Dietary fiber supplements
Stool softeners
Anticholinergics
Mineral oil
Bed rest
Clear liquid diet
Oral antibiotics
Bulk laxatives

Acute Care: Diverticulitis
Antibiotics
NPO status
IV fluids
Possible colon resection for obstruction or hemorrhage
Bed rest
NG suction

CBC, Complete blood count; *IV*, intravenous; *NG*, nasogastric; *NPO*, nothing by mouth.

dominal mass.[50] Elderly patients with diverticulitis may be afebrile, with a normal WBC count and little, if any, abdominal tenderness.

Complications of diverticulitis include perforation with peritonitis, abscess and fistula formation, bowel obstruction, ureteral obstruction, and bleeding. Bleeding can be extensive, but usually stops spontaneously. Diverticulitis is the most common cause of lower GI hemorrhage.[49]

Diagnostic Studies

Initial studies for suspected diverticulosis include a CBC, urinalysis, flat and upright radiographs of the abdomen, and physical examination.[50] Ultrasound and CT scan with contrast are then used to confirm the diagnosis and evaluate the severity of the disease (Table 43-35). A barium enema is used to determine narrowing or obstruction of the colonic lumen. A colonoscopy may be performed to rule out polyps or lesions. A patient with acute diverticulitis should not have a barium enema or colonoscopy because of the possibility of perforation and peritonitis.

NURSING *and* COLLABORATIVE MANAGEMENT
DIVERTICULOSIS AND DIVERTICULITIS

A high-fiber diet, mainly from fruits and vegetables, and decreased intake of fat and red meat are recommended for preventing diverticular disease. High levels of physical activity also seem to decrease the risk.[49] A high-fiber diet is also recommended once diverticular disease is present, although its benefits are unclear (see Table 43-9).

Weight reduction is important for the obese person. Increased intraabdominal pressure should be avoided because it may precipitate an attack. Factors that increase intraabdominal pressure are straining at stool, vomiting, bending, lifting, and tight, restrictive clothing.

In acute diverticulitis, the goal of treatment is to allow the colon to rest and the inflammation to subside. The patient is kept on NPO status and bed rest and is given parenteral fluids. The patient should be observed for signs of possible peritonitis. In acute diverticulitis, broad-spectrum antibiotic therapy is required. The WBC count is monitored. Frequently diverticulitis can be managed in an outpatient setting, and hospitalization is reserved for the elderly or those with severe symptoms.

When the acute attack subsides, oral fluids are given first and then the diet is progressed to semisolids. Ambulation is permitted. At this stage the patient should be observed for a recurrent attack. If the patient has a bowel resection or colostomy, the nursing care is the same as for these procedures.

Although diverticular disease is common, complications are rare. Bowel rest and antibiotic therapy are usually adequate. Surgery is reserved for patients with complications such as an abscess or obstruction that cannot be managed medically.[49] The usual surgical procedures involve resection of the involved colon with either a primary anastomosis if adequate bowel cleansing is feasible or a temporary diverting colostomy. The colostomy is reanastomosed after the colon heals.[50]

The patient should be provided with a full explanation of the condition. Patients who understand the disease process well and adhere to the prescribed regimen are less likely to experience an exacerbation of the disease and its complications.

HERNIAS

A **hernia** is a protrusion of a viscus through an abnormal opening or a weakened area in the wall of the cavity in which it is normally contained. A hernia may occur in any part of the body, but it usually occurs within the abdominal cavity. Hernias that easily return to the abdominal cavity are called reducible. The hernia can be reduced manually or may reduce spontaneously when the person lies down. If the hernia cannot be placed back into the abdominal cavity, it is known as irreducible, or incarcerated. In this situation the intestinal flow may be obstructed. When the hernia is irreducible and the intestinal flow and blood supply are

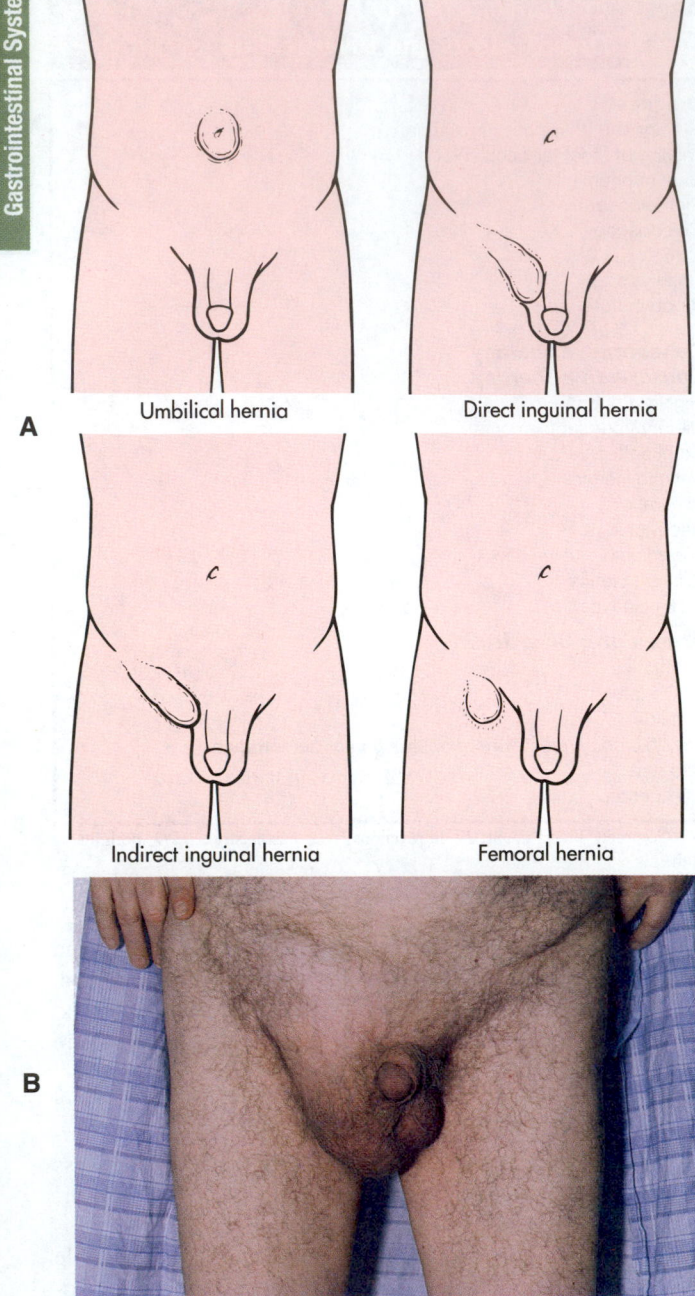

A

Umbilical hernia   Direct inguinal hernia

Indirect inguinal hernia   Femoral hernia

B

FIG. 43-17   A, Types of hernias. **B,** Indirect inguinal hernia.

obstructed, the hernia is strangulated. The result is an acute intestinal obstruction.

Types

The inguinal hernia is the most common type of hernia and occurs at the point of weakness in the abdominal wall where the spermatic cord in men and the round ligament in women emerge (Fig. 43-17). When the protrusion escapes through the inguinal ring and follows the spermatic cord or the round ligament, it is termed an *indirect hernia*. When it escapes through the posterior inguinal wall, it is a *direct hernia*. An inguinal hernia is more common in men.

A femoral hernia occurs when there is a protrusion through the femoral ring into the femoral canal. It occurs below the inguinal

(Poupart's) ligament as a bulge. It becomes strangulated easily and occurs more often in women. The umbilical hernia occurs when the rectus muscle is weak (as with obesity) or the umbilical opening fails to close after birth.

Ventral or incisional hernias are due to weakness of the abdominal wall at the site of a previous incision. They occur most commonly in patients who are obese, have had multiple surgical procedures in the same area, or have had inadequate wound healing because of poor nutrition or infection.

Clinical Manifestations

A hernia may be readily visible, especially when the person tenses the abdominal muscles. There may be some discomfort as a result of tension. If the hernia becomes strangulated, the patient will experience severe pain and symptoms of a bowel obstruction, such as vomiting, cramping abdominal pain, and distention.

NURSING *and* COLLABORATIVE MANAGEMENT
HERNIAS

Diagnosis is based on history and physical examination findings. Surgery is the treatment of choice for hernias and prevents strangulation. Treatment of hernias is by laparoscopic surgery. The surgical repair of a hernia is known as a *herniorrhaphy,* and is usually an outpatient procedure. The reinforcement of the weakened area with wire, fascia, or mesh is known as a *hernioplasty.* Strangulated hernias are treated immediately with resection of the involved area or a temporary colostomy so that necrosis and gangrene do not occur.

Some patients with hernias wear a truss, a pad placed over the hernia and held in place with a belt. The truss is worn to keep the hernia from protruding. If a patient wears a truss, the nurse should check for skin irritation caused by the continual rubbing of the truss against the skin.

After a hernia repair, the patient may have difficulty voiding. Therefore the nurse should observe for a distended bladder. An accurate intake and output record is important. Scrotal edema is a painful complication after an inguinal hernia repair. A scrotal support with application of an ice bag may help relieve pain and edema. Coughing is not encouraged, but deep breathing and turning should be done. If the patient needs to cough or sneeze, the incision should be splinted during coughing, and sneezing should be done with the mouth open. After discharge the patient may be restricted from heavy lifting for 6 to 8 weeks.

Malabsorption Syndrome

Malabsorption results from impaired absorption of fats, carbohydrates, proteins, minerals, and vitamins. The stomach, small intestine, liver, and pancreas regulate normal digestion and absorption. Digestive enzymes ordinarily break down nutrients so that absorption can take place through the intestinal mucosa and nutrients can get into the bloodstream. If there is an interruption in this process at any point, malabsorption may occur. Several problems can cause malabsorption (Table 43-36). They can be classified into malabsorption caused by (1) biochemical or enzyme deficiencies, (2) bacterial proliferation, (3) disruption of small intestine mucosa, (4) disturbed lymphatic and vascular circulation, or (5) surface area loss. Lactose intolerance is the most common malabsorption disorder, followed by IBD, celiac disease, tropical sprue, and cystic fibrosis.

GENDER DIFFERENCES

GENDER DIFFERENCES
Hernia

Men	Women
• Inguinal hernia is more common in men than in women. • The lifetime risk of developing a groin hernia is approximately 25% in men.	• Femoral hernia is more common in women (particularly older women) than in men. • The lifetime risk of developing a groin hernia is less than 5% in women.

TABLE 43-36	Common Causes of Malabsorption

Biochemical or Enzyme Deficiencies
- Lactase deficiency
- Biliary tract obstruction
- Pancreatic insufficiency
- Cystic fibrosis
- Chronic pancreatitis
- Zollinger-Ellison syndrome

Bacterial Proliferation
- Tropical sprue
- Parasitic infection

Small Intestinal Mucosal Disruption
- Celiac disease
- Whipple's disease
- Crohn's disease

Disturbed Lymphatic and Vascular Circulation
- Lymphoma
- Ischemia
- Lymphangiectasia
- Heart failure

Surface Area Loss
- Billroth II gastrectomy
- Short bowel syndrome
- Distal ileal resection, disease, or bypass

TABLE 43-37	Clinical Manifestations of Malabsorption

Manifestations	Pathophysiology
Gastrointestinal	
Weight loss	Malabsorption of fat, carbohydrates, and protein leading to loss of calories; marked reduction in caloric intake or increased use of calories
Diarrhea	Impaired absorption of water, sodium, fatty acids, bile, or carbohydrates
Flatulence	Bacterial fermentation of unabsorbed carbohydrates
Steatorrhea	Undigested and unabsorbed fat
Glossitis, cheilosis, stomatitis	Deficiency of iron, riboflavin, cobalamin, folic acid, and other vitamins
Hematologic	
Anemia	Impaired absorption of iron, cobalamin, and folic acid
Hemorrhagic tendency	Vitamin C deficiency Vitamin K deficiency inhibiting production of clotting factors II, VII, IX, and X
Musculoskeletal	
Bone pain	Osteoporosis from impaired calcium absorption Osteomalacia secondary to hypocalcemia, hypophosphatemia, inadequate vitamin D
Tetany	Hypocalcemia, hypomagnesemia
Weakness, muscle cramps	Anemia, electrolyte depletion (especially potassium)
Muscle wasting	Protein malabsorption
Neurologic	
Altered mental status	Dehydration
Paresthesias	Cobalamin deficiency
Peripheral neuropathy	Cobalamin deficiency
Night blindness	Thiamine deficiency Vitamin A deficiency
Integumentary	
Bruising	Vitamin K deficiency
Dermatitis	Fatty acid deficiency, zinc deficiency, niacin and other vitamin deficiencies
Brittle nails	Iron deficiency
Hair thinning and loss	Protein deficiency
Cardiovascular	
Hypotension	Dehydration
Tachycardia	Hypovolemia, anemia
Peripheral edema	Protein malabsorption, protein loss in diarrhea

The most common clinical manifestation of fat malabsorption is **steatorrhea** (bulky, foul-smelling, yellow-gray, greasy stools with putty-like consistency) (Table 43-37). Steatorrhea does not occur with lactose intolerance.

Screening tests available for malabsorption include qualitative examination of stool for fat (Sudan stain), a 72-hour stool collection for quantitative measurement of fecal fat, and the D-xylose absorption-excretion test, which is a good screening test for carbohydrate absorption. Other diagnostic studies include three different kinds of breath tests: (1) the bile acid breath test, which is used to evaluate bile salt malabsorption or malabsorption from bacterial overgrowth; (2) the triolein breath test, which measures carbon dioxide excretion after ingestion of a radioactive triglyceride; and (3) the excretion of breath hydrogen after ingestion of lactose, which is a sensitive, specific, and noninvasive test for detection of lactase deficiency. The rationale for the hydrogen breath test is that undigested lactose produces hydrogen when metabolized by bacteria in the colon and the hydrogen is excreted via the lungs.

A pancreatic secretion test may be performed to rule out pancreatic insufficiency. Endoscopy may be used to obtain a small bowel biopsy specimen for diagnosis. A small bowel barium enema is often performed to identify abnormal mucosal patterns. Capsule endoscopy can be used to assess the small intestine for malabsorption problems.

Laboratory studies that are frequently ordered include a CBC, measurement of prothrombin time (to see if vitamin K absorption is adequate), serum vitamin A and carotene levels, serum electrolytes, cholesterol, and calcium.

CELIAC DISEASE

Until recently, **celiac disease** was considered a relatively rare intestinal disease that began in childhood and was accompanied by symptoms of diarrhea, malabsorption, and malnutrition. It is now known that it is a common disease that occurs at all ages and can affect multiple body systems besides its primary site in the intestines.[52,53] Celiac sprue and gluten-sensitive enteropathy are other names for celiac disease.[53] It is not the same disease as tropical sprue, a chronic disorder acquired in tropical areas that is characterized by progressive disruption of jejunal and ileal tissue resulting in nutritional difficulties. Tropical sprue is treated with folic acid and tetracycline.

The incidence of celiac disease is thought to be anywhere from 1 in 1500 to 1 in 133 people.[53] Most patients with celiac disease are discovered during screening of high-risk groups.[54] High-risk groups include first- or second-degree relatives of someone with celiac disease and people with disorders associated with the disease. The mean age at diagnosis is the mid-40s. It is slightly more common in women, and symptoms often begin in childhood.[52]

Etiology and Pathophysiology

Three factors necessary for the development of celiac disease are genetic predisposition, gluten ingestion, and an immune-mediated response.[53] About 90% of patients with celiac disease have human leukocyte antigen (HLA) alleles HLA-DQ2, and the other 10% have HLA-DQ8. HLA type does not appear to influence the disease severity, and not everyone with these genetic markers develops the disease.[52]

As with other autoimmune diseases, the tissue destruction that occurs with celiac disease is the result of chronic inflammation. Inflammation is activated by the ingestion of gluten found in wheat, rye, and barley. A portion of the poorly digested gluten, called the gliadin fraction, makes its way from the small intestine's lumen into the lamina propria. Gliadin-containing molecules bind to specific receptors in the lamina propria and stimulate antibody production. The antibodies then activate the release of cytokines, including interferon, interleukin-4, and tumor necrosis factor. The cytokines destroy the microvilli and brush border of the small intestine. This ultimately decreases the amount of surface area available for nutrient absorption. Malabsorption can be so severe that the person develops malnutrition and wasting. Poor calcium and vitamin D absorption can lead to decreased bone density and osteoporosis. Poor nutrition leads to anemia and reproductive problems. The inflammation lasts as long as gluten ingestion continues. Treatment with a gluten-free diet halts the process.[53,54] Most patients recover completely within 3 to 6 months of treatment, but they need to maintain a gluten-free diet for life.[53]

If the disease is untreated and chronic inflammation continues unabated, epithelial cell proliferation at the area of destruction leads to crypt hyperplasia and reduced enterocyte differentiation. This process can lead to lymphoma.[53,54] Adenocarcinoma of the small intestine is also associated with celiac disease.[54]

Clinical Manifestations

Celiac disease was first recognized in infants who had symptoms of foul-smelling diarrhea, abdominal distention, anorexia, wasting, and failure to thrive that appeared at about the time the baby was started on cereal. Adults have different symptoms than the classical symptoms observed in infants. Diarrhea occurs in less than half of all patients with celiac disease. Some people have no symptoms, and the disease is only discovered during screening. Others have atypical symptoms such as decreased bone density and osteoporosis, dental enamel hypoplasia, iron and folate deficiencies, periph-

TABLE 43-38	*NUTRITIONAL THERAPY* Celiac Disease

Examples of Foods to Eat*
- Eggs
- Potatoes
- Butter
- Cheese, cottage cheese
- Meat, fish, poultry (not marinated or breaded)
- Yogurt
- Fresh fruits
- Tapioca
- Corn tortillas
- Flax, corn, and rice
- Soy products
- Gluten-free breads, crackers, pasta, and cereals
- Unflavored milk
- Peanut butter
- Coffee, tea, and cocoa

Examples of Foods to Avoid
- Wheat
- Barley
- Oats
- Rye
- Flour (unless it says gluten-free flour, or is made purely from a non-gluten source, such as rice flour)
- Baked goods, including muffins, cookies, cakes, pies
- Bread, including wheat bread, white bread, "potato" bread
- Pasta, pizza, bagels

*Food labels should be read to detect the presence of gluten stabilizers or ingredients that contain gluten.

eral neuropathy, and reproductive problems.[52,54] A vesicular skin lesion, dermatitis herpetiformis, is sometimes present. Celiac disease is also associated with autoimmune diseases, particularly rheumatoid arthritis, type 1 diabetes mellitus, and thyroid disease. The relationship between celiac disease and other autoimmune diseases is not well understood. However, rheumatoid arthritis symptoms have disappeared in some cases when patients switched to a gluten-free diet.[54]

Early diagnosis and treatment can prevent complications such as cancer (e.g., intestinal lymphoma), osteoporosis, and possibly other autoimmune diseases. Screening is recommended for close relatives of patients known to have the disease, young patients with decreased bone density, those with anemia once other causes are ruled out, and certain autoimmune diseases.[53]

Diagnostic Studies and Collaborative Care

Diagnosis of celiac disease is confirmed by histologic examination of biopsies taken from the duodenum and proximal small intestine. Serologic testing is available and offers good sensitivity and specificity. IgA tissue transglutaminase antibody, using human recombinant protein as the antigen, is currently considered the most reliable serologic test,[54] but a combination of serologic tests may be used.[53] False positives and false negatives are possible, so histologic evidence remains the gold standard for confirming the diagnosis. Biopsies show flattened mucosa and noticeable losses of villi.[53]

Celiac disease should be ruled out during a diagnostic workup of IBS, because the symptoms are similar. Many people spend years seeking treatment for nonspecific complaints before celiac disease is eventually diagnosed (thus the large number of people who are diagnosed in adulthood).

Celiac disease is treated with lifelong avoidance of dietary gluten (Table 43-38). Wheat, barley, oats, and rye products must be avoided. Although pure oats do not contain gluten, oat products can become contaminated with wheat, rye, and barley during the milling process. Gluten is also found in many food additives, preservatives, and stabilizers. A combination of corticosteroids and a gluten-free diet is used to treat individuals with refractory celiac disease who do not respond to the gluten-free diet alone. Maintenance of a gluten-free diet is difficult, particularly when traveling or eating in restaurants. The patient needs to know where to purchase gluten-free products. Patients may need referral for financial assistance, because gluten-free products are more expensive than regular foods. Gluten-free products are sold in health food stores and are available through various Internet sites. The Celiac Sprue Association website *(www.csaceliacs.org)* has recipes and suggestions for maintaining a gluten-free diet. The nurse needs to continuously encourage and motivate patients to continue the gluten-free diet. Patients need to know that the intestinal damage will recur unless they adhere to the diet and that chronic inflammation can lead to complications such as lymphoma.[53]

LACTASE DEFICIENCY

Lactase deficiency is a condition in which the lactase enzyme is deficient or absent. Lactase is the enzyme that breaks down lactose into two simple sugars—glucose and galactose. Primary lactase insufficiency is most commonly due to genetic factors. Certain ethnic or racial groups, especially those with Asian or African ancestry, develop low lactase levels at about age 5. Less common causes include low lactase levels due to premature birth and congenital lactase deficiency, a rare genetic disorder. Lactose malabsorption can also occur when conditions leading to bacterial overgrowth promote lactose fermentation in the small bowel, and when intestinal mucosal damage interferes with absorption.[55] Examples of disease in which the mucosa has been damaged include IBD, gastroenteritis, and celiac disease.

The symptoms of lactose intolerance include bloating, flatulence, cramping abdominal pain, and diarrhea. They may occur within a half hour to several hours after drinking a glass of milk or ingesting a milk product. The diarrhea of lactose intolerance results from fluid secretion into the small intestines, responding to the osmotic action of undigested lactose.

Many lactose-intolerant persons are aware of their milk intolerance and avoid milk and milk products. Lactose intolerance can be diagnosed by a lactose tolerance test or a lactose hydrogen breath test[55] (see p. 1079).

Treatment consists of eliminating lactose from the diet by avoiding milk and milk products and/or replacement of lactase with commercially available preparations. Milk and ice cream have much higher lactose content than cheese. Live culture yogurt is an alternative source of calcium, but the patient needs to be sure that milk products have not been added to the yogurt. A lactose-free diet is given initially and may be gradually advanced to a low-lactose diet as tolerated by the patient. The objective of care is to teach the importance of adherence to the diet. Many lactose-intolerant persons may not exhibit symptoms if lactose is taken in small amounts. In some persons, lactose may be tolerated better if taken with meals. Since avoidance of milk and milk products can

lead to calcium deficiency, supplements may be necessary to prevent osteoporosis. Lactase enzyme (Lactaid) is available commercially as an over-the-counter (OTC) product. It is mixed with milk and breaks down the lactose before the milk is ingested.

SHORT BOWEL SYNDROME

Short bowel syndrome (SBS) results from surgical resection, congenital defect, or disease-related loss of absorption. It is characterized by failure to maintain protein-energy, fluid, electrolyte, and micronutrient balances on a standard diet.[56] Resection of the small intestine may be necessary for bowel infarction because of vascular thrombosis or insufficiency, abdominal trauma, cancer, radiation enteritis, or Crohn's disease.

The length and portions of small bowel resected are associated with the number and severity of symptoms. Resections of up to 50% of the small intestine cause little disturbance of bowel function, especially if the terminal ileum and ileocecal valve remain intact. After large resections, the remaining intestine undergoes adaptive changes that are more pronounced in the ileum. The villi and crypts increase in size, and absorptive capacity of the remaining intestine increases. Intestinal adaptation is enhanced by the presence of food, fiber, bile, and pancreatic secretions in the lumen and continues for up to 2 years. Resection of the ileum, ileocecal valve, or colon results in a rapid intestinal transit and decreased absorption time. Ileal resection causes malabsorption of cobalamin, bile salts, and fat. This results in steatorrhea.

Clinical Manifestations

The predominant manifestations of SBS are diarrhea or steatorrhea. There may be signs of malnutrition and multiple vitamin and mineral deficiencies (e.g., weight loss, cobalamin and zinc deficiency, hypocalcemia). The patient may develop lactase deficiency and bacterial overgrowth. Oxalate kidney stones may form from increased colonic absorption of oxalate.

Collaborative Care

The overall goals are that the patient with SBS will have fluid and electrolyte balance, normal nutritional status, and control of diarrhea. In the period immediately following massive bowel resection, patients receive parenteral nutrition to replace fluid, electrolyte, and nutrient losses to rest the bowel. Proton pump inhibitors are used to decrease gastric acid secretion.

A diet high in carbohydrate and low in fat supplemented with soluble fiber, pectin, the amino acid glutamine, and parenteral growth hormone is often recommended. The patient with SBS is encouraged to eat at least six meals per day to increase the time of contact between food and the intestine. Oral intake can be supplemented with elemental nutrient formulas and tube feeding during the night. For patients with severe malabsorption, parenteral nutrition (see Chapter 40) may be reinstituted. Oral supplements of calcium, zinc, and multivitamins are typically recommended.

Opioid antidiarrheal drugs are the most effective in decreasing intestinal motility (see Table 43-3). For patients with limited ileal resections (<39 in [100 cm]), cholestyramine (Questran) reduces diarrhea resulting from unabsorbed bile acids and increases their excretion in feces. Bile acids stimulate intestinal fluid secretion and reduce colonic fluid absorption.

GASTROINTESTINAL STROMAL TUMORS

Gastrointestinal stromal tumors (GISTs) are the most common mesenchymal tumors in the GI tract. GISTs can involve the stomach, small intestine, or colon. Over half occur in the stomach and the upper small intestine. They are less likely to occur in the esophagus and rectum. Approximately 5000 persons are diagnosed with GISTs each year. At this time there are no known risk factors. However, a familial tendency is present in a small number of patients. These family members inherit a gene mutation that leads to GIST formation.[57]

The manifestations of GISTs depend on the part of the GI tract affected. Early signs and symptoms are often subtle, including early satiety and bloating. Later manifestations may include GI bleeding and obstruction caused by growth of the tumor. Often the GIST is found during evaluation (e.g., endoscopy, x-ray) for other problems such as colorectal or stomach cancer. The diagnosis of GIST is based on histologic examination of biopsied tissue. Endoscopic ultrasound can be used to determine the extent of the tumor.[58]

The main treatment of GIST is surgery. However, the GIST has often metastasized at the time of diagnosis. Targeted drug therapies include imatinib (Gleevec) and sunitinib (Sutent). Imatinib and sunitinib are not curative. The cancer often returns in a period of 2 to 5 years.[59] (Targeted drug therapies are discussed in Chapter 16.)

Anorectal Problems

HEMORRHOIDS

Hemorrhoids are dilated hemorrhoidal veins. They may be internal (occurring above the internal sphincter) or external (occurring outside the external sphincter) (Figs. 43-18 and 43-19). Symptoms of hemorrhoids include rectal bleeding, pruritus, prolapse, and pain. In affected persons, hemorrhoids appear periodically, depending on amount of anorectal pressure.

Etiology and Pathophysiology

Hemorrhoids are thought to develop as a result of shearing forces during defecation. This force damages supporting muscles. When supporting tissues in the anal canal weaken, usually as a result of straining at defecation, venules become dilated. In addition, blood flow through the veins of the hemorrhoidal plexus is impaired. An intravascular clot in the venule results in a thrombosed external hemorrhoid. Hemorrhoids are the most common reason for bleeding with defecation. The amount of blood lost at one time may be small but over time may lead to iron deficiency anemia. Hemorrhoids may be precipitated by many factors, including pregnancy, prolonged constipation, straining in an effort to defecate, heavy lifting, prolonged standing and sitting, and portal hypertension (as found in cirrhosis).

Clinical Manifestations

The classic symptoms of hemorrhoidal disease include bleeding, anal pruritus, prolapse, and pain. The patient with internal hemorrhoids may be asymptomatic. However, when internal hemorrhoids become constricted, the patient will report pain. Internal hemorrhoids can bleed, resulting in blood on toilet paper after defecation or blood on the outside of stool. The patient may report a chronic, dull, aching discomfort, particularly when the hemorrhoids have prolapsed.

External hemorrhoids are reddish blue and seldom bleed or cause pain unless a vein ruptures. Blood clots in external hemor-

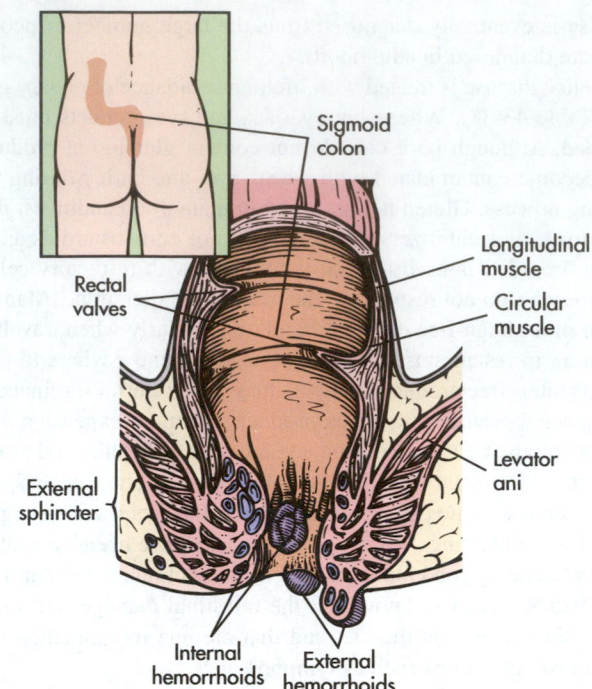

FIG. 43-18   Anatomic structures of the rectum and anus with external and internal hemorrhoids.

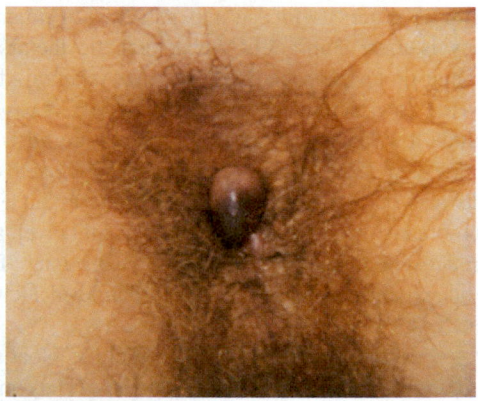

FIG. 43-19   Thrombosed external hemorrhoids.

rhoids cause pain and inflammation, and the hemorrhoids are described as thrombosed. External hemorrhoids cause intermittent pain, pain on palpation, itching, and burning. Patients also report bleeding associated with defecation. Constipation or diarrhea can aggravate these symptoms.

Diagnostic Studies and Collaborative Care

Internal hemorrhoids are diagnosed by digital examination, anoscopy, and sigmoidoscopy. External hemorrhoids can be diagnosed by visual inspection and digital examination. Therapy is directed toward the causes and the patient's symptoms. A high-fiber diet and increased fluid intake prevent constipation and reduce straining, which allows engorgement of the veins to subside. The resulting stool bulk may also decrease stool leakage and therefore itching. Ointments such as Nupercainal; creams, suppositories, and impregnated pads that contain antiinflammatory agents (e.g., hydrocortisone); or astringents and anesthetics (e.g., witch hazel, benzocaine) may be used to shrink the mucous membranes and relieve discomfort. The use of topical corticosteroids such as hydrocortisone agents should be limited to 1 week or less to prevent side effects such as contact dermatitis and mucosal atrophy.[60] Stool softeners may be ordered to keep the stools soft, and sitz baths help relieve pain.

External hemorrhoids are usually managed by conservative therapy unless they become thrombosed. For internal hemorrhoids, nonsurgical approaches (rubber band ligation, infrared coagulation, cryotherapy, laser treatment) can be used. Rubber band ligation is the most widely used technique. An anoscope is inserted so the hemorrhoid can be identified and then ligated with a rubber band. The rubber band around the hemorrhoid constricts circulation, and the tissue becomes necrotic, separates, and sloughs off. There is some local discomfort with this procedure, but no anesthetic is required. Aspirin or acetaminophen is usually given for discomfort. Infrared coagulation can be used to treat bleeding internal hemorrhoids. In this procedure, either infrared or electric current produces local inflammation. Cryotherapy involves rapid freezing of the hemorrhoid. Because this method can result in acute pain, it is used less often.

A hemorrhoidectomy is the surgical excision of hemorrhoids. Surgery is indicated when there is prolapse, excessive pain or bleeding, or large hemorrhoids. In general, hemorrhoidectomy is reserved for patients with severe symptoms related to multiple thrombosed hemorrhoids or marked protrusion. Surgical removal may be done by cautery, clamp, or excision. One surgical approach is to leave the area open so that healing takes place by secondary intention. In another approach the hemorrhoids are removed, the tissue is sutured, and wound healing takes place by primary intention.

NURSING MANAGEMENT
HEMORRHOIDS

Conservative nursing management for the patient with hemorrhoids includes teaching measures to prevent constipation, avoidance of prolonged standing or sitting, proper use of OTC drugs available for hemorrhoidal symptoms, and the need to seek medical care for severe symptoms of hemorrhoids (e.g., excessive pain and bleeding, prolapsed hemorrhoids) when necessary. Sitz baths (15 to 20 minutes) two to three times each day for 7 to 10 days may be helpful to reduce discomfort and swelling associated with hemorrhoids.

Pain caused by sphincter spasm is a common problem after a hemorrhoidectomy. The nurse must be aware that although the procedure is minor, the pain is severe. Opioids are usually given initially. Postoperatively, topical nitroglycerin preparations may be used to decrease pain and subsequent opioid use.

Sitz baths are started 1 to 2 days after surgery. A warm sitz bath provides comfort and keeps the anal area clean. A sponge ring in the sitz bath helps relieve pressure on the area. Initially, the patient should not be left alone because of the possibility of weakness or fainting.

Packing may be inserted into the rectum to absorb drainage. A T-binder may hold the dressing in place. If packing is inserted, it usually is removed on the first or second postoperative day. The nurse should assess for rectal bleeding. The patient may be embarrassed when the dressing is changed, and privacy should be provided. The patient usually dreads the first bowel movement and often resists the urge to defecate. Pain medication may be given before the bowel movement to reduce discomfort.

A stool softener such as docusate (Colace) is usually ordered for the first few postoperative days. If the patient does not have a bowel movement within 2 to 3 days, an oil-retention enema is given. Patients are taught the importance of diet, care of the anal area, symptoms of complications (especially bleeding), and avoidance of constipation and straining. Sitz baths are recommended for 1 to 2 weeks. The health care provider may order a stool softener to be taken for a time. Hemorrhoids may recur. Occasionally, anal strictures develop and dilation is necessary. Regular checkups are important in the prevention of any further problems.

ANAL FISSURE

An **anal fissure** is a skin ulcer or a crack in the lining of the anal wall that is caused by trauma, local infection, or inflammation. Fissures are considered either primary or secondary based on their etiology. Primary fissures usually occur as a result of local trauma associated with defecation or forced trauma such as rape. When there is high pressure in the internal anal sphincter, it can result in ischemia, which can lead to fissuring. Thus conditions that promote constipation are likely to be associated with fissure development. Secondary fissures are due to a variety of conditions, including IBD, prior anal surgery, infection (syphilis, tuberculosis, chlamydia, gonorrhea, herpes simplex virus), and human immunodeficiency virus infection.

The major symptoms are anal pain and bleeding. Pain is especially severe during and after defecation. Bleeding is bright red and usually slight. Constipation results because of fear of pain associated with bowel movements.

Anal fissures are diagnosed through physical examination. Conservative care with fiber supplements, adequate fluid intake, sitz baths, and topical analgesics is successful in about half of all cases, especially if the situation is acute.[61] Topical preparations, including nitroglycerin and calcium channel blockers, are used to decrease rectal anal pressure to allow the fissure to heal without sphincter damage. Local injections of botulin toxin have also been effective in some cases. Pain may be decreased by softening stools with mineral oil or stool softeners.[61] Warm sitz baths (15 to 20 minutes, three times/day) and anal anesthetic suppositories (Anusol) are also ordered.

A lateral internal sphincterotomy is the recommended surgical procedure when conservative treatment fails. Surgical treatment involves excision of the fissure. Problems with incontinence occur in a small number of patients following this procedure. Postoperative nursing care is the same as the care for the patient who has had a hemorrhoidectomy.

ANORECTAL ABSCESS

Anorectal abscesses are collections of perianal pus (Fig. 43-20). They are the result of obstruction of the anal glands, leading to infection and subsequent abscess formation. Abscess formation can occur secondary to anal fissures, trauma, or IBD. The most common causative organisms are *Escherichia coli,* staphylococci, and streptococci. Clinical manifestations include local pain and swelling, foul-smelling drainage, tenderness, and elevated temperature. Sepsis can occur as a complication. Anorectal abscesses are diagnosed by rectal examination.

Surgical therapy consists of drainage of abscesses. If packing is used, it should be impregnated with petroleum jelly, and the area should be allowed to heal by granulation. The packing is changed

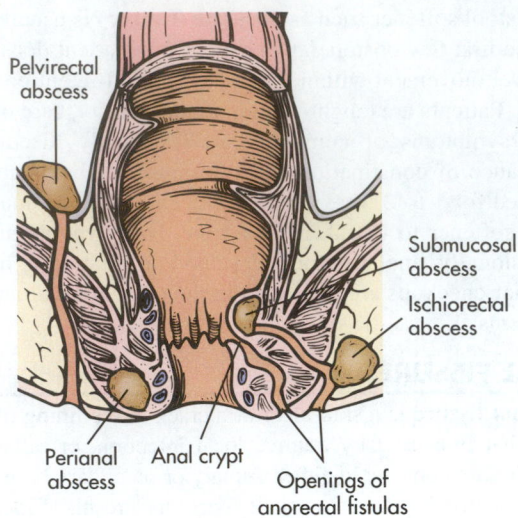

Pelvirectal abscess

Submucosal abscess

Ischiorectal abscess

Perianal abscess

Anal crypt

Openings of anorectal fistulas

FIG. 43-20 Common sites of anorectal abscesses and fistula formation.

every day, and moist, hot compresses are applied to the area. Care must be taken to avoid soiling the dressing during urination or defecation. A low-fiber diet is given. The patient may leave the hospital with the wound still open. Patient teaching includes wound care, the importance of sitz baths, thorough cleaning after bowel movements, and follow-up visits to a health care provider.

ANAL FISTULA

An **anal fistula** is an abnormal tunnel leading from the anus or rectum. It may extend to the outside of the skin, vagina, or buttocks and often precedes an abscess. Anal fistulas are a complication of Crohn's disease.

Feces may enter the fistula and cause an infection. There may be persistent, blood-stained, purulent discharge or stool leakage from the fistula. The patient may need to wear a pad to prevent staining of clothes.

Surgical therapy involves a fistulotomy or a fistulectomy. In a fistulotomy the fistula is opened, and healthy tissue is allowed to granulate. A fistulectomy is an excision of the entire fistulous tract. Gauze packing is inserted, and the wound is allowed to heal by granulation. Care is the same as that given after a hemorrhoidectomy.

PILONIDAL SINUS

A **pilonidal sinus** is a small tract under the skin between the buttocks in the sacrococcygeal area. It is thought to be of congenital origin. It may have several openings and is lined with epithelium and hair, hence the name *pilonidal* ("a nest of hair"). The skin is moist, and movement of the buttocks causes the short, wiry hair to penetrate the skin. The irritated skin becomes infected and forms a pilonidal cyst or abscess. There are no symptoms unless there is an infection. If it becomes infected, the patient complains of pain and swelling at the base of the spine.

The formed abscess requires incision and drainage. The wound may be closed or left open to heal by secondary intention. The wound is packed, and sitz baths are ordered.

Nursing care includes warm, moist heat applications when an abscess is present. The patient is usually more comfortable lying on the abdomen or side. The patient should be instructed to avoid contaminating the dressing when urinating or defecating and to avoid straining whenever possible.

CASE STUDY

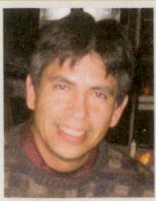

Colorectal Cancer

Patient Profile. Joseph Sandoval, a 58-year-old Native American, is from a Pueblo tribe in northern New Mexico. Mr. Sandoval's wife and family drove 50 miles to take him to the Indian Health Service Hospital because of his deteriorating health.

Subjective Data
- Complains of bright red bleeding during a bowel movement
- Family states that he has become thinner over the past several months and has little appetite
- Describes feeling weak and being easily fatigued; he appears ill
- Complains of abdominal pain and a feeling of fullness
- Bowel pattern has episodes of constipation followed by diarrhea
- No prior screening for colorectal cancer; family history of colorectal cancer is unknown

Objective Data

Physical Examination
- Temperature: 100.4° F (38° C)
- Heart rate is 110 beats/min; BP is 120/74 mm Hg
- Weight: 140 lb (63.6 kg); height: 5 feet 9 inches (172.5 cm)
- Mild palpation over transverse and descending colon elicits pain
- Digital rectal examination reveals a mass

Laboratory Tests
- Double-contrast barium enema shows two medium-sized tumors in the transverse colon
- Hematocrit (Hct): 26%
- Hemoglobin (Hb): 9 g/dl (90 g/L)

Critical Thinking Questions

1. What are the signs and symptoms of colorectal cancer that Mr. Sandoval manifests?
2. What is the significance of Mr. Sandoval's tachycardia?
3. What types of diagnostic information are available from a colonoscopy versus a double-contrast barium enema?
4. What nursing interventions are indicated for Mr. Sandoval at this stage of his illness?
5. What is the priority nursing intervention?
6. What is a culturally sensitive way for the nurse to support Mr. Sandoval and his family in making decisions about his continued health care?
7. Based on the assessment data, write one or more nursing diagnoses. Are there any collaborative problems?

NCLEX EXAMINATION REVIEW QUESTIONS

The number of the question corresponds to the same-numbered objective at the beginning of the chapter.

1. The appropriate collaborative therapy for the patient with acute diarrhea caused by rotavirus is to
   a. increase fluid intake.
   b. administer an antibiotic.

c. administer antimotility drugs.

d. quarantine the patient to prevent spread of the virus.

2. During the assessment of a patient with acute abdominal pain, the nurse should

a. perform deep palpation before auscultation.

b. obtain blood pressure and pulse rate to determine hypervolemic changes.

c. auscultate bowel sounds because hyperactive bowel sounds suggest paralytic ileus.

d. measure body temperature because an elevated temperature may indicate an inflammatory or infectious process.

3. The nurse would increase the comfort of the patient with appendicitis by

a. having the patient lie prone.

b. flexing the patient's right knee.

c. sitting the patient upright in a chair.

d. turning the patient onto his or her left side.

4. In planning care for the patient with Crohn's disease, the nurse recognizes that a major difference between ulcerative colitis and Crohn's disease is that Crohn's disease

a. frequently results in toxic megacolon.

b. causes fewer nutritional deficiencies than does ulcerative colitis.

c. often recurs after surgery, whereas ulcerative colitis is curable with a colectomy.

d. is manifested by rectal bleeding and anemia more frequently than is ulcerative colitis.

5. The nurse performs a detailed assessment of the abdomen of a patient with a possible bowel obstruction, knowing that a manifestation of an obstruction in the large intestine is

a. a largely distended abdomen.

b. diarrhea that is loose or liquid.

c. intermittent, colicky abdominal pain.

d. profuse vomiting that relieves abdominal pain.

6. A patient with metastatic colorectal cancer is scheduled for both chemotherapy and radiation therapy. Patient teaching regarding these therapies for this patient would include an explanation that

a. chemotherapy can be used to cure colorectal cancer.

b. radiation is routinely used as adjuvant therapy following surgery.

c. both chemotherapy and radiation can be used as palliative treatments.

d. the patient should expect few if any side effects from chemotherapeutic agents.

7. The nurse explains to the patient undergoing ostomy surgery that the procedure that maintains the most normal functioning of the bowel is

a. a sigmoid colostomy.

b. a transverse colostomy.

c. a descending colostomy.

d. an ascending colostomy.

8. In contrast to diverticulitis, the patient with diverticulosis

a. has rectal bleeding.

b. often has no symptoms.

c. has localized cramping pain.

d. frequently develops peritonitis.

9. A nursing intervention that is most appropriate to decrease postoperative edema and pain following an inguinal herniorrhaphy is

a. applying a truss to the hernia site.

b. allowing the patient to stand to void.

c. supporting incision during coughing.

d. applying a scrotal support with ice bag.

10. The nurse determines that the goals of dietary teaching have been met when the patient with celiac disease selects from the menu

a. scrambled eggs and sausage.

b. buckwheat pancakes with syrup.

c. oatmeal, skim milk, and orange juice.

d. yogurt, strawberries, and rye toast with butter.

11. Which of the following should a patient be taught after a hemorrhoidectomy?

a. Do not use the Valsalva maneuver.

b. Eat a low-fiber diet to rest the colon.

c. Administer oil-retention enema to empty the colon.

d. Use prescribed pain medication before a bowel movement.

REFERENCES

1. LaMont JT: Patient information: chronic diarrhea. Available at *www.uptodate.com/topic.asp* (accessed January 5, 2006).

2. Posani T: *Clostridium difficile:* causes and interventions, *Crit Care Nurs Clin North Am* 16:547, 2004.

3. Rao S: Pathophysiology of adult fecal incontinence, *Gastroenterology* 126:S14, 2004.

4. Scarlett Y: Medical management of fecal incontinence, *Gastroenterology* 126:S55, 2004.

5. Norton C: Behavioral management of fecal incontinence in adults, *Gastroenterology* 126:S64, 2004.

6. Lesbros-Pantoflickova D, Michetti P, Fried M, et al: Meta-analysis: the treatment of irritable bowel syndrome, *Aliment Pharmacol Ther* 20:1253, 2004.

7. Heitkemper M, Jarrett M: Overlapping conditions in women with irritable bowel syndrome, *Urologic Nurs* 25:25, 2005.

8. Baker DE: Rationale for using serotonergic agents to treat irritable bowel syndrome, *Am J Health Syst Pharm* 62:700, 2005.

9. Johanson JF: Options for patients with irritable bowel syndrome: contrasting traditional and novel serotonergic therapies, *Neurogastroenterol Motil* 16:201, 2004.

10. Tan G, Hammond DC, Gurrala J: Hypnosis and irritable bowel syndrome: a review of efficacy and mechanism of action, *Am J Clin Hypnosis* 47:161, 2005.

11. Blank-Reid C: Abdominal trauma: dealing with the damage, *Nursing* 34:36, 2004.

12. Bristow N: Treatment and management of acute appendicitis, *Nurs Times* 100:34, 2004.

13. Carlson D, Pfadt E: Perforated peptic ulcer, *Nursing* 32:88, 2004.

14. Hersh AS: Ensuring best practice in the treatment of peritonitis and exit site infection, *Nephrol Nurs J* 31:585, 2004.

15. Ohkusa T, Nomura T, Sato N: The role of bacterial infection in the pathogenesis of inflammatory bowel disease, *Intern Med* 43:534, 2004.

16. Mathew CG, Lewis CM: Genetics of inflammatory bowel disease: progress and prospects, *Hum Mol Genet* 13:R161, 2004.

17. Nayar M, Rhodes JM: Management of inflammatory bowel disease, *Postgrad Med J* 80:206, 2004.

18. Palascak-Juif V, Bouvier AM, Cosnes J, et al: Small bowel adenocarcinoma in patients with Crohn's disease compared with small bowel adenocarcinoma de novo, *Inflamm Bowel Dis* 11:828, 2005.

19. Lim W, Hanauer SB: Emerging biologic therapies in inflammatory bowel disease, *Rev Gastroenterol Disord* 4:66, 2004.

20. Broome U, Bergquist A: Primary sclerosing cholangitis, inflammatory bowel disease, and colon cancer, *Semin Liver Dis* 26(1):3, 2006.

21. Crohn's and Colitis Foundation of America, Inc: Available at *www.ccfa.org/research/info* (accessed July 28, 2006).

22. Hara AK, Leighton JA, Heigh RI, et al: Crohn disease of the small bowel: preliminary comparison among CT enterography, capsule endoscopy, small-bowel follow-through, and ileoscopy, *Radiology* 238:128, 2006.

23. Legnani P, Kornbluth A: Video capsule endoscopy in inflammatory bowel disease 2005, *Curr Opin Gastroenterol* 21:438, 2005.

24. Lim W, Hanauer SB: Controversies with aminosalicylates in inflammatory bowel disease, *Rev Gastroenterol Disord* 4:104, 2004.

25. De La Rue SA, Bickston SJ: Evidence-based medications for the treatment of the inflammatory bowel diseases, *Curr Opin Gastroenterol* 22(4):365, 2006.

26. Gionchetti P, Rizzello F, Morselli C, et al: Review article: problematic proctitis and distal colitis, *Aliment Pharmacol Ther* 20:93, 2004.

27. Sandborn WJ: New concepts in anti–tumor necrosis factor therapy for inflammatory bowel disease, *Rev Gastroenterol Disord* 5:10, 2005.

28. Heresbach D, Alexandre JL, Bretagne JF, et al: Crohn's disease in the over-60 age group: a population based study, *Eur J Gastroenterol Hepatol* 16:657, 2004.

29. Helton WS, Fisichella PM: Assessment of intestinal obstruction, *ACS Surgery: Principles and Practice.* Available at *www.medscape.com/viewarticle/482837* (accessed May 30, 2006).

30. Cappel MS: From colonic polyps to colon cancer: pathophysiology, clinical presentation, and diagnosis, *Clin Lab Med* 25(1):135, 2005.
31. Rowley PT: Inherited susceptibility to colorectal cancer, *Annu Rev Med* 56:539, 2005.
32. Forde KA: Colonoscopic screening for colon cancer, *Surg Endosc* 20(Suppl 2):S47, 2006.
33. Abdel-Rahman WM, Mecklin JP, Peltomaki P: The genetics of HNPCC: application to diagnosis and screening, *Crit Rev Oncol Hematol*, 2006 (accessed July 30, 3006).
34. Sansbury LB, Millikan RC, Schroeder JC, et al: Use of nonsteroidal anti-inflammatory drugs and risk of colon cancer in a population-based, case-control study of African Americans and whites, *Am J Epidemiol* 162:548, 2005.
35. Agrawal J, Syngal S: Colon cancer screening strategies, *Curr Opin Gastroenterol* 21:59, 2005.
36. Greenwald BA: Comparison of three stool tests for colorectal cancer screening, *Medsurg Nurs* 14:292, 2005.
37. American Cancer Society: Detailed guide: colon and rectum cancer. How is colorectal cancer staged? Available at *www.cancer.org/docroot/cri/content/cri* (accessed July 30, 2006).
38. Waterston AM, Cassidy J: Adjuvant treatment strategies for early colon cancer, *Drugs* 65(14):1935, 2005.
39. Zerey M, Burns JM, Kercher KW, et al: Minimally invasive management of colon cancer, *Surg Innovat* 13(1):5, 2006.
40. DeSalvo GL, et al: Curative surgery for obstruction from primary left colorectal carcinoma: primary or staged resection? Available at *http://gateway.ut.ovid.com/gw2/ovidweb.cgi* (accessed March 7, 2006).
41. Saltz LB: Metastatic colorectal cancer: is there one standard approach? *Oncology* 19:1147, 2005.
42. Faigel DO, Eisen GM, Baron TH, et al: Preparation of patients for GI endoscopy, *Gastrointest Endosc* 57:446, 2003.
43. Sample CB, Watson M, Okrainec A, et al: Long-term outcomes of laparoscopic surgery for colorectal cancer, *Surg Endosc* 20:30, 2006.
44. Brown H, Randle J: Living with a stoma: a review of the literature, *J Clin Nurs* 14:78, 2005.
45. Wound, Ostomy and Continence Nurses Society (WOCN) position statement. Available at *www.wocn.org/publications/posstate/pdf/stoma* (accessed March 24, 2006).
46. Turnbull BB: The evolution, current status, and regulation of ostomy products in the United States, *J WOCN* 28:18, 2001.
47. Doughty DB: Management of patients with colostomy or ileostomy. Available at *www.updodate.com* (accessed July 30, 2006).
48. O'Shea HS: Teaching the adult ostomy patient, *J WOCN* 28:47, 2001.
49. Kang J, Melville D, Maxwell JDL: Epidemiology and management of diverticular disease of the colon, *Drugs Aging* 21:211, 2004.
50. Whetsone D, Hazey J, Pofahl WE II, et al: Current management of diverticulitis, *Curr Surg* 61:361, 2004.
51. Janes S, Meagher A, Frizelle FA: Elective surgery after acute diverticulitis, *Br J Surg* 92:133, 2005.
52. Green PHR: The many faces of celiac disease: clinical presentation of celiac disease in the adult population, *Gastroenterology* 128:S74, 2005.
53. Young LS, Thomas DJ: Celiac sprue treatment in primary care, *Nurse Pract* 29:42, 2004.
54. Treem WR: Emerging concepts in celiac disease, *Curr Opin Pediatr* 16:552, 2004.
55. Chitkara DK, et al: Lactose intolerance. Available at *www.uptodate.com* (accessed July 30, 2006).
56. O'Keefe SJ, Buchman AL, Fishbein TM, et al: Short bowel syndrome and intestinal failure: consensus definitions and overview, *Clin Gastroenterol Hepatol* 4:6, 2006.
57. American Cancer Society: Available at *www.cancer.org/docroot/CRI/content/CRI* (accessed July 30, 2006).
58. Shinomura Y, Kinoshita K, Tsutsui S, et al: Pathophysiology, diagnosis, and treatment of gastrointestinal stromal tumors, *J Gastroenterol* 40:775, 2005.
59. Wu TJ, Lee LY, Yeh CN, et al: Surgical treatment and prognostic analysis for gastrointestinal stromal tumors (GISTs) of the small intestine: before the era of imatinib mesylate, *BMC Gastroenterol* 6:29, 2006.
60. Bleday R, Breen E: Treatment of hemorrhoids. Available at *www.uptodate.com* (accessed July 30, 2006).
61. American Gastroenterological Association Clinical Practice Committee: AGA guideline: diagnosis and care of patients with anal fissure, *Gastroenterology* 124:233, 2003.

RESOURCES

American Cancer Society
800-ACS-2345
www.cancer.org
American Gastroenterological Association
301-654-2055
Fax: 301-654-5920
www.gastro.org
Email: member@gastro.org
American Society for Gastrointestinal Endoscopy (ASGE)
630-573-0600
www.asge.org
Celiac Sprue Association
877-CSA-4CSA
Email: celiacs@csaciliacs.org
www.csaceliacs.org
Crohn's and Colitis Foundation of America (CCFA)
800-932-2423
Email: info@ccfa.org
www.ccfa.org
Crohn's and Colitis Foundation of Canada (CCFC)
800-387-1479 or 416-920-5035
Email: ccfc@ccfc.ca
www.ccfc.ca
International Ostomy Association
416-633-6783
www.ostomyinternational.org
Society of Gastroenterology Nurses and Associates
800-245-7462 or 312-321-5165
Email: sgna@smithbucklin.com
www.sgna.org
Wound, Ostomy and Continence Nurses Society
WOCN Society National Office
888-224-WOCN (9626)
www.wocn.org

For additional Internet resources, see the website for this book at *http://evolve.elsevier.com/Lewis/medsurg*.

He who dares to teach must never cease to learn.

Richard Henry Dann

Nursing Management
Liver, Pancreas, and Biliary Tract Problems

44

Margaret McLean Heitkemper, Anne Croghan, and Paula Cox-North

LEARNING OBJECTIVES

1. Define jaundice and describe signs and symptoms that may occur with the different types of jaundice.
2. Differentiate among the types of viral hepatitis, including etiology, pathophysiology, clinical manifestations, complications, and collaborative care.
3. Describe the nursing management of the patient with viral hepatitis.
4. Describe the pathophysiology, clinical manifestations, complications, and collaborative care of the patient with nonalcoholic fatty liver disease.
5. Explain the etiology, pathophysiology, clinical manifestations, complications, collaborative care, and nursing management of the patient with cirrhosis of the liver.
6. Describe the clinical manifestations and management of liver cancer.
7. Describe the pathophysiology, clinical manifestations, complications, and collaborative care of acute and chronic pancreatitis.
8. Describe the nursing management of the patient with pancreatitis.
9. Explain the clinical manifestations and collaborative care of the patient with pancreatic cancer.
10. Explain the pathophysiology, clinical manifestations, complications, and collaborative care, including surgical therapy, of gallbladder disorders.
11. Describe the nursing management of the patient undergoing conservative or surgical treatment of cholecystitis and cholelithiasis.

KEY TERMS

acute pancreatitis, p. 1118
ascites, p. 1104
asterixis, p. 1106
cholecystitis, p. 1126
cholelithiasis, p. 1126
chronic pancreatitis, p. 1124
cirrhosis, p. 1101
esophageal varices, p. 1104
gastric varices, p. 1104
hepatic encephalopathy, p. 1104
hepatitis, p. 1088
hepatorenal syndrome, p. 1106
jaundice, p. 1088
nonalcoholic fatty liver disease, p. 1101
paracentesis, p. 1107
portal hypertension, p. 1104
spider angiomas, p. 1102

Electronic Resources

Supplemental content related to Chapter 44 can be found . . .

Companion CD
- Stress-Busting Kit for Nursing Students
- Interactive Case Studies
  - Acute Pancreatitis
  - Cholelithiasis/Cholecystitis
  - Hepatitis
  - Postnecrotic Cirrhosis
- NCLEX Examination Review Questions
- Comprehensive Glossary

Evolve Website **evolve**
http://evolve.elsevier.com/Lewis/medsurg
- Content Updates
- Key Points (Printable and CD/MP3 Download)
- Concept Map Creator
- Expanded Audio Glossary
- Key Term Flash Cards

- Customizable Nursing Care Plans:
  - Acute Pancreatitis
  - Acute Viral Hepatitis
  - Cirrhosis
- Electronic Calculators
- WebLinks

Reviewed by Renee Pozza, RN, PhD, CNS, CFNP, Associate Professor/Associate Dean, School of Nursing, Azusa Pacific University, Azusa, Calif.; and Marian O'Rourke, RN, CCTC, Director, Transplant Administrator, Tulane Abdominal Transplant Institute, Tulane University Hospital and Clinic, New Orleans, La.

JAUNDICE

Jaundice, a yellowish discoloration of body tissues, results from an alteration in normal bilirubin metabolism or flow of bile into the hepatic or biliary duct systems. It is a symptom rather than a disease. Jaundice results when the concentration of bilirubin in the blood becomes abnormally increased. The bilirubin level has to be approximately three times the normal levels (2 to 3 mg/dl [34 to 51 mol/L]) for jaundice to occur. Jaundice can usually first be detected in the sclera and skin (Fig. 44-1).

Most of the body's bilirubin is formed from the breakdown of hemoglobin (from erythrocytes) by macrophages (see Fig. 39-6). This unconjugated (indirect) bilirubin is released into the circulation bound to albumin and is not water soluble. Because it is not water soluble and cannot be filtered by the kidneys, unconjugated bilirubin is not excreted in the urine. In the liver the unconjugated bilirubin is conjugated with glucuronic acid to form conjugated (direct) bilirubin, which is water soluble. Conjugated bilirubin is secreted into bile, which flows through the hepatic and biliary duct system into the small intestine. In the large intestine, bilirubin is converted to stercobilinogen and urobilinogen by bacterial action. Stercobilinogen gives the characteristic brown color to feces. Some urobilinogen is reabsorbed into the portal circulation and returned to the liver. Normally a very small amount of urobilinogen is excreted in urine.

The three types of jaundice are classified as hemolytic, hepatocellular, and obstructive. Diagnostic findings associated with these types of jaundice are shown in Table 44-1.

Hemolytic Jaundice

Hemolytic (prehepatic) jaundice is due to an increased breakdown of red blood cells (RBCs), which produces an increased amount of unconjugated bilirubin in the blood (see Table 44-1). The liver is unable to handle this increased load. Causes of hemolytic jaundice include blood transfusion reactions, sickle cell crisis, and hemolytic anemia.

Hepatocellular Jaundice

Hepatocellular (hepatic) jaundice results from the liver's altered ability to take up bilirubin from the blood or to conjugate or excrete it. Initially both unconjugated and conjugated bilirubin serum levels are increased (see Table 44-1). In hepatocellular disease the hepatocytes are damaged and leak bilirubin, thus increasing levels of conjugated bilirubin. In severe disease, both unconjugated and conjugated bilirubin are elevated as a result of both the inability of hepatocytes to conjugate bilirubin and continued cell leaking of conjugated bilirubin. As the number of unhealthy hepatocytes increases, the ability to conjugate bilirubin will eventually decrease. Because conjugated bilirubin is water soluble, it is excreted in the urine. The most common causes of hepatocellular jaundice are hepatitis, cirrhosis, and hepatic carcinoma.

Obstructive Jaundice

Obstructive (posthepatic) jaundice is due to decreased or obstructed flow of bile through the liver or biliary duct system. The obstruction may be intrahepatic or extrahepatic. Intrahepatic obstructions are due to swelling or fibrosis of the liver's canaliculi and bile ducts. This can be caused by damage from liver tumors, hepatitis, or cirrhosis. Causes of extrahepatic obstruction include common bile duct obstruction from a stone, biliary strictures, sclerosing cholangitis, and carcinoma of the head of the pancreas. Laboratory findings show an elevation of both unconjugated and conjugated bilirubin and urine bilirubin (see Table 44-1). Because bilirubin does not enter the intestines, there is decreased to no fecal or urinary urobilinogen. With complete obstruction, the stools are clay colored.

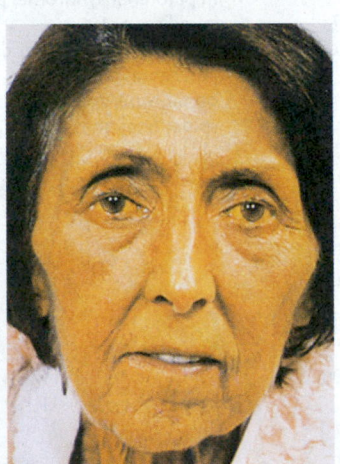

FIG. 44-1   Severe jaundice.

TABLE 44-1	**Diagnostic Findings in Jaundice**		
	Hemolytic	**Hepato-cellular**	**Obstructive**
Serum bilirubin			
Unconjugated (indirect)	↑	↑	Somewhat ↑
Conjugated (direct)	Normal	↑↓	Moderately ↑
Urine bilirubin	Negative	↑	↑
Urobilinogen			
Stool	↑	Normal to ↓	↓
Urine	↑	Normal to ↑	↓

Disorders of the Liver

HEPATITIS

Hepatitis is an inflammation of the liver. Viral hepatitis is the most common cause of hepatitis. The types of viral hepatitis are A, B, C, D, E, and G. Hepatitis may also be caused by drugs (including alcohol), chemicals (see Table 39-6), and autoimmune liver disease. Rarely, hepatitis is caused by bacteria, such as streptococci, salmonellae, and *Escherichia coli.*

Viral hepatitis is a major public health concern in the United States. Approximately 61,000 cases of hepatitis A occur annually in the United States, and 10 million cases occur worldwide. It is nearly universal during childhood in developing countries. Worldwide, nearly 400 million people are infected with the hepatitis B virus (HBV). Of these, approximately 50% to 75% have active viral replication (chronic infection). There are an estimated 73,000 new cases of hepatitis B annually in the United States. Starting in the 1990s and continuing today, the incidence of hepatitis B has decreased overall because of the widespread use of the HBV vaccine. Currently, 1.25 million Americans are chronically infected with HBV, 20% to 30% of whom acquired the infection in childhood.[1]

Worldwide, approximately 170 million people are infected with hepatitis C virus (HCV). In the United States approximately 4 million individuals have antibodies for HCV and 2.7 million are chronically infected. Most are unaware of their infection. Currently, an estimated 30,000 new cases are diagnosed annu-

CULTURAL AND ETHNIC HEALTH DISPARITIES

Disorders of the Liver, Pancreas, and Gallbladder

- Death from cirrhosis occurs more frequently among African Americans than in other ethnic groups.
- Primary liver cancer has a higher incidence among African Americans, Asian Americans, and Eskimos than whites.
- Pancreatic cancer occurs more frequently among African Americans and Asian Americans than whites.
- Whites and Native Americans have a higher incidence of gallbladder disease than African Americans or Asian Americans.

ally.[1] Approximately 20% of patients with chronic HCV will progress to cirrhosis within 20 to 30 years. It is estimated that 8000 to 10,000 individuals in the United States die each year from complications of end-stage liver disease secondary to chronic HCV.[2] The introduction of transfusion blood and blood product testing and safer needle-using practices by injection drug users have resulted in a drop in new cases since the late 1980s. However, because of the 15- to 20-year delay between infection and the clinical appearance of liver damage, it is likely that the long-term effects of HCV infection will pose important health care challenges for the next 20 years. Hepatitis B and C account for 80% of liver cancer cases today.

Persons at risk for HCV infection are also at risk for HBV and human immunodeficiency virus (HIV) infections. Co-infection of HCV and HIV is increasing. Approximately 30% to 40% of HIV-infected patients also have HCV. This high rate of co-infection is primarily related to intravenous (IV) drug use. When patients who are infected with HIV acquire HCV through IV drug use, the rate of HIV/HCV co-infection increases to 50% to 90%.[1] The presence of both HIV and HCV places the patient at greater risk for end-stage liver disease.

Etiology

Viral hepatitis can be caused by one of six major viruses: A, B, C, D, E, and G. Other viruses known to produce liver inflammation and damage include cytomegalovirus, Epstein-Barr virus, herpesvirus, coxsackievirus, and rubella virus.

The only definitive way to distinguish among the various forms of viral hepatitis is by the presence of the antigens and antigenic subtypes and the subsequent development of antibodies to them. Outbreaks of hepatitis are consistently caused by hepatitis A virus (HAV). Approximately 44% of acute viral hepatitis cases in the United States are hepatitis B, 19% are hepatitis C, and 37% are hepatitis A.[1] Infection with hepatitis A or B virus provides immunity to that virus *(homologous immunity)*. However, the patient can still develop another type of viral hepatitis. An individual with hepatitis C can be reinfected with another strain of hepatitis C. Characteristics of hepatitis viruses are summarized in Table 44-2.

Hepatitis A Virus. HAV is an RNA virus that is transmitted through the fecal-oral route. It frequently occurs in small outbreaks caused by fecal contamination of food or drinking water. HAV is found in feces 2 or more weeks before the onset of symptoms and up to 1 week after the onset of jaundice (Fig. 44-2). It is present in the blood only briefly. Anti-HAV (antibody to HAV) immunoglobulin M (IgM) appears in the serum as the stool becomes negative for the virus. Detection of IgM anti-HAV indicates

acute hepatitis, and IgG anti-HAV is an indicator of past infection. The presence of IgG antibody provides lifelong immunity.

The mode of transmission of HAV is predominantly fecal-oral (mainly by ingestion of food or liquid infected with the virus) and rarely parenteral. Poor hygiene, improper handling of food, crowded situations, and poor sanitary conditions are all factors related to hepatitis A. Transmission occurs between family members, institutionalized individuals, children in day-care centers, and from common-source outbreaks. The disease occurs more frequently in underdeveloped countries. Food-borne hepatitis A outbreaks are usually due to contamination of food during preparation by an infected food handler.

There is no chronic carrier state for HAV. The virus is present in feces during the incubation period, so it can be carried and transmitted by persons who have undetectable, subclinical infections. The greatest risk of transmission occurs before clinical symptoms are apparent. HAV can also be transmitted by patients with *anicteric* (nonjaundice) hepatitis A.

Hepatitis B Virus. HBV is a DNA virus that is transmitted perinatally by mothers infected with HBV; percutaneously (e.g., IV drug use, accidental needle-stick punctures); or horizontally by mucosal exposure to infectious blood, blood products, or other body fluids (e.g., semen, vaginal secretions, saliva). Transmission occurs when infected blood or other body fluids enter the body of a person who is not immune to the virus. Approximately 90% of infants infected at birth go on to develop chronic hepatitis B.[1,3] In persons who have HBV, hepatitis B surface antigen (HBsAg) has been detected in almost every body fluid, including vaginal secretions, menstrual fluids, semen, saliva, respiratory secretions, tears, gastric juice, synovial fluid, and cerebrospinal fluid. Infected semen and saliva contain much lower concentrations of HBV than blood, but the virus can be transmitted via these secretions. If gastrointestinal (GI) bleeding occurs, feces can be contaminated with the virus from the blood. There is no evidence that urine, feces (without GI bleeding), breast milk, tears, and sweat are infective. Organ and tissue transplantation is another potential source of infection. In 20% to 30% of patients with acute hepatitis B, there is no readily identifiable risk factor.[1]

Hepatitis B is a sexually transmitted disease. Approximately 30% of HBV cases are related to heterosexual activity (e.g., unprotected sex with an infected person). Male homosexuals (especially those practicing unprotected anal intercourse) are at risk for HBV infection. Although there is a much lower risk of transmission, kissing and sharing of food items may spread the virus via saliva. Other at-risk individuals include those who have household contacts with chronically infected persons, hemodialysis patients, and health care and public safety workers. The HBV can live on a dry surface for at least 7 days. HBV is much more infectious than HIV.

HBV is a complex structure with three distinct antigens: the surface antigen (HBsAg), the core antigen (HBcAg), and the e antigen (HBeAg). The persistence of HBsAg in the serum for 6 to 12 months or longer after infection with the virus indicates a carrier state of hepatitis B. Each antigen has a corresponding antibody that may develop in response to acute viral hepatitis B. These antibodies can be detected in the serum of persons with prior exposure to the virus (Fig. 44-3). The presence of hepatitis B surface antibody (anti-HBs or HBsAB) indicates immunity from the HBV vaccine or from past HBV infection.

Approximately 6% of those infected over age 5 develop chronic HBV. They become chronic HBV carriers and can transmit the virus.[1] In North America, approximately 0.5% of the population are HBV carriers; in parts of Asia, the rate is approxi-

Liver, Pancreas, Gallbladder

TABLE 44-2	Characteristics of Hepatitis Viruses

	Incubation Period	Mode of Transmission	Sources of Infection and Spread of Disease	Infectivity
Hepatitis A virus (HAV)	15-50 days (average 28)	Fecal-oral (fecal contamination and oral ingestion)	Crowded conditions (e.g., day care); poor personal hygiene; poor sanitation; contaminated food, milk, water, and shellfish; persons with subclinical infections; infected food handlers; sexual contact	Most infectious during 2 wk before onset of symptoms; infectious until 1-2 wk after the start of symptoms
Hepatitis B virus (HBV)	45-180 days (average 56-96)	Percutaneous (parenteral)/ permucosal exposure to blood or blood products Sexual contact Perinatal transmission	Contaminated needles, syringes, and blood products; sexual activity with infected partners; asymptomatic carriers Tattoo/body piercing with contaminated needles; bites	Before and after symptoms appear; infectious for 4-6 mo; in carriers continues for patient's lifetime
Hepatitis C virus (HCV)	14-180 days (average 56)	Percutaneous (parenteral)/ mucosal exposure to blood or blood products High-risk sexual contact Perinatal contact	Blood and blood products, needles and syringes, sexual activity with infected partners	1-2 wk before symptoms appear; continues during clinical course; 75%-85% go on to develop chronic hepatitis
Hepatitis D virus (HDV)	2-26 wk; HBV must precede HDV; chronic carriers of HBV are always at risk	Can cause infection only when HBV is present; routes of transmission same as for HBV	Same as HBV	Blood is infectious at all stages of HDV infection
Hepatitis E virus (HEV)	15-64 days (average 26-42 days)	Fecal-oral Outbreaks associated with contaminated water supply in developing countries	Contaminated water; poor sanitation; found in Asia, Africa, and Mexico; not common in United States and Canada	Not known; may be similar to HAV

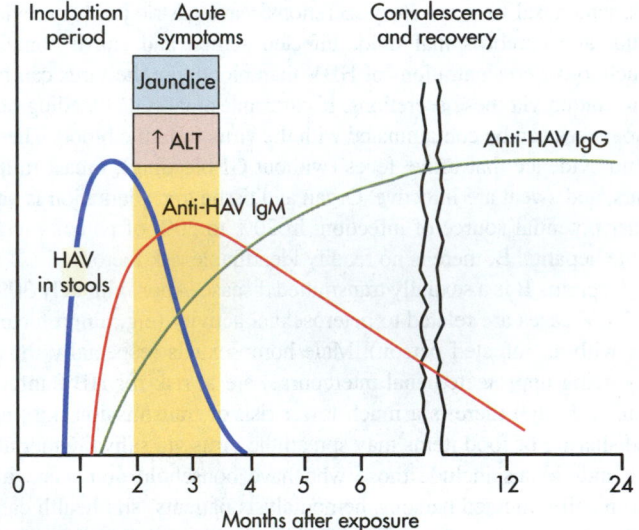

FIG. 44-2 Course of infection with hepatitis A virus (HAV). *ALT,* Alanine aminotransferase; *IgG,* immunoglobulin G; *IgM,* immunoglobulin M.

mately 8% to 10%.[3] The HBsAg level remains detectable in chronic carriers (HBsAg positive on at least two occasions at least 6 months apart). With chronic infection, liver enzyme values may be normal or elevated. Patients with chronic HBV may have a normal liver, low-grade disease, or severe liver disease. Approximately 15% to 25% of chronically infected persons die from chronic liver disease.[2,3]

Hepatitis C Virus. HCV is an RNA virus that is primarily transmitted percutaneously. In the United States and Canada, the most common mode of HCV transmission is the sharing of contaminated needles and paraphernalia among IV drug users. Transmission during blood transfusion has decreased, with trans-

mission occurring in less than 1 per 1 million blood transfusions. The proportion of cases attributed to high-risk sexual behavior (e.g., unprotected sex, multiple partners) has increased in recent years to 20%. However, sexual transmission among monogamous partners is rare. In the United States, 10% of all cases are due to occupational exposure, hemodialysis, and perinatal transmission.[1] Up to 10% of patients with HCV cannot identify a source. A reliable antibody test for HCV was not widely available until 1992. Therefore patients given blood or blood products before then are at risk for chronic HCV infection and should be tested. Additional data are needed regarding the risks of body piercings, tattooing, and intranasal (e.g., cocaine) drug use in the transmission of HCV.

Hepatitis D Virus. Hepatitis D virus (HDV), also called *delta virus,* is a defective single-stranded RNA virus that cannot survive on its own. HDV requires the helper function of HBV to replicate. It can be acquired at the same time as HBV, or a person with HBV can be infected with HDV at a later time. The importance of HDV relates to its clinical virulence. Patients with HBV-HDV co-infection may have more severe acute disease and a greater risk of fulminant hepatitis (2% to 20%) compared with those infected with HBV alone.[1] HDV is transmitted percutaneously, similar to HBV. There is no vaccine for HDV; however, vaccination against HBV reduces the risk of HDV co-infection.

Hepatitis E Virus. Hepatitis E virus (HEV) is an RNA virus that is transmitted by the fecal-oral route. The most common mode of transmission is drinking contaminated water. Hepatitis E occurs primarily in developing countries. There have been reported epidemics in India, Asia, Mexico, and Africa. Only a few cases have been reported in the United States, and these cases have been primarily in persons who had recently traveled to HEV-endemic areas. Currently, no serologic tests to diagnose HEV infection are commercially available in the United States. However, several di-

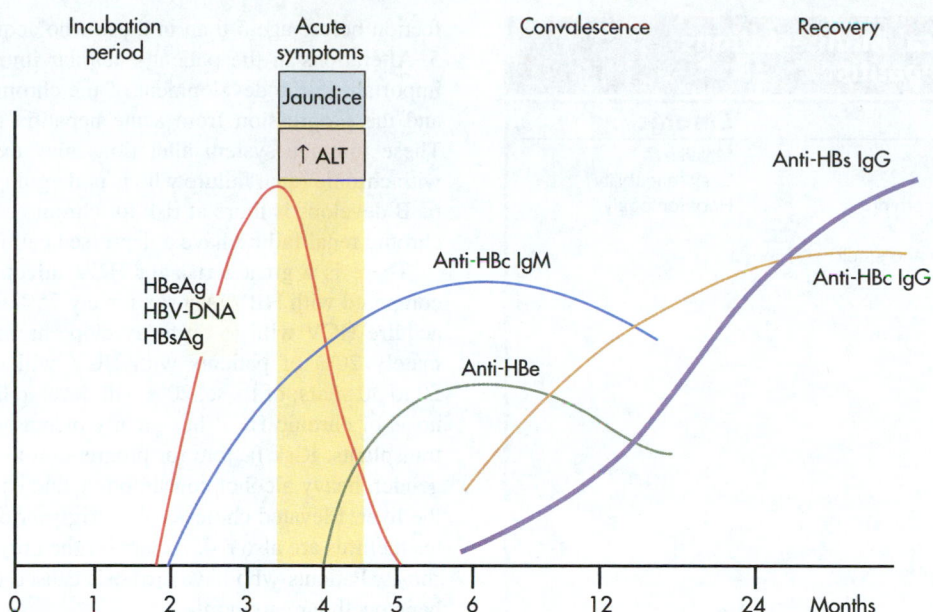

FIG. 44-3 Course of infection with hepatitis B virus (HBV). *ALT,* Alanine aminotransferase; *anti-HBc,* antibody to hepatitis B core antigen; *anti-HBe,* antibody to HBeAg; *anti-HBs,* antibody to HBsAg; *DNA,* deoxyribonucleic acid; *HBeAg,* hepatitis B e antigen; *HBsAg,* hepatitis B surface antigen; *IgG,* immunoglobulin G; *IgM,* immunoglobulin M.

agnostic tests are available in research laboratories to detect IgM and IgG anti-HEV in serum and HEV RNA levels.

Hepatitis G Virus. Hepatitis G virus (HGV) is a poorly characterized parenterally and sexually transmitted virus. HGV coexists with other viral infections, including HBV, HCV, and HIV, but does not appear to cause liver damage by itself.[4] HGV is an RNA virus. It has been found in some blood donors and can be transmitted by blood transfusion.

Pathophysiology

Liver. The pathophysiologic changes in the various types of viral hepatitis are similar. Hepatitis involves widespread inflammation of liver tissue. During acute infection, liver damage is mediated by cytotoxic cytokines and natural killer cells that cause lysis of infected hepatocytes. Liver damage results from hepatic cell necrosis. There is proliferation and enlargement of the Kupffer cells. Inflammation of the periportal areas may interrupt bile flow (cholestasis). With time, liver cells can regenerate in an orderly manner, and if no complications occur, they should resume their normal appearance and function.

Systemic Effects. The antigen-antibody complexes between the virus and its corresponding antibody form a circulating immune complex in the early phases of hepatitis. The circulating immune complexes activate the complement system (see Chapter 13). The clinical manifestations of this activation are rash, angioedema, arthritis, fever, and malaise. *Cryoglobulinemia* (abnormal proteins found in the blood), glomerulonephritis, and vasculitis have also been found secondary to immune complex activation.

Clinical Manifestations

A large number of patients have no symptoms. For example, 30% of patients with acute HBV and 80% of patients with acute HCV will be asymptomatic. For patients who are asymptomatic during the acute phase, the infection may not be detected. The clinical manifestations of viral hepatitis can be classified into acute and chronic phases (Table 44-3).

The acute phase usually lasts from 1 to 4 months. During the incubation period, symptoms may include malaise, anorexia, fatigue, nausea, occasional vomiting, and abdominal (right upper quadrant) discomfort. The anorexia is sometimes severe and may be due to cytokines or other chemicals produced by the infected liver. Weight loss may occur. The patient may find food repugnant and, if a smoker, may have distaste for cigarettes. There is also a decreased sense of smell. Other symptoms may include headache, low-grade fever, arthralgias, and skin rashes. Physical examination may reveal hepatomegaly, lymphadenopathy, and sometimes splenomegaly. This is the period of maximal infectivity for hepatitis A.

The acute phase may be icteric (symptomatic, including jaundice) or anicteric. Jaundice results when bilirubin diffuses into the tissues. The urine may darken because of excess bilirubin being excreted by the kidneys. If conjugated bilirubin cannot flow out of the liver because of obstruction or inflammation of the bile ducts, the stools will be light or clay colored. Pruritus sometimes accompanies the jaundice, especially if cholestasis is present. The pruritus occurs as a result of the accumulation of bile salts beneath the skin.

When jaundice occurs, the fever usually subsides. The GI symptoms usually remain, and some fatigue may continue. The liver is usually enlarged and tender. The convalescent phase following the acute phase begins as jaundice is disappearing and lasts for weeks to months, with an average of 2 to 4 months. During this period the patient's major complaint is malaise and easy fatigability. Hepatomegaly remains for several weeks, but splenomegaly subsides during this period. Relapses may occur.

Almost all cases of acute hepatitis A resolve, although a small number may have a viral relapse in the first 2 to 3 months after the infection. The disappearance of jaundice does not mean the patient has totally recovered. Many HBV infections and the majority of HCV infections result in chronic (lifelong) viral infection. Some patients may be asymptomatic. Others, however, may have intermittent or ongoing malaise, fatigue, myalgias, arthralgias, and hepatomegaly.

TABLE 44-3	Clinical Manifestations of Hepatitis

Acute	Chronic
Anorexia	Malaise
Nausea, vomiting	Easy fatigability
Right upper quadrant discomfort	Hepatomegaly
Constipation or diarrhea	
Decreased sense of taste and smell	
Malaise	
Headache	
Fever	
Arthralgias	
Urticaria	
Hepatomegaly	
Splenomegaly	
Weight loss	
Jaundice	
Pruritus	
Dark urine	
Bilirubinuria	
Light stools	
Fatigue	
Continued hepatomegaly with tenderness	
Weight loss	

General Considerations. Not all patients with viral hepatitis have jaundice. This is termed *anicteric hepatitis.* A high percentage of persons with HAV are anicteric and do not have symptoms.

There is some slight variation in manifestations between the types of hepatitis. In hepatitis A the onset is more acute, and the symptoms are usually mild and flu-like. In hepatitis B the onset is more insidious, and the symptoms are usually more severe. In hepatitis C the majority of cases are asymptomatic or mild. However, HCV has a high rate of persistence and often leads to chronic liver disease.

Complications

Most patients with acute viral hepatitis recover completely with no complications. The overall mortality rate for acute hepatitis is less than 1%. The mortality rate is higher in older adults and those with underlying debilitating illnesses (including chronic liver disease). Complications that can occur include fulminant hepatic failure, chronic hepatitis, cirrhosis of the liver, and hepatocellular carcinoma.

HAV infection can cause fulminant hepatic failure but does not cause chronic hepatitis. HBV can also cause fulminant hepatic failure and results in chronic infection in a small subset of those infected. Chronic HBV is identified by the persistence of HBsAg for longer than 6 months. Patients with chronic HBV are evaluated by assessment of liver function tests, HBV DNA (which measures the level of circulating HBV), and the presence of HBeAg and anti-HBeAg. A liver biopsy may be required to assess for the degree of inflammation and the presence and degree of fibrosis. Fibrosis may progress to cirrhosis in some patients. Chronic hepatitis B is a risk factor for the development of hepatocellular carcinoma with or without the evidence of cirrhosis.

It is not known what factors contribute to the persistence of the virus in some patients. Chronic HBV is more likely to develop in infants born to infected mothers and in those who acquire the in-fection before age 5 than in those who acquire the virus after age 5. Alterations in the patient's cellular immune response may be important in the development of the chronic HBsAg carrier state and the progression from acute hepatitis B to chronic hepatitis. These immune system alterations may explain why the patient with chronic renal failure who is undergoing dialysis when hepatitis B develops is more at risk for chronic hepatitis.[5] (Persons with chronic renal failure have a depressed cellular immune response.)

There is a greater risk for HCV infection to become chronic compared with HBV. Approximately 75% to 85% of patients who acquire HCV will go on to develop chronic infection.[1] Approximately 20% of patients with HCV will develop cirrhosis over 20 to 30 years; of these, 20% will develop liver failure.[6] The prognosis of chronic HCV has greatly increased the demand for liver transplants. Risk factors for progression to cirrhosis include male gender, heavy alcohol consumption, and excess iron deposition in the liver. Elevated cholesterol or triglycerides, obesity, and diabetes mellitus are also risk factors for the progression of HCV to cirrhosis. Patients who have cirrhosis caused by HCV are at risk for hepatocellular carcinoma.

Fulminant Hepatitis. *Fulminant viral hepatitis* results in severe impairment or necrosis of liver cells and potential liver failure. Fulminant viral hepatitis develops in a small percentage of patients. The disorder may occur as a complication of hepatitis B, particularly when it is accompanied by co-infection with HDV. Fulminant hepatitis occurs much less frequently with HCV. Toxic reactions to drugs and congenital metabolic disorders may also cause fulminant hepatitis and liver failure. Hepatocellular failure usually causes death unless liver transplant surgery is performed.

Diagnostic Studies

Tests for the different types of viral hepatitis are presented in Table 44-4. In viral hepatitis, many of the liver function tests show significant abnormalities. The common abnormalities are identified in Table 44-5.

Several tests are available to determine the presence of HCV. Unlike HAV and HBV, antibodies to HCV are not protective and may be an indicator of chronic disease. For the patient who has a positive anti-HCV antibody test by enzyme immunoassay, confirmatory testing is required. To detect active disease (the presence of circulating HCV), HCV RNA polymerase chain reaction (PCR) is performed. This may be particularly helpful in the immunocompromised patient (e.g., patient with HIV) whose antibody production is very low (below the detection level of the antibody tests). In addition, this test may be helpful in identifying the presence of the virus in exposed individuals (e.g., health care workers) before the development of antibodies. Initial testing for HCV includes HCV antibody testing followed by HCV-RNA testing to document viremia if antibody positive. A small number of patients may have a false-positive HCV antibody test. The HCV recombinant immunoblot assay (RIBA), which is a more sensitive antibody test, may be used.

There are 6 genotypes and more than 50 subtypes of HCV. In the United States, 75% of HCV infections are caused by HCV genotype 1, which, unfortunately, is less responsive to treatment than other HCV genotypes. Genotyping has been found to have an important role in managing infection. It is one of the strongest predictors of response to therapy and influences the duration of treatment.[7] Therefore for those patients who test positive for HCV, genotyping of the virus should be determined before drug therapy is started.

TABLE 44-4	**Tests for Viral Hepatitis**	
Virus	**Tests**	**Significance**
A	Anti-HAV IgM	Acute infection
	Anti-HAV IgG	Previous infection and long-term immunity or immunization
B	HBsAg (hepatitis B surface antigen)	Current infection (but not necessarily acute)*
		Positive in chronic carriers
	Anti-HBs (antibody to surface antigen)	Indicates previous infection with hepatitis B or immunization
		Marker of response to vaccine
	HBeAg (hepatitis B e antigen)	Indicates high infectivity; present in acute, active infection
	Anti-HBe (antibody to e antigen)	Indicates previous infection
	HBcAg (hepatitis B core antigen)	Ongoing infection with hepatitis B
	Anti-HBc IgM	Acute infection*
	Anti-HBc IgG (antibody to HB core antigen)	Indicates previous infection or ongoing infection with hepatitis B
		Does not appear after vaccination
	HBV DNA	Indicates active ongoing viral replication
		Best indicator of viral replication
	HBV genotyping	Indicates the genotype of HBV virus
C	Anti-HCV (antibody to hepatitis C)	Marker for acute or chronic infection with HCV
	Enzyme immunoassay (EIA)	Used in initial screening for HCV
	Recombinant immunoblot assay (RIBA)	More sensitive antibody test
	HCV RNA (RNA polymerase chain reaction [PCR] assay)	Indicates active ongoing viral replication
	HCV genotyping	Indicates the genotype of HCV virus
D	Anti-HDV	Present in past or current infection with hepatitis D
	HDV Ag (hepatitis D antigen)	Present within a few days after infection

A, Hepatitis A virus (HAV); *B*, hepatitis B virus (HBV); *C*, hepatitis C virus (HCV); *D*, hepatitis D virus (HDV); *DNA*, deoxyribonucleic acid; *RNA*, ribonucleic acid.
*If positive HBsAg and anti-HBc IgM, it indicates the presence of acute infection.

TABLE 44-5	**Diagnostic Findings in Acute Hepatitis**	
Test	**Abnormal Finding**	**Etiology**
Transaminases (aminotransferases)		
Aspartate aminotransferase (AST)	Increased in acute phase; decreases as jaundice disappears	Liver cell injury
Alanine aminotransferase (ALT)	Increased in acute phase; decreases as jaundice disappears	Liver cell injury
γ-Glutamyl transpeptidase (GGT)	Increased	Liver cell injury
Alkaline phosphatase	Moderately increased	Impaired excretory function of the liver
Serum proteins		
γ-Globulin	Normal or increased	Impaired clearance of the liver
Albumin	Normal or decreased	Liver cell damage
Serum bilirubin (total)	Increased to about 8-15 mg/dl (137-257 μmol/L)	Liver cell damage
Urinary bilirubin	Increased	Conjugated hyperbilirubinemia
Urinary urobilinogen	Increased 2-5 days before jaundice	Diminished reabsorption of urobilinogen
Prothrombin time	Prolonged	Decreased absorption of vitamin K in intestine with decreased production of prothrombin by liver

There are several known genotypes of HBV (e.g., A, B, C). In some centers HBV genotyping is performed before starting treatment. Early evidence suggests that similar to HCV genotyping, HBV genotype may be useful in predicting disease and treatment outcomes.

Physical assessment may reveal hepatic tenderness, hepatomegaly, and splenomegaly. The liver is palpable. A liver biopsy is not indicated in acute hepatitis unless the diagnosis is in doubt. In chronic hepatitis a liver biopsy may be done. Biopsy of liver tissue allows for histologic examination of liver cells and characterization of the degree of inflammation, fibrosis, or cirrhosis that may be present. A patient who has a bleeding disorder may not be an appropriate candidate for biopsy because of the risk of bleeding. In these patients a transjugular biopsy may be an option. Newer techniques (sonograms [Fibroscan]) provide information about the degree of liver scarring, which is sometimes referred to as "stiffness" of the liver.

Collaborative Care

There is no specific treatment or therapy for acute viral hepatitis. Most patients can be managed at home. Emphasis is on measures to rest the body and assist the liver in regenerating (Table 44-6). Adequate nutrients and rest seem to be most beneficial for healing and liver cell regeneration. Emphasis is placed on a well-balanced diet that the patient can tolerate. Rest reduces the metabolic demands on the liver and promotes cell regeneration. Bed rest may be indicated while the patient is symptomatic. The degree of rest ordered depends on the severity of symptoms, but usually alternating periods of activity and rest are adequate. Counseling should include the importance of avoiding alcohol and notification of possible contacts for testing and prophylaxis, if indicated.

Drug Therapy. There are no specific drug therapies for the treatment of acute viral hepatitis. Supportive drug therapy may in-

TABLE 44-6	COLLABORATIVE CARE Viral Hepatitis

Diagnostic
History and physical examination
Liver function studies
    Alanine aminotransferase (ALT)
    Aspartate aminotransferase (AST)
Hepatitis testing
    Anti-HAV—IgM and IgG
    HBsAg
    HBeAg
    Anti-HBs
    Anti-HBc—IgM and IgG
    HBV DNA
    Anti-HCV
    HCV RNA
    Anti-HDV

Collaborative Therapy
Acute and Chronic
High-calorie, high-protein, high-carbohydrate, low-fat diet
Vitamin supplements
Rest—degree of strictness varies
Avoid alcohol intake and drugs detoxified by the liver

Chronic HBV
Pegylated α-interferon (PEG-Intron, Pegasys)
lamivudine (Epivir)
adefovir (Hepsera)
entecavir (Baraclude)
telbivudine (Tyzeka)

Chronic HCV
Pegylated α-interferon (PEG-Intron, Pegasys)
ribavirin (Rebetol, Copegus)

DNA, Deoxyribonucleic acid; *HAV,* hepatitis A virus; *HB,* hepatitis B; *HBeAg,* hepatitis B e antigen; *HBsAg,* hepatitis B surface antigen; *HBV,* hepatitis B virus; *HCV,* hepatitis C virus; *HDV,* hepatitis D virus; *RNA,* ribonucleic acid.

TABLE 44-7	DRUG THERAPY Side Effects of α-Interferon and Ribavirin

α-Interferon	Ribavirin
Flu-like Symptoms	Anemia (hemolytic)
Arthralgia/myalgia	Anorexia
Asthenia (loss of strength)	Cough
Fatigue	Dyspnea
Headache	Insomnia
Fever	Pruritus
Nausea/anorexia	Rash
	Teratogenicity (interferes with
Other Effects	normal fetal development)
Depression or irritability	
Hair thinning	
Insomnia	
Itching/dry skin	
Diarrhea	
Weight loss	
Injection-site reaction	

The long-acting preparations are made by conjugating a conventional interferon with polyethylene glycol (PEG), in a process known as *pegylation.* Therapeutic effects of the pegylated product are due solely to its interferon component. The PEG component serves only to delay elimination of the drug. At this time, two long-acting interferons are available: Pegasys and PEG-Intron. Because of their convenience and superior efficacy, these products are preferred to conventional interferon.

Of those receiving α-interferon, one third will have a significant reduction of serum HBV DNA levels, normalization of ALT levels, and loss of HBV e antigen (HBeAg).[8,9] However, α-interferon treatment is associated with a number of side effects (Table 44-7). These side effects are dose related and tend to decrease in severity with continued treatment.

Nucleoside Analogs. Lamivudine (Epivir), adefovir (Hepsera), entecavir (Baraclude), and telbivudine (Tyzeka) are used in the treatment of chronic HBV when there is evidence of active viral replication. These drugs suppress HBV replication by inhibiting viral DNA synthesis. Lamivudine is taken orally for 1 year. It has beneficial effects in terms of reducing viral load, decreasing liver damage, and decreasing liver enzymes. However, *seroconversion* (loss of HBeAg) occurs in less than 17% to 27% of patients.[9,10]

Drug Alert - *Lamivudine (Epivir)*
• *Use with caution in patients with impaired renal function.*
• *Monitor blood urea nitrogen (BUN) and serum creatinine levels.*

Formulations and dosages for treating HIV and HBV infections differ, and therefore must not be thought of as interchangeable. When lamivudine is stopped, the majority of patients (except those who have seroconverted) have HBV DNA and liver inflammation levels that return to pretreatment levels. Approximately 40% of patients, especially those who take lamivudine for longer than 1 year, develop resistance to the drug.[9,10] Because of resistance, first-line treatment with lamivudine is increasingly limited to pregnant women and immunosuppressed patients. Lamivudine has been used along with HBV immunoglobulin (HBIG) to reduce viral activity in liver transplant patients who have HBV.

Patients with lamivudine-resistant HBV can be treated with adefovir (Hepsera). This drug is taken orally for 1 year and reduces viral load, decreases liver damage, and decreases liver enzymes in

clude antiemetics, such as dimenhydrinate (Dramamine) or trimethobenzamide (Tigan). Phenothiazines should not be used because of their possible cholestatic and hepatotoxic effects. If the patient requires a sedative or hypnotic drug, diphenhydramine (Benadryl) or chloral hydrate may be used.

Chronic Hepatitis B. Drug therapy for chronic HBV is focused on decreasing the viral load, aspartate aminotransferase (AST) and alanine aminotransferase (ALT) levels, the rate of disease progression, and the rate of drug-resistant HBV. Long-term goals are the prevention of cirrhosis and liver cancer. Currently, there are two categories of Food and Drug Administration (FDA)–approved drugs available for suppressing viral activity and decreasing viral load in patients with chronic HBV. However, not all patients respond to the current therapeutic regimens.

α-Interferon. α-Interferon has multiple effects on the viral replication cycle. After binding to receptors on host cell membranes, the drug blocks viral entry into cells, synthesis of viral proteins, and viral assembly and release.

The conventional preparation of α-interferon (Intron A) has a short half-life, and therefore must be administered subcutaneously frequently—at least three times per week. In contrast, the long-acting preparations are administered subcutaneously less frequently—just once per week—making them more convenient. In addition, with the long-acting preparations, blood levels remain high between doses, and therefore clinical responses are better.

approximately two thirds of patients.[10] However, seroconversion occurs in less than 20% of patients. When adefovir is stopped, the majority of patients (except those who have seroconverted) have HBV DNA and liver inflammation levels that return to pretreatment levels. Patients receiving adefovir should be monitored for potential nephrotoxicity. Resistance to adefovir is less than that observed with lamivudine.

> **Drug Alert** - *Adefovir (Hepsera)*
> • *Drug is nephrotoxic.*
> • *Serum creatinine should be monitored, especially in patients at risk such as those having preexisting renal disease or taking nephrotoxic drugs (e.g., cyclosporine, aminoglycosides, vancomycin).*

Entecavir can be used in patients with lamivudine-resistant HBV. This drug is taken orally for approximately 1 year. Entecavir has been shown to reduce viral load, limit liver damage, and decrease liver enzymes in approximately two thirds of patients. However, seroconversion occurs in about 20% of patients. When entecavir is stopped, the majority of patients (except those who have seroconverted) have HBV DNA and liver inflammation levels that return to pretreatment levels. Adefovir and entecavir should not be used in women who are pregnant.

Telbivudine is taken orally once daily. The most common side effects are muscle pain, elevated creatine kinase (an enzyme present in muscle tissue), and upper respiratory tract infections.

Lactic acidosis and severe hepatomegaly with steatosis have been reported with the use of nucleoside analogs. Acute, severe

EVIDENCE-BASED PRACTICE

Does Ethnicity Affect Treatment Outcome in Hepatitis C Patients?

Clinical Question
In patients with hepatitis C (P), do people of nonwhite ethnicities (I) respond differently to treatment (O) than white patients (C)?

Best Available Evidence
• Randomized controlled trial (RCT) and observational trial

Critical Appraisal and Synthesis of Evidence
• One RCT ($n = 390$) and one observational trial ($n = 271$).
• Ethnic groups studied were Asians, whites, Hispanics, and African Americans.
• Treatment efficacy was based on virologic response following α-interferon treatment.

Conclusions
• Treatment outcome was notably influenced by a person's ethnicity.
• Sustained virologic response rate was highest among Asians (61%), followed by whites (39%), Hispanics (23%), and African Americans (14%).

Implications for Nursing Practice
• Instruct African American and Hispanic patients that the natural progression of hepatitis C may differ for them resulting in a lowered treatment response rate.
• Further examination of the effect of ethnicity on varying response rates is warranted given factors such as diet and viral genotype.

Reference for Evidence
Hepburn MJ, Hepburn LM, Cantu NS, et al: Differences in treatment outcome for hepatitis C among ethnic groups, *Am J Med* 117:163, 2004.

PICO: P, Patient population of interest; *I,* intervention or area of interest; *C,* comparison of interest or comparison group; *O,* outcome(s) of interest (see p. 6).

exacerbations of hepatitis B have developed following discontinuation of drugs for hepatitis B. If these drugs are discontinued, liver function should be monitored closely for several months. At this time, a number of new agents are being tested for treating patients with newly diagnosed chronic HBV and lamivudine-resistant HBV.

Chronic Hepatitis C. Drug therapy is directed at eradicating the virus, reducing the viral load, and decreasing progression of the disease.[11] Treatment for HCV includes pegylated α-interferon (PEG-Intron, Pegasys) given with ribavirin (Rebetol, Copegus). Pegylated α-interferon is injected once a week and ribavirin is taken orally twice each week.

Ribavirin, given in combination with α-interferon, has a synergistic effect and has been used to reduce the rate of relapse following α-interferon therapy for HCV. Patients who have advanced fibrosis or cirrhosis can be treated with drug therapy as long as liver decompensation (e.g., ascites, esophageal hemorrhage, jaundice, wasting, encephalopathy) is not present. Ribavirin has a number of side effects, as shown in Table 44-7.

>
> **Drug Alert** - *Ribavirin (Rebetol, Copegus)*
> • *During treatment, pregnancy must be avoided—both by women taking the drug and by women whose male partners are taking the drug.*

Many patients with HIV also have HCV. Patients who have stable HIV and relatively intact immune systems ($CD4^+$ counts $>200/\mu l$) are treated for HCV with the goal of eradicating HCV and enhancing quality of life. However, for those with advanced liver disease, the goal of HCV treatment is to delay disease progression.

The drug treatment of HIV in patients with coexisting HCV requires close attention to liver function. In particular, lymphocyte, white blood cell (WBC), and red blood cell (RBC) counts are monitored. HCV treatment with ribavirin and α-interferon may reduce $CD4^+$ counts, increase leukopenia, and increase the patient's risk for anemia (ribavirin effects). Drug interactions may also occur in patients being treated for both HIV and HCV. Depending on the degree of liver damage, drug therapy for HIV may need to be altered because of the decreased ability of the liver to metabolize the drugs.

Prevention

Hepatitis A. Both hepatitis A vaccine and immune globulin (IG) are used for prevention of hepatitis A. The vaccine is used for preexposure prophylaxis, and IG can be used either before or after exposure. IG provides temporary (1 to 2 months) passive immunity and is effective for preventing hepatitis A if given within 2 weeks after exposure. IG is recommended for persons who do not have anti-HAV antibodies and are exposed as a result of close (household, day-care center) contact with persons who have HAV or food-borne exposure. Because patients with HAV are most infectious just before the onset of symptoms (sometimes referred to as the preicteric phase), those exposed through household contact or food-borne outbreaks should receive IG. Although IG may not prevent infection in all persons, it may modify the illness to a subclinical infection. Persons who have received a dose of HAV vaccine more than 1 month previously or who have a history of laboratory-confirmed HAV infection do not require IG.

There are currently several forms of the HAV vaccine, including Havrix, Vaqta, and Avaxim. HAV vaccine is inactivated hepatitis A virus. Active immunization is an important and effective means of controlling HAV from a public health perspective. Primary immunization consists of a single dose administered intramuscularly (IM) in the deltoid muscle. A booster is recommended any time between

6 and 12 months after the initiation of the primary dose to ensure adequate antibody titers and long-term protection. The primary immunization provides immunity within 30 days after a single dose in more than 95% of those vaccinated. The vaccine may be administered concomitantly with IG for preexposure prophylaxis.

Twinrix, a combined HAV and HBV vaccine, is available for persons over 18 years of age. Immunization consists of three doses, given on a 0-, 1-, and 6-month schedule, the same schedule as that used for the single HBV vaccine. Twinrix may be given to high-risk individuals, including patients with chronic liver disease, users of illicit IV drugs, men who have sex with men, and persons with clotting factor disorders who receive therapeutic blood products. The side effects of the vaccine are mild and are usually limited to soreness and redness at the injection site.

Hepatitis B. Immunization with HBV vaccine is the most effective method of preventing HBV infection. Recommendations from the Centers for Disease Control and Prevention (CDC) Immunization Practices Advisory Committee include making HBV vaccine a part of routine vaccination schedules for all newborns and adolescents. In addition to immunizing newborns and adolescents, it is important to vaccinate adults in the major risk groups, such as IV drug users, household members of a patient with chronic hepatitis B, and those who engage in high-risk sexual behavior. It is hoped that universal vaccination will lead to eventual prevention and control of HBV.

The HBV vaccines (Recombivax HB, Engerix-B) contain HBsAg. The HBsAg is produced using recombinant DNA technology (see Fig. 14-20). Administration of the vaccine promotes synthesis of specific antibodies directed against hepatitis B virus. The vaccine is given in a series of three IM injections in the deltoid muscle. The second dose is administered within 1 month of the first one, and the third one within 6 months of the first. The vaccine is greater than 95% effective. Successful vaccination should result in anti-HBs titers of 10 mIU/ml or greater. It remains to be determined what level of antibody is required to provide protection. Currently, it is not known how frequently boosters (additional doses) are necessary. Only minor adverse reactions have been reported with vaccination, including transient fever and soreness at the injection site. The vaccine is not contraindicated in pregnancy.

For postexposure prophylaxis, the vaccine and hepatitis B immune globulin (HBIG) are used. HBIG contains antibodies to HBV and confers temporary passive immunity. HBIG is prepared from plasma of donors with a high titer of anti-HBs and is expensive. HBIG is recommended for postexposure prophylaxis in cases of needle stick, mucous membrane contact, or sexual exposure and for infants born to mothers who are positive for HBsAg. Preferably it should be given within 24 hours of exposure. The vaccine series should also be started.

Hepatitis C. Currently there is no vaccine to prevent HCV. The CDC does not recommend IG or antiviral agents such as α-interferon for postexposure prophylaxis (e.g., needle-stick exposure from an infected patient) for HCV infection. Following an acute exposure (e.g., needle stick), the person (i.e., the source) should have anti-HCV testing done. For the person exposed to HCV, baseline anti-HCV and ALT levels should be measured. Follow-up testing should be done at 4 to 6 months for anti-HCV and ALT activity. Testing for HCV RNA may be performed at 4 to 6 weeks. Although there is no definitive recommendation, improvements have been seen in reported trials using interferon monotherapy to treat acute HCV.[1]

Nutritional Therapy. Adequate nutrition is important in assisting hepatocytes to regenerate. No special diet is required in the treatment of viral hepatitis. During acute viral hepatitis, adequate calories are important because the patient usually loses weight. If fat content is poorly tolerated because of decreased bile production, it should be reduced. Basically, the specific foods in the diet are dictated by the patient. Vitamin supplements, particularly B-complex vitamins and vitamin K, are frequently used. If anorexia, nausea, and vomiting are severe, IV solutions of glucose or supplemental tube feedings may be used. Fluid and electrolyte balance must be maintained.

NURSING MANAGEMENT
HEPATITIS

■ Nursing Assessment

Subjective and objective data that should be obtained from a person with hepatitis are presented in Table 44-8.

TABLE 44-8	NURSING ASSESSMENT Hepatitis

Subjective Data
Important Health Information
Past health history: Hemophilia; exposure to infected persons; ingestion of contaminated food or water; exposure to benzene, carbon tetrachloride, or other hepatotoxic agents; crowded, unsanitary living conditions; exposure to contaminated needles; recent travel; organ transplant recipient; exposure to new drug regimens, hemodialysis, transfusion of blood or blood products before 1992
Medications: Use and misuse of acetaminophen, phenytoin, halothane, methyldopa

Functional Health Patterns
Health perception–health management: IV drug and alcohol abuse; malaise, distaste for cigarettes (in smokers), high-risk sexual behaviors
Nutritional-metabolic: Weight loss, anorexia, nausea, vomiting; feeling of fullness in right upper quadrant
Elimination: Dark urine; light-colored stools, constipation or diarrhea; skin rashes, hives
Activity-exercise: Fatigue, arthralgias, myalgias
Cognitive-perceptual: Right upper quadrant pain and liver tenderness, headache; pruritus
Role-relationship: Exposure as health care worker, chronic care institution resident, incarceration

Objective Data
General
Low-grade fever, lethargy, lymphadenopathy

Integumentary
Rash, angioedema, jaundice, icteric sclera, injection sites

Gastrointestinal
Hepatomegaly, splenomegaly

Possible Findings
Elevated liver enzyme levels; ↑ serum total bilirubin, hypoalbuminemia, anemia, bilirubin in urine and increased urobilinogen, prolonged prothrombin time, positive tests for hepatitis including anti-HAV IgM, anti-HAV IgG, HBsAg, HBeAg, HBcAg, anti-HBc IgM, HBV DNA, anti-HCV, HCV RNA, anti-HDV; abnormal liver scan; positive liver biopsy

DNA, Deoxyribonucleic acid; *HAV,* hepatitis A virus; *HB,* hepatitis B; *HBcAg,* hepatitis B core antigen; *HBeAg,* hepatitis B e antigen; *HBsAg,* hepatitis B surface antigen; *HBV,* hepatitis B virus; *HCV,* hepatitis C virus; *HDV,* hepatitis D virus; *RNA,* ribonucleic acid.

▪ *Nursing Diagnoses*

Nursing diagnoses for the patient with hepatitis may include, but are not limited to, those presented in NCP 44-1.

▪ *Planning*

The overall goals are that the patient with viral hepatitis will (1) have relief of discomfort, (2) be able to resume normal activities, and (3) return to normal liver function without complications.

▪ *Nursing Implementation*

Health Promotion. Viral hepatitis is a public health problem. The nurse must assume a significant role in the control and prevention of this disease. It is helpful to first understand the epidemiology of the different types of viral hepatitis before considering appropriate control measures.

Hepatitis A. Vaccination is the best protection against HAV. Vaccination is recommended for persons 12 months of age and older who travel to areas with increased rates of hepatitis A, men who have sex with men, injecting and noninjecting drug users, persons with clotting factor disorders (e.g., hemophilia), persons with chronic liver disease, and children living in regions of the United States with consistently increased rates of hepatitis A.[1]

Outbreaks of viral hepatitis are usually due to HAV. In the United States there is usually one major outbreak per decade, the last being in 1995. Preventive measures include personal and environmental hygiene and health education to promote good sanitation (Table 44-9). Hand washing is essential and is probably the most important precaution. Health teaching should include careful hand washing after bowel movements and before eating. When hepatitis A occurs in a food handler, IG should be administered to all other food handlers at the establishment. Patrons may also need to be given IG.

Isolation is not required for hepatitis A. For a patient with hepatitis A, infection control precautions should be used (see Table

---

NURSING CARE PLAN 44-1

Patient with Acute Viral Hepatitis

NURSING DIAGNOSIS **Imbalanced nutrition: less than body requirements** *related to* anorexia, nausea, and reduced metabolism of nutrients by liver *as evidenced by* inadequate food intake, perceived inability to ingest food

PATIENT GOALS
1. Maintains weight appropriate for height
2. Food and fluid intake adequate to meet nutritional needs

OUTCOMES (NOC)	INTERVENTIONS (NIC) and *RATIONALES*
Nutritional Status	**Nutrition Therapy**
• Nutrient intake ____	• Complete a nutritional assessment *to determine baseline nutritional state.*
• Food intake ____	• Monitor food/fluid ingested and calculate daily caloric intake *so appropriate interventions can be planned.*
• Fluid intake ____	• Determine, in collaboration with the dietitian, the number of calories and type of nutrients needed to meet nutrition requirements *so the proper nutritional requirements can be provided.*
• Weight/height ratio ____	
Measurement Scale	• Present food in an attractive, pleasing manner, giving consideration to color, texture, and variety, *to stimulate patient's appetite.*
1 = Severe deviation from normal range	• Provide oral care before meals *to stimulate appetite.*
2 = Substantial deviation from normal range	**Nutrition Management**
3 = Moderate deviation from normal range	• Provide food selection *to increase likelihood of adequate intake.*
4 = Mild deviation from normal range	• Weigh patient at appropriate intervals *to monitor weight loss secondary to poor appetite.*
5 = No deviation from normal range	

NURSING DIAGNOSIS **Activity intolerance** *related to* fatigue and weakness *as evidenced by* verbal report of fatigue or weakness, altered response to activity

PATIENT GOALS
1. Reports ability to perform daily activities with scheduled rest periods
2. Demonstrates gradual increase in activity tolerance

OUTCOMES (NOC)	INTERVENTIONS (NIC) and *RATIONALES*
Energy Conservation	**Energy Management**
• Recognizes energy limitations ____	• Determine patient's physical limitations *for baseline comparison.*
• Reports adequate endurance for activity ____	• Assist patient to schedule rest periods *to prevent stress on liver function.*
• Balances activity and rest ____	• Encourage patient to choose activities that gradually build endurance *so previous activity pattern can be resumed.*
• Organizes activities to conserve energy ____	• Limit environmental stimuli (e.g., light and noise) *to facilitate relaxation.*
Measurement Scale	• Instruct patient/significant other to recognize signs and symptoms of fatigue that require reduction in activity *so patient can be active participant in plan.*
1 = Never demonstrated	• Teach activity organization and time management techniques *to prevent fatigue.*
2 = Rarely demonstrated	• Monitor patient for evidence of excess physical and emotional fatigue *to prevent increasing weakness and fatigue.*
3 = Sometimes demonstrated	
4 = Often demonstrated	
5 = Consistently demonstrated	

ADLs, Activities of daily living.

Continued

NURSING CARE PLAN 44-1

Patient with Acute Viral Hepatitis—cont'd

NURSING DIAGNOSIS   **Ineffective therapeutic regimen management** *related to* lack of knowledge of follow-up care *as evidenced by* frequent questions about transmission of disease, activities allowed, and general follow-up care

PATIENT GOAL   Describes therapeutic regimen with regard to disease process, complications, and management

OUTCOMES (NOC)	INTERVENTIONS (NIC) and *RATIONALES*
Knowledge: Disease Process	**Teaching: Disease Process**
• Description of cause or contributing factors ____	• Explain pathophysiology of the disease and how it relates to anatomy and physiology.
• Description of effects of disease ____	• Describe rationale behind management/therapy/treatment recommendations *so that appropriate follow-up care will be planned and carried out.*
• Description of signs and symptoms of complications ____	• Discuss lifestyle changes that may be required to prevent future complications and/or control the disease process (e.g., avoidance of alcohol, infection control measures).
• Description of measures to minimize disease progression ____	• Instruct patient on which signs and symptoms (e.g., bleeding gums, blood in stools) to report to health care provider *to enable prompt intervention.*
Measurement Scale	• Instruct patient on measures to control/minimize symptoms *to enable liver to repair itself and prevent relapse.*
1 = None	
2 = Limited	
3 = Moderate	
4 = Substantial	
5 = Extensive	

TABLE 44-9   **Preventive Measures for Viral Hepatitis**

Hepatitis A	Hepatitis B and C
General Measures	**Percutaneous Transmission**
Hand washing	Screening of donated blood
Proper personal hygiene	B—HBsAg
Environmental sanitation	C—anti-HCV
Control and screening (signs, symptoms) of food handlers	Use of disposable needles and syringes
Serologic screening while carrying virus	**Sexual Transmission**
Active immunization: HAV vaccine to anyone over age 2	Acute exposure: HBIG administration to sexual partner of HBsAg-positive person
	Administer hepatitis B vaccine series to uninfected sexual partners
Use of Immune Globulin	Use condoms for sexual intercourse
Early administration (1-2 wk after exposure) to those exposed	
Prophylaxis for travelers to areas where hepatitis A is common if not vaccinated with HAV vaccine	**General Measures**
	Hand washing
	Avoid sharing toothbrushes and razors
	HBIG administration for one-time exposure (needle stick, contact of mucous membranes with infectious material)
	Active immunization: HBV vaccine

HAV, Hepatitis A virus; *HBIG*, hepatitis B immune globulin; *HBsAg*, hepatitis B surface antigen; *HBV*, hepatitis B virus; *HCV*, hepatitis C virus.

15-9). A private room is indicated if the patient is incontinent of stool or has poor personal hygiene.

Hepatitis B. The HBV vaccine is the best means of protection. Control and prevention of hepatitis B also focus on identification of possible exposure via percutaneous and sexual trans-

mission (see Table 44-9). The nurse must be aware of the individuals at high risk of contracting HBV and teach methods to reduce risks. These include patients receiving frequent transfusions or hemodialysis, workers in hemodialysis units and laboratories where blood is handled, IV drug users, persons with multiple sexual partners, prisoners, and household members and sexual partners of HBV carriers.

Good hygienic practices, including hand washing and the use of gloves when expecting contact with blood, are important. A condom is advised for sexual intercourse, and the partner should be vaccinated. Razors, toothbrushes, and other personal items should not be shared. Household members of the patient with hepatitis B should be tested and vaccinated if they are HBsAg and antibody negative.

According to CDC guidelines, infection control precautions should be followed for the patient with HBV. This includes the use of disposable needles and syringes, which should be disposed of in puncture-resistant disposal units without recapping, bending, or breaking. (See Table 15-9 for various types of infection control precautions.)

Hepatitis C. No vaccine is currently available for hepatitis C. The primary measures to prevent HCV transmission include screening of blood, organ, and tissue donors; use of infection control precautions; and modification of high-risk behavior. Similar to HBV prevention, the nurse should identify individuals at high risk for contracting HCV and teach methods to reduce risks. Individuals at risk include those who use IV drugs (or have ever used, even once many years earlier); patients who received blood (including blood products) or organ and tissue donation before 1992; patients who are or have been on hemodialysis; workers in hemodialysis units and laboratories in which blood is handled; persons with multiple sexual partners; prisoners; and sexual partners of individuals with HCV. Infection with HCV often coexists with HIV infection.

The use of gloves when expecting contact with blood is important. For those not in long-term, monogamous relationships, a condom is advised for sexual intercourse with an individual with HCV. Razors, toothbrushes, and other personal items should not be shared. Preventive and control measures for hepatitis A, B, and C are summarized in Table 44-9.

Acute Intervention

Jaundice. The nurse should assess for the degree of jaundice. In light-skinned persons the jaundice is usually observed first in the sclera of the eyes and later in the skin. In dark-skinned persons, jaundice is observed in the hard palate of the mouth and inner canthus of the eyes. The urine may have a dark brown or brownish red color because of the presence of bilirubin. Comfort measures to relieve pruritus (if present), headache, and arthralgias are helpful (see NCP 44-1).

Ensuring that the patient receives adequate nutrition is not always easy. The anorexia and distaste for food cause nutritional problems. Dietary assessment must be considered. Small, frequent meals may be preferable to three large ones and may also help prevent nausea. Often, a patient with hepatitis finds that anorexia is not as severe in the morning, so it is easier to eat a good breakfast than a large dinner. Measures to stimulate the appetite, such as mouth care, antiemetics, and attractively served meals in pleasant surroundings, are included in the nursing care plan. Other measures that may be tried to counteract the anorexia are carbonated beverages and avoidance of very hot or very cold foods. Adequate fluid intake (2500 to 3000 ml/day) is important.

Rest. Rest is essential and is an important factor in promoting hepatocyte regeneration. The nurse must assess the patient's response to the rest and activity plan and modify it accordingly. If the patient is on bed rest, measures to prevent skin, respiratory, and circulatory complications should be initiated. Assessment of the liver function tests and symptoms should be used as a guide to activity.

Psychologic and emotional rest is as essential as physical rest. Bed rest may produce anxiety and extreme restlessness in some patients. Diversional activities, such as reading and hobbies, may help the patient.

Ambulatory and Home Care.

Most patients with viral hepatitis will be cared for at home, so the nurse must assess the patient's knowledge of nutrition and provide the necessary dietary teaching. Rest and adequate nutrition are especially important until liver function has returned to normal. The patient is cautioned about overexertion and the need to follow the health care provider's advice about when to return to work. The nurse must also teach the patient and family how to prevent transmission to other family members. The patient should know what symptoms should be reported to the health care provider.

The patient should be assessed for manifestations of complications. Bleeding tendencies with increasing prothrombin time values, symptoms of encephalopathy, or elevated liver function tests indicate problems.

The patient should be instructed to have regular follow-up for at least 1 year after the diagnosis of hepatitis. Because relapses are fairly common with hepatitis B and C, the patient should be instructed about the symptoms of recurrence and the need for follow-up evaluations. All patients with chronic HBV or HCV should avoid alcohol. It is well established that alcohol can make the liver disease worse (progression is accelerated).

A patient who remains positive for HBsAg is a chronic carrier and should never be a blood donor. A patient who tests positive for the HCV antibody should also not donate blood. Because of the shortage of livers available for transplantation, the use of liver tissues from individuals who are HBcAB positive is now being considered for select (HBV naïve) recipients.

The patient who is receiving α-interferon for the treatment of HBV or HCV requires education regarding this drug. Because α-interferon is administered subcutaneously, the patient or family member needs to be taught how to administer the drug. There are numerous side effects with the therapy, including flu-like symptoms (e.g., fever, malaise, fatigue) (see Table 44-7). The health care provider may recommend that acetaminophen be administered 30 to 60 minutes before injection to reduce these symptoms.

■ Evaluation

Expected outcomes for the patient with hepatitis are addressed in NCP 44-1.

Control of Hepatitis in Health Care Personnel

Hepatitis A. Hepatitis A is rarely transmitted from patients to health care personnel. When this does occur, it is associated with patients with undiagnosed hepatitis A who are treated for other problems. Usually these patients are incontinent of feces. The use of infection control precautions should prevent transmission of HAV to health care personnel.

Hepatitis B. Health care workers may be exposed to HBV from needle sticks or blood contamination to mucous membranes or nonintact skin. If a health care worker is exposed to HBV through a needle stick and has not been vaccinated, there is a 6% to 30% chance of infection with HBV.[1] Vaccination is the most effective method to prevent HBV in health care workers. Employers are required by the Occupational Safety and Health Administration to provide free HBV immunization to employees at risk for infection.

The principal mode of transmission of HBV for health care personnel is parenteral. Examples include accidental needle sticks and, rarely, transfusion of contaminated blood or blood products. Because all blood and blood products are tested for HBV and anti-HCV, there is diminishing risk of this mode of transmission. Other forms of transmission include contamination of fresh cutaneous scratches or abrasions, burns, and mucosal surfaces with infective blood, blood products, saliva, or semen.

Hepatitis C. Transmission is usually due to percutaneous needle exposure or other blood exposure and undetected parenteral transmission. Measures to prevent transmission of the viruses from patients to health care personnel are presented in Table 44-10. Very rarely do health care workers infect patients.

TOXIC AND DRUG-INDUCED HEPATITIS

Liver injury and death may occur after the inhalation, parenteral injection, or ingestion of certain chemical substances (see Table 39-6). The two major types of chemical hepatotoxicity are toxic and drug-induced hepatitis. Agents producing toxic hepatitis are generally systemic poisons (e.g., carbon tetrachloride, gold compounds) or are converted in the liver to toxic metabolites (e.g., acetaminophen). Liver necrosis generally occurs within 2 to 3 days of acute exposure to a toxic substance.

Idiosyncratic drug reactions produce drug-induced hepatitis. Such agents as halothane (Fluothane), isoniazid (INH), chlorothiazide (e.g., Diuril), methotrexate, and methyldopa (Aldomet) may

TABLE 44-10	**Measures to Prevent Transmission of Hepatitis Viruses from Patients to Health Care Personnel***

Hepatitis A	**Hepatitis B**	**Hepatitis C**
Always maintain good personal hygiene.	Use infection control precautions.†	Use infection control precautions.†
Wash hands after contact with a patient or removal of gloves.	Wash hands.	Wash hands.
Use infection control precautions.†	Reduce contact with blood or blood-containing secretions.	Reduce contact with blood or blood-containing secretions.
	Handle the blood of patients as potentially infective.	Handle the blood of patients as potentially infective.
	Dispose of needles properly.	Dispose of needles properly.
	Use needleless IV access devices when available.	Use needleless IV access devices when available.
	Administer HBV vaccine to all health care personnel.	

HBV, Hepatitis B virus; *IV*, intravenous.

*A suggested guideline for general practice to prevent the nurse from contracting viral hepatitis from diagnosed and undiagnosed patients and carriers is for the nurse to wear disposable gloves, goggles, and gowns (sometimes) when fecal or blood contamination is likely in handling (1) soiled bedpans, urinals, and catheters and (2) patient's bed linens soiled by body excreta or secretions.

†See Tables 15-8 and 15-9.

produce idiosyncratic reactions because of patient susceptibility (metabolic reactivity) to these agents or immunologically mediated hypersensitivity responses. Liver injury may occur at any time during or shortly after exposure. Some responses occur 2 to 5 weeks after exposure.

Toxic and drug-induced hepatitis are similar to viral hepatitis in the pathophysiologic changes in the liver and the clinical manifestations. The usual presenting clinical findings are anorexia, nausea, vomiting, hepatomegaly, splenomegaly, and abnormal liver function studies. Treatment is largely supportive, as in acute viral hepatitis. Recovery may be rapid if the hepatotoxin is identified and removed. Liver transplantation may be necessary in cases of severe liver damage.

AUTOIMMUNE/METABOLIC/GENETIC LIVER DISEASES

Autoimmune Hepatitis

Autoimmune hepatitis is a chronic inflammatory disorder of the liver of unknown cause. It is characterized by the presence of autoantibodies, high levels of serum immunoglobulins, and frequent association with other autoimmune diseases. The initial signs and symptoms are variable and similar to those of viral hepatitis. Laboratory tests (elevation of liver enzymes) reveal liver inflammation without evidence of viral antigens. Circulating autoantibodies are present in most patients with autoimmune hepatitis. Serologic markers, although not specific for autoimmune hepatitis, are often useful in the diagnosis. These include antinuclear antibodies (ANA) and anti-DNA antibodies. The majority (70% to 80%) of patients with autoimmune hepatitis are women.

The pathogenesis of autoimmune hepatitis is unknown. It is thought to be related to both genetic and environmental factors, including prior viral infections.[12] The disease process involves an autoimmune reaction against normal hepatocytes. The course of the disease is also variable, with the majority of the patients exhibiting chronic hepatitis.

Unlike viral hepatitis, autoimmune hepatitis (in which there is evidence of necrosis and cirrhosis) is treated with corticosteroids or other immunosuppressive agents. Daily treatment with prednisone alone or in combination with azathioprine (Imuran) will induce remission in approximately 80% of patients. If these drugs do not work, other immunosuppressive therapies (e.g., cyclosporine, tacrolimus [Prograf], mycophenolate [CellCept]) are initiated. Liver transplant is indicated for liver failure.

Wilson's Disease

Wilson's disease is a progressive, familial, terminal neurologic disease accompanied by chronic liver disease leading to cirrhosis. It is associated with increased storage of copper. The pattern of inheritance is autosomal recessive. The gene, ATP7B, encodes a protein that is expressed mainly in hepatocytes and affects the transmembrane transport of copper. Absent or reduced function of ATP7B protein leads to decreased hepatocellular excretion of copper into bile. This results in hepatic copper accumulation and cell injury. Wilson's disease occurs worldwide with an average prevalence of 30 individuals per million population.[13]

The hallmark of Wilson's disease is corneal Kayser-Fleischer rings. These are brownish red colored rings that can be seen in the cornea near the limbus on eye examination. Low serum ceruloplasmin levels and measurable copper concentrations from liver biopsy samples are also present. Often in addition to their liver disease, patients will also have neurologic dysfunction, including movement disorders (tremor, involuntary movements), drooling, dysarthria, rigid dystonia, seizures, migraine headaches, and insomnia.

Diagnosis is based on clinical findings, including the corneal findings and presence of neurologic symptoms. Serum ALT and AST levels are elevated, serum ceruloplasmin levels are low, serum uric acid levels are decreased, and urinary copper excretion levels are increased.

The recommended initial treatment of symptomatic patients or those with active disease is with chelating agents such as D-penicillamine or trientine (Syprine) that promote the excretion of urinary copper.[13]

Hemochromatosis

Hemochromatosis (HH) is a systemic disease that affects the liver, heart, pancreas, and endocrine system.[14] It is caused by increased and inappropriate absorption of dietary iron. Prolonged increased iron absorption can lead to complications, including cirrhosis, hepatocellular cancer, diabetes, and heart disease.

The clinical condition of HH begins with clinically insignificant iron accumulation. This progresses to a stage of iron overload without disease at approximately 20 to 40 years of age. If left untreated, this may progress to a stage of iron overload with organ damage (usually around 40 years of age). The degree of iron overload has a direct impact on life expectancy of the individual with HH. The major causes of death are decompensated cirrhosis, hepatocellular carcinoma, diabetes mellitus, and cardiomyopathy. (Hemochromatosis is discussed in Chapter 31.)

Primary Biliary Cirrhosis

Primary biliary cirrhosis (PBC) is a chronic inflammatory condition of the liver. It is characterized by generalized pruritus, hepatomegaly, hyperpigmentation of the skin, and diarrhea of pale, stools. Although the etiology of PBC is not completely understood, it appears that both genetic and environmental factors such as chemical exposure and infection may play a role. In PBC there is a T-cell–mediated attack of the small bile duct epithelial cells resulting in loss of bile ducts and ultimately *cholestasis* (blockage of bile flow). Over time this leads to liver necrosis and cirrhosis. Patients with PBC are at increased risk for hepatocellular cancer.

Approximately 95% of patients diagnosed with PBC are women. The incidence of PBC in the United States is increasing. Women in midlife, ages 30 to 60, are most frequently affected. The disease is associated with other autoimmune disorders such as rheumatoid arthritis, Sjögren's syndrome, and scleroderma.

In the early stages patients may be asymptomatic. Patients may seek treatment from their health care provider for symptoms of fatigue and pruritus. Bleeding associated with hypoprothrombinemia may also be present. Jaundice is a late sign. Osteoporosis is also found in a significant number of patients. Patients may also have signs of fat malabsorption, including low levels of fat-soluble vitamins, which occurs because of decreased bile secretion. Elevated serum alkaline phosphatase levels, antimitochrondrial antibodies (AMA), antinuclear antibodies (ANA), and serum lipid levels are also seen in patients with PBC. Histologic evidence of damage is found on liver biopsy.

The goals of treatment are the suppression of ongoing liver damage, prevention of complications, and symptom management. The only FDA-approved drug for PBC is ursodiol (Actigall). This drug increases the rate of bile acid secretion and appears to have a cytoprotective affect. Complication and symptom management includes a focus on malabsorption, skin disorders such as pruritus and xanthomas (cholesterol deposits in the skin), hyperlipidemia, vitamin deficiencies, anemia, and fatigue. Cholestyramine (Questran) is used to manage pruritus. Patients are monitored for progression to cirrhosis, which is variable across patients. Liver transplantation is a treatment option for end-stage liver disease in patients with PBC.

Nonalcoholic Fatty Liver Disease and Nonalcoholic Steatohepatitis

Nonalcoholic fatty liver disease (NAFLD) is a group of disorders that is characterized by hepatic *steatosis* (accumulation of fat in the liver) that is not associated with other causes such as hepatitis, autoimmune disease, or alcohol. Histologically, cell changes include the presence of fatty changes in the hepatocytes. This accumulation of fat can lead to inflammation and scarring that is called **nonalcoholic steatohepatitis** (NASH). People with NASH can develop advanced scarring called *cirrhosis* with an increased risk for developing liver cancer and liver failure.

The risk for developing NAFLD is directly related to body weight and is a major complication of obesity. NAFLD should be considered in patients with risk factors such as obesity, diabetes, hypertriglyceridemia, severe weight loss (especially in those whose weight loss was recent), and syndromes associated with insulin resistance. Poor diet, tuberculosis, intestinal bypass, and medications (e.g., corticosteroids) can also lead to NAFLD. NAFLD is also considered in patients who have persistently elevated ALT levels and for whom no other cause can be found.

The incidence and prevalence of NAFLD and NASH are unknown. It exists in 15% to 20% of those who are morbidly obese and in 3% to 5% of normal-weight individuals. The highest prevalences of both NAFLD and NASH are found in adults 40 to 49 years of age. NAFLD is also associated with certain medications, including diltiazem (Cardizem), amiodarone (Cordarone), and tamoxifen (Nolvadex). Environmental exposure to certain chemicals, such as organic solvents and dimethylformamide, has also been associated NAFLD. NAFLD can progress to liver fibrosis and cirrhosis.

Clinical Manifestations and Diagnostic Studies. Most patients with NAFLD are asymptomatic. NAFLD is usually diagnosed during the evaluation of other health problems such as hypertension, diabetes, or morbid obesity. For example, in some asymptomatic patients an elevated ALT level is found when liver function tests are performed during the course of monitoring antihyperlipidemic drug therapy. Only a small number of patients exhibit signs of serious liver disease (e.g., ascites, anasarca, variceal hemorrhage). Jaundice occurs late in NAFLD and indicates advanced liver disease.

Elevations in liver function tests (ALT, AST) two to four times higher than normal values are often the first signs of NAFLD. However, elevations may be associated with a number of other liver disorders. With progression of the disease there are reductions in serum albumin and elevations in serum bilirubin and prothrombin. Definitive diagnosis is by liver biopsy and histologic examination of hepatocytes. Ultrasound and computed tomography (CT) scans are also used to diagnose NAFLD.

Collaborative Care. NAFLD can progress to liver cirrhosis. Those who are older, are morbidly obese, or have diabetes are at risk for advanced liver disease. There is no definitive treatment, and therapy is directed at reduction of risk factors. These include treatment of diabetes, reduction in body weight, and elimination of harmful medications.

For those who are overweight, weight reduction is important. Weight loss will improve insulin sensitivity and reduce liver enzyme levels. There is no specific dietary therapy that is recommended. However, a heart-healthy diet as recommended by the American Heart Association is appropriate. Patients should have liver function monitored during weight loss because too-rapid loss of weight is associated with liver failure. Diet changes to induce weight loss are more likely to succeed if behavior-modification therapy is employed. In some cases NAFLD may progress to liver failure, and liver transplantation may be required.

CIRRHOSIS

Cirrhosis is a chronic progressive disease of the liver characterized by extensive degeneration and destruction of the liver parenchymal cells (Fig. 44-4). The liver cells attempt to regenerate, but the regenerative process is disorganized, resulting in abnormal blood vessel and bile duct architecture. The overgrowth of new and fibrous connective tissue distorts the liver's normal lobular structure, resulting in lobules of irregular size and shape with impeded

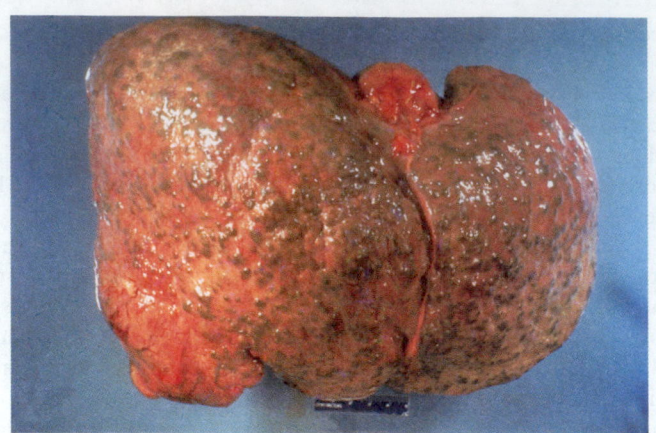

FIG. 44-4 Cirrhosis that developed secondary to alcoholism. The characteristic diffuse nodularity of the surface is due to the combination of regeneration and scarring of the liver.

blood flow. Eventually, irregular, disorganized regeneration; poor cellular nutrition; and hypoxia caused by inadequate blood flow and scar tissue result in decreased functioning of the liver. Cirrhosis may have an insidious, prolonged course.

Cirrhosis is ranked as the ninth leading cause of death in the United States and the fourth leading cause of death in persons between 35 and 54 years of age. The highest incidence occurs between ages 40 and 60, and it is twice as common in men as in women.

Etiology and Pathophysiology

The four types of cirrhosis, in order of incidence, are as follows:

1. *Alcoholic* (previously called *Laënnec's*) *cirrhosis*, also called *portal* or *nutritional cirrhosis,* is usually associated with alcohol abuse. The first change in the liver from excessive alcohol intake is an accumulation of fat in the liver cells. Uncomplicated fatty changes in the liver are potentially reversible if the person stops drinking alcohol. If the alcohol abuse continues, widespread scar formation occurs throughout the liver.
2. *Postnecrotic cirrhosis* is a complication of viral, toxic, or idiopathic (autoimmune) hepatitis. Broad bands of scar tissue form within the liver.
3. *Biliary cirrhosis* is associated with chronic biliary obstruction and infection. There is diffuse fibrosis of the liver with jaundice as the main feature.
4. *Cardiac cirrhosis* results from long-standing, severe right-sided heart failure in patients with cor pulmonale, constrictive pericarditis, and tricuspid insufficiency.

The specific cause of cirrhosis may not be determined in all patients. Excessive alcohol ingestion is the single most common cause of cirrhosis because alcohol has a direct hepatotoxic effect. There continues to be some controversy as to whether the cause is the alcohol or the malnutrition that frequently coexists with chronic ingestion of alcohol. A common problem in alcoholics is protein malnutrition.[15] There have been cases of nutritional cirrhosis resulting from extreme dieting or malnutrition. Environmental factors may also lead to the development of cirrhosis.[16] Some persons may have a predisposition to cirrhosis, regardless of their dietary or alcohol intake.[17]

Approximately 20% of patients with chronic hepatitis C and 10% to 20% of those with chronic hepatitis B will develop cirrhosis. Chronic inflammation and cell necrosis result in fibrosis and, ultimately, cirrhosis. The combination of chronic hepatitis and alcohol ingestion is synergistic in terms of accelerating liver damage.

Biliary causes of cirrhosis include primary biliary cirrhosis (described earlier in this chapter) and primary sclerosing cholangitis. *Primary sclerosing cholangitis* is a chronic inflammatory condition affecting the liver and bile ducts. It is most frequently found in men. The etiology of primary sclerosing cholangitis is unknown. However, it is strongly associated with ulcerative colitis. The chronic inflammation can ultimately progress to cirrhosis and end-stage liver disease.

Clinical Manifestations

Early Manifestations. The onset of cirrhosis is usually insidious. Occasionally there is an abrupt onset of symptoms. GI disturbances are common. Early symptoms include anorexia, dyspepsia, flatulence, nausea and vomiting, and change in bowel habits (diarrhea or constipation). These symptoms occur as a result of the liver's altered metabolism of carbohydrates, fats, and proteins. The patient may complain of abdominal pain described as a dull, heavy feeling in the right upper quadrant or epigastrium. The pain may be due to swelling and stretching of the liver capsule, spasm of the biliary ducts, and intermittent vascular spasm. Other early manifestations are fever, lassitude, slight weight loss, and enlargement of the liver and spleen. The liver is palpable in many patients with cirrhosis.

Later Manifestations. Later symptoms may be severe and result from liver failure and portal hypertension (Fig. 44-5). Jaundice, peripheral edema, and ascites develop gradually. Other late symptoms include skin lesions, hematologic disorders, endocrine disturbances, and peripheral neuropathies (Fig. 44-6). In the advanced stages the liver becomes small and nodular.

Jaundice. Jaundice results from the functional derangement of liver cells and compression of bile ducts by connective tissue overgrowth. Jaundice occurs as a result of the decreased ability to conjugate and excrete bilirubin (hepatocellular jaundice). The jaundice may be minimal or severe, depending on the degree of liver damage. If obstruction of the biliary tract occurs, obstructive jaundice may also occur and is usually accompanied by pruritus. The pruritus is due to an accumulation of bile salts underneath the skin.

Skin Lesions. Various skin manifestations are commonly seen in cirrhosis. **Spider angiomas** (*telangiectasia* or *spider nevi*) are small, dilated blood vessels with a bright red center point and spiderlike branches. They occur on the nose, cheeks, upper trunk, neck, and shoulders. *Palmar erythema* (a red area that blanches with pressure) is located on the palms of the hands. Both of these lesions are attributed to an increase in circulating estrogen as a result of the damaged liver's inability to metabolize steroid hormones.

Hematologic Problems. Hematologic problems include thrombocytopenia, leukopenia, anemia, and coagulation disorders. Thrombocytopenia, leukopenia, and anemia are probably caused by the splenomegaly. Splenomegaly results from backup of blood from the portal vein into the spleen. Overactivity of the enlarged spleen results in increased removal of blood cells from circulation.

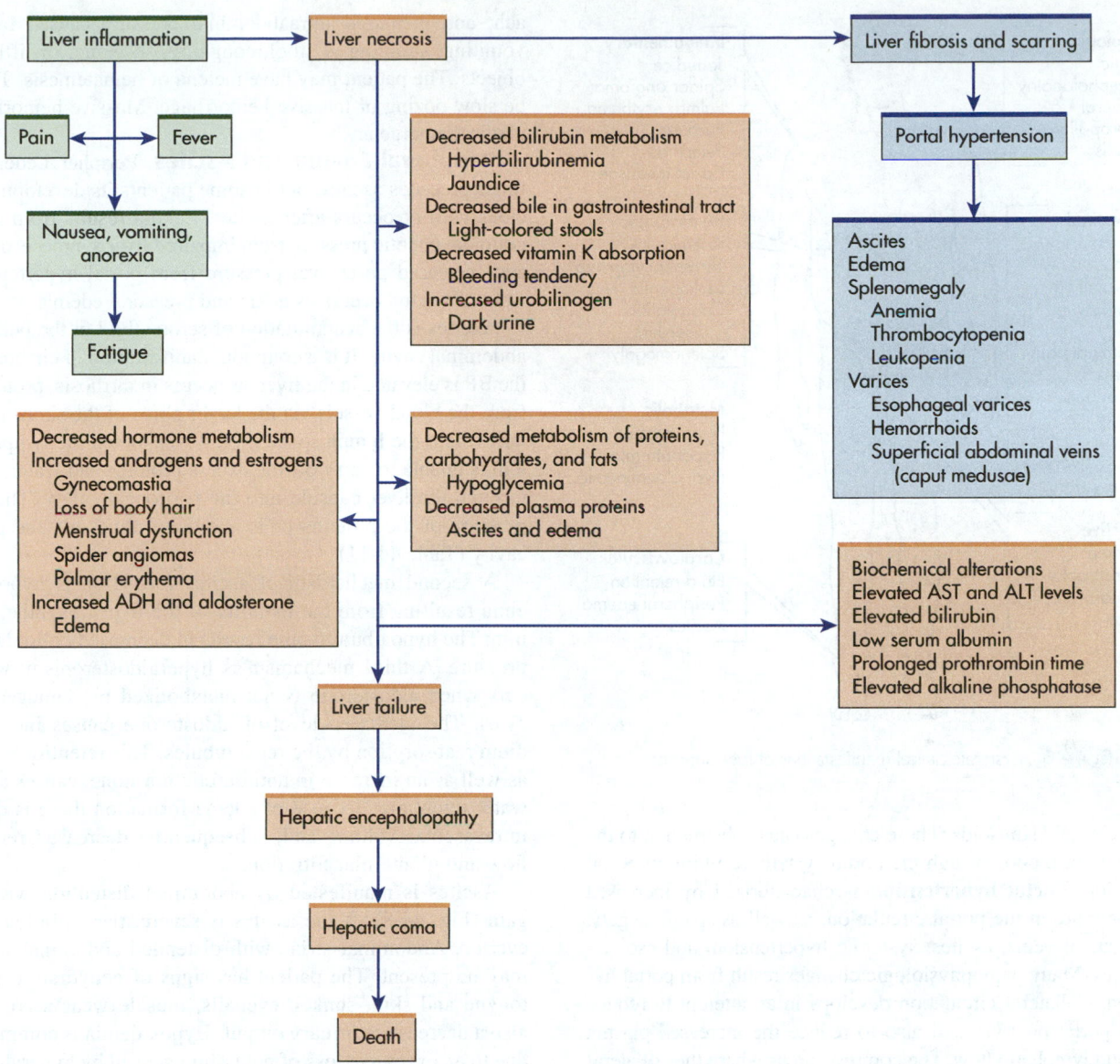

FIG. 44-5 Continuum of liver dysfunction in cirrhosis and resulting manifestations. *ADH,* Antidiuretic hormone; *ALT,* alanine aminotransferase; *AST,* aspartate transaminase.

The anemia is also due to inadequate RBC production and survival. Other factors involved in the anemia relate to poor diet, poor absorption of folic acid, and bleeding from varices.

The coagulation problems result from the liver's inability to produce prothrombin and other factors essential for blood clotting. Coagulation problems are manifested by hemorrhagic phenomena or bleeding tendencies, such as epistaxis, purpura, petechiae, easy bruising, gingival bleeding, and heavy menstrual bleeding.

Endocrine Problems. Several signs and symptoms relating to the metabolism and inactivation of adrenocortical hormones, estrogen, and testosterone occur in cirrhosis. Normally the liver metabolizes these hormones. When the damaged liver is unable to do this, various manifestations occur. In men, gynecomastia, loss of axillary and pubic hair, testicular atrophy, and impotence with loss of libido may occur as a result of increased estrogen levels. In younger women amenorrhea may occur, and in older women there may be vaginal bleeding. The liver fails to metabolize aldosterone

adequately, resulting in hyperaldosteronism with subsequent sodium and water retention and potassium loss.

Peripheral Neuropathy. Peripheral neuropathy is a common finding in alcoholic cirrhosis. It is probably due to a dietary deficiency of thiamine, folic acid, and cobalamin. The neuropathy usually results in mixed nervous system symptoms, but sensory symptoms may predominate. Clinical manifestations of cirrhosis of the liver are numerous and may eventually involve the total body (see Fig. 44-6).

Complications

Major complications of cirrhosis are portal hypertension with resultant esophageal varices, peripheral edema and ascites, hepatic encephalopathy (coma), and hepatorenal syndrome.

Portal Hypertension and Esophageal and Gastric Varices. Because of the structural changes in the liver from the cirrhotic process, there is compression and destruction of the portal and

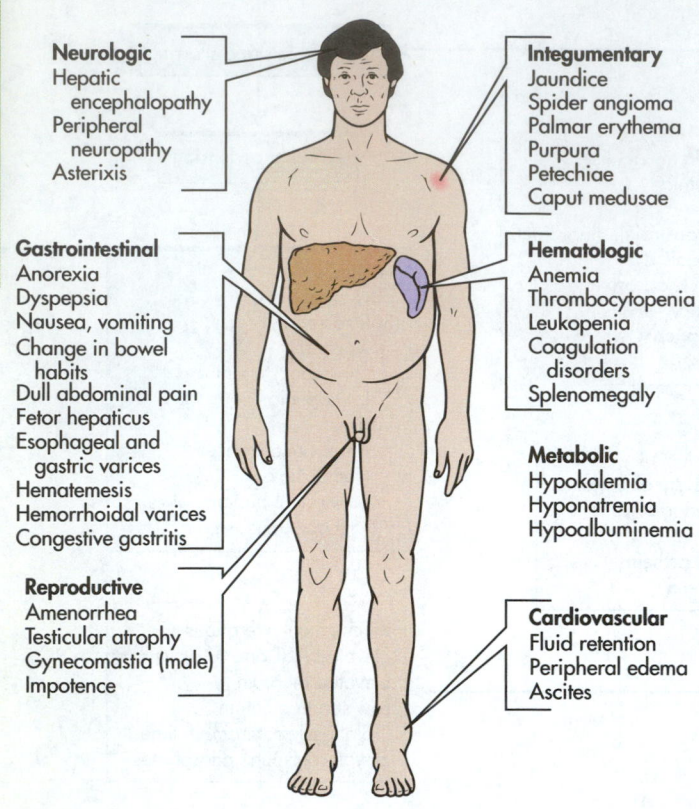

Neurologic
Hepatic
   encephalopathy
Peripheral
   neuropathy
Asterixis

Integumentary
Jaundice
Spider angioma
Palmar erythema
Purpura
Petechiae
Caput medusae

Gastrointestinal
Anorexia
Dyspepsia
Nausea, vomiting
Change in bowel
   habits
Dull abdominal pain
Fetor hepaticus
Esophageal and
   gastric varices
Hematemesis
Hemorrhoidal varices
Congestive gastritis

Hematologic
Anemia
Thrombocytopenia
Leukopenia
Coagulation
   disorders
Splenomegaly

Metabolic
Hypokalemia
Hyponatremia
Hypoalbuminemia

Reproductive
Amenorrhea
Testicular atrophy
Gynecomastia (male)
Impotence

Cardiovascular
Fluid retention
Peripheral edema
Ascites

FIG. 44-6   Systemic clinical manifestations of liver cirrhosis.

hepatic veins and sinusoids. These changes cause obstruction to the normal flow of blood through the portal system, resulting in portal hypertension. **Portal hypertension** is characterized by increased venous pressure in the portal circulation, as well as splenomegaly, large collateral veins, ascites, systemic hypertension, and esophageal varices. Many pathophysiologic changes result from portal hypertension. Collateral circulation develops in an attempt to reduce this high portal pressure and also to reduce the increased plasma volume and lymphatic flow. The common areas where the collateral channels form are in the lower esophagus (the anastomosis of the left gastric vein and the azygos veins), the anterior abdominal wall, the parietal peritoneum, and the rectum. Varicosities may develop in areas where the collateral and systemic circulations communicate, resulting in esophageal and gastric varices, *caput medusae* (ring of varices around the umbilicus), and hemorrhoids.

Esophageal varices are a complex of tortuous veins at the lower end of the esophagus, enlarged and swollen as a result of portal hypertension. **Gastric varices** are located in the upper portion (cardia, fundus) of the stomach. They occur alone or in combination with esophageal varies. Varices occur in two thirds to three fourths of patients with cirrhosis. These collateral vessels contain little elastic tissue and are quite fragile. They tolerate the high pressure poorly, and the result is distended veins that bleed easily. Large varices are more likely to bleed. Esophageal varices are responsible for approximately 80% of variceal hemorrhage. The remaining 20% of varices are due to gastric varices.

Bleeding esophageal varices are the most life-threatening complication of cirrhosis. The varices rupture and bleed in response to ulceration and irritation. Factors producing ulceration and irritation include alcohol ingestion; swallowing of poorly masticated food; ingestion of coarse food; acid regurgitation from the stom-

ach; and increased intraabdominal pressure caused by nausea, vomiting, straining at stool, coughing, sneezing, or lifting heavy objects. The patient may have melena or hematemesis. There may be slow oozing or massive hemorrhage. Massive hemorrhage is a medical emergency.

Peripheral Edema and Ascites. Peripheral edema sometimes precedes ascites, but in some patients its development coincides with or occurs after ascites. Edema results from decreased colloidal oncotic pressure from impaired liver synthesis of albumin and increased portacaval pressure from portal hypertension. Peripheral edema occurs as ankle and presacral edema.

Ascites is the accumulation of serous fluid in the peritoneal or abdominal cavity. It is a common manifestation of cirrhosis. When the BP is elevated in the liver, as occurs in cirrhosis, proteins move from the blood vessels via the larger pores of the sinusoids (capillaries) into the lymph space (Fig. 44-7). When the lymphatic system is unable to carry off the excess proteins and water, they leak through the liver capsule into the peritoneal cavity. The osmotic pressure of the proteins pulls additional fluid into the peritoneal cavity (Table 44-11).

A second mechanism of ascites formation is hypoalbuminemia resulting from the inability of the liver to synthesize albumin. The hypoalbuminemia results in decreased colloidal oncotic pressure. A third mechanism is hyperaldosteronism, which occurs when aldosterone is not metabolized by damaged hepatocytes. The increased level of aldosterone causes increased sodium reabsorption by the renal tubules. This retention of sodium, as well as an increase in antidiuretic hormone, causes additional water retention. Because of edema formation there is decreased intravascular volume and, subsequently, decreased renal blood flow and glomerular filtration.

Ascites is manifested by abdominal distention with weight gain (Fig. 44-8). If the ascites is severe, the umbilicus may be everted. Abdominal striae with distended abdominal wall veins may be present. The patient has signs of dehydration (e.g., dry tongue and skin, sunken eyeballs, muscle weakness). There is also a decrease in urinary output. Hypokalemia is common and is due to an excessive loss of potassium caused by hyperaldosteronism. Low potassium levels can also result from diuretic therapy used to treat the ascites.

Because of alterations in immune function associated with cirrhosis, patients with ascites are at risk for spontaneous bacterial peritonitis. This occurs in approximately 8% to 30% of hospitalized patients with cirrhosis and ascites. The bacteria most frequently found are gram-negative enteric pathogens such as *E. coli.*

Hepatic Encephalopathy. **Hepatic encephalopathy** is a neuropsychiatric manifestation of liver damage. It is considered a terminal complication in liver disease. Hepatic encephalopathy can occur in any condition in which liver damage causes ammonia to enter the systemic circulation without liver detoxification.

The pathogenesis of hepatic encephalopathy is incompletely understood at this time. A number of etiologic factors may be involved. It is basically a disorder of protein metabolism and excretion. The main pathogenic agents appear to be nitrogenous ammonia and aromatic amino acids. A major source of ammonia is the bacterial and enzymatic deamination of amino acids in the intestines. The ammonia that results from this deamination process normally goes to the liver via the portal circulation and is converted to urea, which is then excreted by the kidneys. When the blood is shunted past the liver via the collateral anastomoses or the

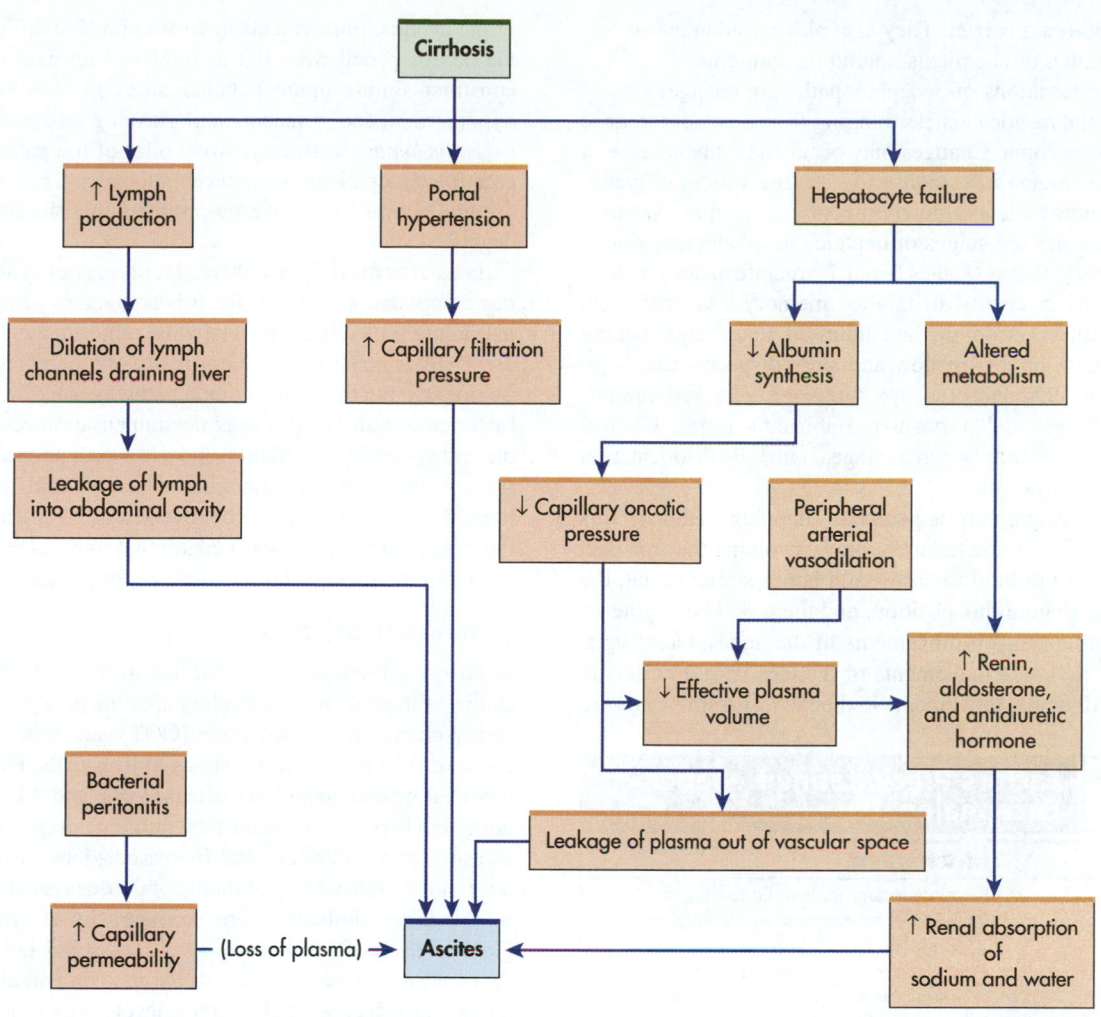

FIG. 44-7 Mechanisms for development of ascites.

TABLE 44-11	**Factors Involved in the Development of Ascites**
Factor	**Mechanism**
Portal hypertension	Increase in resistance of blood flow through liver
Increased flow of hepatic lymph	Leaking of protein-rich lymph from surface of cirrhotic liver, intrahepatic blockage of lymph channels
Decreased serum colloidal oncotic pressure	Impairment of liver synthesis of albumin, loss of albumin into peritoneal cavity
Hyperaldosteronism	Increase in aldosterone secretion stimulated by decreased renal blood flow; decreased liver metabolism of aldosterone
Impaired water excretion	Reduction in renal vascular flow and excessive serum levels of antidiuretic hormone (ADH)

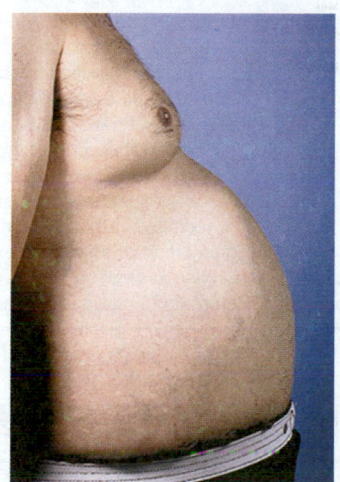

FIG. 44-8 Ascites and gynecomastia associated with cirrhosis of the liver. Photograph was taken after a paracentesis was performed.

liver is unable to convert ammonia to urea, large quantities of ammonia remain in the systemic circulation. The ammonia crosses the blood-brain barrier and produces neurologic toxic manifestations. A number of factors may precipitate hepatic encephalopathy, primarily by increasing the amount of circulating ammonia (Table 44-12). Hepatic encephalopathy is also an outcome of surgical shunt procedures and transjugular intrahepatic portosystemic shunt (TIPS), which are used to reduce portal hypertension.

Another possible contributing factor to hepatic encephalopathy is altered astrocyte function. Astrocytes play a key role in regulation of the blood-brain barrier. They also play a role in the detoxification of a number of chemicals, including ammonia.

Clinical manifestations of encephalopathy are changes in neurologic and mental responsiveness, ranging from sleep disturbance to lethargy to deep coma. Changes may occur suddenly because of an increase in ammonia in response to bleeding varices or gradually as blood ammonia levels slowly increase. A grading system is often used to classify the stages of hepatic encephalopathy (Table 44-13). In the early stages (stages 0 and 1), manifestations include euphoria, depression, apathy, irritability, memory loss, confusion, yawning, drowsiness, insomnia, and agitation. Later stages (stages 2 and 3) are characterized by slow and slurred speech, emotional lability, impaired judgment, hiccups, slow and deep respirations, hyperactive reflexes, and a positive Babinski's reflex. Clinical manifestations of impending coma (stage 4) include disorientation as to time, place, or person.

A characteristic symptom is **asterixis** (flapping tremors). This may take several forms, the most common involving the arms and hands. When asked to hold the arms and hands stretched out, the patient is unable to hold this position, and there will be a series of rapid flexion and extension movements of the hands. Other signs of asterixis are rhythmic movements of the legs with dorsiflexion of the foot and rhythmic movements in the face with strong closure of the eyelids. Impairments in writing involve difficulty in moving the pen or pencil from left to right and *apraxia* (the inability to construct simple figures). Other signs include hyperventilation, hypothermia, and grimacing and grasping reflexes.

Fetor hepaticus (musty, sweet odor of the patient's breath) occurs in some patients with encephalopathy. This odor is from the accumulation of digestive by-products that the liver is unable to degrade.

Hepatorenal Syndrome. **Hepatorenal syndrome** is a serious complication of cirrhosis. It is characterized by functional renal failure with advancing azotemia, oliguria, and intractable ascites. There is no structural abnormality of the kidneys. The etiology is complex, but the final common pathway is likely to be that portal hypertension along with liver decompensation results in splanchnic and systemic vasodilation and decreased arterial blood volume. As a result, renal vasoconstriction occurs, and renal failure follows. This renal failure can be reversed by liver transplantation. In the patient with cirrhosis, hepatorenal syndrome frequently follows diuretic therapy, GI hemorrhage, or paracentesis.[18]

Diagnostic Studies

In cirrhosis there are abnormalities in most of the liver function studies. Enzyme levels, including alkaline phosphatase, AST, ALT, and γ-glutamyl transpeptidase (GGT), are initially elevated because of their release from damaged liver cells. However, in compensated or end-stage liver disease AST and ALT levels may be normal. There is decreased total protein, decreased albumin, increased serum bilirubin, and increased globulin levels. The liver does not synthesize γ-globulins but does synthesize albumin. γ-Globulins (antibodies) are produced by B lymphocytes. The globulin level often increases in cirrhosis and indicates increased synthesis or decreased removal. Fat metabolism abnormalities are reflected by decreased cholesterol levels. The prothrombin time is prolonged, and bilirubin metabolism is altered (Table 44-14). Liver biopsy may be performed to identify liver cell changes and alterations in the lobular structure. Differential analysis of ascitic fluid may be helpful in establishing a diagnosis.

Collaborative Care

At this time there is no specific therapy for cirrhosis. It has long been thought that rest may promote liver cell regeneration by decreasing metabolic demand on the liver. Additional measures are listed in Table 44-15. Management of specific problems associated with cirrhosis is described next.

Ascites. Management of ascites is focused on sodium restriction, diuretics, and fluid removal. The amount of sodium restriction is based on the degree of ascites. Initially the patient

TABLE 44-12	Factors Precipitating Hepatic Encephalopathy
Factor	**Mechanism**
GI hemorrhage	Increase in ammonia in GI tract
Constipation	Increase in ammonia from bacterial action on feces
Hypokalemia	Potassium ions are needed by brain to metabolize ammonia
Hypovolemia	Increase in blood ammonia by causing hepatic hypoxia; impairment of cerebral, hepatic, and renal function because of decreased blood flow
Infection	Increase in catabolism, increase in cerebral sensitivity to toxins
Cerebral depressants (e.g., opioids)	Decrease in detoxification by liver, causing increase in cerebral depression
Metabolic alkalosis	Facilitation of transport of ammonia across blood-brain barrier, increase in renal production of ammonia
Paracentesis	Loss of sodium and potassium ions, decrease in blood volume
Dehydration	Potentiation of ammonia toxicity
Increased metabolism	Increase in workload of liver
Uremia (renal failure)	Retention of nitrogenous metabolites

GI, Gastrointestinal.

TABLE 44-13	Grading Scale for Hepatic Encephalopathy		
Grade	**Level of Consciousness**	**Intellectual Function**	**Neurologic Findings**
0	Insomnia, sleep disturbances	Subtle change in computational skills	Impaired handwriting, tremor
1	Lack of awareness; personality change	Short attention span; mild confusion; depression	Incoordination, asterixis
2	Lethargy, drowsiness, inappropriate behavior	Disoriented	Asterixis, abnormal reflexes
3	Asleep, rousable	Loss of meaningful conversation; marked confusion; incomprehensible speech	Asterixis, abnormal reflexes
4	Not rousable	Absent	Decerebrate; may be responsive to painful stimuli

TABLE 44-14	**Bilirubin Metabolism Abnormalities in Cirrhosis***
Type	**Finding**
Serum bilirubin	
• Unconjugated	↑
• Conjugated	↑↓
Urine bilirubin	↑
Urobilinogen	
• Stool	Normal, ↓
• Urine	Normal, ↑

*Bilirubin metabolism abnormalities occurring with hepatocellular jaundice, the most frequent type of jaundice with cirrhosis.

TABLE 44-15	*COLLABORATIVE CARE* **Cirrhosis of the Liver**

Diagnostic
History and physical examination
Liver function studies
Liver biopsy (percutaneous needle)
Esophagogastroduodenoscopy
Angiography (percutaneous transhepatic portograph)
CT scan, multiphase
Liver ultrasound
Serum electrolytes
Prothrombin time
Serum albumin
CBC
Testing of stool for occult blood
Upper GI barium swallow

Collaborative Therapy
Conservative Therapy
Administration of B-complex vitamins
Rest
Avoidance of alcohol, minimize or avoid aspirin, acetaminophen, and nonsteroidal antiinflammatory agents

Ascites
Administration of 3000-calorie, high-carbohydrate, high-protein, low-fat, low-sodium diet
Diuretics
Paracentesis (if indicated)
Peritoneovenous shunt (if indicated)

Esophageal Varices
β-Adrenergic blockers
vasopressin (Pitressin)
Endoscopic sclerotherapy or ligation
Balloon tamponade
octreotide (Sandostatin)
Surgical shunting procedure
Transjugular intrahepatic portosystemic shunt (TIPS)

Hepatic Encephalopathy
Antibiotics to decrease bacterial flora in GI tract
lactulose (Cephulac)

CBC, Complete blood count; *CT*, computed tomography; *GI*, gastrointestinal.

may be encouraged to limit sodium intake to 2g/day. Patients with severe ascites may need to restrict their sodium intake to 250 to 500 mg/day. Very low sodium intake can result in reduced nutritional intake and subsequent problems associated with malnutrition. The patient is usually not on restricted fluids unless severe ascites develops. There should be accurate assessment and control of fluid and electrolyte balance. Bed rest initially produces diuresis, which increases fluid excretion. Salt-poor albumin may be used to help maintain intravascular volume and adequate urinary output by increasing plasma colloid osmotic pressure.

Diuretic therapy is an important part of management. Often a combination of drugs that work at multiple sites in the nephron is more effective. Spironolactone (Aldactone) is an effective diuretic, even in patients with severe sodium retention. Spironolactone is an antagonist of aldosterone and is potassium sparing. Other potassium-sparing diuretics include amiloride (Midamor) and triamterene (Dyrenium). A high-potency loop diuretic, such as furosemide (Lasix), is frequently used in combination with a potassium-sparing drug. Chlorothiazide (Diuril) or hydrochlorothiazide (HydroDiuril) may also be used, but the thiazide diuretics are not as potent as the loop diuretics.[19]

A **paracentesis** (needle puncture of the abdominal cavity) may be performed to remove ascitic fluid. However, it is reserved for the patient with impaired respiration or abdominal pain caused by severe ascites. It is only a temporary measure because the fluid tends to reaccumulate.

Peritoneovenous Shunt. *Peritoneovenous shunt* is a surgical procedure that provides continuous reinfusion of ascitic fluid into the venous system. One type, the LaVeen peritoneovenous shunt, consists of a tube and a one-way valve. The tube runs from the abdominal cavity through the peritoneum, under the subcutaneous tissue, and into the jugular vein or superior vena cava (Fig. 44-9). The valve opens when the pressure in the peritoneal cavity is 3 to 5 cm H_2O higher than that in the superior vena cava. This allows the ascitic fluid to flow into the venous system. The patient's inspiration increases the intraperitoneal pressure, causing the valve to open. The goal is to increase sodium and water excretion.

Peritoneovenous shunt is not a first-line therapy for ascites because of the number of complications associated with it, including thrombosis formation at the venous tip of the shunt, infection, fluid overload, disseminated intravascular coagulopathy, variceal hemorrhage, and shunt occlusion. In addition, peritoneovenous shunts do not improve patient survival rates. Transjugular intrahepatic portosystemic shunt (TIPS) (discussed later in this section) is used increasingly to alleviate ascites.[20]

Esophageal and Gastric Varices

The main therapeutic goal for esophageal and gastric varices is avoidance of bleeding and hemorrhage. Risk factors for bleeding include variceal size, decreased wall thickness, and degree of liver dysfunction. The patient who has esophageal varices should avoid ingesting alcohol, aspirin, and irritating foods. Upper respiratory infections should be treated promptly, and coughing should be controlled. For patients who have not bled from esophageal or gastric varices, prophylactic treatment with nonselective β-blockers (e.g., propranolol [Inderal]) has been shown to reduce the risk of bleeding, as well as bleeding-related deaths.[15]

Management of bleeding varices includes emergency, therapeutic, and prophylactic interventions. Management that involves a combination of drug therapy and endoscopic therapy is more successful than either approach alone. Drug therapy may include the somatostatin analog octreotide (Sandostatin), vasopressin (VP), nitroglycerin (NTG), and β-adrenergic blockers. Endoscopic therapies include sclerotherapy, ligation of varices, and shunt therapy.

When variceal bleeding occurs, the first step is to stabilize the patient and manage the airway. IV therapy is initiated and may in-

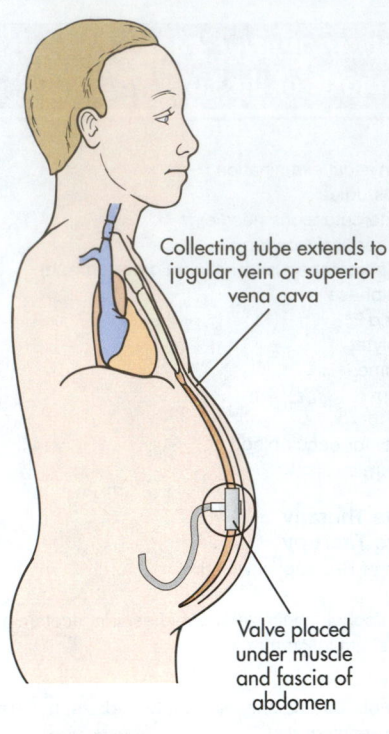

Collecting tube extends to jugular vein or superior vena cava

Valve placed under muscle and fascia of abdomen

FIG. 44-9   Peritoneovenous shunt.

clude administration of blood products. The diagnosis of esophageal or gastric variceal bleeding is made by endoscopic examination as soon as possible. At the time of endoscopy, sclerotherapy or banding of the varices may be performed.

The main goal of drug therapy is to stop bleeding so that treatment measures can be done. Gastric varices are more difficult to manage than esophageal varices. IV administration of VP produces vasoconstriction of the splanchnic arterial bed, decreases portal blood flow, and decreases portal hypertension. However, VP has many side effects, including decreased coronary blood flow and heart rate and increased BP. Because of this, NTG is often given in combination with VP. The NTG reduces the detrimental effects of the VP while enhancing its beneficial effect. VP should be avoided or used cautiously in the older adult because of the risk of cardiac ischemia.

Endoscopic sclerotherapy is a treatment method for both acute and chronic bleeding varices in many institutions. The sclerosing agent (e.g., morrhuate [Scleromate]), introduced via endoscopy, thromboses and obliterates the distended veins.

Another procedure for managing acute variceal bleeding is endoscopic ligation or banding of the varices. A small rubber band (elastic O-ring) is slipped around the base of the varix. Endoscopic variceal ligation can be done using clips instead of the O-rings (endoscopic clipping). Endoscopic ligation is as effective as endoscopic sclerotherapy with fewer complications. A combination of endoscopic sclerotherapy and ligation may be used and seems to be more effective than either treatment alone.

Balloon tamponade may be used in patients with brisk esophageal or gastric variceal hemorrhage that cannot be controlled on initial endoscopy. Balloon tamponade controls the hemorrhage by mechanical compression of the varices. The Minnesota or Sengstaken-Blakemore tube is used for this purpose (Fig. 44-10). These tubes have two balloons: gastric and esophageal. The Sengstaken-Blakemore tube has three lumens: one for the gastric

balloon, one for the esophageal balloon, and one for gastric aspiration. The Minnesota tube has an esophageal aspiration port. When inflated, the gastric and esophageal balloons put mechanical compression on the varices. The gastric balloon anchors the tube in position and also applies pressure to any bleeding gastric varices.

Supportive measures during an acute variceal bleed include administration of fresh frozen plasma and packed RBCs, vitamin K (AquaMEPHYTON), histamine (H_2)–receptor blockers such as cimetidine (Tagamet) or ranitidine (Zantac), and proton pump inhibitors (e.g., pantoprazole [Protonix]). Lactulose (Cephulac) and neomycin administration may be started to prevent hepatic encephalopathy from breakdown of blood and the release of ammonia in the intestine. Antibiotics are given during the hospitalization to prevent bacterial infection.

Long-Term Management. Long-term management of patients who have had an episode of bleeding includes β-adrenergic blockers, repeated sclerotherapy, endoscopic ligation, and portosystemic shunts. There is a high incidence of recurrent bleeding with a high mortality risk with each bleeding episode, so continued therapy is necessary. Repeated endoscopic sclerotherapy and ligation are commonly used.

Propranolol (Inderal) can be given orally to prevent recurrent GI bleeding. It reduces portal venous pressure. This effect is due to reduced cardiac output and, possibly, constriction of splanchnic vessels. However, because it reduces hepatic blood flow, it can enhance the possibility of hepatic encephalopathy.

Shunting Procedures. Surgical and nonsurgical methods of shunting blood away from the varices are available. Shunting procedures tend to be used more after a second major bleeding episode than an initial bleeding episode. *Transjugular intrahepatic portosystemic shunt (TIPS)* is a nonsurgical procedure in which a tract (shunt) between the systemic and portal venous systems is created to redirect portal blood flow (Fig. 44-11). A catheter is placed in the jugular vein and then threaded through the superior and inferior vena cava to the hepatic vein. The wall of the hepatic vein is punctured and the catheter is directed to the portal vein. Stents are positioned along the passageway, overlapping in the liver tissue and extending into both veins.

This procedure reduces portal venous pressure and decompresses the varices, thus controlling bleeding. TIPS does not interfere with future liver transplantation. Limitations of the procedure include the increased risk of hepatic encephalopathy and stenosis of the stent. TIPS is contraindicated in patients with severe hepatic encephalopathy, hepatic carcinoma, and portal vein thrombosis.

Various surgical shunting procedures may be used to decrease portal hypertension by diverting some of the portal blood flow while at the same time allowing adequate liver perfusion. Currently, the surgical shunts most commonly used are the portacaval shunt and the distal splenorenal shunt (Fig. 44-12). Surgical shunts are more likely to be used in emergency situations. Although a prophylactic portacaval shunt decreases bleeding episodes, it does not prolong life. Patients die of hepatic encephalopathy caused by the diversion of the ammonia past the liver and into the systemic circulation. The distal splenorenal shunt (Warren shunt) leaves portal venous flow intact (see Fig. 44-12), so it has a lower incidence of hepatic encephalopathy.[20] However, with time the flow of blood through the liver decreases. Similar to TIPS, surgical stents are also prone to occlusion, necessitating angiography and stent dilation.

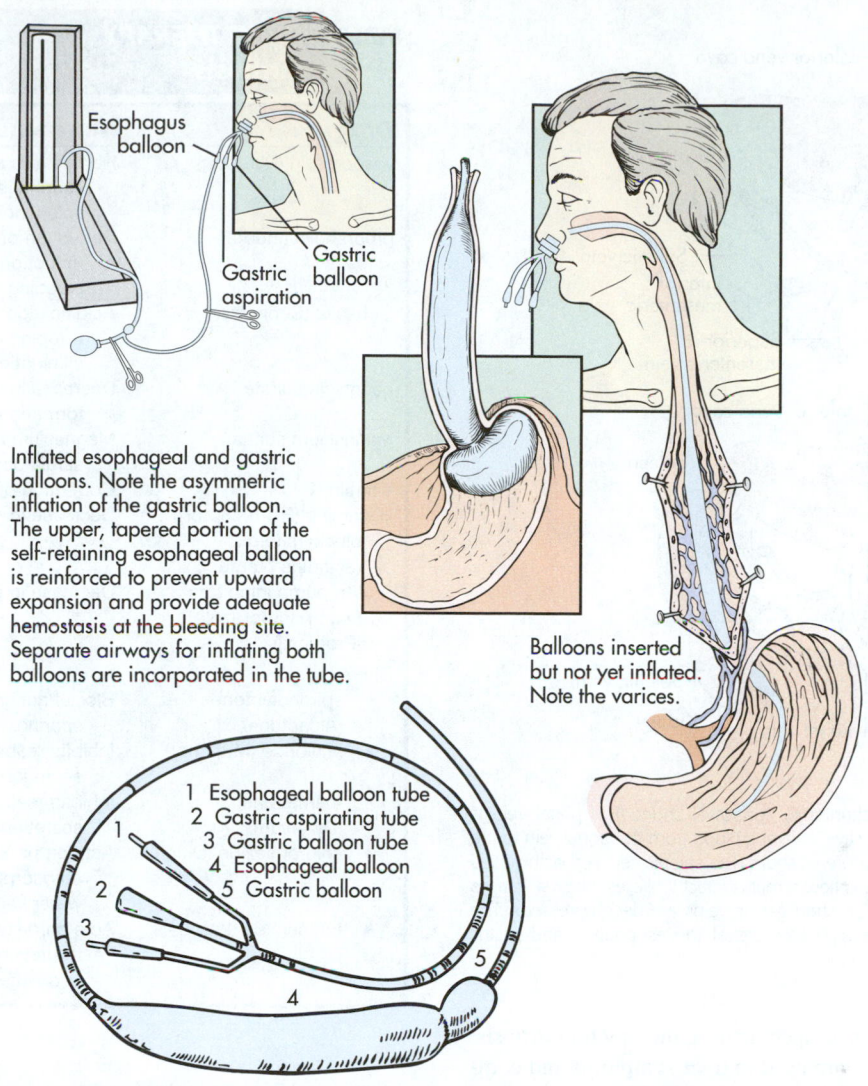

Esophagus balloon

Gastric aspiration

Gastric balloon

Inflated esophageal and gastric balloons. Note the asymmetric inflation of the gastric balloon. The upper, tapered portion of the self-retaining esophageal balloon is reinforced to prevent upward expansion and provide adequate hemostasis at the bleeding site. Separate airways for inflating both balloons are incorporated in the tube.

Balloons inserted but not yet inflated. Note the varices.

1 Esophageal balloon tube
2 Gastric aspirating tube
3 Gastric balloon tube
4 Esophageal balloon
5 Gastric balloon

FIG. 44-10   Esophageal tamponade accomplished with Sengstaken-Blakemore tube.

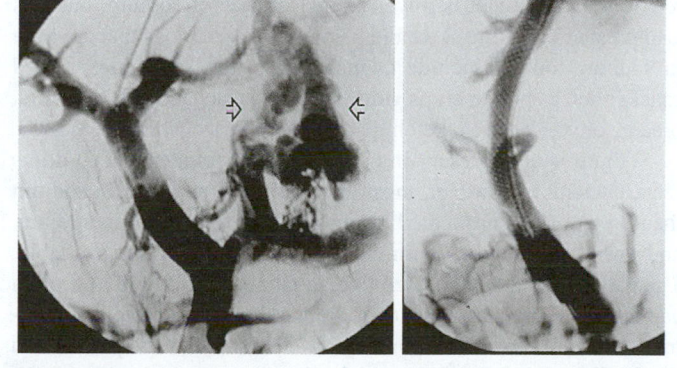

A   B

FIG. 44-11   Total portal diversion after transjugular intrahepatic portosystemic shunt (TIPS). **A,** Portal venogram before TIPS shows filling of large esophageal varices *(arrows)*. **B,** After insertion of a TIPS, flow to varices is eliminated. Intrahepatic portal vein flow is now reversed, with the direction of intrahepatic flow toward the TIPS.

Hepatic Encephalopathy. The goal of management of hepatic encephalopathy is the reduction of ammonia formation. Several measures to reduce ammonia formation in the intestines are used. Lactulose in the colon is split into lactic acid and acetic acid, which decreases the pH from 7.0 to 5.0. The acidic environment discourages bacterial growth. The lactulose traps the ammonia in the gut, and the laxative effect of the drug expels the ammonia from the colon. It is usually given orally but may be given as a retention enema or via a nasogastric (NG) tube. Antibiotics such as neomycin sulfate, which are poorly absorbed from the GI tract, are given orally or rectally. Because neomycin may cause renal toxicity and hearing impairments, lactulose or other antibiotics (metronidazole [Flagyl], vancomycin [Vancocin], rifaximin [Xifaxan]) may be prescribed. These agents reduce the bacterial flora of the colon. Bacterial action on protein in the feces results in ammonia production. Cathartics and enemas are also used to decrease bacterial action. Constipation should be prevented.

Control of hepatic encephalopathy also involves treatment of precipitating causes (see Table 44-12). This includes controlling GI bleeding and removing the blood from the GI tract to decrease the protein in the intestine. Electrolyte, especially hypokalemia, and acid-base imbalances and infections should also be treated.

Liver transplantation may be considered in patients with recurring hepatic encephalopathy and end-stage liver disease. The use of liver transplantation depends on a number of factors, including the cause of the cirrhosis and other systemic medical problems.

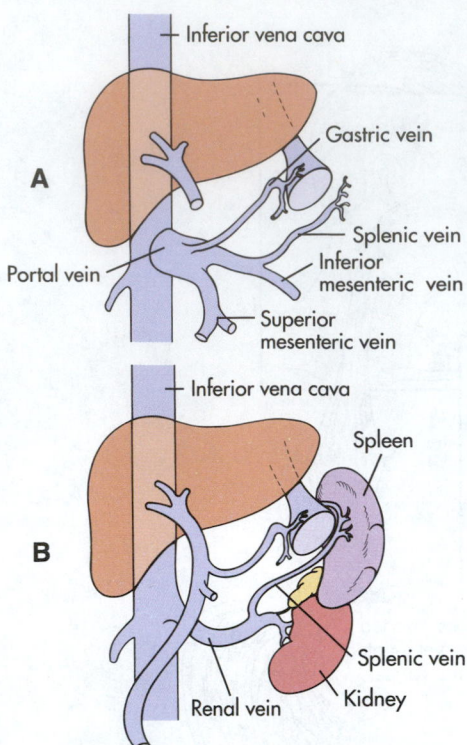

FIG. 44-12 Portosystemic shunts. **A,** Portacaval shunt. The portal vein is anastomosed to the inferior vena cava, diverting blood from the portal vein to the systemic circulation. **B,** Distal splenorenal shunt. The splenic vein is anastomosed to the renal vein. The portal venous flow remains intact while esophageal varices are selectively decompressed. (The short gastric veins are decompressed.) The spleen conducts blood from the high pressure of the esophageal and gastric varices to the low-pressure renal vein.

Drug Therapy. There is no specific drug therapy for cirrhosis. However, a number of drugs are used to treat symptoms and complications of advanced liver disease[21] (Table 44-16).

Nutritional Therapy. The diet for the patient with cirrhosis without complications is high in calories (3000 kcal/day) with high carbohydrate content and moderate to low fat levels.

Low-protein diets were routinely recommended for patients with cirrhosis in hopes of decreasing intestinal ammonia production and preventing exacerbations of hepatic encephalopathy. However, this worsened preexisting protein-calorie malnutrition. Protein restriction may be appropriate in some patients immediately following a severe flare of symptoms (i.e., episodic hepatic encephalopathy). However, protein restriction is rarely justified in patients with cirrhosis and persistent hepatic encephalopathy. Indeed, malnutrition is a more serious clinical problem than hepatic encephalopathy for many of these patients.

Sufficient carbohydrate intake must be provided to maintain a minimum intake of 1500 to 2000 calories to prevent hypoglycemia and catabolism. Glucose polymer (Polycose) is protein free and can be used as a source of calories. It can be given orally or via NG tube. A patient with alcoholic cirrhosis frequently has protein-calorie malnutrition.[15] For the patient with protein malnutrition, enteral formulas such as Hepatic-Aid II Instant Drink may be used. These supplements contain protein from branched-chain amino acids that are metabolized by the muscles. They provide protein that is more easily metabolized by the liver. Parenteral nutrition or tube feedings may be required.

TABLE 44-16	**DRUG THERAPY** Cirrhosis
Drug	**Mechanism of Action**
vasopressin (Pitressin)	Hemostasis and control of bleeding in esophageal varices, constriction of splanchnic arterial bed
propranolol (Inderal)	Reduction of portal venous pressure, reduction of esophageal varices bleeding
lactulose (Cephulac)	Acidification of feces in bowel and trapping of ammonia, causing its elimination in feces
neomycin sulfate	Decrease in bacterial flora, decreasing formation of ammonia
magnesium sulfate	Magnesium replacement; hypomagnesemia occurs with liver dysfunction
Vitamin K	Correction of clotting abnormalities
Histamine (H_2)-receptor blockers (e.g., ranitidine [Zantac])	Decrease in gastric acidity
Proton pump inhibitors (e.g., pantoprazole [Protonix])	Decrease in gastric acidity
Diuretics	
• spironolactone (Aldactone)	Blocks action of aldosterone, potassium sparing
• amiloride (Midamor)	Inhibits reabsorption of sodium and secretion of potassium
• triamterene (Dyrenium)	Inhibits reabsorption of sodium and secretion of potassium
• chlorothiazide (Diuril)	Acts on proximal tubule to decrease reabsorption of sodium and water
• furosemide (Lasix)	Acts on distal tubule and loop of Henle to prevent reabsorption of sodium and water

The patient with ascites and edema is on a low-sodium diet. The degree of sodium restriction varies depending on the patient's condition. The patient needs instruction regarding the degree of restriction. Table salt is a well-known source of sodium, but it is also present in baking soda and baking powder. Foods that are high in sodium content include canned soups and vegetables, salted snacks such as potato chips, nuts, smoked meats and fish, crackers, breads, olives, pickles, ketchup, and beer.

Sodium is also present in many over-the-counter (OTC) drugs (e.g., antacids). However, most antacids are now lower in sodium than previously. Carbonated beverages tend to be high in sodium, and low-sodium and sodium-free carbonated drinks are available. The patient should be advised to read labels. Foods high in protein usually have large amounts of sodium. Alternative protein supplements that are low in sodium may have to be used. The patient and the family need assistance to make the diet more palatable by the use of seasonings such as garlic, parsley, onion, lemon juice, and spices.

NURSING MANAGEMENT
CIRRHOSIS

■ *Nursing Assessment*

Subjective and objective data that should be obtained from an individual with cirrhosis are presented in Table 44-17.

<table>
<tr><td colspan="2">**TABLE 44-17** *NURSING ASSESSMENT* Cirrhosis</td></tr>
</table>

Subjective Data

Important Health Information

Past health history: Previous viral, toxic, or idiopathic hepatitis; chronic biliary obstruction and infection; severe right-sided heart failure

Medications: Adverse reaction to any medication; use of anticoagulants, aspirin, acetaminophen

Functional Health Patterns

Health perception–health management: Chronic alcoholism; weakness, fatigue

Nutritional-metabolic: Anorexia, weight loss, dyspepsia, nausea and vomiting; gingival bleeding

Elimination: Dark urine, decreased urinary output; light-colored or black stools, flatulence, change in bowel habits; dry, yellow skin, bruising

Cognitive-perceptual: Dull, right upper quadrant or epigastric pain; numbness, tingling of extremities; pruritus

Sexuality-reproductive: Impotence, amenorrhea

Objective Data

General

Fever, cachexia, wasting of extremities

Integumentary

Icteric sclera, jaundice, petechiae, ecchymoses, spider angiomas, palmar erythema, alopecia, loss of axillary and pubic hair, peripheral edema

Respiratory

Shallow, rapid respirations, epistaxis

Gastrointestinal

Abdominal distention, ascites, distended abdominal wall veins, palpable liver and spleen, foul breath; hematemesis; black, tarry stools; hemorrhoids

Neurologic

Altered mentation, asterixis

Reproductive

Gynecomastia and testicular atrophy (men), impotence (men), loss of libido (men and women), amenorrhea or heavy menstrual bleeding (women)

Possible Findings

Anemia, thrombocytopenia; leukopenia; ↓ serum albumin, ↓ potassium; abnormal liver function studies; ↑ coagulation studies, ammonia, and bilirubin levels; abnormal abdominal ultrasound and liver scan; positive liver biopsy

---

■ **Nursing Diagnoses**

Nursing diagnoses for the patient with cirrhosis include, but are not limited to, those presented in NCP 44-2.

■ **Planning**

The overall goals are that the patient with cirrhosis will (1) have relief of discomfort, (2) have minimal to no complications (ascites, esophageal varices, hepatic encephalopathy), and (3) return to as normal a lifestyle as possible.

■ **Nursing Implementation**

Health Promotion. The common etiologies of cirrhosis are alcohol, malnutrition, hepatitis, biliary obstruction, and right-sided heart failure. Prevention and early treatment of cirrhosis must focus on the primary cause. Alcoholism must be treated. Patients should be urged to avoid alcohol ingestion, and their efforts should be supported. Adequate nutrition, especially for the alcoholic and other individuals at risk for cirrhosis, is essential to promote liver

regeneration. Acute hepatitis must be identified and treated early so that it does not progress to chronic hepatitis. Biliary disease must be treated so that the stones do not cause obstruction and infection. The underlying cause (e.g., chronic lung disease) of right-sided heart failure must be treated so that the heart failure does not lead to cirrhosis. (The treatment of alcohol dependence is discussed in Chapter 12.)

Acute Intervention. The focus of nursing care for the patient with cirrhosis is on conserving the patient's strength (see NCP 44-2). Rest may enable the liver to restore itself. Complete bed rest may not always be necessary. When the patient requires complete bed rest, measures to prevent pneumonia, thromboembolic problems, and pressure ulcers should be taken. The activity and rest schedule may be modified according to signs of clinical improvement (e.g., decreasing jaundice, improvement in liver function studies). Appropriate nursing care measures to meet the need for rest involve regulation of the physical, emotional, and social climate.

Anorexia, nausea and vomiting, pressure from ascites, and poor eating habits all create problems in maintaining an adequate intake of nutrients. Oral hygiene before meals may improve the patient's taste sensation. Between-meal nourishments should be available so that they can be provided at times when the patient can best tolerate them. Food preferences should be provided whenever possible. The reason for any dietary restrictions should be explained to the patient and family.

Nursing assessment and care should include the patient's physiologic response to cirrhosis. Is jaundice present? Where is it observed—sclera, skin, hard palate? What is the progression of jaundice? If the jaundice is accompanied by pruritus, measures to relieve itching should be carried out. Cholestyramine (Questran) or hydroxyzine (Atarax) may be ordered to help relieve the pruritus. The color of the urine and stools should be noted. With jaundice the urine is often dark brown and foamy when shaken. The stool is gray or tan.

Edema and ascites are frequent manifestations of cirrhosis and require nursing assessments and interventions. Accurate calculation and recordings of intake and output, daily weights, and measurements of extremities and abdominal girth help in the ongoing assessment of the location and extent of the edema. If the patient can assume a kneeling position when abdominal girth measurement is taken, the abdominal fluid will go to the most dependent part of the abdomen. This gives the best measurement of abdominal girth. For many patients, girth must be measured in the standing or lying position. Where the measurements are taken should be recorded and should be a part of the nursing care plan.

When a paracentesis is done, the nurse must have the patient void immediately before the procedure to prevent puncture of the bladder. The patient sits on the side of the bed or is placed in high Fowler's position. Following the procedure the nurse should monitor for hypovolemia and electrolyte imbalances and check the dressing for bleeding and leakage.[22]

Dyspnea is a frequent problem for the patient with ascites. A semi-Fowler's or Fowler's position allows for maximal respiratory efficiency. Pillows can be used to support the arms and chest and may increase the patient's comfort and ability to breathe.

Meticulous skin care is essential because the edematous tissues are subject to breakdown. An alternating–air pressure mattress or other special mattress should be used. A turning schedule (minimum of every 2 hours) must be adhered to rigidly. The abdomen may be supported with pillows. If the abdomen is taut, cleansing

NURSING CARE PLAN 44-2

Patient with Cirrhosis

NURSING DIAGNOSIS   **Imbalanced nutrition: less than body requirements** *related to* anorexia, impaired utilization and storage of nutrients, nausea, and loss of nutrients from vomiting *as evidenced by* lack of interest in food, aversion to eating, reported inadequate food intake

PATIENT GOALS   1. Maintains food and fluid intake adequate to meet nutritional needs
2. Maintains muscle tone and energy provided by nutrients

OUTCOMES (NOC)	INTERVENTIONS (NIC) and *RATIONALES*
Nutritional Status	**Nutrition Management**
• Nutrient intake ____ • Food intake ____ • Fluid intake ____ • Muscle tone ____ • Energy ____	• Monitor recorded intake for nutritional content and calories *to evaluate nutritional status in the presence of fluid retention and edema.* • Ascertain patient's food preferences to increase nutritional appeal for patient *because a low- or no-protein diet can be unpalatable.*
Measurement Scale 1 = Severe deviation from normal range 2 = Substantial deviation from normal range 3 = Moderate deviation from normal range 4 = Mild deviation from normal range 5 = No deviation from normal range	**Nausea Management** • Use frequent oral hygiene *to promote comfort unless it stimulates nausea.* • Encourage eating small amounts of food that are appealing to the nauseated person *to prevent feeling of fullness and maintain nutritional status.* • Teach the use of nonpharmacologic techniques (e.g., biofeedback, hypnosis, relaxation, guided imagery, music therapy, distraction, acupressure) *to manage nausea to avoid use of antiemetic drugs not well metabolized by the liver.*

NURSING DIAGNOSIS   **Impaired skin integrity** *related to* edema, ascites, and pruritus *as evidenced by* complaints of itching; areas of excoriation due to scratching; taut, shiny skin over edematous areas; areas of skin breakdown

PATIENT GOAL   Maintains skin integrity with relief of edema and pruritus

OUTCOMES (NOC)	INTERVENTIONS (NIC) and *RATIONALES*
Tissue Integrity: Skin and Mucous Membranes	**Pruritus Management**
• Skin intactness ____ • Elasticity ____ • Texture ____	• Instruct patient to keep fingernails trimmed short *to prevent excoriation due to pruritus secondary to deposit of bile salts on skin.* • Apply medicated creams and lotions *to relieve itching, avoiding use of systemic drugs that require liver metabolism.*
Measurement Scale 1 = Severely compromised 2 = Substantially compromised 3 = Moderately compromised 4 = Mildly compromised 5 = Not compromised	**Skin Care: Topical Treatments** • Inspect skin of patients at risk of breakdown daily *because edematous tissues are easily traumatized and subject to breakdown.* • Provide support to edematous areas (e.g., pillow under arms and scrotal support). • Turn the immobilized patient at least every 2 hours *to reduce risk of skin breakdown in dependent areas.* • Refrain from using an alkaline soap on the skin *to prevent additional irritation of the skin.*

NURSING DIAGNOSIS   **Dysfunctional family processes: alcoholism** *related to* abuse of alcohol and inadequate coping skills *as evidenced by* deterioration in family relationships, family denial, neglected obligations, inability to accept and receive help appropriately

PATIENT GOALS   1. Family confronts problems and involves family members in decision making
2. Family uses available social support for treatment of alcohol abuse

OUTCOMES (NOC)	INTERVENTIONS (NIC) and *RATIONALES*
Family Coping	**Family Support**
• Seeks family assistance when appropriate ____ • Uses available social support ____ • Involves family members in decision making ____	• Determine the psychologic burden of prognosis for family *to determine appropriate interventions.* • Accept the family's values in a nonjudgmental manner. • Respect and support adaptive coping mechanisms used by family *to facilitate healthy coping.* • Provide opportunities for peer group support. • Refer for family therapy.
Measurement Scale 1 = Never demonstrated 2 = Rarely demonstrated 3 = Sometimes demonstrated 4 = Often demonstrated 5 = Consistently demonstrated	

NURSING CARE PLAN 44-2

Patient with Cirrhosis—cont'd

NURSING DIAGNOSIS   **Excess fluid volume** *related to* portal hypertension and hyperaldosteronism *as evidenced by* weight gain, dependent edema, ascites

PATIENT GOALS   1.   Experiences normalization of fluid balance as a result of medical and nursing interventions
2.   Maintains blood pressure and urinary output within normal limits

OUTCOMES (NOC)

Fluid Overload Severity

* Ascites ____
* Increased abdominal girth ____
* Generalized edema ____
* Increased blood pressure ____
* Increased body weight ____
* Decreased urinary output ____

Measurement Scale

1 = Severe
2 = Substantially
3 = Moderately
4 = Mild
5 = None

INTERVENTIONS (NIC) and *RATIONALES*

Hypervolemia Management

* Weigh patient daily and monitor trends *to evaluate effectiveness of treatment.*
* Administer prescribed diuretics *to prevent fluid retention and promote diuresis.*
* Monitor intake and output *to maintain necessary fluid restrictions and assess renal function.*
* Monitor changes in peripheral edema *to determine patient's response to treatment.*

Fluid/Electrolyte Management

* Provide prescribed diet appropriate for specific fluid or electrolyte imbalance (e.g., low-sodium, fluid-restricted, renal, and no added salt) *to prevent additional fluid retention.*
* Obtain laboratory specimens for monitoring of altered fluid or electrolyte levels (e.g., hematocrit, BUN, protein, sodium, and potassium levels) *to evaluate effectiveness of treatment.*

COLLABORATIVE PROBLEMS

NURSING GOALS

Potential Complication

* Monitor for signs of hemorrhage
* Initiate appropriate medical and nursing interventions

NURSING INTERVENTIONS and *RATIONALES*

Hemorrhage *related to* bleeding tendency secondary to altered clotting factors and rupture of esophageal or gastric varices

* Monitor for hemorrhage by assessing for epistaxis, purpura, petechiae, easy bruising, gingival bleeding, hematuria, heavy menstrual bleeding, hematuria, melena, or frank bleeding from body orifices *because liver disease results in impaired synthesis of clotting factors.*
* Monitor circulatory status: BP, skin color, skin temperature, heart rate and rhythm, presence and quality of peripheral pulses, and capillary refill *for early detection of hypovolemic shock.*
* Provide gentle nursing care *to minimize the risk of tissue trauma.*
* Use smallest-gauge needle possible when giving injections or drawing blood specimens and apply gentle but prolonged pressure to injection sites *to minimize risk of bleeding into tissue.*
* Advise use of soft-bristle toothbrush and avoidance of irritating food *to reduce injury to highly vascular mucous membranes.*
* Teach patient to avoid straining at stool, vigorous blowing of nose, and coughing *to reduce risk of hemorrhage at these sites.*
* Monitor laboratory results (hematocrit, hemoglobin, and prothrombin time) *as indicators of anemia, active bleeding, or impending clotting problems.*

Potential Complication

* Monitor for signs of hepatic encephalopathy
* Report deviation from acceptable parameters
* Carry out appropriate medical and nursing interventions

Hepatic encephalopathy *related to* increased serum levels of ammonia due to inability of liver to convert accumulating ammonia to urea for renal excretion

* Monitor for encephalopathy (assess patient's general behavior, orientation to time and place, speech, blood pH, and ammonia levels) *caused by toxic effects of ammonia on nervous system.*
* Encourage fluids (if not restricted) and administer laxatives and enemas as ordered *to decrease ammonia absorption from the bowel and promote bowel elimination of ammonia.*
* Limit physical activity *because exercise produces ammonia as a by-product of metabolism.*

BP, Blood pressure; *BUN,* blood urea nitrogen.

must be done very gently. This patient tends to move very little because of the abdominal discomfort and dyspnea. Range-of-motion exercises are helpful, and measures such as coughing and deep breathing to prevent respiratory problems should be implemented. The lower extremities may be elevated. If scrotal edema is present, a scrotal support provides some comfort.

When the patient is taking diuretics, the serum levels of sodium, potassium, chloride, and bicarbonate should be monitored. The patient should be observed for signs of fluid and electrolyte imbalance, especially hypokalemia. Hypokalemia may be manifested by cardiac dysrhythmias, hypotension, tachycardia, and generalized muscle weakness. Water excess is manifested by muscle cramping, weakness, lethargy, and confusion.

Observations and nursing care in relation to hematologic disorders (bleeding tendencies, anemia, increased susceptibility to infection) are the same as those for the patient with advanced liver disease (see NCP 44-2).

The nurse must assess the patient's response to altered body image resulting from jaundice, spider angiomas, palmar erythema, ascites, and *gynecomastia* (benign growth of the glandular tissue of the male breast). The patient may experience a great deal of anxiety regarding these changes. The nurse should explain these phenomena and should be a supportive listener. Nursing care with concern and warmth regardless of physical changes helps the patient maintain self-esteem.

Bleeding Varices. If the patient has esophageal and/or gastric varices in addition to cirrhosis, the nurse must observe for any signs of bleeding from the varices, such as hematemesis and melena. If hematemesis occurs, the nurse should assess the patient for hemorrhage, call the physician, and be ready to assist with treatments used to control the bleeding. The patient will be admitted to the intensive care unit (ICU). The patient's airway must be maintained.

Balloon tamponade may be used in patients who have refractory bleeding that is unresponsive to sclerotherapy or ligation. When balloon tamponade is used, the initial nursing task related to insertion of the tube is to explain the use of the tube and how it will be inserted. The balloons should be checked for patency. It is usually the physician's responsibility to insert the tube. It may be inserted via the nose or the mouth (see Fig. 44-10). Then the gastric balloon is inflated with approximately 250 ml of air, and the tube is retracted until resistance (lower esophageal sphincter) is felt. The tube is secured by placement of a piece of sponge or foam rubber at the nostrils (nasal cuff). For continued bleeding the esophageal balloon is then inflated. A sphygmomanometer is used to measure and maintain the desired pressure at 20 to 40 mm Hg. The position of the balloons is verified by x-ray.

Sometimes saline lavage is used to remove blood from the stomach. (Nursing care of upper GI bleeding is discussed in Chapter 42.) This helps prevent the blood from degrading to ammonia, leading to encephalopathy. The esophageal balloon should be deflated every 8 to 12 hours to avoid necrosis. Each lumen must be labeled to avoid confusion. The NG lumen may be connected to suction to remove blood and keep the stomach empty to reduce the risk of aspiration. The most common complication of balloon tamponade therapy is aspiration pneumonia.

Nursing care includes monitoring for complications of rupture or erosion of the esophagus, regurgitation and aspiration of gastric contents, and occlusion of the airway by the balloon. If the gastric balloon breaks or is deflated, the esophageal balloon will slip upward, obstructing the airway and causing asphyxiation. If this happens, the nurse must cut the tube or deflate the esophageal balloon. Scissors should be kept at the bedside. Regurgitation can be minimized by oral and pharyngeal suctioning and by keeping the patient in a semi-Fowler's position.

The patient is unable to swallow saliva because of the inflated esophageal balloon occluding the esophagus. With the Minnesota tube, which has an esophageal aspiration lumen, this problem can be alleviated. The nurse should encourage the patient to expectorate and should provide an emesis basin and tissues. Frequent oral and nasal care provides relief from the taste of blood and irritation from mouth breathing.

Hepatic Encephalopathy. The focus of nursing care of the patient with hepatic encephalopathy is on maintaining a safe environment, sustaining life, and assisting with measures to reduce the formation of ammonia. The nurse should assess (1) the patient's level of responsiveness (e.g., reflexes, pupillary reactions, orientation), (2) sensory and motor abnormalities (e.g., hyperreflexia, asterixis, motor coordination), (3) fluid and electrolyte imbalances, (4) acid-base imbalances, and (5) the effect of treatment measures.

The neurologic status, including an exact description of the patient's behavior, should be assessed and recorded at least every 2 hours. Care of the patient with neurologic problems should be based on the severity of the encephalopathy.

Nursing measures to prevent constipation should be instituted to decrease ammonia production. Drugs, laxatives, and enemas should be given as ordered. Encouragement of fluids may also help if not contraindicated. The patient should not strain at stool because this may cause bleeding of hemorrhoidal varices. Any GI bleeding may worsen the coma. The patient who is taking lactulose should be assessed for diarrhea and excessive fluid and electrolyte losses.

Factors that are known to precipitate coma should be controlled as much as possible. Because exercise produces ammonia as a byproduct of metabolism, the physical activity of the patient must be limited. Hypokalemia should be controlled.

Nutrition is an important consideration in the patient with cirrhosis. Foods and fluids high in carbohydrate should be given because the liver is not synthesizing and storing glucose. The patient may require tube feedings if an adequate diet cannot be ingested.

Ambulatory and Home Care. The patient with cirrhosis may be faced with a prolonged course and the possibility of serious, life-threatening problems and complications. The patient and the family need to understand the importance of continuous health care and medical supervision. They should be taught symptoms of complications and when to seek medical attention. Patients with cirrhosis should avoid activities that place them at risk for contracting viral hepatitis.

Measures to achieve and maintain a remission should be encouraged. These include proper diet, rest, avoidance of potentially hepatotoxic OTC drugs such as acetaminophen, and abstinence from alcohol. Abstinence from alcohol is important and results in improvement in most patients. The nurse must realize the difficulty this poses for some patients. The nurse's own attitude regarding the patient whose cirrhosis is attributed to alcohol abuse should be explored. Care should be given without rejection and moralizing. The patient should be treated with a caring attitude (see Chapter 12).

ETHICAL DILEMMAS
Rationing

Situation

A 43-year-old patient with cirrhosis of the liver is frequently admitted to the hospital. She has been told that her continued drinking will inevitably lead to her death. Now she has been admitted for GI bleeding and needs blood transfusions. She has a rare blood type, and it is frequently difficult to get compatible blood. Should the nurse call an ethics consultation?

Important Points for Consideration

- *Rationing,* or the distribution of scarce resources, is a difficult ethical problem. The needs of an individual patient or group of patients are weighed against the needs of many patients, who may have a greater chance of recovery, and the availability of the needed resources.
- Because alcoholism has both a genetic and a behavioral component, health care providers sometimes view these patients as noncompliant and not deserving of aggressive treatment.
- Whether blood transfusions at this point will alter the course of the patient's disease, extend her life, or improve the quality of her life are important questions to determine if this treatment is medically futile.
- Triage is the basis for rationing decisions. The amount of blood supply available, the number of people needing the blood, and the degree to which their condition can be effectively treated by blood transfusions should provide the justification for treatment decisions.
- An ethics consultation could assist in determining who would receive the greatest benefit from the scarce resource, rather than an individual clinician deciding for a particular patient.

Critical Thinking Questions

1. What are your feelings about patients with diseases, such as substance abuse, that have a behavioral component? Are these patients deserving of aggressive treatment?
2. How would you proceed to make a decision in this case? Would you request an ethics committee consultation?

Cirrhosis is a chronic disease. The patient is affected not only physically but also psychologically, socially, and economically. Major adjustments may be required to make lifestyle changes, especially if alcohol abuse is the primary etiologic factor. The nurse should provide information regarding community support programs, such as Alcoholics Anonymous, for help with alcohol abuse.

Adequate explanations, along with written instructions, related to fluid or possible dietary changes should be given to the patient and the family (Table 44-18). Other health teaching should include instruction about adequate rest periods, how to detect early signs of complications, skin care, drug therapy precautions, observation for bleeding, and protection from infection. Counseling information regarding sexual problems may be needed. Referral to a community or home health nurse may be helpful to ensure adequate patient compliance with prescribed therapy. The emphasis of home care for the patient with cirrhosis should be on helping the patient maintain the highest level of wellness possible and initiate and maintain necessary lifestyle changes.

■ Evaluation

Expected outcomes for the patient with cirrhosis are addressed in NCP 44-2.

TABLE 44-18	*PATIENT AND FAMILY TEACHING GUIDE* Cirrhosis

1. Explain to the patient and family that cirrhosis is a chronic illness and the importance of continuous health care.
2. Teach the patient and family symptoms of complications and when to seek medical attention to enable prompt treatment of complications.
3. Teach the patient to avoid potentially hepatotoxic over-the-counter drugs (see Table 39-6) because the diseased liver is unable to metabolize these drugs.
4. Encourage abstinence from alcohol because continued use of alcohol will increase the risk of liver complications.
5. Instruct the patient to avoid aspirin and control coughing to prevent hemorrhage when esophageal or gastric varices are present.
6. Teach the patient to avoid spicy and rough foods and activities that increase portal pressure, such as straining at stool, coughing, sneezing, and retching and vomiting because hemorrhage is a danger as a result of the inability of the liver to produce clotting factors.

FULMINANT HEPATIC FAILURE

Fulminant hepatic failure, or *acute liver failure,* is a clinical syndrome characterized by severe impairment of liver function associated with hepatic encephalopathy. The most common cause is drugs, usually acetaminophen in combination with alcohol. People who abuse alcohol are particularly susceptible to detrimental effects of acetaminophen on the liver. Other drugs that can cause fulminant hepatitis include isoniazid (INH), halothane (Fluothane), sulfa-containing drugs, and nonsteroidal antiinflammatory drugs (NSAIDs). Drugs can cause liver cell failure by disrupting essential intracellular processes or causing an accumulation of toxic metabolic products.

Viral hepatitis, in particular HBV, is the second most common cause of fulminant hepatic failure. Hepatic failure may also occur with HAV and less frequently with HCV. Mushroom poisoning is also associated with fulminant liver failure. The majority of mushroom poisonings occur with *Amanita phalloides* (also known as "death cap").

Fulminant hepatic failure is characterized by the rapid onset of severe liver dysfunction in someone with no prior history of liver disease. Generally the disease runs its course over 8 weeks, but it can last as long as 26 weeks. With intensive support, survival rates range from 10% to 25%.

Clinical Manifestations and Diagnostic Studies

Manifestations include jaundice, coagulation abnormalities, and encephalopathy. In acute liver failure, changes in mentation are the first clinical sign. Patients with acute liver failure are susceptible to a wide variety of complications. These include cerebral edema, renal failure, hypoglycemia, metabolic acidosis, sepsis, and multiorgan failure.

Fulminant hepatic failure is identified in most patients by laboratory abnormalities and clinical manifestations resulting from hepatic necrosis and fibrosis. Most often, serum bilirubin levels are elevated and the prothrombin time is prolonged. Liver enzyme levels (AST, ALT) are often markedly elevated. Additional laboratory tests include blood chemistries (especially glucose as hypoglycemia may be present and require correction), complete blood counts (CBCs), acetaminophen level and screening for other drugs and toxins, viral hepatitis serologies (especially HAV and HBV), serum ceruloplasmin levels, and autoantibodies (antinuclear and anti–smooth muscle antibodies). Plasma ammonia levels may also be obtained.

A liver biopsy, most often done via the transjugular route because of coagulopathy, may be indicated when conditions such as autoimmune hepatitis, metastatic liver disease, and lymphoma are suspected. In addition, ultrasound and CT are helpful in providing information about the liver size and contour, presence of ascites, tumors, and the patency of the blood vessels.

Collaborative Care

Since fulminant hepatic failure may progress rapidly, with hour-by-hour changes in consciousness, early transfer to the ICU is preferred once the diagnosis is made. Planning for transfer to a transplant center should begin in patients with grade 1 or 2 encephalopathy because they may worsen rapidly. Early transfer is important because the risks involved with patient transport may increase or even preclude transfer once stage 3 or 4 encephalopathy develops (see Table 44-13).

Acute and chronic renal failure is a frequent complication in patients with liver failure and may be due to dehydration, hepatorenal syndrome, or acute tubular necrosis. The frequency of renal failure may be even greater with acetaminophen overdose or other toxins, where direct renal toxicity occurs. Although few patients die of renal failure alone, it often contributes to mortality risk and may predict a poorer prognosis. Efforts should be made to protect renal function by maintaining adequate hemodynamics, by avoiding nephrotoxic agents such as aminoglycosides and NSAIDs, and by the prompt identification and treatment of infection.

Liver transplantation is the treatment of choice for fulminant liver failure. Liver transplant increases survival in 50% to 85% of patients with acute liver failure. Cerebral edema followed by cerebellar herniation and brainstem compression is the most common cause of death. Treatment of cerebral edema is described in Chapter 57.

NURSING MANAGEMENT
FULMINANT HEPATIC FAILURE

Frequent mental status checks should be performed if level of consciousness declines. A quiet environment to minimize agitation should be provided. Additional measures include padding bedrails to avoid injury from possible seizures, close observation to avoid injuries, monitoring of intake and output for renal function, and providing good skin and oral care to avoid breakdown and infection.

Monitoring and management of hemodynamic and renal parameters, as well as glucose, electrolytes, and acid-base status, becomes critical. Frequent neurologic evaluation for signs of elevated intracranial pressure should be conducted. Patients should be positioned with the head elevated at 30 degrees. Efforts should be made to avoid patient stimulation. Maneuvers that cause straining or Valsalva-like movements may increase intracranial pressure (ICP). It may be advisable to use endotracheal lidocaine before endotracheal suctioning. The use of any sedatives is discouraged because of their effects on the evaluation of mental status. Only minimal doses of benzodiazepines should be used, due to their delayed metabolism by the failing liver. ICP should be maintained below 20 to 25 mm Hg if possible; cerebral perfusion pressure (CPP) should be maintained above 50 to 60 mm Hg. Support of systemic BP may be required to maintain adequate CPP.

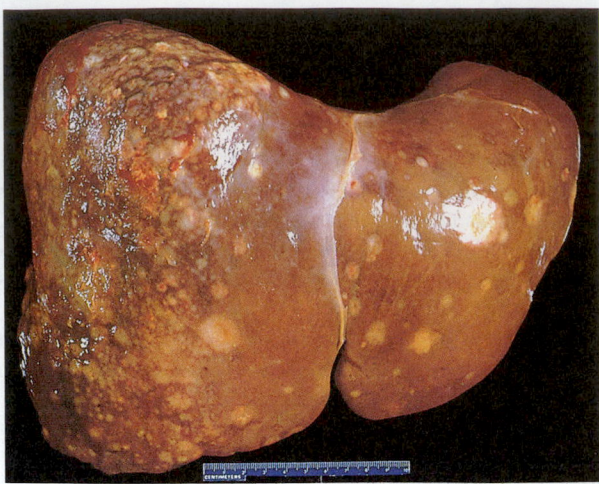

FIG. 44-13   Multiple hepatic metastases from a primary colon cancer.

LIVER CANCER

Primary liver cancer is the fourth most common cancer in the world. In 2006 in the United States there were an estimated 18,500 new cases of liver cancer and 16,200 deaths related to liver cancer.[23] Of these, the majority occur in males. Hepatocellular carcinoma is the most common primary liver cancer. It is the seventh most common cancer in men and ninth in women. The remaining primary tumors are cholangiomas or bile duct carcinomas. About 80% of people with primary liver cancer have cirrhosis of the liver. Cirrhosis is a risk factor regardless of the cause of the cirrhosis. Hepatitis C infection is responsible for about 50% to 60% of all liver cancers, and hepatitis B is responsible for approximately 20%. The incidence of liver cancer is increasing because of the increased incidence of hepatitis C.[23] Liver cancer is very rare in persons under age 40 in the United States.

Metastatic carcinoma of the liver is more common than primary carcinoma (Fig. 44-13). The liver is a common site of metastatic growth because of its high rate of blood flow and extensive capillary network. Cancer cells in other parts of the body are commonly carried to the liver via the portal circulation.

Cancer cells cause the liver to be enlarged and misshapen. Hemorrhage and necrosis in the liver are common. Lesions may be singular or numerous and nodular or diffusely spread over the entire liver. Some tumors infiltrate into other organs such as the gallbladder or into the peritoneum or diaphragm. Primary liver tumors commonly metastasize to the lung.

Clinical Manifestations and Diagnostic Studies

It is difficult to diagnose and differentiate liver cancer from cirrhosis in its early stages because of their similar clinical manifestations (e.g., hepatomegaly, splenomegaly, jaundice, weight loss, peripheral edema, ascites, portal hypertension). Other common manifestations of liver cancer include dull abdominal pain in the epigastric or right upper quadrant region, anorexia, nausea and vomiting, and increased abdominal girth. Patients frequently have pulmonary emboli. Tests used to assist in the diagnosis are a liver scan, CT, magnetic resonance imaging (MRI), magnetic resonance angiography, hepatic angiography, and endoscopic retrograde cholangiopancreatography (ERCP). If performed, liver biopsy is done laparoscopically to decrease the risk of tumor spread. Serum α-fetoprotein (AFP) levels are elevated in approximately 50% to 75% of patients with hepatocellular carcinoma. The level of elevation correlates inversely with prognosis. AFP levels help distinguish primary cancer from metastatic cancer. (AFP is discussed in Chapter 16.)

NURSING *and* COLLABORATIVE MANAGEMENT
LIVER CANCER

Prevention of liver cancer is focused on identification and treatment of chronic viral hepatitis (B and C). Treatment of chronic alcohol ingestion may also lower the risk of liver cancer. Monitoring of viral load, liver function, and histologic changes associated with cirrhosis is an important surveillance measure in at-risk patients.

Treatment of liver cancer depends on the size and number of tumors, presence of spread beyond the liver, and age and overall health of the patient. Overall the management is similar to that for liver cirrhosis. Surgical excision (lobectomy) or liver transplant is sometimes performed if the tumor is localized to one portion of the liver. Surgical resection is possible in only about 15% of patients because the cancer is usually too advanced when the patient is diagnosed. However, surgical interventions offer the best chance for cure of liver cancer. Other treatment options are radiofrequency ablation, cryosurgery (cryoablation), alcohol injection, and chemotherapy and/or chemoembolization.

In *radiofrequency ablation* treatment, a thin needle is inserted through the skin and into the core of the tumor. Then electrical energy is used to create heat in a specific location for a limited amount of time. The end result is destruction of tumor cells. This procedure can be done percutaneously, laparoscopically, or through an open incision. This therapy, although not ideal for all patients, can be used both for tumors (<5 cm in size) that are considered resectable and for palliative purposes. Complications are not common but can include infection, bleeding, dysrhythmias, and skin burn.[24]

Cryoablation is another procedure used for patients whose tumors are considered unresectable but who do not have signs of metastasis. Cryosurgery involves an open surgical approach. Cryoprobes are placed directly into the liver, and liquid nitrogen/argon gas flows through the probe and freezes the liver tissue. The tissue in the area surrounding the probe is destroyed. Cryosurgery is not used for metastatic liver disease.

Percutaneous ethanol injection (PEI) and *percutaneous acetic acid injection* (PAI) are used to treat unresectable liver cancer that has not metastasized outside the liver. This is an outpatient procedure in which a catheter is guided to the liver using ultrasound. Ethanol or acetic acid is injected for six to eight treatments over a 3- to 4-week period, with two to three injections each week. The most common side effect is transient pain following the procedure. Other, less frequent adverse events include intraperitoneal hemorrhage, hepatic insufficiency, bile duct necrosis, hepatic infarction, and transient hypotension.

Chemotherapy is used for patients with hepatocellular cancer who are not likely to benefit from other procedures (e.g., surgery, transplantation, ablation). A variety of chemotherapeutic agents (e.g., 5-fluorouracil [5-FU] and leucovorin) administered either systemically or regionally have been used to treat liver cancer. Sorafenib (Nexavar), a targeted therapy, is used to treat metastatic liver cancer. It inhibits tyrosine kinases, some of which are involved in promoting new blood vessel growth to tumors (see Table 16-17).

Chemoembolization is a minimally invasive procedure frequently performed in the interventional radiology department. In this procedure a catheter is placed in the arteries to the tumor and an embolic agent is administered, often mixed with a chemotherapeutic agent(s). The embolic agent reduces the blood supply, thus allowing greater exposure of liver cells to the chemotherapy drugs.

Nursing intervention for the patient with liver cancer focuses on keeping the patient as comfortable as possible. Because this patient manifests the same problems as any patient with advanced liver disease, the nursing interventions discussed for cirrhosis of the liver apply. (See Chapter 16 for care of the patient with cancer.)

The prognosis for patients with liver cancer is poor. The cancer grows rapidly, and death may occur within 4 to 7 months as a result of hepatic encephalopathy or massive blood loss from GI bleeding.

LIVER TRANSPLANTATION

Liver transplantation has become a practical therapeutic option for many people with end-stage liver disease. It improves the quality of life for end-stage liver disease patients and is an accepted treatment modality for these patients. Liver disease related to chronic viral hepatitis is the leading indication for liver transplantation. Other indications for liver transplantation include congenital biliary abnormalities (biliary atresia), inborn errors of metabolism, hepatic malignancy (confined to the liver), sclerosing cholangitis, fulminant hepatic failure, and chronic end-stage liver disease. Liver transplants are not recommended for the patient with widespread malignant disease. Currently, 17,000 people are waiting for liver transplants; however, only 5000 transplants are performed annually.[25,26]

Liver transplant candidates must go through a rigorous presurgery screening. This is done to ensure the diagnosis of end-stage liver disease, as well as to assess for other comorbid conditions (e.g., cardiovascular disease, chronic kidney disease) that may affect the patient's surgical outcome. The evaluation includes physical examination, laboratory tests (CBC, liver function tests), hemochromatosis evaluation, echocardiogram, endoscopy, liver ultrasound, CT scan, and psychologic testing. Potential recipients should receive counseling regarding cigarette smoking and alcohol abstinence. Contraindications for liver transplant include severe pulmonary hypertension, morbid obesity, and obstructed splanchnic blood flow.

Liver transplantation is performed using both deceased (cadaver) and live donor livers. (See Chapter 14 for a general discussion of organ transplants.) The live liver donor transplant was developed initially for children whose parents wanted to serve as donors. Today liver transplant centers are performing live liver transplant procedures for adults. In this procedure the living person donates a portion of his or her liver to another. The advantages of live organ donation include minimal cold ischemia time for the donated liver. Live liver donation does, however, pose a risk for the donor. Potential complications for the donor include biliary problems, hepatic artery thrombosis, wound infection, postoperative ileus, and pneumothorax.

Approximately 1000 patients die each year while waiting for a liver transplant. Because of the scarcity of available livers, a split organ transplant may be performed. In the split liver transplant, the donor liver is divided into two parts. This allows the liver to be implanted into two recipients. The decision to use a split donor liver is based on the size and health of the donor. The recipients of the split liver generally need to be smaller than the donor. The disadvantage of the split liver procedure is that the recipients receive less liver tissue (one receives 60% and the other 40% of the liver). The success rate associated with split liver transplantation is somewhat lower (e.g., more complications) than that associated with whole organ transplantation.

Postoperative complications of liver transplant include rejection and infection. Rejection is not as major a problem as it is in kidney transplants. The liver seems to be less susceptible to rejection than the kidney. The use of cyclosporine has been a major factor in the success rates of liver transplantation. The mechanism of action and side effects of cyclosporine are discussed in Chapter 14 and Table 14-18. This drug does not cause bone marrow suppression and does not impede wound healing. Other immunosuppressants used include the calcineurin inhibitors (e.g., tacrolimus [Prograf, FK506]), mycophenolate mofetil (CellCept), sirolimus (Rapamune), and corticosteroids (see Table 14-18). Interleukin-2 receptor antagonists such as basiliximab (Simulect) and daclizumab (Zenapax) are being used in combination with other immunosuppressive agents to reduce rejection. Other factors in the improved success rate are advances in surgical techniques, better selection of potential recipients, and improved management of the underlying liver disease before surgery.

Approximately 75% of patients survive more than 3 years following liver transplant. Long-term survival following liver transplantation depends on the cause of liver failure (e.g., localized liver cancer, hepatitis B or C, biliary disease). Patients who have liver disease secondary to viral hepatitis often experience reinfection of the transplanted liver with hepatitis B or C. For patients with HBV, treatment after surgery with HBIG and α-interferon has reduced the rates of reinfection of the graft. Patients with HCV have lower survival rates than other patient groups. Factors that contribute to recurrent HCV include advanced age of donor, HCV genotype 1, high HCV RNA levels before the transplant, and co-infection with other viruses (e.g., cytomegalovirus). Because of adverse effects associated with their use, antiviral therapy after transplant is initiated on an individual basis.[25]

The patient who has had a liver transplant requires highly skilled nursing care, either in an ICU or in some other specialized unit. Postoperative nursing care includes assessing neurologic status; monitoring for signs of hemorrhage; preventing pulmonary complications; monitoring drainage, electrolyte levels, and urinary output; and monitoring for signs and symptoms of infection and rejection. Common respiratory problems are pneumonia, atelectasis, and pleural effusions. The nurse should have the patient use measures such as coughing, deep breathing, incentive spirometry, and repositioning to prevent these complications. Drainage from the Jackson-Pratt drain, NG tube, and T tube should be measured, and the color and consistency of drainage noted. The first 2 months after the surgery are critical for monitoring for infection. Infection can be viral, fungal, or bacterial. Fever may be the only sign of infection. Emotional support and teaching the patient and family are essential.

GERONTOLOGIC CONSIDERATIONS
LIVER DISEASE IN THE OLDER ADULT

The incidence of liver diseases increases with age.[27] With aging there is a decrease in liver volume, a decrease in drug metabolism, and altered hepatobiliary function.[27] There is a decreased ability of the liver to respond to injury, in particular to regenerate following injury. Transplanted livers take longer to regenerate in the older than in the younger adult.

Older patients are particularly vulnerable to drug-induced hepatitis. This is due to several factors, including increased use of prescription and OTC drugs, which can lead to drug interactions and potential drug toxicity. Age-related decreases in liver function

caused by decreased liver blood flow and enzyme activity result in decreased drug metabolism. In addition, with aging there is a decreased ability of the liver to recover from drug-induced injury.

A growing number of older adults have chronic hepatitis C and subsequent cirrhosis.[28] The presence of HCV and elevated liver enzymes may be found during a routine health assessment. Drug therapy for HCV has been shown to be less effective in older adults. Because older adults have more comorbid conditions, liver transplant following liver failure may not be an option.

Lifetime health behaviors may also influence the development of chronic liver disease in the older adult. Chronic alcohol abuse and obesity can contribute to cirrhosis and liver inflammation (NASH) and subsequent liver failure. Because of comorbid cardiovascular and pulmonary diseases, the older adult is less able to tolerate variceal bleeding. In the older adult with liver disease, hepatic encephalopathy may be misdiagnosed as dementia.

Disorders of the Pancreas

ACUTE PANCREATITIS

Acute pancreatitis is an acute inflammatory process of the pancreas. The degree of inflammation varies from mild edema to severe hemorrhagic necrosis. Acute pancreatitis is most common in middle-aged men and women. It affects women and men equally. The severity of the disease varies according to the extent of pancreatic destruction. Some patients recover completely, others have recurring attacks, and chronic pancreatitis develops in others. Acute pancreatitis can be life threatening. The rate of pancreatitis in African Americans is three times higher than in whites.

Etiology and Pathophysiology

Many factors can cause injury to the pancreas. The primary etiologic factors are biliary tract disease (most common cause in women) and alcoholism (most common cause in men). In the United States the most common cause is gallbladder disease (gallstones), followed by chronic alcohol intake. Other, less common causes of acute pancreatitis include trauma (postsurgical, abdominal), viral infections (mumps, coxsackievirus B, HIV), penetrating duodenal ulcer, cysts, abscesses, cystic fibrosis, Kaposi sarcoma, certain drugs (corticosteroids, thiazide diuretics, oral contraceptives, sulfonamides, NSAIDs), metabolic disorders (hyperparathyroidism, hyperlipidemia, renal failure), and vascular diseases.[29] Pancreatitis may occur after surgical procedures on the pancreas, stomach, duodenum, or biliary tract. Pancreatitis can also occur after ERCP. In some cases, the cause is unknown (idiopathic).[30]

The most common pathogenic mechanism is believed to be autodigestion of the pancreas (Fig. 44-14). The etiologic factors cause injury to pancreatic cells or activation of the pancreatic enzymes in the pancreas rather than in the intestine. It is not clear how the activation of pancreatic enzymes occurs. One possible cause is the reflux of bile acids into the pancreatic ducts through an open or distended sphincter of Oddi. This reflux may be due to blockage created by gallstones. Obstruction of pancreatic ducts results in pancreatic ischemia.

Trypsinogen is an inactive proteolytic enzyme produced by the pancreas. Normally it is released into the small intestine via the pancreatic duct. In the intestine it is activated to trypsin by enterokinase. Normally, trypsin inhibitors in the pancreas and plasma bind and inactivate any trypsin that is inadvertently produced. In

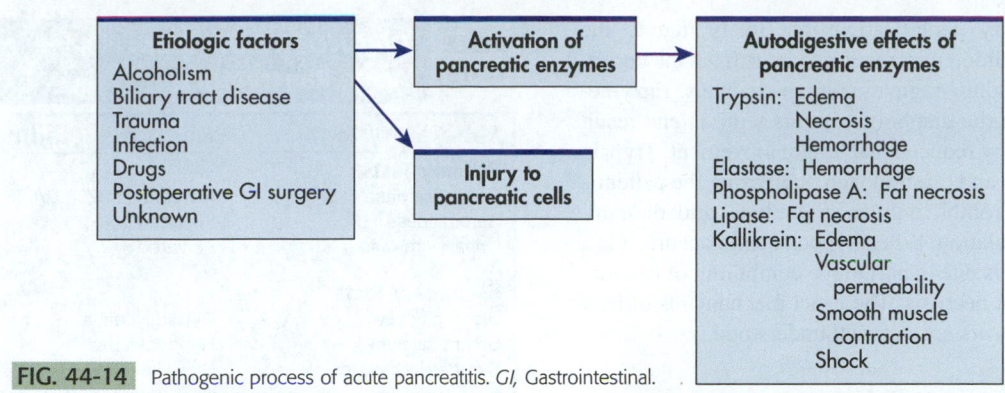

Etiologic factors	Activation of pancreatic enzymes	Autodigestive effects of pancreatic enzymes
Alcoholism Biliary tract disease Trauma Infection Drugs Postoperative GI surgery Unknown	Injury to pancreatic cells	Trypsin: Edema 　　　　Necrosis 　　　　Hemorrhage Elastase: Hemorrhage Phospholipase A: Fat necrosis Lipase: Fat necrosis Kallikrein: Edema 　　　　Vascular 　　　　　permeability 　　　　Smooth muscle 　　　　　contraction 　　　　Shock

FIG. 44-14 Pathogenic process of acute pancreatitis. *GI,* Gastrointestinal.

pancreatitis, activated trypsin is present in the pancreas. This enzyme can digest the pancreas and can activate other proteolytic enzymes such as elastase and phospholipase A.

Elastase and phospholipase A play a major role in autodigestion of the pancreas. Elastase causes hemorrhage by producing dissolution of the elastic fibers of blood vessels. Phospholipase A causes fat necrosis.

The exact mechanism by which chronic alcohol intake predisposes to pancreatitis is not known. It is thought that alcohol increases the production of digestive enzymes in the pancreas and/or increases the sensitivity to the hormone cholecystokinin (CCK). CCK stimulates the production of pancreatic enzymes. Only a small number of chronic alcohol abusers develop pancreatitis. This suggests that environmental and genetic factors may also contribute.

The pathophysiologic involvement of acute pancreatitis ranges from *edematous pancreatitis* (which is mild and self-limiting) to *necrotizing pancreatitis* (also called *severe pancreatitis*) (Fig. 44-15). In necrotizing pancreatitis, permanent decreases in endocrine and exocrine function occur in approximately half of the patients. Those patients with severe pancreatitis are also at high risk of developing pancreatic necrosis,[30] organ failure, and septic complications, resulting in a 25% mortality rate.

Clinical Manifestations

Abdominal pain is the predominant symptom of acute pancreatitis. The pain is usually located in the left upper quadrant, but it may be in the midepigastrium. It commonly radiates to the back because of the retroperitoneal location of the pancreas. The pain has a sudden onset and is described as severe, deep, piercing, and continuous or steady. It is aggravated by eating and frequently has its onset when the patient is recumbent; it is not relieved by vomiting. The pain may be accompanied by flushing, cyanosis, and dyspnea. The patient may assume various positions involving flexion of the spine in an attempt to relieve the severe pain. The pain is due to distention of the pancreas, peritoneal irritation, and obstruction of the biliary tract.

Other manifestations of acute pancreatitis include nausea and vomiting, low-grade fever, leukocytosis, hypotension, tachycardia, and jaundice. Abdominal tenderness with muscle guarding is common. Bowel sounds may be decreased or absent. Ileus may occur and causes marked abdominal distention. The lungs are frequently involved, with crackles present. Intravascular damage from circulating trypsin may cause areas of cyanosis or greenish to yellowbrown discoloration of the abdominal wall. Other areas of ecchymoses are the flanks (*Grey Turner's spots* or *sign,* a bluish flank discoloration) and the periumbilical area (*Cullen's sign,* a bluish periumbilical discoloration). These result from seepage of blood-

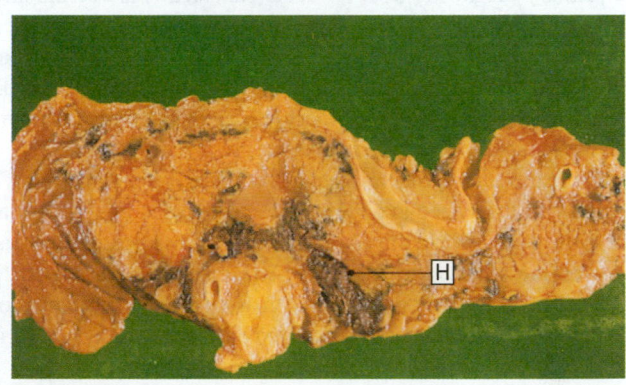

FIG. 44-15 In acute pancreatitis, the pancreas appears edematous and is commonly hemorrhagic *(H).*

stained exudate from the pancreas and may occur in severe cases. Shock may occur due to hemorrhage into the pancreas, toxemia from the activated pancreatic enzymes, or hypovolemia as a result of fluid shift into the retroperitoneal space (massive fluid shifts).

Complications

Two significant local complications of acute pancreatitis are pseudocyst and abscess.[29] A pancreatic **pseudocyst** is a cavity continuous with or surrounding the outside of the pancreas. The pseudocyst is filled with necrotic products and liquid secretions, such as plasma, pancreatic enzymes, and inflammatory exudates. As pancreatic enzymes escape from the pseudocyst, the serosal surfaces next to the pancreas become inflamed, with subsequent formation of granulation tissue leading to encapsulation of the exudate. Manifestations of pseudocyst are abdominal pain, palpable epigastric mass, nausea, vomiting, and anorexia. The serum amylase level frequently remains elevated. These cysts usually resolve spontaneously within a few weeks but may perforate, causing peritonitis, or rupture into the stomach or duodenum. Treatment consists of an internal drainage procedure with an anastomosis between the pancreatic duct and the jejunum.

A pancreatic abscess is a large fluid-containing cavity within the pancreas. It results from extensive necrosis in the pancreas. It may become infected or perforate into adjacent organs. Manifestations of an abscess include upper abdominal pain, abdominal mass, high fever, and leukocytosis. Pancreatic abscesses require prompt surgical drainage to prevent sepsis.

The main systemic complications of acute pancreatitis are pulmonary (pleural effusion, atelectasis, and pneumonia) and cardiovascular (hypotension) complications and tetany caused by hypocalcemia. The pulmonary complications are likely due to the passage of exudate containing pancreatic enzymes from the peritoneal cavity through transdiaphragmatic lymph channels. Enzyme-induced inflammation of the diaphragm occurs with an end result being atelectasis caused by reduced diaphragm movement. Trypsin can activate prothrombin and plasminogen, increasing the patient's risk for intravascular thrombi, pulmonary emboli, and disseminated intravascular coagulation. When hypocalcemia occurs, it is a sign of severe disease. It is due in part to the combining of calcium and fatty acids during fat necrosis. The exact mechanisms of how or why hypocalcemia occurs are not well understood.

Diagnostic Studies

The primary diagnostic tests for acute pancreatitis are serum amylase and lipase (Table 44-19). The serum amylase level is usually elevated early and remains elevated for 24 to 72 hours. Serum lipase level is also elevated in acute pancreatitis and is a helpful complementary test because other disorders (e.g., mumps, cerebral trauma, renal transplantation) may increase serum amylase levels.[31]

During the acute inflammation, other digestive enzymes may be released into the systemic circulation. These include phospholipase A, trypsin, carboxylester lipase, carboxypeptidase A, and co-lipase. However, the measurement of these enzymes does not provide an advantage over serum amylase and lipase.[32] Additional laboratory tests may be done, including urinary amylase, which may persist for several days beyond the elevation of serum amylase.

Normally a timed collection (e.g., a 2-hour collection) is a more dependable measure than a randomly collected urinary specimen. The renal amylase-creatinine clearance test estimates the amount of blood cleared of amylase by the kidney per minute.

Nonenzyme laboratory tests may also be used. Trypsinogen activation peptide (TAP) is produced by the conversion of trypsinogen to active trypsin. Urinary TAP levels may be particularly useful in detection of early acute pancreatitis.[33] Other laboratory abnormalities include hyperglycemia, hyperlipidemia, and hypocalcemia (see Table 44-19). There is a high incidence of hyperlipidemia with recurrent pancreatitis.

Diagnostic evaluation of acute pancreatitis is also directed at determining the cause. An abdominal ultrasound, x-ray, or contrast-enhanced computed tomography (CECT) can be used to identify pancreatic problems. The CECT is the best imaging diagnostic test for pancreatitis and related complications such as pseudocysts and abscesses. Other diagnostic tests include ERCP, endoscopic ultrasound (EUS), magnetic resonance cholangiopancreatography (MRCP), and angiography.

Collaborative Care

Objectives of collaborative care for acute pancreatitis include (1) relief of pain; (2) prevention or alleviation of shock; (3) reduction of pancreatic secretions; (4) control of fluid and electrolyte imbalances; (5) prevention or treatment of infections; and (6) removal of the precipitating cause, if possible[31] (Table 44-20).

Conservative Therapy. Treatment is principally focused on supportive care, including aggressive hydration, pain management, management of metabolic complications, and minimizing pancreatic stimulation. A primary consideration in the treatment of acute pancreatitis is the relief and control of pain. IV morphine may be used. Pain medications may be combined with an antispasmodic agent. However, atropine-like drugs should be avoided when paralytic ileus is present because they may contribute to the problem.

TABLE 44-19	*DIAGNOSTIC STUDIES* Acute Pancreatitis
Laboratory Test	**Abnormal Finding**
Primary Tests	
Serum amylase	Increased (>200 U/L [3.34 μkat/L])
Serum lipase	Elevated
Urinary amylase	Elevated
Secondary Tests	
Blood glucose	Hyperglycemia
Serum calcium	Hypocalcemia
Serum triglycerides	Hyperlipidemia

TABLE 44-20	*COLLABORATIVE CARE* Acute Pancreatitis

Diagnostic
History and physical examination
Serum amylase
Serum lipase
Two-hour urinary amylase and renal amylase clearance
Blood glucose
Serum calcium
Triglycerides
Flat plate of the abdomen
Abdominal ultrasound
Endoscopic ultrasound
Contrast-enhanced CT (CECT) of the pancreas
Magnetic resonance cholangiopancreatography (MRCP)
Endoscopic retrograde cholangiopancreatography (ERCP)
Chest x-ray

Collaborative Therapy
Pain medication (e.g., morphine)
NPO with NG tube to suction
Albumin (if shock present)
IV calcium gluconate (10%) (if tetany present)
Lactated Ringer's solution
ranitidine (Zantac) or omeprazole (Prilosec)
Antibiotics (if necrotizing pancreatitis)

CT, Computed tomography; *IV,* intravenous; *NG,* nasogastric; *NPO,* nothing by mouth.

Other medications that relax smooth muscles (spasmolytics), such as nitroglycerin or papaverine, may be used.

If shock is present, blood volume replacements are used. Plasma or plasma volume expanders such as dextran or albumin may be given. Fluid and electrolyte imbalances are corrected with lactated Ringer's solution or other electrolyte solutions. Central venous pressure readings may be used to assist in determination of fluid replacement requirements. Vasoactive drugs such as dopamine (Intropin) may be used to increase systemic vascular resistance in patients with ongoing hypotension.

It is important to reduce or suppress pancreatic enzymes to decrease stimulation of the pancreas and allow it to rest. This is accomplished in several ways. First, the patient is allowed to take nothing by mouth (NPO). Second, NG suction may be used to reduce vomiting and gastric distention and to prevent gastric acidic contents from entering the duodenum. These measures suppress pancreatic secretion. Certain drugs may also be used for this purpose (Table 44-21).

TABLE 44-21	**DRUG THERAPY** **Acute and Chronic Pancreatitis**

Drug	Mechanism of Action
Acute Pancreatitis	
morphine	Relief of pain
nitroglycerin or papaverine	Relaxation of smooth muscles and relief of pain
Antispasmodics (e.g., dicyclomine [Bentyl], propantheline bromide [Pro-Banthine])	Decrease of vagal stimulation, motility, pancreatic outflow (inhibition of volume and concentration of bicarbonate and enzymatic secretion); contraindicated in paralytic ileus
Carbonic anhydrase inhibitor (acetazolamide [Diamox])	Reduction in volume and bicarbonate concentration of pancreatic secretion
Antacids	Neutralization of gastric hydrochloric (HCl) acid secretion and subsequent decrease in secretion, which stimulates production and secretion of pancreatic secretions
Histamine (H₂)-receptor antagonists (ranitidine [Zantac]); proton pump inhibitors (omeprazole [Prilosec])	Decrease in HCl acid secretion (HCl acid stimulates pancreatic activity)
Chronic Pancreatitis	
pancreatin (Viokase, Pancreatin, Pancrezyme), pancrelipase (Cotazym, Pancrease)	Replacement therapy for pancreatic enzymes
Insulin	Treatment for diabetes mellitus if it occurs or for hyperglycemia

TABLE 44-22	**NURSING ASSESSMENT** **Acute Pancreatitis**

Subjective Data
Important Health Information
Past health history: Biliary tract disease, alcohol use, abdominal trauma, duodenal ulcers, infection, metabolic disorders
Medications: Use of thiazides, nonsteroidal antiinflammatory drugs
Surgery or other treatments: Surgical procedures on the pancreas, stomach, duodenum, or biliary tract; endoscopic retrograde cholangiopancreatography

Functional Health Patterns
Health perception–health management: Alcohol abuse; weakness
Nutritional-metabolic: Nausea and vomiting; anorexia
Activity-exercise: Dyspnea
Cognitive-perceptual: Severe midepigastric or left upper quadrant pain that may radiate to the back, aggravated by food and alcohol intake and unrelieved by vomiting

Objective Data
General
Restlessness, anxiety, low-grade fever

Integumentary
Flushing, diaphoresis, discoloration of abdomen and flanks, cyanosis, jaundice; decreased skin turgor, dry mucous membranes

Respiratory
Tachypnea, basilar crackles

Cardiovascular
Tachycardia, hypotension

Gastrointestinal
Abdominal distention, tenderness, and muscle guarding; diminished bowel sounds

Possible Findings
↑ Serum amylase and lipase, leukocytosis, hyperglycemia, ↑ urine amylase, hyperlipidemia, hypocalcemia, abnormal ultrasound and CT scans of pancreas, abnormal ERCP

CT, Computed tomography; *ERCP,* endoscopic retrograde cholangiopancreatogram.

The inflamed and necrotic pancreatic tissue is a good medium for bacterial growth. Therefore it is important to prevent infections. There is some controversy about the prophylactic use of antibiotics. It is important to monitor the patient closely so that antibiotic therapy can be instituted early if infection occurs.[34]

Peritoneal lavage or dialysis has been used to remove the kinin and phospholipase A–containing exudate from the peritoneal cavity. This has proved beneficial in some cases of severe acute pancreatitis. It prevents early death but has little effect on overall mortality rate.

Surgical Therapy. When the acute pancreatitis is related to the presence of gallstones, an urgent ERCP plus endoscopic sphincterotomy may be performed. This may be followed by laparoscopic cholecystectomy to reduce the potential for recurrence. Surgical intervention may also be indicated when the diagnosis is uncertain and in patients who do not respond to conservative therapy. Surgery is necessary for an abscess, an acute pseudocyst, and severe peritonitis. Percutaneous drainage of a pseudocyst can be performed, and a drainage tube is left in place.

Drug Therapy. Several different drugs may be used in the treatment of both acute and chronic pancreatitis (see Table 44-21). A number of drugs are used in an effort to suppress pancreatic secretion, but these drugs have not proved effective in the management of pancreatitis.

Nutritional Therapy. Initially the patient with acute pancreatitis is on NPO status to reduce pancreatic secretion. Depend-

ing on the severity of the pancreatitis, enteral feedings or parenteral nutrition may be initiated. If IV lipids are ordered, blood triglyceride levels need to be monitored. In cases of moderate to severe pancreatitis, the patient may require enteral feeding via a jejunal feeding tube.[35] If severe nutritional deficiencies exist, parenteral nutrition may be used (see Chapter 40). When food is allowed, small, frequent feedings are given. The diet is usually high in carbohydrate content because that is the least stimulating to the exocrine portion of the pancreas. Intolerance to oral foods is suspected when the patient reports increasing abdominal girth or has elevations in serum amylase and lipase levels. The patient needs to abstain from alcohol. Supplemental fat-soluble vitamins may be given.

NURSING MANAGEMENT
ACUTE PANCREATITIS

■ *Nursing Assessment*

Subjective and objective data that should be obtained from a person with acute pancreatitis are presented in Table 44-22.

■ *Nursing Diagnoses*

Nursing diagnoses for the patient with acute pancreatitis may include, but are not limited to, those presented in NCP 44-3.

NURSING CARE PLAN 44-3

Patient with Acute Pancreatitis

NURSING DIAGNOSIS **Acute pain** *related to* distention of pancreas, peritoneal irritation, obstruction of biliary tract, and ineffective pain and comfort measures *as evidenced by* communication of pain descriptors, guarding behavior, behaviors indicative of pain (e.g., moaning), diaphoresis, changes in blood pressure, pulse, and respiratory rate

PATIENT GOALS
1. Reports adequate pain control
2. Uses nonpharmacologic techniques of pain management to reduce need for pain medication

OUTCOMES (NOC)	INTERVENTIONS (NIC) and *RATIONALES*
Pain Control	**Pain Management**
• Uses analgesics appropriately _____	• Perform a comprehensive assessment of pain to include location, characteristics, onset/duration, frequency, quality, intensity or severity of pain, and precipitating factors *to plan appropriate interventions.*
• Uses nonanalgesic relief measures _____	
• Reported pain controlled _____	• Provide the person optimal pain relief with prescribed analgesics *to ensure more effective relief of pain.*
Measurement Scale	• Evaluate the effectiveness of the pain-control measures used through ongoing assessment of the pain experience *to adjust pain medication administration in order to provide ongoing relief of pain.*
1 = Never demonstrated	
2 = Rarely demonstrated	
3 = Sometimes demonstrated	• Teach the use of nonpharmacologic techniques (e.g., relaxation, guided imagery, hot/cold application, and massage) before, after, and, if possible, during painful activities; before pain occurs or increases; and along with other pain-relief measures *to assist in reducing the restlessness that usually accompanies the pain*
4 = Often demonstrated	
5 = Consistently demonstrated	

NURSING DIAGNOSIS **Deficient fluid volume** *related to* nausea, vomiting, NG suction, and restricted oral intake *as evidenced by* increased fluid output, altered intake, dry skin and mucous membranes, decreased skin turgor

PATIENT GOAL Maintains adequate fluid volume with balanced intake and output, stable weight, and moist mucous membranes

OUTCOMES (NOC)	INTERVENTIONS (NIC) and *RATIONALES*
Fluid Balance	**Vomiting Management**
• Skin turgor _____	• Ensure that effective antiemetic drugs are given to prevent vomiting when possible *to reduce fluid loss by preventing vomiting.*
• Moist mucous membranes _____	
• 24-hour intake and output balance _____	• Measure or estimate emesis volume *as indicators of replacement needs and effectiveness of treatment.*
• Stable body weight _____	**Electrolyte Management: Hypocalcemia**
Measurement Scale	• Monitor for neuromuscular manifestations of hypocalcemia (e.g., tetany, muscle twitching, cramping, grimacing, seizure, altered deep tendon reflexes, and spasm) *to provide appropriate intervention.*
1 = Severely compromised	
2 = Substantially compromised	
3 = Moderately compromised	• Monitor for CNS manifestations of hypocalcemia (e.g., personality disturbances, anxiety, irritability, depression, and psychosis).
4 = Mildly compromised	
5 = Not compromised	

■ *Planning*

The overall goals are that the patient with acute pancreatitis will have (1) relief of pain, (2) normal fluid and electrolyte balance, (3) minimal to no complications, and (4) no recurrent attacks.

■ *Nursing Implementation*

Health Promotion. The major factors involved in health promotion are assessment of the patient for predisposing and etiologic factors and encouragement of early treatment of these factors to prevent occurrence of acute pancreatitis. The nurse should encourage the early diagnosis and treatment of biliary tract disease, such as cholelithiasis. The patient should be encouraged to eliminate alcohol intake, especially if there have been any previous episodes of pancreatitis. Attacks of pancreatitis become milder or disappear with the discontinuance of alcohol use.

Acute Intervention. During the acute phase, it is important to monitor vital signs. Hemodynamic stability may be compromised by hypotension, fever, and tachypnea. IV fluids are or-

dered, and the response to therapy is monitored. Fluid and electrolyte balance is closely monitored. Frequent vomiting, along with gastric suction, may result in decreased chloride, sodium, and potassium levels.

Respiratory failure may develop in the patient with severe acute pancreatitis. It is important that respiratory function be assessed (e.g., lung sounds). If acute respiratory distress syndrome develops, the patient may require intubation and mechanical ventilatory support.

Because hypocalcemia can also occur, the nurse must observe for symptoms of tetany, such as jerking, irritability, and muscular twitching. Numbness or tingling around the lips and in the fingers is an early indicator of hypocalcemia. The patient should be assessed for a positive Chvostek or Trousseau sign (see Fig. 17-15). Calcium gluconate (as ordered) should be given to treat symptomatic hypocalcemia. Hypomagnesemia may also develop, necessitating the observation of serum magnesium levels.[36]

Because abdominal pain is a prominent symptom of pancreatitis, a major focus of nursing care is the relief of pain (see NCP

NURSING CARE PLAN 44-3

Patient with Acute Pancreatitis—cont'd

NURSING DIAGNOSIS **Imbalanced nutrition: less than body requirements** *related to* anorexia, dietary restrictions, nausea, loss of nutrients from vomiting, and impaired digestion resulting in decreased use of nutrients *as evidenced by* weight loss, weakness, fatigue, weight below normal for height and age

PATIENT GOALS 1. Maintains weight appropriate for height
2. Food and fluid intake adequate to meet nutritional needs

OUTCOMES (NOC)	INTERVENTIONS (NIC) and *RATIONALES*
Nutritional Status	*Nutrition Therapy*
• Food intake _____	• Monitor laboratory values *as indicators of patient's response to treatment.*
• Fluid intake _____	• Administer parenteral nutrition to provide carbohydrates, lipids, and amino acids *to prevent negative nitrogen balance.*
• Energy _____	• Provide oral care before meals *to decrease foul taste and odor that inhibit appetite.*
• Weight/height ratio _____	• Ensure availability of progressive therapeutic diet *to avoid overstimulation of the pancreas.*
Measurement Scale	• Provide needed nourishment *within limits of prescribed diet.*
1 = Severe deviation from normal range	*Nutrition Management*
2 = Substantial deviation from normal range	• Weigh patient at appropriate intervals *to monitor nutritional status.*
3 = Moderate deviation from normal range	
4 = Mild deviation from normal range	
5 = No deviation from normal range	

NURSING DIAGNOSIS **Ineffective therapeutic regimen management** *related to* lack of knowledge of preventive measures, diet restrictions, restriction of alcohol intake, and follow-up care *as evidenced by* verbalization of the problem, request for information, inaccurate follow-through on instructions

PATIENT GOALS 1. Describes therapeutic regimen with regard to disease process and management
2. Expresses commitment to lifestyle changes and participation in treatment for alcohol dependence

OUTCOMES (NOC)	INTERVENTIONS (NIC) and *RATIONALES*
Knowledge: Disease Process	*Teaching: Disease Process*
• Description of specific disease process _____	• Appraise patient's current level of knowledge related to specific disease process *to establish baseline for teaching.*
• Description of effects of disease _____	• Explain pathophysiology of the disease and how it relates to anatomy and physiology.
• Description of measures to minimize disease progression _____	• Discuss lifestyle changes that may be required *to prevent future complications and/or control the disease process.*
• Description of signs and symptoms of complications _____	• Instruct the patient on which signs and symptoms to report to health care provider *to prevent recurrence.*
Measurement Scale	• Refer the patient to local community agencies/support groups *for support in treatment of alcohol dependency.*
1 = None	
2 = Limited	
3 = Moderate	
4 = Substantial	
5 = Extensive	

CNS, Central nervous system; *NG,* nasogastric.

44-3). Pain and restlessness can increase the metabolic rate and subsequent stimulation of pancreatic enzymes. Morphine may be used for pain relief. The nurse should ascertain how long the pain medication provides relief. Measures such as comfortable positioning, frequent changes in position, and relief of nausea and vomiting assist in reducing the restlessness that usually accompanies the pain. Assuming positions that flex the trunk and draw the knees up to the abdomen may decrease pain. A side-lying position with the head elevated 45 degrees decreases tension on the abdomen and may help ease the pain.

Nursing measures for the patient who is on NPO status or has an NG tube should be employed. Frequent oral and nasal care to relieve the dryness of the mouth and nose is comforting to the patient. Oral care is essential to prevent parotitis. If the patient is taking anticholinergics to decrease GI secretions, there will be ad-

ditional dryness of the mouth. If the patient is taking antacids to neutralize gastric acid secretion, they should be sipped slowly or inserted in the NG tube.

The nurse should observe for fever and other manifestations of infection in the patient with acute pancreatitis. Respiratory infections are common because the retroperitoneal fluid raises the diaphragm, which causes the patient to take shallow, guarded abdominal breaths. Measures to prevent respiratory infections include turning, coughing, deep breathing, and assuming a semi-Fowler's position.[34]

Other important assessments are observation for signs of paralytic ileus, renal failure, and mental changes. Determination of the blood glucose level should be done to assess damage to the β-cells of the islets of Langerhans in the pancreas.

After pancreatic surgery the patient may require special wound care for an anastomotic leak or a fistula. Measures to prevent skin irritation should be used. These include skin barriers such as Stomahesive, Karaya paste, or Colly-Seel; pouching; and drains. In addition to protecting the skin, pouching also provides a more accurate determination of fluid and electrolyte losses and increases patient comfort. Sterile pouching systems are available. The nurse may want to consult with a clinical specialist or an enterostomal therapy nurse, if available.

Ambulatory and Home Care. After acute pancreatitis, patients may require home care follow-up. The patient may have lost physical and muscle strength. Physical therapy may be needed. Continued care to prevent infection and detect any complications is important. Because frequent doses of opioids may be required for this patient during the acute stage, follow-up for assessment of possible opioid addiction may be indicated. This is a more likely problem with chronic pancreatitis than in the patient with acute pancreatitis. Counseling regarding abstinence from alcohol is important to prevent the patient from experiencing future attacks of acute pancreatitis and development of chronic pancreatitis. Beverages with caffeine should not be consumed. Because smoking and stressful situations can overstimulate the pancreas, they should be avoided.

Dietary teaching should include restriction of fats because they stimulate the secretion of CCK, which then stimulates the pancreas. Carbohydrates are less stimulating to the pancreas and are encouraged. The patient should be instructed to avoid crash dieting and bingeing because they can precipitate attacks.

The patient and the family should be given instructions regarding the recognition and reporting of symptoms of infection, diabetes mellitus, or steatorrhea (foul-smelling, frothy stools). These changes indicate possible ongoing destruction of pancreatic tissue. The nurse should make sure the patient fully understands the prescribed regimen. The importance of taking the required medications and following the recommended diet should be stressed.

■ *Evaluation*

Expected outcomes for the patient with acute pancreatitis are presented in NCP 44-3.

CHRONIC PANCREATITIS

Chronic pancreatitis is a continuous, prolonged, inflammatory, and fibrosing process of the pancreas. The pancreas becomes progressively destroyed as it is replaced with fibrotic tissue. Strictures and calcifications may also occur in the pancreas.

Etiology and Pathophysiology

There are several types of chronic pancreatitis, but they all have a common underlying pathophysiologic disorder. The two major types are *chronic obstructive pancreatitis* and *chronic calcifying pancreatitis*. Chronic pancreatitis may follow acute pancreatitis, but it may also occur in the absence of any history of an acute condition.

Chronic obstructive pancreatitis is associated with biliary disease. The most common cause is inflammation of the sphincter of Oddi associated with cholelithiasis (gallstones). Cancer of the ampulla of Vater, duodenum, or pancreas can also cause this type of chronic pancreatitis.

In chronic calcifying pancreatitis there is inflammation and sclerosis, mainly in the head of the pancreas and around the pancreatic duct. This type of chronic pancreatitis is the most common form. It is also called alcohol-induced pancreatitis. Increases in heavy social drinking have produced a higher incidence in countries in which the disease was previously considered rare. In the United States, chronic pancreatitis is found almost exclusively in individuals who abuse alcohol. There may be a genetic factor that predisposes a person who drinks to the direct toxic effect of the alcohol on the pancreas.

In chronic calcifying pancreatitis the ducts are obstructed with protein precipitates. These precipitates block the pancreatic duct and eventually calcify. This is followed by fibrosis and glandular atrophy. Pseudocysts and abscesses commonly develop.

Clinical Manifestations

As with acute pancreatitis, a major manifestation of chronic pancreatitis is abdominal pain. The patient may have episodes of acute pain, but it usually is chronic (recurrent attacks at intervals of months or years). The attacks may become more and more frequent until they are almost constant, or they may diminish as the pancreatic fibrosis develops. The pain is located in the same areas as in acute pancreatitis but is usually described as a heavy, gnawing feeling or sometimes as burning and cramplike. The pain is not relieved with food or antacids.

Other clinical manifestations include symptoms of pancreatic insufficiency, including malabsorption with weight loss, constipation, mild jaundice with dark urine, steatorrhea, and diabetes mellitus. The steatorrhea may become severe, with voluminous, foul, fatty stools. Urine and stool may be frothy. Some abdominal tenderness may be present.

Chronic pancreatitis is also associated with a variety of complications. These include pseudocyst formation, bile duct or duodenal obstruction, pancreatic ascites or pleural effusion, splenic vein thrombosis, pseudoaneurysms, and pancreatic cancer.

Diagnostic Studies

Confirming the diagnosis of chronic pancreatitis can be challenging. The diagnosis is based on the patient's signs and symptoms, laboratory studies, and imaging. In chronic pancreatitis the levels of serum amylase and lipase may be elevated slightly or not at all, depending on the degree of pancreatic fibrosis. Increased serum bilirubin and increased alkaline phosphatase levels may be present. There is usually mild leukocytosis and an elevated sedimentation rate.

ERCP is used to visualize the pancreatic and common bile ducts. Changes in the pancreatic ductal system, such as gross dilation and microcysts, can be visualized through the use of ERCP. In this procedure an endoscope is orally inserted into the duodenum. The common bile duct and the pancreatic duct are then cannulated. Contrast dye can be injected into the ducts for visualization.

Imaging studies such as CT, MRI, MRCP, transabdominal ultrasound, and EUS are useful in patients with chronic pancreatitis. These procedures show a variety of changes, including calcifications, ductal dilation, pseudocysts, and pancreatic enlargement.

The secretin stimulation test is used to assess the degree of pancreatic function. Because some patients with chronic pancreatitis may have a normal test, it is not useful in the diagnosis. In the normal pancreas secretin stimulates pancreatic bicarbonate (HCO_3^-) secretion. In the stimulation test IV secretin is administered, and gastric-duodenal secretions are collected with a double-lumen tube for separate gastric and duodenal aspiration. In chronic pancreatitis there is reduced volume of secretions and reduced HCO_3^- concentration.

Collaborative Care

When the patient with chronic pancreatitis is experiencing an acute attack, the therapy is identical to that for acute pancreatitis. At other times the focus is on prevention of further attacks, relief of pain, and control of pancreatic exocrine and endocrine insufficiency. It sometimes takes large, frequent doses of analgesics to relieve the pain.

Diet, pancreatic enzyme replacement, and control of the diabetes are measures used to control the pancreatic insufficiency. The diet is bland, low in fat, and high in carbohydrate. The patient does not tolerate fatty, rich, and stimulating foods, and these should be avoided to decrease pancreatic secretions. Alcohol must be totally eliminated.

Pancreatic enzymes such as pancreatin (Viokase) and pancrelipase (Cotazym) contain amylase, lipase, and trypsin and are used to replace the deficient pancreatic enzymes. They are usually enteric coated to prevent their breakdown or inactivation by gastric hydrochloric (HCl) acid. Bile salts are sometimes given to facilitate the absorption of the fat-soluble vitamins (A, D, E, and K) and prevent further fat loss. If diabetes develops, it is controlled with insulin or oral hypoglycemic agents. Acid-neutralizing drugs (e.g., antacids) and acid-inhibiting drugs (e.g., H_2-receptor blockers, proton pump inhibitors, anticholinergics) may be given to decrease HCl acid secretion but have little overall effect on patient outcomes.

Treatment of chronic pancreatitis sometimes requires surgery. When biliary disease is present or if obstruction or pseudocyst develops, surgery may be indicated. Surgical procedures can divert bile flow or relieve ductal obstruction. A choledochojejunostomy diverts bile around the ampulla of Vater, where there may be spasm or hypertrophy of the sphincter. In this procedure the common bile duct is anastomosed into the jejunum. If the pancreatic sphincter is fibrotic, a sphincterotomy enlarges it. Pancreatic drainage procedures relieve ductal obstruction. One type is the Roux-en-Y pancreatojejunostomy, in which the pancreatic duct is opened and an anastomosis is made with the jejunum.

NURSING MANAGEMENT
CHRONIC PANCREATITIS

Except during an acute episode, the focus of nursing management is on chronic care and health promotion. The patient should be instructed to take measures to prevent further attacks. Dietary control, along with consistency of other treatment measures, such as taking pancreatic enzymes, is essential. The pancreatic extracts are usually given with meals or can be given with a snack. The nurse should observe the patient's stools for steatorrhea to help determine the effectiveness of the enzymes. The patient and the family need instructions regarding observation of stools.

If diabetes has developed, the patient will need instruction regarding testing of blood glucose levels and drugs (see Chapter 49). The nurse should make sure that the patient who is taking antacids takes them as ordered to control gastric acidity. Antacids should be taken after meals.

Alcohol must be avoided, and the patient may need assistance with this problem. If the patient has developed a dependence on alcohol, referral to other agencies or resources may be necessary (see Chapter 12).

PANCREATIC CANCER

In 2006 in the United States, it is estimated that 33,700 people were diagnosed with pancreatic cancer, and 32,300 people died of pancreatic cancer.[23] It is the fourth leading cause of death from cancer in the United States and Canada. The risk increases with age, with the peak incidence occurring between 65 and 80 years of age.

Most pancreatic tumors are adenocarcinomas originating from the epithelium of the ductal system. More than half of the tumors occur in the head of the pancreas. As the tumor grows, the common bile duct becomes obstructed, and obstructive jaundice develops. Tumors starting in the body or tail often remain silent until their growth is advanced. The majority of cancers have metastasized at the time of diagnosis. The signs and symptoms of pancreatic cancer are often similar to those of chronic pancreatitis. The prognosis of a patient with cancer of the pancreas is poor. The majority of patients die within 5 to 12 months of the initial diagnosis, and the 5-year survival rate is less than 5%.

Etiology and Pathophysiology

The cause of pancreatic cancer remains unknown. Patients with diabetes mellitus and chronic pancreatitis are at an increased risk for the development of pancreatic cancer. Risk factors for pancreatic cancer include cigarette smoking, family history of pancreatic cancer, high-fat diet, and exposure to chemicals such as benzidine and coke. African Americans have a higher incidence of pancreatic cancer than whites. The most firmly established environmental risk factor is cigarette smoking. Smokers are twice as likely to develop pancreatic cancer as nonsmokers. The risk is related to both duration and amount of cigarettes smoked.[37]

Clinical Manifestations

Common manifestations of pancreatic cancer include abdominal pain (dull, aching), anorexia, rapid and progressive weight loss, nausea, and jaundice. The most common characteristic sign of pancreatic cancer of the head of the pancreas is pain and jaundice. Pruritus may accompany obstructive jaundice. In general, pain is common and is related to the location of malignancy. Extreme, unrelenting pain is related to extension of the cancer into the retroperitoneal tissues and nerve plexuses. The pain is frequently located in the upper abdomen or left hypochondrium and often radiates to the back. It is commonly related to eating, and it also occurs at night. Weight loss is due to poor digestion and absorption caused by lack of digestive enzymes from the pancreas.

Diagnostic Studies

Better diagnostic measures are needed for detection of pancreatic cancer because most of the current methods detect only advanced stages. Transabdominal ultrasound and CT scan are the most commonly used diagnostic imaging techniques for pancreatic diseases, including cancer. CT scan is often the initial study and provides information on metastasis and vascular involvement. MRI and MRCP may also be used for diagnosing and staging pancreatic cancer. ERCP allows visualization of the pancreatic duct and biliary system. When ERCP is used, pancreatic secretions, as well as tissue, can be collected for analysis of different tumor markers. Endoscopic ultrasound (EUS) involves imaging the pancreas with the use of an endoscope positioned in the stomach and duodenum. This procedure also allows for fine-needle aspiration of the tumor.

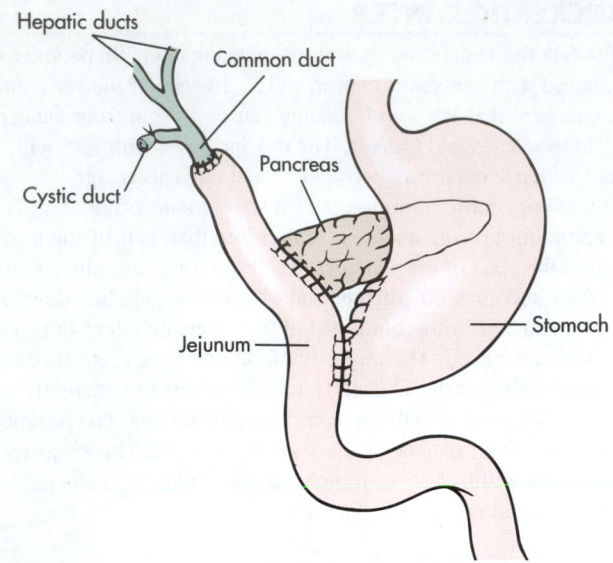

FIG. 44-16 Whipple procedure or radical pancreaticoduodenectomy. This surgical procedure involves resection of the proximal pancreas, adjoining duodenum, distal portion of the stomach, and distal portion of the common bile duct. An anastomosis of the pancreatic duct, common bile duct, and stomach to the jejunum is done.

Tumor markers are used both for establishing the diagnosis of pancreatic adenocarcinoma and for monitoring the response to treatment. Cancer-associated antigen 19-9 (CA 19-9) is elevated in pancreatic cancer and is the most commonly used tumor marker. CA 19-9 can also be elevated in gallbladder cancer, as well as in benign conditions such as acute and chronic pancreatitis, hepatitis, and biliary obstruction.

Collaborative Care

Surgery provides the most effective treatment of cancer of the pancreas. Only 15% to 20% of patients have resectable tumors. The classic surgery is a *radical pancreaticoduodenectomy,* or *Whipple procedure* (Fig. 44-16). This entails resection of the proximal pancreas (proximal pancreatectomy), the adjoining duodenum (duodenectomy), the distal portion of the stomach (partial gastrectomy), and the distal segment of the common bile duct. An anastomosis of the pancreatic duct, common bile duct, and stomach to the jejunum is done. A total pancreatectomy is performed in some institutions for cancers of the head of the pancreas. Sometimes a simple bypass procedure, such as a cholecystojejunostomy to relieve biliary obstruction, may be used as a palliative measure. Some surgeons suggest a more radical resection, such as a total pancreaticoduodenectomy with splenectomy. Biliary stents (e.g., Cotton-Leung stent) can be used as a palliative measure when tumors compress the bile duct.

Radiation therapy alone has little effect on survival, but it is effective for pain relief. External radiation is usually used, but implantation of internal radiation seeds into the tumor has also been used. The current role of chemotherapy in pancreatic cancer is limited. Chemotherapy usually consists of gemcitabine (Gemzar) either alone or in combination with agents such as capecitabine (Xeloda) or erlotinib (Tarceva). Erlotinib is a targeted therapy (see Table 16-17). However, response rates are less than 15% with minor effects on overall survival. Because of the aggressive nature of pancreatic cancer, current emphasis of new experimental chemotherapy is also focused on clinical benefits, including reduction in pain.[38]

NURSING MANAGEMENT
PANCREATIC CANCER

Because the patient with pancreatic cancer has many of the same problems as the patient with pancreatitis, nursing care includes many of the same measures (see NCP 44-3). The nurse should provide symptomatic and supportive nursing care. Medications and comfort measures to relieve pain should be provided before the patient reaches the peak of pain. Psychologic support is essential, especially during times of anxiety or depression.

Adequate nutrition is an important part of the nursing care plan. Frequent and supplemental feedings may be necessary. Measures to stimulate the appetite as much as possible and to overcome anorexia, nausea, and vomiting should be included in the nursing care. Because bleeding can result from impaired vitamin K production, bleeding from body orifices and mucous membranes should be assessed. If the patient is undergoing radiation therapy, the nurse must observe for adverse reactions, such as anorexia, nausea, vomiting, and skin irritation.

The prognosis for a patient with pancreatic cancer is poor. A significant component of the nursing care is helping the patient and the family or significant others through the grieving process. Chapter 11 provides information on palliative and end-of-life care.

Disorders of the Biliary Tract

CHOLELITHIASIS AND CHOLECYSTITIS

The most common disorder of the biliary system is **cholelithiasis** (stones in the gallbladder) (Figs. 44-17 and 44-18). **Cholecystitis** (inflammation of the gallbladder) is usually associated with cholelithiasis. The stones may be lodged in the neck of the gallbladder or in the cystic duct. Cholecystitis may be acute or chronic. These conditions usually occur together.

Gallbladder disease is a common health problem in the United States. It is estimated that 8% to 10% of adults in the United States have cholelithiasis. The actual number is not known because many persons are asymptomatic with stones. *Cholecystectomy* (removal of the gallbladder) ranks among the most common surgical procedures performed in the United States. The incidence of cholelithiasis is higher in women, multiparous women, and persons over 40 years of age. Postmenopausal women on estrogen therapy are at somewhat greater risk of having gallbladder disease than are women who are taking birth control pills. Oral contraceptives alter the character of bile, resulting in increased cholesterol saturation. Other factors that seem to increase the occurrence of gallbladder disease are a sedentary lifestyle, a familial tendency, and obesity. Obesity causes increased secretion of cholesterol in bile. Gallbladder disease is more common in whites than in Asian Americans and African Americans. There is an especially high incidence in the Native American population, particularly in the Navaho and Pima tribes.

Etiology and Pathophysiology

Cholecystitis. Cholecystitis is most commonly associated with obstruction caused by gallstones or biliary sludge. When cholecystitis occurs in the absence of obstruction (acalculous cholecystitis), it is most often in older adults and in patients who

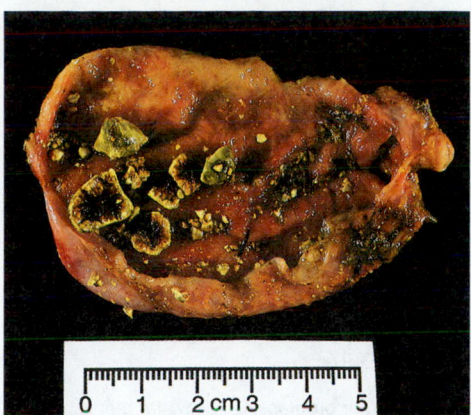

FIG. 44-17   Cholesterol gallstones in a gallbladder that was removed.

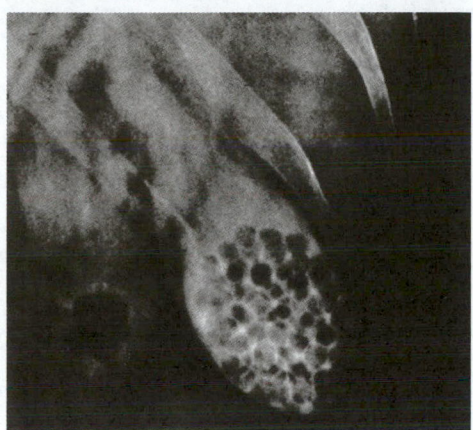

FIG. 44-18   X-ray of a gallbladder with gallstones.

have trauma, extensive burns, or recent surgery.[39] Acalculous cholecystitis can also occur as a result of prolonged immobility and fasting, prolonged parenteral nutrition, and diabetes mellitus. Bacteria reaching the gallbladder via the vascular or lymphatic route, or chemical irritants in the bile, can also produce cholecystitis. *Escherichia coli* are the most common bacteria involved. Streptococci and salmonellae are also common causative bacteria. Other etiologic factors include adhesions, neoplasms, anesthesia, and narcotics.

Inflammation is the major pathophysiologic condition and may be confined to the mucous lining or involve the entire wall of the gallbladder. During an acute attack of cholecystitis the gallbladder is edematous and hyperemic. It may be distended with bile or pus. The cystic duct is also involved and may become occluded. The wall of the gallbladder becomes scarred after an acute attack. Decreased functioning occurs if large amounts of tissue are fibrosed.

Cholelithiasis. The actual cause of gallstones is unknown. Cholelithiasis develops when the balance that keeps cholesterol, bile salts, and calcium in solution is altered so that precipitation of these substances occurs. Conditions that upset this balance include infection and disturbances in the metabolism of cholesterol. It is known that in patients with cholelithiasis the bile secreted by the liver is supersaturated with cholesterol (lithogenic bile). The bile in the gallbladder also becomes supersaturated with cholesterol. When bile is supersaturated with cholesterol, precipitation of cholesterol will occur.

Other components of bile that precipitate into stones are bile salts, bilirubin, calcium, and protein. Mixed cholesterol stones, which are predominantly cholesterol, are the most common gallstones.

The changes in the composition of bile are probably significant in the formation of gallstones. Stasis of bile leads to progression of the supersaturation and changes in the chemical composition of the bile. Immobility, pregnancy, and inflammatory or obstructive lesions of the biliary system decrease bile flow. Hormonal factors during pregnancy may cause delayed emptying of the gallbladder, resulting in stasis of bile.

The stones may remain in the gallbladder or migrate to the cystic duct or to the common bile duct. They cause pain as they pass through the ducts, and they may lodge in the ducts and produce an obstruction. Small stones are more likely to move into a duct and cause obstruction. Table 44-23 depicts the changes and manifestations that occur when the stones obstruct the common bile duct. If the blockage occurs in the cystic duct, the bile can continue to flow into the duodenum directly from the liver. However, when the bile in the gallbladder cannot escape, this stasis of bile may lead to cholecystitis.

Clinical Manifestations

Manifestations of cholecystitis vary from indigestion to moderate to severe pain, fever, and jaundice. Initial symptoms of acute cholecystitis include indigestion and pain and tenderness in the right upper quadrant, which may be referred to the right shoulder and scapula. The pain may be acute and be accompanied by nausea and vomiting, restlessness, and diaphoresis. Manifestations of inflammation include leukocytosis and fever. Physical findings include right upper quadrant tenderness and abdominal rigidity. Symptoms of chronic cholecystitis include a history of fat intolerance, dyspepsia, heartburn, and flatulence.[40]

Cholelithiasis may produce severe symptoms or none at all. Many patients have "silent cholelithiasis." The severity of symptoms depends on whether the stones are stationary or mobile and whether obstruction is present. When a stone is lodged in the ducts or when stones are moving through the ducts, spasms may result. The gallbladder spasms occur in response to the stone. This sometimes produces severe pain, which is termed *biliary colic* even though the pain is rarely colicky; it is more often steady. The pain can be excruciating and accompanied by tachycardia, diaphoresis, and prostration. The severe pain may last up to an hour, and when it subsides there is residual tenderness in the right upper quadrant. The attacks of pain frequently occur 3 to 6 hours after a heavy meal or when the patient lies down. When total obstruction occurs, symptoms related to bile blockage are manifested (see Table 44-23).

TABLE 44-23	Clinical Manifestations Caused by Obstructed Bile Flow

Clinical Manifestation	Etiology
Obstructive jaundice	No bile flow into duodenum
Dark amber urine, which foams when shaken	Soluble bilirubin in urine
No urobilinogen in urine	No bilirubin reaching small intestine to be converted to urobilinogen
Clay-colored stools	Same as above
Pruritus	Deposition of bile salts in skin tissues
Intolerance for fatty foods (nausea, sensation of fullness, anorexia)	No bile in small intestine for fat digestion
Bleeding tendencies	Lack of or decreased absorption of vitamin K, resulting in decreased production of prothrombin
Steatorrhea	No bile salts in duodenum, preventing fat emulsion and digestion

TABLE 44-24	*COLLABORATIVE CARE* Cholelithiasis and Acute Cholecystitis

Diagnostic
History and physical examination
Ultrasound
Liver function studies
WBC count
Serum bilirubin
ERCP

Collaborative Therapy
Conservative Therapy
IV fluid
NPO with NG tube, later progressing to low-fat diet
Antiemetics
Analgesics (e.g., meperidine)
Fat-soluble vitamins (A, D, E, and K)
Anticholinergics (antispasmodics)
Antibiotics (for secondary infection)
ERCP with sphincterotomy (papillotomy)
Extracorporeal shock-wave lithotripsy

Dissolution Therapy
ursodeoxycholic acid (UDCA)
ursodiol (Actigall)
chenodeoxycholic acid (CDCA)

*Surgical Therapy**
Laparoscopic cholecystectomy
Incisional cholecystectomy

ERCP, Endoscopic retrograde cholangiopancreatography; *IV,* intravenous; *NG,* nasogastric; *NPO,* nothing by mouth; *WBC,* white blood cell.
*See Table 44-25.

Complications

Complications of cholecystitis include gangrenous cholecystitis, subphrenic abscess, pancreatitis, *cholangitis* (inflammation of biliary ducts), biliary cirrhosis, fistulas, and rupture of the gallbladder, which can produce bile peritonitis. In older patients and those with diabetes, gangrenous cholecystitis is the most common complication of cholecystitis. Patients who delay seeking health care for cholecystitis are also more likely to develop gangrenous cholecystitis.[38]

Many of the same complications can occur from cholelithiasis, including cholangitis, biliary cirrhosis, carcinoma, and peritonitis. *Choledocholithiasis* (stone in the common bile duct) may occur, producing symptoms of obstruction.

Diagnostic Studies

Ultrasonography is commonly used to diagnose gallstones (see Table 39-12). Ultrasound is 90% to 95% accurate in detecting stones. It is especially useful for patients with jaundice (because it does not depend on liver function) and for patients who are allergic to contrast medium. ERCP allows for visualization of the gallbladder, cystic duct, common hepatic duct, and common bile duct. Bile taken during ERCP is sent for culture to identify possible infecting organisms.[40]

Percutaneous transhepatic cholangiography may be used to diagnose obstructive jaundice and to locate stones within the bile ducts. Laboratory tests reveal an increased WBC count as a result of inflammation. Both the direct and indirect bilirubin levels are elevated, as is the urinary bilirubin level if an obstructive process is present. If the common bile duct is obstructed, no bilirubin will reach the small intestine to be converted to urobilinogen. Serum enzymes, such as alkaline phosphatase, ALT, and AST, may be elevated. The serum amylase is increased if there is pancreatic involvement.

Collaborative Care

Conservative Therapy

Cholecystitis. During an acute episode of cholecystitis, the focus of treatment is on control of pain, control of possible infection with antibiotics, and maintenance of fluid and electrolyte balance

(Table 44-24). Treatment is mainly supportive and symptomatic. If nausea and vomiting are severe, gastric decompression may be used to prevent further gallbladder stimulation. Anticholinergics to decrease secretion and counteract smooth muscle spasms may be administered. Analgesics are given for pain management.[40]

Cholelithiasis. The use of nonsurgical approaches for cholelithiasis has decreased in the last decade because of the increased use of laparoscopic surgical removal.[39] There are two nonsurgical approaches for biliary stone removal. This procedure allows for visualization of the biliary system, as well as the placement of stents and sphincterotomy (papillotomy) if warranted. Endoscopic sphincterotomy is especially effective in removing common bile duct stones (Fig. 44-19). The endoscope is passed to the duodenum. With an electrodiathermy knife attached to the endoscope, the sphincter of Oddi is widened by incision of the sphincter muscle (sphincterotomy). A basket is used to retrieve the stone. The stone may be removed in the basket, but more commonly it is left in the duodenum and will be passed naturally in the stool.

If the stone is too large to pass through the duct, the endoscopist can crush the stone (mechanical lithotripsy). The limitation of this procedure is ERCP-induced acute pancreatitis. In approximately 10% of patients, nonstandard management, including peroral or percutaneous mechanical, electrohydraulic, or laser lithotripsy, will be needed. Other options for cholelithiasis include cholesterol solvents such as methyl tertiary terbutyl ether (MTBE), oral drugs that dissolve stones, endoscopic sphincterotomy, extracorporeal shock-wave lithotripsy (ESWL), and surgery. A direct-contact dissolving agent such as MTBE can be instilled into the gallbladder via a percutaneous catheter. MTBE dissolves cholesterol stones within hours. The gallstones may recur. Oral bile acids are also used to dissolve stones.

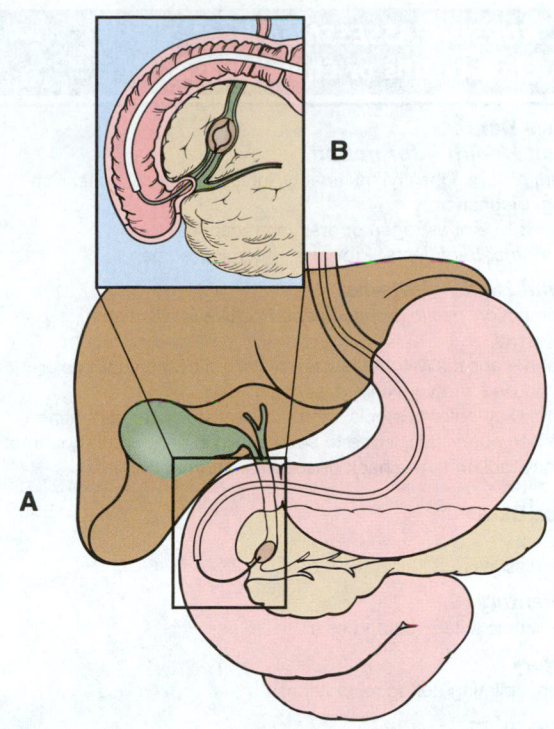

FIG. 44-19   A, During endoscopic sphincterotomy, an endoscope is advanced through the mouth and stomach until its tip sits in the duodenum opposite the common bile duct. **B,** After widening the duct mouth by incising the sphincter muscle, the physician advances a basket attachment into the duct and snags the stone.

TABLE 44-25	Gallbladder Surgery Procedures
Name	**Description**
Cholecystectomy	Removal of gallbladder
Cholecystostomy (usually an emergency)	Incision into gallbladder (usually for removal of stones)
Choledocholithotomy	Incision into common bile duct for removal of stones
Cholecystogastrostomy	Anastomosis between stomach and gallbladder
Cholecystoduodenostomy	Anastomosis between gallbladder and duodenum to relieve obstruction at distal end of common bile duct
Laparoscopic cholecystectomy	Removal of gallbladder via laparoscopy using a dissecting laser

Patient criteria for ESWL include normal gallbladder function, mild symptoms, and small stones (<20 mm). ESWL is less effective in obese patients.[39] In this procedure a biliary lithotriptor uses high-energy shock waves to disintegrate gallstones. Ultrasound is first done to locate the stones and to determine where to direct the shock waves. The shock waves are directed through the abdomen as a water-filled cushion is pressed against the area. It usually takes 1 to 2 hours to disintegrate the stones. After they are broken up, the fragments pass through the common bile duct and into the small intestine. There has been mixed success with ESWL.

Supportive treatment, similar to that given for cholecystitis, may also be necessary. If the stones cause an obstruction, additional treatment consists of replacement of fat-soluble vitamins, administration of bile salts to facilitate digestion and vitamin absorption, and a low-fat diet.

Surgical Therapy. Surgical intervention for cholelithiasis is often indicated and may consist of any one of several procedures (Table 44-25). The procedure of choice for most patients is laparoscopic cholecystectomy. In this procedure the gallbladder is removed through one of four small punctures in the abdomen. A laparoscope, which has a camera attached, is inserted into the abdomen. Two additional punctures are made just below the ribs, one on the right anterior axillary line and the other on the right midclavicular line. These punctures are used for insertion of grasping forceps. (The incision sites may vary.) Using closed-circuit monitors to view the abdominal cavity, the surgeon retracts and dissects the gallbladder and removes it with grasping forceps. This is a safe procedure with minimal morbidity.

Most patients experience minimal postoperative pain and are discharged the day of surgery or the day after. In most cases they are able to resume normal activities and return to work within

1 week. The main complication is injury to the common bile duct. There are few contraindications to laparoscopic cholecystectomy. They include peritonitis, cholangitis, gangrene or perforation of the gallbladder, portal hypertension, and serious bleeding disorders.

On selected patients an open cholecystectomy may be performed. This involves removal of the gallbladder through a right subcostal incision. A T tube is inserted into the common bile duct during surgery when a common bile duct exploration is part of the surgical procedure (Fig. 44-20). This ensures patency of the duct until the edema produced by the trauma of exploring and probing the duct has subsided. It also allows the excess bile to drain while the small intestine is adjusting to receiving a continuous flow of bile.

Transhepatic Biliary Catheter. The transhepatic biliary catheter can be used preoperatively in biliary obstruction and in hepatic dysfunction secondary to obstructive jaundice. It can also be inserted when inoperable liver, pancreatic, or bile duct carcinoma obstructs bile flow. The catheter is used when endoscopic drainage has been unsuccessful. The catheter is inserted percutaneously and allows for decompression of obstructed extrahepatic bile ducts so that bile can flow freely. After insertion, the catheter is connected to a drainage bag. The skin around the catheter insertion site has to be cleansed daily with an antiseptic. It is important to observe for bile leakage at the insertion site. Depending on the reason the catheter was inserted, the patient may be discharged with it in place.

Drug Therapy. The most common drugs used in the treatment of gallbladder disease are analgesics, anticholinergics (antispasmodics), fat-soluble vitamins, and bile salts. Morphine may be used initially for pain management. NSAIDs (e.g., ketorolac [Toradol]) have also been shown to be helpful in pain management. Anticholinergics such as atropine and other antispasmodics may be used to relax the smooth muscle and decrease ductal tone.

If the patient has chronic gallbladder disease or any biliary tract obstruction, fat-soluble vitamins (A, D, E, and K) will probably be given. Bile salts may be administered to facilitate digestion and vitamin absorption.

For treatment of pruritus, cholestyramine (Questran) may provide relief. This is a resin that binds bile salts in the intestine, increasing their excretion in the feces. Cholestyramine is administered in powder form and should be mixed with milk or juice. Side effects include nausea, vomiting, diarrhea or constipation, and skin reactions.

Medical dissolution therapy is recommended for patients with small radiolucent stones who are mildly symptomatic and are

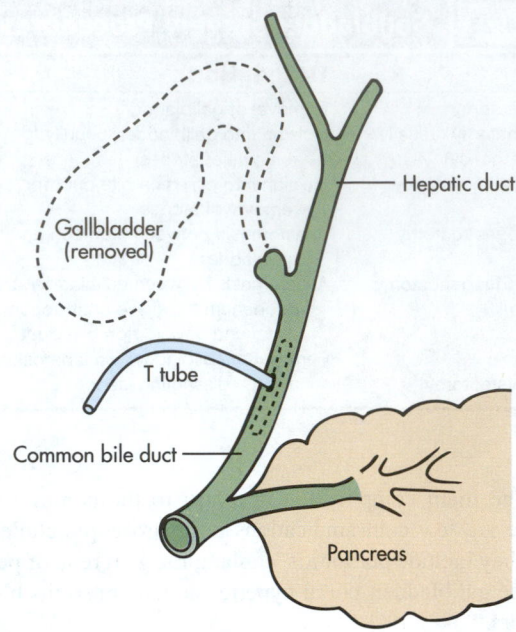

FIG. 44-20   Placement of T tube. *Dotted lines* indicate parts removed.

poor surgical risks. Ursodeoxycholic acid (UDCA), ursodiol (Actigall), and chenodeoxycholic acid (CDCA, chenodiol, Chenix) may be used to dissolve the stones. The main side effects of CDCA are abdominal cramping pain and diarrhea, but these are usually not severe. A more serious side effect is hepatotoxicity. Dissolution of the stones may take anywhere from 6 months to 2 years, and low-dose therapy is recommended to prevent recurrence. The drugs to dissolve the gallstones are not used as much currently because of high use of laparoscopic cholecystectomy.

Nutritional Therapy. The major dietary modification for a patient with cholelithiasis and cholecystitis is a low-fat diet. If obesity is a problem, a reduced-calorie diet is indicated. The low-fat diet decreases stimulation of the gallbladder. Foods that are avoided include dairy products such as whole milk, cream, butter, whole milk cheese, and ice cream; fried foods; rich pastries; gravies; and nuts. Many patients have fewer problems if they eat smaller, more frequent meals.

After a laparoscopic cholecystectomy the patient is instructed to have liquids for the rest of the day and eat light meals for a few days. If an incisional cholecystectomy is done, the patient will progress from liquids to a bland diet once bowel sounds have returned. The amount of fat in the postoperative diet depends on the patient's tolerance of fat. A low-fat diet may be helpful if the flow of bile is reduced (usually only in the early postoperative period) or if the patient is overweight. Sometimes the patient is instructed to restrict fats for 4 to 6 weeks. Otherwise, no special dietary instructions are needed other than to eat nutritious meals and avoid excessive fat intake.

NURSING MANAGEMENT
GALLBLADDER DISEASE

■ *Nursing Assessment*

Subjective and objective data that should be obtained from a person with gallbladder disease are presented in Table 44-26.

TABLE 44-26	*NURSING ASSESSMENT* **Cholecystitis or Cholelithiasis**

Subjective Data
Important Health Information
Past health history: Obesity, multiparity, infection, cancer, extensive fasting, pregnancy
Medications: Use of estrogen or oral contraceptives
Surgery or other treatments: Previous abdominal surgery

Functional Health Patterns
Health perception–health management: Positive family history; sedentary lifestyle
Nutritional-metabolic: Weight loss, anorexia; indigestion, fat intolerance, nausea and vomiting, dyspepsia; chills
Elimination: Clay-colored stools, steatorrhea, flatulence; dark urine
Cognitive-perceptual: Moderate to severe pain in right upper quadrant that may radiate to the back or scapula; pruritus

Objective Data
General
Fever, restlessness

Integumentary
Jaundice, icteric sclera; diaphoresis

Respiratory
Tachypnea, splinting during respirations

Cardiovascular
Tachycardia

Gastrointestinal
Palpable gallbladder, abdominal guarding and distention

Possible Findings
↑ Serum liver enzymes and bilirubin, absence of urobilinogen in urine, ↑ urinary bilirubin; leukocytosis, abnormal gallbladder ultrasound

■ *Nursing Diagnoses*

Nursing diagnoses for the patient with gallbladder disease treated surgically include, but are not limited to, the following:

- Acute pain *related to* surgical procedure
- Ineffective therapeutic regimen management *related to* lack of knowledge of diet and postoperative management

■ *Planning*

The overall goals are that the patient with gallbladder disease will have (1) relief of pain and discomfort, (2) no complications postoperatively, and (3) no recurrent attacks of cholecystitis or cholelithiasis.

■ *Nursing Implementation*

Health Promotion. The nurse should assume responsibility for recognition of predisposing factors of gallbladder disease in general health screening. Ethnic groups in which the disease is more common, such as Native Americans, should be taught initial manifestations and instructed to see their health care provider if these manifestations occur. The patient with chronic cholecystitis does not have acute symptoms and may not seek help until jaundice and biliary obstruction occur. Earlier detection in these patients is beneficial so that they can be managed with a low-fat diet and monitored more closely.

Acute Intervention. Nursing objectives for the patient undergoing conservative therapy include relieving pain, relieving nausea and vomiting, providing comfort and emotional support, maintain-

COMPLEMENTARY AND ALTERNATIVE THERAPIES

Milk Thistle (Silymarin)

Clinical Uses
- Hepatitis (chronic),* cirrhosis*
- Acute viral hepatitis†
- Gallbladder disease‡

Effects
Protects liver cells from toxic damage, antioxidant. May lower blood glucose levels.

Nursing Implications
Generally safe in recommended doses for up to 4 to 6 years. People with allergies to ragweed, marigolds, daisies, and other plants of the Asteraceae family may have mild allergic reactions. Because milk thistle affects liver enzymes, it may alter drug metabolism. It needs to be used cautiously in patients taking medications metabolized by the hepatic cytochrome P450 system. There is insufficient evidence to determine safety during pregnancy or lactation.

Ulbricht CE, Basch EM: *Natural standard herb and supplement reference: evidence-based clinical reviews,* St. Louis, 2005, Mosby.
www.naturalstandard.com.
*Good scientific evidence exists for its use.
†Unclear scientific evidence exists for its use.
‡Use is based on tradition, theory, or limited scientific research.

ing fluid and electrolyte balance and nutrition, making accurate assessments for effectiveness of treatment, and observing for complications.

The patient with acute cholecystitis or cholelithiasis is frequently experiencing severe pain. The medications ordered to relieve the pain should be given as required by the patient and before the pain becomes more severe. The nurse should assess what medications relieve the pain and how much medication is required. Observations for side effects of the medications must be part of the continued assessment. Nursing comfort measures, such as a clean bed, comfortable positioning, and oral care, are appropriate.

Some patients have more severe nausea and vomiting than others. For these patients it may be necessary to use gastric decompression. The elimination of intake of food and fluids also prevents further stimulation of the gallbladder. Oral hygiene, care of nares, accurate intake and output measurements, and maintenance of suction should be a part of the nursing care plan for this patient. For patients with less severe nausea and vomiting, antiemetics are usually adequate. When the patient is vomiting, comfort measures such as frequent mouth rinses should be provided. Any vomitus should be immediately removed from the patient's view.

If pruritus occurs with jaundice, measures to relieve itching are necessary. Such measures include baking soda or Alpha Keri baths; lotions, such as those containing calamine; antihistamines; soft, old linen; and control of the temperature (not too hot and not too cold). The patient's nails should be kept short and clean. Patients should be taught to rub with their knuckles rather than scratch with their nails when they cannot resist scratching.

A significant portion of the nursing care plan for this patient centers on accurate assessment of progression of the symptoms and development of complications. The nurse must be knowledgeable of and observe for signs of obstruction of the ducts by stones. These include jaundice; clay-colored stools; dark, foamy urine; steatorrhea; fever; and increased WBC count.

When symptoms of obstruction are present (see Table 44-23), the nurse must be aware of the possibility of bleeding as a result of decreased prothrombin production. Common sites to observe for bleeding are the mucous membranes of the mouth, nose, gingivae, and injection sites. If injections are given, a small-gauge needle should be used and gentle pressure applied after the injection. The nurse should know the patient's prothrombin time and use this as a guide in the assessment process.

Assessment for infections includes monitoring of vital signs. A temperature elevation with chills and jaundice may indicate choledocholithiasis.

Nursing care of the patient after endoscopic papillotomy includes assessment to detect complications such as pancreatitis, perforation, infection, and bleeding. The patient's vital signs should be monitored. Abdominal pain and fever may indicate pancreatitis. The patient should be on bed rest for several hours and should be NPO until the gag reflex returns.

Postoperative Care. Postoperative nursing care following a laparoscopic cholecystectomy includes monitoring for complications such as bleeding, making the patient comfortable, and preparing the patient for discharge. A common postoperative problem is referred pain to the shoulder because of the CO_2 that was not released or absorbed by the body. The CO_2 can irritate the phrenic nerve and the diaphragm, causing some difficulty breathing. Placing the patient in Sims' position (left side with right knee flexed) helps move the gas pocket away from the diaphragm. Deep breathing should be encouraged, along with movement and ambulation. There is usually minimal pain that can be relieved by NSAIDs or codeine. The patient is allowed clear liquids and can walk to the bathroom to void. Many patients go home the same day, but some will stay overnight.

Postoperative nursing care for incisional cholecystectomy focuses on adequate ventilation and prevention of respiratory complications. Other nursing care is the same as general postoperative nursing care (see Chapter 20).

If the patient has a T tube (see Fig. 44-20), part of the nursing care plan is related to maintaining bile drainage and observation of the T-tube functioning and drainage. The T tube is connected to a closed gravity drainage system. If the Penrose or Jackson-Pratt drain or the T tube is draining large amounts, it is helpful to use a sterile pouching system to protect the skin.

Ambulatory and Home Care. When the patient has conservative therapy, long-term nursing management depends on symptoms and on whether surgical intervention is being planned. Dietary teaching is usually necessary. The diet is usually low in fat, and sometimes a weight-reduction diet is also recommended. The patient may need to take fat-soluble vitamin supplements. The nurse should provide instructions regarding observations that the patient should make indicating obstruction (stool and urine changes, jaundice, and pruritus). Continued health care is important, and its significance should be explained and stressed.

The patient who undergoes a laparoscopic cholecystectomy is discharged soon after the surgery, so home care is important. Teaching is essential (Table 44-27).

After an open-incision cholecystectomy, the patient may be discharged in as soon as 2 to 3 days. The patient should be in-

TABLE 44-27	*PATIENT AND FAMILY TEACHING GUIDE* **Postoperative Laparoscopic Cholecystectomy**

1. Instruct patient to remove the bandages on the puncture site the day after surgery and that he or she can shower.
2. Explain the need to report the following signs and symptoms:
   - Redness, swelling, bile-colored drainage or pus from any incision
   - Severe abdominal pain, nausea, vomiting, fever, chills
3. Explain that normal activities can be resumed gradually.
4. Instruct that returning to work can occur within 1 week of surgery.
5. Instruct to resume usual diet; may need to be a low-fat diet for several weeks following surgery.

structed to avoid heavy lifting for 4 to 6 weeks. Usual sexual activities, including intercourse, can be resumed as soon as the patient feels ready unless given other instructions by the health care provider.

Sometimes the patient is required to remain on a low-fat diet for 4 to 6 weeks. If so, a dietary teaching plan is necessary. A weight-reduction program may be helpful if the patient is overweight. Most patients tolerate a regular diet with no difficulties but should avoid excessive fats.

▪ Evaluation

The overall expected outcomes are that the patient with gallbladder disease will

- appear comfortable and verbalize pain relief
- verbalize knowledge of activity level and dietary restrictions

GALLBLADDER CANCER

Primary cancer of the gallbladder is uncommon. The majority of gallbladder carcinomas are adenocarcinomas. There seems to be a definite relationship between cancer of the gallbladder and chronic cholecystitis and cholelithiasis. The early symptoms of carcinoma of the gallbladder are insidious and are similar to those of chronic cholecystitis and cholelithiasis, which makes diagnosis difficult. Later symptoms are usually those of biliary obstruction.

Diagnosis and staging of gallbladder cancer is done using EUS, transabdominal ultrasound, CT, MRI, and/or MRCP. Unfortunately, gallbladder cancer often is not detected until the disease is advanced. When found early, surgery can be curative. Several factors influence successful surgical outcomes, including the depth of cancer invasion, extent of liver involvement, presence of venous or lymphatic invasion, and lymph node metastasis. Extended cholecystectomy with lymph node dissection has improved the outcomes for patients with gallbladder cancer. When surgery is not an option, endoscopic stenting of the biliary tree to reduce obstructive jaundice may be warranted. Adjuvant therapies, including radiation therapy and chemotherapy, may be used depending on the disease state. Overall, cancer of the gallbladder has a poor prognosis.

Nursing management involves supportive care with special attention to nutrition, hydration, skin care, and pain relief. Many of the nursing care measures used for patients with cholecystitis and cholelithiasis are frequently applied, as well as nursing care measures for the patient with cancer (see Chapter 16).

CRITICAL THINKING EXERCISE

CASE STUDY

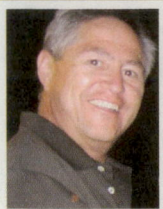

Cirrhosis of the Liver

Patient Profile. Mr. Begay is a 55-year-old Native American man admitted with a diagnosis of cirrhosis of the liver. He has been vomiting for 2 days and noticed blood in the toilet when he vomits.

Subjective Data
- Has had cirrhosis for 12 years
- Acknowledges that he had been drinking heavily for 20 years but has been sober for the past 2 years
- Complains of anorexia, nausea, and abdominal discomfort

Objective Data
Physical Examination
- Thin and malnourished
- Has moderate ascites
- Has jaundice of sclera and skin
- Has 4+ pitting edema of the lower extremities
- Liver and spleen are palpable

Laboratory Values
- Total bilirubin: 15 mg/dl (257 mmol/L)
- Serum ammonia: 220 mcg/dl (122 mmol/L)
- AST: 190 U/L (3.2 μkat/L)
- ALT: 210 U/L (3.5 μkat/L)

Critical Thinking Questions

1. What are possible causes of cirrhosis? What type of cirrhosis does Mr. Begay probably have?
2. Describe the pathophysiologic changes that occur in the liver as cirrhosis develops.
3. List Mr. Begay's clinical manifestations of liver failure. For each manifestation, explain the pathophysiologic basis.
4. Explain the significance of the results of his laboratory values.
5. If Mr. Begay begins to manifest signs and symptoms of hepatic encephalopathy, what would you monitor? What measures should be instituted to control or decrease the ammonia level?
6. What are possible causes of his gastrointestinal bleeding?
7. In the early stages of cirrhosis, what can be done to control the disease?
8. Based on the assessment data presented, write one or more nursing diagnoses. Are there any collaborative problems?

NCLEX EXAMINATION REVIEW QUESTIONS

The number of the question corresponds to the same-numbered objective at the beginning of the chapter.

1. During assessment of a patient with obstructive jaundice, the nurse would expect to find
   a. clay-colored stools.
   b. dark urine and stools.
   c. pyrexia and severe pruritus.
   d. elevated urinary urobilinogen.

2. A patient with hepatitis A is in the acute phase. The nurse plans care for the patient based on the knowledge that
   a. pruritus is a common problem with jaundice in this phase.
   b. the patient is most likely to transmit the disease during this phase.
   c. gastrointestinal symptoms are not as severe in hepatitis A as they are in hepatitis B.
   d. extrahepatic manifestations of glomerulonephritis and polyarteritis are common in this phase.

3. A patient with hepatitis B is being discharged in 2 days. The nurse includes in the discharge teaching plan instructions to
   a. avoid alcohol for 3 weeks.
   b. use a condom during sexual intercourse.
   c. have family members get an injection of immunoglobulin.
   d. follow a low-protein, moderate-carbohydrate, moderate-fat diet.

4. A patient has been told that she has elevated liver enzymes caused by nonalcoholic fatty liver disease (NAFLD). The nurse's teaching plan includes
   a. having genetic testing done.
   b. recommending a heart-healthy diet.
   c. the necessity to reduce weight rapidly.
   d. avoiding alcohol until liver enzymes return to normal.

5. The patient with advanced cirrhosis asks the nurse why his abdomen is so swollen. The nurse's response to the patient is based on the knowledge that
   a. a lack of clotting factors promotes the collection of blood in the abdominal cavity.
   b. portal hypertension and hypoalbuminemia cause a fluid shift into the peritoneal space.
   c. decreased peristalsis in the GI tract contributes to gas formation and distention of the bowel.
   d. bile salts in the blood irritate the peritoneal membranes, causing edema and pocketing of fluid.

6. In planning care for a patient with metastatic cancer of the liver, the nurse includes interventions that
   a. focus primarily on symptomatic and comfort measures.
   b. reassure the patient that chemotherapy offers a good prognosis for recovery.
   c. promote the patient's confidence that surgical excision of the tumor will be successful.
   d. provide information necessary for the patient to make decisions regarding liver transplantation.

7. The nurse explains to the patient with acute pancreatitis that the most common pathogenic mechanism of the disorder is
   a. cellular disorganization.
   b. overproduction of enzymes.
   c. lack of secretion of enzymes.
   d. autodigestion of the pancreas.

8. Nursing management of the patient with acute pancreatitis includes
   a. checking for signs of hypercalcemia.
   b. observing stools for signs of steatorrhea.
   c. providing a diet low in carbohydrates with moderate fat.
   d. monitoring for infection, particularly respiratory infection.

9. A patient with pancreatic cancer is admitted to the hospital for evaluation for treatment. The patient asks the nurse to explain the Whipple procedure the surgeon has described. The nurse's explanation includes the information that a Whipple procedure involves
   a. creating a bypass around the obstruction caused by the tumor by joining the gallbladder to the jejunum.
   b. resection of the entire pancreas and the distal portion of the stomach, with anastomosis of the common bile duct and stomach into the duodenum.
   c. removal of part of the pancreas, part of the stomach, the duodenum, and the gallbladder, with joining of the pancreatic duct, common bile duct, and stomach into the jejunum.
   d. radical removal of the pancreas, duodenum, and spleen, and attaching the stomach to the jejunum, which requires oral supplementation of pancreatic digestive enzymes and insulin replacement therapy.

10. The nursing management of the patient with cholecystitis associated with cholelithiasis is based on the knowledge that
    a. a low-fat diet is recommended.
    b. gallstones once removed tend not to recur.
    c. meperidine is to be avoided in the management of pain.
    d. the disorder can be successfully treated with oral bile salts that dissolve gallstones.

11. Teaching in relation to home management following a laparoscopic cholecystectomy should include
    a. keeping the bandages on the puncture sites for 48 hours.
    b. reporting any bile-colored drainage or pus from any incision.
    c. using over-the-counter antiemetics if nausea and vomiting occur.
    d. emptying and measuring the contents of the bile bag from the T tube every day.

REFERENCES

1. National Center for Infection Control: Hepatitis. Available at *www.cdc.gov/ncidod/diseases/hepatitis* (accessed July 31, 2006).
2. Strader DB, Wright T, Thomas DL, et al: AASLD practice guideline: diagnosis, management, and treatment of hepatitis C, *Hepatology* 39:1147, 2004.
3. Hou J, Liu Z, Gu F: Epidemiology and prevention of hepatitis B virus infection, *Int J Med Sci* 2:50, 2005.
4. Guney C, Kadayifci A, Savas MC, et al: Frequency of hepatitis G virus and transfusion-transmitted virus infection in type II diabetes mellitus, *Int J Clin Pract* 59:206, 2005.
5. Wong PN, Fung TT, Mak SK, et al: Hepatitis B virus in dialysis patients, *J Gastroenterol Hepatol* 20:1641, 2005.
6. Bosch FX, Ribes J, Clevies R, et al: Epidemiology of hepatocellular carcinoma, *Clin Liver Dis* 9:191, 2005.
7. Ghany MG, Doo EC: Management of chronic hepatitis B, *Gastroenterol Clin North Am* 33:563, 2004.
8. Hui AY, et al: Systematic review: treatment of chronic hepatitis B virus infection by pegylated interferon, *Aliment Pharmacol Ther* 22:519, 2005.
9. Perrillo RP: Current treatment of chronic hepatitis B: benefits and limitations, *Semin Liver Dis* 25:S20, 2005.
10. Jacobson IM: Therapeutic options for chronic hepatitis B: considerations and controversies, *Am J Gastroenterol* 101:S1, 2006.
11. Dienstag JL, McHutchinson JG: American Gastroenterological Association medical position statement on the management of hepatitis C, *Gastroenterology* 130:225, 2006.
12. Krawitt EL: Autoimmune hepatitis, *N Engl J Med* 354:54, 2006.
13. Ferenci P: Wilson's disease, *Clin Gastroenterol Hepatol* 3:726, 2005.
14. Zoller H, Cox TM: Hemochromatosis: genetic testing and clinical practice, *Clin Gastroenterol Hepatol* 3:945, 2005.
15. Bergheim I, McClain CJ, Arteel GE: Treatment of alcoholic liver disease, *Dig Dis* 23:275, 2005.
16. Kita H, He XS, Gershwin ME: Autoimmunity and environmental factors in the pathogenesis of primary biliary cirrhosis, *Ann Med* 36:72, 2004.
17. Selmi C, Invernizzi P, Keeffe EB, et al: Epidemiology and pathogenesis of primary biliary cirrhosis, *J Clin Gastroenterol* 38:264, 2004.
18. Sargent S, Martin W: Renal disease. Renal dysfunction in liver cirrhosis, *Br J Med* 15:12, 2006.
19. Sargent S: The management and nursing care of cirrhotic ascites, *Br J Nurs* 8:212, 2006.
20. Sanyal A: Role of transjugular intrahepatic portosystemic shunts in the treatment of variceal bleeding. Available at *www.uptodateonline.com* (accessed July 31, 2006).
21. Oo YH, Neuberger J: Options for treatment of primary biliary cirrhosis, *Drugs* 64:2261, 2004.
22. Sargent S: The management and nursing care of cirrhotic ascites, *Br J Nur* 15(4):212, 2006.
23. American Cancer Society: *Facts and figures, 2006*, Atlanta, 2006. Available at *www.cancer.org* (accessed July 31, 2006).

24. Shea MC: Radiofrequency ablation: putting the heat on liver cancer, *Nursing* 34:32hn1, 2004.

25. Chopra S, Bonis PA: Liver transplantation for hepatitis C virus infection. Available at *www.uptodateonline.com* (accessed July 31, 2006).

26. McCaughan GW, Koorey DJ, Strasser SI: Liver transplantation for viral hepatitis, *Hosp Med* 66:8, 2005.

27. Schmucker DL: Age-related changes in liver structure and function: implications for disease? *Exp Gerontol* 40:650, 2005.

28. Monto A, Patel K, Bostron A, et al: Risks of a range of alcohol intake on hepatitis C–related fibrosis, *Hepatology* 39:826, 2004.

29. Burruss N, Holz S: Understanding acute pancreatitis, *Nursing* 35:32hn1, 2005.

30. Chari S, Vege SS: Etiology of acute pancreatitis. Available at *www.uptodateonline.com* (accessed July 31, 2006).

31. Despins LA, Kivlahan C, Cox KR: Emergency. Acute pancreatitis: diagnosis and treatment of a potentially fatal condition, *Am J Nurs* 105:54, 2005.

32. Chari ST, Vege SS: Clinical manifestations and diagnosis of acute pancreatitis. Available at *www.uptodateonline.com* (accessed July 31, 2006).

33. Al-Bahrani AZ, Ammori BJ: Clinical laboratory assessment of acute pancreatitis, *Clin Chim Acta* 362:26, 2005.

34. Nathens AB, Curtis JR, Beale RJ, et al: Management of the critically ill patient with severe acute pancreatitis, *Crit Care Med* 32:2524, 2004.

35. Binnekade JM: Review: enteral nutrition reduces infections, need for surgical intervention, and length of hospital stay more than parenteral nutrition in acute pancreatitis, *Evid Based Nurs* 8:19, 2005.

36. Hughes E: Continuing professional development. Understanding the care of patients with acute pancreatitis, *Nursing Standard* 18:45, 2004.

37. Lowenfels AB, Maisonneuve P: Epidemiology and risk factors for pancreatic cancer, *Best Pract Res Clin Gastroenterol* 20:197, 2006.

38. Ryan DP: Chemotherapy for advanced pancreatic cancer. Available at *www.uptodateonline.com* (accessed July 31, 2006).

39. Zakko SF, Afdhal NH: Clinical features and diagnosis of acute cholecystitis. Available at *www.uptodateonline.com* (accessed July 31, 2006).

40. Bhattacharya D, Ammori BJ: Contemporary minimally invasive approaches to the management of acute cholecystitis: a review and appraisal, *Surg Laparosc Endosc Percutan Tech* 15:1, 2005.

RESOURCES

American Association for the Study of Liver Diseases (AASLD)
703-299-9766
www.aasld.org

American Gastroenterological Association
301-654-2055
www.gastro.org

American Liver Foundation
800-GO-LIVER (465-4837)
www.liverfoundation.org

American Pancreatic Association
www.american-pancreatic-association.org

Liver Cancer Network
412-359-6738
www.livercancer.com

National Pancreas Foundation
866-726-2737
www.pancreasfoundation.org

Pancreatic Cancer Action Network
877-272-6226
www.pancan.org

For additional Internet resources, see the website for this book at *http://evolve.elsevier.com/Lewis/medsurg.*

Problems of Urinary Function

Section Outline

45 Nursing Assessment
Urinary System, p. 1136

46 Nursing Management
Renal and Urologic Problems, p. 1154

47 Nursing Management
Acute Renal Failure and
Chronic Kidney Disease, p. 1197

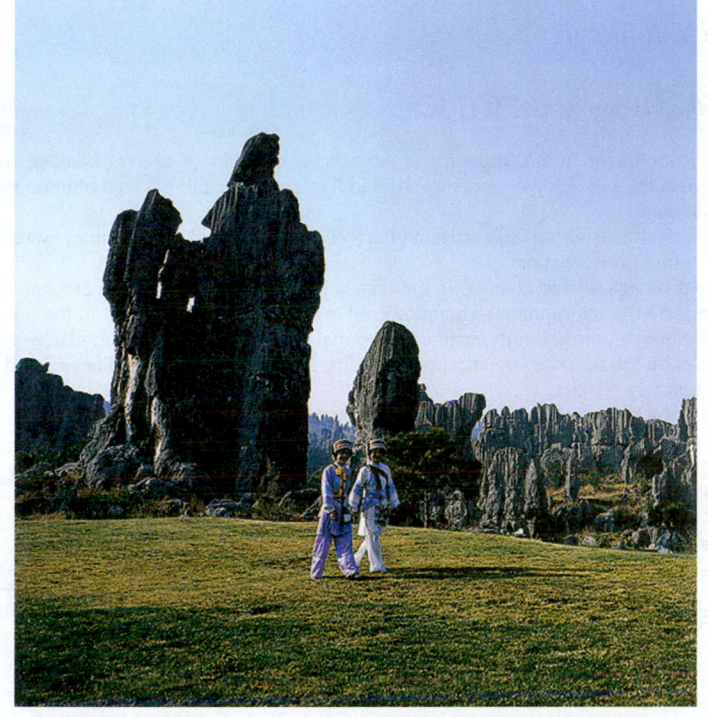

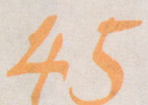

45

Nursing Assessment
Urinary System

Vicki Y. Johnson

LEARNING OBJECTIVES

1. Describe the anatomic location and functions of the kidneys, ureters, bladder, and urethra.
2. Explain the physiologic events involved in the formation and passage of urine from glomerular filtration to voiding.
3. Identify the significant subjective and objective data related to the urinary system that should be obtained from a patient.
4. Describe age-related changes in the urinary system and differences in assessment findings.
5. Describe the appropriate techniques used in the physical assessment of the urinary system.
6. Differentiate normal from common abnormal findings of a physical assessment of the urinary system.
7. Describe the purpose, significance of results, and nursing responsibilities related to diagnostic studies of the urinary system.
8. Describe the normal physical and chemical characteristics of urine.

KEY TERMS

costovertebral angle, p. 1144
creatinine, p. 1151
cystometrogram,* p. 1150
cystoscopy,* p. 1149
glomerular filtration rate, p. 1138
glomerulus, p. 1137
intravenous pyelogram,* p. 1147
nephron, p. 1137
renal arteriogram,* p. 1148
urinalysis, p. 1150
*See Table 45-8 on pp. 1146 to 1150

Electronic Resources

Supplemental content related to Chapter 45 can be found . . .

Companion CD
- Stress-Busting Kit for Nursing Students
- NCLEX Examination Review Questions
- Comprehensive Glossary

Evolve Website *evolve*
http://evolve.elsevier.com/Lewis/medsurg
- Content Updates
- Key Points (Printable and CD/MP3 Download)
- Concept Map Creator
- Expanded Audio Glossary
- Key Term Flash Cards
- Electronic Calculators

- Physical Examination Video Clips:
  - Abdomen: Inspection, Auscultation, and Percussion
  - Abdomen: Palpation
- WebLinks

"Bones can break, muscles can atrophy, glands can loaf, even the brain can go to sleep without immediate danger to survival. But should the kidneys fail . . . neither bone, muscle, gland, nor brain could carry on."[1] This statement underlines the importance of kidneys to our lives. Adequate functioning of the kidneys is essential to the maintenance of a healthy body. If there is complete kidney failure and treatment is not given, death is inevitable.

The urinary system consists of two kidneys, two ureters, a urinary bladder, and a urethra (Fig. 45-1). The bladder provides storage while the ureters and urethra can be thought of as drainage channels for the urine after it is formed by the kidneys.

The kidneys are the principal organs of the urinary system. The primary functions of the kidneys are (1) to regulate the volume and composition of extracellular fluid (ECF) and (2) to excrete waste products from the body. In addition, the kidneys function to control blood pressure, produce erythropoietin, activate vitamin D, and regulate acid-base balance.

STRUCTURES AND FUNCTIONS OF THE URINARY SYSTEM

Kidneys

Macrostructure. The paired kidneys are bean-shaped organs that are retroperitoneal (behind the peritoneum) on either side of the vertebral column at about the level of the twelfth thoracic (T12) vertebra to the third lumbar (L3) vertebra. Each kidney

---

Reviewed by Elizabeth Wheeler, RN, DNS, WHNP, Assistant Professor and Coordinator, Nurse Practitioner Programs, College of Staten Island, City University of New York, Staten Island, N.Y.

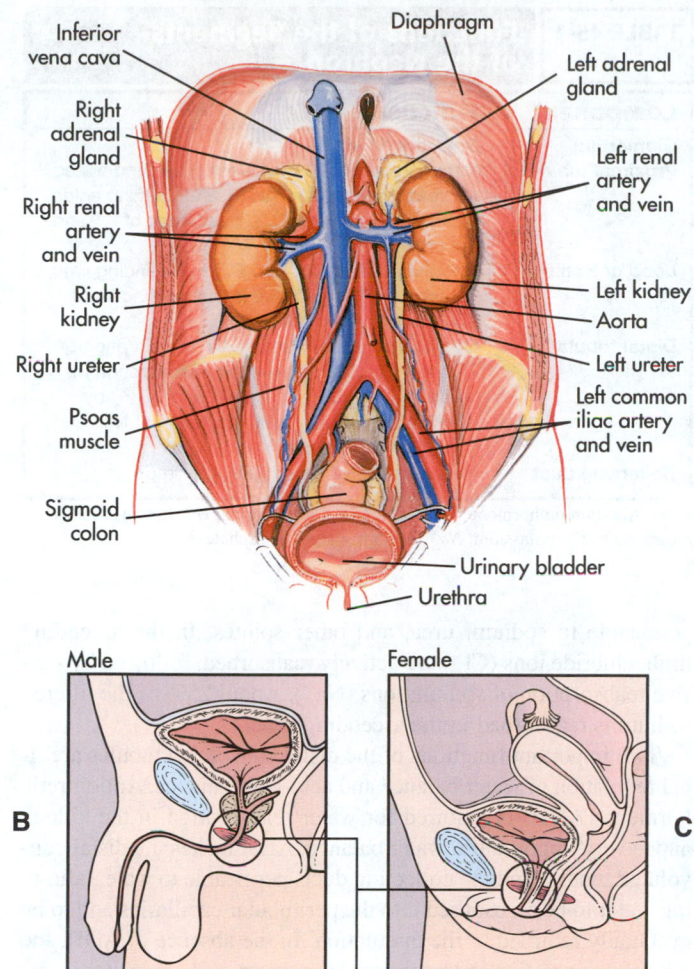

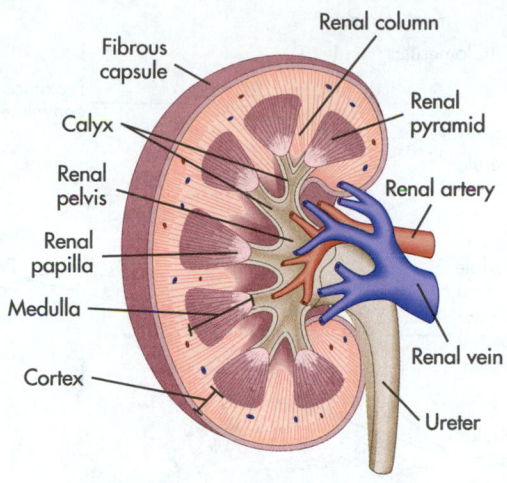

FIG. 45-2 Longitudinal section of the kidney.

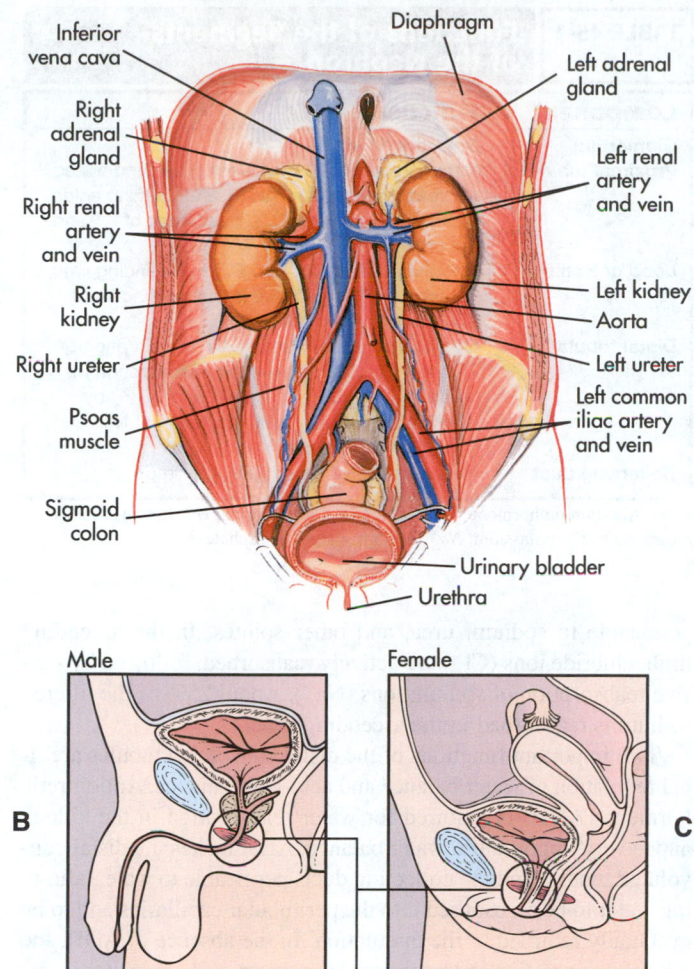

Male Female

Rhabdosphincter

FIG. 45-1 Organs of the urinary system. **A,** Upper urinary tract in relation to other anatomic structures. **B,** Male urethra in relation to other pelvic structures. **C,** Female urethra.

weighs 4 to 6 ounces (115 to 175 g) and is about 5 inches (12 cm) long. The right kidney, at the level of the twelfth rib, is lower than the left. An adrenal gland lies on top of each kidney.

Each kidney is surrounded by a considerable amount of fat and connective tissue that serves to support and maintain its position. The surface of the kidney is covered by a thin, smooth layer of fibrous membrane called the *capsule*. These structures protect the kidney and serve as a shock absorber should the kidney be subjected to a sudden force from a blunt object striking the abdomen or back. The *hilus* on the medial side of the kidney serves as the entry site for the renal artery and nerves, as well as the exit site for the renal vein and ureter.

The parenchyma (actual tissue) of the kidney can be visualized on a longitudinal section of the kidney (Fig. 45-2). The outer layer is termed the *cortex,* and the inner layer is called the *medulla.* The medulla consists of a number of pyramids. The apices of these pyramids are called *papillae,* through which urine passes to enter the calyces. The minor calyces widen and merge to form major calyces, which form a funnel-shaped sac called the *renal pelvis.* The minor and major calyces transport urine to the renal pelvis, from which it drains via the ureter to the bladder. The pelvis of the kidney can store a small volume of urine (3 to 5 ml).

Microstructure. The **nephron** is the functional unit of the kidney. Each kidney contains 800,000 to 1.2 million nephrons.[2] A nephron is composed of a glomerulus, Bowman's capsule, and a tubular system. The tubular system consists of the proximal convoluted tubule, the loop of Henle, the distal convoluted tubule and a collecting tubule (Fig. 45-3). The glomeruli, Bowman's capsule, proximal tubule, and distal tubule are located in the cortex of the kidney. The loop of Henle and the collecting tubules are located in the medulla. Several collecting tubules join to form a single collecting duct. The collecting ducts eventually merge into a pyramid that empties via the papilla into a minor calyx.

Blood Supply. A blood supply of about 1200 ml/min, which is 20% to 25% of the cardiac output, flows to the two kidneys. Blood reaches the kidneys via the renal artery, which arises from the aorta and enters the kidney through the hilus. The renal artery divides into secondary branches and then into still smaller branches, each of which eventually forms an afferent arteriole. The afferent arteriole divides into a capillary network termed the **glomerulus,** which is a tuft of up to 50 capillaries (see Fig. 45-3). The capillaries of the glomerulus eventually unite in the efferent arteriole. This arteriole splits to form a capillary network called the peritubular capillaries, which surround the tubular system. All peritubular capillaries eventually drain into the venous system; the renal vein empties into the inferior vena cava.

Physiology of Urine Formation. The process of urine formation is extremely complex. It represents the outcome of a multistep process of filtration, reabsorption, secretion, and excretion of water, electrolytes, and metabolic waste products. Although urine formation is the result of this process, the primary function of the kidneys is to filter the blood and maintain the body's internal homeostasis.[3]

Glomerular Function. Urine formation begins at the glomerulus, where blood is filtered. The glomerulus is a semipermeable membrane that allows filtration (see Fig. 45-3). The hydrostatic pressure of the blood within the glomerular capillaries causes a portion of blood to be filtered across the semipermeable membrane into Bowman's capsule, where the filtered portion of the blood, the glomerular filtrate, begins to pass down to the tubule. Filtration is more rapid in the glomerulus than in ordinary tissue capillaries because of the porosity of the glomerular membrane. The ultrafiltrate is similar in composition to blood except that it lacks blood

Urinary System

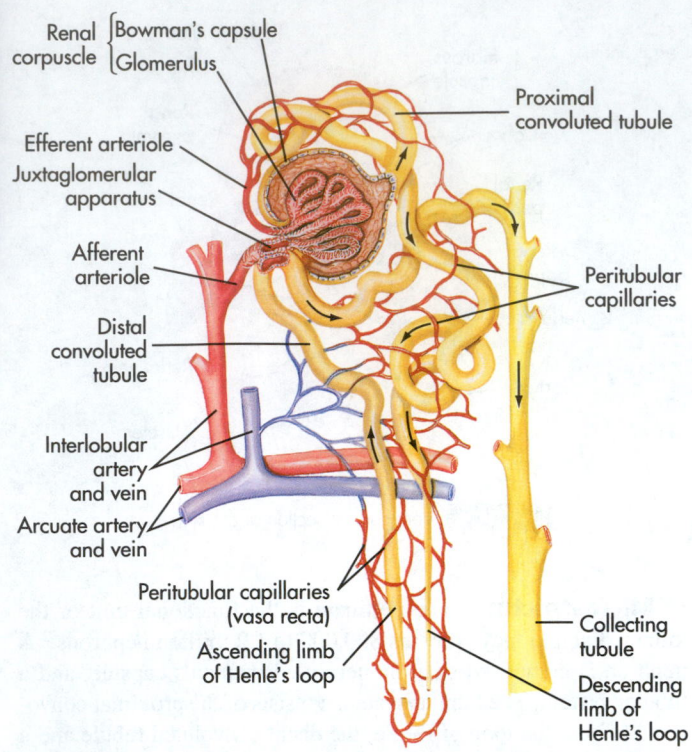

FIG. 45-3 The nephron is the basic functional unit of the kidney. This illustration of a single nephron unit also shows the surrounding blood vessels.

TABLE 45-1	Functions of the Segments of the Nephron
Component	**Function**
Glomerulus	Selective filtration
Proximal tubule	Reabsorption of 80% of electrolytes and water; reabsorption of all glucose and amino acids; reabsorption of HCO_3^-; secretion of H^+ and creatinine
Loop of Henle	Reabsorption of Na^+ and Cl^- in ascending limb; reabsorption of water in descending loop; concentration of filtrate
Distal tubule	Secretion of K^+, H^+, ammonia; reabsorption of water (regulated by ADH); reabsorption of HCO_3^-; regulation of Ca^{2+} and PO_4^{2-} by parathyroid hormone, regulation of Na^+ and K^+ by aldosterone
Collecting duct	Reabsorption of water (ADH required)

ADH, Antidiuretic hormone; Ca^{2+}, calcium; Cl^-, chloride; H^+, hydrogen; HCO_3^-, bicarbonate; K^+, potassium; Na^+, sodium; PO_4^{2-}, phosphate.

cells, platelets, and large plasma proteins. Under normal conditions, the capillary pores are too small to allow the loss of these large blood components. Capillary permeability is increased in many renal diseases, permitting plasma proteins and blood cells to pass into the urine.

The amount of blood filtered by the glomeruli in a given time is termed the **glomerular filtration rate** (GFR). The normal GFR is about 125 ml/min. However, on average, only 1 ml/min is excreted as urine because most glomerular filtrate is reabsorbed by the peritubular capillary network before it reaches the end of the collecting duct.

Tubular Function. Because the glomerular membrane is a selective filtration membrane that filters primarily by size, provision is made for the reabsorption of essential materials and the excretion of nonessential ones (Table 45-1). The tubules and collecting ducts carry out these functions by means of reabsorption and secretion. *Reabsorption* is the passage of a substance from the lumen of the tubules through the tubule cells and into the capillaries. This process involves both active and passive transport mechanisms. Tubular *secretion* is the passage of a substance from the capillaries through the tubular cells into the lumen of the tubule. Reabsorption and secretion occur along the entire length of the tubule, causing numerous changes in the composition of the glomerular filtrate as it moves through the tubules.

In the proximal convoluted tubule, about 80% of the electrolytes are reabsorbed. Normally, all the glucose, amino acids, and small proteins are reabsorbed. For the most part, reabsorption occurs by active transport. Hydrogen ions (H^+) and creatinine are secreted into the filtrate.[3]

The loop of Henle is important in conserving water and thus concentrating the filtrate. In the loop of Henle, reabsorption continues. The descending loop is permeable to water and moderately permeable to sodium, urea, and other solutes. In the ascending limb, chloride ions (Cl^-) are actively reabsorbed, followed by passive reabsorption of sodium ions (Na^+). About 25% of the filtered sodium is reabsorbed in the ascending limb.

Two important functions of the distal convoluted tubules are final regulation of water balance and acid-base balance. Antidiuretic hormone (ADH) is required for water reabsorption in the kidney and is very important in water balance. ADH makes the distal convoluted tubules and the collecting ducts permeable to water, allowing water to be reabsorbed into the peritubular capillaries and to be eventually returned to the circulation. In the absence of ADH, the tubules are practically impermeable to water, and any water in the tubules leaves the body as urine. Decreases in plasma osmolality are detected in the anterior hypothalamus by osmoreceptors. Neural input is sent from the osmoreceptors to other hypothalamic cells called *superoptic nuclei cells*. These cells have axonal extensions that terminate in the posterior pituitary gland and inhibit secretion of ADH. Decreases in cardiovascular pressures (decreased plasma volume) and increases in plasma osmolality cause diminished firing of baroreceptors and stimulation of ADH secretion.[3]

Aldosterone (released from the adrenal cortex) acts on the distal tubule to cause reabsorption of Na^+ and water. In exchange for Na^+, potassium ions (K^+) are excreted. The secretion of aldosterone is influenced by both circulating blood volume and plasma concentrations of Na^+ and K^+.

Acid-base regulation involves reabsorbing and conserving most of the bicarbonate (HCO_3^-) and secreting excess H^+. The distal tubule functions in different ways to maintain the pH of ECF within a range of 7.35 to 7.45 (see Chapter 17).

Atrial natriuretic peptide (ANP) is a hormone secreted from cells in the right atrium in response to atrial distention due to an increase in plasma volume. ANP acts on the kidneys to increase sodium excretion. ANP also inhibits renin, ADH, and the action of angiotensin II on the adrenal glands, thereby suppressing aldosterone secretion. The combined effects of ANP result in the production of a large volume of dilute urine. In addition, secretion of ANP causes relaxation of the afferent arteriole, thus increasing the GFR.[3]

The renal tubules are also involved in calcium balance. Parathyroid hormone (PTH) is released from the parathyroid gland in response to low serum calcium levels. PTH maintains serum Ca^{2+}

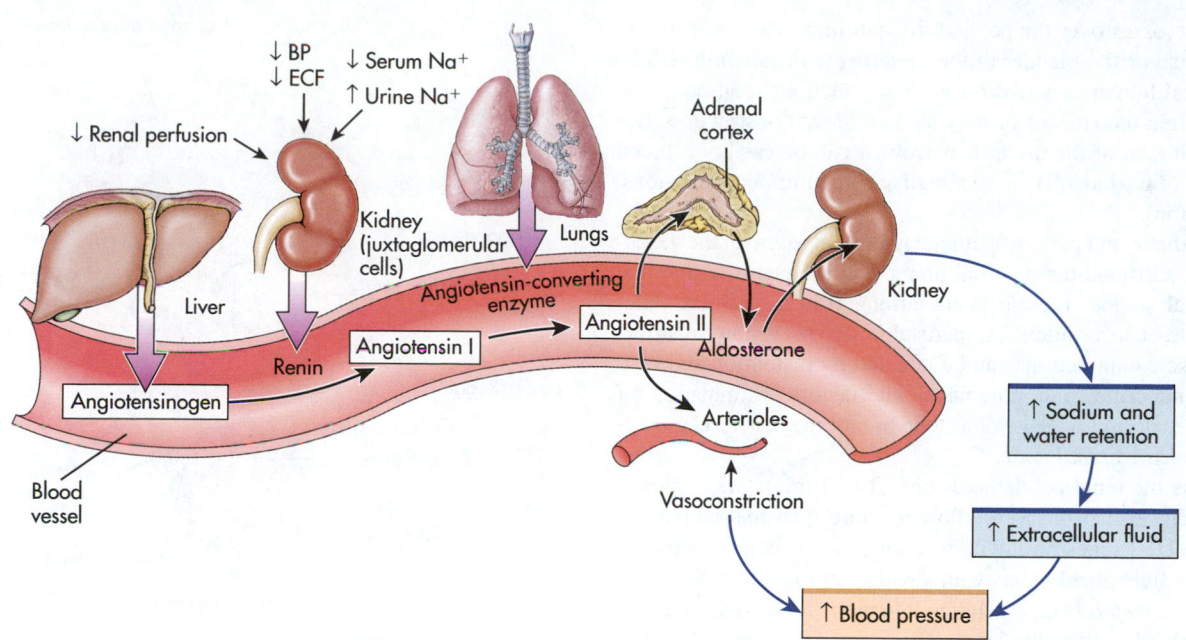

FIG. 45-4   Renin-angiotensin-aldosterone system. *BP,* Blood pressure; *ECF,* extracellular fluid; *Na,* sodium.

levels by causing increased tubular reabsorption of calcium ions (Ca^{2+}) and decreased tubular reabsorption of phosphate ions (PO_4^{2-}). In renal disease, the effects of PTH may have a major effect on bone metabolism.

The basic function of nephrons is to clean or clear blood plasma of unnecessary substances. After the glomerulus has filtered the blood, the tubules select the unwanted from the wanted portions of tubular fluid. The necessary portions are returned to the blood, and the unnecessary portions pass into urine.

Other Functions of the Kidney. In addition to their function in regulating the volume and composition of ECF, the kidneys also have other vital functions, including the production of erythropoietin, activation of vitamin D, and production and secretion of renin.

Erythropoietin is produced and released in response to hypoxia and decreased renal blood flow. Erythropoietin stimulates the production of red blood cells (RBCs) in the bone marrow. A deficiency of erythropoietin occurs in renal failure, leading to anemia.

Vitamin D is a hormone that can be obtained in the diet or synthesized by the action of ultraviolet radiation on cholesterol in the skin. These forms of vitamin D are inactive and require two more steps to become metabolically active. The first step in activation occurs in the liver. The second step occurs in the kidneys. Active vitamin D is essential for the absorption of calcium from the gastrointestinal (GI) tract. The patient with renal failure has a deficiency of the active metabolite of vitamin D and manifests problems of altered calcium and phosphate balance (see Chapter 47).

Renin is important in the regulation of blood pressure. Renin is produced and secreted by juxtaglomerular cells of the kidney (Fig. 45-4). Renin is released into the bloodstream in response to decreased renal perfusion, decreased arterial blood pressure, decreased ECF, decreased serum Na^+ concentration, and increased urinary Na^+ concentration. Renin catalyzes the splitting of the plasma protein angiotensinogen (from the liver) into angiotensin I, which is subsequently converted to angiotensin II by angiotensin-converting enzyme (ACE). ACE is located on the luminal surface

of all blood vessels, with especially high levels in the vessels of the lungs. Angiotensin II stimulates the release of aldosterone from the adrenal cortex, which causes Na^+ and water retention, leading to an increased ECF volume. Angiotensin II also causes increased peripheral vasoconstriction. Release of renin is suppressed by factors opposite to those that cause release. The elevation in blood pressure brought about by the increase in ECF and vasoconstriction and the increase in plasma sodium inhibit further renin release. Excessive renin production caused by impaired renal perfusion may be a contributing factor in the etiology of hypertension (see Chapters 33 and 47).

Prostaglandins (PGs) are synthesized by most body tissues from the precursor, arachidonic acid, in response to appropriate stimuli. PGs, which are involved in the regulation of cell function and host defenses, exert their influence primarily on cells or tissues that are close to the site where they are synthesized. (See Chapter 13 and Fig. 13-5 for a more detailed discussion of PGs.)

In the kidney, PG synthesis (primarily PGE_2 and PGI_2) occurs primarily in the medulla. These PGs have a vasodilating action, thus increasing renal blood flow, and promoting Na^+ excretion. They counteract the vasoconstrictor effect of substances such as angiotensin and norepinephrine. Renal PGs may have a systemic effect in lowering blood pressure by decreasing systemic vascular resistance.[4]

The significance of renal PGs is related to the role of the kidneys in causing hypertension. In renal failure with a loss of functioning tissue, these renal vasodilator factors are also lost, which may be one factor that contributes to hypertension in renal failure (see Chapter 47).

Ureters

The ureters are tubes approximately 10 to 12 inches (25 to 35 cm) long and 0.08 to 0.3 inch (0.2 to 0.8 cm) in diameter that carry urine from the renal pelvis to the bladder (see Fig. 45-1). The narrow area where the ureter joins the renal pelvis is termed the *ureteropelvic junction.* After coursing down along the psoas muscle, the ureter crosses over the pelvic brim and iliac artery and inserts into the base of the bladder at the *ureterovesical junction* (UVJ). The ureteral lumen is narrowest at these junctions; consequently, they are often the sites of urinary stone *(calculi)* obstruction. Because the lumen of the ureter is narrow, it can be easily occluded internally (e.g., calculi) or externally (e.g., tumors, adhesions, inflammation).

Sympathetic and parasympathetic nerves, along with the vascular supply, surround the mucosal lining of the ureter. Circular and longitudinal smooth muscle fibers, arranged in a meshlike outer layer, contract to promote the peristaltic one-way flow of urine. These muscle contractions can be affected by distention and neurologic, endocrine, and pharmacologic factors. Stimulation of these nerves during passage of a stone or clot may cause acute, severe pain termed *renal colic.*

Because the renal pelvis holds only 3 to 5 ml of urine, kidney damage can result from a backflow of more than that amount of urine. The UVJ relies on the ureter's angle of bladder penetration and muscle fiber attachments with the bladder to prevent the backflow of urine *(reflux)* and ascending infection. The distal ureter enters the bladder laterally at its base, courses along obliquely through the bladder wall for about 1.5 cm, and intermingles with muscle fibers of the bladder base. Circular and longitudinal bladder muscle fibers adjacent to the imbedded ureter help secure it. When bladder pressure rises (e.g., during voiding or coughing), muscle fibers that the ureter shares with the bladder base contract first to help promote ureteral lumen closure. The bladder then contracts against its base to further close the UVJ and prevent urine from moving back through the junction.

Bladder

The urinary bladder is a distensible organ positioned behind the symphysis pubis and anterior to the vagina and rectum (Fig. 45-5). Its primary functions are to serve as a reservoir for urine and to help the body eliminate waste products. Normal adult urine output is approximately 1500 ml/day, which varies with food and fluid intake. The volume of urine produced at night is less than half of that formed during the day because of hormonal influences (e.g., ADH). This diurnal pattern of urination is normal. Most people urinate 5 to 6 times during the day and occasionally at night.

The triangular area formed by the two ureteral openings and the bladder neck at the base of the bladder is termed the *trigone.* It is affixed to the pelvis by many ligaments, and it does not change its shape during bladder filling or emptying. The bladder muscle *(detrusor)* is composed of layers of intertwined smooth muscle fibers capable of considerable distention during bladder filling and contraction during emptying. It is affixed to the abdominal wall by an umbilical ligament, termed the *urachus.* Consequently, as the bladder fills, it rises toward the umbilicus. The dome, anterior, and lateral aspects of the bladder expand and contract. When the bladder is empty, it appears as multiple folds within the pelvis.

On the average, 200 to 250 ml of urine in the bladder causes moderate distention and the urge to urinate. When the quantity of urine reaches about 400 to 600 ml, the person feels uncomfortable. Bladder capacity varies with the individual, usually ranging from 600 to 1000 ml. Evacuation of urine is termed *urination, micturition,* or *voiding.*

The bladder has the same mucosal lining as that of the renal pelvis, ureter, and bladder neck. This lining is called transitional

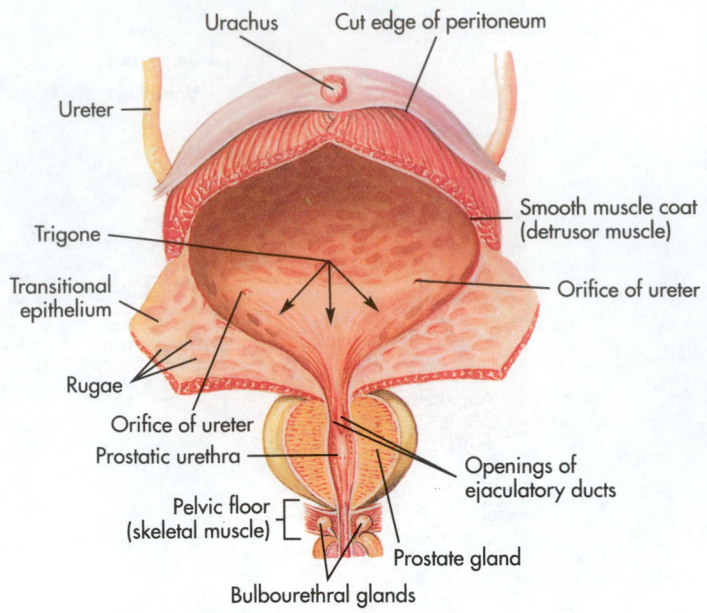

FIG. 45-5 Urinary bladder of a male.

cell epithelium or *urothelium* and is unique to the urinary tract. Transitional cell epithelium is resistant to absorption of urine. Therefore urinary wastes produced by the kidneys do not leak out of the urinary system after they leave the kidneys. Microscopically, transitional cell epithelium is several cells deep. These cells stretch out in the bladder to only a few cells deep as it accommodates filling. As the bladder empties, the epithelium resumes its multicellular layer formation.

Transitional cell tumors that occur in one section of the urinary tract can easily metastasize to other urinary tract areas since the mucosal lining throughout the urinary tract is the same. Malignant cells may move down from upper urinary tract tumors and imbed in the bladder, or large bladder tumors can invade the ureter. Tumor recurrence within the bladder is common. Intact urothelium also has phagocytic properties, although the exact mechanism is unknown.

Urethra

The urethra is a small muscular tube that leads from the bladder neck to the external meatus. The primary function of the urethra is to serve as a conduit for urine from the bladder neck to outside the body during voiding.

The urothelium and submucosal layers are the same as that of the bladder. Smooth muscle fibers from the bladder neck extending down into the urethra are further supported by circular smooth muscle fibers around the urethra. Special C-shaped striated muscle fibers (the rhabdosphincter, or external sphincter) surround a portion of the urethra and voluntarily contract and prevent leaking when bladder pressure increases.

The female urethra is 1 to 2 inches (3 to 5 cm) long and lies behind the symphysis pubis but anterior to the vagina (see Fig. 45-1, *C*). The rhabdosphincter encircles the middle third of the urethra. The short urethra is a contributing factor to the increased incidence of urinary tract infections in women.

The male urethra, which is about 8 to 10 inches (20 to 25 cm) long, originates at the bladder neck and extends the length of the penis (see Fig. 45-1, *B*). It is often separated into three parts. The prostatic urethra extends from the bladder neck through the prostate to the urogenital diaphragm. The membranous urethra passes through the urogenital diaphragm. The rhabdosphincter encircles this portion. Because of the concentrated muscular support, this short portion is not as expandable; consequently, stricture formation in this area after instrumentation is common. The penile urethra continues through the corpus spongiosum, a cavernous penile body, from the urogenital diaphragm to a distal dilated area, the fossa navicularis, before terminating at the meatus.

Urethrovesical Unit

Together, the bladder, urethra, and pelvic floor muscles form what is called the urethrovesical unit. Normal voluntary control of this unit is defined as *continence*. Stimulating and inhibiting impulses are sent from the brain to the thoracolumbar (T11 to L2) and sacral (S2 to S4) areas of the spinal cord to control voiding. Distention of the bladder stimulates stretch receptors within the bladder wall. Impulses are transmitted to the sacral spinal cord and then to the brain, causing a desire to urinate. If the time to void is not appropriate, inhibitor impulses in the brain are stimulated and transmitted back to the thoracolumbar and sacral nerves innervating the bladder. In a coordinated fashion, the detrusor accommodates to the pressure (does not contract) while the sphincter and pelvic floor muscles tighten to resist bladder pressure. If voiding is appropriate, cerebral inhibition is voluntarily suppressed, and impulses are transmitted via the spinal cord for the bladder neck, sphincter, and pelvic floor muscles to relax and for the bladder to contract. The sphincter closes and the detrusor muscle relaxes when the bladder is empty.

Any disease or trauma that affects function of the brain, spinal cord, or nerves that directly innervate the bladder, bladder neck, external sphincter, or pelvic floor can affect bladder function. These conditions include diabetes mellitus, multiple sclerosis, paraplegia, and tetraplegia (quadriplegia). Drugs affecting nerve transmission also can affect bladder function.

GERONTOLOGIC CONSIDERATIONS
EFFECTS OF AGING ON THE URINARY SYSTEM

Anatomic changes in the aging kidney include a 20% to 30% decrease in size and weight between the ages of 30 and 90 years. By the seventh decade of life, 30% to 50% of glomeruli have lost their function. Atherosclerosis has been found to accelerate the decrease of renal size with age. Despite these changes, older individuals maintain body fluid homeostasis unless they encounter diseases or other physiologic stressors.[5]

Physiologic changes in the aging kidney include decreased renal blood flow, due in part to atherosclerosis, resulting in a decreased GFR. Alterations in hormone levels including ADH, aldosterone, and atrial natriuretic peptide (ANP) result in decreased urinary concentrating ability and limitations in excretion of water, sodium, potassium, and acid. Under normal conditions, the aging kidney is able to maintain homeostasis. However, after abrupt changes in blood volume, acid load, or other insults, the kidney may not be able to function effectively because much of its renal reserve has been lost.[6]

Physiologic changes also occur in the aging bladder and urethra. The female urethra, bladder, vagina, and pelvic floor undergo a loss of elasticity, vascularity, and structure. Periurethral striated muscle fibers and muscles supporting the bladder relax. Consequently, older women are more prone to urethral irritation and urethral and bladder infections.[7] Although urinary incontinence in

TABLE 45-2	GERONTOLOGIC DIFFERENCES IN ASSESSMENT — Urinary System	
Gerontologic Changes	**Differences in Assessment Findings**	

Gerontologic Changes	Differences in Assessment Findings
Kidney	
↓ Amount of renal tissue	Less palpable
↓ Number of nephrons and renal blood vessels; thickened basement membrane of Bowman's capsule and glomeruli	↓ Creatinine clearance, ↑ BUN level, ↑ serum creatinine
↓ Function of loop of Henle and tubules	Alterations in drug excretion; nocturia; loss of normal diurnal excretory pattern because of ↓ ability to concentrate urine; less concentrated urine
Ureter, Bladder, and Urethra	
↓ Elasticity and muscle tone	Palpable bladder after urination because of retention
Weakening of urinary sphincter	Stress incontinence (especially during Valsalva maneuver), dribbling of urine after urination
↓ Bladder capacity and sensory receptors	Frequency, urgency, nocturia, overflow incontinence
Estrogen deficiency leading to thin, dry vaginal tissue	Stress or overactive bladder, dysuria
↑ Prevalence of unstable bladder contractions	Overactive bladder
Prostatic enlargement	Hesitancy, frequency, urgency, nocturia, straining to urinate, retention, dribbling

BUN, Blood urea nitrogen.

older women has long been associated with diminished estrogen levels, recent research has found that the incidence of incontinence is higher in menopausal women who use hormone replacement therapy. These new findings may promote changes in therapy for postmenopausal urinary incontinence.[8]

Men's prostates enlarge as they age. Because the prostate surrounds the proximal urethra, increasing prostate size may affect urinary patterns in men, causing hesitancy, retention, slow stream, and bladder infections.

Constipation, a complaint often expressed by the elderly, can also affect urination. Partial urethral obstruction may occur because of the rectum's close proximity to the urethra.

Age-related changes in the urinary system and differences in assessment findings are presented in Table 45-2.

ASSESSMENT OF THE URINARY SYSTEM

Subjective Data
Important Health Information

Past Health History. The patient should be questioned about the presence or history of diseases that are related to renal or other urologic problems. Some of these diseases are hypertension, diabetes mellitus, gout and other metabolic problems, connective tissue disorders (e.g., systemic lupus erythematosus, systemic sclerosis [scleroderma]), skin or upper respiratory infections of

TABLE 45-3	**Potentially Nephrotoxic Agents**	
Antibiotics	**Pharmacologic Agents**	**Other Agents**
amikacin (Amikin)	captopril (Capoten)	gold
amphotericin B	cimetidine (Tagamet)	heavy metals
bacitracin	cisplatin (Platinol)	contrast medium
cephalosporins	cocaine	
gentamicin	cyclosporine	
kanamycin	ethylene glycol	
neomycin	heroin	
polymyxin B	lithium	
streptomycin	methotrexate	
sulfonamides	nitrosoureas (e.g.,	
tobramycin	carmustine)	
(Nebcin)	nonsteroidal antiinflam-	
vancomycin	matory drugs (e.g.,	
	ibuprofen,	
	indomethacin)	
	phenacetin	
	quinine	
	rifampin	
	salicylates (large	
	quantities)	

streptococcal origin, tuberculosis, viral hepatitis, congenital disorders, neurologic conditions (e.g., stroke, back injury), or trauma. Specific urinary problems such as cancer, infections, benign prostatic hyperplasia, and calculi should be noted.

Medications. An assessment of the patient's current and past use of medications is important. This should include over-the-counter drugs, as well as prescription medications and herbs. Drugs affect the urinary tract in several ways. Many drugs are known to be nephrotoxic (Table 45-3). Certain drugs may alter the quantity and character of urine output (e.g., diuretics). A number of drugs such as phenazopyridine (Pyridium) and nitrofurantoin (Macrodantin) change the color of urine. Anticoagulants may cause hematuria. Many antidepressants, calcium channel blockers, antihistamines, and drugs used for neurologic and musculoskeletal disorders affect the ability of the bladder or sphincter to contract or relax normally.

Surgery or Other Treatments. The patient should also be questioned about any previous hospitalizations related to renal or urologic diseases and all urinary problems during past pregnancies. The duration, severity, and patient's perception of any problem and its treatment should be elicited. Past surgeries, particularly pelvic surgeries, or urinary tract instrumentation should be documented. Information should be obtained from the patient about any radiation or chemotherapy treatment for cancer.

Functional Health Patterns. Key questions to ask a patient with problems related to the urinary system are listed in Table 45-4.

Health Perception–Health Management Pattern. The nurse should ask about the patient's general health, particularly when disease affecting the kidneys is suspected. Sometimes responses such as "feeling tired all of the time," changes in weight or appetite, excess thirst, fluid retention, and complaints of headache, pruritus, or blurred vision may be related to abnormal kidney function. Similarly, the elderly patient may report malaise and nonlocalized abdominal discomfort as the only symptoms of a urinary tract infection.[9]

An occupational history should be taken. Exposure to certain chemicals can affect the kidneys and urinary tract system. Phenol and ethylene glycol are examples of nephrotoxic chemicals. Aromatic amines and certain organic chemicals may increase the risk of bladder cancers. Textile workers, painters, hairdressers, and industrial workers have a high incidence of bladder tumors.

A smoking history should be obtained. Cigarette smoking is a major factor in the risk for bladder cancer. Tumors occur 4 times more frequently in cigarette smokers than in nonsmokers.

Places where a patient has lived may be important information to obtain. It has been shown that persons living in certain parts of the United States (Great Lakes, Southwest, Southeast) have a higher than normal incidence of urinary calculi. This may be caused by the higher mineral content of the soil and water. A person living in Middle Eastern countries or Africa can acquire certain parasites that can cause cystitis or bladder cancer.

The presence of certain renal or urologic problems in a family history increases the likelihood of similar problems occurring in the patient. The nurse should ask about family members who have had any of the diseases referred to in the past health history, as well as polycystic renal disease and congenital urinary tract abnormalities, such as Alport syndrome (congenital nephritis).

Nutritional-Metabolic Pattern. The usual quantity and types of fluid a patient drinks are important information related to urinary tract disease. Dehydration may contribute to urinary infections, calculi formation, and renal failure. Large intake of particular foods, such as dairy products or foods high in proteins, may also lead to calculi formation. Asparagus may cause the urine to smell musty, and red urine caused by beet ingestion may be mistaken for bloody urine. Caffeine, alcohol, carbonated beverages, or spicy foods often aggravate urinary inflammatory diseases. Many herbal teas also cause diuresis. An unexplained weight gain may be the result of fluid retention secondary to a renal problem. Anorexia, nausea, and vomiting can dramatically affect fluid status and require careful assessment. Information on vitamin and mineral supplements and herbal therapies should be obtained. The patient may not think of these supplements and therapies when listing over-the-counter drugs; supplements are often considered part of nutritional intake.

Elimination Pattern. Questions about urine elimination patterns are the cornerstone of the health history in the patient with a lower urinary tract disorder. This line of inquiry begins with a question of how the patient manages urine elimination. The majority of patients eliminate urine by spontaneous voiding, and they should be asked about daytime (diurnal) voiding frequency and the frequency of nocturia. Pelvic organ prolapse, particularly advanced anterior vaginal prolapse, may cause suprapubic pressure, frequency, urgency, and incontinence secondary to urinary retention.[10] Patients should also be queried about additional bothersome lower urinary tract symptoms, including urgency, incontinence, or urinary retention. Table 45-5 lists some of the common clinical manifestations of urinary tract disorders. Changes in the color and appearance of urine are often significant and should be evaluated. If blood is visible in the urine, it should be determined if it occurs at the beginning, throughout, or at the end of urination.

Bowel function should also be investigated. Problems with fecal incontinence may signal neurologic causes for bladder problems because of shared nerve pathways. Constipation and fecal impaction can partially obstruct the urethra, causing inadequate bladder emptying, overflow incontinence, and infection.

TABLE 45-4   *HEALTH HISTORY*
Urinary System

Health Perception–Health Management Pattern
- How is your energy level compared with a year ago?
- Do you notice any visual changes?*
- Have you ever smoked? If yes, how many packs per day?

Nutritional-Metabolic Pattern
- How is your appetite?
- Has your weight changed over the past year?*
- Do you take vitamin or mineral supplements?*
- How much and what kinds of fluids do you drink daily?
- How many dairy products and how much meat do you eat?
- Do you drink coffee? Colas?
- Do you eat chocolate?
- Do you spice your food heavily?*

Elimination Pattern
- Are you able to sit through a 2-hr meeting or ride in a car for 2 hr without urinating?
- Do you awaken at night with the desire to urinate? If so, how many times does this occur during an average night?
- Do you ever notice blood in your urine?* If so, at what point in the urination does it occur?
- Do you find it difficult to postpone urination when you feel the urge to urinate?*
- Do you ever leak urine? If so, what causes urine leakage? Do you leak when you cough, walk, run, or lift a heavy object?
- Do you leak if you are unable to reach a toilet right away? Do you ever find that you have leaked without awareness of doing so?
- Do you use special devices or supplies for urine elimination or control?*
- Do you ever have pain when you urinate?* If so, where is the pain?
- How often do you move your bowels?
- Do you ever experience constipation (hardened stools that are difficult to pass or a sensation that you are unable to completely evacuate your bowels)?
- Do you frequently experience diarrhea (high-volume, loose watery stools)? Do you ever have problems controlling your bowels? If so, do you have problems controlling the passage of gas? Watery or liquid stool? Solid stool?

Activity-Exercise Pattern
- Have you noticed any changes in your ability to do your usual daily activities?*
- Do certain activities aggravate your urinary problem?*
- Has your urinary problem caused you to alter or stop any activity or exercise?*
- Do you require assistance in moving or getting to the bathroom?*

Sleep-Rest Pattern
- Do you awaken at night from an urge to urinate?*
- Do you awaken at night from pain or other problems and urinate as a matter of routine before returning to sleep?*
- Do you experience daytime sleepiness and fatigue as a result of nighttime urination?*

Cognitive-Perceptual Pattern
- Describe any pain you have in relation to urination.

Self-Perception–Self-Concept Pattern
- How does your urinary problem make you feel about yourself?
- Do you perceive your body differently since you have developed a urinary problem?

Role-Relationship Pattern
- Does your urinary problem interfere with your relationships with family or friends?*
- Has your urinary problem caused a change in your job status or affected your ability to carry out job-related responsibilities?*

Sexuality-Reproductive Pattern
- Has your urinary problem caused any change in your sexual pleasure or performance?*
- Do you have hygiene problems related to sexual activities that cause you concern?*

Coping–Stress Tolerance Pattern
- Do you feel able to manage the problems associated with your urinary problem? If not, explain.
- What strategies are you using to cope with your urinary problem?

Values-Beliefs Pattern
- Has your present illness affected your belief system?*
- Are your treatment decisions related to your urinary problem in conflict with your value system?*

*If yes, describe.

TABLE 45-5 | Clinical Manifestations of Disorders of the Urinary System

General Manifestations	Manifestations Related to the Urinary System				
	Edema	**Pain**	**Patterns of Urination**	**Urine Output**	**Urine Composition**
Fatigue	Facial (periorbital)	Dysuria	Frequency	Anuria	Concentrated
Headaches	Ankle	Flank or costoverte-	Urgency	Oliguria	Dilute
Blurred vision	Ascites	bral angle	Hesitancy of stream	Polyuria	Hematuria
Elevated blood	Anasarca	Groin	Change in stream		Pyuria
pressure	Sacral	Suprapubic	Retention		Color (red, brown,
Anorexia			Dysuria		yellowish green)
Nausea and vomiting			Nocturia		
Chills			Overactive bladder		
Itching			Incontinence		
Excessive thirst			Stress incontinence		
Change in body			Dribbling		
weight					
Cognitive changes					

The nurse should determine the patient's method of handling a urinary problem. A patient may already be using a catheter or collection device. Sometimes a patient has to assume a particular position to urinate or perform such maneuvers as pressing on the lower abdomen (Credé's method), straining (Valsalva maneuver), or stretching the rectum to empty the bladder.

Activity-Exercise Pattern. The patient's level of activity should be assessed. A sedentary person is more likely to have stasis of urine than an active individual, which can predispose to infection and calculi. Demineralization of bones in a person with limited physical activity can cause increased urine calcium precipitation.

An active person may find that increasing activity aggravates the urinary problem. The patient who has had prostate surgery or who has weakened pelvic floor muscles may leak urine when attempting particular activities such as running. Some men may develop chronic inflammatory prostatitis or epididymitis after heavy lifting or long-distance driving.

Sleep-Rest Pattern. Nocturia is a common and a particularly bothersome lower urinary tract symptom that often leads to sleep deprivation, daytime sleepiness, and fatigue. It occurs in multiple disorders affecting the lower urinary tract, including urinary incontinence, urinary retention, and interstitial cystitis. Nocturia also may be attributable to polyuria owing to renal disease, poorly controlled diabetes mellitus, alcoholism, excessive fluid intake, or obstructive sleep apnea. When asking about nocturia, it is helpful to determine whether it is the desire to urinate that causes the person to arise from sleep or whether pain or some other symptom interrupts sleep and the person urinates as a matter of habit before returning to bed. Up to one episode of nocturia is considered normal in younger adults, and up to two episodes are acceptable among adults age 65 years or older. Sleep problems associated with a urinary disorder should be documented. The older adult may awaken many times during the night to urinate and may need to be assured that this may be normal. However, a complete assessment should be made to rule out any problem.

Cognitive-Perceptual Pattern. Level of mobility, visual acuity, and dexterity are important factors to determine for a patient with urologic problems when managing his or her own care at home, particularly when urine retention or incontinence is a problem. It should be determined if the patient is alert, is able to understand instructions, and can recall the instructions when necessary.

If urinary incontinence is present, a thorough history of the problem should be elicited to assist in determining the type of incontinence. It is important to document what the patient has previously tried to manage the problem. Incontinence is a distressing problem and calls for great sensitivity on the part of the nurse if accurate information is to be obtained.

Pain is a frequent symptom of urinary tract disease. Types of pain associated with renal and urologic problems include dysuria, groin pain, costovertebral pain, and suprapubic pain. Complaints of pain should be assessed and the location, character, and duration documented. The absence of pain when other urinary symptoms exist is also significant. Many urinary tract tumors are painless in the early stages.

Self-Perception–Self-Concept Pattern. Problems associated with the urinary system, such as incontinence, urinary diversion procedures, and chronic fatigue (may indicate anemia), can result in loss of self-esteem and a negative body image. Sensitive questioning may elicit cues to problems in this area.

Role-Relationship Pattern. Urinary problems can affect many aspects of a person's life, including the ability to work and relationships with others. These factors will have important implications for future treatment and management of the patient's condition. The nurse must be alert for indications from the patient.

Urinary system problems may be serious enough to cause problems in job-related and social situations. Chronic dialysis therapy often makes regular employment or full-time homemaking difficult. Concurrent poor health and negative body image can seriously alter existing roles. The nurse should assess this area to plan appropriate interventions.

Sexuality-Reproductive Pattern. The patient should be questioned about the effect of a renal or urologic problem on her or his sexual patterns and satisfaction. Problems related to personal hygiene and fatigue can seriously affect a sexual relationship. Although urinary incontinence is not directly associated with sexual dysfunction, it often has a devastating effect on self-esteem and social and intimate relationships. Counseling of both the patient and partner may be indicated.

Objective Data

Physical Examination

Inspection. The nurse should assess for changes in the following:

Skin: pallor, yellow-gray cast, excoriations, changes in turgor, bruises, texture (e.g., rough, dry skin)

Mouth: stomatitis, ammonia breath odor

Face and extremities: generalized edema, peripheral edema, bladder distention, masses, enlarged kidneys

Abdomen: skin changes described earlier, as well as striae, abdominal contour for midline mass in lower abdomen (may indicate urinary retention) or unilateral mass (occasionally seen in adult, indicating enlargement of one or both kidneys from large tumor or polycystic kidney)

Weight: weight gain secondary to edema; weight loss and muscle wasting in renal failure

General state of health: fatigue, lethargy, and diminished alertness

Palpation. The kidneys are posterior organs protected by the abdominal organs, the ribs, and the heavy back muscles. A landmark useful in locating the kidneys is the **costovertebral angle** (CVA) formed by the rib cage and the vertebral column. The normal-sized left kidney is rarely palpable because the spleen lies directly on top of it. Occasionally the lower pole of the right kidney is palpable.

To palpate the right kidney, the examiner's left (anterior) hand is placed behind and supports the patient's right side between the rib cage and the iliac crest (Fig. 45-6). The right flank is elevated with the left hand, and the right hand is used to palpate deeply for the right kidney. The lower pole of the right kidney may be felt as a smooth, rounded mass that descends on inspiration. If the kidney is palpable, its size, contour, and tenderness should be noted. Kidney enlargement is suggestive of neoplasm or other serious renal pathologic conditions.

The urinary bladder is normally not palpable unless it is distended with urine. If the bladder is full, it may be felt as a smooth, round, firm organ and is sensitive to palpation.

Percussion. Tenderness in the flank area may be detected by fist percussion (kidney punch). This technique is performed by striking the fist of one hand against the dorsal surface of the other hand, which is placed flat along the posterior CVA margin. Normally a firm blow in the flank area should not elicit pain. If CVA

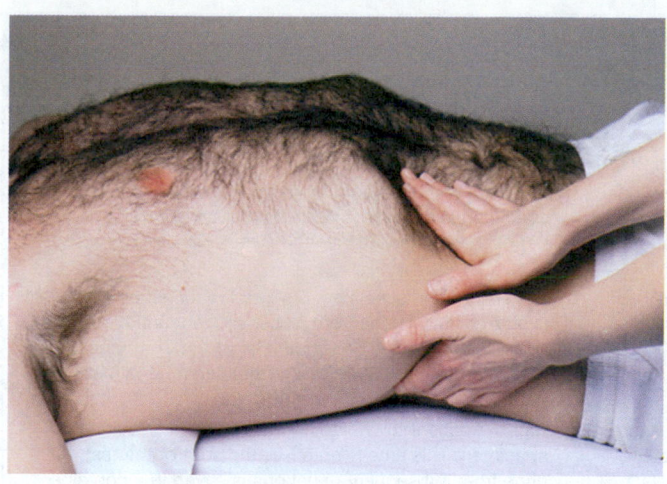

FIG. 45-6 Palpating the right kidney.

TABLE 45-6	**Normal Physical Assessment of the Urinary System**

- No costovertebral angle tenderness
- Nonpalpable kidney and bladder
- No palpable masses

tenderness and pain are present, it may indicate a kidney infection or polycystic kidney disease.

Normally a bladder is not percussible until it contains 150 ml of urine. If the bladder is full, dullness is heard above the symphysis pubis. A distended bladder may be percussed as high as the umbilicus.

Auscultation. The bell of the stethoscope may be used to auscultate over both CVAs and in the upper abdominal quadrants. With this technique, the abdominal aorta and renal arteries are auscultated for a *bruit* (an abnormal murmur), which indicates impaired blood flow to the kidneys.

Table 45-6 shows how to record the normal physical assessment findings of the urinary system. Table 45-7 presents common assessment abnormalities of the urinary system. Normally, assessment findings may vary in the older adult. Table 45-2 shows the age-related changes in the urinary system and differences in assessment findings.

DIAGNOSTIC STUDIES OF THE URINARY SYSTEM

Table 45-8 discusses diagnostic studies common to the urinary system. Diagnostic studies are important in locating and understanding problems of the urinary system. The accuracy of the results is influenced by (1) adherence to the proper procedures re-

Text continued on page 1149.

TABLE 45-7	**COMMON ASSESSMENT ABNORMALITIES** **Urinary System**

Finding	Description	Possible Etiology and Significance
Anuria	Technically no urination (24-hr urine output <100 ml)	Acute renal failure, end-stage renal disease, bilateral ureteral obstruction
Burning on urination	Stinging pain in urethral area	Urethral irritation, urinary tract infection
Chemical cystitis	Painful or difficult urination	Use of spermicides (especially with diaphragm), excessive douching
Dysuria	Painful or difficult urination	Sign of urinary tract infection and interstitial cystitis and wide variety of pathologic conditions
Enuresis	Involuntary nocturnal urinating	Symptomatic of lower urinary tract disorder
Frequency	Increased incidence of urinating	Acutely inflamed bladder, retention with overflow, excess fluid intake
Hematuria	Blood in the urine	Cancer of genitourinary tract, blood dyscrasias, renal disease, urinary tract infection, stones in kidney or ureter, medications (anticoagulants)
Hesitancy	Delay or difficulty in initiating urination	Partial urethral obstruction
Incontinence	Inability to voluntarily control discharge of urine	Neurogenic bladder, bladder infection, injury to external sphincter
Nocturia	Frequency of urination at night	Renal disease with impaired concentrating ability, bladder obstruction, heart failure, diabetes mellitus, finding after renal transplant
Oliguria	Diminished amount of urine in a given time (24-hr urine output of 100-400 ml)	Severe dehydration, shock, transfusion reaction, kidney disease, end-stage renal disease
Pain	Presence over suprapubic area (related to bladder), urethral pain (irritation of bladder neck), flank (CVA) pain	Infection, urinary retention, foreign body in urinary tract, urethritis, pyelonephritis, renal colic or stones
Pneumaturia	Passage of urine containing gas	Fistula connections between bowel and bladder, gas-forming urinary tract infections
Polyuria	Large volume of urine in a given time	Diabetes mellitus, diabetes insipidus, chronic renal failure, diuretics, excess fluid intake
Retention	Inability to urinate even though bladder contains excessive amount of urine	Finding after pelvic surgery, childbirth, catheter removal; urethral stricture or obstruction; neurogenic bladder; postanesthesia
Stress incontinence	Involuntary urination with increased pressure (sneezing or coughing)	Weakness of sphincter control

CVA, Costovertebral angle.

Urinary System

TABLE 45-8	**DIAGNOSTIC STUDIES** **Urinary System**

Study	Description and Purpose	Nursing Responsibility
Urine Studies **Urinalysis**	Urinalysis is a general examination of urine to establish baseline information or provide data to establish a tentative diagnosis and determine whether further studies are to be ordered (see Table 45-9).	Try to obtain first urinated morning specimen. Ensure that specimen is examined within 1 hr of urinating. Wash perineal area if soiled with menses or fecal material.
Creatinine clearance	Creatinine is a waste product of protein breakdown (primarily body muscle mass). Clearance of creatinine by the kidney approximates the GFR. *Normal finding:* 85-135 ml/min	Collect 24-hr urine specimen. Discard first urination when test is started. Save urine from all subsequent urinations for 24 hr. Instruct patient to urinate at end of 24 hr and add specimen to collection. Ensure that serum creatinine is determined during 24-hr period.
Composite urine collection	The purpose of a composite specimen is to examine or measure specific components, such as electrolytes, glucose, protein, 17-ketosteroids, catecholamines, creatinine, and minerals. Composite urine specimens are collected over a period that may range from 2-24 hr.	Instruct the patient to urinate and discard this first urine specimen. This time is noted as the start of the test. All urine from subsequent urinations is saved in a container for the designated period. Finally, at the end of the period, the patient is asked to urinate, and this urine is added to the container. Reminding the patient to save all urine during the study period is critical. Specimens may have to be refrigerated, or preservatives may have to be added to the container used for collecting urine.
Urine culture ("clean catch," "midstream")	Urine culture is done to confirm suspected urinary tract infection and identify causative organisms. *Normally,* bladder is sterile, but urethra contains bacteria and a few WBCs. If properly collected, stored, and handled: <10,000 organisms/ml usually indicates no infection; 10,000-100,000/ml is usually not diagnostic, and test may have to be repeated; >100,000/ml indicates infection.	Use sterile container for collection of urine. Touch only outside of container. For women, separate labia with one hand and clean meatus with other hand, using at least three sponges (saturated with cleansing solution) in a front-to-back motion. For men, retract foreskin (if present) and cleanse glans with at least three cleansing sponges. After cleaning, instruct patient to start urinating and then continue voiding in sterile container. (The initial voided urine flushes out most contaminants in the urethra and perineal area.) Catheterization may be needed if patient is unable to cooperate with this procedure.
Concentration test	Study evaluates renal concentration ability. Concentration is measured by specific gravity readings. *Normal finding:* 1.020-1.035	Instruct patient to fast after given time in evening (in usual procedure). Collect three urine specimens at hourly intervals in morning.
Residual urine	Study determines amount of urine left in bladder after urinating. Finding may be abnormal in problems with bladder innervation, sphincter impairment, BPH, or urethral strictures. *Normal finding:* ≤50 ml urine (increases with age)	If residual urine test is ordered, catheterize patient immediately after urinating or use bladder ultrasound equipment. If a large amount of residual urine is obtained, health care provider may want catheter left in bladder.
Protein determination • Dipstick (Albustix, Combistix)	Dipstick test detects protein (primarily albumin) in urine. *Normal finding:* 0-trace	Dip end of stick in urine and read result by comparison with color chart on label as directed. Grading is from 0 to 4+. Interpret with caution. A positive result may not indicate significant proteinuria; some medications may give false-positive readings.
• Quantitative test for protein	A 12- or 24-hr collection gives a more accurate indication of the amount of protein in urine. Persistent proteinuria usually indicates glomerular renal disease. *Normal finding:* <150 mg/24 hr (<0.15 g/24 hr), consisting mainly of albumin	Perform 12- or 24-hr urine collection.
Urine cytology	Urine can be analyzed to identify abnormal cellular structures that occur with bladder cancer and to follow the progress of bladder cancer.	Specimens may be obtained by voiding, catheterization, or bladder irrigation (bladder washing). The first morning's voided specimen should *not* be used because epithelial cells may change in appearance in urine held in the bladder overnight. As with urinalysis, the specimen should be fresh or brought to the lab within the hour. An alcohol-based fixative is then added to preserve the cellular structure.

BPH, Benign prostatic hypertrophy; *GFR,* glomerular filtration rate; *WBCs,* white blood cells.

TABLE 45-8	**DIAGNOSTIC STUDIES** Urinary System—cont'd

Study	Description and Purpose	Nursing Responsibility
Blood Chemistries		
BUN	BUN is most commonly used to identify presence of renal problems. Concentration of urea in blood is regulated by rate at which kidney excretes urea. *Normal finding:* 10-30 mg/dl (1.8-7.1 mmol/L)	Explain test and watch for postpuncture bleeding. Be aware that, when interpreting BUN, nonrenal factors may cause increase (e.g., rapid cell destruction from infections, fever, GI bleeding, trauma, athletic activity and excessive muscle breakdown, corticosteroid therapy).
Creatinine	Creatinine is more reliable than BUN as a determinant of renal function. Creatinine is end product of muscle and protein metabolism and is liberated at a constant rate. *Normal finding:* 0.5-1.5 mg/dl (44-133 μmol/L). Results are higher in men.	Explain test and watch for postpuncture bleeding.
BUN/creatinine ratio	*Normal finding:* 10:1	
Uric acid	Uric acid study is used as a screening test primarily for disorders of purine metabolism but can indicate kidney disease as well. Values depend on renal function and rate of purine metabolism and dietary intake of food rich in purines. *Normal finding:* 2.5-5.5 mg/dl (149-327 μmol/L) for women; 4.5-6.5 mg/dl (268-387 μmol/L) for men	Explain test and watch for postpuncture bleeding.
Sodium (Na$^+$)	Sodium is main extracellular electrolyte determining blood volume. Usually, values stay within normal range until late stages of renal failure. *Normal finding:* 135-145 mEq/L (135-145 mmol/L)	Explain test and watch for postpuncture bleeding.
Potassium (K$^+$)	Kidneys are responsible for excreting majority of body's potassium. In renal disease, K$^+$ determinations are critical because K$^+$ is one of the first electrolytes to become abnormal. Elevated K$^+$ levels of >6 mEq/L can lead to muscle weakness and cardiac dysrhythmias. *Normal finding:* 3.5-5.0 mEq/L (3.5-5.0 mmol/L)	Explain test and watch for postpuncture bleeding.
Calcium (Ca^{2+})	Calcium is main mineral in bone and aids in muscle contraction, neurotransmission, and clotting. In renal disease, decreased reabsorption of Ca^{2+} leads to renal osteodystrophy. *Normal finding:* 9-11 mg/dl (4.5-5.5 mEq/L, 2.25-2.74 mmol/L)	Explain test and watch for postpuncture bleeding.
Phosphorus	Phosphorus balance is inversely related to Ca^{2+} balance. In renal disease, phosphorus levels are elevated because the kidney is the primary excretory organ. *Normal finding:* 2.8-4.5 mg/dl (0.95-1.45 mmol/L)	Explain test and watch for postpuncture bleeding.
Bicarbonate (HCO$_3^-$)	Most patients in renal failure have metabolic acidosis and low serum HCO$_3^-$ levels. *Normal finding:* 22-26 mEq/L (22-26 mmol/L)	Explain test and watch for postpuncture bleeding.
Radiology Procedures		
Kidneys, ureters, bladder (KUB)	KUB study involves x-ray examination of abdomen and pelvis and delineates size, shape, and position of kidneys. Radiopaque stones and foreign bodies can also be seen.	Perform bowel preparation (if ordered).
Intravenous pyelogram (IVP)	In intravenous pyelogram, x-ray examination visualizes urinary tract after IV injection of contrast material. The presence, position, size, and shape of the kidneys, ureters, and bladder can be evaluated. Cysts, tumors, lesions, and obstructions cause a distortion in the normal appearance of these structures. Patient with significantly decreased renal function should not have IVP because contrast media can be nephrotoxic and worsen renal function.*	Evening before procedure, give cathartic or enema to empty colon of feces and gas. Keep patient on NPO status for 8 hr before procedure. Before procedure, assess patient for iodine sensitivity to avoid anaphylactic reaction. Inform patient that procedure involves lying on table and having serial x-rays taken. Advise the patient that warmth, a flushed face, and a salty taste during injection of contrast material may occur. After procedure, force fluids (if permitted) to flush out contrast material.
Antegrade pyelogram (nephrostogram)	Antegrade pyelogram is an x-ray to evaluate the upper urinary tract when there is allergy to contrast media or decreased renal function and when abnormalities prevent passage of a ureteral catheter. Contrast medium may be injected percutaneously into the renal pelvis or via a nephrostomy tube that is already in place when determining tube function or ureteral integrity after trauma or surgery.*	Explain procedure and prepare patient as for IVP. Watch for signs of complications (e.g., hematuria, infection, hematoma).

BUN, Blood urea nitrogen; *GI,* gastrointestinal; *IV,* intravenous; *NPO,* nothing by mouth.

*N-acetylcysteine (Mucomyst), a renal vasodilator and antioxidant, is sometimes administered to reduce the incidence of contrast-induced nephropathy; it can be given by oral or IV route.

Continued

TABLE 45-8	**DIAGNOSTIC STUDIES** Urinary System—cont'd	

Study	Description and Purpose	Nursing Responsibility
Radiology Procedures—cont'd		
Nephrotomogram	Nephrotomogram is an x-ray taken with rotating tubes. Test delineates segments of the kidney at different levels. Multiple exposures are taken to visualize specific sections of the kidney after IV injection of contrast material.*	Explain procedure and prepare patient as for IVP.
Retrograde pyelogram	Retrograde pyelogram is an x-ray of urinary tract taken after injection of contrast material into kidneys. It may be done if an IVP does not visualize the urinary tract or if the patient is allergic to the contrast material or has decreased renal function. A cystoscope is inserted and ureteral catheters are inserted through it into renal pelvis. Contrast material is injected through catheters.*	Prepare patient as for IVP. Inform patient that pain may be experienced from distention of pelvis and discomfort from cystoscope. Inform patient that anesthesia may be given for procedure. Complications are similar to those for cystoscopy (see cystoscopy later in table).
Renal arteriogram (angiogram)	Purpose of renal arteriogram is to visualize renal blood vessels. Findings can assist in diagnosing renal artery stenosis (Fig. 45-7), additional or missing renal blood vessels, and renovascular hypertension. Can assist in differentiating between renal cyst and renal tumor. Renal arteriograms are also included in the workup of a potential renal transplant donor. A catheter is inserted into the femoral artery and passed up the aorta to the level of the renal arteries (Fig. 45-8). Contrast medium is injected to outline the renal blood supply.*	Prepare patient evening before procedure by giving cathartic or enema. Before injection of contrast material, test for iodine sensitivity. The patient may experience a transient warm feeling along the course of the blood vessel when the contrast material is injected. After procedure, place a pressure dressing over the femoral artery injection site. Observe the site for bleeding. Have patient maintain bed rest with the affected leg straight. Take peripheral pulses in the involved leg every 30-60 min to detect occlusion of blood flow caused by a thrombus. Observe for complications, including thrombus, embolus, local inflammation, and hematoma.
Renal ultrasound	Renal ultrasound is used to detect renal or perirenal masses, in differential diagnosis of renal cysts and solid masses, and in identification of obstructions. Small external ultrasound probe is placed on patient's skin. Conductive gel is applied to the skin. Noninvasive procedure involves passing sound waves into body structures and recording images as they are reflected back. Computer interprets tissue density based on sound waves and displays it in picture form. Can be used safely in patients with renal failure.	Explain procedure to patient. Because radiation exposure is avoided, a number of images can be obtained and repeat studies can be done over a brief period of time. Images can be obtained from both the prone and supine positions. A bowel preparation is not required.
CT scan	CT scan provides excellent visualization of kidneys. Kidney size can be evaluated; tumors, abscesses, suprarenal masses (e.g., adrenal tumors, pheochromocytomas), and obstructions can be detected. Advantage of CT over ultrasound is its ability to distinguish subtle differences in density. Use of IV-administered contrast medium during CT accentuates density of renal tissue and helps differentiate masses.*	Explain procedure to patient. Ask patient about iodine sensitivity. The patient is instructed to lie very still during the procedure while the machine takes precise transaxial images. Sedation may be required if the patient is unable to cooperate.
MRI	MRI is useful for visualization of kidneys. Not proven useful for detecting urinary calculi or calcified tumors. Computer-generated films rely on radiofrequency waves and alteration in magnetic field. *Contraindications:* Presence of implanted ferromagnetic clips or prosthesis, pacemaker, and some cardiac valves.	Explain procedure to patient. Have patient remove all metal objects. Patients with a history of claustrophobia may need to be sedated.
Magnetic resonance angiography	Magnetic resonance angiography allows visualization of renal vasculature. Gadolinium-enhanced studies allow visualization of the renal artery. *Contraindications:* Same as above.	Same as above. Does not require femoral artery puncture.
Cystogram	Cystogram is used to visualize bladder and evaluate vesicoureteral reflux. Also used to evaluate patients with neurogenic bladder and recurrent urinary tract infections. Can also delineate abnormalities of the bladder, such as diverticula, calculi, and tumors. Contrast material is instilled into bladder via cystoscope or catheter.	Explain procedure to patient. If done via cystoscope, follow nursing care related to cystoscopy.
Urethrogram	Urethrogram involves the retrograde injection of contrast material into the urethra to identify strictures, diverticula, or other urethral pathologic conditions. When urethral trauma is suspected, a urethrogram is done before catheterization.	Explain procedure to patient.

CT, Computed tomography; *IV,* intravenous; *IVP,* intravenous pyelogram; *MRI,* magnetic resonance imaging.
*N-acetylcysteine (Mucomyst), a renal vasodilator and antioxidant, is sometimes administered to reduce the incidence of contrast-induced nephropathy; it can be given by oral or IV route.

TABLE 45-8	*DIAGNOSTIC STUDIES* **Urinary System—cont'd**

Study	Description and Purpose	Nursing Responsibility
Radiology Procedures—cont'd		
Voiding cystourethro-gram (VCUG)	Voiding cystourethrogram is a voiding study of the bladder opening (bladder neck) and urethra. The bladder is filled with contrast material. Fluoroscopic films are taken to visualize the bladder and urethra. After urination, another film is taken to assess for residual urine. Can detect abnormalities of the lower urinary tract, urethral stenosis, bladder neck obstruction, and prostatic enlargement.[11]	Explain procedure to patient.
Loopogram	Loopogram is used to detect obstructions, anastomotic leaks, stones, reflux, and other uropathologic features when patient has a urinary pouch or ileal conduit. Because urinary diversions are created with bowel, there is risk of absorption of contrast medium.	Explain procedure to patient. The patient should be closely monitored for reactions to the contrast medium.
Renal Radionuclide Imaging		
Renal scan	Renal scan is to evaluate anatomic structures, perfusion, and function of the kidneys. Radioactive isotopes are injected IV. Radiation detector probes are placed over kidney, and scintillation counter monitors radioactive material in kidney. Radioisotope distribution in kidney is scanned and mapped. Test is useful in showing location, size, and shape of kidney and, in general, assessing blood flow, glomerular filtration, tubular function, and urinary excretion. Abscesses, cysts, and tumors may appear as cold spots because of presence of nonfunctioning tissue. Also used to monitor function of a transplanted kidney.	Requires no dietary or activity restriction. Inform patient that no pain or discomfort should be felt during test.
Renal Biopsy	Renal biopsy is done to obtain renal tissue for examination to determine type of renal disease or to follow progress of renal disease. Technique is usually done as a skin (percutaneous) biopsy through needle insertion into lower lobe of kidney. Can be performed with CT or ultrasound guidance. Absolute contraindications are bleeding disorders, single kidney, and uncontrolled hypertension. Relative contraindications include suspected renal infection, hydronephrosis, and possible vascular lesions.	Type and crossmatch patient for blood. Ensure consent form is signed. *Before:* Ascertain coagulation status through patient history, medication history, CBC, hematocrit, prothrombin time, and bleeding and clotting time. Patient should not be taking aspirin or warfarin (Coumadin). *After:* Apply pressure dressing, and keep on affected side for 30-60 min; bed rest for 24 hr. Vital signs every 5-10 min, first hour. Assess for flank pain, hypotension, ↓ hematocrit, ↑ temperature, chills, urinary frequency, dysuria, and serial urine specimens (gross/microscopic hematuria). Urine dipstick can be used to test for bleeding in urine. Inspect biopsy site for bleeding. Instruct patient to avoid lifting heavy objects for 5-7 days and not to take anticoagulant drugs until allowed by physician.
Endoscopy		
Cystoscopy	Main purpose of cystoscopy is to inspect the interior of the bladder with a tubular lighted scope (cystoscope) (Fig. 45-9). Can be used to insert ureteral catheters, remove calculi, obtain biopsy specimens of bladder lesions, and treat bleeding lesions. Lithotomy position is used. Procedure may be done using local or general anesthesia, depending on needs and condition of patient. Complications include urinary retention, urinary tract hemorrhage, bladder infection, and perforation of the bladder.	*Before:* Force fluids or give IV fluids if general anesthesia is to be used. Ensure consent form is signed. Explain procedure to patient. Give preoperative medication. *After:* Explain that burning on urination, pink-tinged urine, and urinary frequency are expected effects. Observe for bright red bleeding, which is not normal. Do not let patient walk alone immediately after procedure because orthostatic hypotension may occur. Offer warm sitz baths, heat, and mild analgesics to relieve discomfort.

CBC, Complete blood count.

Continued

lated to the study and (2) cooperation of the patient in restricting fluids, collecting urine specimens, lying quietly on the examination table, or following other instructions.

Many radiologic studies require the use of a bowel preparation the evening before the study to clear the lower GI tract of feces and flatus. Because the kidneys lie in a retroperitoneal location, the contents of the colon may obstruct visualization of the urinary tract. If a bowel preparation is not properly done, the study may be unsuccessful and have to be rescheduled. Commonly used bowel preparations include enemas, castor oil, magnesium citrate, and bisacodyl (Dulcolax) tablets or suppositories. Some bowel preparations, such as magnesium citrate and Fleet Enema, are contraindicated in the patient with renal failure. Magnesium cannot be excreted by patients with renal failure (see Chapter 47).

TABLE 45-8	DIAGNOSTIC STUDIES Urinary System—cont'd	

Study	Description and Purpose	Nursing Responsibility
Urodynamics **Urine flow study** (uroflow)	Urine flow study measures urine volume in a single voiding expelled in a period of time. This test is used to (1) assess the degree of outflow obstruction caused by such conditions as benign prostatic hyperplasia or stricture, (2) assess bladder or sphincter dysfunction effects on voiding, and (3) evaluate the effects of treatment for lower urinary tract problems. Graphic displays can illustrate straining and intermittent flow patterns or other abnormal voiding disorders. *Normal maximum flow rate:* Men: 20-25 ml/sec; women: 25-30 ml/sec. Volume voided and the patient's age can affect the flow rate.	Explain procedure to patient. The patient is asked to start the test with a comfortably full bladder, urinate into a special container, and try to empty completely. Measure a residual urine volume immediately after a urine flow study because this will help to identify the degree of chronic urinary retention that is often associated with abnormal flow patterns.
Cystometrogram	Cystometrogram is used to evaluate bladder tone, sensations of filling, and bladder (detrusor) stability. Involves insertion of catheter and instillation of water or saline solution into bladder. Measurements of pressure exerted against bladder wall are recorded. If abdominal pressure is measured, a second tube is inserted into the rectum or vagina. This tube is attached to a small fluid-filled balloon to allow pressure recording.	Explain procedure to patient. During infusion, patient is asked about sensations of bladder filling, usually including first desire (urge) to urinate, a strong desire to urinate, and perception of bladder fullness. Observe patient for manifestations of urinary infection after procedure.
Sphincter electromyography (EMG)	Sphincter electromyography is a recording of electrical activity created when nervous system stimulates motor units within a muscle. By placing needles, percutaneous wires, or patches near the urethra, pelvic floor muscle activity can be assessed. During filling cystometrogram, the sphincter EMG is used to identify voluntary pelvic floor muscle contractions and response of these muscles to bladder filling, coughing, and other provocative maneuvers.	Explain procedure to patient.
Voiding pressure flow study	Voiding pressure flow study combines urinary flow rate, cystometric pressures (intravesical, abdominal, and detrusor pressures), and sphincter EMG for detailed evaluation of micturition. It is completed by assisting the patient to a specialized toilet and allowing the person to urinate while the various pressure tubes and EMG apparatus remain in place.	Explain procedure to patient.
Videourodynamics	Videourodynamics is a combination of filling cystometrogram, sphincter EMG, and/or urinary flow study with anatomic imaging of the lower urinary tract, typically via fluoroscopy. Used in selected cases to identify an obstructive lesion and characterize anatomic changes in bladder and lower urinary tract.	Explain procedure to patient.
Radionuclide cystography (RNC)	Radionuclide cystography is used to detect and grade vesicoureteral reflux. Similar to VCUG, with small dose of radioisotope tracer instilled into the bladder via urethral catheter. More sensitive than VCUG, and radiation dose is 1/1000th that of the VCUG.[12]	Explain procedure to patient as in VCUG.
Whitaker study	Whitaker study is used to measure pressure differential between renal pelvis and bladder. Ureteral obstruction can be assessed. Percutaneous access is gained to renal pelvis by placing a catheter in renal pelvis. A catheter is also placed in bladder. Fluid is perfused through percutaneous tube or needle at a rate of 10 ml/min. Pressure data are then collected. Pressure measurements are combined with fluoroscopic imaging to identify level of obstruction.	Explain procedure to patient.

EMG, Electromyography, *VCUG,* voiding cystourethrogram.

When a patient has repeated diagnostic studies on consecutive days, it is important to prevent dehydration. It is not uncommon to have a patient take nothing by mouth (NPO) after midnight, spend all morning in the x-ray department, be too tired to eat, sleep all afternoon, and be on NPO status after midnight again because of studies scheduled for the next day. Severe dehydration, especially in a diabetic, debilitated, or older patient, may lead to acute renal failure. The nurse is responsible for ensuring that a patient undergoing diagnostic studies is properly hydrated and given adequate nourishment between studies. The nurse should also check with the health care provider regarding the insulin dose for the diabetic patient who is NPO.

Urine Studies

Urinalysis. In evaluating disorders of the urinary tract, one of the first studies done is a **urinalysis** (see Tables 45-8 and 45-9). This test may provide information about possible abnormalities, indicate what further studies need to be done, and supply information on the progression of a diagnosed disorder.

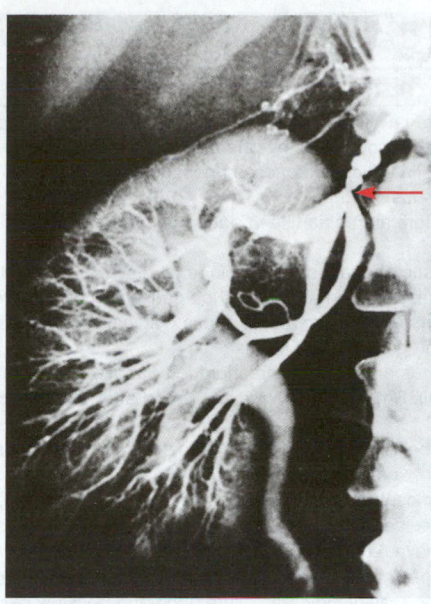

FIG. 45-7 Renal arteriogram showing stenosis of the right renal artery.

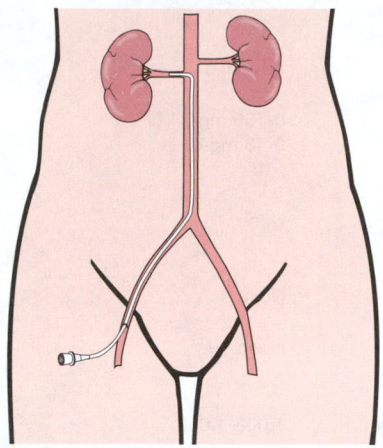

FIG. 45-8 Catheter insertion for a renal arteriogram.

A

B

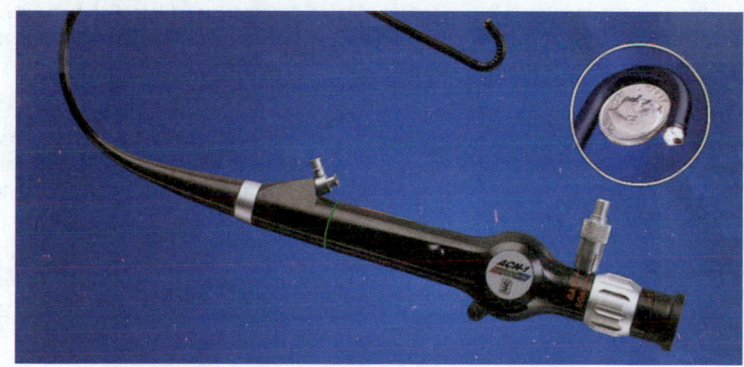

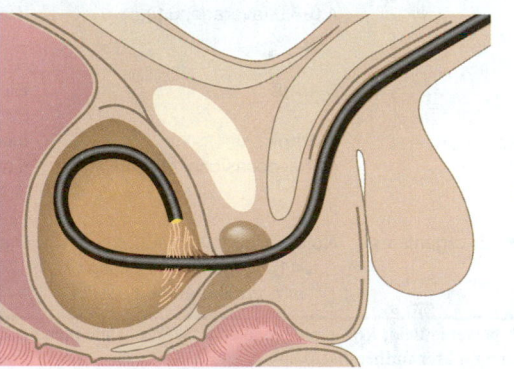

FIG. 45-9 Cystoscopic examination of the bladder in a man. **A,** Flexible Cysto nephroscope. **B,** Scope inserted into bladder.

For a routine urinalysis, a specimen may be collected at any time of the day. However, it is best to obtain the first specimen urinated in the morning. This concentrated specimen is more likely to contain abnormal constituents if they are present in the urine. The specimen should be examined within 1 hour of urinating. If it is not, bacteria multiply rapidly, RBCs hemolyze, *casts* (molds of renal tubules) disintegrate, and the urine becomes alkaline as a result of urea-splitting bacteria. If it is not possible to send the specimen to the laboratory immediately, it should be refrigerated. However, to obtain the best results, the nurse should coordinate specimen collection with routine laboratory hours.

Creatinine Clearance. One of the most common composite indicators used to analyze urinary system disorders is creatinine clearance. **Creatinine** is a waste product produced by muscle breakdown. Urinary excretion of creatinine is a measure of the amount of active muscle tissue in the body, not of body weight.

Therefore people with larger muscle mass have higher values. Because almost all creatinine in the blood is normally excreted by the kidneys, creatinine clearance is the most accurate indicator of renal function. The result of a creatinine clearance test closely approximates that of the GFR.[3] A blood specimen for serum creatinine determination should be obtained during the period of urine collection. Creatinine clearance is calculated as follows:

$$\text{Creatinine clearance} = \frac{\text{Urine creatinine (mg/ml)} \times \text{Urine volume (ml/min)}}{\text{Serum creatinine (mg/ml)}}$$

Creatinine levels remain remarkably constant for each person because they are not significantly affected by protein ingestion, muscular exercise, water intake, or rate of urine production. Normal creatinine clearance values range from 85 to 135 ml/min (see Table 45-8). After age 40, the creatinine clearance rate decreases at a rate of about 1 ml/min/year.

TABLE 45-9	Urinalysis Findings	
Test	**Normal**	**Abnormal Finding and Significance**
Color	Amber yellow	Dark, smoky color suggests hematuria. Yellow-brown to olive-green indicates excessive bilirubin. Orange-red or orange-brown caused by phenazopyridine (Pyridium). Cloudiness of freshly voided urine indicates infection. Colorless urine indicates excessive fluid intake, renal disease, or diabetes insipidus.
Odor	Aromatic	Urine allowed to stand becomes more ammonia-like in odor. In urinary tract infections, urine smells unpleasant.
Protein	0-150 mg/24 hr 0-18 mg/dl	Persistent proteinuria is characteristic of acute and chronic renal disease, especially involving glomeruli. In absence of disease, positive reading may be caused by high-protein diet, strenuous exercise, dehydration, fever, or emotional stress. Vaginal secretions may contaminate urine specimen and give positive reading.
Glucose	None	Glycosuria indicates diabetes mellitus or low renal threshold for glucose reabsorption (if blood glucose level is normal). Small amounts may be found after glucose loading (e.g., glucose tolerance test).
Ketones	None	Altered carbohydrate and fat metabolism indicates diabetes mellitus and starvation. Findings can also be seen in dehydration, vomiting, and severe diarrhea.
Bilirubin	None	Presence of bilirubinuria is as significant as jaundice in detection of liver disorders. Bilirubin may appear in urine before jaundice becomes visible or may be present in persons with hepatic disorders who do not have recognizable jaundice.*
Specific gravity	1.003-1.030	Specific gravity of morning urine specimen reflects maximum concentrating ability of kidney and is 1.025-1.030. Low specific gravity indicates dilute urine and possibly excessive diuresis. High specific gravity indicates dehydration. If it becomes fixed at about 1.010, this indicates renal inability to concentrate urine, suggesting that kidney is progressing to end-stage renal disease.
Osmolality	300-1300 mOsm/kg (300-1300 mmol/kg)	Measurement is a more accurate method than specific gravity for determining diluting and concentrating ability of kidneys. Deviations from normal indicate tubular dysfunction. Findings indicate if kidney has lost ability to concentrate or dilute urine. (Not part of routine urinalysis.)
pH	4.0-8.0 (average, 6.0)	If >8.0, finding may be the result of standing of urine or urinary tract infection because bacteria decompose urea to form ammonia. If <4.0, may indicate respiratory or metabolic acidosis.
RBCs	0-4/hpf	Bleeding in urinary tract is caused by calculi, cystitis, neoplasm, glomerulonephritis, tuberculosis, kidney biopsy, or trauma.
WBCs	0-5/hpf	Increased number of WBCs in urine (pyuria) indicates urinary tract infection or inflammation.
Casts	None–occasional hyaline	Casts are molds of the renal tubules and may contain protein, WBCs, RBCs, or bacteria. Noncellular casts are hyaline in appearance, and a few may be found in normal urine. Casts indicate renal dysfunction or upper urinary tract infections.
Culture for organisms	No organisms in bladder, <10^4 organisms/ml result of normal urethral flora	Bacteria counts >10^5/ml indicate urinary tract infection. Organisms most commonly found in urinary tract infections are *Escherichia coli*, enterococci, *Klebsiella, Proteus,* and streptococci.

hpf, High-powered field; *RBCs,* red blood cells; *WBCs,* white blood cells.
*See Chapter 44 for further discussion.

Urodynamics. *Urodynamics* is a set of tests that is designed to measure urinary tract function. Urodynamic tests study the storage of urine within the bladder and the flow of urine through the urinary tract to the outside of the body. A combination of techniques may be used to provide a detailed assessment of urinary function[11] (see Table 45-8).

NCLEX EXAMINATION REVIEW QUESTIONS

The number of the question corresponds to the same-numbered objective at the beginning of the chapter.

1. A renal stone in the pelvis of the kidney will alter the function of the kidney by interfering with
   a. the structural support of the kidney.
   b. regulation of the concentration of urine.
   c. the entry and exit of blood vessels at the kidney.
   d. collection and drainage of urine from the kidney.
2. A patient with renal disease has oliguria and a creatinine clearance of 40 ml/min. The nurse recognizes that these findings most directly reflect abnormal function of
   a. tubular secretion.
   b. glomerular filtration.

c. capillary permeability.
d. concentration of filtrate.
3. The nurse identifies a risk for urinary calculi in a patient who relates a past health history that includes
   a. adrenal insufficiency.
   b. serotonin deficiency.
   c. hyperaldosteronism.
   d. hyperparathyroidism.
4. Diminished ability to concentrate urine, associated with aging of the urinary system, is attributed to
   a. a decrease in bladder sensory receptors.
   b. a decrease in the number of functioning nephrons.
   c. decreased function of the loop of Henle and tubules.
   d. thickening of the basement membrane of Bowman's capsule.
5. During physical assessment of the urinary system, the nurse
   a. palpates an empty bladder as a small nodule.
   b. uses auscultation over each CVA to detect impaired renal blood flow.
   c. finds a dull percussion sound when 100 ml of urine is present in the bladder.
   d. palpates above the symphysis pubis to determine the level of urine in the bladder.

6. Normal findings expected by the nurse on physical assessment of the urinary system include
   a. nonpalpable left kidney.
   b. auscultation of renal artery bruit.
   c. CVA tenderness elicited by a kidney punch.
   d. palpable bladder to the level of the pubic symphysis.
7. A diagnostic study that indicates renal blood flow, glomerular filtration, tubular function, and excretion is a(n)
   a. IVP.
   b. VCUG.
   c. renal scan.
   d. loopogram.
8. On reading the urinalysis results of a dehydrated patient, the nurse would expect to find
   a. a pH of 8.4.
   b. RBC of 4/hpf.
   c. color: yellow, cloudy.
   d. specific gravity of 1.035.

REFERENCES

1. Smith HW: *Fish to philosopher,* Boston, 1953, Little, Brown.
2. Hallgrimsson B, Benediktsson H, Vize PD: Anatomy and histology of the human urinary system. In Vize PD, Woolf AS, Bard JBL, editors: *The kidney from normal development to congenital disease,* New York, 2003, Academic Press.
3. Eaton DC, Pooler JP: *Vander's renal physiology,* ed 6, New York, 2004, McGraw-Hill.
4. Arima S, Ito S: Role of renal eicosanoids in the control of intraglomerular and systemic blood pressure during development of hypertension. In Suzuki H, Saruta T, editors: *Kidney and blood pressure regulation,* Basel, Switzerland, 2004, Karger.
5. Bax L, van der Graaf Y, Rabelink AJ, et al: Influence of atherosclerosis on age-related changes in renal size and function, *Eur J Clin Invest* 33:34, 2003.
6. Luckey AE, Parsa CJ: Fluid and electrolytes in the aged, *Arch Surg* 138:1046, 2003.
7. Weber AM: Lower urinary tract symptoms: special considerations in frail elderly women. In Weber AM, Brubaker L, Schaffer J, et al, editors: *Office urogynecology: practical pathways in obstetrics and gynecology,* New York, 2004, McGraw-Hill.
8. Hendrix SL, Cochrane BB, Nygaard IE, et al: Effects of estrogen with and without progestin on urinary incontinence, *JAMA* 293:935, 2005.
9. Schaffer J: Urinary tract infection. In Weber AM, Brubaker L, Schaffer J, et al, editors: *Office urogynecology: practical pathways in obstetrics and gynecology,* New York, 2004, McGraw-Hill.
10. Weber AM: Prolapse with lower urinary tract symptoms. In Weber AM, Brubaker L, Schaffer J, et al, editors: *Office urogynecology: practical pathways in obstetrics and gynecology,* New York, 2004, McGraw-Hill.
11. Wen C, Siroky MB: Urodynamic studies. In Siroky MB, Oates RD, Babayan RK, editors: *Handbook of urology: diagnosis and therapy,* ed 3, Philadelphia, 2004, Lippincott, Williams & Wilkins.
12. Powsner RA, Rodman DJ: Radionuclide imaging. In Siroky MB, Oates RD, Babayan RK, editors: *Handbook of urology: diagnosis and therapy,* ed 3, Philadelphia, 2004, Lippincott, Williams & Wilkins.
13. Kshirsager A, Poole C, Mottl A, et al: N-acetylcysteine for the prevention of radiocontrast induced nephropathy: a meta-analysis of prospective controlled trials, *J Am Soc Nephrol* 15:761, 2004.

RESOURCES

Resources for this chapter are listed in Chapter 46 on p. 1196 and Chapter 47 on p. 1232.

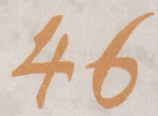

46

Nursing Management
Renal and Urologic Problems

Diane K. Newman

LEARNING OBJECTIVES

1. Describe the pathophysiology, clinical manifestations, collaborative care, and drug therapy of cystitis, urethritis, and pyelonephritis.
2. Explain the nursing management of urinary tract infections.
3. Describe the immunologic mechanisms involved in glomerulonephritis.
4. Explain the clinical manifestations and nursing and collaborative management of acute poststreptococcal glomerulonephritis, Goodpasture syndrome, and chronic glomerulonephritis.
5. Describe the common causes, clinical manifestations, collaborative care, and nursing management of nephrotic syndrome.
6. Compare and contrast the etiology, clinical manifestations, collaborative care, and nursing management of various types of urinary calculi.
7. Explain the common causes and management of renal trauma, renal vascular problems, and hereditary renal problems.
8. Describe the mechanisms of renal involvement in metabolic and connective tissue disorders.
9. Describe the clinical manifestations and collaborative care of kidney cancer and bladder cancer.
10. Describe the common causes and management of bladder dysfunctions, particularly urinary incontinence and urinary retention.
11. Differentiate among ureteral, suprapubic, nephrostomy, urethral, and external catheters with regard to indications for use and nursing responsibilities.
12. Explain the nursing management of the patient undergoing nephrectomy or urinary diversion surgery.

KEY TERMS

calculus, p. 1169
cystitis, p. 1155
glomerulonephritis, p. 1165
Goodpasture syndrome, p. 1166
hydronephrosis, p. 1168
hydroureter, p. 1168
ileal conduit, p. 1189
interstitial cystitis, p. 1163
lithotripsy, p. 1172
nephrolithiasis, p. 1169
nephrosclerosis, p. 1175
nephrotic syndrome, p. 1167
polycystic kidney disease, p. 1176
pyelonephritis, p. 1155
renal artery stenosis, p. 1175
urethritis, p. 1155
urinary incontinence, p. 1180
urinary retention, p. 1180
urosepsis, p. 1155

Electronic Resources

Supplemental content related to Chapter 46 can be found . . .

Companion CD
- Stress-Busting Kit for Nursing Students
- Interactive Case Study: Bladder Cancer with Urinary Diversion
- NCLEX Examination Review Questions
- Comprehensive Glossary

Evolve Website *evolve*
http://evolve.elsevier.com/Lewis/medsurg
- Content Updates
- Key Points (Printable and CD/MP3 Download)
- Concept Map Creator
- Expanded Audio Glossary
- Key Term Flash Cards
- Customizable Nursing Care Plans:
  - Acute Renal Lithiasis
  - Ileal Conduit
  - Urinary Tract Infection

- Patient and Family Instruction Guides in English and Spanish:
  - Changing Your Ileal Conduit Appliances
  - Urinary Tract Infection
- Electronic Calculators
- WebLinks

Reviewed by Donna Walker Hubbard, RN, MSN, CNN, Assistant Professor, University of Mary Hardin Baylor, Belton, Tex.

Renal and urologic disorders encompass a wide spectrum of clinical problems. The diverse causes of these disorders may involve infectious, immunologic, obstructive, metabolic, collagen-vascular, traumatic, congenital, neoplastic, and neurologic mechanisms. This chapter discusses specific disorders of the kidneys, ureters, bladder, and urethra. Acute renal failure and chronic kidney disease are discussed in Chapter 47. Female reproductive problems are discussed in Chapter 54. Male genitourinary problems are discussed in Chapter 55.

Infectious and Inflammatory Disorders of the Urinary System

URINARY TRACT INFECTION

Urinary tract infections (UTIs) are the second most common bacterial disease and the most common bacterial infection in women, with at least one-third of women developing a UTI before the age of 24. During their lifetime, more than half of women will have a UTI, and up to 50% of these will have another infection within a year.[1] Pregnant women are at increased risk for UTIs. UTIs complicate up to 20% of pregnancies and are responsible for 10% of all antepartum admissions.[2] UTIs account for more than 8 million office visits per year and are associated with direct costs of $1.8 billion. More than 100,000 people are hospitalized annually because of UTIs. More than 15% of patients who develop gram-negative bacteremia die, and one third of these cases are caused by bacterial infections originating in the urinary tract.[1,3]

Inflammation of the urinary tract may be attributable to a variety of disorders, but bacterial infection is by far the most common.[1] The bladder and its contents are free from bacteria in the majority of healthy persons. Nevertheless, a minority of otherwise healthy individuals, including many sexually active, young adult women and older women and men, have some bacteria colonizing the bladder. This condition is called *asymptomatic bacteriuria* and does not justify screening or treatment except in pregnant women.[4] In contrast, an infection of the urinary system is diagnosed when bacterial invasion of the urinary tract occurs.

Escherichia coli (Table 46-1) is the most common pathogen causing a UTI, and is primarily seen in women. Bacterial counts of 10^5 colony-forming units per milliliter (CFU/ml) or higher typically indicate a clinically significant UTI. However, counts as low as 10^2 to 10^3 CFU/ml in a person with signs and symptoms are indicative of UTI. Although fungal and parasitic infections may also cause UTIs, they are uncommon. UTIs from these causes are sometimes observed in patients who are immunosuppressed, have diabetes mellitus, or have undergone multiple courses of antibiotic therapy. They also may be seen in persons living in or having traveled to certain third-world countries.

Classification

Several classification systems can be used for UTIs.[1,3] For example, a UTI can be broadly classified as an upper or lower UTI according to its location within the urinary system (Fig. 46-1). Infection of the upper urinary tract (involving the renal parenchyma, pelvis, and ureters) typically causes fever, chills, and flank pain, whereas a UTI confined to the lower urinary tract does not usually have systemic manifestations. Specific terms are used to further delineate the location of a UTI or inflammation. For example, **pyelonephritis** implies

TABLE 46-1	**Common Microorganisms Causing Urinary Tract Infections**
Escherichia coli*	Pseudomonas
Enterococcus	Staphylococcus
Klebsiella	Serratia
Enterobacter	Candida albicans†
Proteus	

*Causes about 80% of cases in persons who do not have urinary tract structural abnormalities or calculi.
†Usually seen in patients who have received broad-spectrum antimicrobial antibiotics and have an indwelling catheter.

CULTURAL AND ETHNIC HEALTH DISPARITIES
Urologic Disorders

- Urinary tract calculi are more common among whites than African Americans.
- Jewish men have a high incidence of uric acid stones.
- Bladder cancer has a higher incidence among white men than African American men.
- In all ethnic groups, bladder cancer affects men about 3 times more often than women.
- Prostate cancer has a higher prevalence in African American men than white men.
- Urinary incontinence is underreported because culturally it is seen as a social hygiene problem causing patient embarrassment.

inflammation (usually due to infection) of the renal parenchyma and collecting system, **cystitis** indicates inflammation of the bladder wall, and **urethritis** means inflammation of the urethra. **Urosepsis** is a UTI that has spread into the systemic circulation and is a life-threatening condition requiring emergency treatment.

Classifying a UTI as complicated or uncomplicated is also useful.[1,3] *Uncomplicated* infections are those that occur in an otherwise normal urinary tract and usually only involve the bladder.[2] *Complicated* infections include those with coexisting presence of obstruction, stones, or catheters; existing diabetes or neurologic diseases; pregnancy-induced changes; or an infection that is recurrent. The individual with a complicated infection is at risk for pyelonephritis, urosepsis, and renal damage.

UTIs can also be classified according to their natural history. An *initial infection* (sometimes called a first or isolated infection) refers to an uncomplicated UTI in a person who has never had an infection or experiences one that is remote from any previous UTI (usually separated by a period of years). In contrast, a *recurrent UTI* is a reinfection caused by a second pathogen in a person who experienced a previous infection that was successfully eradicated. If a recurrent UTI occurs because the original infection is not adequately eradicated, it is classified as unresolved bacteriuria or bacterial persistence. *Unresolved bacteriuria* occurs when bacteria are initially resistant to the antibiotic used to treat an infection, when the antibiotic agent fails to achieve adequate concentrations in the urine or bloodstream to kill bacteria, or when the drug is discontinued before the underlying bacteriuria is completely eradicated. *Bacterial persistence* also may occur when bacteria develop resistance to the antibiotic agent selected for treatment or when a foreign body in the urinary system serves as a harbor or anchor allowing bacteria to survive despite appropriate therapy.[3,5]

Urinary System

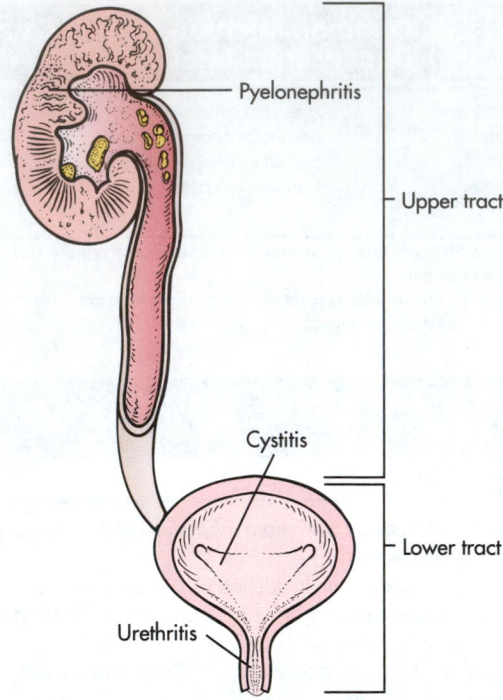

FIG. 46-1 Sites of infectious processes in the urinary tract.

Etiology and Pathophysiology

The urinary tract above the urethra is normally sterile. Several mechanical and physiologic defense mechanisms assist in maintaining sterility and preventing UTIs. These defenses include normal voiding with complete emptying of the bladder, uretero-vesical junction competence, and peristaltic activity that propels urine toward the bladder. Antibacterial characteristics of urine are maintained by an acidic pH (<6.0), high urea concentration, and abundant glycoproteins that interfere with the growth of bacteria. An alteration in any of these defense mechanisms increases the risk of contracting a UTI. Table 46-2 lists predisposing factors to UTIs.

Menopause also appears to be a factor in the incidence of UTI in women. Before menopause, glycogen-rich epithelial cells and the normal bacterial flora *Lactobacillus* keep the vaginal pH acidic (3.5 to 4.5). This acidic environment helps to prevent the overgrowth of organisms that usually only proliferate in a pH above 4.5. In postmenopausal women, lower estrogen levels cause vaginal atrophy, a decrease in vaginal lactobacilli, and an increase in vaginal pH. This leads to an overgrowth of other organisms, specifically *E. coli,* and increases susceptibility to UTIs. Giving women low-dose intravaginal estrogen replacement acidifies the vagina and may be effective in treating recurrent UTI.[6]

The organisms that usually cause UTIs are introduced via the ascending route from the urethra and originate in the perineum. Other less common routes are via the bloodstream or lymphatic system. Most infections are due to gram-negative bacilli normally found in the gastrointestinal (GI) tract, although gram-positive organisms such as streptococci, enterococci, and *Staphylococcus saprophyticus* can also cause urinary infections. A common factor contributing to ascending infection is urologic instrumentation (e.g., catheterization, cystoscopic examinations). Instrumentation allows bacteria that are normally present at the opening of the urethra to enter the urethra or bladder. Sexual intercourse promotes

TABLE 46-2	Predisposing Factors to Urinary Tract Infections

Factors Increasing Urinary Stasis
- Intrinsic obstruction (stone, tumor of urinary tract, urethral stricture, BPH)
- Extrinsic obstruction (tumor, fibrosis compressing urinary tract)
- Urinary retention (including neurogenic bladder and low bladder wall compliance)
- Renal impairment

Foreign Bodies
- Urinary tract calculi
- Catheters (indwelling, external condom catheter, ureteral stent, nephrostomy tube, intermittent catheterization)
- Urinary tract instrumentation (cystoscopy, urodynamics)

Anatomic Factors
- Congenital defects leading to obstruction or urinary stasis
- Fistula (abnormal opening) exposing urinary stream to skin, vagina, or fecal stream
- Shorter female urethra and colonization from normal vaginal flora
- Obesity

Factors Compromising Immune Response
- Aging
- Human immunodeficiency virus infection
- Diabetes mellitus

Functional Disorders
- Constipation
- Voiding dysfunction with detrusor sphincter dyssynergia

Other Factors
- Pregnancy
- Hypoestrogenic state
- Multiple sex partners (women)
- Use of spermicidal agents or contraceptive diaphragm (women)
- Poor personal hygiene

BPH, Benign prostatic hyperplasia.

"milking" of bacteria from the vagina and perineum and may cause minor urethral trauma that predisposes women to UTIs.

Rarely do UTIs result from a hematogenous route, where blood-borne bacteria secondarily invade the kidneys, ureters, or bladder from elsewhere in the body. For a kidney infection to occur from hematogenous transmission, there must be prior injury to the urinary tract, such as obstruction of the ureter, damage caused by stones, or renal scars.

An important source of UTIs is hospital-acquired, or *nosocomial,* infections, which account for 31% of all nosocomial infections.[7] The cause of nosocomial infection is often *E. coli* and, less frequently, *Pseudomonas* organisms. Catheter-acquired urinary tract infections (CAUTIs) are the most common nosocomial infections and are caused by development of bacterial biofilms that are found on the inner surface of the catheter.[8] Most often these infections are underrecognized and undertreated, leading to complications such as renal abscesses, arthritis, epididymitis, periurethral gland infections, and bacteremia.

Clinical Manifestations

Lower urinary tract symptoms (LUTS) are experienced in patients who have UTIs of the upper urinary tracts, as well as those confined to the lower tract.[9] These symptoms are related to either bladder storage or bladder emptying. These symptoms are defined in Table 46-3.

TABLE 46-3	Lower Urinary Tract Symptoms (LUTS)

Emptying Symptoms
Weak urinary stream
Hesitancy—difficulty starting the urine stream resulting in a delay between initiation of urination by relaxation of the urethral sphincter and when urine stream actually begins.
Intermittency—interruption of the urinary stream while voiding.
Postvoid dribbling—urine loss after completion of voiding.
Urinary retention or incomplete emptying—inability to empty urine from the bladder, which can be caused by atonic bladder or obstruction of the urethra. Can be acute or chronic.
Dysuria—difficulty voiding.
Pain on urination

Storage Symptoms
Urinary frequency—an abnormally frequent (usually >8 times in a 24-hr period) desire to void, often of only small quantities (e.g., less than 200 ml).
Urgency—a sudden, strong or intense desire to void immediately, usually accompanied by frequency.
Incontinence—involuntary or unwanted loss or leakage of urine.
Nocturia—waking up 2 or more times at night because of the need or urge to void.
Nocturnal enuresis—complaint of loss of urine during sleep. In children, it is called bedwetting.

These symptoms include dysuria, frequent urination (more often than every 2 hours), urgency, and suprapubic discomfort or pressure. The urine may contain grossly visible blood (hematuria) or sediment, giving it a cloudy appearance. Flank pain, chills, and the presence of a fever indicate an infection involving the upper urinary tract (pyelonephritis). It is important to remember that these symptoms, considered characteristic of a UTI, are often absent in older adults. Older adults tend to experience nonlocalized abdominal discomfort rather than dysuria and suprapubic pain.[10] In addition, they may present with cognitive impairment or generalized clinical deterioration. Because older adults are less likely to experience a fever with a UTI, the value of body temperature as an indicator of a UTI is unreliable. Patients over age 80 years may experience a slight decline in temperature. People with significant bacteriuria may have no symptoms or may have nonspecific symptoms such as fatigue or anorexia.

Multiple factors may produce LUTS similar to a UTI. For example, patients with bladder tumors or those receiving intravesical chemotherapy or pelvic radiation usually experience urinary frequency, urgency, and dysuria. Interstitial cystitis, a chronic inflammatory condition of unknown etiology, also produces urinary symptoms that are sometimes confused with a UTI. (Interstitial cystitis is discussed later in this chapter.)

Diagnostic Studies

Dipstick urinalysis should be obtained initially to identify the presence of nitrites (indicating bacteriuria), white blood cells (WBCs), and leukocyte esterase (an enzyme present in WBCs indicating pyuria). These findings can be confirmed by microscopic urinalysis.[11] Following confirmation of bacteriuria and pyuria, a urine culture may be obtained. A urine culture is indicated in complicated or nosocomial UTIs, persistent bacteria, or frequently recurring UTIs (more than two to three episodes per year). Urine also may be cultured when the infection is unresponsive to empiric therapy or the diagnosis is questionable.

A voided midstream technique yielding a clean-catch urine sample is preferred for obtaining a urine culture in most circumstances. For women, this is done by spreading the labia and wiping the periurethral area from front to back using a moistened, clean gauze sponge (no antiseptic is used as it could contaminate the specimen and cause false positives), keeping the labia spread and collecting the specimen 1 to 2 seconds after voiding starts. For men, the glans penis is wiped around the urethra. The specimen is collected 1 to 2 seconds after voiding begins.

Urine should be refrigerated immediately on collection and should be cultured within 24 hours of refrigeration. However, a specimen obtained by catheterization or suprapubic needle aspiration provides more accurate results and may be necessary when an adequate clean-catch specimen cannot be readily obtained.

A urine culture is accompanied by *sensitivity testing* to determine the bacteria's susceptibility to a variety of antibiotic drugs. The results of this test allow the health care provider to select an antibiotic known to be capable of destroying the bacterial strain producing a UTI in a specific patient.

Imaging studies of the urinary tract are indicated in selected cases. For example, an intravenous pyelogram (IVP) or abdominal computed tomography (CT) scan may be obtained when obstruction of the urinary system is suspected of causing a UTI. In patients with recurrent UTIs, renal ultrasound is the preferred urinary tract imaging technique because it is noninvasive, easy to perform, and relatively inexpensive.

Studies have shown that patients with symptoms can effectively diagnose their own UTIs and self-initiate treatments with the same success rate as physicians.[2,3]

Collaborative Care and Drug Therapy

Once a UTI has been diagnosed, appropriate antimicrobial therapy is initiated. An antibiotic may be selected based on the health care provider's best judgment (empiric therapy) or the results of sensitivity testing. The collaborative care and drug therapy of cystitis are summarized in Table 46-4. Uncomplicated cystitis can be treated by a short-term course of antibiotics, typically for 1 to 3 days. In contrast, complicated UTIs require longer term treatment, lasting 7 to 14 days or even longer.[2,5] Because many residents of long-term care facilities (approximately 30% to 50%), especially females, have chronic asymptomatic bacteriuria, the research-based literature suggests treating only symptomatic UTIs. Therefore continued bacteriuria without clinical symptoms does not warrant repeat or continued antibiotic therapy.[7]

Trimethoprim/sulfamethoxazole (TMP/SMX) or nitrofurantoin (Macrodantin) is often used to empirically treat uncomplicated or initial UTIs. TMP/SMX has the advantages of being relatively inexpensive and being taken twice daily. The disadvantage is that *E. coli* resistance to TMP/SMX is an increasing problem across the United States. Nitrofurantoin is normally given 3 to 4 times daily, but a long-acting preparation (Macrobid) is available that is taken twice daily. However, long-term use of nitrofurantoin can result in pulmonary fibrosis and neuropathies.[3] Ampicillin and amoxicillin are not frequently selected when empirically treating a noncomplicated UTI because they must be administered 3 to 4 times daily. In addition to these agents, the fluoroquinolones (including ciprofloxacin [Cipro], levofloxacin [Levaquin], norfloxacin [Noroxin], ofloxacin [Floxin], and gatifloxacin [Tequin]) may be used to treat complicated UTIs. In patients with UTIs secondary to fungi, amphotericin or fluconazole are preferred therapy.

TABLE 46-4	COLLABORATIVE CARE Urinary Tract Infection

Diagnostic
History and physical examination
Urinalysis—obtain a midstream voided "clean-catch" urine specimen
Urine for culture and sensitivity (if indicated)
Imaging studies of urinary tract (e.g., IVP, cystoscopy) (if indicated)

Collaborative Therapy
Uncomplicated UTI
Antibiotic: trimethoprim-sulfamethoxazole (TMP-SMX) (Bactrim, Septra), or trimethoprim alone in patients with sulfa allergy; nitrofurantoin (Macrodantin, Macrobid)
Adequate fluid intake
Urinary analgesic: phenazopyridine (Pyridium) or combination agent (e.g., Urised)
Counseling about risk of recurrence and reduction of risk factors

Recurrent, Uncomplicated UTI
Repeat urinalysis and consider urine culture and sensitivity testing
Antibiotic: 3- to 5-day treatment regimen of TMP-SMX, nitrofurantoin
Sensitivity-guided antibiotic (ampicillin, amoxicillin, first-generation cephalosporin, fluoroquinolone)
Consider postcoital antibiotic prophylaxis (TMP-SMX, nitrofurantoin, cephalexin)
Advise on pre- and postcoital voiding
Consideration of 3- to 6-month trial of (suppressive) prophylactic antibiotics
Adequate fluid intake
Cranberry or lingonberry juice (200-750 ml or equivalent tablets daily)
Urinary analgesic such as phenazopyridine (Pyridium) or combination agent (e.g., Urised)
Counseling about risk of recurrence and reduction of risk factors
Imaging study of urinary tract in selected cases

IVP, Intravenous pyelogram; *UTI,* urinary tract infection.

Drug Alert - *Nitrofurantoin (Furadantin, Macrodantin)*
• *Avoid sunlight; use sunscreen, wear protective clothing.*
• *Notify health care provider if fever, chills, cough, chest pain, dyspnea, rash, or numbness or tingling of fingers or toes develops.*

A number of over-the-counter (OTC) or prescription drugs may be used in combination with antibiotic agents to relieve the discomfort associated with a UTI. Phenazopyridine (Pyridium) is an OTC drug that provides a soothing effect on the urinary tract mucosa. It also stains the urine a reddish orange that may be mistaken for blood in the urine, and it may permanently stain underclothing. Although this drug is typically effective in relieving the transient acute discomfort associated with a UTI, patients should be advised to avoid long-term use of phenazopyridine because it can produce hemolytic anemia. Combination agents such as Urised (methenamine, phenyl salicylate, methylene blue, benzoic acid, atropine, and hyoscyamine) may also be used to relieve the symptoms associated with a UTI. The patient taking a combination agent such as Urised should be advised that preparations containing methylene blue are expected to tint the urine blue or green.

Prophylactic or *suppressive antibiotics* are sometimes administered to patients who experience repeated UTIs. A low dose of TMP/SMX, nitrofurantoin, or another antibiotic may be administered on a daily basis in an attempt to prevent recurring UTIs, or a single dose may be taken before an event likely to provoke a UTI, such as before having sexual intercourse. Although suppressive therapy is often effective on a short-term basis, this strategy is

---

EVIDENCE-BASED PRACTICE

Are Prophylactic Antibiotics Effective for Recurrent Urinary Tract Infection?

Clinical Question
In women (P), is long-term prophylactic antibiotic use (I) more effective than placebo (C) in preventing recurrent urinary tract infections (O)?

Best Available Evidence
• Systematic review of randomized controlled trials (RCTs)

Critical Appraisal and Synthesis of Evidence
• 10 RCTs (*n* = 430 women) comparing antibiotic use for 6 to 12 months against a placebo for recurrent urinary tract infections (UTI).
• Recurrence is defined as three or more UTI episodes during a 12-month period.
• Antibiotics reduced the number of UTI recurrences in pre- and postmenopausal women with recurrent UTI.
• Antibiotic group had higher incidence of side effects, including vaginal itching, skin rash, and nausea.

Conclusions
Prophylactic antibiotic administration in women who experience recurrent UTIs reduces recurrence.

Implications for Nursing Practice
• Patient treatment preference should be considered when weighing the discomfort of recurrent UTIs and the adverse effects of prophylactic antibiotics.
• UTI prophylaxis for longer than 12 months has not been studied.

Reference for Evidence
Albert X, Huertas I, Pereiró I, et al: Antibiotics for preventing recurrent urinary tract infection in non-pregnant women, *Cochrane Database Syst Rev* 3, 2004.

PICO: P, Patient population of interest; *I,* intervention or area of interest; *C,* comparison of interest or comparison group; *O,* outcome(s) of interest (see p. 6).

limited because of the risk of antibiotic resistance, which ultimately leads to breakthrough infections with increasingly virulent pathogens.[1,3]

NURSING MANAGEMENT
URINARY TRACT INFECTION

■ Nursing Assessment

Subjective and objective data that should be obtained from a patient with a UTI are presented in Table 46-5.

■ Nursing Diagnoses

Nursing diagnoses for the patient with a UTI may include, but are not limited to, those presented in NCP 46-1.

■ Planning

The overall goals are that the patient with a UTI will have (1) relief from bothersome LUTS, (2) prevention of upper urinary tract involvement, and (3) prevention of recurrence.

■ Nursing Implementation

Health Promotion. Health promotion measures include recognizing individuals who are at risk for a UTI. Debilitated persons, older adults, patients with underlying diseases (e.g., cancer, human immunodeficiency virus [HIV], or diabetes mellitus) that compromise host immune responses, and patients treated with immuno-

TABLE 46-5	*NURSING ASSESSMENT* **Urinary Tract Infection**

Subjective Data
Important Health Information
Past health history: Previous urinary tract infections; urinary calculi, stasis, reflux, strictures, or retention; neurogenic bladder; pregnancy; benign prostatic hyperplasia; sexually transmitted disease; bladder cancer
Medications: Use of antibiotics, anticholinergics, antispasmodics
Surgery or other treatments: Recent urologic instrumentation (catheterization, cystoscopy, surgery)

Functional Health Patterns
Health perception–health management: Urinary hygiene practices; lassitude, malaise
Nutritional-metabolic: Nausea, vomiting, and anorexia; chills
Elimination: Urinary frequency, urgency, hesitancy; dysuria, nocturia
Cognitive-perceptual: Suprapubic or low back pain, costovertebral tenderness; bladder spasms, dysuria, burning on urination
Sexuality-reproductive: Multiple sex partners (women), use of spermicidal agents or contraceptive diaphragm (women)

Objective Data
General
Fever, chills, overall clinical deterioration can be seen in elderly

Urinary
Hematuria; cloudy, foul-smelling urine; tender, enlarged kidney

Possible Findings
Leukocytosis; urinalysis positive for bacteria, pyuria, RBCs, and WBCs; positive urine culture; IVP, CT scan, ultrasound, voiding cystourethrogram, and cystoscopy demonstrating abnormalities of urinary tract

CT, Computed tomography; *IVP,* intravenous pyelogram; *RBCs,* red blood cells; *WBCs,* white blood cells.

suppressive drugs or corticosteroids are at high risk for UTIs. Especially for these individuals, health promotion activities can help decrease the frequency of infections and promote early detection of infection. Health promotion activities include teaching preventive measures such as (1) emptying the bladder regularly and completely, (2) evacuating the bowel regularly, (3) wiping the perineal area from front to back after urination and defecation, and (4) drinking an adequate amount of liquid each day. The recommended daily liquid intake for the ambulatory adult is approximately 15 ml per pound of body weight per day. Thus a 150-pound person would require 2250 ml each day. Because the person will obtain approximately 20% of this fluid from food, this leaves 1800 ml obtained by drinking, or just over seven 8-ounce glasses of fluid. Daily intake of cranberry or lingonberry juice or cranberry essence tablets may reduce the risk of UTIs.[12] It is thought that enzymes found in cranberries inhibit attachment of urinary pathogens (especially *E. coli*) to the bladder epithelium. Suppressive antibiotics are not generally recommended to prevent UTIs, but it is important to teach the patient to seek early treatment once symptoms occur.

The nurse can play a major role in the prevention of nosocomial infections. Avoidance of unnecessary catheterization and early removal of indwelling catheters are the most effective means for reducing nosocomial UTIs. All patients undergoing instrumentation of the urinary tract are at risk for developing a nosocomial UTI. Aseptic technique must always be followed during these procedures. Washing hands before and after contact with each patient

and wearing gloves for care involving the urinary system are especially important. When a catheter has been inserted, special measures must be employed as explained in the section on urethral catheterization later in this chapter.

Routine and thorough perineal hygiene is important for all hospitalized patients, especially when a bedpan is used, following a bowel movement, and/or if fecal incontinence is present. Incontinent episodes should be avoided by answering the call light quickly or offering the bedpan or urinal at frequent intervals to the bedridden patient.

Acute Intervention. Acute intervention for a patient with a UTI includes ensuring adequate fluid intake if it is not contraindicated. It is sometimes difficult to get the patient to maintain an adequate fluid intake because the person may think it will worsen the discomfort and frequency associated with a UTI. The patient needs to be told that fluids will increase frequency of urination at first but will also dilute the urine, making the bladder less irritable. Fluids will help flush out bacteria before they have a chance to colonize in the bladder. Caffeine, alcohol, citrus juices, chocolate, and highly spiced foods or beverages should be avoided because they are potential bladder irritants.

Application of local heat to the suprapubic area or lower back may relieve the discomfort associated with a UTI. The patient can be advised to apply a heating pad (turned to its lowest setting) against the back or suprapubic area. A warm shower or sitting in a tub of warm water filled above the waist can also be effective in providing temporary relief.

The patient should be instructed about the prescribed drug therapy, including side effects. The nurse should emphasize the importance of taking the full course of antibiotics. Often patients stop antibiotic therapy once symptoms disappear. This practice can lead to inadequate treatment and recurrence of infection or to bacterial resistance to antibiotics. Sometimes a second drug or a reduced dose of drug is ordered after the initial course to suppress bacterial growth in patients susceptible to recurrent UTI. The patient should be instructed to watch for any changes in the color or consistency of the urine and a decrease in or cessation of symptoms as a sign of the effectiveness of therapy. The patient should be counseled that (1) persistence of bothersome LUTS beyond the antibiotic treatment course, (2) the onset of flank pain, or (3) fever should be reported promptly to a health care provider.

Ambulatory and Home Care. Home care for the patient with a UTI should emphasize the patient's compliance with the drug regimen. The nurse's responsibility is to teach the patient about the need for ongoing care (Table 46-6). This includes taking antimicrobial drugs as ordered, maintaining adequate daily fluid intake, regular voiding (approximately every 3 to 4 hours), urinating before and after intercourse, and temporarily discontinuing the use of a diaphragm (if used).

The patient must understand the need for follow-up care if symptoms do not resolve, worsen, or return once treatment is completed. Recurrent symptoms because of bacterial persistence or inadequate treatment typically occur within 1 to 2 weeks after completion of therapy. If the patient has been compliant with treatment, a relapse indicates the need for further evaluation.

■ *Evaluation*

The expected outcomes for the patient with a UTI are presented in NCP 46-1.

NURSING CARE PLAN 46-1

Patient with a Urinary Tract Infection

NURSING DIAGNOSIS **Impaired urinary elimination** *related to* effects of urinary tract infection (UTI) *as evidenced by* pain and burning on urination; flank, suprapubic, and/or lower back pain; urgency; frequency; nocturia; or hematuria

PATIENT GOALS 1. Experiences normal urinary elimination patterns
2. Reports relief of bothersome urinary tract symptoms

OUTCOMES (NOC)

Urinary Elimination

- Pain with urination _____
- Burning with urination _____
- Urinary frequency _____
- Urgency with urination _____
- Nocturia _____
- Visible blood in urine _____

Measurement Scale

1 = Severe
2 = Substantial
3 = Moderate
4 = Mild
5 = None

INTERVENTIONS (NIC) and RATIONALES

Urinary Elimination Management

- Monitor urinary elimination, including frequency, consistency, odor, volume, and color, *to evaluate elimination status.*
- Obtain midstream voided specimen for culture and sensitivity (as appropriate) *to determine pathogen causing UTI or to monitor effectiveness of treatment.*
- Teach patient to drink eight ounces of liquid with meals, between meals, and in early evening *to prevent dehydration, relieve bladder irritability, and decrease bacterial colonization.*

Pain Management

- Perform a comprehensive assessment of pain to include location, characteristics, onset/duration, frequency, quality, intensity or severity, and precipitating factors *to establish history and baseline pain level.*
- Provide the patient optimal pain relief with prescribed analgesics (such as phenazopyridine [Pyridium]) or combination agents (e.g., Urised) *to promote comfort.*
- Teach the use of nonpharmacologic techniques (e.g., heating pad to suprapubic area or lower back, warm showers) along with other relief measures *to supplement pain medication and increase pain relief.*

NURSING DIAGNOSIS **Ineffective therapeutic regimen management** *related to* lack of knowledge regarding treatment regimen and prevention of recurrent infections *as evidenced by* verbalization of desire to manage treatment of illness and prevent recurrence

PATIENT GOALS 1. Verbalizes knowledge of treatment regimen
2. Expresses intent to carry out treatment regimen

OUTCOMES (NOC)

Knowledge: Treatment Regimen

- Description of specific disease process _____
- Description of rationale for treatment regimen _____
- Description of self-care responsibilities for ongoing treatment _____
- Description of expected effects of treatment _____
- Description of prescribed medications _____

Measurement Scale

1 = None
2 = Limited
3 = Moderate
4 = Substantial
5 = Extensive

INTERVENTIONS (NIC) and RATIONALES

Teaching: Disease Process

- Appraise patient's current level of knowledge related to specific disease process *to plan individualized teaching.*
- Explain pathophysiology of the disease and how it relates to anatomy and physiology.
- Describe rationale behind management/therapy/treatment recommendations *to promote compliance with treatment.*
- Describe possible chronic complications *to emphasize the need for completion of treatment.*

Teaching: Prescribed Medication

- Instruct patient on the purpose and action of each medication.
- Instruct patient on possible adverse effects of each medication *so patient can identify problems.*
- Instruct patient on appropriate actions to take if side effects occur *to prevent serious problems.*

COLLABORATIVE PROBLEM

NURSING GOALS

Potential Complications

- Anticipate potential for urosepsis in patients at risk.
- Report deviations from acceptable parameters.
- Carry out appropriate medical and nursing interventions.

INTERVENTIONS (NIC) and RATIONALES

Urosepsis (bacteriuria and bacteremia) *related to* systemic extension of UTI

- Monitor vital signs and for changes in mental status in patients at risk (immunocompromised, elderly, those with frequent urinary system instrumentation or anatomic abnormalities) *to detect inadequate tissue perfusion.*
- Report abnormalities such as hyper- or hypothermia; decreasing blood pressure; rapid pulse and respirations; and warm, flushed skin *as indicators of septic shock resulting from urosepsis.*
- Monitor platelet levels and coagulation function tests *because alterations indicate bleeding tendencies.*

TABLE 46-6	*PATIENT AND FAMILY TEACHING GUIDE* **Urinary Tract Infection**

The following are important to teach to the patient with a UTI to prevent recurrence:

1. Explain importance of taking all antibiotics as prescribed. Symptoms may improve after 1 to 2 days of therapy, but organisms may still be present.
2. Instruct the patient on appropriate hygiene, including the following:
   - Careful cleansing of perineal region by separating the labia when cleansing
   - Wiping from front to back after urinating
   - Cleansing with warm soapy water after each bowel movement
3. Explain the importance of emptying the bladder before and after sexual intercourse.
4. Instruct the patient to urinate regularly, approximately every 3 to 4 hours during the day.
5. Instruct the patient about the need to maintain adequate fluid intake.
6. Instruct the patient to avoid vaginal douches and/or harsh soaps, bubble baths, powders, and sprays in the perineal area.
7. Advise the patient to report symptoms or signs of recurrent UTI (e.g., fever, cloudy urine, pain on urination, urgency, frequency).
8. Suggest possible use of unsweetened cranberry juice 8 oz three times a day or extract tablets 300 to 400 mg/day for UTI prevention.

UTI, Urinary tract infection.

ACUTE PYELONEPHRITIS

Etiology and Pathophysiology

Pyelonephritis is an inflammation of the renal parenchyma (Fig. 46-2) and collecting system (including the renal pelvis). The most common cause is bacterial infection, but fungi, protozoa, or viruses sometimes infect the kidney.

Urosepsis is a systemic infection arising from a urologic source. Its prompt diagnosis and effective treatment are critical because it can lead to septic shock and death in 15% of cases unless promptly eradicated. Septic shock is the outcome of unresolved bacteremia involving a gram-negative organism.[13] (Septic shock is discussed in Chapter 67.)

Pyelonephritis usually begins with colonization and infection of the lower urinary tract via the ascending urethral route. Bacteria normally found in the intestinal tract, such as *E. coli, Proteus, Klebsiella,* or *Enterobacter* species, frequently cause pyelonephritis. A preexisting factor is often present, such as *vesicoureteral reflux* (retrograde or backward movement of urine from lower to upper urinary tract) or dysfunction of lower urinary tract function such as obstruction from benign prostatic hyperplasia (BPH), a stricture, or urinary stone. In residents of long-term care facilities, urinary tract catheterization and the use of indwelling catheters is a common cause of pyelonephritis and urosepsis.

Acute pyelonephritis commonly starts in the renal medulla and spreads to the adjacent cortex. One of the most important risk factors for acute pyelonephritis is pregnancy-induced physiologic changes in the urinary system.[2] Recurring episodes of pyelonephritis, especially in the presence of obstructive abnormalities, can lead to a scarred, poorly functioning kidney and a condition called *chronic pyelonephritis.*

Clinical Manifestations and Diagnostic Studies

The clinical manifestations of acute pyelonephritis vary from mild fatigue to the sudden onset of chills, fever, vomiting, malaise, flank pain, and the LUTS characteristic of cystitis, including dysuria,

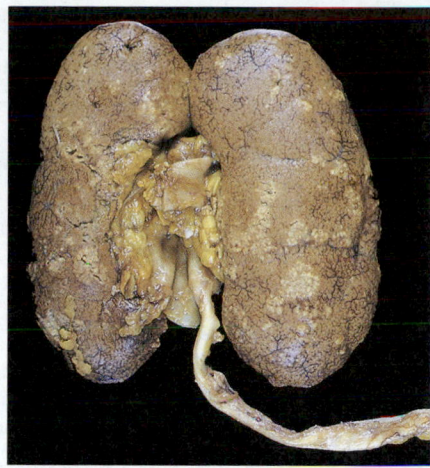

FIG. 46-2 Acute pyelonephritis. Cortical surface shows grayish white areas of inflammation and abscess formation.

urinary urgency, and frequency. *Costovertebral tenderness* (costovertebral angle [CVA] pain) is typically present on the affected side. The clinical manifestations usually subside within a few days, even without specific therapy, but bacteriuria and pyuria usually persist.

Urinalysis shows pyuria, bacteriuria, and varying degrees of hematuria. WBC casts may be found in the urine, indicating involvement of the renal parenchyma. A complete blood count will show leukocytosis and a shift to the left with an increase in immature neutrophils (bands). Urine cultures must be obtained when pyelonephritis is suspected. In patients with more severe illness who are hospitalized, blood cultures are also obtained.

Imaging studies, such as an IVP or CT scan, requiring intravenous (IV) injection of contrast materials are usually not obtained in the early stages of pyelonephritis to prevent the possible spread of infection. Alternatively, ultrasonography of the urinary system may be obtained to identify anatomic abnormalities, hydronephrosis, renal abscesses, or the presence of an obstructing stone. Imaging studies are also used to assess for complications of pyelonephritis such as impaired renal function, scarring, chronic pyelonephritis, or abscesses.

Urosepsis is characterized by bacteriuria and bacteremia (presence of bacteria in blood). If bacteremia is a possibility, close observation and vital sign monitoring are essential. Prompt recognition and treatment of septic shock may prevent irreversible damage or death.

Collaborative Care and Drug Therapy

The diagnostic tests and collaborative therapy of acute pyelonephritis are summarized in Table 46-7. Patients with severe infections or complicating factors such as nausea and vomiting with dehydration require hospital admission.

The patient with mild symptoms may be treated as an outpatient with antibiotics for 14 to 21 days (see Table 46-7). Parenteral antibiotics are often given initially in the hospital to rapidly establish high serum and urinary drug levels. When initial treatment resolves acute symptoms and the patient is able to tolerate oral fluids and drugs, the person may be discharged on a regimen of oral antibiotics for an additional 14 to 21 days. Symptoms and signs typically improve or resolve within 48 to 72 hours after starting therapy.[14]

Relapses may be treated with a 6-week course of antibiotics. Reinfections may be treated as individual episodes of disease or

TABLE 46-7	COLLABORATIVE CARE Acute Pyelonephritis

Diagnostic
History and physical examination
Urinalysis
Urine for culture and sensitivity
Ultrasound (initially) to detect hydronephrosis, IVP, VCUG, radionuclide imaging, CT scan
CBC count with WBC differential
Blood culture (if bacteremia is suspected)
Palpation for flank (costovertebral angle [CVA]) pain

Collaborative Therapy
Mild Symptoms (uncomplicated infection)
Outpatient management or short hospitalization for IV antibiotics
- Empirically selected broad-spectrum antibiotics (ampicillin, vancomycin) combined with an aminoglycoside (e.g., tobramycin [Nebcin], gentamicin [Garamycin])
- Switch to sensitivity-guided therapy (trimethoprim-sulfamethoxazole [Bactrim, Septra]) when results of urine and blood culture are available
Fluoroquinolones (ciprofloxacin [Cipro], ofloxacin [Floxin], norfloxacin [Noroxin], gatifloxacin [Tequin])
Adequate fluid intake
Nonsteroidal antiinflammatory drugs or antipyretic drugs
Urinary analgesics (e.g., phenazopyridine [Pyridium])
Follow-up urine culture and imaging studies

Severe Symptoms
Hospitalization
Parenteral antibiotics
- Empirically selected broad-spectrum antibiotics (e.g., ampicillin, vancomycin) combined with an aminoglycoside (e.g., tobramycin, gentamicin)
- Switch to sensitivity-guided antibiotic therapy when results of urine and blood culture are available
Oral antibiotics when patient tolerates oral intake
Adequate fluid intake (parenteral initially; switch to oral fluids as nausea, vomiting, and dehydration subside)
Nonsteroidal antiinflammatory or antipyretic drugs to reverse fever and relieve discomfort
Urinary analgesics (e.g., to relieve lower urinary tract symptoms)
Follow-up urine culture and imaging studies

CBC, Complete blood count; *CT,* computed tomography; *IVP,* intravenous pyelogram; *VCUG,* voiding cystourethrogram; *WBC,* white blood cell.

managed with long-term antibiotic therapy. Antibiotic prophylaxis may also be used for recurrent infections. The effectiveness of therapy is evaluated in accordance with the presence or absence of bacterial growth on urine culture.

NURSING MANAGEMENT
ACUTE PYELONEPHRITIS

■ Nursing Assessment

Subjective and objective data that should be obtained from a patient with pyelonephritis are presented in Table 46-5.

■ Nursing Diagnoses

Nursing diagnoses for the patient with pyelonephritis include, but are not limited to, those for the patient with UTI (see NCP 46-1).

■ Planning

The overall goals are that the patient with pyelonephritis will have (1) normal renal function, (2) normal body temperature, (3) no complications, (4) relief of pain, and (5) no recurrence of symptoms.

■ Nursing Implementation

Health Promotion. Health promotion and maintenance measures are similar to those for cystitis (see pp. 1158 to 1159). In addition, it is important that the patient receive early treatment for cystitis to prevent ascending infections. Because the patient with structural abnormalities of the urinary tract is at high risk for infection, the need for regular medical care should be stressed to these patients.

Acute Intervention and Home Care. Nursing interventions vary depending on the severity of symptoms. These interventions include teaching the patient about the disease process with emphasis on (1) the need to continue drugs as prescribed, (2) the need for a follow-up urine culture to ensure proper management, and (3) identification of risk for recurrence or relapse (see Table 46-7 and NCP 46-1). In addition to antibiotic therapy, the patient should be encouraged to drink at least eight glasses of fluid every day, even after the infection has been treated. Rest is often indicated to increase patient comfort. The patient with frequent relapses or reinfections may be treated with long-term, low-dose antibiotics. Understanding the rationale for therapy is important to enhance patient compliance.

■ Evaluation

The expected outcomes for the patient with pyelonephritis are presented in NCP 46-1.

CHRONIC PYELONEPHRITIS

Chronic pyelonephritis is a term used to describe a kidney that has become small, atrophic, shrunken and has lost function owing to scarring or fibrosis.[14] It usually occurs as the outcome of recurring infections involving the upper urinary tract. However, it may also occur in the absence of an existing infection, recent infection, or history of UTIs. Alternative terms used to describe this condition include *interstitial nephritis,* chronic atrophic pyelonephritis, or reflux nephropathy (when scarring occurs in the presence of vesicoureteral reflux).

Chronic pyelonephritis is diagnosed by radiologic imaging and histologic testing rather than clinical features. Imaging studies reveal a small, contracted kidney with a thinned parenchyma. The collecting system may be small or hydronephrotic. Pathologic analysis reveals loss of functioning nephrons, infiltration of the parenchyma with inflammatory cells, and fibrosis.

The level of renal function in chronic pyelonephritis varies depending on whether one or both kidneys are affected, the magnitude of scarring, and the presence of coexisting infection. Chronic pyelonephritis often progresses to end-stage renal disease when both kidneys are involved, even if the underlying infection is successfully eradicated. (Nursing and collaborative management of the patient with chronic kidney disease is discussed in Chapter 47.)

URETHRITIS

Urethritis is an inflammation of the urethra. Causes of urethritis include a bacterial or viral infection, *Trichomonas* and monilial infection (especially in women), chlamydia, and gonorrhea (especially in men). Among men, the causes of urethritis are usually sexually transmitted. In men, purulent discharge usually indicates a gonococcal urethritis, whereas a clear discharge typically signifies a nongonococcal urethritis.[15] (Sexually transmitted diseases are discussed in Chapter 53.) Urethritis also produces bothersome LUTS, including dysuria, urgency, and frequent urination, similar to those seen with cystitis.

In women, urethritis is difficult to diagnose. It frequently produces bothersome symptoms as described previously, but urethral discharge may not be present. Cultures on split urine collections (taken at beginning of urine flow and then midstream) or any urethral discharge may confirm a diagnosis of urethral infection.

Treatment is based on identifying and treating the cause and providing symptomatic relief. Drugs used for bacterial infections include sulfamethoxazole with trimethoprim, and nitrofurantoin. Metronidazole (Flagyl) and clotrimazole (Mycelex) may be used for treating *Trichomonas*. Drugs such as nystatin (Mycostatin) or fluconazole (Diflucan) may be prescribed for monilial infections. In chlamydial infections, doxycycline (Vibramycin) may be used. Women with negative urine cultures and no pyuria do not usually respond to antibiotics. Warm sitz baths may temporarily relieve bothersome symptoms. The patient should be instructed to avoid the use of vaginal deodorant sprays, properly cleanse the perineal area after bowel movements and urination, and avoid sexual intercourse until symptoms subside. Patients with sexually transmitted urethritis should be instructed to refer their sex partners for evaluation and testing if they had sexual contact in the 60 days preceding onset of the patient's symptoms or diagnosis.

URETHRAL DIVERTICULA

Urethral diverticula are the result of obstruction and subsequent rupture of the periurethral glands into the urethral lumen with epithelialization (regrowth of tissue) over the opening of the resulting periurethral cavity.[16] Urethral diverticula are seen in women with an incidence of 1% to 5% and are much more common in females than in males. The rare cases reported in males generally have been associated with lower urinary tract congenital anomalies or surgical trauma. The periurethral glands are found along the entire length of the urethra, with the majority draining into the distal third of the urethra. Skene's glands are the largest and most distal of these glands. Urethral diverticula occur mostly in the area of these glands. In many cases, a person may have more than one diverticulum. Causes include urethral trauma from childbearing, urethral instrumentation, or dilation.[17] Infection with gonococcal organisms and normal vaginal flora have been suggested as the causative agents. Urethral diverticula present some of the more challenging diagnostic and reconstructive cases in urology.

Symptoms include dysuria, postvoid dribbling, frequent urination (more often than every 2 hours), urgency, suprapubic discomfort or pressure, dyspareunia, and a feeling of incomplete bladder emptying. Urinary incontinence is frequently seen. However, one of four women may have no symptoms.

The urine may contain gross hematuria or sediment, giving it a cloudy appearance.[17] An anterior vaginal wall mass may be noted on physical examination, which, upon palpation, may be quite tender and express purulent discharge through the urethra. Radiographic studies such as voiding cystourethrography (VCUG) should be used to confirm the diagnosis. Additional studies include ultrasound and magnetic resonance imaging (MRI) to determine the size of the diverticulum in relation to the urethral lumen.

Surgical options include transurethral incision of the diverticular neck, marsupialization (creation of a permanent opening) of the diverticular sac into the vagina (often referred to as a Spence procedure), and surgical excision. Surgical excision of a urethral diverticulum should be performed with caution as the diverticular sac may be adherent to the adjacent urethral lumen, and careless excision of the sac may result in a large urethral defect requiring construction of a neourethra (new urethra). Other important considerations during surgery include identification and closure of the

diverticular neck, complete removal of the mucosal lining of the diverticular sac to prevent recurrence, and a multiple layered closure to prevent postoperative urethrovaginal fistula formation. A complication of the surgery may be stress urinary incontinence.

INTERSTITIAL CYSTITIS/PAINFUL BLADDER SYNDROME

Interstitial cystitis (IC) is a chronic, painful inflammatory disease of the bladder characterized by symptoms of urgency/frequency and pain in the bladder and/or pelvis. *Painful bladder syndrome* (PBS) is suprapubic pain related to bladder filling, accompanied by other symptoms such as frequency, in the absence of UTI or other obvious pathology.[18]

IC/PBS affect as many as 700,000 Americans. The average age at onset is 40 years. The ratio of women to men with IC/PBS is 10:1 to 12:1. Although the etiology of IC/PBS remains unknown, a contributing factor is chronic inflammation with mast cell invasion of the bladder wall (possibly provoked by an infection or an autoimmune disorder). Other etiologic factors include defects of the glycosaminoglycan layer that protects the bladder mucosa from the irritating effects of urine exposure, abnormal constituents in the urine, dysfunction of the sympathetic innervation of the lower urinary tract, and reflex sympathetic dystrophy.[19]

The two primary clinical manifestations that characterize IC/PBS are pain and bothersome LUTS (e.g., frequency, urgency). The pain associated with IC/PBS is usually located in the suprapubic area but may involve the vagina, the labia, or the entire perineal region. It varies from moderate to severe in intensity and is exacerbated by bladder filling, postponing urination, physical exertion, pressure against the suprapubic area, dietary intake of certain foods, or emotional distress. The pain is transiently relieved by urination. Bothersome LUTS are very similar to a UTI, and the condition is often misdiagnosed as a recurring or chronic UTI or, in men, chronic prostatitis. The pain and bothersome voiding symptoms produced by IC/PBS remit and exacerbate over time. Women will report that pain occurs premenstrually and is aggravated by sexual intercourse and/or emotional stress. Some patients experience an onset of symptoms that disappears altogether after a period of weeks to months, whereas others have persistent symptoms over a period of months to years.

IC/PBS is a diagnosis of exclusion. The condition is suspected whenever a patient experiences symptoms of a UTI despite the absence of bacteriuria, pyuria, or a positive urine culture. A careful history and physical examination are necessary to exclude a variety of disorders that may produce somewhat similar symptoms, such as UTI or endometriosis. This evaluation must include at least one negative urine culture during a period of active symptoms. In IC, cystoscopic examination may reveal a small bladder capacity and superficial ulcerations with bladder filling called *glomerulations,* but these findings are frequently absent in PBS. Criteria for diagnosing IC/PBS are presented in Table 46-8.

Collaborative Care and Drug Therapy

Because the etiology of IC/PBS is unknown, no single treatment has been identified that consistently reverses or relieves symptoms. Various therapies have been effective in alleviating or relieving bothersome symptoms in most patients.

Dietary and lifestyle alterations are used to relieve pain and diminish voiding frequency and nocturia.[20] Dietary alterations include elimination of foods and beverages likely to exacerbate the symptoms. A diet low in acidic foods and avoiding beverages such as coffee, tea, and carbonated and alcoholic drinks can be helpful in

TABLE 46-8 | **Criteria for the Diagnosis of Interstitial Cystitis/Painful Bladder Syndrome**

Inclusion Criteria
- Pain during bladder filling that is relieved by voiding
- Bothersome urinary urgency and frequency
- Small bladder capacity on urodynamic testing
- Cystoscopic evidence of ulcerations or glomerulations (*not* specific to interstitial cystitis)

Exclusion Criteria
- Bladder capacity >350 ml on urodynamic testing
- Overactive bladder contractions on urodynamic testing
- Daytime voiding frequency <8 times/day
- Active genital herpes
- History of chemotherapy, particularly if treated with cyclophosphamide (Cytoxan)
- Tubercular cystitis
- History of pelvic radiation
- Bladder tumor

reducing IC/PBS symptoms. Patients may be advised that an OTC dietary supplement called calcium glycerophosphate (Prelief) alkalinizes the urine and can provide relief from the irritating effects of certain foods.[19] This agent may be particularly helpful when dining away from home, where the patient has less control over the preparation of foods. Stress can exacerbate or cause "flare-ups" of IC/PBS symptoms, so basic relaxation techniques (e.g., sitz baths, application of heat or cold to perineum or bladder, stress reduction tapes) may be helpful. Use of lubrication or altering positions may decrease pain associated with sexual intercourse.

Two tricyclic antidepressants, amitriptyline (Elavil) and nortriptyline (Aventyl), are used to reduce the burning pain and urinary frequency. Pentosan (Elmiron) is the only oral agent approved for the treatment of patients with symptoms of IC. It is used to enhance the protective effects of the glycosaminoglycan layer of the bladder and is thought to relieve pain associated with IC/PBS by reducing the irritative effects of urine on the bladder wall.[19] These drugs are effective over time (weeks to months), but they do not provide immediate relief that may be needed when a patient experiences an acute exacerbation of symptoms. For immediate relief, a short course of opioid analgesics may be given.

Several agents may be instilled directly into the bladder through a small catheter. Dimethyl sulfoxide (DMSO) is thought to act by desensitizing pain receptors in the bladder wall. Heparin and hyaluronic acid also may be instilled into the bladder to relieve IC/PBS symptoms. Like pentosan, they are thought to enhance the protective properties of the glycosaminoglycan layer of the bladder.[19] Instillations are often administered with lidocaine, which rapidly desensitizes the bladder wall, rendering the patient better able to tolerate instillation of additional heparin or hyaluronic acid and providing transient relief from pain. Bacille Calmette-Guérin (BCG), an attenuated form of *Mycobacterium bovis,* administered intravesically is a common treatment for IC. The mechanism of action of BCG is unclear, but it may alleviate a possible autoimmune disorder provoking the chronic inflammation characteristic of the disorder.[21]

Distention of the bladder during endoscopic examination relieves IC/PBS-related pain, urgency, and voiding frequency, probably by temporarily disrupting sensory nerve endings in the bladder wall. Several surgical procedures have been used in an attempt to relieve severe, debilitating pain.[18] Surgical urinary diversion,

such as an ileal conduit, is an approach that can be used when other measures fail. Unfortunately, some patients have reported pain within the urinary diversion, possibly indicating that components of the urine may contribute to IC/PBS in certain cases.

NURSING MANAGEMENT
INTERSTITIAL CYSTITIS/PAINFUL BLADDER SYNDROME

Assessment focuses on characterization of the pain associated with IC/PBS. The patient is asked about specific dietary or lifestyle factors known to exacerbate or alleviate pain and about the intensity of the pain.[19] Objective data collection includes a bladder log or voiding diary kept over a period of at least 3 days to determine voiding frequency and patterns of nocturia. A simultaneous pain record may be useful.

Reassurance that IC/PBS is a real condition experienced by others and that it can be effectively treated may relieve the anxiety, anger, guilt, and frustration related to experiences of chronic pain and voiding dysfunction in the absence of a clear-cut diagnosis and treatment strategy. A UTI may occur during the course of IC/PBS management due to diagnostic instrumentation and frequent bladder instillations. A UTI is likely to produce an acute exacerbation of bothersome LUTS and urinary frequency, as well as dysuria (not typically associated with IC/PBS) and odorous urine, possibly with hematuria.

The patient also must be given instruction about the need to maintain good nutrition, particularly in light of the broad dietary restrictions often necessary to control IC-related pain. Specifically, the patient may be advised to take a multivitamin containing no more than the recommended dietary allowance for essential vitamins and to avoid high-potency vitamins because these formulations may irritate the bladder. The patient is also assisted to obtain information from the Interstitial Cystitis Association *(www.ica.org),* which includes recipes and menus for a well-balanced diet that is specifically designed to avoid bladder-irritating foods and beverages.

Elimination of a variety of foods and beverages from the diet that are likely to irritate the bladder typically provides modest to profound relief from symptoms. Typical bladder irritants include caffeine, alcohol, citrus products, aged cheeses, nuts, and foods containing vinegar, curries, or hot peppers, as well as foods or beverages likely to lower urinary pH. In addition, the patient should be taught to self-use Prelief. The patient is advised to avoid clothing that creates suprapubic pressure, including pants with tight belts or restrictive waistlines.[20]

Written educational materials concerning diet, coping with the need for frequent urination, and strategies for coping with the emotional burden of IC/PBS are available from the Interstitial Cystitis Association *(www.ichelp.com).* Providing such materials provides an excellent opportunity for the nurse to introduce the patient to the existence of this patient advocacy group and to the possibility of participating in local support groups when desired.

RENAL TUBERCULOSIS

Renal tuberculosis (TB) is rarely a primary lesion. It is usually secondary to TB of the lung. In a small percentage of patients with pulmonary TB, the tubercle bacilli reach the kidneys via the bloodstream. Onset occurs 5 to 8 years after the primary infection. The patient is often asymptomatic when the kidney is initially infiltrated with bacilli. Sometimes the patient complains of fatigue and develops a low-grade fever. As the lesions ulcerate, infection descends to the bladder and other genitourinary organs, and the patient experiences cystitis, frequent urination, burning on voiding, and epididymitis (in men). Symptoms of a UTI are the first sign in the majority of patients with renal TB. Renal lesions may calcify as they heal. Infrequently, renal colic, lumbar and iliac pain, and hematuria may be present. A diagnosis is based on localization of tubercle bacilli in the urine and on IVP findings.[22]

Long-term complications of renal TB depend on the duration of the disease before treatment. Scarring of the renal parenchyma and the development of ureteral strictures occur. The earlier treatment is initiated, the less likely renal failure will develop. Reduced bladder volume may be irreversible in advanced disease. The patient may require long-term urologic follow-up. (Nursing and collaborative management for the patient with TB is discussed in Chapter 28.)

Immunologic Disorders of the Kidney

GLOMERULONEPHRITIS

Immunologic processes involving the urinary tract predominantly affect the renal glomerulus. The disease process results in **glomerulonephritis** (inflammation of the glomeruli), which affects both kidneys equally and is the third leading cause of renal failure in the United States. Although the glomerulus is the primary site of inflammation, tubular, interstitial, and vascular changes also occur. Glomerulonephritis is divided into a number of classifications, which may describe (1) the extent of damage (diffuse or focal), (2) the initial cause of the disorder (systemic lupus erythematosus, systemic sclerosis [scleroderma], streptococcal infection), or (3) the extent of changes (minimal or widespread).

Etiology and Pathophysiology

Two types of antibody-induced injury can initiate glomerular damage. In the first type, the antibodies have specificity for antigens within the glomerular basement membrane (GBM). These are termed anti-GBM antibodies. Immunoglobulins and complement are deposited along the basement membrane. The mechanism that causes a person to develop antibodies against his or her GBM is not known. Production of autoantibodies (antibodies to one's own tissue) may be stimulated by a structural alteration in the GBM or by a reaction of the basement membrane with an exogenous agent (e.g., hydrocarbon, viruses).[23]

In the second type of immune process, the antibodies react with circulating nonglomerular antigens and are randomly deposited as immune complexes along the GBM. On electron microscopy of renal tissue sections, the deposits appear "lumpy-bumpy." In this immune complex process, the antigens do not come from the glomeruli but rather from either endogenous circulating native deoxyribonucleic acid (DNA) or exogenous sources (e.g., bacteria, viruses, chemicals, drugs). Bacterial products appear to be important in poststreptococcal glomerulonephritis. Viral agents have been recognized in rare cases of glomerulonephritis that developed after hepatitis B or C and rubella (measles).

All forms of immune complex disease are characterized by an accumulation of antigen, antibody, and complement in the glomeruli, which can result in tissue injury. The immune complexes activate complement (see Chapters 13 and 14). Complement activation results in the release of chemotactic factors that attract polymorphonuclear leukocytes, histamine, and other inflammatory mediators. The end result of these processes is glomerular injury.

Clinical Manifestations

Clinical manifestations of glomerulonephritis include varying degrees of hematuria (ranging from microscopic to gross) and urinary excretion of various formed elements, including red blood cells (RBCs), WBCs, and casts. Proteinuria and elevated blood urea nitrogen (BUN) and serum creatinine levels are other manifestations. In most cases, recovery from the acute illness is complete. However, if progressive involvement occurs, the result is destruction of renal tissue and marked renal insufficiency.

The patient's history provides important information related to glomerulonephritis. It is necessary to assess exposure to drugs, immunizations, microbial infections, and viral infections such as hepatitis. It is also important to evaluate the patient for more generalized conditions involving immune disorders, such as systemic lupus erythematosus and systemic sclerosis.

ACUTE POSTSTREPTOCOCCAL GLOMERULONEPHRITIS

Acute poststreptococcal glomerulonephritis (APSGN) is most common in children and young adults, but all age groups can be affected. APSGN develops 5 to 21 days after an infection of the tonsils, pharynx, or skin (e.g., streptococcal sore throat, impetigo) by nephrotoxic strains of group A β-hemolytic streptococci. The person produces antibodies to the streptococcal antigen. Although the specific mechanism is not known, tissue injury occurs as the antigen-antibody complexes are deposited in the glomeruli and complement is activated. Complement activation causes an inflammatory reaction to the injury. The response to the injury is also a decrease in the filtration of metabolic waste products from the blood and an increase in the permeability of the glomerulus to larger protein molecules.

Clinical Manifestations and Complications

The clinical manifestations of APSGN appear as a variety of signs and symptoms. Generalized body edema, hypertension, oliguria, hematuria with a smoky or rusty appearance, and proteinuria may occur. Fluid retention occurs as a result of decreased glomerular filtration. The edema appears initially in low-pressure tissues, such as around the eyes (periorbital edema), but later progresses to involve the total body as ascites or peripheral edema in the legs. Smoky urine indicates bleeding in the upper urinary tract. The degree of proteinuria varies with the severity of the glomerulonephropathy. Hypertension primarily results from increased extracellular fluid volume. The patient with APSGN may have abdominal or flank pain. At times the patient has no symptoms, with the problem found on routine urinalysis.

More than 95% of patients with APSGN recover completely or improve rapidly with conservative management. Accurate recognition and assessment is critical as chronic glomerulonephritis develops in 5% to 15% of the affected persons, and irreversible renal failure occurs in 1% of patients.

Diagnostic Studies

The diagnosis of APSGN is based on a complete history and physical examination and laboratory studies (Table 46-9) to determine the presence or history of a group A β-hemolytic streptococcus in a throat or skin lesion. An immune response to the streptococcus is

TABLE 46-9	**COLLABORATIVE CARE** **Acute Glomerulonephritis**
Diagnostic	History and physical examination Urinalysis CBC with WBC differential BUN, serum creatinine, and albumin Complement levels and ASO titer Renal biopsy (if indicated)
Collaborative Therapy	Rest Sodium and fluid restriction Diuretics Antihypertensive therapy Adjustment of dietary protein intake to level of proteinuria and uremia

ASO, Antistreptolysin-O; *BUN,* blood urea nitrogen; *CBC,* complete blood count; *WBC,* white blood cell.

often demonstrated by assessment of antistreptolysin-O (ASO) titers. The finding of decreased complement components (especially C3 and CH50) indicates an immune-mediated response. A renal biopsy may be performed to confirm the presence of the disease.

Dipstick urinalysis and urine sediment microscopy will reveal the presence of erythrocytes in significant numbers. Erythrocyte casts are highly suggestive of APSGN. Proteinuria may range from mild to severe. Screening blood tests include BUN and serum creatinine to assess the extent of renal impairment.

NURSING and COLLABORATIVE MANAGEMENT
ACUTE POSTSTREPTOCOCCAL GLOMERULONEPHRITIS

The management of APSGN focuses on symptomatic relief (see Table 46-9). Rest is recommended until the signs of glomerular inflammation (proteinuria, hematuria) and hypertension subside. Edema is treated by restricting sodium and fluid intake and by administrating diuretics. Severe hypertension is treated with antihypertensive drugs. Dietary protein intake may be restricted if there is evidence of an increase in nitrogenous wastes (e.g., elevated BUN value). The restriction varies with the degree of proteinuria. (Low-protein, low-sodium, fluid-restricted diets are discussed in Chapter 47.)

Antibiotics should be given only if the streptococcal infection is still present. Corticosteroids and cytotoxic drugs have not been shown to be of value.

One of the most important ways to prevent the development of APSGN is to encourage early diagnosis and treatment of sore throats and skin lesions. If streptococci are found in the culture, treatment with appropriate antibiotic therapy (usually penicillin) is essential. The patient must be encouraged to take the full course of antibiotics to ensure that the bacteria have been eradicated. Good personal hygiene is an important factor in preventing the spread of cutaneous streptococcal infections.

GOODPASTURE SYNDROME

Goodpasture syndrome, an example of cytotoxic (type II) autoimmune disease, is characterized by the presence of circulating antibodies against glomerular and alveolar basement membrane and is a rare autoimmune disease.[24] Although the primary target organ is the kidney, the lungs are also involved. Damage to the kidneys and lungs results when binding of the antibody causes an inflammatory reaction mediated by complement fixation and activation (see Chapters 13 and 14). The causative factors for development of autoantibody production are unknown, although type A influenza viruses, hydrocarbons, penicillamine, and unknown genetic factors may be involved.

Goodpasture syndrome is a rare disease that is seen mostly in young male smokers. The clinical manifestations include flu-like symptoms with pulmonary symptoms that include cough, mild shortness of breath, hemoptysis, crackles, rhonchi, and pulmonary insufficiency. Renal involvement causes hematuria, weakness, pallor, anemia, and renal failure. Pulmonary hemorrhage usually occurs and may precede glomerular abnormalities by weeks or months. Abnormal diagnostic findings include low hematocrit and hemoglobin levels, elevated BUN and serum creatinine levels, hematuria, and proteinuria. Circulating serum anti-GBM antibodies parallel the activity of the renal disease and are diagnostic of this syndrome.

NURSING and COLLABORATIVE MANAGEMENT
GOODPASTURE SYNDROME

Until recently, the prognosis for the patient with Goodpasture syndrome was poor, with a mean survival time of less than 4 months. Current management with corticosteroids, immunosuppressive drugs (e.g., cyclophosphamide [Cytoxan], azathioprine [Imuran]), plasmapheresis (see Chapter 14), and dialysis has reduced the mortality rate to less than 20%.[24]

Plasmapheresis removes the circulating anti-GBM antibodies, and immunosuppressive therapy inhibits further antibody production. Renal transplantation can be attempted after the circulating anti-GBM antibody titer decreases. Although recurrences may develop, the disease is not a contraindication to transplantation. In selected patients with severe pulmonary hemorrhage, bilateral nephrectomy has been helpful. The exact mechanism for improvement has not been determined.

Nursing management appropriate for a critically ill patient who is experiencing symptoms of acute renal failure and respiratory distress is instituted. Death is often secondary to hemorrhage in the lungs and respiratory failure. (Nursing interventions for a patient in acute renal failure are discussed in Chapter 47, and nursing interventions for a patient with respiratory failure are discussed in Chapter 68.) Because this syndrome is rare and primarily affects previously healthy young adults, support and understanding of the patient and family are of major importance. The patient and family need instructions concerning current therapy, drugs, and complications of the disease process.

RAPIDLY PROGRESSIVE GLOMERULONEPHRITIS

Rapidly progressive glomerulonephritis (RPGN) is glomerular disease associated with acute renal failure where there is rapid, progressive loss of renal function over days to weeks. Renal failure may occur within weeks to months in contrast to chronic glomerulonephritis, which develops insidiously and progresses over many years. The manifestations of RPGN are hypertension, edema, proteinuria, hematuria, and RBC casts.

RPGN can occur in a variety of situations: (1) as a complication of inflammatory or infectious disease (e.g., APSGN), (2) as a complication of a multisystemic disease (e.g., systemic lupus erythematosus, Goodpasture syndrome), (3) as an idiopathic disease, or (4) in association with the use of certain drugs (e.g., penicillamine).

Prompt diagnosis and treatment is directed toward correction of fluid overload, hypertension, uremia, and inflammatory injury to the kidney. Treatment includes corticosteroids, cytotoxic agents, and plasmapheresis. Dialysis therapy and transplantation are used as maintenance therapy for the patient with RPGN. Following renal transplantation, RPGN may recur.

CHRONIC GLOMERULONEPHRITIS

Chronic glomerulonephritis is a syndrome that reflects the end stage of glomerular inflammatory disease. Most types of glomerulonephritis and nephrotic syndrome can eventually lead to chronic glomerulonephritis.

The syndrome is characterized by proteinuria, hematuria, and the slow development of uremia (see Chapter 47) as a result of decreasing renal function. Chronic glomerulonephritis progresses insidiously toward renal failure over a few to as many as 30 years.

Chronic glomerulonephritis is often found coincidentally when an abnormality on a urinalysis or elevated blood pressure is detected. It is common to find that the patient has no recollection or history of acute nephritis or any renal problems. A renal biopsy may be performed to determine the exact cause and nature of the glomerulonephritis. However, ultrasound and CT scanning are generally preferred as diagnostic measures.

Treatment is supportive and symptomatic. Hypertension and UTIs should be treated vigorously. Protein and phosphate restrictions may slow the rate of progression of kidney disease. (Management of chronic kidney disease is discussed in Chapter 47.)

NEPHROTIC SYNDROME

Etiology and Clinical Manifestations

Nephrotic syndrome results when the glomerulus is excessively permeable to plasma protein, causing proteinuria that leads to low plasma albumin and tissue edema. Some of the more common causes of nephrotic syndrome are listed in Table 46-10. In adults about one third of patients with nephrotic syndrome will have a systemic disease such as diabetes or systemic lupus erythematosus. The remainder will be categorized as having idiopathic nephrotic syndrome.[25]

The characteristic manifestations include peripheral edema, massive proteinuria, hypertension, hyperlipidemia, and hypoalbuminemia. Characteristic blood chemistries include decreased serum albumin, decreased total serum protein, and elevated serum cholesterol. The increased glomerular membrane permeability found in nephrotic syndrome is responsible for the massive excretion of protein in the urine. This results in decreased serum protein and subsequent edema formation. Ascites and *anasarca* (massive generalized edema) develop if there is severe hypoalbuminemia.

The diminished plasma oncotic pressure from the decreased serum proteins stimulates hepatic lipoprotein synthesis, which results in hyperlipidemia. Initially, cholesterol and low-density lipoproteins are elevated. Later the triglyceride level is also increased. Fat bodies (fatty casts) commonly appear in the urine.

Immune responses, both humoral and cellular, are altered in nephrotic syndrome. As a result, infection is an important cause of morbidity and mortality. Calcium and skeletal abnormalities may occur, including hypocalcemia, blunted calcemic response to parathyroid hormone, hyperparathyroidism, and osteomalacia.

With nephrotic proteinuria, loss of clotting factors can result in a relative hypercoagulable state. Hypercoagulability with thromboembolism is a serious complication of nephrotic syndrome. The renal vein is the most common site for thrombus formation. Pulmonary emboli occur in about 40% of nephrotic patients with thrombosis.

TABLE 46-10	Causes of Nephrotic Syndrome

Primary Glomerular Disease
- Membranous proliferative glomerulonephritis
- Primary nephrotic syndrome
- Focal glomerulonephritis
- Inherited nephrotic disease

Extrarenal Causes
Multisystem Disease
- Systemic lupus erythematosus
- Diabetes mellitus
- Amyloidosis

Infections
- Bacterial (streptococcal, syphilis)
- Viral (hepatitis, human immunodeficiency virus)
- Protozoal (malaria)

Neoplasms
- Hodgkin's lymphoma
- Solid tumors of lungs, colon, stomach, breast
- Leukemias

Allergens (e.g., bee sting, pollen)

Drugs
- penicillamine
- Nonsteroidal antiinflammatory drugs
- captopril (Capoten)
- heroin

Collaborative Care

Treatment of nephrotic syndrome is based in symptom management.[25] The goals are to relieve edema and cure or control the primary disease. Management of the edema includes the cautious use of angiotensin-converting enzyme inhibitors, nonsteroidal antiinflammatory drugs, and a low-sodium (2 to 3 g/day), low- to moderate-protein (0.5 to 0.6 g/kg/day) diet. Dietary salt restrictions are a key to managing edema. In some individuals, thiazide or loop diuretics may be needed. If urine protein loss exceeds 10 g/24 hr, additional dietary protein may be needed.

The treatment of hyperlipidemia is often unsuccessful. However, treatment with lipid-lowering agents, such as colestipol (Colestid) and lovastatin (Mevacor), may result in moderate decreases in serum cholesterol levels. If thrombosis is detected, anticoagulant therapy may be necessary for up to 6 months.

Corticosteroids and cyclophosphamide (Cytoxan) may be used for the treatment of severe cases of nephrotic syndrome. Prednisone has been effective to varying degrees in persons with early-stage nephrosis, membranous glomerulonephritis, proliferative glomerulonephritis, and lupus nephritis. Management of diabetes and treatment of edema are the only measures used for nephrotic syndrome related to diabetes.

NURSING MANAGEMENT
NEPHROTIC SYNDROME

A major nursing intervention for a patient with nephrotic syndrome is related to edema. It is important to assess the edema by weighing the patient daily, accurately recording intake and output, and measuring abdominal girth or extremity size. Comparing this information daily provides the nurse with a tool for assessing the effectiveness of treatment. The edematous skin must be cleaned carefully. Trauma should be avoided, and the effectiveness of diuretic therapy must be monitored.

The patient with nephrotic syndrome has the potential to become malnourished from the excessive loss of protein in the urine. Maintaining a low- to moderate-protein diet that is also low in sodium is not always easy. The patient is usually anorexic. Serving small, frequent meals in a pleasant setting may encourage better dietary intake.

Because the patient is susceptible to infection, measures should be taken to avoid exposure to persons with known infections. The person with nephrotic syndrome is often ashamed of an edematous appearance and needs support in dealing with an altered body image.

RENAL DISEASE AND ACQUIRED IMMUNODEFICIENCY SYNDROME

The patient with HIV infection can have a variety of renal manifestations, ranging from mild fluid and electrolyte abnormalities to progressive renal impairment resulting in end-stage renal disease. The incidence of renal disease associated with HIV infection is about 10% and is highest among IV drug users.

HIV-associated renal syndromes include the following:

1. *Proteinuria and nephrotic syndrome,* which occurs in about 10% of patients with HIV infection. It may be the initial sign of HIV infection in some persons.
2. *HIV-associated nephropathy,* which is characterized by proteinuria, progressive azotemia, absence of hypertension, large kidney size on renal imaging studies, and unusually rapid progression to end-stage renal disease.
3. *Acute renal failure,* which is most commonly seen in the patient with acquired immunodeficiency syndrome (AIDS) who is critically ill with HIV-related infection or malignancy. The natural cause of acute renal failure secondary to AIDS is similar to acute renal failure associated with other acute illnesses (see Chapter 47). Survival and recovery usually depend on the treatment of the primary cause of renal failure and support of renal function by dialysis. (HIV infection is discussed in Chapter 15.)

Obstructive Uropathies

Urinary obstruction refers to any anatomic or functional condition that blocks or impedes the flow of urine (Fig. 46-3). It may be congenital or acquired.

Damaging effects from urinary tract obstruction affect the system above the level of the obstruction. The severity of these effects depends on the location, duration of obstruction, amount of pressure or dilation, presence of urinary stasis, and whether infection is present. Infection increases the risk of irreversible damage.

Although obstruction distal to the prostate in men or the bladder neck in women causes mucosal scarring and a slower urinary stream, it rarely results in major obstructive uropathy because the urethral wall pressure is less than that of the bladder neck and bladder. Urethral obstruction may contribute to outlet resistance and cause lower or upper urinary tract damage when other obstructive or dysfunctional factors are also present. For example, there is an increased risk of compromised renal function in the patient with a spinal cord injury with vesicosphincter dyssynergia.

When obstruction occurs at the level of the bladder neck or prostate, significant bladder changes can occur. Detrusor muscle fibers *hypertrophy* (increase in size) to contract harder to push urine out a narrower pathway. Over a long period, the detrusor loses its ability to compensate for this resistance. Muscle bundles

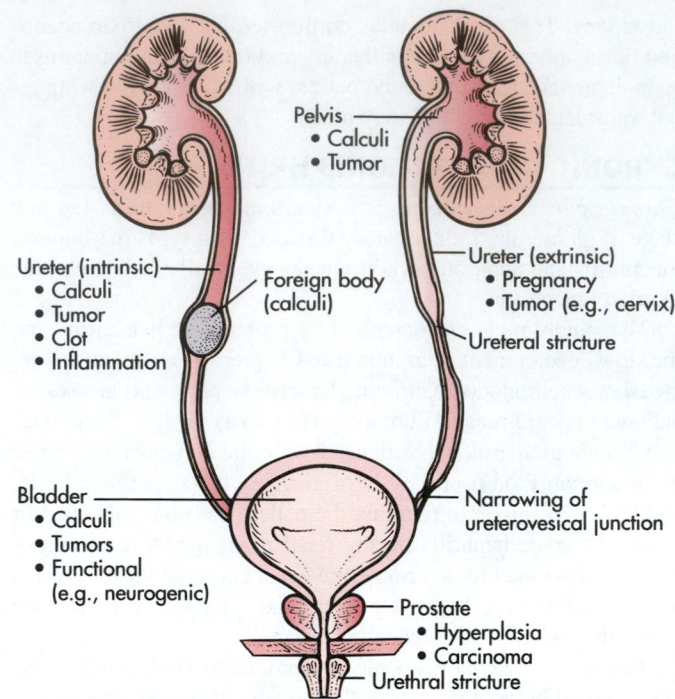

FIG. 46-3   Common causes of urinary tract obstruction.

separate and become less compliant. This separation is called *trabeculation.* Trabeculation is caused by the deposition of collagen in the bladder wall that separates the smooth muscle fascicles. Trabeculation may hasten the decompensation of the detrusor. The areas between these muscle bundles are called *cellules.* Because these areas have no muscle support, the bladder mucosa can herniate between detrusor muscle bundles, forming sacs that drain poorly, called *diverticula.* Residual urine volume can be very high in a noncompensating bladder.

Pressure increases during bladder filling or storage and can be transmitted to the ureter when *bladder outlet obstruction* is present. This pressure overcomes the normal peristaltic pressure and leads to *reflux* (a backflow of urine); ureteral dilation, kinking, and tortuosity; **hydroureter** (dilation of the renal pelvis); vesicoureteral reflux (backflow or backward movement of urine from the lower to upper urinary tracts); and **hydronephrosis** (dilation or enlargement of the renal pelves and calyces) (Fig. 46-4), and consequent chronic pyelonephritis and renal atrophy. If only one kidney is obstructed, the other kidney may try to compensate by hypertrophy, but the ureter will not be dilated on this contralateral side.

Partial obstruction may occur in the ureter or at the ureteropelvic junction (UPJ). If the pressure remains low or moderate, the kidney may continue to dilate with no noticeable loss of function. There is an increased risk of pyelonephritis because of urinary stasis and reflux. If only one kidney is involved and the other kidney is functioning, the patient may be free of symptoms. If both kidneys or only one functioning kidney is involved (e.g., if the patient has only one kidney), alterations in renal function (e.g., increased BUN or serum creatinine levels) are found. If the obstruction progresses, oliguria or anuria develops. Often episodes of oliguria are followed by polyuria if the obstruction is a stone that becomes dislodged. Treatment requires location and relief of the blockage. This can include insertion of a tube (e.g., urethral or ureteral), surgical correction of the disease process, or diversion of the urinary stream above the level of blockage.

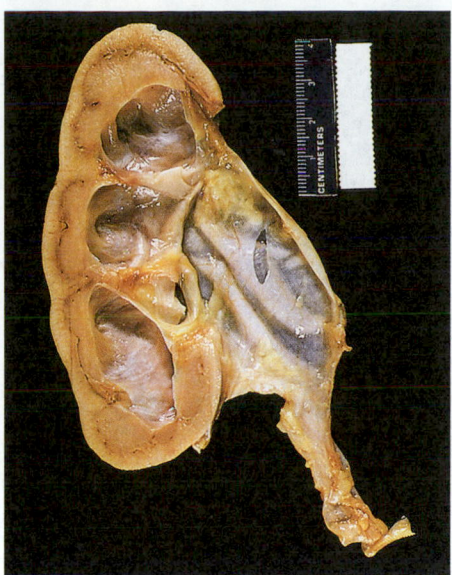

FIG. 46-4   Hydronephrosis of the kidney with marked dilation of the pelvis and calyces and thinning of the renal parenchyma.

TABLE 46-11	Risk Factors for the Development of Urinary Tract Calculi

Metabolic
Abnormalities that result in increased urine levels of calcium, oxaluric acid, uric acid, or citric acid

Climate
Warm climates that cause increased fluid loss, low urine volume, and increased solute concentration in urine

Diet
Large intake of dietary proteins that increases uric acid excretion
Excessive amounts of tea or fruit juices that elevate urinary oxalate level
Large intake of calcium and oxalate
Low fluid intake that increases urinary concentration

Genetic Factors
Family history of stone formation, cystinuria, gout, or renal acidosis

Lifestyle
Sedentary occupation, immobility

GENDER DIFFERENCES
Urinary Tract Calculi

Men	**Women**
• All other urinary calculi disorders are more common in men.	• Struvite stones associated with urinary tract infection are more common in women than in men.

URINARY TRACT CALCULI

Each year an estimated 500,000 people in the United States have **nephrolithiasis** (kidney stone disease). Many of these people require hospitalization. In the United States the incidence of urinary stone disease is highest in the Southeast and Southwest, followed by the Midwest. Except for struvite (magnesium ammonium phosphate) stones associated with UTI, stone disorders are more common in men than in women.[26] The majority of patients are between 20 and 55 years of age. Stone formation is more frequent in whites than in African Americans. The incidence is also higher in persons with a family history of stone formation. Recurrence of stones can occur in up to 50% of patients.[26] Stone formation occurs more often in the summer months, thus supporting the role of dehydration in this process. Stone formation in the kidney also seems to increase in incidence as countries become more industrialized, whereas the incidence of bladder stones decreases.

Etiology and Pathophysiology

Many factors are involved in the incidence and type of stone formation, including metabolic, dietary, genetic, climatic, lifestyle, and occupational influences (Table 46-11). Many theories have been proposed to explain the formation of stones in the urinary tract. No single theory can account for stone formation in all cases. Crystals, when in a supersaturated concentration, can precipitate and unite to form a stone. Keeping urine dilute and free flowing reduces the risk of recurrent stone formation in many individuals. It is known that a mucoprotein is formed (the matrix for the stone) in the kidneys that form stones. Urinary pH, solute load, and inhibitors in the urine affect the formation of stones. The higher the pH (alkaline), the less soluble are calcium and phosphate. The lower the pH (acidic), the less soluble are uric acid and cystine.

Other important factors in the development of stones include obstruction with urinary stasis and urinary tract infection with urea-splitting bacteria (e.g., *Proteus, Klebsiella, Pseudomonas,* and some species of staphylococci). These bacteria cause the urine to become alkaline and contribute to the formation of struvite stones.[27] Infected stones, when they are entrapped in the kidney, may assume a staghorn configuration as they are branched stones that occupy a large portion of the collecting system[28] (Fig. 46-5). Infected stones are frequent in the patient with an external urinary diversion, long-term indwelling catheter, neurogenic bladder, or urinary retention. Genetic factors may also contribute to urine stone formation. Cystinuria is an autosomal recessive disorder. In this disorder there is a marked increased excretion of cystine.

Types

The term **calculus** refers to the stone, and *lithiasis* refers to stone formation. The five major categories of stones are (1) calcium phosphate, (2) calcium oxalate, (3) uric acid, (4) cystine, and (5) struvite (magnesium ammonium phosphate) (Table 46-12). Stone composition may be mixed, although calcium stones are the most common. Calculi can be found in various locations in the urinary tract (Fig. 46-6).

Clinical Manifestations

Urinary stones cause clinical manifestations when they obstruct urinary flow. Common sites of complete obstruction are at the UPJ (the point where the ureter crosses the iliac vessels) and at the ureterovesical junction (UVJ). Symptoms include abdominal or flank pain (usually severe), hematuria, and renal colic (due to increase in peristalsis in the ureters in response to the passage of small stones along the ureters). The pain may be associated with nausea and vomiting. The type of pain is determined by the location of the stone (see Fig. 46-6). If the stone is nonobstructing, pain may be absent. If the obstruction is in a calyx or at the UPJ, the patient may experience dull costovertebral flank pain or even colic. Pain resulting from the pas-

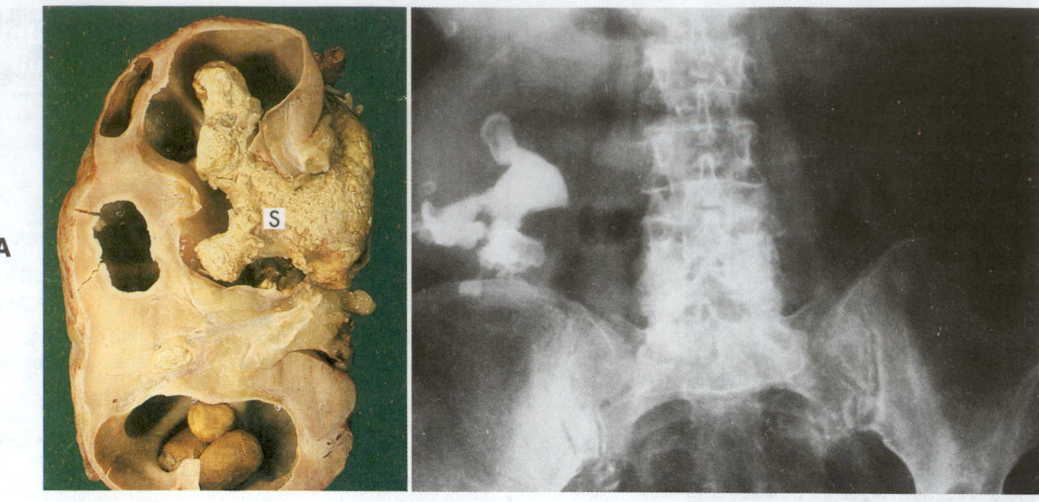

FIG. 46-5 A, Renal staghorn calculus. The renal pelvis is filled with a large calculus that is shaped to its contours, resembling the horns of a stag *(S)*. **B,** Staghorn calculus as seen on an intravenous pyelogram (IVP).

TABLE 46-12	Types of Urinary Tract Calculi			
Urinary Stone	**Incidence (%)**	**Characteristics**	**Predisposing Factors**	**Therapeutic Measures**
Calcium oxalate*	35-40	Small, often possible to get trapped in ureter; more frequent in men than in women	Idiopathic hypercalciuria, hyperoxaluria, independent of urinary pH, family history	Increase hydration. Reduce dietary oxalate.† Give thiazide diuretics. Give cellulose phosphate to chelate calcium and prevent GI absorption. Give potassium citrate to maintain alkaline urine. Give cholestyramine to bind oxalate. Give calcium lactate to precipitate oxalate in GI tract. Reduce daily sodium intake.
Calcium phosphate	8-10	Mixed stones (typically), with struvite or oxalate stones	Alkaline urine, primary hyperparathyroidism	Treat underlying causes and other stones.
Struvite (magnesium ammonium phosphate—$MgNH_4PO_4$)	10-15	Three to four times as common in women as men; always in association with urinary tract infections; large staghorn type (usually)‡	Urinary tract infections (usually *Proteus* organisms)	Administer antimicrobial agents, acetohydroxamic acid. Use surgical intervention to remove stone. Take measures to acidify urine.
Uric acid	5-8	Predominant in men, high incidence in Jewish men	Gout, acid urine, inherited condition	Reduce urinary concentration of uric acid. Alkalinize urine with potassium citrate. Administer allopurinol. Reduce dietary purines.†
Cystine	1-2	Genetic autosomal recessive defect; defective absorption of cystine in GI tract and kidney, excess concentrations causing stone formation	Acid urine	Increase hydration. Give α-penicillamine and tiopronin to prevent cystine crystallization. Give potassium citrate to maintain alkaline urine.

GI, Gastrointestinal.
*Calcium stones can exist as calcium oxalate, calcium phosphate, or a mixture of both. Calcium stones account for the majority of all stones.
†See Table 46-13.
‡See Fig. 46-4.

sage of a calculus down the ureter is intense and colicky. The patient may be in mild shock with cool, moist skin. As a stone nears the UVJ, pain will be felt in the lateral flank and sometimes down into the testicles, labia, or groin. Other clinical manifestations include the presence of urinary infection accompanied by fever and chills.

Diagnostic Studies

Diagnostic studies useful in the evaluation and management of renal lithiasis include urinalysis, urine culture, IVP, retrograde pyelogram, ultrasound, and cystoscopy.[26] A plain film of the abdomen and renal ultrasound will identify larger, radiopaque stones.

An IVP or retrograde pyelogram is used to localize the degree and site of obstruction or to confirm the presence of a radiolucent stone, such as a uric acid or cystine calculus (see Fig. 46-5, *B*). IVP should not be performed in patients with renal failure. Ultrasonography can be used to identify a radiopaque or radiolucent calculus in the renal pelvis, calyx, or proximal ureter. It is less useful when attempting to locate stones trapped in the midureter. A CT scan may be used to differentiate a nonopaque stone from a tumor.

Retrieval and analysis of the stones are important in the diagnosis of the underlying problem contributing to stone formation. The patient's serum calcium, phosphorus, sodium, potassium, bicarbonate,

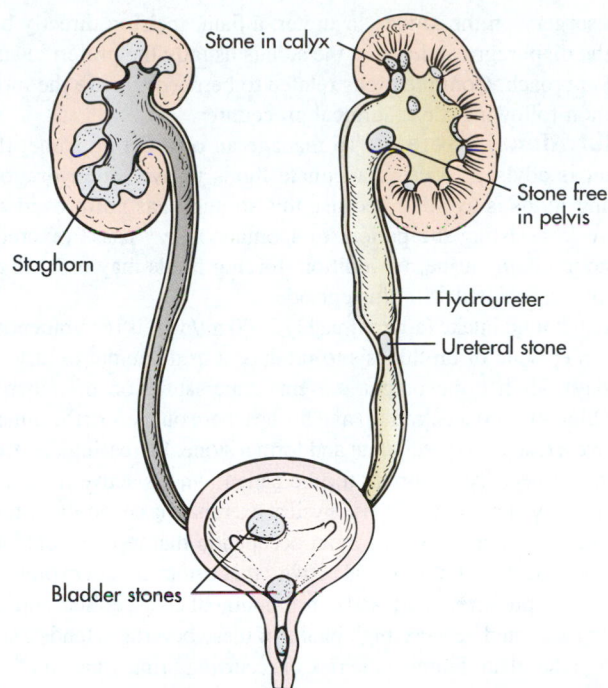

FIG. 46-6 Location of calculi in the urinary tract.

TABLE 46-13	***NUTRITIONAL THERAPY*** **Urinary Tract Calculi**

Depending on the type of calculi, the diet should be modified to decrease foods that are high in the substance that is the cause of the calculi. Listed below are foods that are moderate or high in purine, calcium, or oxalate content.

Purine*
High: Sardines, herring, mussels, liver, kidney, goose, venison, meat soups, sweetbreads
Moderate: Chicken, salmon, crab, veal, mutton, bacon, pork, beef, ham

Calcium
High: Milk, cheese, ice cream, yogurt, sauces containing milk; all beans (except green beans), lentils; fish with fine bones (e.g., sardines, kippers, herring, salmon); dried fruits, nuts; Ovaltine, chocolate, cocoa

Oxalate
High: Dark roughage, spinach, rhubarb, asparagus, cabbage, tomatoes, beets, nuts, celery, parsley, runner beans; chocolate, cocoa, instant coffee, Ovaltine, tea; Worcestershire sauce

*Uric acid is a waste product from purine in food.

uric acid, BUN, and creatinine levels are also measured. A careful history, including previous stone formation, prescribed and OTC medications, dietary supplements, and family history of urinary calculi, is useful. Measurement of urine pH is useful in the diagnosis of struvite stones and renal tubular acidosis (tendency to alkaline or high pH) and uric acid stones (tendency to acidic or low pH). Patients who are recurrent stone formers should undergo a 24-hour urinary measurement of calcium, phosphorus, magnesium, sodium, oxalate, citrate, sulfate, potassium, uric acid, and total volume.[27]

Collaborative Care

Evaluation and management of a patient with renal lithiasis consist of two concurrent approaches.[27] The first approach is directed toward management of the acute attack. This involves treating the symptoms of pain, infection, or obstruction as indicated for the individual patient. At frequent intervals, opioids are typically required for relief of renal colic pain. Many stones pass spontaneously. However, stones larger than 4 mm are unlikely to pass through the ureter, and the patient may require insertion of a ureteral stent to prevent obstruction from passage of stone fragments.

The second approach is directed toward evaluation of the cause of the stone formation and the prevention of further development of stones. Information to be obtained from the patient includes family history of stone formation, geographic residence, nutritional assessment including the intake of vitamins A and D, activity pattern (active or sedentary), history of periods of prolonged illness with immobilization or dehydration, and any history of disease or surgery involving the GI or genitourinary tract.

Therapy for people who are active stone formers requires a concerted management approach, with primary emphasis on teaching and on developing a therapeutic regimen with which the patient can comply. Adequate hydration, dietary sodium restrictions, dietary changes (Table 46-13), and the use of drugs are employed to minimize urinary stone formation. Various drugs are prescribed, depending on the specific problem underlying stone formation. These drugs

prevent stone formation in various ways, including altering urine pH, preventing excessive urinary excretion of a substance, or correcting a primary disease (e.g., hyperparathyroidism).

Treatment of struvite stones requires control of infection. This may be difficult if the stone remains in place. In addition to antibiotics, acetohydroxamic acid may be used in the treatment of kidney infections that result in the continual formation of struvite stones. Acetohydroxamic acid, an inhibitor of the chemical action caused by the persistent bacteria, can be used effectively to retard struvite stone formation.[29] If the infection cannot be controlled, the stone may have to be removed surgically.

Indications for endourologic, lithotripsy, or open surgical stone removal include the following:
1. Stones too large for spontaneous passage
2. Stones associated with bacteriuria or symptomatic infection
3. Stones causing impaired renal function
4. Stones causing persistent pain, nausea, or ileus
5. Inability of patient to be treated medically
6. Patient with one kidney

Endourologic Procedures. If the stone is located in the bladder, a cystoscopy is done to remove small stones. For large stones a *cystolitholapaxy* is done. In this procedure, large stones can be broken up with an instrument called a lithotrite (stone crusher). The bladder is then irrigated and the crushed stones washed out. A *cystoscopic lithotripsy* uses an ultrasonic lithotrite to pulverize stones. Complications associated with these cystoscopic procedures include hemorrhage, retained stone fragments, and infection.

Flexible *ureteroscopes,* inserted via a cystoscope, can be used to remove stones from the renal pelvis and upper urinary tract. Ultrasonic, laser, or electrohydraulic lithotripsy can be used in conjunction with the ureteroscope to pulverize the stone into fragments.

In *percutaneous nephrolithotomy,* a nephroscope is inserted through a sinus tract from the skin into the kidney pelvis. Stones can be fragmented using ultrasound, electrohydraulic, or laser lithotripsy. The stone fragments are removed and the pelvis irrigated. A percutaneous nephrostomy tube is usually left in place to ensure that the ureter is not obstructed. Complications include bleeding, injury to adjacent structures, and infection.

Lithotripsy. **Lithotripsy** is a procedure used to eliminate calculi from the urinary tract. Outcome for lithotripsy is based on stone size, stone location, and stone composition. For example, it is not recommended for patients with staghorn or partial staghorn cystine stones.[28] Lithotripsy techniques include percutaneous ultrasonic lithotripsy, electrohydraulic lithotripsy, laser lithotripsy, and extracorporeal shock-wave lithotripsy.[27] Extracorporeal shock-wave lithotripsy and laser lithotripsy are the most common. In *percutaneous ultrasonic lithotripsy,* an ultrasonic probe is placed in the renal pelvis via a percutaneous nephroscope (inserted through a small incision in the flank) and is positioned against the stone. (The patient is given general or spinal anesthesia for this procedure.) The probe produces ultrasonic waves, which break the stone into sandlike particles. Percutaneous lithotripsy is not used as much as other lithotripsy procedures to treat renal or upper ureteral stones unless the stone is large and other lithotripsy procedures have failed.

The *electrohydraulic lithotripsy* probe is also placed directly on a stone, but it breaks the stone into small fragments that are removed by forceps or by suction. A continuous saline irrigation flushes out the stone particles, and all outflow drainage is strained so that the particles can be analyzed. The calculi can also be removed by forceps or basket extraction. Complications are rare but include hemorrhage, sepsis, and abscess formation. Postoperatively, the patient usually complains of moderate to severe colicky pain. The first few times that the patient urinates, the urine is bright red. As the bleeding subsides, the urine becomes dark red or turns a smoky color. Antibiotics are usually given for 2 weeks to reduce the risk of infection.

Laser lithotripsy probes are used to fragment lower ureteral and large bladder stones. A holmium laser medium is preferred. It fragments stones but does not injure the surrounding tissue.

In *extracorporeal shock-wave lithotripsy (ESWL),* a noninvasive procedure, the patient is anesthetized (spinal or general) and placed in a water bath. Anesthesia is necessary to keep the patient very still during the procedure. Some of the newer generation lithotripters do not require submersion and use other means of initiating shock waves. The lithotripters are categorized as electrohydraulic, electromagnetic, and piezoelectric. The second-generation lithotripters use less power to fragment stones. Lower power reduces a patient's pain, but usually some sedation or analgesia is necessary.

Fluoroscopy or ultrasound is used to focus the lithotripter on the affected kidney, and a high-voltage spark generator produces high-energy acoustic shock waves that shatter the stone without damaging the surrounding tissues. The stone is broken into fine sand, which is excreted into the patient's urine within a few days.

Hematuria is common after lithotripsy procedures. A self-retaining ureteral stent is often placed after the procedure to promote passage of this sand and to prevent obstruction caused by a buildup of sand in the ureter. The stent is removed 1 to 2 weeks after lithotripsy. Because lithotripsy is an outpatient procedure, it offers several advantages including reduced hospital admission, reduced length of hospitalization, and the patient's earlier return to normal activities. Additional treatment, such as surgery, may be necessary if a stone is large and in the mid or distal ureter.

Surgical Therapy. A small group of patients need open surgical procedures, such as the very obese patient or the individual with complex abnormalities in the calyces or at the UPJ. The type of open surgery performed depends on the location of the stone. A *nephrolithotomy* is an incision into the kidney to remove a stone. A *pyelolithotomy* is an incision into the renal pelvis to remove a stone. If the stone is located in the ureter, a *ureterolithotomy* is performed. A *cystotomy* may be indicated for bladder calculi. For open surgery on the kidney or ureter, a flank incision directly below the diaphragm and across the side is usually the preferred surgical approach. Complications related to hemorrhage are the most common following these surgical procedures.

Nutritional Therapy. To manage an obstructing stone, the patient is advised to drink adequate fluids to avoid dehydration. Forcing fluids is avoided because this strategy has not proved effective in assisting the patient to spontaneously "pass" (excrete) the stone via the urine. In addition, forcing fluids may exacerbate the colic associated with this episode.

A high fluid intake (approximately 3000 ml/day) is recommended after an episode of urolithiasis to produce a urine output of at least 2 L/day). High urine output prevents supersaturation of minerals (i.e., dilutes the concentration) and flushes them out before the minerals have a chance to precipitate and form a stone. Increasing the fluid intake is especially important for the patient who is active in sports, lives in a dry climate, performs physical exercise, has a family history of stone formation, or works in an occupation that requires outdoor work or a great deal of physical activity that can lead to dehydration. Water is the preferred fluid, and consumption of colas, coffee, and tea should be limited because high intake of these beverages tends to increase rather than diminish the risk of recurring urinary calculi.[30]

Dietary intervention may be important in the management of urolithiasis. In the past, calcium restriction was routinely implemented for the patient with kidney stones. However, more recent research suggests that a high dietary calcium intake, which was previously thought to contribute to kidney stones, may actually lower the risk by reducing the urinary excretion of oxalate, a common factor in many stones.[31] A low-sodium diet is recommended as high sodium intake increases calcium excretion in the urine. Initial nutritional management should include limiting oxalate-rich foods and thereby reducing oxalate excretion. Foods high in calcium, oxalate, and purines are presented in Table 46-13.

NURSING MANAGEMENT
RENAL CALCULI

■ *Nursing Assessment*

Subjective and objective data that should be obtained from a patient with urinary tract lithiasis are presented in Table 46-14.

■ *Nursing Diagnoses*

Nursing diagnoses for the patient with urinary tract lithiasis include, but are not limited to, those presented in NCP 46-2.

■ *Planning*

The overall goals are that the patient with urinary tract calculi will have (1) relief of pain, (2) no urinary tract obstruction, and (3) an understanding of measures to prevent further recurrence of stones.

■ *Nursing Implementation*

Up to 85% of all patients with renal stones could lower their risk of stone recurrence with changes to lifestyle and dietary habits.[30] A program to prevent stone recurrence always includes adequate fluid intake to produce a urine output of approximately 2 L/day, and it may include measures to alleviate metabolic or secondary risk factors. The nurse should consult with the health care provider concerning recommendations for fluid intake in a given patient. In the moderately active, ambulatory person, this requires the patient to drink about 2000 to 2200 ml/day, with the residual 20% to 30% of fluids gained through consumption of foods. The volume of fluids

TABLE 46-14	*NURSING ASSESSMENT* Urinary Tract Calculi

Subjective Data
Important Health Information
Past health history: Recent or chronic UTI; bed rest; immobilization; previous urinary tract stones, obstruction, or kidney disease with urinary stasis; gout; benign prostatic hyperplasia (BPH); hyperparathyroidism, chronic diarrhea
Medications: Prior use of medication for prevention of stones or treatment of UTI; allopurinol, analgesics, loop diuretics
Surgery or other treatments: External urinary diversion, long-term indwelling urinary catheter

Functional Health Patterns
Health perception–health management: Family history of renal calculi; sedentary lifestyle
Nutritional-metabolic: Nausea, vomiting; dietary intake of purines, excessive calcium ingestion, salt excess, oxalates, phosphates; low fluid intake; chills
Elimination: Decreased urinary output, urinary urgency, frequency, feeling of bladder fullness
Cognitive-perceptual: Acute, severe, colicky pain in flank, back, abdomen, groin, or genitalia; burning on urination, dysuria, anxiety

Objective Data
General
Guarding, back pain, fever, dehydration

Integumentary
Warm, flushed skin or pallor with cool, moist skin (mild shock)

Gastrointestinal
Abdominal distention, absence of bowel sounds

Urinary
Oliguria, hematuria, tenderness on palpation of renal areas, passage of stone or stones

Possible Findings
↑ BUN and serum creatinine levels; RBCs, WBCs, pyuria, crystals, casts, minerals, bacteria on urinalysis; ↑ uric acid, calcium, phosphorus, oxalate, or cystine values on 24-hr urine sample; calculi or anatomic changes on IVP or KUB x-ray; direct visualization of obstruction on cystoureteroscopy

BUN, Blood urea nitrogen; *IVP,* intravenous pyelogram; *KUB,* kidneys, ureters, bladder; *RBCs,* red blood cells; *UTI,* urinary tract infection; *WBCs,* white blood cells.

will be higher in the highly active patient who works outdoors or who regularly engages in demanding athletic activities. In contrast, fluid intake will be less for the very sedentary or immobile person. Preventive measures related to the person who is on bed rest or is relatively immobile for a prolonged time include maintaining an adequate fluid intake, turning the patient every 2 hours, and helping the patient to sit or stand, if possible, to maximize urinary flow.[32]

Additional preventive measures focus on reducing metabolic or secondary risk factors. For example, dietary restriction of purines may be helpful to the patient at risk for developing uric acid stones. Reduced intake of oxalates may be indicated in the person with recurring calcium oxalate calculi. The patient is taught the dosage, scheduling, and potential side effects of drugs used to reduce the risk of stone formation. Selected patients may be taught to self-monitor urinary pH, or they may be asked to measure urinary output.

Pain management and patient comfort are primary nursing responsibilities when managing an obstructing stone and renal colic (see NCP 46-2). It is important to ensure that the patient retrieves any spontaneously passed stones. All urine voided by the patient should be strained through gauze or a special urine strainer in an effort to detect the stone. The high fluid intake necessary for stone prevention is avoided, but consumption should be adequate to meet daily needs and avoid dehydration. Ambulation is generally encouraged to promote the movement of the stone from the upper to the lower urinary tract, but the patient should not walk unattended when experiencing acute colic, particularly if opioid analgesics are being used.

■ Evaluation

The expected outcomes for the patient with urinary calculi are presented in NCP 46-2.

STRICTURES

A **stricture** is a narrowing of the lumen of the ureter or urethra.

Ureteral Strictures

Ureteral strictures can affect the entire length of the ureter, from the UPJ to the UVJ. These strictures are usually an unintended result of surgical intervention, usually secondary to adhesions or scar forma-

---

NURSING CARE PLAN 46-2

Patient with Acute Renal Lithiasis

NURSING DIAGNOSIS   **Acute pain** *related to* effects of renal stone and inadequate pain control or comfort measures *as evidenced by* complaints of pain, facial grimacing, restlessness

PATIENT GOAL   Reports satisfactory pain relief

OUTCOMES (NOC)	INTERVENTIONS (NIC) and *RATIONALES*
Pain Control	*Pain Management*
• Uses analgesics appropriately ____ • Uses nonanalgesic relief measures ____ • Reports uncontrolled symptoms to health care professional ____ • Reports pain controlled ____ **Measurement Scale** 1 = Never demonstrated 2 = Rarely demonstrated 3 = Sometimes demonstrated 4 = Often demonstrated 5 = Consistently demonstrated	• Perform a comprehensive assessment of pain to include location, characteristics, onset/duration, frequency, quality, intensity or severity, and precipitating factors *to plan appropriate interventions.* • Ensure that patient receives attentive analgesic care *as renal colic is a severe type of pain.* • Implement use of PCA, if appropriate, *to permit patient control of analgesic dosing.* • Use pain control measures before pain becomes severe *to prevent breakthrough pain that is difficult to control.* • Teach use of nonpharmacologic techniques for patient to use in lieu of or in conjunction with analgesics *to obtain pain relief.* • Institute and modify pain control measures on the basis of patient's response.

PCA, Patient-controlled analgesia.

NURSING CARE PLAN 46-2

Patient with Acute Renal Lithiasis—cont'd

NURSING DIAGNOSIS **Impaired urinary elimination** *related to* trauma or blockage of ureters or urethra *as evidenced by* decreased urinary output, hematuria

PATIENT GOAL Maintains free flow of urine with minimal hematuria

OUTCOMES (NOC)	INTERVENTIONS (NIC) and *RATIONALES*
Urinary Elimination	**Urinary Elimination Management**
• Elimination pattern ____	• Monitor urinary elimination, including frequency, consistency, odor, volume, and color, *to evaluate patency of urinary system and degree of hematuria.*
• Urine amount ____	• Teach patient to drink eight ounces of liquid with meals, between meals, and in early evening *to provide fluids for hydration but not to an excess that may increase renal colic.*
• Urine color ____	• Teach patient signs and symptoms of urinary tract infection *as infection may result from renal stones.*
• Adequate fluid intake ____	
Measurement Scale	
1 = Severely compromised	
2 = Substantially compromised	
3 = Moderately compromised	
4 = Mildly compromised	
5 = Not compromised	

NURSING DIAGNOSIS **Ineffective therapeutic regimen management** *related to* lack of knowledge regarding disease process, prevention of recurrence, diet, and fluid requirements *as evidenced by* questions about how to prevent future renal stones

PATIENT GOAL Verbalizes understanding of disease process and measures to prevent recurrence

OUTCOMES (NOC)	INTERVENTIONS (NIC) and *RATIONALES*
Knowledge: Illness Care	**Teaching: Disease Process**
• Description of recommended diet ____	• Appraise the patient's current level of knowledge related to specific disease process *to plan appropriate teaching.*
• Description of specific disease process ____	• Describe the disease process.
• Description of treatment regimen ____	• Identify possible etiologies *to decrease or avoid recurrence.*
Measurement Scale	• Describe rationale behind management/therapy/treatment recommendations *to increase compliance.*
1 = None	**Teaching: Prescribed Diet**
2 = Limited	• Explain the purpose of the diet *to increase compliance with the diet.*
3 = Moderate	• Assist patient to accommodate food preferences into the prescribed diet.
4 = Substantial	
5 = Extensive	

tion. Depending on its severity, ureteral obstruction can threaten the function of the kidney. Clinical manifestations of a ureteral stricture include mild to moderate colic; this pain may be of moderate to severe intensity if the patient consumes a large volume of fluids (such as alcohol) over a brief period. Infection is unusual unless a calculus or foreign object such as a stent or nephrostomy tube is present.

The discomfort and obstruction of a ureteral stricture may be temporarily bypassed by placing a stent under endoscopic control or by diverting urinary flow via a nephrostomy tube inserted into the renal pelvis of the affected kidney. Definitive correction requires dilation with a balloon or catheter. If the stricture is severe or recurs after initial balloon or catheter dilation, it may be incised under endoscopic control *(endoureterotomy)*. In selected cases, an open surgical approach may be required to excise the stenotic area and reanastomose the ureter to the contralateral ureter *(ureteroureterostomy)* or to the renal pelvis. Alternatively, distal ureteral strictures may be managed by an *ureteroneocystostomy* (reimplantation of the ureter into the bladder wall).

Urethral Stricture

A *urethral stricture* is the result of fibrosis or inflammation of the urethral lumen.[33] Causes of urethral strictures include trauma, urethritis (particularly following gonococcal infection), iatrogenic

(following surgical intervention or repeated catheterizations), or a congenital defect in the canalization of the urethra. Once the process of inflammation and fibrosis begins, the lumen of the urethra narrows, and its compliance (ability to close or open in response to bladder filling or micturition) is compromised. Meatal stenosis, a narrowing of the urethral opening, is also common. A urethral stricture creates symptoms when it creates voiding dysfunction or bladder outlet obstruction.[33]

Clinical manifestations associated with a urethral stricture include a diminished force of the urinary stream, straining to void, sprayed stream, postvoid dribbling, or a split urine stream. The patient may report feelings of incomplete bladder emptying with urinary frequency and nocturia. Moderate to severe obstruction of the bladder outlet may lead to acute urinary retention. The patient may report a history of urethritis, difficulty with insertion of a urinary catheter, or trauma involving the penis or perineum. However, many patients are unable to recall any such events, thus leading to a diagnosis of an idiopathic stricture. A history of a UTI is not uncommon, particularly if the stricture involves the distal urethra. Retrograde urethrography (RUG) and voiding cystourethrography (VCUG) will identify stricture length, location, and caliber.[33]

Initial management of a stricture may be based on dilation. A metal instrument (urethral sound) may be placed, or a series of progressively enlarging stents (filiforms and followers) can be placed into the urethra to expand its lumen in a stepwise fashion.[34] While initially successful, recurring stenosis is frequent. Recurrences may be managed by teaching the patient to repeatedly dilate the urethra by self-catheterization using a soft (coudé-tip, red rubber) catheter every few days. Alternatively, an endoscopic or open surgical procedure (*urethroplasty*) may be completed to provide a more durable solution to an obstructive urethral stricture. Shorter strictures may be managed by resection of the fibrotic area with primary reanastomosis. Longer strictures may require autotransplantation of a substitute segment such as a skin flap.

Renal Trauma

A continual increase in the incidence of traumatic renal injuries is related to an increase in violent crimes and injuries and in the mechanization and speed of transportation. The majority of incidents occur in men younger than 30 years of age. Blunt trauma is the most common cause. Injury to the kidney should be considered in multiple or sports injuries, traffic accidents, and falls. It is especially likely when the patient injures the abdomen, flank, or back as the kidney is injured in 5% of abdominal trauma cases, making it the most susceptible genitourinary organ.[35] Penetrating injuries may result from violent encounters (e.g., gunshot or stabbing incidents) or from iatrogenic injuries.

Clinical findings include a history of trauma to the area of the kidneys. Gross or microscopic hematuria may be present. Diagnostic studies include urinalysis, IVP with cystography, and ultrasound, CT, or MRI evaluation. Renal arteriography may also be used. Both the injured kidney and the noninvolved kidney should be evaluated to provide information for further management.

The severity of renal trauma depends on the extent of the injury. Treatments range from bed rest, fluids, and analgesia to surgical exploration and repair or nephrectomy.

Nursing interventions vary with the type and extent of associated injuries. Specific interventions related to renal trauma include monitoring for shock, which can occur in penetrating injury. The nurse should ensure increased fluid intake, provide comfort measures, monitor intake and output, observe for hematuria, determine the presence of myoglobinuria, assess the cardiovascular status, and monitor potentially nephrotoxic antibiotics.

Renal Vascular Problems

Vascular problems involving the kidney include (1) nephrosclerosis, (2) renal artery stenosis, and (3) renal vein thrombosis.

NEPHROSCLEROSIS

Nephrosclerosis consists of sclerosis of the small arteries and arterioles of the kidney. There is decreased blood flow, which results in patchy necrosis of the renal parenchyma. Ischemic necrosis and destruction of glomeruli with subsequent fibrosis also occur.

Benign nephrosclerosis usually occurs in adults 30 to 50 years of age. It is caused by vascular changes resulting from hypertension and from the atherosclerosis process. Atherosclerotic vascular changes account for most of the loss of renal function associated with aging. There is a direct relation between the degree of nephrosclerosis and the severity of hypertension. The patient with benign nephrosclerosis may have normal renal function in the early stages. The only detectable abnormality may be hypertension.

Accelerated nephrosclerosis, or *malignant nephrosclerosis,* is associated with malignant hypertension, a complication of hypertension characterized by a sharp increase in blood pressure (BP) with a diastolic pressure greater than 130 mm Hg. The patient is usually a young adult, with a male-to-female predominance of 2:1. Renal insufficiency progresses rapidly.

Treatment for benign nephrosclerosis is the same as that for essential hypertension (see Chapter 33). Malignant nephrosclerosis is treated with aggressive antihypertensive therapy (see Chapter 33). The availability and use of antihypertensive agents have improved the prognosis for the patient with benign and malignant nephrosclerosis. Renal dysfunction and renal failure constitute two of the major complications of hypertension. The prognosis for the patient with untreated or refractory malignant hypertension is poor, with the major cause of death related to renal failure.

RENAL ARTERY STENOSIS

Renal artery stenosis is a partial occlusion of one or both renal arteries and their major branches. It can be due to atherosclerotic narrowing or fibromuscular hyperplasia. Renal artery stenosis accounts for 1% to 2% of all cases of hypertension.

When hypertension develops rather abruptly, renal artery stenosis should be considered as a possible cause, especially in the patient under 30 or over 50 years of age and in the patient with no familial history of hypertension. This contrasts with the age distribution for essential hypertension, which is 30 to 50 years of age. A renal arteriogram is the best diagnostic tool for identifying renal artery stenosis.

The goals of therapy are control of BP and restoration of perfusion to the kidney. Percutaneous transluminal renal angioplasty is the procedure of first choice, especially in older patients who are poor surgical risks. Surgical revascularization of the kidney is indicated when blood flow is decreased enough to cause renal ischemia or when evidence indicates that renovascular hypertension is present and surgical intervention may result in the patient becoming normotensive. The surgical procedure usually involves anastomoses between the kidney and another major artery, usually the splenic artery or aorta. In selected cases of unilateral renal involvement with high renin production, unilateral nephrectomy may be indicated.

RENAL VEIN THROMBOSIS

Renal vein thrombosis may occur unilaterally or bilaterally. Trauma, extrinsic compression (e.g., tumor, aortic aneurysm), renal cell carcinoma, pregnancy, contraceptive use, and nephrotic syndrome are associated with renal vein thrombosis.

The patient has symptoms of flank pain, hematuria, or fever or has nephrotic syndrome. Anticoagulation (e.g., heparin, warfarin [Coumadin]) is important in treatment because there is a high incidence of pulmonary emboli. Corticosteroids may be used for the patient with nephrotic syndrome. Surgical thrombectomy may be performed instead of or along with anticoagulation.

Hereditary Renal Diseases

Hereditary renal diseases involve developmental abnormalities of the renal parenchyma. These abnormalities are either isolated or part of more complex malformation syndromes. The majority of inherited structural abnormalities are cystic. However, cysts may also develop as a result of obstructive uropathies, metabolic derangements, or neurologic diseases. Cysts may be evaluated to rule out any tumor content.

POLYCYSTIC KIDNEY DISEASE

Polycystic kidney disease (PKD) is the most common life-threatening genetic disease in the world, affecting 600,000 people in the United States and 12.5 million people worldwide. PKD accounts for 10% to 15% of chronic kidney disease. There are two forms of hereditary PKD; it may be manifested in childhood or adulthood. The childhood form of PKD is a rare autosomal recessive disorder that is often rapidly progressive (see the Genetics in Clinical Practice box).

The adult form of PKD is an autosomal dominant disorder (see Fig. 14-4). If one parent has the disease, there is 50% chance that the disease will pass to the child. It is latent for many years and is usually manifested between 30 and 40 years of age. However, PKD has also been found in newborns. It involves both kidneys and occurs in both men and women. The cortex and the medulla are filled with large, thin-walled cysts that are several millimeters to several centimeters in diameter (Fig. 46-7, *A*). The cysts enlarge and destroy surrounding tissue by compression. They are filled with fluid and may contain blood or pus. Upon autopsy, PKD kidneys look like they are filled with golf balls.

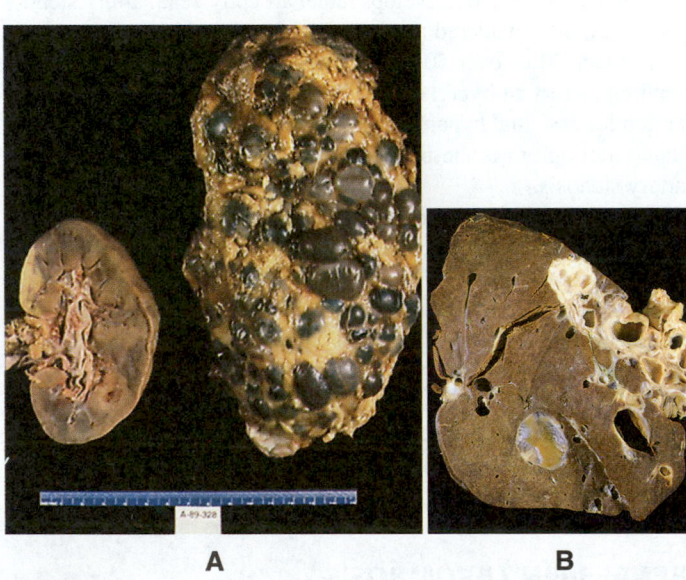

FIG. 46-7   **A,** Comparison of polycystic kidney with normal kidney. **B,** Cysts in the liver.

Clinical Manifestations

Early in the disease there are generally no symptoms. Symptoms appear when the cysts begin to enlarge. Often the first manifestations are hypertension, hematuria (from rupture of cysts), or a feeling of heaviness in the back, side, or abdomen. Sometimes the first manifestations are a UTI and/or urinary calculi. Chronic pain is one of the most common problems for people with PKD. In some people the pain can be constant and quite severe. On physical examination, palpable bilateral enlarged kidneys are often found (Fig. 46-8).

PKD is not just a kidney disorder. Other organs can be affected, including the liver, heart, and intestines. This results in liver cysts (Fig. 46-7, *B*), abnormal heart valves, aneurysms, and diverticulosis.

Diagnosis is based on clinical manifestations, family history, IVP, ultrasound (best screening measure), or CT scan. Usually the disease progresses to end-stage renal failure, although some individuals have relatively mild disease and die from unrelated problems. Loss of kidney function to the point of end-stage renal disease occurs by age 60 in 50% of patients.[36]

Collaborative Care

There is no specific treatment for PKD. A major aim of treatment is to prevent infections of the urinary tract and/or to treat them with appropriate antibiotics if they occur. Nephrectomy may be neces-

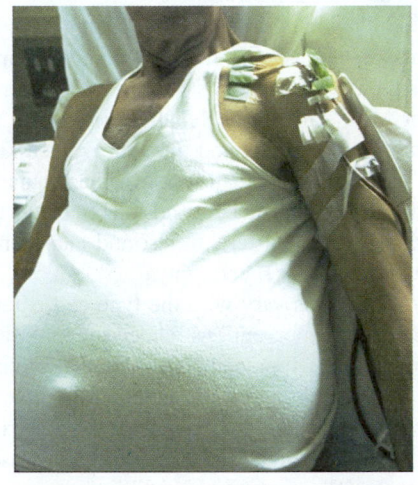

FIG. 46-8   Male with a 24-pound polycystic kidney.

GENETICS IN CLINICAL PRACTICE
Polycystic Kidney Disease

	Adult	Child
Genetic basis	• Autosomal dominant	• Autosomal recessive
Incidence	• 1 in 400-500	• 1 in 10,000-40,000
Gene location	• *ADPKD1* gene on chromosome 16 (about 18%) and *ADPKD2* on chromosome 4 (about 20%). *ADPKD3* gene location not identified.	• *PKHD1* gene on chromosome 6
Genetic testing	• DNA testing available	• DNA testing available*
Age of onset	• Third to fourth decade of life	• Infancy or childhood
Clinical implications	• Multisystem involvement • Systemic hypertension occurs in 60%-80% of patients • Families at risk should be screened	• Up to 30%-50% of affected newborns die shortly after birth. • If infant survives the newborn period, chances of survival are good but about one third will need dialysis or transplantation by age 10.

*Genetic testing is also available on fertilized embryos prior to implantation. This allows embryos free of the disorder to be placed into the uterus; embryos that test positive can be destroyed.

sary if pain, bleeding, or infection becomes a chronic, serious problem. Kidney transplant remains the only cure.

When the patient begins to experience progressive renal failure, the interventions are determined by the remaining renal function. Nursing measures are those used for management of end-stage renal disease (see Chapter 47). They include diet modification, fluid restriction, drugs (e.g., antihypertensives), assisting the patient to accept the chronic disease process, and assisting the patient and family to deal with financial concerns and other issues related to the hereditary nature of the disease.

The patient who has adult PKD often has children by the time the disease is diagnosed. The patient will need appropriate counseling regarding plans for having more children. In addition, genetic counseling resources should be provided for the children.

MEDULLARY CYSTIC DISEASE

Medullary cystic disease is a hereditary disorder that occurs in two forms. The *autosomal recessive form* is associated with renal failure before age 20; the *autosomal dominant form* is associated with renal failure after age 20. Most cysts are located in the medulla. The kidneys are asymmetric in shape and are significantly scarred. There are defects in the concentration ability of the kidneys. Polyuria, progressive renal failure, severe anemia, metabolic acidosis, and poor sodium conservation are common. Hypertension can be a terminal event. Genetic counseling may be helpful in family planning. Treatment measures are those related to end-stage renal disease (see Chapter 47).

ALPORT SYNDROME

Alport syndrome is also known as *chronic hereditary nephritis.* Two forms of the disease exist: (1) classic Alport syndrome, which is inherited as a sex-linked disorder with hematuria, sensorineural deafness, and deformities of the anterior surface of the lens, and (2) nonclassic Alport syndrome, which is inherited as an autosomal trait that causes hematuria but not deafness or lens deformities. Men are affected earlier and more severely than women. The disease is often diagnosed in the first decade of life. The basic defect is a mutation in a gene for collagen that results in altered synthesis of the GBM. The patient most commonly has hematuria and progressive uremia. Treatment is supportive. Corticosteroids and cytotoxic drugs are not effective. The disease does not recur after kidney transplantation.

Renal Involvement in Metabolic and Connective Tissue Diseases

Various metabolic and connective tissue disease processes may have an effect on renal function. The pathophysiologic effects on the renal parenchyma are not always specific to each process. The clinical course of renal involvement is that of chronic progressive nephropathy, which can result in uremia and death. Management includes treatment of the primary disorder along with symptomatic relief of renal involvement. If renal involvement progresses to end-stage renal disease, management includes dialysis or transplantation (see Chapter 47). Nursing interventions include teaching the patient about the primary disease process, the renal involvement, and the resulting need to comply with dietary and fluid restrictions and drug regimens.

Diabetic nephropathy is the primary cause of end-stage renal failure in the United States. Diabetes mellitus may affect the kid-

neys in several ways. Microangiopathic changes in diabetes consist of diffuse glomerulosclerosis, involving thickening of the GBM, and nodular glomerulosclerosis (Kimmelstiel-Wilson syndrome), which is characterized by nodular lesions. Nodular glomerulosclerosis is reasonably specific for type 1 diabetes mellitus. The diabetic patient prone to glomerulonephropathy (e.g., the presence of trace proteinuria or retinopathy) requires careful monitoring of glucose levels and insulin requirements. (Diabetes mellitus is discussed in Chapter 49.)

Gout is a syndrome of acute attacks of arthritis caused by hyperuricemia (see Chapter 65). Monosodium urate crystals deposited in joints are responsible for the syndrome. Renal disease may develop as a result of damage caused by deposition of uric acid crystals in the renal interstitium and tubules.

Amyloidosis is a group of disorders manifested by impaired organ function from the infiltration of tissues with a hyaline substance (amyloid). The hyaline bodies consist largely of protein. Kidney involvement is common in amyloidosis. Proteinuria is often the first clinical manifestation.

Systemic lupus erythematosus is a connective tissue disorder characterized by the involvement of several tissues and organs, particularly the joints, skin, and kidneys. (Systemic lupus erythematosus is discussed in Chapter 65.) Clinical manifestations of lupus nephritis are similar to those of other forms of glomerulonephritis. Renal failure frequently occurs in systemic lupus erythematosus and has a poor prognosis.

Systemic sclerosis (scleroderma) is a disease of unknown etiology characterized by widespread alterations of connective tissue and by vascular lesions in many organs (see Chapter 65). In the kidney, vascular lesions are associated with fibrosis. An immune complex mechanism has been postulated as a possible etiologic factor. The severity of renal involvement varies. The patient who develops severe renal lesions has a poor prognosis.

Urinary Tract Tumors

KIDNEY CANCER

In the United States, over 39,000 new cases of kidney cancer are diagnosed each year and about 12,800 people die from kidney cancer.[37] **Kidney cancers** arise from the cortex or pelvis (and calyces). Tumors arising from both areas may be benign or malignant. However, malignant tumors are more frequent. Renal cell carcinoma (adenocarcinoma) is the most common type (Fig. 46-9). Adenocarcinoma occurs twice as often in men as in women and is typically discovered when the person is 50 to 70 years old. Cigarette smoking is the most significant risk factor for the development of renal cell carcinoma. An increased incidence has also been seen in first-degree relatives. Other risk factors are obesity, hypertension, and exposure to asbestos, cadmium, and gasoline.[37] The risk is also increased for those who have acquired cystic disease of the kidney associated with end-stage renal disease (see Chapter 47).

Clinical Manifestations and Diagnostic Studies

There are no characteristic early symptoms, and many patients with kidney cancer go undetected due to lack of symptoms. Many kidney cancers are diagnosed as incidental findings on imaging studies used to evaluate symptoms for often unrelated conditions. Kidney tumors can cause symptoms by compressing, stretching, or invading structures near or within the kidney. The most common

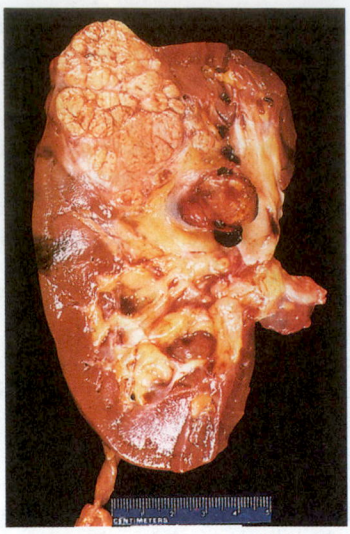

FIG. 46-9   Renal cell carcinoma. Cross section shows yellowish cancer in one pole of kidney. The tumor also involves the dilated thrombosed renal vein.

TABLE 46-15	Robson's System of Staging Renal Carcinoma
Stage	**Description**
I	Limitation to renal capsule
II	Spreading to perirenal fat but confined within fascia; includes metastasis to adrenal gland
III	Regional lymph node involvement, tumor thrombus in renal vein or vena cava, involvement of renal vein or vena cava
IV	Presence of distant metastases

presenting manifestations are hematuria, flank pain, and a palpable mass in the flank or abdomen. Other clinical manifestations include weight loss, fever, hypertension, and anemia. The most common sites of metastases include the lungs, liver, and long bones. About 30% of patients have metastasis at the time of diagnosis. Local extension of kidney cancer into the renal vein and vena cava is common (see Fig. 46-9).

Several studies are used to diagnose kidney cancer. IVP with nephrotomography is the primary examination by which most masses are detected and evaluated. Ultrasound examinations have improved the ability to differentiate between a solid mass or tumor and a cyst, which is important as the majority (90%) of masses detected on imaging are cysts. Angiography, percutaneous needle aspiration, CT, and MRI are also used in the diagnosis of renal tumors. Small renal tumors are found earlier because of the increased use of CT scans and MRI. Radionuclide isotope scanning is used to detect metastases.

NURSING and COLLABORATIVE MANAGEMENT
KIDNEY CANCER

Robson's system of staging renal carcinoma is presented in Table 46-15. The treatment of choice is a radical nephrectomy for patients with stage I or II tumors and selected stage III tumors. It can be performed by the standard open approach or laparoscopically. Radical nephrectomy is the removal of the kidney, adrenal gland, surrounding fascia, part of the ureter, and draining lymph nodes.[38] (The pre- and postoperative care following nephrectomy is discussed later in this chapter on p. 1188.) Radiation therapy is used palliatively in inoperable cases and when there are metastases to bone or lungs.

Chemotherapy using 5-fluorouracil (5-FU), floxuridine (FUDR), and gemcitabine (Gemzar), is used to treat metastatic disease. However, renal cell carcinoma is refractory to most chemotherapy drugs. Biologic therapy, including α-interferon and interleukin-2 (IL-2), is used in the treatment of metastatic disease.[37] (The use of α-interferon and IL-2 is discussed in Chapter 16.) Targeted therapy, including sunitinib (Sutent) and sorafenib (Nexavar), is used to treat metastatic kidney cancer. Sunitinib is

a tyrosine kinase inhibitor that works at multiple targets to deprive tumor cells of the blood and nutrients needed for growth. Sorafenib targets enzymes involved in cancer growth and formation of blood vessels that supply nutrients to cancer cells (see Chapter 16, Fig. 16-21, Table 16-17).

Patients with early-stage kidney cancer can expect a 60% to 70% 5-year survival after undergoing radical nephrectomy. The 5-year survival rate for patients with metastatic disease is only 3% to 10% at 5 years. However, patients with metastatic disease often remain stable for a prolonged period of time.

BLADDER CANCER

About 61,000 new cases of bladder cancer are diagnosed annually, and about 13,000 deaths related to bladder cancer occur every year. Bladder cancer accounts for nearly 1 in every 20 cancers diagnosed in the United States.[39] The most frequent malignant tumor of the urinary tract is transitional cell carcinoma of the bladder. Most bladder tumors are papillomatous growths within the bladder (Fig. 46-10, *A*). Cancer of the bladder is most common between the ages of 60 and 70 years and is at least three times as common in men as in women. Risk factors for bladder cancer include cigarette smoking, exposure to dyes used in the rubber and cable industries, and chronic abuse of phenacetin-containing analgesics. Women treated with radiation for cervical cancer and patients receiving cyclophosphamide (Cytoxan) also have increased risk, but the reason is unknown.

Individuals with chronic, recurrent renal calculi (often bladder) and chronic lower UTIs have an increased risk of squamous cell cancer of the bladder. Patients who have indwelling catheters for long periods can also develop bladder cancer.

Clinical Manifestations and Diagnostic Studies

Microscopic or gross, painless hematuria (chronic or intermittent) is the most common clinical finding. Bladder irritability with dysuria, frequency, and urgency may also occur. When cancer is suspected, urine specimens for cytology can be obtained to determine the presence of neoplastic or atypical cells. Exfoliated cells from the epithelial surface of the bladder can readily be detected in voided specimens. Other urine tests assess for specific factors associated with bladder cancer, such as bladder tumor antigens. Bladder cancers can be detected using IVP, ultrasound, CT, or MRI. However, the presence of cancer is confirmed by cystoscopy and biopsy. Cystoscopy is the most reliable test for detecting the presence of bladder tumors.[40]

The clinical staging of carcinoma of the bladder is determined by the depth of invasion of the bladder wall and surrounding tissue. The Jewett-Strong-Marshall classification system broadly classifies bladder cancer as superficial (carcinoma in situ [CIS], O, A), invasive (B1, B2, C), or metastatic (D1 to D4) disease. Pathologic grading systems are also used to classify the malignant potential of tumor

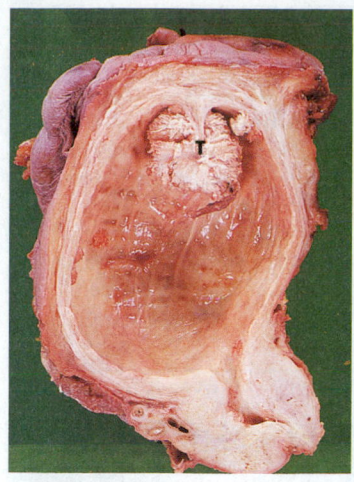 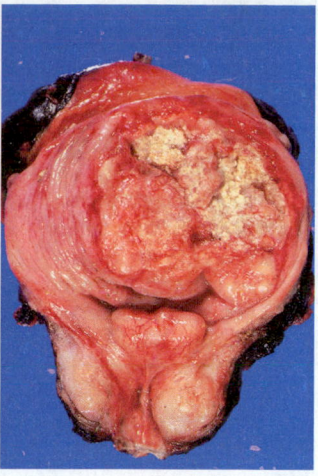

FIG. 46-10 **A,** A papillary transitional cell carcinoma is seen arising from the dome of the bladder as a cauliflower-like lesion. **B,** Opened bladder showing a bladder cancer at an advanced stage. The yellow areas represent ulcerations and necrosis.

TABLE 46-16	COLLABORATIVE CARE Bladder Cancer

Diagnostic
History and physical examination
Urinalysis
Urine cytology studies
Intravenous pyelogram (IVP)
Cystoscopy with biopsy
Ultrasound
CT scan

Collaborative Therapy
Surgical treatment
- Transurethral resection with fulguration
- Laser photocoagulation
- Open loop resection with fulguration
- Cystectomy (segmental, partial, or radical)

Radiation therapy
Intravesical immunotherapy
- Bacille Calmette-Guérin (BCG)
- α-interferon (Roferon-A, Intron A)

Intravesical chemotherapy
- thiotepa (Thioplex)
- valrubicin (Valstar)

Systemic chemotherapy

CT, Computed tomography.

cells, indicating a scale from well-differentiated to anaplastic categories (see Fig. 46-10, *B*). Eighty percent of bladder tumors are "superficial," meaning they do not invade the bladder wall. These low-stage, low-grade bladder cancers are the most responsive to treatment that includes instillation of intravesical chemotherapy and transurethral resection of the bladder tumor (TURBT).[39] Although patients with superficial tumors are more easily cured, periodic surveillance is important as two thirds of patients have tumor recurrence with 5 years and nearly 95% have recurrence by 15 years.

NURSING *and* COLLABORATIVE MANAGEMENT
BLADDER CANCER

Collaborative care of bladder cancer is outlined in Table 46-16.

■ *Surgical Therapy*

Surgical therapies include a variety of procedures. *Transurethral resection with fulguration* (electrocautery) is used for the diagnosis and treatment of superficial lesions with a low recurrence rate. This procedure is also used to control bleeding in the patient who is a poor operative risk or who has advanced tumors. With this technique, the tumor mass is excised by means of a blade inserted through the cystoscope. The remaining portions of the tumor are cauterized.

A second technique, *laser photocoagulation,* is also used to treat superficial bladder cancers. This procedure can be repeated a number of times for recurrence. The advantages of laser include bloodless destruction of the lesion, minimal risk of perforation, and lack of need for a urinary catheter. The primary disadvantage is destruction of the tumor, so pathologic evaluation for grading and staging cannot be completed.

A third technique used is *open loop resection* (snaring of polyp types of lesion) *with fulguration.* It is used for the control of bleeding, for large superficial tumors, and for multiple lesions. Treatment of large lesions entails a segmental resection of the bladder (*segmental cystectomy*).

Postoperative management of the patient who has had any of these surgical procedures includes instructions to drink a large volume of fluid each day for the first week following the procedure and to avoid intake of alcoholic beverages. The patient is

taught to self-monitor the urine. It is anticipated to be pink during the first several days after the procedure, but it should not be bright red or contain blood clots. Approximately 7 to 10 days following tumor resection or ablation, the patient may observe dark red or rust-colored flecks in the urine. These are anticipated and represent scabs from the healing tumor resection sites. Opioid analgesics may be required for a brief period after the procedure, along with stool softeners. The patient can be encouraged to take a 15- to 20-minute sitz bath 2 to 3 times a day to promote muscle relaxation and to reduce the risk of urinary retention. The nurse should also help the patient and family cope with fears about cancer, surgery, and sexuality and should emphasize the importance of regular follow-up care. Follow-up cystoscopies are required every 3 to 6 months for 3 years and at least yearly thereafter.[41]

When the tumor is invasive or when it involves the trigone (the area where the ureters insert into the bladder) and the patient is free from metastasis beyond the pelvic area, a partial or radical cystectomy with urinary diversion is the treatment of choice (see the following section on urinary diversion). A *partial cystectomy* includes resection of that portion of the bladder wall containing the tumor, along with a margin of normal tissue. A *radical cystectomy* involves removal of the bladder, prostate, and seminal vesicles in men and the bladder, uterus, cervix, urethra, and ovaries in women.

■ *Radiation Therapy and Chemotherapy*

Radiation therapy is used with cystectomy or as the primary therapy when the cancer is inoperable or when surgery is refused. Increasingly, radiation therapy is being combined with systemic chemotherapy. Sometimes combination systemic chemotherapy is used for bladder cancer, usually preoperatively or before radiation therapy, or is used to treat distant metastases. Chemotherapy drugs used in treating invasive bladder cancer include cisplatin (Platinol), vinblastine (Velban), doxorubicin (Adriamycin), and methotrexate (Folex).

■ *Intravesical Therapy*

Chemotherapy with local instillation of chemotherapeutic or immune-stimulating agents can be delivered directly into the bladder by a urethral catheter.[39] Protocols vary, but *intravesical therapy* is usually initiated at weekly intervals for 6 to 12 weeks. The chemotherapeutic agents are instilled directly into the patient's bladder and retained for about 2 hours. The patient's bladder must be empty prior to instillation. The patient's position may be changed every 15 minutes for maximum contact in all areas of the bladder, especially if the tumor occurred on the bladder dome. The use of maintenance therapy after the initial induction regimen may be beneficial.

BCG, a weakened strain of *Mycobacterium bovis,* is the treatment of choice for carcinoma in situ. BCG stimulates the immune system rather than acting directly on cancer cells in the bladder. When BCG fails, α-interferon in addition to BCG may be used. Other treatments that can be used when BCG fails include thiotepa (Thioplex), an alkylating agent, and valrubicin (Valstar), an antineoplastic antibiotic.[42]

Most patients have irritative voiding symptoms and hemorrhagic cystitis following intravesical therapy. Thiotepa can significantly reduce WBC and platelet counts in some individuals when absorbed into the circulation from the bladder wall. BCG may cause flu-like symptoms, increased urinary frequency, hematuria, or systemic infection. Other side effects usually associated with chemotherapy, such as nausea, vomiting, and hair loss, are not experienced with intravesical chemotherapy.

Nursing responsibilities include encouraging the patient to increase the daily fluid intake and to quit smoking, assessing the patient for secondary UTI, and stressing the need for routine urologic follow-up.[41] The patient may have fears or concerns about sexual activity or bladder function that will need to be addressed.

Urinary Incontinence and Retention

Urinary incontinence (UI) is an uncontrolled leakage of urine.[43] Approximately 17 million people living in the United States suffer from UI. Among young adult to middle-aged women, prevalence is 30% to 40% and it increases to 30% to 50% in elderly women. In contrast, UI in men tends to be considerably lower, ranging from 1% to 5% in young adult men and increasing to 9% to 34% in elderly men.[44] The prevalence of incontinence is higher among older women and older men, but it is not a natural consequence of aging. Although UI has traditionally been viewed as a social or hygienic problem, it is now known to affect quality of life, as well as contribute to serious health problems in older adults.[43]

Anything that interferes with bladder or urethral sphincter control can result in UI. Causes can include confusion or depression, infection, atrophic vaginitis, urinary retention, restricted mobility, fecal impaction, or drugs. (Table 46-17 presents a list of drugs that can affect the lower urinary tract.) Patients may have more than one type of incontinence,[43,45] as described in Table 46-18.

Urinary retention is the inability to empty the bladder despite micturition or the accumulation of urine in the bladder because of an inability to urinate.[46] In certain cases, it is associated with urinary leakage or postvoid dribbling, called *overflow UI. Acute urinary retention* is the total inability to pass urine via micturition; it is a medical emergency. *Chronic urinary reten-*

TABLE 46-17 **DRUG THERAPY**
Drugs Influencing Lower Urinary Tract Function

Medication Class/Examples	Effect
Alcohol	Polyuria, frequency, urgency, sedation, delirium
α-Adrenergic receptor agonists (pseudoephedrine [Sudafed], ephedrine)	Urethral constriction and urinary retention (males)
α-Adrenergic receptor antagonists (prazosin [Minipress], terazosin [Hytrin], doxazosin [Cardura])	Urethral relaxation and stress urinary incontinence (SUI) in females
ACE inhibitors (captopril [Capoten], lisinopril [Zestril], enalapril [Vasotec])	Cough triggering stress urinary incontinence
Anticholinergics (H₁-antihistamines, antiparkinsonian agents)	Urinary retention, overflow incontinence, fecal impaction
Tricyclic antidepressants	Anticholinergic effect, α-adrenergic receptor antagonist effect
β-Adrenergic receptor antagonists (propranolol [Inderal], metoprolol [Toprol, Lopressor], atenolol [Tenormin])	Urinary retention
Calcium channel blockers (verapamil [Calan], diltiazem [Cardizem], nifedipine [Procardia])	Urinary retention, fecal impaction
Opioids	Urinary retention, fecal impaction, sedation, delirium
Sedative-hypnotics	Sedation, delirium, muscle relaxation
Diuretics (loop diuretics such as furosemide [Lasix])	Polyuria, frequency, urgency
Methylxanthines (caffeine, theophylline)	Polyuria, bladder irritation
Neuroleptics (thioridazine [Mellaril], chlorpromazine [Thorazine])	Anticholinergic effect, sedation

ACE, Angiotensin-converting enzyme.

| TABLE 46-18 | Types of Urinary Incontinence |

Type and Description	Causes	Treatment
Stress Incontinence* Sudden increase in intraabdominal pressure causes involuntary passage of urine. Can occur during coughing, laughing, sneezing, or physical activities such as heavy lifting, exercising. Leakage usually in small amounts and may not be daily.	Found most commonly in women with relaxed pelvic floor musculature (from delivery, use of instrumentation during vaginal delivery, or multiple pregnancies). Structures of the female urethra atrophy when estrogen decreases. Prostate surgery for BPH or prostate cancer.	Pelvic floor muscle exercises (e.g., Kegel exercises), weight loss if patient is obese, cessation of smoking, topical estrogen products, external condom catheters or penile clamp in men, surgery Urethral inserts, patches, or bladder neck support devices (e.g., incontinence pessary) to correct underlying problem
Urge Incontinence* Condition occurs randomly when involuntary urination is preceded by urinary urgency. Seen with overactive bladder symptoms of urgency and frequency. Leakage is periodic but frequent and usually in large amounts. Nocturnal frequency and incontinence are common.	Condition is caused by uncontrolled contraction or overactivity of detrusor muscle. Bladder escapes central inhibition and contracts reflexively. Conditions include central nervous system disorders (e.g., cerebrovascular disease, Alzheimer's disease, brain tumor, Parkinson's disease), bladder disorders (e.g., carcinoma in situ, radiation effects, interstitial cystitis), interference with spinal inhibitory pathways (e.g., malignant growth in spinal cord, spondylosis), and bladder outlet obstruction, conditions of unknown etiology.	Treatment of underlying cause, behavioral interventions including bladder retraining with urge suppression, decrease in dietary irritants, bowel regularity, and pelvic floor muscle exercises Anticholinergic drugs (e.g., oxybutynin [Ditropan XL, Oxytrol], tolterodine [Detrol, Detrol LA], trospium chloride [Sanctura], solifenacin [VESIcare], and darifenacin [Enablex]); imipramine (Tofranil) at bedtime; calcium channel blockers External condom catheters Vaginal estrogen creams
Overflow Incontinence Condition occurs when the pressure of urine in overfull bladder overcomes sphincter control. Leakage of small amounts of urine is frequent throughout the day and night. Urination may also occur frequently in small amounts. Bladder remains distended and is usually palpable.	Disorder is caused by bladder or urethral outlet obstruction (bladder neck obstruction, urethral stricture, pelvic organ prolapse) or by underactive detrusor muscle caused by myogenic or neurogenic factors (e.g., herniated disk, diabetic neuropathy). May also occur after anesthesia and surgery (especially procedures such as hemorrhoidectomy, herniorrhaphy, cystoscopy). Neurogenic bladder (flaccid type).	Urinary catheterization to decompress bladder Implementation of Credé's or Valsalva maneuver α-adrenergic blocker (doxazosin [Cardura], terazosin [Hytrin], tamsulosin [Flomax], alfuzosin [Uroxatral]) 5α-reductase inhibitors (e.g., finasteride [Proscar]) to decrease outlet resistance bethanechol (Urecholine) to enhance bladder contractions Intravaginal device such as a pessary to support prolapse Intermittent catheterization Surgery to correct underlying problem
Reflex Incontinence Condition occurs when no warning or stress precedes periodic involuntary urination. Urination is frequent, is moderate in volume, and occurs equally during the day and night.	Spinal cord lesion above S2 interferes with central nervous system inhibition. Disorder results in detrusor hyperreflexia and interferes with pathways coordinating detrusor contraction and sphincter relaxation.	Treatment of underlying cause Bladder decompression to prevent ureteral reflux and hydronephrosis Intermittent self-catheterization diazepam (Valium) or baclofen (Lioresal) to relax external sphincter Prophylactic antibiotics Surgical sphincterotomy
Incontinence After Trauma or Surgery Vesicovaginal or urethrovaginal fistula may occur in women. Alteration in continence control in men involves proximal urethral sphincter (bladder neck and prostatic urethra) and distal urethral sphincter (external striated muscle).	Fistulas may occur during pregnancy, after delivery of baby, as a result of hysterectomy or invasive cancer of cervix, or after radiation therapy. Incontinence is found as postoperative complication after transurethral, perineal, or retropubic prostatectomy.	Surgery to correct fistula Urinary diversion surgery to bypass urethra and bladder External condom catheter Penile clamp Placement of artificial implantable sphincter
Functional Incontinence Loss of urine resulting from cognitive, functional, or environmental factors.	Elderly often have problems that affect balance and mobility.	Modifications of environment or care plan that facilitate regular, easy access to toilet and promote patient safety (e.g., better lighting, ambulatory assistance equipment, clothing alterations, timed voiding, different toileting equipment)

BPH, Benign prostatic hyperplasia.

*Patients can have a combination of stress and urge incontinence that is referred to as mixed incontinence.

tion is defined as incomplete bladder emptying despite urination. The postvoid residual (PVR) volumes in patients with chronic urinary retention vary widely. Normal PVR is between 50 and 75 ml, and findings over 100 ml indicate the need to repeat the measurement. An abnormal PVR in the elderly patient is a measurement of ≥200 ml obtained on two separate occasions and requires further evaluation.[47] Even smaller volumes may justify evaluation when the patient has lower urinary tract symptoms suggestive of UTIs or these small volumes occur in a context of recurring UTIs.

Urinary retention is caused by two different dysfunctions of the urinary system: bladder outlet obstruction and deficient detrusor (bladder muscle) contraction strength. Obstruction leads to urinary retention when the blockage is sufficiently severe so that the bladder can no longer evacuate its contents despite a detrusor contraction. A common cause of obstruction in men is an enlarged prostate. Deficient detrusor contraction strength leads to urinary retention when the muscle is no longer able to contract with enough force or for a sufficient period of time to completely empty the bladder.

Common causes of deficient detrusor contraction strength are neurologic diseases affecting sacral segments 2, 3, and 4; long-standing diabetes mellitus; overdistention; chronic alcoholism; and drugs (e.g., anticholinergic drugs).

Diagnostic Studies

The basic evaluation for UI and urinary retention includes a focused history, physical assessment, and a bladder log or voiding record whenever possible.[48] Information should be obtained on the onset of UI, factors that provoke urinary leakage, and associated conditions. The nurse should pay special attention to factors known to produce transient UI, particularly when a relatively sudden onset of urine loss is reported. The physical examination begins with an assessment of general health and functional issues associated with urinary function, including mobility, dexterity, and cognitive function. A pelvic examination includes careful inspection of the perineal skin for signs of erosion or rashes related to UI and existence of pelvic organ prolapse. Local innervation and pelvic floor muscle strength should also be evaluated, including a digital examination of the pelvic floor muscle to determine weakness or tension. Whenever possible, the patient is asked to keep a bladder log or voiding diary documenting the timing of urinations, episodes of urinary leakage, and frequency of nocturia for a period of 1 to 7 days.[49] This record can be kept by nursing staff if the person is in an inpatient or long-term care facility.

A urinalysis is used to identify possible factors contributing to transient UI or urinary retention (e.g., UTI, diabetes mellitus). A PVR urine must be measured in the patient undergoing evaluation for urinary retention and UI. The PVR volume is obtained by asking the patient to urinate, followed by catheterization within a relatively brief period (preferably 10 to 20 minutes). Alternatively, an ultrasound can be used to estimate the residual volume. The use of a portable ultrasound scanner (BladderScan) permits noninvasive identification of clinically significant residual urine with an accuracy rate of more than 90%. Ultrasound scanners avoid catheterization with its associated discomfort and risk of UTI. They are being used by bedside nurses as the standard of care in all care settings to noninvasively diagnose, treat, and manage bladder disorders.[47]

Urodynamic testing is indicated in selected cases of UI and urinary retention. Imaging studies of the upper urinary tract (e.g., ultrasound, IVP) are obtained when retention or UI is associated with UTIs or when there is evidence of upper urinary tract involvement.[48]

Collaborative Care: Urinary Incontinence

An estimated 80% of incontinence can be cured or significantly improved. Transient, reversible factors are corrected initially, followed by management of the type of UI (see Table 46-18). In general, less invasive treatments are attempted before more invasive methods (e.g., surgery) are used. Nevertheless, the choice of the initial treatment is highly individualized and based on patient preference, the type and severity of UI, and associated anatomic defects.

Several behavioral therapies may be employed to improve urinary incontinence.[50-52] These interventions are outlined in Table 46-19. Pelvic floor muscle training (Kegel exercises) is used to manage stress, urge, or mixed UI (Table 46-20). Biofeedback is used to assist the patient to identify, isolate, contract, and relax the pelvic muscles (see the Complementary and Alternative Therapies box below).

Drug Therapy. Drug therapy varies according to the UI type (Table 46-21). Drugs have a very limited role in the management of stress UI. α-Adrenergic agonists can be used to increase bladder sphincter tone and urethral resistance. Unfortunately, they exert a limited beneficial effect, and they are associated with adverse effects including exacerbation of hypertension and tachycardia. Drugs play a more central role in the management of urge or reflex UI. Anticholinergic drugs and newer, more specific, muscarinic receptor antagonists relax the bladder muscle and inhibit overactive detrusor contractions.[53] There are several preparations of these drugs, including immediate and extended-release tolterodine (Detrol, Detrol LA) and immediate, extended-release, and transdermal oxybutynin (Ditropan XL, Oxytrol transdermal system), twice-daily trospium chloride (Sanctura), extended-release solifenacin (VESIcare), and darifenacin (Enablex). Efficacy is similar for these medications, and side effects include dry mouth, dry eyes, constipation, blurred vision, and somnolence.

Drug Alert - *Tolterodine (Detrol)*
- *Overdosage can result in severe anticholinergic effects, including GI cramping, diaphoresis, blurred vision, and urinary urgency.*

COMPLEMENTARY AND ALTERNATIVE THERAPIES
Biofeedback for Urinary Incontinence

Clinical Uses
Kegel exercises help to strengthen the pelvic floor muscles. Biofeedback instruments help to isolate muscle groups in the pelvis.

Effects
Sensors for biofeedback are placed in the vagina or rectum or on the skin outside of the anus. These sensors measure electrical signals produced when pelvic floor muscles contract. Biofeedback training develops an awareness of and control of the pelvic floor muscles.

Nursing Implications
If done correctly, pelvic floor exercise is effective treatment for mild to moderate urinary incontinence and other conditions related to pelvic floor weakness or tension. Unfortunately, many women do not do these exercises correctly. Biofeedback is a technique to make sure that these exercises are done correctly. Most insurance companies cover the cost of biofeedback.

TABLE 46-19	Interventions for Urinary Incontinence

Intervention	Description
Lifestyle Modifications	Self-management strategies to reduce or eliminate risk factors, including: 　Smoking cessation 　Weight reduction 　Good bowel regimen 　Reduction of bladder irritants such as caffeine 　Fluid modifications for those with urge incontinence
Scheduling Voiding Regimens	
• Timed voiding	Toileting on a fixed schedule (typically every 2-3 hr during waking hours).
• Habit retraining	Scheduled toileting with adjustments of voiding intervals (longer or shorter) based on the individual's voiding pattern.
• Prompted voiding	Scheduled toileting that requires prompts to void from a caregiver (typically every 3 hr). Used in conjunction with operant conditioning techniques for rewarding individuals for maintaining continence and appropriate toileting.
• Bladder retraining and urge-suppression strategies	Scheduled toileting with progressive voiding intervals. Includes teaching of urge-control strategies using relaxation and distraction techniques, self-monitoring, use of reinforcement techniques, and other strategies such as conscious contraction of pelvic floor muscles.
Pelvic Floor Muscle Rehabilitation	
• Pelvic floor muscle (Kegel) exercises or training	See Table 46-20.
• Vaginal weight training	Active retention of increasing vaginal weights at least twice a day. Typically used in combination with pelvic floor muscle exercises.
• Biofeedback	See Complementary and Alternative Therapies box on the facing page.
• Electrical stimulation	Application of low-voltage electric current to sacral and pudendal afferent fibers through vaginal, anal, or surface electrodes. Used to inhibit bladder overactivity and improve awareness, contractility, and efficiency of pelvic muscle contraction.
Anti-Incontinence Devices	
• Intravaginal support devices (pessaries and bladder neck support prostheses)	Devices support bladder neck, relieve minor pelvic organ prolapse, and change pressure transmission to the urethra.
• Intraurethral occlusive device (urethral plug)	Single-use device that is worn in the urethra to provide mechanical obstruction to prevent urine leakage. Removed for voiding.
• Penile compression device	Mechanical fixed compression applied to the penis to prevent any flow or leakage via the urethra. Must be released hourly to void.
Containment Devices	
• External collection devices	External catheter (condom) systems (i.e., penile sheaths) direct urine into a drainage bag. Most commonly used by men.
• Absorbent products	Variety of reusable and disposable pads and pant systems.

Surgical Therapy. Surgical techniques also vary according to the type of UI.[54] Surgical correction of stress UI may reposition the urethra and/or create a backboard of support or otherwise stabilize the urethra and bladder neck to be more receptive to changes in intraabdominal pressure. Another technique for stress UI augments the urethral resistance of the intrinsic sphincter unit with a sling or periurethral injectables.[45] Consensus as to the best surgical procedure is lacking. Few data are available on complications, treatment of complications, or frequency and effectiveness of additional treatment. Retropubic colposuspension and pubovaginal sling placement, with overall cure rates in the 80% to 90% range, appear to be most effective overall. Typically, both procedures are performed through low transverse incisions. Complications specific to the retropubic suspensions include postoperative voiding dysfunction, urgency, and vaginal prolapse.

Placement of a suburethral sling, using autologous fascia, cadaveric fascia, or a synthetic material, is also used to correct stress UI in women. Complications include vascular and bowel injury, urinary retention, mesh/sling erosion, and infection, urgency, and bladder perforation. Suburethral slings are less invasive outpatient procedures that have success rates comparable to colposuspensions/slings and are associated with a more rapid return to normal

activity. An artificial urethral sphincter can be used in men with intrinsic sphincter deficiency and severe stress UI.

Alternatively, one of several bulking agents can be injected underneath the mucosa of the urethra to correct stress UI in women or men.[54] Bulking agents include glutaraldehyde cross-linked bovine collagen (GAX collagen), small silicone beads (Durasphere), or polytetrafluoroethylene (Teflon). Because of the risk of migration of Teflon particles, GAX collagen or Durasphere injections are most commonly used today. Although treatment with suburethral compounds avoids the risk associated with open surgery, reinjection after a period of several years is typically required.

NURSING MANAGEMENT
URINARY INCONTINENCE

The nurse must recognize both the physical and the emotional problems associated with UI. The patient's dignity, privacy, and feelings of self-worth must be maintained or enhanced. This often includes a two-step approach comprising containment devices to manage existing urinary leakage and a definitive plan of management designed to reduce or resolve the factors leading to UI.

TABLE 46-20	*PATIENT TEACHING GUIDE*
	Pelvic Floor Muscle or Kegel Exercises

What Is the Pelvic Floor Muscle?

Your pelvic floor muscle provides support for your bladder and rectum and, in women, the vagina and the uterus. If it weakens or is damaged, it cannot support these organs and their position can change. This causes problems with the normal bladder and rectal function. If you have a weak pelvic floor muscle, you might want to do special exercises to make the muscle stronger, prevent unwanted urine leakage, and lessen urinary urgency.

Woman

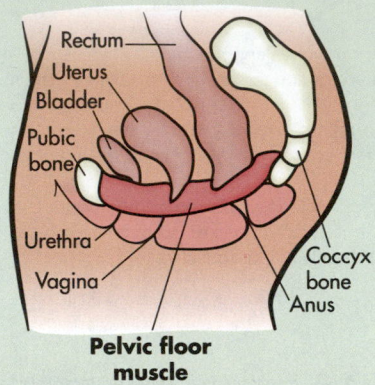

Man

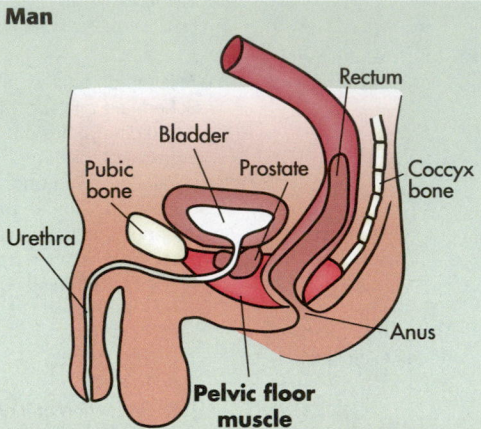

Finding the Pelvic Floor Muscle

Without tensing the muscles of your leg, buttocks, or abdomen, imagine that you are trying to control the passing of gas or pinching off a stool. Or imagine you are in an elevator full of people and you feel the urge to pass gas. What do you do? You tighten or pull in the ring of muscle around your rectum—your pelvic floor muscle. You should feel a lifting sensation in the area around the vagina or a pulling in of your rectum.

How to Do the Exercises

There are two different kinds of exercises—short squeezes and long squeezes.
1. To do the *short squeezes,* tighten your pelvic floor muscle quickly, squeeze hard for 2 seconds, and then relax the muscle. Also, when you have strong urinary urges, try to tighten your pelvic floor muscle quickly and hard several times in a row until the urge passes.
2. To do the *long squeezes,* tighten the muscle for 5 to 10 seconds before you relax.
Do both of these exercises 40 to 50 times each day.

When to Do These Exercises

You can do these exercises anytime and anywhere. You can do these exercises in any position, but sitting or lying down may be the easiest.

How Long Does It Take Before I Notice a Change?

After 4 to 6 weeks of doing these exercises, you should start to see less urine leakage and urinary urgency.

Courtesy of Diane Newman.

Management options are reviewed in Table 46-18. They include lifestyle interventions such as teaching the patient about consumption of an adequate volume of fluids and reduction or elimination of bladder irritants (particularly caffeine and alcohol) from the diet. The patient is advised to maintain a regular, flexible schedule of urination (usually every 2 to 3 hours while awake). In addition, patients are strongly advised to quit smoking because this habit increases the risk of stress UI. Patients should also be counseled about the relationship among constipation, UI, and urinary retention. Aggressive management of constipation, beginning with ensuring adequate fluid intake, increasing dietary fiber, light exercise, and judicious use of stool softeners, is recommended. (The management of constipation is discussed in Chapter 43.)

Behavioral treatments include scheduled voiding regimens (timed voiding, habit training, and prompted voiding), bladder retraining, and pelvic floor muscle training (see Table 46-19). A patient teaching guide for pelvic floor muscle exercise is found in Table 46-20.

The nurse should assess strategies the patient uses to contain UI and offer advice concerning alternative devices when indicated. When attempting to manage UI, many women use feminine hygiene pads, and many men and women use household products such as rags, paper towels, or folded toilet tissue.[6] Unfortunately, none of these products are adequately designed to wick urine away from the skin, prevent soiling of clothing, and reduce or eliminate odor. Instead, the nurse should provide information on products specifically designed to contain urine. For example, patients with mild to moderate UI often benefit from incontinent pads containing superabsorbent material, which is specifically designed to absorb many times its weight in water. Patients with higher volume urine loss or those with both urinary and fecal incontinence may benefit from disposable or reusable incontinence protective underwear, briefs, or pad/pant systems designed for more severe cases.

In inpatient or long-term care facilities, nursing management of UI includes maximizing toilet access. This assistance may take the form of offering the urinal or bedpan or assisting the patient to the bathroom every 2 to 3 hours or at scheduled times. The nurse ensures that patient toilets are accessible to patients and that adequate privacy occurs to allow effective urine elimination.

■ *Collaborative Care: Urinary Retention*

Behavioral therapies also may be used in the management of urinary retention.[46] Scheduled toileting and double voiding may be effective in chronic urinary retention with moderate PVR volumes. *Double voiding* is an attempt to maximize bladder evacuation. The patient is asked to urinate, sit on the toilet for 3 to 4 minutes, and urinate again before exiting the bathroom. For acute or chronic urinary retention, catheterization may be required. Ideally, intermittent catheterization is used to manage urinary retention. It allows the patient to remain free of an indwelling catheter with its associated risk of UTI and urethral irritation. Despite these potential advantages, an indwelling catheter is preferred in certain cases (e.g., the patient who is unwilling or unable to perform intermittent catheterization). An indwelling catheter is also used when urethral obstruction renders intermittent catheterization uncomfortable or unfeasible.

Drug Therapy. Several drugs may be administered to promote bladder evacuation. For the patient with obstruction at the level of the bladder neck, an α-adrenergic blocker may be prescribed. These drugs relax the smooth muscle of the bladder neck, the prostatic urethra, and possibly the dual-innervated rhabdosphincter, diminishing urethral resistance. Examples of α-adrenergic blocking agents are listed in Table 46-21. They are indicated in patients with BPH, bladder neck dyssynergia, or detrusor sphincter dyssynergia.

Surgical Therapy. Surgical interventions are often useful when managing urinary retention caused by obstruction. Transurethral or open surgical techniques are used to treat benign or malignant prostatic enlargement, bladder neck contracture, urethral strictures, or dyssynergia of the bladder neck in selected patients. Pelvic reconstruction using an abdominal or transvaginal approach can be used to correct bladder outlet obstruction in women with severe pelvic organ prolapse.

Unfortunately, surgery plays little role in the management of urinary retention caused by deficient detrusor contraction strength. Attempts to create a bladder stimulator (implanted device capable of stimulating micturition) have proved largely unsuccessful because of the difficulty in achieving a coordinated detrusor contraction associated with pelvic muscle and striated sphincter relaxation.

NURSING MANAGEMENT
URINARY RETENTION

Acute urinary retention is a medical emergency that requires prompt recognition and bladder drainage. The nurse should insert a catheter (as prescribed) unless otherwise directed. A catheter with a retention balloon is used in anticipation of the need for an indwelling catheter.

The patient with acute urinary retention (as well as the patient predisposed to these episodes) should be taught strategies to minimize risk, including avoiding intake of large volumes of fluid over a brief period. Instead, the patient is advised to drink small volumes throughout the day. The patient is advised to warm up before attempting urination when chilled and to avoid large volumes of alcohol intake because it leads to polyuria and a diminished awareness of the need to urinate until the bladder is distended. A patient who is unable to urinate is advised to drink a cup of coffee or brewed tea containing caffeine to create or maximize urinary urgency and to sit in a tub of warm water or take a warm shower and attempt to urinate while in the bathtub or shower. The patient can be reassured that he or she can easily bathe immediately following bladder evacuation. If this does not lead to successful urination, the patient is advised to seek immediate care.

Patients with chronic urinary retention may be managed by behavioral methods, indwelling or intermittent catheterization, surgery, or drugs.[46] Scheduled toileting and double voiding are the primary behavioral interventions used for chronic retention. Scheduled

TABLE 46-21	**DRUG THERAPY** Voiding Dysfunction*
Drug Class and Mechanism of Action	**Drug**
Muscarinic Receptor Antagonists and Anticholinergics	
Reduce overactive bladder contractions in urge urinary incontinence and overactive bladder	oxybutynin (Ditropan IR, Ditropan XL, Oxytrol transdermal system)
	tolterodine (Detrol, Detrol LA)
	trospium chloride (Sanctura)
	solifenacin (VESIcare)
	darifenacin (Enablex)
	hyoscyamine (Levsin, Levbid)
	dicyclomine (Bentyl)
	flavoxate (Urispas)
	propantheline (Pro-Banthīne)
α-Adrenergic Antagonists	
Reduce urethral sphincter resistance to urinary outflow	doxazosin (Cardura)
	terazosin (Hytrin)
	tamsulosin (Flomax)
	alfuzosin (Uroxatral)
5α-Reductase Inhibitors	
Androgen suppression that results in epithelial atrophy and a decrease in total prostate size	finasteride (Proscar)
	dutasteride (Avodart)
α-Adrenergic Agonists	
Increase urethral resistance	phenylpropanolamine
Tricyclic Antidepressants	
Reduce sensory urgency and burning pain of interstitial cystitis	imipramine (Tofranil)
Reduce overactive bladder contractions	amitriptyline (Elavil)
Calcium Channel Blockers	
Reduce smooth muscle contraction strength	nifedipine (Adalat)
May reduce burning pain of interstitial cystitis	diltiazem (Cardizem)
	verapamil (Calan, Isoptin)
Hormone Replacement Therapy	
Local application reduces urethral irritation and increases host defenses against UTI	Estrogen cream (Premarin, Estrace)
	Estrogen vaginal ring (Estring)
	Estrogen vaginal tablets (Vagifem)

UTI, Urinary tract infection.
*The type of drug therapy depends on the type of incontinence.

toileting is used to reduce rather than expand bladder capacity. In this case, patients are asked to void every 3 to 4 hours regardless of the desire to urinate. This intervention is particularly useful in the patient with chronic overdistention, diabetes mellitus, or chronic alcoholism characterized by a large bladder capacity and diminished or delayed sensations of bladder filling and urgency.

INSTRUMENTATION

Reasons for short-term urinary catheterization are listed in Table 46-22. Two reasons that are not indications for catheterization are (1) routine acquisition of a urine specimen for laboratory analysis and (2) convenience of the nursing staff or the patient's family. Increased prevalence of complications seen with long-term use (>30 days) of indwelling catheters include bladder spasms, periurethral

TABLE 46-22	Indications for Urinary Catheterization

Indwelling Catheter
- Relief of urinary retention caused by lower urinary tract obstruction, paralysis, or inability to void
- Bladder decompression preoperatively and operatively for lower abdominal or pelvic surgery
- Facilitation of surgical repair of urethra and surrounding structures
- Splinting of ureters or urethra to facilitate healing after surgery or other trauma in area
- Accurate measurement of urinary output in critically ill patient
- Measurement of residual urine after urination (referred to as postvoid residual [PVR]) if portable ultrasound not available
- Contamination of stage III or IV pressure ulcers with urine that has impeded healing, despite appropriate personal care for the incontinence (indwelling)
- Terminal illness or severe impairment, which makes positioning or clothing changes uncomfortable, or which is associated with intractable pain (indwelling)

Straight (In-and-Out) Catheter
- Study of anatomic structures of urinary system
- Urodynamic testing
- Collection of sterile urine sample in selected situations
- Instillation of medications into bladder

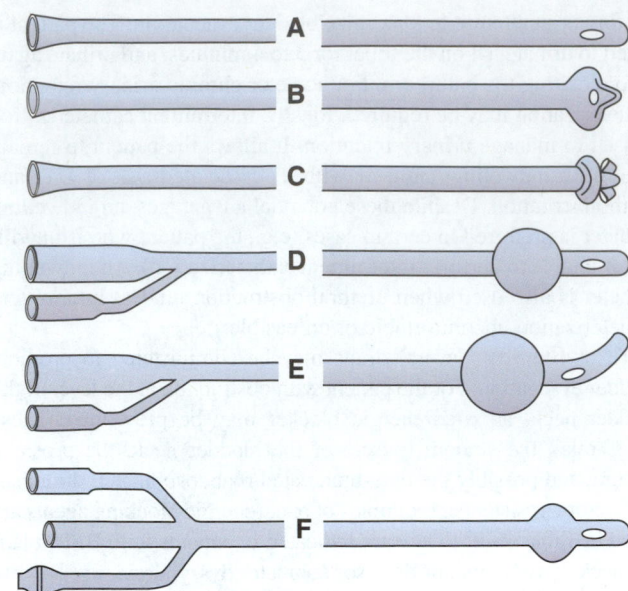

FIG. 46-11 Different types of commonly used catheters. **A,** Simple urethral catheter. **B,** Mushroom-tipped Pezzar catheter (can be used for suprapubic catheterization). **C,** Winged-tip Malecot catheter. **D,** Indwelling catheter with inflated balloon. **E,** Indwelling Tiemann catheter with coudé tip. **F,** Three-way indwelling catheter (the third lumen is used for irrigation of the bladder).

abscess, pain, urosepsis, UTIs, urethral trauma/erosion, fistula/stricture formation, and stones.[55] The risks of nosocomial infection are too high to allow catheterization of a patient for the convenience of hospital personnel or family members. Catheterization for sterile urine specimens may occasionally be indicated when patients have a history of complicated UTI. These specimens have to be as free of contaminants as possible. A catheter should be the final means of providing the patient with a dry environment for prevention of skin breakdown and protection of dressings or skin lesions.

Urinary catheterization is commonly used in the management of the hospitalized patient. However, it is not without serious risks. The urinary tract is the most common site of nosocomial infections. Urinary catheterization is a major cause of UTIs.[56] Scrupulous aseptic technique is mandatory when a urinary catheter is inserted. After insertion, maintenance and protection of the closed drainage system are major nursing responsibilities. Irrigation of the catheter should not be routinely performed and should be done only with medical direction.[55]

While the patient has a catheter in place, nursing actions should include maintaining patency of the catheter, managing fluid intake, providing for the comfort and safety of the patient, and preventing infection. Attention should be given to the psychologic implications of urinary drainage. Concerns of the patient can include embarrassment related to exposure of the body, an altered body image, and fear concerning the care of the catheter that results in increased dependency.

Catheter material includes Teflon-coated latex (polytetrafluoro-ethylene-[PTFE]), 100% silicone elastomer, and hydrogel-coated silicone. Catheters coated with silver or antimicrobial agents may lead to fewer UTIs in short-term catheter use.[57]

Catheters vary in construction materials, tip shape (Fig. 46-11), and size of the lumen. A coudé-tip catheter is commonly used in men. Catheters are sized according to the French scale. Each French unit (F) equals 0.33 mm of diameter. The diameter measured is the internal diameter of the catheter. The size used varies with the size of the individual and the purpose of catheterization. In women, urethral catheter sizes 14 F to 16 F are the most common; in men, sizes 14 F to 18 F are used. Balloon sizes are either 5 ml (instilled with 5 ml of sterile water) or 30 ml (instilled with 30 ml sterile water).[55] The primary problem resulting from too large a catheter is tissue erosion secondary to excessive pressure on the meatus or urethra. Four routes are used for urinary tract catheterization: urethral, ureteral, suprapubic, and via a nephrostomy tube.

Urethral Catheterization

The most common route of catheterization is insertion of the catheter through the external meatus into the urethra, past the internal sphincter, and into the bladder. Principles that should be considered in the management of the patient with an indwelling urethral catheter include the following:[55,58]

1. The catheterized patient, particularly the person who is ambulatory, should receive appropriate instruction regarding catheter care.
2. A sterile, closed drainage system should always be used in short-term catheterization. The distal urinary catheter and the proximal drainage tube should not be disconnected except for necessary catheter irrigation. Unobstructed downhill flow must be maintained. The collecting bag should be emptied regularly (when urine drainage reaches 400 ml) and kept below the level of the bladder. A poorly functioning catheter should be replaced. The leg bag should not be used for the short-term patient in the hospital setting because the risk of bacterial infection is great when the catheter is disconnected and the drainage bags are exchanged.
3. Perineal care (1 to 2 times per day and when necessary) should include cleaning of the meatus-catheter junction with soap and water. Lotion or powder should not be used near the catheter.

4. All catheters should be anchored using some type of securement device. It is recommended that the catheter be anchored to the upper thigh in women and to the lower abdomen in men to prevent catheter movement and urethral tension.

5. Sterile technique must be used whenever the collecting system is opened. Catheter irrigation is performed only when blood clots are suspected. If frequent irrigations are necessary in short-term catheterization for catheter patency, a triple-lumen catheter may be preferable, permitting continuous irrigations within a closed system.

6. Small volumes of urine for culture can be aspirated from the catheter sampling port by means of a sterile syringe and a 21-gauge needle. The puncture site must first be prepared with a tincture of iodine or alcohol solution.

7. When the patient is catheterized for less than 2 weeks, routine catheter change is not necessary. For long-term use of an indwelling catheter, catheter replacement should be based on patient assessment and not on a routine changing schedule.

8. With long-term use of a catheter, a leg bag may be used. If the collection bag is reused, it should be washed in soap and water and rinsed thoroughly. When not reused immediately, it should be filled with $1/2$ cup of vinegar and drained. The vinegar is effective against *Pseudomonas* and other organisms and eliminates odors.

9. Remove the catheter at the earliest moment possible. Intermittent catheterization and external catheters are alternatives that may be associated with less bacteriuria and/or UTIs than chronic indwelling urethral catheters.

Ureteral Catheters

The ureteral catheter is placed through the ureters into the renal pelvis. The catheter is inserted either (1) by being threaded up the urethra and bladder to the ureters under cystoscopic observation or (2) by surgical insertion through the abdominal wall into the ureters. The ureteral catheter is used after surgery to splint the ureters and to prevent them from being obstructed by edema. The urine volume from the ureteral catheter should be recorded separately from other urinary catheters. The patient is usually kept on bed rest while a ureteral catheter is in place until specific orders indicate that ambulation is permissible. The self-retaining ureteral catheter is often inserted after a lithotripsy procedure or when ureteral obstruction from adjacent tumors or fibrosis threatens renal function. The double-J ureteral catheter is often used and allows the patient to ambulate. One end coils up in the kidney pelvis, while the other coils in the bladder.

The placement of the ureteral catheter should be checked frequently, and tension on the catheter should be avoided. The catheter drains urine from the renal pelvis, which has a capacity of 3 to 5 ml. If the volume of urine in the renal pelvis increases, tissue damage to the pelvis will result from pressure. Therefore the ureteral catheter should not be clamped. If the physician orders irrigation of the ureteral catheter, strict aseptic technique is required. If output is decreased, the physician should be notified immediately. Drainage should be checked often (at least every 1 to 2 hours). It is normal for some urine to drain around the ureteral catheter into the bladder. Accurate recording of urine output from both the ureters and the urethral catheter is essential. Some-

times a ureteral catheter may be used as a stent and is not expected to drain. It is important to check with the physician as to the type of catheter and what to expect.

Suprapubic Catheters

Suprapubic catheterization is the simplest and oldest method of urinary diversion. The two methods of insertion of a suprapubic catheter into the bladder are (1) through a small incision in the abdominal wall and (2) by the use of a trocar. A suprapubic catheter is placed while the patient is under general anesthesia for another surgical procedure or at the bedside with a local anesthetic. The catheter may be sutured into place. The nursing responsibility includes taping the catheter to prevent dislodgment. The care of the tube and catheter is similar to that of the urethral catheter. A pectin-base skin barrier (e.g., Stomahesive) is effective around the insertion site in protecting the skin from breakdown.

The suprapubic catheter is used in temporary situations such as bladder, prostate, and urethral surgery. The suprapubic catheter is also used long term in selected patients (e.g., male tetraplegic patient who tends to form penoscrotal fistulas).

A suprapubic catheter is prone to poor drainage because of mechanical obstruction of the catheter tip by the bladder wall, sediment, and clots. Nursing interventions to ensure patency of the tube include (1) preventing tube kinking by coiling the excess tubing and maintaining gravity drainage, (2) having the patient turn from side to side, and (3) milking the tube.[59] If these measures are not effective, the catheter is irrigated with sterile technique after a physician's order has been obtained.

If the patient experiences bladder spasms that are difficult to control, urinary leakage may result. Oxybutynin (Ditropan or Oxytrol transdermal system) or other oral antispasmodics or belladonna and opium (B&O) suppositories may be prescribed to decrease bladder spasms.

Nephrostomy Tubes

The nephrostomy tube (catheter) is inserted on a temporary basis to preserve renal function when complete obstruction of a ureter is present. It is inserted directly into the pelvis of the kidney and attached to connecting tubing for closed drainage. The principle is the same as with the ureteral catheter; that is, the catheter should never be kinked, compressed, or clamped. If the patient complains of excessive pain in the area or if there is excessive drainage around the tube, the catheter should be checked for patency. If irrigation is ordered, strict aseptic technique is required. No more than 5 ml of sterile saline solution is gently instilled at one time to prevent overdistention of the kidney pelvis and renal damage. Infection and secondary stone formation are complications associated with the insertion of a nephrostomy tube.

Intermittent Catheterization

An alternative approach to a long-term indwelling catheter is *intermittent catheterization,* often referred to as "straight" catheterization or "in-and-out" catheterization.[55] It is being used with increasing frequency in conditions characterized by neurogenic bladder (e.g., spinal cord injuries, chronic neurologic diseases) or bladder outlet obstruction in men. This type of catheterization is used in the oliguric and anuric phases of acute renal failure to reduce the possibility of infection from an indwelling catheter. Intermittent catheterization is also used postoperatively, after a surgical procedure for female incontinence, or following radioactive seed implantation into the prostate for cancer. The main goal of intermittent catheterization is to prevent urinary retention, stasis, and compromised blood supply to the bladder caused by prolonged pressure.

The technique consists of inserting a urethral catheter into the bladder every 3 to 5 hours. Some patients do intermittent catheterization only once or twice a day to measure residual urine and to ensure an empty bladder. Two main catheter designs are available: those that have a hydrophilic coating (which becomes slippery when immersed in water to aid insertion) and those with no coating (polyvinyl chloride [PVC]). The hydrophilic catheter was introduced in the United States in the past decade and is indicated for single use.[55] Some catheters show a marked propensity to "stick" to the wall of the urethra depending on differences in the slipperiness of catheter coatings. The design of single-use, self-lubricating, silicone-coated (closed-sterile) systems is useful for patients who have recurrent UTIs or need to catheterize while at work or during travel. Patients should be instructed to wash and rinse the catheter and their hands with soap and water before and after catheterization. Lubricant is necessary for men and may make catheterization more comfortable for women. The catheter may be inserted by the patient or the care provider. The bladder is emptied and the catheter is removed. The catheter can be dried and placed in a carrying pouch or purse or folded in a paper towel until it is next needed. In general, patients should change the catheter every 7 days.[60]

Sterile technique is used for catheterization in the hospital or long-term care facility. For home care, a clean technique that includes good hand washing with soap and water is used. There has been no significant increase in infection with the use of an appropriate clean technique as compared with sterile technique. The patient is taught to observe for signs of UTI so that treatment can be instituted early. If indicated, some patients are placed on a regimen of prophylactic antibiotics. Urethral damage from intermittent catheterization in men is similar to problems seen with indwelling catheterization. Complications include urethritis, urethral sphincter damage (especially if there is a forceful catheterization against a closed sphincter), urethral stricture, and creation of a false passage.[55]

Surgery of the Urinary Tract

RENAL AND URETERAL SURGERY

The most common indications for nephrectomy are a renal tumor, polycystic kidneys that are bleeding or severely infected, massive traumatic injury to the kidney, and the elective removal of a kidney from a donor. Surgery involving the ureters and kidneys is most commonly performed to remove calculi that become obstructive, correct congenital anomalies, and divert urine when necessary.

Preoperative Management

The basic needs of the patient undergoing renal and ureteral surgery are similar to those of any patient who experiences surgery (see Chapters 18 through 20). In addition, it is especially important preoperatively to ensure adequate fluid intake and a normal electrolyte balance. The patient should be told that there will probably be a flank incision on the affected side and that surgery will require a hyperextended, side-lying position. This position frequently causes the patient to experience muscle aches after surgery. If a nephrectomy is planned, the patient must be assured that one working kidney is sufficient to maintain normal renal function.

Postoperative Management

Specific postoperative needs of a patient are related to urine output, respiratory status, and abdominal distention.

Urine Output. In the immediate postoperative period, urine output should be determined at least every 1 to 2 hours. Drainage from various catheters should be recorded separately. The catheter or tube should not be clamped or irrigated without a specific order. The total urine output should be at least 0.5 ml/kg/hr. It is also important to assess for urine drainage on the dressing and to estimate the amount. Daily weighing of the patient is important. The same scale should be used and properly balanced, and the patient should wear similar clothing and dressings each time.

It is important to observe and monitor the color and consistency of urine. Urine with increased amounts of mucus, blood, or sediment may occlude the drainage tubing or catheter.

Respiratory Status. Renal surgery is often performed through a flank incision just below the diaphragm and often involves removal of the twelfth rib. Postoperatively, it is important to ensure adequate ventilation. The patient is often reluctant to turn, cough, and deep breathe because of the incisional pain. Adequate pain medication should be given to ensure the patient's comfort and ability to perform coughing and deep-breathing exercises. Frequently, additional respiratory devices such as an incentive spirometer are used every 2 hours while the patient is awake. In addition, early and frequent ambulation assists in maintaining adequate respiratory function.

Abdominal Distention. Abdominal distention is present to some degree in most patients who have had surgery on their kidneys or ureters. It is most commonly due to paralytic ileus caused by manipulation and compression of the bowel during surgery. Oral intake is restricted until bowel sounds are present (usually 24 to 48 hours after surgery). IV fluids are given until the patient can take oral fluids. Progression to a regular diet follows.

Laparoscopic Nephrectomy

Laparoscopic nephrectomy can be performed in selected situations to remove a diseased kidney. Laparoscopic nephrectomy can also be used to obtain a kidney from a living donor to be transplanted into a person with end-stage renal disease. In contrast to the open incision of about 7 inches (18 cm) required in a conventional nephrectomy, a laparoscopic nephrectomy is performed using five puncture sites. One incision is to view the kidney and another is to dissect it. The laparoscope contains a miniature camera so that the surgeons can watch what they are doing on a video monitor. Once dissected, the kidney is maneuvered into a nylon impermeable sack, and its contents can then be safely removed from the patient. Compared with conventional nephrectomy, the laparoscopic approach is less painful and requires no sutures or staples, involves a shorter hospital stay, and has a much faster recovery.

URINARY DIVERSION

Urinary diversion may be performed with and without cystectomy. Urinary diversion procedures are performed to treat cancer of the bladder, neurogenic bladder, congenital anomalies, strictures, trauma to the bladder, and chronic infections with deterioration of renal function. Numerous urinary diversion techniques and bladder substitutes are possible, including an incontinent urinary diversion, a continent urinary diversion catheterized by the patient, or an orthotopic bladder so that the patient voids urethrally.[61] Types of these surgical procedures are presented in Table 46-23 and Fig. 46-12.

TABLE 46-23	Types of Urinary Diversion Surgery Requiring Collection Devices			
Type	**Description**	**Advantages**	**Disadvantages**	**Special Considerations**
Ileal Conduit	Ureters are implanted into part of ileum or colon that has been resected from intestinal tract. Abdominal stoma is created.	Relatively good urine flow with few physiologic alterations	External appliance necessary to continually collect urine	Surgical procedure is more complex. Postoperative complications may be increased. Reabsorption of urea by ileum occurs. Meticulous attention is necessary to care for stoma and collecting device.
Cutaneous ureterostomy	Ureters are excised from bladder and brought through abdominal wall, and stoma is created. Ureteral stomas may be created from both ureters, or ureters may be brought together and one stoma created.	No need for major surgery as required with ileal conduit	External appliance necessary because of continuous urine drainage; possibility of stricture or stenosis of small stoma	Periodic catheterizations may be required to dilate stomas to maintain patency.
Nephrostomy	Catheter is inserted into pelvis of kidney. Procedure may be done to one or both kidneys and may be temporary or permanent. It is most frequently done in advanced disease as palliative procedure.	No need for major surgery	High risk of renal infection; predisposition to calculus formation from catheter	Nephrostomy tube may have to be changed every month. Catheter must never be clamped.

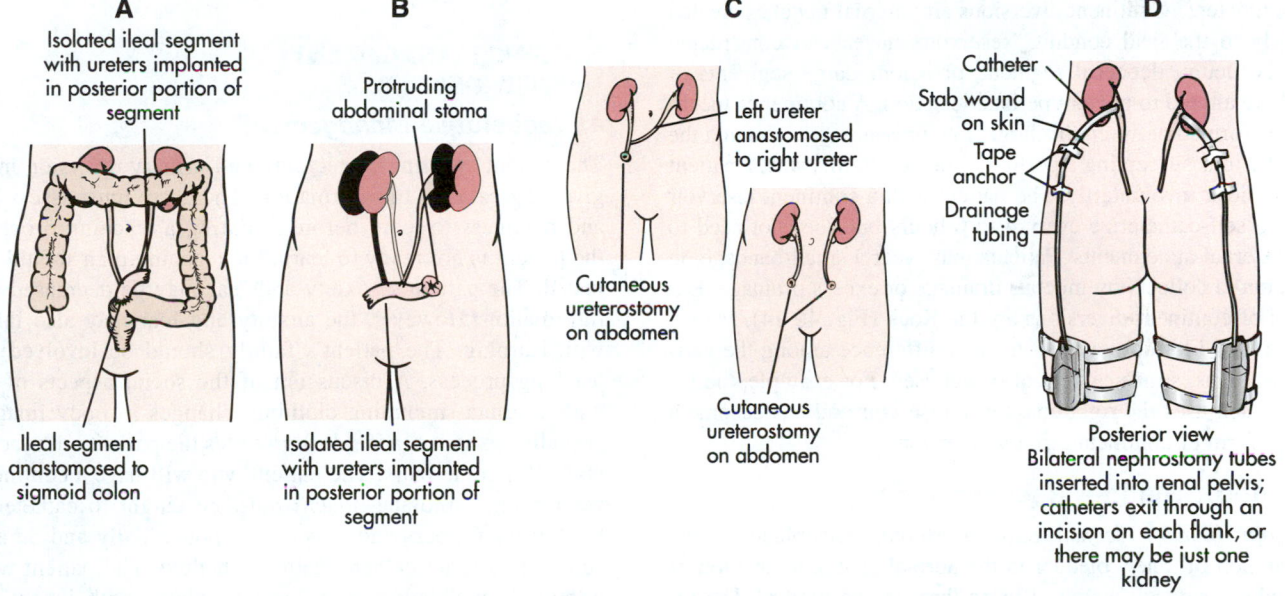

FIG. 46-12   Methods of urinary diversion. **A,** Ureteroileosigmoidostomy. **B,** Ileal loop (or ileal conduit). **C,** Ureterostomy (transcutaneous ureterostomy and bilateral cutaneous ureterostomies). **D,** Nephrostomy.

Incontinent Urinary Diversion

Incontinent urinary diversion is diversion to the skin, requiring an appliance. The simplest form is the cutaneous ureterostomy, but scarring and strictures of the ureter have led to the use of ileal or colonic conduits. The most commonly performed incontinent urinary diversion procedure is the **ileal conduit** (ileal loop). In this procedure a 6- to 8-inch (15- to 20-cm) segment of the ileum is converted into a conduit for urinary drainage. The colon (colon conduit) can be used instead of the ileum. The ureters are anastomosed into one end of the conduit, and the other end of the bowel is brought out through the abdominal wall to form a stoma (Fig. 46-13). Although the segment of bowel remains supported by the mesentery, it is completely isolated from the intestinal tract. The bowel is anastomosed and continues to function normally. Because there is no valve and no voluntary control over the stoma, drops of urine flow from the stoma every few seconds, requiring the use of a permanent external collecting device. The visible stoma and the need for external collection devices are obvious disadvantages of this procedure. The lifelong care and dealing with the stoma and collection devices may be psychologically difficult. These problems have stimulated the increasing use of continent diversions and orthotopic bladder substitutes.

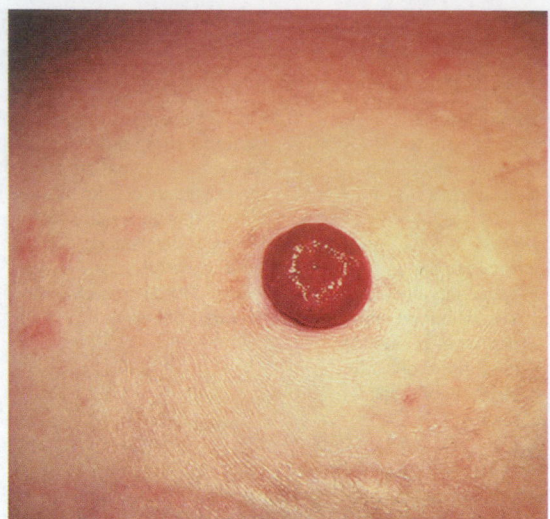

FIG. 46-13   Ideal urinary stoma. It is symmetric, has no skin breakdown, and protrudes about 1.5 cm; the mucosa is a healthy red and the configuration is flat when the patient is upright and supine.

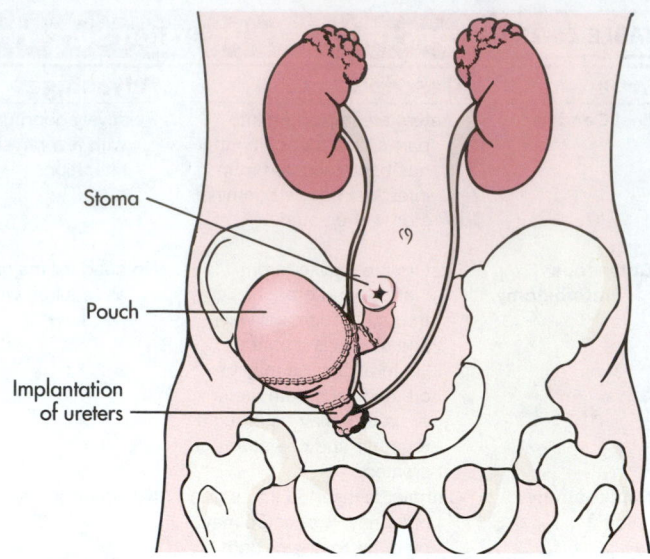

FIG. 46-14   Creation of a Kock pouch with implantation of ureters into one intussuscepted portion of the pouch and creation of a stoma with the other intussuscepted portion.

Continent Urinary Diversions

A *continent urinary diversion* is an intraabdominal urinary reservoir that can be catheterized or that has an outlet controlled by the anal sphincter.[61] Continent diversions are internal pouches created similarly to the ileal conduit. Reservoirs have been constructed from the ileum, ileocecal segment, or colon. Large segments of bowel are altered to prevent peristaltic action. A continence mechanism is formed between this large, low-pressure reservoir and the stoma by intussuscepting a portion of bowel. In this way, a patient does not leak involuntarily. The patient with a continent reservoir needs to self-catheterize every 4 to 6 hours but does not need to wear external attachments. Patients may wear a small bandage on the stoma to collect any mucous drainage or excess drainage. Examples of continent diversions are the Kock (Fig. 46-14), Mainz, Indiana, and Florida pouches. A main difference among the various diversions is the segment of bowel used. For example, the Indiana pouch uses the right colon as a reservoir and has become a popular form of continent urinary diversion.

Orthotopic Bladder Reconstruction

Orthotopic bladder reconstruction or orthotopic neobladder is the construction of a new bladder in the normal anatomic position of the bladder, with discharge of urine through the urethra. The reconstruction or neobladder can be derived from various segments of the intestines to create a low-pressure reservoir. An isolated segment of the distal ileum is often preferred. Various procedures include the hemi-Kock pouch, the Studer pouch, and the W-shaped ileoneobladder. In these procedures the bowel is surgically reshaped to become a neobladder.[62] The ureters and urethra are sutured into the neobladder. Orthotopic bladder reconstruction has become a more viable option for both men and women if cancer does not involve the bladder neck or urethra. Ideal candidates for this procedure are those with normal renal and liver function, longer than 1- to 2-year life expectancy, adequate motor skills, and no history of inflammatory bowel disease or colon cancer. Obese patients and patients with inflammatory bowel disease are not good candidates for this procedure. The advantage of orthotopic bladder substitution is that it allows for natural micturition. Incon-

tinence is a possible problem with this technique, and intermittent catheterization may be required.

NURSING MANAGEMENT
URINARY DIVERSION

■ *Preoperative Management*

The patient awaiting cystectomy and urinary diversion must be given a great deal of information. The nurse must assess ability and readiness to learn before initiating a teaching program. If the patient is not ready to learn, the teaching plan should be adjusted. The patient's anxiety and fear may be decreased by the information. However, the anxiety and fear may also interfere with learning. The patient's family should be involved in the teaching process. A discussion of the social aspects of living with a stoma (including clothing, changes in body image and sexuality, exercise, and odor) provides the patient with facts that may allay some fears. The patient who will have a continent diversion (e.g., Indiana pouch) must be taught to catheterize at least every 6 hours and irrigate the pouch daily and be able to adhere to a strict catheterization schedule. The patient with an orthotopic neobladder may have problems with incontinence. Concerns about the effect on sexual activities should be discussed. The enterostomal therapy nurse should be involved in the preoperative phase of the patient's care. A visit from an ostomate or enterostomal therapy nurse can be helpful. Additional interventions are presented in NCP 46-3.

■ *Postoperative Management*

Nursing interventions during the postoperative period (see NCP 46-3 for care after an ileal conduit) should be planned to prevent surgical complications such as postoperative atelectasis and shock (see Chapter 20). After pelvic surgery, there is an increased incidence of thrombophlebitis, small bowel obstruction, and UTI.[63] With removal of part of the bowel, the incidence of paralytic ileus and small bowel obstruction is increased, the patient is kept on nothing-by-mouth (NPO) status, and a nasogastric tube is necessary for a few days.

NURSING CARE PLAN 46-3

Patient with an Ileal Conduit

NURSING DIAGNOSIS **Anxiety** *related to* effects of ileal conduit on lifestyle and relationships and lack of knowledge regarding surgical procedure *as evidenced by* frequent questions about surgical procedure, restlessness

PATIENT GOALS
1. Reports decreased anxiety regarding the effects of surgery on lifestyle
2. Verbalizes understanding of surgical procedure and postoperative expectations

OUTCOMES (NOC)

Anxiety Self-Control

- Seeks information to reduce anxiety ____
- Uses effective coping strategies ____
- Uses relaxation techniques to reduce anxiety ____

Measurement Scale

1 = Never demonstrated
2 = Rarely demonstrated
3 = Sometimes demonstrated
4 = Often demonstrated
5 = Consistently demonstrated

INTERVENTIONS (NIC) and *RATIONALES*

Anxiety Reduction

- Provide factual information concerning diagnosis, treatment, and prognosis *to reduce fear of the unknown and convey a caring attitude.*
- Encourage verbalization of feelings, perceptions, and fears *to help patient recognize anxiety and promote problem solving.*
- Assist patient to articulate a realistic description of an upcoming event *to reduce anxiety and promote decision making.*
- Instruct patient in use of relaxation techniques *to promote coping.*

NURSING DIAGNOSIS **Disturbed body image** *related to* effects of change in body function on lifestyle or relationships *as evidenced by* negative feelings about self, refusal to look at or touch stoma or participate in self-care, expression of concern about effect on family and lifestyle

PATIENT GOALS
1. Verbalizes acceptance of changes in body appearance and function
2. Participates in care of ileal conduit

OUTCOMES (NOC)

Body Image

- Description of affected body part ____
- Willingness to touch affected body part ____
- Satisfaction with body function ____
- Adjustment to changes in physical appearance ____
- Adjustment to changes in body function ____

Measurement Scale

1 = Never positive
2 = Rarely positive
3 = Sometimes positive
4 = Often positive
5 = Consistently positive

INTERVENTIONS (NIC) and *RATIONALES*

Body Image Enhancement

- Help patient determine extent of actual changes in the body or its level of functioning *to assist with issues and misconceptions and plan appropriate interventions.*
- Monitor whether patient can look at changed body part *to assess readiness to participate in self-care.*
- Assist patient to separate physical appearance from feelings of personal worth *to provide support and convey a sense of worth.*
- Facilitate contact with individuals with similar changes in body image *to provide patient with realistic experiences related to ostomy care.*
- Identify support groups available to patient *as these resources may provide new information and suggestion of ways to modify lifestyle.*

NURSING DIAGNOSIS **Risk for impaired skin integrity** *related to* need for chronic use of external appliance on skin or ill-fitting appliance

PATIENT GOAL Maintains intact, healthy skin around stoma

OUTCOMES (NOC)

Tissue Integrity: Skin and Mucous Membranes

- Skin lesions ____
- Skin scaling ____
- Erythema ____

Measurement Scale

1 = Severe
2 = Substantial
3 = Moderate
4 = Mild
5 = None

INTERVENTIONS (NIC) and *RATIONALES*

Ostomy Care

- Apply appropriately fitting ostomy appliance *to protect the skin from urine exposure.*
- Monitor stoma/surrounding tissue healing and adaptation to ostomy equipment *to ensure prompt identification of problems.*
- Change/empty ostomy bag *to prevent urine leakage onto the skin.*

Skin Care: Topical Treatments

- Refrain from using alkaline soap on the skin around the stoma *to prevent alkaline accumulation on the skin.*

Continued

NURSING CARE PLAN 46-3

Patient with an Ileal Conduit—cont'd

NURSING DIAGNOSIS   **Ineffective therapeutic regimen management** *related to* lack of knowledge regarding stoma and appliance care *as evidenced by* expression of concern about how to manage ileal conduit, frequent questions, or inaccurate responses regarding stoma care

PATIENT GOALS   1. Demonstrates correct removal and application of ostomy appliance and maintenance of ostomy pouch
          2. Describes all factors involved in the care and maintenance of the ileal conduit

OUTCOMES (NOC)	INTERVENTIONS (NIC) and *RATIONALES*
Knowledge: Ostomy Care	**Ostomy Care**
• Description of purpose of ostomy ____	• Instruct patient/significant other in the use of ostomy equipment and care *to promote self-care.*
• Description of skin care around ostomy ____	• Have patient/significant other demonstrate use of equipment *to evaluate performance and correct any deficiencies.*
• Description of procedure to change/empty ostomy pouch ____	• Provide support and assistance while patient develops skill in caring for stoma/surrounding tissue *to give support and convey acceptance of the altered body function.*
• Description of complications related to stoma/skin ____	• Instruct patient on measures to reduce odor.
• Description of need for adequate fluid intake ____	• Instruct patient how to monitor for complications (e.g., mechanical breakdown, chemical breakdown, rash, leaks, dehydration, infection) *to obtain early treatment of complications.*
• Description of odor control mechanisms ____	
	Teaching: Psychomotor Skill
Measurement Scale	• Provide written information/diagrams *to enhance learning and to provide references for future use.*
1 = None	• Provide frequent feedback to patient on what he/she is doing correctly and incorrectly, *so that bad habits are not formed.*
2 = Limited	
3 = Moderate	
4 = Substantial	
5 = Extensive	

NURSING DIAGNOSIS   **Ineffective sexuality pattern** *related to* perceived or actual effects of surgery on sexual activity *as evidenced by* verbalizing concerns about sexuality and unwillingness to discuss sexual issues with partner

PATIENT GOAL   Reports satisfaction with sexual practices

OUTCOMES (NOC)	INTERVENTIONS (NIC) and *RATIONALES*
Sexual Functioning	**Sexual Counseling**
• Expresses comfort with sexual expression ____	• Discuss the effect of the illness/health situation on sexuality *so patient will know the effect of this surgery on sexual activities/practices.*
• Expresses self-esteem ____	• Provide factual information about sexual myths and misinformation that patient may verbalize.
• Communicates comfortably with partner ____	• Introduce patient to positive role models who have successfully conquered a similar problem *to reassure patient that problems can be overcome.*
Measurement Scale	
1 = Never demonstrated	
2 = Rarely demonstrated	
3 = Sometimes demonstrated	
4 = Often demonstrated	
5 = Consistently demonstrated	

NURSING DIAGNOSES

Acute pain, Ineffective breathing pattern, Risk for imbalanced fluid volume*

COLLABORATIVE PROBLEMS

Hemorrhage, Paralytic ileus, Thromboembolism*

*Postoperative care of the patient with an ileal conduit includes nursing diagnoses for the postoperative patient found in Nursing Care Plan 20-1: Postoperative Patient, pp. 383 to 386.

Specific attention should be given to preventing injury to the stoma and maintaining urine output. Mucus is present in the urine because it is secreted by the intestines as a result of the irritating effect of the urine. The patient should be told that this is a normal occurrence. A high fluid intake is encouraged to "flush" the ileal conduit or continent diversion.

When an ileal conduit is created, the skin around the stoma requires meticulous care. Alkaline encrustations with dermatitis may occur when alkaline urine comes in contact with exposed skin (Fig.

46-15). Other common peristomal skin problems include yeast infections, product allergies, and shearing-effect excoriations. Changing appliances (pouches) is described in Table 46-24. A properly fitting appliance is essential to prevent skin problems. The appliance should be about 0.1 inch (0.2 cm) larger than the stoma. It is normal for the stoma to shrink within the first few weeks after surgery. The urine is kept acidic to prevent alkaline encrustations.

Patients with a neobladder may have postoperative urinary retention and require catheterization.[63] It may take up to 6 months

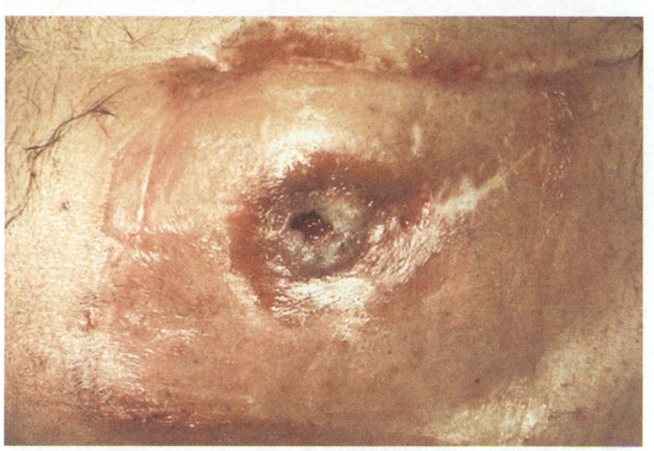

FIG. 46-15   Ammonia salt encrustation secondary to alkaline urine.

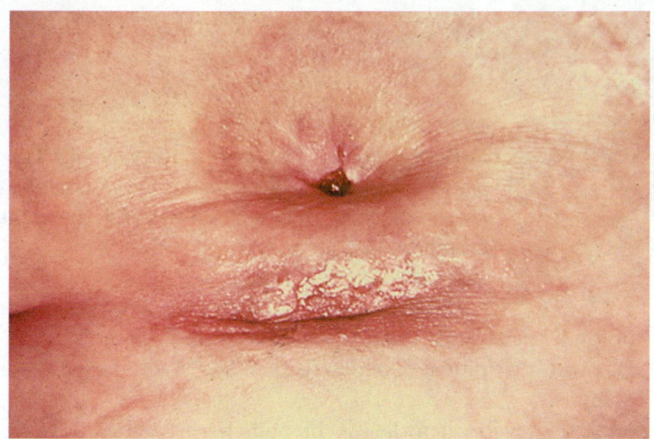

FIG. 46-16   Retracted urinary stoma with pressure sore from faceplate above stoma.

TABLE 46-24	*PATIENT AND FAMILY TEACHING GUIDE* **Changing Ileal Conduit Appliances**

Temporary Appliance	**Permanent Appliance***
1. Cut hole in pouch to fit over stoma (pouch 3.2 mm [⅛ inch] larger than stoma). 2. Remove old pouch. 3. Clean area gently and remove old adhesive. 4. Wash area with warm water. 5. Place wick (rolled-up 4 × 4–inch pad) over stoma to keep area dry during rest of procedure. 6. Dry skin around stoma. 7. Apply tincture of benzoin or other skin protectant around stoma to area where pouch will be placed. 8. Apply pouch by first smoothing its edges toward side and lower portion of body. 9. Remove wick and complete application of bag. 10. If patient is usually in bed, apply bag so that it lies toward side of body. 11. If patient is ambulatory, apply bag so that it lies vertically. 12. Connect drainage tubing to pouch. 13. Keep drainage pouch on same side of bed as stoma.	1. Keep appliance in place for 2-14 days. 2. Change appliance when fluid intake has been restricted for several hours. 3. Have patient sit or stand in front of mirror. 4. Moisten edge of faceplate with adhesive solvent and gently remove. 5. Clean skin with adhesive solvent. 6. Wash skin with warm water. (Patient may shower.) 7. Dry skin and inspect. 8. Place wick (rolled-up 4 × 4–inch pad) over stoma to keep skin free of urine. 9. Apply skin cement to faceplate and skin. 10. Place appliance over stoma. 11. Wash removed appliance with soap and lukewarm water; soak in distilled vinegar; rinse with lukewarm water and air dry.

*Many disposable appliances with self-adhesive backing are used as permanent appliances.

for them to regain daytime bladder control but nocturnal enuresis is seen in 25% of patients. Patients empty their neobladders by relaxing their outlet sphincter muscles and bearing down with their abdominal muscles. As there is no longer neurologic feedback between reservoir and brain, the patient should not expect a normal desire to void. To avoid bladder overdistension, patients should void at least every 2 to 4 hours, sit during voiding, and practice pelvic floor muscle relaxation to aid voiding. Follow-up studies include a "pouchogram" 3 to 4 weeks after surgery to assess for extravasations. The presence of extravasations indicates that the reservoir's suture lines are not yet healed.

Acceptance of the surgery and of alterations in body image is needed to ensure the patient's best adjustment. Meeting and sharing feelings with similar patients can enhance a patient's adjustment to a urinary diversion. Concerns of the patient include fear that the stoma will be offensive to others and will interfere with sexual, personal, professional, and recreational activities. The patient should know that few activities, if any, will be restricted as a result of the urinary diversion.

Discharge planning after an ileal conduit includes teaching the patient symptoms of obstruction or infection and care of the ostomy. The patient with an ileal conduit is fitted for a permanent appliance 7 to 10 days after surgery and may need to be refitted at a later time, depending on the degree of stoma shrinkage. Appliances are made of a variety of products, including natural and synthetic rubbers, plastics, and metals. Most appliances have a faceplate that adheres to the skin, a collecting pouch, and an opening to drain the pouch. The faceplate may be secured to the skin with glues, adhesives, or adhering synthetic wafers. Some appliances do not require adhesives, but their design relies on pressure to keep the pouch in place. If improperly fitted or applied, the faceplate may cause skin problems (Fig. 46-16). The patient needs information on where to purchase supplies, emergency telephone numbers, location of ostomy clubs, and follow-up visits with an enterostomal therapist. Physician follow-up is imperative to monitor and correct homeostatic abnormalities and to prevent complications and renal function deterioration.

CRITICAL THINKING EXERCISE

CASE STUDY

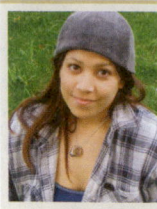

Urinary Tract Infection

Patient Profile. Suzanna, a 28-year-old Hispanic woman, was seen in the nurse practitioner's office for a history of painful, frequent urination.

Subjective Data
- Has had a history of painful, frequent urination with passage of small volumes of urine for 3 days
- Has had intermittent fever, chills, and back pain during these 3 days
- Was frightened when she saw blood in her urine
- Reports that this is her third attack of painful urination and back pain in 4 months
- Is anxious because her father died of kidney cancer
- Remembers having many UTIs as a child

Objective Data
Physical Examination
- Complains of bilateral flank pain and abdominal tenderness to palpation
- Temperature is 100.4° F (38° C)

Diagnostic Study
- Urinalysis: pyuria and hematuria

Critical Thinking Questions

1. What are the most common organisms that cause UTIs?
2. What factors predispose a patient to a UTI?
3. What is the difference between upper and lower UTIs?
4. What are the priority nursing interventions for Suzanna?
5. Why might she be having recurrent bouts of UTIs? What other diagnostic tests may be indicated?
6. What can the nurse do to help Suzanna prevent another UTI?
7. Based on the data presented, write one or more appropriate nursing diagnoses. Are there any collaborative problems?

NCLEX EXAMINATION REVIEW QUESTIONS

The number of the question corresponds to the same-numbered objective at the beginning of the chapter.

1. In teaching a patient with pyelonephritis about the disorder, the nurse informs the patient that the organisms that cause pyelonephritis most commonly reach the kidneys through
   a. the bloodstream.
   b. the lymphatic system.
   c. a descending infection.
   d. an ascending infection.
2. The nurse teaches the female patient who has frequent UTIs that she should
   a. take tub baths with bubble bath.
   b. urinate before and after sexual intercourse.
   c. take prophylactic sulfonamides for the rest of her life.
   d. restrict fluid intake to prevent the need for frequent voiding.
3. The immunologic mechanisms involved in glomerulonephritis include
   a. tubular blocking by precipitates of bacteria and antibody reactions.
   b. deposition of immune complexes and complement along the GBM.
   c. thickening of the GBM from autoimmune microangiopathic changes.
   d. destruction of glomeruli by proteolytic enzymes contained in the GBM.
4. One of the most important roles of the nurse in relation to acute poststreptococcal glomerulonephritis is to
   a. promote early diagnosis and treatment of sore throats and skin lesions.
   b. encourage patients to request antibiotic therapy for all upper respiratory infections.
   c. teach patients with APSGN that long-term prophylactic antibiotic therapy is necessary to prevent recurrence.
   d. monitor patients for respiratory symptoms that indicate that the disease is affecting the alveolar basement membrane.
5. The edema that occurs in nephrotic syndrome is due to
   a. increased hydrostatic pressure caused by sodium retention.
   b. decreased aldosterone secretion from adrenal insufficiency.
   c. increased fluid retention caused by decreased glomerular filtration.
   d. decreased colloidal osmotic pressure caused by loss of serum albumin.
6. A patient is admitted to the hospital with severe renal colic caused by renal lithiasis. The nurse's first priority in management of the patient is to
   a. administer opioids as prescribed.
   b. obtain supplies for straining all urine.
   c. encourage fluid intake of 3 to 4 L/day.
   d. keep the patient NPO in preparation for surgery.
7. The nurse recommends genetic counseling for the children of a patient with
   a. nephrotic syndrome.
   b. chronic pyelonephritis.
   c. malignant nephrosclerosis.
   d. adult-onset polycystic renal disease.
8. The nurse encourages strict diabetic control in the patient prone to diabetic nephropathy knowing that the renal tissue changes that may occur in this condition include
   a. uric acid calculi and nephrolithiasis.
   b. renal sugar-crystal calculi and cysts.
   c. lipid deposits in the glomeruli and nephrons.
   d. thickening of the GBM and glomerulosclerosis.
9. The nurse identifies a risk factor for kidney and bladder cancer in a patient who relates a history of
   a. aspirin use.
   b. tobacco use.
   c. chronic alcohol abuse.
   d. use of artificial sweeteners.
10. In planning nursing interventions to increase bladder control in the patient with urinary incontinence, the nurse includes
    a. teaching the patient to use Kegel exercises.
    b. clamping and releasing a catheter to increase bladder tone.
    c. teaching the patient biofeedback mechanisms to suppress the urge to void.
    d. counseling the patient concerning choice of incontinence containment device.

11. A patient with a ureterolithotomy returns from surgery with a nephrostomy tube in place. Postoperative nursing care of the patient includes
    a. encouraging the patient to drink fruit juices and milk.
    b. forcing fluids of at least 2 to 3 L/day after nausea has subsided.
    c. irrigating the nephrostomy tube with 10 ml of normal saline solution as needed.
    d. notifying the physician if nephrostomy tube drainage is more than 30 ml/hr.

12. A patient has had a cystectomy and ileal conduit diversion performed. Four days postoperatively, mucous shreds are seen in the drainage bag. The nurse should
    a. notify the physician.
    b. notify the charge nurse.
    c. irrigate the drainage tube.
    d. chart it as a normal observation.

REFERENCES

1. Griebling TL: Urologic Diseases in America Project: trends in resource use for urinary tract infections in women, *J Urol* 173:1281, 2005.
2. Nickel JC: Management of urinary tract infections: historical perspective and current strategies: Part 2—modern management, *J Urol* 173:27, 2005.
3. U.S. Preventive Services Task Force Recommendation Statement. Screening for asymptomatic bacteriuria: recommendation statement, *Am Fam Physician* 71:1575, 2005.
4. Mehnert-Kay SA: Diagnosis and management of uncomplicated urinary tract infections, *Am Fam Physician* 72:451, 2005.
5. Sheffield JS, Cunningham FG: Urinary tract infection in women, *Obstet Gynecol* 106:1085, 2005.
6. Newman DK: *Managing and treating urinary incontinence,* Baltimore, Md, 2002, Health Professions Press.
7. Liu H, Mulholland SG: Appropriate antibiotic treatment of genitourinary infections in hospitalized patients, *Am J Med* 118:145, 2005.
8. Trautner BW, Darouiche RO: Catheter-associated infections: pathogenesis affects prevention, *Arch Intern Med* 164:842, 2004.
9. Kuritzky L: Role of primary care clinicians in the diagnosis and treatment of LUTS and BPH, *Rev Urol* 6:S53, 2004.
10. Woods A: Managing UTIs in older adults, *Nursing* 35(3):12, 2005.
11. Wallace M, Sadocsky R: What clinicians should know about urinalysis, *Clin Advisor* April:39, 2005.
12. Lynch DM: Cranberry for prevention of urinary tract infections, *Am Fam Physician* 70:2175, 2004.
13. Loeb S, Vardi I, Nadler RB: Contemporary issues of urosepsis, *Contemp Urol* 17(7):35, 2005.
14. Schaefer AJ: Infections of the urinary tract. In Wein AJ, Kavoussi LR, Novick AC, et al, editors: *Campbell-Walsh urology,* ed 9, Philadelphia, 2007, Elsevier.
15. Nickel P, Naher H: Nongonococcal urethritis, *Curr Probl Dermatol* 24:97, 1996.
16. Dmochowski R: Urethral diverticula. In Wein AJ, Kavoussi LR, Novick AC, et al, editors: *Campbell-Walsh urology,* ed 9, Philadelphia, 2007, Elsevier.
17. Rufford J, Cardozo L: Urethral diverticula: a diagnostic dilemma, *BJU Int* 94:1044, 2004.
18. Hanno P, et al: Painful bladder syndrome. In Abrams P, Cardozo L, Khoury S, et al, editors: *Incontinence: proceedings from the 3rd International Consultation on Incontinence,* Plymouth, UK, 2004, International Consultation on Urological Diseases.
19. Page S, Rosenberg M, Hazzard M: Interstitial cystitis: current diagnostic and management strategies, *Adv Nurse Pract* 13(12):18, 2005.
*20. Baldwin CM: The impact of self-care practices on treatment of interstitial cystitis, *Urol Nurs* 24:107, 2004.
*21. Mayer R, Propert KJ, Peters KM, et al: A randomized controlled trial of intravesical bacillus Calmette-Guerin for treatment of refractory interstitial cystitis, *J Urol* 173:1186, 2005.
22. Lambie SH, Cassidy MJ: Minimal change nephropathy and renal tuberculosis, *Clin Nephrol* 60:439, 2003.
23. Lau KK, Wyatt RJ: Glomerulonephritis, *Adolesc Med Clin* 16(1):67, 2005.
24. Bergs L: Goodpasture syndrome, *Crit Care Nurse* 25(5):50, 2005.
25. Schwarz A: New aspects of the treatment of nephrotic syndrome, *J Am Soc Nephrol* 12(Suppl 17):S44, 2001.
26. Colella J, Kochis E, Galli B, et al: Urolithiasis/nephrolithiasis: what's it all about? *Urol Nurs* 25:427, 2005.
27. Delvecchio FC, Preminger GM: Medical management of stone disease, *Curr Opin Urol* 13:229, 2003.
28. Preminger GM, Assimos DG, Lingeman JE, et al: Chapter 1: AUA Guideline on management of staghorn calculi: diagnosis and treatment recommendations, *J Urol* 173:1991, 2005.
29. Straub M, Hautmann RE: Developments in stone prevention, *Curr Opin Urol* 15:119, 2005.
30. Curhan GC, Willett WC, Knight EL, et al: Dietary factors and the risk of incident kidney stones in younger women: Nurses' Health Study II, *Arch Intern Med* 164:885, 2004.
31. Kreig C: The role of diet in the prevention of common kidney stones, *Urol Nurs* 25:427, 2005.
32. Champion J, Longhorn S: Urinary tract stones. In Fillingham S, Douglas J, editors: *Urological nursing,* London, 2004, Bailliere Tindall.
33. Peterson AC, Webster GD: Management of urethral stricture disease: developing options for surgical intervention, *BJU Int* 94:971, 2004.
34. Chew BH, Knudsen BE, Denstedt JD: The use of stents in contemporary urology, *Curr Opin Urol* 14:111, 2004.
35. Rosenstein D, McAninch JW: Urologic emergencies, *Med Clin North Am* 88:495, 2004.
36. Arnold HL, Harrison SA: New advances in evaluation and management of patients with polycystic liver disease, *Am J Gastroenterol* 100:2569, 2005.
37. Cohen HT, McGovern MD: Renal-cell carcinoma, *N Engl J Med* 353:2477, 2005.
38. Galli B, Munver R: Laparoscopic radical nephrectomy in renal cell carcinoma, *Urol Nurs* 25:83, 2005.
39. Lamm DL, McGee WR, Hale K: Bladder cancer: current optimal intravesical treatment, *Urol Nurs* 25:323, 2005.
40. Gray M, Sims TW: NMP-22 for bladder cancer screening and surveillance, *Urol Nurs* 24:171, 2004.
41. Moyad MA: Bladder cancer prevention. Part 1: what do I tell my patients about lifestyle changes and dietary supplements? *Curr Opin Urol* 13:363, 2003.
42. Boyd LA: Intravesical bacillus Calmette-Guerin for treating bladder cancer, *Urol Nurs* 23:189, 2003.
43. Newman DK: Urinary incontinence, *J Adv Nurs* 6:19, 2004.
44. Wyman JA: Treatment of urinary incontinence in men and older women, *Am J Nurs* 103(3 Suppl):26, 2003.
45. Newman DK: Stress urinary incontinence in women, *Am J Nurs* 103(8):46, 2003.
46. Wareing M: Urinary retention: issues of management and care, *Emerg Nurse* 11(8):24, 2004.
47. Newman DK, Gaines T, Snare E: Innovation in bladder assessment: use of technology in extended care, *J Gerontol Nurs* 31(12):33, 2005.
48. Newman DK: Assessment of the patient with an overactive bladder, *J Wound Ostomy Continence Nurs* 32(3 Suppl 1):S5, 2005.
49. Sampselle CM: Teaching women to use a voiding diary, *Am J Nurs* 103(11):62, 2003.
50. Newman DK: Therapeutic strategies for managing stress urinary incontinence in women, *Am J Nurs Pract Suppl,* May:23, 2004.
51. Newman DK: Behavioral treatments. In Vasavada SP, Appell A, Sand PK, et al, editors: *Female urology, urogynecology, and voiding dysfunction,* New York, 2005, Marcel Dekker.
52. Newman DK: Lifestyle interventions. In Bourcier AP, McGuire EJ, Abrams P, editors: *Pelvic floor disorders,* Philadelphia, 2004, Saunders.
53. Taylor P: Pharmacologic management of overactive bladder, *J Wound Ostomy Continence Nurs* 32(3 Suppl 1):S16, 2005.
54. Smith AL, Moy ML: Modern management of women with stress urinary incontinence, *Ostomy Wound Manage* 50(12):32, 2004.
55. Newman DK: Incontinence products and devices for the elderly, *Urol Nurs* 24:316, 2004.
56. Warren JW: Nosocomial urinary tract infections. In Mandel G, Bennett J, Dolin R, editors: *Principles and practice of infectious diseases,* ed 6, Philadelphia, 2005, Churchill Livingstone.
57. Newman DK, Fader M, Bliss DZ: Managing incontinence using technology, devices and products, *Nurs Res* 53(6 Suppl):S42, 2004.

*Nursing research–based reference.

58. Niel-Weise BS, van den Broek PJ: Urinary catheter policies for short-term bladder drainage in adults, *Cochrane Database Syst Rev* 3: CD004203, 2006.

59. Robinson J: Suprapubic catheterization: challenges in changing catheters, *Br J Community Nurs* 10:461, 2005.

60. Heard L, Buhrer R: How do we prevent UTI in people who perform intermittent catheterization? *Rehabil Nurs* 30:44, 2005.

61. Beitz JM: Continent diversions: the new gold standards of ileoanal reservoir and neobladder, *Ostomy Wound Manage* 50(9):26, 2004.

62. Perimenis P, Koliopanou E: Postoperative management and rehabilitation of patients receiving a ileal orthotopic bladder substitution, *Urol Nurs* 24:383, 2004.

63. Farnham SB, Cookson MS: Surgical complications of urinary diversions, *World J Urol* 22:157, 2004.

RESOURCES

American Association of Kidney Patients
800-749-2257 or 813-636-8100
Email: *info@aakp.org*
www.aakp.org

American Nephrology Nurses Association
888-600-2662 or 856-256-2320
Email: *anna@ajj.com*
www.annanurse.org

Bladder Health Council

American Urological Association
800-828-7866 or 410-689-3990
Email: *admin@afud.org*
www.afud.org

Interstitial Cystitis Association
800-435-7422 or 301-610-5300
www.ichelp.org

Kestrel Incontinence Product Sourcebook
Kestrel Health Information
802-453-2955
www.kestrelhealthinfo.com/incontinence_sourcebook.html

National Association for Continence (NAFC)
800-BLADDER (252-3337) or 843-377-0900
www.nafc.org

National Kidney and Urologic Diseases Information Clearinghouse
800-891-5390
Email: *nkudic@info.niddk.nih.gov*
www.kidney.niddk.nih.gov

National Kidney Foundation
800-622-9010 or 212-889-2210
Email: *info@kidney.org*
www.kidney.org

Polycystic Kidney Disease Foundation
800-753-2873 or 816-931-2600
Email: *pkdcure@pkdcure.org*
www.pkdcure.org

Society of Urological Nurses and Associates
888-827-7862
www.suna.org

United Ostomy Association of America
800-826-0826
www.uoa.org

Wound, Ostomy and Continence Nurses Society
888-224-9626
www.wocn.org

Also see Resources for Chapter 47 on p. 1232.

For additional Internet resources, see the website for this book at *http://evolve.elsevier.com/Lewis/medsurg.*

Nursing Management

Acute Renal Failure and Chronic Kidney Disease

47

Terran R. Mathers

LEARNING OBJECTIVES

1. Differentiate between acute renal failure and chronic kidney disease.
2. Differentiate among the causes of prerenal, intrarenal, and postrenal acute renal failure.
3. Describe the clinical course of reversible acute renal failure.
4. Explain the collaborative care and nursing management of a patient with acute renal failure.
5. Describe the systemic manifestations of chronic kidney disease.
6. Explain the conservative collaborative care for and the related nursing management of the patient with chronic kidney disease.
7. Differentiate between peritoneal dialysis and hemodialysis in terms of purpose, indications, advantages and disadvantages, and nursing responsibilities.
8. Describe common vascular access sites used for hemodialysis.
9. Compare dialysis and renal transplantation as methods of treatment for end-stage renal disease.
10. Describe the nursing management of patients in the preoperative, intraoperative, and postoperative stages of kidney transplantation.
11. Discuss the potential long-term problems of the patient with a kidney transplant.

KEY TERMS

acute renal failure, p. 1197
azotemia, p. 1197
chronic kidney disease, p. 1204
continuous ambulatory peritoneal dialysis, p. 1218
continuous renal replacement therapy, p. 1224
dialysis, p. 1216
end-stage renal disease, p. 1204
hemodialysis, p. 1216
oliguria, p. 1198
peritoneal dialysis, p. 1216
renal osteodystrophy, p. 1208
uremia, p. 1198

Electronic Resources

Supplemental content related to Chapter 47 can be found ...

Companion CD
- Stress-Busting Kit for Nursing Students
- Interactive Case Studies:
  - Glomerulonephritis and Chronic Kidney Disease
  - Kidney Transplant
- NCLEX Examination Review Questions
- Comprehensive Glossary

Evolve Website *evolve*
http://evolve.elsevier.com/Lewis/medsurg
- Content Updates
- Key Points (Printable and CD/MP3 Download)
- Concept Map Creator
- Expanded Audio Glossary
- Key Term Flash Cards

- Customizable Nursing Care Plan: Chronic Kidney Disease
- Electronic Calculators
- WebLinks

Renal failure is the partial or complete impairment of kidney function resulting in an inability to excrete metabolic waste products and water, as well as causing functional disturbances of all body systems. Renal failure is classified as acute or chronic. Acute renal failure (ARF) has a rapid onset. Although ARF is potentially reversible, the mortality rate for intrarenal ARF remains at about 50% despite advances in treatment over the last 30 years.[1]

Chronic kidney disease (CKD) usually develops slowly over months to years and necessitates the initiation of dialysis or transplantation for long-term survival. The focus in CKD has changed from treating a terminally ill patient to caring for a person with a manageable chronic disease that requires effective monitoring and interventions over a long period of time. The change in focus is the result of technologic advances, improved surgical techniques, effective immunosuppressive therapy, and the collaboration of professionals and industry leaders whose efforts are changing the outcomes of patients with CKD.

ACUTE RENAL FAILURE

Acute renal failure is a clinical syndrome characterized by a rapid loss of renal function with progressive **azotemia** (an accumulation of nitrogenous waste products such as urea nitrogen and creatinine

Reviewed by Darryl E. Reid, Sr., RN, MSN, Clinical Informatics Nurse, Dialysis Nurse, South Texas Veterans Health Care System, Audie Murphie Division, San Antonio, Tex.

in the blood). Electrolyte and fluid status also changes, but only a few symptoms may be seen in patients at this stage.[2]

Uremia is the condition in which renal function declines to the point that symptoms develop in multiple body systems. ARF is often associated with **oliguria,** which is a decrease in urinary output to less than 400 ml/day. In about 50% of the cases there is normal or increased urinary output (nonoliguria). Patients with nonoliguria usually have fewer complications and recover more quickly.[3] Patients with oliguric ARF do not have as good an outcome.[2]

ARF usually develops over hours or days with progressive elevations of blood urea nitrogen (BUN), creatinine, and potassium with or without oliguria. Most commonly, ARF follows severe, prolonged hypotension or hypovolemia or exposure to a nephrotoxic agent. Five percent to 7% of all hospitalized patients are affected.[4]

Etiology and Pathophysiology

The causes of ARF are multiple and complex. They are categorized according to similar pathogenesis into prerenal, intrarenal (or intrinsic), and postrenal causes (Table 47-1 and Fig. 47-1).

Prerenal causes leading to ARF are due to factors external to the kidneys that reduce renal blood flow and lead to decreased glomerular perfusion and filtration. Hypovolemia, decreased cardiac output, decreased peripheral vascular resistance, and vascular obstruction can all decrease the effective circulating volume of the blood. Oliguria occurs as the kidneys respond to the decreased blood flow by activating the renin-angiotensin-aldosterone system (see Fig. 45-4). This compensation by the kidneys results in sodium and water conservation. Decreased renal perfusion also decreases clearance of wastes (azotemia). As decreased perfusion continues, the kidneys lose their ability to engage in compensatory mechanisms and intrarenal damage to renal tissue occurs. The result is low urine output due to the kidneys' inability to excrete water, a rise in BUN and serum creatinine proportionate to each other (ratio of >10:1), and the inability of the kidneys to conserve sodium. Prerenal conditions can lead to intrarenal disease if renal ischemia is prolonged. Prerenal conditions account for approximately 60% to 70% of the cases of intrarenal disease.[2]

Intrarenal causes of ARF include conditions that cause direct damage to the renal tissue (parenchyma), resulting in impaired nephron function. The damage by intrarenal causes usually results from prolonged ischemia, nephrotoxins (e.g., aminoglycoside antibiotics, contrast media), hemoglobin released from hemolyzed red blood cells (RBCs), or myoglobin released from necrotic muscle cells. Nephrotoxins can cause obstruction of intrarenal structures by crystallization or actual damage to the epithelial cells of the tubules. Hemoglobin and myoglobin block the tubules and cause renal vasoconstriction. Primary renal diseases such as acute glomerulonephritis and systemic lupus erythematosus may also cause ARF.

Acute tubular necrosis (ATN) is an intrarenal condition caused by ischemia, nephrotoxins, or pigments[3] (Fig. 47-2). Ischemic and

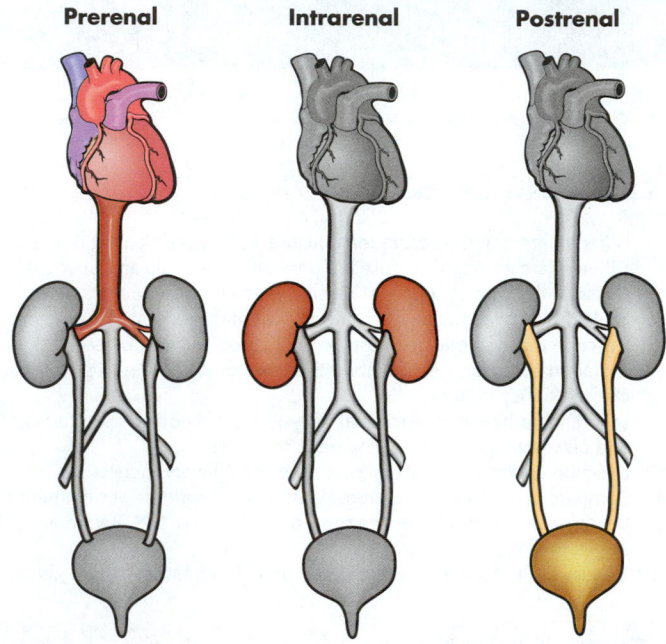

Prerenal   **Intrarenal**   **Postrenal**

FIG. 47-1   Prerenal, intrarenal, and postrenal causes of acute renal failure.

TABLE 47-1	**Common Causes of Acute Renal Failure**

Prerenal	**Intrarenal**	**Postrenal**

• Hypovolemia
  Dehydration
  Hemorrhage
  GI losses (diarrhea, vomiting)
  Excessive diuresis
  Hypoalbuminemia
  Burns
• Decreased cardiac output
  Cardiac dysrhythmias
  Cardiogenic shock
  Heart failure
  Myocardial infarction
• Decreased peripheral vascular resistance
  Anaphylaxis
  Neurologic injury
  Septic shock
• Decreased renovascular blood flow
  Bilateral renal vein thrombosis
  Embolism
  Hepatorenal syndrome
  Renal artery thrombosis
	• Prolonged prerenal ischemia
	• Nephrotoxic injury
	  Drugs (aminoglycosides [gentamicin, amikacin], amphotericin B)
	  Radiocontrast agents
	  Hemolytic blood transfusion reaction
	  Severe crush injury
	  Chemical exposure (ethylene glycol, lead, arsenic, carbon tetrachloride)
	• Interstitial nephritis
	  Allergies (antibiotics [sulfonamides, rifampin], non-steroidal antiinflammatory drugs, ACE inhibitors)
	  Infections (bacterial [acute pyelonephritis], viral [CMV], fungal [candidiasis])
	• Acute glomerulonephritis
	• Thrombotic disorders
	• Toxemia of pregnancy
	• Malignant hypertension
	• Systemic lupus erythematosus
		• Benign prostatic hyperplasia
		• Bladder cancer
		• Calculi formation
		• Neuromuscular disorders
		• Prostate cancer
		• Spinal cord disease
		• Strictures
		• Trauma (back, pelvis, perineum)

ACE, Angiotensin-converting enzyme; *CMV,* cytomegalovirus; *GI,* gastrointestinal.

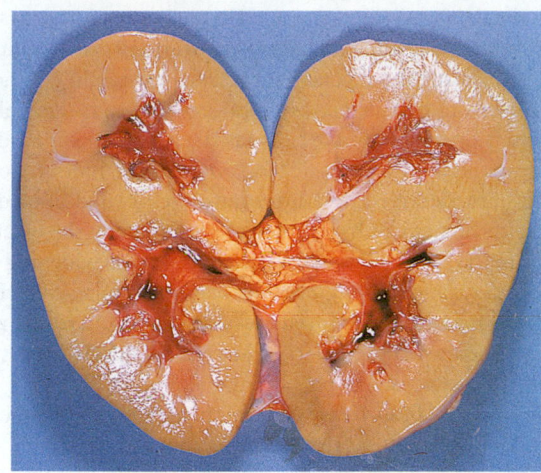

FIG. 47-2   Acute tubular necrosis. In acute tubular necrosis, the kidneys are swollen and pale.

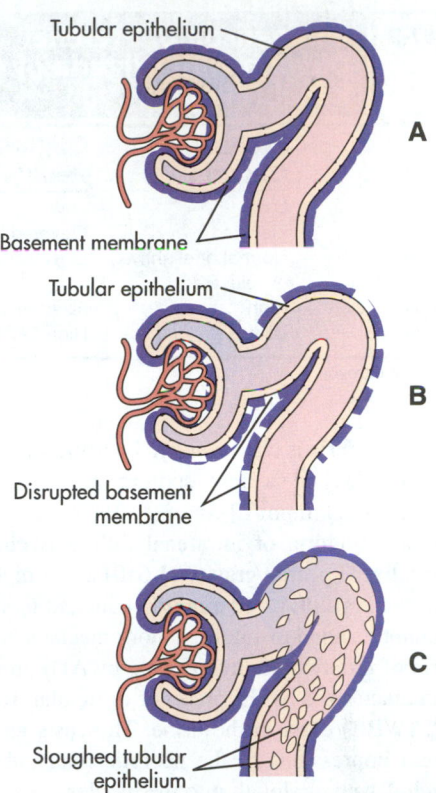

FIG. 47-3   Nephron destruction in acute renal failure. **A,** Normal nephron. **B,** Damage from renal ischemia results in patchy necrosis of the tubule. The lumen may also be blocked by casts. **C,** Damage from nephrotoxic agents.

nephrotoxic ATN are responsible for 90% of intrarenal ARF cases.[1] Severe renal ischemia causes a disruption in the basement membrane and patchy destruction of the tubular epithelium. Nephrotoxic agents cause necrosis of tubular epithelial cells, which slough off and plug the tubules, but usually leave the basement membrane intact (Fig. 47-3). ATN is potentially reversible if the basement membrane is not destroyed and the tubular epithelium regenerates.

Possible pathologic processes involved in ATN include the following:

1. Hypovolemia and decreased renal blood flow stimulate renin release, which activates the renin-angiotensin-aldosterone system (see Chapter 45, Fig. 45-4) and results in constriction of the peripheral arteries and the renal afferent arterioles. With decreased renal blood flow, there is decreased glomerular capillary pressure and glomerular filtration rate (GFR), as well as tubular dysfunction and, ultimately, oliguria.
2. Ischemia alters glomerular epithelial cells and decreases glomerular capillary permeability. This reduces the GFR, which significantly reduces blood flow and leads to tubular dysfunction.
3. When tubules are damaged, interstitial edema occurs, and necrotic epithelial cells accumulate in the tubules. The debris lowers the GFR by obstructing the tubules and increasing intratubular pressure.
4. Glomerular filtrate leaks back into plasma through holes in the damaged tubular membranes, which decreases intratubular fluid flow.

Postrenal causes involve mechanical obstruction of urinary outflow. As the flow of urine is obstructed, urine refluxes into the renal pelvis, impairing kidney function. The most common causes are benign prostatic hyperplasia, prostate cancer, calculi, trauma, and extrarenal tumors. Postrenal causes of ARF account for less than 5% of the cases.[1] Azotemia can be reversed if the outflow obstruction is relieved before damage to the kidney occurs. Outflow obstructions that are not corrected will damage renal parenchyma and cause ARF.

Clinical Course

Prerenal and postrenal situations that have not yet resulted in intrarenal damage usually resolve quickly with correction of the cause. However, if parenchymal damage has occurred due to either pre-

renal or postrenal causes, or when parenchymal damage occurs directly, as with ATN or other intrarenal causes, ARF occurs and has a prolonged course of recovery. Clinically, ARF may progress through four phases: initiating, oliguric, diuretic, and recovery. In some situations, the patient does not recover from ARF, and chronic kidney disease (CKD) results, eventually requiring dialysis or a kidney transplant.[5]

Initiating Phase. This begins at the time of the insult and continues until the signs and symptoms become apparent. It can last hours to days.

Oliguric Phase. The most common initial manifestation of ARF is oliguria caused by a reduction in the GFR. Oliguria usually occurs within 1 to 7 days of the causative event. If the cause is ischemia, oliguria may occur within 24 hours. When nephrotoxic drugs are involved, the onset may be delayed for as long as a week. About 50% of the patients will not demonstrate oliguria, making the initial diagnosis more difficult.[1] The duration of the oliguric phase lasts on average about 10 to 14 days but can last months in some cases. The longer the oliguric phase lasts, the poorer the prognosis for recovery of complete renal function.

It is important to distinguish prerenal oliguria from the oliguria of intrarenal ARF (Table 47-2). In prerenal oliguria there is no damage to the renal tissue. The oliguria is caused by a decrease in circulating blood volume (e.g., as a result of severe dehydration, decreased cardiac output, burns) and is usually reversible. With a decrease in circulating blood volume, autoregulatory mechanisms that increase angiotensin II, aldosterone, norepinephrine, and antidiuretic hormone attempt to preserve blood flow to essential organs. Vasoconstriction occurs along with sodium and water reten-

TABLE 47-2	Comparison of Prerenal Oliguria with Oliguria of Acute Renal Failure	
	Prerenal Oliguria	**Oliguria of Acute Renal Failure**
Urine output	Low	Low
BUN	Elevated	Elevated
Serum creatinine	Normal or slightly elevated	Elevated
Urine specific gravity	High	Fixed at 1.010
Urine sodium	Low	High

BUN, Blood urea nitrogen.

tion. Prerenal oliguria is characterized by urine with a high specific gravity (>1.025) and a low sodium concentration (<10 to 20 mEq/L [10 to 20 mmol/L]).

In contrast, oliguria of intrarenal failure is characterized by urine with a fixed specific gravity (1.010) and a high sodium concentration (>40 mEq/L [>40 mmol/L]), indicating that the injured tubules cannot respond to autoregulatory mechanisms. In addition, the oliguria of intrarenal failure caused by ATN from ischemia or toxins is characterized by the presence of tubular, RBC, and white blood cell (WBC) casts in the urine. The casts are formed from mucoprotein impressions of the necrotic renal tubular epithelial cells, which detach or slough into the tubules.

In addition to oliguria, other changes during the oliguric phase include fluid and electrolyte abnormalities and uremia. The nurse must be alert for the signs and symptoms of these changes.

Urinary Changes. Urinary output decreases to less than 400 ml/24 hr for about 50% of the patients. A urinalysis may show casts, RBCs, WBCs, a specific gravity fixed at around 1.010, and urine osmolality at about 300 mOsm/kg (300 mmol/kg). This is the same specific gravity and osmolality as for plasma, reflecting tubular damage with a loss of concentrating ability by the kidney. Proteinuria may be present if the renal failure is related to glomerular membrane dysfunction.

Fluid Volume Excess. When urinary output decreases, fluid retention occurs. The severity of the symptoms depends on the extent of the fluid overload. The neck veins may become distended with a bounding pulse. Edema and hypertension may develop. Fluid overload can eventually lead to heart failure (HF), pulmonary edema, and pericardial and pleural effusions.

Metabolic Acidosis. In renal failure, the kidneys cannot synthesize ammonia, which is needed for hydrogen ion excretion, or excrete acid products of metabolism. The serum bicarbonate level decreases because bicarbonate is used up in buffering hydrogen ions. In addition, defective reabsorption and regeneration of bicarbonate occurs. The patient may develop Kussmaul respirations (rapid, deep respirations) to increase the excretion of carbon dioxide. Lethargy and stupor will occur if treatment is not started.

Sodium Balance. Damaged tubules cannot conserve sodium. Consequently, the urinary excretion of sodium may increase, resulting in normal or below-normal levels of serum sodium. Excessive intake of sodium should be avoided because it can lead to volume expansion, hypertension, and HF. Uncontrolled hyponatremia or water excess can lead to cerebral edema.

Potassium Excess. The serum potassium levels increase because the normal ability of the kidneys to excrete 80% to 90% of the body's potassium is impaired. If the ARF is caused by massive tissue

trauma, the damaged cells release additional potassium into the extracellular fluid. Bleeding and blood transfusions cause cellular destruction, releasing more potassium into the extracellular fluid. Acidosis worsens hyperkalemia as hydrogen ions enter the cells and potassium is driven out of the cells into the extracellular fluid.

When potassium levels exceed 6 mEq/L (6 mmol/L) or dysrhythmias are identified, treatment must be initiated immediately. Before clinical signs of hyperkalemia are apparent, the electrocardiogram (ECG) will show tall, peaked T waves; widening of the QRS complex; and, ST segment depression. Progressive changes in the ECG that are related to increasing potassium levels are depicted in Chapter 17, Fig. 17-14. The cardiac muscle is very intolerant of acute increases in potassium.

Hematologic Disorders. Several hematologic disorders are seen in ARF. Anemia occurs because renal failure results in impaired erythropoietin production. The anemia may be compounded by platelet abnormalities that can lead to bleeding from multiple sources (i.e., intestines, brain). WBCs are also altered, causing immunodeficiency. This leaves the patient susceptible to numerous systemic and local infections. The two most common causes of death in patients with ARF are infection and cardiorespiratory complications.[2]

Calcium Deficit and Phosphate Excess. A low serum calcium level results from decreased gastrointestinal (GI) absorption of calcium. To absorb calcium from the GI tract, activated vitamin D is necessary. Only functioning kidneys can activate vitamin D, allowing absorption to occur. When hypocalcemia occurs, the parathyroid gland secretes parathyroid hormone (PTH), which stimulates bone demineralization, thereby releasing calcium from the bones. Phosphate is released as well, leading to elevated serum phosphate levels. Hyperphosphatemia also results from decreased phosphate excretion by the kidneys. Normally plasma calcium is found ionized or free (physiologically active form) or bound to protein. In renal failure, it is unusual for hypocalcemia to be symptomatic. The reason for this is that, in the acidotic state associated with renal failure, more calcium is in the ionized form rather than bound to protein. However, a low ionized calcium level can lead to tetany (see Chapter 17).

Waste Product Accumulation. The kidneys are the primary excretory organs for urea, an end product of protein metabolism, and creatinine, an end product of endogenous muscle metabolism. The BUN and serum creatinine levels are elevated in kidney failure. An elevated BUN level must be interpreted with caution because dehydration, corticosteroids, and catabolism resulting from infections, fever, severe injury, or GI bleeding can also elevate BUN. The best serum indicator of renal failure is creatinine because it is not significantly altered by other factors. Measuring creatinine clearance with a 24-hour urine study or using radioactive tracer is the best method for assessing renal function. But clinically, serum creatinine is most commonly used.

Neurologic Disorders. Neurologic changes can occur as the nitrogenous waste products accumulate in the brain and other nervous tissue. The symptoms can be as mild as fatigue and difficulty concentrating, then escalate to seizures, stupor, and coma.

Eventually all body systems become involved in the uremia of ARF (Table 47-3). The extrarenal manifestations are generally similar to those found in the patient with chronic uremia, discussed later in this chapter (see Fig. 47-5).

Diuretic Phase. The diuretic phase of ARF begins with a gradual increase in daily urine output of 1 to 3 L/day, but may

TABLE 47-3	Manifestations of Acute Renal Failure
Body System	**Clinical Manifestations**
Urinary	↓ Urinary output
	Proteinuria
	Casts
	↓ Specific gravity
	↓ Osmolality
	↑ Urinary sodium
Cardiovascular	Volume overload
	Heart failure
	Hypotension (early)
	Hypertension (after development of fluid overload)
	Pericarditis
	Pericardial effusion
	Dysrhythmias
Respiratory	Pulmonary edema
	Kussmaul respirations
	Pleural effusions
Gastrointestinal	Nausea and vomiting
	Anorexia
	Stomatitis
	Bleeding
	Diarrhea
	Constipation
Hematologic	Anemia (development within 48 hr)
	↑ Susceptibility to infection
	Leukocytosis
	Defect in platelet functioning
Neurologic	Lethargy
	Seizures
	Asterixis
	Memory impairment
Metabolic	↑ BUN
	↑ Creatinine
	↓ Sodium
	↑ Potassium
	↓ pH
	↓ Bicarbonate
	↓ Calcium
	↑ Phosphate

BUN, Blood urea nitrogen.

reach 3 to 5 L or more. Although urine output is increasing, the nephrons are still not fully functional. The high urine volume is caused by osmotic diuresis from the high urea concentration in the glomerular filtrate and the inability of the tubules to concentrate the urine. In this phase the kidneys have recovered their ability to excrete wastes, but not to concentrate the urine. Hypovolemia and hypotension can occur from massive fluid losses.

At this stage the uremia may still be severe, as reflected by low creatinine clearances, elevated serum creatinine and BUN levels, and persistent signs and symptoms. Because of the large losses of fluid and electrolytes, the patient must be monitored for hyponatremia, hypokalemia, and dehydration. The diuretic phase may last 1 to 3 weeks. Near the end of this phase, the patient's acid-base, electrolyte, and waste product (BUN, creatinine) values begin to normalize.

Recovery Phase. The recovery phase begins when the GFR increases, allowing the BUN and serum creatinine levels to plateau and then decrease. Although the major improvements occur in the first 1 to 2 weeks of this phase, renal function may take up to 12 months to stabilize.

The outcome of ARF is influenced by the patient's overall health, the severity of renal failure, and the number and type of complications. Some individuals do not recover and progress to chronic kidney disease. The older adult patient is less likely to recover full kidney function than the younger patient. Among the individuals who recover, the majority achieves clinically normal kidney function with no complications (e.g., hypertension).

Diagnostic Studies

A thorough history is essential for diagnosing the etiology of ARF. Prerenal causes should be considered when there is a history of dehydration, blood loss, or severe heart disease. Intrarenal causes may be suspected if the patient has been taking potentially nephrotoxic drugs or has a recent history of prolonged hypotension or hypovolemia. Postrenal causes are suggested by a history of changes in the urinary stream, stones, benign prostatic hyperplasia, or cancer of the bladder or prostate.

Urinalysis is an important diagnostic test. Urine sediment containing abundant cells, casts, or proteins suggests intrarenal disorders. The urine osmolality, sodium content, and specific gravity help in differentiating the causes of ARF. Urine sediment may be normal in both prerenal and postrenal ARF. Hematuria, pyuria, and crystals may be seen with postrenal conditions.

To establish a diagnosis of ARF, other testing may be required. A renal ultrasound is often the first test done. It is useful for evaluating for possible renal disease and obstruction of the urinary collection system. A renal scan can assess renal blood flow, tubular function, and the integrity of the collecting system. A computed tomography (CT) scan and magnetic resonance imaging (MRI) can identify lesions and masses, as well as obstructions and vascular anomalies. A renal biopsy can be very useful in the diagnosis of intrarenal causes of ARF.

Collaborative Care

Because ARF is potentially reversible, the primary goals of treatment are to eliminate the cause, manage the signs and symptoms, and prevent complications while the kidneys recover (Table 47-4). The first step is to determine if there is adequate intravascular volume and cardiac output to ensure adequate perfusion of the kidneys. Diuretic therapy is often administered along with volume expanders to prevent fluid overload. Diuretic therapy usually includes loop diuretics (e.g., furosemide [Lasix], bumetanide [Bumex]), or an osmotic diuretic (e.g., mannitol).[6] If ARF is already established, forcing fluids and diuretics will not be effective and may, in fact, be harmful. Conservative therapy may be all that is necessary until renal function improves. The general trend is to initiate early and frequent dialysis to minimize symptoms and prevent complications.

Fluid intake must be closely monitored during the oliguric phase. The general rule for calculating the fluid restriction is to add all losses for the previous 24 hours (e.g., urine, diarrhea, emesis, blood) plus 600 ml for insensible losses (e.g., respiration, diaphoresis). For example, if a patient excreted 300 ml of urine on Tuesday with no other losses, the fluid restriction on Wednesday would be 900 ml.

Hyperkalemia is one of the most serious complications in ARF because it can cause life-threatening cardiac dysrhythmias. The various therapies used to treat elevated potassium levels are listed in Table 47-5. Both insulin and sodium bicarbonate temporarily shift potassium into the cells, but it will eventually shift back out. Calcium

TABLE 47-4	COLLABORATIVE CARE Acute Renal Failure

Diagnostic
History and physical examination
Identification of precipitating cause
Serum creatinine and BUN levels
Serum electrolytes
Urinalysis
Renal ultrasound
Renal scan (as indicated)
CT scan or MRI (as indicated)
Retrograde pyelogram (as indicated)

Collaborative Therapy
Treatment of precipitating cause
Fluid restriction (600 ml plus previous 24-hr fluid loss)
Nutritional therapy
- Adequate protein intake (0.6-2 g/kg/day) depending on degree of catabolism
- Potassium restriction
- Phosphate restriction
- Sodium restriction
Measures to lower potassium (if elevated)*
Calcium supplements or phosphate-binding agents
Parenteral nutrition (if indicated)†
Enteral nutrition (if indicated)†
Initiation of dialysis (if necessary)
Continuous renal replacement therapy (if necessary)

BUN, Blood urea nitrogen; *CT*, computed tomography; *MRI*, magnetic resonance imaging.
*See Table 47-5.
†Renal formulations of these two forms of nutrition are available.

TABLE 47-5	Therapies to Treat Elevated Potassium Levels

1. Regular Insulin Administration IV
Potassium moves into cells when insulin is given. Glucose is given concurrently to prevent hypoglycemia. When effects of insulin diminish, potassium shifts back out of cells.

2. Sodium Bicarbonate
Therapy can correct acidosis and causes shift of potassium into cells.

3. Calcium Gluconate IV
Therapy is given IV and generally used in advanced cardiac toxicity. Calcium raises the threshold for excitation, resulting in dysrhythmias.

4. Dialysis
Hemodialysis can bring potassium levels to normal within 30 minutes to 2 hours.

5. Sodium Polystyrene Sulfonate (Kayexalate)
Cation-exchange resin is administered by mouth or retention enema. When resin is in the bowel, potassium is exchanged for sodium. Therapy removes 1 mEq of potassium per gram of drug. It is mixed in water with sorbitol to produce osmotic diarrhea, allowing for evacuation of potassium-rich stool from body.

6. Dietary Restriction
Daily potassium intake is limited to 40 mEq.

IV, Intravenous.

gluconate raises the threshold at which dysrhythmias will occur. Only sodium polystyrene sulfonate (Kayexalate) and dialysis actually remove potassium from the body. The nurse must be cautious, however; sodium polystyrene sulfonate should never be given to a patient with a paralytic ileus because bowel necrosis can occur.

The most common indications for dialysis in ARF include (1) volume overload, resulting in compromised cardiac and/or pulmonary status; (2) elevated potassium level with ECG changes; (3) metabolic acidosis (serum bicarbonate level <15 mEq/L [15 mmol/L]); (4) BUN level >120 mg/dl (43 mmol/L); (5) significant change in mental status; and (6) pericarditis, pericardial effusion, or cardiac tamponade. Laboratory values are only rough parameters, and clinical assessment is the most important guide in determining the need for dialysis.

If dialysis is required, two options are available: hemodialysis (HD) and peritoneal dialysis (PD). HD is the method of choice when rapid changes are required in a short period of time. It is technically more complicated because specialized staff and equipment and a vascular access are required. It also requires anticoagulation therapy to prevent the patient's blood from clotting when the blood contacts the foreign membrane material in the dialysis circuit. Rapid fluid shifts during HD may cause hypotension. HD is preferred for the hypercatabolic patient and for the individual who has had abdominal or thoracic trauma or surgery. PD is much simpler than HD, but it carries the risk of peritonitis, is less efficient in the catabolic patient, and requires longer treatment times. PD may be preferred for the individual with intracranial bleeding or cardiovascular instability. (HD and PD are discussed later in this chapter.)

Continuous renal replacement therapy (CRRT) may also be used in the treatment of ARF. (CRRT is discussed later in this chapter.) In the hemodynamically unstable patient, CRRT provides gradual removal of excess fluid and solutes. It is technically similar to HD and requires extracorporeal blood circulation via cannulation of two veins or an artery and a vein. Blood removed from the artery or vein passes through a hemofilter where solutes and water are removed, and then the blood is returned to the patient. CRRT runs continuously and requires at least 12 to 24 hours to accomplish what can be done with 3 to 4 hours of HD. Larger amounts of fluid may be removed than with intermittent HD. CRRT is the preferred treatment in the hemodynamically unstable patient with mild to moderate ARF with fluid overload.

Nutritional Therapy. The challenge of nutritional management in renal failure is to provide adequate calories to prevent catabolism despite the restrictions required to prevent electrolyte and fluid disorders and azotemia. If the patient does not receive adequate nutrition, catabolism of body protein will occur.[4] This process causes increased urea, phosphate, and potassium levels. Adequate energy should be primarily from carbohydrate and fat sources to prevent ketosis from endogenous fat breakdown and gluconeogenesis from muscle protein breakdown. The daily caloric intake should be about 30 to 35 kcal/kg of body weight. Protein intake is adjusted according to the patient's condition, but is generally 0.6 g/kg per day to control nitrogenous waste production and limit starvation ketosis.[2] Essential amino acid supplements (e.g., Amin-Aid) can be given for amino acid and caloric supplementation.

Potassium and sodium are regulated in accordance with plasma levels. Sodium is restricted as needed to prevent edema, hypertension, and HF. Dietary fat intake is increased so that the patient receives at least 30% to 40% of total calories from fat. Fat emulsion intravenous (IV) infusions can also be given as a nutritional supplement and provide a good source of nonprotein calories (see Chapter 40). If a patient cannot maintain adequate oral intake, enteral nutrition is the preferred route for nutritional support[7] (see Chapter 40). When the GI tract is not functional, parenteral nutrition is necessary for the provision of adequate nutrition. The patient treated with parenteral nutrition may need daily HD or CRRT to remove the excess fluid. Concentrated formulas are available to minimize fluid volume.

NURSING MANAGEMENT
ACUTE RENAL FAILURE

■ Nursing Assessment

An assessment of the patient in ARF includes the specific manifestations presented in Table 47-3. It is important to monitor the vital signs and fluid intake and output. The urine should be examined for color, specific gravity, glucose, protein, blood, or sediment. The patient's general appearance should be assessed, including skin color, edema, neck vein distention, and bruises.

If the patient is receiving dialysis, the access site should be observed for signs of inflammation. The patient's mental status and level of consciousness should also be evaluated. The oral mucosa should be examined for dryness and inflammation. The lungs should be auscultated for crackles and rhonchi or diminished breath sounds. The heart should be monitored for the presence of an S_3, other murmurs, or a pericardial friction rub. ECG readings should be assessed for the presence of dysrhythmias. Laboratory values and diagnostic test results should be reviewed. All of the previous data are essential for developing a collaborative plan of care.

■ Nursing Diagnoses

Nursing diagnoses and potential complications for the patient with ARF include, but are not limited to, the following:

- Excess fluid volume *related to* renal failure and fluid retention
- Risk for infection *related to* invasive lines, uremic toxins, and altered immune responses secondary to kidney failure
- Imbalanced nutrition: less than body requirements *related to* altered metabolic state and dietary restrictions
- Disturbed thought processes *related to* effects of uremic toxins on central nervous system (CNS)
- Fatigue *related to* anemia, metabolic acidosis, and uremic toxins
- Anxiety *related to* disease process, therapeutic interventions, and uncertainty of prognosis
- Potential complication: dysrhythmias *related to* electrolyte imbalances
- Potential complication: metabolic acidosis *related to* inability to excrete H^+, impaired HCO_3^- reabsorption, and decreased synthesis of ammonia

■ Planning

The overall goals are that the patient with ARF will (1) completely recover without any loss of kidney function, (2) maintain normal fluid and electrolyte balance, (3) have decreased anxiety, and (4) comply with and understand the need for careful follow-up care.

■ Nursing Implementation

Health Promotion. Prevention of ARF is essential because of the high mortality rate and is primarily directed toward identifying and monitoring high-risk populations, controlling exposure to nephrotoxic drugs and industrial chemicals, and preventing prolonged episodes of hypotension and hypovolemia. In the hospital,

the factors that increase the risk for developing ARF are advanced age, massive trauma, major surgical procedures, extensive burns, cardiac failure, sepsis, obstetric complications, or baseline renal insufficiency caused by hypertension or diabetes mellitus. Careful monitoring of intake and output and fluid and electrolyte balance is essential. Extrarenal losses of fluid from vomiting, diarrhea, and hemorrhage and increased insensible losses must be assessed and recorded. Prompt replacement of significant fluid losses will help prevent ischemic tubular damage associated with trauma, burns, and extensive surgery. Intake and output records and the patient's weight provide valuable indicators of fluid volume status. Aggressive diuretic therapy for the patient with fluid overload resulting from any cause can lead to inadequate renal vascular perfusion.

Streptococcal infections must be identified and treated with antibiotics. Compliance with the antibiotic regimen is critical to eliminate the source of infection and prevent complications such as acute poststreptococcal glomerulonephritis and rheumatic heart disease.

For the older adult or diabetic patient who is undergoing diagnostic studies requiring IV contrast media, special attention must be given to prevent a nephrotoxic injury secondary to the dye. There is evidence that, if patients with renal impairment (GFR <50 ml/min) receive acetylcysteine (Mucomyst) or sodium bicarbonate infusion prior to radiocontrast-media procedures along with adequate hydration, contrast-induced nephropathy is reduced.[8] Patients with urinary tract infections need prompt treatment and careful follow-up care. Chemotherapeutic drugs that cause hyperuricemia also can put a patient at risk for renal injury.

The individual who is taking drugs that are potentially nephrotoxic (see Table 45-3) must have renal function monitored. Nephrotoxic drugs should be used sparingly in the high-risk patient. When these drugs must be used, they should be given in the smallest effective doses for the shortest possible periods. The patient should be cautioned about the abuse of over-the-counter analgesics (especially nonsteroidal antiinflammatory drugs [NSAIDs]) because some of these may worsen renal function in the patient with borderline renal insufficiency by decreasing glomerular pressure. Angiotensin-converting enzyme (ACE) inhibitors can also decrease perfusion pressure and cause hyperkalemia. If other measures such as diet modification, diuretics, and sodium bicarbonate cannot control the hyperkalemia, the ACE inhibitor needs to be discontinued.[9] Industrial and agricultural chemicals and products (organic solvents, insecticides, cleaning agents) must be monitored regularly to assess their safety for employees and the general population.

Acute Intervention. The patient with ARF is critically ill and suffers not only from the effects of renal disease but also from the effects of comorbid diseases or conditions (e.g., diabetes, cardiovascular disease) that also affect renal function. The nurse must focus on the patient as a total person with many physical and emotional needs. Usually the changes caused by ARF come on suddenly. Both the patient and the family need assistance in understanding that the functioning of the whole body can be disrupted by renal failure but that these changes are generally reversible with time.

The nurse has an important role in managing fluid and electrolyte balance during the oliguric and diuretic phases. Observing and recording accurate intake and output are essential. Daily weights measured with the same scale at the same time each day allow for the evaluation and detection of excessive gains or losses of body fluid (1 kg is equivalent to 1000 ml of fluid). The nurse must be knowledgeable about the common signs and symptoms of hypervolemia (in the oliguric phase) or hypovolemia (in the diuretic phase), potassium and sodium disturbances, and other electrolyte imbalances that may occur in ARF (see Chapter 17). Hyperkalemia is a leading cause of death in the oliguric phase of ARF. Most typically, hyperkalemia is manifested by dysrhythmias and impairment of neuromuscular function, including muscle weakness, abdominal cramps, flaccid paralysis, and absence of deep tendon reflexes. Cardiac conduction abnormalities to watch for include a prolonged PR interval, prolonged QRS interval, peaked T wave, and depressed ST segment.

Because infection is the leading cause of death overall in ARF, meticulous aseptic technique is critical. The patient should be protected from other individuals with infectious diseases. The nurse should be alert for local manifestations of infection (e.g., swelling, redness, pain) as well as systemic manifestations (e.g., malaise, leukocytosis) because an elevated temperature may not be present. Patients with renal failure have a blunted febrile response to an infection (e.g., pneumonia). If antibiotics are used to treat an infection, the type, frequency, and dosage must be carefully considered because the kidneys are the primary route of excretion for many antibiotics. Nephrotoxic drugs (see Table 45-3) should not be used unless there is no other alternative.

Respiratory complications, especially pneumonitis, can be prevented. Humidified oxygen; incentive spirometry; coughing, turning, and deep breathing; and ambulation are measures the nurse can use to help maintain adequate respiratory ventilation.

Skin care and measures to prevent pressure ulcers should be performed because the patient usually develops edema, as well as decreased muscle tone. Mouth care is important to prevent stomatitis, which develops when ammonia (produced by bacterial breakdown of urea) in saliva irritates the mucous membranes.

Ambulatory and Home Care. Recovery from ARF is highly variable and depends on the underlying illness, the general condition and age of the patient, the length of the oliguric phase, and the severity of nephron damage. Good nutrition, rest, and activity are necessary. The diet should be high in calories. Protein and potassium intake should be regulated in accordance with renal function. Follow-up care and regular evaluation of renal function are necessary. The patient should be taught the signs and symptoms of recurrent kidney disease. Measures to prevent the recurrence of ARF must be emphasized.

The long-term convalescence of 3 to 12 months may cause psychosocial and financial hardships for the family, and appropriate counseling, social work, and psychiatrist/psychologist referrals should be made as indicated. If the kidneys do not recover, the patient will eventually need dialysis or transplantation.

■ Evaluation

The expected outcomes are that the patient with ARF will
- regain and maintain normal fluid and electrolyte balance
- comply with the treatment regimen
- experience no infectious complications
- have complete recovery

GERONTOLOGIC CONSIDERATIONS
ACUTE RENAL FAILURE

The older adult is more susceptible than the younger adult to ARF as the number of functioning nephrons decreases with age. Impaired function of other organ systems, such as cardiovascular disease or diabetes mellitus, can increase the risk of developing ARF.

The aging kidney is less able to compensate for changes in fluid volume, solute load, and cardiac output. Common causes of ARF in the older adult include dehydration, hypotension, diuretic therapy, aminoglycoside therapy, obstructive disorders (e.g., prostatic hyperplasia), surgery, infection, and radiocontrast agents.

Diuretics may not be the best treatment for older adults with ARF because these drugs may actually worsen outcomes.[6] The overall prognosis after an episode of ARF is generally worse in the older adult, with a mortality rate 5% to 25% higher than that of younger adults. The higher mortality rate usually results from infection, GI hemorrhage, or myocardial infarction. Research continues in the effort to determine what treatment is most appropriate for older adults to decrease mortality rate. Several studies indicate that serum cystatin C, a nonglycosolated protein produced by nucleated cells, is a better indicator of renal function than serum creatinine. As a result, it shows promise as a more accurate predictor of mortality risk in older adults from all causes, particularly cardiovascular disease.[10]

CHRONIC KIDNEY DISEASE

Chronic kidney disease (CKD) involves progressive, irreversible loss of kidney function. It is defined as either the presence of kidney damage or glomerular filtration rate (GFR) <60 ml/min for 3 months or longer. (Normal GFR is about 125 ml/min and is reflected by urine creatinine clearance measurements.) Kidney damage is defined as either pathologic abnormalities or markers of damage, including abnormalities in blood or urine tests or imaging studies. Disease staging based on the decreasing GFR is shown in Table 47-6. As indicated in this table, the last stage of kidney failure (**end-stage renal disease** [ESRD]) occurs when the GFR is less than 15 ml/min. At this point, renal replacement therapy (dialysis or transplantation) is required. Although there are many different causes of CKD (Fig. 47-4), the end result is a systemic disease involving every body organ. (Diseases of the renal system that affect the kidney are discussed in Chapter 46.)

The kidneys have remarkable functional reserve. Up to 80% of the GFR (reflected in creatinine clearance measurements) may be lost with few obvious changes in the functioning of the body. A person is born with about 2 million nephrons and can survive without dialysis until almost 90% of the nephrons are lost. In the majority of cases the individual passes through the early stages of CKD without recognizing the disease state because the remaining nephrons hypertrophy to compensate. The prognosis and course of CKD are highly variable depending on the etiology, pa-

---

CULTURAL AND ETHNIC HEALTH DISPARITIES
Chronic Kidney Disease

- Chronic kidney disease has a disproportionate impact on minority populations, especially African Americans and Native Americans.
- A history of hypertension and diabetes mellitus is also more common in these African Americans and Native Americans.
- The rate of chronic kidney disease is 6 times higher among Native Americans with diabetes than among other ethnic groups with diabetes.
- The risk of chronic kidney disease as a complication of hypertension is significantly increased in African Americans.
- African Americans live longer and have better outcomes on chronic dialysis than whites.

TABLE 47-6	Stages and Descriptions of Chronic Kidney Disease*		
	Description	**GFR (ml/min/1.73 m²)**	**Action†**
	At increased risk for CKD	≥90 (with CKD risk factors)	Screening CKD risk reduction
Stage 1	Kidney damage with normal or ↑ GFR	≥90	Diagnosis and treatment Treatment of comorbid conditions CVD risk reduction
Stage 2	Kidney damage with mild ↓ GFR	60-89	Estimation of progression
Stage 3	Moderate ↓ GFR	30-59	Evaluation and treatment of complications
Stage 4	Severe ↓ GFR	15-29	Preparation for renal replacement therapy
Stage 5	Kidney failure	<15 (or dialysis)	Renal replacement (if uremia present)

Source: National Kidney Foundation: *Kidney Disease Outcomes Quality Initiative: clinical practice guidelines for chronic kidney disease: evaluation, classification, and stratification,* New York, 2000, National Kidney Foundation; also available at *www.kidney.org/professionals/kdoqi/guidelines_updates/doqi-nut.html* (accessed April 26, 2006). *CKD,* Chronic kidney disease; *CVD,* cardiovascular disease; *GFR,* glomerular filtration rate.
*Chronic kidney disease is defined as either kidney damage or GFR <60 ml/min/1.73 m² for ≥3 months. Kidney damage is defined as pathologic abnormalities or markers of damage, including abnormalities in blood or urine tests or imaging studies. Stages 1 to 5 identify patients who have chronic kidney disease.
†Includes actions from preceding stages.

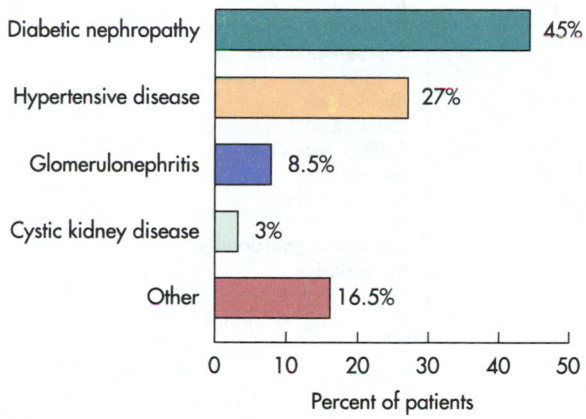

FIG. 47-4   Incidence of primary renal disease leading to end-stage renal disease (data from United States Renal Data Systems).

HEALTHY PEOPLE

Prevention and Detection of Chronic Kidney Disease

- Early detection and treatment are the primary methods for reducing chronic kidney disease
- Monitor blood pressure to detect elevations so treatment can be started early
- Ensure proper diagnosis and treatment of diabetes mellitus as it is the leading cause of chronic kidney disease
- Treat hypertension appropriately and aggressively as it is the second leading cause of chronic kidney disease

---

tient's condition and age, and adequacy of health care follow-up. Some individuals live normal, active lives with compensated renal failure, whereas others may rapidly progress to ESRD (stage 5).

According to the United States Renal Data Systems report in 2005, over 102,000 new patients were placed on some form of renal replacement therapy (93,276 hemodialysis; 6690 peritoneal dialysis; 2068 transplants). Over 452,000 people with ESRD were being treated (298,101 hemodialysis; 25,825 peritoneal dialysis; and 128,131 transplant). The number of patients with ESRD is expected to reach 660,000 by 2010. Each year about 70,000 people die from causes related to renal failure. At least 40 million Americans are at risk for CKD. In the United States the leading causes of ESRD are diabetes mellitus and hypertension[11] (see Fig. 47-4).

In the most recent statistics available for Canada, in 1 year over 4800 new patients started some form of renal replacement therapy, with a total of 17,116 (80% hemodialysis; 20% peritoneal dialysis) individuals being treated for ESRD. Fifty-eight percent of the total number of single-organ transplants were kidneys (1044 in 2003). The primary causes for renal failure in Canada are diabetes mellitus and glomerulonephritis.[12]

In 1972, Title XVIII of the Social Security Act recognized CKD as a disability. As such, approximately 93% of individuals of any age who have ESRD are eligible for financial assistance for treatment through Medicare. Medicare pays for 80% of eligible charges, with the remaining amount being paid for by state or private insurance, or

out-of-pocket. The Center for Medicare and Medicaid Services (CMS) continues to assess coverage for patients with CKD as polices regarding reimbursement continue to change.[13]

Since 1973 many deaths have been prevented through the use of maintenance dialysis and renal transplantation. Most patients are treated with dialysis because (1) there is a lack of donated organs, (2) some patients are physically or mentally unsuitable for transplantation, or (3) some patients do not want transplants. With the advancement of medical science, an increasing number of individuals are receiving maintenance dialysis, including the elderly and those with complex medical problems. Every patient with ESRD, regardless of age, should be offered dialysis unless it is medically contraindicated or the patient refuses treatment.

The National Kidney Foundation has been active in recent years in preventing and managing CKD at all stages. Currently, the Foundation's *Kidney Disease Outcomes Quality Initiative (K/DOQI)* has as its goal the development of clinical practice guidelines to manage patients in earlier stages of kidney disease by slowing disease progression, detecting/treating complications, and managing cardiovascular risk factors. CKD has been defined and classified into stages, and updates and new practice guidelines continue to evolve from this initial project.[14] CKD has also been a focus of *Healthy People 2010* initiatives since 2000[15] (Healthy People Box).

Clinical Manifestations

As renal function progressively deteriorates, every body system becomes affected. The clinical manifestations are a result of retained substances, including urea, creatinine, phenols, hormones,

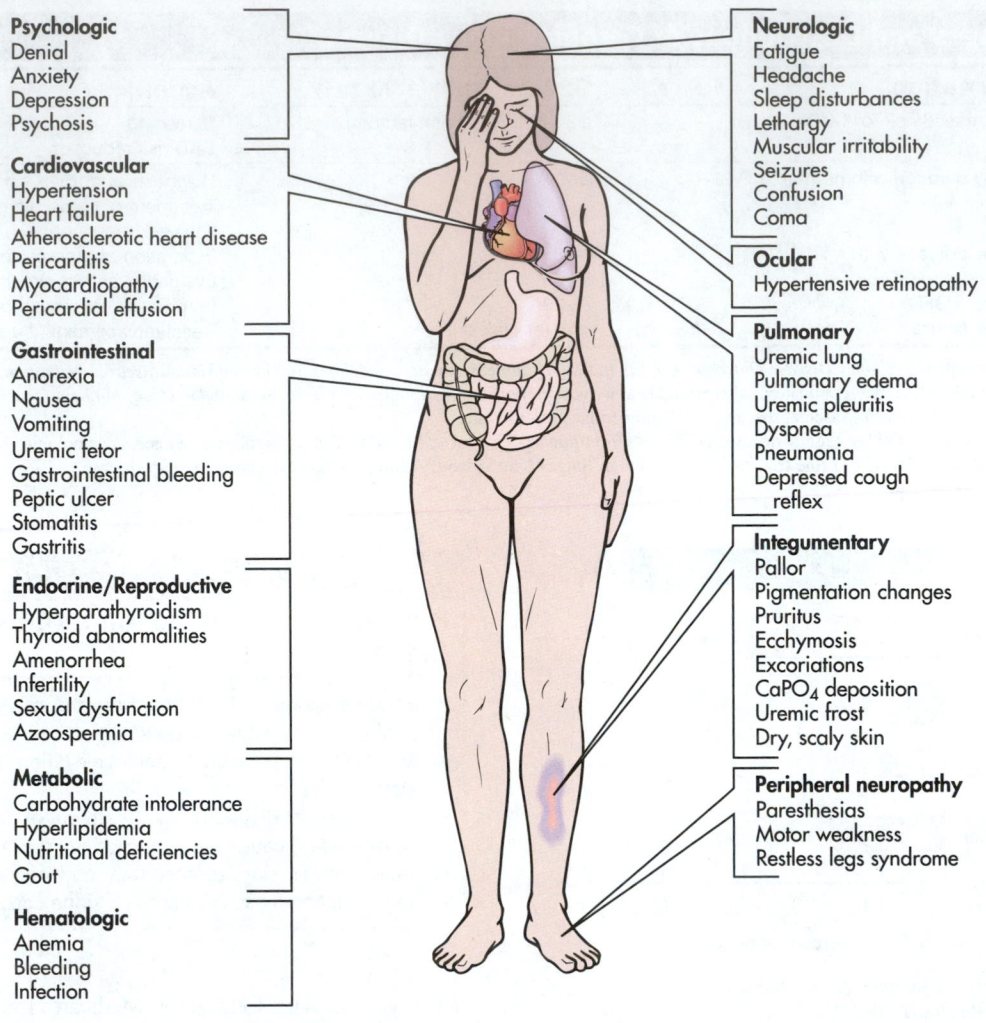

Psychologic
Denial
Anxiety
Depression
Psychosis

Cardiovascular
Hypertension
Heart failure
Atherosclerotic heart disease
Pericarditis
Myocardiopathy
Pericardial effusion

Gastrointestinal
Anorexia
Nausea
Vomiting
Uremic fetor
Gastrointestinal bleeding
Peptic ulcer
Stomatitis
Gastritis

Endocrine/Reproductive
Hyperparathyroidism
Thyroid abnormalities
Amenorrhea
Infertility
Sexual dysfunction
Azoospermia

Metabolic
Carbohydrate intolerance
Hyperlipidemia
Nutritional deficiencies
Gout

Hematologic
Anemia
Bleeding
Infection

Neurologic
Fatigue
Headache
Sleep disturbances
Lethargy
Muscular irritability
Seizures
Confusion
Coma

Ocular
Hypertensive retinopathy

Pulmonary
Uremic lung
Pulmonary edema
Uremic pleuritis
Dyspnea
Pneumonia
Depressed cough
   reflex

Integumentary
Pallor
Pigmentation changes
Pruritus
Ecchymosis
Excoriations
$CaPO_4$ deposition
Uremic frost
Dry, scaly skin

Peripheral neuropathy
Paresthesias
Motor weakness
Restless legs syndrome

FIG. 47-5 Clinical manifestations of chronic uremia.

electrolytes, water, and many other substances. *Uremia* is a syndrome that incorporates all the signs and symptoms seen in the various systems throughout the body in CKD (Fig. 47-5). It is important to recognize that the manifestations of uremia vary among patients, according to the cause of the kidney disease, comorbid conditions, age, and degree of compliance with the prescribed medical regimen. Many patients are very tolerant of the changes that occur because they develop gradually.

Urinary System. In the early stage of renal insufficiency, polyuria results from the inability of the kidneys to concentrate urine. This happens most often at night, and the patient must arise several times to urinate (nocturia). Because of the decrease in renal concentrating ability, the specific gravity of urine gradually becomes fixed at around 1.010 (the osmolar concentration of plasma). As CKD worsens, oliguria develops and eventually anuria (urine output <100 ml/24 hr) occurs. If the patient is still producing urine, proteinuria, casts, pyuria, and hematuria could be present depending on the cause of the kidney disease.

Metabolic Disturbances

Waste Product Accumulation. As the GFR decreases, the BUN and serum creatinine levels increase. The BUN is increased not only by the kidney failure but also by protein intake, fever, corticosteroids, and catabolism. For this reason, serum creatinine and creatinine clearance determinations are consid-

ered more accurate indicators of kidney function than BUN.[16] As the BUN increases, nausea, vomiting, lethargy, fatigue, impaired thought processes, and headaches become common as a result of the effects of waste products on the central nervous and GI systems.

The serum creatinine level in an older adult patient with ESRD will be lower than in a younger person with the same degree of renal dysfunction. Decreased muscle mass and decreased muscle activity from aging account for this finding because creatinine is an end product of muscle metabolism.

Altered Carbohydrate Metabolism. Defective carbohydrate metabolism is caused by impaired glucose use resulting from cellular insensitivity to the normal action of insulin. The exact nature of this insulin resistance is unclear, but it may be related to circulating insulin antagonists, alterations in hormone receptors, or abnormalities of transport mechanisms. Moderate hyperglycemia, hyperinsulinemia, and abnormal glucose tolerance tests may be seen. Insulin and glucose metabolism may improve (but not to normal values) after the initiation of dialysis.

Patients with diabetes who become uremic may require less insulin than before the onset of CKD. This is because insulin, which is dependent on the kidneys for excretion, remains in circulation longer. The insulin dosing must be individualized and glucose levels monitored carefully.[17]

Elevated Triglycerides. Hyperinsulinemia stimulates hepatic production of triglycerides. Almost all patients with uremia develop hyperlipidemia, with elevated very-low-density lipoproteins (VLDLs), normal or decreased low-density lipoproteins (LDLs), and decreased high-density lipoproteins (HDLs). The altered lipid metabolism is related to decreased levels of the enzyme lipoprotein lipase that is important in the breakdown of lipoproteins. Hyperlipidemia is a definite risk factor for accelerated atherosclerosis (see Chapter 34), and it can worsen atherosclerotic changes in diabetics with ESRD.[18]

The serum level of triglycerides does not usually decrease after dialysis is started. For patients receiving long-term peritoneal dialysis (PD), the level frequently becomes higher as a result of the increased amounts of glucose absorbed from the peritoneal dialysate fluid. Elevated glucose levels lead to increased insulin levels. Insulin stimulates the liver to produce triglycerides.

Electrolyte and Acid-Base Imbalances

Potassium. Hyperkalemia is the most serious electrolyte disorder associated with kidney disease. Fatal dysrhythmias can occur when the serum potassium level reaches 7 to 8 mEq/L (7 to 8 mmol/L). Hyperkalemia results from the decreased excretion by the kidneys, the breakdown of cellular protein, bleeding, and metabolic acidosis. Potassium may also come from the food consumed, dietary supplements, drugs, and IV infusions.

Sodium. Sodium may be normal or low in renal failure. Because of impaired sodium excretion, sodium along with water is retained. If large quantities of body water are retained, dilutional hyponatremia occurs. Sodium retention can contribute to edema, hypertension, and heart failure. Sodium intake must be individually determined but is generally restricted to 2 g/day.

Calcium and Phosphate. Calcium and phosphate alterations are discussed in the section on ARF (p. 1200) and in the section on the musculoskeletal system (p. 1208).

Magnesium. Magnesium is primarily excreted by the kidneys. Hypermagnesemia is generally not a problem unless the patient is ingesting magnesium (e.g., milk of magnesia, magnesium citrate, antacids containing magnesium). Clinical manifestations of hypermagnesemia can include absence of reflexes, decreased mental status, cardiac dysrhythmias, hypotension, and respiratory failure.

Metabolic Acidosis. Metabolic acidosis results from the impaired ability of the kidneys to excrete the acid load (primarily ammonia) and from defective reabsorption and regeneration of bicarbonate. The average adult produces 80 to 90 mEq of acid per day. This acid is normally buffered by bicarbonate. In renal failure, plasma bicarbonate, which is an indirect measure of acidosis, usually falls to a new steady state at around 16 to 20 mEq/L (16 to 20 mmol/L). The decrease in plasma bicarbonate reflects its use in buffering metabolic acids. It generally does not progress below this level because hydrogen ion production is usually balanced by buffering from demineralization of the bone (the phosphate buffering system). Although Kussmaul respiration is uncommon in CKD, this breathing pattern can reduce the severity of acidosis by increasing carbon dioxide excretion (see Chapter 17).

Hematologic System

Anemia. A normocytic or normochromic anemia is associated with CKD. The anemia is due to decreased production of the hormone erythropoietin by the kidneys, caused by the decrease of functioning renal tubular cells.[19] Erythropoietin normally stimulates precursor cells in the bone marrow to produce RBCs (erythropoiesis). Other factors contributing to anemia are nutritional deficiencies, decreased RBC life span, increased hemolysis of RBCs, frequent blood samplings, and bleeding from the GI tract. For patients receiving maintenance hemodialysis (HD), blood loss in the dialyzer may also contribute to the anemic state. Elevated levels of parathyroid hormone (PTH) (produced to compensate for low serum calcium levels) can inhibit erythropoiesis, shorten survival of RBCs, and cause bone marrow fibrosis, which can result in decreased numbers of hematopoietic cells.

Sufficient iron stores are needed for erythropoiesis. Many patients with renal failure are iron deficient and require oral iron supplements. Folic acid, which is essential for RBC maturation, is dialyzable. If it is not adequately replaced in the diet or by supplements, megaloblastic anemia resulting from folic acid deficiency may develop in a patient receiving chronic HD.

Bleeding Tendencies. The most common cause of bleeding in uremia is a qualitative defect in platelet function. This dysfunction is caused by impaired platelet aggregation and impaired release of platelet factor III. In addition, alterations in the coagulation system with increased concentrations of both factor VIII and fibrinogen are found in the serum of these patients (see Chapter 30). The altered platelet function, hemorrhagic tendencies, and GI bleeding can usually be corrected with regular HD or PD.

Infection. Infectious complications are caused by changes in leukocyte function and altered immune response and function. There is a diminished inflammatory response because of an altered chemotactic response by both neutrophils and monocytes. This impairment significantly decreases the accumulation of WBCs at the site of injury or infection. Both cellular and humoral immune responses are suppressed. Characteristic clinical findings include lymphopenia, lymphoid tissue atrophy (especially of the thymus), decreased antibody production, and suppression of the delayed hypersensitivity response. Other factors contributing to the increased risk of infection include malnutrition, hyperglycemia, and external trauma (e.g., catheters, needle insertions into vascular access sites).

Increased Incidence of Cancer. There is a significant increase in the incidence of neoplasms in the patient with renal failure who has not had a transplant compared with the general population. Lung, breast, uterus, colon, prostate, and skin malignancies are most commonly found.

Cardiovascular System. The most common cardiovascular abnormality is hypertension, which is usually present pre-ESRD and is aggravated by sodium retention and increased extracellular fluid volume.[19] In some individuals, increased renin production contributes to hypertension (see Fig. 45-4).

The vascular changes from long-standing hypertension and the accelerated atherosclerosis from elevated triglyceride levels are responsible for many cardiovascular complications (e.g., myocardial infarction, stroke). These are leading causes of death for patients receiving long-term dialysis. Diabetes mellitus is a contributing risk factor for the development of vascular problems.

Left ventricular hypertrophy resulting from long-standing hypertension, extracellular fluid volume overload, and anemia leads to cardiomyopathy and heart failure. Pulmonary and peripheral edema can occur.

Cardiac dysrhythmias may result from hyperkalemia, hypocalcemia, and decreased coronary artery perfusion. Uremic pericarditis can develop and occasionally progresses to pericardial effusion and cardiac tamponade. Pericarditis is manifested by a friction rub, chest pain, and low-grade fever.[19]

In addition to direct cardiovascular effects, hypertension can cause retinopathy, encephalopathy, and nephropathy. Because of the many effects of hypertension, blood pressure (BP) control becomes a positive patient outcome in the management of CKD.[19]

Respiratory System. Respiratory changes include Kussmaul breathing (to compensate for metabolic acidosis), dyspnea from fluid overload, pulmonary edema, uremic pleuritis (pleurisy), pleural effusion, and a predisposition to respiratory infections, which may be related to decreased pulmonary macrophage activity. The sputum is thick and tenacious. The cough reflex is depressed. "Uremic lung," or uremic pneumonitis, is typically found in CKD and shows up as interstitial edema on chest x-ray. This condition usually responds to vigorous fluid removal during dialysis treatments.

Gastrointestinal System. Every part of the GI system is affected as a result of inflammation of the mucosa caused by excessive urea. Mucosal ulcerations, found throughout the GI tract, are caused by the increased ammonia produced by bacterial breakdown of urea. Stomatitis with exudates and ulcerations, a metallic taste in the mouth, and *uremic fetor* (a urinous odor of the breath) are commonly found. Anorexia, nausea, and vomiting caused by irritation of the GI tract by waste products contribute to weight loss and malnutrition. Diabetic gastroparesis can compound these problems for patients with diabetes. GI bleeding is also a risk because of mucosal irritation coupled with the platelet defect. Diarrhea may occur because of hyperkalemia and altered calcium metabolism. Constipation may be due to the ingestion of iron salts and/or calcium-containing phosphate binders (e.g., calcium acetate [PhosLo]). Constipation can be made worse by the limited fluid intake and inactivity.

Neurologic System. Neurologic changes are expected as renal failure progresses. They are attributed to increased nitrogenous waste products, electrolyte imbalances, metabolic acidosis, and axonal atrophy and demyelination of nerve fibers.[20] High levels of waste products have been implicated in axonal damage.

In renal failure a general depression of the CNS results in lethargy, apathy, decreased ability to concentrate, fatigue, irritability, and altered mental ability. Seizures and coma may result from a rapidly increasing BUN and hypertensive encephalopathy.

Peripheral neuropathy is initially manifested by a slowing of nerve conduction to the extremities. The patient complains of restless legs syndrome (described in Chapter 59) and may describe it as "bugs crawling inside the leg." Paresthesias are most often experienced in the feet and legs and may be described by the patient as a burning sensation. Eventually, motor involvement may lead to bilateral footdrop, muscular weakness and atrophy, and loss of deep tendon reflexes. Muscle twitching, jerking, *asterixis* (hand-flapping tremor), and nocturnal leg cramps also occur. In patients with diabetes, uremic neuropathy is compounded by the neuropathy associated with diabetes mellitus.

The treatment for neurologic problems is dialysis or transplantation. Altered mental status is often the signal that dialysis must be initiated. Dialysis should improve the general CNS symptoms and may slow or halt the progression of neuropathies. However, motor neuropathy may not be reversible.

Musculoskeletal System. **Renal osteodystrophy** is a syndrome of skeletal changes found in CKD that is a result of alterations in calcium and phosphate metabolism[19] (Fig. 47-6). Normally the calcium/phosphate ratio maintains the electrolytes in a soluble state. When calcium levels decline, the parathyroid

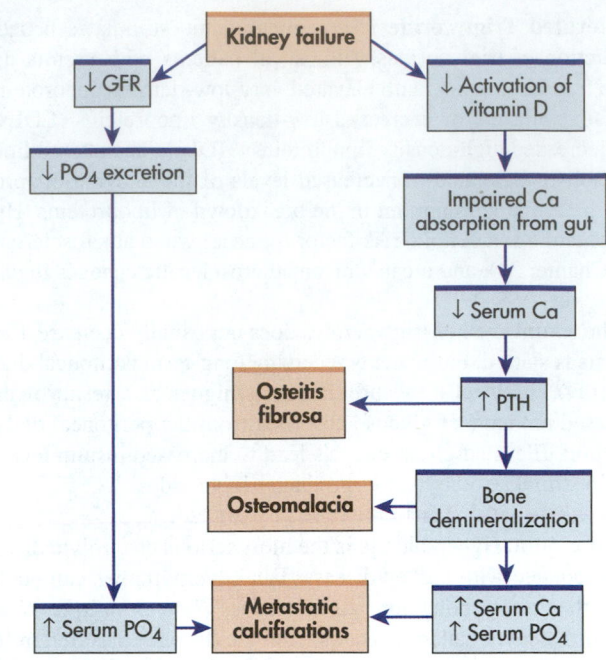

FIG. 47-6 Mechanisms of renal osteodystrophy. *GFR,* Glomerular filtration rate.

glands release PTH. PTH stimulates the kidneys to activate vitamin D, which promotes absorption of calcium from the bowel. PTH also increases calcium resorption by the kidney, phosphate excretion by the kidney, and release of calcium from the bone. Calcium and phosphate levels return to normal and secretion of PTH is reversed.

However, in CKD, as the GFR decreases, urinary phosphate excretion is impaired, and the serum phosphate levels increase. The kidneys fail to activate vitamin D, calcium absorption is impaired, and serum calcium decreases. Low serum calcium and high serum phosphate stimulate the release of PTH, which causes resorption of calcium and phosphate from the bone. This release increases serum calcium, as well as serum phosphate. The excess phosphate binds with calcium, leading to the formation of insoluble metastatic calcifications that are deposited throughout the body. Common sites are the muscles, lungs, skin and subcutaneous tissue, GI tract, and eyes.[21] "Uremic red eye" is caused by the irritation from deposits in the eye. Metastatic calcifications in the arteries of the fingers and toes may cause gangrene. Intracardiac calcifications can disrupt the conduction system and cause cardiac arrest.

Two types of renal osteodystrophy are associated with ESRD:
1. *Osteomalacia.* This condition of demineralization results from slow bone turnover and defective mineralization of newly formed bone.[21] It can be a result of PTH suppression from high calcium intake (through diet, calcium-based phosphate binders), high vitamin D dosage, and the presence of diabetes mellitus. It may also be caused by aluminum accumulation due to the inability of the kidneys to excrete aluminum.
2. *Osteitis fibrosa cystica.* This condition results from decalcification of the bone and replacement of bone tissue with fibrous tissue. Osteitis fibrosa is primarily a result of markedly elevated levels of PTH (secondary hyperparathyroidism) that cause bone resorption and softening.[21]

Both forms of renal osteodystrophy weaken the bones and increase the risk of fractures.[22]

Integumentary System. The most noticeable change in the integumentary system is a yellow-gray discoloration of the skin. This change is a result of the absorption and retention of urinary pigments that normally give the characteristic color to urine. The skin also appears pale as a result of anemia and is dry and scaly because of a decrease in oil and sweat gland activity. Decreased perspiration results from a decrease in the size of the sweat glands.

Pruritus most commonly results from a combination of the dry skin, calcium-phosphate deposition in the skin, and sensory neuropathy. The itching may be so intense that it can lead to bleeding or infection secondary to scratching. Uremic frost is a rare condition in which urea crystallizes on the skin and is usually seen only when BUN levels are extremely high. It occurs when a patient refuses dialysis or is withdrawn from dialysis.

The hair is dry and brittle and may fall out. The nails are thin, brittle, and ridged. Petechiae and ecchymoses may be present and are due to platelet abnormalities.

Reproductive System. Both sexes characteristically experience infertility and a decreased libido. Women usually have decreased levels of estrogen, progesterone, and luteinizing hormone, causing anovulation and menstrual changes (usually amenorrhea). Menses and ovulation may return after dialysis is started. Men experience loss of testicular consistency, decreased testosterone levels, and low sperm counts. Sexual dysfunction in both sexes may also be caused by anemia, which causes fatigue and decreased libido. In addition, peripheral neuropathy can cause impotence in men and anorgasmy in women. Additional factors that may cause changes in sexual function are psychologic problems (e.g., anxiety, depression), physical stress, and side effects of drugs.

Sexual function may improve with maintenance dialysis and may become normal with successful transplantation. Pregnant dialysis patients have been able to carry a fetus to term, but there is significant risk to the mother and infant. Pregnancy in transplant patients is more common, but there is also a risk to both the mother and fetus.

Endocrine System. Many patients with CKD exhibit some clinical manifestations of hypothyroidism. Tests of thyroid function may yield low to low-normal levels for serum triiodothyronine (T_3) and thyroxine (T_4) levels. Neither the clinical significance nor the exact cause of these findings is known.

Psychologic Changes. Personality and behavioral changes, emotional lability, withdrawal, and depression are commonly observed. Fatigue and lethargy contribute to the feeling of illness. The changes in body image caused by edema, integumentary disturbances, and access devices (e.g., fistulas, catheters) lead to further anxiety and depression. Decreased ability to concentrate and slowed mental activity can give the appearance of dullness and disinterest in the environment. There are also significant changes in lifestyle, occupation, family responsibilities, and financial status that must be dealt with by the patient. Long-term survival depends on drugs, dietary restrictions, dialysis, and possibly transplantation. The patient will also grieve the loss of renal function. This can be a prolonged process for some individuals.

Diagnostic Studies

Adverse outcomes of CKD can often be prevented or delayed through early detection and treatment. Because persistent proteinuria is usually the first indication of kidney damage, screen-

TABLE 47-7	COLLABORATIVE CARE Conservative Therapy of Chronic Kidney Disease

Diagnostic
History and physical examination
Identification of reversible renal disease
Renal ultrasound
Renal scan
CT scan
Renal biopsy
BUN, serum creatinine, and creatinine clearance levels
Serum electrolytes
Protein-to-creatinine ratio in first morning voided specimen
Urinalysis and urine culture
Hematocrit and hemoglobin levels

Collaborative Therapy
Correction of extracellular fluid volume overload or deficit
Nutritional therapy*
Erythropoietin therapy
Calcium supplementation, phosphate binders, or both
Antihypertensive therapy
Measures to lower potassium†
Adjustment of drug dosages to degree of renal function

BUN, Blood urea nitrogen; *CT,* computed tomography.
*See Tables 47-8 and 47-9.
†See Table 47-5.

ing for CKD involves a dipstick evaluation of protein in the urine. A person with persistent proteinuria (1+ protein on standard dipstick testing two or more times over a 3-month period) should have further assessment of risk factors and a diagnostic workup with blood and urine tests. A urine test for albumin-to-creatinine ratio provides an accurate estimate of the protein and albumin excretion rate. A ratio greater than 300 mg albumin per 1 gram creatinine signals CKD.[23] Serum creatinine values, rather than urine creatinine clearance tests, are used to estimate GFR and stage CKD. A urinalysis can detect RBCs, WBCs, protein, casts, and glucose. Imaging of the kidneys to exclude obstruction and note size of the kidneys is usually achieved by ultrasound. Other diagnostic studies as noted in Table 47-7 help establish the diagnosis and cause of CKD.

Collaborative Care: Conservative Therapy of Chronic Kidney Disease

When a patient is diagnosed as having CKD, conservative therapy is attempted before maintenance dialysis begins (see Table 47-7). Every effort is made to detect and treat potentially reversible causes of renal failure (e.g., cardiac failure, dehydration, infections, nephrotoxins, urinary tract obstruction, glomerulonephritis, renal artery stenosis). A renal biopsy may be necessary to provide a definitive diagnosis. The goals of conservative therapy are to preserve existing renal function, treat the clinical manifestations, prevent complications, and provide for the patient's comfort. Through early recognition, diagnosis, and appropriate treatment, it has been shown that the progression of renal disease can be slowed, quality of life maintained, and outcomes for these individuals improved. A focus on stages 1 through 4 (see Table 47-6) prior to the need for dialysis (stage 5) includes the control of hyperkalemia, hypertension, hyperparathyroid disease, anemia, hyperglycemia, and dyslipidemia.[24] If hypothyroidism is present, it is also treated. Laboratory analysis, drug and nutritional therapy, and supportive care are essential components of the conservative treatment plan. The following section focuses primarily on the drug and nutritional aspects of care.

Drug Therapy

Hyperkalemia. There are multiple strategies for managing hyperkalemia (see Table 47-5). Every effort is made to control hyperkalemia with the restriction of high-potassium foods and drugs. Acute hyperkalemia may require treatment with IV glucose and insulin or IV 10% calcium gluconate. Sodium polystyrene sulfonate (Kayexalate), a cation-exchange resin, is commonly used to lower potassium levels in stage 4 and can be administered on an outpatient basis.[9] The patient should be told to expect some diarrhea because this preparation contains sorbitol, a sugar alcohol that has an osmotic laxative action that ensures evacuation of the potassium from the bowel. It should never be given to a patient with a hypoactive bowel (paralytic ileus) because fluid shifts could lead to bowel necrosis. As sodium polystyrene sulfonate exchanges sodium ions for potassium ions, the patient should be observed for sodium and water retention.[9] If life-threatening dysrhythmias are present, dialysis may be required to remove excess potassium.

Hypertension. The progression of CKD can be delayed by controlling hypertension. (Control and treatment of hypertension is discussed in Chapter 33.) It is recommended that the target BP be less than 130/80 mm Hg for patients with CKD.[25] Treatment of hypertension includes (1) weight loss (if obese), (2) therapeutic lifestyle changes (i.e., exercise, avoidance of alcohol, smoking cessation), (3) diet recommendations[26] (DASH Diet; see Table 33-7), and (4) administration of antihypertensive drugs.

The antihypertensive drugs most commonly used are diuretics (e.g., furosemide [Lasix]), β-adrenergic blockers (e.g., metoprolol [Lopressor]), calcium channel blockers (e.g., nifedipine [Procardia]), angiotensin-converting enzyme (ACE) inhibitors (e.g., captopril [Capoten], enalapril [Vasotec]), and angiotensin receptor blocker (ARB) agents (e.g., losartan [Cozaar]). Prescribed medications are dependent on whether the patient with CKD is diabetic or nondiabetic. Diuretics and β-adrenergic blockers are the recommended initial therapy for nondiabetics. The ACE inhibitors and ARBs are used with diabetics and those with nondiabetic proteinuria because they decrease proteinuria and delay the progression of CKD.[25,26] However, they must be used cautiously when ESRD occurs because they can further decrease the GFR and increase serum potassium levels.

The BP should periodically be measured in supine, sitting, and standing positions to effectively monitor the effect of antihypertensive drugs. The patient and family should be taught how to monitor the BP at home and what readings require immediate intervention. BP control is essential to slow atherosclerotic changes that could further impair renal function.

Renal Osteodystrophy. The National Kidney Foundation's *K/DOQI Bone Metabolism Clinical Practice Guidelines* for bone metabolism and disease in CKD provide information for the clinician to assist in the care of patients with renal osteodystrophy.[27] Interventions include limiting dietary phosphorus, administering phosphate binders, supplementing vitamin D, and controlling hyperparathyroidism.[22]

Phosphate intake is generally restricted to less than 1000 mg/day, but dietary control alone is usually inadequate. Calcium-based phosphate binders such as calcium carbonate (e.g., Tums) and calcium acetate (e.g., PhosLo) are used to bind phosphate in the bowel, which is then excreted in the stool. Giving a calcium-based binder when serum phosphate levels are still high ($\geq$6 mg/dl [1.98 mmol/L]) may cause the formation of systemic calcium-phosphate deposits. Sevelamer hydrochloride (Renagel) is a phosphate binder that does not contain either calcium or aluminum. It has the added benefits of lowering cholesterol and LDLs.[27] The newest drug that reduces serum phosphorus, lanthanum carbonate (Fosrenol), does not contain either calcium or aluminum. An added benefit is that it is a chewable tablet.[28]

Phosphate binders should be administered with each meal to be effective because most phosphate is absorbed within 1 hour after eating. Constipation is a frequent side effect of phosphate binders and may necessitate the use of stool softeners.

Because dementia (aluminum toxicity) and bone disease (osteomalacia) are associated with excessive absorption of aluminum, aluminum preparations such as Alu-Cap, Amphojel, Basaljel, and ALternaGEL should be used with caution in patients with renal impairment. Magnesium-containing antacids (Maalox, Mylanta) should not be used because magnesium is dependent on the kidneys for excretion.

Hypocalcemia is often a problem because of the inability of the GI tract to absorb calcium in the absence of vitamin D. If hypocalcemia persists in the setting of controlled serum phosphate levels and supplemental calcium, the active form of vitamin D should be given. It is commercially available in oral preparations such as calcitriol (Rocaltrol) and in an IV preparation (Calcijex). Paricalcitol (Zemplar) and doxercalciferol (Hectorol) are synthetic vitamin D_2 analogs.[27] It is important that the serum phosphate level is lowered before administering calcium or vitamin D because these drugs may contribute to soft tissue calcification if both calcium and phosphate levels are elevated. Hypercalcemia may occur with calcium and vitamin D supplementation and is associated with increased cardiac calcifications and mortality in ESRD patients. If hypercalcemia occurs, dosages of vitamin D and calcium-based phosphate binders should be reduced, and dietary calcium restricted. Non–calcium-based phosphate binders could also be substituted.

Calcimimetic agents are a new class of drugs used to control secondary hyperparathyroidism. Cinacalcet (Sensipar) increases the sensitivity of the calcium receptors in the parathyroid glands. As a result, the parathyroid glands detect calcium at lower serum levels and decrease PTH secretion. Cinacalcet is currently only used for patients on dialysis, but its role in treatment of renal osteodystrophy at earlier stages is under investigation.[29]

If renal osteodystrophy remains severe despite conservative therapy, a subtotal parathyroidectomy may be performed to decrease the synthesis and secretion of PTH. In some situations a total parathyroidectomy is performed, and some parathyroid tissue is transplanted into the forearm. The transplanted cells produce PTH as needed. If production of PTH becomes excessive, some of the cells can be removed from the forearm using local anesthesia.

The most common methods for evaluating the status of the bone disease are skeletal x-rays, bone scans, bone biopsy, and bone densitometry. PTH and alkaline phosphatase levels should also be measured. Alkaline phosphatase is elevated when there is demineralization of the bone but can also be increased by liver disease.

Anemia. The most important cause of anemia is a decreased production of erythropoietin due to the decrease in the number of functioning renal tubular cells.[19] K/DOQI guidelines recommend that hemoglobin levels should be 11 to 12 g/dl and hematocrit should be 33% to 36% for patients with CKD.[19] With the use of recombinant deoxyribonucleic acid (DNA) technology (see Chapter 14, Fig. 14-20), erythropoietin (epoetin alfa [Epogen, Procrit]) is produced and available for treatment of anemia. It can be administered intravenously or subcutaneously and has proven to be very effective. A significant increase in hemoglobin and hematocrit levels is usually not seen for 2 to 3 weeks. The patient who is receiving epoetin alfa has improved cardiac performance and exercise tolerance and an enhanced quality of life. Darbepoetin alfa (Aranesp) is a newer and longer acting erythropoietin product for subcutaneous and IV use that requires fewer injections.

A common adverse effect of exogenous erythropoietin is the development or acceleration of hypertension. The underlying mechanism is related to the hemodynamic changes (e.g., increased whole blood viscosity) that occur as the anemia is corrected. Another side effect of erythropoietin therapy is the development of functional iron deficiency resulting from the increased demand for iron to support erythropoiesis. Oral iron supplements are recommended if the plasma ferritin concentrations fall below 100 ng/ml.[19] Most patients with CKD receive oral iron supplements. Noncompliance may be an issue because of GI side effects such as gastric irritation and constipation. Orally administered iron should not be taken at the same time as phosphate binders because calcium binds the iron, preventing its absorption. The patient should be advised that iron may make the stool dark in color. Parenteral iron sucrose injection (Venofer) or sodium ferric gluconate complex in sucrose injection (Ferrlecit) is used if iron deficiencies persist in spite of oral iron intake. Supplemental folic acid (1 mg daily) is usually given because it is needed for RBC formation and is removed by dialysis.

Blood transfusions should be avoided in treating anemia unless the patient experiences an acute blood loss or has symptomatic anemia (i.e., dyspnea, excess fatigue, tachycardia, palpitations, chest pain). Undesirable effects of transfusions are the suppression of erythropoiesis as a result of a decrease in the hypoxic stimulus and the possibility of iron overload because each unit of blood contains about 250 mg of iron.

Dyslipidemia. A common problem of progressive CKD is that of dyslipidemia, a primary risk factor for cardiovascular disease. Recommendations for patients with CKD include a goal of lowering LDLs below 100 mg/dl (2.6 mmol/L) and maintaining a triglyceride level below 200 mg/dl (2.25 mmol/L).[18] Statins (HMG-CoA reductase inhibitors) are the most effective drugs for lowering LDL cholesterol levels (see Chapter 34). Fibrates (fibric acid derivatives) are the most effective drugs available for lowering triglyceride levels, and can also increase HDLs.[30] Specific drugs of these classes that are used depend on the individual patient response and physician recommendation.

Complications of Drug Therapy. Many drugs are partially or totally excreted by the kidneys. Delayed and decreased elimination lead to an accumulation of drugs and the potential for drug toxicity. Drug doses and frequency of administration must be adjusted based on the severity of the kidney disease. Increased sensitivity may result as drug levels increase in the blood and tissues. Drugs of particular concern include digitalis preparations, antibiotics, and pain medication.[31]

Digitalis preparations are excreted largely by the kidneys. While loading doses may not need to be changed, maintenance doses and frequency of digoxin (Lanoxin) may have to be adjusted. Many patients require only 0.125 mg every other day. Dialysis does not affect body levels of digoxin, but it does affect potassium levels. Hypokalemia can potentiate the action of digitalis.

Aminoglycosides, penicillin in high doses, and tetracyclines are potentially nephrotoxic and require dose and frequency adjustments. The frequency and dose of vancomycin (Vancocin) and gentamicin (Garamycin) must be decreased because they are dependent on the kidney for excretion. These drugs can accumulate to toxic levels if appropriate adjustments are not made.

Meperidine (Demerol) should never be administered to a patient with CKD because the liver metabolizes it to normeperidine, which is dependent on the kidneys for excretion. If normeperidine accumulates, seizures can result. Other pain medications may be given, but less frequently and in smaller doses (e.g., oxycodone with acetaminophen, morphine sulfate).

Patients should be advised to avoid nonsteroidal antiinflammatory drugs (NSAIDs). These drugs block the synthesis of the renal prostaglandins that promote vasodilation. This can worsen renal hypoperfusion. Many NSAIDs are available over the counter, so it is essential that the patient be cautioned. Acetaminophen may be substituted.

Nutritional Therapy

Protein Restriction. The current diet is designed to be as normal as possible to maintain good nutrition (Table 47-8). Calorie-protein malnutrition is a potential and serious problem that results from altered metabolism, anemia, proteinuria, anorexia, and nausea. Additional factors leading to malnutrition include depression and complex diets that restrict protein, phosphorus, potassium, and sodium. Frequent monitoring of laboratory parameters, especially serum albumin and ferritin, and anthropometric measurements are necessary to evaluate nutritional status. All patients with CKD should be referred to a dietitian for nutritional education and guidance.[22]

Dietary protein is restricted because urea nitrogen and creatinine are end products of protein metabolism. For the patient who is not undergoing dialysis, one guide is to restrict protein intake to 0.6 to 0.75 g/kg of ideal body weight (IBW) per day when the creatinine clearance is less than 25 ml/min. Some treatment centers use a routine 40-g protein diet. Because this diet is deficient in vitamins and water-soluble vitamins are lost through dialysis, supplemental multivitamins are prescribed.

Protein restriction may reduce the decline of renal function in the patient with chronic renal insufficiency. A low-protein (0.6 to 0.8 g/kg of body weight per day), low-phosphorus diet supplemented with amino acids and their ketoanalogues can slow the progression of renal failure.[32] Keto acids of essential amino acids are a dietary supplement. The rationale for using this treatment is that, in the body, nonessential amino acids transfer amine groups to the essential keto acids synthesizing essential amino acids. The nitrogen present in nonessential amino acids is used, and the total nitrogen intake is kept to an absolute minimum. Keto acid supplements are available in liquid preparations. Modest protein restriction (0.6 to 0.8 g/kg/day) appears to be a relatively safe therapeutic option for patients with moderate renal insufficiency. For patients with more severe renal insufficiency, low-protein diets should be used with caution because these patients are at risk for developing malnutrition.

Once the patient starts dialysis, protein intake can be increased to 1.2 to 1.3 g/kg of IBW per day. Dietary protein guidelines for PD differ from those for HD because excessive amounts of protein are lost in the dialysate. During PD protein intake must be high enough to compensate for the losses so that the nitrogen balance is maintained. The recommended protein intake is at least 1.2 g/kg of IBW per day and can be increased depending on the individual

Urinary System

| | **TABLE 47-8** | **_NUTRITIONAL THERAPY_**
Daily Requirements for the Patient with Chronic Kidney Disease | | |

	Pre–End-Stage Renal Disease	Hemodialysis	Peritoneal Dialysis	Comments
Fluid allowance	As desired	Urine output plus 500-1000 ml	Unrestricted if weight and blood pressure controlled and residual renal function	
Calories	30-35 kcal/kg IBW or aBW$_{ef}$	30-35 kcal/kg IBW or aBW$_{ef}$ if ≥ age 60 35 kcal/kg IBW or aBW$_{ef}$ if < age 60	25-35 kcal/kg IBW or aBW$_{ef}$ (includes kcal from dialysate glucose absorption)	If patient <90% or >115% of medium standard weight, use aBW$_{ef}$
Protein	0.6-1.0 g/kg IBW or aBW$_{ef}$ based on creatinine clearance, GFR, urinary protein losses	1.1-1.4 g/kg IBW or aBW$_{ef}$	1.2-1.3 g/kg IBW or aBW$_{ef}$	At least 50% from high biologic value animal or plant protein
Fat	For lipid abnormalities: fats, cholesterol, and CHO adjusted per severity of risk factors	For lipid abnormalities: fats, cholesterol, and CHO adjusted per severity of risk factors	For lipid abnormalities: fats, cholesterol, and CHO adjusted per severity of risk factors	
Sodium	Individualized or 1-3 g/day	Individualized or 2-3 g/day	Individualized based on blood pressure and weight or 2-4 g/day	
Potassium	Individualized per laboratory values	Individualized, approximately 40 mg/kg IBW or aBW$_{ef}$ (approximately 2-3 g/day)	Restricted only by laboratory values	
Phosphorus	Individualized or 8-12 mg/kg IBW or aBW$_{ef}$	Individualized, approximately ≤17 mg/kg IBW or aBW$_{ef}$ (approximately 800-1200 mg/day)	Individualized, approximately ≤17 mg/kg IBW or aBW$_{ef}$	May require phosphate binder
Calcium	Individualized per calcium, phosphorus, and PTH laboratory values and use of vitamin D; approximately 1000-1500 mg/day	Individualized per calcium, phosphorus, and PTH laboratory values and use of vitamin D; approximately 1000-1500 mg/day	Individualized per calcium, phosphorus, and PTH laboratory values and use of vitamin D; approximately 1000-1500 mg/day	Supplement may be needed to maintain normal serum levels
Vitamin C	Supplements should not exceed 100 mg/day to prevent hyperoxalemia	Supplements should not exceed 100 mg/day to prevent hyperoxalemia	Supplements should not exceed 100 mg/day to prevent hyperoxalemia	
Vitamin A	Supplement not recommended	Supplement not recommended	Supplement not recommended	
Iron	Supplement recommended if receiving erythropoietin	Supplement recommended if receiving erythropoietin	Supplement recommended if receiving erythropoietin	

Sources: National Kidney Foundation: _Kidney Disease Outcomes Quality Inititiative: clinical practice guidelines for nutrition in chronic renal failure,_ New York, 2000, National Kidney Foundation; also available at _www.kidney.org/professionals/kdoqi/guidelines_updates/doqi-nut.html_ (accessed April 26, 2006); Grodner M, Long S, DeYoung S: _Foundations and clinical applications of nutrition,_ ed 3, St Louis, 2004, Mosby.
aBW$_{ef}$, Adjusted edema-free body weight; _CHO,_ carbohydrate; _GFR,_ glomerular filtration rate; _IBW,_ ideal body weight; _PTH,_ parathyroid hormone.

needs of the patient. At least 50% of protein intake should have high biologic value containing all of the essential amino acids (e.g., eggs, milk, meat, poultry).[32]

Sufficient calories from carbohydrates and fat are needed to minimize catabolism of body protein and to maintain body weight. Therefore an appropriate amount of carbohydrates and fats are prescribed to maintain an intake of 30 to 35 kcal/kg of body weight per day (see Table 47-8 for specific guidelines).

For patients with malnutrition or inadequate caloric intake, commercially prepared products that are high in calories and low in protein, sodium, and potassium are available. Liquid and powder preparations include Nepro, Microlipid, SumaCal, Suplena, and Polycose. Products containing only the essential amino acids (Amin-Aid) can also be used as dietary supplements.

Water Restriction. Water intake depends on the daily urine output. Generally, 600 ml (from insensible loss) plus an amount equal to the previous day's urine output is allowed for a patient with CKD who is not receiving dialysis. Foods that are liquid at room temperature (e.g., gelatin, ice cream) should be counted as fluid intake. The fluid allotment should be spaced throughout the day so that the patient does not become thirsty. For the chronic HD patient, fluid intake is adjusted so that weight gains are no more than 1 to 3 kg between dialyses.

Sodium and Potassium Restriction. The sodium and potassium restriction depends on the ability of the kidneys to excrete these electrolytes. Sodium-restricted diets may vary from 2 to 4 g depending on the degree of edema and hypertension. Sodium and salt should not be equated because the sodium content in 1 g of sodium chloride is equivalent to 400 mg of sodium. The patient should be instructed to avoid high-sodium foods such as cured meats, pickled foods, canned soups and stews, frankfurters, cold cuts, soy sauce, and salad dressings (see Chapter 35, Tables 35-11 through 35-13). Most salt substitutes should not be used because they contain potassium chloride.

TABLE 47-9	*NUTRITIONAL THERAPY* High-Potassium* Foods	
Fruits	**Vegetables**	**Other Foods**
Apricot, raw (2 medium) dried (5 halves)	Acorn squash	Bran/bran products
Avocado (¼ whole)	Artichoke	Chocolate (1.5-2 oz)
Banana (½ whole)	Bamboo shoots	Granola
Cantaloupe	Baked beans	Milk, all types
Dates (5 whole)	Butternut squash	(1 cup)
Dried fruits	Refried beans	Molasses (1 tbs)
Figs, dried	Beets, fresh then boiled	Nutritional supple-
Grapefruit juice	Black beans	ments: Use only
Honeydew	Broccoli, cooked	under the direc-
Kiwi (1 medium)	Brussels sprouts	tion of physician
Mango (1 medium)	Chinese cabbage	or dietitian
Nectarine (1 medium)	Carrots, raw	Nuts and seeds (1 oz)
Orange (1 medium)	Dried beans and peas	Peanut butter (2 tbs)
Orange juice	Greens, except kale	Salt substitutes/Lite
Papaya (½ whole)	Hubbard squash	Salt
Pomegranate (1 whole)	Kohlrabi	Salt-free broth
Pomegranate juice	Lentils	Yogurt
Prunes	Legumes	
Prune juice	Mushrooms, canned	
Raisins	Parsnips	
	Potatoes, white and sweet	
	Pumpkin	
	Rutabagas	
	Spinach, cooked	
	Tomatoes/tomato products	
	Vegetable juices	

Source: National Kidney Foundation: Potassium and your CKD diet. Available at *www.kidney.org/atoz/atozItem.cfm?id=103* (accessed June 30, 2006).
*Contain at least 200 mg/portion; portion = ½ cup unless otherwise noted.

Dietary restrictions for potassium range from about 2 to 4 g (39 mg = 1 mEq). Some PD patients do not need potassium restrictions. Some foods with high potassium content that should be avoided are oranges, bananas, melons, tomatoes, prunes, raisins, deep green and yellow vegetables, beans, and legumes (Table 47-9).

Phosphate Restriction. Phosphate should be limited to approximately 1000 mg/day. Foods that are high in phosphate include dairy products (e.g., milk, ice cream, cheese, yogurt) or foods containing dairy products (pudding). Most foods that are high in phosphate are also high in calcium. Restricting phosphate will restrict calcium intake.

NURSING MANAGEMENT
CONSERVATIVE THERAPY OF CHRONIC KIDNEY DISEASE

■ Nursing Assessment

The nurse should obtain a complete history of any existing renal disease or family history of renal disease because some kidney disorders have a hereditary basis. Genetics has been a focus of kidney diseases for quite some time, especially those classified as single gene disorders (e.g., Alport syndrome, focal segmental glomerulosclerosis, immunoglobulin A [IgA] nephropathy, polycystic kidney disease, and Wilms' tumor). Other disorders that can lead to CKD are chromosomal disorders (e.g., Down syndrome, Turner syndrome) and multifactorial disorders (e.g., diabetes mellitus, hypertension, systemic lupus erythematosus).[33] Because many drugs are potentially nephrotoxic, both current and past use of

prescription and over-the-counter drugs and herbal preparations must be reviewed.

The nurse should assess the patient's dietary habits and discuss any problems regarding intake. The height and weight should be measured, and any recent weight changes evaluated.

Clinical manifestations of CKD are apparent in multiple body systems (see Fig. 47-5). Fatigue, lethargy, and pruritus are often the early symptoms of CKD. Hypertension and proteinuria are often the first signs.

Support systems should be assessed. The chronicity of renal disease and the long-term nature of treatment modalities affect every area of a person's life, including family relationships, social and work activities, self-image, and emotional state. The choice of treatment modality may be related to support systems available to the patient. Recognition that CKD is a lifelong illness will facilitate the care.

■ Nursing Diagnoses

Nursing diagnoses for CKD may include, but are not limited to, those presented in NCP 47-1.

■ Planning

The overall goals are that a patient with CKD will (1) demonstrate knowledge and ability to comply with the therapeutic regimen, (2) participate in decision making for the plan of care and future treatment modality, (3) demonstrate effective coping strategies, and (4) continue with activities of daily living within physiologic limitations.

■ Nursing Implementation

Health Promotion. Individuals at risk for CKD must be identified. These include people with a history (or a family history) of renal disease, hypertension, diabetes mellitus, and repeated urinary tract infection. These individuals should have regular checkups including serum creatinine, BUN, and urinalysis. They should be advised that any changes in urine appearance (color, odor), frequency, or volume must be reported to the health care provider. If a patient must be prescribed a potentially nephrotoxic drug, it is important to monitor renal function with serum creatinine and BUN.

Individuals identified as at risk need to take measures to prevent or delay the progression of CKD. These include glycemic control for patients with diabetes (see Chapter 49), BP control, and early and definitive treatment of urinary tract infections.

Acute Intervention. The specific nursing management of the patient with CKD is detailed in NCP 47-1. It is important to teach the patient and family because diet, drugs, and follow-up medical care are the responsibilities of the patient[34] (Table 47-10). The patient should check a daily weight; learn to take daily BPs; and be able to identify signs and symptoms of fluid overload, hyperkalemia, and other electrolyte imbalances. The patient and family must understand the importance of strict dietary adherence. The dietitian should meet with the patient and family on a regular basis for diet planning. A diet history and consideration of cultural variations will facilitate diet planning and adherence.

The patient needs a complete understanding of the drugs, the dosages, and the common side effects. It may be helpful to make a list of the drugs and the times of administration that can be posted in the home. The patient must be instructed to avoid certain over-the-counter drugs such as NSAIDs and magnesium-

Urinary System

NURSING CARE PLAN 47-1

Patient with Chronic Kidney Disease

NURSING DIAGNOSIS **Excess fluid volume** *related to* inability of kidneys to excrete fluid and excessive fluid intake *as evidenced by* edema, hypertension, bounding pulse, weight gain, shortness of breath, pulmonary edema

PATIENT GOAL Maintains an acceptable body weight and fluid balance with fluid and sodium restrictions or with peritoneal dialysis or hemodialysis treatments

OUTCOMES (NOC)

Kidney Function

- 24-hour intake and output balance _____
- Blood urea nitrogen _____
- Serum creatinine _____
- Serum electrolytes _____

Measurement Scale

1 = Severely compromised
2 = Substantially compromised
3 = Moderately compromised
4 = Mildly compromised
5 = Not compromised

- Weight gain _____
- Hypertension _____

Measurement Scale

1 = Severe
2 = Substantial
3 = Moderate
4 = Mild
5 = None

INTERVENTIONS (NIC) and *RATIONALES*

Hypervolemia Management

- Monitor respiratory pattern for symptoms of respiratory difficulty (e.g., dyspnea, tachypnea, and shortness of breath) *that are indicators of fluid excess.*
- Weigh patient daily and monitor trends.
- Provide appropriate diet *to help control edema and hypertension.*
- Instruct patient and/or family on measures instituted to treat the hypervolemia (e.g., daily weights, fluid restrictions) *to help monitor and control fluid overload and related hypertension.*

Hemodialysis Therapy/Peritoneal Dialysis Therapy

- Draw blood sample and review blood chemistries (e.g., BUN, serum creatinine, serum sodium, potassium, and PO_4 levels) before treatment *to evaluate response.*
- Record baseline vital signs: weight, temperature, pulse, respirations, and blood pressure, *to evaluate response to therapy.*
- Institute and discontinue dialysis according to protocol.
- Adjust filtration pressure to remove an appropriate amount of fluid.
- Work collaboratively with patient to adjust length of dialysis, diet regulations, fluid limitations, and medications to regulate fluid and electrolyte shifts between treatments.

NURSING DIAGNOSIS **Risk for injury** *related to* alterations in bone structure due to decreased calcium absorption, retention of phosphate, and altered vitamin D metabolism

PATIENT GOALS 1. Experiences no injuries
2. Describes interventions to reduce risk of fractures

OUTCOMES (NOC)

Physical Injury Severity

- Skin abrasions _____
- Bruises _____
- Extremity fractures _____
- Hip fractures _____
- Impaired mobility _____

Measurement Scale

1 = Severe
2 = Substantial
3 = Moderate
4 = Mild
5 = None

INTERVENTIONS (NIC) and *RATIONALES*

Electrolyte Management: Hypocalcemia

- Monitor trends in serum levels of calcium (e.g., ionized calcium) *to provide early intervention if necessary.*
- Monitor for electrolyte imbalances associated with hypocalcemia (e.g., hyperphosphatemia, hypomagnesemia, and alkalosis) *to determine degree of bone demineralization and potential risk for fracture.*
- Administer appropriate prescribed calcium salt (e.g., calcium carbonate, calcium chloride, and calcium gluconate).
- Provide adequate intake of vitamin D (e.g., vitamin supplement and organ meats) to facilitate GI absorption of calcium *to prevent and/or treat the bone demineralization.*

Teaching: Disease Process

- Instruct patient on measures to control/minimize symptoms (e.g., taking calcium and vitamin D supplements).
- Discuss lifestyle changes that may be required to prevent future complications (e.g., fall risk reduction) and/or control the disease process *to reduce the risk of unsafe practices that might result in a traumatic or pathologic fracture.*

NURSING CARE PLAN 47-1

Patient with Chronic Kidney Disease—cont'd

NURSING DIAGNOSIS   **Imbalanced nutrition: less than body requirements** *related to* restricted intake of nutrients (especially protein), nausea, vomiting, anorexia, and stomatitis *as evidenced by* loss of appetite and weight

PATIENT GOALS   1. Maintains an acceptable weight with no more than a 10% weight loss
2. Maintains serum albumin, creatinine, and hemoglobin and hematocrit within normal limits

OUTCOMES (NOC)

Nutritional Status

- Nutrient intake _____
- Food intake _____
- Weight/height ratio _____
- Energy _____
- Muscle tone _____

Measurement Scale

1 = Severe deviation from normal range
2 = Substantial deviation from normal range
3 = Moderate deviation from normal range
4 = Mild deviation from normal range
5 = No deviation from normal range

INTERVENTIONS (NIC) and RATIONALES

Nutritional Monitoring

- Monitor for nausea and vomiting *to intervene as necessary.*
- Monitor trends in weight loss and gain *to detect changes in status.*
- Monitor albumin, total protein, hemoglobin, and hematocrit levels *as indicators of nutritional status, and response to treatments.*
- Monitor caloric and nutrient intake *to detect changes.*

Nutrition Therapy

- Provide oral care before meals *to prevent stomatitis, remove bad taste, and increase patient's appetite.*
- Refer for diet teaching and planning *to ensure adequate intake within prescribed diet restrictions.*
- Provide needed nourishment within limits of prescribed diet *to promote adequate nutrition.*

NURSING DIAGNOSIS   **Grieving** *related to* loss of kidney function *as evidenced by* expression of feelings of sadness, anger, inadequacy, hopelessness

PATIENT GOALS   1. Demonstrates effective coping strategies
2. Reports that life is worth living

OUTCOMES (NOC)

Acceptance: Health Status

- Recognizes reality of health situation _____
- Pursues information about health _____
- Adjusts to change in health status _____
- Makes decisions about health _____
- Reports sense of life being worth living _____

Measurement Scale

1 = Never demonstrated
2 = Rarely demonstrated
3 = Sometimes demonstrated
4 = Often demonstrated
5 = Consistently demonstrated

INTERVENTIONS (NIC) and RATIONALES

Grief Work Facilitation

- Listen to expressions of grief *to convey a caring attitude and foster a relationship and/or to determine how patient is handling the situation.*
- Identify sources of community support for continued grief work.

Coping Enhancement

- Assist patient to solve problems in a constructive manner *to help facilitate the grieving process.*
- Encourage family involvement *to enable them to assist the patient and foster their support and understanding.*
- Assist patient to grieve and work though the losses of chronic illness and/or disability.

NURSING DIAGNOSIS   **Risk for infection** *related to* suppressed immune system, access sites, and malnutrition secondary to dialysis and uremia

PATIENT GOALS   1. Experiences no infections
2. Describes self-care practices to decrease the risk for infection

OUTCOMES (NOC)

Infection Severity

- Purulent drainage _____
- Pyuria _____
- Fever _____
- Pain/tenderness _____
- White blood count elevation _____

Measurement Scale

1 = Severe
2 = Substantial
3 = Moderate
4 = Mild
5 = None

INTERVENTIONS (NIC) and RATIONALES

Infection Protection

- Monitor for systemic and localized signs and symptoms of infection (e.g., pain on urination, hematuria, cloudy urine, chills, fever) *to ensure early identification and treatment.*
- Screen all visitors for communicable disease.
- Limit number of visitors *to decrease risk of infection.*

Infection Control

- Ensure aseptic handling of all IV lines *to prevent the introduction of organisms.*
- Wash hands before and after each patient care activity *to prevent transmission of pathogens.*
- Teach patient and family about signs and symptoms of infection and when to report them to the health care provider *to obtain early treatment.*

TABLE 47-10	*PATIENT AND FAMILY TEACHING GUIDE* Chronic Kidney Disease

1. Explain dietary (protein, sodium, potassium, phosphate) and fluid restrictions.
2. Encourage discussion of difficulties in modifying diet and fluid intake.
3. Explain signs and symptoms of electrolyte imbalance, especially high potassium.
4. Teach alternative ways of reducing thirst, such as sucking on ice cubes, lemon, or hard candy.
5. Explain the rationale for prescribed drugs and common side effects. Examples:
   * Phosphate binders (including calcium supplements used as phosphate barriers) should be taken with meals.
   * Calcium supplements prescribed to treat hypocalcemia directly should be taken on an empty stomach (but not at the same time as iron supplements).
   * Iron supplements should be taken between meals.
6. Explain the importance of reporting any of the following:
   * Weight gain greater than 4 lb (2 kg)
   * Increasing BP
   * Shortness of breath
   * Edema
   * Increasing fatigue or weakness
   * Confusion or lethargy
7. Encourage patient and family to share concerns about lifestyle changes, living with a chronic illness, and decisions about type of dialysis or transplantation.

BP, Blood pressure.

based laxatives and antacids. The patient should also be aware that meperidine and ACE inhibitors may be harmful because of renal insufficiency.

Motivating patients to assume the primary role in the management of their disease is essential. The period of conservative management provides an opportunity to evaluate each patient's ability to manage the disease. This knowledge will be helpful when determining the treatment modality.

Ambulatory and Home Care. The length of time that a patient can receive conservative therapy is highly variable and depends on the progression of renal failure and the presence of other comorbid conditions. When conservative therapy is no longer effective, HD, PD, and transplantation are the available treatment options.

While the patient is receiving conservative therapy, the decision regarding future therapies should be made. This should be done before complications such as mental status changes, bleeding, progressive neuropathies, and fluid overload occur.[34]

The patient and family need a clear explanation of what is involved in dialysis and transplantation. If alternative treatments are presented early in the course of therapy, there will be an opportunity to carefully consider choices. Providing information about the treatment options will allow the patient to be active in the decision-making process and give a sense of control over life-altering decisions. The patient should be informed that, if dialysis is chosen, the option of transplantation still remains. It should be emphasized that, if a transplanted organ fails, the patient can return to dialysis. The patient should also be counseled that re-transplantation is also an option.

■ *Evaluation*

The expected outcomes for the patient with CKD are presented in NCP 47-1.

Dialysis

Dialysis is the movement of fluid and molecules across a semipermeable membrane from one compartment to another. Clinically, dialysis is a technique in which substances move from the blood through a semipermeable membrane and into a dialysis solution (dialysate). It is used to correct fluid and electrolyte imbalances and to remove waste products in renal failure. It can also be used to treat drug overdoses. The two methods of dialysis available are **peritoneal dialysis** (PD) and **hemodialysis** (HD) (Table 47-11). In PD the peritoneal membrane acts as the semipermeable membrane. In HD an artificial membrane (usually made of cellulose-based or synthetic materials) is used as the semipermeable membrane and is in contact with the patient's blood.[35]

Dialysis is begun when the patient's uremia can no longer be adequately managed conservatively. Generally dialysis is initiated when the GFR (or creatinine clearance) is less than 15 ml/min. This criterion can vary widely in different clinical situations, and the physician will determine when to start dialysis based on the patient's clinical status. Certain uremic complications, including encephalopathy, neuropathies, uncontrolled hyperkalemia, pericarditis, and accelerated hypertension, indicate a need for immediate dialysis.

General Principles of Dialysis

Solutes and water move across the semipermeable membrane from the blood to the dialysate or from the dialysate to the blood in accordance with concentration gradients. The principles of diffusion, osmosis, and ultrafiltration are involved in dialysis (Fig. 47-7). *Diffusion* is the movement of solutes from an area of greater concentration to an area of lesser concentration. In renal failure, urea, creatinine, uric acid, and electrolytes (potassium, phosphate) move from the blood to the dialysate with the net effect of lowering their concentration in the blood. RBCs, WBCs, and plasma proteins are too large to diffuse through the pores of the membrane. Bacteria and viruses that may be present in the dialysate are too large to migrate through the pores into the blood.

Osmosis is the movement of fluid from an area of lesser to an area of greater concentration of solutes. Glucose is added to the dialysate and creates an osmotic gradient across the membrane, pulling excess fluid from the blood.

Ultrafiltration (water and fluid removal) results when there is an osmotic gradient or pressure gradient across the membrane. In PD, excess fluid is removed by increasing the osmolality of the dialysate (osmotic gradient) with the addition of glucose. In HD, the gradient is created by increasing pressure in the blood compartment (positive pressure) or decreasing pressure in the dialysate compartment (negative pressure). Extracellular fluid moves into the dialysate because of the pressure gradient. The excess fluid is removed by creating a pressure differential between the blood and the dialysate solution with a combination of positive pressure in the blood compartment or negative pressure in the dialysate compartment.

PERITONEAL DIALYSIS

Although PD was first used in 1923, it did not come into widespread use for chronic treatment until the 1970s with the development of soft, pliable peritoneal solution bags and the introduction of the concept of continuous PD. In the United States, approximately 10% of patients receiving dialysis treatments are on PD.[11] In recent years the use of PD to treat CKD has decreased in the United States.

TABLE 47-11	Comparison of Peritoneal Dialysis and Hemodialysis			
Peritoneal Dialysis (PD)		**Hemodialysis (HD)**		
Advantages	**Disadvantages**	**Advantages**	**Disadvantages**	
Immediate initiation in almost any hospital	Bacterial or chemical peritonitis	Rapid fluid removal	Vascular access problems	
Less complicated than hemodialysis	Protein loss into dialysate	Rapid removal of urea and creatinine	Dietary and fluid restrictions	
Portable system with CAPD	Exit site and tunnel infections	Effective potassium removal	Heparinization may be necessary	
Fewer dietary restrictions	Self-image problems with catheter placement	Less protein loss	Extensive equipment necessary	
Relatively short training time	Hyperglycemia	Lowering of serum triglycerides	Hypotension during dialysis	
Usable in the patient with vascular access problems	Aggravated hyperlipidemia	Home dialysis possible	Added blood loss that contributes to anemia	
Less cardiovascular stress	Surgery for catheter placement	Temporary access can be placed at bedside	Specially trained personnel necessary	
Home dialysis possible	Contraindication in the patient with multiple abdominal surgeries, trauma, unrepaired hernia		Surgery for permanent access placement	
Preferable for the diabetic patient	Specially trained personnel needed		Self-image problems with permanent access	
	Catheter can migrate			

CAPD, Continuous ambulatory peritoneal dialysis.

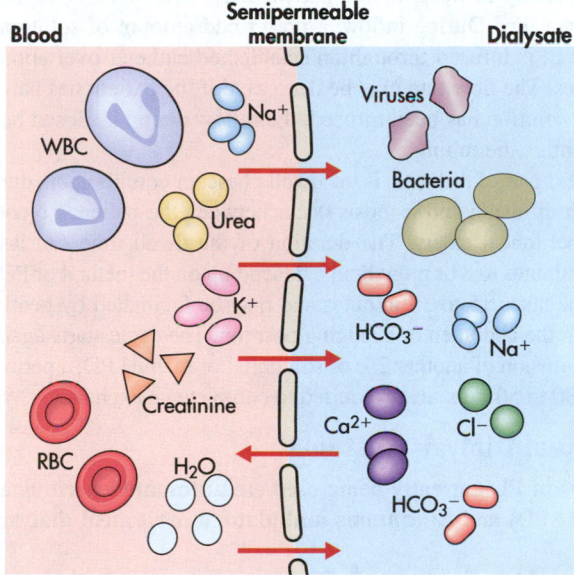

FIG. 47-7 Osmosis and diffusion across a semipermeable membrane.

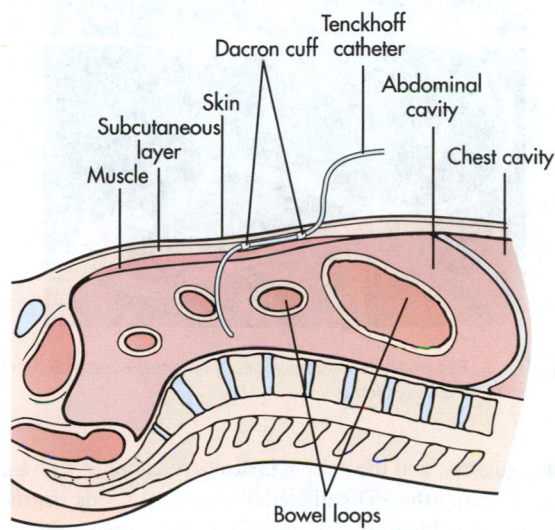

FIG. 47-8 Tenckhoff catheter used in peritoneal dialysis.

Catheter Placement

Peritoneal access is obtained by inserting a catheter through the anterior abdominal wall (Fig. 47-8). The prototype of the catheter that is used was developed by Tenckhoff in 1968 and is made of silicone rubber tubing. The catheters are about 60 cm long and have two Dacron cuffs on the subcutaneous and peritoneal portions of the catheter that act as anchors and prevent the migration of microorganisms down the shaft from the skin. Within a few weeks, fibrous tissue grows into the Dacron cuff, holding the catheter in place and preventing bacterial penetration into the peritoneal cavity. The tip of the catheter rests in the peritoneal cavity and has many perforations spaced along the distal end of the tubing to allow fluid to flow in and out of the catheter. Bent or "swan-neck" catheters with curled, "pigtail" ends are preferred because they prevent catheter migration and kinking and allow for easier fills and drains. There are numerous variations of the peritoneal catheter (Fig. 47-9).

The technique for catheter placement varies. Although it is possible to place a permanent catheter in the peritoneal cavity at the bedside with a trocar, it is usually done via surgery so that its placement can be directly visualized, minimizing potential complications. Preparation of the patient for catheter insertion includes

emptying the bladder and bowel, weighing the patient, and obtaining a signed consent form.

In the nonsurgical (bedside) approach, an area approximately 2 cm below the umbilicus is numbed with a local anesthetic, and a small stab wound is made. A stylet is inserted, and the abdomen is distended with dialysis solution. The catheter is then placed into the peritoneal cavity. When the patient feels pressure in the rectal area and has the urge to defecate, the catheter is in place.

In the surgical approach, a midline umbilical incision is made, and a small puncture is made to one side of and below this incision. The distal end of the catheter is placed in the peritoneum, and it is tunneled under the skin to the puncture site. The tunnel helps prevent peritonitis. After the catheter is inserted, the skin is cleaned with an antiseptic solution, and a sterile dressing is applied. Complications of catheter insertion include perforation of the bladder, the bowel, or a blood vessel and the introduction of bacteria.

The catheter is connected to a sterile tubing system and secured to the abdomen with tape. The catheter is irrigated immediately with heparinized dialysate (usually 500 ml) to clear blood and fibrin from it. Prophylactic antibiotics may also be instilled. The irrigations may continue for 12 to 24 hours using small volumes of dialysate. This procedure helps prevent catheter occlusion that can lead to poor drainage and inflow. Catheter placement is usually

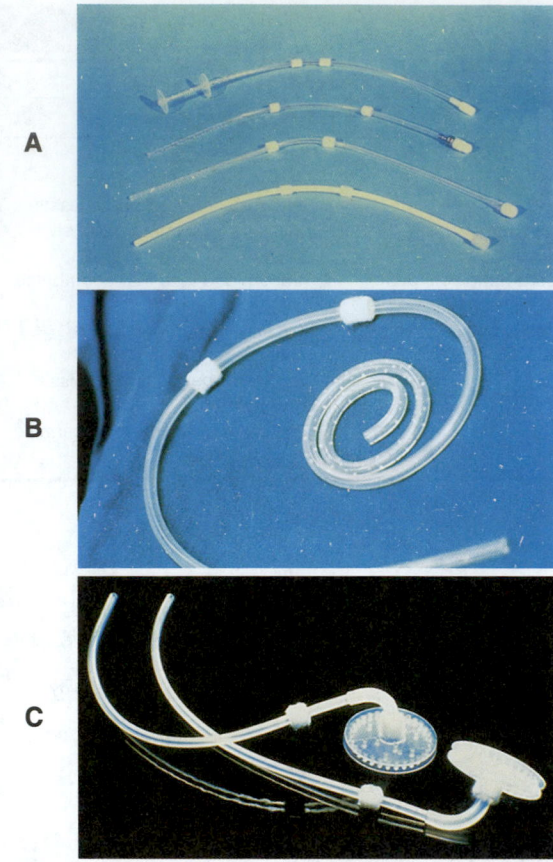

FIG. 47-9   **A,** Peritoneal catheters used for peritoneal dialysis. **B,** Bent neck, curled catheters. **C,** Disc catheters.

same-day surgery, and the patient is discharged home with a sterile dressing covering the PD catheter. The patient needs instructions on keeping the dressing dry, avoiding accidentally pulling the catheter, and receiving follow-up care.

Before the start of PD, it is preferable to allow a waiting period of 7 to 14 days for proper sealing of the catheter and for tissue to grow into the cuffs. However, some centers start dialysis 5 to 7 days after catheter insertion. About 2 to 4 weeks after catheter implantation, the exit site should be clean, dry, and free of redness and tenderness (Fig. 47-10). Once the catheter incision site is healed, the patient may shower and then pat the catheter and exit site dry. Daily catheter care includes the application of an antiseptic solution and a clean dressing, as well as examination of the catheter site for signs of infection.

Dialysis Solutions and Cycles

Dialysis solutions are available commercially in 1- or 2-L (and sometimes smaller or larger volume) plastic bags (Dianeal, Inpersol) with glucose concentrations of 1.5%, 2.5%, and 4.25%. The electrolyte composition is similar to that of plasma. Using dry heat, the dialysis solution is warmed to body temperature to increase peritoneal clearance, prevent hypothermia, and enhance comfort.

Ultrafiltration (fluid removal) during PD depends on osmotic forces, with glucose being the most effective osmotic agent currently available. However, the problems arising from high rates of peritoneal glucose absorption, such as obesity, hypertriglyceridemia, and difficult control of blood glucose levels in the diabetic patient, have led to a search for alternative osmotic agents, including amino acid solutions. Many of these agents are currently under investigation.

The three phases of the PD cycle are *inflow* (fill), *dwell* (equilibration), and *drain.* The three phases are called an *exchange.* The patient dialyzing at home will receive about four exchanges per day. An acutely ill hospitalized patient may receive 12 to 24 exchanges per day. During inflow, a prescribed amount of solution, usually 2 L, is infused through an established catheter over about 10 minutes. The flow rate may be decreased if the patient has pain. After the solution has been infused, the inflow clamp is closed before air enters the tubing.

The next part of the cycle is the dwell phase, or equilibration, during which diffusion and osmosis occur between the patient's blood and the peritoneal cavity. The duration of the dwell time can last 20 to 30 minutes to 8 or more hours, depending on the method of PD. Drain time takes 15 to 30 minutes and may be facilitated by gently massaging the abdomen or changing position. The cycle starts again with the infusion of another 2 L of solution. For manual PD, a period of about 30 to 50 minutes is required to complete an exchange.

Peritoneal Dialysis Systems

Two types of PD currently being used are **automated peritoneal dialysis** (APD) and **continuous ambulatory peritoneal dialysis** (CAPD).

Automated Peritoneal Dialysis. An automated device called a cycler is used to deliver the dialysate for APD (Fig. 47-11). The automated cycler times and controls the fill, dwell, and drain phases. The machine cycles four or more exchanges per night with 1 to 2 hours per exchange. Alarms and monitors are built into the system to make it safe for the patient to dialyze while sleeping. The patient disconnects from the machine in the morning and usually

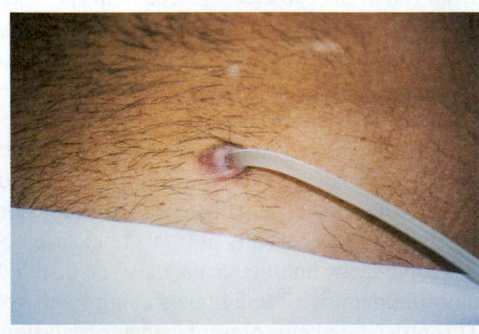

FIG. 47-10   Peritoneal catheter exit site.

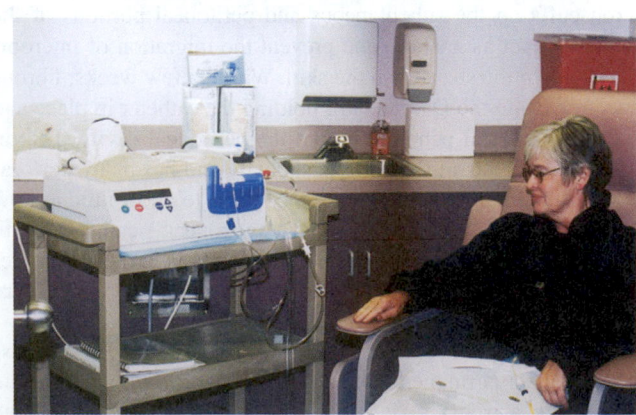

FIG. 47-11   Automated peritoneal dialysis cycler, which can be used while the patient is sleeping or for hospitalized patients who require frequent exchanges.

leaves fluid in the abdomen during the day. One to two daytime manual exchanges may also be prescribed to ensure adequate dialysis. It is difficult to achieve the required solute and fluid clearance with solely nighttime APD. Older cyclers were quite large. With new technology cyclers are now about the size of a VCR or DVD player and have longer tubing to allow greater mobility.

Continuous Ambulatory Peritoneal Dialysis. CAPD is carried out manually by exchanging 1.5 to 3 L (usually 2 L) of peritoneal dialysate at least 4 times daily, with dwell times of 4 to 10 hours. For example, one schedule starts the exchanges at 7 AM, 12 noon, 5 PM, and 10 PM. In this procedure the person instills 2 L of dialysate from a collapsible plastic bag into the peritoneal cavity through a disposable plastic tube.

Technical advances in CAPD systems allow the bag and line to be disconnected after the instillation of the fluid, decreasing the risk of peritonitis. After the equilibration period, the line is reconnected to the catheter, the dialysate (effluent) is drained from the peritoneal cavity, and a new 2-L bag of dialysate solution is infused (Fig. 47-12). It is critical in PD to maintain aseptic technique to avoid peritonitis. Several tubing connections and devices are commercially available to help maintain an aseptic system.

Contraindications for PD include the following:
1. History of multiple abdominal surgical procedures or chronic abdominal pathologic conditions (e.g., pancreatitis, diverticulitis)
2. Recurrent abdominal wall or inguinal hernias
3. Obesity with large abdominal wall and fat deposits
4. Preexisting vertebral disease (e.g., chronic back problems)
5. Severe obstructive pulmonary disease

Complications of Peritoneal Dialysis

Exit Site Infection. Infection of the peritoneal catheter exit site is most commonly caused by *Staphylococcus aureus* or *S. epidermidis* (from skin flora). Superficial exit site infections caused by these organisms are generally resolved with antibiotic therapy. Clinical manifestations of an exit site infection include redness at the site, tenderness, and drainage. If not treated immediately, subcutaneous tunnel infections usually result in abscess formation and may cause peritonitis, necessitating catheter removal.

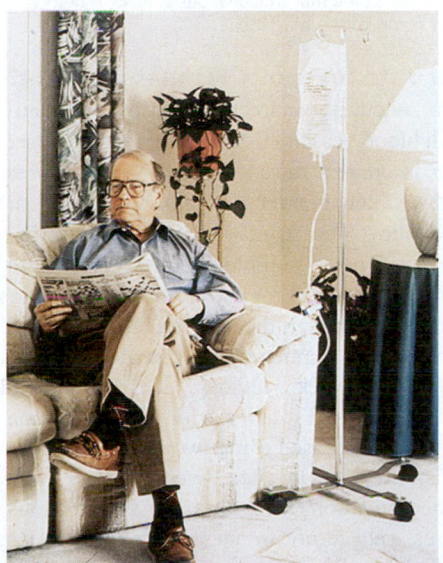

FIG. 47-12   Infusion period for a continuous ambulatory peritoneal dialysis patient.

Peritonitis. Peritonitis results from contamination of the dialysate or tubing or from progression of an exit site or tunnel infection. Less commonly, peritonitis results from bacteria in the intestine crossing over into the peritoneal cavity. Peritonitis is usually caused by *S. aureus* or *S. epidermidis*. The primary clinical manifestation of peritonitis is a cloudy peritoneal effluent that has a WBC count of over 100 cells/µl (particularly neutrophils). GI manifestations may also be present, including diffuse abdominal pain, diarrhea, vomiting, abdominal distention, and hyperactive bowel sounds. Fever may or may not be present. Cultures, Gram stain, and a WBC differential of the peritoneal effluent are used to confirm the diagnosis of peritonitis. Antibiotics can be given orally, intravenously, or intraperitoneally. The patient is usually treated on an outpatient basis. Repeated infections may require the removal of the peritoneal catheter and termination of PD. The formation of adhesions in the peritoneum can result from repeated infections and interferes with the peritoneal membrane's ability to act as a dialyzing surface.

Abdominal Pain. Although not severe, pain is a common complication. It may be caused by intraperitoneal irritation from the low pH of the dialysate solution (which usually subsides in 1 to 2 weeks) or peritonitis. Pain can also occur when the tip of the catheter touches the bladder, bowel, or peritoneum. A change in the position of the catheter should correct this problem. Accidental infusion of air or infusing the dialysate too rapidly may cause referred pain in the shoulder. If the infusion rate is decreased, the pain usually subsides.

Outflow Problems. When outflow is less than 80% of inflow immediately after catheter placement, it may be caused by a kink in the tunnel segment of the catheter, omentum wrapped around the catheter, or migration of the catheter out of the pelvic region. Persistent outflow problems may require radiologic or surgical manipulation of the catheter. Outflow problems after the catheter has settled into place are often the result of a full colon. Bowel evacuation frequently relieves the problem.

Hernias. Because of increased intraabdominal pressure secondary to the dialysate infusion, hernias can develop in predisposed individuals such as multiparous women and older men. However, in most situations after hernia repair, PD can be resumed after several days using small dialysate volumes and keeping the patient supine.

Lower Back Problems. Increased intraabdominal pressure can cause or aggravate lower back pain. The lumbosacral curvature is increased by intraperitoneal infusion of dialysate. Orthopedic binders and a regular exercise program for strengthening the back muscles have been beneficial for some patients.

Bleeding. Effluent drained after the first few exchanges may be pink or slightly bloody because of the trauma of catheter insertion. Bloody effluent over several days or the new appearance of blood in the effluent can indicate active intraperitoneal bleeding. If this occurs, the BP and hematocrit should be checked. Blood may also be present in the effluent of women who are menstruating or ovulating, and this requires no intervention.

Pulmonary Complications. Atelectasis, pneumonia, and bronchitis may occur from repeated upward displacement of the diaphragm, resulting in decreased lung expansion. The longer the dwell time, the greater the likelihood of pulmonary problems. Frequent repositioning and deep-breathing exercises can help. When lying in bed, elevation of the head of the bed may prevent these problems.

Protein Loss. The peritoneal membrane is permeable to plasma proteins, amino acids, and polypeptides. These substances are lost in the dialysate fluid. The amount of loss may be as much as 5 to 15 g/day. This loss may increase up to 40 g/day during episodes of peritonitis as the membrane becomes more permeable. Positive nitrogen balance can be maintained with adequate protein intake.

Carbohydrate and Lipid Abnormalities. Dialysate glucose is absorbed via the peritoneum and may be as much as 100 to 150 g/day. Continuous absorption of glucose results in increased insulin secretion and increased plasma insulin levels. The hyperinsulinemia stimulates hepatic production of triglycerides.

Encapsulating Sclerosing Peritonitis and Loss of Ultrafiltration. *Encapsulating sclerosing peritonitis* is a term applied to the development of a thick fibrous membrane that surrounds and compresses the bowel for unknown reasons. Intestinal obstruction and strangulation are common complications. This condition generally necessitates changing the patient to HD because of the loss of ultrafiltration. Loss of ultrafiltration is associated with rapid glucose absorption.

Effectiveness of and Adaptation to Chronic Peritoneal Dialysis

The technique is associated with a short training program, independence, and ease of traveling.[36] Clinically, the patient receiving PD does as well as the patient receiving HD and sometimes better. There are fewer dietary restrictions, and greater mobility is possible than with conventional HD. The major disadvantage is the possibility of developing peritonitis. As further improvements in techniques are made (e.g., improved connecting and sterilizing devices, in-line filters, improved catheters), the incidence of peritonitis should decrease.

PD is especially indicated for the individual who has vascular access problems or responds poorly to the hemodynamic stresses of HD (e.g., the older adult patient with diabetes and cardiovascular disease). The diabetic patient with ESRD does better with PD than with HD. The advantages of PD for the diabetic patient include better BP control, less hemodynamic instability because fluid shifts are gradual, better control of blood glucose by using intraperitoneal insulin (which can often eliminate the need for subcutaneous insulin), and prevention of retinal hemorrhage because heparin is not required as it is in HD.

HEMODIALYSIS

In 1943, Willem Kolff in the Netherlands performed the first successful dialysis on a human using a rotating-drum dialyzer. He initiated dialysis treatment in the United States in 1948.[35] Tremendous technologic advances have been made in HD since then, allowing for safer, shorter treatments using sophisticated equipment.

Vascular Access Sites

Obtaining vascular access is one of the most difficult problems associated with HD. To carry out HD, a very rapid blood flow is required, and access to a large blood vessel is essential. The types of vascular access in current use include arteriovenous fistulas (AVFs) and grafts (AVGs), temporary and semipermanent catheters, subcutaneous ports, and shunts.

Shunts. In the past external shunts were used, but today they are rarely used except with continuous renal replacement therapy (CRRT) because of the numerous complications (e.g., infection, thrombosis) associated with them. The shunt consists of a U-shaped Silastic tube divided at the midpoint, and each of the two ends is placed in an artery and a vein (Fig. 47-13, *A*).

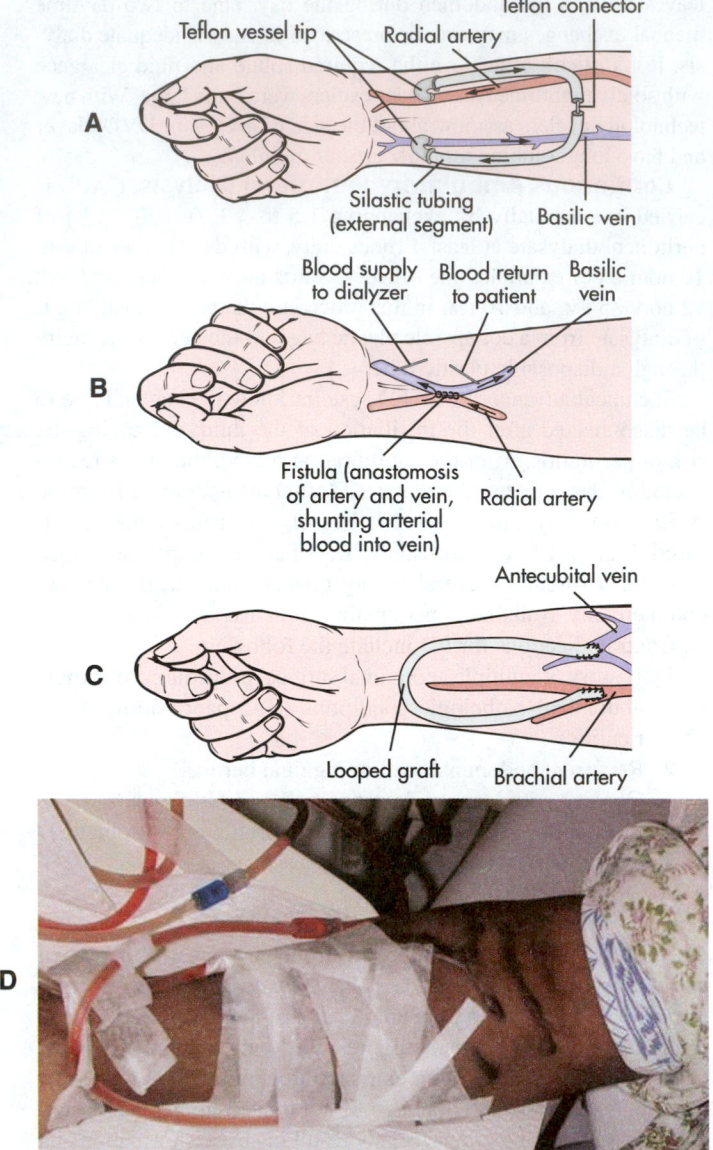

FIG. 47-13 Vascular access for hemodialysis. **A,** External shunt. **B,** Internal arteriovenous fistula. **C,** Internal arteriovenous graft. **D,** A hemodialysis graft while connected to a hemodialysis machine.

Internal Arteriovenous Fistulas and Grafts. In 1966 the use of the subcutaneous internal arteriovenous native (using the person's own blood vessels) fistula was introduced (see Fig. 47-13, *B*). An AVF is created most commonly in the forearm with an anastomosis between an artery (usually radial or ulnar) and a vein (usually cephalic). The fistula provides for arterial blood flow through the vein. The arterial blood flow is essential to provide the rapid blood flow required for HD. The increased pressure of the arterial blood flow through the vein makes the vein dilate and become tough, making it amenable to repeated venipuncture in approximately 4 to 6 weeks, although it is recommended that the AVF be placed at least 3 months prior to the initiation of hemodialysis. The vein is accessed using two large-gauge needles.

Native fistulas have the best overall patency rates and least number of complications (e.g., thrombosis, infections) of all vascular accesses, yet are not frequently used. Several reasons have been identified for the infrequent placement of AVFs, including late referrals; lack of surgical expertise; less surgery reimbursement, although the procedure is more complicated and time consuming than the placement of a graft (described in the next paragraph); and staff inexperience with cannulation and care for fistulas.[37] In 2004, the Centers for Medicare and Medicaid Services launched a national initiative called "Fistula First" to encourage the increased placement and use of native AVFs. However, AVFs may not be possible in patients with a history of severe hypertension, peripheral vascular disease, diabetes, prolonged IV drug use, or previous multiple IV procedures in the forearm. For these individuals a synthetic graft is usually required.

Arteriovenous grafts (AVGs) are made of synthetic materials (polytetrafluoroethylene [PTFE], Teflon) and form a "bridge" between the arterial and venous blood supplies. Grafts are placed under the skin and are surgically anastomosed between an artery (usually brachial) and a vein (usually antecubital) (see Fig. 47-13, *C*). An interval of 2 to 4 weeks is usually necessary to allow the graft to heal, but some centers may use it earlier. The graft is accessed using two large-gauge needles and the graft material is self-healing, closing over puncture sites with sufficient pressure to also stop the bleeding when needles are removed. Because grafts are made of artificial materials, they are easily infected and are thrombogenic.

The needles used are 14 to 16 gauge and are inserted into the fistula or graft to obtain vascular access. One needle is placed to pull blood from the circulation to the HD machine, and the other needle is used to return the dialyzed blood to the patient. The needles are attached via tubing to dialysis lines. Normally, a *thrill* can be felt by palpating the area of anastomosis, and a *bruit* can be heard with a stethoscope. The bruit and thrill are created by arterial blood rushing into the vein.

Blood pressure measurements, insertion of IVs, and venipuncture should never be performed on the affected extremity. These special precautions are taken to prevent infection and clotting of the vascular access. The AVF is much less likely to clot and become infected than a graft. Thrombosis in AVGs is common but can often be corrected with interventional radiology techniques or a surgical procedure. AVGs can cause the development of distal ischemia (*steal syndrome*) because too much of the arterial blood is being shunted or "stolen" from the distal extremity. This is usually seen soon after surgery and may require surgical correction. Aneurysms can also develop at the fistula site and can rupture if left untreated. AVG infections are not uncommon, and immediate treatment is essential to salvage the graft and prevent bacteremia. Severe AVG infections may necessitate graft removal.

Temporary Vascular Access. In some situations when immediate vascular access is required, percutaneous cannulation of the internal jugular or femoral vein is performed. In the past the subclavian vein was often cannulated, but the central stenosis that can occur with this approach has made it the option of last resort. A flexible Teflon, silicone rubber, or polyurethane catheter is inserted at the bedside into one of these large veins and provides access to circulation without surgery (Fig. 47-14, *A*). The catheters usually have a double external lumen with an internal septum separating the two internal segments (Fig. 47-14, *B*). One lumen is used for blood removal and the other for blood return. Temporary catheters in the jugular or subclavian veins can be left in place for 1 to 3 weeks. Femoral vein cannulas can remain in place for up to 1 week.

Jugular vein cannulation is associated with a low incidence of thrombosis. That is the primary reason this method is preferred over subclavian cannulation. Short-term jugular vein access with stiff catheters may be uncomfortable and restrict neck movement.

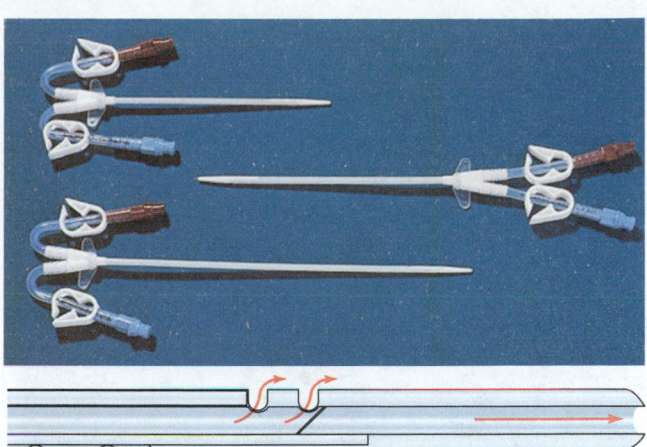

FIG. 47-14   Temporary double-lumen vascular access catheter for acute hemodialysis. **A,** Soft, flexible dual-lumen tube is attached to a Y hub. **B,** The distance between the arterial intake and the venous return lumina typically provides recirculation rates of 5% or less.

Bent catheters can ease this problem (see Fig. 47-14, *A*). In addition to vessel thrombosis and stenosis, subclavian vein cannulation has been associated with pneumothorax, brachial plexus neuropathies, and hemothorax. Both types of catheter placements pose the risk of infection.

Disadvantages of femoral vessel cannulation include the following: (1) the catheter can remain in place only a short time, (2) the location encourages catheter kinking, and (3) the groin is not a clean site. Potential complications of femoral catheterization are femoral vein thrombosis with pulmonary emboli (especially if the treatment is prolonged), infections, immobility, and inadvertent blood vessel punctures with hematoma formation. The patient must be on bed rest while the femoral catheter is in place to prevent trauma to the vessel.

For all temporary catheters, no drugs should be administered or blood withdrawn via the catheter by nondialysis staff. This is to minimize the risk of infection, catheter loss, and accidental injection of heparin. Trained dialysis staff will instill heparin into the lumens of the catheter at the end of each treatment to ensure patency and withdraw it before the next treatment. Should patency be incapacitated as shown by an inability to withdraw blood, instillation of a medication as prescribed by a physician to restore function may be necessary (e.g., alteplase [Cathflo Activase]). Semipermanent, soft, flexible Silastic double-lumen catheters (Davol, Bard, PermCath) are being used more often. These catheters can be used as temporary access while awaiting fistula placement and development or as long-term access when other forms of access have failed. This type of catheter exits on the upper chest wall and is tunneled subcutaneously to the internal or external jugular vein (Fig. 47-15). The catheter tip rests in the right atrium. It has one or two subcutaneous Dacron cuffs that prevent infection from tracking along the catheter and anchor the catheter, eliminating the need for sutures.

Several new semipermanent silicone and polyurethane catheters are now available. The aim of all of the new catheters is to increase blood flow rates while decreasing rates of infection and catheter loss from clotting or the development of fibrin sheaths on the catheter exterior. The Tesio catheters involve two tunneled cuffed catheters that are placed through separate tunnels. Both catheter

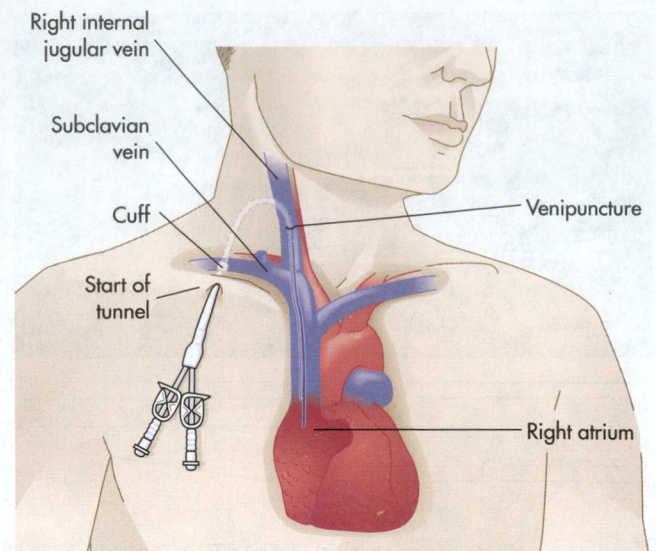

FIG. 47-15 Right internal jugular placement for a tunneled, cuffed semipermanent catheter.

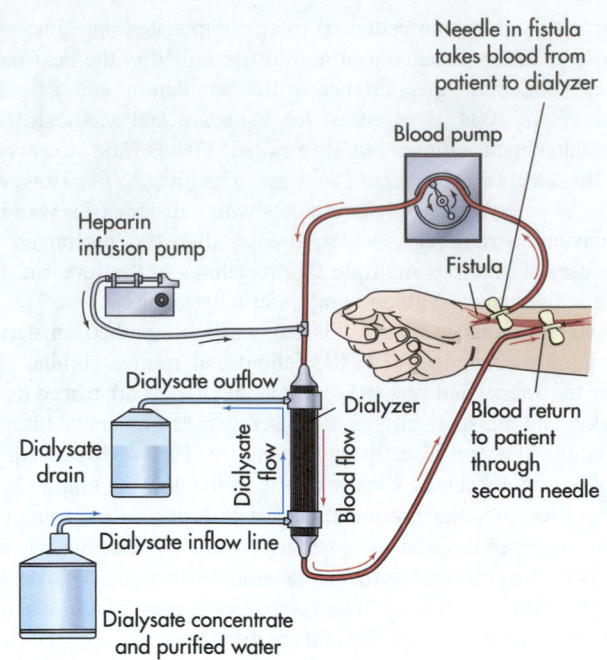

FIG. 47-16 Components of a hemodialysis system. Blood is removed via a needle inserted in a fistula or via catheter lumen. It is propelled to the dialyzer by a blood pump. Heparin is infused either as a bolus predialysis or through a heparin pump continuously to prevent clotting. Dialysate is pumped in and flows in the opposite direction of the blood. The dialyzed blood is returned to the patient through a second needle or catheter lumen. Old dialysate and ultrafiltrate are drained and discarded.

tips are in the right atrium. The Ash Split catheter is a single-tunneled cuffed catheter, but the internal and external lumens are split into two lumens. The separate catheters or lumens are thought to improve blood flows. A system called LifeSite uses two subcutaneous implanted ports that are accessed using 14-gauge needles. The implanted ports are attached to internal silicone catheters that are usually tunneled into the internal or external jugular vein.

Advance planning is essential for management of the patient with renal failure who is approaching end-stage disease and dialysis. Several months before the estimated start of dialysis, a permanent dialysis access should be created to allow time for healing and maturation. If dialysis is required before the permanent access is ready for use, then a temporary access should be placed.

Dialyzers

The dialyzer is a long plastic cartridge that contains thousands of parallel hollow tubes or fibers (Fig. 47-16). The fibers are the semipermeable membrane made of cellulose-based or other synthetic materials. The blood is pumped into the top of the cartridge and is dispersed into all of the fibers. Dialysis fluid (*dialysate*) is pumped into the bottom of the cartridge and bathes the outside of the fibers with dialysis fluid. Ultrafiltration, diffusion, and osmosis occur across the pores of this semipermeable membrane. When the dialyzed blood reaches the end of the thousands of semipermeable fibers, it converges into a single tube that returns it to the patient. Dialyzers available differ in regard to surface area, membrane composition and thickness, clearance of waste products, and removal of fluid.

Procedure

To initiate chronic dialysis in a patient with an AVG or AVF, two needles are placed in the fistula or graft. If the patient has a catheter, the two blood lines are attached to the two catheter lumens. The needle closer to the fistula or the red catheter lumen is used to pull blood from the patient and send it to the dialyzer with the assistance of a blood pump. The dialyzer and blood lines are usually primed with up to 1000 ml of saline solution to eliminate air from the system. Heparin is added to the blood as it flows into the dialyzer because any time blood contacts a foreign substance, it has a tendency to clot. When the blood enters the extracorporeal circuit,

it is propelled through the top of the dialyzer by a blood pump at a flow rate of 200 to 500 ml/min, while the dialysate (warmed to body temperature) circulates in the opposite direction at a rate of 300 to 900 ml/min. Blood is returned from the dialyzer to the patient through the second needle or blue catheter lumen.

In addition to the dialyzer, there is a dialysate delivery and monitoring system (see Fig. 47-16). This system pumps the dialysate through the dialyzer, countercurrent to the blood flow. Adjustments can be made for ultrafiltration by creating positive pressure on the blood side or negative pressure on the dialysate side or by a combination of both. The newest dialysis delivery systems have ultrafiltration controllers that equalize negative and positive pressures for the removal of the precise amount of fluid per hour. The dialysis system has alarm systems to warn of blood leaking into the dialysate or air leaking into the blood; alterations in dialysate temperature, concentration, or pressure; and extremes in BP readings.

Dialysis is terminated by flushing the dialyzer with saline solution to return all blood through the access. The needles are then removed from the patient, and firm pressure is applied to the venipuncture sites until the bleeding stops. On occasion the access site can begin to bleed again. If this occurs, pressure should be reapplied, but not so firmly that flow is occluded because this could cause thrombosis. For patients with a catheter, the blood lines are clamped and removed from the catheter lumens.

Before beginning treatment, the nurse must complete an assessment that includes fluid status (weight, BP, peripheral edema, lung and heart sounds), condition of vascular access, temperature, and general skin condition. The difference between the last postdialysis weight and the present predialysis weight determines the ultrafiltration or the amount of weight to be removed. Ideally, no more than 1 to 1.5 kg should be gained between treatments to avoid causing hypotension associated with the removal of larger volumes of fluid. Many patients gain 2 to 3 kg between treatments, and this volume usually can be removed if their BP is not labile. While the patient is on dialysis, vital signs should be taken at least every 30 to 60 minutes because rapid changes may occur in the BP.

Most maintenance dialysis units use reclining chairs that allow for elevation of the feet if hypotension develops. Most people sleep, read, talk, or watch television during dialysis. Treatments usually last 3 to 5 hours and are done three times per week to achieve adequate clearance and maintain fluid balance.

New trends in HD include the use of daily dialysis and nocturnal dialysis. In daily HD, the patient dialyzes for 2 to 3 hours Monday through Friday. The patient receiving nocturnal dialysis can sleep while dialyzing. Each nocturnal treatment lasts 6 to 8 hours and the patient dialyzes up to six times per week. The rationale for daily dialysis and nocturnal dialysis is that either one provides better clearances and weight control than the conventional HD regimen of three times per week. Neither daily nor nocturnal dialysis is widely available for outpatients in the United States.

Settings for Hemodialysis. HD can be done in an inpatient (hospital) or outpatient (clinic or hospital) setting. Inpatient dialysis is used for treating hospitalized patients. In outpatient (in-center) dialysis the patient comes to the unit for treatment (Fig. 47-17). The patient may choose to do self-care with backup support from trained personnel if needed. Self-care patients put in the dialysis needles, set up the machine, and monitor the course of the treatment.

HD can also be done at home, yet less than 1.3% of patients receiving HD do so.[38] One of the main advantages of home HD is that it allows greater freedom in choosing dialysis times. Daily home HD has shown some promise in the overall improvement of patient status: fluid management, control of blood pressure, improved nutritional status, and better uremic clearance.[38] However, this is not a method of treatment often supported by dialysis centers. For home dialysis, PD tends to be the treatment of choice because it is less technically demanding, it requires less specialized equipment, and no water treatment system is needed.

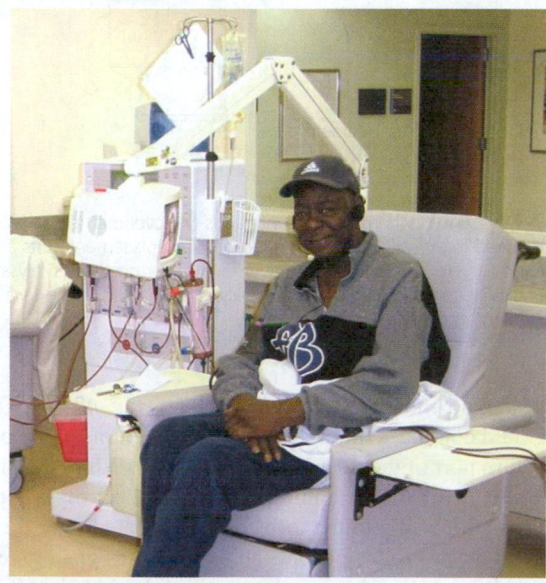

FIG. 47-17   Patient receiving in-center hemodialysis.

Complications of Hemodialysis

Hypotension. Hypotension that occurs during HD primarily results from rapid removal of vascular volume (hypovolemia), decreased cardiac output, and decreased systemic intravascular resistance. The drop in BP during dialysis may precipitate lightheadedness, nausea, vomiting, seizures, vision changes, and chest pain from cardiac ischemia. The usual treatment for hypotension includes decreasing the volume of fluid being removed and infusion of 0.9% saline solution (100 to 300 ml). If a patient experiences recurrent hypotensive episodes, a reassessment may have to be done of dry weight and BP drugs. BP drugs should be held before dialysis if there are frequent episodes of hypotension during dialysis.

Muscle Cramps. Painful muscle cramps are a common problem. They result from rapid removal of sodium and water or from neuromuscular hypersensitivity. Treatment includes reducing the ultrafiltration rate and infusing hypertonic saline or a normal saline bolus.

Loss of Blood. Blood loss may result from blood not being completely rinsed from the dialyzer, accidental separation of blood tubing, dialysis membrane rupture, or bleeding after the removal of needles at the end of dialysis. If a patient has received too much heparin or has clotting problems, there can be significant postdialysis bleeding. It is essential to rinse back all blood, to closely monitor heparinization to avoid excess anticoagulation, and to hold firm but nonocclusive pressure on access sites until the risk of bleeding has passed.

Hepatitis. The causes of hepatitis B and C in dialysis patients include blood transfusions or the lack of adherence to precautions used to prevent the spread of infection. As blood is now screened for hepatitis B and C, blood is an unlikely source of infection. IV drug abuse and unprotected sex can also contribute to the incidence of hepatitis in the dialysis population. The incidence of hepatitis B has decreased with frequent testing for hepatitis B surface antigen in patients, isolation of dialysis patients who are positive for hepatitis B, the use of disposable equipment, the hepatitis B vaccine, and infection control precautions. All patients and personnel in dialysis units should receive hepatitis B vaccine.

Currently, hepatitis C is responsible for the majority of cases of hepatitis in dialysis patients. (Hepatitis is discussed in more detail in Chapter 44.) The Centers for Disease Control and Prevention does not recommend isolation of the HD patient who has hepatitis C. Infection control precautions are mandated in the care of the patient with hepatitis C to protect the patient and staff. (Infection control precautions are discussed in Chapter 15 and Tables 15-8 and 15-9.) Currently, no vaccine is available for hepatitis C.

Sepsis. Sepsis is most often related to infections of vascular access sites. Bacteria can also be introduced during the dialysis treatment as a result of poor technique or interruption of blood tubing or dialyzer membranes. Bacterial endocarditis can occur because of the frequent and prolonged access to the vascular system. Aseptic technique is essential to prevent this problem. Nurses must monitor patients for signs and symptoms of sepsis such as fever, hypotension, and an elevated WBC.

Disequilibrium Syndrome. *Disequilibrium syndrome* develops as a result of very rapid changes in the composition of the extracellular fluid. Urea, sodium, and other solutes are removed more rapidly from the blood than from the cerebrospinal fluid and the brain. This creates a high osmotic gradient in the brain resulting in the shift of fluid into the brain, causing cerebral edema. Manifestations include nausea, vomiting, confusion, restlessness, headaches, twitching and jerking, and seizures. The rapid changes in osmolality may cause muscle cramps and worsen hypotension. Treatment consists of slowing or stopping dialysis and infusing hypertonic saline solution, albumin, or mannitol to draw fluid from the brain cells back into the systemic circulation. It is more commonly observed in the initial treatment of the patient when the BUN level is high. First dialysis treatment sessions are purposely short with limited total solute removal to prevent this rare syndrome.

Effectiveness of and Adaptation to Hemodialysis

HD is still an imperfect technique to treat ESRD. It cannot fully replace the metabolic and hormonal functions of the kidneys. It can ease many of the symptoms of CKD and, if started early, can prevent certain complications. It does not alter the accelerated atherosclerosis.

The yearly death rate of patients receiving maintenance dialysis has increased to 22%.[11] The major reason for this is the increased proportion of older adult patients who are now receiving dialysis as maintenance therapy. The majority of deaths are caused by cardiovascular disease (stroke or myocardial infarction). Infectious complications are the second leading cause of death.

Individual adaptation to maintenance HD varies considerably. Initially many patients feel positive about the dialysis because it makes them feel better and keeps them alive, but there is often great ambivalence about whether it is worthwhile. Dependence on a machine is a reality, and some have dreams about being tied to the machine. In response to their illness, dialysis patients may demonstrate noncompliance, depression, and suicidal tendencies. The primary nursing goals are to help the patient regain or maintain positive self-esteem and control of his or her life and to continue to be productive in society.

CONTINUOUS RENAL REPLACEMENT THERAPY

Continuous renal replacement therapy (CRRT) is an alternative or adjunctive method for treating ARF. It provides a means by which uremic toxins and fluids are removed, while acid-base status and electrolytes are adjusted slowly and continuously from a hemodynamically unstable patient. The patients selected are usually those who do not respond to dietary interventions and pharmacologic agents. CRRT is contraindicated if a patient has life-threatening manifestations of uremia (hyperkalemia, pericarditis) that require rapid resolution.[39] CRRT can be used in conjunction with HD.

Various types of CRRT are available, differentiated by whether arterial and/or venous access is required and if a blood pump is needed (Table 47-12). Due to technologic advances with automated and volumetric equipment that includes a blood pump, CRRT most commonly uses the venovenous approaches of continuous venovenous hemofiltration (CVVH) and continuous venovenous hemodialysis (CVVHD). These approaches are the focus of this discussion of CRRT.

Vascular access for CVVH or CVVHD is achieved through the use of a double-lumen catheter (as used in HD, noted in Fig. 47-14) placed in the femoral, jugular, or subclavian vein. Venous access necessitates the use of a blood pump to propel the blood through the circuit. A highly permeable, hollow fiber hemofilter removes plasma water and nonprotein solutes, which are collectively termed *ultrafiltrate*. The ultrafiltration rate (UFR) may range from 0 to 500 ml/hr. Under the influence of hydrostatic pressure and osmotic pressure, water and nonprotein solutes pass out of the filter into the extracapillary space and drain through the ultrafil-

TABLE 47-12	Types of Continuous Renal Replacement Therapies		
Therapies		**Abbreviation**	**Purpose**
Venous Access Therapies (Venovenous [VV])			
Continuous venovenous ultrafiltration		CVVU	Solute loss via convection
Continuous venovenous hemofiltration*		CVVH	Solute loss via convection; hemodilution using replacement fluid
Continuous venovenous hemodialysis*		CVVHD	Solute loss via convection and diffusion
Arterial Access Therapies (Arteriovenous [AV])			
Slow continuous ultrafiltration		SCUF	Fluid removal via ultrafiltration
Continuous arteriovenous hemofiltration		CAVH	Ultrafiltration and convective losses occur; replacement fluid used
Continuous arteriovenous hemodialysis		CAVHD	Fluid removal via ultrafiltration and osmosis

*Most commonly used therapies.

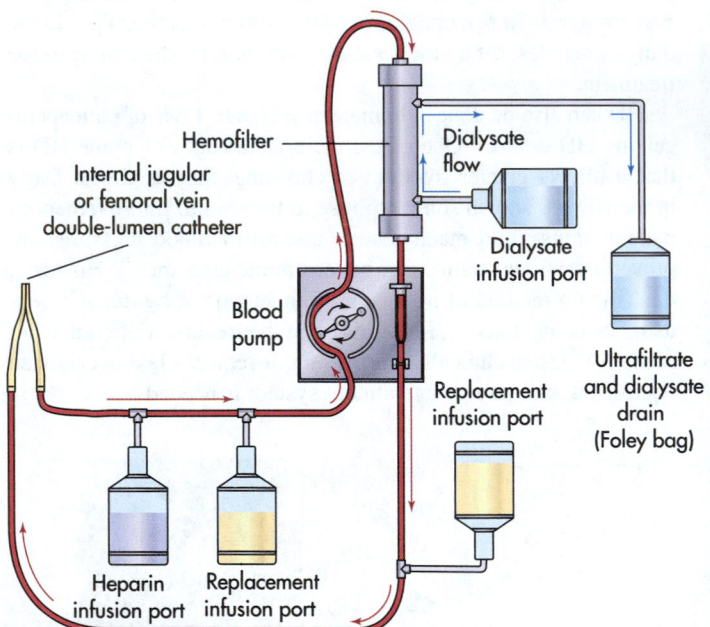

FIG. 47-18 Basic schematic of continuous venovenous therapies. Blood pump is required to pump blood through the circuit. Replacement ports are used for CVVH and CVVHD only and can be given prefilter or postfilter. Dialysate port is used for CVVHD only. Regardless of modality, ultrafiltrate is drained via the ultrafiltration drain port.

trate port into a collection device (Foley bag) (Fig. 47-18). The remaining fluid continues through the filter and returns to the patient via the return port of the double-lumen catheter. While the ultrafiltrate drains out of the hemofilter, fluid and electrolyte replacements can be infused into the infusion port located after the filter as the blood returns to the patient. This fluid is designed to replace volume and solutes such as sodium, chloride, bicarbonate, and glucose. It will also further dilute intravascular fluid, decreasing the concentration of unwanted solutes such as BUN, creatinine, and potassium. The infusion rate of replacement fluid is determined by the degree of fluid and electrolyte imbalance. Replacement fluid may also be infused into the infusion port before the hemofilter. This method allows for greater clearance of urea and can decrease filter clotting.

Anticoagulation is a consideration to prevent blood clotting during CRRT. Heparin may be infused as a bolus at the initiation of CRRT or through the heparin infusion port before the hemofilter. Heparin dosage is based on the patient's activated clotting time (ACT), partial prothrombin time (PTT), or prothrombin time (PT).

Several features of CRRT differ from HD:

1. It is continuous rather than intermittent. Large volumes of fluid can be removed over days (24 hours to >2 weeks) versus hours (3 to 4 hours).
2. Solute removal can occur by *convection* (no dialysate required) in addition to osmosis and diffusion.
3. It causes less hemodynamic instability (e.g., hypotension).
4. It does not require constant monitoring by a specialized HD nurse but does require a trained intensive care unit (ICU) nurse.
5. It does not require complicated HD equipment, but a blood pump is needed for venovenous therapies.

Regardless of whether the modality is arteriovenous or venovenous, the approaches can be customized to the patient needs and have equivalent outcomes. The *ultrafiltration therapies* (SCUF and CVVU) are strictly for ultrafiltration or fluid removal. There is some convective loss of solutes, but no diffusion or osmosis is involved.

The *hemofiltration therapies* (CAVH and CVVH) involve the introduction of replacement fluids. Large volumes of fluid may be removed hourly (200 to 800 ml), and then a portion of this fluid is replaced. The type of fluid replacement is dependent on the stability and individualized needs of the patient. Ultrafiltration and convective losses occur, and solute concentrations in the blood are diluted with the replacement fluid.

The *hemodialysis therapies* (CAVHD and CVVHD) use dialysate. Peritoneal dialysate bags are attached to the distal end of the hemofilter, and the fluid is pumped countercurrent to the blood flow (see Fig. 47-18). As in dialysis, diffusion of solutes and ultrafiltration via hydrostatic pressure and osmosis occur. This is an ideal treatment for a patient who needs both fluid and solute control but cannot tolerate the rapid fluid shifts associated with HD.

CRRT can be continued as long as 30 to 40 days, but the hemofilter should be changed every 24 to 48 hours because of loss of filtration efficiency or potential for clotting. The ultrafiltrate should be clear yellow, and specimens may be obtained for evaluation of serum chemistries. If the ultrafiltrate becomes bloody or blood tinged, a possible rupture in the filter membrane should be suspected, and treatment suspended immediately to prevent blood loss and infection.

The nurse responsible for the care of the patient with ARF who is receiving CRRT may be a critical care nurse or a nephrology nurse specialist, working in collaboration with other health care providers. Specific nursing interventions include obtaining weights and monitoring and documenting laboratory values daily to ensure adequate fluid and electrolyte balance. Hourly intake/output measurements, vital signs, and hemodynamic status are essential. Although reductions in central venous pressure and pulmonary artery pressure are expected, there should be little change in mean arterial pressure or cardiac output. Patency of the CRRT system is assessed and maintained, and the patient's vascular access site is cared for to prevent infection. Treatment is discontinued and the needle(s) removed once the patient's ARF is resolved or there is a decision to withdraw treatment due to patient deterioration.

KIDNEY TRANSPLANTATION

Major progress has been made in organ transplantation since the first kidney transplant was performed in 1954 in Boston between identical twins. The advances made in organ procurement and preservation, surgical techniques, tissue typing and matching, understanding of the immune system, immunosuppressant therapy, and prevention of and treatment for graft rejection have dramatically increased the success of organ transplantation (see the general discussion of organ transplantation in Chapter 14, p. 236 to 238).

The disparity between the supply and demand for organs is significant. To put this in perspective, consider the fact that over 300,000 patients are receiving either HD or PD. Over 66,000 patients are currently awaiting deceased donor kidney transplants, yet only 19,549 kidneys were transplanted in 2004. This was a 7.0% increase since 2003. Over 6990 living donor kidney transplants were transplanted in 2004. Transplantation from a deceased donor usually requires a prolonged waiting period with differences depending on age, gender, and race, as well as the availability of a matching blood type. Blood types B and O have the longest waiting times.[40]

Kidney transplantation is extremely successful, with 1-year graft survival rates of about 90% for deceased donor transplants and 95% for live donor transplants.[40] An advantage of kidney transplantation

---

ETHICAL DILEMMAS
Payment for Organs

Situation
You are caring for Rosie, a 45-year-old woman, who has been receiving dialysis for nearly 10 years. She tells you she is on a waiting list for a kidney transplant but cannot deal with the long wait anymore. Recently she heard from a friend about the ability to purchase a kidney and have the transplant operation in India. Rosie asks what you think about this option and what you would recommend.

Important Points for Consideration
* It is currently illegal in the United States and several other countries to be involved, either directly or indirectly, in the buying or selling of organs.
* In the United States alone it is estimated that 3000 people die annually awaiting kidney transplant due to the lack of available kidneys for donation.
* The large unregulated black market in kidneys in developing countries places people at increased risk of morbidity and mortality.
* Wealthy people are at an advantage of being able to purchase organs on the black market, while the poor are disadvantaged and this may increase their health risk.
* Compensation for sperm and egg donation as well as surrogate mothers is already an acceptable practice legally and ethically.
* A carefully regulated compensation system could remove the advantage of wealth and add important protections for the poor, thus enhancing informed consent.

Critical Thinking Questions
1. How can you provide information to help ensure that the patient makes a truly informed decision?
2. How can nurses be involved in shaping or changing health policy that may benefit the public?
3. What resources can be enlisted to support Rosie to reduce the feeling that there are no other options available?

when compared with dialysis is that it reverses many of the pathophysiologic changes associated with renal failure when normal kidney function is restored. It also eliminates the dependence on dialysis and the accompanying dietary and lifestyle restrictions. Transplantation is also less expensive than dialysis after the first year.

Recipient Selection

Appropriate recipient selection is important for a successful outcome. Candidacy is determined by a variety of medical and psychosocial factors that vary among transplant centers. A careful evaluation is completed in an attempt to identify and minimize potential complications after transplantation. Certain patients, particularly those with cardiovascular disease and diabetes mellitus, are considered high risk and must be carefully evaluated and then monitored closely after the transplantation. Some patients who are approaching ESRD can receive a transplant before dialysis is required if they have a living donor. This approach is most advantageous for patients with diabetes, who have a much higher mortality rate on dialysis than nondiabetics.

Contraindications to transplantation include disseminated malignancies, refractory or untreated cardiac disease, chronic respiratory failure, extensive vascular disease, chronic infection, and unresolved psychosocial disorders (e.g., noncompliance with medical regimens, alcoholism, drug addiction). The presence of hepatitis B or C is not a contraindication to transplantation.

Surgical procedures may be required before transplantation based on the results of the recipient evaluation. Coronary artery bypass may be indicated for advanced coronary artery disease. Cholecystectomy may be necessary for patients with a history of gallstones, biliary obstruction, or cholecystitis. On rare occasions, bilateral nephrectomies may be done for patients with refractory hypertension, recurrent urinary tract infections, or grossly enlarged kidneys resulting from polycystic kidney disease. In general, the recipient's own kidneys do not need to be removed prior to receiving a kidney transplant.

Histocompatibility Studies

Histocompatibility studies, including HLA testing and cross-matching, are discussed in Chapter 14 on p. 237.

Donor Sources

Kidneys for transplantation may be obtained from compatible–blood-type deceased donors, blood relatives, emotionally related (close and distant) living donors (e.g., spouses, distant cousins, etc.), and altruistic living donors who are known (friends) and unknown to the recipient. Expanding the living donor pool is one of the best possibilities for decreasing the size of the waiting list and reducing wait times for people needing a deceased donor.

Live Donors. Live donors must undergo an extensive multidisciplinary evaluation to be certain that they are in good health and have no history of disease that would place them at risk for developing kidney failure or operative complications. Psychosocial and financial evaluations are done as well. Crossmatches are done at the time of the evaluation and about a week before the transplantation to ensure that no antibodies to the donor are present or that the antibody titer is below the allowed level. Advantages of a live donor kidney include better patient and graft survival rates regardless of histocompatibility match, immediate organ availability, immediate function because of minimal cold time (kidney out of body and not getting blood supply), and the opportunity to have the recipient in the best possible medical condition because the surgery is elective.

The donor will see a nephrologist for a complete history and physical and laboratory and diagnostic studies. Laboratory studies include a 24-hour urine study for creatinine clearance and total protein, complete blood count, and chemistry and electrolyte profiles. Hepatitis B and C, human immunodeficiency virus (HIV), and cytomegalovirus (CMV) testing are done to assess for the presence of any transmissible diseases. An ECG and chest x-ray are also done. A renal ultrasound and a renal arteriogram or three-dimensional CT are performed to ensure that the blood vessels supplying each kidney are adequate and that there are no anomalies and to determine which kidney will be removed.

A transplant psychologist or social worker will determine if the individual is emotionally stable and able to deal with the issues related to organ donation. All donors must be informed about the risks and benefits of donation, the potential short-term and long-term complications, and what can be expected during the hospitalization and recovery phases. Although the cost of the evaluation and surgery are covered by the recipient's insurance, there is no compensation available for lost wages during the posthospitalization recovery period. This period can last 6 weeks or longer. The laparoscopic donor nephrectomy procedure is minimally invasive with fewer risks and shorter recovery time.

ETHICAL DILEMMAS
Allocation of Resources

Situation
A transplant nurse coordinator is considering her feelings about two patients who are being evaluated for placement on the deceased (cadaveric) kidney transplant waiting list. One patient is a 40-year-old African American school teacher. She is married and has two children. The other patient is a 22-year-old unemployed white male who is actively using cocaine. He misses three to four dialysis treatments per month and does not take his antihypertensive medications consistently.

Important Points for Consideration
- It is tempting to believe that nurses can be neutral, basing allocation of scarce resources on need rather than worth. However, it is sometimes difficult to withhold value judgments.
- Psychologic, physiologic, and adherence factors are included in the assessment process for eligibility for organ transplantation.
- In kidney transplantation, the organ is transplanted into the patient who has received the most points based on a scoring system, regardless of the health care provider's opinion of the patient's worth. If a patient is denied transplant candidacy on this basis, he or she must be given a chance to change or improve the problem or condition in a specified period of time.
- The national organ procurement system is designed to be unbiased about the patient in all respects. Once a patient is placed on the list for transplantation, that patient is deemed of no greater or lesser worth than any other patient.
- Since organ donation is voluntary and altruistic in the United States, any concerns that the system of procurement and transplantation is not fair may negatively affect the pool of available organs.

Critical Thinking Questions
1. What does the 2001 American Nurses Association (ANA) Code of Ethics say about how nurses should view patients?
2. What are your feelings about which of the patients should receive the next available organ?

In a limited number of transplant centers, plasmapheresis is being used to remove antibodies from the recipient in situations where there is an ABO incompatibility or positive crossmatch between the donor and recipient. (Crossmatching is discussed in Chapter 14.) This allows transplant candidates to receive kidneys from live donors with blood types that have traditionally been considered incompatible. Following the transplant, the patient undergoes additional plasmapheresis treatments.

Deceased Donors. Deceased (cadaver) kidney donors are relatively healthy individuals who have suffered an irreversible brain injury. The most common causes of injury are cerebral trauma from motor vehicle accidents or gunshot wounds, intracerebral or subarachnoid hemorrhage, and anoxic brain damage caused by cardiac arrest. The brain-dead donor must have effective cardiovascular function and be supported on a ventilator to preserve the organs. The age range of most suitable kidney donors is from 2 to 70 years. The age of the donor is less important than the quality of kidney function. The donor must be free of active IV drug abuse, severe hypertension, long-standing diabetes mellitus, malignancies, sepsis, and communicable diseases, including HIV, hepatitis B and C, syphilis, and tuberculosis. Permission from the donor's legal next of kin is required after brain death is determined even if the donor carried a signed donor card.[41]

The kidneys are removed and preserved. They can be preserved for up to 72 hours, but most transplant surgeons prefer to transplant kidneys before the cold ischemic time (time outside of the body when being transported from the deceased donor to the recipient) reaches 24 hours. Experience has shown that prolonged cold time increases the likelihood that the kidney will not function immediately, and the transplant recipient will require dialysis until the acute tubular necrosis (ATN) from the extended cold time resolves.

Deceased donor kidneys are distributed by the United Network for Organ Sharing using an objective computerized point system. The ABO group, HLA typing, age, antibody level, and length of time waiting are entered into the national computer for each candidate when he or she is listed. When a donor becomes available, the donor's HLA data, ABO type, and other key information are compared with the data of all patients awaiting transplantation locally and nationwide. Points are given for how close the HLA match is, how long the patient has been waiting, if the antibody level is unusually high, and if the recipient is less than 19 years old. Extra points are given for high antibody levels because this can severely limit the number of donors with which the patient will not have a positive crossmatch. The kidney is offered to the recipient with the most points in the local area. If there are no patients in the local area who are suitable, the organ is then offered in the region and then in the nation. When a kidney arrives at the recipient's transplant center, a final crossmatch is done and must be negative for the deceased donor transplantation to proceed. (Crossmatching is discussed in Chapter 14.)

The only exception to the previous plan is if a patient needs an emergency transplant or if a donor and recipient do not mismatch on any of the six HLA antigens (zero antigen mismatch). In these situations, the patient meeting either one of these criteria goes to the top of the list. Emergency transplants are given priority because the patient is facing imminent death if not transplanted (e.g., a patient who had no vascular access sites left and can no longer dialyze). Zero antigen mismatches are given priority because statistically these grafts have much better survival rates. If a zero antigen mismatch patient is identified nationally, one of the donor kidneys must be sent to that recipient's transplant center regardless of location.

Surgical Procedure

Live Donor. The donor nephrectomy is performed by a urologist or transplant surgeon. The donor's surgery begins an hour or two before the recipient's surgery is started. The recipient is surgically prepared for the kidney transplant in a nearby operating room. For a conventional nephrectomy, the donor is placed in the lateral decubitus position on the operating table so that the flank is presented laterally. An incision is made at the level of the eleventh rib. The rib may have to be removed to provide adequate visualization of the kidney. After removal of the kidney, it is flushed with a chilled, sterile electrolyte solution and prepared for immediate transplant into the recipient. The nephrectomy takes about 3 hours. The short cold ischemic time is the primary reason for the success of living donor transplants.

Laparoscopic donor nephrectomy is an alternative to a conventional nephrectomy. (Laparoscopic nephrectomy is discussed in Chapter 46.) This procedure is now being used as the primary method of live kidney procurement. The laparoscopic approach significantly decreases the hospital stay, pain, operative blood loss, debilitation, and length of time off work. For these reasons, the number of people willing to donate a kidney has increased significantly.[42]

Kidney Transplant Recipient. The transplanted kidney is usually placed extraperitoneally in the iliac fossa. The right iliac fossa is preferred to facilitate anastomoses and minimize the occurrence of ileus.

Before any incisions are made, a urinary catheter is placed into the bladder. An antibiotic solution is instilled to distend the bladder and decrease the risk of infection. A crescent-shaped incision is made extending from the iliac crest to the symphysis pubis (Fig. 47-19). The peritoneum is left intact. The iliac and hypogastric vessels are dissected free.

Rapid revascularization is critical to prevent ischemic injury to the kidney. The donor artery is anastomosed to the recipient's internal iliac (hypogastric) or external iliac artery. The donor vein is anastomosed to the recipient's external iliac vein. Kidney transplants with living donors can be technically more difficult because the blood vessel lengths can be shorter than in deceased donor transplants.

When the anastomoses are complete, the clamps are released, and blood flow to the kidney is reestablished. The kidney should become firm and pink. Urine may begin to flow from the ureter immediately. Mannitol or furosemide (Lasix) may be administered to promote diuresis.

The donor ureter in most cases is then tunneled through the bladder submucosa before entering the bladder cavity and being sutured in place. This approach is called *ureteroneocystostomy*. This allows the bladder wall to compress the ureter as it contracts for micturition, thereby preventing reflux of urine up the ureter into the transplanted kidney. The transplant surgery takes approximately 3 to 4 hours.

NURSING MANAGEMENT
KIDNEY TRANSPLANT RECIPIENT

The successful recovery and rehabilitation of the recipient are made possible with careful nursing assessment, diagnosis, intervention, and evaluation of all body systems. With a hospital length of stay averaging 4 to 5 days, discharge planning and teaching needs must be identified and addressed early in the hospital course.

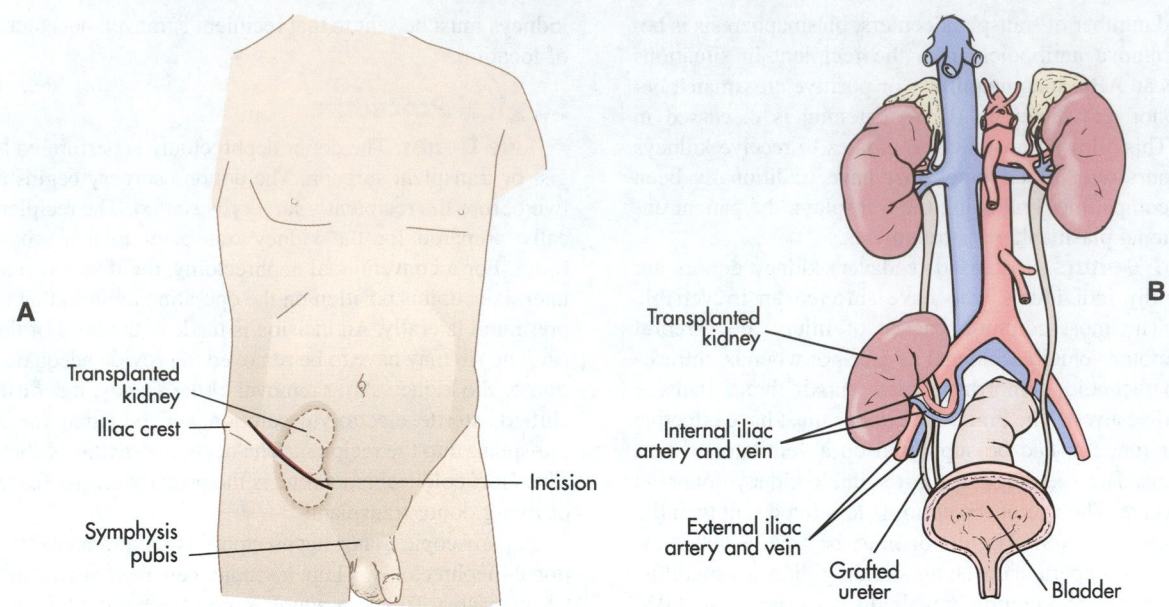

FIG. 47-19   **A,** Surgical incision for a renal transplant. **B,** Surgical placement of transplanted kidney.

■ Preoperative Care

Nursing care of the patient in the preoperative phase includes emotional and physical preparation for surgery. Because the patient and family may have been waiting years for the kidney transplant, a review of the operative procedure and what can be expected in the immediate postoperative recovery period is necessary. It is important to stress that there is a chance the kidney may not function immediately, and dialysis may be required for days to weeks. The need for immunosuppressive drugs and measures to prevent infection must be reviewed.

To ensure the patient is in optimal physical condition for surgery, an ECG, chest x-ray, and laboratory studies are ordered. Dialysis may be required before surgery for any significant abnormality such as fluid overload or hyperkalemia. A patient on PD must empty the peritoneal cavity of all dialysate solution before going to surgery. Because dialysis may be required after transplantation, the patency of the vascular access must be maintained. The vascular access extremity should be labeled "dialysis access, no procedures" to prevent use of the affected extremity for BP measurement, blood drawing, or IV infusions.

■ Postoperative Care

Live Donor. The usual postoperative care for the donor is similar to that following conventional or laparoscopic nephrectomy (see Chapter 46). Close monitoring of renal function to assess for impairment and of the hematocrit to assess for bleeding is essential. The creatinine should be less than 1.4 mg/dl, and the hematocrit should not fall more than 3 to 6 points. The donor who has had a conventional nephrectomy experiences greater pain than that of the donor who had a laparoscopic procedure. Generally, all donors have more pain than their recipients. Conventional donors are ready to be discharged from the hospital in 4 or 5 days and can usually return to work in 6 to 8 weeks. Laparoscopic donors are able to be discharged from the hospital in 2 to 4 days and can return to work in 4 to 6 weeks. The donor is seen by the surgeon 1 to 2 weeks after discharge.

Nurses caring for the living donor need to acknowledge the precious gift that this person has given. The donor has taken physi-cal, emotional, and financial risks to assist the recipient. It is vital that they not be forgotten postoperatively. The donor will need even greater support if the donated organ does not work immediately or for some reason fails.

Recipient. The first priority during this period is maintenance of fluid and electrolyte balance. In many centers, kidney transplant recipients spend the first 12 to 24 hours in the ICU because of the close monitoring required.[43] Very large volumes of urine may be produced soon after the blood supply to the transplanted kidney is reestablished. This diuresis is due to (1) the new kidney's ability to filter BUN, which acts as an osmotic diuretic; (2) the abundance of fluids administered during the operation; and (3) initial renal tubular dysfunction, which inhibits the kidney from concentrating urine normally. Urine output during this phase may be as high as 1 L/hr and gradually decreases as the BUN and serum creatinine levels return toward normal. Urine output is replaced with fluids milliliter for milliliter hourly for the first 12 to 24 hours. Central venous pressure readings are essential for monitoring postoperative fluid status. Dehydration must be avoided to prevent subsequent renal hypoperfusion and renal tubular damage. Electrolyte monitoring to assess for the hyponatremia and hypokalemia often associated with rapid diuresis is critical. Treatment with potassium supplements or 0.9% normal saline solution infusion may be indicated. IV sodium bicarbonate may also be required if the patient develops metabolic acidosis from delayed kidney function.

ATN can occur because of prolonged cold ischemic times and the use of marginal donors. The ischemic damage from extended cold times causes ATN. While the patient is in ATN, dialysis is required to maintain fluid and electrolyte balance. Some patients have high-output ATN with the ability to excrete fluid, but not metabolic wastes or electrolytes. Other patients have oliguric or anuric ATN. These patients are at risk for fluid overload in the immediate postoperative period and must be assessed closely for the need for dialysis. The period of ATN can last anywhere from days to weeks, with gradually improving kidney function. Most patients with ATN will be discharged from the hospital on dialysis. This is extremely discouraging for the patient, who will need reassurance that renal function usually improves. Dialysis will be discontinued when urine output increases and serum creatinine and BUN begin to normalize.

A sudden decrease in urine output in the early postoperative period is a cause for concern. It may be due to dehydration, rejection, a urine leak, or obstruction. A common cause of early obstruction is a blood clot in the urinary catheter. Catheter patency must be maintained as the catheter remains in the bladder for 3 to 5 days to allow the bladder anastomosis to heal. If blood clots are suspected, gentle catheter irrigation with an order from the health care provider can reestablish patency.

Postoperative teaching should include the prevention and treatment of rejection, infection, and complications of surgery and the purpose and side effects of immunosuppression. Patients should be aware that rejection is a common occurrence during the first 3 months after transplant. Frequent blood tests and clinic visits help detect rejection early. Patient education to ensure a smooth transition from hospital to home is an integral part of the nursing care.[43]

Immunosuppressive Therapy

The goal of immunosuppression is to adequately suppress the immune response to prevent rejection of the transplanted kidney while maintaining sufficient immunity to prevent overwhelming infection. Immunosuppressive therapy is discussed in Chapter 14 and in Table 14-18.

Complications of Transplantation

Complications of renal replacement therapies, including PD, HD, and kidney transplantation, are compared in Table 47-13.

Rejection. Rejection is one of the major problems following kidney transplantation. Rejection can be hyperacute, acute, or chronic. These types of rejection are discussed in Chapter 14 on pp. 237 to 238. Patients with chronic rejection should be put on the transplant list in the hope that they can be retransplanted before dialysis is required.

Infection. Infection remains a significant cause of morbidity and mortality after transplantation. The transplant recipient is at risk for infection because of suppression of the body's normal defense mechanisms by surgery, immunosuppressive drugs, and the effects of ESRD. Underlying systemic illness such as diabetes mellitus or systemic lupus erythematosus, malnutrition, and older age can further compound the negative effects on the immune response. At times the signs and symptoms of infection can be subtle. Nurses caring for transplant recipients must be astute in their observation and assessment because prompt diagnosis and treatment of infections will improve patient outcomes.

The most common infections observed in the first month after transplantation are similar to those acquired by any postoperative patient, such as pneumonia, wound infections, IV line and drain infections, and urinary tract infections. Fungal and viral infections are not uncommon because of the patient's immunosuppressed state. Fungal infections can include *Candida, Cryptococcus, Aspergillus,* and *Pneumocystis jiroveci.* Fungal infections are difficult to treat, require prolonged treatment periods, and often involve the administration of nephrotoxic drugs. Transplant recipients usually receive prophylactic antifungal drugs to prevent these infections, such as clotrimazole (Mycelex), fluconazole (Diflucan), and trimethoprim/sulfamethoxazole (Bactrim).

Viral infections, including CMV, Epstein-Barr virus, herpes simplex virus (HSV), varicella-zoster virus, and polyomavirus (e.g., BK virus), can be primary or reactivation of existing disease. Primary infections occur as new infections after transplantation from an exogenous source such as the donated organ or a blood transfusion. Reactivation occurs when a virus exists in a patient and becomes reactivated after transplantation because of immunosuppression.

CMV is one of the most common viral infections. If a recipient has never had CMV and receives an organ from a donor with a history of CMV, antiviral prophylaxis will be administered (e.g., ganciclovir [Cytovene], valganciclovir [Valcyte]). If a primary active CMV infection is diagnosed or there is symptomatic reactivation of CMV, IV ganciclovir will be given along with an immune globulin that contains CMV antibodies. To prevent HSV infections, oral acyclovir (Zovirax) is given for several months after the transplant.

Cardiovascular Disease. Transplant recipients have an increased incidence of atherosclerotic vascular disease. Cardiovascular disease is the leading cause of death after renal transplantation.[44] Hypertension, hyperlipidemia, diabetes mellitus, smoking, rejection, infections, and increased homocysteine levels can all contribute to cardiovascular disease. Immunosuppressants can worsen hypertension and hyperlipidemia. It is important that the patient be taught to control risk factors such as elevated cholesterol, triglycerides, and blood glucose and weight gain. Adherence to the prescribed antihypertensive regimen is essential not only to prevent cardiovascular events but also to prevent damage to the new kidney. (Hypertension is discussed in Chapter 33.)

TABLE 47-13	Complications of Renal Replacement Therapy and Transplantation		
Peritoneal Dialysis (PD)	**Hemodialysis (HD)**	**Transplantation**	
Exit site infection	Hypotension	Rejection of transplant:	
Peritonitis	Muscle cramps	Hyperacute	
Abdominal pain	Exsanguination	Acute	
Catheter outflow	Hepatitis	Chronic	
Hernias	Sepsis	Susceptibility to infection	
Lower back pain	Disequilibrium syndrome	Cardiovascular disease	
Blood in effluent drainage		Malignancies	
Pulmonary difficulties:		Recurrence of renal disease	
Atelectasis		Corticosteroid-related complications	
Pneumonia			
Bronchitis			
Protein loss			
Carbohydrate abnormalities			
Lipid abnormalities			
Encapsulating sclerosing peritonitis			

Malignancies. The overall incidence of malignancies in kidney transplant recipients is about 6%, which is 100 times greater than in the general population. The primary cause of this increased incidence is the immunosuppressive therapy. Not only do immunosuppressants suppress the immune system, but they also suppress the ability to fight infection and the production of abnormal cells such as cancer cells. The malignancies include cancer of the skin, lips, kidney, hepatobiliary system, vulva, and perineum; lymphomas; and Kaposi sarcoma and other sarcomas. Regular screening for cancer is an important part of the transplant recipient's preventive care. The patient must also be advised to avoid sun exposure by using protective clothing and sunscreens to minimize the incidence of skin cancers.[45]

Recurrence of Original Renal Disease. Recurrence of the original disease that destroyed the native kidneys occurs in some kidney transplant recipients. It is most common with certain types of glomerulonephritis, IgA nephropathy, diabetic nephropathy, and focal segmental sclerosis. Disease recurrence can result in the loss of a functioning kidney transplant. Patients must be advised before transplantation if they have a disease known to recur.

Corticosteroid-Related Complications. Aseptic necrosis of the hips, knees, and other joints can result from chronic corticosteroid therapy and renal osteodystrophy. Other significant problems related to corticosteroids include peptic ulcer disease, glucose intolerance and diabetes, cataracts, hyperlipidemia, and an increased incidence of infections and malignancies. In the first year after transplantation, corticosteroid doses are usually decreased to 5 to 10 mg/day. The use of tacrolimus and cyclosporine has allowed for the corticosteroid doses to be much lower than they were in the past. Some patients have been successfully withdrawn from corticosteroids within 2 years after transplantation, thus eliminating these problems. Vigilant monitoring for side effects of corticosteroids and early treatment is essential.

GERONTOLOGIC CONSIDERATIONS
CHRONIC KIDNEY DISEASE

The incidence of CKD in the United States and Canada is increasing most rapidly in older patients. Recent data indicate that, of all the patients who have CKD, approximately 35% are 65 or older.[11] The most common diseases leading to renal failure in older people are hypertension and diabetes. Due to this, Medicare and non-Medicare expenditures can be expected to increase as this CKD population ages with accompanying comorbid conditions.

The care of this older population is particularly challenging, not only because of the normal physiologic changes of aging that occur but also because of the disabilities, chronic diseases, and number of comorbid conditions that develop.[46] Physiologic changes of clinical importance in the older CKD patient include diminished cardiopulmonary function, bone loss, immunodeficiency, altered protein synthesis, impaired cognition, and altered drug metabolism. Malnutrition is common in these patients for a variety of reasons, including lack of mobility, lack of understanding of basic nutritional requirements, social isolation, physical disability, impaired cognitive function, and malabsorption problems.[47]

When conservative therapy for CKD is no longer effective, the older patient needs to consider the best treatment modality based on his or her physical and emotional health, personal preferences, and availability of support. PD allows the patient to be more mobile and to enjoy an increased sense of control over the illness. PD

causes less hemodynamic instability than HD but does require self-care or assistance from another person, which may not always be available.

Most individuals 65 years of age and older select treatment with HD, specifically in-center, because of a lack of assistance in the home and reluctance to manage the technology of dialysis. Establishing vascular access for HD may be somewhat of a concern for an older patient because of atherosclerotic changes. Although transplantation is an option, elderly patients must be carefully screened to ensure that the benefits outweigh the risks. A living donor is preferable so that there is not a prolonged waiting time.

The most common cause of death in the elderly ESRD patient is cardiovascular disease (MI, stroke), followed by withdrawal from dialysis. If a competent patient decides to withdraw from dialysis, it is essential to support the patient and family. Ethical issues (see the Ethical Dilemmas box) to be considered in this situation include patient competency, benefit versus burden of treatment, and futility of treatment. Withdrawal from treatment is not a failure if the patient is well informed and comfortable with the decision.

The increasing number of elderly, debilitated ESRD patients receiving dialysis has raised a number of ethical concerns about the use of scarce resources in a population with a limited life expectancy.[46] Substantial evidence exists showing success of dialysis (especially PD) in the elderly. Quality of life has also been reported to be good to excellent in many older ESRD patients receiving dialysis. There appears to be no justification for excluding the older adult from dialysis programs. Rationing dialysis on the basis of age alone is not supported based on current outcome and quality-of-life data.

CRITICAL THINKING EXERCISE

CASE STUDY

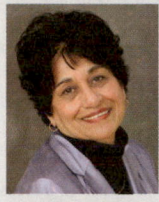

Case Study photo
©iStockphoto.com/
Michael Blackburn.

Chronic Kidney Disease

Patient Profile. Juanita, a 46-year-old Native American school teacher, has been treated for type 2 diabetes mellitus since the age of 30. She has been monitored by her nephrologist for the past several years for manifestations of progressive chronic kidney disease. Eight weeks ago she had an arteriovenous fistula created in preparation for starting hemodialysis. Over the past week she has experienced anorexia, nausea, vomiting, problems with concentration, and pruritus.

Subjective Data
- Complains of swelling in her feet and hands
- Has gained 10 lb (4.5 kg) in the past 2 weeks
- Complains of dyspnea and weakness when walking

Objective Data

Laboratory Data
- Creatinine clearance: 8.2 ml/min
- Serum creatinine: 12.8 mg/dl (1132 mmol/L)
- BUN: 125 mg/dl (45 mmol/L)
- Potassium: 6 mEq/L (6 mmol/L)
- Hematocrit: 20%

Chest X-ray
- Pulmonary edema

Critical Thinking Questions

1. Explain the basic pathophysiologic changes that resulted in the development of her diabetic nephropathy.
2. What are the indications for dialysis in this patient?
3. Identify the abnormal diagnostic study results and why each would occur.
4. Explain why Juanita developed each of her clinical manifestations.
5. What are important nursing interventions for Juanita and her family?
6. Based on the assessment data provided, write one or more nursing diagnoses. Are there any collaborative problems?

NCLEX EXAMINATION REVIEW QUESTIONS

The number of the question corresponds to the same-numbered objective at the beginning of the chapter.

1. A patient is admitted to the hospital with chronic kidney disease. The nurse understands that this condition is characterized by
   a. progressive irreversible destruction of the kidneys.
   b. a rapid decrease in urinary output with an elevated BUN.
   c. an increasing creatinine clearance with a decrease in urinary output.
   d. prostration, somnolence, and confusion with coma and imminent death.
2. Prerenal causes of ARF include
   a. prostate cancer and calculi formation.
   b. hypovolemia and myocardial infarction.
   c. acute glomerulonephritis and neoplasms.
   d. septic shock and nephrotoxic injury from drugs.
3. During the oliguric phase of ARF, the nurse monitors the patient for
   a. hypernatremia and CNS depression.
   b. pulmonary edema and ECG changes.
   c. Kussmaul respirations and hypotension.
   d. urine with high specific gravity and low sodium concentration.
4. If a patient is in the diuretic phase of ARF, the nurse must monitor for which serum electrolyte imbalances?
   a. Hyperkalemia and hyponatremia
   b. Hyperkalemia and hypernatremia
   c. Hypokalemia and hyponatremia
   d. Hypokalemia and hypernatremia
5. A systemic effect of chronic kidney disease that is usually reversed by the initiation of dialysis is
   a. anemia.
   b. hyperlipidemia.
   c. psychologic changes.
   d. nausea and vomiting.
6. Measures indicated in the conservative therapy of chronic kidney disease include
   a. decreased fluid intake, carbohydrate intake, and protein intake.
   b. increased fluid intake, decreased carbohydrate intake and protein intake.
   c. decreased fluid intake and protein intake, increased carbohydrate intake.
   d. decreased fluid intake and carbohydrate intake, increased protein intake.
7. One of the major disadvantages of peritoneal dialysis is that
   a. hypotension is a constant problem because of continuous fluid removal.
   b. blood loss can be extensive because of the use of heparin to keep the catheter patent.
   c. solutes are removed more rapidly from the blood than from the CNS, causing disequilibrium syndrome.
   d. high glucose concentrations of the dialysate necessary for ultrafiltration cause carbohydrate and lipid abnormalities.
8. To assess the patency of a newly placed arteriovenous graft for dialysis, the nurse should
   a. irrigate the graft daily with low-dose heparin.
   b. monitor for any increase in BP in the affected arm.
   c. listen with a stethoscope over the graft for the presence of a bruit.
   d. frequently monitor the pulses and neurovascular status distal to the graft.
9. A patient in ESRD receiving hemodialysis is considering asking a relative to donate a kidney for transplantation. In assisting the patient to make a decision about treatment, the nurse informs the patient that
   a. successful transplantation usually provides better quality of life than that offered by dialysis.
   b. if rejection of the transplanted kidney occurs, no further treatment for the renal failure is available.
   c. the immunosuppressive therapy that is required following transplantation causes fatal malignancies in many patients.
   d. hemodialysis replaces the normal functions of the kidneys and patients do not have to live with the continual fear of rejection.
10. Following a kidney transplantation, the nurse teaches the patient that signs of rejection include
    a. fever, weight loss, increased urinary output, increased BP.
    b. fever, weight gain, increased urinary output, increased BP.
    c. fever, weight loss, increased urinary output, decreased BP.
    d. fever, weight gain, decreased urinary output, increased BP.
11. Most of the long-term problems that occur in the patient with a kidney transplant are a result of
    a. chronic rejection.
    b. immunosuppressive therapy.
    c. recurrence of the original renal disease.
    d. failure of the patient to follow the prescribed regimen.

Urinary System

REFERENCES

1. Brady H, et al: Acute renal failure. In Brenner BM, editor: *The kidney,* Philadelphia, 2004, Saunders.
2. Needham E: Management of acute renal failure, *Am Fam Physician* 72:1739, 2005.
3. Campbell D: How acute renal failure puts the brakes on kidney function, *Nursing* 33(1):59, 2003.
4. Singri N, Ahya S, Levin M: Acute renal failure, *JAMA* 289:747, 2003.
5. Redmond R, McDevitt M, Barnes S: Acute renal failure: recognition and treatment in ward patients, *Nurs Stand* 18:46, 2004.
6. O'Neill P: Your patient relies on dialysis: does he need tube feeding too?, *Nursing* 34(10):32hn6, 2004.
*7. Cantarivuch F, Rangoonwala B, Lorenz H, et al: High dose furosemide for established ARF: a prospective, randomized, double-blind, placebo-controlled, multicenter trial, *Am J Kidney Dis* 44:402, 2004.
*8. Kay J, Chow WH, Chan TM, et al: Acetylcysteine for prevention of acute deterioration of renal function following elective coronary angiography and intervention: a randomized controlled trial, *JAMA* 289:553, 2003.
9. Campoy S, Elwell R: Pharmacology and CKD: how chronic kidney disease and its complications alter drug response, *Am J Nurs* 105(9):60, 2005.
*10. Shilipak M, Sarnak MJ, Katz R, et al: Cystatin C and the risk of death and cardiovascular events among elderly persons, *N Engl J Med* 352:2049, 2005.
11. United States Renal Data System: *USRDS 2005 annual data report: atlas of end-stage renal disease,* Bethesda, Md, 2005, National Institute of Diabetes and Digestive and Kidney Diseases.
12. Canadian Organ Replacement Register: *CORR annual report 2002–2003,* Canadian Institute for Health Information. Available at *www.cihi. ca/corr/* (accessed June 30, 2006).
13. U.S. Department of Health and Human Resources: ESRD—general information, Centers for Medicare and Medicaid Services, 2005. Available at *www.cms.hhs.gov/ESRDGeneralInformation* (accessed June 28, 2006).
14. National Kidney Foundation: *Kidney disease outcomes quality initiative 2000,* New York, 2000, National Kidney Foundation.
15. U.S. Department of Health and Human Resources: *Healthy people 2010,* U.S. Department of Health and Human Resources, 2000. Available at *www.healthypeople.gov/* (accessed June 30, 2006).
16. Snively C, Gutierrez C: Chronic kidney disease: prevention and treatment of common complications, *Am Fam Physician* 70:1921, 2004.
17. Stevens LA, Levey AS: Measurement of kidney function, *Med Clin North Am* 89:457, 2005.
18. Benner D: K/DOQI gets to the heart of managing dyslipidemias in patients with CKD, *Nephrol Nurs J* 32:337, 2005.
19. Pendse S, Singh AK: Complications of chronic kidney disease: anemia, mineral metabolism, and cardiovascular disease, *Med Clin North Am* 89:549, 2005.
20. Krishman AV, Phoon RK, Pussell BA, et al: Altered motor nerve excitability in end-stage kidney disease, *Brain* 128(Pt 9):2164, 2005.
21. Goodman WG: Calcium and phosphorus metabolism in patients who have chronic kidney disease, *Med Clin North Am* 89:631, 2005.
22. Legg V: Complications of chronic kidney disease, *Am J Nurs* 105(6):40, 2005.
23. Castner D, Douglas C: Now onstage: chronic kidney disease, *Nursing* 35(12):58, 2005.
24. Zandi-Nejad K, Brenner BM: Strategies to retard the progression of chronic kidney disease, *Med Clin North Am* 89:489, 2005.
25. Chobanian A, Bakris G, Black H, et al: The seventh report of the Joint National Committee on Prevention, Detection, Evaluation, and Treatment of High Blood Pressure: the JNC 7 report, *JAMA* 289:2560, 2003.
26. National Kidney Foundation: K/DOQI clinical practice guidelines on hypertension and antihypertensive agents in chronic kidney disease, *Am J Kidney Dis* 43(5 Suppl 1):S1, 2004.
27. National Kidney Foundation: K/DOQI clinical practice guidelines for bone metabolism and disease in chronic kidney disease, *Am J Kidney Dis* 43:4, 2004.
28. Shire U.S. Inc: *Fosrenal facts, 2005,* Shire U.S. Inc. Available at *www. fosrenol.com/HCP/Facts/Default.aspx* (accessed June 28, 2006).
29. Brommage D, Gallgano C: The role of cinacalcet in treating secondary hyperparathyroidism, *Nephrol Nurs J* 32:229, 2005.
30. Agarwal R, Curley TM: The role of statins in chronic kidney disease, *Am J Med Sci* 330:69, 2005.
31. Gabardi S, Abramson S: Drug dosing in chronic kidney disease, *Med Clin North Am* 89:649, 2005.
32. Kopple J: National Kidney Foundation K/DOQI clinical practice guidelines for nutrition in chronic renal failure, *Am J Kidney Dis* 37(Suppl 2): S66, 2001.
33. Rabetoy C: Acute renal failure. In Molzahn A, Butera E, editors: *Contemporary nephrology nursing: principles and practice,* Pitman, NJ, 2006, American Nephrology Nurses' Association.
34. Burrows-Hudson S: Chronic kidney disease: an overview, *Am J Nurs* 105(2):40, 2005.
35. Rosner MH: Hemodialysis for the non-nephrologist, *South Med J* 98:785, 2005.
36. Saxena R: Peritoneal dialysis: a viable renal replacement therapy option, *Am J Med Sci* 330:110, 2005.
37. Newmann M: Fistula First initiative pushes for new standards in access care, *Nephrol News* 18:43, 2004.
38. Harwood L, Leitch R: Home dialysis therapies, *Nephrol Nurs J* 33:46, 2006.
39. Kaplow R, Richard B: Continuous renal replacement therapies: a more gentle blood filtering technique allows for fewer complications, *Am J Nurs* 102(11):26, 2002.
40. United Network for Organ Sharing: *2005 Annual report: the US scientific registry of transplant recipients and the organ procurement and transplantation network,* Bethesda, Md, 2005, U.S. Department of Health and Human Services.
41. Merion RM, Ashby VB, Wolfe RA, et al: Deceased-donor characteristics and the survival benefit of kidney transplantation, *JAMA* 294:2726, 2005.
42. Salazar A, Pelletier R, Yilmaz S, et al: Use of a minimally invasive donor nephrectomy program to select technique for live donor nephrectomy, *Am J Surg* 189(5):558, 2005.
43. Barone CP, Martin-Watson AL, Barone GW: The postoperative care of the adult renal transplant recipient, *Medsurg Nurs* 13:296, 2004.
44. McCarley PB, Salai PB: Cardiovascular disease in chronic kidney disease, *Am J Nurs* 105(4):40, 2005.
45. Hollenbeak CS, Todd MM, Billingsley EM, et al: Increased incidence of melanoma in renal transplantation recipients, *Cancer* 104:1962, 2005.
46. Brown WW: The geriatric dialysis patient. In Henrick WL, editor: *Principles and practice of dialysis,* ed 2, Baltimore, 2003, Lippincott Williams & Wilkins.
47. Durose CL, Holdsworth M, Watson V, et al: Knowledge of dietary restrictions and the medical consequences of noncompliance by patients on hemodialysis are not predictive of dietary compliance, *J Am Diet Assoc* 104(1):35, 2004.

RESOURCES

American Association of Kidney Patients (AAKP)
800-749-2257
www.aakp.org
American Nephrology Nurses Association
888-600-ANNA (2662) or 856-256-2320
www.annanurse.org
American Organ Transplant Association
281-493-2047
www.a-o-t-a.org
International Society of Nephrology (ISN)
www.isn-online.org
International Transplant Nurses Society
412-343-ITNS
www.itns.org
Kidney Transplant/Dialysis Association, Inc.
781-641-4000
http://users.rcn.com/ktda1
National Kidney Disease Education Program
www.nkdep.nih.gov
National Kidney Foundation
800-622-9010 or 212-889-2210
www.kidney.org
RenalWEB Patient Education
www.renalweb.com/topics/patiented/patiented.htm
United Network for Organ Sharing
888-TX-INFO-1 or 804-330-8541
www.unos.org
United States Renal Data System
www.usrds.org/adr.htm

For additional Internet resources, see the website for this book at *http://evolve. elsevier.com/Lewis/medsurg.*

*Nursing research–based reference.

Problems Related to Regulatory and Reproductive Mechanisms

Section Outline

48 **Nursing Assessment**
Endocrine System, p. 1234

49 **Nursing Management**
Diabetes Mellitus, p. 1253

50 **Nursing Management**
Endocrine Problems, p. 1290

51 **Nursing Assessment**
Reproductive System, p. 1323

52 **Nursing Management**
Breast Disorders, p. 1343

53 **Nursing Management**
Sexually Transmitted Diseases, p. 1366

54 **Nursing Management**
Female Reproductive Problems, p. 1381

55 **Nursing Management**
Male Reproductive Problems, p. 1414

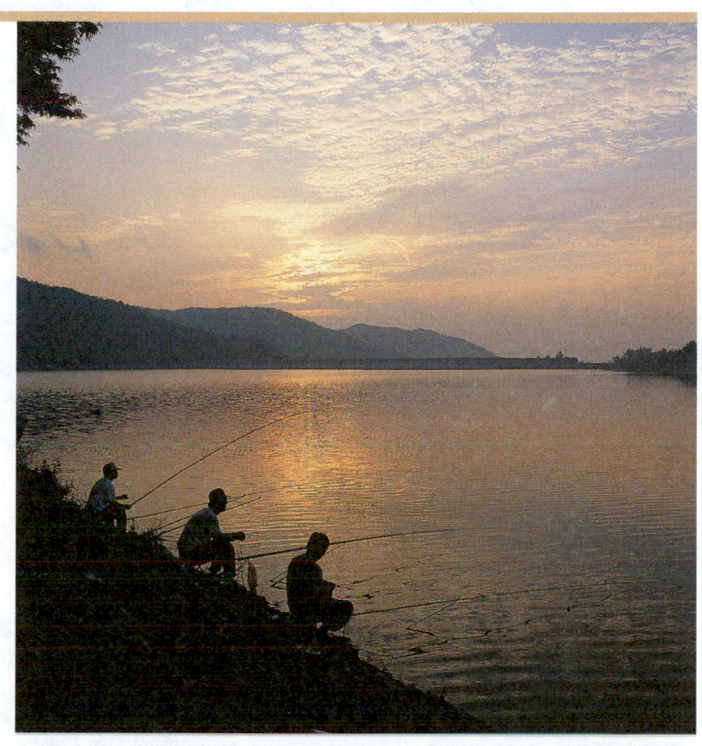

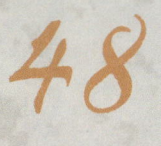

Nursing Assessment
Endocrine System

JoAnne Konick-McMahan

LEARNING OBJECTIVES

1. Identify the common characteristics and functions of hormones.
2. Identify the locations of the endocrine glands.
3. Describe the functions of hormones secreted by the pituitary, thyroid, parathyroid, and adrenal glands and the pancreas.
4. Describe the locations and roles of hormone receptors.
5. Identify the significant subjective and objective assessment data related to the endocrine system that should be obtained from a patient.
6. Describe the appropriate technique used in the physical assessment of the thyroid gland.
7. Describe age-related changes in the endocrine system and differences in assessment findings.
8. Differentiate normal from common abnormal findings in the assessment of the endocrine system.
9. Describe the purpose, significance of results, and nursing responsibilities related to diagnostic studies of the endocrine system.

KEY TERMS

aldosterone, p. 1241
antidiuretic hormone, p. 1239
catecholamines, p. 1241
corticosteroid, p. 1241
cortisol, p. 1241
growth hormone, p. 1239
hormone, p. 1235
insulin, p. 1241
islets of Langerhans, p. 1241
negative feedback, p. 1237
thyroxine, p. 1240
tropic hormones, p. 1239

Electronic Resources

Supplemental content related to Chapter 48 can be found . . .

Companion CD
- Stress-Busting Kit for Nursing Students
- NCLEX Examination Review Questions
- Comprehensive Glossary

Evolve Website *evolve*
http://evolve.elsevier.com/Lewis/medsurg
- Content Updates
- Key Points (Printable and CD/MP3 Download)
- Concept Map Creator
- Expanded Audio Glossary
- Key Term Flash Cards
- Electronic Calculators

- Physical Examination Video Clips:
  - Abdomen: Inspection, Auscultation, and Percussion
  - Abdomen: Palpation
- WebLinks

The endocrine system and the nervous system are two of the primary communicating and coordinating systems in the body. The nervous system communicates through nerve impulses; the endocrine system communicates through chemical substances known as hormones, and it plays a role in reproduction, growth and development, and regulation of energy. The endocrine system is composed of glands or glandular tissues that produce, store, and secrete hormones that travel through the blood to specific target cells throughout the body.

The endocrine glands include the hypothalamus, pituitary, thyroid, parathyroids, adrenals, pancreas, ovaries, testes, and pineal (Fig. 48-1). The pineal gland, which secretes melatonin, is involved in stimulating gonadal function.[1] In addition to the endocrine glands, other body organs secrete hormones. For example, the kidneys secrete erythropoietin, the heart secretes atrial natriuretic peptide, and the gastrointestinal tract secretes numerous peptide hormones (e.g., gastrin). These hormones are discussed in their respective assessment chapters.

Reviewed by Phyllis L. Christianson, MN, ANCC, ARNP, Senior Lecturer, Department of Behavioral Nursing and Health Systems, School of Nursing, University of Washington, Seattle, Wash.; and Coleen R. Elmers, RN, MSN, Staff Development Education, Baptist Health System, San Antonio, Tex.

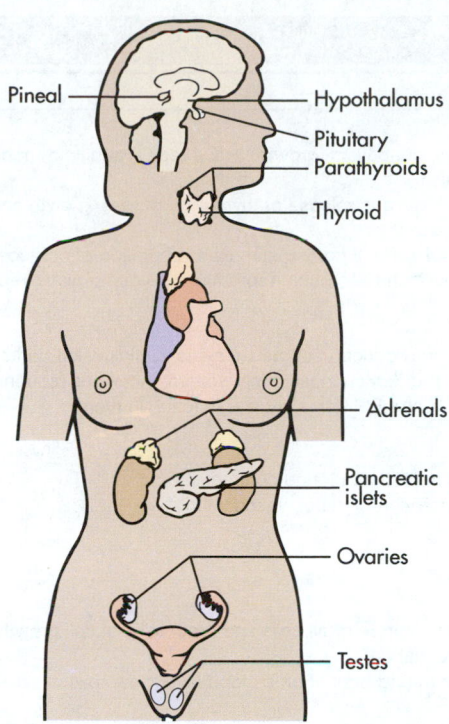

FIG. 48-1 Location of the major endocrine glands. The parathyroid glands lie on the posterior surface of the thyroid.

STRUCTURES AND FUNCTIONS OF THE ENDOCRINE SYSTEM

Glands

The organs of the endocrine system are referred to as *glands*. Endocrine glands produce chemical substances called *hormones* and secrete them into blood, where they eventually affect specific target tissues. A **target tissue** is the body tissue or organ that the hormone has its effect on. For example, the thyroid (gland) synthesizes thyroxine (the hormone), which influences all body tissues (*target tissue*). It is important to note that not all glands in the body belong to the endocrine system. There are two types of glands—*exocrine glands* and *endocrine glands*. Exocrine glands secrete their substances into ducts that then empty into a body cavity or onto a surface (e.g., skin). For example, salivary glands produce saliva, which is secreted through salivary ducts into the mouth. By contrast, endocrine glands do not have ducts. They secrete their substances directly into the blood.

Hormones

Classifications and Functions. A **hormone** is a chemical substance synthesized and secreted by a specific organ or tissue. Most hormones have common characteristics, including (1) secretion in small amounts at variable but predictable rates, (2) circulation through the blood, and (3) binding to specific cellular receptors either in the cell membrane or within the cell.

Hormones are classified by their chemical structure: *lipid-soluble hormones* and *water-soluble* (protein-based) *hormones*. Lipid-soluble hormones include steroid hormones (all hormones produced by the adrenal cortex and sex glands) and thyroid hormones. All other hormones are water soluble.[2] The differences in solubility become important in understanding how the hormone interacts with the target cell.

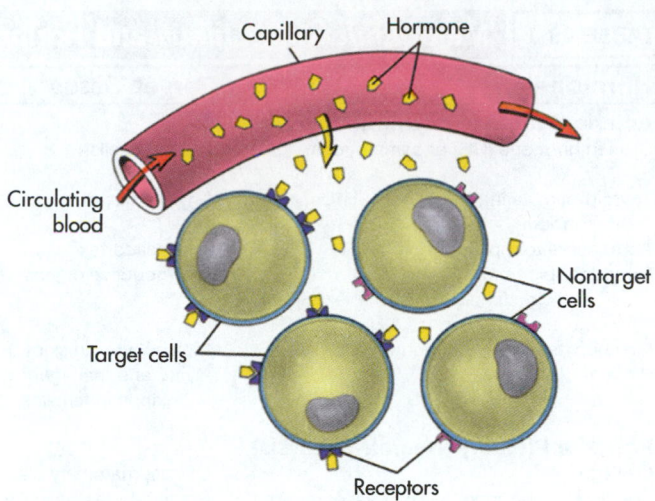

FIG. 48-2 The target cell concept. Hormones act only on cells that have receptors specific to that hormone, because the shape of the receptor determines which hormone can react with it. This is an example of the lock-and-key model of biochemical reactions.

Hormones control a number of physiologic activities. Important hormonal functions are related to reproduction, response to stress and injury, electrolyte balance, energy metabolism, growth, maturation, and aging. Hormones also play a role in nervous system function. Some hormones have a regulatory effect on nervous tissue. For example, catecholamines are hormones when they are secreted by the adrenal medulla, but act as neurotransmitters when secreted by nerve cells in the brain and peripheral nervous system. When epinephrine travels through the blood, it is a hormone and affects target tissues. When it travels across synaptic junctions, it acts as a neurotransmitter.

Hormones can also influence behavior.[3] For example, excess growth hormone, cortisol, and parathyroid hormone can cause mood swings. Depression has been associated with adrenal insufficiency and hypothyroidism. Table 48-1 summarizes the major hormones, glands, or tissues from which they are synthesized, target organs or tissues, and functions.

Hormone Transport. Hormones are carried by the blood to other sites in the body where their actions are exerted. Some hormones (e.g., steroid and thyroid hormones) are not water soluble. Therefore these types of hormones are bound to plasma proteins for transport in the blood. Although hormones are inactive when bound to plasma proteins, they can be released when appropriate and immediately exert their action at the target tissue. Water-soluble hormones (e.g., protein hormones, catecholamines) circulate freely in the blood and are not dependent on proteins for transport.

Targets and Receptors. As mentioned, hormones exert their effects on target tissue. The hormone recognizes the target tissue through receptors (the site that interacts with the hormone) on or within cells of the target tissue. The specificity of hormone–target cell interaction is determined by receptors in a "lock-and-key" type of mechanism. Thus a hormone will act only on cells that have a receptor specific for that hormone (Fig. 48-2). It is important to note that there are two types of receptors: those that are within the cell (e.g., steroid and thyroid hormone receptors) and those that are on the cell membrane (e.g., protein-type hormone receptors). The location of the receptor sites affects the mechanism of action for the hormone.

Steroid Hormone Receptors. Steroid and thyroid hormone receptors are located inside the cell. Because these hormones are

Endocrine System

TABLE 48-1	Major Endocrine Glands and Hormones

Hormones	Target Tissue	Functions
Anterior Pituitary (Adenohypophysis)		
Growth hormone (GH) or somatotropin	All body cells	Promotes protein anabolism (growth, tissue repair) and lipid mobilization and catabolism
Thyroid-stimulating hormone (TSH) or thyrotropin	Thyroid gland	Stimulates synthesis and release of thyroid hormones, growth and function of thyroid gland
Adrenocorticotropic hormone (ACTH)	Adrenal cortex	Fosters growth of adrenal cortex; stimulates secretion of corticosteroids
Gonadotropic hormones	Reproductive organs	Stimulate sex hormone secretion, reproductive organ growth, reproductive processes
• Follicle-stimulating hormone (FSH)		
• Luteinizing hormone (LH)		
Melanocyte-stimulating hormone (MSH)	Melanocytes in skin	Increases melanin production in melanocytes to make skin darker in color
Prolactin	Ovary and mammary glands in females	Stimulates milk production in lactating women; increases response of follicles to LH and FSH; has unclear function in men
Posterior Pituitary (Neurohypophysis)		
Oxytocin	Uterus; mammary glands	Stimulates milk secretion, uterine contractility
Antidiuretic hormone (ADH) or vasopressin	Renal tubules, vascular smooth muscle	Promotes reabsorption of water, vasoconstriction
Thyroid		
Thyroxine (T_4)	All body tissues	Precursor to T_3
Triiodothyronine (T_3)	All body tissues	Regulates metabolic rate of all cells and processes of cell growth and tissue differentiation
Calcitonin	Bone tissue	Regulates calcium and phosphorus blood levels; decreases serum Ca^{2+} levels
Parathyroids		
Parathyroid hormone (PTH) or parathormone	Bone, intestine, kidneys	Regulates calcium and phosphorus blood levels; promotes bone demineralization and increases intestinal absorption of Ca^{2+}; increases serum Ca^{2+} levels
Adrenal Medulla		
Epinephrine (adrenaline)	Sympathetic effectors	Response to stress; enhances and prolongs effects of sympathetic nervous system
Norepinephrine	Sympathetic effectors	Response to stress; enhances and prolongs effects of sympathetic nervous system
Adrenal Cortex		
Corticosteroids (e.g., cortisol, hydrocortisone)	All body tissues	Promotes metabolism, response to stress
Androgens (e.g., testosterone, androsterone) and estrogen	Reproductive organs	Promotes masculinization in men, growth and sexual activity in women
Mineralocorticoids (e.g., aldosterone)	Kidney	Regulates sodium and potassium balance and thus water balance
Pancreas (Islets of Langerhans)		
Insulin (from beta cells)	General	Promotes movement of glucose out of blood and into cells
Glucagon (from alpha cells)	General	Promotes movement of glucose from glycogen (glycogenolysis) and into blood
Somatostatin	Pancreas	Inhibits insulin and glucagon secretion
Pancreatic polypeptide	General	Influences regulation of pancreatic exocrine function and metabolism of absorbed nutrients
Gonads		
Women: Ovaries		
Estrogen	Reproductive system, breasts	Stimulates development of secondary sex characteristics, preparation of uterus for fertilization and fetal development; stimulates bone growth
Progesterone	Reproductive system	Maintains lining of uterus necessary for successful pregnancy
Men: Testes		
Testosterone	Reproductive system	Stimulates development of secondary sex characteristics, spermatogenesis

lipid soluble, they pass through the target cell membrane by passive diffusion and bind to receptor sites located in the cytoplasm or nucleus of the target cell.[4] Intracellular hormone-receptor complexes, such as those seen in steroid hormone action, bind to specific sites on deoxyribonucleic acid (DNA) to stimulate or inhibit the synthesis of messenger ribonucleic acid (mRNA). When new mRNA is synthesized, it migrates to the cytoplasm, where it stimu-

lates the synthesis of new protein. These new proteins produce specific effects in the target cell (Fig. 48-3).

Protein Hormone Receptors. Protein hormone action is a two-step process. The receptor is located in the target cell membrane; thus the hormone itself acts as a "first messenger." The hormone-receptor interaction stimulates the production of a "second messenger" such as cyclic adenosine monophosphate (cAMP). cAMP

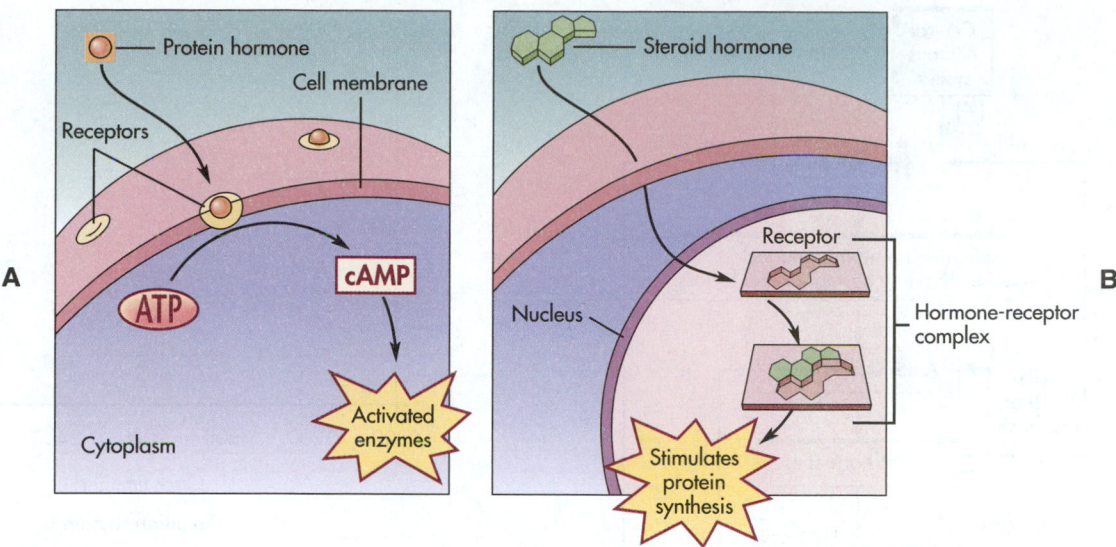

FIG. 48-3 **A,** Protein hormones bind to receptors located on the surface of the cell membrane. The hormone-receptor interaction stimulates the formation of cAMP, thereby activating various cell processes. **B,** Steroid hormones penetrate the cell membrane and interact with intracellular receptors. The hormone-receptor complex activates the cell by stimulating protein synthesis.

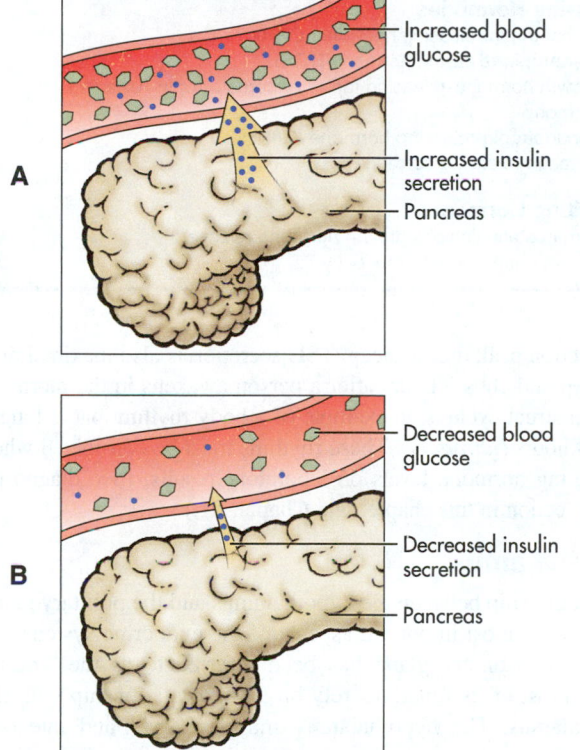

FIG. 48-4 Feedback mechanism between blood glucose and insulin. **A,** Increased blood glucose stimulates increased insulin secretion from the pancreas. **B,** As blood glucose levels decline, insulin secretion decreases.

works by activating enzymes to regulate intracellular activity (see Fig. 48-3).

Regulation of Hormonal Secretion.
The regulation of endocrine activity is controlled by specific mechanisms of varying levels of complexity. These mechanisms stimulate or inhibit hormone synthesis and secretion and include simple feedback, complex feedback, nervous system control, and physiologic rhythms.

Simple Feedback. The regulation of hormone levels in the blood depends on a highly specialized mechanism called *feedback*.

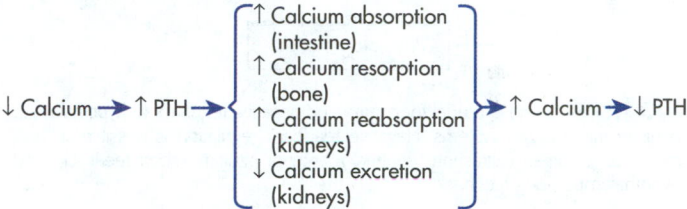

FIG. 48-5 Feedback mechanism between parathyroid hormone (PTH) and calcium.

Feedback is based on the blood level of a particular substance. This substance may be a hormone or other chemical compound regulated by, or responsive to, a hormone. With **negative feedback,** the most common type of feedback system, the gland responds by increasing or decreasing the secretion of a hormone based on feedback from various factors. Negative feedback is similar to the functioning of a thermostat in which cold air in a room activates the thermostat to release heat, and hot air turns off the thermostat to prevent more warm air from entering the room.

The pattern of insulin secretion is a physiologic example of negative feedback between glucose and insulin. Elevated blood glucose levels stimulate the secretion of insulin from the pancreas. As blood glucose levels decrease, the stimulus for insulin secretion also decreases (Fig. 48-4). The homeostatic mechanism is considered negative feedback because it reverses the change in blood glucose level. Another example of negative feedback is the relationship between calcium and parathyroid hormone (PTH). Low blood levels of calcium stimulate the parathyroid gland to release PTH, which acts on bone, the intestine, and kidneys to increase blood calcium levels. The increased blood calcium levels then inhibit further PTH release (Fig. 48-5).

Positive feedback is a second method of regulation of hormone secretion. The positive feedback mechanism increases the target organ action beyond normal. The action of oxytocin in childbirth is an example. The hormone oxytocin from the posterior pituitary stimulates and increases uterine contractions. Oxytocin's release is stimulated by pressure receptors in the vagina. As the fetus enters the vagina during childbirth, the pressure receptors sense increased

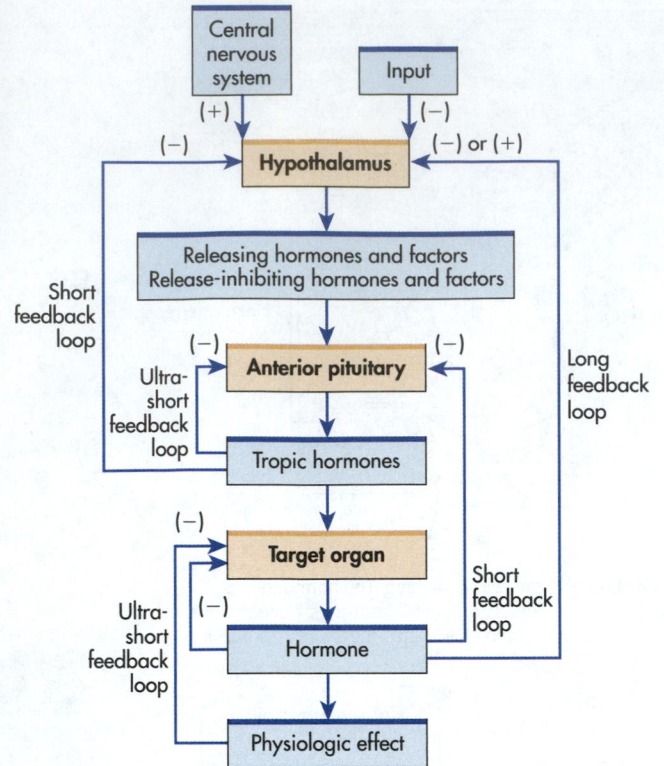

FIG. 48-6   General model for control and negative feedback to hypothalamus-pituitary target organ systems. Negative feedback regulation is possible at three levels: target organ (ultrashort feedback), anterior pituitary (short feedback), and hypothalamus (long feedback).

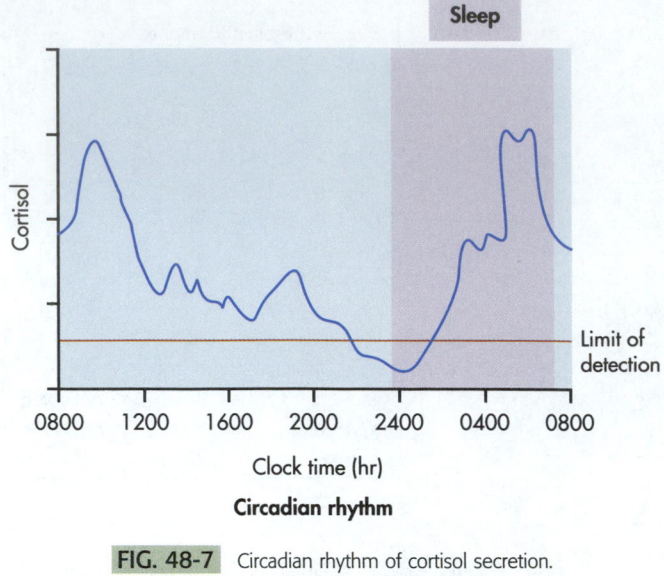

FIG. 48-7   Circadian rhythm of cortisol secretion.

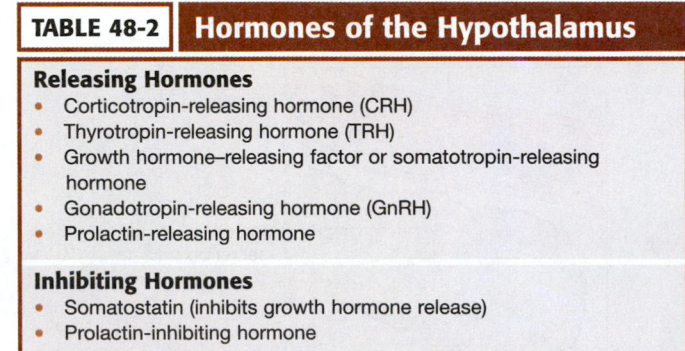

TABLE 48-2	**Hormones of the Hypothalamus**

Releasing Hormones
- Corticotropin-releasing hormone (CRH)
- Thyrotropin-releasing hormone (TRH)
- Growth hormone–releasing factor or somatotropin-releasing hormone
- Gonadotropin-releasing hormone (GnRH)
- Prolactin-releasing hormone

Inhibiting Hormones
- Somatostatin (inhibits growth hormone release)
- Prolactin-inhibiting hormone

pressure and signal the brain to release more oxytocin. Oxytocin release leads to stronger uterine contractions. With birth, the stimulus to the pressure receptors in the vagina ends, thus leading to decreased oxytocin secretion.

Complex Feedback. *Complex feedback* involves communication via hormones among several glands to turn on or turn off target organ hormone secretion. An example of this is regulation of thyroid hormones (Fig. 48-6). The synthesis and release of thyroid-stimulating hormone (TSH) or thyrotropin from the anterior pituitary is stimulated by thyrotropin-releasing hormone (TRH), which is secreted by the hypothalamus. The thyroid hormones, T_3 and T_4, have an inhibitory effect on the secretion of both TRH from the hypothalamus and TSH from the anterior pituitary.

Nervous System Control. In addition to chemical regulation, some endocrine glands are directly affected by the activity of the nervous system. Pain, emotion, sexual excitement, and stress can stimulate the nervous system to modulate hormone secretion. Neural involvement is initiated by the central nervous system (CNS) and implemented by the sympathetic nervous system (SNS). For example, stress is sensed by the CNS, and the SNS secretes catecholamines that increase heart rate and blood pressure to deal with stress more effectively. (Effects of stress are discussed in Chapter 9.)

Rhythms. Another regulatory mechanism affecting many hormonal secretions involves the rhythms of secretions. These rhythms originate in brain structures. A common physiologic rhythm is the *circadian rhythm,* in which a hormone level fluctuates predictably during a 24-hour period.[5] These rhythms may be related to sleep-wake or dark-light cycles. For example, cortisol rises early in the day, declines toward evening, and rises again toward the end of sleep to peak by morning (Fig. 48-7). Growth hormone (GH) and prolac-

tin secretion peak during sleep. TSH secretion is also maximal during sleep and ebbs 3 hours after a person awakens in the morning. The menstrual cycle is an example of a body rhythm that is longer than 24 hours *(ultradian).* These rhythms must be considered when interpreting hormone levels on laboratory results. (See diagnostic studies section in this chapter and Chapter 51.)

Hypothalamus

The relationship between the hypothalamus and the pituitary gland is one of the most important aspects of the endocrine system. Although the pituitary gland has been referred to as the "master gland," most of its functions rely on an interrelationship with the hypothalamus. The hypothalamus and pituitary gland integrate communication between nervous and endocrine systems.

The hypothalamus is located in the most central part of the diencephalon area of the brain (see Fig. 48-1). Although it is really part of the brain, the hypothalamus secretes many hormones. Two important groups of hormones from the hypothalamus are *releasing* hormones and *inhibiting* hormones.[6] The function of these hormones is to either stimulate (release) or inhibit the secretion of hormones from the anterior pituitary (Table 48-2).

The hypothalamus also contains neurons, which receive input from the brainstem and limbic system. These neurons influence the limbic system, brainstem, and spinal cord. This creates a circuit to facilitate the coordination of the endocrine system, ANS, and expression of complex behavioral responses, such as anger and feelings of fear and pleasure.

Pituitary

The pituitary gland (also called the hypophysis) is very small—about the size of a pea. It is located in the sella turcica under the hypothalamus at the base of the brain above the sphenoid bone (see Fig. 48-1). The pituitary is connected to the hypothalamus by the infundibular (hypophyseal) stalk. This stalk serves as a communication mechanism between the hypothalamus and the pituitary. The pituitary consists of two parts, the *anterior* (adenohypophysis) and the *posterior* (neurohypophysis) lobes. Hormones secreted from each of these pituitary lobes serve very different functions.

Anterior Pituitary. The anterior lobe accounts for 80% of the gland by weight. As mentioned previously, the anterior pituitary is regulated by the hypothalamus through releasing and inhibiting hormones. These hypothalamic hormones reach the anterior pituitary through a network of capillaries known as the *hypothalamus-hypophyseal portal system.* The releasing and inhibiting hormones in turn affect the secretion of six hormones from the anterior pituitary (Fig. 48-8; see Table 48-2).

Tropic Hormones. Several hormones secreted by the anterior pituitary are referred to as **tropic hormones.** These are hormones that control the secretion of hormones by other glands. Thyroid-stimulating hormone (TSH) stimulates the thyroid gland to secrete thyroid hormones. Adrenocorticotropic hormone (ACTH) stimulates the adrenal cortex to secrete corticosteroids. Follicle-stimulating hormone (FSH)

stimulates secretion of estrogen and the development of ova in the female and sperm development in the male. Luteinizing hormone (LH) stimulates ovulation in the female and secretion of sex hormones in both the male and female.

Growth Hormone. Growth hormone (GH) has effects on all body tissues. GH, as its name suggests, affects the growth and development of skeletal muscles and long bones, affecting a person's size and height. It also has numerous biologic actions, including a role in protein, fat, and carbohydrate metabolism.[7]

Prolactin. Prolactin is a hormone that stimulates breast development necessary for lactation after childbirth. Prolactin is also referred to as lactogenic hormone.

Posterior Pituitary. The posterior pituitary is composed of nerve tissue and is essentially an extension of the hypothalamus. The communication between the hypothalamus and posterior pituitary occurs through nerve tracts known as the *median eminence.* The hormones secreted by the posterior pituitary, **antidiuretic hormone** (ADH) and oxytocin, are actually produced in the hypothalamus. These hormones travel down the nerve tracts from the hypothalamus to the posterior pituitary and are stored until their release is triggered by the appropriate stimuli (see Fig. 48-8).

Antidiuretic Hormone. The major physiologic role of ADH is regulation of fluid volume by stimulating reabsorption of water in the renal tubules. ADH, also called vasopressin, is also a potent vasoconstrictor.

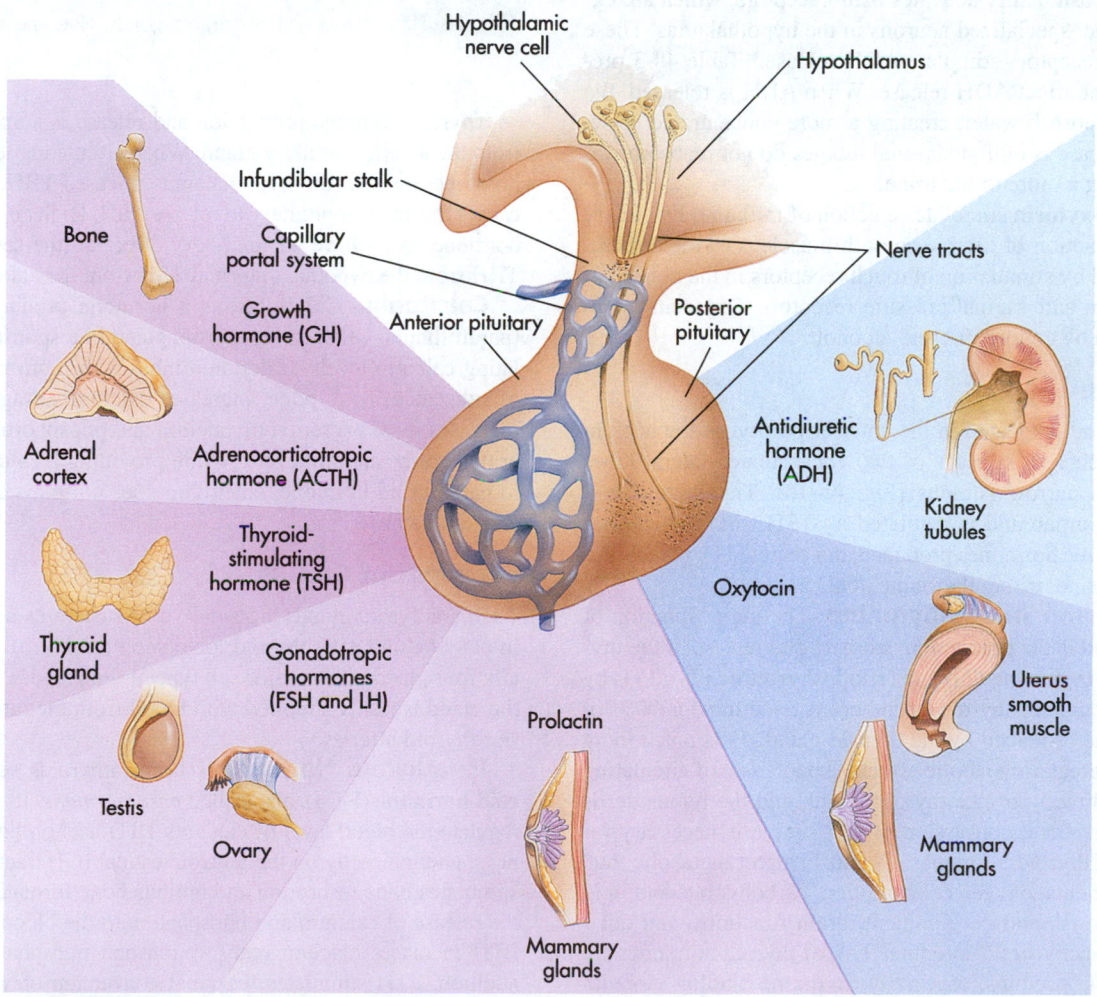

FIG. 48-8 Relationship between the hypothalamus, pituitary, and target organs. The hypothalamus communicates with the anterior pituitary via a capillary system and with the posterior pituitary via nerve tracts. The anterior and posterior pituitary hormones are shown with their target tissues.

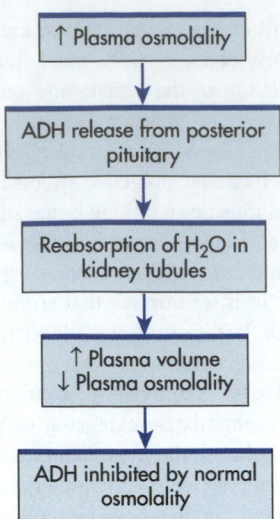

FIG. 48-9 Relationship of plasma osmolality to antidiuretic hormone (ADH) release and action.

TABLE 48-3	Factors Affecting ADH Release	
Stimulate ADH Release		**Inhibit ADH Release**
Increased plasma osmolality		Decreased plasma osmolality
Decreased fluid volume		Increased fluid volume
Hypotension		β-Adrenergic agonists
Pain		Alcohol
Nausea and vomiting		

ADH, Antidiuretic hormone.

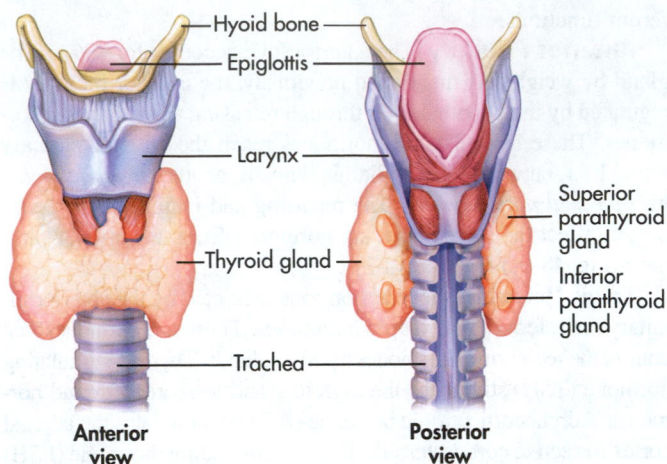

FIG. 48-10 Thyroid and parathyroid glands. Note the surrounding structures.

The most important stimulus to ADH secretion is *plasma osmolality* (a measure of solute concentration of circulating blood) (Fig. 48-9). Plasma osmolality will increase when there is a decrease in extracellular fluid or an increase in solute concentration. The increased plasma osmolality activates osmoreceptors, which are extremely sensitive, specialized neurons in the hypothalamus. These activated osmoreceptors stimulate ADH release.[8] Table 48-3 presents factors that affect ADH release. When ADH is released, the renal tubules reabsorb water, creating a more concentrated urine. When ADH release is inhibited, renal tubules do not reabsorb water, thus creating a more dilute urine.

Oxytocin. Oxytocin stimulates ejection of milk into mammary ducts and contraction of uterine smooth muscle. Oxytocin secretion is increased by stimulation of touch receptors in the nipples of lactating women and vaginal pressure receptors. Oxytocin secretion is inhibited by endorphins and alcohol.

Thyroid Gland

The thyroid gland is located in the anterior portion of the neck in front of the trachea. It consists of two encapsulated lateral lobes connected by a narrow isthmus (Fig. 48-10). The thyroid is a highly vascular organ and is regulated by TSH from the anterior pituitary. The three hormones produced and secreted by the thyroid gland are thyroxine, triiodothyronine, and calcitonin.

Thyroxine and Triiodothyronine. The major function of the thyroid gland is the production, storage, and release of the thyroid hormones, **thyroxine** (T_4) and **triiodothyronine** (T_3). T_4 is by far the most abundant thyroid hormone, accounting for 90% of thyroid hormone produced by the thyroid gland. T_3 is much more potent and has greater metabolic effects. About 20% of circulating T_3 is secreted directly by the thyroid gland, and the remainder is obtained by peripheral conversion of T_4.[9] Iodine is necessary for the synthesis of thyroid hormones. T_4 and T_3 affect metabolic rate, caloric requirements, oxygen consumption, carbohydrate and lipid metabolism, growth and development, brain functions, and other nervous system activities. More than 99% of thyroid hormones are bound to plasma proteins, especially thyroxine-binding globulin synthesized by the liver. Only the unbound "free" hormones are biologically active.

Thyroid hormone production and release is stimulated by TSH from the anterior pituitary gland. When circulating levels of thyroid hormone are low, the hypothalamus releases TRH, which in turn causes the anterior pituitary to release TSH. High circulating thyroid hormone levels have an inhibitory effect on the secretion of both TRH from the hypothalamus and TSH from the anterior pituitary.

Calcitonin. Calcitonin is a hormone produced by C cells (parafollicular cells) of the thyroid gland in response to high circulating calcium levels. Calcitonin inhibits calcium *resorption* (loss of substance) from bone, increases calcium storage in bone, and increases renal excretion of calcium and phosphorus, thereby lowering serum calcium levels. While providing a countermechanism to parathyroid hormone, calcitonin does not play a critical role in calcium balance.[10]

Parathyroid Glands

The parathyroid glands are small, oval structures usually arranged in pairs behind each thyroid lobe (see Fig. 48-10). There are usually four glands. The major cell type of the glands is epithelial, and the gland is richly supplied with blood from the inferior and superior thyroid arteries.

Parathyroid Hormone. The parathyroids secrete **parathyroid hormone** (PTH), also called *parathormone*. Its major role is to regulate the blood level of calcium. PTH acts on bone, on the kidneys, and indirectly on the gastrointestinal (GI) tract. In bone, PTH stimulates bone resorption and inhibits bone formation, resulting in the release of calcium and phosphate into the blood. In the kidney, PTH increases calcium reabsorption and phosphate excretion. In addition, PTH stimulates the renal conversion of vitamin D to its most active form (1,25-dihydroxyvitamin D_3). This active vitamin D then enhances the intestinal absorption of calcium.

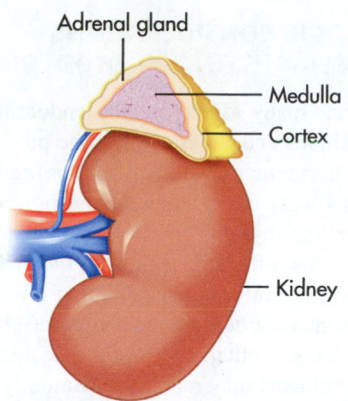

FIG. 48-11 The adrenal gland is composed of the adrenal cortex and the adrenal medulla.

PTH is not under pituitary and hypothalamic control. The secretion of this hormone is directly regulated by a feedback system (see Fig. 48-5). When the serum calcium level is low, PTH secretion increases; when the serum calcium level rises, PTH secretion falls. In addition, high levels of active vitamin D inhibit PTH and low levels of magnesium stimulate PTH secretion.

Adrenal Glands

The adrenal glands are small, paired, highly vascularized glands located on the upper portion of each kidney. Each gland consists of two parts, the medulla and the cortex (Fig. 48-11). Each part has distinct functions, and the glands act independently from one another.

Adrenal Medulla. The adrenal medulla is the inner part of the gland and consists of sympathetic postganglionic neurons. The medulla secretes the catecholamines epinephrine (the major hormone [75%]), norepinephrine (25%), and dopamine. **Catecholamines,** usually considered neurotransmitters, are hormones when secreted by the adrenal medulla, because they are released into the circulation and transported to their target organs. Catecholamines exert their effects after binding to adrenergic receptors on cells, and they have widespread effects on all body systems. Catecholamines are an essential part of the body's response to stress (see Chapter 9).

Adrenal Cortex. The adrenal cortex is the outer part of the adrenal gland. It secretes more than 50 steroid hormones, which are classified as glucocorticoids, mineralocorticoids, and androgens. Cholesterol is the precursor for steroid hormone synthesis. Glucocorticoids (e.g., cortisol) are named for their effects on glucose metabolism. Mineralocorticoids (e.g., aldosterone) are essential for the maintenance of fluid and electrolyte balance. Adrenal androgens are produced and secreted in small but significant amounts. The term **corticosteroid** refers to any of the hormones synthesized by the adrenal cortex (excluding androgens).

Cortisol. Cortisol, the most abundant and potent glucocorticoid, is necessary to maintain life. One major function of cortisol is the regulation of blood glucose concentration. Cortisol increases blood glucose through stimulation of hepatic gluconeogenesis (conversion of amino acids to glucose) and inhibiting protein synthesis. Cortisol also decreases peripheral glucose use in the fasting state. Additionally, glucocorticoids stimulate lipolysis in adipose tissue, thereby mobilizing glycerol and free fatty acids.

Another major effect of glucocorticoids is their antiinflammatory action and supportive actions in response to stress. A marked increase in the rate of cortisol secretion by the adrenal cortex aids the body in coping more effectively with stressful situations (see Chapter 9). Cortisol decreases the inflammatory response by stabilizing the membranes of cellular lysosomes and preventing increased capillary permeability. The lysosomal stabilization reduces the release of proteolytic enzymes and thereby their destructive effects on surrounding tissue. Cortisol can also inhibit production of prostaglandins, thromboxanes, and leukotrienes (see Chapter 13, Fig. 13-5) and alter the cell-mediated immune response.

Cortisol helps maintain vascular integrity and fluid volume. It has a mineralocorticoid effect because it can bind to mineralocorticoid receptors.

Cortisol is secreted in a diurnal pattern (see Fig. 48-7). The major control of cortisol is by means of a negative feedback mechanism that involves the secretion of corticotropin-releasing hormone (CRH) from the hypothalamus. CRH stimulates the secretion of ACTH by the anterior pituitary. Cortisol levels are also increased by surgical stress, burns, infection, fever, acute anxiety, and hypoglycemia.

Aldosterone. Aldosterone is a potent mineralocorticoid that maintains extracellular fluid volume. It acts at the renal tubule to promote renal reabsorption of sodium and excretion of potassium and hydrogen ions. Aldosterone synthesis and secretion are stimulated by angiotensin II, hyponatremia, and hyperkalemia and inhibited by atrial natriuretic peptide and hypokalemia.

Adrenal Androgens. The third class of steroids synthesized and secreted by the adrenal cortex are the androgens. Normally, the adrenal cortex secretes small amounts of androgens. Adrenal androgens stimulate pubic and axillary hair growth and sex drive in females. In females, androgens are converted to estrogen in the peripheral tissues. In postmenopausal women the major source of estrogen is from the peripheral conversion of adrenal androgen to estrogen. The effects of adrenal androgen in men are negligible in comparison with testosterone secreted by the testes.

Pancreas

The pancreas is a long, tapered, lobular, soft gland located behind the stomach and anterior to the first and second lumbar vertebrae. The pancreas has both exocrine and endocrine functions. The hormone-secreting portion of the pancreas is referred to as the **islets of Langerhans.** The islets account for less than 2% of the gland and consist of four types of hormone-secreting cells: alpha, beta, delta, and F cells. Alpha cells produce and secrete the hormone glucagon. Insulin is produced and secreted by beta cells. Somatostatin is produced and secreted by the delta cells. Pancreatic polypeptide is secreted by the F (or PP) cells.

Glucagon. Glucagon is synthesized and released from pancreatic alpha cells in response to low levels of blood glucose, protein ingestion, and exercise. Glucagon increases blood glucose by stimulating glycogenolysis, gluconeogenesis, and ketogenesis. Usually, glucagon and insulin function in a reciprocal manner to maintain normal blood glucose levels. The exception is after ingestion of a high-protein, carbohydrate-free diet, in which case both hormones are secreted. In this instance, glucagon counteracts the inhibitory effect of insulin on gluconeogenesis, and normal blood glucose levels are maintained.

Insulin. Insulin is the principal regulator of the metabolism and storage of ingested carbohydrates, fats, and proteins. Insulin facilitates glucose transport across cell membranes in most tissues. However, the brain, nerves, the lens of the eye, hepatocytes, erythrocytes, and cells in the intestinal mucosa and kidney tubules are not dependent on insulin for glucose uptake. An increased blood glucose level is the major stimulus for insulin synthesis and secretion. Other stimuli to insulin secretion are increased amino acid levels and vagal stimulation. Insulin secretion is usually inhibited by low blood glucose levels, glucagon, somatostatin, hypokalemia, and catecholamines (Table 48-4).

A major effect of insulin on glucose metabolism occurs in the liver, where the hormone enhances glucose incorporation into glycogen and triglycerides by altering enzymatic activity and inhibiting gluconeogenesis. Another major effect occurs in peripheral tissues where insulin facilitates glucose transport into cells, transport of amino acids across muscle membranes and their synthesis into protein, and transport of triglycerides into adipose tissue. Thus insulin is a storage, or *anabolic,* hormone.

The endocrine system is concerned with the regulation of body processes and the maintenance of internal homeostasis despite vastly changing substrates, as is seen in glucose homeostasis after food ingestion. After a meal, insulin is responsible for the storage of nutrients (anabolism). In the fasting state (during which ingested glucose is not readily available), hormones such as catecholamines, cortisol, and glucagon break down stored complex fuels (catabolism) to provide simple glucose as fuel for energy.

GERONTOLOGIC CONSIDERATIONS
EFFECTS OF AGING ON THE ENDOCRINE SYSTEM

Normal aging has many effects on the endocrine system (Table 48-5). These include (1) decreased hormone production and secretion, (2) altered hormone metabolism and biologic activity, (3) decreased responsiveness of target tissues to hormones, and (4) alterations in circadian rhythms.

Assessment of the effects of aging on the endocrine system is difficult because the subtle changes of aging often mimic manifestations of endocrine disorders. Some endocrine changes associated with aging are obvious; others are subtle. The nurse must be aware that endocrine problems may manifest differently in an older adult than in a younger person. Older adults may have multiple comorbidities and take multiple medications that alter the body's usual response to endocrine dysfunction. Symptoms of endocrine dysfunction such as fatigue, constipation, or mental impairment in the older adult are often missed because they are attributed solely to aging. It is important that the nurse consider age-related endocrine changes when assessing the older adult.[2]

ASSESSMENT OF THE ENDOCRINE SYSTEM

Hormones affect every body tissue and system, causing great diversity in the signs and symptoms of endocrine dysfunction. Therefore assessment of the endocrine system is often difficult and requires keen clinical skills to detect manifestations of disorders. Endocrine dysfunction may result from deficient or excessive hormone secretion, transport abnormalities, an inability of the target tissue to respond to a hormone, or inappropriate stimulation of the target-tissue receptor.

Endocrine disorders may have specific or nonspecific (vague) clinical manifestations. Specific signs and symptoms such as the classic "polys" (polyuria, polydipsia, and polyphagia) in diabetes mellitus make the assessment easier. Nonspecific signs and symptoms such as tachycardia, palpitations, fatigue, or altered mood are more problematic. Nonspecific changes should alert the health care provider to the possibility of an endocrine disorder. The most

TABLE 48-4	Factors Influencing Insulin Secretion
Stimulate Secretion	**Inhibit Secretion**
• ↑ Glucose levels	• ↓ Glucose levels
• ↑ Amino acid levels	• ↓ Amino acid levels
• ↑ Gastrointestinal hormone levels	• ↓ Potassium levels
• ↑ Vagal stimulation	• ↑ Corticosteroid hormone levels
• ↑ Fats	• ↑ Catecholamine levels
	• ↑ Somatostatin levels
	• ↑ Glucagon levels (usually)
	• ↑ Insulin levels

TABLE 48-5	*GERONTOLOGIC DIFFERENCES IN ASSESSMENT* Endocrine System	
Gland	**Changes**	**Clinical Significance**
Thyroid	Atrophy of thyroid gland; TSH and T_3 secretion is decreased	Increased incidence of hypothyroidism with aging; however, most older adults maintain adequate thyroid function
Parathyroid	Increased basal level of PTH and increased secretion	Increased calcium resorption from bone; hypercalcemia, hypercalciuria
Adrenal cortex	Adrenal cortex becomes more fibrotic and slightly smaller Higher plasma levels of cortisol Decreased plasma levels of adrenal androgens and aldosterone	Unknown; possibly contributes to a decreased response to sodium restriction and upright posture
Adrenal medulla	Increased secretion and basal level of norepinephrine; no change in plasma epinephrine levels with aging Decreased β-adrenergic receptor response to norepinephrine	Decreased responsiveness to β-adrenergic agonists and receptor blockers May partly explain increased incidence of hypertension with aging
Pancreas	Increase in fibrosis and fatty deposits in pancreas Increased glucose intolerance and decreased sensitivity to insulin	May partly contribute to increased incidence of diabetes mellitus with advanced aging
Gonads	*Women:* decline in estrogen secretion	Women experience symptoms associated with menopause and have increased risk for atherosclerosis and osteoporosis
	Men: decline in testosterone secretion	Men may or may not experience symptoms

PTH, Parathyroid hormone; *TSH,* thyroid-stimulating hormone; T_3, triiodothyronine.

common nonspecific symptoms, fatigue and depression, often are accompanied by other manifestations such as changes in energy level, alertness, sleep patterns, mood, affect, weight, skin, hair, personal appearance, and sexual function.

Subjective Data

The lack of clear-cut manifestations of endocrine problems requires a conscientious and detailed health history. A careful health history will yield data to help sort out possible causes and the effect of the problem on the person's life (Table 48-6).

Important Health Information

Past Health History. During an assessment, the patient should be questioned about the general state of health and if there have been any changes. In addition, the patient or significant other should be specifically questioned about previous or current endocrine abnormalities and abnormal patterns of growth and development.

Medications. The patient should be questioned about the use of all medications (both prescription and over-the-counter drugs) and the use of herbs and dietary supplements. The patient should be asked the reason for taking the drug, dose, and the length of time taken. The patient should specifically be asked about the use of hormone replacements. Information that the patient is currently taking hormone replacements such as insulin, thyroid, or corticosteroids (e.g., prednisone) helps direct the nurse regarding possible problems associated with the use of these agents. For example, corticosteroids may cause glucose intolerance in the susceptible patient by increasing glycogenolysis and insulin resistance. The side and adverse effects of many nonhormone medications can contribute to problems affecting endocrine function. For example, many drugs can affect blood glucose levels (see Chapter 49, Table 49-8).

Surgery or Other Treatments. The nurse should inquire about previous hospitalizations, surgery, chemotherapy, and radiation therapy (especially of the neck). Surgery of the brain or a severe

---

TABLE 48-6	HEALTH HISTORY Endocrine System

Health Perception–Health Management
- What is your usual day like?
- Have you noticed any changes in your ability to perform your usual activities compared with last year? 5 years ago?*

Nutritional-Metabolic
- What is your weight and height?
- How much do you want to weigh?
- Have there been any changes in your appetite or weight?*
- Have you noticed any changes in the distribution of the hair anywhere on your body?*
- Have you noticed any changes in the color of your skin, particularly on your face, neck, hands, or body creases?*
- Has the texture of your skin changed? For example, does it seem thicker and drier than it used to?*
- Have you noticed any difficulty swallowing, or are your shirts more difficult to button?*
- Do you feel more nervous than you used to? Do you notice your heart pounding, or that you sweat when you do not think you should be sweating?
- Do you have difficulty holding things because of shakiness of your hands?*
- Do you feel that most rooms are too hot or too cold? Do you frequently have to put on a sweater, or feel as though you need to open windows when others in the room seem comfortable?*

Elimination
- Do you have to get up at night to urinate? If so, how many times? Do you keep water by your bed at night?
- Have you ever had a kidney stone?*
- Describe your usual bowel pattern. Have you noted any bowel changes?*
- Do you use anything, such as laxatives, to help you move your bowels?*

Activity-Exercise
- What is your usual activity pattern during a typical day?
- Do you have a planned exercise program? If yes, what is it and have you had to make any changes in this routine lately? If so, why and what kinds of changes?
- Do you experience fatigue with or without activity?*

Sleep-Rest
- How many hours do you sleep at night? Do you feel rested on awakening?
- Are you ever awakened by sweating during the night?*
- Do you have nightmares?*

Cognitive-Perceptual
- How is your memory? Have you noticed any changes?
- Have you experienced any blurring or double vision?*
- When was your last eye examination?

Self-Perception–Self-Concept
- Have you noticed any changes in your physical appearance or size?*
- Are you concerned about your weight?*
- Do you feel you are able to do what you think you should be capable of doing? If not, why not?
- Does your health problem affect how you feel about yourself?*

Role-Relationship
- Are you married? Do you have any children? Do you think you are able to take care of your family, home? If no, why not?
- Where do you work? What kind of work do you do? Are you able to do what is expected of you and what you expect of yourself?

Sexuality-Reproductive
Women
- When did you start to menstruate? Was this earlier or later than other women in your family? Do you have scant, heavy, or irregular menstrual flows?
- How many children have you had? How much did they weigh at birth? Were you told you had diabetes during any pregnancy?*
- Were you able to nurse your children if you wanted to?
- Are you attempting to get pregnant but cannot?*

Men
- Have you noticed any changes in your ability to have an erection?*
- Are you trying to have children but cannot?*

Coping–Stress Tolerance
- What kind of stressors do you have?
- How do you deal with stress or problems?
- What is your support system? To whom do you turn when you have a problem?

Value-Belief
- Do you think medicine should still be taken even though you feel OK?
- Do any of your prescribed therapies cause any conflict in your value-belief system?*

*If yes, describe.

blow to the head could have resulted in pituitary or hypothalamic alterations.

Functional Health Patterns

Health Perception–Health Management Pattern. Inquiry should be made about the patient's general health care and health care behaviors. Such an inquiry might result in the identification of vague, nonspecific symptoms that could suggest an endocrine problem.

Heredity can play a major role in the occurrence of endocrine problems. The patient should be questioned about the following conditions in family members: diabetes mellitus or insipidus; hyperthyroidism or hypothyroidism, goiter; hypertension or hypotension; obesity; infertility; growth problems; *pheochromocytoma* (neoplastic tumor of the adrenal medulla or sympathetic ganglia); autoimmune diseases (e.g., Addison's disease); and adrenal hyperplasia. Asking the question "Are there any other members of your family who have, or have had, a similar problem?" will assist in uncovering evidence of a familial tendency.

Nutritional-Metabolic Pattern. Because a major function of the endocrine system is regulating metabolism and maintaining homeostasis, the patient with endocrine dysfunction will often experience alterations in nutritional-metabolic patterns. Reported changes in appetite and weight can indicate endocrine dysfunction. Weight loss with increased appetite may indicate hyperthyroidism or diabetes mellitus, particularly type 1. Weight loss with decreased appetite may indicate hypopituitarism, hypocortisolism, or *gastroparesis* (decreased gastric motility and emptying due to autonomic neuropathy) from diabetes mellitus. Weight gain may indicate hypothyroidism and, if the weight gain is concentrated in the truncal area, hypercortisolism. In addition, weight gain in a genetically susceptible patient may increase the risk for type 2 diabetes mellitus.

Difficulty swallowing or a change in neck size may indicate a thyroid disorder or inflammation. Questions related to increased sympathetic nervous system activity (e.g., nervousness, palpitations, sweating, tremors) may assist the nurse in identifying a thyroid disorder or pheochromocytoma. Heat or cold intolerance may indicate hyperthyroidism or hypothyroidism, respectively.

The patient should also be asked about changes to his or her skin or hair. Hair distribution and skin and hair color and texture can all indicate endocrine dysfunction. Hair loss can indicate hypopituitarism, hypothyroidism, hypoparathyroidism, or increased testosterone and other androgens. Increased body hair may indicate hypercortisolism. Decreased skin pigmentation can occur in hypopituitarism, hypothyroidism, and hypoparathyroidism, whereas increased skin pigmentation, particularly in sun-exposed areas, can indicate hypocortisolism. A patient with hypothyroidism or excess growth hormone may complain of coarse, leathery skin. A patient with hyperthyroidism may comment about fine, silky hair.

Elimination Pattern. Because maintenance of fluid balance is a major role of the endocrine system, questions related to elimination patterns may uncover endocrine dysfunction. For example, increased thirst and urination can indicate diabetes mellitus or insipidus. The patient should be asked about the frequency and consistency of bowel movements. Frequent defecation may indicate hyperthyroidism. Large-volume, watery stools or fecal incontinence may indicate autonomic neuropathy of diabetes mellitus. Constipation is also seen in patients with diabetes mellitus, as well as in hypothyroidism, hypoparathyroidism, and hypopituitarism.

Activity-Exercise Pattern. The nurse should ask about energy levels, particularly as compared with the patient's past energy level. Fatigue and hyperactivity are two common problems associated with endocrine problems. The major effect of endocrine dysfunction on the activity-exercise pattern is an inability to maintain previous activity levels.

Sleep-Rest Pattern. It is important that the nurse obtain a detailed sleep history. Sleep disturbances are frequently seen in endocrine dysfunction. The patient with diabetes mellitus or insipidus will complain of nocturia, which can severely disrupt normal sleep patterns. The patient with type 1 diabetes mellitus on a tight glucose control regimen who complains of sweating or nightmares may be experiencing hypoglycemia. The hyperthyroid patient may complain of inability to sleep, as may one with hypercortisolism. The patient with hypothyroidism, hypocortisolism, or hypopituitarism may tell the nurse of sleeping all the time, yet still being fatigued.

Cognitive-Perceptual Pattern. A patient with an endocrine dysfunction will frequently manifest apathy and depression. The nurse can question both the patient and significant other to determine if any cognitive changes are present. Memory deficits and an inability to concentrate are common in endocrine disorders. A patient report of visual changes such as blurring or double vision could be an indication of endocrine problems.

Self-Perception–Self-Concept Pattern. Endocrine disorders may affect the patient's self-perception because of associated physical changes affecting appearance. Changes in weight, size, and level of fatigue should be determined. The chronicity of many endocrine disorders and need for continued therapy can affect the patient's self-perception. The patient can be asked to describe the effects of the present illness on self-perception.

Role-Relationship Pattern. The nurse should ask whether there have been any changes in the patient's ability to maintain roles at home, at work, or in the community. Often the patient with an endocrine disorder will be unable to sustain life's roles. However, in most cases the patient can be advised that, with adequate management, previous roles can be resumed. This can be very reassuring for the patient and family.

Sexuality-Reproductive Pattern. The development of abnormal secondary sex characteristics (e.g., facial hair in a woman or decreased need for shaving in a man) should be documented. Problems with menstruation and pregnancy in a woman may indicate an endocrine disorder. Consequently, a detailed history of menstruation and pregnancy should be obtained. Menstrual irregularities are seen in disorders of the ovaries and in disorders of the pituitary, thyroid, and adrenal glands. A female patient with a history of large babies may have had undiagnosed gestational diabetes, which may put her at a higher risk to develop diabetes mellitus. A history of inability to lactate may indicate a pituitary disorder.

Male sexual dysfunction is also frequently seen in endocrine disorders. It usually takes the form of impotence, although retrograde ejaculation can occur. Infertility in either sex warrants a full reproductive and endocrine workup.

Coping–Stress Tolerance Pattern. Stressors of all kinds affect the endocrine system. Areas that can cause a great deal of stress should be investigated. These would include job stresses, role stresses, and financial stresses. Usual coping patterns and support systems are also discussed. The nurse then determines whether previous coping patterns are still successful and if support systems are meeting the patient's current needs.

Value-Belief Pattern. When dealing with a patient with a chronic condition, identification of the patient's value-belief patterns can assist the health care team to identify appropriate regimens. This is particularly important in a condition such as diabetes mellitus, which may require major lifestyle changes for successful management. Other endocrine disorders, such as hypothyroidism or hypocortisolism, can be easily managed with oral medication taken faithfully. Identification of a patient's ability to make lifestyle changes or take daily medication (and increase this medication as indicated) is an important nursing function.

Objective Data

Most endocrine glands are inaccessible to direct examination. With the exception of the thyroid and male gonads, the glands are deeply encased in the body, protected against injury and trauma. However, assessment can be accomplished using a variety of objective data. It is imperative that the nurse understand the actions of hormones so that the function of a gland can be assessed by monitoring the target tissue.

Physical Examination. It is important to keep in mind that the endocrine system affects every body system. Clinical manifestations of endocrine function vary significantly depending on the gland involved. Specific clinical findings for the various endocrine problems are discussed in Chapters 49 and 50. Regardless of the type of endocrine dysfunction, the following general examination procedure should be followed.

Vital Signs. A full set of vital signs is taken at the beginning of the examination. Variations in temperature may be associated with thyroid dysfunction. Cardiovascular changes such as tachycardia, bradycardia, hypotension, or hypertension may be seen with a variety of endocrine-related problems.

Height and Weight. Assessment of the endocrine system includes a history of growth and development patterns, weight distribution and changes, and comparisons of these factors with normal findings. Growth pattern abnormalities suggest problems associated with growth hormone. Changes in weight also may be associated with endocrine dysfunction. Thyroid disorders and diabetes mellitus are examples of endocrine disorders that can affect body weight. Body mass index (BMI) is a height-to-weight ratio used to assess nutritional status (see Chapter 41, Fig. 41-4).

It may also be helpful to compare the patient's current body weight with her or his usual body weight in order to assess changes. Weight change (%) is calculated by dividing the current body weight by usual body weight and multiplying by 100. Weight change greater than 5% in 1 month, 7.5% in 3 months, or 10% in 6 months is considered severe.[11]

Mental-Emotional Status. Throughout the examination the patient's orientation, alertness, memory, affect, personality, anxiety, and appropriateness of dress and speech pattern should be objectively assessed. Endocrine disorders can commonly cause changes in mental and emotional status.

Integument. The nurse should note the color and texture of the skin, hair, and nails. The overall skin color should be noted, as well as pigmentation and possible ecchymosis. Hyperpigmentation of the skin (particularly on the knuckles, elbows, knees, genitalia, and palmar creases) is a classic finding in Addison's disease, but also is seen with ACTH-producing tumors and acromegaly.[12] The skin should be palpated for skin texture and presence of moisture. The hair distribution should be examined not only on the head, but also on the face, trunk, and extremities. The appearance and texture of the hair should be examined. Dull, brittle hair; excessive hair growth; or hair loss may indicate endocrine dysfunction.

Head. The size and contour of the head should be inspected. Facial features should be symmetric. Eyes should be inspected for position, symmetry, shape and eye movement, opacity over the lens, lid lag, and edema. Visual acuity should also be checked because changes may be associated with a pituitary tumor. In the mouth, the nurse should inspect the buccal mucosa and the condition of teeth, malocclusion and mottling, tongue size, and *fasciculations* (localized, uncoordinated, uncontrollable twitching of a single muscle group).

Neck. When inspecting the thyroid gland, observation should be made first in the normal position (preferably with side lighting), then in slight extension, and then as the patient swallows some water. The trachea should be midline and the neck should appear symmetric. Any unusual bulging over the thyroid area should be noted. If there is no noticeable enlargement of the thyroid gland, palpation can be done. (Because palpation can trigger the release of thyroid hormones, palpation should be deferred in the patient with a visibly enlarged thyroid gland.) When an enlarged thyroid is noted, the lateral lobes should be auscultated with the stethoscope bell to determine the presence of a bruit.

The thyroid gland is difficult to palpate. Thyroid palpation requires considerable practice, as well as validation by a more experienced examiner. Water should always be available for the patient to swallow as part of this examination. There are two acceptable approaches to thyroid palpation: anterior or posterior. For anterior palpation the nurse stands in front of the patient, with the patient's neck flexed. The nurse places the thumb horizontally with the upper edge along the lower border of the cricoid cartilage. The thumb is then moved over the isthmus as the patient swallows water. The fingers are then placed laterally to the anterior border of the sternocleidomastoid muscle, and each lateral lobe is palpated before and while the patient swallows water.

For posterior palpation the examiner stands behind the patient. With the thumbs of both hands resting on the nape of the patient's neck, the nurse uses the index and middle fingers of both hands to feel for the thyroid isthmus and for the anterior surfaces of the lateral lobes. To facilitate the examination of each lobe and to relax the neck muscles, the nurse asks the patient to flex the neck slightly forward and to the right. The thyroid cartilage is displaced to the right by the left hand and fingers. The nurse palpates with the right hand after placing the thumb deep and behind the sternocleidomastoid muscle with the index and middle fingers in front of it; the area is palpated with the right hand (Fig. 48-12). While this is done, the patient is asked to

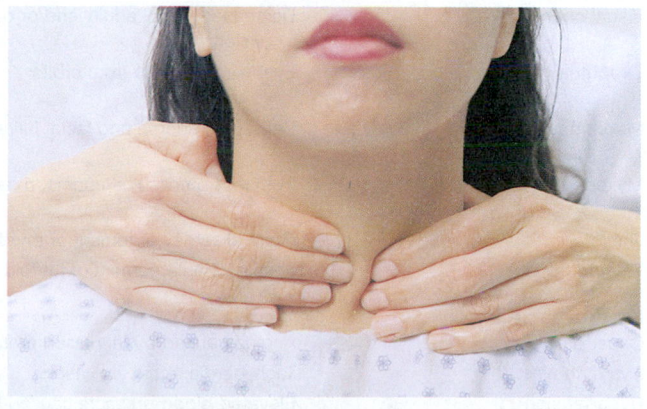

FIG. 48-12 Posterior palpation of the thyroid gland.

swallow water. This procedure is then repeated on the left side. The thyroid is palpated for its size, shape, symmetry, and tenderness and for any nodules.

In a normal person the thyroid is often not palpable. If palpable, it usually feels smooth, with a firm consistency, and is not tender with gentle pressure. Nodules, enlargement, asymmetry, or hardness is abnormal, and the patient should be referred for further evaluation.

Thorax. The thorax should be inspected for shape and characteristics of the skin. The presence of gynecomastia in men should be noted. Lung sounds and heart sounds are auscultated, noting the presence of adventitious lung sounds or extra heart sounds.

Abdomen. There are no specific abdominal examination findings for endocrine dysfunction other than skin characteristics and hyperactive or hypoactive bowel sounds.

Extremities. The size, shape, symmetry, and general proportion of hand and feet size should be assessed. The skin should be inspected for changes in pigmentation and presence of lesions and edema. Muscle strength should be evaluated, as well as deep tendon reflexes. In the upper extremities, the presence of tremors is assessed by placing a piece of paper on the outstretched fingers, palm down.

Genitalia. The hair distribution pattern should be inspected. A diamond pattern in women is an abnormal finding and may indi-cate endocrine dysfunction. For males, the testes should be palpated; for females, any clitoral enlargement should be noted.

Common assessment abnormalities related to the endocrine system are presented in Table 48-7.

DIAGNOSTIC STUDIES OF THE ENDOCRINE SYSTEM

Accurately performed laboratory tests and radiologic examinations contribute to the diagnosis of an endocrine problem. Laboratory tests usually involve blood and urine testing. Ultrasound may be used as a screening tool to localize endocrine growths such as thyroid nodules. Radiologic tests include regular x-ray, computed tomography (CT), and magnetic resonance imaging (MRI). With all diagnostic testing, the nurse is responsible for explaining the procedure to the patient and family. Diagnostic studies common to the endocrine system are presented in Table 48-8.

Laboratory Studies

Laboratory studies used to diagnose endocrine problems may include direct measurement of the hormone level, or they may involve an indirect indication of gland function by evaluating blood or urine components affected by the hormone (e.g., electrolytes).

TABLE 48-7	COMMON ASSESSMENT ABNORMALITIES Endocrine System	
Finding	**Description**	**Possible Etiology and Significance**
Integument		
Hyperpigmentation	Darkening of the skin, particularly in creases and skinfolds	Addison's disease caused by increased secretion of melanocyte-stimulating hormone
Striae	Purplish red marks below the skin surface—usually seen on abdomen, breasts, and buttocks	Cushing syndrome
Changes in skin texture	Thick, cold, dry skin	Hypothyroidism
	Thick, leathery, oily skin	Growth hormone excess (acromegaly)
	Warm, smooth, moist skin	Hyperthyroidism
Changes in hair distribution	Hair loss	Hypothyroidism, hyperthyroidism, decreased pituitary secretion
	Diminished axillary and pubic hair	Cortisol deficiency
	Hirsutism (excessive facial hair on women)	Cushing syndrome, prolactinoma (a pituitary tumor)
Skin ulceration	Areas of ulcerated skin, most commonly found on the legs and feet	Peripheral neuropathy and peripheral vascular disease are contributory factors in the development of diabetic foot ulcers
Edema	Generalized edema	Mucopolysaccharide accumulation in tissue in hypothyroidism
Head, Neck		
Visual changes	Decreased visual acuity and/or decreased peripheral vision	Pituitary gland enlargement/tumor leads to pressure on optic nerve
Exophthalmos	Eyeball protrusion from orbits	Occurs in hyperthyroidism as result of fluid accumulation in eye and retroorbital tissue
Moon face	Periorbital edema and facial fullness	Cushing syndrome as a result of increased cortisol secretion
Myxedema	Puffiness, periorbital edema, masklike affect	Hydrophilic mucopolysaccharides infiltrate dermis in patients with hypothyroidism
Goiter	Generalized enlargement of thyroid gland	Hyperthyroidism, hypothyroidism, iodine deficiency
Thyroid nodule(s)	Localized enlargement of thyroid gland(s)	May be benign or malignant
Cardiovascular		
Chest pain	Angina caused by increased metabolic demands	Hyperthyroidism
Dysrhythmias	Tachycardia, atrial fibrillation	Hypothyroidism, hyperthyroidism, pheochromocytoma
Hypertension	Elevated blood pressure caused by increased metabolic demands and catecholamines	Hyperthyroidism, pheochromocytoma, Cushing syndrome

ADH, Antidiuretic hormone.

Hormones with fairly constant basal levels (e.g., T_4) require only a single measurement. Notation of sample time on the laboratory slip and sample is important for hormones with circadian or sleep-related secretion (e.g., cortisol). Evaluation of other hormones may require multiple blood sampling such as in suppression (e.g., dexamethasone) and stimulation (e.g., glucose tolerance) tests. In these situations, it is often necessary to obtain intravenous access to administer medications and fluids and to draw multiple blood samples.

Pituitary Studies. Disorders associated with the pituitary gland can manifest in a wide variety of ways because of the number of hormones produced. There are many diagnostic studies that evaluate these hormones either directly or indirectly. The studies used to assess function of the anterior pituitary hormones relate to GH, prolactin, FSH, LH, TSH, and ACTH.

Thyroid Studies. A number of tests are available to evaluate thyroid function. The most sensitive and accurate laboratory test is measurement of TSH; thus it is often recommended as a first diagnostic test for evaluation of thyroid function.[13] Common additional tests ordered in the presence of abnormal TSH include total T_4, free T_4, and total T_3. Free T_4 is the unbound thyroxine and is a more accurate reflection of thyroid function than total T_4. Less common tests that help in the differentiation of various types of thyroid disease include T_3, free T_3 resin uptake, thyroid autoantibodies, thyroid scanning, ultrasound, and biopsy. These tests are done to help differentiate various types of thyroid disorders.

Parathyroid Studies. The only hormone secreted by the parathyroid glands is PTH. Because the function of PTH is to regulate serum calcium and phosphate levels, abnormalities in PTH se-

TABLE 48-7	*COMMON ASSESSMENT ABNORMALITIES* Endocrine System—cont'd	

Finding	Description	Possible Etiology and Significance
Musculoskeletal		
Changes in muscular strength or muscle mass	Generalized weakness and/or fatigue	Common symptoms associated with many endocrine problems, including pituitary, thyroid, parathyroid, and adrenal dysfunctions; diabetes mellitus; diabetes insipidus
	Decreased muscle mass	Specifically seen in those with growth hormone deficiency and in Cushing syndrome secondary to protein wasting
Enlargement of bones and cartilage	Coarsening of facial features; increases in size of hands and feet over a period of several years	Gradual enlargement and thickening of bony tissue occurs with growth hormone excess in adults as seen in acromegaly
Nutrition		
Changes in weight	Weight loss	Hyperthyroidism caused by increases in metabolism, diabetic ketoacidosis
Altered glucose levels	Weight gain	Hypothyroidism, Cushing syndrome
	Increased serum glucose	Diabetes mellitus, Cushing syndrome, growth hormone excess
Neurologic		
Lethargy	State of mental sluggishness or somnolence	Hypothyroidism
Tetany	Intermittent involuntary muscle spasms usually involving the extremities	Severe calcium deficiency that can occur with hypoparathyroidism
Seizure	Sudden involuntary contraction of muscles	Consequence of a pituitary tumor; fluid and electrolyte imbalance associated with excessive ADH secretion; complications of diabetes mellitus; severe hypothyroidism
Increased deep tendon reflexes	Hyperreflexia	Hyperthyroidism, hypoparathyroidism
Gastrointestinal		
Constipation	Passage of infrequent hard stools	Hyperthyroidism, hypothyroidism; hyperparathyroidism caused by calcium imbalances
Reproductive		
Changes in reproductive function	Menstrual irregularities, decreased libido, decreased fertility, impotence	Reproductive function is significantly affected by various endocrine abnormalities, including pituitary hypofunction, growth hormone excess, thyroid dysfunction, and adrenocortical dysfunction
Other		
Polyuria	Excessive urinary output	Diabetes mellitus (secondary to hyperglycemia) or diabetes insipidus (associated with decreased ADH)
Polydipsia	Excessive thirst	Extreme water losses in diabetes mellitus (with severe hyperglycemia) and diabetes insipidus
Decreased urine output	ADH leads to reabsorption of water from kidney tubules	Syndrome of inappropriate antidiuretic hormone (SIADH)
Thermoregulation	Cold insensitivity	Hypothyroidism caused by a slowing of metabolic processes
	Heat intolerance	Hyperthyroidism caused by excessive metabolism

TABLE 48-8	*DIAGNOSTIC STUDIES* **Endocrine System**	

Study	**Purpose and Description***	**Nursing Responsibility**
Pituitary Studies *Serum Studies* **Growth hormone** (GH) (Somatotropin)	Evaluates GH secretion. Used to identify GH deficiency or GH excess. GH levels are affected by time of day, food intake, and stress. GH should be <5 ng/ml (5.0 mcg/L) in men and <10 ng/ml (10.0 mcg/L) in women. Values >50 ng/ml (50.0 mcg/L) suggest acromegaly.	Make sure that patient has been fasting and has not recently been emotionally or physically stressed. Indicate patient fasting status and recent activity level on the laboratory slip. Send blood sample to laboratory immediately.
Somatomedin C (insulin-like growth factor 1 [IGF-1])	Evaluates GH secretion. Provides a more accurate reflection of mean plasma concentration of GH because it is not subject to circadian rhythm and fluctuations. *Normal values* are 135-250 ng/ml; low levels indicate GH deficiency, high levels indicate GH excess.	Overnight fasting is preferred but not necessary.
Growth hormone stimulation test	Needed to adequately diagnose GH deficiency. Measures GH secretion in response to stimulation (insulin, arginine). For insulin, baseline blood levels for GH, glucose, and cortisol are obtained. Insulin is then administered intravenously; blood samples for GH are obtained 30, 60, and 90 min after insulin is administered; blood glucose levels are monitored at 15- to 30-min intervals. Blood glucose should drop to less than 40 mg/dl for effective testing. GH level should rise twofold to threefold over baseline levels. Response is subnormal or absent in GH deficiency.	Ensure patient/family understands this procedure. Patient must be NPO after midnight. Water is permitted on morning of the test. IV access is established for administration of medications and frequent blood sampling. Nurse must continually assess for hypoglycemia and hypotension. A 50% dextrose and 5% dextrose IV solution should be kept at the bedside in case severe hypoglycemia occurs.
Gonadotropin levels • Follicle-stimulating hormone (FSH) • Luteinizing hormone (LH)	Useful in distinguishing primary gonadal problems from pituitary insufficiency. Normal levels vary according to age and gender. In women, there are marked differences during menstrual cycle and in postmenopausal period. Levels are low in pituitary insufficiency and high in primary gonadal failure. *FSH* *Female:* Follicular phase: 2-15 mIU/ml Midcycle: 8-40 mIU/ml Luteal phase: 2-15 mIU/ml Postmenopause: 50-250 mIU/ml *Male:* 2-15 mIU/ml *LH* *Female:* Follicular phase: 1.68-15 IU/L Ovulatory peak: 21.9-56.6 IU/L Postmenopause: 14.2-52.3 IU/L *Male:* 1.24-7.8 IU/L	There is no special preparation of the patient. Only one blood tube is needed for both FSH and LH. Note on the laboratory slip time of menstrual cycle or whether she is postmenopausal.
Water deprivation test	Used to differentiate causes of polyuria, including central diabetes insipidus (DI), nephrogenic DI, syndrome of inappropriate antidiuretic hormone (SIADH), and psychogenic polydipsia. ADH or vasopressin is administered intravenously or subcutaneously. In normal patients and those with psychogenic DI, urine osmolality and plasma osmolality are normal after ADH administration. In patients with central DI, urine osmolality increases after ADH administration. In patients with nephrogenic DI, there is no or minimal response to ADH.	Caution: Severe dehydration may occur with central or nephrogenic DI during this test. Preparation: If urine output is less than 4000 ml/24 hr, have patient discontinue fluids after midnight. If urine output is greater than 4000 ml/24 hr, begin fluid restriction as test starts. The test lasts 6 hours, usually from 6 AM to 12 noon. Obtain baseline weight and urine and plasma osmolality. Assess urine hourly for volume and specific gravity. Send hourly samples for urine osmolality. Draw sample for plasma osmolality when urine osmolality increases less than 30 mOsm/kg. If serum osmolality is greater than 288 mOsm/kg, patient is dehydrated and vasopressin should be administered. Administer 5 units of vasopressin (ADH) subcutaneously. Obtain urine osmolality 30-60 min after injection. Compare with baseline and preinjection values. Discontinue test and rehydrate if patient's weight drops more than 2 kg at any time. Rehydrate with oral fluids. Check orthostatic BP and pulse after rehydration to ensure adequate fluid volume.

BP, Blood pressure; *IV,* intravenous; *NPO,* nothing by mouth.
*Note: Assay methods vary. Always check laboratory normals.

TABLE 48-8	DIAGNOSTIC STUDIES — Endocrine System—cont'd

Study	Purpose and Description	Nursing Responsibility
Pituitary Studies—cont'd *Serum Studies—cont'd* **Prolactin level**	Evaluates prolactin levels. Decreased levels in postpartum women attempting to nurse may be associated with Sheehan syndrome. *Normal values:* Males: <20 ng/ml (<20 mcg/L) Females (nonlactating): <25 ng/ml (<25 mcg/L) Levels above normal reflect potential pituitary tumor.	Draw blood within 3-4 hr after patient awakens. Specimen must be sent to the laboratory immediately. If there is a delay, the specimen is placed on ice.
Radiology **Magnetic resonance imaging** (MRI)	Examination of choice for radiologic evaluation of the pituitary gland and hypothalamus. Useful in identification of tumors involving the hypothalamus or pituitary.	Inform patient of the need to lie as still as possible during the test; explain that tests are painless and noninvasive.
Thyroid Studies *Serum Studies* **Thyroid-stimulating hormone** (TSH)	Measures levels for TSH. *Normal values* are 0.3-5.4 μU/ml (0.3-5.4 mU/L). Considered the most sensitive method for evaluating thyroid disease. Generally recommended as first diagnostic test for thyroid dysfunction.	Explain blood draw procedure to the patient. No specific preparations are necessary.
Thyroxine (T_4), **total**	Measures total serum level of T_4. Useful in evaluating thyroid function and monitoring thyroid therapy. *Normal values* are 5-12 mcg/dl (64-154 nmol/L).	See above.
Triiodothyronine (T_3)	Measures serum levels of T_3. Helpful in diagnosing hyperthyroidism if T_4 levels are normal. *Normal values:* Ages 20-50: 70-204 ng/dl (1.1-3.1 nmol/L) Ages >50: 40-180 ng/dl (0.6-2.8 nmol/L)	See above.
Free T_4	Measures active component of total T_4. *Normal values* are 0.8-2.3 ng/dl (10-30 pmol/L). Because level remains constant, this is considered a better indication of thyroid function than total T_4.	See above.
T_3 resin uptake (T_3RU)	Indirectly measures binding capacity of thyroid-binding globulin. *Normal values* are 25%-35%.	See above.
Radiology **Ultrasound**	Evaluates thyroid nodule(s) to determine if fluid filled (cystic) or solid tumor.	Explain that gel and a transducer will be used over the neck. The test will last 15 min. Neither fasting nor sedation is required.
Radioactive iodine uptake (RAIU)	Provides direct measure of thyroid activity. Useful for evaluation of functional activity of solitary thyroid nodules. Patient is given radioactive iodine either orally or intravenously. The uptake by the thyroid gland is measured with a scanner at several time intervals such as 2-4 hr and at 24 hr. The values of RAIU are expressed in percentage of uptake. For 2-4 hr *normal values* are 3%-19%; for 24 hr, they are 11%-30%.	Check for iodine allergy. Fasting usually not required. Patient should not have supplemental iodine for several weeks before the test. Thyroid medications interfere with test results.
Thyroid scan	Used to evaluate nodules of the thyroid. Radioactive isotopes are given orally or intravenously. Scanner passes over thyroid and makes graphic record of radiation emitted. Normal thyroid scan reveals homogeneous pattern with symmetric lobes. Benign nodules appear as warm spots because they take up the radionuclide; malignant tumors appear as cold spots because they tend not to take up the radionuclide.	Explain procedure to the patient; be sure patient understands that radioactive iodine taken orally is harmless. No special preparation is required.
Parathyroid hormone (PTH)	Measures PTH level in serum. Normal range depends on assay used (check with laboratory). This study must be interpreted in terms of concomitantly drawn serum calcium level.	Fasting specimen preferred. Inform patient that blood sample will be drawn. Sample must be kept on ice. Observe venipuncture site for bleeding or hematoma formation.

Continued

TABLE 48-8	*DIAGNOSTIC STUDIES* Endocrine System—cont'd	

Study	Purpose and Description	Nursing Responsibility
Parathyroid Studies *Serum Studies* Total serum calcium	Measures total serum calcium to help detect bone and parathyroid disorders. Hypercalcemia can indicate primary hyperparathyroidism, and hypocalcemia can indicate hypoparathyroidism. *Normal value:* 9.0-11.0 mg/dl or 4.5-5.5 mEq/L (2.25-2.74 mmol/L).	Inform patient that blood sample will be drawn. Observe venipuncture site for bleeding or hematoma formation. Ensure that prolonged tourniquet application does not cause falsely elevated values.
Ionized calcium	Free form of calcium unaffected by variable serum albumin levels. *Normal value:* 4.5-5.5 mg/dl or 2.25-2.75 mEq/L (1.13-1.38 mmol/L).	See above.
Serum phosphate	Measures inorganic phosphorus. Hyperphosphatemia indicates primary hypoparathyroidism or secondary causes (e.g., renal failure); hypophosphatemia indicates hyperparathyroidism. Phosphorus and calcium levels are inversely related. *Normal value:* 2.8-4.5 mg/dl (0.90-1.45 mmol/L).	Fasting preferred. Inform patient that blood sample will be drawn. Observe venipuncture site for bleeding or hematoma formation.
Adrenal Studies *Serum Studies* Cortisol	Measures amount of total cortisol in serum and evaluates status of adrenal cortex function. *Normal values:* 5-23 mcg/dl (138-635 nmol/L) at 8 AM, 3-13 mcg/dl (83-359 nmol/L) at 4 PM.	Cortisol has diurnal variation—levels are higher in the morning than in the evening. Sample should be drawn in the morning—evening samples may also be ordered. Mark time of blood draw on laboratory slip. Patient anxiety should be minimized.
Aldosterone	Aldosterone levels are drawn to evaluate for hyperaldosteronism. *Normal values:* female adults 5-30 ng/dl (0.14-0.8 nmol/L) (upright posture) and 3-10 ng/dl (0.08-0.30 nmol/L) (supine position).	Usually morning blood sample is preferred. Indicate patient position (supine, sitting, standing) during venipuncture.
Adrenocoroticotropic hormone (ACTH, corticotropin)	Measures the plasma level of ACTH. Although ACTH is a pituitary hormone, it controls adrenal cortex secretion and thus helps determine if underproduction or overproduction of cortisol is caused by dysfunction of the adrenal gland or pituitary gland. *Normal values:* morning: <80 pg/ml (18 pmol/L); evening: <50 pg/ml (<11 pmol/L).	Patient should be NPO after midnight before morning blood draw. Minimize stress. Diurnal levels correspond with variation of cortisol levels; that is, levels are higher in morning, lower in evening. ACTH is very unstable; blood tube must be placed on ice and sent to laboratory immediately.
ACTH stimulation with cosyntropin	Used to evaluate adrenal function. After baseline samples are drawn, 250 mg cosyntropin (synthetic ACTH) is given as IV or IM bolus; samples are drawn 30 and 60 min after bolus. Baseline ACTH sample is often drawn in case results are abnormal. Plasma cortisol at 60 min should be (1) greater than baseline and (2) >20 mcg/dl.	Obtain baseline cortisol level at beginning of cosyntropin infusion. Inject cosyntropin with a plastic syringe and collect blood samples in plastic heparinized tubes. Administer test with continuous-infusion method. Monitor site and rate of IV infusion. Ensure sample collection at appropriate times.
ACTH suppression (dexamethasone suppression)	Assesses adrenal function and is especially helpful if hyperactivity is suspected. Useful in evaluation of Cushing syndrome. Dexamethasone (Decadron) 2 mg is given at 11 PM to suppress secretion of corticotropin-releasing hormone. Plasma cortisol sample is drawn at 8 AM. Cortisol level <5 mcg/dl (138 nmol/L) indicates normal adrenal response (50% decrease in cortisol production).	Ensure that patient has fasted. Inform patient that blood sample will be taken. Observe venipuncture site for bleeding and hematoma formation. Do not test acutely ill patients; those under stress are not tested. ACTH may override suppression. Screen patient for drugs such as estrogen and glucocorticoids, which may give false-positive results. Ensure accurate timing of medication and sample collection.

FBS, Fasting blood sugar; *IM,* intramuscular.

cretion are reflected in the calcium and phosphate levels. For this reason, diagnostic tests for the parathyroid gland typically include PTH, serum calcium, and serum phosphate levels.

Adrenal Studies. Diagnostic tests associated with the adrenal glands focus on the three types of hormones secreted: glucocorticoids, mineralocorticoids, and androgens. These hormone levels can be measured both in blood plasma and in urine. If urine studies are done, these will usually be done as 24-hour urine collection. The major advantage of a 24-hour urine sample is that the short-term fluctuations in hormone levels seen in plasma samples are eliminated.[14]

Pancreatic Studies. The tests found in Table 48-8 are used to evaluate the metabolism of glucose. They are important in the diagnosis and management of diabetes. (Diagnostic studies for diabetes are also discussed in Chapter 49.)

TABLE 48-8	*DIAGNOSTIC STUDIES* Endocrine System—cont'd	
Study	**Purpose and Description**	**Nursing Responsibility**
Adrenal Studies—cont'd *Urine Studies* 17-Ketosteroids	Measures androgen metabolites in urine and evaluates adrenocortical and gonadal function. *Normal values: Men:* 6-20 mg/day (20-70 μmol/day) *Women:* 6-16 mg/day (21-55 μmol/day).	Instruct patient regarding 24-hr urine collection. Tell patient that specimen must be kept refrigerated or iced during collection. Determine whether preservative is required for method used.
Aldosterone	Measures urinary aldosterone level to evaluate adrenal function. Useful in determining therapy for hypertension. *Normal values:* 2-26 mcg/24 hr (5.5-72 nmol/day).	Ensure that patient is on unrestricted diet with normal salt intake and no medication for 3 wk before collection. Instruct patient regarding 24-hr urine collection.
Free cortisol	Measures free (unbound) cortisol. Preferred test to evaluate hypercortisolism. *Normal values:* <100 mcg/24 hr (276 nmol/day).	Instruct patient about 24-hr urine collection and avoidance of stressful situations and excessive physical exercise. Some drugs (e.g., reserpine, diuretics, phenothiazines, amphetamines) may elevate levels. Ensure that patient is on low-sodium diet.
Vanillylmandelic acid	Measures urinary excretion of catecholamine metabolite and is helpful in diagnosing pheochromocytoma. *Normal values* are <6.8 mg/24 hr (35 μmol/day); pheochromocytoma is indicated with values of 10-250 mg/24 hr (51-126 μmol/day).	Keep 24-hr urine collection at pH of less than 3.0 with hydrochloric acid as preservative. Keep on ice. Know that newer methods are not affected by dietary intake. Consult with laboratory or physician about patient discontinuing any drugs 3 days before urine collection.
Radiology Computed tomography (CT)	Abdominal CT is the radiologic examination of choice for the adrenal gland. Used to detect tumor and size of tumor mass or metastatic spread. Oral and/or IV contrast medium may be used.	Inform patient of procedure. Patient must lie still during the procedure. If IV contrast is used, check for iodine allergy.
Pancreatic Studies *Serum Studies* **Fasting blood glucose level**	Measures circulating glucose level. *Normal values* for adults are 70-100 mg/dl (3.9-5.5 mmol/L)	Patient should fast for at least 4-8 hr—water intake is permitted. If patient has an IV infusion containing dextrose, test is not considered valid.
Oral glucose tolerance	The 2-hr test is used to diagnose diabetes mellitus if FBS is equivocal. Patient drinks 75 g of glucose; samples for glucose are drawn immediately and at 30, 60, and 120 min. *Normal values* are <200 mg/dl (11.1 mmol/L) at 30, 60, and 90 min and <140 mg/dl (7.8 mmol/L) at 120 min. The 5-hr test is used to evaluate hypoglycemia. Patient drinks 100 g of glucose; samples of glucose are drawn immediately and at 30, 60, 90, 120, 180, 240, and 300 min. Baseline cortisol level test is done if patient becomes symptomatic. Patients with reactive hypoglycemia have adrenergic symptoms and glucose <60 mg/dl (3.3 mmol/L) between 30 min and 5 hr after glucose ingestion.	Ensure that tests are not done on patients who are malnourished, confined to bed for over 3 days, or severely stressed. Instruct patient to refrain from smoking and caffeine and to fast for 12 hr before test. Ensure that patient's diet 3 days before test included 150-300 g of carbohydrate with intake of at least 1500 cal/day. Screen for estrogens, phenytoin (Dilantin), and corticosteroids, and check for hypokalemia, which may impair glucose tolerance. Simultaneously monitor glucose levels with capillary glucose monitoring.
Capillary glucose monitoring	Used to give immediate glucose values with glucose oxidase or electrochemical methods. Capillary values (whole blood) are usually 10%-15% less than serum values.	Obtain large drop of blood from clean finger, touch strip to drop of blood (not finger), time accurately, and compare colors in good lighting, if using visual method. Use digital readout if available. Use automatic finger-puncture device if available. Be sure to change section of device that touches patients' fingers between patients.
Glycosylated hemoglobin (Hb A1C)	Measures degree of glucose control during previous 3 mon (life span of hemoglobin molecule). *Normal values* are 4%-6% (values vary widely; check with laboratory).	Inform patient that fasting is not necessary and that blood sample will be drawn. Observe venipuncture site for bleeding or hematoma formation.
Urine Studies Glucose	Estimate amount of glucose in urine by using an enzymatic method. Dipstick is dipped into the urine and read for color changes after 1 min. *Normal* results will show negative glucose in the urine.	Use freshly voided urine specimen collected at appropriate time. Know that many different drugs alter glucose readings and that errors are great if directions for timing are not followed exactly. Follow package directions.

Continued

TABLE 48-8	*DIAGNOSTIC STUDIES* Endocrine System—cont'd	
Study	**Purpose and Description**	**Nursing Responsibility**
Pancreatic Studies—cont'd **Urine Studies—cont'd** Ketones	Measures amount of acetone excreted in urine as a result of incomplete fat metabolism. Tested with a dipstick as described above. Normal value is negative or trace ketone. Positive result can indicate lack of insulin and diabetic acidosis.	Use freshly voided urine specimen. Test is often done with glucose test. Directions must be followed exactly. Certain drugs can produce false-positive and false-negative results.
Radiology Computed tomography (CT)	Abdominal CT is the radiologic examination of choice for pancreas. Used to identify tumors or cysts. Oral and/or IV contrast medium may be ordered.	Inform patient of procedure. Patient must lie still during the procedure. If IV contrast is used, check for iodine allergy.

NCLEX EXAMINATION REVIEW QUESTIONS

The number of the question corresponds to the same-numbered objective at the beginning of the chapter.

1. A characteristic common to all hormones is that they
   a. circulate in the blood bound to plasma proteins.
   b. influence cellular activity of specific target tissues.
   c. accelerate the metabolic processes of all body cells.
   d. enter cells to alter the cell's metabolism or gene expression.

2. A patient is receiving radiation therapy for cancer of the kidney. The nurse monitors the patient for signs and symptoms of damage to the
   a. pancreas.
   b. thyroid gland.
   c. adrenal glands.
   d. posterior pituitary gland.

3. A patient has a serum sodium level of 152 mEq/L (152 mmol/L). The normal hormonal response to this situation is
   a. release of ADH.
   b. release of renin.
   c. secretion of aldosterone.
   d. secretion of corticotropin-releasing hormone.

4. All cells in the body are believed to have intracellular receptors for
   a. insulin.
   b. glucagon.
   c. growth hormone.
   d. thyroid hormone.

5. When obtaining subjective data from a patient during assessment of the endocrine system, the nurse asks specifically about
   a. energy level.
   b. intake of vitamin C.
   c. employment history.
   d. frequency of sexual intercourse.

6. An appropriate technique to use during physical assessment of the thyroid gland is
   a. asking the patient to hyperextend the neck during palpation.
   b. percussing the neck for dullness to define the size of the thyroid.
   c. having the patient swallow water during inspection and palpation of the gland.
   d. using deep palpation to determine the extent of a visibly enlarged thyroid gland.

7. Endocrine disorders often go unrecognized in the older adult because
   a. symptoms are often attributed to aging.
   b. older adults rarely have identifiable symptoms.
   c. endocrine disorders are relatively rare in the older adult.
   d. older adults usually have subclinical endocrine disorders that minimize symptoms.

8. An abnormal finding by the nurse during an endocrine assessment would be
   a. blood pressure of 100/70.
   b. excessive facial hair on a woman.
   c. soft, formed stool every other day.
   d. 5 lb weight gain over last 6 months.

9. A patient has a total serum calcium level of 3 mg/dl (1.5 mEq/L). If this finding reflects hypoparathyroidism, the nurse would expect further diagnostic testing to reveal
   a. decreased serum PTH.
   b. increased serum ACTH.
   c. increased serum glucose.
   d. decreased serum cortisol levels.

REFERENCES

1. Aron DC, Findling JW, Tyrrell JB: Hypothalamus and pituitary gland. In Greenspan FS, Gardner DG: *Basic and clinical endocrinology*, New York, 2004, McGraw-Hill.
2. Eliopoulos C: *Gerontological nursing*, Philadelphia, 2005, Lippincott Williams & Wilkins.
3. Baxter JD, Ribeiro RC, Webb P: Introduction to endocrinology. In Greenspan FS, Gardner DG: *Basic and clinical endocrinology*, New York, 2004, McGraw-Hill.
4. Greenspan FS: The thyroid gland. In Greenspan FS, Gardner DG: *Basic and clinical endocrinology*, New York, 2004, McGraw-Hill.
5. Aron DC, Findling JW, Tyrell JB: Glucocorticoids and adrenal androgens. In Greenspan FS, Gardner DG: *Basic and clinical endocrinology*, New York, 2004, McGraw-Hill.
6. Guillemin R: Hypothalamic hormones a.k.a. hypothalamic releasing factors, *J Endocrinol* 184:11, 2005.
7. Styne D: Growth. In Greenspan FS, Gardner DG: *Basic and clinical endocrinology*, New York, 2004, McGraw-Hill.
8. Dadeppo A, Johnson KL: Shock states. In Wagner KD, Johnson K, Kidd PS: *High acuity nursing*, Upper Saddle River, NJ, 2006, Prentice Hall.
9. Streetman DD, Ujjaini K: Diagnosis and treatment of Graves' disease, *Am J Nurse Pract* 8:27, 2004.
10. Shoback D, Marcus R, Bihle D: Metabolic bone disease. In Greenspan FS, Gardner DG: *Basic and clinical endocrinology*, New York, 2004, McGraw-Hill.
11. Wilson SF, Giddens JF: *Health assessment for nursing practice*, St Louis, 2005, Elsevier Mosby.
12. Jarvis C: *Physical examination and health assessment*, St Louis, 2004, Elsevier Saunders.
13. American Association of Clinical Endocrinologists: Medical guidelines for clinical practice for the evaluation and treatment of hyperthyroidism and hypothyroidism, *Endocrine Practice* 8:457, 2002.
14. Pagana KD, Pagana TJ: *Diagnostic and laboratory test reference*, ed 3, St Louis, 2006, Elsevier Mosby.

RESOURCES

Resources for this chapter are listed in Chapter 49 on p. 1289 and Chapter 50 on p. 1322.

To handle yourself, use your head; to handle others, use your heart.

Donald Laird

Nursing Management
Diabetes Mellitus

49

Nancy C. Robbins, Cory A. Shaw, and Sharon L. Lewis

LEARNING OBJECTIVES

1. Describe the pathophysiology and clinical manifestations of diabetes mellitus.
2. Describe the differences between type 1 and type 2 diabetes mellitus.
3. Describe the collaborative care of the patient with diabetes mellitus.
4. Describe the role of nutrition and exercise in the management of diabetes mellitus.
5. Describe the nursing management of a patient with newly diagnosed diabetes mellitus.
6. Describe the nursing management of the patient with diabetes mellitus in the ambulatory and home care settings.
7. Identify the pathophysiology and clinical manifestations of acute and chronic complications of diabetes mellitus.
8. Explain the collaborative care and nursing management of the patient with acute and chronic complications of diabetes mellitus.

KEY TERMS

diabetes mellitus, p. 1253
diabetic ketoacidosis, p. 1278
diabetic nephropathy, p. 1285
diabetic neuropathy, p. 1285
glycemic index, p. 1267
hyperosmolar hyperglycemic syndrome, p. 1280
insulin resistance, p. 1256
lipodystrophy, p. 1263
prediabetes, p. 1255
Somogyi effect, p. 1263

Electronic Resources

Supplemental content related to Chapter 49 can be found . . .

Companion CD
- Stress-Busting Kit for Nursing Students
- Interactive Case Studies:
  - Diabetic Ketoacidosis
  - Type 2 Diabetes Mellitus
- NCLEX Examination Review Questions
- Comprehensive Glossary

Evolve Website *evolve*
http://evolve.elsevier.com/Lewis/medsurg
- Content Updates
- Key Points (Printable and CD/MP3 Download)
- Concept Map Creator
- Expanded Audio Glossary
- Key Term Flash Cards
- Customizable Nursing Care Plan: Diabetes Mellitus
- Patient and Family Instruction Guides in English and Spanish:
  - Exercise Guidelines for Patients with Diabetes Mellitus

- Foot Care for Patients with Diabetes or Peripheral Vascular Problems
- Insulin Administration
- Management of Diabetes Mellitus
- Self-Monitoring of Blood Glucose (SMBG)
- Electronic Calculators
- WebLinks

Diabetes Mellitus

Diabetes mellitus is a chronic multisystem disease related to abnormal insulin production, impaired insulin utilization, or both. Diabetes mellitus is a serious health problem throughout the world and its prevalence is increasing rapidly. In the United States an estimated 20.8 million people, or 7% of the population, have diabetes mellitus, and 41 million more people have prediabetes. More than 2 million Canadians have diabetes. Over 6 million people with diabetes mellitus are not diagnosed, and these individuals are unaware that they have the disease. Diabetes mellitus is the fifth leading cause of death in the United States, but it is likely to be underreported.[1] The annual cost of diabetes exceeds $132 billion, with $92 billion in direct medical costs.[2]

Reviewed by Carolyn M. Lowe, RN, BSN, CDE, Diabetes Educator, St. Luke's Baptist Hospital, San Antonio, Tex.; Brenda Michel, RN, EdD, Professor of Nursing, Lincoln Land Community College, Springfield, Ill., and Diabetes Educator, Southern Illinois University School of Medicine, Springfield, Ill.; and Diana Kristin Smith, RN, MSN, CDE, APRN-BC, Diabetes Clinical Nurse Specialist, Christiana Care Health System, Wilmington, Del.

The long-term complications of diabetes are what make it such a devastating disease. Diabetes is the leading cause of adult blindness, end-stage renal disease, and nontraumatic lower limb amputations. It is also a major contributing factor for heart disease and stroke. Adults with diabetes have heart disease death rates two to four times higher than adults without diabetes. The risk for stroke is also two to four times higher among people with diabetes. In addition, about 73% of adults with diabetes have hypertension.[2]

Etiology and Pathophysiology

Current theories link the causes of diabetes, singly or in combination, to genetic, autoimmune, viral, and environmental factors (e.g., stress). Regardless of its cause, diabetes is primarily a disorder of glucose metabolism related to absent or insufficient insulin supplies and/or poor utilization of the insulin that is available.

Although the American Diabetes Association (ADA) recognizes 11 different classifications of the disease, most of these types are rarely encountered in routine nursing practice. The two most common types of diabetes are classified as type 1 or type 2 diabetes mellitus (Table 49-1). Gestational diabetes, prediabetes, and secondary diabetes are other classifications of diabetes commonly seen in clinical practice (discussed later in this chapter).

Normal Insulin Metabolism. Insulin is a hormone produced by the β cells in the islets of Langerhans of the pancreas. Under normal conditions, insulin is continuously released into the bloodstream in small pulsatile increments (a basal rate), with increased release (bolus) when food is ingested (Fig. 49-1). The action of released insulin lowers blood glucose and facilitates a stable, normal glucose range of approximately 70 to 120 mg/dl (3.9 to 6.66 mmol/L). The average amount of insulin secreted daily by an adult is approximately 40 to 50 U, or 0.6 U/kg of body weight.

Other hormones (glucagon, epinephrine, growth hormone, and cortisol) work to oppose the effects of insulin and are often referred to as *counterregulatory hormones.* These hormones work to increase blood glucose levels by stimulating glucose production and output by the liver, and by decreasing the movement of glucose into the cells. Insulin and these counterregulatory hormones provide a sustained but regulated release of glucose for energy during food intake and periods of fasting and usually maintain blood glucose levels within the normal range. An abnormal production of any or all of these hormones may be present in diabetes.

Insulin is released from the pancreatic β cells as its precursor, proinsulin, and is then routed through the liver. Proinsulin is composed of two polypeptide chains, chain A and chain B, which are linked by the C-peptide chain. Insulin is formed when enzymes cleave C off, leaving the A and B chains. The presence of C peptide in serum and urine is a useful indicator of β-cell function.

Insulin promotes glucose transport from the bloodstream across the cell membrane to the cytoplasm of the cell. The rise in plasma insulin after a meal stimulates storage of glucose as glycogen in liver and muscle, inhibits gluconeogenesis, enhances fat deposition in adipose tissue, and increases protein synthesis. The fall in insulin level during normal overnight fasting facilitates the release of stored glucose from the liver, protein from muscle, and fat from adipose tissue. For this reason insulin is known as the *anabolic* or storage hormone.

Skeletal muscle and adipose tissue have specific receptors for insulin and are considered insulin-dependent tissues. Other tissues

CULTURAL AND ETHNIC HEALTH DISPARITIES
Diabetes Mellitus

- The highest incidence of diabetes is among Native Americans, 15% of whom are treated for diabetes.
- Pima Indians in Arizona have the highest rate of diabetes in the world, with 50% of adults having diabetes.
- Complications of diabetes are more common in Native Americans and African Americans than in whites.
- Complications from diabetes are the major causes of death in most Native American populations.
- The rate of end-stage renal failure is six times higher among Native Americans than among other people with diabetes.
- Amputation rates among Native Americans are three to four times higher than in other populations with diabetes.
- The incidence of diabetes is higher among African Americans and Hispanics than whites, with 10% of Hispanics and 13% of African Americans having diabetes.
- Type 2 diabetes tends to affect a younger-age population in nonwhites than in whites.

TABLE 49-1	**Characteristics of Type 1 and Type 2 Diabetes Mellitus**	
Factor	**Type 1 Diabetes Mellitus**	**Type 2 Diabetes Mellitus**
Age at onset	More common in young persons but can occur at any age	Usually age 35 yr or older but can occur at any age; Incidence is increasing in children
Type of onset	Signs and symptoms abrupt, but disease process may be present for several years	Insidious, may go undiagnosed for years
Prevalence	Accounts for 5%-10% of all types of diabetes	Accounts for 90% of all types of diabetes
Environmental factors	Virus, toxins	Obesity, lack of exercise
Primary defect	Absent or minimal insulin production	Insulin resistance, decreased insulin production over time, and alterations in production of adipokines
Islet cell antibodies	Often present at onset	Absent
Endogenous insulin	Minimal or absent	Possibly excessive; adequate but delayed secretion or reduced utilization; secretions diminish over time
Nutritional status	Thin, catabolic state	Obese or possibly normal
Symptoms	Thirst, polyuria, polyphagia, fatigue, weight loss	Frequently none, fatigue, recurrent infections
Ketosis	Prone at onset or during insulin deficiency	Resistant except during infection or stress
Nutritional therapy	Essential	Essential
Insulin	Required for all	Required for some
Vascular and neurologic complications	Frequent	Frequent

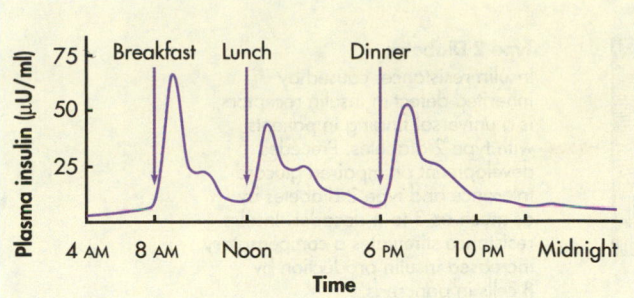

FIG. 49-1   Normal endogenous insulin secretion. In the first hour or two after meals, insulin concentrations rise rapidly in blood and peak at about 1 hour. After meals, insulin concentrations promptly decline toward preprandial values as carbohydrate absorption from the gastrointestinal tract declines. After carbohydrate absorption from the gastrointestinal tract is complete and during the night, insulin concentrations are low and fairly constant, with a slight increase at dawn.

(e.g., brain, liver, blood cells) do not directly depend on insulin for glucose transport but require an adequate glucose supply for normal function. Although liver cells are not considered insulin-dependent tissue, insulin receptor sites on the liver facilitate the hepatic uptake of glucose and its conversion to glycogen.

Type 1 Diabetes Mellitus. Formerly known as "juvenile onset" or "insulin-dependent" diabetes, *type 1 diabetes mellitus* most often occurs in people who are under 30 years of age, with a peak onset between ages 11 and 13, but it can occur at any age. The rate of type 1 diabetes is highest in Finland, Scandinavia, and Scotland; lower in southern Europe and the Middle East; and very low in Asia.[3] Typically, it is seen in people with a lean body type, although it can occur in people who are overweight.

Etiology and Pathophysiology. Type 1 diabetes is the end result of a long-standing process in which the body's own T cells attack and destroy pancreatic beta (β) cells, which are the source of the body's insulin. In addition, autoantibodies to the islet cells cause a reduction of 80% to 90% of normal β-cell function before hyperglycemia and other manifestations occur (Fig. 49-2). A genetic predisposition and exposure to a virus are factors that may contribute to the pathogenesis of immune-related type 1 diabetes. Occasionally, type 1 diabetes may be caused by nonimmune factors of unknown (idiopathic) etiologies. This type of diabetes is known as type 1B diabetes. When type 1 diabetes is caused by an immune mechanism, the disease is known as type 1A.

Predisposition to type 1 diabetes is believed to be related to human leukocyte antigens (HLAs). (See Chapter 14 for a discussion of HLAs and disease associations.) Theoretically, when an individual with certain HLA types is exposed to viral infections, the β cells of the pancreas are destroyed, either directly or through an autoimmune process. The HLA types associated with an increased risk for type 1 diabetes include HLA-DR3 and HLA-DR4 (see Genetics in Clinical Practice box).

Onset of Disease. Type 1 diabetes is associated with a long preclinical period. The islet cell autoantibodies responsible for β-cell destruction are present for months to years before the onset of symptoms. Manifestations of type 1 diabetes develop when the person's pancreas can no longer produce insulin. Once this occurs, the onset of symptoms is usually rapid, and the patient comes to the emergency department with impending or actual ketoacidosis. The patient usually has a history of recent and sudden weight loss, as well as the classic symptoms of *polydipsia* (excessive thirst), *polyuria* (frequent urination), and *polyphagia* (excessive hunger).

The individual with type 1 diabetes requires a supply of insulin from an outside source (*exogenous insulin*), such as an injection, in order to sustain life. Without insulin, the patient will develop **diabetic ketoacidosis** (DKA), a life-threatening condition resulting in metabolic acidosis. Newly diagnosed patients with type 1 diabetes often experience a remission, or "honeymoon period," soon after treatment is initiated. During this time, the patient requires very little injected insulin because β-cell mass remains sufficient for glucose control as the progressive destruction continues to occur. Eventually, as more β cells are destroyed, blood glucose levels increase, more insulin is needed, and the honeymoon period ends. The honeymoon period usually lasts 3 to 12 months, after which the person will require insulin on a permanent basis.

Prediabetes. **Prediabetes,** also known as **impaired glucose tolerance** (IGT) or **impaired fasting glucose,** is a condition in which blood glucose levels are higher than normal (>100 mg/dl [5.56 mmol/L] but <126 mg/dl [7.0 mmol/L] when fasting) but not high enough for a diagnosis of diabetes (Fig. 49-3). Most people with prediabetes are at increased risk for developing type 2 diabetes, and if no preventive measures are taken, they will usually develop it within 10 years.

Long-term damage to the body, especially the heart and blood vessels, may already be occurring in patients with prediabetes. People with prediabetes usually do not have symptoms. Individuals with prediabetes should test their blood glucose regularly and watch for the symptoms of diabetes, such as polyuria, polyphagia, or polydipsia.

If action is taken to manage blood glucose, patients with prediabetes can delay or prevent the development of type 2 diabetes. Maintaining a healthy weight, exercising regularly, and eating a healthy diet have all been found to reduce the risk of developing diabetes in people with prediabetes.

Type 2 Diabetes Mellitus. *Type 2 diabetes mellitus* is, by far, the most prevalent type of diabetes, accounting for over 90% of patients with diabetes. Type 2 diabetes usually occurs in people over 35 years of age, and 80% to 90% of patients are overweight at the time of diagnosis. However, because of the epidemic of childhood obesity, type 2 diabetes is now being seen in children. It has a tendency to run in families and probably has a genetic basis (see Genetics in Clinical Practice box).

Prevalence of type 2 diabetes increases with age, with about half of the people diagnosed being older than 55. In the past, type 2 diabetes was known as "adult-onset" diabetes. This term is no longer considered appropriate because the disease is now being seen in an increasing number of children, adolescents, and young adults.

Prevalence of type 2 diabetes is greater in some ethnic populations. African Americans, Asian Americans, Hispanic Americans, and Native Americans have a higher rate of this type of diabetes than whites. Native Americans and Alaska Natives have the highest rate of type 2 diabetes in the world, with occurrence in 15% of the population. Hispanic groups that share genes with the Native American population, such as Mexican Americans, have a higher prevalence of type 2 diabetes than Hispanic groups that have had little contact with native groups, such as Cuban Americans.[4]

Etiology and Pathophysiology. In type 2 diabetes, the pancreas usually continues to produce some *endogenous* (self-made) insulin. However, the insulin that is produced is either insufficient for the needs of the body and/or is poorly utilized by the tissues. In contrast, there is a virtual absence of endogenous insulin in type 1 diabetes. The presence of endogenous insulin is the major pathophysiologic distinction between type 1 and type 2 diabetes.

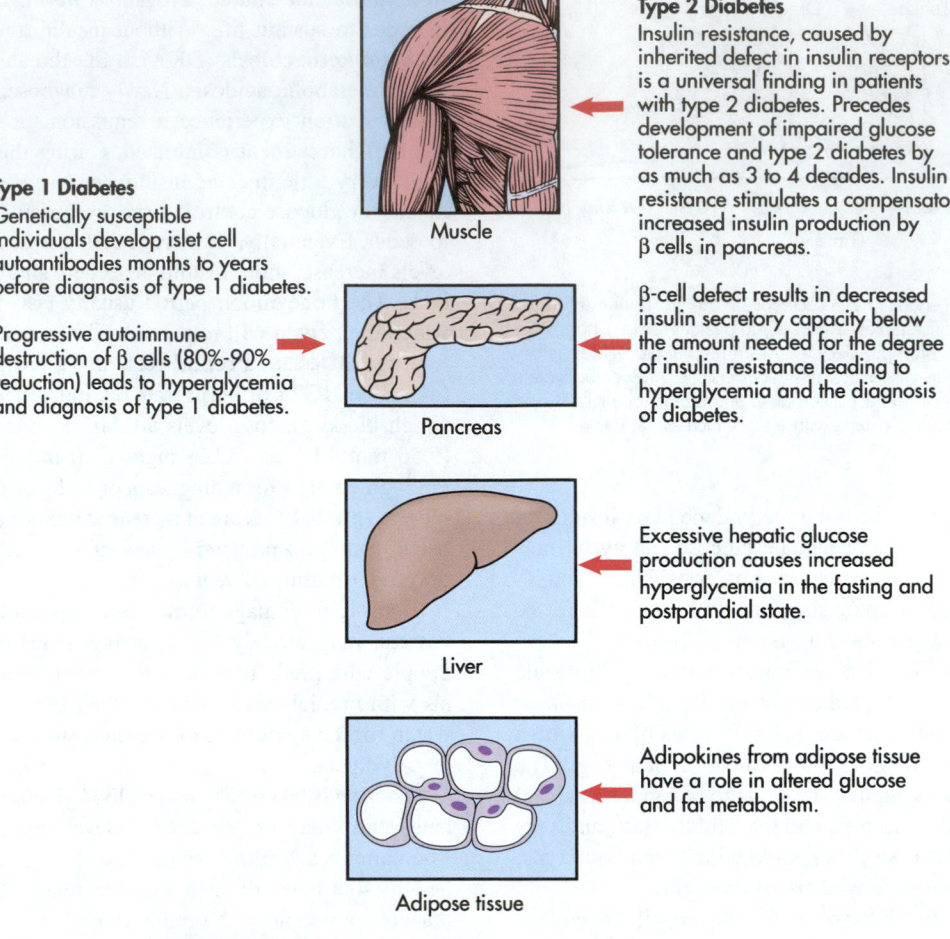

Type 1 Diabetes
Genetically susceptible individuals develop islet cell autoantibodies months to years before diagnosis of type 1 diabetes.

Progressive autoimmune destruction of β cells (80%-90% reduction) leads to hyperglycemia and diagnosis of type 1 diabetes.

Type 2 Diabetes
Insulin resistance, caused by inherited defect in insulin receptors, is a universal finding in patients with type 2 diabetes. Precedes development of impaired glucose tolerance and type 2 diabetes by as much as 3 to 4 decades. Insulin resistance stimulates a compensatory increased insulin production by β cells in pancreas.

β-cell defect results in decreased insulin secretory capacity below the amount needed for the degree of insulin resistance leading to hyperglycemia and the diagnosis of diabetes.

Muscle

Pancreas

Excessive hepatic glucose production causes increased hyperglycemia in the fasting and postprandial state.

Liver

Adipokines from adipose tissue have a role in altered glucose and fat metabolism.

Adipose tissue

FIG. 49-2   Altered mechanisms in type 1 and type 2 diabetes mellitus.

GENETICS IN CLINICAL PRACTICE

Types 1 and 2 Diabetes Mellitus

	Type 1 Diabetes Mellitus	Type 2 Diabetes Mellitus
Genetic basis	• Associations between specific human leukocyte antigens (HLA-DR3, HLA-DR4) • As many as 20 genes (and maybe more) influence susceptibility	• Majority of cases are polygenic • Monogenic genes have been identified including maturity-onset diabetes of the young (MODY) types 1-6*
Incidence	• Accounts for about 5%-10% of cases in the United States	• Accounts for about 90% of cases in the United States
Risk to offspring	• Risk to offspring of diabetic mothers is only 1%-4% • Risk to offspring of diabetic fathers is 5%-6% • Identical twin concordance is 30%-40%	• Risk to offspring is 8%-14% • Identical twin concordance is 60%-75%
Clinical implications	• Disease is a result of complex interaction of genetic, autoimmune, and environmental factors	• Disease is a result of complex genetic interactions, which are modified by environmental factors such as body weight and exercise

*MODY is a kind of type 2 diabetes that accounts for 1% to 5% of people with diabetes and is a result of a defect in a single gene.

A multitude of factors contribute toward the development of type 2 diabetes. The most powerful risk factor is believed to be obesity, specifically abdominal and visceral adiposity. Also, genetic mutations that lead to insulin resistance and a higher risk for obesity have been found in many people with type 2 diabetes. It is likely that multiple genes are involved in this complex, multifactorial disorder (see Genetics in Clinical Practice box).

Four major metabolic abnormalities have a role in the development of type 2 diabetes (see Fig. 49-2). The first factor is **insulin resistance** in glucose and lipid metabolism, which is a condition in which body tissues do not respond to the action of insulin. This is due to insulin receptors that are either unresponsive to the action of insulin and/or insufficient in number. Most insulin receptors are located on skeletal muscle, fat, and liver cells. When insulin is not

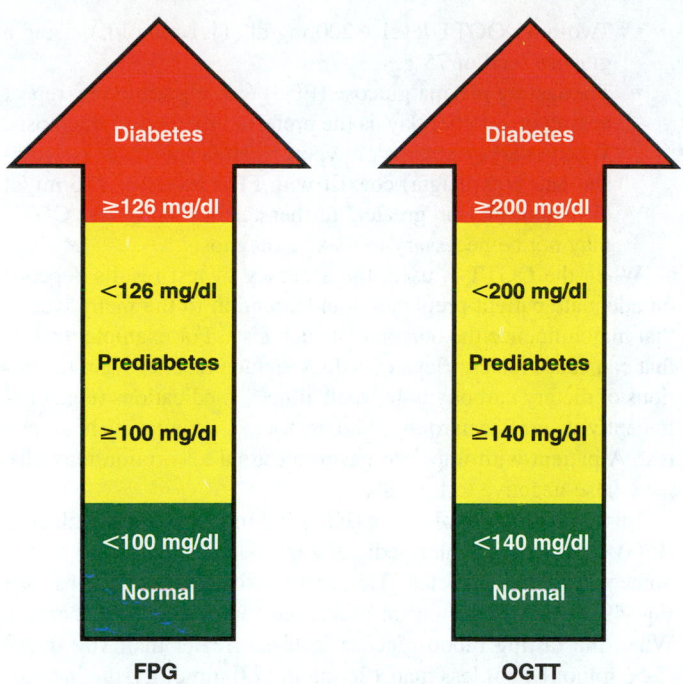

FIG. 49-3 The glucose continuum. *FPG,* Fasting plasma glucose; *OGTT,* oral glucose tolerance test.

properly used, the entry of glucose into the cell is impeded, resulting in hyperglycemia. In the early stages of insulin resistance, the pancreas responds to high blood glucose by producing greater amounts of insulin (if β-cell function is normal). This creates a temporary state of hyperinsulinemia that coexists with the hyperglycemia.

A second factor in the development of type 2 diabetes is a marked decrease in the ability of the pancreas to produce insulin, as the β cells become fatigued from the compensatory overproduction of insulin or when β-cell mass is lost. The underlying basis for the failure of β cells to adapt is unknown. However, it may be linked to the adverse effects of chronic hyperglycemia or high circulating free fatty acids.

A third factor is inappropriate glucose production by the liver. Instead of properly regulating the release of glucose in response to blood levels, the liver does so in a haphazard way that does not correspond to the body's needs at the time. However, this is not considered a primary factor in the development of type 2 diabetes.

A fourth factor is alteration in the production of hormones and cytokines by adipose tissue (adipokines). Adipokines appear to play a role in glucose and fat metabolism and are likely to contribute to the pathophysiology of type 2 diabetes. The two main adipokines believed to affect insulin sensitivity are adiponectin and leptin. Fig. 49-2 depicts the altered mechanisms in type 1 and type 2 diabetes.

Individuals with metabolic syndrome are at an increased risk for the development of type 2 diabetes. *Metabolic syndrome* is a cluster of abnormalities that act synergistically to greatly increase the risk for cardiovascular disease and diabetes. Metabolic syndrome is characterized by insulin resistance, elevated insulin levels, high levels of triglycerides, decreased levels of high-density lipoproteins (HDLs), increased levels of low-density lipoproteins (LDLs), and hypertension (see Table 41-10). Risk factors for metabolic syndrome include, but are not limited to, central obesity, sedentary lifestyle, urbanization/Westernization, and certain eth-

EVIDENCE-BASED PRACTICE

Can Weight Loss Interventions Affect the Clinical Outcome of Patients with Prediabetes?

Clinical Question

In patients who are prediabetic (P), do weight loss interventions (I) decrease the incidence of developing diabetes (O) compared with no intervention (C)?

Best Available Evidence

Systematic review of randomized controlled trials (RCTs)

Critical Appraisal and Synthesis of Evidence

- Nine RCTs (n = 5168) were reviewed.
- Dietary, physical, and behavioral interventions were used.
- For those in the intervention group, 1-year follow-up averaged a 3.3% weight loss, with a similar loss at 2 years.
- The incidence of developing diabetes was significantly lower in intervention groups compared with controls at 3-6 years of follow-up.

Conclusions

- Dietary, physical, and behavioral interventions produced significant weight loss in prediabetic individuals.
- A significant decrease in the development of diabetes was also noted.

Implications for Nursing Practice

- Inform prediabetic patients about their risk for developing diabetes and the effect of weight loss on lowering their risk status.
- Encourage and instruct prediabetic patients in modifying their diet and increasing physical activity.

Reference for Evidence

Norris SL, Zhang X, Avenell A, et al: Long-term non-pharmacological weight loss interventions for adults with pre-diabetes, Cochrane Metabolic and Endocrine Disorders Group, *Cochrane Database of Systematic Reviews* 4, 2005.

PICO: P, Patient population of interest; *I,* intervention or area of interest; *C,* comparison of interest or comparison group; *O,* outcome(s) of interest (see p. 6).

nicities (Native Americans, Hispanics, and African Americans). Overweight individuals with metabolic syndrome can prevent or delay the onset of diabetes through a program of weight loss and regular physical activity. Metabolic syndrome is discussed in further detail in Chapter 41.

Onset of Disease. Disease onset in type 2 diabetes is usually gradual. The person may go for many years with undetected hyperglycemia that might produce few, if any, symptoms. If the patient with type 2 diabetes has marked hyperglycemia (e.g., 500 to 1000 mg/dl [27.6 to 55.1 mmol/L]), a sufficient endogenous insulin supply may prevent DKA from occurring. However, osmotic fluid and electrolyte loss related to hyperglycemia may become severe and lead to hyperosmolar coma. (Complications of diabetes are discussed later in this chapter.)

Gestational Diabetes. *Gestational diabetes* develops during pregnancy and occurs in about 4% of pregnancies in the United States. It is detected at 24 to 28 weeks of gestation, usually following an oral glucose tolerance test (OGTT). Women with gestational diabetes have a higher risk for cesarean delivery, perinatal death, and neonatal complications. Although most women with gestational diabetes will have normal glucose levels within 6 weeks postpartum, their risk for developing type 2 diabetes in 5 to 10 years is increased. Nutritional therapy is considered to be the first-line therapy. If nutritional therapy alone does not achieve de-

Diabetes

sirable fasting blood glucose levels, insulin therapy is usually indicated. Gestational diabetes and management of the pregnant patient with diabetes is a specialized area not covered in detail in this chapter. The reader is advised to consult an obstetric text for information about this area.

Secondary Diabetes. Diabetes occurs in some people because of another medical condition or due to the treatment of a medical condition that causes abnormal blood glucose levels. Conditions that may cause secondary diabetes can result from damage to, injury to, interference with, or destruction of the pancreas. These include Cushing syndrome, hyperthyroidism, recurrent pancreatitis, cystic fibrosis, hemochromatosis, and the use of parenteral nutrition. Commonly used medications that can induce diabetes in some people include corticosteroids (prednisone), thiazides, phenytoin (Dilantin), and atypical antipsychotics (e.g., clozapine [Clozaril]). Secondary diabetes usually resolves when the underlying condition is treated. (Drugs that can alter blood glucose levels are listed in Table 49-8 later in this chapter.)

Clinical Manifestations

Type 1 Diabetes Mellitus. Because the onset of type 1 diabetes is rapid, the initial manifestations are usually acute. The classic symptoms are *polyuria, polydipsia,* and *polyphagia.* The osmotic effect of glucose produces the manifestations of polydipsia and polyuria. Polyphagia is a consequence of cellular malnourishment when insulin deficiency prevents utilization of glucose for energy. Weight loss may occur as the body cannot get glucose and turns to other energy sources, such as fat and protein. Weakness and fatigue may also be experienced, as body cells lack needed energy from glucose. Ketoacidosis, a complication associated with untreated type 1 diabetes, is associated with additional clinical manifestations that are discussed later in this chapter.

Type 2 Diabetes Mellitus. The clinical manifestations of type 2 diabetes are often nonspecific, although it is possible that an individual with type 2 diabetes will experience some of the classic symptoms associated with type 1. Some of the more common manifestations associated with type 2 diabetes include fatigue, recurrent infections, recurrent vaginal yeast or monilia infections, prolonged wound healing, and visual changes. Unfortunately, the clinical manifestations appear so gradually that an individual may blame the symptoms on another cause, such as lack of sleep or increasing age, and before the person knows it, he or she may have complications.

Complications

Complications of diabetes are discussed in detail later in this chapter.

Diagnostic Studies

Regardless of the type, the diagnosis of diabetes mellitus can be made through one of three methods. Whichever method is used, diagnosis of diabetes must be confirmed on a subsequent day by any of the three methods.[5] These methods and their criteria for diagnosis are as follows:

- Fasting plasma glucose level ≥126 mg/dl (7.0 mmol/L). *Fasting* is defined as no caloric intake for at least 8 hours.
- Random, or casual, plasma glucose measurement ≥200 mg/dl (11.1 mmol/L), plus manifestations of diabetes, such as polyuria, polydipsia, and unexplained weight loss. *Casual* is defined as any time of day without regard to the time of the last meal.

- Two-hour OGTT level ≥200 mg/dl (11.1 mmol/L), using a glucose load of 75 g.
- The fasting plasma glucose (FPG) test, confirmed by repeat testing on another day, is the preferred method of diagnosis. When overt symptoms of hyperglycemia (polyuria, polydipsia, and polyphagia) coexist with FPG levels of 126 mg/dl (7.0 mmol/L) or greater, further testing using the OGTT may not be necessary to make a diagnosis.[4]

When the OGTT is used, the accuracy of test results depends on adequate patient preparation and attention to the many factors that may influence the outcome of such tests. For example, factors that can cause falsely elevated values include recent severe restrictions of dietary carbohydrate, acute illness, medications (e.g., contraceptives, corticosteroids), and restricted activity such as bed rest. A patient with impaired gastrointestinal absorption may also have false-negative test results.

Impaired glucose tolerance (IGT) and impaired fasting glucose (IFG) represent an intermediate stage between normal glucose homeostasis and diabetes. This stage is called prediabetes (see Fig. 49-3 and discussion on prediabetes earlier in this chapter). When the fasting blood glucose level is greater than 100 mg/dl (5.56 mmol/L) but less than 126 mg/dl (7.0 mmol/L), the individual is considered to have IFG. Similarly, IGT is classified as a 2-hour plasma glucose level higher than normal but lower than that considered diagnostic for diabetes mellitus (between 140 and 199 mg/dl [7.82 and 11.2 mmol/L]).[4]

Measurement of glycosylated hemoglobin, also known as the *hemoglobin A1C* (A1C) test, is useful in determining glycemic levels over time. A1C tests are used by diabetic patients and health care providers to monitor success of treatment and to make changes in treatment modalities. It is not used as a diabetes diagnostic test. The test works by showing the amount of glucose that has been attached to hemoglobin molecules over their life span. When blood glucose is elevated over time, the amount of glucose attached to the hemoglobin molecule increases and remains attached to the red blood cell (RBC) for the life of the cell (approximately 120 days). Therefore a glycosylated hemoglobin test indicates the overall glucose control for the previous 90 to 120 days.[4]

All patients with diabetes should have regular assessments of A1C done. Major studies have demonstrated that people with diabetes who can maintain near-normal A1C levels over time have a greatly reduced risk for the development of retinopathy, nephropathy, and neuropathy. For people with diabetes, the ideal A1C goal is 7.0% or less according to the American Diabetes Association.[4] The American College of Endocrinology recommends an A1C of less than 6.5%. Diseases affecting RBCs (e.g., sickle cell anemia) can affect the A1C results and should be taken into consideration in the interpretation of this test result.

Collaborative Care

The goals of diabetes management are to reduce symptoms, promote well-being, prevent acute complications of hyperglycemia, and prevent or delay the onset and progression of long-term complications. These goals are most likely to be met when the patient is able to maintain blood glucose levels as near to normal as possible. Diabetes is a chronic disease that requires daily decisions about food intake, blood glucose testing, medication, and exercise. Patient teaching, which enables the patient to become the most active participant in his or her own care, is essential for a successful treatment plan. Nutritional therapy, drug therapy, exercise, and self-monitoring

EVIDENCE-BASED PRACTICE

Can Group-Based Educational Programs Improve the Health of Diabetic Patients?

Clinical Question
In patients with diabetes (P), will involvement in group-based education (I) as compared with routine care (C) improve their clinical outcomes (O)?

Best Available Evidence
Systematic review of randomized controlled trials (RCTs)

Critical Appraisal and Synthesis of Evidence
- Eleven RCTs (n = 1532) of adults with type 2 diabetes who were in regular group educational sessions led by a health care professional were reviewed.
- Follow-up sessions were conducted at 6 months, 1 year, and 2 years.
- Glycosylated hemoglobin (A1C) was decreased in those who received group education at 6, 12, and 24 months.
- Improvements were also noted in fasting blood glucose, body weight, diabetes knowledge, systolic blood pressure, and need for diabetes medication in those who received group education.

Conclusions
- Individuals enrolled in group-based education improved their diabetic health.
- One out of every five individuals attending group-based education was able to reduce his or her diabetes medication.

Implications for Nursing Practice
- Encourage patients to attend group-based educational programs to learn self-management strategies for diabetes.
- If group-based educational programs are not available, teach the important skills of diabetes management in a one-on-one environment.

Reference for Evidence
Deakin T, McShane CE, Cade JE, et al: Group based training for self-management strategies in people with type 2 diabetes mellitus, Cochrane Metabolic and Endocrine Disorders Group, *Cochrane Database of Systematic Reviews* 4, 2005.

PICO: P, Patient population of interest; *I*, intervention or area of interest; *C*, comparison of interest or comparison group; *O*, outcome(s) of interest (see p. 6).

TABLE 49-2

COLLABORATIVE CARE
Diabetes Mellitus

Diagnostic
History and physical examination
Blood tests, including fasting blood glucose, postprandial blood glucose, glycosylated hemoglobin (A1C), lipid profile, blood urea nitrogen and serum creatinine, electrolytes, TSH
Urine for complete urinalysis, microalbuminuria, and acetone (if indicated)
Funduscopic examination—dilated eye examination
Neurologic examination, including monofilament test for sensation to lower extremities
ECG
Blood pressure
Monitoring of weight
Doppler scan (if indicated)
Dental examination
Foot (podiatric) examination

Collaborative Therapy
Nutritional therapy (see Table 49-9)
Exercise therapy (see Tables 49-10 and 49-11)
Drug therapy
- Insulin (see Fig. 49-3 and Tables 49-3 and 49-4)
- Oral and other agents (see Table 49-7)
- Enteric-coated aspirin (325 mg)
- Angiotensin-converting enzyme (ACE) inhibitors (see Table 33-8)
- Antihyperlipidemic drugs (if indicated) (see Table 34-6)
Self-monitoring of blood glucose (SMBG)
Patient and family teaching and follow-up programs

ECG, Electrocardiogram; *TSH,* thyroid-stimulating hormone.

---

of blood glucose are the tools used in the management of diabetes (Table 49-2). The two major types of glucose-lowering agents (GLAs) used in the treatment of diabetes are insulin and oral agents (OAs). All individuals with type 1 diabetes require insulin. For some people with type 2 diabetes, a regimen of proper nutrition, regular physical activity, and maintenance of desirable body weight will be sufficient to attain an optimal level of blood glucose control. For the majority, however, drug therapy will be necessary.

Drug Therapy: Insulin

Exogenous (injected) insulin is needed when a patient has inadequate insulin to meet specific metabolic needs. People with type 1 diabetes require exogenous insulin to survive and may need up to four to five injections per day to adequately control blood glucose levels. People with type 2 diabetes, who are usually controlled with diet, exercise, and/or OAs, may require exogenous insulin temporarily during periods of severe stress such as illness or surgery.[6] However, since type 2 diabetes is a progressive disease, over time the combination of nutritional therapy, exercise, and OAs may no longer control blood glucose levels. At that point exogenous insulin will be added as a permanent part of the management plan. People with type 2 diabetes may need one, two, three, or four injections per day to adequately control their blood glucose levels.

Types of Insulin. In the past, insulin was made from beef and pork pancreas, but these forms of insulin are no longer available. Today, only human insulin is used. Human insulin is not directly harvested from human organs. Instead, it is prepared through the use of genetic engineering. The insulin is derived from common bacteria (e.g., *Escherichia coli*) or yeast cells using recombinant DNA technology (see Chapter 14, Fig. 14-20).

Insulins differ in regard to onset, peak action, and duration (Fig. 49-4) and are categorized as rapid-acting, short-acting, intermediate-acting, and long-acting insulin. The specific properties of each type of insulin are matched with the patient's diet and activity. Various combinations of these insulins can be used to tailor treatment to the patient's specific pattern of blood glucose levels, lifestyle, eating, and activity patterns. Different types of insulin are listed in Table 49-3. All insulin preparations start with regular insulin as a base. By adding zinc, acetate buffers, and protamine to insulin in various ways, the onset of activity, peak, and duration times can be manipulated. Zinc and protamine are added to make the intermediate-acting NPH (Neutral Protamine Hagedorn). These additives can cause an allergic reaction at the injection site.

Insulin Regimens. Examples of insulin regimens ranging from one injection per day to four injections per day are presented in Table 49-4. The exogenous insulin regimen that most closely mimics endogenous insulin production is the basal-bolus regimen, which uses rapid- and short-acting (bolus) insulin before meals and long-acting (basal) background insulin once a day. Other, less intense regimens can also give good glucose control for many people. Ideally, regimens should be mutually selected by the pa-

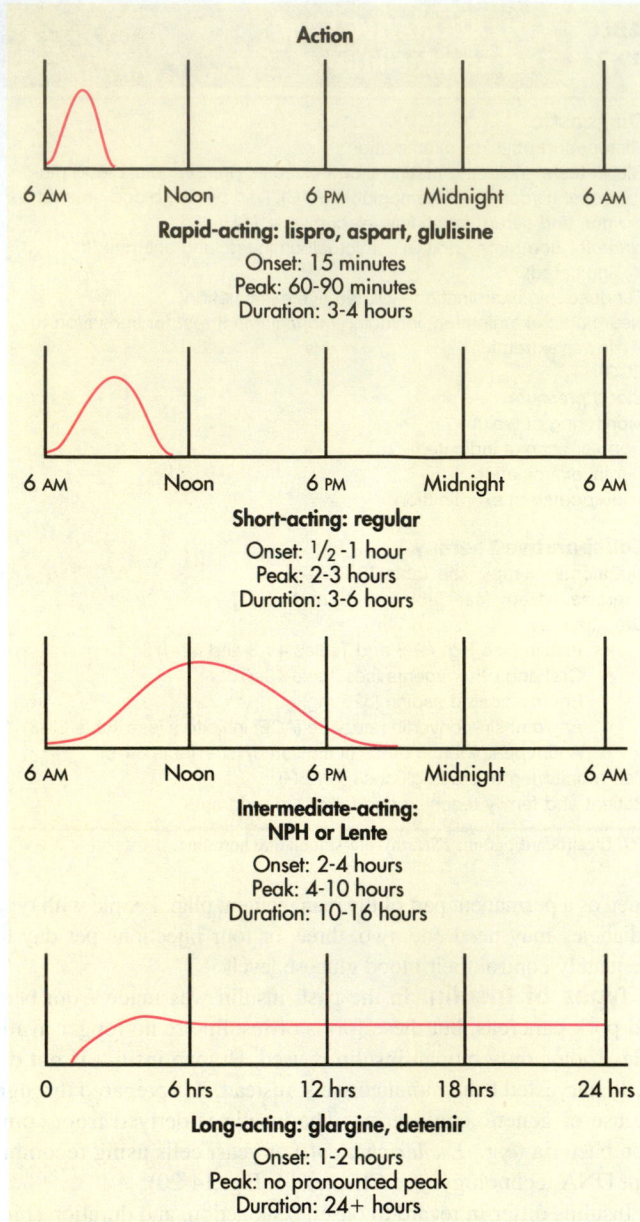

Action

Rapid-acting: lispro, aspart, glulisine
Onset: 15 minutes
Peak: 60-90 minutes
Duration: 3-4 hours

Short-acting: regular
Onset: 1/2-1 hour
Peak: 2-3 hours
Duration: 3-6 hours

**Intermediate-acting:
NPH or Lente**
Onset: 2-4 hours
Peak: 4-10 hours
Duration: 10-16 hours

Long-acting: glargine, detemir
Onset: 1-2 hours
Peak: no pronounced peak
Duration: 24+ hours

FIG. 49-4   Commercially available insulin preparations showing onset, peak, and duration of action.

TABLE 49-3	*DRUG THERAPY* Types of Insulin

Classification	Examples, Clarity of Solution
Rapid-acting insulin	lispro (Humalog), clear aspart (NovoLog), clear glulisine (Apidra), clear
Short-acting insulin	regular (Humulin R, Novolin R, ReliOn R), clear
Intermediate-acting insulin	NPH (Humulin N, Novolin N, ReliOn N), cloudy
Long-acting insulin	glargine (Lantus), clear detemir (Levemir), clear
Combination therapy (premixed)	NPH/regular 70/30* (Humulin 70/30, Novolin 70/30, ReliOn 70/30), cloudy NPH/regular 50/50* (Humulin 50/50), cloudy lispro protamine/lispro 75/25* (Humalog Mix 75/25), cloudy aspart protamine/aspart 70/30* (NovoLog Mix 70/30), cloudy

*These numbers refer to percentages of each type of insulin.

absorption. Because timing an injection 30 to 45 minutes before a meal is difficult for people to incorporate into their lifestyles, the rapid-acting insulins are often preferred by people who take insulin with meals.[8]

Long-Acting (Basal) Background Insulin. In addition to mealtime insulin, people with type 1 diabetes must also use long-acting basal (background) insulin to control blood glucose levels in between meals and overnight. Without 24-hour background insulin, people with type 1 diabetes are more prone to developing diabetic ketoacidosis. Many people with type 2 diabetes who use mealtime insulin injections also require long-acting insulin to adequately control blood glucose levels. Insulin glargine (Lantus) and detemir (Levemir) are long-acting insulins that are released steadily and continuously, and for most people do not have a peak of action (see Fig. 49-4). They are used for once-daily subcutaneous administration at bedtime or in the morning for patients with type 1 and type 2 diabetes mellitus who require basal (long-acting) insulin. Because they lack peak action time, the risk for hypoglycemia from these insulins is greatly reduced. Glargine and detemir must not be diluted or mixed with any other insulin or solution.[8,9] When patients use glargine insulin, they need to be instructed that they should not prefill the syringes with insulin and store them for future use.

Combination Therapy. For those who do not want to use more than one or two injections per day, two different insulin types can be mixed in the same syringe. Although this may be more appealing to the patient, it may not achieve the kind of blood glucose control that can be achieved with basal-bolus therapy. Short- or rapid-acting insulin is often mixed with intermediate-acting insulin to provide both mealtime and basal coverage without having to administer two separate injections. Patients may mix the two types of insulin themselves or may use a commercially premixed formula (see Table 49-3). These offer convenience to patients and are especially helpful to those who lack the visual, manual, or cognitive skills to mix insulin themselves. However, the convenience of these formulas sacrifices the potential for optimal blood glucose control, because there is less opportunity for flexible dosing based

tient and the health care provider.[7] The criteria for selection are based on the desired and feasible levels of glycemic control and the patient's lifestyle. If a less intense regimen is not giving the person optimal control, a more intense approach should be encouraged by the health care provider.

Mealtime Insulin (Bolus). To control postmeal blood glucose levels, the timing of rapid- and short-acting insulin in relation to meals is crucial. Rapid-acting synthetic insulin analogs, which include lispro (Humalog), aspart (NovoLog), and glulisine (Apidra), have an onset of action of approximately 15 minutes and should be injected 0 to 15 minutes before the meal. The rapid-acting analogs most closely mimic natural insulin secretion in response to a meal. Short-acting regular insulin has an onset of action of 30 to 60 minutes and should be injected 30 to 45 minutes before a meal to ensure that the onset of action coincides with meal

TABLE 49-4	*DRUG THERAPY* Insulin Regimens		

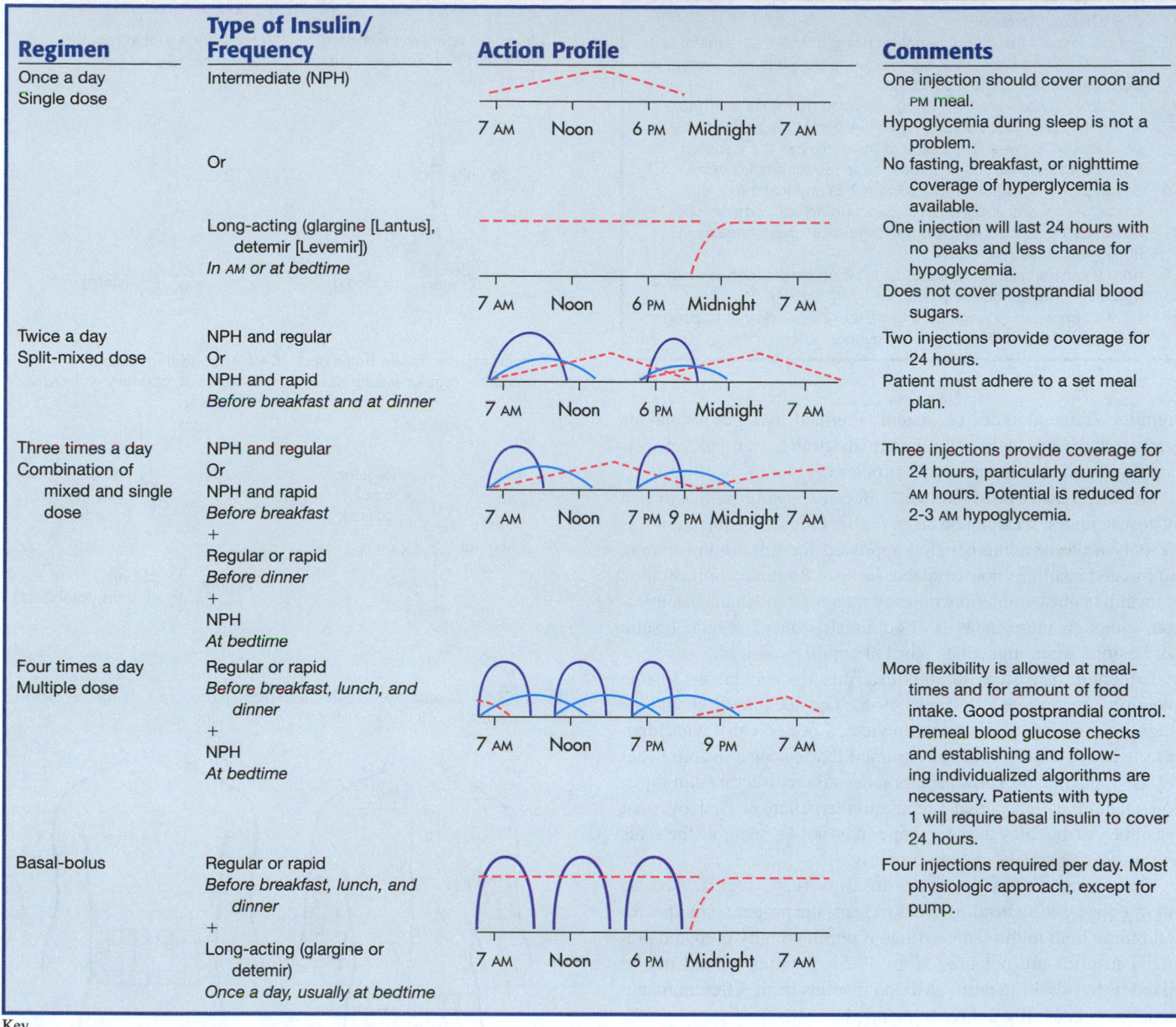

Regimen	Type of Insulin/ Frequency	Action Profile	Comments
Once a day Single dose	Intermediate (NPH)		One injection should cover noon and PM meal. Hypoglycemia during sleep is not a problem. No fasting, breakfast, or nighttime coverage of hyperglycemia is available.
	Or		
	Long-acting (glargine [Lantus], detemir [Levemir]) *In AM or at bedtime*		One injection will last 24 hours with no peaks and less chance for hypoglycemia. Does not cover postprandial blood sugars.
Twice a day Split-mixed dose	NPH and regular Or NPH and rapid *Before breakfast and at dinner*		Two injections provide coverage for 24 hours. Patient must adhere to a set meal plan.
Three times a day Combination of mixed and single dose	NPH and regular Or NPH and rapid *Before breakfast* + Regular or rapid *Before dinner* + NPH *At bedtime*		Three injections provide coverage for 24 hours, particularly during early AM hours. Potential is reduced for 2-3 AM hypoglycemia.
Four times a day Multiple dose	Regular or rapid *Before breakfast, lunch, and dinner* + NPH *At bedtime*		More flexibility is allowed at mealtimes and for amount of food intake. Good postprandial control. Premeal blood glucose checks and establishing and following individualized algorithms are necessary. Patients with type 1 will require basal insulin to cover 24 hours.
Basal-bolus	Regular or rapid *Before breakfast, lunch, and dinner* + Long-acting (glargine or detemir) *Once a day, usually at bedtime*		Four injections required per day. Most physiologic approach, except for pump.

Key

—————— Rapid-acting (lispro, aspart, glulisine) insulin.
—————— Short-acting (regular) insulin.
- - - - - - Intermediate-acting (NPH) or long-acting (glargine, detemir) insulin.

on need. Patients may also use other types of insulin in combination (i.e., long-acting and rapid-acting insulin), but these combinations must be administered separately.

Storage of Insulin. As a protein, insulin requires special storage considerations. Heat and freezing alter the insulin molecule. Insulin vials that the patient is currently using may be left at room temperature for up to 4 weeks unless the room temperature is higher than 86° F (30° C) or below freezing (less than 37° F [2° C]). Prolonged exposure to direct sunlight should be avoided. Extra insulin should be stored in the refrigerator. The same principles apply for a patient who is traveling. Insulin can be stored in a thermos or cooler to keep it cool (not frozen) if the patient is traveling in hot climates.

Prefilled syringes are stable for up to 30 days when stored in the refrigerator. This may be beneficial to patients who are sight impaired or who lack the manual dexterity to fill their own syringes at home. In these cases family members, friends, and caregivers may prefill syringes on a periodic basis. Syringes prefilled with a cloudy solution should be stored in a vertical position with the needle pointed up to avoid clumping of suspended insulin binders in the needle. When stored properly, prefilled syringes with mixed insulins should maintain potency for 30 days. Likewise, commercially prepared mixtures may be prefilled and stored for later use. Some insulin combinations are not appropriate for prefilling and storage because the mixture can alter the onset, action, and/or peak times of either of the types. Pharmacy references should be consulted as needed when mixing and

TABLE 49-5	*PATIENT AND FAMILY TEACHING GUIDE* **Insulin Therapy**

1. Wash hands thoroughly.
2. Always inspect insulin bottle before using it. Make sure that it is of proper type and concentration, expiration date has not passed, and top of bottle is in perfect condition.
3. If insulin solutions are NPH or combination therapies (see Table 49-3), they are cloudy solutions. The insulin bottle needs to be gently rolled between the palms of hands to mix the insulin.
4. Prepare insulin injection in same manner as for any injection.
5. Select proper injection site (see Fig. 49-6) and inject following procedure for any subcutaneous injection. In sites where subcutaneous tissue is adequate, inject commercial insulin needles at 90-degree angle.
6. After injecting insulin, leave needle in place for 5 seconds to ensure that all insulin has been injected.
7. Hold alcohol pad in place for a few seconds but do not massage.
8. Destroy and dispose of single-use syringe safely.

1 Wash hands.
2 Gently rotate NPH insulin bottle.
3 Wipe off tops of insulin vials with alcohol sponge.
4 Draw back amount of air into the syringe that equals total dose.

5 Inject air equal to NPH dose into NPH vial. Remove syringe from vial.

6 Inject air equal to regular dose into regular vial.

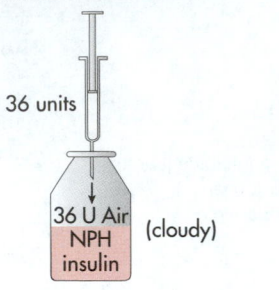
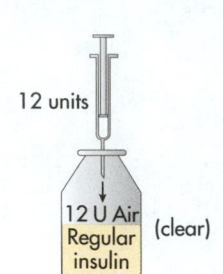

7 Invert regular insulin bottle and withdraw regular insulin dose.

8 Without adding more air to NPH vial, carefully withdraw NPH dose.

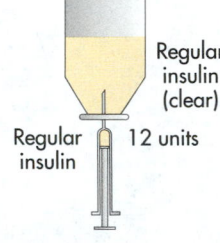
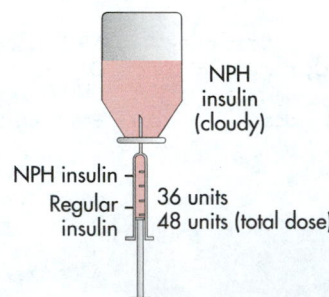

FIG. 49-5 Mixing insulins. This step-order process avoids the problem of contaminating regular insulin with intermediate-acting insulin.

prefilling different types of insulin. Prefilled syringes should be gently rolled between the palms before injection to warm the refrigerated insulin and to resuspend the particles.[8]

Administration of Insulin. Because insulin is inactivated by gastric juices, it cannot be taken orally. Previously, injection was the only route of administration approved for self-administration, but inhaled insulin is now available for use. Routine administration of insulin is most commonly done by means of subcutaneous injection, although intravenous (IV) administration of regular insulin can be done when immediate onset of action is desired.

Injection. The steps in administering a subcutaneous insulin injection are outlined in Table 49-5. The technique should be taught to new insulin users and reviewed periodically with long-term users. It should never be assumed that because insulin is being used, the patient knows and practices the correct insulin injection technique. Inaccurate preparation is often caused by poor eyesight. Air bubbles in the syringe may not be seen, or the scale on the syringe may be read improperly.

The patient receiving mixed insulins (e.g., regular and an intermediate-acting insulin) needs to learn the proper technique for combining both in the same syringe if commercially prepared pre-mixed insulins are not used (Fig. 49-5). Insulins should not be mixed if they differ in purity. Mixing insulins from different manufacturers is generally not recommended.

The speed with which peak serum concentrations are reached varies with the anatomic site for injection. The fastest absorption is from the abdomen, followed by the arm, thigh, and buttock. Appropriate sites for insulin injection are noted in Fig. 49-6, although the abdomen is the preferred site. The patient should be cautioned about injecting into a site that is to be exercised. For example, the patient should not inject insulin into the thigh and then go jogging. Exercise of the area containing the injection site, together with the increased body heat and circulation generated by the exercise, may increase the rate of absorption and speed the onset of insulin action.

Before purified human insulins were widely used, patients were advised to rotate anatomic injection sites to prevent *lipodystrophy,* a condition that produces lumps and dents in the skin from repeated injection in the same spot. The use of human insulin reduces the risk for lipodystrophy. Because of this, and because rotating sites causes variability in insulin absorption, rotation of injection sites to different anatomic sites is no longer the recom-

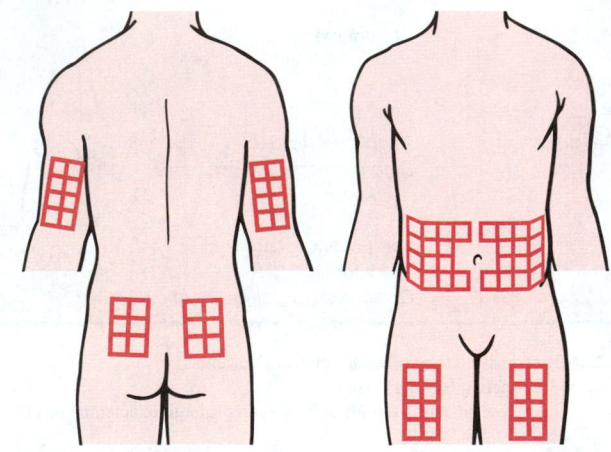

FIG. 49-6 Injection sites for insulin.

mended practice. Instead, patients are advised to rotate the injection within one particular site, such as the abdomen. Sometimes it is helpful to think of the entire abdomen as a checkerboard, with each half inch square representing an injection site as the patient rotates sites systematically across the board.

Most commercial insulin is available as U100, indicating that 1 ml contains 100 U of insulin. U100 insulin must be used with a U100-marked syringe. Disposable plastic insulin syringes are available in a variety of sizes, including 1, 0.5, and 0.3 ml. The 0.5-ml size may be used for doses of 50 U or less, and the 0.3-ml syringe can be used for doses of 30 U or less. Smaller syringes offer a num-

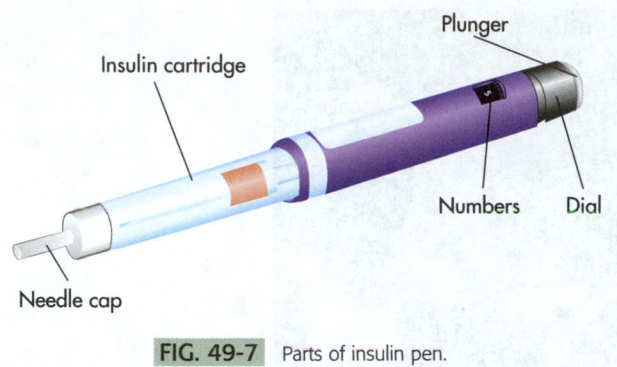

Plunger

Insulin cartridge

Numbers   Dial

Needle cap

FIG. 49-7 Parts of insulin pen.

ber of advantages. The major benefit is increased accuracy and reliability when delivering smaller doses because wider line markings are easier to see. Patients should be cautioned to check dosage lines carefully when changing syringe types because some use a scale of 1 U increments and others use a scale of 2 U increments.

Recapping should *only* be done by the person using the syringe. The nurse must never recap a needle that has been used by a patient. The use of an alcohol swab on the site before self-injection is no longer recommended. Routine hygiene such as washing with soap and rinsing with water is adequate. This applies primarily to patient self-injection technique. When injection occurs in a health care facility, policy may dictate site preparation with alcohol to prevent nosocomial infection. Injection should be performed at a 45- to 90-degree angle, depending on the thickness of the patient's fat pad.

An insulin pen is a compact portable device that serves the same function as a needle and syringe but is handier to use (Fig. 49-7). The pen is loaded with an insulin cartridge. Advantages of insulin pens are that they are less "medical" looking and contain all the necessary parts in one piece. However, before each use a needle has to be attached and then discarded after each use. Some insulin pens also serve as a blood glucose monitor.

Alternative Delivery Methods. Continuous subcutaneous insulin infusion can be administered using an **insulin pump,** a small battery-operated device that resembles a standard paging device in size and appearance (Fig. 49-8). Usually worn on the belt or under clothing, the pump is connected via plastic tubing to a catheter inserted into the subcutaneous tissue in the abdominal wall. Every 2 to 3 days the insertion site must be changed to avoid site infection and to promote good insulin absorption. The pump is then refilled with insulin and reprogrammed. The device is programmed to deliver a continuous infusion of rapid-acting or short-acting (regular) insulin 24 hours a day, known as the "basal rate." At mealtime, the user programs the pump to deliver a bolus infusion of insulin appropriate to the amount of carbohydrate ingested and to bring down high pre-meal blood glucose, if necessary. A major advantage of the insulin pump is the potential for tight glucose control. In addition, basal insulin can be decreased for increased exercise. This is possible because insulin delivery becomes very similar to the normal physiologic pattern. Pumps also offer the benefit of a more normal lifestyle, allowing users more flexibility with meal and activity patterns. The insertion site should be checked daily for redness and swelling. A disadvantage of the insulin pump is the increased frequency of blood glucose monitoring. Insulin pump users must frequently check their blood glucose, often four to six times a day or more.[10]

One alternative to the insulin pump is **intensive insulin therapy,** which consists of multiple daily insulin (MDI) injections together with frequent self-monitoring of blood glucose. The goal is to achieve a near-normal glucose level of 80 to 120 mg/dl (4.45 to 6.7 mmol/L) before meals. The Diabetes Control and Complications Trial (DCCT) demonstrated that people with type 1 diabetes who have tight glucose control through intensive management develop fewer and less severe complications.[4] Studies have shown comparable control outcomes in patients receiving intensive therapy and patients with an insulin pump. The disadvantages of MDI are that three or more injections are needed daily. Intermediate- or long-acting insulins (e.g., NPH, glargine) are used as the basal component with rapid- or short-acting insulin for boluses. Individuals using intensive insulin therapy management need to check their glucose as often as four to six times a day.

Inhaled Insulin. An alternative to injectable insulin is inhaled insulin (Exubera). Exubera is a rapid-acting, dry-powder form of insulin that is inhaled through the mouth into the lungs before eating via a specially designed inhaler. In type 1 diabetes, inhaled insulin may be added to longer-acting insulins as a replacement for short-acting insulin taken with meals. In type 2 diabetes, inhaled insulin may be used alone, along with oral medications, or with longer-acting insulins.

Like insulin, hypoglycemia is a side effect of Exubera, and patients should carefully monitor their glucose regularly. Other side effects associated with Exubera therapy include cough, shortness of breath, sore throat, and dry mouth. Exubera is not to be used if a patient smokes or has recently quit smoking (within the last 6 months). Exubera is not recommended for patients with asthma, bronchitis, or emphysema. Baseline tests for lung function are recommended after the first 6 months of treatment and every year thereafter, even if there are no pulmonary symptoms.[11]

Problems with Insulin Therapy. Hypoglycemia, allergic reactions, lipodystrophy, and Somogyi effect are problems associated with insulin therapy. Hypoglycemia is discussed in detail later in this chapter. (Guidelines for assessing patients treated with insulin are presented in Table 49-6.)

Allergic Reactions. Local inflammatory reactions to insulin may occur, such as itching, erythema, and burning around the injection site. Local reactions may be self-limiting within 1 to 3 months or may improve with a low dose of antihistamine. A true insulin allergy is rare. It is manifested by a systemic response with urticaria and possibly anaphylactic shock. Zinc or protamine used as preservatives in the insulin and the latex or rubber stoppers on the vials have been implicated in insulin reactions.

Lipodystrophy. Lipodystrophy (atrophy of subcutaneous tissue) may occur if the same injection sites are used frequently. It is best prevented by rotation of injection sites. Hypertrophy, a thickening of the subcutaneous tissue, eventually regresses if the patient does not use the site for at least 6 months. The use of hypertrophied sites may result in erratic insulin absorption.

Somogyi Effect and Dawn Phenomenon. The **Somogyi effect** is a rebound effect in which an overdose of insulin induces hypoglycemia. Usually occurring during the hours of sleep, the Somogyi effect produces a decline in blood glucose level in response to too much insulin. Counterregulatory hormones are released, stimulating lipolysis, gluconeogenesis, and glycogenolysis, which in turn produce rebound hyperglycemia and ketosis. The danger of this effect is that when blood glucose levels are measured in the morning, hyperglycemia is apparent and the patient (or the health care professional) may increase the insulin dose. The Somogyi effect is associated with the occurrence of undetected hypoglycemia during sleep, although it can happen at any time.

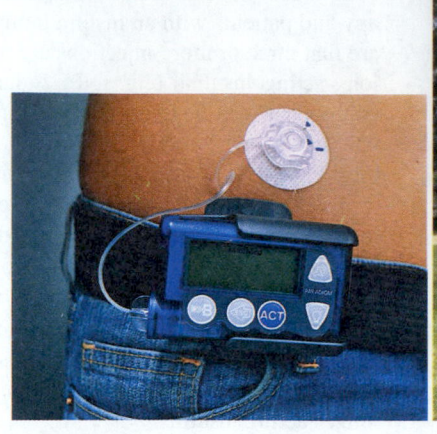

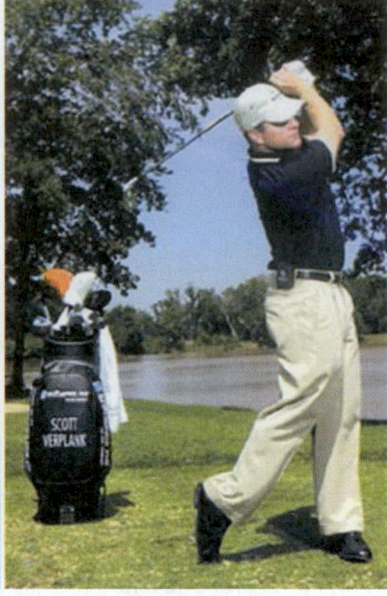

FIG. 49-8 **A,** Medtronic MiniMed insulin pump. **B,** Professional golfer Scott Verplank wearing his Medtronic MiniMed pump.

TABLE 49-6	Assessing the Patient Treated with Glucose-Lowering Agents

For Patient with Newly Diagnosed Diabetes or for Reevaluation of Medication Regimen

Cognitive	Is patient or responsible other able to understand why insulin or OAs are being used as part of diabetes management?
	Is patient or responsible other able to understand concepts of asepsis, combining insulins, insulin-OA actions, and side effects?
	Is patient able to remember to take >1 dose/day?
	Does patient take medications at right times in relation to meals?
Psychomotor	Is patient or responsible other physically able to prepare and administer accurate doses of the medication?
Affective	What emotions and attitudes are patient and responsible others displaying in regard to diagnosis of diabetes and insulin or OA treatment?

For Follow-up of GLA-Treated Patient

Effectiveness of therapy	Is patient having symptoms of hyperglycemia?
	Does blood glucose record show good or poor control?
	Is glycosylated hemoglobin consistent with glucose records?
Side effects of therapy	Is atrophy or hypertrophy present at injection sites?
	Has patient had hypoglycemic episodes? If so, how often? What time of day?
	Are there complaints of nightmares, night sweats, or early morning headaches?
	Has patient had skin rash or GI upset since taking OAs?
Self-management behaviors	If patient is having hypoglycemic episodes, how are those episodes managed?
	Has patient analyzed episodes to determine reason for hypoglycemic episodes?
	How much insulin or OA is the patient taking and at what time of day? Is patient adjusting insulin or OA dose? Under what circumstances and by how much?
	Has exercise pattern changed?
	Is patient adhering to the meal plan? Are meals taken at times corresponding to peak insulin action?

GI, Gastrointestinal; *GLA,* glucose-lowering agent; *OA,* oral agent.

The patient may report headaches on awakening and may recall night sweats or nightmares. If the Somogyi effect is suspected as a cause for early morning high blood glucose, the patient may be advised to check blood glucose levels between 2:00 and 4:00 AM to determine if hypoglycemia is present at that time. If it is, the insulin dosage affecting the early morning blood glucose is reduced.

The *dawn phenomenon* is characterized by hyperglycemia that is present on awakening in the morning due to the release of counterregulatory hormones in the predawn hours. It has been suggested that growth hormone and cortisol are possible factors in this occurrence. The dawn phenomenon affects the majority of people

with diabetes and tends to be most severe when growth hormone is at its peak in adolescence and young adulthood.

Careful assessment is required to document each phenomenon because the treatment for each differs. The treatment for Somogyi effect is less insulin. The treatment for dawn phenomenon is an adjustment in the timing of insulin administration or an increase in insulin. The assessment must include insulin dose, injection sites, and variability in the time of meals or insulin administration. In addition, the patient is asked to measure and document bedtime, nighttime (between 2:00 and 4:00 AM), and morning fasting blood glucose levels on several occasions. If the predawn levels are below 60 mg/dl (3.3 mmol/L) and signs and symptoms of hypoglycemia are present, the insulin dosage should be reduced. If the 2:00 to 4:00 AM blood glucose is high, the insulin dosage should be increased. In addition, the patient should be counseled on appropriate bedtime snacks.

Drug Therapy: Oral Agents

Oral agents (OAs) are not insulin, but they work to improve the mechanisms by which insulin and glucose are produced and used by the body. OAs work on the three defects of type 2 diabetes: (1) insulin resistance, (2) decreased insulin production, and (3) increased hepatic glucose production. OAs may be used in combination with agents from other classes or with insulin to achieve blood glucose targets. Guidelines for assessing patients receiving OAs are shown in Table 49-6.

Currently, five classes of oral medications are available to improve diabetes control for patients with type 2 diabetes.[12] These agents are listed in Table 49-7.

Sulfonylureas. Sulfonylureas include glipizide (Glucotrol, Glucotrol XL), glyburide (Micronase, DiaBeta, Glynase), and glimepiride (Amaryl). They are frequently the drugs of choice in treating type 2 diabetes because of the decreased chance of prolonged hypoglycemia. The primary action of the sulfonylureas is to increase insulin production from the pancreas. Therapy with sulfonylureas may be more effective early in the course of type 2 diabetes. About 10% of patients will experience decreased effectiveness of these medications after prolonged use.[8]

Meglitinides. Like the sulfonylureas, repaglinide (Prandin) and nateglinide (Starlix) increase insulin production from the pancreas. But because they are more rapidly absorbed and eliminated, they offer a reduced potential for hypoglycemia. When taken just before meals, pancreatic insulin production increases during and after the meal, mimicking the normal blood glucose response to eating. Patients should be instructed to take meglitinides anytime from 30 minutes before each meal right up to the time of the meal. They should not be taken if a meal is skipped.

Biguanides. Metformin (Glucophage) is a biguanide glucose-lowering agent. It can be used alone or with sulfonylureas, other OAs, or insulin to treat type 2 diabetes. The primary action of metformin is to reduce glucose production by the liver. It also enhances insulin sensitivity at the tissue level and improves glucose transport into the cells. Besides being an effective blood glucose–lowering agent, metformin has other advantages. Unlike sulfonylureas and insulin, metformin does not promote weight gain. It also has beneficial effects on plasma lipids. Metformin is also used in the prevention of type 2 diabetes in those with prediabetes, especially individuals who are obese and have a genetic predisposition toward diabetes. Combination therapy that combines metformin with another drug is available as one tablet. These combinations include metformin with glyburide (Glucovance), with rosiglitazone (Avandamet), and with glipizide (Metaglip).[13]

α-Glucosidase Inhibitors. Also known as "starch blockers," these drugs work by slowing down the absorption of carbohydrate in the small intestine. Acarbose (Precose) and miglitol (Glyset) are the available drugs in this class. Taken with the first bite of each main meal, they are most effective in lowering postprandial blood glucose. Effectiveness of these medications is measured by checking 2-hour postprandial glucose levels. Medications from this class are not effective against fasting hyperglycemia.[13]

Thiazolidinediones. Sometimes referred to as "insulin sensitizers," these agents include pioglitazone (Actos) and rosigli-

tazone (Avandia). They are most effective for people who have insulin resistance. They improve insulin sensitivity, transport, and utilization at target tissues. Because they do not increase insulin production, thiazolidinediones will not cause hypoglycemia when used alone, but the risk is still present when a thiazolidinedione is used in combination with a sulfonylurea or an insulin. Patients taking these medications may experience a secondary benefit of improved lipid profiles and blood pressure levels.[14]

> *Drug Alert* - *Thiazolidinediones*
> • *Can cause edema.*
> • *Do not use in patients with heart failure.*

Dipeptidyl Peptidase-4 (DDP-4) Inhibitor. Dipeptidyl peptidase-4 (DDP-4) inhibitors make up the newest class of glucose-lowering drugs. This class of drugs includes sitagliptin (Januvia) and vildagliptin (Galvus). The incretin hormones are normally inactivated by DDP-4. These medications inhibit DDP-4, thus slowing the inactivation of incretin hormones. Incretin hormones are released by the intestines throughout the day but levels increase in response to a meal. Incretins are part of the physiologic process that regulates glucose homeostasis. When glucose levels are normal or elevated, incretins increase insulin synthesis and release from the pancreas, as well as decrease hepatic glucose production.

Sitagliptin and vildagliptin manage type 2 diabetes by increasing and prolonging incretin levels. These drugs are glucose-dependent (i.e., they respond to the presence of elevated glucose and result in insulin release only when needed), therefore they lower the potential for hypoglycemia. The main benefit of these drugs over other medications for diabetes with similar effects is the absence of weight gain as a side effect. These drugs may be taken alone or in combination with metformin or thiazolidinediones.

Drug Therapy: Other Agents

Amylin Analog. Amylin is a hormone secreted by the β cells of the pancreas. It is normally co-secreted with insulin in response to food intake. Pramlintide (Symlin) is a synthetic analog of human amylin. It is indicated for type 1 diabetics and type 2 diabetics who have not achieved glucose control despite taking insulin at mealtimes. Pramlintide is an adjunct to insulin therapy, and not a replacement for it. When taken concurrently with insulin, it provides for better glucose control. Pramlintide works to control diabetes by three mechanisms of action: (1) it slows gastric emptying, (2) it reduces postprandial glucagon secretion, and (3) it increases satiety, thereby leading to decreased caloric intake. Pramlintide is administered subcutaneously into the thigh or abdomen. It cannot be injected into the arm because absorption from this site is too variable. The drug cannot be mixed with insulin.[15]

> *Drug Alert* - *Pramlintide (Symlin)*
> • *Can cause severe hypoglycemia when used with insulin.*
> • *Usually occurs within 3 hr following injection.*

The concurrent use of pramlintide and insulin increases the risk of severe hypoglycemia during the 3 hours after injection. Severe hypoglycemia is possible, especially in patients with type 1 diabetes. Patients should be instructed to eat a meal with at least 250 calories and keep fast-acting sugar on hand in the event that hypoglycemia develops. When pramlintide is used, the bolus dose of insulin should be reduced.

Incretin Mimetic. Exenatide (Byetta) is a synthetic peptide that stimulates the release of insulin from the pancreatic

TABLE 49-7	*DRUG THERAPY* Diabetes Mellitus		

Type	Route of Administration	Mechanism of Action	Side Effects
Sulfonylureas glipizide (Glucotrol, Glucotrol XL) glyburide (Micronase, DiaBeta, Glynase) glimepiride (Amaryl)	Oral Oral Oral	Stimulate release of insulin from pancreatic islets; decrease glycogenolysis and gluconeogenesis; enhance cellular sensitivity to insulin	Weight gain, hypoglycemia
Meglitinides repaglinide (Prandin) nateglinide (Starlix)	Oral Oral	Stimulate a rapid and short-lived release of insulin from the pancreas	Weight gain, hypoglycemia
Biguanide metformin (Glucophage, Glucophage XR, Riomet, Fortamet)	Oral	↓ Rate of hepatic glucose production; augments glucose uptake by tissues, especially muscles	Diarrhea, lactic acidosis Needs to be held for 48 hours after administration of IV contrast media
α-Glucosidase Inhibitors acarbose (Precose) miglitol (Glyset)	Oral Oral	Delay absorption of glucose from GI tract	Gas, abdominal pain, diarrhea
Thiazolidinediones pioglitazone (Actos) rosiglitazone (Avandia)	Oral Oral	↑ Glucose uptake in muscle; ↓ endogenous glucose production	Weight gain, edema Not recommended for patients with heart failure
Dipeptidyl Peptidase-4 (DDP-4) Inhibitors sitagliptin (Januvia) vildagliptin (Galvus)	Oral	Enhances the incretin system, stimulates release of insulin from pancreatic β cells, and ↓ hepatic glucose production	Upper respiratory tract infection, sore throat, headache, diarrhea
Combination Therapy Glucovance Avandamet Metaglip Duetact	Oral Oral Oral Oral	Combination of metformin and glyburide Combination of rosiglitazone and metformin Combination of metformin and glipizide Combination of pioglitazone and glimepiride	Nausea, diarrhea, abdominal pain, lactic acidosis, weight gain, hypoglycemia
Incretin Mimetic exenatide (Byetta)	Subcutaneous	Stimulates release of insulin; ↓ glucagon secretion; ↑ satiety; ↓ gastric emptying	Nausea, vomiting, hypoglycemia, diarrhea, headache
Amylin Analog pramlintide (Symlin)	Subcutaneous; only in abdomen or thigh	↓ Gastric emptying; ↓ glucagon secretion; ↓ endogenous glucose output from liver; ↑ satiety	Hypoglycemia, nausea, vomiting, decreased appetite, headache

β cells. It simulates one of the incretin hormones found to be decreased in people with type 2 diabetes. The actions created by exanatide are similar to those performed by the incretin hormone it mimics.

Its other major mechanisms of action are (1) suppression of glucagon secretion from the pancreatic β cells, which reduces glucose output from the liver; (2) reduction of food intake by increasing satiety, thereby reducing caloric intake; and (3) slowing of gastric emptying. It is not indicated for use with insulin. It is an adjunct therapy for patients with type 2 diabetes who have not achieved optimal glucose control on oral agents.[16] Exenatide is administered using a subcutaneous injection.

Other Drugs Affecting Blood Glucose Levels. Both the patient and the health care provider must be aware of drug interactions that can potentiate hypoglycemic and hyperglycemic effects. For example, β-adrenergic blockers can mask symptoms of hypoglycemia and prolong the hypoglycemic effects of insulin. Thia-

zide and loop diuretics can potentiate hyperglycemia by inducing potassium loss, although low-dose therapy with a thiazide is usually considered safe. A list of medications that may influence glycemic control is presented in Table 49-8.

Nutritional Therapy

Although nutritional therapy is the cornerstone of care for the person with diabetes, it is also the most challenging for many people. Achieving nutritional goals requires a coordinated team effort that takes into account the behavioral, cognitive, socioeconomic, cultural, and religious aspects of the person. Because of these complexities, it is recommended that a diabetes nurse educator and a registered dietitian, with expertise in diabetes management, be members of the team.

Guidelines from the American Diabetes Association (ADA) indicate that within the context of an overall healthy eating plan, a person with diabetes can eat the same foods as a person who does

TABLE 49-8	*DRUG THERAPY* **Blood Glucose Level Effects**

Glucose-Lowering Effect	Glucose-Raising Effect
acetaminophen (Tylenol)	acetazolamide (Diamox)
allopurinol (Zyloprim)	arginine
α-glucosidase inhibitors	asparaginase (Elspar)
anabolic steroids	caffeine in large doses
β-adrenergic blockers	barbiturates
biguanides	calcitonin
chloramphenicol	calcium channel blockers
clofibrate (Atromids)	cholestyramine (Questran)
insulin	clonidine (Catapres)
monoamine oxidase inhibitors	corticosteroids
phenylbutazone	cyclosporine
potassium salts	ethacrynic acid (Edecrin)
probenecid	morphine
salicylates in large doses	epinephrine
sulfonylureas	furosemide (Lasix)
thiazolidinediones	glucagon
tricyclic antidepressants	glucose
urinary acidifiers	glycerin
	glycerol
	levodopa
	lithium
	niacin
	marijuana
	nicotine
	nifedipine (Procardia)
	oral contraceptives
	phenobarbital
	phenothiazines
	phenytoin (Dilantin)
	rifampin
	tacrolimus (Prograf)
	thiazide diuretics
	urinary alkalizing agents

not have diabetes. This means that the same principles of good nutrition that apply to the general population also apply to the person with diabetes. The U.S. Department of Agriculture (USDA) Food Pyramid (see Chapter 40, Fig. 40-1 and Table 40-1) summarizes and illustrates nutritional guidelines and nutrient needs. It is also appropriate in guiding the food choices of people with diabetes. Tools used to measure the effectiveness of nutritional therapy include blood glucose, Hb A1C and lipid values, tests of renal status, and clinical measurements such as body weight and blood pressure.[17] Table 49-9 describes nutritional therapy for type 1 and type 2 diabetes.

According to the ADA, the overall goal of nutritional therapy is to assist people with diabetes in making healthy nutritional choices, eating a varied diet, and maintaining exercise habits that will lead to improved metabolic control. Additional specific goals include the following:[18]

1. Maintain blood glucose levels to as near normal as safely possible to prevent or reduce the risk for complications of diabetes.
2. Achieve lipid profiles and blood pressure levels that reduce the risk for cardiovascular disease.
3. Modify lifestyle as appropriate for the prevention and treatment of obesity, dyslipidemia, cardiovascular disease, and nephropathy.
4. Improve health through healthy food choices and physical activity.

5. Address individual nutritional needs while taking into account personal and cultural preferences and respecting the individual's willingness to change.

Type 1 Diabetes Mellitus. Meal planning should be based on the individual's usual food intake and balanced with insulin and exercise patterns. The insulin regimen should be developed with the patient's eating habits and activity pattern in mind. Day-to-day consistency in timing and amount of food eaten is important for those individuals using conventional, fixed insulin regimens. Patients using rapid-acting insulin can make adjustments in dosage before the meal based on the current blood glucose level and the carbohydrate content of the meal. Intensified insulin therapy, such as multiple daily injections or the use of an insulin pump, allows considerable flexibility in food selection and can be adjusted for deviations from usual eating and exercise habits.

Type 2 Diabetes Mellitus. The emphasis for nutritional therapy in type 2 diabetes should be placed on achieving glucose, lipid, and blood pressure goals. Because 80% to 90% of people with type 2 diabetes are overweight, caloric and fat reduction is a goal.[19]

There is no one proven strategy or method that can be uniformly recommended. A nutritionally adequate meal plan with a reduction of total fat, especially saturated fats, and simple sugars can bring about decreased calorie and carbohydrate consumption. Spacing meals is another strategy that can be adopted to spread nutrient intake throughout the day. A weight loss of 5% to 7% of body weight often improves glycemic control, even if desirable body weight is not achieved. Weight loss is best attempted by a moderate decrease in calories and an increase in caloric expenditure. Regular exercise and learning new behaviors and attitudes can help facilitate long-term lifestyle changes. Monitoring of blood glucose levels, Hb A1C, lipids, and blood pressure provide feedback on how well the goals of nutritional therapy are being met.

Food Composition. Diabetes has been called a disease of carbohydrate metabolism, but it is actually a general metabolic disorder involving three energy nutrients: carbohydrates, fats, and proteins. Therefore the nutrient balance of a diabetic diet is essential to maintenance of blood glucose levels. The nutritional energy intake should be constantly balanced with the energy output of the individual, taking into account exercise and metabolic body work. The following are general recommendations for nutrient balance, but each patient's individual meal plan should be constructed with her or his lifestyle and health goals in mind.[20]

Carbohydrates. In the diabetic meal plan, carbohydrates and monounsaturated fats should provide 45% to 65% of the total energy intake each day. Low-carbohydrate diets are not recommended for diabetes management. Carbohydrates include sugars, starches, and fiber. Foods containing carbohydrates from whole grains, fruits, vegetables, and low-fat milk should be included as part of a healthy meal plan.[21]

Glycemic index (GI) is the term used to describe the rise in blood glucose levels after a person has consumed a carbohydrate-containing food. A GI of 100 refers to the response of 50 g of glucose or white bread in a normal person without diabetes. All other food with an equivalent carbohydrate value is measured against this standard. For example, the GI of an apple is 52, regular milk 27, baked potato 93, cornflake cereal 119, and baked beans 69.

The GI of carbohydrates should be considered when choosing them in a meal plan. Foods with a high GI (e.g., potatoes, white

TABLE 49-9	**NUTRITIONAL THERAPY** Diabetes Mellitus	

Factor	Type 1 Diabetes Mellitus	Type 2 Diabetes Mellitus
Total calories	Increase in caloric intake possibly necessary to achieve desirable body weight and restore body tissues	Reduction in caloric intake desirable for overweight or obese patient
Effect of diet	Diet and insulin necessary for glucose control	Diet alone possibly sufficient for glucose control
Distribution of calories	Equal distribution of carbohydrates through meals or adjustment of carbohydrates for insulin activity	Equal distribution recommended; low-fat diet desirable; consistency of carbohydrate at meals desirable
Consistency in daily intake	Necessary for glucose control	Desirable for weight reduction and moderation of blood glucose levels
Uniform timing of meals	Crucial for NPH insulin programs; flexibility with multidose rapid-acting insulin	Desirable but not essential, unless using insulin or sulfonylureas
Intermeal and bedtime snacks	Frequently necessary	Is based on patient's eating habits and preferences; may be necessary if using insulin or sulfonylurea
Nutritional supplement for exercise programs	Carbohydrates 20 g/hr for moderate physical activities	May be necessary if patient controlled on sulfonylurea or insulin

bread) will cause a sharp rise in blood glucose, whereas those with a low GI (e.g., brown rice), steadily increase blood glucose over a longer period of time. Although the GI affects blood glucose, the total amount of carbohydrates is more important than the source.[19]

With all individuals, dietary fiber should be included as part of a healthy meal plan. There is no reason that those with diabetes should consume more or less fiber than the person who does not have diabetes.

Nutritive and nonnutritive sweeteners may be included in a healthy meal plan in moderation. Nonnutritive sweeteners include the sugar substitutes saccharine, aspartame, sucralose, and acesulfame-K.[20]

Fats. Fat should compose no more than 25% to 30% of the meal plan's total calories, with less than 7% of calories from saturated fats. Less than 300 mg/day of cholesterol and limited trans fats are also recommended as part of a healthy meal plan. Decreasing fat and cholesterol intake assists in reducing the risk for cardiovascular disease. Individuals with elevated LDL are advised to lower their saturated fat intake to 7% and cholesterol to under 200 mg/day.[20]

Protein. Protein should contribute less than 10% of the total energy consumed in those with diabetes. Protein intake for the diabetic patient should be significantly lower than the general population. Moderate to high protein intake generally is not recommended because of high saturated fat content and unnecessary stress on the kidneys to excrete excess nitrogen.[18]

Alcohol. Alcohol is high in calories, has no nutritive value, and promotes hypertriglyceridemia. In addition, it has detrimental effects on the liver (see Chapter 44). The inhibitory effect of alcohol on glucose production by the liver can cause severe hypoglycemia in patients on insulin or oral hypoglycemic medications that increase insulin secretion. Patients should be cautioned to honestly discuss the use of alcohol with their health care providers because its use can make blood glucose more difficult to control.

Moderate alcohol consumption can sometimes be safely incorporated into the meal plan if blood glucose levels are well controlled and if the patient is not on medications that will cause adverse effects. Moderate consumption is defined as one drink per day for women and two drinks per day for men. A patient can reduce the risk for alcohol-induced hypoglycemia by eating carbohydrates when drinking alcohol. The patient with diabetes should drink alcohol with food, use sugar-free mixes, and drink dry, light wines.[4]

Patient Teaching. Most often, the dietitian initially teaches the principles of the nutrition therapy prescription. Whenever possible, nurses should be prepared to work with dietitians as part of an interdisciplinary diabetes care team. In some instances, access to a dietitian is not possible for patients with limited insurance coverage or who live in remote areas. In these cases, nurses often assume responsibility for teaching basic dietary management to patients with diabetes.

The MyPyramid guide is an appropriate basic teaching tool for people with diabetes (see Chapter 40, Fig. 40-1 and Table 40-1). The stripes across the pyramid help the patient visualize the recommended amounts of foods that should be eaten from each group on a daily basis. Although MyPyramid is intended for the general public, the principles of food variation, moderate use of fats and sugars, and emphasis on exercise are also applicable to the diabetic meal plan.

An alternative method of presenting the basics of meal planning is to use what is known as the *plate method*. This simple method helps the patient visualize the amount of vegetables, starch, and meat that should fill a 9-inch plate. For each meal one half of the plate is filled with nonstarchy vegetables, one fourth is filled with a starch, and one fourth is filled with a protein. A glass of nonfat milk and a small piece of fresh fruit complete the meal. Assuming low-fat and nonfat foods are selected, following the plate method will provide 1200 to 1400 calories per day and a properly balanced meal plan.[22]

Teaching should include the patient's family and significant others whenever possible. It is most effective to direct teaching efforts to the person who will be cooking. It is important, however, that the responsibility for maintaining a diabetic diet not fall to someone other than the patient with diabetes. Reliance on another person to make health decisions fosters dependence and should be avoided except in special situations.

In an acute health care facility, the nutritional needs of the diabetic patient vary slightly from the normal meal plans. Previously, standardized calorie-level meal patterns were used, but new alternatives are now being used, such as the consistent-carbohydrate diabetes meal plan. Under this system, meal plans are not created using calorie level, but instead are created with consistent carbohydrate content. For example, every day each breakfast contains the same amount of carbohydrates as the previous day; the same method is used for lunch and dinner.[23]

Exercise

Regular, consistent exercise is considered an essential part of diabetes and prediabetes management. Exercise increases insulin receptor sites in the tissue and can have a direct effect on lowering the blood glucose levels. It also contributes to weight loss, which also decreases insulin resistance. The therapeutic benefits of regular physical activity may result in a decreased need for diabetes medicines in order to reach target blood glucose goals. Regular exercise may also help reduce triglyceride and LDL cholesterol levels, increase HDL, reduce blood pressure, and improve circulation.[24]

Any new exercise program in the diabetic patient should be started only after medical clearance and should be started slowly with gradual progression toward the desired goal. Patients who use insulin, sulfonylureas, or meglitinides are at increased risk for hypoglycemia when there is an increase in physical activity, especially if the patient exercises at the time of peak drug action or if food intake has not been sufficient to maintain adequate blood glucose levels. This can also occur if a normally sedentary patient with diabetes has an unusually active day. The glucose-lowering effects of exercise can last up to 48 hours after the activity, so it is possible for hypoglycemia to occur for that long after the activity. It is recommended that patients who use medications that can cause hypoglycemia schedule exercise about 1 hour after a meal or that they have a 10 to 15 g carbohydrate snack and check their blood glucose before exercising. Several small carbohydrate snacks can be taken every 30 minutes during exercise to prevent hypoglycemia. Patients using medications that place them at risk for hypoglycemia should always carry a fast-acting source of carbohydrate, such as glucose tablets or hard candies, when exercising. Table 49-10 gives guidelines on the number of calories burned per hour for different activities.

Although exercise is generally beneficial to blood glucose levels, strenuous activity can be perceived by the body as a stress, causing a release of counterregulatory hormones that result in a temporary elevation of blood glucose. As a result, hyperglycemia may occur in cases of poorly controlled type 2 diabetes or in patients with type 1 diabetes who exercise at a time of day when insulin action is waning. Some patients may have to inject a small bolus of rapid-acting or regular insulin if the blood glucose level is

elevated before exercising to prevent progressive hyperglycemia. Furthermore, patients should exercise with caution if the blood glucose is greater than 300 mg/dl and there are no ketones, or if the blood glucose is greater than 250 mg/dl and ketones are present in the urine.[25] Additional information about exercise and diabetes that is important for both the patient and the health care provider is provided in the patient and family teaching guide (Table 49-11).

Monitoring Blood Glucose

Self-monitoring of blood glucose (SMBG) is a cornerstone of diabetes management. By providing a current blood glucose reading, SMBG enables the patient to make self-management decisions regarding diet, exercise, and medication. SMBG is also important for detecting episodic hyperglycemia and hypoglycemia.

Portable blood glucose monitors (meters) are used at the hospital bedside and by patients who perform SMBG. A wide variety of blood glucose monitors are available (Fig. 49-9). Disposable lancets are usually used to obtain a small drop of capillary blood (usually from a finger stick) that is placed onto a reagent strip. After a specified time, the monitor displays a digital reading of the blood glucose. The technology of SMBG is a rapidly changing field with newer and more convenient systems being introduced every year (Fig. 49-10). Newer systems allow the user to collect blood from alternative sites such as the forearm or palm, but will not register rapidly changing blood glucose readings. Therefore finger sticks are still recommended if symptoms of low blood glucose are present.

Invasive approaches to glucose monitoring include the (1) Dexcom STS System and the (2) Medtronic Paradigm REAL-Time System (see Fig. 49-10). Using a sensor inserted under the skin, both systems display glucose values continuously with updated

TABLE 49-10	Activities that Affect Caloric Expenditure

Light Activity (100-200 kcal/hr)	**Moderate Activity** (200-350 kcal/hr)	**Vigorous Activity** (400-900 kcal/hr)
Driving a car	Active housework	Aerobic exercise
Fishing	Bicycling (light)	Bicycling (vigorous)
Light housework	Bowling	Hard labor
Secretarial work	Dancing	Ice skating
Teaching	Gardening	Outdoor sports
Walking casually	Golf	Running
	Roller skating	Soccer
	Walking briskly	Tennis
		Wood chopping

TABLE 49-11	**PATIENT AND FAMILY TEACHING GUIDE** **Exercise for Patients with Diabetes Mellitus**

1. Exercise does not have to be vigorous to be effective. The blood glucose–reducing effects of exercise can be attained with exercise such as brisk walking.
2. The exercises selected should be enjoyable to foster regularity.
3. The exercise session should have a warm-up period and a cool-down period. The exercise program should be started gradually and increased slowly.
4. Exercise is best done after meals, when the blood glucose level is rising.
5. Exercise plans should be individualized for each patient and monitored by the health care provider.
6. It is important to self-monitor blood glucose levels before, during, and after exercise to determine the effect exercise has on blood glucose level at particular times of the day.
   - Before exercise, if blood glucose is less than 100 mg/dl, eat a 10-15 g carbohydrate snack. After 15 to 30 minutes, retest blood glucose levels. Do not exercise if less than 100 mg/dl.
   - Before exercise, if blood glucose is over 250 mg/dl, delay exercise or if patient insists on exercising, reduce the intensity and duration by half.
   - Recheck blood glucose at the end of the exercise program.
7. Be alert to the possibility of delayed exercise-induced hypoglycemia, which may occur several hours after the completion of exercise.
8. Taking a glucose-lowering medication does not mean that planned or spontaneous exercise cannot occur.
9. It is important to compensate for extensive planned and spontaneous activity by monitoring blood glucose level to make adjustments in the insulin dose (if taken) and food intake.

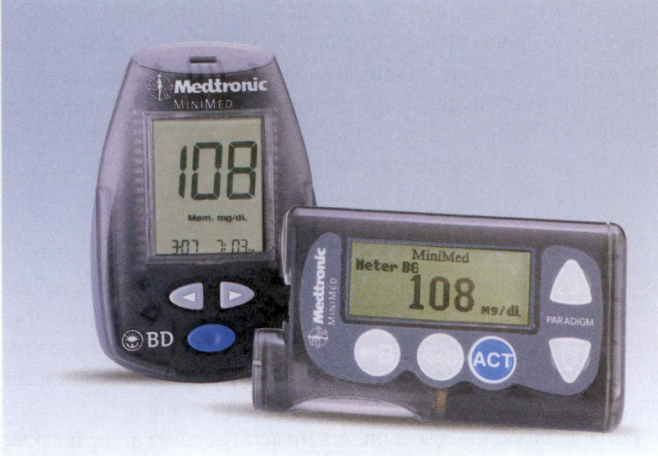

FIG. 49-9 Blood glucose monitors are used to measure blood glucose levels. Certain glucose monitors, such as Medtronic's Paradigm Link Blood Glucose Monitor *(on the left)*, can transmit wirelessly a glucose value to a "smart" insulin pump *(on the right)*. The insulin pump calculates complex math based on these measures and recommends insulin dosages to patients.

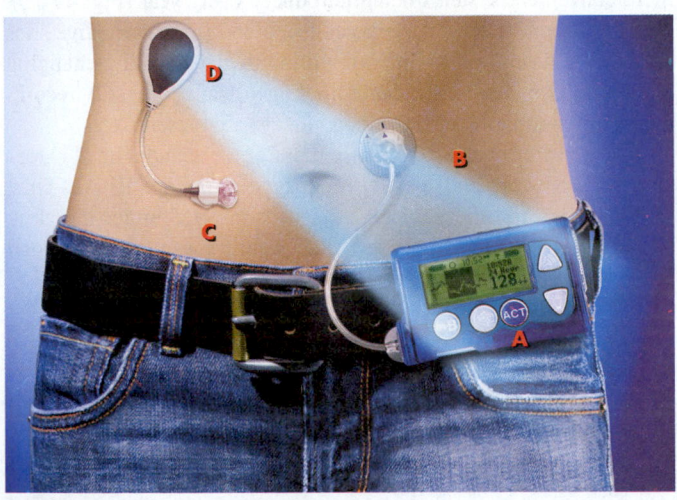

FIG. 49-10 The MiniMed Paradigm insulin pump *(A)* delivers insulin into a cannula *(B)* that sits under the skin. Continuous glucose monitoring occurs through a tiny sensor *(C)* inserted under the skin. Sensor data are sent continuously to the transmitter *(D)*. The transmitter sends data to the insulin pump through wireless technology.

values occurring every 5 minutes. The sensor is inserted by the patient using an automatic insertion device. Data are sent from the sensor to a transmitter, which displays the glucose value on either an insulin pump (Medtronic Paradigm REAL-Time system) or a pager-like receiver (Dexcom STS system). These systems assist the patient and health care provider to identify trends and track patterns. These data are particularly useful for the management of insulin therapy. The patient is alerted during episodes of hypoglycemia and hyperglycemia, allowing corrective action to be taken quickly. Both systems still require fingerstick measurements using a blood glucose monitor to calibrate the sensor and to make treatment decisions.

Noninvasive approaches to blood glucose monitoring have also been developed. The G2 Biographer from GlucoWatch is a device worn on the wrist and is available by prescription. It pulls glucose through the skin using low electric current. It then measures glucose

TABLE 49-12	**PATIENT AND FAMILY TEACHING GUIDE** **Self-Monitoring of Blood Glucose (SMBG)**

1. Wash hands in warm water. It is not necessary to clean the site with alcohol, and it may interfere with test results. Finger should be dry before puncturing it.
2. If it is difficult to obtain an adequate drop of blood for testing, warm the hands in warm water or let the arms hang dependently for a few minutes before the finger puncture is made.
3. If the puncture is made on the finger, use the side of the finger pad rather than near the center. Fewer nerve endings are along the side of the finger pad. If an alternative site is used (e.g., forearm), special equipment may be needed. Refer to manufacturer's instructions for alternative site use, except during hypoglycemic episodes.
4. The puncture should be only deep enough to obtain a sufficiently large drop of blood. Unnecessarily deep punctures may cause pain and bruising.
5. Follow monitor instructions for testing the blood.
6. Record results. Compare to personal target blood glucose goals.

levels for 13 hours and sends an alarm if the reading is abnormal. However, this device is intended to detect trends and patterns and is not currently recommended for use in making decisions about insulin dosages. Another device, Pendra, is already in use in Europe and measures glucose using radio rays directed at the skin.

The blood glucose level reported by a laboratory is sometimes higher than the patient's home glucose monitor or the hospital's portable monitor. This is because some monitors give capillary blood glucose values from whole blood (via finger stick), whereas venous samples taken in the laboratory provide plasma readings. Plasma samples, or venous samples, are approximately 10% to 12% higher. Some monitors are automatically calibrated to give a "plasma" test result (although whole blood was used for the sample) so that the home readings can be more readily compared with laboratory values. The literature accompanying a monitor will identify if that particular monitor is calibrated to give plasma or whole blood readings.

Instructions for using a blood glucose monitor also accompany each product. Because errors in monitoring technique can cause errors in management strategies, thorough patient training is crucial. Initial training should be followed up at regular intervals with reassessment. In addition, patients must be taught to use and interpret calibration and control solutions that are a part of each blood glucose monitoring kit.[26] Table 49-12 lists the steps that should be taught to the patient learning to perform SMBG.

The chief advantage of SMBG is that it supplies immediate information about blood glucose levels that can be used to make adjustments in food intake, activity patterns, and medication dosages. It also produces accurate records of daily glucose fluctuations and trends, as well as alerting the patient to acute episodes of hyperglycemia and hypoglycemia. Furthermore, it provides patients with a tool for achieving and maintaining specific glycemic goals. SMBG is recommended for all insulin-treated patients with diabetes. Other patients with diabetes frequently use SMBG to help achieve and maintain glycemic goals, as well as monitor for acute fluctuations in blood glucose.

The frequency of monitoring depends on several factors, including the patient's glycemic goals, the type of diabetes that the patient has, the patient's ability to perform the test independently, and the patient's willingness to test. Patients with type 1 diabetes typically test four times per day (before meals and at bedtime).

Those using an insulin pump may test more frequently. Patients with type 2 diabetes will have more variable and individualized testing regimens.

Testing is most often done before meals, but certain situations warrant more frequent monitoring. For example, the patient should be instructed to test blood glucose before and after exercise to determine its effects on metabolic control. This is especially important in the patient with type 1 diabetes. Blood glucose testing should also be performed whenever hypoglycemia is suspected so that immediate action can be taken if necessary. When the person with diabetes is ill, the blood glucose should be tested at 4-hour intervals to determine the effects of this stressor on the blood glucose level. Also, testing after meals helps a person see how effectively he or she judged what was eaten.[27]

SMBG is an empowering tool that allows the patient to be an active partner in the treatment of diabetes. Achieving the desired level of patient participation does require time and effort from the health care professional. The nurse involved in this aspect of management should anticipate a close working relationship with patients as they refine their techniques and learn appropriate decision making about managing their diabetes. A patient who is visually impaired, cognitively impaired, or limited in manual dexterity needs careful evaluation of the degree to which SMBG can be performed independently. Nurses working in home health and outpatient settings may need to identify caregivers who can assume this responsibility. Adaptive devices are available to help patients with certain limitations. These include talking meters and other equipment for the visually impaired, as well as devices to stabilize insulin vials and syringes for those with limitations affecting dexterity.

Pancreas Transplantation

Pancreas transplantation can be used as a treatment option for patients with type 1 diabetes mellitus. Most commonly it is done for patients who have end-stage renal disease and who have had or plan to have a kidney transplant. Kidney and pancreas transplants are often performed together, or a pancreas may be transplanted following a kidney transplant. Pancreas transplants alone are rare. If renal failure is not present, the ADA recommends that pancreas transplantation should only be considered for patients who exhibit the following three criteria: (1) a history of frequent, acute, and severe metabolic complications (e.g., hypoglycemia, hyperglycemia, ketoacidosis) requiring medical attention; (2) clinical and emotional problems with exogenous insulin therapy that are so severe as to be incapacitating; and (3) consistent failure of insulin-based management to prevent acute complications.

Successful pancreas transplantation can improve the quality of life of people with diabetes, primarily by eliminating the need for exogenous insulin, frequent blood glucose measurements, and many of the dietary restrictions imposed by the disorder. Transplantation can also eliminate the acute complications commonly experienced by patients with type 1 diabetes (e.g., hypoglycemia, hyperglycemia). However, pancreas transplantation is only partially successful in reversing the long-term renal and neurologic complications of diabetes.

Patients who undergo pancreas transplantation require lifelong immunosuppression to prevent rejection of the graft. Complications can result from immunosuppressive therapy. (Immunosuppressive therapy is discussed in Chapter 14.)

Pancreatic islet cell transplantation is another potential treatment measure. During this procedure, the islets are harvested from a single pancreas and infused into the portal vein of the recipient. With only the islets transplanted, pain and recovery time are diminished compared with whole pancreas transplants. Research is continuing to investigate the best ways to implant the islet cells and to prevent their rejection.

CULTURALLY COMPETENT CARE
DIABETES MELLITUS

Because culture can have a strong influence on dietary preferences and meal preparation practices, culturally competent care has special relevance for the care of the patient with diabetes. This is especially pertinent when considering the prevalence of diabetes in certain cultural groups. Certain ethnic groups, such as Hispanics, Native Americans, and African Americans, have a high prevalence of diabetes when compared with the general population. The increased prevalence can be attributed to genetic predisposition, environmental factors, and dietary choices.

The influences of culture on food choices and meal planning should be explored with the patient as part of the health history. When giving diet instructions, efforts should be made to consider the food preferences of the cultural group. Nutritional resources specifically designed for members of different cultural groups are available from the American Diabetes Association (see Resources at the end of the chapter).

NURSING MANAGEMENT
DIABETES MELLITUS

■ *Nursing Assessment*

Table 49-13 provides initial subjective and objective data that should be obtained from a person with diabetes mellitus. After the initial assessment, periodic patient assessments should be done on a regular basis.

■ *Nursing Diagnoses*

Nursing diagnoses related to diabetes mellitus may include, but are not limited to, those found in NCP 49-1.

■ *Planning*

The overall goals for the patient with diabetes mellitus include the following: (1) to be an active participant in the management of the diabetes regimen; (2) to experience few or no episodes of acute hyperglycemic or hypoglycemic emergencies; (3) to maintain blood glucose levels at normal or near-normal levels; (4) to prevent, minimize, or delay the occurrence of chronic complications of diabetes; and (5) to adjust lifestyle to accommodate the diabetes regimen with a minimum of stress.

■ *Nursing Implementation*

Health Promotion. The role of the nurse in health promotion and maintenance relates to the identification, monitoring, and education of the patient at risk for the development of diabetes mellitus. Obesity is the number one predictor of type 2 diabetes mellitus. The Diabetes Prevention Program found that a modest weight loss of 5% to 7% of body weight and regular exercise of 30 minutes five times a week lowered the risk of developing type 2 diabetes up to 58%.[28]

The ADA recommends routine screening for diabetes for all overweight adults over age 45. If normal, it should be repeated at

TABLE 49-13 · NURSING ASSESSMENT
Diabetes Mellitus

Subjective Data
Important Health Information

Past health history: Mumps, rubella, coxsackievirus or other viral infections; recent trauma, infection, or stress; pregnancy, gave birth to infant >9 lb; chronic pancreatitis; Cushing syndrome, acromegaly; family history of type 1 or type 2 diabetes mellitus

Medications: Use of and compliance with insulin or OAs; use of corticosteroids, diuretics, phenytoin (Dilantin)

Surgery or other treatments: Any recent surgery

Functional Health Patterns

Health perception–health management: Positive family history; malaise; date of last eye and dental examination

Nutritional-metabolic: Obesity; weight loss (type 1), weight gain (type 2); thirst, hunger; nausea and vomiting; poor healing especially involving the feet, compliance with diet in patients with previously diagnosed diabetes

Elimination: Constipation or diarrhea; frequent urination, nocturia, urinary incontinence; skin infections

Activity-exercise: Muscle weakness, fatigue

Cognitive-perceptual: Abdominal pain, headache; blurred vision; numbness or tingling of extremities; pruritus

Sexuality-reproductive: Impotence; frequent vaginal infections; decreased libido

Coping–stress tolerance: Depression, irritability, apathy

Value-belief: Commitment to lifestyle changes involving diet, medication, and activity patterns

Objective Data
Eyes

Soft, sunken eyeballs; vitreal hemorrhages, cataracts

Integumentary

Dry, warm, inelastic skin; pigmented lesions (on legs); ulcers (especially on feet), loss of hair on toes

Respiratory

Rapid, deep respirations (Kussmaul respirations)

Cardiovascular

Hypotension; weak, rapid pulse

Gastrointestinal

Dry mouth, vomiting, fruity breath

Neurologic

Altered reflexes, restlessness, confusion, stupor, coma

Musculoskeletal

Muscle wasting

Possible Findings

Serum electrolyte abnormalities; fasting blood glucose level ≥126 mg/dl (7 mmol/L); glucose tolerance test ≥200 mg/dl (11.1 mmol/L); leukocytosis; ↑ blood urea nitrogen, creatinine, triglycerides, cholesterol, LDL, VLDL; ↓ HDL; glycosylated hemoglobin ≥6%; glycosuria; ketonuria; albuminuria; acidosis

HDL, High-density lipoprotein; *LDL,* low-density lipoprotein; *OA,* oral agent; *VLDL,* very-low-density lipoprotein.

TABLE 49-14 · Criteria for Testing for Diabetes in Asymptomatic, Undiagnosed Individuals

Testing* for diabetes should be considered in all individuals at age 45 years and above, especially in those with a BMI ≥25 kg/m² and, if normal, should be repeated at 3-year intervals.

Testing* should be considered at a younger age or be carried out more frequently in individuals who are overweight (BMI ≥25 kg/m²) and have additional risk factors:

*   Have a first-degree relative with diabetes
*   Are habitually physically inactive
*   Are members of a high-risk ethnic population (African American, Hispanic, Native American, Asian American, Pacific Islander)
*   Have delivered a baby weighing >9 lb or have been diagnosed with gestational diabetes mellitus
*   Are hypertensive (≥140/90 mm Hg)
*   Have an HDL cholesterol level ≤35 mg/dl (0.90 mmol/L) and/or a triglyceride level ≥250 mg/dl (2.82 mmol/L)
*   On previous testing, had impaired glucose tolerance or increased fasting glucose
*   Have been diagnosed with polycystic ovary syndrome
*   Have a history of vascular disease
*   Have other clinical conditions associated with insulin resistance (e.g., acanthosis nigricans)

American Diabetes Association Clinical Practice Recommendations, Standards of Medical Care, *Diabetes Care* 29:S4, 2006.
BMI, Body mass index; *HDL,* high-density lipoprotein.
*Testing may include fasting plasma glucose (FPG) or oral glucose tolerance test (OGTT). The FPG is the recommended diagnostic test because of its ease of administration, convenience, acceptability to patients, and lower cost.

history. A diabetes risk test is available at *www.diabetes.org/risk-test.jsp.* A high score may indicate that a person has prediabetes or is at risk for prediabetes.

Acute Intervention. Acute situations involving the patient with diabetes include hypoglycemia, diabetic ketoacidosis (DKA), and hyperosmolar hyperglycemic syndrome (HHS). Nursing management for these situations is discussed in more detail later in this chapter. Other areas of acute intervention relate to management during stress, such as during acute illness and surgery.

Stress of Acute Illness and Surgery. Both emotional and physical stress can increase the blood glucose level and result in hyperglycemia. Because it is impossible to avoid stress totally in life, certain situations may require more intense management, such as extra insulin, to maintain glycemic goals and avoid hyperglycemia.

Acute illness, injury, and surgery are situations that may evoke a counterregulatory hormone response resulting in hyperglycemia. Even minor illnesses such as a viral upper respiratory infection or the flu can cause this. When patients with diabetes are ill, they should continue with the regular meal plan while increasing the intake of noncaloric fluids, such as broth, water, diet gelatin, and other decaffeinated beverages. They should also continue taking oral agents and insulin as prescribed and check blood glucose at least every 4 hours. If the glucose is greater than 240 mg/dl (13.3 mmol/L), urine should be tested for ketones every 3 to 4 hours. Patients should report moderate to large ketone levels to the health care provider.

When the illness causes the patient to eat less than normal, she or he should continue to take oral hypoglycemic medications and/or insulin as prescribed while supplementing food intake with carbohydrate-containing fluids. Examples include soups, juices, and regular decaffeinated soft drinks.[28] The health care provider

3-year intervals. The FPG is the preferred method for screening in clinical settings, although the OGTT is also suitable.[29] Testing should be considered at a younger age or be carried out more frequently in individuals who meet the criteria listed in Table 49-14. It is important to know where an individual is on the glucose continuum (see Fig. 49-3).

There are many factors that put an individual at an increased risk for diabetes. These include age, ethnicity (being Native American, Hispanic, African American, Asian American, Pacific Islander), obesity, having a baby that weighs more than 9 pounds, and family

NURSING CARE PLAN 49-1
Patient with Diabetes Mellitus

NURSING DIAGNOSIS   **Ineffective therapeutic regimen management** *related to* insufficient knowledge *as evidenced by* continued hyperglycemia, inaccurate statements regarding diabetes and its management, and stated confusion regarding the pathophysiology of diabetes

PATIENT GOALS   1. Verbalizes key elements of the therapeutic regimen, including knowledge of disease and treatment plan
2. Describes self-care measures that may prevent or decrease progression of chronic complications

OUTCOMES (NOC)

Knowledge: Diabetes Management

- Description of insulin function _____
- Description of role of diet in controlling blood glucose level _____
- Description of role of exercise in controlling blood glucose level _____
- Description of hyperglycemia and related symptoms _____
- Description of hypoglycemia and related symptoms _____
- Description of procedures to be followed in treating hyperglycemia _____
- Description of procedures to be followed in treating hypoglycemia _____
- Description of impact of acute illness on blood glucose level _____
- Description of when to seek help from health care professional _____

Measurement Scale

1 = None
2 = Limited
3 = Moderate
4 = Substantial
5 = Extensive

INTERVENTIONS (NIC) and *RATIONALES*

Teaching: Disease Process

- Appraise the patient's current level of knowledge related to specific disease process *to determine the scope and extent of required teaching.*
- Describe the disease process.
- Discuss rationale behind management/therapy/treatment recommendations *to enable patient to better understand rationale behind treatment regimen and lifestyle changes.*
- Instruct patient on measures to prevent/minimize symptoms *to promote management of disease.*
- Discuss lifestyle changes that may be required to prevent future complications and/or control the disease process *to encourage patient to actively participate in determining changes that will be acceptable.*
- Describe possible chronic complications *to increase awareness of the long-term effects of inadequate control of disease process.*
- Instruct the patient on which signs and symptoms to report to health care provider *to ensure prompt treatment.*
- Refer the patient to local community agencies/support groups *to provide continuing support and education.*

NURSING DIAGNOSIS   **Imbalanced nutrition: more than body requirements** *related to* intake in excess of activity expenditure or medication coverage *as evidenced by* hyperglycemia, weight gain

PATIENT GOAL   Maintains a balance of nutrition, activity, and insulin availability that results in normal blood glucose levels and optimum weight

OUTCOMES (NOC)

Diabetes Self-Management

- Uses diary to monitor blood glucose over time _____
- Treats symptoms of hyperglycemia _____
- Follows recommended diet _____
- Participates in recommended exercise program _____
- Uses effective weight control strategies _____
- Maintains optimum weight _____
- Seeks health care if blood glucose levels fluctuate outside recommended parameters _____
- Demonstrates correct procedure for insulin administration _____
- Performs treatment regimen as prescribed _____

Measurement Scale

1 = Never demonstrated
2 = Rarely demonstrated
3 = Sometimes demonstrated
4 = Often demonstrated
5 = Consistently demonstrated

INTERVENTIONS (NIC) and *RATIONALES*

Teaching: Prescribed Diet

- Determine patient's/significant other's feelings/attitude toward prescribed diet and expected degree of dietary compliance *to determine readiness to learn.*
- Assist the patient to accommodate food preferences into the prescribed diet *to improve compliance.*
- Refer patient to dietitian/nutritionist *to provide continuing diet education and evaluation.*

Teaching: Prescribed Activity/Exercise

- Inform the patient of the purpose for, and the benefits of, the prescribed activity/exercise *to improve commitment to activity.*
- Instruct the patient how to monitor tolerance of the activity/exercise *to prevent injury.*
- Assist the patient to incorporate activity/exercise regimen into daily routine/lifestyle *because it is an integral part of diabetes control.*

Hyperglycemia Management

- Monitor for signs and symptoms of hyperglycemia: polyuria, polydipsia, polyphagia, weakness, lethargy, malaise, blurring of vision, or headache *to alert patient to glucose/insulin imbalance and need for treatment.*
- Anticipate situations in which insulin requirements will increase (e.g., intercurrent illness) *to allow patient to adjust insulin dosage appropriately and avoid undue fatigue.*
- Facilitate adherence to diet and exercise regimen *to promote diabetes control.*
- Restrict exercise when blood glucose levels are >250 mg/dl, especially when ketones are present, *to decrease the body's requirement for already unavailable glucose.*

Continued

Diabetes

NURSING CARE PLAN 49-1

Patient with Diabetes Mellitus—cont'd

NURSING DIAGNOSIS   **Risk for injury** *related to* decreased tactile sensation, episodes of hypoglycemia

PATIENT GOALS   1.   Experiences no injury resulting from decreased sensation in feet
2.   Experiences no injury resulting from hypoglycemia

OUTCOMES (NOC)

Risk Control

- Acknowledges risk factors _____
- Modifies lifestyle to reduce risk _____
- Avoids exposure to health threats _____
- Monitors health status changes _____

Measurement Scale

1 = Never demonstrated
2 = Rarely demonstrated
3 = Sometimes demonstrated
4 = Often demonstrated
5 = Consistently demonstrated

INTERVENTIONS (NIC) and *RATIONALES*

Teaching: Foot Care

- Provide information regarding the relationship between neuropathy, injury, and vascular disease and the risk for ulceration and lower extremity amputation in persons with diabetes *to promote commitment to care.*
- Caution about potential sources of injury to the feet (e.g., heat, cold, cutting corns or calluses, chemicals, use of strong antiseptics or astringents, use of adhesive tape, and going barefoot or wearing thongs or open-toe shoes).
- Instruct individual to inspect inside of shoes daily for foreign objects, nail points, torn linings, and rough areas *to avoid injury by factors that are not felt.*

Hypoglycemia Management

- Monitor for signs and symptoms of hypoglycemia *to alert patient to glucose/insulin imbalance and need for treatment.*
- Determine patient's recognition of hypoglycemia signs and symptoms *to assess learning needs.*
- Instruct patient to have simple carbohydrate available at all times *to treat hypoglycemia.*
- Instruct patient to obtain and carry/wear appropriate emergency identification *to facilitate treatment by others.*

NURSING DIAGNOSIS   **Risk for peripheral neurovascular dysfunction** *related to* vascular effects of diabetes

PATIENT GOALS   1.   Verbalizes effects of diabetes on peripheral artery circulation
2.   Implements measures to increase peripheral circulatory status

OUTCOMES (NOC)

Tissue Perfusion: Peripheral

- Capillary refill, toes _____
- Sensation _____
- Skin color _____
- Skin integrity _____
- Extremity skin temperature _____
- Pedal pulse rate (right) _____
- Pedal pulse rate (left) _____

Measurement Scale

1 = Severely compromised
2 = Substantially compromised
3 = Moderately compromised
4 = Mildly compromised
5 = Not compromised

INTERVENTIONS (NIC) and *RATIONALES*

Circulatory Care: Arterial Insufficiency

- Perform a comprehensive appraisal of peripheral circulation (e.g., check peripheral pulses, edema, capillary refill, color, and temperature) *to establish baseline findings.*
- Inspect skin for arterial ulcers or tissue breakdown *to provide treatment to prevent infection and additional necrosis.*
- Protect the extremity from injury (e.g., sheepskin under feet and lower legs, footboard/bed cradle at foot of bed; well-fitted shoes) *to prevent conditions that favor skin breakdown.*
- Maintain adequate hydration *to decrease blood viscosity.*
- Encourage the patient to exercise as tolerated *to increase peripheral circulation.*
- Instruct the patient on factors that interfere with circulation (e.g., smoking, restrictive clothing, exposure to cold temperatures, crossing of legs and feet).
- Instruct the patient on proper foot care.

---

should be notified promptly if the patient is unable to keep any fluids or food down. The patient should understand that medication for diabetes, including insulin, should not be withheld during times of illness because counterregulatory mechanisms often increase the blood glucose level dramatically. Food intake is also important during this time because the body requires extra energy to deal with the stress of the illness. Extra insulin may be necessary to meet this demand and to prevent the onset of DKA in the patient with type 1 diabetes.[30]

During the intraoperative period adjustments in the diabetes regimen can be planned to ensure glycemic control. The patient is given IV fluids and insulin immediately before, during, and after surgery when there is no oral intake. The patient with type 2 diabetes who has been on oral agents should understand that this is a temporary measure and it should not be interpreted as a worsening of diabetes. Patients who are undergoing surgery or any radiologic procedures that involve the use of a contrast medium are instructed to hold their metformin the day of surgery or the procedure. They will also be instructed not to resume the metformin until 48 hours after the surgery or the procedure and after their serum creatinine has been checked and is normal.[31]

The nurse caring for an unconscious surgical patient receiving insulin must be alert for hypoglycemic signs such as sweating, tachycardia, and tremors. Frequent monitoring of blood glucose will prevent episodes of severe hypoglycemia in this patient.

Ambulatory and Home Care. Successful management of diabetes requires ongoing interaction among the patient, the family, and the health care team. It is important that a diabetes nurse educator be involved in the care of the patient and the family. This person provides expertise in many areas of specialized care needs.

Because diabetes is a complex chronic condition, a great deal of patient contact takes place in outpatient and home settings. The major goal of patient care in these settings is to enable the patient or caregiver to reach an optimal level of independence in self-care activities. Unfortunately, many patients with diabetes face challenges in reaching these goals. Diabetes increases the risk for other chronic conditions that can affect self-care activities. These include visual impairment, lower extremity problems that affect mobility, and other functional limitations related to cerebrovascular disease. Therefore important nursing functions are to assess the ability of patients and caregivers in such activities as SMBG and insulin injection techniques. Assistive devices for self-administration of insulin include syringe magnifiers, vial stabilizers, and dosing aids for the visually impaired. In some cases, the nurse will make referrals to others who can help the patient achieve the self-care goal. These may include an occupational therapist, a social worker, a home health aide, or a dietitian.

A diagnosis of diabetes affects the patient in many profound ways. Patients with diabetes must continually contend with lifestyle choices that affect the food they eat, the activity they engage in, and demands on their time and energy. In addition, they face the potential of becoming victim to the devastating complications of this disease. Careful assessment of what it means to the patient to have diabetes should be the starting point of patient teaching. The nurse can help patients make adjustments by displaying an attitude that is supportive and nonjudgmental. The goals of teaching should be mutually determined by the patient and the nurse based on individual needs, as well as therapeutic requirements.

The patient's support system must be identified. If this is the family, they need to be involved in teaching so they can care for the patient when self-care is no longer possible. The family and significant others need to be encouraged to provide emotional support and encouragement as the patient deals with the reality of living with a chronic disease.

Insulin Therapy. Nursing responsibilities for the patient receiving insulin include proper administration, assessment of the patient's response to insulin therapy, and education of the patient regarding administration, adjustment to, and side effects of insulin (see Table 49-5). Table 49-6 lists guidelines for the nurse assessing a patient using glucose-lowering agents, including insulin and OAs.

Assessment of the patient who is new to insulin must include an evaluation of his or her ability to manage this therapy safely. This includes the ability to understand the interaction of insulin,

diet, and activity and to be able to recognize and treat the symptoms of hypoglycemia appropriately. If the patient does not have the cognitive skills to do these things, another responsible person must be identified and trained. The patient or caregiver must also have the cognitive and manual skills needed to prepare and inject the insulin. If the patient or family lacks these, additional resources will be needed to assist the patient.

Many patients are fearful when they first begin using insulin. Some patients find it difficult to self-inject because they are afraid of needles or the pain associated with an injection. Some are afraid they will hurt themselves by giving too much or too little insulin. And in some cases, the patient believes that using insulin is a "last-ditch" effort and that he or she is now in the final stages of the disease process. Therefore it is important to explore the patient's underlying fears before beginning the teaching.

Follow-up assessment of the patient who has been using insulin therapy includes an inspection of injection sites for signs of lipodystrophy and other reactions, review of insulin preparation and injection technique, a history pertaining to the occurrence of hypoglycemic episodes, and the patient's method for handling hypoglycemic episodes. A review of the patient's recorded blood glucose tests is also important in assessing overall glycemic control.

Oral Agents. Nursing responsibilities for the patient taking OAs are similar to those for the patient taking insulin. Proper administration, assessment of the patient's use of and response to the OA, and education of the patient and the family about OAs are all part of the nurse's function.

The nurse's assessment can be extremely valuable in determining the most appropriate OA for a patient. Factors such as the patient's mental status, eating habits, home environment, attitude toward diabetes, and medication history all play a significant role in determining the most appropriate OA for the individual patient. For example, frail older adults who live alone are at high risk for severe hypoglycemia because low blood glucose is frequently undetected and/or untreated in this population. This is especially true if the patient has a short-term memory deficit. In these cases, an OA that does not cause hypoglycemia, or a shorter-acting OA, would be most appropriate.

Patient teaching is an essential nursing function when caring for the patient who uses OAs for blood glucose control. Some patients may assume that their diabetes is not a serious condition if they are taking only a pill for glycemic control. Therefore the patient should be instructed that these agents will help keep blood glucose controlled and will help prevent serious long- and short-term complications of diabetes. Patients should be instructed that OAs are used in addition to diet and activity as therapy for diabetes and that they should continue with their meal and activity plans. Patients should not take extra pills if overeating has occurred, unless specifically instructed to do so by their health care provider. If the patient uses sulfonylureas and meglitinides, instructions should be given with regard to prevention, symptom recognition, and management of hypoglycemia.

The patient should also be instructed to contact a health care provider if periods of illness or extreme stress occur. During such a period, insulin therapy may be required to prevent or treat hyperglycemic symptoms and avoid an acute hyperglycemia emergency.

Personal Hygiene. The potential for microvascular complications and infections requires diligent skin and dental hygiene practices on the part of the patient. Because of the susceptibility to periodontal disease, daily brushing and flossing should be encouraged in addition to regular visits to the dentist. When dental work must be done, the dentist should be informed that the patient has diabetes.

Routine care should include regular bathing, with particular emphasis given to foot care. Problems associated with the feet and lower extremities are presented later in this chapter. If cuts, scrapes, or burns occur, they should be treated promptly and monitored carefully. The area should be washed, and a nonabrasive or nonirritating antiseptic ointment may be applied. The area should be covered with a dry, sterile pad. If the injury does not begin to heal within 24 hours or if signs of infection develop, the health care provider should be notified immediately.

Medical Identification and Travel. The patient should be instructed to carry medical identification at all times indicating that he or she has diabetes. Police, paramedics, and many private citizens are aware of the need to look for this identification when working with sick or unconscious persons. Every person with diabetes should wear a medical alert bracelet or necklace. An identification card (Fig. 49-11) can supply valuable information, such as the name of the health care provider and the type and dose of insulin or OA.

Travel for a patient with diabetes requires advance planning. The patient should have a full set of diabetes care supplies in the carry-on luggage when traveling by plane, train, or bus. This includes blood glucose monitoring equipment, insulin, and syringes. When syringes and lancing devices are carried onto a commercial airliner, insulin vials, insulin pumps, insulin pens, and other supplies should be accompanied by the professional printed pharmaceutical labels. In addition, a letter from the prescribing health care provider indicating medical necessity may prevent delays at security checkpoints. Screeners should be notified if an insulin pump is used so they can inspect it while it is on the body, rather than remove it.

For patients who use insulin or an OA that can cause hypoglycemia, snack items and a quick-acting carbohydrate source for treating hypoglycemia should be included in the carry-on luggage. Extra insulin should be available in case a bottle breaks or gets lost. In addition, the patient should carry a full day's supply of food in the event of cancelled flights, delayed meals, or closed restaurants. If the patient is planning a trip out of the country, it is wise to have a letter from the health care provider explaining that the patient has diabetes and requires all the materials, particularly syringes, for ongoing health care.

Some travel involves time changes such as traveling coast to coast or across the international date line. The patient should contact the health care provider to plan an appropriate insulin schedule. Many patients find it easier and more predictable to take only rapid-acting or regular insulin every 4 to 6 hours to cover insulin needs while on long airplane trips instead of trying to anticipate the peak of intermediate insulin and the availability of meals. During travel, most patients find it helpful to keep watches set to the time of the city of origin until they reach their destination. The key to travel when taking insulin is to know the type of insulin being taken, its onset of action, the anticipated peak time, and meal times.

Patient and Family Teaching. The goals of diabetes self-management education are to enable the patient to become the most active participant in his or her care, while matching the level of self-management to the ability of the individual patient. Patients who actively manage their diabetes care have better outcomes than those who do not. For this reason, an educational approach that facilitates informed decision making on the part of the patient is

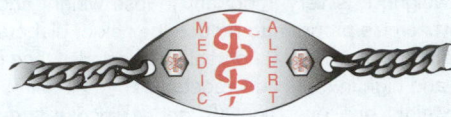

> **I am a DIABETIC**
>
> If unconscious or behaving abnormally, I may be having a reaction associated with diabetes or its treatment.
>
> If I can swallow, give me a sweet drink, orange juice, Lifesavers, or lowfat milk.
>
> If I do not recover promptly, call a physician or send me to the hospital.
>
> If I am unconscious or cannot swallow, do not attempt to give me anything by mouth, but call 911 or send me to the hospital immediately.

FIG. 49-11   Medical alerts. A patient with diabetes should carry a card and wear a bracelet or necklace that indicates diabetes. If the patient with diabetes is unconscious, these measures will ensure prompt and appropriate attention.

COMPLEMENTARY AND ALTERNATIVE THERAPIES

Herbs that May Affect Glucose

Effects

In traditional medical systems many herbs are used to manage diabetes. Many of these herbs are being studied for their effect on blood glucose. The following herbs may lower blood glucose levels: aloe vera, bilberry, bitter melon, fenugreek, fish oils, garlic, ginseng, *Gymnema,* horse chestnut seed extract, marshmallow, milk thistle, and nopal (prickly pear cactus). In other cultures, these and other herbs are often used in combination to manage hyperglycemia. Some herbs, such as burdock, may raise blood glucose levels.

Nursing Implications

It is very important that any patients with diabetes mellitus consult with their health care provider before using herbs or nutritional supplements. Patients who use herbs should monitor their blood glucose levels carefully and regularly.

---

widely advocated. Sometimes this is referred to as the *empowerment approach* to education.

Unfortunately, patients can encounter a variety of physical, psychologic, and emotional barriers when it comes to effectively managing their diabetes. These barriers may include feelings of inadequacy about one's own abilities, unwillingness to make the necessary behavioral changes, ineffective coping strategies, and cognitive deficits. If the patient is not able to manage the disease, a family member may be able to assume part of this role. If the patient or the family cannot make decisions related to diabetes management, the nurse may refer the patient to a social worker or other resources within the community. These resources can assist the patient and the family in outlining a feasible treatment program that meets their capabilities. Patient and health care provider resources are listed at the end of this chapter.

An assessment of the patient's knowledge of diabetes and lifestyle preferences is useful in planning a teaching program. Tables 49-15 and 49-16 present guidelines to use for patient and family teaching. The nurse should assess the patient's knowledge base frequently so that gaps in knowledge or incorrect or inaccurate ideas can be quickly corrected.

The ADA and the American Association of Diabetes Educators offer pamphlets, booklets, and a bimonthly magazine called

TABLE 49-15 PATIENT AND FAMILY TEACHING GUIDE
General Guidelines for the Management of Diabetes Mellitus

Disease Process
- Include an introduction about the pancreas and the islets of Langerhans.
- Describe how insulin is made and what affects its production.
- Discuss the relationship of insulin and glucose.

Physical Activity
- Discuss the importance of regular exercise on the management of blood glucose, improvement of cardiovascular function, and general health.

Menu Planning
- Educate the patient on the importance of a well-balanced diet as part of a diabetes management plan.
- Explain the impact of carbohydrates on the glycemic index and blood glucose levels.

Medication Compliance
- Ensure that the patient is well educated on the proper use of insulin (see Table 49-5) and oral agents.
- Account for a patient's physical limitation or inabilities for self-medication. If necessary, involve the family or caregiver in proper use of medication.
- Discuss all side effects and safety issues regarding medication.

Monitoring Blood Glucose
- Teach how to correctly monitor blood glucose levels.
- Include when blood glucose levels should be checked, how to record them, and if necessary, how to adjust insulin levels accordingly.

Risk Reduction
- Ensure that the patient understands and appropriately responds to the signs and symptoms of hypoglycemia and hyperglycemia (see Table 49-17).
- Stress the importance of proper foot care (see Table 49-22), regular eye examinations, and consistent glucose monitoring.
- Inform the patient about the effect that stress can have on blood glucose.

Psychosocial
- Advise the patient of resources that are available to facilitate the adjustment and answer questions about living with a chronic condition such as diabetes (see Resources at end of chapter).

TABLE 49-16 PATIENT AND FAMILY TEACHING GUIDE
Instructions for Patients with Diabetes Mellitus

Do

Blood Glucose
- Monitor your blood glucose at home and record results in a log.
- Take your insulin or OA as prescribed.
- Obtain a hemoglobin A1C blood test every 3-6 months as an indicator of your long-term blood glucose control.
- Carry some form of glucose at all times so you can treat hypoglycemia quickly.
- Instruct family members in the use of glucagon administration in the case of emergencies due to hypoglycemia.

Exercise
- Learn how exercise and food affect your blood glucose levels.
- Begin a medically supervised exercise program.

Diet
- Have an individualized meal plan created by a dietitian.
- Follow your diet, eating regular meals at regular times.
- Eat slowly and chew food thoroughly.
- Choose foods low in saturated fats.
- Limit the amount of alcohol you drink.
- Learn your cholesterol level.

Other Guidelines
- Obtain an annual eye examination by an ophthalmologist.
- Obtain annual urine testing for protein.
- Examine your feet at home.
- Wear comfortable, well-fitting shoes to help prevent foot injury. Break in new shoes gradually.
- Always carry identification that says you have diabetes.
- Have other medical problems treated, especially high blood pressure and high cholesterol.
- Know the symptoms of hypoglycemia and hyperglycemia.
- Quit smoking.

Don't

- Skip doses of your insulin, especially when you are sick.
- Run out of insulin.
- Enroll in a fad diet.
- Rub the area where insulin was administered.

- Forget that exercise will lower your blood glucose level.
- Exercise if your blood glucose levels are very elevated. This may lead to a temporary worsening of your blood glucose levels.

- Drink excessive amounts of alcohol because this may lead to unpredictable low blood glucose reactions.
- Eat fried foods.
- Drink regular soda or lots of fruit juice.

- Smoke.
- Apply hot or cold directly to your feet.
- Go barefoot.
- Ignore the symptoms of hypoglycemia and hyperglycemia.
- Put oil or lotion between your toes.

OA, Oral agent.

TABLE 49-17	Comparisons of Hyperglycemia and Hypoglycemia	

Hyperglycemia	Hypoglycemia
Manifestations*	
Elevated blood glucose†	Blood glucose <70 mg/dl (3.9 mmol/L)
Increase in urination	Cold, clammy skin
Increase in appetite followed by lack of appetite	Numbness of fingers, toes, mouth
Weakness, fatigue	Rapid heartbeat
Blurred vision	Emotional changes
Headache	Headache
Glycosuria	Nervousness, tremors
Nausea and vomiting	Faintness, dizziness
Abdominal cramps	Unsteady gait, slurred speech
Progression to DKA or HHS	Hunger
	Changes in vision
	Seizures, coma
Causes	
Illness, infection	Alcohol intake without food
Corticosteroids	Too little food—delayed, omitted, inadequate intake
Too much food	Too much diabetic medication
Too little or no diabetes medication	Too much exercise without compensation
Inactivity	Diabetes medication or food taken at wrong time
Emotional, physical stress	Loss of weight without change in medication
Poor absorption of insulin	Use of β-adrenergic blockers interfering with recognition of symptoms
Treatment	
Physician's attention	Immediate ingestion of 15-20 g of simple carbohydrates
Continuance of diabetes medication as ordered	Ingestion of another 15-20 g of simple carbohydrates in 15 min if no relief obtained
Check blood glucose frequently. Check urine for ketones. Record results	Contacting of health care provider if no relief obtained
Hourly drinking of fluids	Discussion with health care provider about medication dosage
Preventive Measures	
Taking prescribed dose of medication at proper time	Taking prescribed dose of medication at proper time
Accurate administration of insulin/OA	Accurate administration of insulin/OA
Maintenance of diet	Ingestion of all recommended foods at proper time
Maintenance of good personal hygiene	Provision of compensation for exercise
Adherence to sick-day rules when ill	Ability to recognize and know symptoms and treat them immediately
Checking of blood for glucose as ordered	Carrying of simple carbohydrates
Contacting of health care provider regarding ketonuria	Education of friends, family, fellow employees about symptoms and treatment
Wearing of diabetic identification	Checking blood glucose as ordered
	Wearing medical alert (diabetic) identification

DKA, Diabetic ketoacidosis; *HHS,* hyperosmolar hyperglycemic syndrome; *OA,* oral agent.
*There is usually a gradual onset of symptoms in hyperglycemia and a rapid onset in hypoglycemia.
†Specific clinical manifestations related to elevated levels of blood glucose vary according to the patient.

Diabetes Forecast. Affiliates of the ADA are located in all states, and most can be reached by dialing 1-800-DIABETES. The ADA also publishes materials and sponsors conferences for health care professionals concerned with diabetes education, research, and management of patients. This organization also gives recognition to education programs that meet the national standards of diabetes education and can provide a list of these programs. Drug companies manufacturing diabetes-related products also have free educational materials for patients and health care providers.

■ *Evaluation*

The expected outcomes for the patient with diabetes mellitus are addressed in NCP 49-1.

Acute Complications of Diabetes Mellitus

The acute complications of diabetes mellitus arise from events associated with hyperglycemia and insufficient insulin. A problem that may arise from too much insulin or an excessive dose of an OA is *hypoglycemia* (also referred to as *insulin reaction* or *low blood glu-*

cose). It is important for the health care provider to be able to distinguish between hyperglycemia and hypoglycemia because hypoglycemia worsens rapidly and constitutes a serious threat if action is not immediately taken. Table 49-17 compares the manifestations, causes, management, and prevention of hyperglycemia and hypoglycemia.

DIABETIC KETOACIDOSIS

Etiology and Pathophysiology

Diabetic ketoacidosis (DKA), also referred to as *diabetic acidosis* and *diabetic coma,* is caused by a profound deficiency of insulin and is characterized by hyperglycemia, ketosis, acidosis, and dehydration. It is most likely to occur in people with type 1 diabetes but may be seen in type 2 in conditions of severe illness or stress when the pancreas cannot meet the extra demand for insulin. Precipitating factors include illness and infection, inadequate insulin dosage, undiagnosed type 1 diabetes, poor self-management, and neglect.

When the circulating supply of insulin is insufficient, glucose cannot be properly used for energy so that the body breaks down fat stores as a secondary source of fuel (Fig. 49-12). Ketones are acidic by-products of fat metabolism that can cause serious prob-

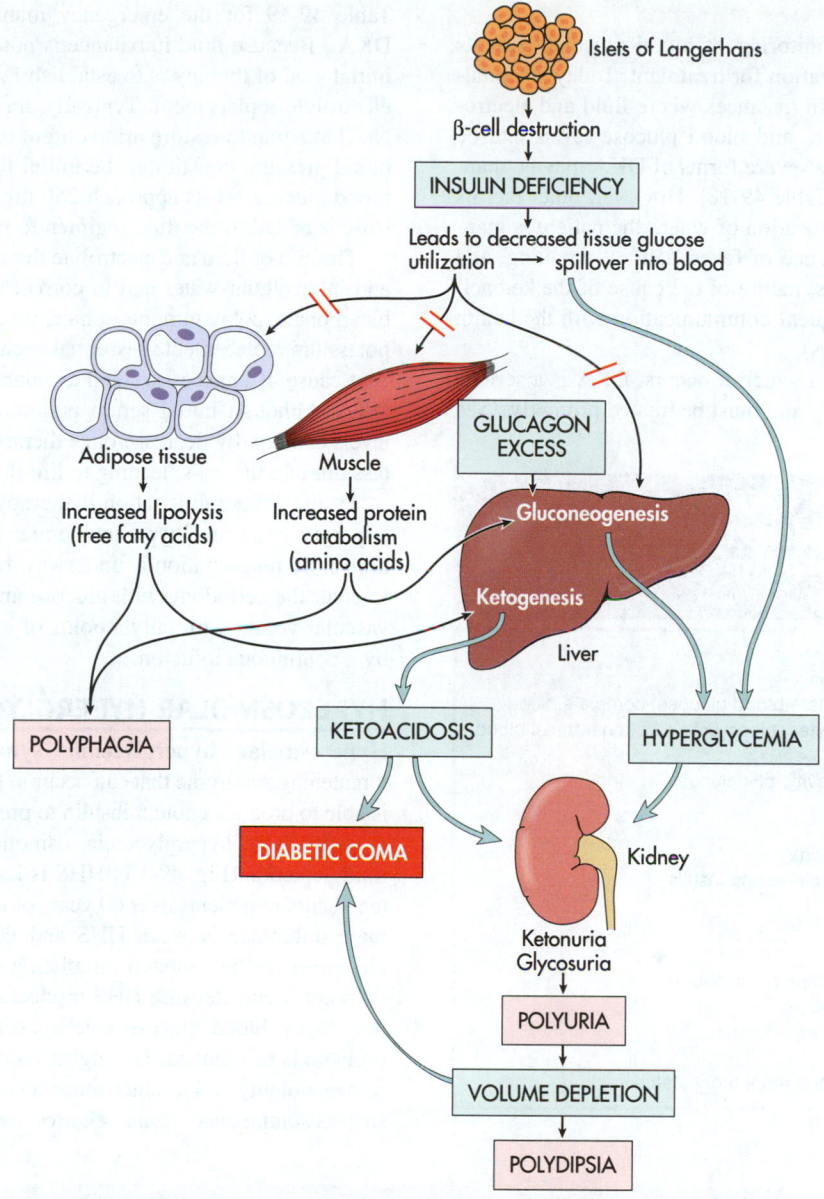

Islets of Langerhans

β-cell destruction

INSULIN DEFICIENCY

Leads to decreased tissue glucose
utilization → spillover into blood

Adipose tissue

Muscle

GLUCAGON
EXCESS

Increased lipolysis
(free fatty acids)

Increased protein
catabolism
(amino acids)

Gluconeogenesis

Ketogenesis

Liver

POLYPHAGIA

KETOACIDOSIS

HYPERGLYCEMIA

DIABETIC COMA

Kidney

Ketonuria
Glycosuria

POLYURIA

VOLUME DEPLETION

POLYDIPSIA

FIG. 49-12   Metabolic events leading to diabetic ketoacidosis and diabetic coma.

lems when they become excessive in the blood. Ketosis alters the pH balance, causing metabolic acidosis to develop. Ketonuria is a process that begins when ketone bodies are excreted in the urine. During this process, electrolytes become depleted as cations are eliminated along with the anionic ketones in an attempt to maintain electrical neutrality.

Insulin deficiency impairs protein synthesis and causes excessive protein degradation. This results in nitrogen losses from the tissues. Insulin deficiency also stimulates the production of glucose from amino acids (from proteins) in the liver and leads to further hyperglycemia. Because there is a deficiency of insulin, the additional glucose cannot be used and the blood glucose level rises further, adding to the osmotic diuresis. Untreated, this leads to severe depletion of sodium, potassium, chloride, magnesium, and phosphate. Vomiting caused by the acidosis results in more fluid and electrolyte losses. Eventually, hypovolemia followed by shock will ensue.

Renal failure may eventually occur from hypovolemic shock. This causes the retention of ketones and glucose, and the acidosis progresses. Untreated, the patient becomes comatose as a result of

dehydration, electrolyte imbalance, and acidosis. If the condition is not treated, death is inevitable.

Clinical Manifestations

Signs and symptoms of DKA include manifestations of dehydration such as poor skin turgor, dry mucous membranes, tachycardia, and orthostatic hypotension. Early symptoms may include lethargy and weakness. As the patient becomes severely dehydrated, the skin becomes dry and loose, and the eyeballs become soft and sunken. Abdominal pain is another symptom of DKA that may be accompanied by anorexia and vomiting. Finally, Kussmaul respirations (rapid, deep breathing associated with dyspnea) are the body's attempt to reverse metabolic acidosis through the exhalation of excess carbon dioxide. Acetone is noted on the breath as a sweet, fruity odor. (See Chapter 17 for a discussion of respiratory compensation of metabolic acidosis.) Laboratory findings include a blood glucose level above 300 mg/dl (16.7 mmol/L), arterial blood pH below 7.30, serum bicarbonate level less than 15 mEq/L (15 mmol/L), and ketones in the blood and urine.[32]

Collaborative Care

Before the advent of self-monitoring of blood glucose, patients with DKA required hospitalization for treatment. Today, hospitalization may not be required. In instances where fluid and electrolyte imbalances are not severe and blood glucose levels can be safely monitored at home, less severe forms of DKA may be managed on an outpatient basis (Table 49-18). However, other factors must be considered as to the location of where the patient is managed. These include the presence of fever, nausea, vomiting, and diarrhea; altered mental status; nature of the cause of the ketoacidosis; and availability of frequent communication with the health care provider (every few hours).

Regardless of the setting in which it occurs, DKA is a serious condition that proceeds rapidly and must be treated promptly. (See Table 49-19 for the emergency management of a patient with DKA.) Because fluid imbalance is potentially life threatening, the initial goal of therapy is to establish IV access and begin fluid and electrolyte replacement. Typically, an infusion of 0.45% or 0.9% NaCl at a rate to restore urine output to 30 to 60 ml/hr and to raise blood pressure constitutes the initial fluid therapy regimen. When blood glucose levels approach 250 mg/dl (13.9 mmol/L), 5% dextrose is added to the fluid regimen to prevent hypoglycemia.[33]

The aim of fluid and electrolyte therapy is to replace extracellular and intracellular water and to correct deficits of sodium, chloride, bicarbonate, potassium, phosphate, magnesium, and nitrogen. Early potassium replacement is essential because hypokalemia is a significant cause of unnecessary and avoidable death during treatment of DKA. Although initial serum potassium may be normal or high, levels can rapidly decrease once therapy starts as insulin drives potassium into the cells, leading to life-threatening hypokalemia.

IV insulin administration is therapy directed toward correcting hyperglycemia and hyperketonemia. Insulin therapy is withheld until fluid resuscitation is underway, because insulin allows water to enter the cell along with glucose and can lead to a depletion of vascular volume. Initially a bolus of insulin is delivered, followed by a continuous infusion.

HYPEROSMOLAR HYPERGLYCEMIC SYNDROME

Hyperosmolar hyperglycemic syndrome (HHS) is a life-threatening syndrome that can occur in the patient with diabetes who is able to produce enough insulin to prevent DKA but not enough to prevent severe hyperglycemia, osmotic diuresis, and extracellular fluid depletion (Fig. 49-13). HHS is less common than DKA. It often occurs in patients over 60 years of age with type 2 diabetes. The main difference between HHS and DKA is that the patient with HHS usually has enough circulating insulin so that ketoacidosis does not occur. Because HHS produces fewer symptoms in the earlier stages, blood glucose levels can climb quite high before the problem is recognized. The higher blood glucose levels increase serum osmolality and produce more severe neurologic manifestations, such as somnolence, coma, seizures, hemiparesis, and aphasia. HHS

TABLE 49-18	**COLLABORATIVE CARE** **Diabetic Ketoacidosis (DKA) and Hyperosmolar Hyperglycemic Syndrome (HHS)**

Diagnostic
History and physical examination
Blood studies, including immediate blood glucose, complete blood count, ketones, pH, electrolytes, blood urea nitrogen, arterial blood gases
Urinalysis, including specific gravity, pH, glucose, acetone

Collaborative Therapy
Administration of intravenous fluids
Intravenous administration of rapid-acting insulin
Electrolyte replacement
Assessment of mental status
Recording of intake and output
Central venous pressure monitoring (if indicated)
Assessment of blood glucose levels
Assessment of blood and urine for ketones
ECG monitoring
Assessment of cardiovascular and respiratory status

ECG, Electrocardiogram.

TABLE 49-19	**EMERGENCY MANAGEMENT** **Diabetic Ketoacidosis**

Etiology	Assessment Findings	Interventions
• Undiagnosed diabetes mellitus • Inadequate treatment of existing diabetes mellitus • Insulin not taken as prescribed • Infection • Change in diet, insulin, or exercise regimen	• Dry mouth • Thirst • Abdominal pain • Nausea and vomiting • Gradually increasing restlessness, confusion, lethargy • Flushed, dry skin • Eyes appear sunken • Breath odor of ketones • Rapid, weak pulse • Labored breathing (Kussmaul respirations) • Fever • Urinary frequency • Serum glucose >300 mg/dl (16.7 mmol/L) • Glucosuria and ketonuria	**Initial** • Ensure patent airway. • Administer oxygen via nasal cannula or non-rebreather mask. • Establish IV access with large-bore catheter. • Begin fluid resuscitation with 0.9% NaCl solution 1 L/hr until BP stabilized and urine output 30-60 ml/hr. • Begin continuous regular insulin drip 0.1 U/kg/hr. • Identify history of diabetes, time of last food, and time/amount of last insulin injection. **Ongoing Monitoring** • Monitor vital signs, level of consciousness, cardiac rhythm, oxygen saturation, and urine output. • Assess breath sounds for fluid overload. • Monitor serum glucose and serum potassium. • Administer potassium to correct hypokalemia. • Administer sodium bicarbonate if severe acidosis (pH <7.0).

BP, Blood pressure; *IV,* intravenous.

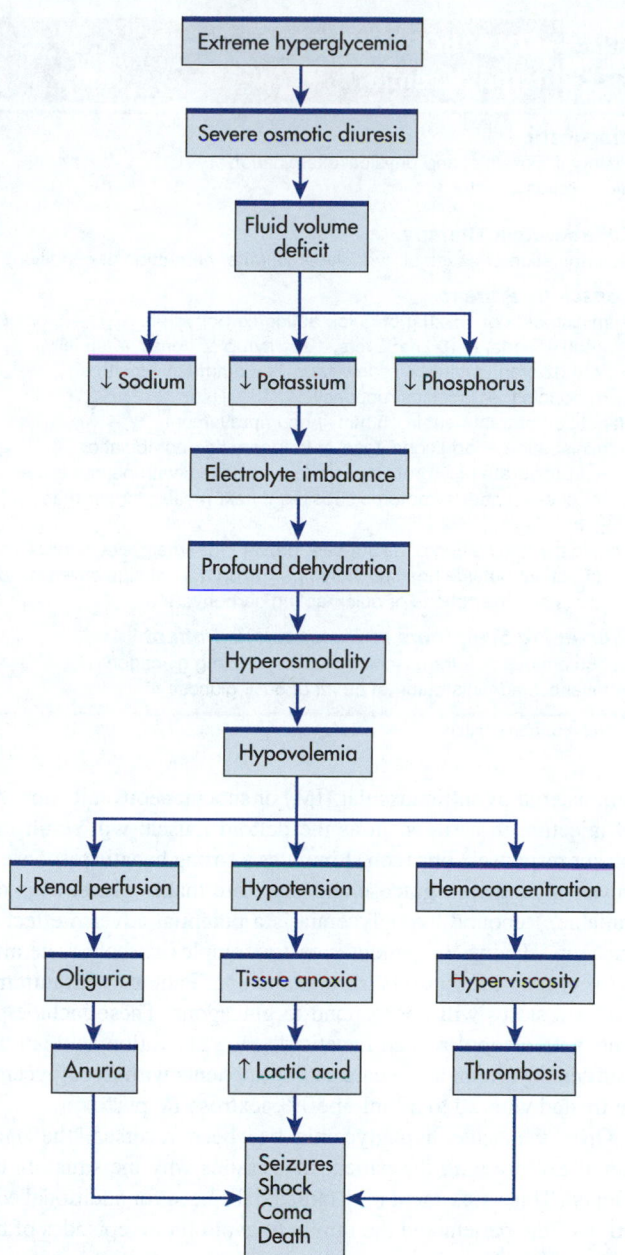

FIG. 49-13 Pathophysiology of hyperosmolar hyperglycemic syndrome (HHS).

is often related to impaired thirst sensation and/or a functional inability to replace fluids. There is usually a history of inadequate fluid intake, increasing mental depression, and polyuria. Laboratory values in HHS include blood glucose greater than 400 mg/dl (22.25 mmol/L) and a marked increase in serum osmolality. Ketone bodies are absent or minimal in both blood and urine.

Collaborative Care

HHS constitutes a medical emergency and has a high mortality rate. Therapy is similar to that for the treatment of DKA and includes immediate IV administration of either 0.9% or 0.45% NaCl at a rate that is dependent on cardiac status and the degree of fluid volume deficit. Regular insulin is given by IV bolus, followed by an infusion after fluid replacement therapy is instituted to aid in reducing the hyperglycemia. When blood glucose levels fall to approximately 250 mg/dl (13.9 mmol/L), IV fluids containing glucose are administered to prevent hypoglycemia. Electrolytes are

monitored and replaced as needed. Hypokalemia is not as significant in HHS as it is in DKA, although fluid losses may result in milder potassium deficits that require replacement. Vital signs, intake and output, tissue turgor, laboratory values, and cardiac monitoring are assessed to monitor the efficacy of fluid and electrolyte replacement. Patients with renal or cardiac compromise require special monitoring to avoid fluid overload during fluid replacement. This includes monitoring of serum osmolality and frequent assessment of cardiac, renal, and mental status.[33]

The management for both DKA and HHS is similar, except that HHS requires greater fluid replacement (see Table 49-18). Once the patient is stabilized, attempts to detect and correct the underlying precipitating cause should be initiated.

NURSING MANAGEMENT
DIABETIC KETOACIDOSIS AND HYPEROSMOLAR HYPERGLYCEMIC SYNDROME

When hospitalized, the patient is closely monitored with appropriate blood and urine tests. The nurse is responsible for monitoring blood glucose and urine for output and ketones, as well as using laboratory data to direct care.

Areas that must be monitored are administration of IV fluids to correct dehydration, administration of insulin therapy to reduce blood glucose and serum acetone, administration of electrolytes to correct electrolyte imbalance, assessment of renal status, assessment of the cardiopulmonary status related to hydration and electrolyte levels, and monitoring of the level of consciousness.

The nurse must also monitor the signs of potassium imbalance resulting from hypoinsulinemia and osmotic diuresis (see Chapter 17). When treatment for hyperglycemia is begun with insulin, serum potassium levels may decrease rapidly as potassium moves into the cells once insulin becomes available. This movement of potassium into and out of extracellular fluid influences cardiac functioning. Cardiac monitoring is a useful aid in detecting hyperkalemia and hypokalemia because characteristic changes indicating potassium excess or deficit are observable on electrocardiogram (ECG) tracings (see Chapter 17, Fig. 17-14). Vital signs should be assessed often to determine the presence of fever, hypovolemic shock, tachycardia, and Kussmaul respirations.

HYPOGLYCEMIA

Hypoglycemia, or low blood glucose, occurs when there is too much insulin in proportion to available glucose in the blood. This causes the blood glucose level to drop to less than 70 mg/dl (3.9 mmol/L). Because the brain requires a constant supply of glucose in sufficient quantities to function properly, hypoglycemia can affect mental functioning. Common manifestations of hypoglycemia include confusion, irritability, diaphoresis, tremors, hunger, weakness, and visual disturbances. Manifestations of hypoglycemia can mimic alcohol intoxication. Untreated hypoglycemia can progress to loss of consciousness, seizures, coma, and death.

Hypoglycemic unawareness is a condition in which a person does not experience the warning signs and symptoms of hypoglycemia, increasing his or her risk for dangerously low blood glucose levels. This is often related to autonomic neuropathy of diabetes that interferes with the secretion of counterregulatory hormones that produce these symptoms. Elderly patients and patients who use β-adrenergic blockers are also at risk for hypoglycemic unawareness. It is usually not safe for patients with risk factors for hypoglycemic unawareness to aim for tight blood glucose control, because a major drawback of intensive treatment is hypoglycemia. These patients are usually managed with blood glucose goals that are somewhat higher than those of patients who are able to detect and manage the onset of hypoglycemia.

Hypoglycemic symptoms may occur when a very high blood glucose level falls too rapidly (e.g., a blood glucose level of 300 mg/dl [16.7 mmol/L] falling quickly to 180 mg/dl [10 mmol/L]). Although the blood glucose level is above normal by definition and measurement, the sudden metabolic shift can evoke hypoglycemic symptoms. Too vigorous management of hyperglycemia with insulin can induce this type of situation.

Causes of hypoglycemia are often related to a mismatch in the timing of food intake and the peak action of insulin or oral hypoglycemic agents that increase endogenous insulin secretion. The balance between blood glucose and insulin can be disrupted by the administration of too much insulin or medication, the ingestion of too little food, delaying the time of eating, and performing unusual amounts of exercise. Insulin reactions can occur at any time, but most reactions occur when the OA or insulin is at its peak of action or when the patient's daily routine is disrupted without adequate adjustments in diet, medications, and activity. Although hypoglycemia is more common with insulin therapy, it can occur with OAs and may be severe and persist for an extended time because of the longer duration of action.

NURSING *and* COLLABORATIVE MANAGEMENT
HYPOGLYCEMIA

With effective treatment, hypoglycemia can usually be quickly reversed. At the first sign of hypoglycemia, the blood glucose should be checked if possible (Table 49-20). If it is below 70 mg/dl (3.9 mmol/L), the patient should immediately begin treatment for hypoglycemia. If the blood glucose is above 70 mg/dl (3.9 mmol/L), other causes of the signs and symptoms should be investigated. If the patient has manifestations of hypoglycemia and monitoring equipment is not available, hypoglycemia should be assumed and treatment should be initiated.

Hypoglycemia is treated by ingesting 15 to 20 g of a simple (fast-acting) carbohydrate, such as 4 to 6 oz of fruit juice or regular soft drink or 8 oz of low-fat milk. Commercial products such as gels or tablets containing specific amounts of glucose are convenient for carrying in a purse or pocket to be used in such situations.

Treatment with sweet foods that also contain fat, such as candy bars, cookies, and ice cream, should be avoided because the fat in them will slow down the absorption of the sugar and delay the response to treatment. Overtreatment with large quantities of quick-acting carbohydrates should also be avoided so that a rapid fluctuation to hyperglycemia does not occur. A prompt but moderate approach is best. Blood glucose should be checked about 15 minutes following the initial treatment for hypoglycemia, and treatment should be repeated if the blood glucose remains below 70 mg/dl (3.9 mmol/L). Once the blood glucose is greater than 70 mg/dl (3.9 mmol/L), the patient should eat the regularly scheduled meal or a snack to prevent hypoglycemia from recurring. Good snacks include low-fat peanut butter, bread, or cheese and crackers. Blood glucose should also be checked again about 45 minutes after treatment to ensure that hypoglycemia is not recurring.

If there is no significant improvement in the patient's condition after two to three doses of 15 g of simple carbohydrate, or if the patient is not alert enough to swallow, 1 mg of glucagon may be

TABLE 49-20	**COLLABORATIVE CARE** **Hypoglycemia**

Diagnostic
History (if possible) and physical examination
Blood glucose—stat

Collaborative Therapy
Determination of cause of hypoglycemia (after correction of condition)

Conscious Patient
Administration of 15-20 g of quick-acting carbohydrate (e.g., 4-6 oz of regular soda, 8-10 LifeSavers, 1 tbs syrup or honey, 4 tsp jelly, 4-6 oz orange juice, 8 oz low-fat milk, commercial dextrose products [per label instructions])
Repetition of treatment in 15 min (if no improvement)
Administration of additional food of longer-acting combination carbohydrate plus protein or fat (e.g., crackers with peanut butter or cheese) after symptoms subside, if next meal is longer than 1 hr away
Immediate notification of health care provider or emergency service (if patient outside hospital) if symptoms do not subside after two to three administrations of quick-acting carbohydrate

Worsening Symptoms or Unconscious Patient
Subcutaneous or intramuscular injection of 1 mg glucagon
Intravenous administration of 50 ml of 50% glucose

stat (statim), Immediately.

administered by intramuscular (IM) or subcutaneous injection. An IM injection in a site such as the deltoid muscle will result in a quicker response. Glucagon stimulates a strong hepatic response to convert glycogen to glucose and therefore makes glucose rapidly available. Rebound hypoglycemia is a potential adverse effect of glucagon. Having the patient ingest a complex carbohydrate after recovery may prevent this from happening. Patients with minimal glycogen stores will not respond to glucagons. These include patients with alcohol-related hepatic disease, starvation, and adrenal insufficiency. In an acute care setting, patients with hypoglycemia are treated with 20 to 50 ml of 50% dextrose IV push.

Once the acute hypoglycemia has been reversed, the nurse should explore with the patient the reasons why the situation developed. This assessment may indicate the need for additional education of the patient and the family to avoid future episodes of hypoglycemia. The danger of hypoglycemic reactions must be stressed because memory and learning impairment can result from repeated episodes of severe hypoglycemia.

Chronic Complications
of Diabetes Mellitus

Chronic complications of diabetes are primarily those of end-organ disease from damage to blood vessels (**angiopathy**) secondary to chronic hyperglycemia (Fig. 49-14). Angiopathy is one of the leading causes of diabetes-related deaths, with about 65% of deaths due to cardiovascular disease and stroke.[34] These chronic blood vessel dysfunctions are divided into two categories: *macrovascular complications* and *microvascular complications.*

Several theories exist as to how and why chronic hyperglycemia damages cells and tissues. Possible causes include (1) the accumulation of damaging by-products of glucose metabolism, such as sorbitol, which is associated with damage to nerve cells; (2) the formation of abnormal glucose molecules in the basement membrane of small blood vessels such as those that circulate to the eye

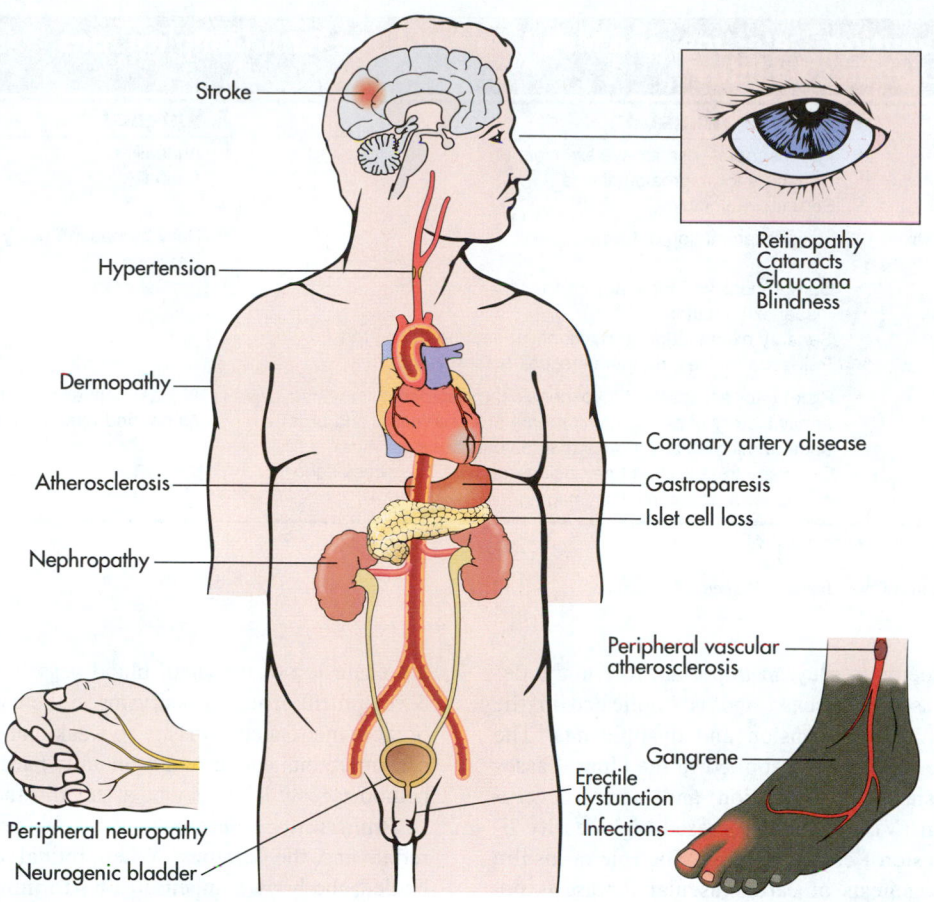

FIG. 49-14   Long-term complications of diabetes mellitus.

and kidney; and (3) a derangement in red blood cell function that leads to a decrease in oxygenation to the tissues.

The Diabetes Control and Complications Trial (DCCT), a landmark study in diabetes management, demonstrated that in patients with type 1 diabetes the risk for microvascular complications could be significantly reduced by keeping blood glucose levels as near to normal as possible for as much of the time as possible (*tight glucose control*).[35] These results found that the subjects who maintained tight glucose control reduced their risk for the development of retinopathy and nephropathy, some of the most common microvascular complications.

Based on the findings of the DCCT, the ADA issued recommendations for the management of diabetes that included treatment goals to maintain blood glucose levels as near to normal as possible. Specific targets for individual patients must take into account the risk for severe or undetected hypoglycemia as a side effect of tight glucose control.

The United Kingdom Prospective Diabetes Study (UKPDS) demonstrated that intensive treatment of type 2 diabetes can also significantly lower the risk for developing diabetes-related eye, kidney, and neurologic problems. The findings from this study included a 25% reduction of microvascular disease in subjects who maintained long-term glycemic control.[36]

Because of the devastating effects of long-term complications, patients with diabetes require scheduled and ongoing monitoring for the detection and prevention of chronic complications. The ADA recommendations for ongoing evaluation are listed in Table 49-21. It is imperative that patients understand the importance of participating in regular follow-up examinations.[29]

Macrovascular Complications

Macrovascular complications are diseases of the large and medium-size blood vessels that occur with greater frequency and with an earlier onset in people with diabetes. Although atherosclerotic plaque formation is believed to have a genetic origin, its development seems to be promoted by the altered lipid metabolism common to diabetes. Tight glucose control may help delay the atherosclerotic process.[36] Macrovascular diseases include cerebrovascular, cardiovascular, and peripheral vascular disease. Adults with diabetes have a two to four times increased risk of heart and cerebrovascular disease compared to those without diabetes.[36] Although genetic makeup cannot be altered, a patient with diabetes can diminish other risk factors associated with macrovascular complications, such as obesity, smoking, hypertension, high fat intake, and sedentary lifestyle. Smoking, which is detrimental to health in general, is especially injurious to people with diabetes. Smoking significantly increases the risk for blood vessel disease in people with diabetes and increases the risk for cardiovascular disease, stroke, and lower extremity amputation.

Blood pressure control reduces the risk of cardiovascular disease (heart disease or stroke) among persons with diabetes by 33% to 50% and the risk of microvascular complications (eye, kidney, and nerve problems) by approximately 33%. In general, for every 10 mm Hg reduction in systolic blood pressure, the risk for any complications related to diabetes is reduced by 12%. Improved control of cholesterol or blood lipids (e.g., HDL, LDL, and triglycerides) can reduce cardiovascular complications by 20% to 50%.[1,2] (Hypertension is discussed in Chapter 33 and coronary artery disease is discussed in Chapter 34.)

TABLE 49-21	Prevention, Detection, and Monitoring of Long-Term Complications of Diabetes Mellitus*	

Complication	Type of Examination	Frequency
Retinopathy	• Funduscopic—dilated eye examination	• Annually
Nephropathy	• Urinalysis for microalbuminuria	• Annually
	• Serum creatinine	
Neuropathy (foot and lower extremities)	• Visual examination of foot	• Daily by patient; every visit by health care provider
	• Comprehensive foot examination: Visual examination Sensory examination with monofilament and tuning fork Palpation (pulses, temperature, callus formation)	• Annually
Cardiovascular disease	• Risk factor assessment (hypertension, dyslipidemia, smoking, family history of premature coronary artery disease, and presence of microalbuminuria or macroalbuminuria)	• At least annually
	• Exercise stress testing (may include stress ECG, stress echocardiogram, stress nuclear imaging)	• As needed based on risk factors

Source: Standards of Medical Care, *Diabetes Care* 29:S4, 2006.
ECG, Electrocardiogram.
*Based on the recommendations of the American Diabetes Association.

Insulin resistance seems to play an important role in the development of cardiovascular disease and is implicated in the pathogenesis of essential hypertension and dyslipidemia. The term *insulin resistance syndrome* is applied to the clinical association of insulin resistance, hypertension, and increased very-low-density lipoprotein (VLDL) and decreased high-density lipoprotein (HDL) cholesterol concentrations. The role of insulin resistance in the pathogenesis of cardiovascular disease is not well understood, but it seems to combine with dyslipidemia in contributing to greater risk of cardiovascular disease in patients with diabetes mellitus. All patients with diabetes should be screened for dyslipidemia at the time diabetes is diagnosed. These abnormalities typically include an elevated triglyceride level and reduced HDL cholesterol.[37]

Microvascular Complications

Microvascular complications result from thickening of the vessel membranes in the capillaries and arterioles in response to conditions of chronic hyperglycemia. They differ from the macrovascular complications in that they are specific to diabetes. Although microangiopathy can be found throughout the body, the areas most noticeably affected are the eyes (retinopathy), the kidneys (nephropathy), and the skin (dermopathy). Thickening of the basement membrane has been found in some persons with diabetes before or at the time of diagnosis or before the onset of symptoms of diabetes mellitus. However, clinical manifestations usually do not appear until 10 to 20 years after the onset of diabetes.

DIABETIC RETINOPATHY

Etiology and Pathophysiology

Diabetic retinopathy refers to the process of microvascular damage to the retina as a result of chronic hyperglycemia in patients with diabetes. After 15 years with diabetes mellitus, nearly all patients with type 1 diabetes and 80% with type 2 diabetes will have some degree of retinal disease. Diabetic retinopathy is estimated to be the most common cause of new cases of blindness in people ages 20 to 74 years.[29]

Retinopathy can be classified as nonproliferative or proliferative. In *nonproliferative retinopathy,* the most common form, partial occlusion of the small blood vessels in the retina causes the development of microaneurysms in the capillary walls. The walls of these microaneurysms are so weak that capillary fluid leaks out, causing retinal edema and eventually hard exudates or intraretinal hemorrhages. Vision may be affected if the macula is involved.

Proliferative retinopathy, the most severe form, involves the retina and the vitreous. When retinal capillaries become occluded, the body compensates by forming new blood vessels to supply the retina with blood, a pathologic process known as *neovascularization.* These new vessels are extremely fragile and hemorrhage easily, producing vitreous contraction. Eventually light is prevented from reaching the retina as the vessels become torn and bleed into the vitreous cavity. The patient sees black or red spots or lines. If these new blood vessels pull the retina while the vitreous contracts, causing a tear, partial or complete retinal detachment will occur. If the macula is involved, vision is lost. Without treatment, more than half of patients with proliferative diabetic retinopathy will be blind.

Collaborative Care

The earliest and most treatable stages of diabetic retinopathy often produce no changes in the vision. Because of this, the patient with diabetes must have regular dilated eye examinations by an ophthalmologist or a specially trained optometrist at the time of diagnosis and annually thereafter for early detection and treatment.

The most common forms of treatment for diabetic retinopathy are early photocoagulation of the retina, cryotherapy, and vitrectomy. Photocoagulation by laser destroys the ischemic areas of the retina that produce growth factors that encourage neovascularization, thereby preventing further visual loss.[29] (Photocoagulation is discussed in Chapter 22.)

Cryotherapy is sometimes used to treat peripheral areas of the retina that cannot be reached with lasers or when retinal hemorrhage prevents complete photocoagulation. In this procedure, topical anesthesia is used so that a cryoprobe can be placed directly on the surface of the eye. When the probe is properly located, its tip creates a frozen area that extends through the external tissue through the eyeball until it reaches a specific point on the retina. Multiple points on the retina can be treated in this way. (Cryotherapy is discussed in Chapter 22.)

Vitrectomy is the aspiration of blood, membrane, and fibers from the inside of the eye through a small incision just behind the cornea. Vitrectomy is indicated when there is vitreal hemorrhage that does not clear in 6 months or when there is threatened or actual retinal detachment.[38] (Vitrectomy is discussed in Chapter 22.)

Persons with diabetes are also prone to other visual problems. Glaucoma occurs as a result of the occlusion of the outflow channels secondary to neovascularization. This type of glaucoma is difficult to treat and often results in blindness. Cataracts develop at an earlier age and progress more rapidly in people with diabetes.

NEPHROPATHY

Diabetic nephropathy is a microvascular complication associated with damage to the small blood vessels that supply the glomeruli of the kidney. It is the leading cause of end-stage renal disease (ESRD) in the United States. The risk of nephropathy is about the same in patients with either type 1 or type 2 diabetes. Risk factors for the development of diabetic nephropathy include hypertension, genetic predisposition, smoking, and chronic hyperglycemia. Results of the DCCT and UKPDS studies have demonstrated that kidney disease can be significantly reduced when near-normal blood glucose control is achieved and maintained.[34,35]

Tight blood glucose control is critical to the prevention and delay of diabetic nephropathy. Hypertension will significantly accelerate the progression of nephropathy. Therefore aggressive blood pressure management is indicated for all patients with diabetes. Angiotensin-converting enzyme (ACE) inhibitor drugs (e.g., lisinopril [Prinivil, Zestril]) are commonly prescribed for patients with diabetes because they are effective blood pressure–lowering agents with few side effects. In addition, ACE inhibitors are often prescribed for patients with diabetes even when they are not hypertensive. This is because drugs in this class have a protective effect on the kidney that prevents the progression of diabetic nephropathy independent of hypertension control. Angiotensin II receptor antagonists (e.g., losartan [Cozaar]) may also be used for their kidney-protective benefits.[39] (See Chapter 33 for a discussion of hypertension and Chapter 47 for a discussion of renal failure.)

Standards for the prevention and detection of nephropathy in patients with diabetes include yearly screening for the presence of microalbuminuria (MAU) in the urine and serum creatinine. The presence of MAU detects kidney damage at an earlier stage than the standard dipstick test for urine protein. Serum creatinine measurements provide an estimation of the glomerular filtration rate and thus the degree of kidney function.[40]

NEUROPATHY

Diabetic neuropathy is nerve damage that occurs because of the metabolic derangements associated with diabetes mellitus. About 60% to 70% of patients with diabetes have some degree of neuropathy, with neurologic complications occurring equally in type 1 and type 2 diabetes. The most common type of neuropathy affecting persons with diabetes is sensory neuropathy. This can lead to the loss of protective sensation in the lower extremities, and, coupled with other factors, this significantly increases the risk for complications that result in a lower limb amputation. More than 60% of nontraumatic amputations in the United States occur in people with diabetes.[1]

Etiology and Pathophysiology

The pathophysiologic processes of diabetic neuropathy are not well understood. Several theories exist, including metabolic, vascular, and autoimmune elements. The prevailing theory suggests that persistent hyperglycemia leads to an accumulation of sorbitol and fructose in the nerves that causes damage by an unknown mechanism. The result is reduced nerve conduction and demyelinization. Ischemia in blood vessels damaged by chronic hyperglycemia that supply the peripheral nerves is also implicated in the development of diabetic neuropathy. Neuropathy can precede, accompany, or follow the diagnosis of diabetes.

Classification

The two major categories of diabetic neuropathy are *sensory neuropathy*, which affects the peripheral nervous system, and *autonomic neuropathy*. Each of these types can take on several forms.

Sensory Neuropathy. The most common form of sensory neuropathy is distal symmetric neuropathy, which affects the hands and/or feet bilaterally. This is sometimes referred to as "stocking-glove neuropathy." Characteristics of distal symmetric neuropathy include loss of sensation, abnormal sensations, pain, and paresthesias. The pain, which is often described as burning, cramping, crushing, or tearing, is usually worse at night and may occur only at that time. The paresthesias may be associated with tingling, burning, and itching sensations. The patient may report a feeling of walking on pillows or numb feet. At times the skin becomes so sensitive (hyperesthesia) that even light pressure from bedsheets cannot be tolerated. Complete or partial loss of sensitivity to touch and temperature is common. Foot injury and ulcerations can occur without the patient ever having pain (Fig. 49-15). Neuropathy can also cause atrophy of the small muscles of the hands and feet, causing deformity and limiting fine movement.

Control of blood glucose is the only treatment for diabetic neuropathy. It is effective in many, but not all, cases. Drug therapy may be used to treat neuropathic symptoms, particularly pain. Medications commonly used include topical creams (e.g., capsaicin [Zostrix]), tricyclic antidepressants (e.g., amitriptyline [Elavil]), selective serotonin and norepinephrine reuptake inhibitors (e.g., duloxetine [Cymbalta]), and antiseizure medications (e.g., gabapentin [Neurontin]). Capsaicin is a moderately effective topical cream made from chili peppers. It depletes the accumulation of pain-mediating chemicals in the peripheral sensory neurons. The cream is applied three to four times a day. There is usually an increase in symptoms at the start of therapy, which is followed by relief of pain in 2 to 3 weeks. Tricyclic antidepressants are also moderately effective in treating the symptoms of diabetic neuropathy. They work by inhibiting the reuptake of norepinephrine and serotonin, which are neurotransmitters that are believed to play a role in the transmission of pain through the spinal cord.[41] Duloxetine is thought to relieve pain by increasing the levels of serotonin and norepinephrine, which improves the body's ability to regulate pain. The exact mechanism of action of gabapentin is unknown.

Autonomic Neuropathy. Autonomic neuropathy can affect nearly all body systems and lead to hypoglycemic unawareness, bowel incontinence and diarrhea, and urinary retention. Delayed gastric emptying *(gastroparesis)* is a complication of autonomic neuropathy that can produce anorexia, nausea, vomiting, gastroesophageal reflux, and persistent feelings of fullness. Gastroparesis can trigger hypoglycemia by delaying food absorption. Cardiovascular abnormalities associated with autonomic neuropathy are postural hypotension, resting tachycardia, and painless myocardial infarction. A patient with postural hypotension should be instructed to change from a lying or sitting position slowly.

Diabetes can affect sexual function in men and women. Erectile dysfunction in diabetic men is well recognized and common,

Diabetes

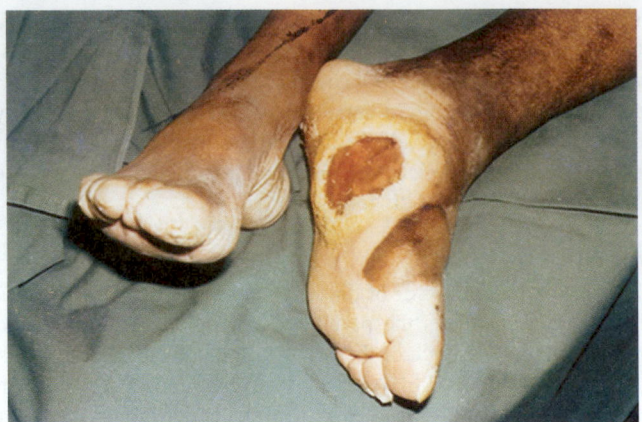

FIG. 49-15   Neuropathy: neurotrophic ulceration.

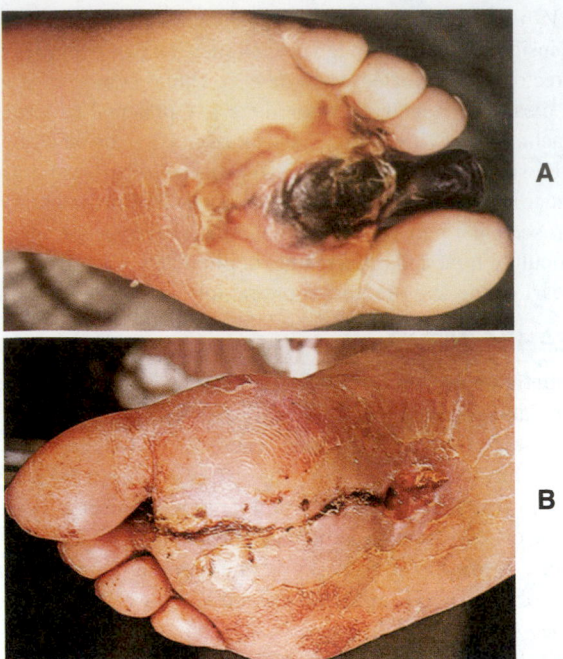

FIG. 49-16   The necrotic toe developed as a complication of diabetes. **A,** Before amputation. **B,** After amputation.

often being the first manifestation of autonomic failure. Erectile dysfunction associated with diabetes mellitus is believed to result from damage to the sacral parasympathetic nerves. Determining whether this problem is of organic or psychologic origin is an important part of the assessment. Decreased libido is a problem with some women with diabetes. Monilial and nonspecific vaginitis are also common. Organic erectile dysfunction or sexual dysfunctioning in either the male or the female patient requires sensitive therapeutic counseling for both the patient and the patient's partner.[42] (See Chapter 55 for a further discussion of erectile dysfunction.)

A neurogenic bladder may develop as sensation in the inner bladder wall decreases, causing urinary retention. A patient with retention has infrequent voiding, difficulty in voiding, and a weak stream of urine. Emptying the bladder every 3 hours in a sitting position helps prevent stasis and subsequent infection. Tightening the abdominal muscles during voiding and using the Credé maneuver (mild massage downward over the lower abdomen and bladder) may also help with complete bladder emptying. Cholinergic agonist drugs such as bethanechol (Urecholine) may be used. The patient may also have to learn self-catheterization (see Chapter 46).

COMPLICATIONS OF FEET AND LOWER EXTREMITIES

Foot complications are the most common cause of hospitalization in the person with diabetes.[43] The development of diabetic foot complications is a multifactoral process.[44] They result from a combination of microvascular and macrovascular diseases that place the patient at risk for injury and serious infection that may lead to amputation (Fig. 49-16). Sensory neuropathy and peripheral arterial disease (PAD) are risk factors, and clotting abnormalities, impaired immune function, and autonomic neuropathy also play important roles. Smoking is deleterious to the health of lower extremity blood vessels and increases the risk for amputation.

Sensory neuropathy is a major risk factor for lower extremity amputation in the person with diabetes. Loss of protective sensation (LOPS) often prevents the patient from becoming aware that a foot injury has occurred. Improper footwear and injury from stepping on foreign objects while barefoot are common causes of undetected foot injury in the person with LOPS. Because the primary risk factor for lower extremity amputation is LOPS, annual screening using a *monofilament* is an extremely important preventive measure. This is done by applying a thin, flexible filament to

several spots on the plantar surface of the foot and asking the patient to report if it is felt. Insensitivity to a 10-g Semmes-Weinstein monofilament has been shown to greatly increase the risk for diabetic foot ulcers that can lead to amputation. If the patient has LOPS, aggressive measures must be taken to teach the patient how to prevent foot ulceration. These measures include the selection of proper footwear, including prescription shoes. Other measures are to carefully avoid injury to the foot, to practice diligent skin and nail care, to inspect the foot thoroughly each day, and to treat small problems promptly.[43]

PAD increases the risk for amputation by causing a reduction in blood flow to the lower extremities. When blood flow is decreased, oxygen, white blood cells, and vital nutrients are not available to the tissues. Therefore wounds take longer to heal and the risk for infection increases. Signs of PAD include intermittent claudication, pain at rest, cold feet, loss of hair, delayed capillary filling, and dependent rubor (redness of the skin that occurs when the extremity is in a dependent position). The disease is diagnosed by history, Doppler findings, and angiography. Management includes control or reduction of risk factors, particularly smoking, high cholesterol intake, and hypertension. Bypass or graft surgery is indicated in some patients. Proper care of the feet is essential for the patient with PAD. Guidelines for patient teaching are listed in Table 49-22. (PAD is discussed in Chapter 38.)

The Doppler instrument is used to diagnose the presence or degree of PAD. Similar to an electronic stethoscope, this device amplifies sound. The procedure is noninvasive and can measure blood pressure in the lower extremities and blood flow velocity. It can indicate areas of stenosis or occlusion and is useful as an indicator of the need for additional vascular tests.

Proper care of a diabetic foot ulcer is critical to prevention of infections. A topical gel of recombinant platelet-derived growth factor, becaplermin (Regranex), can be used to assist with the healing of a foot ulcer. If a foot ulcer is unresponsive to conventional therapy for 3 weeks and no underlying structures are ex-

TABLE 49-22	***PATIENT AND FAMILY TEACHING GUIDE*** Foot Care

1. Wash feet daily with a mild soap and warm water. Test water temperature with hands first.
2. Pat feet dry gently, especially between toes.
3. Examine feet daily for cuts, blisters, swelling, and red, tender areas. Do not depend on feeling sores. If eyesight is poor, have others inspect feet.
4. Use lanolin on feet to prevent skin from drying and cracking. Do not apply between toes.
5. Use mild foot powder on sweaty feet.
6. Do not use commercial remedies to remove calluses or corns.
7. Cleanse cuts with warm water and mild soap, covering with clean dressing. Do not use iodine, rubbing alcohol, or strong adhesives.
8. Report skin infections or nonhealing sores to health care provider immediately.
9. Cut toenails evenly with rounded contour of toes. Do not cut down corners. The best time to trim nails is after a shower or bath.
10. Separate overlapping toes with cotton or lamb's wool.
11. Avoid open-toe, open-heel, and high-heel shoes. Leather shoes are preferred to plastic ones. Wear slippers with soles. Do not go barefoot. Shake out shoes before putting on.
12. Wear clean, absorbent (cotton or wool) socks or stockings that have not been mended. Colored socks must be colorfast.
13. Do not wear clothing that leaves impressions, hindering circulation.
14. Do not use hot water bottles or heating pads to warm feet. Wear socks for warmth.
15. Guard against frostbite.
16. Exercise feet daily either by walking or by flexing and extending feet in suspended position. Avoid prolonged sitting, standing, and crossing of legs.

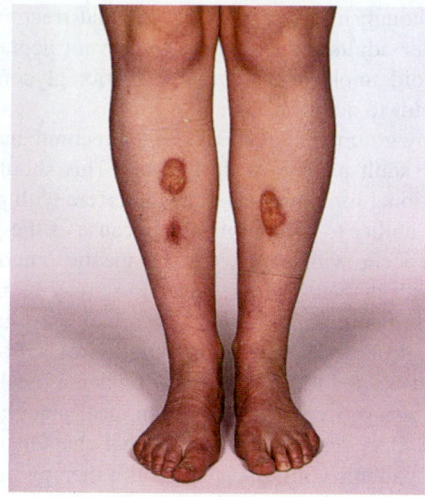

FIG. 49-17 Necrobiosis lipoidica diabeticorum.

posed, Apligraf may be used. Apligraf is a human skin equivalent that is used to accelerate the closure of nonhealing wounds. With Apligraf, since the skin does not have to be harvested from another body site, the patient only has one wound to heal, not two.[43,45]

Neuropathic arthropathy, or *Charcot foot,* results in ankle and foot changes that ultimately lead to joint dysfunction and footdrop. These changes occur gradually and promote an abnormal distribution of weight over the foot, further increasing the chances of developing a foot ulcer as new pressure points emerge. Neuropathic ulcers resemble a "BB shot" or "punched out" wound and are usually painless. Infection is a danger and necessitates the long-term use of antibiotics and weeks of avoidance of weight bearing on the affected limb.

INTEGUMENTARY COMPLICATIONS

The skin is often affected in patients with diabetes. *Acanthosis nigricans* is a dark, coarse, thickened skin predominantly seen in flexures and on the neck. Diabetic dermatopathy is red-brown flat-topped papules. *Necrobiosis lipoidica diabeticorum,* associated with type 1 diabetes, usually appears as red-yellow lesions, with atrophic skin that becomes shiny and transparent revealing tiny blood vessels under the surface (Fig. 49-17). Because the thin skin is prone to injury, special care must be taken to protect affected areas from injury and ulceration. This condition is not common, but it may appear before other clinical signs or symptoms of diabetes. It is more frequently seen in young women. *Granuloma annulare,* associated mainly with type 1 diabetes, is probably autoimmune in nature and forms partial rings of papules, often on the dorsal surface of hands and feet.

INFECTION

A patient with diabetes is more susceptible to infections than other patients. The mechanisms for this phenomenon include a defect in the mobilization of inflammatory cells and an impairment of phagocytosis by neutrophils and monocytes. Recurring or persistent infections such as *Candida albicans,* as well as boils and furuncles, in the undiagnosed patient often lead the health care provider to suspect diabetes. Loss of sensation (neuropathy) may delay the detection of an infection.

Persistent glycosuria may predispose to bladder infections, especially in patients with a neurogenic bladder. Decreased circulation resulting from angiopathy can prevent or delay the immune response. Antibiotic therapy has prevented infection from being a major cause of death in diabetic patients. The treatment of infections must be prompt and vigorous.

GERONTOLOGIC CONSIDERATIONS
DIABETES MELLITUS

The prevalence of diabetes increases with age. A major reason for this is that the process of aging is associated with a reduction in β-cell function, decreased insulin sensitivity, and altered carbohydrate metabolism.[46] Aging is also associated with a number of conditions that are more likely to be treated with medications that impair insulin action (e.g., corticosteroids, antihypertensives, phenothiazines). Undiagnosed and untreated diabetes is more common in the elderly, partly because many of the normal physiologic changes of aging resemble those of diabetes, such as visual changes and decreased glomerular filtration.

Although good glycemic control is important to people of all ages with diabetes, several factors are taken into account when determining glycemic goals for an older adult. One is that hypoglycemic unawareness is more common in this age-group, making these patients more likely to suffer adverse consequences from blood glucose–lowering therapy. They may also have delayed psychomotor function that could interfere with the ability to treat hypoglycemia. Other factors to consider in establishing glycemic goals for the older patient include the patient's own desire for treatment and other coexisting medical problems such as cognitive impairment. Compounding the challenge, diabetes has been found to contribute to a greater rate of decline of cognitive function. Although it is generally agreed that treatment is indicated for older adults with diabetes to prevent acute complications and avoid unpleasant symptoms, strict glycemic control may be difficult to achieve.[47]

As with any group, diet and exercise are recommended as therapy for older adult patients with diabetes. This should take into account functional limitations that may interfere with physical activity and the ability to prepare meals. Because of the physiologic changes that occur with aging, the therapeutic outcome for the older adult with diabetes who receives OAs may be altered. The sulfonylurea drugs (e.g., glyburide [Micronase]) are usually well tolerated. Meglitinides have a short duration of action. Because patients are instructed to only take a pill when a meal is eaten, it reduces their risk of hypoglycemia when meal planning is inconsistent. Other OAs described earlier in this chapter may also be used in older patients with diabetes. Insulin therapy may be instituted if OAs are not effective. However, it is important to recognize that older adults are more likely to have limitations in manual dexterity and visual acuity, both of which are necessary for accurate insulin administration.[46]

Patient teaching should be based on the individual's needs, using a slower pace with simple printed or audio materials. It is important to include family or a support person in the teaching. The patient education issues for the older patient include those related to vision, mobility, mental status, functional ability, financial and social situation, the effect of multiple medications, eating habits, the potential for undetected hypoglycemia, and quality-of-life issues.

CRITICAL THINKING EXERCISE

CASE STUDY

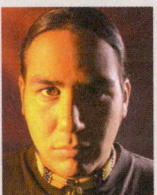

Diabetic Ketoacidosis

Patient Profile. John, a 34-year-old Native American man, was admitted to the emergency department after he was found unconscious in his apartment by his wife.

Subjective Data (Provided by Wife)
- Was diagnosed with diabetes mellitus 12 months ago
- Was taking 48 U of insulin daily: 12 U of regular insulin plus 20 U of NPH before breakfast, 8 U of regular insulin before dinner, and 8 U of NPH at bedtime
- Has history of flu for 1 week with vomiting and anorexia
- Stopped taking insulin 2 days ago when he was unable to eat

Objective Data
Physical Examination
- Breathing is deep and rapid
- Acetone smell on breath
- Skin flushed and dry

Diagnostic Studies
- Blood glucose level of 730 mg/dl (40.5 mmol/L)
- Blood pH of 7.26

Critical Thinking Questions

1. Briefly explain the pathophysiology of the development of diabetic ketoacidosis (DKA) in this patient.
2. What clinical manifestations of DKA does this patient exhibit?

3. What factors precipitated this patient's DKA?
4. What is the priority nursing intervention for John?
5. What distinguishes this case history from one of hyperosmolar hyperglycemic syndrome (HHS) or hypoglycemia?
6. What teaching should be done with this patient and his family?
7. What role should John's wife have in the management of his diabetes?
8. Based on the assessment data presented, write one or more appropriate nursing diagnoses. Are there any collaborative problems?

NCLEX EXAMINATION REVIEW QUESTIONS

The number of the question corresponds to the same-numbered objective at the beginning of the chapter.

1. The polydipsia and polyuria related to diabetes mellitus are primarily caused by
   a. the release of ketones from cells during fat metabolism.
   b. fluid shifts resulting from the osmotic effect of hyperglycemia.
   c. damage to the kidneys from exposure to high levels of glucose.
   d. changes in RBCs resulting from attachment of excessive glucose to hemoglobin.
2. When a patient with type 2 diabetes mellitus is admitted to the hospital with pneumonia, the nurse recognizes that the patient
   a. must receive insulin therapy to prevent the development of ketoacidosis.
   b. has islet cell antibodies that have destroyed the ability of the pancreas to produce insulin.
   c. has minimal or absent endogenous insulin secretion and requires daily insulin injections.
   d. may have sufficient endogenous insulin to prevent ketosis but is at risk for development of hyperosmolar hyperglycemic nonketotic syndrome.
3. Effective collaborative management of diabetes includes
   a. using insulin with all patients to achieve glycemic goals.
   b. relying on the health care provider as the central figure in the program for good control.
   c. relying solely on nutritional therapy as the initial treatment modality for all patients with diabetes.
   d. aiming for a balance of diet, activity, and medications together with appropriate monitoring and patient and family teaching.
4. The nurse assists the patient with nutritional therapy of diabetes with the knowledge that a "diabetic diet" is designed
   a. to be used only for type 1 diabetes.
   b. for use during periods of high stress.
   c. to normalize blood glucose by elimination of sugar.
   d. to help normalize blood glucose through a balanced diet.
5. In teaching a newly diagnosed type 1 diabetic "survival skills," the nurse includes information about
   a. weight loss measures.
   b. elimination of sugar from diet.
   c. need to reduce physical activity.
   d. self-monitoring of blood glucose.
6. An appropriate teaching measure for the patient with diabetes mellitus related to care of the feet is to
   a. use heat to increase blood supply.
   b. avoid softening lotions and creams.
   c. inspect all surfaces of the feet daily.
   d. use iodine to disinfect cuts and abrasions.

7. A diabetic patient has a serum glucose level of 824 mg/dl (45.7 mmol/L) and is unresponsive. Following assessment of the patient, the nurse suspects diabetic ketoacidosis rather than hyperosmolar hyperglycemic syndrome based on the finding of
   a. polyuria.
   b. severe dehydration.
   c. rapid, deep respirations.
   d. decreased serum potassium.

8. Which of the following is not an appropriate therapy for patients with diabetes mellitus?
   a. Use of diuretics to treat renal problems
   b. Use of ACE inhibitors to treat renal problems
   c. Use of laser photocoagulation to treat retinopathy
   d. Use of regular insulin for a patient with type 2 diabetes during the intraoperative period

REFERENCES

1. American Diabetes Association: Total prevalence of diabetes and prediabetes. Available at *www.diabetes.org.*
2. National Diabetes, Digestive, and Kidney Disease Website: National diabetes statistics. Available at *www.nih.gov.*
3. Drury P, Gatling W: *Your questions answered: diabetes,* Edinburgh, 2005, Churchill Livingstone.
4. American Diabetes Association: *American diabetes association complete guide to diabetes,* Alexandria, Va., 2005, American Diabetes Association.
5. Kumar V, Abbas AK, Fausto N: *Robbins and Cotran's pathologic basis of disease,* ed 7, Philadelphia, 2005, Elsevier Saunders.
6. American Diabetes Association: Resource guide 2005: insulin. Available at *www.diabetes.org.*
7. Riddle MC: Glycemic management of type 2 diabetes: an emerging strategy with oral agents, insulins, and combinations, *Endocrinol Metab Clin North Am* 34:77, 2004.
8. Lehne RA: *Pharmacology for nursing care,* ed 6, St Louis, 2007, Saunders.
9. Rosenstock J, Dailey G, Massi-Benedetti M, et al: Reduced hypoglycemia risk with insulin glargine, *Diabetes Care* 28:950, 2005.
10. Diabetes Health Online: Insulin administration. Available at *diabetes.healthcentersonline.com.*
11. Nektar Therapeutics: Nektar reports that FDA advisory committee recommends approval of Exubera for use in adults with type 1 and type 2 diabetes, September 2005. Available at *www.nektar.com.*
12. American Diabetes Association: Resource guide 2005: oral agents for type 2. Available at *www.diabetes.org.*
13. Funnell MM, Barlage DL: Managing diabetes with "agent oral," *Nursing* 34:36, 2004.
14. Viberti G: Thiazolidinediones—benefits on microvascular complications of type 2 diabetes, *J Diabetes Complications* 19:168, 2005.
15. Laustsen G: Symlin for adults with type 1 and type 2 diabetes, *Nurse Pract* 30:55, 2005.
16. Poon T, Nelson P, Shen L: Enatide improves glycemic control and reduces body weight in subjects with type 2 diabetes: a dose-ranging study, *Diabetes Technology and Therapeutics* 7:467, 2005.
17. Moore MC: *Pocket guide to nutritional assessment and care,* ed 5, St Louis, 2005, Elsevier.
18. American Diabetes Association: Position statement: nutrition principles and recommendations in diabetes, *Diabetes Care* 27(suppl):36, 2004.
19. Vaughan L: Dietary guidelines for the management of diabetes, *Nurs Stand* 19:56, 2005.
20. Nix S: *Williams' basic nutrition and diet therapy,* ed 12, St Louis, 2005, Mosby.
21. Grodner M, Long S, DeYoung S: *Foundations and clinical applications of nutrition: a nursing approach,* ed 3, St Louis, 2004, Mosby.
22. American Diabetes Association: Diabetes meal plans and a healthy diet. Available at *www.diabetes.org.*
23. American Diabetes Association: Diabetes nutrition recommendations for health care institutions, *Diabetes Care* 27(suppl):55, 2004.
24. Hawley JA: Exercise as a therapeutic intervention for the prevention and treatment of insulin resistance, *Diabetes/Metabolism Research Reviews* 20:383, 2004.
25. Hopkins D: Exercise-induced and other daytime hypoglycemic events in patients with diabetes: prevention and treatment, *Diabetes Res Clin Pract* 65(suppl):35, 2004.
26. Fain JA: Blood glucose meters: different strokes for different folks, *Nursing* 34:48, 2004.
27. Mulcahy K, American Diabetes Association, Lumber T: *Diabetes ready reference guide for health care professionals,* Alexandria, Va., 2004, American Diabetes Association.
28. Diabetes Prevention Program Research Group: Reduction in the incidence of type 2 diabetes with lifestyle intervention or metformin, *N Engl J Med* 346:393, 2002.
29. American Diabetes Association: Position statement: standards of medical care in diabetes, *Diabetes Care* 28(suppl):4, 2005.
30. American Diabetes Association: *Complete nurse's guide to diabetes care,* Alexandria, Va., 2005, American Diabetes Association.
31. Glucophage (metformin hydrochloride tablets) prescribing information, Bristol-Myers Squibb Company, revised 2004.
32. Guthrie RA, Guthrie DW: Pathophysiology of diabetes mellitus, *Crit Care Nurse Q* 27:113, 2004.
33. Moore T: Diabetic emergencies in adults, *Nurs Stand* 18:45, 2004.
34. Centers for Disease Control and Prevention/National Center for Chronic Disease Prevention and Health Promotion: National diabetes fact sheet, 2002. Available at *www.cdc.gov/diabetes/pubs/estimates.htm.*
35. Diabetes Control and Complications Trial Research Group: The effect of intensive treatment of diabetes on the development and progression of long-term complications in insulin-dependent diabetes mellitus, *N Engl J Med* 329:977, 1993.
36. American Diabetes Association: Position statement: implications of the United Kingdom Prospective Diabetes Study, *Diabetes Care* 25(suppl 1):28, 2002.
37. American Diabetes Association: Dyslipidemia management in adults with diabetes, *Diabetes Care* 27(suppl):68, 2004.
38. Helbig H, Sutter FKP: Surgical treatment of diabetic retinopathy, *Graefe's Arch Clin Exp Ophthalmol* 242:704, 2004.
39. Willoughby D, Burriss P: Protecting the kidneys of patients with diabetes, *Clin Nurse Spec* 19:150, 2005.
40. Gross JL, Canani LH, DeAzevedo MJ: Diabetic nephropathy: diagnosis, prevention, and treatment, *Diabetes Care* 28:164, 2005.
41. Adriaensen H, Plaghki L, Mathieu C, et al: Critical review of oral drug treatments for diabetic neuropathic pain—clinical outcomes based on efficacy and safety data from placebo-controlled and direct comparative studies, *Diabetes/Metabolism Research Reviews* 21:231, 2005.
42. Sinnreich M, Taylor BV, Dyck PJB: Diabetic neuropathies: classification, clinical features, and pathophysiological basis, *Neurologist* 11:63, 2005.
43. Sieggreen MY: Stepping up care for diabetic foot ulcers, *Nursing* 35:36, 2005.
44. Boulton AJM, Kirsner RS, Vileikyte L: Neuropathic diabetes foot ulcers, *N Engl J Med* 351:48, 2004.
45. Kiemele LJ, Takahashi PY: Practical wound management in long-term care, *Ann Long-Term Care* 12:25, 2004.
46. Sakharova OV, Inzucchi SE: Treatment of diabetes in the elderly: addressing its complexities in this high-risk group, *Postgrad Med* 118:19, 2005.
47. Pinkstaff SM: Aging with diabetes—an underappreciated cause of progressive disability and reduced quality of life, *Clin Geriatr* 12:45, 2004.

RESOURCES

American Association of Diabetes Educators
800-338-3633
www.aadenet.org
American Diabetes Association
800-DIABETES (342-2383)
www.diabetes.org
Council for the Advancement of Diabetes Research and Education
888-771-1297
www.cadre-diabetes.org
Diabetes at Work
www.diabetesatwork.org
Diabetes Monitor
www.diabetesmonitor.com
National Diabetes Education Program
301-496-3583
www.ndep.nih.gov
National Diabetes Education Program's Better Diabetes Care
www.betterdiabetescare.nih.gov
National Diabetes Information Clearinghouse
www.diabetes.niddk.nih.gov
Neuropathy Association
212-692-0662
www.neuropathy.org
For additional Internet resources, see the website for this book at *http://evolve.elsevier.com/Lewis/medsurg.*

What we see depends mainly on what we look for.

Sir John Lubbock

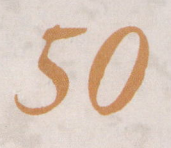

50

Nursing Management
Endocrine Problems

JoAnne Konick-McMahan

LEARNING OBJECTIVES

1. Describe the pathophysiology, clinical manifestations, collaborative care, and nursing management of the patient with an imbalance of hormones produced by the anterior pituitary gland.
2. Describe the pathophysiology, clinical manifestations, collaborative care, and nursing management of the patient with an imbalance of hormones produced by the posterior pituitary gland.
3. Describe the pathophysiology, clinical manifestations, collaborative care, and nursing management of the patient with thyroid dysfunction.
4. Describe the pathophysiology, clinical manifestations, collaborative care, and nursing management of the patient with an imbalance of the hormone produced by the parathyroid glands.
5. Describe the pathophysiology, clinical manifestations, collaborative care, and nursing management of the patient with an imbalance of hormones produced by the adrenal cortex.
6. Describe the pathophysiology, clinical manifestations, collaborative care, and nursing management of the patient with an excess of hormones produced by the adrenal medulla.
7. Describe the side effects of corticosteroid therapy.
8. List common nursing assessments, interventions, rationales, and expected outcomes related to patient teaching for management of chronic endocrine problems.

KEY TERMS

acromegaly, p. 1291
Cushing syndrome, p. 1312
diabetes insipidus, p. 1296
exophthalmos, p. 1299
goiter, p. 1297
Graves' disease, p. 1299
hyperparathyroidism, p. 1308
hyperthyroidism, p. 1299
hypoparathyroidism, p. 1311
hypopituitarism, p. 1293
hypothyroidism, p. 1305
myxedema, p. 1305
pheochromocytoma, p. 1320
thyroiditis, p. 1298
thyrotoxicosis, p. 1299

Electronic Resources

Supplemental content related to Chapter 50 can be found . . .

Companion CD
• Stress-Busting Kit for Nursing Students
• Interactive Case Studies:
  • Addison's Disease
  • Cushing Syndrome
  • Hyperthyroidism
• NCLEX Examination Review Questions
• Comprehensive Glossary

Evolve Website *evolve*
http://evolve.elsevier.com/Lewis/medsurg
• Content Updates
• Key Points (Printable and CD/MP3 Download)
• Concept Map Creator
• Expanded Audio Glossary
• Key Term Flash Cards
• Customizable Nursing Care Plans:
  • Hyperthyroidism
  • Hypothyroidism
  • Cushing Syndrome

• Patient and Family Instruction Guide in English and Spanish: Corticosteroid Therapy
• Electronic Calculators
• WebLinks

Reviewed by Cynthia L. Donell, RN, MSN, Medical Surgical Nursing Instructor, The Reading Hospital School of Nursing, The Reading Hospital and Medical Center, Reading, Pa.; and Coleen R. Elmers, RN, MSN, Staff Development Educator, Baptist Health System, San Antonio, Tex.

Disorders of the Anterior Pituitary Gland

GROWTH HORMONE EXCESS

Etiology and Pathophysiology

Growth hormone (GH), an anabolic hormone, promotes protein synthesis and mobilizes glucose and free fatty acids. GH is produced by the anterior pituitary and stimulates the liver to produce insulin-like growth factor–1 (IGF-1), also known as somatomedin C. IGF-1 stimulates the growth of bones and soft tissues. Normally IGF-1 signals the anterior pituitary to reduce GH production. Overproduction of GH is almost always caused by a benign pituitary tumor (adenoma). The pituitary tumor secretes GH despite elevated IGF-1 levels, leading to the unwanted growth of bones and other soft tissue. Overproduction of GH also causes elevation of blood glucose through insulin antagonism. Prolonged elevated glucose levels associated with an elevation in GH leads to glucose intolerance.

In children, the excessive secretion of GH results in *gigantism*. When the onset of GH excess occurs before closure of the epiphyses, the long bones are still capable of longitudinal growth. The excessive growth seen is usually proportional. These children may grow as tall as 8 feet (240 cm) and weigh more than 300 lb (136 kg).

In adults, excessive secretion of GH results in acromegaly. **Acromegaly** is characterized by an overgrowth of the bones and soft tissues. Because the problem develops after epiphyseal closure in adults, the bones are unable to grow longer. Instead, the bones increase in thickness and width. Acromegaly is relatively rare. Only 3 out of every 1 million adults in the United States is diagnosed with this disease each year, with a prevalence of 70 out of every 1 million individuals.[1] Both genders are affected equally.

Clinical Manifestations

Manifestations of acromegaly begin gradually, usually in the 20s and 30s. Typically there is an average of 7 to 9 years between the initial onset of symptoms and final diagnosis. Individuals experience enlargement of the hands and feet. The fingertips develop a tufted or clubbed-like appearance. The enlargement of the bones and cartilage may cause symptoms that range from mild joint pain to deforming, crippling arthritis. Changes in physical appearance occur, with thickening and enlargement of bony and soft tissues on the face and head (Fig. 50-1). Enlargement of the mandible causes the jaw to jut forward. The paranasal and frontal sinuses enlarge, as does the bony tissue of the forehead. Enlargement of soft tissue around the eyes, nose, and mouth results in a coarsening of facial features. Enlargement of the tongue results in speech difficulties,

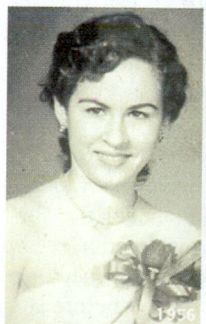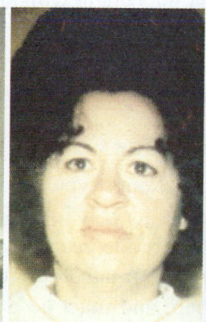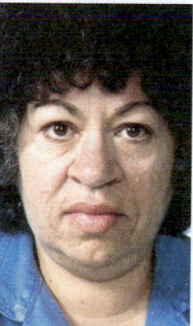

FIG. 50-1 Progressive development of facial changes associated with acromegaly.

and the voice deepens as a result of hypertrophy of the vocal cords.

Sleep apnea may also occur and is related to upper airway narrowing and obstruction resulting from increased amounts of pharyngeal soft tissues.[2] The skin becomes thick, leathery, and oily. Persons with acromegaly may also experience peripheral neuropathy and proximal muscle weakness. Women may develop menstrual disturbances. Individuals with acromegaly are more likely to develop polyps in the colon and colon cancer.

The enlarged pituitary tumor gland can exert pressure on surrounding structures within the brain, leading to visual disturbances and headaches. Because GH mobilizes stored fat for energy, it increases free fatty acid levels in the blood and predisposes the patient to atherosclerosis. The hormone also antagonizes the action of insulin and causes hyperglycemia. Manifestations of diabetes mellitus may occur, including polydipsia and polyuria. Prolonged secretion of GH leads to glucose intolerance.

Left untreated, acromegaly can lead to a number of changes in the body. Effects on the cardiovascular system include cardiomegaly, left ventricular hypertrophy, angina pectoris, and hypertension. For this reason, disease of the cardiovascular system is associated with increased mortality rates in these individuals. Other systems that undergo changes include the respiratory, gastrointestinal, genitourinary, musculoskeletal, and nervous systems.

Diagnostic Studies

In addition to the history and physical examination, a diagnosis of acromegaly requires evaluation of plasma IGF-1 levels, IGF binding protein–3 (IGFBP-3) levels, and GH response to an oral glucose challenge. A single measurement of serum GH is of limited value in the diagnosis of acromegaly because GH levels normally fluctuate. IGF-1 levels are more constant and thus provide a more reliable measure than GH levels. The definitive test for acromegaly is the oral glucose challenge test. Normally, GH concentration falls during an oral glucose tolerance test. In acromegaly, growth hormone levels do not fall below 1 ng/ml.[3]

Magnetic resonance imaging (MRI) is indicated for identifying and determining the extent of spread of the pituitary tumor into surrounding tissue. High-resolution computed tomography (CT) scanning with contrast media may also be used to localize the tumor. A complete ophthalmologic examination, including visual fields, is typically done because the tumor (especially a macroadenoma larger than 10 mm) may cause pressure on the optic chiasm or optic nerves.

Collaborative Care

The therapeutic goal in acromegaly is to return the patient's GH levels to normal. This is accomplished by surgery, radiation, drug therapy, or a combination of these therapies. The prognosis depends on age at onset, age when treatment is initiated, and tumor size. Individuals with large pituitary tumors invading the dura, bone, or cavernous sinus (80% of patients diagnosed with acromegaly) require multiple therapies. Usually, bone growth can be arrested and soft tissue hypertrophy can be reversed. However, sleep apnea and diabetic and cardiac complications may persist in spite of treatment.

Surgical Therapy. Surgery (hypophysectomy) is the treatment of choice and offers the best hope for a cure, especially for smaller tumors (microadenomas smaller than 10 mm). The majority of surgeries done to remove pituitary tumors associated with

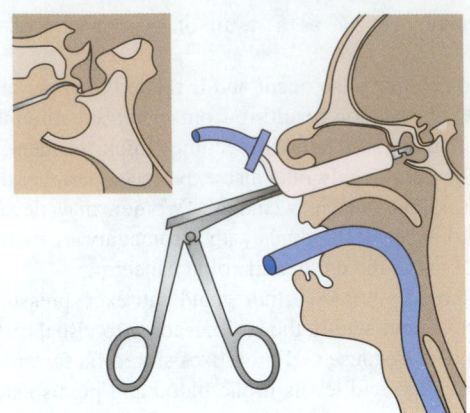

FIG. 50-2 Surgery on the pituitary gland is most commonly performed with the transsphenoidal approach. An incision is made in the inner aspect of the upper lip and gingiva. The sella turcica is entered through the floor of the nose and sphenoid sinuses.

acromegaly are accomplished with the *transsphenoidal* approach.[4] The goal of transsphenoidal surgery is to remove only the tumor that is causing GH secretion (Fig. 50-2). This procedure produces an immediate reduction in GH levels followed by a drop in IGF-1 levels within a few weeks.

Although most of these procedures are effective, some patients (especially those with larger tumors or those with GH levels greater than 45 ng/ml) do not obtain a cure with the surgery and require adjuvant radiation or drug therapy.[5] In some cases, the entire pituitary gland is removed during surgery *(hypophysectomy),* resulting in a permanent absence of pituitary hormones. Rather than replacing the pituitary (tropic) hormones, which requires parenteral administration, the essential hormones produced by target organs (glucocorticoids, thyroid hormone, and sex hormones) can be given orally. Hormone replacement must then be continued throughout life.

Radiation Therapy. Radiation therapy is considered when surgery has failed to produce complete remission. External radiation can successfully reduce GH levels in 30% to 70% of patients, but the primary disadvantage is the long delay (5 to 10 years) for GH levels to normalize. Because of the length of time it takes to achieve GH reduction, radiation therapy is usually offered in combination with drugs that reduce GH levels. Radiation has also been used to reduce the size of a tumor before surgery. The patient may experience local skin changes, alopecia, or oral complications. Hypopituitarism commonly results from radiation therapy and requires hormone replacement therapy.

Stereotactic radiosurgery (gamma surgery, proton beam, linear accelerator [linac]) may be used for small, surgically inaccessible pituitary tumors or in place of conventional radiation (see Chapter 57). This procedure consists of a single dose of radiation delivered to one site from multiple angles. It is used to occlude blood vessels supplying the tumor and results in cell death. Focused radiotherapy may lead to earlier GH reduction than conventional radiotherapy.[5]

Drug Therapy. Three types of drugs are used in the treatment of acromegaly: somatostatin analogs, GH receptor antagonists, and dopamine agonists. These drugs reduce GH levels and can be used as initial treatment or as adjunct therapy to surgery or radiation. The most common drug used for acromegaly is octreotide (Sandostatin), a somatostatin analog that reduces GH levels to within the normal range in many patients. Octreotide is given by subcutaneous injection three times a week. Two long-acting analogs, octreotide (Depot, Sandostatin LAR) and lanreotide SR (Ipstyl), are now available as intramuscular (IM) injections given every 2 to 4 weeks. Pegvisomant is a GH receptor antagonist (Somavert) and is considered an alternative to somatostatin analogs. This drug is used for patients who have received surgery or radiation therapy, but still have hypersecretion of GH. It is not considered appropriate for primary treatment because this agent only blocks hormone action rather than acting on the tumor itself. Dopamine agonists (cabergoline [Dostinex]) may also be used in the treatment of acromegaly to suppress GH secretion. Dopamine agonists may be tried first because they are less expensive than the other two classes of drugs, but they are often not effective.[5]

Somatropin (Omnitrope), recombinant human growth hormone, is now available for long-term replacement therapy in adults with growth hormone deficiency of either childhood or adult onset. It is given daily as a subcutaneous injection (preferably in the evening). Gradual dosage increases at 4- to 8-week intervals up to a maximum of 0.08 mg/kg/week may be given based on patient tolerance. Mild to moderate side effects include fluid retention and myalgia.

NURSING MANAGEMENT
GROWTH HORMONE EXCESS

■ *Nursing Assessment*

The nurse needs to assess for signs and symptoms of abnormal tissue growth and evaluate changes in the physical size of each patient. The adult should be questioned about increases in hat, ring, glove, and shoe sizes. Photographs are helpful to evaluate any changes. Because physical changes occur slowly and over a long period of time, it is possible that the individual is not even aware of such changes.

■ *Nursing Diagnoses*

Nursing diagnoses for the patient with GH excess include, but are not limited to, the following:
- Disturbed body image *related to* enlargement of the hands, feet, jaw, and soft body tissue
- Deficient fluid volume *related to* polyuria
- Insomnia *related to* soft tissue swelling
- Disturbed sensory perception (visual) *related to* enlarged pituitary gland

■ *Planning*

The overall goals are that the patient with GH excess will (1) cope effectively with altered body image, (2) maintain adequate fluid volume, (3) experience restful sleep patterns, (4) develop no complications, and (5) obtain long-term follow-up care.

■ *Nursing Implementation*

Acute Intervention. Patients typically have many questions and concerns regarding surgery. It is important for the nurse to offer reassurance and to provide accurate information regarding this process. The individual treated surgically will need skilled neurosurgical nursing care and must be prepared before surgery for postoperative care. The patient should be instructed to avoid vigorous coughing, sneezing, and straining at stool (Valsalva maneuver) to prevent cerebrospinal fluid leakage from the point at which the sella turcica was entered.

After surgery in which a transsphenoidal approach has been used, the head of the patient's bed should be elevated at a 30-degree angle at all times. This elevation avoids pressure on the sella turcica and decreases headaches, a frequent postoperative problem. Monitoring neurologic status, including pupillary response, should be done in order to detect neurologic complications.

Any clear nasal drainage should be sent to the laboratory to be tested for glucose. A glucose level greater than 30 mg/dl (1.67 mmol/L) indicates cerebrospinal fluid leakage from an open connection to the brain. If this happens, the patient is at an increased risk for meningitis. Complaints of persistent and severe generalized or supraorbital headache may indicate cerebrospinal fluid leakage into the sinuses. A cerebrospinal fluid leak usually resolves within 72 hours when treated with head elevation and bed rest. If the leak persists, daily spinal taps may be done to reduce pressure to below-normal levels and allow the fossa to heal. Intravenous (IV) antibiotics are usually administered when there is a cerebrospinal fluid leak to prevent meningitis. If the leak does not respond to treatment in 72 hours, surgical intervention may be required.

Mild analgesia is given for headaches. The nurse should perform mouth care every 4 hours to keep the surgical area clean and free of debris and to promote patient comfort. Toothbrushing should be avoided for at least 10 days to prevent disrupting the suture line and to avoid discomfort.

If stereotactic radiosurgery is used, the patient is usually moved from the specialized radiation center to the neurosurgical nursing unit for overnight observation. The patient will be in a stereotactic head frame. Vital signs, neurologic status, and fluid volume status must be carefully monitored. Possible complications include increased headaches, seizures, nausea, and vomiting. The patient with a history of seizures is at increased risk for seizures for at least 24 hours after the procedure. All staff should be instructed in removing a stereotactic frame in case of an emergency. The patient may experience discomfort at the pin sites. Pin-site care should be done according to institutional policy. Family members can be instructed in pin-site care if the patient is discharged the day after the procedure.

A possible postoperative complication is transient diabetes insipidus (DI). This may occur because of the loss of antidiuretic hormone (ADH), which is stored in the posterior lobe of the pituitary gland, or cerebral edema related to manipulation of the pituitary during surgery. To assess for DI, urine output and serum and urine osmolarity must be closely monitored. Clinical manifestations and treatment of DI are discussed in more detail later in this chapter.

Ambulatory and Home Care. If a hypophysectomy is performed or the pituitary is damaged, hormone replacement will be necessary. ADH, cortisol, and thyroid hormone replacement will be needed. Because these medications need to be taken for life, careful patient teaching is essential when replacement of these hormones is necessary.

Because surgery may result in permanent hormone deficiencies and possible decreased fertility, the patient needs assistance in working through the grieving process associated with these losses. The need for continued drug therapy reduces the patient's perception of independence and requires considerable emotional adjustment. The nurse must consider the emotional impact of a hypophysectomy when counseling the patient and planning the educational program related to hormone replacement. Serial photographs to show improvement may be helpful. Psychologic support from the nurse and from the patient's family and friends is needed to promote positive mental health outcomes for the patient with acromegaly.

The teaching plan should include self-administration of subcutaneous injection if prescribed. Cost issues related to the expense of ongoing medication, as well as other therapies, may be another area for nursing intervention.

■ *Evaluation*

The expected outcomes are that the patient with GH excess will
- experience no complications postoperatively
- know how and when to take hormone replacements (if indicated)
- state symptoms requiring immediate attention and appropriate actions
- state the importance of long-term follow-up

EXCESSES OF OTHER TROPIC HORMONES

An excess of tropic hormones and the overproduction of a single anterior pituitary hormone usually produces a syndrome related to hormone excess from the target organ. For example, if adrenocorticotropic hormone (ACTH) is increased, Cushing's disease results; if thyroid-stimulating hormone (TSH) levels are excessive, hyperthyroidism develops.

Prolactinomas (prolactin-secreting adenomas) are the most frequently occurring pituitary tumor. Common manifestations experienced by women with prolactinomas include galactorrhea, ovulatory dysfunction (anovulation, infertility), menstrual dysfunction (oligomenorrhea or amenorrhea), decreased libido, and hirsutism. In men, impotence and decreased libido and sperm density may result. The affected patient may also experience headaches and visual problems. The visual problems are secondary to pressure on the optic chiasm. Because prolactinomas do not typically progress in size, drug therapy is usually the first-line treatment. Dopamine agonists such as bromocriptine (Parlodel), cabergoline (Dostinex), and pergolide (Permax) have successfully been used to treat this disorder. Surgery using the transsphenoidal approach (discussed previously) may be considered depending on size and extent of the tumor. The use of radiation for treatment of prolactinomas has been somewhat limited. It is mainly used in those patients who have failed to respond to medical or surgical therapy.

HYPOFUNCTION OF THE PITUITARY GLAND

Hypopituitarism is a rare disorder that involves a decrease in one or more of the pituitary hormones. The anterior pituitary gland secretes ACTH, TSH, follicle-stimulating hormone (FSH), luteinizing hormone (LH), GH, and prolactin; the posterior pituitary gland secretes ADH and oxytocin. A deficiency of only one pituitary hormone is referred to as *selective hypopituitarism*. Total failure of the pituitary gland results in deficiency of all pituitary hormones—a condition referred to as *panhypopituitarism*. The most common hormone deficiencies associated with hypopituitarism involve GH and gonadotropins (e.g., LH, FSH).

Etiology and Pathophysiology

The most common cause of pituitary hypofunction is a pituitary tumor. Autoimmune disorders, infections, pituitary infarction (Sheehan syndrome), or destruction of the pituitary gland (as a result of trauma, radiation, and surgical procedures) also can cause hypopituitarism. *Sheehan syndrome* is a postpartum condition of pituitary necrosis and hypopituitarism that occurs after circulatory collapse from uterine hemorrhaging.

Hormone deficiencies involving anterior pituitary hormones lead to end-organ failure; thus the effects of hypopituitarism depend on the specific pituitary hormone or hormones that are lacking. For example, infertility may be the first indication of pituitary hypofunction associated with a pituitary tumor. Deficiencies of TSH and ACTH are life threatening. ACTH deficiency causes a tendency toward shock and may result in an episode of acute adrenal insufficiency (refractory and life-threatening shock from sodium and water depletion). (Adrenal shock is discussed later in this chapter.)

Clinical Manifestations

The signs and symptoms associated with pituitary hypofunction vary with the degree and speed of onset of pituitary dysfunction and are related to hyposecretion of the target glands and/or a growing pituitary tumor. Common symptoms associated with a space-occupying lesion include headaches, visual changes (decreased peripheral vision or decreased visual acuity), *anosmia* (loss of the sense of smell), and seizures.

Adults with GH deficiency often have subtle nonspecific clinical findings. They have truncal obesity and decreased muscle mass causing reduced strength, decreased energy, and reduced exercise capability. They may have a flat affect or appear depressed. Impaired psychologic well-being is a common finding associated with GH deficiency in adults.

FSH and LH deficiencies in the adult woman are first manifested as menstrual irregularities, diminished libido, and changes in secondary sex characteristics (e.g., decreased breast size). Men with FSH and LH deficiencies experience testicular atrophy, diminished spermatogenesis, loss of libido, impotence, and decreased facial hair and muscle mass.

A deficiency of ACTH and cortisol often produces a nonspecific clinical picture. Signs and symptoms may include weakness, fatigue, headache, dry and pale skin, and diminished axillary and pubic hair. Individuals may have postural hypotension, fasting hypoglycemia, diminished tolerance for stress, and poor resistance to infection.

The clinical presentation of an individual with thyroid hormone deficiency associated with hypopituitarism is similar to (although usually milder than) what is seen with primary hypothyroidism. Common symptoms include cold intolerance, constipation, fatigue, lethargy, and weight gain. (Hypothyroidism is discussed in greater detail later in this chapter.)

Diagnostic Studies

In addition to conducting a history and physical examination, diagnostic studies are useful in the diagnosis and treatment of hypopituitarism. Radiologic tests such as MRI and CT are used to determine the presence of a pituitary tumor. The laboratory tests for hypopituitarism vary widely, but generally involve the direct measurement of pituitary hormones or an indirect determination of the hormone level. Diagnostic tests are also used to evaluate the effectiveness of therapy. See Chapter 48 for more information regarding diagnostic studies.

Collaborative Care

The treatment for hypopituitarism consists of surgery or radiation for tumor removal, followed by lifelong hormone replacement. Surgery and radiation therapy for pituitary tumors are discussed earlier in this chapter. Hormone replacement therapy is carried out with the appropriate hormone needed (e.g., GH, corticosteroids, thyroid hormone, and sex hormones). Hormone replacement therapies for thyroid hormone and corticosteroids are discussed later in this chapter.

Somatropin (Genotropin, Humatrope) is used for GH replacement therapy. Adults with GH deficiency respond well to GH replacement

and experience increased energy, increased lean body mass, a feeling of well-being, and improved body image. The side effects most commonly reported by adults include swelling in the feet and hands, pain in the joints, and headache. Somatropin is given as a subcutaneous injection daily or one or two times per month in adults.[6] The dosing is variable because it is adjusted based on relief of symptoms, IGF-1 levels, and the development of adverse effects.

Although gonadal deficiency is not life threatening, replacement therapy is offered to improve sexual function and general well-being. Replacement therapy is contraindicated in individuals with certain medical conditions, such as breast cancer, phlebitis, and pulmonary embolism in women and prostate cancer in men. Estrogen and progesterone replacement therapy may be indicated for hypogonadal women to treat hot flashes, vaginal dryness, and decreased libido. Hormone replacement for women is discussed in greater detail in Chapter 54. Testosterone is used to treat men with gonadotropin deficiency. The benefits achieved with testosterone therapy include a return of male secondary sex characteristics, improvement in libido, and increased muscle mass, bone mass, and bone density. Hormone replacement for men is discussed in greater detail in Chapter 55.

NURSING MANAGEMENT
HYPOFUNCTION OF THE PITUITARY GLAND

A primary nursing role in anterior pituitary insufficiency is assessment and recognition of the signs and symptoms associated with hypopituitarism. Nursing management is directed at providing interventions associated with problems that result from hormone deficiency. The nurse also plays a pivotal role in teaching the patient about diagnostic procedures, the disease process, and collaborative care options. Because of the need for lifelong hormonal therapy, patient teaching is important regarding hormonal administration, side effects, and follow-up therapy.

Disorders Associated with Antidiuretic Hormone Secretion

The two primary conditions associated with ADH secretion are a result of either overproduction or underproduction of ADH. Overproduction or oversecretion of ADH results in a condition known as *syndrome of inappropriate antidiuretic hormone* (SIADH). Underproduction or undersecretion of ADH results in a condition referred to as *diabetes insipidus* (DI).

ADH, also referred to as *arginine vasopressin* (AVP), is synthesized in the hypothalamus and then transported and stored in the posterior pituitary gland. It plays a major role in the regulation of water balance and osmolarity (see Chapter 48).

SYNDROME OF INAPPROPRIATE ANTIDIURETIC HORMONE

Etiology and Pathophysiology

SIADH occurs when ADH is released despite normal or low plasma osmolality (Fig. 50-3). SIADH results from an abnormal production or sustained secretion of ADH and is characterized by fluid retention, serum hypoosmolality, dilutional hyponatremia, hypochloremia, concentrated urine in the presence of normal or increased intravascular volume, and normal renal function. This syndrome occurs more commonly in older adults. SIADH has vari-

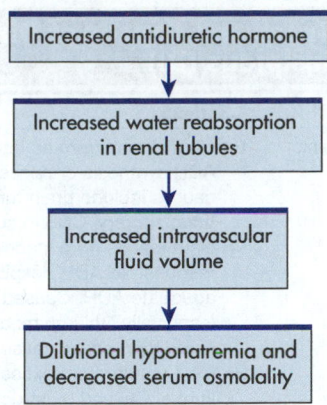

FIG. 50-3 Pathophysiology of syndrome of inappropriate antidiuretic hormone (SIADH).

TABLE 50-1	**Causes of Syndrome of Inappropriate Antidiuretic Hormone (SIADH)**

Malignant Tumors
- Small cell carcinoma of the lung
- Pancreatic cancer
- Lymphoid cancers (Hodgkin's lymphoma, non-Hodgkin's lymphoma, lymphocytic leukemia)
- Thymus cancer
- Prostate cancer
- Colorectal cancer

Central Nervous System Disorders
- Head injury (skull fracture, subdural hematoma, subarachnoid hemorrhage)
- Cerebrovascular injury
- Brain tumors
- Infection (encephalitis, meningitis)
- Cerebral atrophy
- Guillain-Barré syndrome
- Systemic lupus erythematosus

Drug Therapy
- carbamazepine (Tegretol)
- chlorpropamide (Diabinese)
- General anesthesia agents
- Opioids
- Oxytocin
- Thiazide diuretics
- SSRI antidepressants
- Tricyclic antidepressants
- Antineoplastic agents (vincristine [Oncovin], vinblastine [Velban], cyclophosphamide [Cytoxan])

Miscellaneous Conditions
- Hypothyroidism
- Lung infection (pneumonia, tuberculosis, lung abscess)
- Chronic obstructive pulmonary disease
- Positive pressure mechanical ventilation
- HIV
- Adrenal insufficiency

HIV, Human immunodeficiency virus; *SSRI*, selective serotonin reuptake inhibitor.

ous causes (Table 50-1). The most common cause is malignancy, especially small cell lung cancer. These cancerous cells are capable of producing, storing, and releasing ADH.[7] SIADH tends to be self-limiting when caused by head trauma or drugs but is chronic in nature when associated with tumors or metabolic diseases.

Clinical Manifestations

Excess ADH increases the permeability of the distal tubule and collecting duct, which leads to the reabsorption of water into the circulation. Consequently, extracellular fluid volume expands, plasma osmolality declines, the glomerular filtration rate increases, and sodium levels decline (dilutional hyponatremia). Hyponatremia causes muscle cramps and weakness. Initially, thirst, dyspnea on exertion, fatigue, and dulled sensorium may be evident. The patient with SIADH will experience low urinary output and increased body weight.[8] As the serum sodium level falls (usually less than 120 mEq/L [120 mmol/L]), manifestations become more severe and include vomiting, abdominal cramps, muscle twitching, and seizures. As plasma osmolality and serum sodium levels continue to decline, cerebral edema may occur, leading to lethargy, anorexia, confusion, headache, seizures, and coma.

Diagnostic Studies

The diagnosis of SIADH is made by simultaneous measurements of urine and serum osmolality. The dilutional hyponatremia is indicated by a serum sodium less than 134 mEq/L, serum osmolality less than 280 mOsm/kg (280 mmol/kg), and a urine specific gravity greater than 1.005. A serum osmolality much lower than the urine osmolality indicates the inappropriate excretion of concentrated urine in the presence of dilute serum.

Collaborative Care

Once SIADH is diagnosed, treatment is directed at the underlying cause. Medications that stimulate the release of ADH should be avoided or discontinued (see Table 50-1). The immediate treatment goal is to restore normal fluid volume and osmolality. If symptoms are mild and serum sodium is greater than 125 mEq/L (125 mmol/L), the only treatment may be restriction of fluids to 800 to 1000 ml per day. This restriction should result in gradual, daily reductions in weight, a progressive rise in serum sodium concentration and osmolality, and symptomatic improvement.

In cases of severe hyponatremia (less than 120 mEq/L), especially in the presence of neurologic symptoms such as seizures,

intravenous hypertonic saline solution (3% to 5%) may be administered. Hypertonic saline requires a very slow infusion rate on an infusion pump to avoid too-rapid a rise in sodium. A diuretic such as furosemide (Lasix) may be used to promote diuresis, but only if the serum sodium is at least 125 mEq/L (125 mmol/L), because it may promote further loss of sodium. Because furosemide increases potassium, calcium, and magnesium losses, supplements may be needed. A fluid restriction of 500 ml per day is also indicated for those with severe hyponatremia.

In chronic SIADH, water restriction of 800 to 1000 ml per day is recommended. Because this degree of restriction may not be tolerated, demeclocycline (Declomycin) and lithium may be administered. These agents block the effect of ADH on the renal tubules, thereby allowing a more dilute urine.

NURSING MANAGEMENT
SYNDROME OF INAPPROPRIATE ANTIDIURETIC HORMONE

An appropriate nursing assessment (Table 50-2) should be conducted for those at risk and those who have confirmed SIADH. Specifically, the nurse should be alert for low urinary output with

TABLE 50-2	Nursing Assessment and Management: Syndrome of Inappropriate Antidiuretic Hormone (SIADH)

Assessment
- Frequent vital signs
- Frequent intake (oral and parenteral) and output
- Frequent measurement of urine specific gravity
- Daily weights
- Level of consciousness
- Observe for signs of hyponatremia (e.g., decreased neurologic function, seizures, nausea and vomiting, muscle cramping)
- Monitor heart and lung sounds

Management
- Restrict total fluid intake to no more than 1000 ml/day (including that taken with medications)
- Position head of bed flat or with no more than 10 degrees of elevation to enhance venous return to heart and increase left atrial filling pressure, reducing ADH release
- Protect from injury (e.g., assist with ambulation, bed alarm) because of potential alterations in mental status
- Seizure precautions
- Frequent turning, positioning, and range-of-motion exercise (if patient is bedridden)
- Frequent oral hygiene
- Provide distractions to decrease the discomfort of thirst related to fluid restrictions
- Provide support for patient and significant others regarding diagnosis and any mental status changes

ADH, Antidiuretic hormone.

a high specific gravity, a sudden weight gain without edema, or a serum sodium decline. Nursing management of acute onset of SIADH is presented in Table 50-2.

When SIADH is chronic, the patient must learn to self-manage treatment regimens. Fluids are restricted to 800 to 1000 ml per day. Ice chips or sugarless chewing gum can help decrease thirst. If drinking liquids is an aspect of socialization, the patient should be assisted in planning fluid intake so liquid allowances are saved for social occasions. The patient may be treated with a diuretic to remove excess fluid volume. The diet should be supplemented with sodium and potassium, especially if diuretics are prescribed. Solutions of these electrolytes must be well diluted to prevent gastrointestinal (GI) irritation or damage. They are best taken at mealtime to allow mixing with and dilution by food. The patient should be taught the symptoms of fluid and electrolyte imbalances, especially those involving sodium and potassium, so that responses to treatment can be monitored (see Chapter 17).

DIABETES INSIPIDUS

Etiology and Pathophysiology

Diabetes insipidus (DI) is associated with a deficiency of production or secretion of ADH or a decreased renal response to ADH. The decrease in ADH results in fluid and electrolyte imbalances caused by increased urinary output and increased plasma osmolality (Fig. 50-4). Depending on the cause, DI may be transient or a chronic lifelong condition.

There are several classifications of DI (Table 50-3). *Central DI* (also known as *neurogenic DI*) occurs when any organic lesion of the hypothalamus, infundibular stem, or posterior pituitary interferes with ADH synthesis, transport, or release.

TABLE 50-3	Types and Causes of Diabetes Insipidus (DI)

Types	Causes
Central DI (neurogenic)	Problem results from an interference with ADH synthesis or release. Multiple causes include brain tumor, head injury, brain surgery, CNS infections.
Nephrogenic DI	Problem results from inadequate renal response to ADH despite presence of adequate ADH. Caused by drug therapy (especially lithium), renal damage, or hereditary renal disease.
Psychogenic DI	Problem results from excessive water intake. Caused by structural lesion in thirst center or psychologic disorder.

ADH, Antidiuretic hormone; *CNS,* central nervous system.

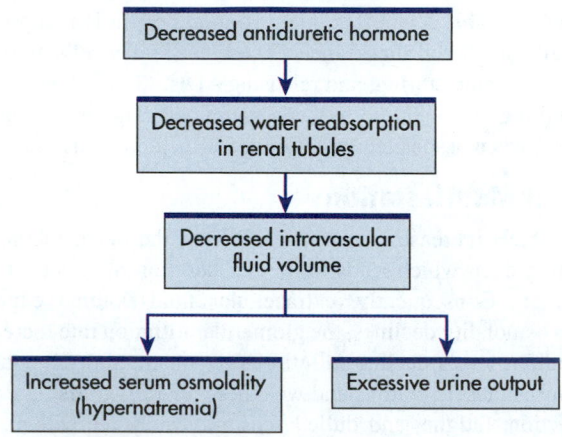

FIG. 50-4   Pathophysiology of diabetes insipidus (DI).

Nephrogenic DI describes a condition in which there is adequate ADH, but there is a decreased response to ADH in the kidney. Lithium is one of the most common causes of drug-induced nephrogenic DI. Hypokalemia and hypercalcemia may also lead to nephrogenic DI.

Psychogenic DI, a less common condition, is associated with excessive water intake. This can be caused by a structural lesion in the thirst center or may be caused by psychiatric problems.

Clinical Manifestations

DI is characterized by increased thirst (polydipsia) and increased urination (polyuria) (see Fig. 50-4). The primary characteristic of DI is the excretion of large quantities of urine (5 to 20 L per day) with a very low specific gravity (<1.005) and urine osmolality of <100 mOsm/kg (<100 mmol/kg). Serum osmolality is elevated (usually greater than 295 mOsm/kg [295 mmol/kg]) as a result of hypernatremia due to pure water loss in the kidney. Most patients compensate for fluid loss by drinking great amounts of water so that serum osmolality is normal or only moderately elevated. The patient may be fatigued from nocturia and may experience generalized weakness.

Central DI usually occurs suddenly with excessive fluid loss. After intracranial surgery, DI usually has a triphasic pattern: the acute phase, with abrupt onset of polyuria; an interphase, in which urine volume apparently normalizes; and a third phase, in which central DI is permanent. The third phase is usually apparent within

10 to 14 days postoperatively. Central DI that results from head trauma is usually self-limiting and improves with treatment of the underlying problem. DI following cranial surgery is more likely to be permanent. Although the clinical manifestations of nephrogenic DI are similar, the onset and amount of fluid losses are less dramatic than with central DI.

If oral fluid intake cannot keep up with urinary losses, severe fluid volume deficit results. This deficit is manifested by weight loss, constipation, poor tissue turgor, hypotension, tachycardia, and shock. In addition, the patient shows central nervous system (CNS) manifestations, ranging from irritability and mental dullness to coma. These manifestations are related to increasing serum osmolality and hypernatremia. Because of the polyuria, severe dehydration and hypovolemic shock may occur.

Diagnostic Studies

Because DI may be central, nephrogenic, or psychogenic in origin, identification of the cause is the initial step. A complete history and physical is done. Psychogenic DI is associated with overhydration and hypervolemia rather than with dehydration and hypovolemia seen in other forms of DI. A water deprivation test is usually done to confirm the diagnosis of central DI. Before a water deprivation test is done, the patient's baseline weight, pulse, urine and plasma osmolalities, urine specific gravity, and blood pressure (BP) are obtained. All fluids are withheld for 8 to 16 hours. The patient may be anxious and should be reassured that the test will be stopped if fluid volume deficit becomes severe. The patient should be observed throughout the test because of the craving to drink. During the test, the patient's BP, weight, and urine osmolality are assessed hourly. The test continues until urine osmolalities stabilize (hourly increase less than 30 mOsm/kg [30 mmol/kg] in 3 consecutive hours) or body weight declines by 3%, or orthostatic hypotension develops. ADH is then given, and urine osmolality is measured 1 hour later. In central DI, the rise in urinary osmolality after vasopressin exceeds 9%. Individuals with nephrogenic DI will have no response.[9]

Collaborative Care

Determining and treating the primary cause is central to the collaborative management of DI. The therapeutic goal is maintenance of fluid and electrolyte balance.

For central DI, fluid and hormonal replacement is the cornerstone of treatment. In acute DI, hypotonic saline or dextrose 5% in water (D_5W) is administered intravenously (IV), and titrated to replace urinary output. Hormone replacement is necessary because of the lack of ADH production or secretion. Desmopressin acetate (DDAVP), an analog of ADH, is the hormone replacement of choice for central DI. DDAVP can be administered orally, IV, or as a nasal spray. Several other drugs are available for ADH replacement, including aqueous vasopressin (Pitressin), vasopressin tannate, and lysine vasopressin (Diapid). Several drugs can be used for the treatment of partial central DI, including chlorpropamide (Diabinese) and carbamazepine (Tegretol). Chlorpropamide, thought to potentiate the action of ADH and stimulate endogenous release, is considered the most consistently effective and safest of these agents.

Hormone replacement and chlorpropamide have little effect in the treatment of nephrogenic DI because the kidney is unable to respond to ADH. Instead, the treatment revolves around dietary measures (low-sodium diet) and thiazide diuretics. Limiting sodium intake to no more than 3 g per day is thought to help decrease urine output. Thiazide diuretics (e.g., hydrochlorothiazide [Hydro-

Diuril], chlorothiazide [Diuril]) are able to slow the glomerular filtration rate, and allow the kidney to reabsorb more water in the loop of Henle and distal tubules. When a low-sodium diet and thiazide drug use are not effective, indomethacin (Indocin) may be prescribed. Indomethacin, a nonsteroidal antiinflammatory agent, helps increase renal responsiveness to ADH.

NURSING MANAGEMENT
DIABETES INSIPIDUS

Nursing management of the patient with DI includes early detection, maintenance of adequate hydration, and patient teaching for long-term management.

During acute central DI, the nurse administers fluids and hormone replacement. Fluids are replaced orally or IV, depending on the patient's condition and ability to drink copious amounts of fluids. Adequate fluids should be kept at the bedside. If IV glucose solutions are used, serum glucose should be monitored because hyperglycemia and glucosuria can lead to osmotic diuresis, which increases the fluid volume deficit. Accurate records of intake and output, urine specific gravity, and daily weights are mandatory in the assessment of fluid volume status.

Nursing interventions also include the administration of DDAVP. The patient should be assessed for weight gain, headache, restlessness, and signs of hyponatremia and water intoxication. The adequacy of treatment is assessed by monitoring fluid intake and output and by urine specific gravity. The health care provider should be notified immediately if the individual with DI develops increased urine volume with a low specific gravity, because this indicates need for increased dosing of DDAVP.

The patient with chronic DI who requires long-term ADH replacement needs instruction in self-management. DDAVP can be taken orally or intranasally. Nasal irritation may occur due to nasal administration. Headache, nausea, and other signs of hyponatremia may indicate overdosage. Failure to improve may indicate underdosage. The patient should be instructed to report any of these symptoms. Patients taking DDAVP should be instructed to monitor their weight daily. Increases in weight may indicate fluid retention. The need for close follow-up including laboratory studies is an essential part of the teaching plan.

Disorders of the Thyroid Gland

The thyroid hormones, thyroxine (T_4) and triiodothyronine (T_3), regulate energy metabolism and growth and development. Disorders of the thyroid gland include enlargement, benign and malignant nodules, inflammation, and hyperfunctioning and hypofunctioning (Fig. 50-5).

THYROID ENLARGEMENT

Goiter is hypertrophy and enlargement of the thyroid gland caused by excess TSH stimulation, which in turn can be caused by inadequate circulating thyroid hormones. Goiter may also be caused by

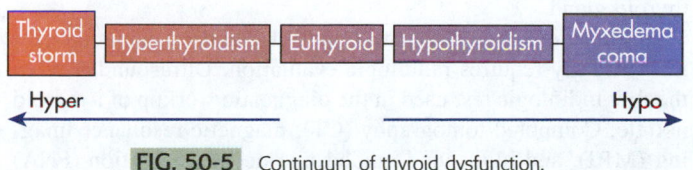

FIG. 50-5   Continuum of thyroid dysfunction.

TABLE 50-4	Drugs That Are Goitrogens

Thyroid Inhibitors
• propylthiouracil (PTU)
• methimazole (Tapazole)
• Iodine in large doses

Others
• Sulfonamides
• Salicylates
• p-Aminosalicylic acid
• phenylbutazone (Butazolidin)
• lithium
• amiodarone (Cordarone)

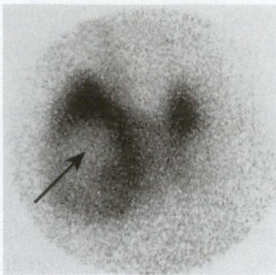

FIG. 50-7 A large "cold" nodule on the thyroid gland (arrow) detected by a scan.

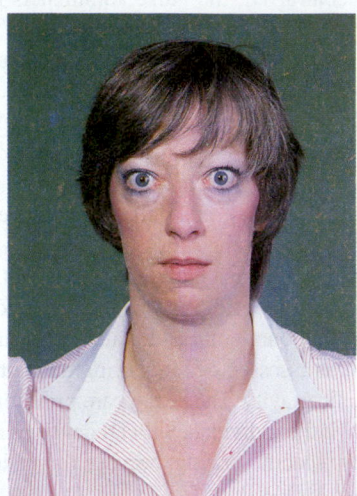

FIG. 50-6 Exophthalmos and goiter of Graves' disease.

growth-stimulating immunoglobulins and other growth factors. *Goitrogens* (foods or drugs that contain thyroid-inhibiting substances) can cause goiter (Table 50-4) but usually only in the individual who lives in an iodine-deficient area (endemic goiter). A goiter is also commonly found in patients with Graves' disease (Fig. 50-6).

TSH and T₄ levels are measured to determine whether a goiter is associated with hyperthyroidism, hypothyroidism, or normal thyroid function. Thyroid antibodies are measured to assess for thyroiditis. Treatment with thyroid hormone may prevent further thyroid enlargement. Surgery to remove large goiters may be necessary.

THYROID NODULES

A thyroid nodule, a palpable deformity of the thyroid gland, may be benign or malignant. Benign nodules are usually not dangerous, but they can cause tracheal compression if they become too large. Malignant tumors of the thyroid gland are not common. The American Cancer Society estimates that 30,180 new cases of thyroid cancer occur per year.[10] The major sign of *thyroid cancer* is the presence of a hard, painless nodule or nodules on an enlarged thyroid gland.

Nodular enlargement of the thyroid gland or palpation of a mass usually requires radiologic evaluation. Ultrasound is often the first radiologic test used in the diagnostic workup of a thyroid nodule. Computed tomography (CT), magnetic resonance imaging (MRI), and ultrasound-guided fine-needle aspiration (FNA)

are other diagnostic options. FNA is indicated when a tissue sample for pathologic examination is necessary. FNA is considered one of the most effective methods to identify malignancy.[11] A thyroid scan may also be done to evaluate for possible malignancy. The scan shows whether nodules on the thyroid are "hot" or "cold." Thyroid tumors may or may not take up radioactive iodine. Tumors that take up the radioactive iodine are called "hot" nodules and are nearly always benign. If the nodule does not take up the radioactive iodine, it appears as "cold" and has a higher risk of being malignant (Fig. 50-7). An increase in the level of serum calcitonin may also be helpful in diagnosis, because increased levels are associated with a certain type (medullary) of thyroid cancer.

Surgical removal of the tumor is usually indicated in the treatment of thyroid cancer. Surgical procedures may range from unilateral total lobectomy with removal of the isthmus to total thyroidectomy with bilateral lobectomy. Many thyroid cancers are TSH dependent, and thyroid hormone in hyperphysiologic doses is often prescribed to inhibit pituitary secretion of TSH. Radiation therapy may also be indicated to prolong survival.

Nursing care for the patient with thyroid tumors is similar to care for the patient who has undergone thyroidectomy and also includes general nursing measures for the patient with cancer (see Chapter 16).

THYROIDITIS

Thyroiditis is an inflammatory process in the thyroid that can have several causes. *Subacute granulomatous thyroiditis* (de Quervain's thyroiditis), which causes thyrotoxicosis, is thought to be caused by a viral infection. *Acute thyroiditis* is due to bacterial or fungal infection. Subacute and acute forms of thyroiditis have an abrupt onset and the thyroid gland is painful. *Chronic autoimmune thyroiditis* (Hashimoto's thyroiditis) can lead to hypothyroidism. *Hashimoto's thyroiditis* is a chronic autoimmune disease in which thyroid tissue is replaced by lymphocytes and fibrous tissue. It is the most common cause of goiterous hypothyroidism in the United States. *Silent painless thyroiditis* is a form of lymphocytic thyroiditis with a variable onset. In women, this condition may occur in the postpartum period and usually resolves within 3 to 12 months. It is believed to be an autoimmune disease and may be early Hashimoto's thyroiditis.[11]

T₄ and T₃ are initially elevated in subacute, acute, and silent thyroiditis but may become depressed with time. TSH levels are low and then elevated. Thyroid hormone levels are usually low in chronic Hashimoto's thyroiditis, and TSH is high. Suppression of radioactive iodine uptake (RAIU) is seen in subacute and silent thyroiditis. Antithyroid antibodies are present in Hashimoto's thyroiditis.

Recovery from thyroiditis may be complete in weeks or months without treatment. If the condition is bacterial in origin, treatment may include specific antibiotics or surgical drainage. In the subacute and acute forms, salicylates and nonsteroidal antiinflammatory drugs are used. If there is no response to these drugs in 50 hours, corticosteroids are given. Propranolol (Inderal) or atenolol (Tenormin) may be used for the cardiovascular symptoms from a hyperthyroid condition. Thyroid hormone replacement is indicated if the patient is hypothyroid.

Nursing care of the patient with thyroiditis depends, in part, on the therapeutic management. Education regarding treatment and encouraging compliance are important for all types of thyroiditis. The patient should be instructed to remain under close health care supervision so that progress can be monitored and to report any change in symptoms to the health care provider.

The patient with thyroiditis of an autoimmune origin may be susceptible to other autoimmune diseases such as Addison's disease, pernicious anemia, premature gonadal failure, or Graves' disease. The patient should be taught the signs and symptoms of these disorders, particularly Addison's disease. A patient receiving thyroid hormone replacement must be taught the expected side effects of these drugs and measures to manage them. This information is covered in greater detail later in this chapter. The patient treated surgically needs care similar to that given to the person undergoing thyroidectomy.

HYPERTHYROIDISM

Hyperthyroidism is hyperactivity of the thyroid gland with sustained increase in synthesis and release of thyroid hormones. The term **thyrotoxicosis** refers to the physiologic effects or clinical syndrome of hypermetabolism that results from excess circulating levels of T_4, T_3, or both. Hyperthyroidism and thyrotoxicosis usually occur together as in Graves' disease. However, in some forms of thyroiditis, thyrotoxicosis may occur without hyperthyroidism.[12]

Hyperthyroidism occurs in women more than men, with the highest frequency in persons 20 to 40 years old. The most common form of hyperthyroidism is Graves' disease. Other causes include toxic nodular goiter, thyroiditis, exogenous iodine excess, pituitary tumors, and thyroid cancer.

Etiology and Pathophysiology

Graves' Disease. **Graves' disease** is an autoimmune disease of unknown etiology marked by diffuse thyroid enlargement and excessive thyroid hormone secretion. Precipitating factors such as insufficient iodine supply, infection, and stressful life events may interact with genetic factors to cause Graves' disease.

Graves' disease accounts for 75% of the cases of hyperthyroidism. The patient develops antibodies to the TSH receptor. These antibodies attach to the receptors and stimulate the thyroid gland to release T_3, T_4, or both. The excessive release of thyroid hormones leads to the clinical manifestations associated with thyrotoxicosis. The disease is characterized by remissions and exacerbations, with or without treatment. It may progress to destruction of the thyroid tissue, causing hypothyroidism.

Toxic Nodular Goiters. Nodular goiters are thyroid hormone–secreting nodules that function independent of TSH stimulation. If these nodules are associated with hyperthyroidism, they are termed *toxic*. There may be multiple nodules (multinodular goiter) or a single nodule (solitary autonomous nodule). The nodules are usually benign follicular adenomas. Toxic nodular goiters occur equally in

---

GENDER DIFFERENCES
Endocrine Problems

Men	Women
• Ectopic ACTH production is more common in men.	• Hyperthyroidism occurs more commonly in women than men. • Hypothyroidism affects more women than men. • Graves' disease affects four to eight times as many women as men.

ACTH, Adrenocorticotropic hormone.

---

men and women. Although they can appear at any age, the frequency of toxic multinodular goiter is greatest in people over 40 years of age. Small solitary autonomous nodules do not usually secrete enough thyroid hormone to cause clinical thyrotoxicosis. However, larger nodules (greater than 3 cm) may result in clinical disease.

Clinical Manifestations

The clinical manifestations of hyperthyroidism are related to the effect of thyroid hormone excess. Excess circulating thyroid hormone directly increases metabolism. It also increases tissue sensitivity to stimulation by the sympathetic nervous system.

Palpation of the thyroid gland may reveal a goiter. When the thyroid gland is excessively large, a goiter may be noted on inspection. Auscultation of the thyroid gland may reveal bruits, a reflection of increased blood supply. Another common finding associated with hyperthyroidism is *ophthalmopathy,* a term used to describe abnormal eye appearance or function. A classic finding in Graves' disease is **exophthalmos**, a protrusion of the eyeballs from the orbits (see Fig. 50-6). Exophthalmos is a type of infiltrative ophthalmopathy that is due to impaired venous drainage from the orbit, which causes increased fat deposits and fluid (edema) in the retroorbital tissues. Due to increased pressure, the eyeballs are forced outward and protrude. This sign is seen in 20% to 40% of patients with Graves' disease. It is usually bilateral but can be unilateral or asymmetric. In noninfiltrative ophthalmopathy, the upper lids are usually retracted and elevated, with the sclera visible above the iris. When the eyelids do not close completely, the exposed corneal surfaces become dry and irritated. Serious consequences, such as corneal ulcers and eventual loss of vision, can occur.

Other manifestations of thyroid hyperfunction are summarized in Table 50-5. A patient with advanced disease may exhibit many of the manifestations, including *acropachy* (Fig. 50-8), whereas a patient in the early stages of hyperthyroidism may exhibit only weight loss and increased nervousness. Symptoms in the elderly patient with this disorder can be very different (referred to as *apathetic hyperthyroidism*) and may include anorexia, apathy, lassitude, depression, weight loss, atrial fibrillation, and confusion.[13] Table 50-6 compares features of hyperthyroidism in younger and older adult patients.

Complications

Thyrotoxic crisis (also called *thyroid storm*) is an acute, rare condition in which all hyperthyroid manifestations are heightened. Although it is considered a life-threatening emergency, death is

TABLE 50-5	Clinical Manifestations: Thyroid Hormone Dysfunction		
Hypofunction	**Hyperfunction**	**Hypofunction**	**Hyperfunction**
Cardiovascular System		**Musculoskeletal System**	
Increased capillary fragility	Systolic hypertension	Fatigue	Fatigue
Decreased rate and force of contraction	Increased rate and force of cardiac contractions	Weakness	Muscle weakness
Varied changes in blood pressure	Bounding, rapid pulse	Muscular aches and pains	Proximal muscle wasting
Cardiac hypertrophy	Increased cardiac output	Slow movements	Dependent edema
Distant heart sounds	Cardiac hypertrophy	Arthralgia	Osteoporosis
Anemia	Systolic murmurs		
Tendency to develop heart failure, angina, myocardial infarction	Dysrhythmias	**Nervous System**	
	Palpitations	Apathy	Difficulty in focusing eyes
	Atrial fibrillation (more common in the older adult)	Lethargy	Nervousness
	Angina	Fatigue	Fine tremor (of fingers and tongue)
		Forgetfulness	Insomnia
		Slowed mental processes	Lability of mood, delirium
Respiratory System		Hoarseness	Restlessness
Dyspnea	Increased respiratory rate	Slow, slurred speech	Personality changes of irritability, agitation
Decreased breathing capacity	Dyspnea on mild exertion	Prolonged relaxation of deep tendon muscles	Exhaustion
		Stupor, coma	Hyperreflexia of tendon reflexes
Gastrointestinal System		Paresthesias	Depression, fatigue, apathy (in the older adult)
Decreased appetite	Increased appetite, thirst	Anxiety, depression	Lack of ability to concentrate
Nausea and vomiting	Weight loss	Polyneuropathy	Stupor, coma
Weight gain	Increased peristalsis		
Constipation	Diarrhea, frequent defecation		
Distended abdomen	Increased bowel sounds	**Reproductive System**	
Enlarged, scaly tongue	Splenomegaly	Prolonged menstrual periods or amenorrhea	Menstrual irregularities
	Hepatomegaly	Decreased libido	Amenorrhea
		Infertility	Decreased libido
Integumentary System			Impotence in men
Dry, thick, inelastic, cold skin	Warm, smooth, moist skin		Gynecomastia in men
Thick, brittle nails	Thin, brittle nails detached from nail bed (onycholysis)		Decreased fertility
Dry, sparse, coarse hair	Hair loss (may be patchy)		
Poor turgor of mucosa	Clubbing of fingers (thyroid acropachy) (see Fig. 50-8)	**Other**	
Generalized interstitial edema	Palmar erythema	Increased susceptibility to infection	Intolerance to heat
Puffy face	Fine silky hair	Increased sensitivity to opioids, barbiturates, anesthesia	Increased sensitivity to stimulant drugs
Decreased sweating	Premature graying (in men)	Intolerance to cold	Elevated basal temperature
Pallor	Diaphoresis	Decreased hearing	Lid lag, stare
	Vitiligo	Sleepiness	Eyelid retraction
	Pretibial myxedema (infiltrative dermopathy)	Goiter	Exophthalmos
			Goiter
			Rapid speech

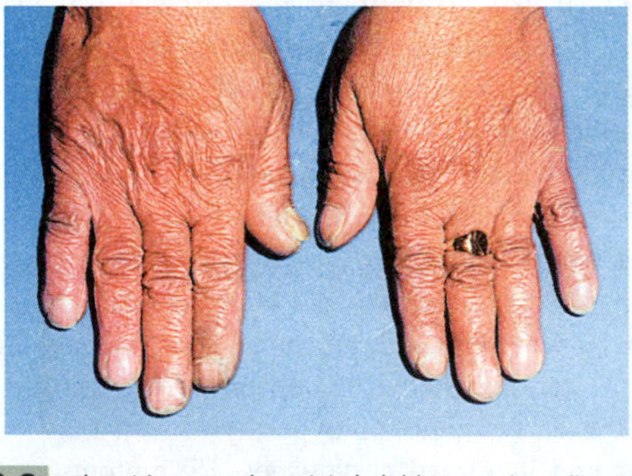

FIG. 50-8   Thyroid acropachy. Digital clubbing and swelling of fingers.

rare when treatment is vigorous and initiated early. The physiologic factor or factors that initiate thyrotoxic crisis are unknown. The cause is thought to be stressors (e.g., infection, trauma, surgery) in a patient with preexisting hyperthyroidism, either diagnosed or undiagnosed. Heart and nerve tissues become more sensitive to catecholamines due to more binding sites for epinephrine and norepinephrine.

Manifestations include severe tachycardia, heart failure, shock, hyperthermia (up to 105.3° F [40.7° C]), restlessness, agitation, seizures, abdominal pain, nausea, vomiting, diarrhea, delirium, and coma. Treatment is aimed at reducing circulating thyroid hormone levels and the clinical manifestations of this disorder by appropriate drug therapy. Supportive therapy is directed at managing respiratory distress, fever reduction, fluid replacement, and elimination or management of the initiating stressor(s).

Diagnostic Studies

The two primary laboratory findings used to confirm the diagnosis of hyperthyroidism are decreased TSH levels and elevated free thyroxine (free T_4) levels. Total T_3 and T_4 may also be assessed, but these are not as useful. Measurements of total T_3 and T_4 measure both free and bound (to protein) hormone levels. The free hormone is the only form of the hormone that is biologically active.

The RAIU test is used to differentiate Graves' disease from other forms of thyroiditis. The patient with Graves' disease will show a diffuse, homogeneous uptake of 35% to 95%, whereas the patient with thyroiditis will show an uptake of less than 2%. The

TABLE 50-6	Comparison of Hyperthyroidism in Younger and Older Adults	
	Younger Adult	**Older Adult**
Common causes	Graves' disease in >90% of cases	Graves' disease or toxic nodular goiter
Common symptoms	Nervousness, irritability, weight loss, heat intolerance, warm, moist skin	Anorexia, weight loss, apathy, lassitude, depression, confusion
Goiter	Present in >90% of cases	Present in about 50% of cases
Ophthalmopathy	Exophthalmos present in 20%-40% of cases	Exophthalmos less common
Cardiac features	Tachycardia and palpitations common, but without heart failure	Angina, dysrhythmia (especially atrial fibrillation), heart failure may occur

TABLE 50-7 COLLABORATIVE CARE Hyperthyroidism

Diagnostic
History and physical examination
Ophthalmologic examination
ECG
Laboratory tests
- Serum free T_4, TSH levels
- TRH stimulation test
Radioactive iodine uptake (RAIU)

Collaborative Therapy
Drug Therapy
Antithyroid drugs
- propylthiouracil (PTU)
- methimazole (Tapazole)
Iodine
β-Adrenergic blockers (e.g., propranolol [Inderal])

Radiation Therapy
Radioactive iodine

Surgical Therapy
Subtotal thyroidectomy

Nutritional Therapy
High-calorie diet
High-protein diet
Frequent meals

ECG, Electrocardiogram; *TRH,* thyrotropin-releasing hormone; *TSH,* thyroid-stimulating hormone.

person with a nodular goiter will have an uptake in the high-normal range (Table 50-7).

Collaborative Care

The overall goal in the treatment of hyperthyroidism is to block the adverse effects of thyroid hormones and stop their oversecretion. The three primary treatment options for the patient with hyperthyroidism are antithyroid medications, radioactive iodine therapy, and subtotal thyroidectomy (see Table 50-7). In general, the treatment of choice in nonpregnant adults in the United States is radioactive iodine therapy. However, the choice of treatment is influenced by the patient's age and preferences, severity of the disorder, and complicating features (including pregnancy). If surgery is to be performed, the patient is usually given antithyroid drugs and iodine to produce a euthyroid state and possibly β-adrenergic blockers to relieve symptoms preoperatively.

Drug Therapy. Drugs used in the treatment of hyperthyroidism include antithyroid drugs, iodine, and β-adrenergic blockers. These drugs are useful in the treatment of thyrotoxic states, but they are not considered curative. Radiation therapy or surgery may ultimately be required.

Antithyroid Drugs. The first-line antithyroid drugs are propylthiouracil (PTU) and methimazole (Tapazole). These drugs inhibit the synthesis of thyroid hormones. PTU also blocks peripheral conversion of T_4 to T_3. Although there is individual variation, improvement usually begins 1 to 2 weeks after the start of therapy. Good results are usually seen within 4 to 8 weeks. Therapy is usually continued for 6 to 15 months to allow for spontaneous remission, which occurs in 20% to 40% of individuals with hyperthyroidism. These drugs are not curative.[14] The major disadvantages of these drugs are patient noncompliance and a high rate of recurrence of hyperthyroidism when the drugs are discontinued. PTU lowers hormone levels more quickly but must be taken three times per day. Tapazole is administered in a single daily dose. Indications for the use of antithyroid drugs include Graves' disease in the young patient, hyperthyroidism during pregnancy, and the need to achieve a euthyroid state before surgery or radiation therapy.

Iodine. Iodine is used with other antithyroid drugs to prepare the patient for thyroidectomy or for treatment of thyrotoxic crisis. The administration of iodine in large doses rapidly inhibits

synthesis of T_3 and T_4 and blocks the release of these hormones into circulation. It also decreases the vascularity of the thyroid gland, making surgery safer and easier. The maximal effect of iodine is usually seen within 1 to 2 weeks. Because there is a reduction in the therapeutic effect, long-term iodine therapy is not effective in controlling hyperthyroidism. Iodine is available in the form of saturated solution of potassium iodide (SSKI) and Lugol's solution.

β-Adrenergic Blockers. β-Adrenergic blockers are used for symptomatic relief of thyrotoxicosis that results from increased β-adrenergic receptor stimulation caused by excess thyroid hormones. Propranolol (Inderal) is usually administered with other antithyroid agents and rapidly provides symptomatic relief. Atenolol (Tenormin) is the preferred β-adrenergic blocker for use in the hyperthyroid patient with asthma or heart disease.

Radioactive Iodine Therapy. Radioactive iodine (RAI) therapy is the treatment of choice for most nonpregnant adults. (A pregnancy test is done on all women who experience menstrual cycles before initiation of therapy.) RAI damages or destroys thyroid tissue, thus limiting thyroid hormone secretion. RAI has a delayed response, and the maximum effect may not be seen for 2 to 3 months. For this reason, the patient is usually treated with antithyroid drugs and propranolol before and during the first 3 months after the initiation of RAI until the effects of radiation become apparent. Although RAI is usually effective, there is a high incidence of posttreatment hypothyroidism (80% of adequately treated individuals), resulting in the need for lifelong thyroid hormone replacement.

Surgical Therapy. Thyroidectomy is indicated for individuals who have been unresponsive to antithyroid therapy, for individuals with very large goiters causing tracheal compression, and for individuals with a possible malignancy. Additionally, this surgery may be done when an individual is not a good candidate for RAI.[14] One advantage thyroidectomy has over RAI is a more rapid reduction in T_3 and T_4 levels. A *subtotal thyroidectomy* is the preferred surgical procedure and involves the removal of a significant portion of the thyroid gland. For subtotal thyroidectomy to be effective, approximately 90% of thyroid tissue must be removed. If too much tissue is taken, the gland will not regenerate after surgery and hypothyroidism will result.

Endoscopic thyroidectomy is a minimally invasive procedure. It is an appropriate procedure for patients with small nodules (less than 3 cm) where there is no evidence of malignancy. Advantages of endoscopic thyroidectomy over open thyroidectomy include less scarring, less pain, and a faster return to normal activity.

Before surgery, antithyroid drugs, iodine, and β-adrenergic blockers may be administered to achieve a euthyroid state and to control symptoms. Iodine reduces vascularization of the gland, reducing the risk of hemorrhage. Postoperative complications include hypothyroidism, damage to or inadvertent removal of parathyroid glands causing hypoparathyroidism and hypocalcemia, hemorrhage, injury to the recurrent or superior laryngeal nerve, thyrotoxic crisis, and infection.

Nutritional Therapy. The potential for nutritional deficits is high when an increased metabolic rate is present. A high-calorie diet (4000 to 5000 kcal/day) may be ordered to satisfy hunger and prevent tissue breakdown. This can be accomplished with six full meals a day and snacks high in protein, carbohydrates, minerals, and vitamins, particularly vitamin A, thiamine, vitamin B_6, and vitamin C. The protein content should be 1 to 2 g/kg of ideal body weight. Increased carbohydrates should compensate for an altered metabolism, while providing energy and lessening the use of body stored protein. Highly seasoned and high-fiber foods should be avoided because they stimulate the already hyperactive GI tract. Substitutes should be provided for caffeine-containing liquids such as coffee, tea, and cola because the stimulating effects of these fluids increase restlessness and sleep disturbances. A dietitian should be consulted for guidance in meeting the nutritional needs of a patient with hyperthyroidism.

NURSING MANAGEMENT
HYPERTHYROIDISM

▪ Nursing Assessment

Subjective and objective data that should be obtained from an individual with hyperthyroidism are presented in Table 50-8.

▪ Nursing Diagnoses

Nursing diagnoses for the patient with hyperthyroidism include, but are not limited to, those presented in NCP 50-1.

▪ Planning

The overall goals are that the patient with hyperthyroidism will (1) experience relief of symptoms, (2) have no serious complications related to the disease or treatment, (3) maintain nutritional balance, and (4) cooperate with the therapeutic plan.

▪ Nursing Implementation

Acute Intervention. Individuals who have hyperthyroidism are usually treated in an outpatient setting. However, patients who develop acute thyrotoxicosis (thyroid storm) or those who undergo thyroidectomy require hospitalization and acute care.

TABLE 50-8	*NURSING ASSESSMENT* Hyperthyroidism

Subjective Data
Important Health Information
Past health history: Preexisting goiter; recent infection or trauma, immigration from iodine-deficient area, autoimmune disease
Medications: Use of thyroid hormones, herbal therapies that may contain thyroid hormone

Functional Health Patterns
Health perception–health management: Positive family history of thyroid or autoimmune disorders
Nutritional-metabolic: Insufficient iodine intake; weight loss; increased appetite, thirst; nausea
Elimination: Diarrhea; polyuria; sweating
Activity-exercise: Dyspnea on exertion; palpitations; muscle weakness, fatigue
Sleep-rest: Insomnia
Cognitive-perceptual: Chest pain; nervousness; heat intolerance; pruritus
Sexuality-reproductive: Decreased libido; impotence; gynecomastia (in men); amenorrhea (in women)
Coping–stress tolerance: Emotional lability, irritability, restlessness, personality changes, delirium

Objective Data
General Observation
Agitation, rapid speech and body movements; hyperthermia, enlarged or nodular thyroid gland

Eyes
Exophthalmos, eyelid retraction; infrequent blinking

Integumentary
Warm, diaphoretic, velvety skin; thin, loose nails; fine, silky hair and hair loss; palmar erythema; clubbing; white pigmentation of skin (vitiligo), diffuse edema of legs and feet

Respiratory
Tachypnea

Cardiovascular
Tachycardia, bounding pulse, systolic murmurs, dysrhythmias, hypertension

Gastrointestinal
Increased bowel sounds; hepatosplenomegaly

Neurologic
Hyperreflexia; diplopia; fine tremors of hands, tongue, eyelids; stupor; coma

Musculoskeletal
Muscle wasting

Reproductive
Menstrual irregularities, infertility; impotence, gynecomastia in men

Possible Diagnostic Findings
↑ T_3, ↑ T_4; ↑ T_3 resin uptake; ↓ serum thyroid-stimulating hormone (TSH); chest x-ray showing enlarged heart; ECG findings of tachycardia, atrial fibrillation

ECG, Electrocardiogram.

Acute Thyrotoxicosis. Acute thyrotoxicosis is a systemic syndrome that requires aggressive treatment, often in an intensive care unit. The nurse needs to administer medications (previously discussed) that block thyroid hormone production. Nursing management also includes provisions for supportive therapy. Having an understanding of the major organ response to the hypermetabolic state is a critical aspect of nursing management. Supportive therapy includes monitoring for cardiac dysrhythmias and decompensation, ensuring adequate oxygenation, and administering IV fluids

NURSING CARE PLAN 50-1

Patient with Hyperthyroidism

NURSING DIAGNOSIS   **Activity intolerance** *related to* fatigue, exhaustion, and heat intolerance secondary to hypermetabolism *as evidenced by* complaints of weakness, inability to perform usual activities, short attention span, memory lapses, dyspnea, tachycardia, irritability

PATIENT GOALS   1.   Achieves a program of activity that balances physical activity with energy-conserving activities
2.   Reports increased tolerance to activity with less weakness and fatigue

OUTCOMES (NOC)	INTERVENTIONS (NIC) and *RATIONALES*
Activity Tolerance	**Energy Management**
• Pulse rate with activity ____	• Monitor patient for evidence of excess physical and emotional fatigue *because hyperthyroidism results in protein catabolism, overactivity, and increased metabolism leading to exhaustion.*
• Respiratory rate with activity ____	• Monitor cardiorespiratory response to activity (e.g., tachycardia, other dysrhythmias, dyspnea, diaphoresis, pallor, blood pressure [BP], and respiratory rate) *because tachycardia and BP elevations can indicate excessive activity.*
• Ease of performing activities of daily living (ADLs) ____	
• Ease of breathing with activity ____	• Assist with regular physical activities (e.g., ambulation, transfers, turning, and personal care) *to make certain patient's daily needs are met.*
Endurance	• Assist the patient to understand energy conservation principles (e.g., the requirement for restricted activity or bed rest) *to avoid fatiguing patient.*
• Performance of usual routine ____	• Assist the patient to schedule rest periods.
• Concentration ____	• Avoid care activities during scheduled rest periods *to promote adequate rest periods.*
Measurement Scale	
1 = Severely compromised	
2 = Substantially compromised	
3 = Moderately compromised	
4 = Mildly compromised	
5 = Not compromised	

NURSING DIAGNOSIS   **Imbalanced nutrition: less than body requirements** *related to* hypermetabolism and inadequate diet *as evidenced by* complaints of weight loss; less than optimal body weight

PATIENT GOALS   1.   Maintains weight appropriate for height
2.   Consumes food and fluid adequate to meet nutritional needs
3.   Corrects nutritional deficiencies

OUTCOMES (NOC)	INTERVENTIONS (NIC) and *RATIONALES*
Nutritional Status	**Nutrition Management**
• Nutrient intake ____	• Ascertain patient's food preferences *to determine extent of the problem and plan appropriate interventions.*
• Food intake ____	• Provide patient with high-protein, high-calorie, nutritious finger foods and drinks that can be easily consumed *because hyperthyroidism increases metabolic rate with resulting need to prevent muscle breakdown and weight loss.*
• Weight/height ratio ____	
Nutritional Status: Biochemical Measures	• Weigh patient at appropriate intervals *to evaluate effectiveness of nutritional plan.*
• Serum albumin ____	• Assist the patient in receiving help from appropriate community nutritional programs.
Measurement Scale	**Nutrition Therapy**
1 = Severe deviation from normal range	• Monitor laboratory values (e.g., BUN, albumin) *to evaluate protein levels to determine extent of protein malnutrition.*
2 = Substantial deviation from normal range	
3 = Moderate deviation from normal range	
4 = Mild deviation from normal range	
5 = No deviation from normal range	

BUN, Blood urea nitrogen.

to replace fluid and electrolyte losses. This is especially important in the patient who develops vomiting and diarrhea.

A calm, quiet room should be provided because increased metabolism causes sleep disturbances. Providing for adequate rest may be a challenge because of the patient's irritability and restlessness. Specific interventions may include (1) placing the patient in a cool room, away from very ill patients and noisy, high-traffic areas; (2) using light bed coverings and changing the linen frequently if the patient is diaphoretic; (3) encouraging and assisting with exercise involving large muscle groups (tremors can interfere with small-muscle coordination) to allow the release of

nervous tension and restlessness; and (5) establishing a supportive, trusting relationship to help the patient cope with aggravating events and lessen anxiety.

If exophthalmos is present, there is a potential for corneal injury related to irritation and dryness. The patient may also have orbital pain. Nursing interventions to relieve eye discomfort and prevent corneal ulceration include applying artificial tears to soothe and moisten conjunctival membranes. Salt restriction may help reduce periorbital edema. Elevation of the patient's head promotes fluid drainage from the periorbital area; the patient should sit upright as much as possible. Dark glasses reduce glare and prevent irritation from smoke, air currents, dust, and dirt. If the eyelids cannot be closed, they should be lightly taped shut for sleep. To maintain flexibility, the patient should be taught to exercise the intraocular muscles several times a day by turning the eyes in the complete range of motion. Good grooming can be helpful in reducing the loss of self-esteem that can result from an altered body image. If the exophthalmos is severe, corticosteroids, radiation of retroorbital tissues, orbital decompression, or corrective lid or muscle surgery may be used.

Thyroid Surgery. When subtotal thyroidectomy is the treatment of choice, the patient must be adequately prepared to avoid postoperative complications. The signs and symptoms of thyrotoxicosis must be alleviated as much as possible, and cardiac problems must be controlled before surgery. If iodine is used to relieve hyperthyroid symptoms, it should be mixed with water or juice, sipped through a straw, and administered after meals. The patient must be assessed for signs of iodine toxicity such as swelling of buccal mucosa and other mucous membranes, excessive salivation, nausea and vomiting, and skin reactions. If toxicity occurs, iodine administration should be discontinued and the physician notified.

Preoperative teaching should include comfort and safety measures in which the patient can participate. Coughing, deep breathing, and leg exercises should be practiced and their importance explained. The patient should be taught how to support the head manually while turning in bed, because this maneuver minimizes stress on the suture line after surgery. Range-of-motion exercises of the neck should be practiced. The nurse should explain routine postoperative care such as IV infusions. The patient should be told that talking is likely to be difficult for a short time after surgery.

The hospital room must be prepared before the patient's return from surgery. Oxygen, suction equipment, and a tracheostomy tray should be readily available. A tracheostomy tray is required in case airway obstruction occurs. Although this rarely occurs, it is an emergency situation the nurse must be prepared for. Recurrent laryngeal nerve damage leads to vocal cord paralysis. If there is paralysis of both cords, spastic airway obstruction will occur, requiring an immediate tracheostomy.

Respiration may also become difficult because of excess swelling of the neck tissues, hemorrhage, hematoma formation, and laryngeal stridor. *Laryngeal stridor* (harsh, vibratory sound) may occur during inspiration and expiration as a result of edema of the laryngeal nerve. Laryngeal stridor may also be related to tetany, which occurs if the parathyroid glands are removed or damaged during surgery leading to hypocalcemia. To treat tetany, IV calcium salts such as calcium gluconate or gluceptate should be available.

After a thyroidectomy the nurse should do the following:

1. Assess the patient every 2 hours for 24 hours for signs of hemorrhage or tracheal compression such as irregular breathing, neck swelling, frequent swallowing, sensations of fullness at the incision site, choking, and blood on the anterior or posterior dressings.
2. Place the patient in a semi-Fowler position and support the patient's head with pillows, and avoid flexion of the neck and any tension on the suture lines.
3. Monitor vital signs. Complete the initial assessment by checking for signs of tetany secondary to hypoparathyroidism (e.g., tingling in toes, fingers, or around the mouth;

muscular twitching; apprehension) and by evaluating difficulty in speaking and hoarseness. Trousseau's sign and Chvostek's sign should be monitored for 72 hours (see Chapter 17, Fig. 17-15). Some hoarseness is to be expected for 3 to 4 days after surgery because of edema.

4. Control postoperative pain by giving medication.

If postoperative recovery is uneventful, the patient is ambulated within hours after surgery, is permitted to take fluid as soon as tolerated, and eats a soft diet the day after surgery.

The appearance of the incision may be highly distressing to the patient. The patient can be reassured that the scar will fade in color and eventually look like a normal neck wrinkle. A scarf, jewelry, a high collar, or other covering can effectively camouflage the scar.

Ambulatory and Home Care

Postoperative Care. Discharge teaching for the patient following surgery is an important aspect of nursing care. The patient and family need to be aware that thyroid hormone balance should be monitored periodically to ensure that normal function has returned. Most patients experience a period of relative hypothyroidism soon after surgery because of the substantial reduction in the size of the thyroid. However, the remaining tissue usually hypertrophies, recovering the capacity to produce the hormone needed by the body, but this takes time. The administration of thyroid hormone is avoided because exogenous hormone inhibits pituitary production of TSH and delays or prevents the restoration of normal gland function and thyroid tissue regeneration.

Caloric intake must be reduced substantially below the amount that was required before surgery to prevent weight gain. Adequate iodine is necessary to promote thyroid function, but excesses can inhibit the thyroid. Seafood once or twice a week or normal use of iodized salt should provide sufficient intake. Regular exercise helps stimulate the thyroid gland and should be encouraged. High environmental temperature should be avoided because it inhibits thyroid regeneration.

Regular follow-up care is necessary. The patient should be seen biweekly for a month and then at least semiannually to assess for the development of hypothyroidism. If a complete thyroidectomy has been performed, the patient needs instruction in lifelong thyroid replacement. Failure of thyroid function is considered the end stage of Graves' disease. The patient should be taught the signs and symptoms of progressive thyroid failure and instructed to seek medical care if these develop. Hypothyroidism is relatively easy to manage with oral administration of thyroid replacement.

Radioactive Iodine Therapy. Radioactive iodine therapy is administered on an outpatient basis and is the therapy of choice for the nonpregnant adult. Because the therapeutic dose of radioactive iodine is low, no radiation safety precautions are necessary. The patient should be instructed that radiation thyroiditis and parotiditis are possible and may cause dryness and irritation of the mouth and throat. Relief may be obtained with frequent sips of water, ice chips, or the use of a salt and soda gargle three or four times per day. This gargle is made by dissolving 1 teaspoon of salt and 1 teaspoon of baking soda in 2 cups of warm water. The discomfort should subside in 3 to 4 days. Because of the high frequency of hypothyroidism after radioactive iodine therapy, the patient and family should be taught the symptoms of hypothyroidism and instructed to seek medical help if these symptoms occur.

■ *Evaluation*

The expected outcomes are that the patient with hyperthyroidism will

- experience relief of symptoms
- have no serious complications related to the disease or treatment
- cooperate with the therapeutic plan

HYPOTHYROIDISM

Etiology and Pathophysiology

Hypothyroidism is one of the most common medical disorders in the United States, affecting 10% of women and 3% of men over 65 years of age.[12] **Hypothyroidism** results from insufficient circulating thyroid hormone as a result of a variety of abnormalities. Hypothyroidism can be primary (related to destruction of thyroid tissue or defective hormone synthesis) or secondary (related to pituitary disease with decreased TSH secretion or hypothalamic dysfunction with decreased thyrotropin-releasing hormone [TRH] secretion). It may also be transient, related to thyroiditis or discontinuance of thyroid hormone therapy.

Iodine deficiency is the most common cause of hypothyroidism worldwide and is most prevalent in iodine-deficient areas of the world. In areas where iodine intake is adequate, such as the United States, the most common cause of primary hypothyroidism in the adult is atrophy of the thyroid gland. This atrophy is the end result of Hashimoto's thyroiditis and Graves' disease. These autoimmune diseases destroy the thyroid gland. Hypothyroidism also may develop due to treatment for hyperthyroidism, specifically the surgical removal of the thyroid glands or radioactive iodine therapy.[15] Drugs such as amiodarone (contains iodine) and lithium (blocks hormone production) are known to produce hypothyroidism.

Hypothyroidism that develops in infancy (termed **cretinism**) is caused by thyroid hormone deficiencies during fetal or early neonatal life. All infants in the United States are screened for decreased thyroid function at birth.

Clinical Manifestations

All hypothyroid states have certain features in common, regardless of the cause. Manifestations vary depending on the severity and the duration of thyroid deficiency, as well as the patient's age at onset of the deficiency.

Hypothyroidism has systemic effects characterized by an insidious and nonspecific slowing of body processes. The clinical presentation can range from a patient with no symptoms to a patient with classic symptoms and physical changes easily detected on examination. Unless hypothyroidism occurs after thyroidectomy or thyroid ablation, or during treatment with antithyroid drugs, the onset of symptoms may occur over months to years. The severity of symptoms depends on the degree of thyroid hormone deficiency and the long-term physiologic effects of thyroid hormone deficiency. Long-term effects may involve any body system but are more pronounced in the neurologic, cardiovascular, GI, reproductive, and hematologic systems.

The adult with hypothyroidism often is fatigued and lethargic, and experiences personality and mental changes. The mental changes seen in hypothyroidism include impaired memory, slowed speech, decreased initiative, and somnolence. Many individuals with hypothyroidism appear depressed. Although the patient with hypothyroidism sleeps long periods of time, the stages of sleep are altered.

Hypothyroidism is associated with decreased cardiac output and decreased cardiac contractility. Thus the patient may experience low exercise tolerance and shortness of breath on exertion. In the patient with a preexisting cardiovascular condition, hypothyroidism may cause significant hemodynamic compromise.

Anemia is a common feature of hypothyroidism. Erythropoietin levels may be low or normal. Oxygen demand is decreased, and there is a hypocellular bone marrow. The result is a low hematocrit. Other hematologic problems are related to cobalamin, iron, and folate deficiencies. The patient may bruise easily. Increased serum cholesterol and triglyceride levels and the accumulation of mucopolysaccharides in the intima of small blood vessels can result in coronary atherosclerosis. This accumulation is seldom symptomatic (i.e., characterized by angina) because of the decreased myocardial oxygen consumption that has been observed in hypothyroidism.

GI motility is also decreased in hypothyroidism, and achlorhydria (absence or decrease of hydrochloric acid) is common. Constipation, which is a common complaint, may progress to obstipation and, rarely, to intestinal obstruction. The underlying metabolic disease makes the individual a high-risk candidate for intestinal surgery.

Other physical changes include cold intolerance, hair loss, dry and coarse skin, brittle nails, hoarseness, muscle weakness and swelling, and weight gain. Weight gain is most likely a result of decreased metabolic rate.

Patients with severe long-standing hypothyroidism may display **myxedema**, the accumulation of hydrophilic mucopolysaccharides in the dermis and other tissues (Fig. 50-9). This mucinous edema causes the characteristic facies of hypothyroidism (i.e., puffiness, periorbital edema, and masklike affect). Individuals with hypothyroidism may describe an impaired self-image in regard to their disabilities and altered appearance.

Women with hypothyroidism frequently complain of menorrhagia. Some affected individuals have been treated for menorrhagia for years and may have undergone hysterectomy before the hypothyroidism was diagnosed. In addition, anovulatory cycles with subsequent infertility may occur.

In the older adult, the typical manifestations of hypothyroidism (including fatigue, cold and dry skin, hoarseness, hair loss, constipation, and cold intolerance) may be attributed to normal aging.

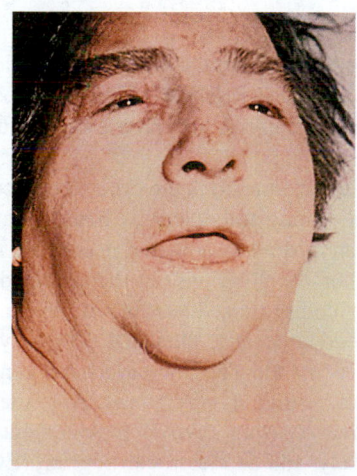

FIG. 50-9 Common features of myxedema. Dull, puffy skin; coarse, sparse hair; periorbital edema; and prominent tongue.

TABLE 50-9	**COLLABORATIVE CARE** Hypothyroidism

Diagnostic
History and physical examination
Serum TSH and free T$_4$
Serum T$_3$ and T$_4$
TRH stimulation test

Collaborative Therapy
Thyroid hormone replacement (e.g., levothyroxine)
Monitor thyroid hormone levels and adjust dosage (if needed)
Nutritional therapy to promote weight loss
Patient and family teaching (see Table 50-10)

TRH, Thyrotropin-releasing hormone; *TSH,* thyroid-stimulating hormone.

For this reason, the patient's symptoms may not raise suspicion of an underlying condition. Older adults who have confusion, lethargy, and depression should be evaluated for thyroid disease.

Complications

The mental sluggishness, drowsiness, and lethargy of hypothyroidism may progress gradually or suddenly to a notable impairment of consciousness or coma. This situation, termed *myxedema coma,* constitutes a medical emergency. Myxedema coma can be precipitated by infection, drugs (especially opioids, tranquilizers, and barbiturates), exposure to cold, and trauma. It is characterized by subnormal temperature, hypotension, and hypoventilation. For the patient to survive, vital functions must be supported and IV thyroid hormone replacement must be administered.

Diagnostic Studies

The most common and reliable laboratory tests used to evaluate thyroid function are those that measure TSH and free T$_4$.[16] These values, correlated with symptoms gathered from the history and physical examination, confirm the diagnosis. Serum TSH levels help determine the cause of hypothyroidism. Serum TSH is high when the defect is in the thyroid and low when it is in the pituitary or hypothalamus. An increase in TSH after TRH injection suggests hypothalamic dysfunction, whereas no change suggests anterior pituitary dysfunction (Table 50-9). Other abnormal laboratory findings are elevated cholesterol and triglycerides, anemia, and increased creatine kinase.

Collaborative Care

The overall treatment in a patient with hypothyroidism is restoration of a euthyroid state as safely and rapidly as possible with hormone replacement therapy. A low-calorie diet is indicated to promote weight loss.

Levothyroxine (Synthroid) is the drug of choice to treat hypothyroidism. In the young and otherwise healthy patient, the maintenance replacement dose is adjusted according to the patient's response and laboratory findings. In the older adult patient and the person with compromised cardiac status, a smaller initial dose is recommended because the usual dose may increase myocardial oxygen demand. The increased oxygen demand may cause angina and cardiac dysrhythmias. Any chest pain experienced by a patient starting thyroid replacement should be reported immediately, and an electrocardiogram (ECG) and serum cardiac enzyme tests must be performed.

Drug Alert - *Levothyroxine (Synthroid)*
• *Carefully monitor patients with cardiovascular disease.*
• *Monitor heart rate and report pulse of 100 beats/min or greater.*
• *Promptly report chest pain, weight loss, nervousness, tremors, insomnia.*

In the patient without side effects, the dose is increased at 4- to 6-week intervals. It is important that the patient take replacement medication regularly. Lifelong thyroid replacement therapy is usually required.

Multiple levothyroxine preparations are currently available. Controversy regarding the equal value of thyroid hormone from brand to brand exists. Individuals using levothyroxine should be cautioned by the health care team to have serum TSH checked 4 to 6 weeks after changing levothyroxine preparation.

Liotrix is a synthetic mix of levothyroxine (T$_4$) and liothyronine (T$_3$) in a 4:1 combination. Liotrix has a faster onset of action with a peak of 2 to 3 days, as opposed to levothyroxine, with a peak of 1 to 3 weeks. Liotrix may be used in acutely ill individuals with hypothyroidism.

NURSING MANAGEMENT
HYPOTHYROIDISM

■ *Nursing Assessment*

Careful assessment may reveal early and subtle changes that indicate dysfunction. Assessment of the patient who is suspected of having hypothyroidism should include questions about weight gain, mental changes, fatigue, slowed and slurred speech, cold intolerance, skin changes such as increased dryness or thickening, constipation, and dyspnea. In addition, the nurse should question the patient about the recent introduction of iodine-containing medications. The patient should be assessed for bradycardia; distended abdomen; dry, thick, cold skin; thick, brittle nails; paresthesias; and muscular aches and pains.

■ *Nursing Diagnoses*

Nursing diagnoses for the patient with hypothyroidism may include, but are not limited to, those presented in NCP 50-2.

■ *Planning*

The overall goals are that the patient with hypothyroidism will (1) experience relief of symptoms, (2) maintain a euthyroid state, (3) maintain a positive self-image, and (4) comply with lifelong thyroid replacement therapy.

■ *Nursing Implementation*

Health Promotion. There is currently no consensus regarding thyroid function screening. Although hypothyroidism is relatively common, particularly among women over age 50, there does not appear to be strong justification to screen the general population.[17] Research suggests that high-risk populations should be screened for subclinical (asymptomatic) thyroid disease. High-risk individuals include those with a family history of thyroid disease, those with a history of neck radiation, women over 50, and postpartum women.

Acute Intervention. Most individuals with hypothyroidism do not require acute nursing care, because most are managed on an outpatient basis. The patient who develops myxedema coma requires acute nursing care, often in an intensive care setting. Mechanical respiratory support and cardiac monitoring are frequently necessary.

NURSING CARE PLAN 50-2

Patient with Hypothyroidism

NURSING DIAGNOSIS   **Imbalanced nutrition: more than body requirements** *related to* calorie intake in excess of metabolic rate *as evidenced by* hypometabolism and weight gain

PATIENT GOALS   1.   Attains weight appropriate for height
2.   Maintains low-calorie diet that meets nutritional needs

OUTCOMES (NOC)	INTERVENTIONS (NIC) and *RATIONALES*
Weight Control	**Weight Reduction Assistance**
• Demonstrates progress toward target weight ____	• Determine patient's desire and motivation to reduce weight or body fat.
• Balances exercise with caloric intake ____	• Plan an exercise program, taking into consideration the patient's limitations.
• Maintains optimal daily caloric intake ____	• Chart progress toward reaching final goal, and post in strategic location.
• Achieves optimum weight ____	• Encourage use of internal rewards system when goals are accomplished.
• Maintains optimum weight ____	**Teaching: Prescribed Diet**
Measurement Scale	• Instruct the patient how to plan appropriate meals (e.g., low calorie, include snacks) *because eating frequently will prevent feelings of hunger and overeating.*
1 = Never demonstrated	• Explain the purpose of the diet *so patient will be more agreeable to dietary restrictions.*
2 = Rarely demonstrated	• Provide written meal plans.
3 = Sometimes demonstrated	**Nutrition Management**
4 = Often demonstrated	• Determine, in collaboration with dietitian, number of calories and type of nutrients needed to meet nutrition requirements.
5 = Consistently demonstrated	• Monitor recorded intake for nutritional content and calories.
	• Weigh patient at appropriate intervals.

NURSING DIAGNOSIS   **Constipation** *related to* gastrointestinal hypomotility *as evidenced by* irregular, hard stools

PATIENT GOAL   Experiences regular, soft formed stools that are easy to pass

OUTCOMES (NOC)	INTERVENTIONS (NIC) and *RATIONALES*
Bowel Elimination	**Constipation/Impaction Management**
• Stool soft and formed ____	• Encourage increased fluid intake (e.g., 2-3 L of fluids per day) *to maintain soft stool.*
• Comfort of stool passage ____	• Instruct patient/family on high-fiber diet *to increase knowledge of how to increase fecal mass.*
• Passage of stool without aids ____	• Monitor bowel movements, including frequency, consistency, shape, volume, and color, *to plan appropriate interventions.*
Measurement Scale	• Suggest use of laxatives/stool softeners *to stimulate GI motility.*
1 = Severely compromised	
2 = Substantially compromised	
3 = Moderately compromised	
4 = Mildly compromised	
5 = Not compromised	

Continued

The nurse will administer thyroid hormone replacement therapy and all other medications IV because the paralytic ileus associated with myxedema coma causes unreliable absorption of oral medications. If the patient is hyponatremic, hypertonic saline may be administered until the serum sodium reaches at least 130 mEq/L (130 mmol/L). The nurse should monitor core temperature because the patient with myxedema coma is often hypothermic.

For assessment of the patient's progress, vital signs, body weight, fluid intake and output, and visible edema should be monitored. Cardiac assessment is especially important because the cardiovascular response to the hormone determines the medication regimen. Energy level and mental alertness should be noted. These should increase within 2 to 14 days and continue to rise steadily to normal levels.

Ambulatory and Home Care. Patient teaching is imperative for the patient with hypothyroidism. A patient and family teaching guide is provided in Table 50-10. Initially the hypothyroid patient needs more time to comprehend all of the necessary information. It is important to provide written instructions, repeat the information often, and assess the patient's comprehension level.

The need for lifelong drug therapy must be stressed. The patient should be instructed in expected and unexpected side effects. Specifically, the signs and symptoms of hypothyroidism or hyperthyroidism that indicate hormone imbalance should be included in the teaching plan. Toxic symptoms should be clearly defined. Table 50-4 lists signs of hyperthyroidism that are the same as the toxic symptoms of thyroid hormone replacement.

The patient must be taught to contact a health care provider immediately if signs of overdose appear, such as orthopnea, dyspnea, rapid pulse, palpitations, nervousness, or insomnia. The patient with diabetes mellitus should test his or her capillary blood glucose at least daily because return to the euthyroid state frequently

NURSING CARE PLAN 50-2

Patient with Hypothyroidism—cont'd

NURSING DIAGNOSIS   **Activity intolerance** *related to* decreased metabolic rate and mucin deposits in joints and interstitial spaces *as evidenced by* generalized weakness and muscle and joint stiffness

PATIENT GOALS   1. Participates in self-care activities of daily living with minimal discomfort and fatigue
2. Reports increased energy and endurance

OUTCOMES (NOC)	INTERVENTIONS (NIC) and *RATIONALES*

Energy Conservation

- Balances activity and rest ____
- Organizes activities to conserve energy ____
- Recognizes energy limitations ____
- Reports adequate endurance for activity ____
- Uses energy conservation techniques ____

Measurement Scale

1 = Never demonstrated
2 = Rarely demonstrated
3 = Sometimes demonstrated
4 = Often demonstrated
5 = Consistently demonstrated

Activity Therapy

- Assist to choose activities consistent with physical, psychologic, and social capabilities.
- Facilitate activity substitution when patient has limitations in time, energy, or movement.

Energy Management

- Determine patient's physical limitations *to determine extent of problem and plan appropriate interventions.*
- Monitor patient for evidence of excess physical and emotional fatigue.
- Monitor patient's oxygen response (e.g., pulse rate, cardiac rhythm, respiratory rate) to self-care or nursing activities *to determine effect of activities and plan activity increases.*
- Encourage alternate rest and activity periods *to prevent fatigue.*
- Teach activity organization and time-management techniques *to prevent fatigue.*
- Promote bed rest/activity limitation (e.g., increase number of rest periods) *to improve patient's tolerance and comfort level.*
- Plan activities for periods when the patient has the most energy *to allow maximum participation.*

NURSING DIAGNOSIS   **Disturbed thought process** *related to* hypometabolism *as evidenced by* forgetfulness, memory loss, somnolence, and personality changes

PATIENT GOAL   Demonstrates cognitive orientation with correction of hormone deficiency

OUTCOMES (NOC)	INTERVENTIONS (NIC) and *RATIONALES*

Cognition

- Comprehends the meaning of events and situations ____
- Attentiveness ____
- Demonstrates recent memory ____
- Cognitive orientation ____

Measurement Scale

1 = Severely compromised
2 = Substantially compromised
3 = Moderately compromised
4 = Mildly compromised
5 = Not compromised

Reality Orientation

- Monitor for changes in sensation and orientation *to determine appropriate interventions.*
- Inform patient of person, place, and time *to decrease confusion.*
- Provide a low-stimulation environment for patient in whom disorientation is increased by overstimulation.
- Speak to patient in slow, distinct manner with appropriate volume *to allow patient to understand.*
- Use environmental cues (e.g., signs, pictures, clocks, calendars) *to maintain orientation to time and day.*

Anxiety Reduction

- Explain all procedures, including sensations likely to be experienced during the procedure, *to reduce anxiety and frustration.*

---

increases insulin requirements. In addition, thyroid preparations potentiate the effects of anticoagulants and decrease the effect of digitalis compounds. Thus the patient should be taught the toxic signs and symptoms of these medications and should remain under close medical observation until stable.

It is sometimes difficult for the patient to recognize signs of overdosage or underdosage of drug therapy. Therefore a family member or friend should be included in the instruction process. Handouts for the patient should be written in understandable language and should accompany verbal instruction. The handouts should be reviewed with the patient and family to assess understanding, and information should be clarified when necessary.

With treatment, striking transformations occur in both appearance and mental function. Most adults return to a normal state. Cardiovascular conditions and (occasionally) psychosis may persist despite corrections of the hormonal imbalance. Relapses occur if treatment is interrupted.

■ Evaluation

The expected outcomes are that the patient with hypothyroidism will

- have relief from symptoms
- maintain a euthyroid state as evidenced by normal thyroid hormone and TSH levels
- adhere to lifelong therapy

Disorders of Parathyroid Glands

HYPERPARATHYROIDISM

Etiology and Pathophysiology

Hyperparathyroidism is a condition involving an increased secretion of parathyroid hormone (PTH). PTH helps regulate calcium and phosphate levels by stimulating bone resorption of calcium, renal tubular reabsorption of calcium, and activation of vitamin D. Thus

TABLE 50-10	*PATIENT AND FAMILY TEACHING GUIDE* Hypothyroidism

1. Patient and family must understand the importance of thyroid replacement therapy. It is especially important to emphasize the need for lifelong replacement, the need to continually take the medication, and the need for regular follow-up care. Self-care practices to prevent complications should also be emphasized.
2. Emphasize the need for a comfortable, warm environment because of intolerance to cold.
3. Teach measures to prevent skin breakdown. Soap should be used sparingly and lotion applied to skin.
4. Caution the patient, especially older adults, to avoid sedatives. If they must be used, suggest that the lowest dose be used. Family members should closely monitor mental status, level of consciousness, and respirations.
5. Discuss with the patient measures to minimize constipation. Suggestions should include a gradual increase in activity and exercise, increased fiber in diet, use of stool softeners, and maintenance of a regular bowel elimination time. Use of enemas should be avoided because they produce vagal stimulation, which can be hazardous if cardiac disease is present.

ETHICAL DILEMMAS
Alternative Healers

Situation
The nurse is caring for a Hispanic woman with thyroid disease. Thyroid replacement therapy is the planned treatment. The patient's cultural healer tells her not to take the medication and suggests that she should begin an herbal regimen instead. Should the nurse intervene?

Important Points for Consideration
- Culturally competent nursing care should incorporate the patient's cultural and religious values and beliefs.
- Patient autonomy, the patient's right to choose a treatment plan, should be respected.
- Having adequate, understandable information about available treatment options and their possible consequences facilitates an informed choice.

Critical Thinking Questions
1. What information should the nurse obtain from the patient? What information should the nurse provide for the patient?
2. How should the nurse proceed? Should the nurse try to incorporate the healer's herbal regimen into the plan of care while attempting to persuade the woman of the need for thyroid replacement therapy?

oversecretion of PTH is associated with increased serum calcium levels. Hyperparathyroidism affects approximately 1% of the general population and is more common in women than men.[18,19]

Hyperparathyroidism is classified as primary, secondary, or tertiary. *Primary hyperparathyroidism* is due to an increased secretion of PTH leading to disorders of calcium, phosphate, and bone metabolism. The most common cause is a benign tumor (adenoma) in the parathyroid gland. Primary hyperparathyroidism usually occurs between 30 and 70 years of age. Peak incidence is in the 40s and 50s. Patients who have previously undergone head and neck radiation may have an increased risk of developing a parathyroid adenoma.

Secondary hyperparathyroidism appears to be a compensatory response to conditions that induce or cause hypocalcemia, the main stimulus of PTH secretion. Disease conditions associated with secondary hyperparathyroidism include vitamin D deficiencies, malabsorption, chronic renal failure, and hyperphosphatemia. *Tertiary hyperparathyroidism* occurs when there is hyperplasia of the parathyroid glands and a loss of negative feedback from circulating calcium levels. Thus there is autonomous secretion of PTH, even with normal calcium levels. This condition is observed in the patient who has had a kidney transplant after a long period of dialysis treatment for chronic kidney disease (see Chapter 47).

Excessive levels of circulating PTH usually lead to hypercalcemia and hypophosphatemia, creating a multisystem effect (Table 50-11). In the bones, decreased bone density, cyst formation, and general weakness can occur as a result of the effect of PTH on osteoclastic (bone resorption) and osteoblastic (bone formation) activity. In the kidneys, the excess calcium cannot be reabsorbed, leading to increased levels of calcium in the urine (hypercalciuria). This urinary calcium, along with a large amount of urinary phosphate, can lead to calculi formation.[20] In addition, PTH stimulates the synthesis of a biologically active form of vitamin D, a potent stimulator of calcium transport in the intestine. In this way, PTH indirectly increases GI absorption of calcium, which further contributes to the high serum calcium levels.

Clinical Manifestations and Complications

Clinical manifestations of hyperparathyroidism range from the asymptomatic individual (who is diagnosed through testing for unrelated problems) to the patient with overt symptoms. Clinical manifestations are associated with hypercalcemia and are shown in Table 50-11. The major manifestations include weakness, loss of appetite, constipation, increased need for sleep, emotional disorders, and shortened attention span. Major signs include loss of calcium from bones (osteoporosis), fractures, and kidney stones (nephrolithiasis). Neuromuscular abnormalities are characterized by muscle weakness, particularly in the proximal muscles of the lower extremities. Asymptomatic cases are often identified with routine calcium screening. Serious complications of hyperparathyroidism are renal failure; pancreatitis; cardiac changes; and long bone, rib, and vertebral fractures.

Diagnostic Studies

PTH, as measured by radioimmunoassay, is elevated with hyperparathyroidism. Serum calcium levels usually exceed 10 mg/dl (2.50 mmol/L). Because of its inverse relation with calcium, the serum phosphorus level is usually below 3 mg/dl (0.1 mmol/L).

Elevations in other laboratory tests include urine calcium, serum chloride, uric acid, creatinine, amylase (if pancreatitis is present), and alkaline phosphatase (in the presence of bone disease). Bone density measurements may also be used to detect bone loss. Conversely, individuals found to have bone loss on a screening dual-energy x-ray absorptiometry (DEXA) scan should be tested for hypercalcemia.[19] MRI, CT, and/or ultrasound may be used for localization of the adenoma.

Collaborative Care

The treatment objectives are to relieve symptoms and prevent complications caused by excess PTH. The choice of therapy depends on the urgency of the clinical situation, the degree of hypercalcemia, and the underlying cause of the disorder.

Surgical Therapy. The most effective treatment of primary and secondary hyperparathyroidism is surgical intervention. Parathyroidectomy leads to a rapid reduction of chronically high calcium levels. Criteria for surgery include serum calcium levels

TABLE 50-11	Clinical Manifestations: Parathyroid Dysfunction	
System	**Hypofunction**	**Hyperfunction**
Cardiovascular	Decreased contractility of heart muscle	Dysrhythmias
	Decreased cardiac output	Shortened QT interval on ECG
	Prolongation of QT and ST intervals on ECG	Hypertension
	Dysrhythmias	
Gastrointestinal	Abdominal cramps	Vague abdominal pain
	Fecal incontinence (in older adult)	Anorexia
	Malabsorption	Nausea and vomiting
		Constipation
		Pancreatitis
		Peptic ulcer disease
		Cholelithiasis
		Weight loss
Integumentary	Dry, scaly skin	Skin necrosis
	Hair loss on scalp and body	Moist skin
	Brittle nails, transverse ridging	
	Changes in developing teeth, lack of tooth enamel	
Musculoskeletal	Fatigue	Skeletal pain
	Weakness	Backache
	Painful muscle cramps	Weakness, fatigue
	Skeletal x-ray changes, osteosclerosis	Pain on weight bearing
	Soft tissue calcification	Osteoporosis
	Difficulty in walking	Pathologic fractures of long bones
		Compression fractures of spine
		Decreased muscle tone, muscle atrophy
Neurologic	Personality changes	Personality disturbances
	Psychiatric manifestations of depression, anxiety, psychosis	Emotional irritability
	Irritability	Memory impairment
	Memory impairment	Psychosis, depression
	Headache, increased intracranial pressure	Delirium, confusion, coma
	Seizures	Poor coordination
	Positive Chvostek's sign or Trousseau's phenomenon	Hyperactive deep-tendon reflexes
	Tremor	Abnormalities of gait
	Paresthesias of lips, hands, feet	Psychomotor retardation
	Hyperactive deep-tendon reflexes	Headache
	Disorientation, confusion (in older adult)	Paresthesias
Renal	Urinary frequency	Hypercalciuria
	Urinary incontinence	Kidney stones (nephrolithiasis)
		Urinary tract infections
		Polyuria
Other	Eye changes, including lenticular opacities, cataracts, papilledema	Corneal calcification on slit-lamp examination

ECG, Electrocardiogram.

greater than 12 mg/dl (3.0 mmol/L), hypercalciuria (greater than 400 mg/day), markedly reduced bone mineral density, overt symptoms (e.g., neuromuscular effects, nephrolithiasis), or those under age 50. Surgery involves partial or complete removal of the parathyroid glands. The most commonly used procedure involves an endoscope and is done on an outpatient basis. Successful removal of the parathyroid glands is facilitated by intraoperative PTH assay, nuclear scanning with sestamibi, and a radio-guided probe.[21]

Autotransplantation of normal parathyroid tissue in the forearm or near the sternocleidomastoid muscle is usually done. This allows PTH secretion to continue with normalization of calcium levels. If autotransplantation is not possible, or if it fails, the patient will need to take calcium supplements for life.

Nonsurgical Therapy. If the patient does not meet the criteria for surgical intervention, or if the patient is elderly or at increased surgical risk from other health problems, a conservative management approach is used. This includes an annual examination with tests for serum PTH, calcium, phosphorus, and alkaline phosphatase levels; renal function; x-rays to assess for metabolic bone loss; and measurement of urinary calcium excretion. Continued ambulation and the avoidance of immobility are critical aspects of management. Dietary measures also include maintenance of a high fluid intake and a moderate calcium intake.

Phosphorus is usually supplemented unless contraindicated by an increased risk for urinary calculi formation. Several drugs currently used in the treatment of hyperparathyroidism are helpful in lowering calcium levels, but do not, in themselves, treat the underlying problem. Bisphosphonates (e.g., alendronate [Fosamax]) inhibit osteoclastic bone resorption and rapidly normalize serum calcium levels. Estrogen or progestin therapy can reduce serum and urinary calcium levels in the postmenopausal woman and may retard demineralization of the skeleton. Oral phosphate may be used to inhibit the calcium-absorbing effects of vitamin D in the intestine. Phosphates should only be used if the patient has normal renal function and low serum phosphate levels. Diuretics may be given to increase the urinary excretion of calcium.

Calcimimetic agents (e.g., cinacalcet [Sensipar]) are a new class of drugs that increase the sensitivity of the calcium receptor on the parathyroid gland, resulting in decreased PTH secretion and calcium blood levels, thus sparing calcium stores in the bone. Drugs in this class are currently approved for secondary hyperparathyroidism in individuals with chronic kidney disease on dialysis, and patients with parathyroid cancer.[22] Cinacalcet is under investigation for use in primary hyperparathyroidism.

NURSING MANAGEMENT
HYPERPARATHYROIDISM

Nursing care for the patient following a parathyroidectomy is similar to that for a patient after thyroidectomy. The major postoperative complications are associated with hemorrhage and fluid and electrolyte disturbances. *Tetany,* a condition of neuromuscular hyperexcitability associated with sudden decrease in calcium levels, is another concern. It is usually apparent early in the postoperative period but may develop over several days. Mild tetany, characterized by unpleasant tingling of the hands and around the mouth, may be present but should decrease over time. If tetany becomes more severe (e.g., muscular spasms or laryngospasms develop), IV calcium may be given. IV calcium gluconate or gluceptate should be readily available for patients following parathyroidectomy in the event that acute tetany occurs.

Intake and output are monitored to evaluate fluid status. Calcium, potassium, phosphate, and magnesium levels are assessed frequently, as well as Chvostek's and Trousseau's signs (see Chapter 17, Fig. 17-15). Mobility is encouraged to promote bone calcification.

If surgery is not performed, treatment to relieve symptoms and prevent complications is initiated. The nurse can assist the patient with hyperparathyroidism to adapt the meal plan to his or her lifestyle. A referral to a dietitian may be useful. Because immobility can aggravate the bone loss, the nurse needs to stress to the patient the importance of an exercise program. The patient should be encouraged to keep the regular appointments, and the tests being performed should be explained. The patient should also be instructed in the symptoms of hypocalcemia or hypercalcemia and to report these should they occur. Hypocalcemia and hypercalcemia are discussed in Chapter 17.

HYPOPARATHYROIDISM

Etiology and Pathophysiology

Hypoparathyroidism, a condition associated with inadequate circulating PTH, is uncommon. It is characterized by hypocalcemia resulting from a lack of PTH to maintain serum calcium levels. PTH resistance at the cellular level may also occur (pseudohypoparathyroidism). This is caused by a genetic defect resulting in hypocalcemia in spite of normal or high PTH levels and is often associated with hypothyroidism and hypogonadism.

The most common cause of hypoparathyroidism is iatrogenic. This may include accidental removal of the parathyroid glands or damage to the vascular supply of the glands during neck surgery (e.g., thyroidectomy, radical neck surgery). Idiopathic hypoparathyroidism resulting from the absence, fatty replacement, or atrophy of the glands is a rare disease that usually occurs early in life and may be associated with other endocrine disorders. Affected patients may have antiparathyroid antibodies. Severe hypomagnesemia also leads to a suppression of PTH secretion.[23]

Clinical Manifestations

The clinical features of acute hypoparathyroidism are due to hypocalcemia (see Table 50-11). Sudden decreases in calcium concentration cause tetany. This state is characterized by tingling of the lips, fingertips, and occasionally feet and increased muscle tension leading to paresthesias and stiffness. Painful tonic spasms of smooth and skeletal muscles (particularly of the extremities and face), dysphagia, a constricted feeling in the throat, and laryngospasms are also present. Chvostek's sign and Trousseau's sign are usually positive. Respiratory function may be severely compromised by accessory muscle spasm and laryngospasm-induced airway obstruction. Patients are usually anxious and apprehensive. Abnormal laboratory findings include decreased serum calcium and PTH levels and increased serum phosphate levels. Other causes of chronic hypocalcemia include chronic kidney disease, vitamin D deficiency, and hypomagnesemia.

NURSING and COLLABORATIVE MANAGEMENT
HYPOPARATHYROIDISM

The primary management objectives for a patient with hypoparathyroidism are to treat acute complications such as tetany, maintain normal serum calcium levels, and prevent long-term complications. Emergency treatment of tetany requires the administration of IV calcium.

IV calcium chloride, calcium gluconate, or calcium gluceptate should be given slowly. Calcium must be infused slowly because high blood levels can cause hypotension, serious cardiac dysrhythmias, or cardiac arrest. Thus ECG monitoring is indicated when calcium is administered. The patient who takes digoxin is particularly vulnerable. IV calcium can cause venous irritation and inflammation. Extravasation may cause cellulitis, necrosis, and tissue sloughing. IV patency should be assessed before administration.

Rebreathing may partially alleviate acute neuromuscular symptoms associated with hypocalcemia such as generalized muscle cramps or mild tetany. The patient who can cooperate should be instructed to breathe in and out of a paper bag or breathing mask. This reduces carbon dioxide excretion from the lungs, increases carbonic acid levels in the blood, and lowers the pH.

A lower pH (acidic environment) enhances the degree of ionization of calcium causing an increase in the proportion of total body calcium available in the active form. This will then temporarily relieve the manifestations of hypocalcemia.

The patient with hypoparathyroidism needs instruction in the management of long-term drug therapy and nutrition. PTH replacement is not a recommended drug therapy because of the expense and the need for parenteral administration. Oral calcium supplements of at least 1.5 to 3 g/day in divided doses are usually prescribed.

Vitamin D is used in chronic and resistant hypocalcemia to enhance intestinal calcium absorption and bone resorption. Preferred preparations are dihydrotachysterol (Hytakerol) and 1,25-dihydroxycholecalciferol (calcitriol [Rocaltrol]). These drugs raise calcium levels rapidly and are quickly metabolized. Rapid metabolism is desired because vitamin D is a fat-soluble vitamin and toxicity can cause irreversible renal impairment. Ergocalciferol (Calciferol), the least expensive of the vitamin D preparations, may also be prescribed. A high-calcium meal plan includes foods such as dark green vegetables, soybeans, and tofu. The patient should be told that foods containing oxalic acid (e.g., spinach, rhubarb), phytic acid (e.g., bran, whole grains), and phosphorus reduce calcium absorption. The patient should be instructed about the need for lifelong treatment and follow-up care including the monitoring of calcium levels three to four times a year.

Disorders of the Adrenal Cortex

There are three main classifications of adrenal cortex steroid hormones: glucocorticoid, mineralocorticoid, and androgen. Glucocorticoids regulate metabolism, increase blood glucose levels, and are critical in the physiologic stress response. In humans the primary glucocorticoid is cortisol. Mineralocorticoids regulate sodium and potassium balance. The primary mineralocorticoid is aldosterone. Androgens contribute to growth and development in both genders and to sexual activity in adult women. The term *corticosteroid* refers to any one of these three types of hormones produced by the adrenal cortex.

CUSHING SYNDROME

Etiology and Pathophysiology

Cushing syndrome is a spectrum of clinical abnormalities caused by an excess of corticosteroids, particularly glucocorticoids. Several conditions can cause Cushing syndrome (Table 50-12). The most common cause is iatrogenic administration of exogenous corticosteroids (e.g., prednisone). Approximately 85% of the cases of endogenous Cushing syndrome are due to an adrenocorticotropic hormone (ACTH)–secreting pituitary tumor (Cushing's disease). Other causes of Cushing syndrome include adrenal tumors and ectopic ACTH production by tumors (usually of the lung or pancreas) outside of the hypothalamic-pituitary-adrenal axis. Cushing's disease and primary adrenal tumors are more common in women in the 20- to 40-year-old age-group; ectopic ACTH production is more common in men.

Clinical Manifestations

The clinical manifestations of Cushing syndrome can be seen in most body systems and are related to excess levels of corticosteroids (Table 50-13). Although manifestations of glucocorticoid excess usually predominate, symptoms of mineralocorticoid and androgen excess may also be seen.

Corticosteroid excess causes pronounced changes in physical appearance (Fig. 50-10). Weight gain, the most common feature, results from the accumulation of adipose tissue in the trunk, face, and cervical spine area[24] (Fig. 50-11). Transient weight gain from sodium and water retention may be present because of the mineralocorticoid effects of cortisol. Hyperglycemia occurs because of glucose intolerance (associated with cortisol-induced insulin resistance) and increased gluconeogenesis by the liver.

Protein wasting is caused by the catabolic effects of cortisol on peripheral tissue. Muscle wasting leads to muscle weakness, especially in the extremities. A loss of protein matrix in the bone leads to osteoporosis with subsequent pathologic fractures (e.g., vertebral compression fractures) and bone and back pain. The loss of collagen makes the skin weaker and thinner, and therefore more easily bruised. Catabolic processes predominate, and wound healing is delayed. Mood disturbances (irritability, anxiety, euphoria), insomnia, irrationality, and occasionally psychosis may occur.

Mineralocorticoid excess may cause hypertension (secondary to fluid retention), whereas adrenal androgen excess may cause pronounced acne, virilization in women, and feminization in men. Menstrual disorders and hirsutism in women and gynecomastia and impotence in men are seen more commonly in adrenal carcinomas.

The clinical presentation is the first indication of Cushing syndrome. Of particular importance are (1) centripetal (truncal) obesity

---

TABLE 50-12	**Causes of Cushing Syndrome**

- Prolonged administration of high doses of corticosteroids
- ACTH-secreting pituitary tumor (Cushing's disease)
- Cortisol-secreting neoplasm within the adrenal cortex that can be either carcinoma or adenoma
- Excess secretion of ACTH from carcinoma of the lung or other malignant growth outside the pituitary or adrenal glands

ACTH, Adrenocorticotropic hormone.

or generalized obesity; (2) "moon facies" (fullness of the face) with facial plethora; (3) purplish red striae, which are usually depressed below the skin surface, on the abdomen, breast, or buttocks (Fig. 50-12); (4) hirsutism in women; (5) menstrual disorders in women; (6) hypertension; and (7) unexplained hypokalemia.

Diagnostic Studies

When Cushing syndrome is suspected, a 24-hour urine collection for free cortisol is done. Urine cortisol levels of 50 to 100 mcg/day in adults indicate Cushing syndrome.[25] If these results are borderline, a high-dose dexamethasone suppression test is done (see Table 48-8). False-positive results can occur in patients with depression, those under acute stress, and those who are active alcoholics. Plasma cortisol (the primary glucocorticoid) levels may be elevated, with loss of diurnal variation. CT scanning and MRI of the pituitary and adrenal glands may be used.

Plasma ACTH levels may be low, normal, or elevated depending on the underlying problem. High or normal levels indicate ACTH-dependent Cushing's disease, whereas low or undetectable levels indicate an adrenal or exogenous etiology. Other findings on diagnostic tests associated with, but not diagnostic of, Cushing syndrome include leukocytosis, lymphopenia, eosinopenia, hyperglycemia, glycosuria, hypercalciuria, and osteoporosis. Hypokalemia and alkalosis are seen in ectopic ACTH syndrome and adrenal carcinoma.

Collaborative Care

The primary goal of treatment for Cushing syndrome is to normalize hormone secretion. The specific treatment is dependent on the underlying cause (Table 50-14). If the underlying cause is a pituitary adenoma, the standard treatment is surgical removal of the pituitary tumor using the transsphenoidal approach.[26] (The transsphenoidal approach is discussed earlier in this chapter.) Radiation to the pituitary adenoma may be necessary if surgical outcomes are not optimal or if the patient is not a good surgical candidate. Adrenalectomy is indicated for Cushing syndrome caused by adrenal tumors or hyperplasia. Occasionally, bilateral adrenalectomy is necessary.

Laparoscopic adrenalectomy is used unless a known or suspected malignant adrenal tumor is present. An open surgical adrenalectomy is used for adrenal cancer. Patients with ectopic ACTH-secreting tumors are managed by treating the primary neoplasm.

Drug therapy is used when surgery is contraindicated or as an adjunct to surgery. The goal of drug therapy is the inhibition of adrenal function. Mitotane (Lysodren) suppresses cortisol production, alters peripheral metabolism of cortisol, and decreases plasma and urine corticosteroid levels. This drug essentially results in a "medical adrenalectomy." Metyrapone, ketoconazole (Nizoral), and aminoglutethimide (Cytadren) are used to inhibit cortisol synthesis. Common side effects of these agents include

TABLE 50-13 | **Clinical Manifestations: Adrenocortical Hormone Dysfunction**

System	Hypofunction (Addison's Disease)	Hyperfunction (Cushing Syndrome)
Glucocorticoids		
General appearance	Weight loss	Truncal (centripetal) obesity, thin extremities, rounding of face (moon face), fat deposits on back of neck and on shoulders ("buffalo hump")
Integumentary	Bronzed or smoky hyperpigmentation of face, neck, hands (especially creases), buccal membranes, nipples, genitalia, and scars (if pituitary function normal); vitiligo, alopecia	Thin, fragile skin; purplish red striae; petechial hemorrhages; bruises; florid cheeks (plethora); acne; poor wound healing
Cardiovascular	Hypotension, tendency to develop refractory shock, vasodilation	Hypervolemia, hypertension, edema of lower extremities
Gastrointestinal	Anorexia, nausea and vomiting, cramping abdominal pain, diarrhea	Increase in secretion of pepsin and hydrochloric acid, anorexia
Urinary		Glycosuria, hypercalciuria, kidney stones
Musculoskeletal	Fatigability	Muscle wasting in extremities, proximal muscle weakness, fatigue, osteoporosis, awkward gait, back and joint pain, weakness, fractures
Immune	Tendency toward coexisting autoimmune diseases	Inhibition of immune response, suppression of allergic response, inhibition of inflammation
Hematologic	Anemia, lymphocytosis	Leukocytosis, lymphopenia, polycythemia, increased coagulability
Fluids and electrolytes	Hyponatremia, hypovolemia, dehydration, hyperkalemia	Sodium and water retention, edema, hypokalemia
Metabolic	Hyponatremia, insulin sensitivity, fever	Hyperglycemia, negative nitrogen balance, dyslipidemia
Emotional	Neurasthenia, depression, exhaustion or irritability, confusion, delusions	Psychic stimulation, euphoria, irritability, hypomania to depression, emotional lability
Mineralocorticoids		
Fluid and electrolytes	Sodium loss, decreased volume of extracellular fluid, hyperkalemia, salt craving	Marked sodium and water retention, tendency toward edema, marked hypokalemia, alkalosis
Cardiovascular	Hypovolemia, tendency toward shock, decreased cardiac output, decreased heart size	Hypertension, hypervolemia
Androgens		
Integumentary	Decreased axillary and pubic hair (in women)	Hirsutism, acne, hyperpigmentation
Reproductive	No effect in men, decreased libido in women	Menstrual irregularities and enlargement of clitoris (in females); gynecomastia and testicular atrophy (in males)
Musculoskeletal	Decrease in muscle size and tone	Muscle wasting and weakness

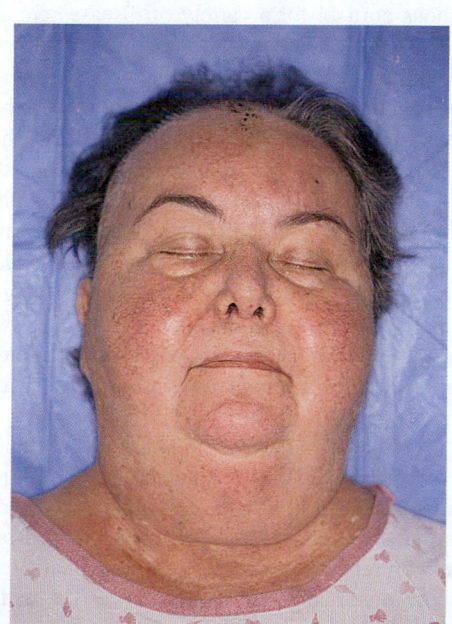

FIG. 50-10   Cushing syndrome. Facies include a rounded face ("moon face") with thin, reddened skin. Hirsutism may also be present.

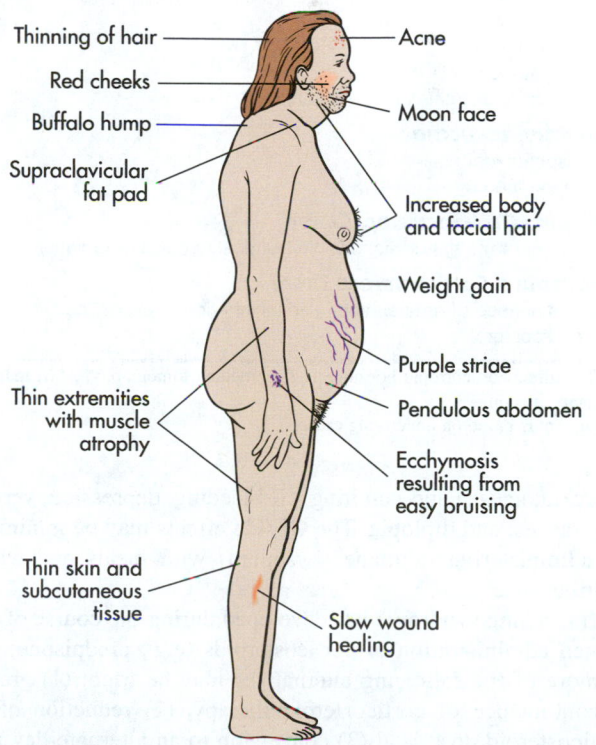

Thinning of hair
Red cheeks
Buffalo hump
Supraclavicular fat pad
Thin extremities with muscle atrophy
Thin skin and subcutaneous tissue

Acne
Moon face
Increased body and facial hair
Weight gain
Purple striae
Pendulous abdomen
Ecchymosis resulting from easy bruising
Slow wound healing

FIG. 50-11   Common characteristics of Cushing syndrome.

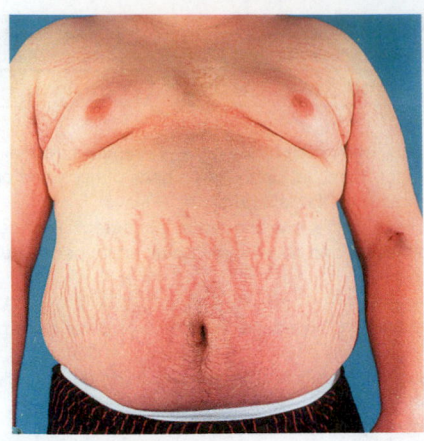

FIG. 50-12   Cushing syndrome. Truncal obesity; broad, purple striae; and easy bruising (left antecubital fossa).

TABLE 50-14	**COLLABORATIVE CARE** **Cushing Syndrome**

Diagnostic
History and physical examination
Mental status examination
Plasma cortisol levels for diurnal variations
Plasma ACTH level
Complete blood count
Blood chemistries for sodium, potassium, glucose
Dexamethasone suppression test
24-hr urine for free cortisol
Examination of visual field
CT scan, MRI

Collaborative Therapy*
Adrenocortical Adenoma, Carcinoma, or Hyperplasia
Adrenalectomy (open or laparoscopic)
Drug therapy
- mitotane (Lysodren)
- metyrapone
- ketoconazole (Nizoral)
- aminoglutethimide (Cytadren)

Pituitary Adenoma
Transsphenoidal resection
Radiation therapy

Ectopic ACTH-Secreting Tumor
Treatment of the tumor responsible (surgical removal or radiation)

Exogenous Corticosteroid Therapy
Discontinuance of or alteration in administration of exogenous corticosteroids

ACTH, Adrenocorticotropic hormone; *CT*, computed tomography; *MRI*, magnetic resonance imaging.
*Treatment is based on underlying cause.

anorexia, nausea and vomiting, GI bleeding, depression, vertigo, skin rashes, and diplopia. The GI side effects may be minimized by administering mitotane (Lysodren) with meals and with a bedtime snack.

If Cushing syndrome has developed during the course of prolonged administration of corticosteroids (e.g., prednisone), one or more of the following alternatives may be tried: (1) gradual discontinuance of corticosteroid therapy, (2) reduction of the corticosteroid dose, and (3) conversion to an alternate-day regimen.[27] Gradual tapering of the corticosteroids is necessary to

avoid potentially life-threatening adrenal insufficiency. An alternate-day regimen is one in which twice the daily dosage of a shorter-acting corticosteroid is given every other morning to minimize hypothalamic-pituitary-adrenal suppression, growth suppression, and altered appearance. This regimen is not used when the corticosteroids are given as endocrine replacement therapy.

NURSING MANAGEMENT
CUSHING SYNDROME

▪ *Nursing Assessment*

Subjective and objective data that should be obtained from a patient with Cushing syndrome are presented in Table 50-15.

▪ *Nursing Diagnoses*

Nursing diagnoses for the patient with Cushing syndrome may include, but are not limited to the following:
- Risk for infection *related to* lowered resistance to stress and suppression of immune system
- Imbalanced nutrition: more than body requirements *related to* increased appetite, high caloric content of foods, and inactivity
- Disturbed self-esteem *related to* altered body image and emotional lability
- Impaired skin integrity *related to* excess corticosteroids, immobility, and altered skin fragility

▪ *Planning*

The overall goals are that the patient with Cushing syndrome will
- experience relief of symptoms
- have no serious complications
- maintain a positive self-image
- actively participate in the therapeutic plan

▪ *Nursing Implementation*

Health Promotion. Health promotion is focused on identifying patients at risk for Cushing syndrome. Patients receiving long-term, exogenous cortisol for a variety of diseases are at risk. Patient teaching related to the medication use and monitoring of side effects are important preventive measures.

Acute Intervention. The patient with Cushing syndrome is seriously ill. Because the therapy has many side effects, the focus of assessment is on signs and symptoms of hormone and drug toxicity and complicating conditions (e.g., cardiovascular disease, diabetes mellitus, and infection). Nursing assessment should include monitoring of vital signs, daily weight, glucose, possible infection (especially pain, loss of function, and purulent drainage, because other signs and symptoms of inflammation such as fever and redness may be minimal or absent), and signs and symptoms of abnormal thromboembolic phenomena, such as sudden chest pain, dyspnea, or tachypnea.

Another important focus of nursing care is emotional support. Changes in appearance such as centripetal obesity, multiple bruises, hirsutism in women, and gynecomastia in men can be distressing. The patient may feel unattractive, repulsive, or unwanted. The nurse can help by remaining sensitive to the patient's feelings and offering respect and unconditional acceptance. The patient can be reassured that the physical changes and much of the emotional lability will resolve when hormone levels return to normal.

TABLE 50-15	**NURSING ASSESSMENT** Cushing Syndrome

Subjective Data

Important Health Information

Past health history: Pituitary tumor (Cushing's disease); adrenal, pancreatic, or pulmonary neoplasms; GI bleeding; frequent infections

Medications: Use of corticosteroids

Functional Health Patterns

Health perception–health management: Malaise
Nutritional-metabolic: Weight gain, anorexia
Elimination: Polyuria; prolonged wound healing, easy bruising
Activity-exercise: Weakness, fatigue
Sleep: Insomnia, poor sleep quality
Cognitive-perceptual: Headache; back, joint, bone, and rib pain; poor concentration and memory
Self-perception–self-concept: Negative feelings regarding changes in personal appearance
Sexuality-reproductive: Amenorrhea, impotence, decreased libido
Coping–stress tolerance: Anxiety, mood disturbances, emotional lability, psychosis

Objective Data

General

Truncal obesity, supraclavicular fat pads, buffalo hump, moon facies

Integumentary

Plethora; hirsutism of body and face, thinning of head hair; thin, friable skin; acne; petechiae; purpura; hyperpigmentation; purplish red striae on breasts, buttocks, and abdomen; edema of lower extremities

Cardiovascular

Hypertension

Musculoskeletal

Muscle wasting, thin extremities, awkward gait

Reproductive

Gynecomastia, testicular atrophy (in men), enlarged clitoris (in women)

Possible Findings

Hypokalemia, hyperglycemia, dyslipidemia; polycythemia, granulocytosis, lymphocytopenia, eosinopenia; ↑ plasma cortisol; high, low, or normal ACTH levels; abnormal dexamethasone suppression test; ↑ urine free cortisol, 17-ketosteroids; glycosuria, hypercalciuria; osteoporosis on x-ray

ACTH, Adrenocorticotropic hormone; *GI,* gastrointestinal.

If treatment involves surgical removal of a pituitary adenoma, an adrenal tumor, or one or both adrenal glands, nursing care will have an additional focus on preoperative and postoperative care.

Preoperative Care. Before surgery the patient should be brought to optimal physical condition. Hypertension and hyperglycemia must be controlled, and hypokalemia must be corrected with diet and potassium supplements before surgery. A high-protein diet helps correct the protein depletion. Preoperative teaching will depend on the type of surgical approach planned (hypophysectomy or adrenalectomy), but should include information regarding the postoperative care the patient should anticipate. In the postoperative period (for both open and laparoscopic adrenalectomy), patients will probably have a nasogastric tube, a urinary catheter, IV therapy, central venous pressure monitoring, and leg sequential compression devices to prevent emboli. Preoperative management for the patient undergoing a hypophysectomy is discussed earlier in this chapter.

Postoperative Care. Surgery on the adrenal glands poses risks beyond those of other types of operations. Because these glands are highly vascular, the risk of hemorrhage is increased. The manipulation of glandular tissue during surgery may release large amounts of hormone into the circulation, producing marked fluctuations in the metabolic processes affected by these hormones. Postoperatively, BP, fluid balance, and electrolyte levels tend to be unstable because of these hormone fluctuations.

High doses of corticosteroids (e.g., hydrocortisone [Solu-Cortef]) are administered IV during surgery and for several days afterward to ensure adequate responses to the stress of the procedure. If large amounts of endogenous hormone have been released into the systemic circulation during surgery, the patient is likely to develop hypertension, increasing the risk of hemorrhage. High levels of corticosteroids also increase susceptibility to infection and delay wound healing.

Any rapid or significant changes in BP, respirations, or heart rate should be reported. Fluid intake and output are monitored carefully and assessed for potential imbalances. The critical period for circulatory instability ranges from 24 to 48 hours after surgery. IV corticosteroids are given, and the dose and rate of flow are adjusted to the patient's clinical manifestations and fluid and electrolyte balance. Oral doses are given as tolerated. The IV line may be kept in place after IV corticosteroids are withdrawn to keep a line open for quick administration of corticosteroids or vasopressors. Morning urine levels of cortisol (obtained at the same time each morning) are measured to evaluate the effectiveness of the surgery.

If corticosteroid dosage is tapered too rapidly after surgery, acute adrenal insufficiency may develop. Vomiting, increased weakness, dehydration, and hypotension may indicate hypocortisolism. In addition, the patient may complain of painful joints, pruritus, or peeling skin and may experience severe emotional disturbances. These signs and symptoms should be reported so that drug doses can be adjusted as necessary. The nurse must constantly be alert for signs of corticosteroid imbalance. After surgery the patient is usually maintained on bed rest until the BP stabilizes. The nurse must be alert for subtle signs of postoperative infections because the usual inflammatory responses are suppressed. Meticulous care must be used when changing the dressing and during any other procedures that necessitate access to body cavities, circulation, or areas under the skin so that infection is prevented. A nursing care plan for the patient with Cushing syndrome is available on the website at *http://evolve.elsevier.com/Lewis/medsurg.*

Ambulatory and Home Care. Discharge instructions are based on the patient's lack of endogenous corticosteroids and resulting inability to react to stressors physiologically. Consider a visiting nurse referral, especially for older adults, because of the need for ongoing evaluation and educational needs. Patients should wear medical alert bracelets at all times and carry medical identification and instructions in a wallet or purse. Exposure to extremes of temperature, infections, and emotional disturbances should be avoided as much as possible. Stress may produce or precipitate acute adrenal insufficiency because the remaining adrenal tissue cannot meet an increased hormonal demand. Many patients can be taught to adjust their corticosteroid replacement therapy in accordance with their stress levels. The nurse should consult with each patient's health care provider to determine the parameters for dosage changes if this plan is feasible. If the patient cannot adjust his or her own medication or if weakness, fainting, fever, or nausea and vomiting occur, the patient should contact the health care provider for a possible adjustment in corticosteroid dosage. Lifetime replacement therapy is required by many patients. However, it may take several months to adjust the hormone dose satisfactorily, and patients should be prepared for this.

■ *Evaluation*

The expected outcomes are that the patient with Cushing syndrome will

- experience no signs or symptoms of infection
- attain weight appropriate for height
- report increased acceptance of appearance
- demonstrate healing of skin and maintenance of intact skin

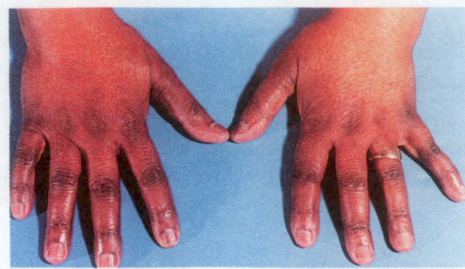

FIG. 50-13   Hyperpigmentation typically seen in Addison's disease.

ADRENOCORTICAL INSUFFICIENCY

Etiology and Pathophysiology

Adrenocortical insufficiency (hypofunction of the adrenal cortex) may be from a primary cause (known as **Addison's disease**) or a secondary cause (lack of pituitary ACTH secretion). In Addison's disease, all three classes of adrenal corticosteroids (glucocorticoids, mineralocorticoids, and androgens) are reduced. In secondary adrenocortical insufficiency, corticosteroids and androgens are deficient but mineralocorticoids rarely are. ACTH deficiency may be caused by pituitary disease or suppression of the hypothalamic-pituitary axis as a result of the administration of exogenous corticosteroids.

The most common cause of Addison's disease in industrialized nations is an autoimmune response. Adrenal tissue is destroyed by antibodies against the patient's own adrenal cortex. Susceptibility genes for Addison's disease are beginning to be identified.[28] Often, other endocrine conditions are present and Addison's disease is considered a component of *polyendocrine deficiency syndrome.* Tuberculosis causes Addison's disease worldwide, but this is now rare in North American and industrialized nations. Other causes include infarction, fungal infections (e.g., histoplasmosis), acquired immunodeficiency syndrome (AIDS), and metastatic cancer. Iatrogenic Addison's disease may be due to adrenal hemorrhage, often related to anticoagulant therapy, antineoplastic chemotherapy, ketoconazole (Nizoral) therapy for AIDS, or bilateral adrenalectomy. Adrenal insufficiency most often occurs in adults less than 60 years of age and affects both genders equally. Addison's disease, if caused by an autoimmune response, is most common in white females.

Clinical Manifestations

Because manifestations do not tend to become evident until 90% of the adrenal cortex is destroyed, the disease is often advanced before it is diagnosed. The manifestations have a very slow (insidious) onset and include progressive weakness, fatigue, weight loss, and anorexia as primary features. Skin hyperpigmentation, a striking feature, is seen primarily in sun-exposed areas of the body, at pressure points, over joints, and in creases, especially palmar creases (Fig. 50-13). It is most likely due to increased secretion of β-lipotropin (which contains melanocyte-stimulating hormone [MSH]) or ACTH. These tropic hormones are increased because of decreased negative feedback and subsequent low corticosteroid levels. Other frequent manifestations are orthostatic hypotension, hyponatremia, hyperkalemia, nausea and vomiting, and diarrhea. Irritability and depression may also occur in primary adrenal hypofunction.

Patients with secondary adrenocortical hypofunction may have many signs and symptoms in common with patients with Addison's disease but are characteristically not hyperpigmented because ACTH and related peptide levels are low.

Complications

Patients with adrenocortical insufficiency are at risk for an acute adrenal insufficiency *(addisonian crisis),* a life-threatening emergency caused by insufficient adrenocortical hormones or a sudden sharp decrease in these hormones. Addisonian crisis is triggered by stress (e.g., from infection, surgery, trauma, hemorrhage, or psychologic distress); the sudden withdrawal of corticosteroid hormone replacement therapy (which is often done by a patient who lacks knowledge of the importance of replacement therapy); after adrenal surgery; or following sudden pituitary gland destruction.

During acute adrenal insufficiency, severe manifestations of glucocorticoid and mineralocorticoid deficiencies are exhibited, including hypotension (particularly postural), tachycardia, dehydration, hyponatremia, hyperkalemia, hypoglycemia, fever, weakness, and confusion. Hypotension may lead to shock. Circulatory collapse associated with adrenal insufficiency is often unresponsive to the usual treatment (vasopressors and fluid replacement). GI manifestations include severe vomiting, diarrhea, and pain in the abdomen. Pain may also occur in the lower back or legs.

Diagnostic Studies

In addition to clinical features, a diagnosis of Addison's disease can be made when cortisol levels are subnormal or fail to rise over basal levels with an ACTH-stimulation test. A failure of cortisol levels to rise in response to ACTH stimulation indicates primary adrenal disease. A positive response to ACTH stimulation indicates a functioning adrenal gland and points to a probable diagnosis of pituitary disease (see Table 48-8).

Other abnormal laboratory findings include hyperkalemia, hypochloremia, hyponatremia, hypoglycemia, anemia, and increased blood urea nitrogen levels. Urine levels of free cortisol are low. An ECG may show low voltage and peaked T waves caused by hyperkalemia. CT scans and MRI are used to localize tumors or identify adrenal calcifications or enlargement (Table 50-16).

Collaborative Care

Treatment of adrenocortical insufficiency is focused on management of the underlying cause when possible. The mainstay of treatment for adrenocortical insufficiency is replacement therapy (see Table 50-16). Hydrocortisone, the most commonly used form of replacement therapy, has both glucocorticoid and mineralocorticoid properties. During situations associated with physiologic stress, glucocorticoid dosage must be increased to prevent addisonian crisis. Mineralocorticoid replacement with fludrocortisone acetate (Florinef) is administered daily with increased salt in the diet.

Addisonian crisis is a life-threatening emergency requiring aggressive management. Treatment must be directed toward shock management and high-dose hydrocortisone replacement. Large

TABLE 50-16	*COLLABORATIVE CARE* Addison's Disease

Diagnostic
History and physical examination
Plasma cortisol levels
Serum electrolytes
ACTH-stimulation test
CT scan, MRI

Collaborative Therapy
Daily glucocorticoid (e.g., hydrocortisone) replacement (two thirds on awakening in morning, one third in late afternoon)*
Daily mineralocorticoid in morning*
Salt additives for excess heat or humidity
Increased doses of cortisol for stress situations (e.g., surgery, hospitalization)

ACTH, Adrenocorticotropic hormone; *CT*, computed tomography; *MRI*, magnetic resonance imaging.
*For conditions of normal daily stress in individuals with usual daytime activity.

TABLE 50-17	*PATIENT AND FAMILY TEACHING GUIDE* Addison's Disease

The following should be included in a teaching plan for the patient and family:
1. Names, dosages, and actions of drugs
2. Symptoms of overdosage and underdosage
3. Conditions requiring increased medication (e.g., trauma, infection, surgery, emotional crisis)
4. Course of action to take relative to changes in medication
   - Increase in dose of corticosteroid
   - Administration of large dose of corticosteroid intramuscularly, including demonstration and return demonstration
   - Consultation with health care provider
5. Prevention of infection and need for prompt and vigorous treatment of existing infections
6. Need for lifelong replacement therapy
7. Need for lifelong medical supervision
8. Need for medical identification device

volumes of 0.9% saline solution and 5% dextrose are administered to reverse hypotension and electrolyte imbalances until BP returns to normal.

NURSING MANAGEMENT
ADDISON'S DISEASE

■ *Nursing Implementation*

Acute Intervention. When the patient with Addison's disease is hospitalized, whether for diagnosis, an acute crisis, or some other health problem, frequent nursing assessment is necessary. Vital signs and signs of fluid volume deficit and electrolyte imbalance should be assessed every 30 minutes to 4 hours for the first 24 hours depending on the patient's instability. In addition, daily weights, diligent corticosteroid administration, protection against exposure to infection, and complete assistance with daily hygiene should be practiced. The patient should be protected from noise, light, and environmental temperature extremes. The patient cannot cope with these stresses because of the inability to produce corticosteroids.

If the hospitalization was due to adrenal crisis, the patient usually responds by the second day and can start oral corticosteroid replacement. Because discharge frequently occurs before the maintenance dose of corticosteroids is reached, the patient should be instructed on the importance of keeping scheduled follow-up appointments.

Ambulatory and Home Care. The nurse has an important role in the long-term management of Addison's disease. The serious nature of the disease and the need for lifelong replacement therapy necessitate a well-organized and carefully presented teaching plan. Table 50-17 outlines the major areas that must be included in the teaching plan.

Glucocorticoids are usually given in divided doses, two thirds in the morning and one third in the afternoon. Mineralocorticoids are given once daily, preferably in the morning. This dosage schedule reflects normal circadian rhythm in endogenous hormone secretion and decreases the side effects associated with corticosteroid replacement therapy. Because the aim of replacement therapy is to return to normal hormone levels, nursing care is focused on helping the patient maintain hormone balance while managing the medication regimen.

Because the patient with Addison's disease is unable to tolerate physical or emotional stress without additional exogenous corticosteroids, long-term care revolves around recognizing the need for extra medication and techniques for stress management. The need for corticosteroid hormone is proportional to stress levels. Examples of situations requiring corticosteroid adjustment are fever, influenza, extraction of teeth, and rigorous physical activity, such as playing tennis on a hot day or running a marathon. Doses of glucocorticoids are usually doubled when minor stress occurs (e.g., a respiratory infection, dental work) and tripled when major stress occurs (e.g., divorce, loss of parent). When in doubt, it is better to err on the side of overreplacement. If vomiting or diarrhea occurs, as may happen with influenza, the health care provider must be notified immediately because electrolyte replacement may be necessary. In addition, these manifestations may be early indicators of crisis. Overall, patients who take their medications consistently can anticipate a normal life expectancy.

Patients must be taught the signs and symptoms of corticosteroid deficiency and excess (Cushing syndrome) and to report these signs to their health care provider so the dose can be adjusted to each patient's need. It is critical that the patient wear an identification bracelet (Medic Alert) and carry a wallet card stating the patient has Addison's disease so that appropriate therapy can be initiated in case of an unexpected stressful event. The patient should be instructed about and given handouts related to other medications that can cause a need to increase glucocorticoid dosage (e.g., phenytoin [Dilantin], barbiturates, rifampin [Rifadin], and antacids). In addition, estrogen inhibits steroid metabolism. Patients using mineralocorticoid therapy (Florinef) should be instructed how to take their BP, instructed to increase salt intake, and given parameters to report to their health care provider. Changes may indicate a need for dosage adjustment.

The patient should carry an emergency kit at all times. The kit should consist of 100 mg of IM hydrocortisone, syringes, and instructions for use. The patient and significant others should be instructed in how to give an IM injection in case the replacement therapy cannot be taken orally. The patient should verbalize instructions, practice IM injections with saline, and have written instructions as to when to alter the dose.[29]

CORTICOSTEROID THERAPY

Cortisol and related glucocorticoids are used to relieve the signs and symptoms associated with many diseases (Table 50-18). The long-term administration of corticosteroids in therapeutic doses often leads to serious complications and side effects (Table 50-19).

Endocrine System

TABLE 50-18	*DRUG THERAPY* Diseases and Disorders Treated with Corticosteroids

Hormone Replacement
Adrenal insufficiency
Congenital adrenal hyperplasia

Therapeutic Effect
Allergic Reactions
- Anaphylaxis
- Bee stings
- Contact dermatitis
- Drug reactions
- Serum sickness
- Urticaria

Collagen Diseases
- Giant cell arteritis
- Mixed connective tissue disorders
- Polymyositis
- Polyarteritis nodosa
- Rheumatoid arthritis
- Systemic lupus erythematosus

Inflammation

Gastrointestinal Diseases
- Inflammatory bowel disease
- Celiac disease

Endocrine Diseases
- Hypercalcemia
- Hashimoto's thyroiditis
- Thyroid storm

Immunosuppression (after Organ Transplantation)

Liver Diseases
- Alcoholic hepatitis
- Autoimmune hepatitis

Nephrotic Syndrome

Neurologic Disease
- Prevention of cerebral edema and increased intracranial pressure
- Head trauma

Pulmonary Diseases
- Aspiration pneumonia
- Asthma
- Chronic obstructive pulmonary disease

Skin Diseases

Malignancies, Leukemia, Lymphoma

TABLE 50-19	*DRUG THERAPY* Side Effects of Corticosteroids

- Hypokalemia may develop.
- Predisposition to peptic ulcer disease.
- Skeletal muscle atrophy and weakness occurs.
- Mood and behavior changes may be observed.
- Glucose intolerance predisposes to diabetes mellitus.
- Fat from extremities is redistributed to trunk and face.
- Hypocalcemia related to anti–vitamin D effect may occur.
- Healing is delayed. At increased risk for wound dehiscence.
- Susceptibility to infection is increased. Infection develops more rapidly and spreads more widely.
- Suppression of pituitary ACTH synthesis occurs. Corticosteroid deficiency is likely if hormones are withdrawn abruptly. Taper corticosteroid doses.
- Increased blood pressure occurs because of excess blood volume and potentiation of vasoconstrictor effects. Hypertension predisposes to heart failure.
- Protein depletion decreases bone formation, density, and strength. Predisposes to pathologic fractures, especially compression fractures of the vertebrae (osteoporosis).

ACTH, Adrenocorticotropic hormone.

For this reason, corticosteroid therapy is not recommended for minor chronic conditions. Therapy should be reserved for diseases in which there is a risk of death or permanent loss of function, and conditions in which short-term therapy is likely to produce remission or recovery. The potential benefits of treatment must always be weighed against the risks.

Effects of Corticosteroid Therapy

There are multiple effects of corticosteroid therapy. Although these actions can prove to be beneficial and therapeutic in some situations, they can also contribute to adverse effects as well. The expected effects of corticosteroid therapy include the following:

1. *Antiinflammatory action.* Corticosteroids decrease the number of circulating lymphocytes, monocytes, and eosinophils. They enhance the release of polymorphonuclear leukocytes from bone marrow, inhibit the accumulation of leukocytes at the site of inflammation, and inhibit the release of substances involved in the inflammatory response (e.g., kinins, prostaglandins, histamine) from the leukocytes. As a result,

manifestations of inflammation, including redness, tenderness, heat, swelling, and local edema, are suppressed.

2. *Immunosuppression.* Corticosteroids cause atrophy of lymphoid tissue, suppress the cell-mediated immune responses, and decrease the production of antibodies.

3. *Maintenance of normal BP.* Corticosteroids potentiate the vasoconstrictor effect of norepinephrine and act on the renal tubules to increase sodium reabsorption and enhance potassium and hydrogen excretion. Retention of sodium (and subsequently water) increases blood volume and helps maintain BP. Mineralocorticoids have a direct effect on sodium reabsorption in the distal tubule of the kidney and as a result increase sodium and water retention.

4. *Carbohydrate and protein metabolism.* Corticosteroids antagonize the effects of insulin and can induce glucose intolerance by increasing hepatic glycogenolysis and insulin resistance. They also stimulate the breakdown of protein for gluconeogenesis, which can lead to skeletal muscle wasting. Although corticosteroids mobilize free fatty acids and redistribute fat in cushingoid patterns, the mechanism for this process is unknown.

Complications Associated with Corticosteroid Therapy

A beneficial effect in one situation may be a harmful one in another. For example, the vasopressive effect of the hormone is critical in enabling the organism to function in stressful situations but can produce hypertension when used for drug therapy. Suppression of inflammation and the immune response may help save the lives of the victim of anaphylaxis and the transplant recipient, but it causes reactivation of latent tuberculosis and greatly reduces resistance to other infections and cancers. In addition, corticosteroids inhibit the antibody response to vaccines. Specific side effects related to corticosteroid therapy are listed in Table 50-19.

 Drug Alert - *Corticosteroids*
- *Instruct patient not to discontinue abruptly.*
- *Monitor for signs of infection.*
- *Instruct diabetics to closely monitor blood glucose.*

TABLE 50-20	*PATIENT AND FAMILY TEACHING GUIDE* **Corticosteroid Therapy**

The nurse needs to teach the patient and family the following:

1. Plan a diet high in protein, calcium (at least 1500 mg/day), and potassium but low in fat and concentrated simple carbohydrates such as sugar, honey, syrups, and candy.
2. Identify measures to ensure adequate rest and sleep, such as daily naps and avoidance of caffeine late in the day.
3. Develop and maintain an exercise program to help maintain bone integrity.
4. Recognize edema and ways to restrict sodium intake to less than 2000 mg/day if edema occurs.
5. Monitor glucose levels and recognize symptoms and signs of hyperglycemia (e.g., polydipsia, polyuria, blurred vision) and glycosuria (glucose in the urine). The patient should be instructed to report hyperglycemic symptoms or capillary glucose levels greater than 120 mg/dl (10 mmol/L) or urine positive for glucose.
6. Notify health care provider if experiencing postprandial heartburn or epigastric pain that is not relieved by antacids.
7. See an eye specialist yearly to assess development of possible cataracts.
8. Use safety measures such as getting up slowly from bed or a chair and use good lighting to avoid accidental injury.
9. Maintain good hygiene practices and avoid contact with persons with colds or other contagious illnesses to avoid infection.
10. Inform all health care providers about long-term corticosteroid use.
11. May need increased doses of corticosteroids in times of physical and emotional stress.
12. Never abruptly stop the corticosteroids because this could lead to addisonian crisis and possible death.

NURSING *and* COLLABORATIVE MANAGEMENT
CORTICOSTEROID THERAPY

Many patients receive corticosteroid therapy, in particular glucocorticoid therapy, for nonendocrine reasons (see Table 50-18). Thorough instruction is necessary to ensure patient compliance. When corticosteroids are used as nonreplacement therapies, they are taken once daily or once every other day. They should be taken early in the morning with food to decrease gastric irritation. Because exogenous corticosteroid administration may suppress endogenous ACTH and therefore endogenous cortisol (suppression is time and dose dependent), the danger of abrupt cessation of corticosteroid therapy must be emphasized to patients and significant others. Steroids taken for longer than 1 week will suppress adrenal production, and oral steroids should be tapered. Nurses must ensure that increased doses of steroid are prescribed in acute care or home care situations with increased physical or emotional stress.

Because patients often receive corticosteroid treatment for prolonged periods of time (greater than 3 months), corticosteroid-induced osteoporosis is an important concern.[30] Therapies to reduce the resorption of bone may include increased calcium intake, vitamin D supplementation, bisphosphonates (e.g., alendronate [Fosamax]), and institution of a low-impact exercise program. Further instruction and interventions to minimize the side effects and complications of corticosteroid therapy are shown in Table 50-20.

HYPERALDOSTERONISM
Etiology and Pathophysiology

Hyperaldosteronism is characterized by excessive aldosterone secretion. The main effects of aldosterone are sodium retention and potassium and hydrogen ion excretion. Thus the hallmark of this disease is hypertension with hypokalemic alkalosis. *Primary hyperaldosteronism* (PA) is most commonly caused by a small solitary adrenocortical adenoma. Occasionally multiple lesions are involved and are associated with bilateral adrenal hyperplasia. PA affects both genders equally and occurs most frequently between 30 and 50 years of age. It is estimated that approximately 1% of cases of hypertension are caused by PA. *Secondary hyperaldosteronism* occurs in response to a nonadrenal cause of elevated aldosterone levels such as renal artery stenosis, renin-secreting tumors, and chronic kidney disease.

Clinical Manifestations

Elevated levels of aldosterone are associated with sodium retention and elimination of potassium. Sodium retention leads to hypernatremia, hypertension, and headache. Edema does not usually occur because the rate of sodium excretion increases, which prevents more severe sodium retention. The potassium wasting leads to hypokalemia, which causes generalized muscle weakness, fatigue, cardiac dysrhythmias, glucose intolerance, and metabolic alkalosis that may lead to tetany.

Diagnostic Studies

The diagnosis of hyperaldosteronism should be suspected in all hypertensive patients with hypokalemia who are not being treated with diuretics. PA is associated with elevated plasma aldosterone levels, elevated sodium levels, decreased serum potassium levels, and decreased plasma renin activity. Adenomas are localized by means of a CT scan or MRI. If a tumor is not found, plasma 18-hydroxycorticosterone is measured after overnight bed rest. A level >50 ng/dl indicates an adenoma.

NURSING *and* COLLABORATIVE MANAGEMENT
PRIMARY HYPERALDOSTERONISM

The preferred treatment for PA is surgical removal of the adenoma (adrenalectomy). Although this surgery can be done as an open procedure, laparoscopic adrenalectomy is increasingly performed because of the benefits this minimally invasive surgery offers.[31] Before surgery, patients should be treated with a low-sodium diet, potassium-sparing diuretics (spironolactone [Aldactone], eplerenone [Inspra]), and antihypertensive agents to normalize serum potassium levels and BP. Spironolactone and eplerenone block the binding of aldosterone to the mineralocorticoid receptor in the terminal distal tubules and collecting ducts of the kidney, thus increasing the excretion of sodium and water and retention of potassium. Oral potassium supplements and sodium restrictions are also necessary. Potassium supplementation and a potassium-sparing diuretic should not be started simultaneously because of the danger of hyperkalemia.

Patients with bilateral adrenal hyperplasia are treated with spironolactone; amiloride (Midamor), which is another potassium-sparing diuretic; or aminoglutethimide (Cytadren), which blocks aldosterone synthesis. Calcium channel blockers may also be used to control BP. Dexamethasone may also be used to decrease the hyperplasia. A new drug that is available for the treatment of hyperaldosteronism is eplerenone (Inspra). Eplerenone is the first agent of a new class of drugs known as selective aldosterone receptor antagonists.

Nursing care includes careful assessment for signs of fluid and electrolyte balance (especially potassium) and cardiovascular status.

BP should be monitored frequently before and after surgery because unilateral adrenalectomy is successful in controlling hypertension in only 80% of patients with adenoma. Patients receiving maintenance therapy with spironolactone or amiloride need instruction about the possible side effects of gynecomastia, impotence, and menstrual disorders, as well as knowledge about the signs and symptoms of hypokalemia and hyperkalemia. Patients should be taught how to monitor their own BP and the need for frequent monitoring. The need for continued health supervision should be stressed.

Disorders of the Adrenal Medulla

PHEOCHROMOCYTOMA

Etiology and Pathophysiology

Pheochromocytoma is a rare condition characterized by a tumor of the adrenal medulla that produces excessive catecholamines (epinephrine, norepinephrine). Pheochromocytoma can occur at any age and in either gender, but it is found most commonly in young to middle-aged adults. In most cases affecting adults, the tumor is benign, encapsulated, unilateral, and solitary. Occasionally, bilateral tumors are found. The secretion of excessive catecholamines results in severe hypertension. If undiagnosed and untreated, pheochromocytoma may lead to diabetes mellitus, cardiomyopathy, and death.

Clinical Manifestations

The most striking clinical features of pheochromocytoma include severe, episodic hypertension accompanied by the classic manifestations of severe, pounding headache, tachycardia with palpitations, profuse sweating, and unexplained abdominal or chest pain. Attacks of episodic hypertension are due to sympathetic nervous system stimulation and are often accompanied by anxiety. Attacks may be provoked by many medications, including antihypertensives, opioids, radiologic contrast media, and tricyclic antidepressants. The duration of the attacks may vary from a few minutes to several hours.

Diagnostic Studies

Although pheochromocytoma is associated with a number of symptoms, the diagnosis is often missed. Pheochromocytoma is an uncommon cause of hypertension, accounting for only 0.1% of all cases of hypertension. This condition should be considered in patients who do not respond to traditional hypertensive treatments.

The measurement of urinary fractionated metanephrines (catecholamine metabolites), as well as fractionated catecholamines and creatinine, usually done as a 24-hour urine collection, is the simplest and most reliable test. Values are elevated in at least 95% of persons with pheochromocytoma.[32] A less sensitive test that measures vanillylmandelic acid (VMA) may also be done using a 24-hour urine sample. Plasma catecholamines are also elevated. It is preferable to measure serum catecholamines during an "attack." CT scans and MRI are used for tumor localization.

NURSING *and* COLLABORATIVE MANAGEMENT
PHEOCHROMOCYTOMA

The primary treatment consists of surgical removal of the tumor. Preoperatively, calcium channel blockers such as nicardipine (Cardene) are used to control BP and other excess catecholamine symptoms. Sympathetic blocking agents such as phenoxybenzamine (Dibenzyline) and prazosin (Minipress) may be administered to reduce BP and alleviate other symptoms of catecholamine excess along with the calcium channel blockers. Sympathetic blocking agents may result in orthostatic hypotension. The patient must be advised to make postural changes cautiously. β blockers are also used (e.g., propranolol [Inderal]) to decrease tachycardia and other dysrhythmias.

Surgery is more commonly done via laparoscopic adrenalectomy than via open abdominal incision. Complete removal of the adrenal tumor cures the hypertension in the majority of individuals, but hypertension persists in approximately 10% to 30% of patients. For these individuals, BP management involves standard antihypertensive drug therapy. If surgery is not an option, metyrosine is used to diminish catecholamine production by the tumor and simplify chronic management.

Case finding is an important nursing function. Any patient with hypertension accompanied by symptoms of sympathoadrenal discharge should be referred to a health care provider for definitive diagnosis. An important part of the nursing assessment is observation of the patient for the classic triad of symptoms of pheochromocytoma (severe pounding headache, tachycardia, and profuse sweating). BP should be monitored immediately if the patient is experiencing an "attack." The nurse should be prepared to check BP when any of the drugs that might precipitate an attack are given.

The nurse should attempt to make the patient with pheochromocytoma as comfortable as possible. All diagnostic samples should be collected appropriately. Capillary blood glucose levels should be monitored to assess for diabetes mellitus. Patients need rest, nourishing food, and emotional support during this period.

Preoperative and postoperative care is similar to that for any patient undergoing adrenalectomy except that BP fluctuations from catecholamine excesses tend to be severe and must be carefully monitored. Because hypertension may persist even when the tumor is removed, the nurse should stress the importance of follow-up care and routine BP monitoring. If metyrosine is being used, the patient should be instructed to rise slowly and hold onto a secure object, because this medication can cause orthostatic hypotension.

CRITICAL THINKING EXERCISE

CASE STUDY

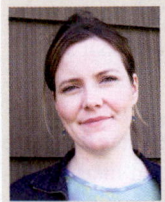

*Case Study photo
©iStockphoto.com/
Lanica Klein.*

Graves' Disease

Patient Profile. Elizabeth Minton, a 43-year-old white woman, was admitted to the hospital with a high fever. Following an endocrine workup, she was diagnosed as having Graves' disease.

Subjective Data
• Reports recent job loss because of inability to cope with job stress
• Reports symptoms including fatigue, unintentional weight loss, insomnia, palpitations, and heat intolerance

Objective Data
Physical Examination
• Has a fever of 104° F (40° C)
• Has BP of 150/78, pulse of 118, and respiratory rate of 24
• Has hot, moist skin
• Has fine tremors of the hands
• Has 4+ deep tendon reflexes and muscle strength of 1 to 2

Collaborative Care
- Subtotal thyroidectomy planned for 2 months later
- Started on propylthiouracil (PTU) and propranolol (Inderal)

Critical Thinking Questions

1. What is the etiology of Elizabeth's symptoms?
2. What diagnostic studies were probably ordered? What would the results have been to establish the diagnosis of Graves' disease?
3. Why was surgery delayed?
4. What is the purpose of drug therapy for Elizabeth?
5. What are the patient's immediate learning needs and her learning needs preoperatively and postoperatively? What teaching strategies would the nurse use if Elizabeth could not read?
6. What are the nursing interventions for successful long-term management of this patient after the subtotal thyroidectomy? How would nursing interventions change if Elizabeth was 70 years old?
7. Based on the assessment data presented, write one or more appropriate nursing diagnoses pertinent to this patient while hospitalized. Are there any collaborative problems?

NCLEX EXAMINATION REVIEW QUESTIONS

The number of the question corresponds to the same-numbered objective at the beginning of the chapter.

1. Following a hypophysectomy for acromegaly, postoperative nursing care should focus on
   a. frequent monitoring of serum and urine osmolarity.
   b. parenteral administration of a GH-receptor antagonist.
   c. keeping the patient in a recumbent position at all times.
   d. patient education regarding the need for lifelong ACTH, TSH, FSH, and LH hormone replacement.
2. A patient with a head injury develops SIADH. Symptoms the nurse would expect to find include
   a. hypernatremia and edema.
   b. low urinary output and thirst.
   c. muscle spasticity and hypertension.
   d. weight gain and decreased glomerular filtration rate.
3. The health care provider prescribes levothyroxine for a patient with hypothyroidism. Following teaching regarding this medication, the nurse determines that further instruction is needed when the patient says,
   a. "I can expect the medication dose may need to be increased."
   b. "I can expect to return to normal function with the use of this drug."
   c. "I will only need to take this medication until my symptoms are improved."
   d. "I will report any chest pain or difficulty breathing to the doctor right away."
4. Following thyroid surgery, the nurse suspects damage or removal of the parathyroid glands when the patient develops
   a. muscle weakness and weight loss.
   b. hyperthermia and severe tachycardia.
   c. hypertension and difficulty swallowing.
   d. laryngeal stridor and tingling in the hands and feet.

5. An important nursing intervention when caring for a patient with Cushing syndrome is to
   a. restrict protein intake.
   b. observe for signs of hypotension.
   c. administer medication in equal doses.
   d. protect the patient from exposure to infection.
6. After an adrenalectomy for pheochromocytoma, the patient is most likely to experience
   a. hypokalemia.
   b. hyperglycemia.
   c. marked sodium and water retention.
   d. marked fluctuations in blood pressure.
7. To control the side effects of corticosteroid therapy, the nurse teaches the patient who is taking corticosteroids to
   a. increase calcium intake to 1500 mg/day.
   b. perform glucose monitoring for hypoglycemia.
   c. obtain immunizations due to high risk of infections.
   d. avoid abrupt position changes because of orthostatic hypotension.
8. The nurse teaches the patient that the best time to take corticosteroids for replacement purposes is
   a. once a day at bedtime.
   b. every other day on awakening.
   c. on arising and in the late afternoon.
   d. at consistent intervals every 6 to 8 hours.

REFERENCES

1. *Atlas of pathophysiology*, Philadelphia, 2006, Lippincott Williams & Wilkins.
2. AACE Acromegaly Guidelines Task Force: AACE Medical Guidelines for Clinical Practice for the diagnosis and treatment of acromegaly, *Endocr Prac* 10:213, 2004.
3. American Association for Clinical Chemistry: Growth hormone, in *Lab Tests Online*, 2005. Available at *www.labtestsonline.org* (accessed April 12, 2006).
4. Aron DC, Findling JW, Tyrrell JB: Hypothalamus and pituitary gland. In Greenspan FS, Gardner DG, editors: *Basic and clinical endocrinology*, New York, 2004, McGraw-Hill.
5. Cook M: Optimal treatment and patient care: nursing perspectives, 2005. Available at *www.acromegalyonline.com* (accessed April 13, 2006).
6. Karch AM: *Nursing drug guide*, Philadelphia, 2005, Lippincott Williams & Wilkins.
7. Johnson AL, Criddle LM: Pass the salt: indications for and implications of using hypertonic saline, *Crit Care Nurse* 24:36, 2005.
8. Held-Warmkessel J: Managing critical complications of cancer, *Nursing* 35:58, 2005.
9. Robinson A: Posterior pituitary—diabetes insipidus. In Goldman L, Ausiello D, editors: *Cecil textbook of medicine*, ed 22, St Louis, 2004, Saunders.
10. Jemal A, Siegel R, Ward E, et al: Cancer statistics, 2006, *CA Cancer J Clin* 56:106, 2006.
11. Neale D: Thyroid disease in pregnancy, *Obstet Gynecol Clin North Am* 31:893, 2004.
12. Greenspan FS: Thyroid diseases. In Greenspan FS, Gardner DG, editors: *Basic and clinical endocrinology*, New York, 2004, McGraw-Hill.
13. Stanley M, Blair KA, Beare PG: *Gerontological nursing: promoting successful aging with older adults*, Philadelphia, 2005, FA Davis.
14. Holcomb S: Detecting thyroid disease, *Nursing*. Available at *www.nursing2005.com* (accessed April 14, 2006).
15. Connery LE: Assessment and therapy of selected endocrine disorders, *Anesthesiol Clin North Am* 22:93, 2004.
16. Demers LM: Thyroid disease: pathophysiology and diagnosis, *Clin Lab Med* 24:19, 2004.
17. U.S. Preventive Services Task Force: Screening for thyroid disease: recommendation statement. Available at *www.ahrg.gov/clinic* (accessed April 19, 2006).
18. Clayton BD, Stock YN, Harroun R: *Basic pharmacology for nurses*, ed 14, St Louis, 2007, Mosby.

19. AACE/AAES Task Force on Primary Hyperparathyroidism: The American Association of Clinical Endocrinologists and the American Association of Endocrine Surgeons position statement on the diagnosis and management of primary hyperparathyroidism, *Endocr Prac* 11:49, 2005.

20. Manicor N: Primary hyperparathyroidism: a case study, *J Peri Anesth Nurs* 19:334, 2004.

21. Shaha A: Parathyroid re-exploration, *Otolaryngol Clin North Am* 37:833, 2004.

22. U.S. Food and Drug Administration Talk Paper: FDA approves first in a new class of drugs to treat hyperparathyroidism associated with renal failure and in patients with parathyroid cancer. Available at *www.fda.gov/bbs/topics* (accessed April 18, 2006).

23. Chew S, Leslie D: *Clinical endocrinology and diabetes,* London, 2006, Elsevier Churchill Livingstone.

24. Findling J, Raff H: Screening and diagnosis of Cushing's syndrome, *Endocrinol Metab Clin North Am* 34:385, 2005.

25. National Institute of Diabetes and Digestive and Kidney Diseases: Cushing's syndrome. Available at *www.niddk.nih.gov/health/endo/pubs/cushings* (accessed April 19, 2006).

26. Aron DC, Findling MD, Tyrrell JB: Glucocorticoids and adrenal androgens. In Greenspan FS, Gardner DG, editors: *Basic and clinical endocrinology,* New York, 2004, McGraw-Hill.

27. Torrey S: Recognition and management of adrenal emergencies, *Emerg Med Clin North Am* 23:687, 2005.

28. Lovas K, Husebye ES: Addison's disease, *Lancet* 365:2058, 2005.

29. National Institute of Diabetes and Digestive and Kidney Diseases: Addison's disease: adrenal insufficiency. Available at *www.niddk.nih.gov/health/endo/pubs/addison* (accessed April 19, 2006).

30. Rhen T, Cidlowski J: Antiinflammatory action of glucocorticoids—new mechanisms for old drugs, *N Engl J Med* 353:1711, 2005.

31. Ramacciato G, Paolo M, Pietromaria A, et al: Ten years of laparoscopic adrenalectomy: lesson learned from 104 procedures, *Am Surg* 71:321, 2005.

32. Vaughan ED: Diseases of the adrenal gland, *Med Clin North Am* 88:443, 2004.

RESOURCES

American Association of Clinical Endocrinologists (AACE)
904-353-7878
www.aace.com

American Society for Bone and Mineral Research
202-367-1161
www.asbmr.org

American Thyroid Association
703-998-8890
www.thyroid.org

Endocrine Nurses Society (ENS)
301-941-0249
www.endo-nurses.org

Endocrine Society
301-941-0200
www.endo-society.org

Pituitary Network Association
805-499-9973
www.pituitary.com

Thyroid Federation International
613-544-8364
www.thyroid-fed.org

For additional Internet resources, see the website for this book at *http://evolve.elsevier.com/Lewis/medsurg.*

Don't go where the path may lead, go instead where there is no path and leave a trail.

Ralph Waldo Emerson

Nursing Assessment
Reproductive System

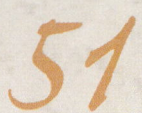

51

Shannon Ruff Dirksen

LEARNING OBJECTIVES

1. Describe the structures and functions of the male and female reproductive systems.
2. Explain the functions of the major hormones essential for the functioning of the male and female reproductive systems.
3. Describe the physiologic changes of a man and of a woman during the stages of sexual response.
4. Describe age-related changes in the male and female reproductive systems and differences in assessment findings.
5. Identify significant subjective and objective data related to the male and female reproductive systems and information about sexual function that should be obtained from a patient.
6. Describe noninvasive techniques used in the physical assessment of the male and female reproductive systems.
7. Differentiate normal from abnormal findings obtained from a physical assessment of the male and female reproductive systems.
8. Describe the purpose, significance of results, and nursing responsibilities related to diagnostic studies of the male and female reproductive systems.

KEY TERMS

amenorrhea, p. 1330
clitoris, p. 1327
ductus deferens, p. 1324
dyspareunia, p. 1334
epididymis, p. 1324
gonads, p. 1324
menarche, p. 1329
menopause, p. 1330
menstrual cycle, p. 1329
mons pubis, p. 1327
nulliparous, p. 1325
spermatogenesis, p. 1324

Electronic Resources

Supplemental content related to Chapter 51 can be found . . .

Companion CD
- Stress-Busting Kit for Nursing Students
- NCLEX Examination Review Questions
- Animations:
  - Lymphatic Drainage of the Breast
  - The Menstrual Cycle
- Video Clips:
  - Inspection and Palpation—Standing Position (Male)—1
  - Inspection and Palpation—Standing Position (Male)—2
  - Inspection: Female Breasts—Sitting Position
  - Inspection: External Genitalia (Female)
  - Inspection: Speculum Examination (Female)
  - Palpation: Bimanual Examination (Female)
  - Palpation: Female Breasts—Supine Position
  - Palpation: Inguinal Hernia Evaluation (Male)
- Comprehensive Glossary

Evolve Website **evolve**
http://evolve.elsevier.com/Lewis/medsurg
- Content Updates
- Key Points (Printable and CD/MP3 Download)
- Concept Map Creator
- Expanded Audio Glossary
- Key Term Flash Cards
- Physical Examination Video Clips:
  - Breasts
  - Breasts and Heart

- Abdominal Reflexes, Abdominal Muscles, and Inguinal Area
- Genitalia and Rectum (Female)
- Rectum and Prostate Gland (Male)
- Electronic Calculators
- WebLinks

Reviewed by Janice J. Hoffman, RN, PhD, Instructor, School of Nursing, Johns Hopkins University, Baltimore, Md.

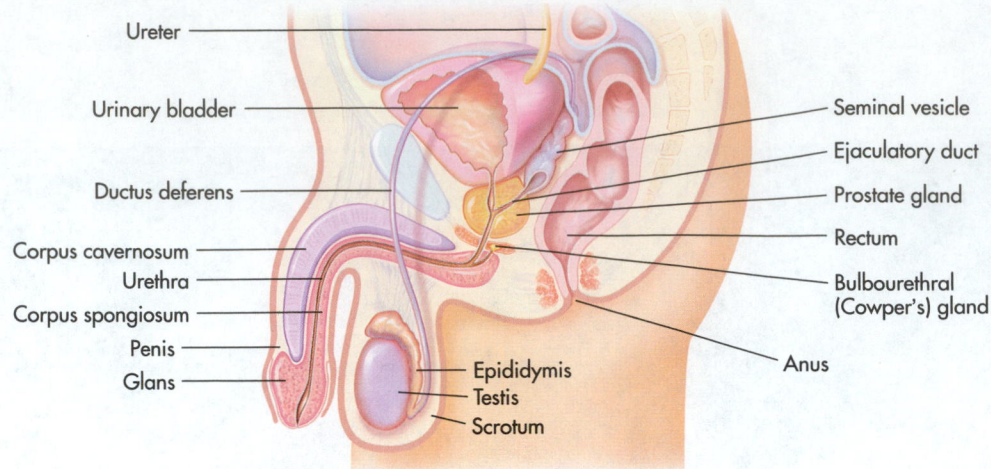

FIG. 51-1 External and internal male sex organs.

STRUCTURES AND FUNCTIONS OF THE MALE AND FEMALE REPRODUCTIVE SYSTEMS

The reproductive system of both males and females consists of primary (or essential) organs and secondary (or accessory) organs. The primary reproductive organs are referred to as **gonads.** The female gonads are the ovaries; the male gonads are the testes. The primary responsibility of the gonads is secretion of hormones and production of gametes (ova and sperm). Secondary or accessory organs are responsible for transporting and nourishing the ova and sperm, as well as preserving and protecting the fertilized eggs.

Male Reproductive System

The three primary roles of the male reproductive system are (1) production and transportation of sperm, (2) deposition of sperm in the female reproductive tract, and (3) secretion of hormones. The primary reproductive organs in the male are the testes. Secondary reproductive organs include ducts (epididymis, ductus deferens, ejaculatory duct, and urethra), sex glands (prostate gland, Cowper's glands, and seminal vesicles), and the external genitalia (scrotum and penis)[1] (Fig. 51-1).

Testes. The paired testes are ovoid, smooth, firm organs measuring 3.5 to 5.5 cm long and 2 to 3 cm wide. They are within the scrotum, which is a loose protective sac composed of a thin outer layer of skin over a tough connective tissue layer. Within the testes, coiled structures known as seminiferous tubules form *spermatozoa* (immature sperm). The process of sperm production is called **spermatogenesis.** Interstitial cells of the testes lie between the seminiferous tubules and produce the male sex hormone testosterone.

Ducts. Sperm formed in the seminiferous tubules move through a series of ducts. These ducts transport the sperm from the testes to the outside of the body. As sperm exit the testes they enter and pass through the epididymis, ductus deferens, ejaculatory duct, and urethra.

The **epididymis** is a comma-shaped structure located on the posterior-superior aspect of each testis within the scrotum (Figs. 51-1 and 51-2). It is a very long, tightly coiled structure that measures about 20 feet in length.[1] The epididymis transports the sperm as they mature. Sperm exit the epididymis through a long, thick tube known as the ductus deferens.

The **ductus deferens** (also known as the *vas deferens*) is continuous with the epididymis within the scrotal sac. It travels upward through the scrotum and continues through the inguinal ring

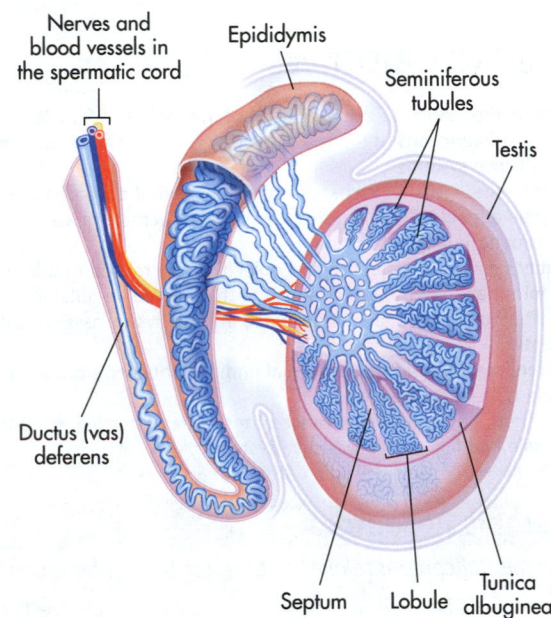

FIG. 51-2 Seminiferous tubules, testis, epididymis, and ductus (vas) deferens.

into the abdominal cavity. The spermatic cord is composed of a connective tissue sheath that encloses the ductus deferens, arteries, veins, nerves, and lymph vessels as it ascends up through the inguinal canal (see Fig. 51-2). In the abdominal cavity, the ductus deferens travels up, over, and behind the bladder. Posterior to the bladder the ductus deferens joins the seminal vesicle to form the ejaculatory duct (see Fig. 51-1).

The ejaculatory duct passes downward through the prostate gland, connecting with the urethra. The urethra extends from the bladder, through the prostate, and ends in a slitlike opening (the meatus) on the ventral side of the *glans,* the tip of the penis. During the process of ejaculation, sperm travels through the urethra and out of the penis.

Glands. The seminal vesicles, prostate gland, and Cowper's (bulbourethral) glands are the accessory glands of the male reproductive system. These glands produce and secrete seminal fluid (semen), which surrounds the sperm and forms the *ejaculate.*

The seminal vesicles lie posterior to the bladder and between the rectum and the bladder. The ducts of the seminal vesicles fuse with the ductus deferens to form the ejaculatory ducts that enter the prostate gland. The prostate gland lies beneath the bladder. Its posterior surface is in contact with the rectal wall. The prostate normally measures 2 cm wide and 3 cm long and is divided into the right and left lateral lobes and an anteroposterior median lobe. Cowper's glands lie on each side of the urethra and slightly posterior to it, just below the prostate. The ducts of these glands enter directly into the urethra.

The secretion from the seminal vesicles and prostate makes up most of the fluid in the ejaculate. By comparison, the seminal vesicles and Cowper's glands contribute a minimum amount of fluid to the ejaculate. These various secretions serve as a medium for the transport of sperm and create an alkaline, nutritious environment that promotes sperm motility and survival.

External Genitalia. The external genitalia consist of the penis and the scrotum. The penis consists of a shaft, and the tip is known as the glans. The glans is covered by a fold of skin, the prepuce (or foreskin), that forms at the junction of the glans and the shaft of the penis. In circumcised men the prepuce has been removed. The broadened segment of the glans at the junction is the corona. The shaft of the penis consists of erectile tissue composed of the corpus cavernosum, the corpus spongiosum, the fibrous sheath that encases the erectile tissue, and the urethra. The skin covering the penis is thin, loose, and essentially hairless.

Female Reproductive System

The three primary roles of the female reproductive system are (1) production of ova (eggs), (2) secretion of hormones, and (3) protection and facilitation of the development of the fetus in a pregnant female. Like the male, the female has primary and secondary reproductive organs. The primary reproductive organs in the female are the paired ovaries. Secondary reproductive organs include ducts (fallopian tubes), the uterus, the vagina, sex glands (Bartholin's glands and breasts), and the external genitalia (vulva).

Pelvic Organs

Ovaries. The ovaries are usually located on either side of the uterus, just behind and below the fallopian (uterine) tubes (Figs.

51-3 and 51-4). The ovaries are firm and solid, approximately 1.5 cm wide, and 3 cm long. Their functions include *ovulation,* as well as secretion of the two major reproductive hormones, estrogen and progesterone. The outer zone of the ovary contains follicles with germ cells, or *oocytes.* Each follicle contains a primordial (immature) oocyte surrounded by granulosa and theca cells. These two layers protect and nourish the oocyte until the follicle reaches maturity and ovulation occurs. However, not all follicles reach maturity. In a process termed *atresia,* most of the primordial follicles become smaller and are reabsorbed by the body; thus the number of follicles declines from 2 million to 4 million at birth to approximately 300,000 to 400,000 at menarche. This number continues to decrease throughout a woman's reproductive years. Fewer than 500 oocytes are actually released by ovulation during the reproductive years of the normal healthy woman.

Fallopian Tubes. Normally, each month during a woman's reproductive years, one ovarian follicle reaches maturity, and the ovum is ovulated, or expelled, from the ovary through the stimulus of the gonadotropic hormones, follicle-stimulating hormone (FSH) and luteinizing hormone (LH). The ovum then travels up a fallopian tube where fertilization by sperm may occur, if they are present. An ovum can be fertilized up to 72 hours after its release.

The distal ends of the fallopian tubes consist of fingerlike projections called *fimbriae* that "massage" the ovaries at ovulation to help extract the mature ovum. The tubes, which average 4.8 inches (12 cm) in length, extend from the fimbriae to the superior lateral borders of the uterus. Fertilization usually takes place within the outer one third of the fallopian tubes.

Uterus. The uterus is a pear-shaped, hollow, muscular organ (see Figs. 51-3 and 51-4). It is located between the bladder and the rectum. In the mature **nulliparous** (never pregnant) female, the uterus is approximately 6 to 8 cm long and 4 cm wide. The uterine walls consist of an outer serosal layer, the perimetrium; a middle muscular layer, the myometrium; and an inner mucosal layer, the endometrium.

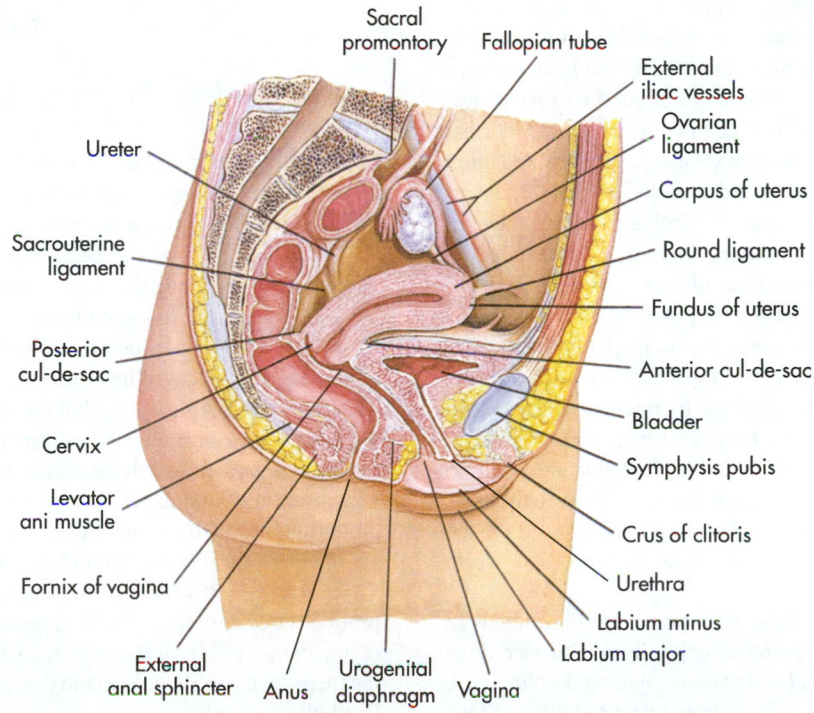

FIG. 51-3   Female reproductive tract and related organs.

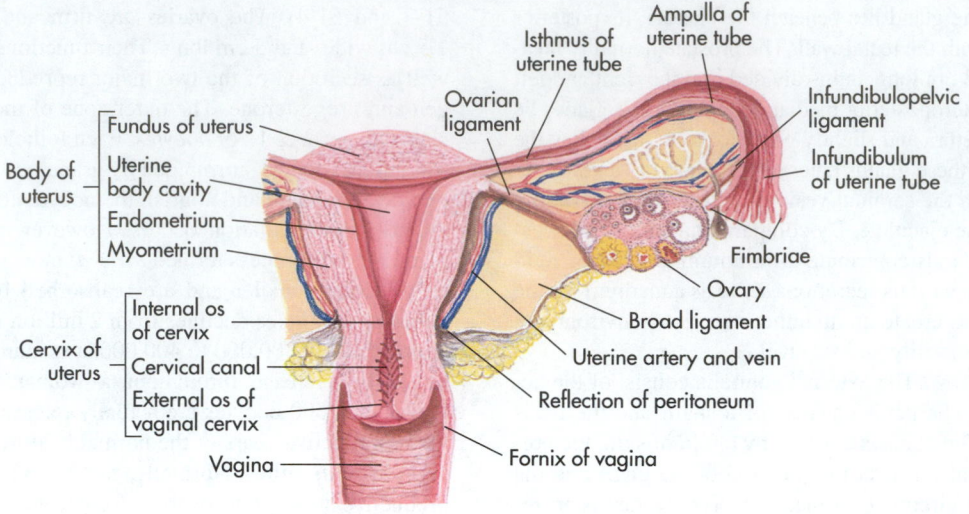

FIG. 51-4 Female reproductive tract: anterior view.

The uterus consists of the fundus, body (or corpus), and cervix (see Fig. 51-4). The body makes up about 80% of the uterus and connects with the cervix at the isthmus, or neck. The cervix is the lower portion of the uterus that projects into the anterior wall of the vaginal canal. It makes up about 15% to 20% of the uterus in the nulliparous female. The cervix consists of the *ectocervix*, the outer portion that protrudes into the vagina, and the *endocervix,* the canal in the opening of the cervix. The ectocervix is covered with squamous epithelial cells, which give it a smooth, pinkish appearance. The endocervix contains a lining of columnar epithelial cells, which give it a rough, reddened appearance. The junction at which the two types of epithelial cells meet is termed the *squamocolumnar junction* and contains the optimal types of cells needed for an accurate Papanicolaou (Pap) test to screen for malignancies.

The cervical canal is 2 to 4 cm long and is relatively tightly closed. The cervix, however, allows sperm to enter the uterus and also allows menses to be expelled. The columnar epithelium, under hormonal influence, provides elasticity at labor for the cervix to stretch to allow for the passage of a fetus during the birth process. The entrance of sperm into the uterus is facilitated by mucus produced by the cervix under the influence of estrogen. Under normal conditions, the cervical mucus becomes watery, stretchy, and more abundant at ovulation. This mucus, referred to as *spinnbarkeit,* is considered "fertile mucus" because it facilitates the passage of sperm into the uterus. The postovulatory cervical mucus, under the influence of progesterone, is thick and inhibits sperm passage.

The anterior and posterior peritoneal covering of the uterus is called the *broad ligament.* It separates the uterus from the bladder and the rectum but does not provide support for the uterus or the *adnexa* (ovaries and tubes). The cardinal ligaments, which extend from the isthmus of the uterus to the pelvic wall, also offer only minimal support. The round ligament, which extends anteriorly to the labia majora, provides some support but is easily weakened by pregnancy. The firmest support for the uterus is provided by the uterine sacral ligaments, which pull the uterus back and away from the vaginal orifice.

Vagina. The vagina is a tubular structure 3 to 4 inches (8 to 10 cm) long that is lined with squamous epithelium. The secretions of the vagina consist of cervical mucus, desquamated epithelium, and, during sexual stimulation, a direct transudate secretion. These

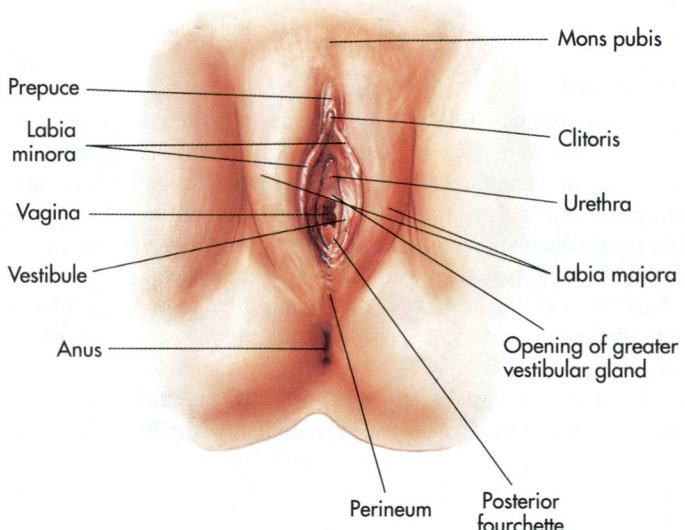

FIG. 51-5 External female genitalia.

fluids help protect against vaginal infection. The muscular and erectile tissue of the vaginal walls allows enough dilation and contraction to accommodate the passage of the fetus during labor, as well as penetration of the penis during intercourse. The anterior vaginal wall lies along the urethra and bladder. The posterior vaginal wall is adjacent to the rectum.

Pelvis. The female pelvis consists of four bones (two pelvic bones, sacrum, coccyx) held together by several strong ligaments. The sections of these bones that lie below the iliopectineal line are very important during birth and are often a factor determining the ability of a woman to deliver a child vaginally. Knowledge of these bones and the landmarks that they form in the pelvis allows the practitioner to estimate pelvic measurements and the potential for a woman's pelvis to accommodate the birth of a full-term fetus.

External Genitalia. The external portion of the female reproductive system (Fig. 51-5), commonly called the *vulva,* consists of the mons pubis, labia majora, labia minora, clitoris, urethral meatus, ducts of Skene's glands, vaginal introitus (opening), and Bartholin's glands.

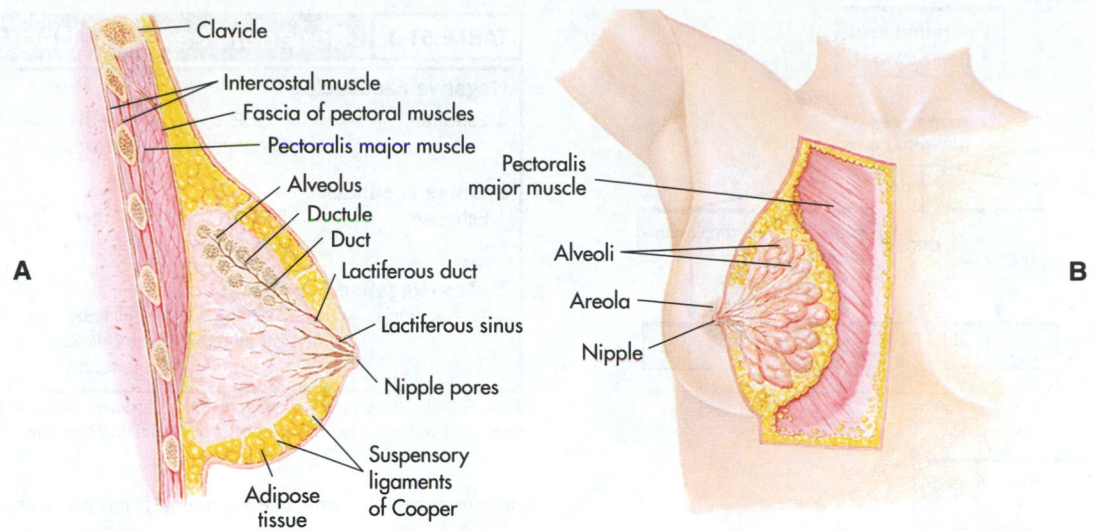

FIG. 51-6 The female breast. **A,** Sagittal section of a lactating breast. Notice how the glandular structures are anchored to the overlying skin and to the pectoral muscle by suspensory ligaments of Cooper. Each lobule of glandular tissue is drained by a lactiferous duct that eventually opens through the nipple. **B,** Anterior view of a lactating breast. In nonlactating breasts, the glandular tissue is much less prominent with adipose tissue comprising most of each breast.

The **mons pubis** is a fatty layer lying over the pubic bone. It contains coarse hair that lies in a triangular pattern. (The male hair pattern is diamond shaped.) The labia majora are folds of adipose tissue that form the outer borders of the vulva. These hair-covered folds contain sweat glands and sebaceous glands. The hairless labia minora form the borders of the vaginal orifice and extend anteriorly to enclose the clitoris.[2]

The *vestibule* is a boat-shaped fossa between the labia minora, extending from the clitoris at the anterior end to the vaginal opening at the posterior end. The perineum is the area between the vagina and the anus. The vaginal introitus is surrounded by thin membranous tissue called the *hymen*. In the adult woman, the hymen usually appears as folds or hymenal tags and separates the external genitalia from the vagina. Although all females have this structure, there is wide anatomic variation in its morphology. At the posterior aspect of the vagina, a tense band of mucous membrane connecting the posterior ends of the labia minora is referred to as the *posterior fourchette.*

The **clitoris** is erectile tissue that becomes engorged during sexual excitation. It lies anterior to the urethral meatus and the vaginal orifice and is usually covered by the prepuce, or hood.[2] Clitoral stimulation is an important part of sexual activity for many women.

Ducts of the Skene's glands lie alongside the urinary meatus and are thought to help lubricate the urinary meatus.[3] The Bartholin's glands, located at the posterior and lateral aspects of the vaginal orifice, secrete a thin, mucoid material believed to contribute slightly to lubrication during sexual intercourse. These glands are not usually palpable unless sebaceous-like cysts form or in the presence of an infection, such as a sexually transmitted disease (STD).

Breasts. The breasts are a secondary sex characteristic that develops during puberty in response to estrogen and progesterone. Cyclic hormonal changes lead to regular changes in breast tissue to prepare it for lactation when fertilization and pregnancy occur. The breasts are also considered a major organ of sexual stimulation.

The breasts extend from the second to the sixth ribs, with the tail reaching the axilla (Fig. 51-6). The fully mature breast is dome

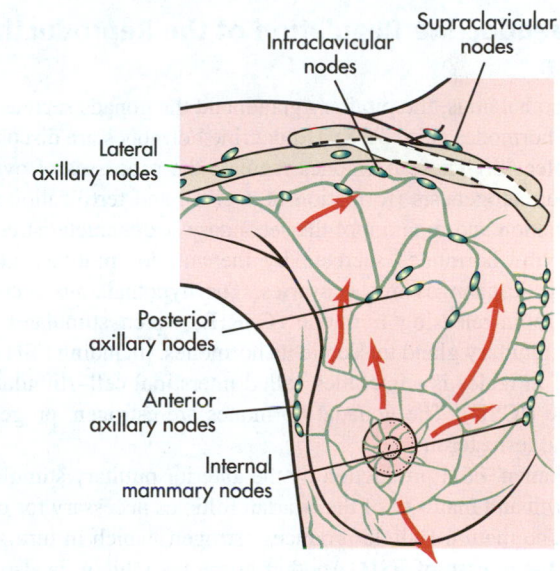

FIG. 51-7 Lymphatic drainage of the breast. *Arrows* indicate direction of drainage.

shaped and contains a pigmented center termed the *areola*. The areolar region contains Montgomery's tubercles, which are similar to sebaceous glands and assist in lubricating the nipple. During lactation, the alveoli, or acini, secrete milk. The milk then flows into a ductal system and is transported to the lactiferous sinuses. The nipple contains 15 to 20 tiny openings through which the milk flows during breastfeeding. The fibrous and fatty tissue that supports and separates the channels of the mammary duct system is primarily responsible for the varying sizes and shapes of the breasts in different individuals.

The breast's rich lymphatic network drains primarily into the axillary, infraclavicular, and supraclavicular channels (Fig. 51-7). Superficial lymph nodes are located in the axilla and are accessible to examination. This system is often responsible for the metastasis of a malignant tumor from the breast to other parts of the body.

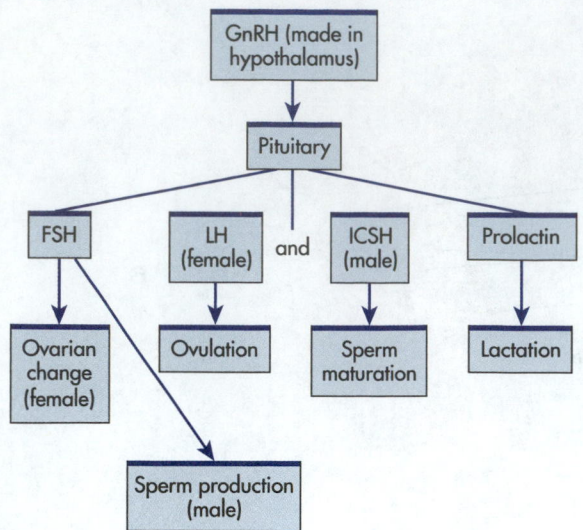

FIG. 51-8   Hypothalamic-pituitary-gonadal axis. Only the major pituitary hormone actions are depicted. *FSH,* Follicle-stimulating hormone; *GnRH,* gonadotropin-releasing hormone; *ICSH,* interstitial cell–stimulating hormone; *LH,* luteinizing hormone.

Neuroendocrine Regulation of the Reproductive System

The hypothalamus, the pituitary gland, and the gonads secrete numerous hormones (Fig. 51-8). (Endocrine hormones are discussed in Chapter 48.) These hormones regulate the processes of ovulation, spermatogenesis (formation of sperm), and fertilization and the formation and function of the secondary sex characteristics. In women, the hormones secreted by the anterior pituitary gland cause cyclic changes in the ovaries. The hypothalamus secretes gonadotropin-releasing hormone (GnRH), which stimulates the anterior pituitary gland to secrete its hormones, including FSH and LH. LH in males is sometimes called interstitial cell–stimulating hormone (ICSH). The gonadal hormones are estrogen, progesterone, and testosterone.

In women, FSH production by the anterior pituitary stimulates the growth and maturity of the ovarian follicles necessary for ovulation. The mature follicle produces estrogen, which in turn suppresses the release of FSH. Another hormone, inhibin, is also secreted by the ovarian follicle and inhibits both GnRH and FSH secretion. In men, FSH stimulates the seminiferous tubules to produce sperm.

LH contributes to the ovulatory process because it causes follicles to complete maturation and undergo ovulation. It also causes the development of a ruptured follicle, or the area on the ovum where the ovum exited during ovulation. The ruptured follicle develops into a corpus luteum from which progesterone is secreted. Progesterone maintains the rich vascular state of the uterus (secretory phase) in preparation for fertilization and implantation. In men, LH or ICSH is responsible for the production of testosterone by the interstitial cells of the testes and thus is essential for the full maturation of sperm. Prolactin has no known function in men. In women, prolactin stimulates the development and growth of the mammary glands. During lactation, it initiates and maintains milk production.

The gonadal hormones, estrogen and progesterone, are produced by the ovaries in women. Small amounts of an estrogen

TABLE 51-1   Gonadal Feedback Mechanisms

Negative Feedback

↓ Estrogen → ↑ GnRH (hypothalamus) → ↑ FSH (pituitary) → ↑ Estrogen (ovaries)

Positive Feedback

↑ Estrogen → ↑ GnRH (hypothalamus) → ↑ LH (pituitary)

Testes (Negative Feedback)

↓ Testosterone → ↑ GnRH (hypothalamus) → ↑ FSH and ICSH (pituitary) → ↑ Testosterone (testes)

FSH, Follicle-stimulating hormone; *GnRH,* gonadotropin-releasing hormone; *ICSH,* interstitial cell–stimulating hormone; *LH,* luteinizing hormone.

precursor are also produced in the adrenal cortices. Estrogen is essential to the development and maintenance of the secondary sex characteristics, the proliferative phase of the menstrual cycle immediately after menstruation, and the uterine changes essential to pregnancy. The role and importance of estrogen in men are not well understood. In men, estrogen is produced predominantly in the adrenal cortex.

Progesterone plays a major role in the menstrual cycle but most specifically in the secretory phase. Like estrogen, progesterone is involved in the bodily changes associated with pregnancy. Adequate progesterone is necessary to maintain an implanted egg.

The major gonadal hormone of men, testosterone, is produced by the testes. Testosterone is responsible for the development and maintenance of secondary sex characteristics, as well as for adequate spermatogenesis. Androgens are produced in females by the adrenal glands and ovaries in small amounts.

The circulating levels of gonadal hormones are controlled primarily by a negative feedback process. Receptors within the hypothalamus and pituitary are sensitive to the circulating blood levels of the hormones (Table 51-1). Increased levels of hormones stimulate a hypothalamic response to decrease the high circulating levels. Likewise, low circulating levels provoke a hypothalamic response that increases the low circulating levels. For example, if the circulating level of testosterone in men is low, the hypothalamus is stimulated to secrete GnRH. This stimulates the anterior pituitary to secrete greater amounts of FSH and ICSH, which in turn causes an increase in the production of testosterone. The high levels of testosterone then stimulate a decrease in the production of GnRH and thus of FSH and ICSH.

In women, however, there is a slight variation. The circulating levels are controlled through a combination of both a negative and a positive feedback system. A negative feedback control mechanism exists similar to that described previously. When circulating estrogen levels are low, the hypothalamus is stimulated to increase its production of GnRH. GnRH stimulates the pituitary to secrete greater amounts of FSH and LH, resulting in higher levels of estrogen production by the ovaries. Reciprocally higher levels of circulating estrogen result in a decreasing secretion of GnRH and thus a decrease in the secretion of FSH by the pituitary.

There is also a positive feedback control mechanism in women. Thus with increasing levels of circulating estrogen, a greater level of GnRH is produced, resulting in an increased level of LH from

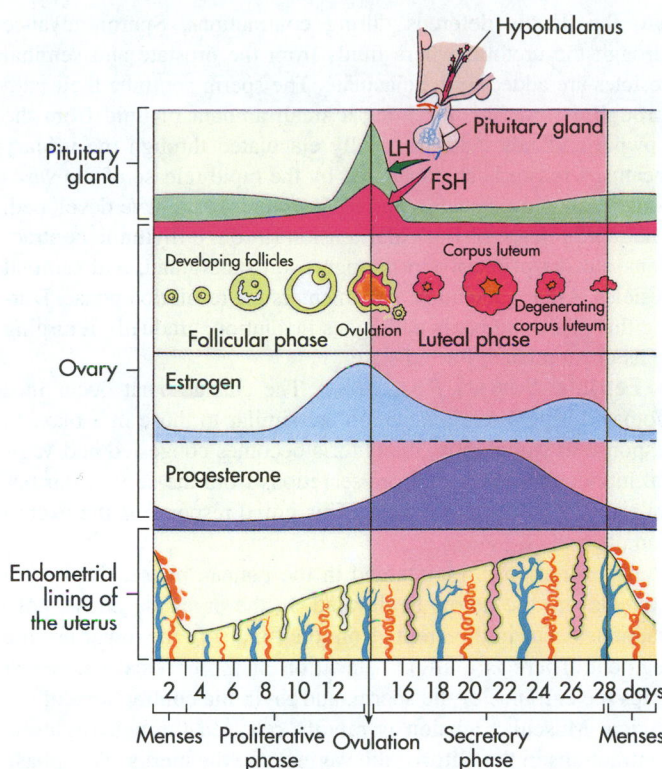

FIG. 51-9 Events of the menstrual cycle. The various lines depict the changes in blood hormone levels, the development of the follicles, and the changes in the endometrium during the cycle. *FSH,* Follicle-stimulating hormone; *LH,* luteinizing hormone.

the pituitary. Likewise, lowered levels of estrogen result in a lowered level of LH.

Menarche

Menarche is the first episode of menstrual bleeding, indicating that a female has reached puberty. Although normal onset can be as early as 10 years of age in some individuals, menarche usually occurs at approximately 12 to 13 years of age.[4] As puberty approaches, there are changes associated with the elevated rate of estrogen and progesterone secretion by the ovaries. These changes include the development of breast buds and pubic hair, and later the development of axillary hair. During this time, there is a decrease in the sensitivity of the hypothalamic-pituitary axis that allows for increased secretion of FSH and LH and a resultant increase in estrogen. It is during this time that the adult pattern of gonadotropin secretion occurs, resulting in the menstrual cycle. Menstrual cycles are often irregular for the first 1 to 2 years following menarche because of *anovulatory cycles* (cycles without ovulation).[4]

Menstrual Cycle

The major functions of the ovaries are ovulation and the secretion of hormones. These functions are accomplished during the normal **menstrual cycle,** a monthly process mediated by the hormonal activity of the hypothalamus, pituitary gland, and ovaries. Menstruation occurs during each month in which an egg is not fertilized (Fig. 51-9). The endometrial cycle is divided into three phases labeled in relation to uterine and ovarian changes: (1) the *proliferative* or *follicular phase,* (2) the *secretory* or *luteal phase,* and (3) the *menstrual* or *ischemic phase.*

TABLE 51-2	**PATIENT AND FAMILY TEACHING GUIDE** **Characteristics of Menstruation**	

Characteristic	Patient Teaching
Menarche Occurs between ages 9 and 16 yr; average age at onset is 12 or 13 yr.	See health care provider regarding possible endocrine or developmental abnormality when delayed.
Interval Usually is 21-35 days, but regular cycles as short as 17 days or as long as 45 days are considered normal if pattern is consistent for individual.	Keep written record to identify own pattern of menstrual cycle. Expect some irregularity in perimenopausal period. Be aware that drugs (phenothiazines, opioids, contraceptives) and stressful life events can result in missed periods.
Duration Menstrual flow generally lasts 2-8 days.	Realize that pattern is fairly constant but that wide variations do exist.
Amount Menstrual flow varies from 20-80 ml per menses; average is 30 ml; amount varies among women and in the same woman at different times; it is usually heaviest first 2 days.	Count pads or tampons used per day. The average tampon or pad, when completely saturated, absorbs 20-30 ml. Very heavy flow is indicated by complete soaking of two pads in 1-2 hr. Flow increases and then gradually decreases in perimenopausal period. IUD or drugs such as anticoagulants and thiazides can produce heavy menses.
Composition Menstrual discharge is mixture of endometrium, blood, mucus, and vaginal cells; it is dark red and less viscous than blood and usually does not clot.	Clots indicate heavy flow or vaginal pooling.

IUD, Intrauterine device.

The length of the menstrual cycle ranges from 20 to 40 days, the average being 28 days.

The menstrual cycle begins on the first day of menstruation, which usually lasts 3 to 7 days. Table 51-2 includes characteristics of the menstrual cycle and related patient teaching. During this time, estrogen and progesterone levels are low, but FSH levels begin to increase. During the follicular phase, a single follicle matures fully under the stimulation of FSH. (The mechanism that ensures that usually only one follicle reaches maturity is not known.) The mature follicle stimulates estrogen production, causing a negative feedback with resulting decreased FSH secretion.

Although the initial stage of follicular maturation is stimulated by FSH, complete maturation and ovulation occur only with the presence of LH. When estrogen levels peak on about the twelfth day of the cycle, there is a surge of LH, which triggers ovulation a day or two later. After ovulation (maturation and release of an ovum), LH promotes the development of the corpus luteum.

The fully developed corpus luteum continues to secrete estrogen and initiates progesterone secretion. If fertilization occurs, high levels of estrogen and progesterone continue to be secreted as a result of the continued activity of the corpus luteum from stimulation by human chorionic gonadotropin (hCG). If fertilization does not take place, menstruation occurs because of a decrease in estrogen production and progesterone withdrawal.

During the follicular phase, the endometrial lining of the uterus also undergoes change. As larger amounts of estrogen are produced, the endometrial lining undergoes proliferative changes, and there is an increase in cellular growth, including an increase in the length of blood vessels and glandular tissue.

With ovulation and the resulting increased levels of progesterone, the luteal (or secretory) phase begins. In this phase, the blood vessels begin to coil, increasing the surface area of the vascular supply. The glandular tissues mature and secrete a glycogen-rich substance, and the glandular ducts dilate. If the corpus luteum regresses (when fertilization does not occur) and estrogen and progesterone levels fall, the endometrial lining can no longer be supported. As a result, the blood vessels contract, and tissue begins to slough (fall away). This sloughing results in the menses and the start of the menstrual phase.

Menopause

Menopause is the physiologic cessation of menses associated with declining ovarian function.[5] It is usually considered complete after 1 year of **amenorrhea** (absence of menstruation). (Menopause is discussed in Chapter 54.)

Phases of the Sexual Response

The sexual response is a complex interplay of psychologic and physiologic phenomena and is influenced by a number of variables, including daily stress, illness, and crisis. The changes that occur during sexual excitement are similar for men and women. Masters and Johnson described the sexual response in terms of the excitement, plateau, orgasmic, and resolution phases.[6]

Male Sexual Response. The penis and the urethra are essential to the transport of sperm into the vagina and the cervix during intercourse. This transport is facilitated by penile erection in response to sexual stimulation during the excitement phase. Erection results from the filling of the large venous sinuses within the erectile tissue of the penis. In the flaccid state the sinuses hold only a small amount of blood, but during the erection stage they are congested with blood. Because the penis is richly endowed with sympathetic, parasympathetic, and pudendal nerve endings, it is readily stimulated to erection. The loose skin of the penis becomes taut as a result of the intense venous congestion. This erectile tautness allows for easy insertion into the vagina.

As the man reaches the plateau phase, the erection is maintained, and a small increase in diameter occurs as a result of a slight increase in vasocongestion. There is also an increase in testicle size. Sometimes a change in color occurs in the glans penis, which becomes more reddish-purple.

The subsequent contraction of the penile and urethral musculature during the orgasmic phase propels the sperm outward through the meatus. In this process, termed *ejaculation,* sperm are released

into the ductus deferens during contractions. Sperm advance through the urethra, where fluids from the prostate and seminal vesicles are added to the ejaculate. The sperm continue their path through the urethra, receiving a small amount of fluid from the Cowper's glands, and are finally ejaculated through the urinary meatus. Orgasm is characterized by the rapid release of the vasocongestion and muscular tension (myotonia) that have developed. The rapid release of muscular tension (through rhythmic contractions) occurs primarily in the penis, prostate gland, and seminal vesicles. After ejaculation, a man enters the resolution phase. During this phase the penis undergoes involution, gradually returning to its unstimulated, flaccid state.

Female Sexual Response. The changes that occur in a woman during sexual excitation are similar to those in a man. In response to stimulation, the clitoris becomes congested and vaginal lubrication increases from secretions from the cervix, Bartholin's glands, and vaginal walls. This initial response is the excitation phase.

As excitation is maintained in the plateau phase, the vagina expands and the uterus is elevated. In the orgasmic phase, contractions occur in the uterus from the fundus to the lower uterine segment. There is a slight relaxation of the cervical os, which helps the entrance of the sperm, and rhythmic contractions of the vagina. Muscular tension is rapidly released through rhythmic contractions in the clitoris, the vagina, and the uterus. This phase is followed by a resolution phase in which these organs return to their preexcitation state. However, women do not have to go through the resolution (refractory) recovery state before they can be orgasmic again. They can be multiorgasmic without resolution between orgasms.

GERONTOLOGIC CONSIDERATIONS
EFFECTS OF AGING ON THE REPRODUCTIVE SYSTEMS AND THE SEXUAL RESPONSE

With advancing age, changes occur in the male and female reproductive systems. In women many of these changes are related to the altered estrogen production that is associated with menopause. A reduction in circulating estrogen along with an increase in androgens in postmenopausal women is associated with breast and genital atrophy, reduction in bone mass, and increased rate of atherosclerosis.[7] The decrease in estrogen also contributes to dry, friable vaginal mucosa, causing many women to experience dyspareunia. A gradual hormonal decline in elderly men also occurs and is sometimes referred to as male menopause.[8] Manifestations of hormonal decline in men can be physical, psychologic, or sexual. Some of the changes include an increase in prostate size, decreased testosterone level, decreased sperm production, decreased muscle tone of the scrotum, and a decrease in the size and firmness of the testicles. Erectile dysfunction and sexual dysfunction occur in some men as a result of these changes.[9] Age-related changes in the reproductive systems and differences in assessment findings are presented in Table 51-3.

Gradual changes resulting from advancing age occur in the sexual responses of men and women (Table 51-4). These changes occur at different rates and to varying degrees. The cumulative effects of these changes, as well as the negative social attitude toward sexuality in older adults, can affect the sexual practices of people in this age-group. Nurses have an important role in providing accurate and unbiased information about sexuality and age.

TABLE 51-3	*GERONTOLOGIC DIFFERENCES IN ASSESSMENT* Reproductive Systems

Changes	Differences in Assessment Findings
Male	
Penis	
Decreased subcutaneous fat, decreased skin turgor	Easily retractable foreskin (if uncircumcised); decrease in size; fewer sustained erections
Testes	
Decreased testosterone production	Decrease in size; change in position (lower); increase in firmness
Prostate	
Benign hyperplasia	Enlargement
Breasts	
Enlargement	Gynecomastia (abnormal enlargement)
Female	
Breasts	
Decreased subcutaneous fat, increased fibrous tissue, decreased skin turgor	Less resilient, looser, more pendulous tissue; decreased size; duct around nipple may feel like stringy strand
Vulva	
Decreased skin turgor	Atrophy; decreased amount of pubic hair; decreased size of clitoris and labia
Vagina	
Atrophy of tissue, decreased muscle tone, pH becomes alkaline	Pale and dry mucosa; relaxation of outlets; mucosa thins; vagina narrower and shorter; increased potential for infection
Urethra	
Decreased muscle tone	Cystocele (protrusion of bladder through vaginal wall)
Uterus	
Decreased thickness of myometrium	Decrease in size; uterine prolapse
Ovaries	
Decreased ovarian function	Nonpalpable ovaries; decreased size

TABLE 51-4	**Effects of Aging on Sexual Function**

Men
- Increased stimulation necessary for erection
- Force of ejaculation decreased
- Decreased ability to attain erection
- Decreased size and rigidity of the penis at full erection
- Decreased libido and interest in sex

Women
- Decreased vaginal lubrication
- Decreased sensitivity with labia shrinking and more clitoris exposed
- Difficulty in maintaining arousal
- Difficulty in achieving orgasm after stimulation
- Decreased libido and interest in sex

Nurses should emphasize the normalcy of sexual activity in older adults. Counseling may be necessary to help older patients accommodate to these normal physiologic changes.

ASSESSMENT OF THE MALE AND FEMALE REPRODUCTIVE SYSTEMS

Subjective Data

Important Health Information. In addition to general health information, the nurse needs to elicit information specifically relating to the reproductive system. Reproduction and sexual issues are often considered extremely personal and private. The nurse must develop trust to elicit such information. A professional demeanor is important when taking a reproductive or sexual history. The nurse needs to be sensitive, ask gender-neutral questions, and maintain an awareness of a patient's culture and beliefs. It is helpful if the nurse begins with the least sensitive information (e.g., menstrual history) before asking questions about more sensitive issues such as sexual practices or STDs.

Past Health History. The past health history should include information about major illnesses, hospitalizations, immunizations, and surgeries. The nurse should also inquire about any infections involving the reproductive system, including STDs. Women should also have a complete obstetric and gynecologic history taken.

Common pediatric illnesses that affect reproductive function are mumps and rubella. The occurrence of mumps in young men has been associated with an increase in sterility. Bilateral testicular atrophy can occur secondary to mumps-related orchitis. In the health history the nurse should ask if male patients have had mumps, have been immunized with mumps vaccine, or have any indications of sterility.

Rubella is of primary concern to women of childbearing age. If rubella occurs during the first 3 months of pregnancy, the possibility of congenital anomalies is increased.[10] For this reason, nurses should encourage immunization for all women of childbearing age who have not been immunized for rubella or have not already had the disease. However, women should not be immunized if they are already pregnant. Women are also advised not to conceive for at least 3 months after immunization. Rubella immunity can be determined by antibody titers.

The nurse should also question the patient regarding current health status and the presence of any acute or chronic health problems. Problems in other body systems are often related to problems with the reproductive system. Questions relating to possible endocrine disorders, particularly diabetes mellitus (DM), hypothyroidism, and hyperthyroidism, must be asked, because these disorders directly interfere with women's menstrual cycles and with sexual performance. Men who have DM may experience erectile dysfunction and retrograde ejaculation. In women with uncontrolled DM, pregnancy and the use of oral contraceptives may constitute significant risks to health. Many other chronic illnesses such as cardiovascular disease, respiratory disorders, anemia, cancer, and kidney and urinary tract disorders may affect the reproductive system and sexual functioning.

A history of a stroke should be determined. In men, strokes may cause physiologic or psychologic erectile dysfunction. Men who have suffered a myocardial infarction (MI) may experience erectile dysfunction because of the fear of precipitating another MI resulting from sexual activity. This same concern is shared by the woman both as a partner of someone who has had an MI and as the person recovering from an MI. Although most patients have concerns about sexual activity following an MI, many are not comfortable expressing these concerns to the nurse. The nurse must be sensitive to this concern. In women, a history of cardiovascular disease (e.g., hypertension, thrombophlebitis, angina) causes a higher incidence of morbidity and mortality with pregnancy or oral contraceptive use.

Medications. A list of all prescription and over-the-counter medications that the patient is taking should be documented, including reason for the medication, the dosage, and the length of time that the medication has been taken. All drugs taken by female patients should be evaluated for possible teratogenic effects in women of childbearing age. The patient should be asked about the use of herbal products and dietary supplements.

Particularly relevant in the assessment of the reproductive system is the use of diuretics (sometimes prescribed for premenstrual edema), psychotropic agents (which may interfere with sexual performance), and antihypertensives (some of which may cause erectile dysfunction). Thus patients who use drugs such as amlodipine (Norvasc), lisinopril (Prinivil), propranolol (Inderal), and clonidine (Catapres) must be closely assessed for these problems.[11] The nurse must also note the use of drugs such as alcohol, marijuana, barbiturates, amphetamines, or phencyclidine hydrochloride (PCP; also called "angel dust"), which can have serious behavioral or physiologic effects on the functioning of the reproductive system.

In women, the use of oral contraceptives or other hormones should be noted. The long-term use of both estrogen and progesterone in hormone replacement therapy (HRT) increases the risk of cardiovascular disease, stroke, and breast cancer in postmenopausal women.[12] The short-term use of HRT appears to be appropriate for women experiencing moderate-to-severe menopausal symptoms. (HRT is discussed in Chapter 54.)

A history of cholecystitis and hepatitis is important information because these conditions may be contraindications for the use of oral contraceptives; cholecystitis is often aggravated by oral contraceptives, and chronic active inflammation of the liver generally precludes the use of estrogen products because they are metabolized by the liver. Chronic obstructive pulmonary disease may be a contraindication to oral contraceptive use because progesterone thickens respiratory secretions.

Surgery or Other Treatments. Any surgical procedures should be noted in the health history. Surgical procedures involving the reproductive system are listed in Table 51-5. Therapeutic or spontaneous abortions should also be documented.

Functional Health Patterns. The key questions to ask a patient with a reproductive problem are presented in Table 51-6.

Health Perception–Health Management Pattern. Two of the primary focuses of this health pattern are the patient's perception of his or her own health and measures that the patient takes to maintain health. Specifically, it is important to ask about self-examination practices and screenings. Monthly breast self-examination (BSE), mammography according to age-specific guidelines (see Chapter 52), and routine Pap tests are integral to a woman's health. Testicular self-examination (TSE) should be practiced by all men, starting in adolescence. Regular prostate examination should be encouraged as well. The American Cancer Society recommends that men over age 50 have digital rectal examination (DRE) and prostate-specific antigen (PSA) test yearly.[13]

Family history is also a component of this health pattern. The nurse should inquire about a history of cancer, particularly cancer

TABLE 51-5	Surgeries of the Reproductive Systems
Surgery	**Description**
Male	
Herniorrhaphy	Repair of hernia
Orchiectomy	Removal of one or both testes
Prostatectomy	Removal of prostate gland
Repair of testicular torsion	Correction of axial rotation of spermatic cord, which cuts off blood supply to the testicle, epididymis, and other structures
Varicocelectomy	Repair of varicose vein of scrotum
Vasectomy	Removal of part of ductus (vas) deferens; can be an elective procedure for sterilization or contraception
Female	
Cryosurgery	Use of subfreezing temperature to destroy tissue, especially in treatment of abnormal cells
Dilation and curettage	Dilation of uterus and scraping of endometrium, performed to diagnose disease of uterus, correct heavy or prolonged vaginal bleeding, or empty uterus of products of conception; also used in the treatment of infertility to correlate state of endometrium and time of cycle
Hysterectomy	Removal of uterus
Mastectomy	Removal of one or both breasts
Oophorectomy	Removal of one or both ovaries
Repair of cystocele	Correction of protrusion of urinary bladder through vaginal wall
Repair of rectocele	Correction of protrusion of rectum into vagina
Salpingectomy	Removal of one or both fallopian tubes
Tubal sterilization	Ligation of fallopian tubes

of the reproductive organs. Having a first-degree relative who has had cancer of the breast, ovaries, uterus, or prostate significantly increases the risk of cancer for the patient. Determination of a familial tendency for diabetes mellitus, hypothyroidism, hyperthyroidism, hypertension, stroke, angina, myocardial infarction, endocrine disorders, or anemia is also important.

Assessment of the reproductive system is incomplete without a knowledge of the patient's lifestyle choices. The nurse should know whether a woman uses cigarettes, alcohol, caffeine, or other drugs because these substances can be detrimental to both mother and fetus. Cigarette smoking may delay conception and can also increase the risk of morbidity in women using oral contraceptives. Early menopause is also associated with smoking in women. These substances may also adversely affect the sperm count in men and cause erectile dysfunction or decreased libido.

The nurse must determine if the patient is allergic to sulfonamides, penicillin, rubber, or latex. Sulfonamides and penicillin are used frequently in the treatment of reproductive and genitourinary problems such as vaginitis and gonorrhea. Rubber and latex are commonly used in diaphragms and condoms. An allergy to these substances precludes their use as contraceptive methods.

Nutritional-Metabolic Pattern. Anemia is a common problem in women in their reproductive years, particularly during pregnancy and the postpartum period. The adequacy of the diet should be evaluated with this condition in mind.

A thorough nutritional and psychologic history should be taken to assess for the presence of an eating disorder. Anorexia can cause

TABLE 51-6	*HEALTH HISTORY* **Reproductive System**

Health Perception–Health Management
- How would you describe your overall health?
- *Women:* Explain how you examine your breasts. Have you had a Pap test or mammogram recently? If so, what were the results and dates of these tests?
- *Men:* Explain how you examine your testes. Have you had a prostate examination recently? If so, what were the results and date of this examination?
- Describe the health of your family members. Any history of breast, uterine, ovarian, or prostate cancer?
- Do you use tobacco products, alcohol, or drugs?*

Nutritional-Metabolic
- Describe what you usually eat and drink.
- Have you experienced any changes in weight?*
- How do you feel about your current weight?
- Do you take any nutritional supplements such as calcium or vitamins?*
- Do you have any dietary restrictions?*

Elimination
- Do you experience problems with urination (e.g., pain, burning, dribbling, incontinence, frequency)?*
- Have you had bladder infections? If so, when? How often?
- Do you experience problems with bowel movements?* Do you use laxatives?*

Activity-Exercise
- What activities do you typically do each day?
- Do you have enough energy for your desired activities?
- Can you dress yourself? Feed yourself? Walk without help?

Sleep-Rest
- How many hours do you typically sleep each night?
- Do you feel rested after sleep?
- Do you experience any problems associated with sleeping?*

Cognitive-Perceptual
- Are you able to read and write?
- Do you experience problems with dizziness?*
- Do you experience pain? If yes, where?
- Do you experience pain during sexual activity or intercourse?*

Self-Perception–Self-Concept
- How would you describe yourself?
- Have there been any recent changes that have made you feel differently about yourself?*
- Are you experiencing any problems that are affecting your sexuality?*

Role-Relationship
- Describe your living arrangements. Who do you live with?
- Do you have a significant other? If yes, is this relationship satisfying?
- Are you experiencing any role-related problems in your family?* At work?*
- What are the relationships among your family members?

Sexuality-Reproductive
- Are you sexually active? If so, how many partners do you have?
- What kind of sex do you engage in (e.g., oral, vaginal, rectal)?
- How do you protect yourself against sexually transmitted disease and unwanted pregnancy?
- Are you satisfied with your present means of sexual expression? If no, explain.
- Have you experienced any recent changes in your sexual practices?*
- *Women:* Date of last menstruation, description of menstrual flow, problems with menstruation, age of menarche, age of menopause.
- *Women:* Pregnancy history—number of times pregnant, number of living children, number of miscarriages/abortions.

Coping–Stress Tolerance
- Have there been any major changes in your life within the last couple of years?*
- What is stressful in your life right now?
- How do you handle health problems when they occur?

Value-Belief
- What beliefs do you have about your health and illnesses?
- Do you use home remedies?*
- Is religion an important part of your life?*
- Do you feel that any of your personal beliefs or values may be compromised because of your treatment?*

*If yes, describe.

amenorrhea and the subsequent problems, such as osteoporosis, that are related to menopause. The nurse has the opportunity to help prevent the debilitating condition of osteoporosis. From early adolescence, women can be counseled regarding adequate calcium and vitamin D intake to prevent osteoporosis. The patient's daily calcium intake should be estimated to determine whether there is a need for supplementation. Folic acid intake for women in their reproductive years should be evaluated because a deficiency can result in spina bifida and other neural tube defects in the fetus.[14]

Elimination Pattern. Many gynecologic problems can result in genitourinary problems. Stress and urge incontinence are common in older women because of relaxation of the pelvic musculature caused by multiple births or advancing age. Vaginal infections predispose patients to chronic or recurrent urinary tract infections. The proximity of the reproductive organs and the genitourinary tract makes metastasis of malignant tumors to this site a possibility to be considered. Benign prostatic hyperplasia is a common problem of older men. It can alter normal urination, causing retention and difficulty in initiating the urinary stream.

Activity-Exercise Pattern. The amount, type, and intensity of activity and exercise should be documented. Lack of stress on bones secondary to lack of exercise is an important factor in the development of osteoporosis. Weight-bearing exercise decreases the risk of osteoporosis in women. Women who engage in excessive exercise may experience amenorrhea. This may result from decreased estrogen related to a low percentage of body fat because estrogen is stored in fat cells. Anemia can result in fatigue and activity intolerance and can interfere with satisfactory performance of the activities of daily living.

Sleep-Rest Pattern. Sleep patterns may be affected during the postpartum period and also while raising young children. The hot flashes and sweating often present during perimenopause can cause serious sleep interruption when the woman is awakened in a drenching sweat. The need to change her nightgown and bedding further disrupts her sleep. Insomnia is also a common complaint of perimenopausal women. Daytime fatigue often results from such nighttime awakenings. In men, sleep disturbances may be caused by frequent urination at night associated with prostate enlargement.

Cognitive-Perceptual Pattern. Pelvic pain is associated with various gynecologic disorders such as pelvic inflammatory disease, ovarian cysts, and endometriosis. **Dyspareunia** (painful intercourse) can be particularly problematic for a woman. The pain associated with intercourse can make her reluctant to participate in sexual activity and strain her relationship with her sexual partner. The woman should be referred to her health care provider if dyspareunia is present.

Self-Perception–Self-Concept Pattern. The reproductive changes of aging such as pendulous breasts and vaginal dryness in women and decreased size of the penis in men may lead to emotional distress. The subtle changes associated with sexuality and advancing age may alter the self-concept of many persons.

Role-Relationship Pattern. The nurse needs to obtain information regarding the family structure and occupation. Questions regarding recent changes in work-related relationships or family conflicts should be asked. It is important to ascertain the patient's role in the family as a starting point in determining family dynamics.

Roles and relationships are affected by changes within the family. The addition of a new baby into the family may change family dynamics. Role-relationship patterns change as children begin their careers and move away from home. Another change occurs when people retire.

Sexuality-Reproductive Pattern. The extent and depth of the interview about a patient's sexuality depend primarily on the expertise of the interviewer and on the needs and the willingness of the patient. Before taking a sexual history, interviewers should assess their own comfort with their sexuality, because any discomfort in questioning becomes obvious to the patient. Interviews must be carried out in an environment that provides reassurance, confidentiality, and a nonjudgmental attitude. It is best to begin with the least sensitive areas and then move to more sensitive areas.

For women, it is important to obtain a menstrual and an obstetric history. The menstrual history includes the first day of the last menstrual period, description of menstrual flow, age of menarche, and, if applicable, age at menopause. Menstrual history data are used in the detection of pregnancy, infertility, and numerous other gynecologic concerns. Changes in the usual menstrual pattern must be explicitly described to determine whether the change is transient and unimportant or connected with a more serious gynecologic problem. *Metrorrhagia* (spotting or bleeding between menstruations), *menorrhagia* (excessive menstrual bleeding), *amenorrhea* (lack of menstruation), and *postcoital bleeding* are examples of such problems. Changes in menstrual patterns associated with the use of contraceptive pills, intrauterine devices (IUDs), birth control patches, vaginal rings, subdermal estrogen-only implant (Norplant), or medroxyprogesterone (Depo-Provera) injections must be identified. Contraceptive pills usually decrease the amount and duration of flow, whereas some IUDs may cause an increase in the amount and duration. Some IUDs also increase the severity of dysmenorrhea. However, newer IUDs contain progestin and may be therapeutic. The obstetric history includes the number of pregnancies, full-term births, preterm births, and live births. Other obstetric information should include information about any ectopic pregnancies or abortions, either spontaneous or therapeutic. Any problems that occurred with pregnancy should be documented.

A sexual history should include information regarding sexual activity, beliefs, and practices. Sexual preference (heterosexual, homosexual, bisexual), the frequency and type of sexual activity (penile-vaginal, penile-rectal, recipient rectal, oral), and the number of partners and protective measures against STD and pregnancy should be explored. The patient's knowledge of safe sexual practices should be determined. A history of multiple sex partners and unprotected sex increases the risk of contracting an STD. For a woman, this can increase the risk of pelvic inflammatory disease, which can compromise her ability to become pregnant.

Table 51-7 outlines specific questions for a sexual history. It should be noted that only a skilled interviewer should approach some of the questions presented in Table 51-7, and then only with discretion and sensitivity to cultural differences.[9]

Both men and women should be asked about their general satisfaction with sexuality. The patient's satisfaction with the opportunities for sexual gratification is important information that should be elicited. The patient should be questioned about sexual beliefs and practices and whether orgasm is achieved. Any unexplained change in sexual practices or performance should be explored. Problems of the reproductive system can cause physiologic or psychologic problems that can lead to painful intercourse, erectile dysfunction, sexual dysfunction, or infertility. Both the cause and the effect of such problems should be determined.

Coping–Stress Tolerance Pattern. The stress related to situations such as pregnancy or menopause may cause an increased dependence on support systems. It is essential for the nurse to ascertain who the support people are in the patient's life. The diagnosis of an STD can cause stress for the patient and the partner. Ways to manage this stress should be explored.

Value-Belief Pattern. Sexual and reproductive functioning is closely related to cultural, religious, moral, and ethical values. The nurse should be aware of his or her own beliefs in these areas and should recognize and sensitively react to the patient's personal beliefs associated with reproductive and sexuality issues.

Objective Data

Physical Examination: Male. The examination of the male external genitalia includes inspection and palpation. An examination may be performed with the patient lying or standing. The standing position is generally preferred. The examiner should

TABLE 51-7	Sexual History Format

- Are you currently in a relationship that involves sexual intercourse? If yes, do you have one or multiple partners?
- How frequently do you engage in sexual activities? Are you and your partner(s) satisfied with the sexual relationship?
- How many sexual partners have you had in the past 6 months?
- Do you prefer relationships with men, women, or both? (If the patient is gay or lesbian, inquire if he or she is in a significant relationship.)
- Has your sex life changed during the past year? If yes, how?
- Have you ever had a sexually transmitted disease? If yes, what?
- What are you doing to protect yourself from sexually transmitted diseases? If protection is used, what type? Do you use protection every time you have intercourse?
- Are you currently using any birth control measures? If yes, what type? How long have you been using this product? How effective do you feel this has been?
- Have you ever been in a relationship with anyone who hurt you? Have you ever been forced into sexual acts as a child or an adult?
- How often have you experienced erectile dysfunction (male) or difficulty with vaginal lubrication (female) or pain with intercourse?

Adapted from Wilson SF, Giddens JF: *Health assessment for nursing practice*, ed 3, St Louis, 2005, Mosby.

be seated in front of the standing patient. Gloves should be used during examination of the male genitalia.

Pubis. The nurse observes the distribution and general characteristics of the pubic hair and the skin. Normally, the hair is in a diamond-shaped pattern. The hair is usually coarser than scalp hair. The absence of hair is not a normal finding. The skin is also evaluated.

Penis. The nurse notes the size and skin texture of the penis and any lesions, scars, or swelling. The location of the urethral meatus, as well as the presence or absence of a foreskin, should be noted. If present, the foreskin should be retracted to note cleanliness and replaced over the glans after observation. The glans is compressed to note any discharge and its amount, color, and odor if present. The nurse also palpates the penile shaft for tenderness or masses and observes the ventral and dorsal aspects.

Scrotum and Testes. This part of the examination in usually not performed by the nurse generalist. The nurse with advanced skills would start by performing a complete skin examination by lifting each testis to inspect all sides of the scrotal sac. Palpation of the scrotum is done to note changes in consistency or the presence of masses. It is important to note if the testes are descended. The left testis usually hangs lower than the right. An undescended testis is a major risk factor for testicular cancer, as well as a potential cause of male infertility.

Inguinal Region and Spermatic Cord. This part of the examination is usually not performed by the nurse generalist. The examiner with advanced skills would first inspect the skin overlying the inguinal regions for rashes or lesions. The patient should be asked to bear down or cough. While he is straining, the inguinal area should be inspected for the presence of a bulge. No bulging should be seen.

Examination of the inguinal area continues with palpation. The right and left inguinal rings should be palpated using the index finger or middle finger. The finger should be inserted into the lower aspect of the scrotum and should follow the spermatic cord upward through the triangular, slitlike opening of the inguinal ring. At this point, the patient should be asked to bear down and cough. The nurse determines whether the strain produces a bulging of the intestines through the ring, indicating the presence of a hernia, a condition that requires follow-up. The inguinal lymph nodes should also be palpated. Enlargement of the lymph nodes (termed *lymphadenopathy*) could suggest a pelvic organ infection or malignancy.

Anus and Prostate. The anal sphincter and perineal regions are inspected for lesions, masses, and hemorrhoids. A digital rectal examination (DRE) is required for all men who have symptoms of prostate trouble, such as difficulty in initiating urination and the urge to void frequently. This examination should be performed annually for all men over 50 years of age.

Physical Examination: Female. Physical examination of women often begins with inspection and palpation of the breasts and then proceeds to the abdomen and genitalia. Examination of the abdomen provides an opportunity to detect pain or any masses that may involve the genitourinary system. Abdominal examination is discussed in Chapter 39.

Breasts. Breasts are examined first by visual inspection. The nurse, with the patient seated, observes the breasts for symmetry, size, shape, skin color, vascular patterns, dimpling, and the presence of unusual lesions. The patient is asked to put her arms at her sides, arms overhead, lean forward, and press hands on hips. The nurse observes for any abnormalities during these maneu-

vers. The axillae and the clavicular areas are then palpated for enlarged lymph nodes.

After the patient assumes a supine position, a pillow is placed under the back on the side to be examined. The patient is asked to put her arm above and behind her head. These maneuvers flatten breast tissue and make palpation easier. The breast is then palpated in a systematic fashion using a vertical line, a clockwise, or a spoke approach. The nurse should use the distal finger pads for palpation. The tail of Spence should be included in the examination because this area and the upper outer quadrant are the areas where most breast malignancies develop. Finally, the nurse should palpate the area around the areolae for masses. The nipple should be compressed to determine the presence of discharge or any masses. The color, consistency, and odor of any discharge should be documented.

External Genitalia. The nurse uses gloves for examination of the external genitalia. The mons pubis, labia majora, labia minora, posterior fourchette, perineum, and anal region are inspected for characteristics of skin, hair distribution, and contour. Lesions, inflammation, swelling, and discharge are noted. The nurse must separate the labia to fully inspect the clitoris, urethral meatus, and vaginal orifice.

Internal Pelvic Examination. During the speculum examination, the nurse observes the walls of the vagina and the cervix for inflammation, discharge, polyps, and suspicious growths. During this examination, it is possible to obtain a Pap test and collect cells for culture and microscopic examination. After the speculum examination, a bimanual examination is performed to allow assessment of the size, shape, and consistency of the uterus, ovaries, and tubes. The tubes are not normally palpable.

Pelvic and bimanual examinations are considered advanced skills and are not usually within the scope of the nurse generalist.[15] For this reason, these parts of the examination are not included in this text.

Table 51-8 provides an example of a recording format for the physical assessment findings for the male and female reproductive systems. Tables 51-9 through 51-11 summarize common assessment abnormalities of the breasts, female reproductive system, and male reproductive system, respectively.

TABLE 51-8	**Normal Physical Assessment of the Reproductive System**
Male	**Female**
	Breasts Symmetric without dimpling. Nipples soft; no drainage, retraction, or lesions noted. No masses or tenderness; no lymphadenopathy.
External Genitalia Diamond-shaped hair distribution. Penis circumcised, no lesions or discharge noted. Scrotum symmetric, no masses, descended testes. No inguinal hernia.	**External Genitalia** Triangular hair distribution. Genitalia dark pink, no lesions, redness, swelling, or inflammation in perineal region. No vaginal discharge noted. No tenderness with palpation of Skene's ducts and Bartholin's glands.
Anus No hemorrhoids, fissures, or lesions noted.	**Anus** No hemorrhoids, fissures, or lesions noted.

TABLE 51-9	COMMON ASSESSMENT ABNORMALITIES Breast	

Finding	Description	Possible Etiology and Significance
Nipple inversion or retraction	Recent onset, erythematous, pain, unilateral Recent onset (usually within past year), unilateral presentation, lack of tenderness	Abscess, inflammation, cancer Neoplasm
Nipple secretions		
• Galactorrhea (female)	Milky, no relationship to lactation, unilateral or bilateral or intermittent or consistent presentation	Drug therapy, particularly phenothiazines, tricyclic antidepressants, methyldopa; hypofunction or hyperfunction of thyroid or adrenal glands; tumors of hypothalamus or pituitary gland; excessive estrogen; prolonged suckling or breast foreplay
• Galactorrhea (male)	Milky, bilateral presentation	Chorioepithelioma of testes, manifestation of pituitary tumor
• Purulent	Gray-green or yellow color; frequent unilateral presentation; association with pain, erythema, induration, nipple inversion Same as above but usually without nipple inversion	Puerperal (after birth) mastitis (inflammatory condition of breast) or abscess Infected sebaceous cyst
• Serous discharge	Clear appearance, unilateral or bilateral or intermittent or consistent presentation	Intraductal papilloma
• Dark green or multicolored discharge	Thick, sticky, and frequently bilateral	Ductal ectasia (dilation of mammary ducts)
• Serosanguineous or bloody drainage	Unilateral presentation	Papillomatosis (widespread development of nipple-like growths), intraductal papilloma, carcinoma (male and female)
Scaling or irritation of nipple	Unilateral or bilateral presentation, crusting, possible ulceration	Paget's disease, eczema, infection
Nodules, lumps, or masses	Multiple, bilateral, well-delineated, soft or firm, mobile cysts; pain; premenstrual occurrence Rubbery consistency, fluid-filled interior, pain Soft, mobile, well-delineated cyst, absence of pain Erythema, tenderness, induration Usually singular, hard, irregularly shaped, poorly delineated, nonmobile	Fibrocystic changes Ductal ectasia Lipoma, fibroadenoma Infected sebaceous cysts, abscesses Neoplasm
Dimpling of breast	Unilateral, recent onset, no pain	Neoplasm

TABLE 51-10	COMMON ASSESSMENT ABNORMALITIES Female Reproductive System	

Finding	Description	Possible Etiology and Significance
Vulvar discharge	Plaque-like consistency, frequent itching and inflammation, lack of odor or yeast-like smell Grayish color, copious flow, frothy appearance, vulvar irritation Grayish green or yellow color; malodorous or "fishy" odor Bloody color	Candidiasis (*Candida* or yeast infection), vaginitis Bacterial vaginosis infection *Trichomonas vaginalis* *Chlamydia trachomatis* or *Neisseria gonorrhoeae* infection, menstruation, trauma, cancer
Vulvar erythema	Bright or beefy red color, itching Reddened base, painful vesicles or ulcerations Macules or papules, itching	*Candida albicans,* allergy, chemical vaginitis Genital herpes Chancroid (STD), contact dermatitis, scabies, pediculosis
Vulvar growths	Soft, fleshy growth; nontender Flat and warty appearance, nontender Same as either of above, possible pain Reddened base, vesicles, and small erosions; pain Indurated, firm ulcers; lack of pain	Condyloma acuminatum Condyloma latum Neoplasm Lymphogranuloma venereum, genital herpes, chancroid Chancre (syphilis), granuloma inguinale
Abdominal pain or tenderness	Intermittent or consistent tenderness in right or left lower quadrant Periumbilical location, consistent occurrence	Salpingitis (infection of fallopian tube), ectopic pregnancy, ruptured ovarian cyst, PID, tubal or ovarian abscess Cystitis, endometritis (inflammation of endometrium), ectopic pregnancy

PID, Pelvic inflammatory disease; *STD*, sexually transmitted disease.

TABLE 51-11	COMMON ASSESSMENT ABNORMALITIES
	Male Reproductive System

Finding	Description	Possible Etiology and Significance
Penile growths or masses	Indurated, smooth, disklike appearance; absence of pain; singular presentation	Chancre
	Papular to irregularly shaped ulceration with pus, lack of induration	Chancroid
	Ulceration with induration and nodularity	Cancer
	Flat, wartlike nodule	Condyloma latum
	Elevated, fleshy, moist, elongated projections with single or multiple projections	Condyloma acuminatum
	Localized swelling with retracted, tight foreskin	Paraphimosis (inability to replace foreskin to its normal position after retraction), trauma
Vesicles, erosions, or ulcers	Painful, erythematous base; vesicular or small erosions	Genital herpes, balanitis (inflammation of glans penis), chancroid
	Painless, singular, small erosion with eventual lymphadenopathy	Lymphogranuloma venereum, cancer
Scrotal masses	Localized swelling with tenderness, unilateral or bilateral presentation	Epididymitis (inflammation of epididymis), testicular torsion, orchitis (mumps)
	Swelling, tenderness	Incarcerated hernia
	Unilateral or bilateral presentation; swelling without pain; translucent, cordlike or wormlike appearance	Hydrocele (accumulation of fluid in outer covering of testes), spermatocele (firm, sperm containing cyst of epididymis), varicocele (dilation of veins that drain testes), hematocele (accumulation of blood within scrotum)
	Firm, nodular testes or epididymis; frequent unilateral presentation	Tuberculosis, cancer
Penile discharge	Clear to purulent color, minimal to copious flow	Urethritis or gonorrhea, *Chlamydia trachomatis* infection, trauma
Penile or scrotal erythema	Macules and papules	Scabies, pediculosis
Inguinal masses	Bulging unilateral presentation during straining	Inguinal hernia
	Shotty, 1-3 cm nodules	Lymphadenopathy

DIAGNOSTIC STUDIES OF THE REPRODUCTIVE SYSTEMS

Table 51-12 summarizes the most commonly used diagnostic studies in the assessment of the reproductive systems and the nurse's responsibility regarding these diagnostic tests.

Urine Studies

Pregnancy Testing. Occurrence of pregnancy is generally validated by measuring human chorionic gonadotropin (hCG) in the urine. A solution containing monoclonal antibodies specific for hCG is mixed with a small amount of urine. The presence of hCG causes a change in color of the tested urine.

Home pregnancy test kits use the same assay principle described in the preceding paragraph. Positive results are based on the presence of hCG in urine. Some tests can detect pregnancy as early as the first day following a missed menstrual period. These tests are 98% accurate if the test is performed exactly per instructions. A second test is recommended within a week if the first test is negative (assuming menses has not yet occurred).[16]

Hormone Studies. Although estrogen studies are performed on urine, the results are frequently inaccurate because of variable estrogen levels during the normal cycle and the difficulty in estimating the day of the cycle in women with irregular menses. Adrenal androgens are precursors of estrogens and can be measured in the urine of both men and women. FSH can be measured in a 24-hour urine specimen. Increased and decreased FSH levels can

indicate gonadal failure resulting from pituitary dysfunction. For more information regarding hormone studies, see Chapter 48.

Blood Studies

Hormone Studies. Serum assays for hCG can detect pregnancy before a woman misses her menstrual period.[16] The prolactin assay is used primarily in the workup of a patient with amenorrhea. High levels of prolactin are normally associated with low levels of estrogen, such as those that occur during lactation. However, the same finding can occur with pituitary adenomas, especially with otherwise unexplained galactorrhea (excessive secretion of breast milk). Serum progesterone and estradiol are sometimes measured in assessment of ovarian function, particularly for amenorrhea. In addition, hormonal blood studies are essential components of a thorough fertility workup.

Tumor Markers. Biologic tumor markers are substances associated with malignant disease. Measurement of these markers is useful in monitoring therapy (marker levels rise as disease progresses and fall with disease regression) because marker levels may rise months before new disease or metastasis is evident. α-Fetoprotein (AFP) and hCG are sometimes used as tumor markers for testicular malignancy. A specific tumor antigen such as prostate-specific antigen (PSA) is another type of tumor marker frequently used for prostate cancer.[13]

Serology Tests for Syphilis. The Venereal Disease Research Laboratory (VDRL) test and the rapid plasma reagin (RPR) detect

TABLE 51-12	*DIAGNOSTIC STUDIES* **Male and Female Reproductive Systems**	

Study	Description and Purpose	Nursing Responsibility
Urine Studies		
hCG	Used to detect pregnancy. Also used to detect hydatidiform mole and chorioepithelioma (in men and women).	Obtain thorough menstrual history from patient, including birth control methods. Determine presence or absence of presumptive signs of pregnancy (e.g., breast changes, increased whitish vaginal discharge).
Testosterone levels	Tumors and developmental anomalies of the testes can be detected.	Instruct patient to collect 24-hr urine specimen. Keep it refrigerated.

Follicle-stimulating hormone (FSH) **assay**	Indicates gonadal failure because of pituitary dysfunction.
	Female:
	    Follicular phase: 2-5 IU/24 hr
	    Midcycle: 8-40 IU/24 hr
	    Luteal phase: 2-10 IU/24 hr
	    Postmenopause: 35-100 IU/24 hr
	Male: 2-15 IU/24 hr
		Instruct patient to collect 24-hr urine specimen. Indicate phase of menstrual cycle, if menopausal, and if on oral contraceptives or hormones.

Blood Studies		
Prolactin Assay	Detects pituitary dysfunction that can cause amenorrhea.	Observe venipuncture site for bleeding or hematoma formation.
Prostate-specific antigen (PSA)	Used to detect prostate cancer. Also a sensitive test for monitoring response to therapy. Normal finding is <4 ng/ml (<4 mcg/L).	No food or fluid restrictions. Collect 5 ml of blood. Observe venipuncture site for bleeding.
Serum hCG assay	Used to detect pregnancy; can also be used as a tumor marker for testicular malignancy. Also used to detect hydatidiform mole and chorioepithelioma (in men and women). *Males and nonpregnant females:* <5 mIU/ml	Instruct patient to have blood drawn in laboratory. Elicit where she is in her menstrual cycle, whether she has missed menses, and if so, how late she is.
Serum testosterone levels	Ascertain whether elevated androgens are due to testicular, adrenal, or ovarian dysfunction or pituitary tumors. Serum testosterone is also drawn to assess male infertility and tumors of the testicle or ovary. *Male:* 300-1200 ng/dl (10.4-41.6 nmol/L) *Female:* 25-90 ng/dl (0.87-3.1 nmol/L)	Collect health history to eliminate potential sources of interference with accuracy of results (e.g., use of corticosteroids or barbiturates, presence of hypothyroidism or hyperthyroidism).

Serum progesterone	Frequently used to detect functioning corpus luteum cyst.
	Female:
	    Follicular phase: <50 ng/dl (1.6 nmol/L)
	    Luteal phase: 200-2500 ng/dl (6.4-79.5 nmol/L)
	    Postmenopause: <40 ng/dl (1.28 nmol/L)
	Male: 10-50 ng/dl (0.32-1.6 nmol/L)
		Observe venipuncture site for bleeding or hematoma formation. Include last menstrual period and trimester of pregnancy because progesterone levels vary with gestation.

Serum estradiol	Measures ovarian function. Particularly useful in assessing estrogen-secreting tumors and states of precocious female puberty. Normal values depend on laboratory that performs test. May be used to confirm perimenopausal status. Increased serum estradiol levels in men may be indicative of testicular tumors.	Observe venipuncture site for bleeding or hematoma formation.

Serum FSH	Indicates gonadal failure due to pituitary dysfunction; used to validate menopausal status.
	Female:
	    Follicular phase: 2-15 mIU/ml
	    Midcycle: 8-40 mIU/ml
	    Luteal phase: 2-15 mIU/ml
	    Postmenopause: 50-250 mIU/ml
	Male: 2-15 mIU/ml
		No food or fluid restrictions required. State phase of menstrual cycle, if menopausal, or if on oral contraceptive or hormones.

Venereal disease research laboratory (VDRL) (flocculation)	Nonspecific antibody tests used to screen for syphilis. Positive readings can be made within 1-2 wk after appearance of primary lesion (chancre) or 4-15 wk after initial infection.	Observe venipuncture site for bleeding or hematoma formation.

hCG, Human chorionic gonadotropin.

TABLE 51-12	*DIAGNOSTIC STUDIES* **Male and Female Reproductive Systems—cont'd**

Study	Description and Purpose	Nursing Responsibility
Blood Studies—cont'd		
Rapid plasma reagin (RPR) (agglutination)	Nonspecific antibody test used to screen for syphilis.	Obtain data to determine presence or absence of problems such as hepatitis, pregnancy, and autoimmune diseases that may interfere with the accuracy of results.
Fluorescent treponemal antibody absorption (FTA-Abs)	Detects syphilis antibodies. Also detects early syphilis with great accuracy. Usually performed if results of VDRL and RPR are questionable.	Inform patient that blood sample will be drawn. Observe venipuncture site for bleeding or hematoma formation.
Cultures and Smears		
Dark-field microscopy	Direct examination of specimen obtained from potential syphilitic lesion (chancre) is performed to detect *Treponema pallidum.*	Avoid direct skin contact with open lesion.
Wet mounts	Direct microscopic examination of specimen of vaginal discharge is performed immediately after collection. Determines presence or absence and number of *Trichomonas* organisms, bacteria, white and red blood cells, and candidal buds or hyphae. Other clues or causes of inflammation or infection may be determined.	Explain procedure and purpose to patient. Instruct patient not to douche before examination. Prepare for collection of specimens (glass slide, 10%-20% potassium hydroxide [KOH] solution, sodium chloride [NaCl] solution, and cotton-tipped applicators).
Cultures	Specimens of vaginal, urethral, or cervical discharge are cultured and used to assess presence of gonorrhea or chlamydia. Rectal and throat cultures may also be taken, depending on data obtained from sexual history.	Obtain specific contact and sexual history inclusive of oral and rectal intercourse. Instruct against douching before examination. Obtain urethral specimen from men before they void. Instruct women who are sexually active with multiple partners to have at least a yearly culture for gonorrhea and chlamydia. Instruct sexually active men to have any discharge evaluated immediately to rule out gonorrhea strains that do not cause classic symptoms of dysuria.
Gram stain	Used for rapid detection of gonorrhea. Presence of gram-negative intracellular diplococci generally warrants initiation of treatment. Not highly accurate for women. Has also been shown as accurate alternative for *Chlamydia* testing.	Same as above.
Cytologic Studies		
Papanicolaou (Pap) test	Microscopic study of exfoliated cells via special staining and fixation technique detects abnormal cells. Cells most commonly studied are those obtained directly from the endocervix and ectocervix.	Instruct women who are sexually active and who are over age 18 to have Pap smears according to American Cancer Society guidelines. Instruct patients not to douche for at least 24 hr before examination. Collect careful menstrual and gynecologic history.
Nipple discharge test	Cytologic study of nipple discharge is performed.	Indicate whether hormonal preparations or other drugs are being taken, breastfeeding, or history of amenorrhea. Instruct patient during demonstration of breast self-examination or examination of breasts that nipple discharge should always be evaluated.
Radiologic Studies		
Mammography	X-ray image of breast tissue on radiographic film is used to assess breast tissue.	Instruct patient about advantages of the examination. Instruct regarding American Cancer Society recommendations for screening (see Chapter 52).
• Screening • Diagnostic	Used to detect benign and malignant masses. Performed when patient has suspicious clinical symptoms or abnormality is found on screening mammogram. Additional views of affected breast are taken.	
Ultrasound (transabdominal and transvaginal)	Measures and records high-frequency sound waves as they pass through tissues of variable density. In women, it is very useful in detecting masses greater than 3 cm, such as ectopic pregnancies, IUDs, ovarian cysts, and hydatidiform moles. In men, it is used to detect testicular torsion or masses.	Instruct patient that a full bladder may be required depending on the reason for the study.

IUDs, Intrauterine devices.

Continued

TABLE 51-12	*DIAGNOSTIC STUDIES* Male and Female Reproductive Systems—cont'd

Study	Description and Purpose	Nursing Responsibility
Radiologic Studies—cont'd		
Computed tomography (CT) of pelvis	Pelvic CT is used to detect tumors within the pelvis.	Inform patient of procedure. Patient must lie still during the procedure. If IV contrast medium is used, check for iodine allergy.
Magnetic resonance imaging (MRI)	Radio waves and magnetic field are used to view soft tissue. Useful if there is an abnormal mammogram or breast dysplasia. Also used to diagnose abnormalities in the female and male reproductive systems.	Screen patient for metal parts and pacemaker. Inform patient that the procedure is painless. Patient must lie still during the procedure.
Invasive Procedures		
Breast biopsy	Histologic examination of excised breast tissue is performed, either by needle aspiration or excisional biopsy.	Before surgery, instruct patient about operative procedures and sedation. After surgery, perform wound care and instruct patient about breast self-examination.
Hysterosalpingogram	Involves instillation of contrast media through cervix into uterine cavity and subsequently through and out fallopian tubes. Spot x-ray images are taken to detect abnormalities of uterus and its adnexa (ovaries and tubes) as contrast medium progresses through them. Test may be most useful in diagnostic assessment of fertility (e.g., to detect adhesions near ovary, an abnormal uterine shape, blockage of tubal pathways).	Inform patient about procedure and that it may be fairly uncomfortable. Determine possibility of iodine allergy.
Colposcopy	Direct visualization of cervix with binocular microscope that allows magnification and study of cellular dysplasia and vascular and tissue abnormalities of cervix. Used as a follow-up study for abnormal Pap smears and for examination of women exposed to DES in utero. Biopsy of cervix may be taken during examination. Valuable in decreasing number of false-negative cervical biopsies.	Instruct patient about this outpatient procedure. Inform patient that this examination is similar to speculum examination. Explain purpose of procedure and prepare patient for it.
Conization	Cone-shaped sample of squamocolumnar tissue of cervix is removed for direct study.	Explain purpose and method of procedure and that it requires use of surgical facilities and anesthesia. Instruct patient to rest for at least 3 days after procedure. Also discuss necessity for 3 wk follow-up check.
Loop electrosurgical excision of transformation zone (LEETZ)	Excision of cervical tissue via an electrosurgical instrument.	Explain purpose and method of procedure and that it may be done in the physician's office for further diagnostic testing.
Loop electrosurgical excision procedure (LEEP)	Same as above.	Same as above.
Culdotomy, culdoscopy, and culdocentesis	Culdotomy is an incision made through posterior fornix of cul-de-sac and allows visualization of peritoneal cavity (i.e., uterus, tubes, and ovaries). Culdoscope can then be used to study these structures closely. This technique is valuable in fertility evaluations. Withdrawal of fluid (culdocentesis) allows examination of fluid characteristics.	Explain purpose and method of procedure. Prepare patient for vaginal operation with preoperative instruction and sedation. Perform assessment of bleeding and discomfort after surgery.
Laparoscopy (peritoneoscopy)	Allows visualization of pelvic structures via fiberoptic scopes inserted through small abdominal incisions. Instillation of carbon dioxide into cavity improves visualization. This technique is used in diagnostic assessment of uterus, tubes, and ovaries. Can be used in conjunction with tubal sterilization.	Explain purpose and method of procedure. Before surgery, instruct patient about procedure, prepare abdomen, and reassure patient about sedation. Tell patient to rest for 1-3 days after surgery. Inform patient of probability of shoulder pain because of air in the abdomen.
Dilation and curettage (D&C)	The operative procedure dilates cervix and allows curetting of endometrial lining. This test is used in assessment of abnormal bleeding patterns and cytologic evaluation of lining.	Before surgery, instruct patient about procedure and sedation. Perform postoperative assessment of degree of bleeding (frequent pad check during first 24 hr).

DES, Diethylstilbestrol.

Continued

| TABLE 51-12 | *DIAGNOSTIC STUDIES* **Male and Female Reproductive Systems—cont'd** |

Study	Description and Purpose	Nursing Responsibility
Fertility Studies		
Semen analysis	Semen is assessed for volume (2-5 ml), viscosity, sperm count (>20 million/ml), sperm motility (60% motile), and percent of abnormal sperm (60% with normal structure).	Instruct patient to bring in fresh specimen within 2 hr after ejaculation.
Basal body temperature assessment	This measurement indicates indirectly whether ovulation has occurred. (Temperature rises at ovulation and remains elevated during secretory phase of normal menstrual cycle.)	Instruct woman to take her temperature using special basal temperature thermometer (calibrated in tenths of degrees) every morning before getting out of bed. Tell woman to record temperature on graph.
Huhner test or Sims-Huhner	Mucus sample of cervix is examined within 2-8 hr after intercourse. Total number of sperm is assessed in relation to number of live sperm. This test is performed to determine whether cervical mucus is "hostile" to passage of sperm from vagina into uterus.	Instruct couples to have intercourse at estimated time of ovulation and be present for test within 2-8 hr after intercourse.
Endometrial biopsy	Small curette is used to obtain piece of endometrial lining to assess endometrial changes common to progesterone secretion after ovulation.	Tell patient that test must be performed postovulation. Explain that procedure should cause only short period of uterine cramping.
Hysterosalpingogram	Same as operative procedures.	Same as operative procedures.
Serum progesterone	Same as blood studies.	Same as blood studies.

the presence of antibodies in the serum of patients infected with syphilis. These tests are inexpensive and reliable but have high levels of false-positive results. The fluorescent treponemal antibody absorption (FTA-Abs) test is highly reliable and should be used after a positive VDRL or RPR, even if it is weakly positive or questionable.[16]

Cultures and Smears

Cultures and smears are most frequently employed in the diagnosis of STD. Specimens for cultures and smears are most commonly taken from the vagina, endocervix, and rectum for females and the urethra and rectum for males. For a culture, the specimen is placed on a special culture medium; a smear involves rubbing the specimen on a slide for direct examination. Gram stain smears have been shown to be effective in the diagnosis of chlamydia infection. A nucleic acid amplification test (NAAT) can screen for both gonorrhea and chlamydia from a wide variety of samples, including vaginal, endocervical, urine, and urethral specimens. Dark-field microscopy involves the direct examination of a specimen obtained from a syphilitic chancre for the diagnosis of syphilis.

Cytologic Studies

Cytology involves the study of cells under microscopic examination. The Pap test is a screening test to detect abnormal cells obtained from the cervix or vagina. It is performed by obtaining cells from the cervical canal, preferably the endocervix, as well as from the vagina. The cells are placed in a fixative for examination by a cytologist for cellular abnormalities. A Pap test (also called a smear) should be done at least once every 3 years beginning 3 years after first sexual intercourse, but no later than age 21. Women ages 65 to 70 may decide to stop having Pap tests after having no abnormal Pap tests in the last 10 years.[17] However, this decision needs to be made in collaboration with their health care provider. Women who have had a total hysterectomy (uterus and cervix removed) do not need to be screened for cervical cancer unless the surgery was done for cervical precancer or cancer.[18]

Cytologic study is also indicated for nipple discharge. Cytologic examination discharge can detect the presence of malignant cells as opposed to a discharge associated with infection.

Radiologic Studies

Mammography. Mammography has become one of the most frequently used diagnostic tools in assessment of the reproductive system. It is used to detect breast masses. Mammography can detect breast masses before they are palpable. Mammography and screening guidelines for mammography are discussed in Chapter 52.

Ultrasound. Ultrasound has many applications for diagnostic study. Pelvic ultrasound is used to obtain images of the pelvic organs. Transvaginal ultrasound is used to visualize the female genital tract. These types of ultrasound are also used to detect pregnancy in the uterus, ectopic pregnancy, ovarian cysts, and other pelvic masses. Breast ultrasound is useful in the detection of fluid-filled masses. In men, ultrasound is used to detect testicular masses and testicular torsion. Transrectal ultrasound is useful in locating prostate tumors.

Pelvic Computed Tomography and Magnetic Resonance Imaging. Pelvic computed tomography (CT) and magnetic resonance imaging (MRI) are used to detect primary or metastatic tumors of the reproductive organs. Contrast media may be used in conjunction with the CT procedure.

NCLEX EXAMINATION REVIEW QUESTIONS

The number of the question corresponds to the same-numbered objective at the beginning of the chapter.

1. A normal reproductive function that may be altered in a patient who undergoes a prostatectomy is
   a. sperm production.
   b. production of testosterone.
   c. production of seminal fluid.
   d. release of sperm from the epididymis.

2. Estrogen production by the mature ovarian follicle causes
   a. decreased secretion of FSH and LH.
   b. increased production of GnRH and FSH.
   c. release of GnRH and increased secretion of LH.
   d. decreased release of FSH and decreased progesterone production.

3. Male orgasm is the result of
   a. clitoral swelling and increased vaginal lubrication.
   b. vaginal enlargement and secretion with penile insertion.
   c. clitoral swelling, vaginal lubrication, and uterine elevation.
   d. rapid release of vasocongestion and muscular tension in the reproductive structures.

4. An age-related finding noted by the nurse during assessment of the older woman's reproductive system is
   a. gynecomastia.
   b. increased vaginal discharge.
   c. decreased amount of pubic hair.
   d. soft, nontender, fleshy vulvar lesions.

5. Significant information about a patient's past medical history related to the reproductive system should include
   a. extent of sexual activity.
   b. general satisfaction with sexuality.
   c. previous sexually transmitted diseases.
   d. self-image and relationships with others.

6. The examination technique used to evaluate the prostate involves
   a. palpation.
   b. percussion.
   c. inspection.
   d. auscultation.

7. An abnormal finding noted during physical assessment of the male reproductive system is
   a. slight clear urethral discharge.
   b. the glans covered with prepuce.
   c. rubbery feeling of the testes on palpation.
   d. urethral meatus on the ventral side of the glans.

8. The screening criteria for assessing prostate cancer include a
   a. baseline ultrasound of the prostate at age 40.
   b. baseline ultrasound of the prostate at age 50.
   c. yearly digital rectal examination for men over age 30.
   d. yearly digital rectal examination for men over age 50.

REFERENCES

1. Thibodeau GA, Patton KT: *Structure and function of the body*, ed 12, St Louis, 2004, Mosby.
2. Scott JR et al, editors: *Danforth's obstetrics and gynecology*, ed 9, Philadelphia, 2003, Lippincott Williams & Wilkins.
3. McCance KL, Huether SE: *Pathophysiology: the biologic basis for disease in adults and children*, ed 5, St Louis, 2006, Mosby.
4. Strickland J, Harel Z: Approach to the adolescent girl as she transits from irregular to regular menstrual cycles, *J Pediatr Adolesc Gynecol* 18:193, 2005.
5. Smith P: Menopause assessment, treatment and patient education, *Nurs Pract* 30:32, 2005.
6. Masters WH, Johnson E: *Human sexual response*, Boston, 1966, Little, Brown.
7. Lobo R: Menopause. In Goldman L, editor: *Cecil textbook of medicine*, ed 22, St Louis, 2004, Saunders.
8. Charlton R: Aging male syndrome, andropause, androgen decline or midlife crisis? *J Men's Health Gender* 1:55, 2004.
9. Sadovsky R, Althof S: Men's sexual issues, *Clin Fam Pract* 6:863, 2004.
10. Ford-Jones L, Ryan G: Implications for the fetus of maternal infections in pregnancy. In Cohen J, Powderly W, editors: *Infectious diseases*, ed 2, St Louis, 2004, Elsevier.
11. *Mosby's 2005 drug reference*, St Louis, 2005, Mosby.
12. Aschenbrenner D: HRT reconsidered, *Am J Nurs* 104:51, 2004.
13. American Cancer Society: Prostate cancer screening guidelines. Available at *www.cancer.org* (accessed June 23, 2005).
14. de Jong–Van den Berg LT: Trends and predictors of folic acid awareness and periconceptual use in pregnant women, *Am J Obstet Gynecol* 192:121, 2005.
15. Wilson S, Giddens JF: *Health assessment for nursing practice*, ed 3, St Louis, 2005, Mosby.
16. Chernecky C, Berger B: *Laboratory tests and diagnostic procedures*, ed 4, St Louis, 2004, Saunders.
17. Saslow D et al: American Cancer Society guidelines for the early detection of cervical dysplasia and cancer, *CA Cancer J Clin* 52:342, 2002. Available at *www.caonline.amcancersoc.org* (accessed June 26, 2005).
18. U.S. Preventive Services Task Force: *Screening for cervical cancer: recommendations and rationale*, Rockville Md, Agency for Healthcare Research and Quality, 2003. Available at *www.ahrq.gov* (accessed June 26, 2005).

RESOURCES

Resources for this chapter are listed in Chapter 54 on p. 1413 and Chapter 55 on p. 1439.

Now is no time to think of what we do not have. Think of what you can do with what there is.

Ernest Hemingway

Nursing Management
Breast Disorders

52

Cynthia Matthews

LEARNING OBJECTIVES

1. Discuss screening guidelines for the early detection of breast cancer.
2. Assess breast tissue by inspection and palpation using appropriate examination techniques.
3. Describe the types, causes, clinical manifestations, collaborative care, and nursing management of common benign breast disorders.
4. Identify the risk factors for breast cancer.
5. Describe the pathophysiology, clinical manifestations, and collaborative care of breast cancer.
6. Identify the types of, indications for, and complications of surgical interventions for breast cancer.
7. Explain the physical and psychologic preoperative and postoperative aspects of nursing management for the patient undergoing a mastectomy.
8. Describe the indications for reconstructive breast surgery; types, potential risks, and complications of reconstructive breast surgery; and nursing management after reconstructive breast surgery.

KEY TERMS

fibroadenoma, p. 1347
fibrocystic changes, p. 1346
galactorrhea, p. 1347
gynecomastia, p. 1347
lumpectomy, p. 1352
lymphedema, p. 1352
mammoplasty, p. 1361
mastalgia, p. 1345
mastectomy, p. 1351
mastitis, p. 1345
Paget's disease, p. 1350

Electronic Resources

Supplemental content related to Chapter 52 can be found . . .

Companion CD
- Stress-Busting Kit for Nursing Students
- Interactive Case Study: Breast Cancer
- NCLEX Examination Review Questions
- Comprehensive Glossary

Evolve Website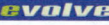
http://evolve.elsevier.com/Lewis/medsurg
- Content Updates
- Key Points (Printable and CD/MP3 Download)
- Concept Map Creator
- Expanded Audio Glossary
- Key Term Flash Cards

- Customizable Nursing Care Plan: Mastectomy or Lumpectomy
- Electronic Calculators
- WebLinks

Breast disorders are a significant health concern for women. Although most breast pain is of a benign nature, in a woman's lifetime there is a one in seven chance that she will be diagnosed with breast cancer.[1] Whether benign or malignant, intense feelings of shock, fear, and denial often accompany the initial discovery of a lump or change in the breast. These feelings can be associated both with the fear of death and with the possible loss of a breast. Throughout history, the female breast has been regarded as a symbol of beauty, femininity, sexuality, and motherhood. The potential loss of a breast, or part of a breast, may be devastating for many women because of the significant psychologic, social, sexual, and body image implications associated with it. The most frequently encountered breast disorders in women are fibrocystic changes, breast cancer, fibroadenoma, intraductal papilloma, and ductal ectasia. In men, gynecomastia is the most common breast disorder.

ASSESSMENT OF BREAST DISORDERS

It is critical that breast disorders be detected early, diagnosed accurately, and treated promptly. Guidelines established in the United States by the American Cancer Society (ACS) and the National Cancer Institute (NCI) for breast cancer screening offer specific guidance for older women, women who have serious health problems, and women at increased risk. Screening guidelines for the early detection of breast cancer include the following.[2]

Reviewed by Karen K. Swenson, RN, PhD(c), AOCN, Oncology Research Manager, Park Nicollet Institute, St. Louis Park, Minn.

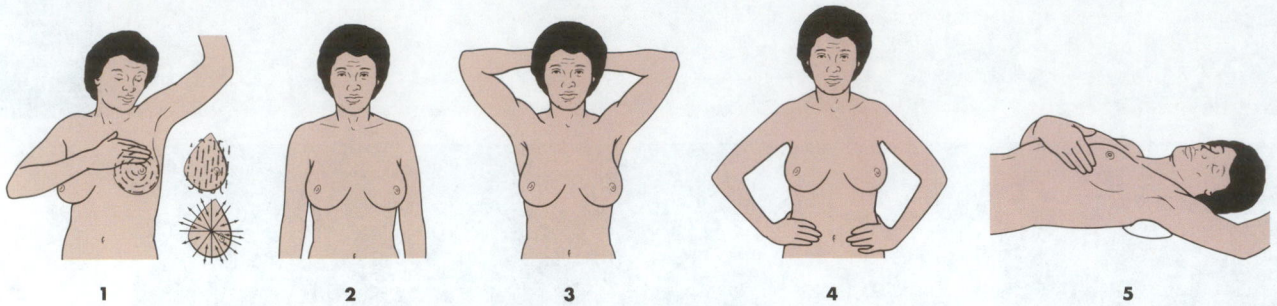

FIG. 52-1 Breast self-examination and patient instruction. *1,* While in the shower or bath, when the skin is slippery with soap and water, examine your breasts. Use the pads of your second, third, and fourth fingers to firmly press every part of the breast. While examining your left breast, use your right hand, and use your left hand to examine your right breast. Using the pads of the fingers on your left hand, examine the entire breast using small circular motions in a spiral or in an up-and-down motion so that the entire breast area is examined. Repeat the procedure using your right hand to examine your left breast. Repeat pattern of palpation under the arm. Check for any lump, hard knot, or thickening of the tissue. *2,* Look at your breasts in a mirror. Stand with your arms at your sides. *3,* Raise your arms overhead and check for any changes in the shape of your breasts, dimpling of the skin, or any changes in the nipple. *4,* Next, place your hands on your hips and press down firmly, tightening the pectoral muscles. Observe for asymmetry or changes, keeping in mind that your breasts probably do not exactly match. *5,* While lying down, feel your breasts as described in step 1. When examining your right breast, place a folded towel under your right shoulder and put your right hand behind your head. Repeat the procedure while examining your left breast.

1. Yearly mammograms starting at age 40 and continuing for as long as a woman is in good health.
2. Clinical breast examination (CBE) about every 3 years for women between ages 20 and 30 and every year for women beginning at age 40.
3. Women should report any breast changes promptly to their health care provider. Breast self-examination (BSE) is an option for women starting at age 20.
4. Women at increased risk (family history, genetic tendency, past breast cancer) should talk with their health care provider about the benefits and limitations of starting mammography screening earlier, having additional tests (e.g., breast ultrasound), or having more frequent examinations.

In recent years there has been some controversy regarding the value of BSE and its role in reducing mortality rates from breast cancer in women.[3] While the benefit of BSE in reducing breast cancer deaths is currently being reviewed, BSE remains a useful technique in helping women become self-aware of how their breasts normally look and feel. The nurse should teach women beginning at age 20 the benefits and limitations of BSE, and the importance of reporting any new breast changes (e.g., nipple discharge, finding a lump) to their health care provider.[4]

Techniques for teaching BSE should include allowing time for the woman to ask questions about the procedure and to perform a return demonstration. At every periodic health examination the health care provider should ask the woman who is performing BSE to demonstrate her technique. For women who choose to do BSE, the technique has been established by the ACS (available at *www.cancer.org*) and the NCI (Fig. 52-1). BSE should be done monthly when the breasts are not tender. For women who are having regular menstrual periods this would be right after the period. If the period is irregular, the same day each month should be picked so it is easy to remember. For women taking oral contraceptives the first day of a new package may be a helpful reminder. Postmenopausal women and women who have had hysterectomies often use the monthly date of a birthday or the first day of the month.

Diagnostic Studies

Several techniques can be used to screen for breast disease or provide a diagnosis of a suspicious physical finding. *Mammography* is a method used to visualize the internal structure of the breast using

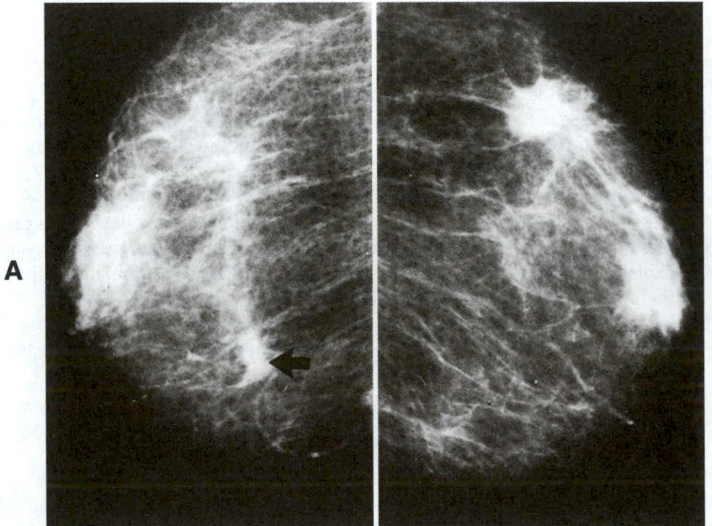

FIG. 52-2 Mammogram showing bilateral invasive ductal carcinoma. **A,** Left breast. The larger mass was palpable. The smaller right mass was not palpable *(arrow).* **B,** Right breast. Multiple masses are shown.

x-rays (Fig. 52-2). This simple, safe procedure can detect tumors and cysts that cannot be felt by palpation. Mammography has significantly improved the early and accurate detection of breast malignancies. Improved imaging techniques have also reduced the radiation that accompanies mammography to insignificant levels.

Digital mammography is a newer technique in which x-ray images are digitally coded into a computer. This allows for a clearer and more accurate image than conventional mammography x-ray film.

The minimum size of a tumor detectable by physical examination is 1 cm. It may take 10 years or longer for a tumor to grow to this size. Mammography can detect smaller masses depending on the equipment and whether malignant calcifications are present.

Calcifications are the most easily recognized mammogram abnormality. These deposits of calcium crystals form in the breast for many reasons, such as inflammation, trauma, and aging. Although most calcifications are benign, they also may be associated with preinvasive cancer.[5]

A comparison of current and prior mammograms may show early cancer tissue changes. Because some tumors metastasize late in the preclinical course, early detection by mammography allows for early treatment and the prevention of metastasis of these smaller lesions. In younger women mammography is less sensitive because of the greater density of breast tissue, resulting in more false-negative results.[6] About 10% to 15% of all breast cancers cannot be seen on mammography and are detected only by palpation. Suspicious masses should be biopsied even if mammogram findings are unremarkable.

Ultrasound is another diagnostic procedure that can be used to differentiate a benign tumor from a malignant tumor. It is particularly useful in women with fibrocystic changes whose breasts are very dense. Unlike a mammogram, an ultrasound will not detect microcalcifications.

Magnetic resonance imaging (MRI) may be used as a more sensitive nonspecific screening tool for women at high risk for breast cancer, or in women whose mammography or ultrasound is suspicious for malignancy. Limitations to MRI use include its high cost and greater rate of false positives when compared with mammography.[7]

A definitive diagnosis of a suspicious area is often made by means of histologic examination of biopsied tissue. Biopsy techniques include fine-needle aspiration (FNA) biopsy, stereotactic or ultrasound core biopsy, and open surgical biopsy.

FNA biopsy is performed by inserting a needle into the lesion and aspirating cellular fluid into a syringe. Three or four passes are usually made. FNA and cytologic evaluation may be helpful in making a diagnosis and planning treatment. It should be done only if an experienced cytologist is available and all suspicious lesions read as negative are followed with a more definitive biopsy procedure. If the aspirated specimen is positive for malignancy, the patient can be given this information at the same visit.

Stereotactic and ultrasound core biopsy are reliable diagnostic techniques for obtaining a biopsy of an abnormality seen on a mammogram. In this procedure mammography is used to locate the lesion. The skin is anesthetized, and a small skin incision is made to allow the entrance of a biopsy gun device. The gun is fired

and removes a core sample of the lesion. This is repeated several times, and the core samples are sent for pathologic analysis. This technique has several advantages over an open surgical biopsy, including minimal scarring, the use of local anesthesia, outpatient procedure, reduced cost, and shorter recovery time.[8]

Benign Breast Disorders

MASTALGIA

Mastalgia (breast pain) is the most common breast-related complaint in women. It affects up to 70% of all women at some time in their lives.[9] The most common form is *cyclic mastalgia,* which coincides with the menstrual cycle. It is described as diffuse breast tenderness or heaviness. Breast pain may last 2 to 3 days or most of the month. The pain is related to hormonal sensitivity. The symptoms often decrease with menopause. *Noncyclic mastalgia* has no relationship to the menstrual cycle and can continue into menopause. It may be constant or intermittent throughout the month and last for several years. Symptoms include a burning, aching, or soreness in the breast. The etiology of the pain may be due to trauma, fat necrosis, or ductal ectasia.

Mammography is frequently done to exclude cancer and provide information on the etiology of mastalgia. Some relief may occur with caffeine and dietary fat reduction; taking vitamins E, A, and B complex and gamma-linolenic acid (evening primrose oil); and the continual wearing of a support bra. Hormonal therapy may be recommended, including oral contraceptives and danazol (Danocrine).

BREAST INFECTIONS

Mastitis

Mastitis is an inflammatory condition of the breast that occurs most frequently in lactating women (Table 52-1). *Lactational mastitis* manifests as a localized area that is erythematous, painful, and

TABLE 52-1	Selected Benign Breast Disorders	
Disorder	**Risk Factors**	**Clinical Manifestations**
Lactation mastitis	Lactating woman Occurs spontaneously in approximately 2% of all postpartum lactating mothers (both primipara and multipara), usually 2-4 wk after birth	Warm to touch Indurated Usually unilateral Most common etiology is *Staphylococcus aureus*
Nonlactation mastitis	Rare condition Usually women in late adolescence or middle age	Palpable mass Usually an obscure organism Should rule out syphilis or tuberculosis
Fibrocystic changes	Most common between ages 35 and 50	Not usually discrete masses, nodularity instead; usually accompanied by cyclic pain and tenderness; mass(es) usually cyclic in occurrence (movable, soft)
Cysts	Most common between ages 30 and 50	Palpable mass (movable, soft); may have multiple microcysts
Fibroadenoma	Peak age range between ages 15 and 25 Most occur before age 30 Most common among African American women	Often bilateral Palpable mass (movable, firm) Most common size at diagnosis is 2-3 cm Rapid growth Accounts for 2%-3% of all breast masses
Fat necrosis	50% report previous history of trauma to breast	Usually a hard, tender, mobile, indurated mass with irregular borders
Intraductal papilloma	Affects women ages 40-60	Usually associated with serous, serosanguineous, or bloody nipple discharge on affected side
Ductal ectasia	Perimenopausal woman—most common in women in their 50s Previous lactation Inverted nipples	Fixation of nipple Usually accompanied by nipple discharge of thick gray material Often associated with breast pain

tender to palpation. Fever is usually present. The infection develops when organisms, usually staphylococci, gain access to the breast through a cracked nipple. In its early stages, mastitis can be cured with antibiotics. Breastfeeding should continue unless an abscess is forming or a purulent drainage is noted. The mother may wish to use a nipple shield or to hand-express milk from the involved breast until the pain subsides. The woman should see her health care provider promptly to begin a course of antibiotic therapy. Any breast that remains red, tender, and not responsive to antibiotics requires follow-up care and evaluation for inflammatory breast cancer.

Lactational Breast Abscess

If lactational mastitis persists after several days of antibiotic therapy, a lactational breast abscess may have developed. In this condition the skin may become red and edematous over the involved breast, often with a corresponding palpable mass, and the patient may have an elevated temperature. Antibiotics alone constitute insufficient treatment for a breast abscess. Ultrasound-guided drainage of the abscess or surgical incision and drainage are necessary. The drainage is cultured, sensitivities are obtained, and therapy with an appropriate antibiotic is begun. Often the woman will find it necessary to express and discard milk from the affected breast until the abscess is resolved.

FIBROCYSTIC CHANGES

Fibrocystic changes in the breast constitute a benign condition characterized by changes in breast tissue (Fig. 52-3). The changes include the development of excess fibrous tissue, hyperplasia of the epithelial lining of the mammary ducts, proliferation of mammary ducts, and cyst formation. These changes produce pain by nerve irritation from edema in the connective tissue and by fibrosis from pinching of the nerve. The use of the term *fibrocystic disease* is incorrect because the cluster of problems is actually an exaggerated response to hormonal influence. It has been suggested that the term *fibrocystic condition* or *fibrocystic complex* be used. Fibrocystic changes do not increase the risk of breast cancer for the majority of patients. Masses or nodularities can appear in both breasts and are often found in the upper, outer quadrants and usually occur bilaterally. It is the most frequently occurring breast disorder.

Fibrocystic changes occur most frequently in women between 35 and 50 years of age but often begin in women as young as

20 years of age. Pain and nodularity often increase over time but tend to subside after menopause unless high doses of estrogen replacement are used. The cause of these fibrocystic changes is thought to be heightened responsiveness of breast tissue and stroma to circulating estrogen and progesterone.[10] Fibrocystic changes most commonly occur in women with premenstrual abnormalities, nulliparous women, women with a history of spontaneous abortion, nonusers of oral contraceptives, and women with early menarche and late menopause. Symptoms related to fibrocystic changes often worsen in the premenstrual phase and subside after menstruation.

Manifestations of fibrocystic breast changes include one or more palpable lumps that are usually round, well delineated, and freely movable within the breast (see Table 52-1). Some lumps are fibrous and do not contain cysts. There may be accompanying discomfort ranging from tenderness to pain. The lump is usually observed to increase in size and perhaps in tenderness before menstruation. Cysts may enlarge or shrink rapidly. Nipple discharge associated with fibrocystic breasts is often milky, watery-milky, yellow, or green.

Mammography may be helpful in distinguishing fibrocystic changes from breast cancer. However, in some women the breast tissue is so dense that it is difficult to obtain a worthwhile mammogram study. In these situations, ultrasound may be more useful in differentiating a cystic mass from a solid mass.

NURSING *and* COLLABORATIVE MANAGEMENT
FIBROCYSTIC CHANGES

With the initial discovery of a discrete mass in the breast by a woman or her health care provider, aspiration or surgical biopsy may be indicated. A wait of 7 to 10 days may be planned if the nodularity is recurrent to note changes as the menstrual cycle changes. With large or frequent cysts, surgical removal may be favored over repeated aspiration. An excisional biopsy should be done (1) if no fluid is found on aspiration, (2) if the fluid that is found is hemorrhagic, or (3) if a residual mass remains. This surgery is performed in an office or day surgery unit.

Biopsies in women with fibrocystic disease may be indicated for women with an increased risk for breast cancer. Atypical hyperplasia discovered by breast biopsy increases a woman's risk of developing breast cancer later in life.

The woman with cystic changes should be encouraged to return regularly for follow-up examinations throughout her life. She may also be taught BSE to self-monitor the problem. Severe fibrocystic changes may make palpation of the breast more difficult. Any new lumps or changes in the breasts should be evaluated. Changes in symptoms should be reported and investigated.

Many types of treatment have been suggested for a fibrocystic condition. These include the use of a good support bra, dietary therapy (low-salt diet, restriction of methylxanthines such as coffee and chocolate), vitamin E therapy, analgesics, danazol (Danocrine), diuretics, hormone therapy, and antiestrogen therapy. Because stress can be a contributing factor in breast discomfort, efforts should also be directed toward the reduction of stress. Although many of these treatments have not been scientifically proven to be beneficial, many women report less discomfort with these nonsurgical measures. Danazol has been used for patients with severe pain. It decreases follicle-stimulating hormone (FSH) and luteinizing hormone (LH), resulting in reduced estrogen pro-

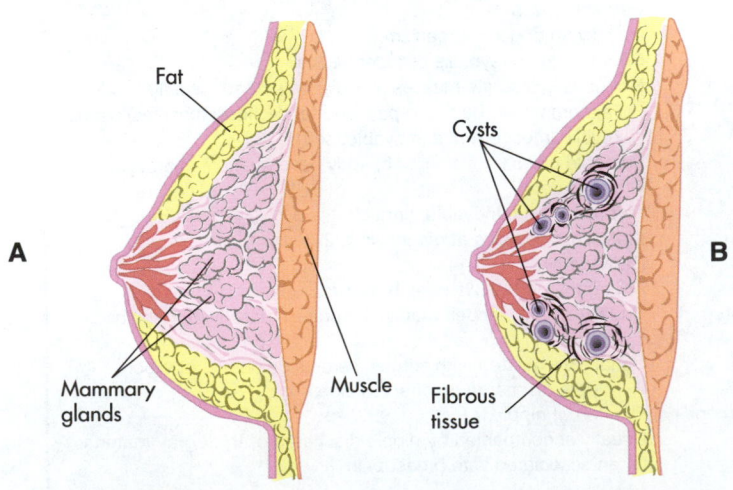

FIG. 52-3   **A,** Normal breast tissue. **B,** Fibrocystic breast tissue.

A

Fat

Mammary glands

Muscle

Cysts

B

Fibrous tissue

duction and subsequent decreased pain and nodularity.[11] The androgenic side effects of danazol (acne, edema, hirsutism) often make this therapy intolerable for many women.

The role of the nurse in the care of the patient with fibrocystic breast changes is primarily one of teaching. A woman with fibrocystic breasts should be told that she may expect recurrence of the cysts in one or both breasts until menopause and that cysts may enlarge or become painful just before menstruation. Additionally, she should be reassured that cysts do not "turn into" cancer. Any new lump that does not respond in a cyclic manner over 1 to 2 weeks should be examined by a health care provider promptly.

FIBROADENOMA

Fibroadenoma is a common cause of discrete benign breast lumps in young women. It generally occurs in women between 15 and 25 years of age. It is the most frequent cause of breast masses in women under 25 years of age. Fibroadenomas tend to develop more frequently and at a younger age in African American women.[12] The possible cause of fibroadenoma may be increased estrogen sensitivity in a localized area of the breast. Fibroadenomas are usually small (but can be large [2 to 3 cm]), painless, round, well delineated, and very mobile. They may be soft but are usually solid, firm, and rubbery in consistency. There is no accompanying retraction or nipple discharge. The lump is often painless. The fibroadenoma may appear as a single unilateral mass, although multiple bilateral fibroadenomas have been reported. Growth is slow and often ceases when size reaches 2 to 3 cm. Size is not affected by menstruation. However, pregnancy can stimulate dramatic growth. Fibroadenomas are rarely associated with cancer.

NURSING *and* COLLABORATIVE MANAGEMENT FIBROADENOMA

Fibroadenomas are easily detected by physical examination and are often visible on mammography and ultrasound. Definitive diagnosis, however, requires biopsy and tissue examination by a pathologist. Treatment of fibroadenomas can include surgical excision, which is not urgent in women less than 25 years of age. In women over 35 years of age all new lesions should be evaluated by breast ultrasound and possible biopsy. Fibroadenomas are not reduced by radiation and are not affected by hormone therapy.

As an alternative to surgery, tumor removal can be accomplished using *cryoablation* after an established diagnosis of a fibroadenoma. In this procedure a cryoprobe is inserted into the tumor using ultrasound guidance. Extremely cold gas is piped into the tumor. The frozen tumor dies and gradually shrinks.

The nurse frequently has the opportunity to counsel a young woman with fibroadenomas. During this contact the benign nature of the lesion should be stressed and follow-up examinations should be encouraged.

NIPPLE DISCHARGE

Nipple discharge may occur spontaneously or as a result of nipple manipulation. A milky secretion is due to inappropriate lactation (termed **galactorrhea**) as a result of such problems as drug therapy, endocrine problems, and neurologic disorders. Nipple discharge may also be idiopathic.

Secretions can also be serous, grossly bloody, or brown to green. These may be caused by either benign or malignant disease.

A slide can be made of the secretion to detect specific disease. Diseases associated with nipple discharge include malignancies, cystic disease, intraductal papilloma, and ductal ectasia. Treatment depends on identification of the cause.[13] In most cases, nipple discharge is not related to malignancy. If galactorrhea is accompanied by amenorrhea, various gynecologic endocrinopathies should be explored.

Intraductal Papilloma

An **intraductal papilloma** is a benign, wartlike growth found in the mammary ducts, usually near the nipple. Typically, there is an associated bloody nipple discharge, a mass, or both. Intraductal papillomas usually affect women 40 to 60 years of age. A single duct or several ducts may be involved. Treatment includes excision of the papilloma and the involved duct or duct system.

Ductal Ectasia

Ductal ectasia is a benign breast disease of perimenopausal and postmenopausal women involving the ducts in the subareolar area. It usually involves several bilateral ducts. Nipple discharge is the primary symptom. This discharge is multicolored and sticky. Ductal ectasia is initially painless but may progress to burning, itching, and pain around the nipple, as well as swelling in the areolar area. Inflammatory signs are often present, the nipple may retract, and the discharge may become bloody in more advanced disease. Ductal ectasia is not associated with malignancy. If an abscess develops, warm compresses and antibiotics are usually effective treatments. Therapy consists of close follow-up examinations or surgical excision of the involved ducts.

GYNECOMASTIA IN MEN

Gynecomastia, a transient, noninflammatory enlargement of one or both breasts, is the most common breast problem in men (Fig. 52-4). The condition is usually temporary and benign. Gynecomastia in itself is not an established risk factor for breast cancer. The most common cause of gynecomastia is a disturbance of the normal ratio of active androgen to estrogen in plasma or within the breast itself.

Gynecomastia may also be a manifestation of other problems. It is seen accompanying developmental abnormalities of the male reproductive organs. It may also accompany organic diseases, including testicular tumors, cancer of the adrenal cortex, pituitary adenomas, hyperthyroidism, and liver disease.[14] Gynecomastia

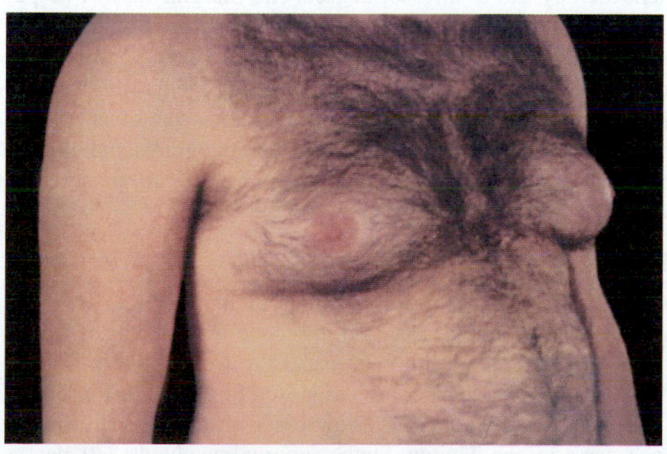

FIG. 52-4   Gynecomastia.

may occur as a side effect of drug therapy, particularly with administration of estrogens and androgens, digitalis, isoniazid (INH), ranitidine (Zantac), and spironolactone (Aldactone). Use of heroin and marijuana can also cause gynecomastia.

Pubertal Gynecomastia

Pubertal gynecomastia caused by increased estrogen production is seen most often in boys between ages 13 and 17. It is usually limited, although occasionally the localized hyperplasia may measure 2 to 3 cm in size. Pubertal gynecomastia is almost always self-limiting, and disappears within 4 to 6 months of onset. Parents and the affected boy should be reassured that in almost all cases this is a normal physiologic phenomenon that will disappear spontaneously and will require no treatment. Rarely, unilateral gynecomastia in the young male may be marked and fail to regress. This is the only indication for surgical intervention (i.e., mastectomy).

Senescent Gynecomastia

Senescent gynecomastia occurs in 40% of older men. A probable cause is the elevation in plasma estrogen in older adult men as the result of increased conversion of androgens to estrogens in peripheral circulation. Although initially unilateral, the tender, firm, centrally located enlargement may become bilateral. When gynecomastia is characterized by a discrete, circumscribed mass, it must be diagnosed to differentiate it from the rarer breast cancer in males. Senescent hyperplasia requires no treatment and generally regresses within 6 to 12 months.

GERONTOLOGIC CONSIDERATIONS
AGE-RELATED BREAST CHANGES

Loss of subcutaneous fat and structural support and atrophy of mammary glands often result in pendulous breasts in the postmenopausal woman. The nurse should encourage older women to wear a well-fitting bra. Adequate support can improve physical appearance and reduce pain in the back, shoulders, and neck. It can also prevent *intertrigo* (dermatitis caused by friction between opposing surfaces of skin). Surgical lifting of sagging breasts is possible and may be desirable when reconstruction after a mastectomy is performed.

The decrease in glandular tissue in older women makes a breast mass easier to palpate. This decreased density is probably age related and occurs even with women on hormone replacement therapy, but to a lesser degree. Rib margins may be palpable in the older adult woman and can be confused with a mass. As a woman becomes more familiar with her own breasts and is reassured about her findings, the anxiety about this finding should decrease. The nurse should encourage the older woman to continue BSE and to have annual mammograms and clinical examinations because the incidence of breast cancer increases with age.

BREAST CANCER

Breast cancer is the most common malignancy in American women except for skin cancer. It is second only to lung cancer as the leading cause of death from cancer in women. Over 211,000 new cases of breast cancer are diagnosed in women in the United States each year. About 1700 new cases are diagnosed in men.[1] Each year in the United States, approximately 40,870 deaths (40,410 women and 460 men) occur related to breast cancer. The

---

CULTURAL AND ETHNIC HEALTH DISPARITIES
Breast Cancer

- African American women have lower survival rates from breast cancer than white women, even when diagnosed at an early stage.
- White women have a higher incidence of breast cancer than nonwhites.
- Breast cancer incidence and mortality rates are lower among Hispanic and Asian/Pacific Islander women than among white and African American women.
- Breast cancer is the most commonly diagnosed cancer among Hispanic women.
- Hispanic women, especially Mexican Americans, have the lowest rate of cancer screening of any ethnic group.
- Hispanic women are more likely to be diagnosed at a later stage of breast cancer than white women.

---

incidence rate of breast cancer is slowly increasing, with a slight decline in the number of deaths related to breast cancer. The largest decreases have been noted in younger women, including both African American and white women.

Patients diagnosed with localized breast cancer with no axillary node involvement have a 5-year survival rate of 98%. Conversely, only 6% of patients diagnosed with advanced-stage breast cancer with metastases to distant sites will survive 5 years or more.[15]

Etiology and Risk Factors

Although the etiology is not completely understood, a number of factors are thought to relate to the cause of breast cancer. Heredity or genetically related susceptibility is considered to play a role. Hormonal regulation of the breast is related to the development of breast cancer, but the mechanisms are poorly understood. Sex hormones may act as tumor promoters if initiating agents have induced malignant changes. Additional factors include weight gain during adulthood, dietary fat intake, obesity, and alcohol intake.[15] Environmental factors such as radiation exposure may also play a role.

Some factors that place a woman at higher risk for breast cancer have been identified (Table 52-2). Women are at far greater risk than men because 99% of breast cancers occur in women. Increasing age also increases the risk of developing breast cancer. The incidence of breast cancer in women under 25 years of age is very low and increases gradually until age 60. After age 60 the incidence increases dramatically. Family history is an important risk factor, especially if the involved family member also had ovarian cancer, was premenopausal, had bilateral breast cancer, and/or is a first-degree relative (i.e., mother, sister, daughter). Having any first-degree relative with breast cancer increases a woman's risk of breast cancer 1.5 to 3 times, depending on age. Data from the Women's Health Initiative study has shown that the use of combined hormone replacement therapy (estrogen plus progesterone) increases the risk of breast cancer while also increasing the risk of having a larger, more advanced breast cancer at diagnosis.[16] The use of estrogen replacement therapy alone (for women who have had a prior hysterectomy) does not currently appear to increase breast cancer risk.[17] A link may exist between recent oral contraceptive use and increased risk of breast cancer for women under age 35.[18]

TABLE 52-2	Risk Factors for Breast Cancer

Increased Risk	Comments
Female	Women account for 99% of breast cancer cases.
Age 50 or over	Majority of breast cancers are found in postmenopausal women. After age 60 great increase in incidence.
Family history	Breast cancer in a first-degree relative, particularly when premenopausal or bilateral, increases risk. Gene mutations (BRCA-1 or BRCA-2) play a role in 5%-10% of breast cancer cases.
Personal history of breast cancer, colon cancer, endometrial cancer, ovarian cancer	Personal history significantly increases risk of breast cancer, risk of cancer in other breast, and recurrence.
Early menarche (before age 12); late menopause (after age 55)	A long menstrual history increases the risk of breast cancer.
First full-term pregnancy after age 30; nulliparity	Prolonged exposure to unopposed estrogen increases risk for breast cancer.
Benign breast disease with atypical epithelial hyperplasia, lobular carcinoma in situ	Atypical changes in breast biopsy increase the risk of breast cancer.
Weight gain and obesity after menopause	Fat cells store estrogen.
Exposure to ionizing radiation	Radiation damages DNA (e.g., prior treatment for Hodgkin's lymphoma).

Risk factors appear to be cumulative and interacting. Therefore the presence of other risk factors may greatly increase the overall risk, especially for those with a positive family history. Identification of risk factors indicates an increased need for careful clinical surveillance of the patient and participation in cancer screening measures. However, most women who develop breast cancer have none of the identifiable risk factors.

As many as 5% to 10% of all breast cancer patients may have inherited a specific genetic abnormality contributing to the development of their breast cancer. The first genetic alteration to be identified was in the tumor suppressor gene, p53. The BRCA-1 gene, located on chromosome 17, is a tumor suppressor gene that inhibits tumor development when functioning normally. Women who have BRCA-1 mutations have a 40% to 80% lifetime chance of developing breast cancer.[19] The BRCA-2 gene, located on chromosome 11, is another tumor suppressor gene. Women with a mutation of this gene have a similar risk of breast cancer. Mutations in BRCA genes may cause as many as 10% to 40% of all inherited breast cancers. As many as 1 in 200 to 400 women in the United States may be carriers for these genetic abnormalities. These women are also at high risk for developing ovarian cancer. Routine screening for genetic abnormalities in women without evidence of a strong family history of breast cancer is not warranted.

In women with BRCA-1 or BRCA-2 mutations, prophylactic bilateral oophorectomy can decrease the risk of breast cancer and ovarian cancer.[20] In deciding whether to undergo this surgical procedure, women should take into account how long they wish to maintain fertility. In addition, they should receive counseling about the risks and benefits of prophylactic oophorectomy.

A woman who has a high risk of developing breast cancer (i.e., related to factors such as family history and prior tissue biopsies) may choose (in consultation with her physician) to undergo prophylactic bilateral mastectomy. This surgery may reduce a women's breast cancer risk by 90%.[21]

Women with hereditary (non-BRCA) breast cancer have a higher risk of developing a secondary primary breast cancer in the unaffected breast. These women may also choose to have the unaffected breast removed prophylactically at the time of initial surgery for breast cancer or at a later time.

Predisposing risk factors for breast cancer in men include states of hyperestrogenism, a family history of breast cancer, and radiation exposure. A thorough examination of the male breast should be a routine part of a physical examination for all men.

GENETICS IN CLINICAL PRACTICE
Breast Cancer

Genetic Basis
- Mutations in genes BRCA-1 and BRCA-2
- Autosomal dominant transmission

Incidence
- Approximately 5% to 10% of breast cancers are related to BRCA-1 and BRCA-2 gene mutations.
- Women with BRCA-1 and BRCA-2 gene mutations have a 40% to 80% lifetime risk of developing breast cancer.
- BRCA-1 and BRCA-2 gene mutations are associated with early-onset breast cancer.
- Family history of both breast and ovarian cancer increases the risk of having a BRCA mutation.

Genetic Testing
- DNA testing is available for BRCA-1 and BRCA-2.

Clinical Implications
- Bilateral oophorectomy reduces the risk of breast cancer in women with BRCA-1 and BRCA-2 mutations.
- Genetic counseling and testing for BRCA mutations should be considered for women whose personal or family history puts them at high risk for a genetic predisposition to breast cancer.

Pathophysiology

Various types of breast cancer have been identified based on their histologic characteristics and growth patterns (Table 52-3). The main components of the breast are lobules (milk-producing glands) and ducts (milk passages that connect the lobules and the nipple). In general, breast cancer arises from the epithelial lining of the ducts (ductal carcinoma) or from the epithelium of the lobules (lobular carcinoma). Breast cancers may be invasive or in situ. Most breast cancers arise from the ducts and are invasive.

The natural history of breast cancer varies considerably from patient to patient. Cancer growth rate can range from slow to rapid. Factors that affect cancer prognosis are size, axillary node involvement (the more nodes involved, the worse the prognosis), tumor differentiation, *human epidermal growth factor receptor 2* (HER-2) status, and estrogen and progesterone receptor status. (HER-2 is a transmembrane receptor that helps regulate cell growth. In many patients with breast cancer it is overexpressed.) The histologic type

TABLE 52-3	Types of Breast Cancer
Type	**Frequency of Occurrence**
Infiltrating ductal carcinoma	63%-68%
• Colloid (mucinous)	
• Inflammatory	
• Paget's disease	
• Medullary	
• Papillary	
• Tubular	
Infiltrating lobular carcinoma	10%-15%
Noninvasive	22%
• Ductal carcinoma in situ	

of breast cancer seems to have little prognostic significance once the cancer has metastasized.

Noninvasive Breast Cancer. The increased use of screening mammography has led to more women being diagnosed with noninvasive breast cancer. An estimated 22% of all diagnosed breast cancer cases are noninvasive. These intraductal cancers include *ductal carcinoma in situ* (DCIS) and *lobular carcinoma in situ* (LCIS). DCIS tends to be unilateral and most likely would progress to invasive breast cancer (usually infiltrating ductal cell carcinoma) if left untreated.

Although the management of DCIS can be controversial, patients should discuss all treatment options with their physician, including local excision, mastectomy with breast reconstruction, breast-conserving treatment (lumpectomy), radiation therapy, and/or tamoxifen (Nolvadex).

The term *lobular carcinoma in situ* is somewhat misleading. Although LCIS is a risk factor for developing breast cancer, it is not known to be a premalignant lesion. No treatment is necessary for LCIS. Tamoxifen may be given as a chemoprevention agent in some patients.

Paget's Disease. **Paget's disease** is a rare breast malignancy characterized by a persistent lesion of the nipple and areola with or without a palpable mass. (This is different from Paget's disease of the bone, which is discussed in Chapter 64.) Itching, burning, bloody nipple discharge with superficial erosion, and ulceration may be present. Diagnosis of Paget's disease is confirmed by pathologic examination of the erosion. Nipple changes are often diagnosed as an infection or dermatitis, which can lead to treatment delays. The treatment of Paget's disease is a simple or modified radical mastectomy. Prognosis is good when the cancer is confined to the nipple. The nursing care for the patient with Paget's disease is the same as the care for a patient with breast cancer.

Inflammatory Breast Cancer. *Inflammatory breast cancer,* the most malignant form of all breast cancers, is rare. It is an aggressive and fast-growing cancer. The skin of the breast looks red, feels warm, and has a thickened appearance that is often described as resembling an orange peel (peau d'orange). Sometimes the breast develops ridges and small bumps that look like hives. The inflammatory changes, often mistaken for an infection, are caused by cancer cells blocking lymph channels. Metastases occur early and widely. Radiation therapy, chemotherapy, and hormone therapy are more likely to be used for treatment than surgery.

Clinical Manifestations

Breast cancer is detected as a lump or mammographic abnormality in the breast. It occurs most often in the upper, outer quadrant of the breast because it is the location of most of the glandular

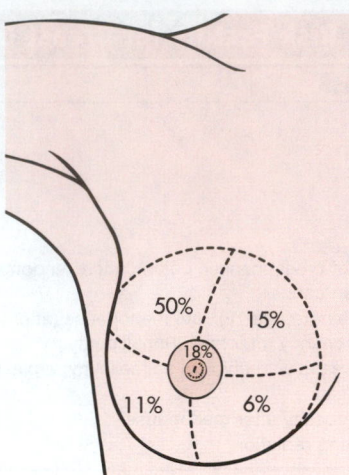

FIG. 52-5   Distribution of where breast cancer occurs.

tissue (Fig. 52-5). The rate at which the lesion grows varies considerably. Slow-growing lesions are often associated with a lower mortality rate. If palpable, breast cancer is characteristically hard, and may be irregularly shaped, poorly delineated, nonmobile, and nontender.

A small percentage of breast cancers cause nipple discharge. The discharge is usually unilateral and may be clear or bloody. Nipple retraction may occur. Peau d'orange may occur due to the plugging of the dermal lymphatics. In large cancers, infiltration, induration, and dimpling (pulling in) of the overlying skin may also be noted.

Complications

The main complication of breast cancer is recurrence (Table 52-4). Recurrence may be local or regional (skin or soft tissue near the mastectomy site, axillary or internal mammary lymph nodes) or distant (most commonly involving the bone, lung, brain, and liver). However, metastatic disease can be found in any distant site.

Widely disseminated or metastatic disease involves the growth of colonies of cancerous breast cells in parts of the body distant from the breast. Metastases primarily occur through the lymphatics, principally those of the axilla (see Chapter 51, Fig. 51-7). However, the cancer can spread to other parts of the body without invading the axillary nodes even when the primary breast tumor is small. Even in node-negative breast cancer, there is a possibility of distant metastasis.

Diagnostic Studies

In addition to studies used to diagnose breast cancer (see earlier discussion in this chapter), other tests are useful in predicting the risk of recurrence or metastatic breast disease. These tests include axillary lymph node status, tumor size, estrogen and progesterone receptor status, and cell proliferative indices. Many of these diagnostic studies are useful prognostic indicators of the disease.

Axillary lymph node involvement is one of the most important prognostic factors in breast cancer.[22] An axillary lymph node dissection is often performed to determine if cancer has spread to the axilla on the side of the breast cancer. The more nodes involved, the greater the risk of recurrence. Patients with four or more positive nodes have the greatest risk of recurrence.

TABLE 52-4	Common Sites of Breast Cancer Recurrence and Metastasis
Site	**Clinical Presentation**
Local Recurrence	
Skin	Firm, discrete nodules; occasionally pruritic, usually painless
Regional Recurrence	
Lymph nodes	Enlarged nodes in axilla or supraclavicular area, usually nontender
Distant Metastasis	
Skeletal	Localized pain of gradually increasing intensity, percussion tenderness at involved sites, pathologic fracture caused by involvement of bone cortex
Spinal cord	Progressive back pain, localized and radiating
Brain	Headache described as "different," unilateral sensory loss, focal muscular weakness, hemiparesis, incoordination (ataxia)
Pulmonary (including lung nodules and pleural effusions)	Shortness of breath, tachypnea, nonproductive cough (not present in all patients)
Liver	Abdominal distention; right lower quadrant abdominal pain sometimes with radiation to scapular area; nausea and vomiting, anorexia, weight loss; weakness and fatigue; hepatomegaly, ascites, jaundice; peripheral edema; elevated liver enzymes
Bone marrow	Anemia; infection; increased bleeding, bruising, petechiae; weakness and fatigue; mild confusion, light-headedness; dyspnea

TABLE 52-5	COLLABORATIVE CARE Breast Cancer

Diagnostic
History, including risk factors
Physical examination, including breast and lymphatics
Mammography
Ultrasound
Biopsy
MRI (if indicated)

Staging Workup
Complete blood count, platelet count
Calcium and phosphorus levels
Liver function tests
Chest x-ray
Bone scan (if indicated)
CT scan of chest, abdomen, pelvis (if indicated)
MRI (if indicated)

Collaborative Therapy
Surgery
  • Breast-conserving (lumpectomy) with sentinel lymph node biopsy/dissection and/or axillary lymph node dissection
  • Modified radical mastectomy (may include reconstruction)
Radiation therapy
  • Primary radiotherapy
  • Adjuvant radiotherapy
  • High-dose brachytherapy
  • Palliative radiotherapy
Chemotherapy
  • Adjuvant chemotherapy
  • Chemotherapy for recurrent disease
Hormonal therapy (see Table 52-8)
Biologic and targeted therapy

CT, Computed tomography; *MRI,* magnetic resonance imaging.

Lymphatic mapping and *sentinel lymph node dissection* (SLND) helps the surgeon identify the lymph node(s) that drain first from the tumor site *(sentinel node).*[22] A radioisotope and/or blue dye is injected into the tumor site, and intraoperatively, it is determined in which sentinel lymph nodes (SLNs) the radioisotope and/or blue dye is located. A local incision is made in the axilla, and the surgeon dissects the blue-stained and/or the radioactive SLNs. Generally with an SLND, one to four axillary lymph nodes are removed. The nodes are then sent for a frozen section pathologic analysis. If the SLNs are negative, no further axillary surgery is required. If the SLNs are positive, a complete axillary dissection is usually done. SLND has been associated with lower morbidity rates and greater accuracy as compared with complete axillary node dissection.[23]

Tumor size is a valuable prognostic variable: the larger the tumor, the poorer the prognosis. The wide variety of histologic types of breast cancer explains the heterogeneity of the disease. In general, the more well differentiated the tumor, the less aggressive it is. Poorly differentiated tumors appear morphologically disorganized and are more aggressive.

Another diagnostic test useful both for treatment decisions and prediction of prognosis is estrogen and progesterone receptor status. Receptor-positive tumors (1) commonly show histologic evidence of being well differentiated, (2) frequently have a *diploid* (more normal) DNA content and low proliferative indices, (3) have a lower chance for recurrence, and (4) are frequently hormone dependent and responsive to hormonal therapy.

Receptor-negative tumors (1) are often poorly differentiated histologically, (2) have a high incidence of *aneuploidy* (abnormally high or low DNA content) and higher proliferative indices, (3) frequently recur, and (4) are usually unresponsive to hormonal therapy.

Ploidy status correlates with tumor aggressiveness. Diploid tumors have been shown to have a significantly lower risk of recurrence than aneuploid tumors.

Cell-proliferative indices indirectly measure the rate of tumor cell proliferation. The percent of tumor cells in the synthesis (S) phase of the cell cycle (see Chapter 16, Fig. 16-1) is another important prognostic indicator. Patients with cells that have high S-phase fractions have a higher risk for recurrence and earlier cancer death.

Another prognostic indicator is the marker HER-2. Overexpression of this receptor has been associated with a greater risk for recurrence and a poorer prognosis in breast cancer. Between 25% and 30% of metastatic breast cancers produce excessive HER-2. High numbers of HER-2 receptors are associated with unusually aggressive tumor growth.[24] The presence of this marker assists in the selection and sequence of chemotherapy and predicting a patient's response to treatment.

Collaborative Care

Historically, a **mastectomy** (removal of breast, pectoral muscles, axillary lymph nodes, and all fat and adjacent tissue) was the standard of care. Presently a wide range of treatment options is available to both the patient and the health care providers attempting to make critical decisions about what treatment to select (Table 52-5).

Reproductive System

TABLE 52-6	Staging of Breast Cancer		
Stage	**Tumor Size**	**Lymph Node Involvement**	**Metastasis**
I	<2 cm	No	No
II			
A	No evidence of tumor, ranges to 5 cm	No, or 1-3 axillary nodes and/or internal mammary nodes	No
B	Ranging from 2 to >5 cm	No, or 1-3 axillary nodes and/or internal mammary nodes	No
III			
A	No evidence of tumor ranging to >5 cm	Yes, 4-9 axillary nodes and/or internal mammary nodes	No
B	Any size with extension to chest wall or skin	Yes, 4-9 axillary nodes and/or internal mammary lymph nodes	No
C	Any size	Yes, 10 or more axillary nodes, internal mammary nodes, or infraclavicular nodes	No
IV	Any size	Any type of nodal involvement	Yes

Adapted from Singletary SE, Allred C, Ashley P, et al: Revision of the American Joint Committee on Cancer staging system for breast cancer, *J Clin Oncol* 20:3628, 2002.

Prognostic factors are considered when treatment decisions are made about a specific breast cancer. Some of these factors also enter into the staging of breast cancer. The most widely accepted staging method for breast cancer is the American Joint Committee on Cancer's TNM system.[25] This system uses tumor size (T), nodal involvement (N), and presence of metastasis (M) to determine the stage of disease. The stage of a breast cancer describes its size and the extent to which it has spread (Table 52-6).

The stages range from I to IV, with stage I being very small tumors (less than 2 cm) with no lymph node involvement and no metastasis. Further classification within these stages depends on the size of the tumor and the number of lymph nodes involved. Stage IV indicates the presence of metastatic spread, regardless of tumor size or lymph node involvement.

The therapeutic regimen is often dictated by the clinical stage classification of the cancer. (Side effects and appropriate nursing management of general treatment modalities for cancer are discussed in Chapter 16.)

In spite of the advent of new prognostic indicators such as determination of DNA content and analysis of cell-cycle phases, the single most powerful prognostic factor related to local recurrence or metastasis after primary therapy is still the presence or absence of malignant cells in lymph nodes.

Surgical Therapy. Breast conservation surgery with radiation therapy and modified radical mastectomy with or without reconstruction are currently the most common options for resectable breast cancer. Most women diagnosed with early-stage breast cancer (tumors smaller than 4 to 5 cm) are candidates for either treatment choice. The overall survival rate with lumpectomy and radiation is about the same as that with modified radical mastectomy.[26]

Axillary Node Dissection. Axillary lymph node dissection (ALND) on the same side as the breast cancer is often performed, and until recently was the standard of care for invasive breast cancer. A typical ALND generally involves the removal of 12 to 20 nodes. Recently sentinel lymph node dissection (SLND) has replaced ALND for patients who do not have malignant cells identified in their sentinel nodes. If one or more sentinel lymph nodes contain malignant cells, generally an ALND is recommended. Examination of the lymph nodes provides prognostic information and helps determine further treatment (chemotherapy, hormone therapy, or both).

Lymphedema (accumulation of lymph in soft tissue) can occur as a result of the excision or radiation of lymph nodes.[27] When the axillary nodes cannot return lymph fluid to the central circulation, the fluid accumulates in the arm, causing obstructive pressure on the veins and venous return (Fig. 52-6). The patient may experi-

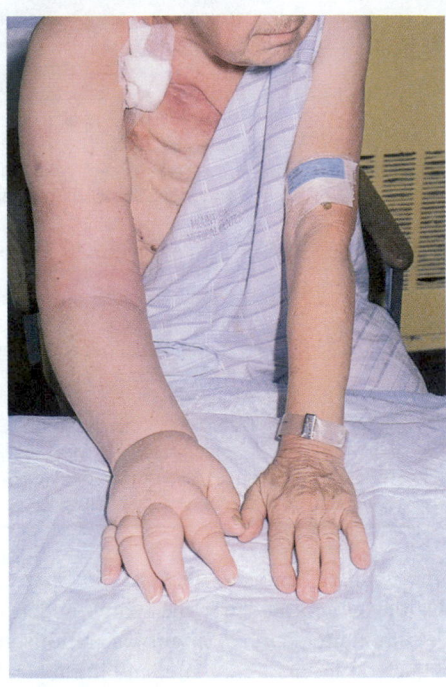

FIG. 52-6   Lymphedema. Accumulation of lymph fluid in the tissue after cancer treatment.

ence heaviness, pain, impaired motor function in the arm, and numbness and paresthesia of the fingers as a result of lymphedema. Cellulitis and progressive fibrosis can result from lymphedema. Although lymphedema is not always preventable, it can be controlled somewhat after surgery or radiation[28] (see discussion later in chapter).

Breast Conservation Surgery. Breast conservation surgery (also called **lumpectomy**) involves the removal of the entire tumor along with a margin of normal tissue. Following surgery, radiation therapy is delivered to the entire breast, ending with a boost to the tumor bed. If there is evidence of systemic disease, chemotherapy may be given before radiation therapy. Contraindications to breast conservation surgery include breast size too small in relation to the tumor size to yield an acceptable cosmetic result, masses and calcifications that are multifocal (within the same breast quadrant), masses that are multicentric (in more than one quadrant), diffuse calcifications in more than one quadrant, or central location of tumor near the nipple.

One of the main advantages of breast conservation surgery and radiation is that it preserves the breast, including the nipple. The goal of the combined surgery and radiation is to maximize the benefits of both cancer treatment and cosmetic outcome while minimizing risks. Disadvantages of this surgery include the increased cost of the surgery plus radiation over surgery alone and the possible side effects of radiation. Table 52-7 describes treatment options, side effects, complications, and patient issues related to the most common surgical procedures currently used to treat breast cancer.

Modified Radical Mastectomy. A modified radical mastectomy includes removal of the breast and axillary lymph nodes, but it preserves the pectoralis major muscle. This surgery would be selected over breast conservation therapy if the tumor is too large to excise with good margins and attain a reasonable cosmetic result. Some patients may select this surgical procedure over lumpectomy when presented with the choice of either procedure.

When a modified radical mastectomy is performed, the patient has the option of breast reconstruction. If the patient chooses to have reconstructive surgery, it can be performed immediately following the mastectomy or it can be delayed until postoperative recovery is complete (as long as 6 months).

Follow-up Care. After surgery, the woman must be followed up for the rest of her life at regular intervals. Most women have professional examinations every 6 months for 2 years and then annually thereafter. In addition, the woman should practice monthly BSE on both breasts or the remaining breast and the mastectomy site. The most common site of local recurrence of breast cancer is at the surgical site. The woman should also have yearly mammography of the remaining breast or breast tissue.

Postmastectomy Pain Syndrome. *Postmastectomy pain syndrome* can occur in patients following a mastectomy or an axillary node dissection. Common symptoms include chest and upper arm pain, tingling down the arm, numbness, shooting or pricking pain, and unbearable itching that persist beyond the normal 3-month healing time. The pain syndrome is caused by a number of factors, including injury to nerves and tissue as a result of surgery, radiation therapy, chemotherapy, or secondary neuroma development. The most common theory for its onset is the injury to intercostobrachial nerves, which are sensory nerves that exit chest wall muscles and provide sensation to the shoulder and upper arm.

Treatments include nonsteroidal antiinflammatory drugs, antidepressants, topical lidocaine patches, EMLA (eutectic mixture of local anesthetics: lidocaine and prilocaine), and antiseizure drugs (e.g., gabapentin [Neurontin]). Other possible treatment modalities include imagery, biofeedback, physical therapy to prevent "frozen shoulder" syndrome as a result of inadequate movement, and psychologic counseling with a person trained in the management of chronic pain syndromes.

Adjuvant Therapy. The decision to recommend adjuvant (additional) therapy after surgery depends on the stage of the disease (number of involved nodes and tumor size), menstrual status and age, cancer cell characteristics, presence or absence of estrogen and/or receptors, progesterone, and other preexisting health problems that can complicate treatment. Adjuvant therapies include radiation therapy after breast conservation surgery and systemic therapies such as chemotherapy and hormonal therapy.[26]

Radiation Therapy. Radiation therapy may be used for breast cancer as (1) primary treatment to prevent local breast recur-

TABLE 52-7	Surgical Procedures for Breast Cancer			
Procedures	**Description**	**Side Effects**	**Potential Complications**	**Patient Issues**
Modified radical mastectomy	Removal of breast, preservation of pectoralis muscle, axillary lymph node dissection (ALND)	Chest wall tightens Phantom breast sensations Arm swelling Sensory changes	Short-term: skin flap necrosis, seroma, hematoma, infection Long-term: sensory loss, muscle weakness, lymphedema	Loss of breast Incision Body image Need for prosthesis Impaired arm mobility
Breast conservation surgery (lumpectomy) with radiation therapy	Wide excision of tumor, sentinel lymph node dissection (SLND) and/or ALND, radiation therapy	Breast soreness Breast edema Skin reactions Arm swelling Sensory changes in breast and arm Fatigue	Short-term: moist desquamation,* hematoma, seroma, infection Long-term: fibrosis, lymphedema,† myositis, pneumonitis,* rib fractures*	Prolonged treatment* Impaired arm mobility† Change in texture and sensitivity of breast
Tissue expansion and breast implants	Expander used to slowly stretch tissue; saline gradually injected into reservoir over weeks to months Insertion of implant under musculofascial layer of chest wall	Discomfort Chest wall tightness	Short-term: skin flap necrosis, wound separation, seroma, hematoma, infection Long-term: capsular contractions, displacement of implant	Body image Prolonged physician visits to expand implants Additional surgeries for nipple construction, symmetry
Musculocutaneous flap procedures	A musculocutaneous flap (muscle, skin, blood supply) is transposed from latissimus dorsi to transverse rectus abdominis to chest wall‡	Pain related to two surgical sites and extensive surgery	Short-term: delayed wound healing, infection, skin flap necrosis, abdominal hernia, hematoma	Prolonged postoperative recovery

*Specific to radiation therapy.
†If ALND (less likely with SLND).
‡Concurrent with mastectomy.

rences after breast conservation surgery, (2) adjuvant treatment following mastectomy to prevent local and nodal recurrences, and (3) palliative treatment for pain caused by local recurrence and metastases.

Primary Radiation Therapy. When radiation therapy is the primary treatment, it is usually performed after local excision of the breast mass. The breast (and the regional lymph nodes in some cases) is radiated daily over the course of approximately 5 to 6 weeks. An external beam of radiation is used to deliver an approximate total dose of 4500 to 5000 cGy (4500 to 5000 rads; 1 rad = 1 cGy). A "boost" treatment to the full breast may also be given, either before or after therapy has been completed. The boost is a dose of radiation delivered to the area in which the original tumor was located. It can be given by external beam and usually adds 10 treatments to the total number given. Fatigue, skin changes, and breast edema may be temporary side effects of external beam radiation therapy. Radiation of the axilla is also effective in decreasing the incidence of axillary recurrence. Chemotherapy may be used systemically to enhance the local effects of radiation. (Nursing management of the patient receiving radiation therapy is discussed in Chapter 16.)

The decision to use radiation therapy after mastectomy is based on the probability of the presence of local residual cancer cells (related to size of cancer and number of involved lymph nodes). Radiating the area will not prevent the appearance of distant metastasis at a later date. The site of radiation therapy (lymph nodes, chest wall, or both) depends on the degree of possible spread of the cancer.

High-Dose Brachytherapy. Brachytherapy (internal radiation) is a procedure that is an alternative to traditional radiation treatment for early-stage breast cancer. For many years, internal radiation therapy has primarily been delivered using a multicatheter implant method that requires many catheters to be placed in the breast. After placement, a radioactive seed is delivered into each catheter to treat the target area.

One of the latest advances in the treatment of breast cancer and currently the most widely practiced method of brachytherapy is balloon brachytherapy. Traditional radiation treatments can take 5 to 6 weeks. In contrast, high-dose brachytherapy using the balloon catheter may require only 5 days.

The MammoSite® technique uses a balloon catheter to insert radioactive seeds into the breast after the tumor is removed (Fig. 52-7). Radiation is emitted by a tiny radioactive seed attached by a wire on the way to an afterloader, a computer-controlled machine. The seed travels through the MammoSite applicator into the inflated balloon. Where the seed goes and how much radiation it releases is carefully determined.[29] The radiation dose is focused on the area of the breast at highest risk for tumor recurrence.

The MammoSite system is a minimally invasive method of delivering internal radiation therapy. Radiation therapy with the MammoSite is performed over a 1- to 5-day period on an outpatient basis. Patients typically receive treatments twice a day for 5 days.

The MammoSite may also be used as a boost therapy in conjunction with external radiation. A boost is a procedure that delivers additional therapy directly to the area of the breast at highest risk for tumor recurrence.

No source of radiation remains in the body between treatments or after the final treatment is over. The tiny radioactive seed is inserted only during treatment and then removed. Neither the MammoSite nor the liquid inside is radioactive in any way. Once the final session is completed, the balloon is deflated and the MammoSite system is easily removed.

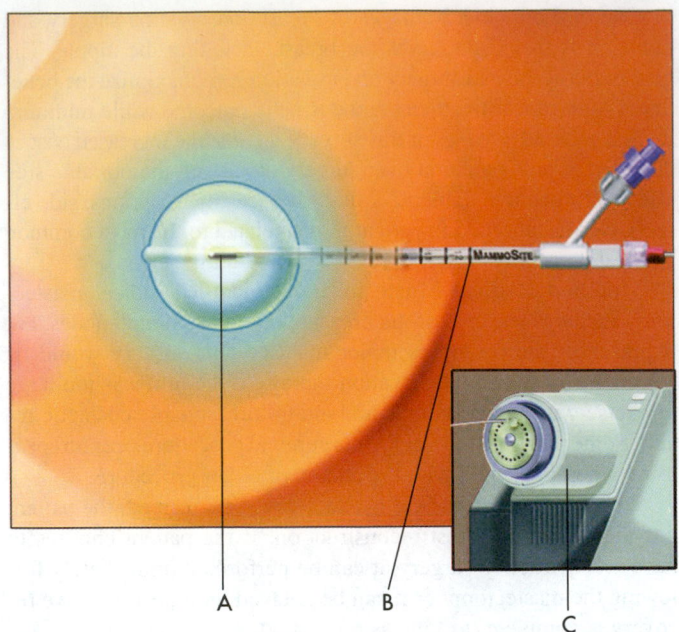

A   B   C

FIG. 52-7   High-dose brachytherapy for breast cancer. The MammoSite® system involves the insertion of a single small balloon catheter (B) at the time of the lumpectomy or shortly thereafter into the tumor resection cavity—the space that is left after the surgeon removes the tumor. A tiny radioactive seed (A) is inserted into the balloon, connected to a machine called an afterloader (C), and delivers the radiation therapy.

Palliative Radiation Therapy. In addition to reducing the primary tumor mass with a resultant decrease in pain, radiation therapy is also used to stabilize symptomatic metastatic lesions in such sites as bone, soft tissue organs, brain, and chest. Radiation therapy relieves pain and is often successful in controlling recurrent or metastatic disease for long periods.

Systemic Therapy. The goal of systemic therapy is to destroy tumor cells that may have spread undetected to distant sites. Systemic therapy as an adjuvant to primary local treatment (in the absence of demonstrable metastases) can decrease the rate of recurrence and increase the length of survival. Because of the high risk for recurrent disease, nearly all women with evidence of node involvement, particularly those who are hormone-receptor negative, will have some type of systemic therapy. Certain women, particularly those with a larger tumor or a more aggressive type of tumor, are known to be at higher risk for recurrent or metastatic disease. These women are often recommended for systemic therapy even when no evidence of node involvement is found. Weighing the different risk factors to determine the need for adjuvant therapy in a node-negative patient is a complex process.

Chemotherapy. Chemotherapy refers to the use of cytotoxic drugs to destroy cancer cells. Breast cancer is one of the solid tumors that is the most responsive to chemotherapy.

In some patients, chemotherapy is given preoperatively. Preoperative chemotherapy can decrease the size of the primary tumor, possibly permitting less extensive surgery. Breast cancer survival rates are not altered when comparing preoperative chemotherapy to postoperative chemotherapy.[30]

The use of combinations of drugs is clearly superior to the use of a single drug. The benefit of combination treatment results from the use of drugs that have different actions on cell growth and division. The more common combination-therapy protocols are

(1) cyclophosphamide (Cytoxan), methotrexate, and 5-fluorouracil (5-FU), referred to as CMF; (2) doxorubicin (Adriamycin) and cyclophosphamide, referred to as AC, with or without the addition of a taxane such as paclitaxel (Taxol) or docetaxel (Taxotere); or (3) cyclophosphamide, epirubicin (Ellence) or doxorubicin (Adriamycin), and 5-FU, referred to as CEF or CAF, respectively. Docetaxel, capecitabine (Xeloda), and an albumin-bound form of paclitaxel (Abraxane) are used in women whose metastatic breast cancer has not responded to standard chemotherapy. Vinorelbine (Navelbine), a relatively new chemotherapeutic drug for treating metastatic breast cancer, is well tolerated with fewer and milder side effects than other chemotherapy drugs.

> **Drug Alert** - Doxorubicin (Adriamycin)
> • Monitor for signs of cardiotoxicity and heart failure (e.g., dysrhythmias, electrocardiogram changes).
> • Instruct patient not to have immunizations without physician's approval.
> • Instruct patient to avoid contact with those who recently received live virus vaccine.

Because healthy cells are also affected by chemotherapy, a variety of side effects accompany this treatment modality. The incidence and severity of predictable and commonly observed side effects will be influenced by the specific drug combination, drug schedule, and dose of the drug or drugs. Usually, body organs with rapidly growing cells are the most strongly affected. The most common side effects involve the gastrointestinal tract, bone marrow, and hair follicles, resulting in nausea, anorexia, weight loss, bone marrow suppression and subsequent fatigue, and alopecia (hair loss).

Hormonal Therapy. Estrogen can promote the growth of breast cancer cells if the cells are estrogen receptor positive. Hormonal therapy removes or blocks the source of estrogen, thus promoting tumor regression.[31]

Two advances have increased the use of hormone therapy in breast cancer. First, hormone receptor assays, which are reliable diagnostic tests, have been developed to identify women who are likely to respond to hormone therapy. Both estrogen and progesterone receptor status of the tumor can be determined. The importance of these assays is their ability to predict whether hormonal therapy is a treatment option for women with breast cancer, either at the time of initial therapy or if the cancer recurs. Second, drugs have been developed that can inactivate the hormone-secreting glands as effectively as surgery or radiation. Premenopausal and perimenopausal women are more likely to have tumors that are not hormone dependent, whereas women who are postmenopausal are more likely to have hormone-dependent tumors. Chances of tumor regression are significantly greater in women whose tumors contain estrogen and progesterone receptors.

Estrogen deprivation can occur by destroying the ovaries by surgery or radiation therapy or drug therapy (Table 52-8). Hormonal therapy can (1) block or destroy the estrogen receptors or (2) suppress estrogen synthesis through inhibiting aromatase, an enzyme needed for endogenous estrogen synthesis.[31] Hormonal therapy may be used as an adjuvant to primary treatment or in patients with recurrent or metastatic cancer.

Tamoxifen (Nolvadex) has been the hormonal agent of choice in estrogen receptor–positive women with all stages of breast cancer for the past 30 years.[32] Tamoxifen, an antiestrogen drug, blocks the estrogen receptor sites of malignant cells and thus inhibits the growth-stimulating effects of estrogen. It is commonly used in advanced and

TABLE 52-8	**DRUG THERAPY** Hormonal Therapy for Breast Cancer	
Mechanism of Action	**Examples**
Blocks estrogen receptors	tamoxifen (Nolvadex) toremifene (Fareston)
Destroys estrogen receptors	fulvestrant (Faslodex)
Prevents production of estrogen by inhibiting aromatase	anastrozole (Arimidex) letrozole (Femara) exemestane (Aromasin) aminoglutethimide (Cytadren)

early-stage breast cancer and to treat recurrent disease. Tamoxifen may also be used to prevent breast cancer in high-risk individuals. Side effects of tamoxifen are minimal but include hot flashes, mood swings, vaginal discharge, and other effects commonly associated with decreased estrogen. It also increases the risk of blood clots, cataracts, stroke, and endometrial cancer in postmenopausal women.

> **Drug Alert** - Tamoxifen (Nolvadex)
> • Decreased visual acuity, corneal opacity, and retinopathy can occur in women receiving high doses (240-320 mg/day for >17 months); may be irreversible.
> • Instruct patient to immediately report decreased visual acuity.
> • Monitor for signs of deep vein thrombosis, pulmonary embolism, and stroke, including shortness of breath, leg cramps, and weakness.

Toremifene (Fareston) is an antiestrogen agent similar to tamoxifen. It is indicated in the treatment of metastatic breast cancer in postmenopausal women. Fulvestrant (Faslodex) may be given to women with advanced breast cancer who no longer respond to tamoxifen. This drug slows cancer progression by destroying estrogen receptors in the breast cancer cells. Fulvestrant is given intramuscularly on a monthly basis. Side effects include fatigue, hot flashes, and nausea.

Aromatase inhibitor drugs, which interfere with the enzyme that synthesizes endogeneous estrogen, are used in the treatment of breast cancer in postmenopausal women. These drugs include anastrozole (Arimidex), letrozole (Femara), exemestane (Aromasin). Aromatase inhibitors do not block the production of estrogen by the ovaries. Thus they are of little benefit in premenopausal women.

Clinical trials have demonstrated greater disease-free survival when aromatase inhibitors are given after tamoxifen treatment has ended.[32] They also appear to be as effective as tamoxifen in preventing breast cancer recurrence and perhaps more effective in preventing contralateral disease (disease in the other breast). Aromatase inhibitors have fewer side effects than tamoxifen. They only rarely cause blood clots and they do not cause endometrial cancer. Because they block the production of estrogen in postmenopausal women, osteoporosis and bone fractures may occur. These drugs have also been associated with night sweats, nausea, arthralgias, and myalgias.[31]

Raloxifene (Evista), a drug used to prevent bone loss, may also reduce the risk of breast cancer without stimulating endometrial growth. Raloxifene acts as an estrogen antagonist at the hormone-sensitive tissues of breast cancer and bone. (Raloxifene is discussed in the section on osteoporosis in Chapter 64.)

Additional drugs that may be used to suppress hormone-dependent breast tumors include megestrol acetate (Megace), diethylstilbestrol (DES), and fluoxymesterone (Halotestin). Less common hormone-deprivation strategies include bilateral oophorectomy, adrenalectomy, and hypophysectomy.

Biologic and Targeted Therapy. Trastuzumab (Herceptin) is a monoclonal antibody to HER-2. After the antibody attaches to the antigen, it is taken into the cells and eventually kills them. It can be used alone or in combination with other chemotherapy, such as docetaxel (Taxotere), to treat patients with metastatic breast cancer whose tumors overexpress HER-2. Women who overexpress HER-2 typically have a poorer prognosis. The drug can be used for treatment at any stage of disease following surgery or diagnosis of metastatic disease. (The use of biologic and targeted therapies is discussed in Chapter 16.)

> **Drug Alert** - *Trastuzumab (Herceptin)*
> • Use with caution in women with preexisting heart disease.
> • Monitor for signs of ventricular dysfunction and heart failure.

Angiogenesis inhibitors that prevent the formation of blood vessels into newly developing tumors are also being investigated for use in patients with breast cancer. In early clinical trials, bevacizumab (Avastin), which is an angiogenesis inhibitor, has been used in combination with chemotherapy. It has been shown to extend the survival of women with newly diagnosed advanced breast cancer. This drug has already been approved for use by the U.S. Food and Drug Administration (FDA) for patients with colorectal cancer.

CULTURALLY COMPETENT CARE
BREAST CANCER

Breast cancer does not respect the boundaries of ethnicity or culture. However, there are differences in various ethnic groups related to breast cancer (see Cultural and Ethnic Health Disparities box on p. 1348). Cultural considerations may involve cultural gender roles, health beliefs, religion, and family structure. Other differences may be due to dietary factors and insufficient use of early detection procedures such as clinical breast examinations and mammograms.

Cultural values strongly influence how women respond to and cope with breast cancer and treatment. Nurses must take into account how health behaviors are influenced by cultural norms and, in particular, the cultural value of breasts and the cultural factors related to the disease of breast cancer. A possible reason that some women may delay treatment after they have discovered a large breast lump is their belief in fatalism—an acceptance of disease as inevitable fate or "God's will."

NURSING MANAGEMENT
BREAST CANCER

■ Nursing Assessment

Many factors need to be considered when a nurse is assessing a patient with a breast problem. The history of the breast disorder assists in establishing the diagnosis. The presence of nipple discharge, pain, rate of growth of the lump, breast asymmetry, and correlation with the menstrual cycle should all be investigated.

The size and location of the lump or lumps should be carefully documented. The physical characteristics of the lesion, such as consistency, mobility, and shape, should be assessed. If nipple discharge is present, the color and consistency should be noted, as well as whether it occurs from one or both breasts.

Subjective and objective data that should be obtained from an individual suspected of having or diagnosed as having breast cancer are presented in Table 52-9.

TABLE 52-9	NURSING ASSESSMENT Breast Cancer

Subjective Data
Important Health Information
Past health history: Benign breast disease with atypical changes; previous unilateral breast cancer; menstrual history (early menarche with late menopause); pregnancy history (nulliparity or first full-term pregnancy after age 30); previous endometrial, ovarian, or colon cancer; hyperestrogenism and testicular atrophy (in men)

Medications: Use of hormones, especially as postmenopausal hormone replacement therapy and in oral contraceptives, infertility treatments

Surgery or other treatments: Exposure to excessive radiation (e.g., lymphoma or thyroid radiation)

Functional Health Patterns
Health perception–health management: Family history of breast cancer (especially mother or sister); positive mammography history; palpable change found on BSE; alcohol use

Nutritional-metabolic: Obesity; anorexia (possible indicator of metastasis); dietary habits

Cognitive-perceptual: Headache, back, arm, or bone pain (possible indicators of metastasis)

Sexuality-reproductive: Unilateral nipple discharge (clear, milky, or bloody); change in breast contour, size, or symmetry

Coping–stress tolerance: Psychologic stress

Self-perception–self-concept: Anxiety regarding threat to self-esteem

Physical activity: Level of usual activity

Objective Data
General
Axillary and supraclavicular lymphadenopathy

Integumentary
Firm, discrete nodules at mastectomy site (possible indicator of local recurrence); peripheral edema (possible indicator of metastasis)

Respiratory
Pleural effusions (possible indicator of metastasis)

Gastrointestinal
Hepatomegaly, jaundice; ascites (possible indicators of liver metastasis)

Reproductive
Hard, irregular, nonmobile breast lump most often in upper, outer sector, possibly fixated to fascia or chest wall; nipple inversion or retraction, erosion; edema ("orange peel"), erythema, induration, infiltration, or dimpling (in later stages)

Possible Findings
Finding of mass or change in tissue on breast examination; positive results of mammography or ultrasonography; positive results of FNA or surgical biopsy or similar results with a needle biopsy

BSE, Breast self-examination; *FNA,* fine-needle aspiration.

■ Nursing Diagnoses

Nursing diagnoses related to the care of a patient diagnosed with breast cancer vary. Following diagnosis and before a treatment plan has been selected, the following diagnoses would apply:

• Decisional conflict *related to* lack of knowledge about treatment options and their effects
• Fear *related to* diagnosis of breast cancer
• Disturbed body image *related to* anticipated physical and emotional effects of treatment modalities

If a mastectomy or lumpectomy is planned, the nursing diagnoses may include, but are not limited to, those presented in NCP 52-1.

NURSING CARE PLAN 52-1

Patient after Mastectomy or Lumpectomy*

NURSING DIAGNOSIS   **Acute pain** *related to* surgical procedure *as evidenced by* verbalization of pain at operative area

PATIENT GOALS   1. Uses pain control measures appropriately
2. Reports progressive reduction in pain

OUTCOMES (NOC)	INTERVENTIONS (NIC) and *RATIONALES*
Pain Control	**Pain Management**
• Uses nonanalgesic relief measures ____ • Uses analgesics appropriately ____ • Reports pain controlled ____ **Measurement Scale** 1 = Never demonstrated 2 = Rarely demonstrated 3 = Sometimes demonstrated 4 = Often demonstrated 5 = Consistently demonstrated	• Perform a comprehensive assessment of pain to include location, characteristics, onset/duration, frequency, quality, and intensity or severity of pain *to plan appropriate interventions.* • Explore with patient factors that relieve/worsen pain. • Teach the use of nonpharmacologic techniques (e.g., distraction, imagery, and relaxation) *to use along with or in place of analgesics.* • Use pain control measures before pain becomes severe *to prevent pain from becoming out of control.* **Positioning** • Immobilize or support the arm *to prevent tension on suture line.*

NURSING DIAGNOSIS   **Anxiety** *related to* a situational crisis and unpredictable outcome secondary to a diagnosis of cancer *as evidenced by* insomnia, crying, and questioning of prognosis

PATIENT GOAL   Demonstrates effective use of coping strategies that provide reduction of anxiety

OUTCOMES (NOC)	INTERVENTIONS (NIC) and *RATIONALES*
Coping	**Coping Enhancement**
• Uses available social support ____ • Uses effective coping strategies ____ • Reports increase in psychologic comfort ____ • Reports decrease in physical symptoms of stress ____ **Measurement Scale** 1 = Never demonstrated 2 = Rarely demonstrated 3 = Sometimes demonstrated 4 = Often demonstrated 5 = Consistently demonstrated	• Encourage verbalization of feelings, perceptions, and fears *to promote successful resolution of fear and establish effective coping mechanisms.* • Encourage the family to verbalize feelings *because their fear about the diagnosis and outcome can decrease their effectiveness as a support system.* • Provide factual information concerning diagnosis, treatment, and prognosis *to help decrease feelings of the unknown.* • Encourage an attitude of realistic hope as a way of dealing with feelings of helplessness *because hope is associated with better physical health.*

NURSING DIAGNOSIS   **Disturbed body image** *related to* perceived effects of mastectomy *as evidenced by* verbalization of concern about appearance and feelings of loss of femininity, and refusal to view incision

PATIENT GOALS   1. Discusses feelings about and the meaning of changes in physical appearance
2. Identifies community resources and self-help groups available for support

OUTCOMES (NOC)	INTERVENTIONS (NIC) and *RATIONALES*
Body Image	**Body Image Enhancement**
• Willingness to touch affected part ____ • Satisfaction with body appearance ____ • Adjustment to changes in physical appearance ____ • Willingness to use strategies to enhance appearance ____ **Measurement Scale** 1 = Never positive 2 = Rarely positive 3 = Sometimes positive 4 = Often positive 5 = Consistently positive	• Identify support groups available to patient *so that social support will be available.* • Assist patient to separate physical appearance from feelings of personal worth. • Facilitate contact with individuals with similar change in body image (e.g., Reach to Recovery) *to serve as a role model and provide hope for recovery and a normal future.* • Assist patient to discuss changes caused by illness or surgery *to promote grief work and maintain support from family/friends.* • Assist patient to identify actions that will enhance appearance (e.g., prosthesis, breast reconstruction).

ADLs, Activities of daily living.

*For the patient who has a lumpectomy, many of the specific interventions in this care plan relate to the patient who has also had an axillary node dissection.

Continued

Reproductive System

NURSING CARE PLAN 52-1

Patient after Mastectomy or Lumpectomy—cont'd

NURSING DIAGNOSIS   **Ineffective therapeutic regimen management** *related to* lack of knowledge regarding disease process and postoperative care *as evidenced by* frequent questions about disease and treatment, follow-up care

PATIENT GOALS   1. Demonstrates care of incision site
2. Explains disease process and measures to minimize disease progression

OUTCOMES (NOC)	INTERVENTIONS (NIC) and *RATIONALES*

Knowledge: Treatment Regimen

*   Description of breast cancer disease process ____
*   Description of rationale for treatment regimen ____
*   Description of self-care responsibilities for ongoing treatment ____
*   Description of benefits of disease management ____

Measurement Scale

1 = None
2 = Limited
3 = Moderate
4 = Substantial
5 = Extensive

Teaching: Procedure/Treatment

*   Instruct the patient on how to participate during the procedure (e.g., taking care of incision, applying new dressing, emptying drains, performing return demonstration) *to become self-sufficient in own care.*
*   Include family/significant other as needed.

Teaching: Disease Process

*   Review patient's knowledge about condition *to determine what teaching is needed.*
*   Instruct patient on which signs and symptoms to report to health care provider (e.g., skin changes at surgical site, new changes in breast or chest wall).

Breast Examination

*   Instruct patient about the importance of regular self-examination and advise regular mammograms *because they are recommended screening techniques for identification of local recurrence after mastectomy and for assessing other breast.*

NURSING DIAGNOSIS   **Impaired physical mobility** *related to* weakness and muscle loss *as evidenced by* limitation in movement of upper extremity on surgical side

PATIENT GOALS   1. Identifies activities that can reduce postoperative edema and mobility
2. Demonstrates appropriate hand and arm exercises

OUTCOMES (NOC)	INTERVENTIONS (NIC) and *RATIONALES*

Coordinated Movement

*   Steadiness of movement ____
*   Strength of muscle contraction (affected side) ____
*   Movement in desired direction (affected side) ____

Measurement Scale

1 = Severely compromised
2 = Substantially compromised
3 = Moderately compromised
4 = Mildly compromised
5 = Not compromised

Exercise Therapy: Joint Mobility

*   Determine limitations of joint movement and effect on function *to plan appropriate interventions.*
*   Initiate pain control measures before beginning exercise *to promote participation in exercise plan.*
*   Perform passive or assisted range-of-motion exercises *to prevent contractures and muscle shortening, maintain muscle tone, and improve lymph and blood circulation.*

Exercise Therapy: Muscle Control

*   Incorporate ADLs into exercise protocol *to reduce dependent behaviors, raise self-esteem, and maintain mobility of affected arm.*
*   Use motor activities that require attention to and use of both sides of the body *to prevent guarding of operative side and loss of function.*

COLLABORATIVE PROBLEM

NURSING GOALS	NURSING INTERVENTIONS and *RATIONALES*

Potential Complication

*   Monitor for signs of lymphedema
*   Report deviations from acceptable parameters
*   Carry out appropriate medical and nursing interventions

Lymphedema *related to* impaired lymphatic drainage and lack of knowledge of preventive measures

*   Assess woman for signs of lymphedema such as edema in hand and/or arm on operative side, heaviness, and/or localized pain *to enable early diagnosis and intervention to prevent and treat the complication.*
*   Instruct patient about self-care strategies and precautions to reduce risk of lymphedema *so patient will be an active, informed participant in self-care.*
*   Do not perform venipunctures or take blood pressure measurements on affected arm *to reduce risk of constriction, infection, and lymphedema in affected arm.*
*   Avoid dependent arm position *to allow proper wound healing and decrease stress to incision site.*
*   Use elastic sleeve if ordered *to apply mechanical pressure to reduce fluid collection in affected arm and promote venous return.*

■ Planning

The overall goals are that the patient with breast cancer will (1) actively participate in the decision-making process related to treatment options, (2) fully comply with the therapeutic plan, (3) manage the side effects of adjuvant therapy, and (4) be satisfied with the support provided by significant others and health care providers.

■ Nursing Implementation

Acute Intervention. The time between the diagnosis of breast cancer and the selection of a treatment plan is a difficult period for the woman and her family. Although the primary care provider has discussed treatment options, the woman often relies on the nurse to clarify and expand on these options. During this time, the woman may be very self-focused, verbalizing her conflict and indecision frequently. Appropriate nursing interventions during this period include exploring the woman's usual decision-making patterns, helping the woman accurately evaluate the advantages and disadvantages of the options, providing information relevant to the decision, and supporting the patient once the decision is made.

During this period the woman may exhibit signs of distress or tension, such as tachycardia, increased muscle tension, sleep disturbances, and restlessness, whenever she focuses on the decision to be made. The nurse should assess the woman's body language, motor activity, and affect during periods of high stress and indecision so that appropriate interventions can be carried out.

Regardless of the surgery planned, the patient must be provided with sufficient information to ensure informed consent. Some patients seek extensive, detailed information, whereas others avoid information. Sensitivity to an individual's need for information is essential. Teaching in the preoperative phase includes instruction in turning, coughing, and deep breathing; a review of postoperative exercises; a pain management plan; and an explanation of the recovery period from the time of surgery until discharge.

The woman who has breast conservation surgery usually has an uneventful postoperative course with only a moderate amount of pain. If an axillary lymph node dissection (ALND) has been done or if a woman has had a mastectomy, drains are often left in place and patients are discharged home with them. Patients and their families need to be taught how to manage the drainage tubes at home.

Restoring arm function on the affected side after mastectomy and axillary lymph node dissection is one of the most important goals of nursing activities. The woman should be placed in a semi-Fowler position with the arm on the affected side elevated on a pillow. Flexing and extending the fingers should begin in the recovery room with progressive increases in activity encouraged. (Information pertaining to arm exercises and care applies to women who have had an ALND after lumpectomy or total mastectomy.) Postoperative arm and shoulder exercises are instituted gradually at the surgeon's direction (Fig. 52-8). These exercises are designed to prevent contractures and muscle shortening, maintain muscle tone, and improve lymph and blood circulation. The difficulty and pain encountered by the woman in performing the previously simple tasks included in the exercise program may cause frustration and depression. The goal of all exercise is a gradual return to full range of motion within 4 to 6 weeks.

Postoperative discomfort can be minimized by administering analgesics about 30 minutes before initiating exercises. When

showering is appropriate, the flow of warm water over the involved shoulder often has a soothing effect and reduces joint stiffness. Whenever possible, the same nurse should work with the woman so that progress can be monitored and problems can be identified.

Measures to prevent or reduce lymphedema after ALND must be used by the nurse and taught to the woman. The affected arm should never be dependent, even while the person is sleeping. Blood pressure readings, venipunctures, and injections should not be done on the affected arm. Elastic bandages should not be used in the early postoperative period because they inhibit collateral lymph drainage. The woman must be instructed to protect the arm on the operative side from even minor trauma such as a pinprick or sunburn. If trauma to the arm occurs, the area should be washed thoroughly with soap and water. A topical antibiotic ointment and a bandage or other sterile dressing should be applied. The surgeon must be advised of the trauma, and the site of injury must be observed closely for evidence of inflammation. The patient must

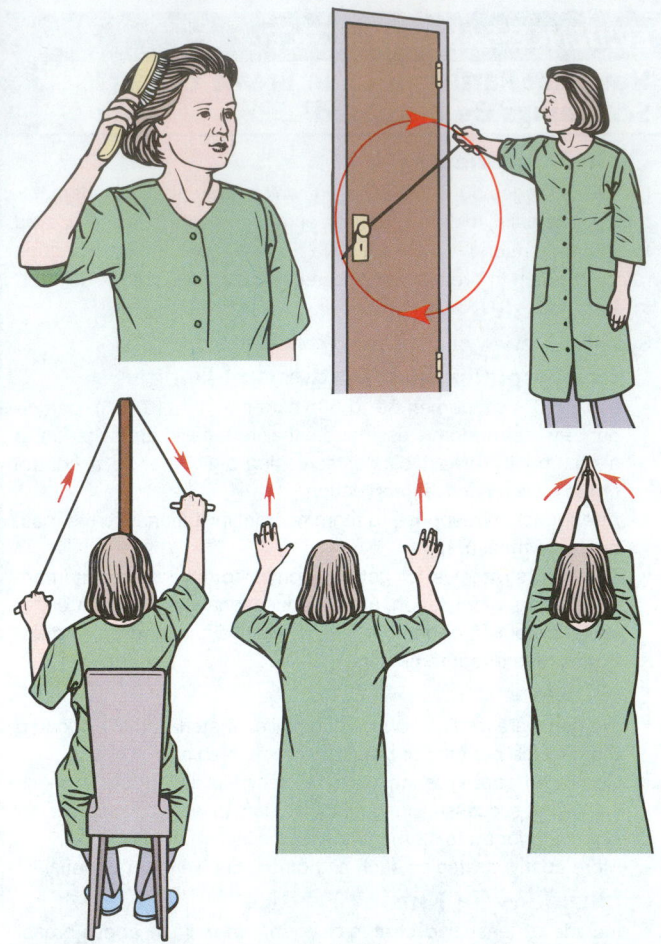

FIG. 52-8   Postoperative exercises for the patient with a mastectomy or lumpectomy with axillary lymph node dissection.

know and understand that she is at risk of developing lymphedema for the rest of her life.

When lymphedema is acute (see Fig. 52-6), an intermittent pneumatic compression sleeve may be prescribed. This device applies mechanical massage to the arm and facilitates lymph drainage up toward the heart.[33] Manual massage is also effective in mobilizing subcutaneous accumulations of fluid. Elevation of the arm so that it is level with the heart, diuretics, and isometric exercises may be recommended to reduce the fluid volume in the arm. The patient may need to wear a fitted elastic pressure gradient sleeve during waking hours to maintain maximum volume reduction and preventively during air travel.

Psychologic Care. Throughout interactions with a woman with breast cancer, the nurse must keep in mind the extensive psychologic impact of the disease. All aspects of care must include sensitivity to the woman's efforts to cope with a life-threatening disease. An open relationship in which the woman can express her fears and feelings is essential. The nurse can help meet the woman's psychologic needs by doing the following:

1. Assisting her to develop a positive but realistic attitude
2. Helping her identify sources of support and strength to her, such as her partner, family, and spiritual practices
3. Encouraging her to verbalize her anger and fears about her diagnosis and the impact it will have on her life and her family

4. Promoting open communication of thoughts and feelings between the patient and her family
5. Providing accurate and complete answers to questions about her disease, treatment options, and reproductive or lactation issues (if appropriate)
6. Offering information about community resources, such as Reach to Recovery, Y-Me, CanSurmount, Encore, and local support organizations and groups

The nurse can promote the woman's recovery by arranging a visit from a woman who had similar treatment, such as a Reach to Recovery volunteer, if the service is available. The Reach to Recovery program of the American Cancer Society is a rehabilitation program for women who have had breast surgery. It is designed to help them meet their psychologic, physical, and cosmetic needs. The volunteers, who are all women who have had breast cancer, can answer questions about what to expect at home, how to tell people about the surgery, and what prosthetic devices are available. If a Reach to Recovery volunteer is not available, it is the nurse's responsibility to be knowledgeable about the needs of the woman after breast surgery. The American Cancer Society and the National Cancer Institute can provide excellent materials to assist the nurse in meeting the special needs of women with breast cancer.

The professional staff must never underestimate the tremendous psychologic impact that a diagnosis of cancer and subsequent breast surgery can have on a woman and her family.[28] Emotional complications are common. The nurse's accepting, concerned attitude can do a great deal to relieve the feelings of anger and depression experienced by many patients.

Ambulatory and Home Care. The nurse should explain the follow-up routine to the patient and emphasize the importance of an annual mammography and breast self-awareness. Referral to a mental health provider to address individual and family support in addition to coping needs may be indicated. Immediately after surgery, symptoms that should be reported to the clinician include fever, inflammation at the surgical site, erythema, postoperative constipation, and unusual swelling. Other changes to report in the future are new back pain, weakness, shortness of breath, and confusion. If adjuvant therapy is to be used, the woman should have specific instructions about appointment times and treatment locations and management of side effects.

For women who have had a mastectomy, the nurse should stress the importance of wearing a well-fitting prosthesis. A variety of products are available to meet the specific needs of the individual woman. After surgery a temporary camisole prosthesis may be used. A well-trained salesperson can help the woman select a suitable, more permanent weighted prosthesis and bra, generally at 6 weeks postoperatively. There are both physical and psychologic advantages to the use of a prosthesis. The return of a normal external appearance is especially important to most women.

The implications of the loss of a breast on the sexual identity and relationships of the woman vary. A preoperative sexual assessment provides helpful baseline data that the nurse can use to plan postoperative interventions. Often the husband, sexual partner, or family members may need assistance in dealing with their emotional reactions to the diagnosis and surgery for them to act as effective means of support for the patient. There are no physical reasons for a mastectomy to prevent sexual satisfaction. The woman taking tamoxifen may have a decreased sexual drive or vaginal dryness. She may need to use lubrication to prevent

COMPLEMENTARY AND ALTERNATIVE THERAPIES
Imagery

Imagery, or visualization, is the process of using mental images to create a desired state.

Clinical Uses
Imagery has many uses, including pain control, cancer treatment, asthma, menstrual disorders, GI disorders, arthritis, hypertension, and headaches.

Effects
Promote relaxation, decrease stress, lower BP, relieve pain, reduce side effects of chemotherapy, improve immune function, enhance performance, and enhance wound healing. This behavioral intervention has few side effects.

Nursing Implications
Imagery should be individualized, using an individual's dominant sensory mode (visual, auditory, and kinesthetic are most common) and avoiding images that are individually distressing. People can invent their own forms of imagery or use those that have been created by others. Imagery is well suited as a self-care technique because almost anyone can use it. Additional information on imagery can be found at *www.healthjourneys.com* and in Chapter 9.

discomfort during intercourse. If difficulty in adjustment or other problems develop, counseling may be necessary to deal with the emotional component of a mastectomy and the diagnosis of cancer.

Depression and anxiety may occur with the continued stress and uncertainty of a cancer diagnosis. A woman's self-esteem and identity may also be threatened. Special nursing interventions are necessary in terms of both psychologic support and self-care teaching, if a recurrence of cancer is found. The support of family and friends and participation in a cancer support group are important aspects of care that are often helpful in improving quality of life and have been found to have a clinically significant impact on survival.

■ *Evaluation*

The expected outcomes for the patient after a mastectomy or lumpectomy are presented in NCP 52-1.

GERONTOLOGIC CONSIDERATIONS
BREAST CANCER

A major risk for breast cancer is increasing age, and more than half of all breast cancers are diagnosed in women who are age 65 or older. About 48% of women diagnosed with metastatic disease are 65 years or older.[34]

Older women are less likely to have mammograms. Screening and treatment decisions for breast cancer should be based on a woman's general health status rather than biologic age. This is important because tolerance to treatment and long-term prognosis is influenced more by a patient's health status than biologic age. In addition to comorbidities and life expectancy, treatment decisions for the older woman with breast cancer should be based on an assessment of nutritional and functional status, vision, gait, and balance, and the presence of delirium, dementia, and/or depression.

Breast cancer treatment is similar between older and younger patients, including the use of surgery, radiation therapy, chemotherapy, and hormonal therapy when appropriate. For healthy older women, breast cancer survival rates are similar to those of younger women when matched by cancer stage.[34]

MAMMOPLASTY

Mammoplasty is the surgical change in the size or shape of the breast. It may be done electively for cosmetic purposes to either enlarge or reduce the size of the breasts. It may also be done to reconstruct the breast after a mastectomy.

Health care providers should remain nonjudgmental toward women who desire mammoplasty. The desire to alter the appearance of the breasts has special significance for each woman as she attempts to alter or re-create her body image. It is important for the nurse to be aware of the cultural value placed on the breast by the woman. It is important that the woman have a realistic idea about what mammoplasty can accomplish and about possible complications, such as hematoma formation, hemorrhage, and infection. If an implant is involved, capsular contracture and loss of the implant are possible.

Breast Augmentation

In augmentation mammoplasty (the procedure to enlarge the breasts), an implant is placed in a surgically created pocket between the capsule of the breast and the pectoral fascia, or ideally under the pectoral muscle. Most implants are silicone envelopes filled with a fluid such as dextran, saline, or silicone. Because of their resemblance to the human breast, implants filled with silicone gel were the most widely used. In 1992 the Food and Drug Administration (FDA) suspended the routine use of silicone gel implants in response to potential hazards related to silicone leakage and possible health hazards. However, in 2006 the FDA approved the use of silicone gel implants for breast reconstruction.[35] The postapproval studies will continue to collect data on the safety and effectiveness of these implants.

In the United States saline-filled implants are usually used. Saline-filled implants are silicone shells filled with normal saline. Soybean oil implants are an alternative form of implant. This implant has an outer shell of silicone that is filled with highly refined soybean oil. A major advantage of soybean implants is that it is easier for x-rays to penetrate the implant, so better visualization of the underlying breast tissue is possible with mammography.

Breast Reduction

For some women, large breasts can be a source of pain and embarrassment. They can interfere with normal daily activities such as walking, typing, and driving a car. Overly large breasts can interfere with self-esteem and self-image and can lead to back, shoulder, and neck problems, including degenerative nerve changes. They may make stylish dressing more difficult. Reduction in the size of the breasts can have positive effects on both the psychologic and the physical health of the patient. Reduction mammoplasty is performed by resecting wedges of tissue from the upper and lower quadrants of the breast. The excess skin is removed, and the areola and nipple are relocated on the breast. Lactation can usually be accomplished if massive amounts of tissue are not removed and the nipples are left connected during surgery.

NURSING MANAGEMENT
BREAST AUGMENTATION AND REDUCTION

Breast augmentation and breast reduction may be done in the outpatient surgical area, or it may involve overnight hospitalization. General anesthesia is used. Drains are generally placed in the surgical site to prevent hematoma formation and then removed 2 to 3 days after surgery or when drainage is under 20 ml per day. The drainage must be examined for color and odor to detect postoperative infection or hemorrhage. The woman's temperature should also be monitored. Dressings should be changed as necessary and prescribed using sterile technique. After surgery the woman should be assured that the appearance of the breast will improve when healing is completed. Depending on physician instructions, the patient may be instructed to wear a bra that provides good support continuously for 2 to 3 days after breast reduction or augmentation. Depending on the extent of the operation, most women can resume normal activities within 2 to 3 weeks. Strenuous exercise may not be appropriate until several weeks later.

Breast Reconstruction

Breast reconstructive surgery may be done simultaneously with a mastectomy or some time afterward to achieve symmetry and to restore or preserve body image. The timing of reconstructive surgery should be individualized based on the psychologic needs of the patient. Immediate breast reconstruction after mastectomy is commonly performed. The advantages to immediate reconstruction are only one surgical procedure, one anesthesia induction, and one recovery period. Also, surgery takes place before the development of scar tissue or adhesions. Early reconstruction does not delay or influence further treatment or adversely affect predicted survival.

Indications. The main indication for breast reconstruction is to improve the woman's self-image and regain a sense of normality. Present techniques cannot restore lactation, nipple sensation, or erectility. Therefore the erotic functions of the breast are not present. Although the breast will not fully resemble its premastectomy appearance, the reconstructed appearance usually represents an improvement over the mastectomy scar (Fig. 52-9). The contour of the breast is restored without the use of an external prosthesis.

Types of Reconstruction

Breast Implants and Tissue Expansion. Breast implants are placed in a pocket under the pectoralis muscle, which protects the implant and provides soft tissue coverage over the implant. Implants can be placed either at the time of mastectomy or later. Because many mastectomy patients have insufficient tissue, simple placement of an implant may lead to small breast reconstruction that is tight or firm. Autologous tissue reconstruction may then be recommended.

A tissue expander can be used to stretch the skin and muscle at the mastectomy site before inserting implants (Fig. 52-10). The use of tissue expanders and breast implants is the most common breast reconstruction technique currently used. Placement of the expander can be performed at the time of mastectomy or at a later date. The tissue expander, which is minimally inflated at the time of surgery, is gradually filled by weekly injections of sterile water or saline solution, which stretch the skin and muscle. Once the tissue is adequately stretched and the anticipated breast size is reached, the expander is surgically removed and a permanent implant is inserted. Some expanders are designed to remain in place and become the implant, eliminating the need for a second surgical procedure. Tissue expansion does not work well in individuals with extensive scar tissue from surgery or radiation therapy.

The body's natural response to the presence of a foreign substance is the formation of a fibrous capsule around the implant.[35] If excessive capsular formation occurs as a result of infection, hematoma, trauma, or reaction to a foreign body, a contracture can develop, resulting in a deformed breast. Surgeons differ in their approaches to the prevention of contracture formation, although gentle manual massage around the implant is routine. Prevention of the problems that cause excessive capsule formation is critical. Other postoperative complications include skin ulceration, hypertrophic scar formation, intercostal neuralgia, and wound infection.

Musculocutaneous Flap Procedure. If insufficient muscle is left after mastectomy or if the chest wall has been radiated, the person's own tissue may be used to repair the soft tissue defects. Musculocutaneous flaps are most often taken from the back (latissimus dorsi muscle) or the abdomen (transverse rectus abdominis muscle). In the latissimus dorsi musculocutaneous flap, a block of skin and muscle from the patient's back is used to replace tissue removed during mastectomy. A small implant may be needed beneath the flap to gain reasonable breast shape and size. A disadvantage of this technique is an additional scar on the back.

The *transverse rectus abdominis musculocutaneous* (TRAM) flap is the most frequently used flap operation. The rectus abdominis muscles are paired flat muscles running from the rib cage down to the pubic bone. Arteries running inside the muscle provide branches at many levels, and these branches supply the fat and skin across a large expanse of the abdomen. With this technique the surgeon elevates a large block of tissue from the

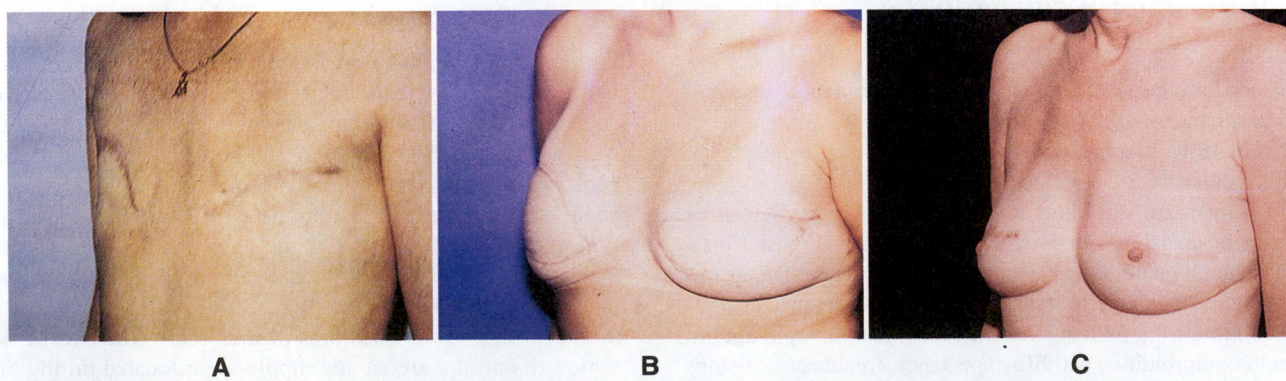

A **B** **C**

FIG. 52-9 **A,** Appearance of chest following bilateral mastectomy. **B,** Postoperative breast reconstruction before nipple-areolar reconstruction. **C,** Postoperative breast reconstruction after nipple-areolar reconstruction.

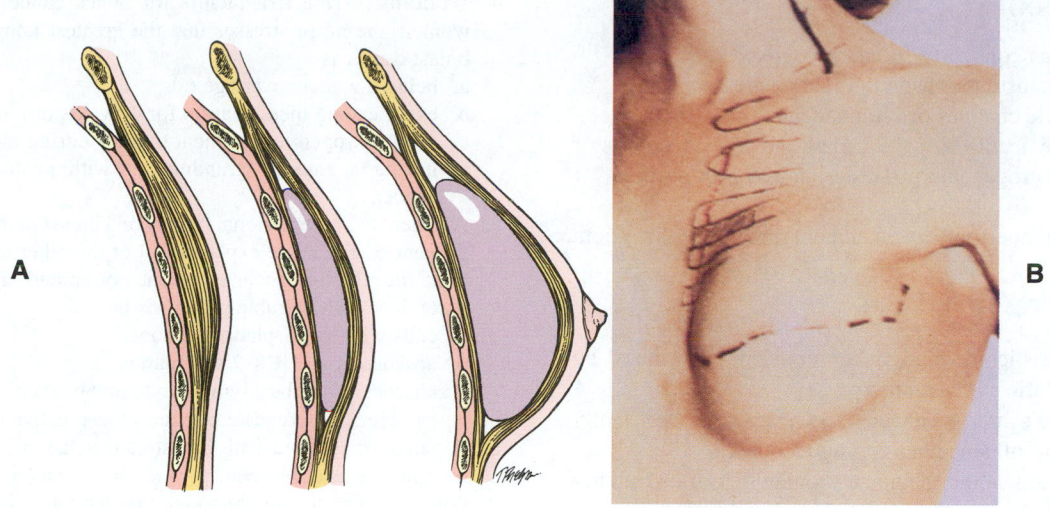

FIG. 52-10 **A,** Tissue expander with gradual expansion. **B,** Tissue expander in place after mastectomy.

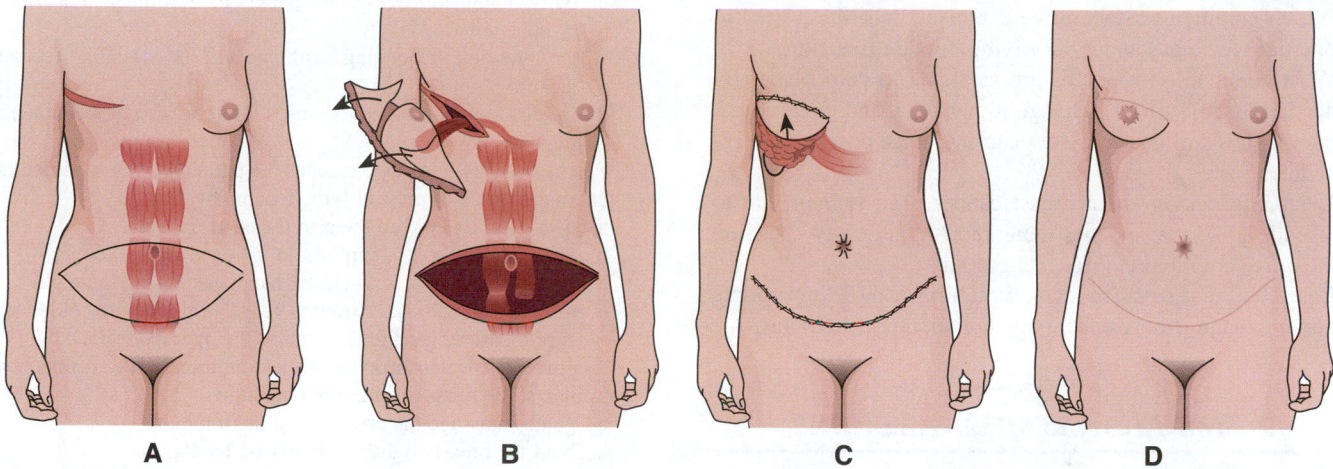

FIG. 52-11 TRAM flap. **A,** TRAM flap is planned. **B,** The abdominal tissue, while attached to the rectus muscle, nerve, and blood supply, is tunneled through the abdomen to the chest. **C,** The flap is trimmed to shape the breast. The lower abdominal incision is closed. **D,** Nipple and areola are reconstructed after the breast is healed.

lower abdominal area, but leaves it attached to the rectus muscle (Fig. 52-11). This tissue is then tunneled or placed as "free flaps" under the skin up to the area where the breast will be reconstructed. Then it is molded and fashioned to form a breast. The abdominal incision is closed, giving the patient a result that is similar to having an abdominoplasty. This surgical procedure can last 2 to 8 hours, with recovery taking 4 to 6 weeks. Complications include bleeding, hernia, and infection. An implant may be used in addition to the flap if the flap does not provide the desired cosmetic result alone.

Nipple-Areolar Reconstruction. The majority of patients who have breast reconstruction also have nipple-areolar reconstruction. Nipple reconstruction gives the reconstructed breast a much more natural appearance. Nipple-areolar reconstruction is usually done a few months after breast reconstruction. Tissue to construct a nipple may be taken from the opposite breast or from a small flap of tissue on the reconstructed breast mound. The areola may be grafted from the labia, skin in the area of the groin, or lower abdominal skin, or it may be tattooed with a permanent pigmented dye. In some patients a small implant may be placed under the completed nipple-areolar reconstruction to add additional projection.

CRITICAL THINKING EXERCISE

CASE STUDY

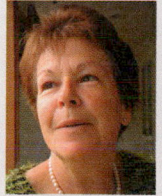

Case Study photo ©iStockphoto.com/ Jessica Jones Photography.

Breast Cancer

Patient Profile. Marie K., a 59-year-old divorced white woman, found a large lump in the upper, outer quadrant of her left breast while showering. She states, "My breasts are lumpy but this feels different."

Subjective Data
• Has family history of breast cancer—mother diagnosed at age 60 and sister diagnosed at age 55
• Had onset of menarche at age 11
• Has two daughters, ages 33 and 37
• Has no prior history of breast cancer
• On combined hormone replacement therapy for 12 years
• Last mammogram and CBE 2 years ago
• States she is afraid she has cancer

Objective Data
• Palpable, firm, fixed, 1.5-cm mass in upper, outer quadrant of left breast

Continued

CRITICAL THINKING EXERCISE—cont'd

- Left breast lesion confirmed by mammogram
- Ultrasound demonstrates suspicious shadowing
- No skin or nipple changes or lymphadenopathy
- Ultrasound core needle biopsy of mass indicates diagnosis of breast cancer; estrogen and progesterone receptor positive

Collaborative Care
- Scheduled for lumpectomy and sentinel lymph node dissection

Critical Thinking Questions

1. What characteristics of malignancy could be determined by palpation of Marie's breast mass?
2. What in Marie's breast cancer experience with her family members might influence her coping response?
3. What information would the nurse provide to Marie about her initial treatment?
4. What are the possible complications the patient may face after a lumpectomy?
5. Which common postoperative exercises will Marie need to practice if she has an axillary lymph node dissection?
6. What community resources are available to help Marie and her family adjust to the change in her body and to cope with the diagnosis of cancer? How can the nurse access these resources?
7. What information about breast cancer risks is important to provide to Marie and her daughters? What early detection measures are important for them to know?
8. Based on the assessment data, write one or more appropriate nursing diagnoses. Are there any collaborative problems?

NCLEX EXAMINATION REVIEW QUESTIONS

The number of the question corresponds to the same-numbered objective at the beginning of the chapter.

1. An occupational health nurse is planning a program on breast cancer screening guidelines for women in the company. To best promote learning and adherence of the participants, the nurse includes
   a. a movie that demonstrates the procedure of BSE.
   b. distribution of detailed written instructions for use at home.
   c. an assessment of learning needs and readiness to learn the guidelines.
   d. explanations emphasizing the value of early detection of breast cancer.

2. The nurse teaches a patient who wants to perform BSE that the technique involves both the palpation of the breast tissue and
   a. palpation of cervical lymph nodes.
   b. hard squeezing of the breast tissue.
   c. a mammogram to evaluate breast tissue.
   d. inspection of the breasts for any changes.

3. In teaching a patient with painful fibrocystic breast changes about the condition, the nurse explains that
   a. all discrete breast lumps must be biopsied to rule out malignant changes.
   b. the symptoms will probably subside following menopause unless hormone replacement is used.
   c. restrictions of coffee and chocolate and supplements of vitamin E may relieve the discomfort for some patients.
   d. the lumps will become progressively larger and more painful, eventually necessitating surgical removal.

4. While discussing risk factors for breast cancer with a group of women, the nurse stresses that the greatest known risk factor for breast cancer is
   a. being a woman over age 60.
   b. experiencing menstruation for 40 years or more.
   c. using estrogen replacement therapy during menopause.
   d. having a paternal grandmother with postmenopausal breast cancer.

5. A patient has an excisional biopsy of a breast nodule that is positive for cancer. The nurse explains that of the other tests done to determine the risk for cancer recurrence or spread, the result that supports the most favorable prognosis is
   a. cells with low S-phase fractions.
   b. absence of an HER-2 cell marker.
   c. absence of axillary lymph node involvement.
   d. estrogen and progesterone receptor–positive tumors.

6. A patient diagnosed with breast cancer has been scheduled for a modified radical mastectomy with an axillary lymph node dissection. Postoperative nursing care that would assist in restoring arm function on the affected side would include
   a. the use of heating pads or blankets to increase circulation.
   b. daily applications of ice packs to minimize the risk of lymphedema.
   c. compression bandaging with sleeves or stocking for acute swelling.
   d. frequent and sustained exercises with the arm in the dependent position.

7. Postoperatively, the nurse teaches the patient with a modified radical mastectomy to prevent lymphedema by
   a. using a sling to keep the arm flexed at the side.
   b. exposing the arm to sunlight to increase circulation.
   c. wrapping the arm with elastic bandages during the night.
   d. avoiding unnecessary trauma (e.g., venipuncture, blood pressure measurement) to the arm on the operative side.

8. To prevent capsular formation following breast reconstruction with implants, the nurse teaches the patient to
   a. gently massage the area around the implant.
   b. bind the breasts tightly with elastic bandages.
   c. exercise the arm on the affected side to promote drainage.
   d. avoid strenuous exercise until implant healing has occurred.

REFERENCES

1. Jemal A et al: Cancer statistics 2005, *CA Cancer J Clin* 55:10, 2005.
2. Smith R et al: American Cancer Society guidelines for breast cancer screening: update 2003, *CA Cancer J Clin* 53:141, 2003.
3. Smith R, Cokkinides V, Eyre H: American Cancer Society guidelines for the early detection of cancer 2005, *CA Cancer J Clin* 55:31, 2005.
4. American Cancer Society: Role of breast self-examination changes in guidelines. Available at *www.cancer.org* (accessed July 4, 2005).
5. Jackson V: Diagnostic mammography, *Radiol Clin North Am* 42:853, 2004.
6. National Cancer Institute: PDQ: breast cancer screening—screening by mammography. Available at *http://cis.nci.nih.gov/cancertopics* (accessed July 6, 2005).
7. Engstrom P: The pros and cons of breast MRI, *Cancer Updates, Research, and Education (CURE)* 3:70, 2004.
8. Cleveland Clinic: Minimally invasive breast biopsy—stereotactic breast biopsy. Available at *www.clevelandclinic.org/breastcenter/services* (accessed July 6, 2005).
9. Harris J: Breast pain, *Pract Nurse* 29:36, 2005.
10. Inglehart D, Keelin C: Diseases of the breast. In Townsend C, editor: *Sabiston textbook of surgery*, ed 7, St Louis, 2004, Elsevier.
11. *Saunders nursing drug handbook*, St Louis, 2005, Saunders.
12. McCance KL, Huether SE, editors: *Pathophysiology: biologic basis for disease in adults and children*, ed 5, St Louis, 2006, Mosby.
13. Leung A, Pacaud D: Diagnosis and management of galactorrhea, *Am Fam Physician* 70:534, 2004.
14. Jarvis C: *Physical examination and health assessment*, ed 4, St Louis, 2004, Saunders.

15. American Cancer Society: *Breast cancer facts and figures 2003-2004,* Atlanta, 2003, American Cancer Society.

16. Chlebowski R et al: Influence of estrogen plus progestin on breast cancer and mammography in healthy postmenopausal women: the Women's Health Initiative Randomized Trial, *JAMA* 289:3253, 2003.

17. Women's Health Initiative Steering Committee: Effects of conjugated equine estrogen in postmenopausal women with hysterectomy, *JAMA* 291:1712, 2005.

18. National Cancer Institute: Cancer facts: oral contraceptives and cancer risk. Available at *http://cis.nci.nih.gov/fact* (accessed July 6, 2005).

19. Hollingsworth A et al: Current comprehensive assessment and management of women at increased risk for breast cancer, *Am J Surg* 187:349, 2004.

20. Dowdy SC: Surgical risk reduction: prophylactic salpingo-oophorectomy and prophylactic mastectomy, *Am J Obstet Gynecol* 191:1113, 2004.

21. Metcalfe K, Semple J, Narod S: Time to reconsider subcutaneous mastectomy for breast cancer prevention, *Lancet Oncol* 6:431, 2005.

*22. Baron R et al: Eighteen sensations after breast cancer surgery: a two-year old comparison of sentinel lymph node biopsy and axillary lymph node dissection, *Oncol Nurs Forum* 31:691, 2004.

23. Hughes M: Obesity and lymphatic mapping with sentinel lymph node biopsy in breast cancer, *Am J Surg* 187:52, 2004.

24. Hobday T, Perez E: Molecularly targeted therapies for breast cancer, *Cancer Control* 12:73, 2005.

25. American Joint Committee on Cancer: *Manual for staging of cancer,* ed 4, Philadelphia, 1992, Lippincott.

26. Mirshahidi H, Abraham J: Managing early breast cancer, *Postgrad Med* 116:23, 2004.

*27. Brown J: A clinically useful method for evaluating lymphedema, *Clin J Oncol Nurs* 8:35, 2004.

28. Sammarco A: Enhancing the quality of life of survivors of breast cancer, *Ann Long-Term Care* 12:40, 2004.

29. Thomson N et al: MammoSite radiation therapy system, *Clin J Oncol Nurs* 9:375, 2005.

30. Rouzier M et al: Breast conserving surgery after neoadjuvant anthracycline-based chemotherapy for large breast cancer tumors, *Cancer* 101:918, 2004.

31. Viale P: Aromatase inhibitor agents in breast cancer: evolving practices in hormonal therapy treatment, *Oncol Nurs Forum* 32:343, 2005.

32. Kudchadkar R, O'Regan R: Aromatase inhibitors as adjuvant therapy for postmenopausal patients with early stage breast cancer, *CA Cancer J Clin* 55:145, 2005.

33. Muscari E: Lymphedema: responding to our patient's needs, *Oncol Nurs Forum* 31:905, 2004.

34. Siebel MF, Muss HB: The influence of aging on the early detection, diagnosis, and treatment of breast cancer, *Curr Oncol Rep* 7:23, 2005.

35. U.S. Food and Drug Administration: Breast implant consumer handbook 2004. Available at *www.fda.gov/cdrh/breastimplants* (accessed July 9, 2005).

*Nursing research–based reference.

RESOURCES

American Cancer Society
800-ACS-2345
www.cancer.org

American Society of Plastic Surgeons
Plastic Surgery Education Foundation
888-475-2784
www.plasticsurgery.org

Living Beyond Breast Cancer
Survivors' helpline: 888-753-5222
610-645-4567
www.lbbc.org

National Alliance of Breast Cancer Organizations
888-80-NABCO
212-889-0606
www.nabco.org

National Breast Cancer Coalition
202-296-7477
www.natlbcc.org

National Cancer Institute
800-4-CANCER
www.nci.nih.gov

National Coalition for Cancer Survivorship (NCCS)
301-650-9127
www.canceradvocacy.org

National Lymphedema Network (NLN)
800-541-3259
510-208-3200
www.lymphnet.org

OncoLink (cancer information site)
University of Pennsylvania Cancer Center
www.oncolink.upenn.edu

Oncology Nursing Society
866-257-4667
www.ons.org

Sisters Network: A National Support Group for African American Breast Cancer Patients
713-781-0255
www.sistersnetworkinc.org

Susan G. Komen Breast Cancer Foundation
Helpline: 1-800-I'm Aware
972-855-1600
www.komen.org

Y-Me National Breast Cancer Organization
English: 800-221-2141
Spanish: 800-986-9505
www.Y-me.org

For additional Internet resources, see the website for this book at *http://evolve.elsevier.com/Lewis/medsurg.*

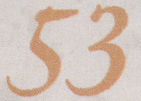

Questioning means longing to know the truth deeply, and insisting that we can.

Sharon Salzberg

53

Nursing Management
Sexually Transmitted Diseases

Shari Goldberg

LEARNING OBJECTIVES

1. Identify the factors contributing to the high incidence of sexually transmitted diseases.
2. Explain the etiology, clinical manifestations, complications, and diagnostic abnormalities of gonorrhea, syphilis, chlamydial infections, genital herpes, and genital warts.
3. Compare primary genital herpes with recurrent genital herpes.
4. Explain the collaborative care and drug therapy of gonorrhea, syphilis, chlamydial infections, genital herpes, and genital warts.
5. Identify the nursing assessment and nursing diagnoses for patients who have a sexually transmitted disease.
6. Describe the nursing role in the prevention and control of sexually transmitted diseases.
7. Describe the nursing management of patients with sexually transmitted diseases.

KEY TERMS

chancres, p. 1369
chlamydial infections, p. 1371
genital herpes, p. 1373
gonorrhea, p. 1367
lymphogranuloma venereum, p. 1373
sexually transmitted diseases, p. 1366
syphilis, p. 1369
venereal diseases, p. 1366

Electronic Resources

Supplemental content related to Chapter 53 can be found . . .

Companion CD
- Stress-Busting Kit for Nursing Students
- NCLEX Examination Review Questions
- Comprehensive Glossary

Evolve Website *evolve*
http://evolve.elsevier.com/Lewis/medsurg
- Content Updates
- Key Points (Printable and CD/MP3 Download)
- Concept Map Creator
- Expanded Audio Glossary

- Key Term Flash Cards
- Electronic Calculators
- WebLinks

Sexually Transmitted Diseases

Sexually transmitted diseases (STDs) are infectious diseases transmitted most commonly through sexual contact (Table 53-1). Historically they have been referred to as **venereal diseases.** Many of the agents causing STDs are easily inactivated by drying, heating, and washing. These infections can be bacterial (gonorrhea, chlamydia, syphilis) or viral (genital herpes, genital warts). Most infections start as lesions on the genitalia and other sexually exposed mucous membranes. Wide dissemination to other areas of the body can then occur. A latent or subclinical phase is present with all STDs. This can lead to a long-term persistent infection and the transmission of disease from an asymptomatic (but infected) person to another contact person. Different STDs can coexist within one person. For example, if a person has gonorrhea, chlamydial infection may also be present.

In the United States all cases of gonorrhea and syphilis, and in most states chlamydial infection, must be reported to the state or local public health authorities. In spite of this requirement, there are many unreported cases of these infections. An estimated 65 million Americans are currently infected with one or more STDs.[1] Every year an additional 19 million Americans are newly infected with an STD.[2] Diseases that are associated with sexual transmission can also be contracted by other routes such as through blood, blood products, and autoinoculation.

The more commonly diagnosed STDs are discussed in this chapter. Human immunodeficiency virus (HIV) infection and related problems are discussed in Chapter 15. Hepatitis B infection and related problems are discussed in Chapter 44.

Reviewed by Dana Rosdahl, RN, PhD, APRN-BC, Assistant Professor, College of Nursing, Arizona State University, Phoenix, Ariz.

TABLE 53-1	Microorganisms Responsible for Diseases Transmitted by Sexual Activity
Organism	**Disease**
Chlamydia trachomatis	Nongonococcal urethritis (NGU), cervicitis, lymphogranuloma venereum
Cytomegalovirus (CMV)	Encephalitis, esophagitis, retinitis, pneumonitis in immunocompromised patients
Hepatitis B virus	Hepatitis B
Herpes simplex virus (HSV)	Genital herpes
Human immunodeficiency virus (HIV)	HIV infection, acquired immunodeficiency syndrome (AIDS)
Human papillomavirus (HPV)	Genital warts
Poxvirus	Molluscum contagiosum
Neisseria gonorrhoeae	Gonorrhea
Treponema pallidum	Syphilis

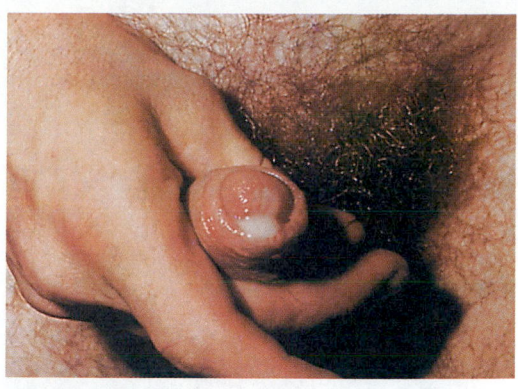

FIG. 53-1 Gonococcal urethritis. Profuse, purulent drainage.

Factors Affecting Incidence of Sexually Transmitted Diseases

Many contributing factors are related to the current STD rates. Earlier reproductive maturity and increased longevity have resulted in a longer sexual life span. The increase in the total population has resulted in an increase in the number of susceptible hosts. Other factors include greater sexual freedom, lack of barrier methods (e.g., condoms) during sexual activity, and an increased emphasis in the media on sexuality. In addition, increased leisure time, more national and international travel, and urbanization have brought together people with varying social behaviors and value systems.[1]

Changes in the methods of contraception are also reflected in the incidence of STDs. The condom is considered to be the best form of protection against STDs.[3] Although condom use has increased, condoms are still not used frequently in the general population. Commonly used oral contraceptives cause the secretions of the cervix and the vagina to become more alkaline. This change produces a more favorable environment for the growth of organisms that cause STDs at these sites. Women who take oral contraceptives may have a lower risk of pelvic inflammatory disease (PID) as a result of the ability of the cervical mucus to act as a barrier against bacteria. However, the proliferation of chlamydia, the leading cause of nongonococcal PID, may be enhanced by oral contraceptive use. Whether or not intrauterine device (IUD) users are at increased risk of PID is controversial, but it is clear that IUDs confer no protection against STDs. Long-acting contraceptives such as levonorgestrel (Norplant) and medroxyprogesterone (Depo-Provera) also confer no protection against STDs.

Bacterial Infections

GONORRHEA

Gonorrhea is the second most frequently reported STD in the United States (chlamydial infections are the most common).[4] Following a 74% decline in the reported rate of gonorrhea from 1975 to 1997, gonorrhea rates remained stable, then from 2000 to 2004 decreased 11.8%. In 2004, over 330,000 cases of gonorrhea were reported in the United States.[4] Gonorrhea rates are highest in ado-

lescents of all racial and ethnic groups, in people living in the southern part of the United States, and among African Americans. Most states have enacted laws that permit examination and treatment of minors without parental consent.

Etiology and Pathophysiology

Gonorrhea is caused by *Neisseria gonorrhoeae,* a gram-negative diplococcus. The disease is spread by direct physical contact with an infected host, usually during sexual activity (vaginal, oral, or anal). Mucosa with columnar epithelium is susceptible to gonococcal infection. This tissue is present in the genitalia (urethra in men, cervix in women), the rectum, and the oropharynx. Neonates can develop a gonococcal infection during delivery from an infected mother. The delicate gonococcus is easily killed by drying, heating, or washing with an antiseptic solution. Consequently, indirect transmission by instruments or linens is rare. The incubation period is 3 to 8 days. The disease confers no immunity to subsequent reinfection. Gonococcal infection elicits an inflammatory response, which, if left untreated, leads to the formation of fibrous tissue and adhesions. This fibrous scarring is subsequently responsible for many complications in women such as strictures and tubal abnormalities, which can lead to tubal pregnancy, chronic pelvic pain, and infertility.

Clinical Manifestations

Men. The initial site of infection in men is usually the urethra. Symptoms of urethritis consist of dysuria and profuse, purulent urethral discharge developing 2 to 5 days after infection (Fig. 53-1). Painful or swollen testicles may also occur. Men generally seek medical evaluation early in the disease because their symptoms are usually obvious and distressing. It is unusual for men with gonorrhea to be asymptomatic.

Women. Many women who contract gonorrhea are asymptomatic or have minor symptoms that are often overlooked, making it possible for them to remain a source of infection. A few women may complain of vaginal discharge, dysuria, or frequency of urination. Changes in menstruation may be a symptom, but these changes are often disregarded by the woman. After the incubation period, redness and swelling occur at the site of contact, which is usually the cervix or urethra (Fig. 53-2). A greenish-yellow purulent exudate often develops with a potential for abscess formation. The disease may remain local or can spread by direct tissue extension to the uterus, fallopian tubes, and ovaries. Although the vulva and vagina are uncommon sites for a gonorrheal infection, they may become involved when little or no estrogen is

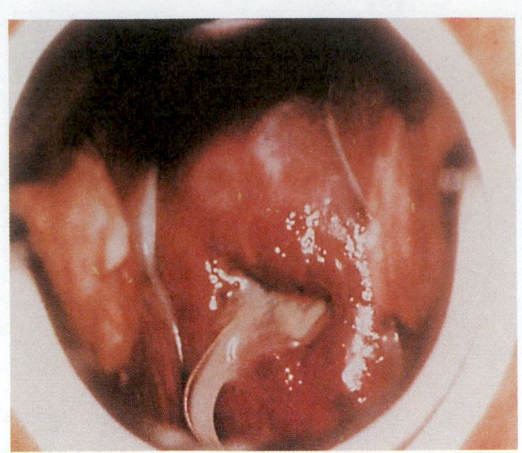

FIG. 53-2 Endocervical gonorrhea. Cervical redness and edema with discharge.

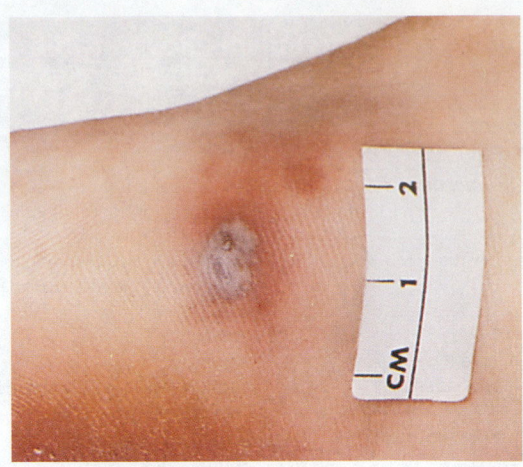

FIG. 53-3 Disseminated gonococcal infection. Skin lesion with gray, necrotic center on erythematous base.

present, as is the case in prepubertal girls and postmenopausal women. Because the vagina acts as a natural reservoir for infectious secretions, transmission is often more efficient from men to women than it is from women to men.

General. Anorectal gonorrhea may be present and is usually caused by anal intercourse. Symptoms may include soreness, itching, and discharge of the anus. Most patients with anorectal infections and infections in the throat have few symptoms. A small percentage of individuals develop gonococcal pharyngitis resulting from orogenital sexual contact. When the gonococcus can be demonstrated by a laboratory culture, individuals of either gender are infectious to their sexual partners.

Complications

Because men often seek treatment early in the course of the disease, they are less likely to develop complications. The complications that do occur in men are prostatitis, urethral strictures, and sterility from orchitis or epididymitis. Because women who are asymptomatic seldom seek treatment, complications are more common and usually constitute the reason for seeking medical attention. Pelvic inflammatory disease (PID), Bartholin's abscess, ectopic pregnancy, and infertility are the main complications of gonorrhea in women. A small percentage of infected persons, mainly women, may develop a disseminated gonococcal infection (DGI). In DGI the appearance of skin lesions, fever, arthralgia, arthritis, or endocarditis usually causes the patient to seek medical help (Fig. 53-3).

Eye Infections in Newborns. Almost all states have a health department regulation or law requiring the instillation of a prophylactic drug such as erythromycin (0.5%) ophthalmic ointment or silver nitrate (0.1%) aqueous solution into the eyes of all newborns in a single application. The incidence of gonorrheal eye infections in newborns *(ophthalmia neonatorum)* is therefore relatively rare today.[5] Untreated infected infants develop permanent blindness.

Diagnostic Studies

For men, a presumptive diagnosis of gonorrhea is made if there is a history of sexual contact with a new or infected partner followed within a few days by a urethral discharge. Typical clinical manifestations, combined with a positive finding in a Gram-stained smear of

the purulent discharge from the penis, gives an almost certain diagnosis. A culture of the discharge is indicated for men whose smears are negative in the presence of strong clinical evidence. A nonculture test is now available that can test for both *N. gonorrhoeae* and *Chlamydia trachomatis*. This nucleic acid amplification test (NAAT) (using ligase or polymerase chain reaction) has sensitivity similar to culture, and testing can be done on a wide variety of samples, including vaginal, endocervical, urethral, and urine specimens. Other nonculture testing procedures include enzyme immunoassays (EIAs) and direct fluorescent antibody (DFA) tests.

Making a diagnosis of gonorrhea in women on the basis of symptoms is difficult because most women are symptom free or have complaints that may be confused with other conditions. Smears and purulent discharge do not establish a diagnosis of gonorrhea because the female genitourinary tract normally harbors a large number of organisms that resemble *N. gonorrhoeae*. A culture must be performed to confirm the diagnosis. Although the cervix is the most common site of sampling, specimens for culture may also be taken from the urethra, anus, or oropharynx to confirm the diagnosis.[6]

Collaborative Care

Drug Therapy. Because of a short incubation period and high infectivity, treatment is generally instituted without awaiting culture results, even in the absence of any signs or symptoms.[1] The treatment of gonorrhea in the early stage is curative. The most common treatment for gonorrhea is a single intramuscular (IM) dose of ceftriaxone (Rocephin). Other medications that may be used in the treatment of gonorrhea include cefixime (Suprax), ciprofloxacin (Cipro), ofloxacin (Floxin), and levofloxacin (Levaquin) (Table 53-2). Resistance to the fluoroquinolones, such as ciprofloxacin (Cipro), has been reported and is a cause for concern, although it is still somewhat rare. The high frequency (up to 20% in men and 40% in women) of coexisting chlamydial and gonococcal infections has led to the addition of azithromycin (Zithromax) or doxycycline (Vibramycin) to the treatment regimen. Patients with coexisting syphilis are likely to be cured by the same drugs used for gonorrhea.

Drug Alert - *Doxycycline (Vibramycin)*
• *Avoid unnecessary exposure to sunlight.*
• *Do not take with antacids, iron products, or dairy products.*

TABLE 53-2	COLLABORATIVE CARE Gonorrhea

Diagnostic
History and physical examination
Gram-stained smears of urethral or endocervical exudate
Culture for *Neisseria gonorrhoeae*
Nucleic acid amplification test (NAAT) to detect *N. gonorrhoeae*
Testing for other STDs (syphilis, HIV, chlamydia)

Collaborative Therapy
Uncomplicated gonorrhea: cefixime (Suprax) 400 mg orally in a single dose or ceftriaxone (Rocephin) 125 mg IM in a single dose or ciprofloxacin (Cipro) 500 mg orally in a single dose or ofloxacin (Floxin) 400 mg orally in a single dose or levofloxacin (Levaquin) 250 mg orally in a single dose
If chlamydial infection is not ruled out: azithromycin (Zithromax) 1 g orally in a single dose or doxycycline (Vibramycin) 100 mg orally twice a day for 7 days
Patients who are allergic to cephalosporins or quinolones should be treated with spectinomycin 2 g IM in a single dose
Patients who have uncomplicated gonorrhea and who are treated with any of the above therapies may not need to return to confirm that they are cured
Case finding
Treatment of sexual contacts
Instruction on abstinence from sexual intercourse and alcohol
Reexamination if symptoms persist or recur after completion of treatment

Modified from Centers for Disease Control and Prevention: STD treatment guidelines, *www.cdc.gov/STD/treatment*.
HIV, Human immunodeficiency virus; *IM*, intramuscular; *STD*, sexually transmitted disease.

All sexual contacts of patients with gonorrhea must be evaluated and treated to prevent reinfection after resumption of sexual relations. The "ping-pong" effect of reexposure, treatment, and reinfection can cease only when infected partners are treated simultaneously. Additionally, the patient should be counseled to abstain from sexual intercourse and alcohol during treatment. Sexual intercourse allows the infection to spread and can delay complete healing. Alcohol has an irritant effect on the healing urethral walls. Men should be cautioned against squeezing the penis to look for further discharge. Reinfection, rather than treatment failure, is the main cause for infections identified after treatment has ended.

SYPHILIS

The incidence of **syphilis** reported in the United States in 2000 was at its lowest rate since reporting started in 1941.[7] However, an increase in syphilis rates was noted from 2001 to 2004. In 2004, the total number of cases was 7980. The increased rate is mainly due to men who have sex with men.[7] The rates increased in whites, African Americans, Hispanics, and Asians.

Etiology and Pathophysiology

The causative organism of syphilis is *Treponema pallidum*, a spirochete. This bacterium is thought to enter the body through very small breaks in the skin or mucous membranes. Its entry is facilitated by the minor abrasions that often occur during sexual intercourse. Syphilis is a complex disease in which many organs and tissues of the body can become infected by *T. pallidum*. The infection causes the production of antibodies that also react with normal tissues.

After a short period of protection, the antibody levels decrease, and a person is susceptible to reinfection.[8] Not all people who are exposed to syphilis acquire the disease; about one third become infected after intercourse with an infected person. In addition to sexual contact, syphilis may be spread through contact with infectious lesions and sharing of needles among intravenous (IV) drug users. *T. pallidum* is extremely fragile and easily destroyed by drying, heating, or washing. The incubation period for syphilis ranges from 10 to 90 days (average 21 days). Congenital syphilis is transmitted from an infected mother to the fetus in utero after the tenth week of pregnancy. An infected pregnant woman has a high risk of a stillbirth (baby born dead) or having a baby who dies shortly after birth. Rates of congenital syphilis declined 8.8% from 2002 to 2003.[9]

There is an association between syphilis and HIV infection. Persons at high risk for acquiring syphilis are also at an increased risk for acquiring HIV. Often, both infections may be present in the same person. The presence of syphilitic lesions on the genitals enhances HIV transmission. HIV-infected patients with syphilis appear to be at greatest risk for clinically significant central nervous system (CNS) involvement and may require more intensive treatment with penicillin than do other patients with syphilis. Therefore the evaluation of all patients with syphilis should also include testing for HIV with the patient's consent.

Clinical Manifestations

Syphilis has a variety of signs and symptoms that can mimic a number of other diseases. Consequently, compared with other STDs, it is more difficult to recognize syphilis. If it is not treated, specific clinical stages are characteristic of the progression of the disease (Table 53-3). In the *primary stage* of the bacterial invasion (Fig. 53-4), **chancres** appear. These are painless indurated lesions on the penis, vulva, lips, mouth, vagina, and rectum. They frequently occur 10 to 90 days after inoculation. The chancre lasts 3 to 6 weeks, eventually healing on its own. During this time the draining of the microorganisms into the lymph nodes causes regional lymphadenopathy. Genital ulcers may also be present. Without treatment the infection progresses to the secondary stage.

The *secondary stage* of syphilis is systemic. The stage begins a few weeks after the chancres are first seen, and blood-borne bacteria spread to all major organ systems. Manifestations characteristic of the secondary stage can include flu-like symptoms, such as fever, sore throat, headaches, fatigue, and generalized adenopathy. Cutaneous eruptions can also occur (Fig. 53-5), and include a bilateral, symmetric rash that typically begins on the trunk and also involves the palms and soles; mucous patches in the mouth, tongue, or cervix; and *condylomata lata* (moist, weeping papules) in the anal and genital area.

The *latent* or *hidden stage* of syphilis follows the secondary stage and is a period during which the immune system is able to suppress the infection. The latent stage can be further divided into an early stage, in which the infection has been acquired in the preceding year, and a late stage, in which the infection has been present for greater than 1 year. There are no signs or symptoms of syphilis during this time. During the latent stage, the diagnosis is established by a positive specific treponemal antibody test for syphilis together with a normal cerebrospinal fluid (CSF) examination and the absence of clinical manifestations on physical examination and chest x-rays. About 70% of untreated patients with latent syphilis never develop clinically evident, third-stage syphilis, but the occurrence of a spontaneous cure of syphilis is doubtful.[10]

The *third stage* of syphilis (also called *late* or *tertiary* syphilis) is the most severe stage of the disease. Because antibiotics can

TABLE 53-3	Stages of Syphilis		
Clinical Stage	**Characteristic Findings**	**Communicability**	**Duration of Stage**
Primary	Chancre	Exudate from chancre highly infectious; blood is infectious	3-8 wk
Secondary	Cutaneous lesions, condylomata lata, alopecia, systemic symptoms (malaise, arthralgia, headache, occasionally liver and kidney dysfunction), regional adenopathy 6-12 wk after chancre	Exudate from skin and mucous membrane lesions highly infectious	1-2 yr
Latent	Absence of signs or symptoms	Noninfectious after 4 yr, possible placental transmission	Throughout life or progression to late stage
Late*	Appearance 3-20 yr after initial infection	Noninfectious	Chronic (without treatment), possibly fatal
Benign	Gummas (chronic, destructive lesions affecting any organ of body, especially skin, bone, liver, mucous membranes)	Spinal fluid possibly containing organism	
Cardiovascular	Aortic valve insufficiency or saccular aneurysm of thoracic aorta, aortitis		
Neurosyphilis	General paresis (personality changes from minor to psychotic, tremors, physical and mental deterioration) Tabes dorsalis (ataxia, areflexia, paresthesias, lightning pains, damaged joints) Speech disturbances		

*Several forms such as cardiovascular and neurosyphilis occur together in approximately 25% of untreated cases.

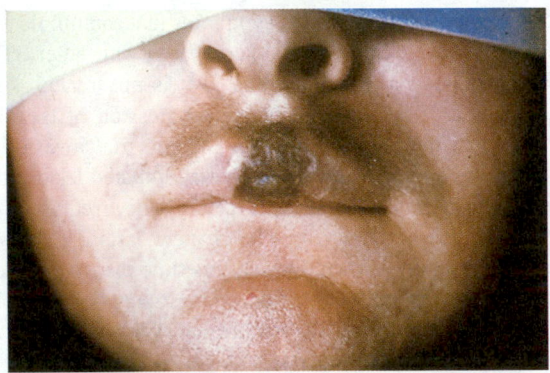

FIG. 53-4   Primary syphilis chancre on upper lip.

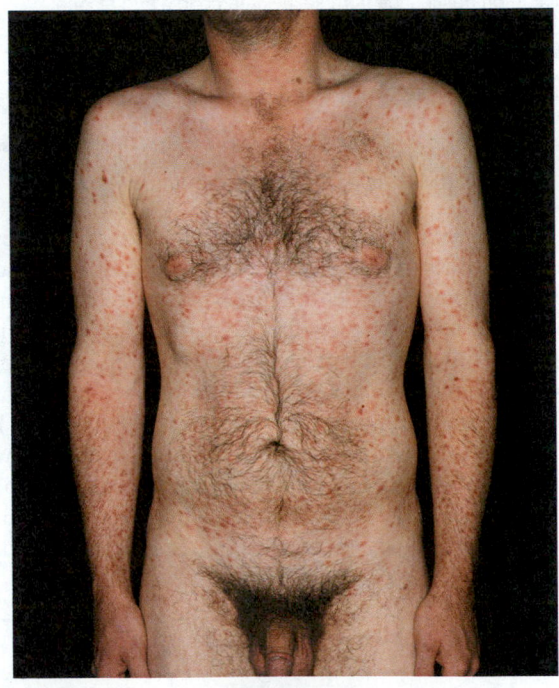

FIG. 53-5   Secondary syphilis. Bilateral, symmetric cutaneous lesions.

cure syphilis, manifestations of late syphilis are rare. However, when it does occur, it is responsible for significant morbidity and mortality rates. The pathogenesis of the manifestations of this stage is unclear. *Gummas* (destructive skin, bone, and soft tissue nodular lesions associated with late syphilis) are probably caused by a severe hypersensitivity reaction to the microorganism. Within the cardiovascular system late syphilis may cause aneurysms, heart valve insufficiency, and heart failure. Within the CNS the presence of *T. pallidum* in CSF may cause manifestations of *neurosyphilis* (general paresis) (see Table 53-3).

Complications

Complications of the disease occur mostly in late syphilis. The gummas of benign late syphilis may produce irreparable damage to bone, liver, or skin but seldom result in death. In cardiovascular syphilis, the resulting aneurysm may press on structures such as the intercostal nerves, causing pain. The possibility of a rupture exists as the aneurysm increases in size. Scarring of the aortic valve results in aortic valve insufficiency and eventually heart failure.

Neurosyphilis is responsible for degeneration of the brain with mental deterioration. Evidence of other neurologic deficits may be present. Problems related to sensory nerve involvement are a result

of *tabes dorsalis* (progressive locomotor ataxia). There may be sudden attacks of pain anywhere in the body, which can confuse the diagnosis with other conditions. Loss of vision and sense of position in the feet and legs can also occur. Walking may become even more difficult as joint stability is lost. (Late syphilis is also discussed in Chapter 59.)

Diagnostic Studies

The first step in diagnosis is to obtain a detailed and accurate sexual history. A physical examination should be done to identify any suspicious lesions, as well as to note other significant signs and symptoms.

TABLE 53-4	COLLABORATIVE CARE Syphilis

Diagnostic
History and physical examination
Dark-field microscopy
Nontreponemal and/or treponemal serologic testing
Testing for other STDs (HIV, gonorrhea, chlamydia)

Collaborative Therapy
Appropriate drug therapy (see Table 53-5)
Confidential counseling and testing for HIV infection
Case finding
Surveillance
- Repeat of quantitative nontreponemal tests at 3, 6, and 12 mo
- Examination of cerebrospinal fluid at 1 yr if treatment involves alternative antibiotics or treatment failure has occurred

HIV, Human immunodeficiency virus; *STD,* sexually transmitted disease.

TABLE 53-5	DRUG THERAPY Syphilis	

Stage	Type of Penicillin	Other Antibiotics*
Early syphilis (primary, secondary, and early latent)	2.4 million U IM of penicillin G benzathine (Bicillin) in a single dose	doxycycline (Vibramycin) 100 mg orally twice a day for 2 wk, or tetracycline 500 mg orally four times a day for 2 wk
Re-treatment, if needed	7.2 million U of Bicillin total, given as three doses of 2.4 million U IM of Bicillin each, at 1-wk intervals	
Late latent syphilis	7.2 million U total of Bicillin given as three doses of 2.4 million U IM of Bicillin each at 1-wk intervals	doxycycline or tetracycline given for 4 wk at same dosage/ routes as early syphilis
Tertiary syphilis		
Gumma, cardiovascular	Same as for re-treatment and late latent stage	Same as for late latent stage
Neurosyphilis	Aqueous crystalline penicillin G 18-24 U IV daily, given as 3-4 million U every 4 hr for 10-14 days	procaine penicillin G 2.4 million U IM once daily plus probenecid (Benemid) 500 mg orally four times a day; both drugs given for 10-14 days

Modified from Centers for Disease Control and Prevention: STD treatment guidelines, *www.cdc.gov/STD/treatment.*
IM, Intramuscular; *IV,* intravenous.
*Given when penicillin is contraindicated.

The presence of spirochetes on dark-field microscopy and direct fluorescent antibody tests of lesion exudate or tissue can confirm a clinical diagnosis of syphilis. However, syphilis is more commonly diagnosed by a serologic test. Tests for syphilis may be classified as those performed for screening and those performed for confirmation of a positive screening test. Nonspecific antitreponemal antibodies can be detected by tests such as the Venereal Disease Research Laboratory (VDRL) test and the rapid plasma reagin (RPR) test. These nontreponemal tests are suitable for screening purposes and usually become positive 10 to 14 days after the appearance of a chancre. The fluorescent treponemal antibody absorption (FTA-Abs) test and the *T. pallidum* particle agglutination (TP-PA) test detect specific antitreponemal antibodies and are suitable for confirming the diagnosis.

False-negative and false-positive test results do occur with the nontreponemal tests (VDRL, RPR). A false-negative result may be obtained during primary syphilis if the test is done before the individual has had time to produce antibodies. A false-positive finding may occur with other diseases or conditions such as hepatitis, infectious mononucleosis, after smallpox vaccination, collagen diseases (e.g., systemic lupus erythematosus), pregnancy, or aging. Positive nontreponemal test results should be confirmed by more specific treponemal tests to rule out other causes. In the CSF, changes such as increased white blood cell count, increased total protein, and a positive treponemal antibody test are diagnostic of asymptomatic neurosyphilis.

If a patient is treated with antibiotics early in the course of the disease on the basis of the history and the symptoms, the serologic testing may not indicate the presence of syphilis. Once a person has positive serologic findings for syphilis, indicating the presence of antibodies, these findings may remain positive for an indefinite period in spite of successful treatment.

Collaborative Care

Drug Therapy. Management of syphilis is aimed at eradication of all syphilitic organisms (Table 53-4). However, treatment cannot reverse damage that is already present in the late stage of the disease. Penicillin G benzathine (Bicillin) or aqueous procaine penicillin G remains the treatment of choice for all stages of syphilis. To date, after four decades of use, there is no evidence to suggest a decrease in the effectiveness of penicillin against *T. pallidum.* Table 53-5 describes therapy for the various stages of syphilis and

is in accordance with U.S. Public Health Service recommendations. All stages of syphilis should be treated. Patients having persistent or recurring symptoms after drug therapy has ended should be re-treated. All patients with neurosyphilis must be carefully monitored, with periodic serologic testing, clinical evaluation at 6-month intervals, and repeat CSF examinations for at least 3 years. Specific management is based on the symptoms.

During pregnancy, IM penicillin G is effective in preventing the transmission of syphilis from mother to fetus.[2] It is also effective in treating fetal infection.

CHLAMYDIAL INFECTIONS

Chlamydial infections are the most commonly reported STD in the United States today. In 2004, there were 929,462 cases of genital *C. trachomatis* infections reported in the United States. This represents a 5.9% increase compared with the rate of the previous year. The incidence of chlamydia is three times higher in women than men, which may be due to the larger numbers of women screened for this disease.[11] In Canada, chlamydia is also the most commonly reported STD, with a rate increase of 60% between 1997 and 2002. More than two thirds of the total reported cases were attributed to women.[12] Underreporting is substantial because most people are asymptomatic and do not seek testing. Chlamydial

TABLE 53-6	Risk Factors for Chlamydial Infection

- Women and adolescents
- New or multiple sexual partners
- Sexual partners who have had multiple partners
- History of STDs and cervical ectopy
- Coexisting STDs
- Inconsistent or incorrect use of condom

Data from U.S. Preventive Services Task Force: Screening for chlamydial infection: recommendations and rationale, *Am J Prev Med* 20(3 suppl):90, 2001. *STDs,* Sexually transmitted diseases.

infections are a major contributor to PID, ectopic pregnancy, infertility among women, and nongonococcal urethritis in men.

Etiology and Pathophysiology

Chlamydial infections are caused by *Chlamydia trachomatis,* a gram-negative bacterium. Chlamydia can be transmitted during vaginal, anal, or oral sex. Numerous different serotypes, or strains, of *C. trachomatis* cause urogenital infections (e.g., nongonococcal urethritis [NGU] in men and cervicitis in women), ocular trachoma, and lymphogranuloma venereum. Chlamydial infections can cause fallopian tube damage, a leading cause for ectopic pregnancy and failure to conceive.[13]

By age 30, it is estimated that at some time during their lives 50% of all sexually active women have had a chlamydial infection. Women with chlamydia may also be at high risk for acquiring HIV from an infected partner.

Because chlamydial infections are closely associated with gonococcal infections, clinical differentiation may be difficult. In men, urethritis, epididymitis, and proctitis may occur in both diseases. In women, bartholinitis, cervicitis, and salpingitis (inflammation of the fallopian tube) can occur in both chlamydial and gonococcal infections. Therefore both infections are usually treated concurrently even without diagnostic evidence. The incubation period of 1 to 3 weeks for chlamydial infection is longer than that for gonorrhea, and the symptoms are often milder. The high incidence of recurrence may be because of failure to treat the sexual partners of infected persons. Table 53-6 lists the risk factors for chlamydial infection. Because of the high prevalence of asymptomatic infections, screening of high-risk populations is needed to identify those infected.

Clinical Manifestations and Complications

Chlamydia is known as a silent disease because symptoms may be absent or minor in most infected women and in many men. As with gonorrhea, chlamydial infections result in a superficial mucosal infection that can become more invasive. Signs and symptoms in men include urethritis (dysuria, urethral discharge), proctitis (rectal discharge and pain during defecation), and epididymitis (unilateral scrotal pain, swelling, tenderness, fever) (Fig. 53-6). Signs and symptoms in women include cervicitis (mucopurulent discharge, hypertrophic ectopy [area that is edematous and bleeds easily]), urethritis (dysuria, frequent urination, pyuria), bartholinitis (purulent exudate), dyspareunia (pain with intercourse), PID (abdominal pain, nausea, vomiting, fever, malaise, abnormal vaginal bleeding, menstrual abnormalities), and perihepatitis (fever, nausea, vomiting, right upper quadrant pain).

Complications often develop from poorly managed, inaccurately diagnosed, or undiagnosed chlamydial infections. The infection is often not diagnosed until complications appear. Complications in

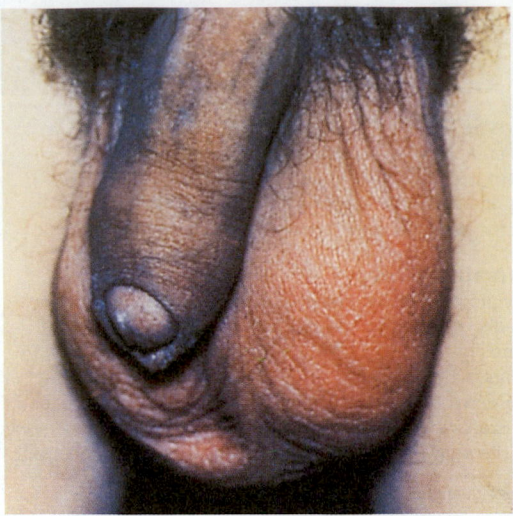

FIG. 53-6 Chlamydial epididymitis. Red, swollen scrotum.

TABLE 53-7	*COLLABORATIVE CARE* Chlamydial Infection

Diagnostic
History and physical examination
Nucleic acid amplification test (NAAT) to detect chlamydia
Direct fluorescent antibody (DFA) test for chlamydia
Enzyme immunoassay (EIA) for chlamydia antigen
Testing for other STDs (gonorrhea, HIV, syphilis)
Culture for chlamydia

Collaborative Therapy
doxycycline (Vibramycin) 100 mg twice a day for 7 days or azithromycin (Zithromax) 1 g in a single dose
Alternative regimen: erythromycin, ofloxacin (Floxin), or levofloxacin (Levaquin)
Instruction on abstinence from sexual intercourse for 7 days after treatment
Treatment of all sexual partners

HIV, Human immunodeficiency virus; *STDs,* sexually transmitted diseases.

men may result in epididymitis, with possible infertility and reactive arthritis (a systemic condition characterized by urethritis, conjunctivitis, arthritis, and mucocutaneous lesions). Complications from chlamydial infections in women may result in PID, which can lead to chronic pelvic pain and infertility. For this reason the Centers for Disease Control and Prevention (CDC) recommends that all females younger than 25 years of age be routinely screened for chlamydia at their annual gynecologic examination. The CDC further advises annual screening of all women older than 25 years of age with one or more risk factors for the disease.[2]

Diagnostic Studies and Collaborative Care

Chlamydial infections in men can be diagnosed by excluding gonorrhea. The cervical or urethral discharge appears to be less purulent, watery, and painful in chlamydial infections than in gonorrhea. Table 53-7 outlines collaborative care for chlamydial infections.

Cell culture can be used to detect chlamydia. However, the most common diagnostic tests include the nucleic acid amplification test (NAAT), the direct fluorescent antibody (DFA) test, and enzyme immunoassay (EIA). These tests do not require special handling of specimens and are easier to perform than cell cultures. Amplification

EVIDENCE-BASED PRACTICE

Which Male Condom Has More Breakage During Intercourse?

Clinical Question

In sexually active, heterosexual couples (P), do nonlatex male condoms (I) or latex male condoms (C) have higher rates of breakage during intercourse (O)?

Best Available Evidence

Systematic review of randomized controlled trials (RCTs)

Critical Appraisal and Synthesis of Evidence

- Randomized crossover trials ($n = 7$) with 1590 couples and three randomized parallel trials ($n = 1635$ couples).
- Clinical breakage was higher for the nonlatex condoms than for the latex condoms.
- Lack of experience with condom use may have increased number of condom failures and subject attrition.

Conclusions

- Nonlatex condoms are more likely to break than latex condoms.
- Nonlatex condoms are preferred over latex condoms and are useful in cases of latex sensitivity and allergy.

Implications for Nursing Practice

- Educate patients about higher risk for breakage of nonlatex condoms as compared to latex condoms.
- Explore if nonlatex condom users have greater compliance with condom use.
- Conduct RCTs comparing latex and nonlatex condoms for their effectiveness in reducing transmission of human immunodeficiency virus and sexually transmitted diseases.

Reference for Evidence

Gallo MF, Grimes DA, Schulz KF: Non-latex versus latex male condoms for contraception, *Cochrane Database of Systematic Reviews* 1, 2003.

PICO: P, Patient population of interest; *I,* intervention or area of interest; *C,* comparison of interest or comparison group; *O,* outcome(s) of interest (see p. 6).

---

tests are the most sensitive diagnostic methods available and require fewer organisms. In addition, these tests can be used with urine samples rather than urethral and cervical swabs.

Drug Therapy. When diagnosed, chlamydia can be easily treated and cured. Chlamydial infections respond to treatment with doxycycline (Vibramycin) or azithromycin (Zithromax).[14] For doxycycline, the dosage is 100 mg two times a day for 7 days. Azithromycin (1 g in a single dose) offers the advantage of ease of administration. Alternative regimens include erythromycin, ofloxacin (Floxin), and levofloxacin (Levaquin). Patients treated for chlamydia should abstain from sexual intercourse for 7 days after treatment and until all sexual partners have completed a full course of treatment.[6] Follow-up care should include advising the patient to return if the symptoms persist or recur, treating sexual partners, and encouraging the use of condoms during all sexual contacts.

Lymphogranuloma Venereum

Lymphogranuloma venereum (LGV) is an STD caused by specific strains of *C. trachomatis*. LGV is rare in the United States, but it is endemic in other areas of the world, including Africa, Asia, South America, and the Caribbean. The peak incidence of LGV is during the ages of 20 to 30 years old, generally the time of greatest sexual activity.

The strain of *C. trachomatis* that causes LGV is transmitted through intercourse or through contact with exudate from active lesions. LGV begins as a small, painless genital lesion and spreads via the lymph nodes of the genital-rectal areas. It may also spread systemically through the bloodstream and enter the CNS. Penile, vulvar, and anal infection can lead to inguinal and femoral lymphadenopathy. Marked inflammation occurs, resulting in necrosis, *buboes* (greatly enlarged, inflamed lymph nodes), abscesses of inguinal lymph nodes, and infection of surrounding tissue. Healing occurs by fibrosis after several weeks or months and can result in chronic scarring, which damages the lymph nodes and disrupts nodal function.

Constitutional symptoms that occur during the stage of regional lymphadenopathy include fever, chills, headache, *meningismus* (meningitis-like symptoms), anorexia, myalgia, and arthralgia. Complications of untreated anorectal infection include strictures, fissures, constipation, perirectal abscesses, and rectovaginal and perianal fistulas. LGV is generally treated with doxycycline (Vibramycin), 100 mg orally twice a day, for 21 days. Also effective is erythromycin 500 mg orally four times a day for 21 days. Buboes may require aspiration to prevent inguinal and femoral ulcerations from occurring. Sexual partners should also be treated.

Viral Infections

GENITAL HERPES

Genital herpes is not a reportable disease in most states, and its true incidence is difficult to determine. Approximately 1.7 million new cases of herpes simplex virus type 2 (HSV-2) are acquired each year, and more than 50% of these cases are asymptomatic or unrecognized. The CDC estimates that at least 45 million people in the United States have had genital HSV infection.[2] Since the late 1970s the prevalence of HSV-2 has risen by 30%.

Etiology and Pathophysiology

The herpes simplex virus (HSV) enters through the mucous membranes or breaks in the skin during contact with an infected person. HSV then reproduces inside the cell and spreads to the surrounding cells. The virus next enters the peripheral or autonomic nerve endings and ascends to the sensory or autonomic nerve ganglion, where it often becomes dormant. Viral reactivation (recurrence) may occur when the virus descends down to the initial site of infection, either the mucous membranes or skin. When a person is infected with HSV, the virus usually persists within the individual for life. Transmission of HSV occurs through direct contact with skin or mucous membranes when an infected individual is symptomatic or through asymptomatic viral shedding.[15]

Two different strains of HSV cause infection. In general, HSV type 1 (HSV-1) causes infection above the waist, involving the gingivae, the dermis, the upper respiratory tract, and the CNS. HSV type 2 (HSV-2) most frequently infects the genital tract and the perineum (i.e., locations below the waist). However, either strain can cause disease on the mouth or the genitals. The majority of genital herpes cases are from HSV-2 infection. The incidence of genital herpes caused by HSV-1 is on the rise. However, current reports indicate that at least 15% of genital herpes cases in the United States are now caused by HSV-1.

Clinical Manifestations

In the *primary (initial) episode* of genital herpes the patient may complain of burning or tingling at the site of inoculation. Multiple small, vesicular lesions may appear on the penis, scrotum, vulva, perineum, perianal region, vagina, or cervix. The vesicles contain

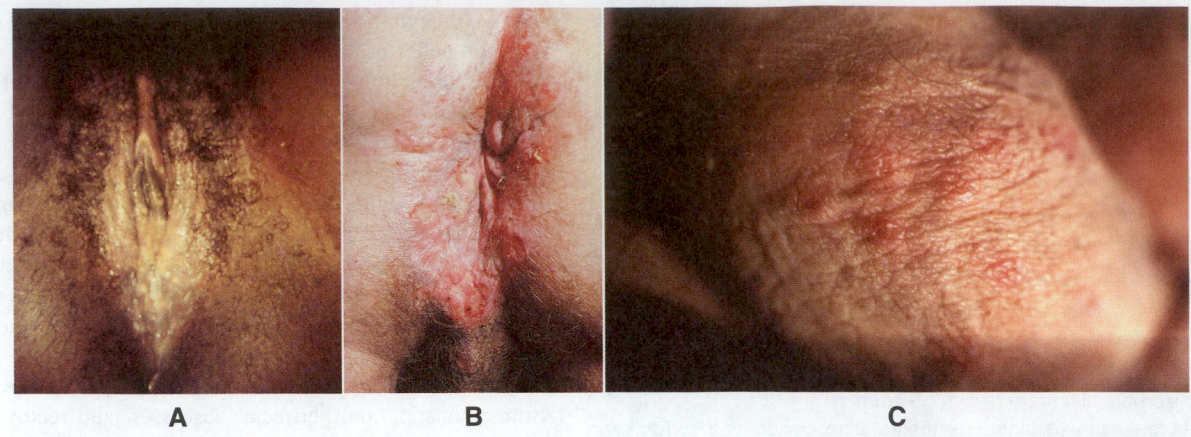

FIG. 53-7 Unruptured vesicles of herpes simplex virus type 2 (HSV-2). **A,** Vulvar area. **B,** Perianal area. **C,** Penile herpes simplex, ulcerative stage.

large quantities of infectious viral particles (Fig. 53-7). The lesions rupture and form shallow, moist ulcerations. Finally, crusting and epithelialization of the erosions occur. Primary infections tend to be associated with local inflammation and pain, accompanied by systemic manifestations of fever, headache, malaise, myalgia, and regional lymphadenopathy.

Urination may be painful from the urine touching active lesions. Urinary retention may occur as a result of HSV urethritis or cystitis. A purulent vaginal discharge may develop with HSV cervicitis. The duration of symptoms is longer and the frequency of complications is greater in women. Primary lesions are generally present for 17 to 20 days, but new lesions sometimes continue to develop for 6 weeks. The lesions heal spontaneously unless secondary infection occurs.

Recurrent genital herpes occurs in about 50% to 80% of individuals during the year following the primary episode. Stress, fatigue, sunburn, and menses are commonly noted trigger factors. Many patients can predict a recurrence by noticing the early prodromal symptoms of tingling, burning, and itching at the site where the lesions will eventually appear. The symptoms of recurrent episodes are less severe, and the lesions usually heal within 8 to 12 days. With time the recurrent lesions will generally occur less frequently.

Women with recurrent symptomatic genital herpes can shed the virus up to 1% of the time even when no visible lesions are present. Suppressive therapy with antiviral agents can reduce but not eradicate asymptomatic shedding.[16] Barrier forms of contraception, especially condoms, used during asymptomatic periods may decrease transmission of the virus. When lesions are present, the patient should avoid sexual activity altogether because even barrier protection is not satisfactory in eliminating disease transmission.

Complications

Although most infections are of a relatively benign nature, complications of genital herpes may involve the CNS, causing aseptic meningitis and lower motor neuron damage. Neuron damage may result in atonic bladder, impotence, and constipation. Another complication is *autoinoculation* of the virus to extragenital sites such as the lips, breasts, and, most commonly, the fingers (herpetic whitlow) (Fig. 53-8).

Herpes Simplex Virus Keratitis. HSV infection of the eye usually resolves within 1 to 2 weeks, but it can progress, resulting in the development of ulcers. It is the most common cause of

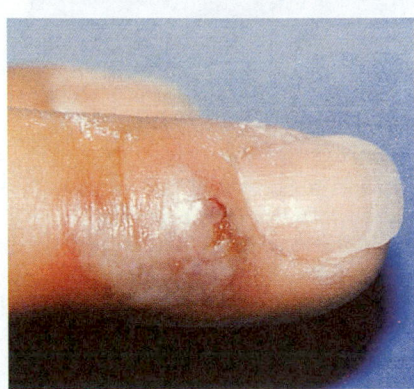

FIG. 53-8 Autoinoculation of herpes simplex virus (HSV), herpetic whitlow.

corneal ulceration and blindness in the United States.[17] Symptoms include blurred vision, acute pain, and conjunctivitis. Recurrent attacks may result in scarring of the cornea and vision impairment. The primary treatment is topical antiviral agents (e.g., trifluridine [Viroptic]) and systemic acyclovir (Zovirax). The ulcer may need to be debrided. Despite treatment, attacks can last for weeks and recurrences are common. Corneal transplantation may be needed to replace an opacified cornea.

Herpes Simplex Virus Infection in Pregnancy. Women with a primary episode of HSV near the time of delivery have the highest risk of transmitting genital herpes to the neonate. The risk of transmission is lowest for women who acquire HSV early in the pregnancy or have a history of recurrent HSV. An active genital lesion at the time of delivery is usually an indication for cesarean section delivery because most infections to neonates occur during birth.

Diagnostic Studies

A diagnosis of genital herpes is usually based on the patient's symptoms and history. The diagnosis can be confirmed through isolation of the virus from active lesions by means of tissue culture. Once the lesions begin to heal, cultural sensitivity declines. Cultures are frequently more positive in primary infection versus recurrent infection. Because viral cultures may result in a false-negative result, the CDC recommends a serologic test for HSV-2 in addition to a viral culture. Highly accurate serologic tests are available for the diagnosis of HSV-2. These type-specific immunoassays for HSV infection test for the presence

TABLE 53-8	*COLLABORATIVE CARE* Genital Herpes

Diagnostic
History and physical examination
Viral isolation by tissue culture
Antibody assay for specific HSV viral type

Collaborative Therapy
Primary Infection
acyclovir (Zovirax) 400 mg three times a day or acyclovir 200 mg five times a day or famciclovir (Famvir) 250 mg three times a day or valacyclovir (Valtrex) 1 g twice a day; all drugs are given orally for 7 to 10 days

Recurrent Episodic Infection
acyclovir 400 mg three times a day or acyclovir 200 mg five times a day or acyclovir 800 mg twice a day or famciclovir 125 mg twice a day or valacyclovir 500 mg twice a day or valacyclovir 1 g once a day; drugs are given orally for 5 days
Attempt to identify trigger mechanisms
Yearly Pap test
Abstinence from sexual contact while lesions are present; however, virus may be shed without lesions
Symptomatic care
Confidential counseling and testing for HIV

Suppressive Therapy for Frequent Recurrence
acyclovir 400 mg two times a day or famciclovir 250 mg twice a day or valacyclovir 500 mg twice a day or valacyclovir 1 g once a day

Severe Infection
acyclovir 5 to 10 mg/kg IV every 8 hours for 2 to 7 days or until clinical improvement, followed by oral antiviral therapy to complete at least 10 days of treatment

Modified from Centers for Disease Control and Prevention: STD treatment guidelines, *www.cdc.gov/STD/treatment.*
HIV, Human immunodeficiency virus; *HSV,* herpes simplex virus.

of antibodies to HSV and determine the presence of a chronic HSV infection.

Collaborative Care

Drug Therapy. Three antiviral agents are available for the treatment of HSV: acyclovir (Zovirax), valacyclovir (Valtrex), and famciclovir (Famvir). These drugs inhibit herpetic viral replication and are prescribed for primary and recurrent infections (Table 53-8). Acyclovir, valacyclovir, and famciclovir are also used to suppress frequent recurrences (more than six episodes per year). Although not a cure, these drugs shorten the duration of viral shedding and the healing time of genital lesions and reduce outbreaks by 75%.[2] Continued use of oral acyclovir as suppressive therapy for up to 5 years is safe and effective for persons with frequent or severe recurrences. Adverse reactions are mild and include headache, occasional nausea and vomiting, and diarrhea. The safety of these drugs for treatment of pregnant women has not been established. Acyclovir ointment appears to have no clinical benefit in the treatment of recurrent lesions, either in speed of healing or in resolution of pain, and is not commonly recommended. IV acyclovir is reserved for severe or life-threatening infections in which hospitalization is required for the treatment of disseminated infections, CNS infections (meningitis), or pneumonitis. Nephrotoxicity has been observed with high-dose IV use. Clinical trials are examining the effectiveness of a vaccine for HSV-2.

Symptomatic Care. Symptomatic treatment such as good genital hygiene and the wearing of loose-fitting cotton undergarments should be encouraged. The lesions should be kept clean and

dry. To ensure complete drying of the perineal area, women may use a hair dryer set on a cool setting. Frequent sitz baths may soothe the area and reduce inflammation. Drying agents such as colloidal oatmeal (Aveeno) and aluminum salts (Burow's solution) may provide some relief from the burning and itching. Techniques to reduce pain on urination include pouring a pitcher of water onto the perineal area while voiding to dilute the urine, and voiding in a warm tub of water or shower. Pain may require a local anesthetic such as lidocaine (Xylocaine) or systemic analgesics such as codeine and aspirin. Sexual transmission of HSV has been documented during asymptomatic periods, and the use of barrier methods, especially condoms, should be encouraged.

GENITAL WARTS

Genital warts (*condylomata acuminata*) are caused by the human papillomavirus (HPV). There are over 100 types of papillomaviruses, and about 40 of these affect the genital tract. Visible genital warts are usually caused by HPV types 6 and 11. These types can also cause warts on the anus, urethra, and vagina. Other HPV types in the genital region (e.g., types 16, 18, 31, 33, and 35) are associated with vaginal, anal, and cervical dysplasia. HPV is a highly contagious STD seen frequently in young, sexually active adults. An estimated 20 million Americans are currently infected with HPV.[1] Infection with HPV is the most common STD in the United States.[18] Most individuals who have HPV infection do not know they are infected because symptoms are often not present.

Minor trauma during intercourse can cause abrasions that allow HPV to enter the body. The epithelial cells infected with HPV undergo transformation and proliferation to form a warty growth. The incubation period of the virus is generally 3 to 4 months, but may be longer. Prevention is hampered by a high proportion of asymptomatic infections and lack of curative treatment. In most states, genital warts are not a reportable disease.

Clinical Manifestations and Complications

Genital warts are discrete single or multiple papillary growths that are white to gray and pink-flesh colored. They may grow and coalesce to form large, cauliflower-like masses. Most patients have from 1 to 10 genital warts. In men, the warts may occur on the penis and scrotum, around the anus, or in the urethra. In women, the warts may be located on the vulva, vagina, or cervix and in the perianal area (Fig. 53-9). There are usually no other signs or symptoms. Itching may occur with anogenital warts. Bleeding on defecation may occur with anal warts.

During pregnancy, genital warts tend to grow rapidly. An infected mother may transmit the condition to her newborn. Cesarean delivery is not routinely indicated unless the birth canal becomes blocked by massive warts.

HPV infection has been linked with cervical and vulvar cancer in women and with anorectal and squamous cell carcinoma of the penis in men. Some HPV types appear to be harmless and self-limiting (e.g., types 6 and 11 commonly found in genital warts), whereas others are thought to have oncogenic (cancer-causing) potential (e.g., types 16 and 18). Up to two thirds of the early lesions caused by HPV are undetectable by visual examination.

Diagnostic Studies and Collaborative Care

A diagnosis of genital warts can be made on the basis of the gross appearance of the lesions. However, the warts may be confused with condylomata lata of secondary syphilis, carcinoma, or benign neoplasms. Serologic and cytologic testing should be done to rule

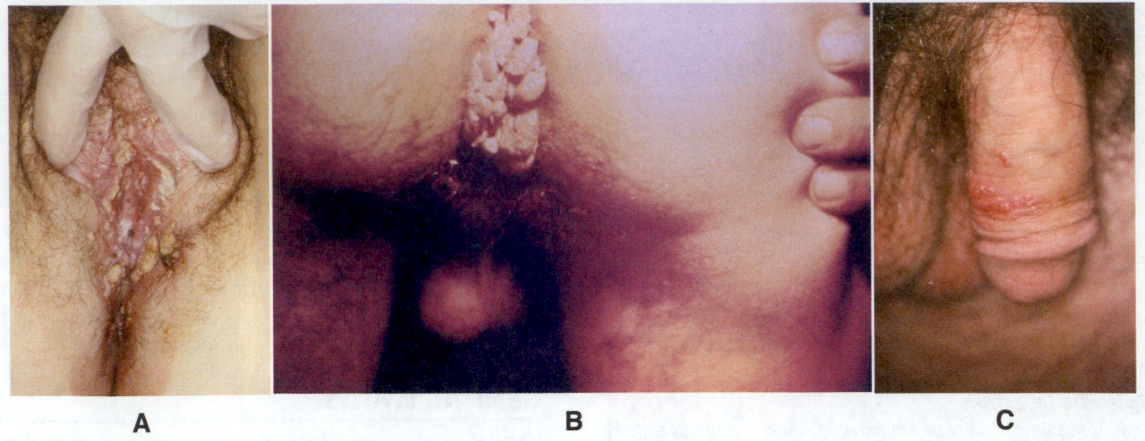

FIG. 53-9   Genital warts. **A,** Severe vulvular warts. **B,** Perineal wart. **C,** Multiple genital warts of the glans penis.

out these conditions. The HPV DNA test helps to determine if women with abnormal Papanicolaou (Pap) test results need further follow-up. The HPV DNA test can also identify women who are infected with the high-risk HPV strains associated with cervical cancer.[19] Currently, HPV cannot be confirmed by culture.

The primary goal when treating visible genital warts is the removal of symptomatic warts. The removal may or may not decrease infectivity. Genital warts are difficult to treat and often require multiple office visits with a variety of treatment modalities. Many patients will have a course of therapy rather than one treatment. The therapy should be modified if a patient has not improved after three treatments or if the warts have not completely disappeared after six treatments. Treatment consists of chemical or ablative (removal with laser or electocautery) methods. One common treatment is the use of 80% to 90% trichloroacetic acid (TCA) or bichloroacetic acid (BCA) applied directly to the wart surface. Petroleum jelly is applied to the surrounding normal skin to minimize irritation before a small amount of TCA is applied to the wart with a cotton swab. A sharp stinging pain is often felt with initial acid contact, but this quickly subsides. TCA is not washed off after treatment. It can be used in pregnant women.

Podophyllin resin (10% to 25%), a cytotoxic agent, is recommended therapy for small external genital warts. When podophyllin is used, it is applied carefully to each wart, with normal tissue being avoided, and is then thoroughly washed off in 1 to 4 hours. This substance encourages the sloughing off of skin containing viral particles. Podophyllin has local (e.g., pain, burning) and systemic (e.g., nausea, dizziness, leukopenia, respiratory distress) toxic symptoms. It is contraindicated in pregnant women. In general, warts located on moist surfaces respond better to topical treatment (e.g., TCA, podophyllin) than do warts on drier surfaces.

Patient-managed treatment is also an option. Podofilox (5%) liquid and gel are available by prescription (Condylox and Condylox Gel). The patient applies the solution or gel for 3 successive days followed by 4 days of no treatment. Treatment can be repeated for up to 4 weeks or until resolution of the lesions. Imiquimod (5%) cream (Aldara) is an immune response modifier that is applied once daily at bedtime, three times a week for up to 16 weeks. None of these treatments is recommended for use during pregnancy or lactation.

If the warts do not regress with any of these therapies, treatments such as cryotherapy with liquid nitrogen, electrocautery, laser therapy, intralesional use of alpha-interferon, and surgical excision may be indicated.[20] Because treatment does not destroy the virus, merely the infected tissue, recurrences and reinfection are possible, and careful long-term follow-up is advised. A vaccine is now available to prevent cervical cancer, precancerous genital lesions, and genital warts due to human papillomavirus (HPV) types 6, 11, 16, and 18. The vaccine is given in three doses over a 6-month period and has minimal side effects.[21]

NURSING MANAGEMENT
SEXUALLY TRANSMITTED DISEASES

■ **Nursing Assessment**

Subjective and objective data that should be obtained from a person with an STD are presented in Table 53-9.

■ **Nursing Diagnoses**

Nursing diagnoses for the patient with an STD include, but are not limited to, the following:

- Risk for infection *related to* lack of knowledge about mode of transmission, inadequate personal and genital hygiene, and failure to practice precautionary measures
- Anxiety *related to* impact of condition on relationships, disease outcome, and lack of knowledge of disease
- Ineffective health maintenance *related to* lack of knowledge about disease process, appropriate follow-up measures, and possibility of reinfection

■ **Planning**

The overall goals are that the patient with an STD will (1) demonstrate understanding of the mode of transmission of STDs and the risk posed by STDs, (2) complete treatment and return for appropriate follow-up, (3) notify or assist in notification of sexual contacts about their need for testing and treatment, (4) abstain from intercourse until infection is resolved, and (5) demonstrate knowledge of safer sex practices.

■ **Nursing Implementation**

Health Promotion. Many approaches to curtailing the spread of STDs have been advocated and have met with varying degrees of success. Nurses should be prepared to discuss practices with all patients, not only those who are perceived to be at risk. These "safe" sex practices include abstinence, monogamy with an uninfected partner, avoidance of certain high-risk sexual practices, and

TABLE 53-9	**NURSING ASSESSMENT** Sexually Transmitted Diseases

Subjective Data
Important Health Information
Past health history: Contact with individuals with STDs, multiple sexual partners, pregnancy
Medications: Use of oral contraceptives; allergy to any antibiotics, especially penicillin

Functional Health Patterns
Health perception–health management: Shared needles during IV drug use; malaise
Nutritional-metabolic: Nausea, vomiting, anorexia; pharyngitis, oral lesions, itching at infected site; chills; alopecia
Elimination: Dysuria, urinary frequency, retention; urethral discharge; tenesmus, proctitis
Cognitive-perceptual: Arthralgia; headache; painful, burning lesions
Sexuality-reproductive: Dyspareunia; vaginal discharge, menstrual abnormalities; presence of genital or perianal lesions

Objective Data
General
Fever, lymphadenopathy (generalized or inguinal)

Integumentary
Syphilis: Primary—painless, indurated genital, oral, or perianal lesions; secondary—bilateral, symmetric rash on palms, soles, or entire body, mucous patches on mouth or tongue, alopecia
Genital herpes: Painful genital or anal vesicular lesions
Genital warts: Single or multiple gray or white genital or anal warts (possibly becoming massive)

Gastrointestinal
Purulent rectal discharge (indicator of gonorrhea), rectal lesions, proctitis

Urinary
Urethral discharge, erythema

Reproductive
Cervical discharge, lesions, inflamed Bartholin's glands

Possible Findings
Gonorrhea: Positive Gram stain, smears, cultures, and DNA amplification for *N. gonorrhoeae*
Syphilis: Positive findings on VDRL and RPR, spirochetes on dark-field microscopy
Chlamydia: Positive culture or DNA amplification for *Chlamydia* organism
Genital herpes: Positive tissue culture for HSV-2; positive HSV-2 antibody titer

HSV-2, Herpes simplex virus type 2; *IV,* intravenous; *RPR,* rapid plasma reagin; *STDs,* sexually transmitted diseases; *VDRL,* Venereal Disease Research Laboratory.

TABLE 53-10	**PATIENT TEACHING GUIDE** Sexually Transmitted Diseases

1. Instruct patient in hygienic measures, such as washing and urinating after intercourse to flush out some organisms.
2. Explain the importance of taking all antibiotics as prescribed. Symptoms will improve after 1-2 days of therapy, but organisms may still be present.
3. Teach patient about the need for treatment of sexual partners with antibiotic to prevent transmission of disease.
4. Instruct patient to abstain from sexual intercourse during treatment and to use condoms when sexual activity is resumed to prevent spread of infection and prevent reinfection.
5. Explain the importance of follow-up examination and reculture at least once after treatment if appropriate to confirm complete cure and prevent relapse.
6. Allow patient and partner to verbalize concerns to clarify areas that need explanation.
7. Instruct patient about symptoms of complications and need to report problems to ensure proper follow-up and early treatment of reinfection.
8. Explain precautions to take, such as being monogamous; asking potential partners about sexual history; avoiding sex with partners who use IV drugs or who have visible oral, inguinal, genital, perineal, or anal lesions; using condoms; and voiding and washing genitalia and surrounding area after coitus to reduce the occurrence of reinfection.
9. Inform patient regarding state of infectivity to prevent a false sense of security, which might result in careless sexual practices and poor personal hygiene.

HEALTHY PEOPLE

Health Impact of Practicing Responsible Sexual Behavior

- Greatly reduces the risk of contracting sexually transmitted diseases, including infection from human immunodeficiency virus, gonorrhea, chlamydia, syphilis, and herpes
- Greatly reduces the risk of spreading viruses such as human papillomavirus that potentially causes cervical cancer

use of condoms and other barriers to limit contact with potentially infectious body fluids or lesions. Sexual abstinence is a certain method of avoiding all STDs, but few adults consider this a feasible alternative to sexual expression. Limiting sexual intimacies outside of a well-established monogamous relationship can reduce the risk of contracting an STD. A patient teaching guide related to the patient with an STD is presented in Table 53-10.

All sexually active women should be screened for cervical cancer. Women with a history of STDs are at greater risk for cervical cancer than women without this history. Pap tests are discussed in Chapter 54.

Measures to Prevent Infection. An inspection of the sexual partner's genitals before coitus is recommended. The presence of discharge, sores, blisters, or rash should be viewed with concern. A patient who is aware of specific signs and symptoms of infection can intelligently make the decision to continue the sexual interaction with modifications or elect not to have sexual relations. The patient should remember that, when engaging in sex, there is exposure to the infections of everyone with whom the partner has ever had sex. Men should be told that some protection is provided if they void immediately following intercourse and wash their genitalia and the adjacent areas with soap and water. Women may also benefit from postcoital voiding and washing. However, it should not be assumed that this provides adequate protection against STDs after exposure to infection. Spermicidal jellies and creams have not been shown to reduce the risk of contracting STDs. These same barriers can serve as supplementary lubrication, thereby decreasing irritation and friction and chances for development of a minor laceration that could serve as an entry point for the organism.

Proper use of a latex condom provides a highly effective mechanical barrier to infection. The condom should be undamaged and correctly in place throughout all phases of sexual activity. A deterrent to condom usage is alcohol and drug use. Studies continue to document that IV drug users do not consistently use condoms. Use of barrier contraceptives requires planning and motivation, both of which are impaired with alcohol or drug ingestion. The patient should be given specific verbal and written instructions on the proper use of condoms (see Chapter 15, Fig. 15-7 and Table 15-17). The objections to condom usage, such as interference with spontaneity and the presence of a barrier, should be discussed by the partners. Information about the mechanics of sexual arousal and incorporating a condom into lovemaking can help in overcoming patient or partner resistance to its use. Female condoms are lubricated polyurethane sheaths designed for vaginal use (see Chapter 15, Fig. 15-8 and Table 15-18).

Sexual contact with persons known or suspected to have HIV infection should be avoided (see Chapter 15). Among couples with one infected partner, consistent and scrupulous condom use can reduce transmission to the uninfected partner. A sexually active homosexual man can reduce risk by minimizing the number of sexual contacts. Unprotected anal intercourse and other high-risk behaviors should be eliminated, and condoms should be used if sexual contact continues.

The nurse can initiate an interview to establish the patient's risk for contracting an STD. Questions to ask include number of partners, type of birth control used, use of condoms, history of an STD, use of IV drugs, and sexual preference. Patient education can be planned based on the response to these questions. Interpersonal skills necessary for this interview include respect, compassion, and a nonjudgmental attitude. Counseling should be tailored to the individual patient.

Screening Programs. Screening programs that are used to detect infected patients can also help prevent certain STDs. For many years, there have been various screening programs to find cases of syphilis. With the decline of infection rates across the United States, many states have eliminated laws requiring premarital testing for syphilis. Many institutions offer voluntary prenatal HIV and syphilis testing and counseling for pregnant women.

Screening programs have been developed and implemented for detection of gonorrhea and chlamydia. These programs are targeted to women because women are more likely to have asymptomatic gonorrhea and thereby serve as sources of infection. Routine gonorrheal and chlamydial testing during pelvic examinations and prenatal visits are being performed as a major part of these programs. Mass application of screening programs for genital chlamydial infections, genital herpes, and HPV infections (warts) may also be possible with the advent of rapid, cost-effective tests.

Case Finding. Interviewing and case finding are other processes used to control STDs. These activities are directed toward locating and examining all contacts of each known patient with an STD as soon after sexual exposure as possible so that effective treatment can be initiated. Trained interviewers may often find cases even if they are supplied with only limited information. The caseworkers, who are often nurses, are aware of the social implications of these diseases and the need for discretion. Sexual contacts are often not informed about the origin of the information naming them as a contact so that greater cooperation and privacy is ensured.

Educational and Research Programs. Nurses can actively encourage their communities to provide better education about STDs for their citizens.[22] Teenagers, who are known to have a high incidence of infection, should be a prime target for such educational programs. Hotline services, school nurses, nurse practitioners, nurse midwives, and outreach programs sponsored by the

ETHICAL DILEMMAS
Confidentiality

Situation
A nurse in a clinic gives the positive results of a test for chlamydia to a patient and advises her to tell her sexual partners that she has this disease. The patient refuses to tell her boyfriend because he will know that she has had sex with another partner. Should the nurse contact the boyfriend?

Important Points for Consideration
- Nurses and other health care professionals have both a legal and an ethical obligation to maintain confidentiality of patient information. If confidentiality is violated, trust is eroded and patients may not share privileged information that is essential to plan effective care.
- Health care providers have an obligation to maintain confidentiality unless there is a risk to the health or life of innocent third parties. Each state has requirements for reporting communicable diseases and other health-related data.
- The nurse's primary obligation is to the patient seeking care. However, there are long-term health consequences for this patient, as well as the public in general.
- Patient teaching is one way to establish a partnership with this woman. Information should be shared about the effects of the disease being untreated, the consequences of reinfection, and the results that the disease may have on others who may not know they are infected. The patient can then be encouraged to inform her partners of the diagnosis for the good of everyone.

Critical Thinking Questions
1. What are your state's requirements for reportable conditions?
2. Should the nurse contact the boyfriend?
3. In your opinion, what is the best way to balance the needs of an individual patient with those of the general public?

CDC in the United States and Canada's Health Protection Branch are effective. Knowledge and understanding can decrease the STD epidemic. A highly effective vaccine for the HPV strains which cause genital warts and cervical cancer is now available (see Chapter 54). In addition, efforts are being made to develop vaccines for syphilis, gonorrhea, genital herpes, and HIV. The development of effective vaccines is viewed by many clinicians as a prerequisite for eradication of STDs.

Acute Intervention
Psychologic Support. The diagnosis of an STD may be met with a variety of emotions, such as shame, guilt, anger, and a desire for vengeance. The nurse should provide counseling and try to help the patient verbalize feelings. Couples in marital or committed relationships are confronted with an added problem when an STD is diagnosed. The implication of sexual activity by one of the partners with a person outside the relationship must be faced. Other concerns relative to their relationship are present, and the acute problem may serve as an incentive for further problem solving. Support and counseling for the couple are needed. A referral for professional counseling to explore the ramifications of an STD in their relationship may be indicated.

A patient who has genital herpes is faced with the fact that repeated infections can occur and that no cure is available. This can be frustrating and disruptive to the patient's physical, emotional, social, and sexual lives. Helping the patient identify and avoid any factors that may precipitate the condition is indicated. Informing the patient that the incidence and severity of recurrences will decrease over time may provide some support.

HPV infections involve a prolonged course of treatment. The patient can become frustrated and distressed because of frequent office visits, associated costs, potential for unpleasant side effects as a result of treatment, and effects of the infection on future health and sexual relationships. Tremendous support and a willingness to listen to the patient's concerns are needed.

Compliance and Follow-up. A nurse working in public health facilities, clinics, or other outpatient settings may care for a patient with an STD more often than a nurse in a hospital. This nurse is in a position to explain and interpret treatment measures such as the purpose and possible side effects of prescribed drugs and the need for follow-up care.

Frequently, single-dose treatment for gonorrhea, chlamydia, and syphilis helps prevent the problems associated with noncompliance with drug therapy. The patient requiring multiple-dose therapy should be given special instructions in completing the prescribed regimen and should be informed about problems resulting from noncompliance. All patients should return to the treatment center for a repeat culture from the infected sites or for serologic testing at designated times to determine the effectiveness of the treatment. Informing the patient that cures are not always obtained on the first treatment can reinforce the need for a follow-up visit. The patient should also be advised to inform sexual partners of the need for testing and treatment, regardless of whether they are free of symptoms or experiencing symptoms.

Hygiene Measures. The patient with an STD should have certain hygiene measures emphasized. An important measure is frequent hand washing and bathing. Bathing and cleaning of the involved areas can provide local comfort and prevent secondary infection. Douching may spread the infection or undermine local immune responses and is therefore contraindicated. The synthetic materials used in most undergarments frequently increase or exacerbate local irritations by trapping moisture. Cotton undergarments provide better absorption and are cooler and more comfortable for the patient with an STD.

Sexual Activity. Sexual abstinence is indicated during the communicable phase of the disease. If sexual activity occurs before treatment of the patient has been completed, the use of condoms may prevent the spread of infection and reinfection. Condom usage after treatment should be encouraged to prevent future exposure to infection. The patient can also choose to relate to a partner in an intimate way that avoids both coitus and oral-genital contact. It is important to note that even single-dose treatments can take up to 1 week to be effective and thus the patient is infective during this period.

Ambulatory and Home Care. Because many STDs are cured with a single dose or short course of antibiotic therapy, many persons are casual about the outcome of these diseases. The consequences of this attitude can include delays in treatment, noncompliance with instructions, and subsequent development of complications. The complications are serious and costly. They can result in disfigurement and destruction of important tissues and organs.

Surgery and prolonged therapy are indicated for many patients with disease-related complications. Major surgical procedures such as resection of an aneurysm or aortic valve replacement may be necessary to treat cardiovascular problems caused by syphilis. Pelvic surgery and procedures to correct fertility problems secondary to an STD may include lysis of adhesions, dilation of strictures, reconstructive tuboplasty, and in vitro fertilization.

■ Evaluation

Expected outcomes for the patient with an STD are that the patient will

- describe modes of transmission
- use appropriate hygienic measures
- experience no reinfection
- demonstrate compliance with follow-up protocol

CRITICAL THINKING EXERCISE

CASE STUDY

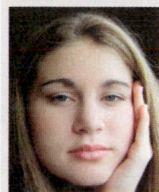

Chlamydia and Gonorrhea

Patient Profile. Rebecca Warren is a 17-year-old white female who visits the outpatient "teen clinic" for the first time seeking birth control pills. She had sexual intercourse for the first time 8 weeks ago.

Case Study photo ©iStockphoto.com/ Roberta Osborne.

Subjective Data

- Her partner does not use a condom or spermicide with intercourse
- Her last menstrual period was 2 weeks ago
- Denies any symptoms
- Interested in using oral contraceptives
- Very nervous

Objective Data

- Cervical ectopy noted during Pap test
- Mucopurulent cervical discharge
- Urine pregnancy test is negative
- Nucleic acid amplification test is positive for *Chlamydia trachomatis* and *Neisseria gonorrhoeae*

Collaborative Care

- Doxycycline 100 mg bid for 7 days
- Ceftriaxone 250 mg IM once

Critical Thinking Questions

1. What were Rebecca's risk factors for acquiring chlamydia and gonorrhea?
2. What complications could have occurred if Rebecca's infections had not been detected?
3. What impact is her diagnosis likely to have on Rebecca's self-image? On her relationship with her sexual partner?
4. What instructions should Rebecca receive to ensure successful treatment? To prevent reinfection? To prevent further transmission of the infection?
5. What is the priority nursing intervention for Rebecca?
6. What does she need to know about other STDs? What other testing would you recommend?
7. Based on the assessment data presented, write one or more nursing diagnoses. Are there any collaborative problems?

NCLEX EXAMINATION REVIEW QUESTIONS

The number of the question corresponds to the same-numbered objective at the beginning of the chapter.

1. The individual with the lowest risk for sexually transmitted pelvic inflammatory disease is a woman who
   a. uses oral contraceptives.
   b. uses barrier methods of contraception.
   c. uses an intrauterine device for contraception.
   d. uses a Norplant implant or injectable Depo-Provera for contraception.

2. While obtaining subjective assessment data from a woman reported as a sexual contact of a man with chlamydia, the nurse understands that symptoms of chlamydial infection in women
   a. are frequently absent.
   b. are similar to those of genital herpes.
   c. include a macular palmar rash in the later stages.
   d. may involve chancres inside the vagina that are not visible.

3. A primary HSV infection differs from recurrent HSV episodes in that
   a. it is of shorter duration than recurrent episodes.
   b. only primary infections are sexually transmissible.
   c. systemic manifestations such as fever and myalgia are more common.
   d. transmission of the virus to a fetus is less likely during primary infection.

4. The nurse explains to a patient with gonorrhea that treatment will include both ceftriaxone and doxycycline because
   a. most patients do not respond to ceftriaxone alone.
   b. coverage with more than one antibiotic prevents reinfection.
   c. no single agent successfully eradicates all strains of gonorrhea.
   d. the high rate of coexisting chlamydia and gonorrhea indicates dual coverage.

5. A patient with an STD who is most likely to have a nursing diagnosis of disturbed body image that hinders future sexual relationships is the patient with
   a. syphilis.
   b. gonorrhea.
   c. chlamydia.
   d. genital warts.

6. Teaching by the nurse to prevent infection and transmission of STDs would include an explanation of
   a. the appropriate use of oral contraceptives.
   b. sexual positions that can be used to avoid infection.
   c. sexual practices that are considered high-risk behaviors.
   d. the necessity of annual Pap tests for patients with HPV.

7. An appropriate nursing intervention to provide emotional support to a patient with an STD is to
   a. offer information on how safe sexual practices can prevent STDs.
   b. use concerned listening when the patient expresses negative feelings.
   c. reassure the patient that the disease is highly curable with appropriate treatment.
   d. help the patient who received an STD from his or her sexual partner in forgiving the partner.

REFERENCES

1. Blair M: Sexually transmitted diseases: an update, *Urol Nurs* 24:6, 2004.
2. Centers for Disease Control and Prevention: Sexually transmitted diseases treatment guidelines, 2006. Available at *www.cdc.gov/STD/treatment* (accessed October 5, 2006).
3. Harvey S, Henderson J, Branch M: Protecting against both pregnancy and disease: predictors of dual method use among a sample of women, *Woman Health* 39:25, 2004.
4. Centers for Disease Control and Prevention, Division of STD Prevention: *Sexually transmitted disease surveillance—gonorrhea, 2006.* Available at *www.cdc.gov/std/stats/gonorrhea.htm.*
5. U.S. Preventive Services Task Force: Screening for gonorrhea: recommendation statement, Agency for Healthcare Research and Quality, 2005. Available at *www.guideline.gov/summary* (accessed June 13, 2005).
6. Uphold CR, Graham MV: *Clinical guidelines in family practice,* ed 4, Gainesville, Fla., 2003, Barmarrae.
7. Centers for Disease Control and Prevention, Division of STD Prevention: *Sexually transmitted disease surveillance—syphilis, 2006.* Available at *www.cdc.gov/std/stats/syphilis.htm*
8. Jacobs R: Infectious diseases—spirochetal. In Tierney L et al, editors: *Current medical diagnosis and treatment,* ed 44, New York, 2005, Lange/McGraw-Hill.
9. Centers for Disease Control and Prevention, Division of Sexually Transmitted Diseases: *Trends in reportable sexually transmitted diseases in the United States, 2003—national data on chlamydia, gonorrhea, syphilis,* Atlanta, 2003.
10. Lukehart SA, Holmes KK: Syphilis. In Fauci AS et al, editors: *Harrison's principles of internal medicine,* ed 16, New York, 2005, McGraw-Hill.
11. Centers for Disease Control and Prevention, Division of STD prevention: *Sexually transmitted disease surveillance—chlamydia 2006.* Available at *www.cdc.gov/std/stats/chlamydia.htm.*
12. Health Canada: 2002 Canadian sexually transmitted infections (STI) surveillance report, Public Agency of Canada, June 2005. Available at *www.phuc-aspc.gc.ca.*
13. Goldenberg R, Culhane J, Johnson D: Maternal infection and adverse fetal and neonatal outcomes, *Clin Perinatol* 32:523, 2005.
14. Stevens-Simon C: *Chlamydia trachomatis.* In Rakel R et al, editors: *Conn's current therapy,* ed 57, St Louis, 2005, Elsevier.
15. Roe VA: Living with genital herpes: how effective is antiviral therapy, *J Perinatal Neonatal Nurs* 18:3, 2004.
16. Goade D: Genital herpes. In Cohen J, Powderly W, editors: *Infectious diseases,* ed 2, St Louis, 2004, Elsevier.
17. Van Loon A, Cleator G, Klapper P: Herpes viruses. In Cohen J, Powderly W, editors: *Infectious diseases,* ed 2, St Louis, 2004, Elsevier.
18. Grimshaw L: How to recognize and manage HPV infections, *Clin Advisor* 8:24, 2005.
19. Falsetti D: HPV infection and cervical cancer risk, *Am J Nurs Pract* 9:21, 2005.
20. Kodner CM, Nasraty S: Management of genital warts, *Am Fam Physician* 70:12, 2004.
21. U.S. Food and Drug Administration: *FDA licenses new vaccine for prevention of cervical cancer and other diseases in females caused by human papillomavirus.* Available at *www.fda.gov/bbs/topics/NEWS/2006* (accessed August 28, 2006).
22. Oumeish O, Oumeish I: Community understanding and prevention of sexually transmitted diseases, *Clin Dermatol* 22:533, 2004.

RESOURCES

Centers for Disease Control and Prevention STD/HIV/AIDS Hotline
800-342-2437 (800-342-AIDS)
Herpes Resource Center
919-361-8400
www.ashastd.org
www.iwannaknow.org (for teens)
Sexuality Information and Education Council of the United States
212-819-9770
www.siecus.org
For additional Internet resources, see the website for this book at *http://evolve.elsevier.com/Lewis/medsurg.*

Patience is the companion of wisdom.

Saint Augustine

Nursing Management
Female Reproductive Problems

54

Nancy J. MacMullen and Laura Dulski

LEARNING OBJECTIVES

1. Identify the etiologies of infertility and the strategies for diagnosis and treatment of the infertile woman.
2. Discuss the nursing management of women who experience a spontaneous or an induced termination of a pregnancy.
3. Describe the etiology, clinical manifestations, and nursing and collaborative management of menstrual problems and abnormal vaginal bleeding.
4. Identify the risk factors, clinical manifestations, and collaborative care of ectopic pregnancy.
5. Discuss the changes related to menopause and the nursing and collaborative management of the patient with menopausal symptoms.
6. Differentiate among the common problems that affect the vulva, vagina, and cervix and the related nursing and collaborative management.
7. Describe the assessment, collaborative care, and nursing management of women with pelvic inflammatory disease.
8. Describe the clinical manifestations, complications, collaborative care, and nursing management of endometriosis.
9. Describe the clinical manifestations and collaborative care of benign tumors of the female reproductive system.
10. Identify the clinical manifestations, diagnostic studies, collaborative care, and surgical therapy for cervical, endometrial, ovarian, and vulvar cancers.
11. Describe the preoperative and postoperative nursing management for the patient requiring surgery of the female reproductive system.
12. Describe common problems that occur with cystoceles, rectoceles, and fistulas and the related nursing and collaborative management.
13. Identify the clinical manifestations of sexual assault and the appropriate nursing and collaborative management of the patient who has been sexually assaulted.

KEY TERMS

abortion, p. 1383
amenorrhea, p. 1387
cystocele, p. 1408
dysmenorrhea, p. 1386
ectopic pregnancy, p. 1389
endometriosis, p. 1396
hysterectomy, p. 1398
infertility, p. 1382
leiomyomas, p. 1398
menopause, p. 1390
menorrhagia, p. 1387
metrorrhagia, p. 1387
oligomenorrhea, p. 1387
pelvic inflammatory disease, p. 1395
perimenopause, p. 1390
postmenopause, p. 1390
premenstrual syndrome (PMS), p. 1385
rectocele, p. 1408
sexual assault, p. 1409
uterine prolapse, p. 1407

Electronic Resources

Supplemental content related to Chapter 54 can be found . . .

Companion CD
- Stress-Busting Kit for Nursing Students
- Interactive Case Study: Endometrial Cancer
- NCLEX Examination Review Questions
- Comprehensive Glossary

Evolve Website *evolve*
http://evolve.elsevier.com/Lewis/medsurg
- Content Updates
- Key Points (Printable and CD/MP3 Download)
- Concept Map Creator
- Expanded Audio Glossary
- Key Term Flash Cards

- Customizable Nursing Care Plan: Abdominal Hysterectomy
- Electronic Calculators
- WebLinks

Reviewed by Maureen Chrzanowski, RN, MSN, CNM, FNP, Certified Menopause Clinician, Practicing Nurse Midwife, Family Nurse Practitioner, Associates in OB/GYN and Infertility, Grand Rapids, Mich., and Faculty, Kirkhof College of Nursing, Grand Valley State University, Allendale, Mich.

INFERTILITY

Infertility is the inability to achieve a pregnancy after at least 1 year of regular intercourse without contraception.[1] Approximately 15% of couples in North America are infertile. Assessment and therapy measures can be invasive, expensive, and lengthy. Understandably, infertility can constitute a physical and an emotional crisis.

Etiology and Pathophysiology

Infertility may be caused by either female, male, or combined factors. Conditions that cause male infertility are discussed in Chapter 55. In up to 20% of the couples evaluated, the cause of infertility may not be identified.[1] The most frequent female causes of infertility include factors associated with ovulation (anovulation or inadequate corpus luteum), tubal obstruction or dysfunction (endometriosis or damage from pelvic infection), and uterine or cervical factors (fibroid tumors or structural anomalies). Risk factors for infertility include tobacco and illicit drug use, infection of the reproductive tract, and specific occupational and environmental exposures. In women the risk for infertility increases with age.[1] In particular, the probability of becoming pregnant begins decreasing at age 35 and decreases even further after age 40.

Diagnostic Studies

A detailed history and a general physical examination of the woman and her partner provide the basis for selecting diagnostic studies (Table 54-1). The possibility of medical, genetic, or gynecologic diseases is explored before tests are performed to determine problems affecting general health, as well as fertility. These tests include hormone levels, ovulatory studies, tubal patency studies, and postcoital studies.

    Ovulatory Studies. A basal body temperature record is kept to determine whether there is regular ovulation (Fig. 54-1). The woman is instructed to take and graph her temperature, referred to as basal body temperature, on awakening before any activity. The same site (e.g., oral, rectal) for taking the temperature should be used each time. Any cause for variation, such as sleeplessness or illness, should be noted. As ovulation approaches, the production of estrogen increases. This may cause a drop in temperature. When ovulation occurs, progesterone is produced, causing a rise in temperature. The temperature graph thus helps detect ovulation and suggests the timing of intercourse if pregnancy is desired. Rigid adherence to a schedule for intercourse can produce psychologic stress sufficient to inhibit sexual relations.

    Ovulation prediction kits are now available for use by women at home. These kits are generally used daily to measure luteinizing hormone (LH) levels in urine samples. Ovulation occurs about 28 to 36 hours after the first rise of LH, so intercourse can be timed accordingly. Other tests for ovulation include cervical and vaginal smears, endometrial biopsy, and plasma progesterone levels.

    Tubal Patency Studies. Tubal factors (occlusion or deformity) are assessed most commonly by means of hysterosalpingogram. This procedure consists of the radiographic visualization of the uterus and tubes by injecting a radiopaque dye through the cervix. Tubal patency, shape, position, and any distortions of the endometrial cavity can be determined. Laparoscopy may be used when hysterosalpingogram is contraindicated or other pelvic pathology appears likely.

    Postcoital Studies. Examination of the cervical mucus can reveal whether it undergoes favorable changes at ovulation, enabling penetration, survival, and normal motility of the sperm. A postcoital test can determine whether the cervical environment is favorable for the sperm. The couple is asked to have intercourse about the time ovulation is expected and 2 to 12 hours before the office visit. Douching or bathing should be avoided before the test.

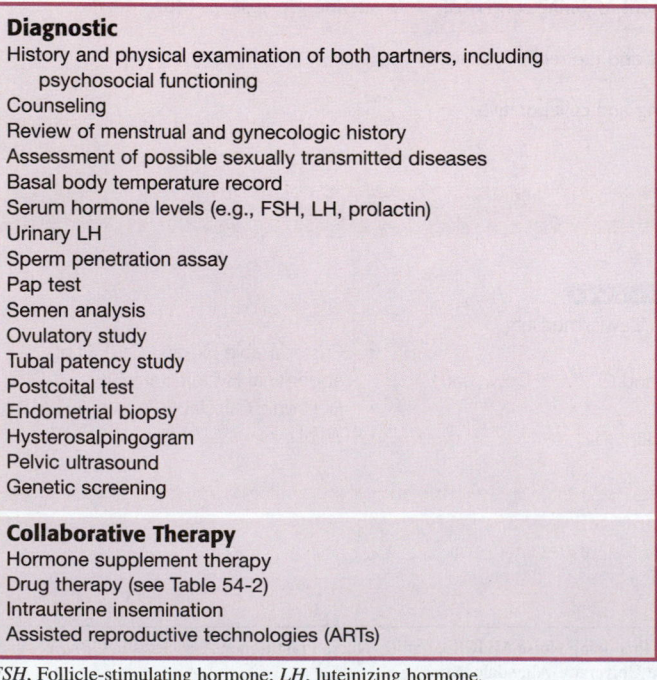

TABLE 54-1	COLLABORATIVE CARE Infertility

Diagnostic
History and physical examination of both partners, including psychosocial functioning
Counseling
Review of menstrual and gynecologic history
Assessment of possible sexually transmitted diseases
Basal body temperature record
Serum hormone levels (e.g., FSH, LH, prolactin)
Urinary LH
Sperm penetration assay
Pap test
Semen analysis
Ovulatory study
Tubal patency study
Postcoital test
Endometrial biopsy
Hysterosalpingogram
Pelvic ultrasound
Genetic screening

Collaborative Therapy
Hormone supplement therapy
Drug therapy (see Table 54-2)
Intrauterine insemination
Assisted reproductive technologies (ARTs)

FSH, Follicle-stimulating hormone; *LH,* luteinizing hormone.

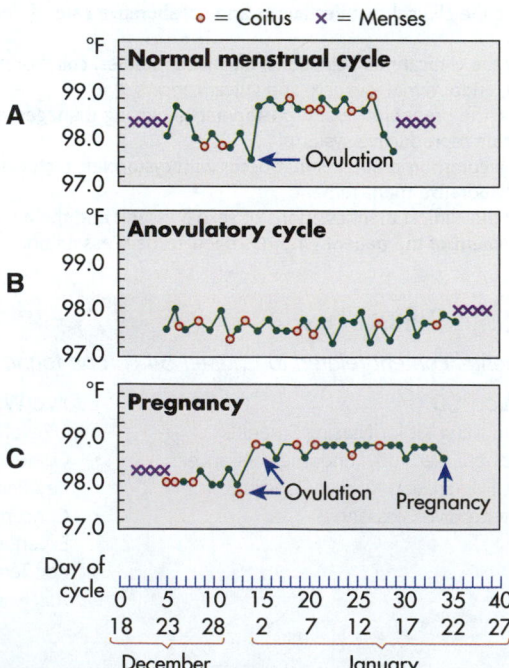

FIG. 54-1 Basal body temperature chart. **A,** Typical biphasic temperature curve indicative of ovulation and normal progesterone effect. **B,** Irregular monophasic curve characteristic of anovulatory cycles. **C,** Ovulatory curve with sustained temperature elevation following conception and the first missed period.

The cervical and vaginal secretions are aspirated and examined for the number and motility of sperm present. Other screening tests for infertility include semen analysis, endometrial biopsy, and pelvic ultrasound.

NURSING and COLLABORATIVE MANAGEMENT
INFERTILITY

The management of infertility problems depends on the cause. If infertility is secondary to an alteration in ovarian function, supplemental hormone therapy to restore and maintain ovulation may be attempted.[2] Drug therapy used to treat infertility is presented in Table 54-2. Chronic cervicitis and inadequate estrogenic stimulation are cervical factors causing infertility. Antibiotic therapy is indicated for cervicitis. Inadequate estrogenic stimulation is treated by the administration of estrogen.

When a couple has not succeeded in conceiving while under infertility management, an option is intrauterine insemination with sperm from the partner or a donor. If this technique does not succeed, assisted reproductive technologies (ARTs) may be used. ARTs include in vitro fertilization (IVF), gamete intrafallopian transfer (GIFT), zygote intrafallopian transfer (ZIFT), donor gametes, and embryo cryopreservation. IVF is the removal of mature oocytes from the woman's ovarian follicle via laparoscopy, followed by in vitro fertilization of the ova with the partner's sperm. When fertilization and cleavage have occurred, the resulting embryos are transferred into the woman's uterus. The procedure requires 2 to 3 days to complete and is used in cases of fallopian tube obstruction, diminished sperm count, and unexplained infertility. Frequently, multiple attempts are needed for successful implantation. IVF is financially costly and emotionally stressful. However, it has become a recognized and accepted method of therapy for infertile couples.

With the increasing sophistication of ART, couples have an increased potential for pregnancy. However, the use of ART often poses many ethical, legal, and social concerns.

Nurses can assist women experiencing infertility by providing information about the physiology of reproduction, infertility evaluation, and addressing the psychologic and social distress that can accompany infertility. Reducing psychologic stress can improve the emotional climate, making it more conducive to achieving a pregnancy.

The nurse has a major responsibility for teaching and providing emotional support throughout infertility testing and treatment. Feelings of anger, frustration, grief, and helplessness may heighten as additional diagnostic tests are performed. Infertility can generate great tension in a marriage as the couple exhausts financial and emotional resources. Few insurance carriers cover the high cost of infertility testing or expensive infertility treatment. Recognizing and taking steps to deal with the psychologic factors that surface can assist the couple to better cope with the situation. Couples should be encouraged to participate in a support group for infertile couples, as well as individual therapy.

ABORTION

An **abortion** is the loss or termination of a pregnancy before the fetus has developed to a state of viability. Abortions are classified as *spontaneous* (those occurring naturally) or *induced* (those occurring as a result of mechanical or medical intervention). *Miscarriage* is the common term for the unintended loss of a pregnancy. *Habitual recurrent abortion* is a history of three or more aborted pregnancies or miscarriages in succession.

Spontaneous Abortion

Spontaneous abortion is the natural loss of pregnancy before 20 weeks of gestation. Fetal chromosomal anomalies account for 50% of miscarriages before 8 weeks of gestation. Other causes of spontaneous abortions include endocrine abnormalities, maternal infection, acquired anatomic abnormalities (e.g., uterine fibroids, endometriosis), immunologic factors, and environmental factors. About 10% to 15% of all pregnancies end as a result of spontaneous abortion.[3]

Uterine cramping coupled with vaginal bleeding often indicates a spontaneous abortion. Cramping is usually absent if the vaginal bleeding is caused by other conditions, such as polyps. Serial serum β–human chorionic gonadotropin hormone (β-hCG) and vaginal ultrasound examination of the pelvis are the most reliable indicators of early pregnancy viability. The gestational sac can be visualized using ultrasound as early as 6 weeks of gestation.

Treatment for a possible spontaneous abortion is limited. Although bed rest and avoiding vaginal intercourse are often recommended, there is no evidence that these measures improve the outcome. The woman is advised to report any bleeding to her health care provider. An estimated 80% of these women proceed to abortion regardless of treatment. If the products of conception do not pass completely or bleeding becomes excessive, a *dilation and cu-*

TABLE 54-2	*DRUG THERAPY* Infertility
Drug	**Mechanism of Action**
Selective Estrogen Receptor Modulator	
clomiphene (Clomid, Serophene)	Stimulates hypothalamus to ↑ production of GnRH, which ↑ release of LH and FSH; end result is stimulation of ovulation.
Menotropin (Human Menopausal Gonadotropin)	
Pergonal Repronex Humegon	Product made of equal amounts of FSH and LH that promotes the development and maturation of follicles in the ovaries.
Follicle-Stimulating Hormone Agonists	
urofollitropin (Fertinex, Bravelle) follitropin (Gonal-f, Follistim)	Stimulate follicle growth and maturation by mimicking the actions of the body's natural FSH.
GnRH Antagonists	
cetrorelix (Cetrotide) ganirelix (Antagon)	Prevent premature LH surges and premature ovulation in women undergoing ovarian stimulation.
GnRH Agonists	
leuprolide (Lupron) nafarelin (Synarel)	Suppress release of LH and FSH with continuous use. May also be used in the treatment of endometriosis.
Human Chorionic Gonadotropin (hCG)	
Pregnyl Profasi Novarel	Induces ovulation by stimulating the release of eggs from follicles.

FSH, Follicle-stimulating hormone; *GnRH*, gonadotropin-releasing hormone; *LH*, luteinizing hormone.

Reproductive System

TABLE 54-3	**Methods for Inducing Abortion**			
Method	**Length of Pregnancy**	**Procedure**	**Advantages**	**Disadvantages**
Early Abortion				
Menstrual extraction	Usually up to 2 wk after first missed period	Catheter is inserted through cervix into uterus, and suction is applied. Endometrium and contents of uterus are aspirated.	Low cost, simple, done at outpatient facility without anesthesia or cervical dilation, minimal trauma	Continuation of pregnancy possible, potential for uterine injury and bleeding
Suction curettage	Up to 14 wk	Cervix is usually dilated, uterine aspirator is introduced, and suction is applied, removing endometrial tissue and implanted pregnancy.	Outpatient procedure, most often involving local anesthesia, 1- to 2-day recovery period	Infection, uterine perforation possible
Dilation and evacuation (D&E)	10-16 wk (approximate)	Cervix is dilated, and products of conception are removed by vacuum cannula and the use of other instruments as needed.	Safe and effective procedure for more advanced pregnancy, outpatient procedure with general anesthesia, 2-day recovery period	More psychologic trauma, more expensive, greater risk with general anesthesia and more invasive procedure
mifepristone (Mifeprex) (RU-486) with misoprostol (Cytotec)	Up to 7 wk	Mifepristone is administered orally. Misoprostol (prostaglandin) is administered orally or intravaginally 2 days later.	Effective, does not require surgical procedure	Very expensive, prolonged bleeding, sepsis possible
methotrexate with misoprostol	Up to 7 wk	Methotrexate is administered intramuscularly. Misoprostol is given intravaginally 5-7 days later.	Safe, effective, does not require surgical procedure	Not considered as effective as mifepristone, prolonged bleeding possible
Late Abortion				
Instillation of drugs • Hypertonic saline solution	After 16 wk	About 200 ml of amniotic fluid is withdrawn, and a similar amount of 20% normal saline solution is injected. Uterus is irritated and begins to contract within 12-36 hr. Contractions may be assisted with IV oxytocin.	Inexpensive, readily available, feticidal	Hypernatremia, infection, hemorrhage, disseminated intravascular coagulation, more emotional trauma because of time required
• Prostaglandins (carboprost [Hemabate], dinoprostone [Prostin E$_2$, Cervidil])	After 16 wk	Amniocentesis is done, and prostaglandin is inserted into amniotic sac, resulting in stimulation of smooth muscle of uterus. Expulsion of uterine contents occurs within 24 hr.	Fast induction, no need for surgery	Nausea and vomiting, abdominal cramps, cervical laceration, possible delivery of live fetus, high cost
Hysterotomy	16-20 wk	Miniature cesarean section is performed. Incision is made into uterus and contents are removed.	Concurrent sterilization procedure possible	More difficult and expensive in time and money, surgical incision with possible complications

IV, Intravenous.

rettage (D&C) procedure is generally performed. The D&C involves dilating the uterine cervix and scraping the endometrium of the uterus to empty the uterus of the products of conception.

Women who are experiencing bleeding and cramping during pregnancy may be admitted to the hospital. Nurses need to attend to both the physical and the emotional needs of patients. Vital signs and estimated blood loss are monitored. Any tissue or blood clots that might contain tissue are examined for products of conception. Women are very distressed and experience both physical and emotional pain. Nurses should use comfort measures to provide the needed physical and mental rest. Arranging for someone to stay with the patient provides important emotional support. The nurse should be aware of the grieving process that results from the loss of a pregnancy. Support of the patient and her family is essential.

Induced Abortion

Induced abortion is an intentional or elective termination of a pregnancy. Induced abortion is done for personal reasons (at the request of the woman) and for medical reasons. Several techniques are used to induce abortion, including menstrual extraction, suction curettage, dilation and evacuation (D&E), and drug therapy. Deciding which technique to use to terminate a pregnancy depends on the gestational age (length of the pregnancy) and the woman's condition. Suction curettage may be performed up to 14 weeks of gestation and accounts for more than 90% of abortion procedures.[3] Table 54-3 lists current methods for induced abortion.

Drug therapy is another method to induce abortion (medical abortion) early in pregnancy. These agents must be given within the first 49 days of pregnancy (day 1 being the first day of the last

Situation

A recently married, 39-year-old woman is informed that the results of her amniocentesis indicate her fetus has major chromosomal abnormalities and is expected to have severe physical and mental disabilities. The patient has no children, but her husband has three children from a previous marriage. She asks the nurse what she should do. How would the nurse respond?

Important Points for Consideration

* Decisions about whether to continue a pregnancy with a child who has severe disabilities are extremely personal and emotional. The woman and her husband will need support and information to explore their options and their values.
* Pregnancy counseling is warranted about the woman's choices, her feelings about the pregnancy, her desire to have a child with her husband, her concerns about raising a child with severe disabilities, her feelings about abortion, and concerns about possible future pregnancies.
* Patient autonomy ensures that a woman decide for herself whether or not to continue a pregnancy.
* The Supreme Court decision in 1973, Roe v Wade, legalized abortion in the United States. In the first trimester, abortion is a private matter between a woman and her physician. In the second trimester, the state may regulate abortion services for safety reasons. In the third trimester, abortions may only be performed when the life or health of the woman is endangered by the pregnancy.
* The role of the health care professional in these difficult situations is to provide education and support, and to facilitate a decision consistent with the patient's values.

Critical Thinking Questions

1. How would your feelings about abortion affect your ability to care for this patient?
2. How would you proceed in this case?

menstrual period). Mifepristone (Mifeprex) (also known as RU-486) works by blocking progesterone, a hormone needed for pregnancy to continue. It is given in combination with misoprostol (Cytotec), an agent that produces uterine contractions resulting in expulsion of the products of conception. In rare cases, fatal bacterial infections have been associated with mifepristone.[4]

Methotrexate, also given in combination with misoprostol, is another option for medically induced abortions. Methotrexate induces abortion because of its toxicity to trophoblastic tissue; misoprostol induces uterine contractions.

Once the decision is made to have an abortion, the woman and her significant others need support and acceptance. The patient should be prepared for what to expect both emotionally and physically. Grief and sadness are normal emotions after an abortion. The patient needs to understand the procedure, including instructions for preprocedure and postprocedure care. The nurse's caring attitude can be a positive factor in the patient's experience.

Follow-up care includes instructions on signs and symptoms of possible complications, including abnormal vaginal bleeding, severe abdominal cramping, fever, and foul drainage. Avoiding intercourse and vaginal insertions until reexamination should be stressed. The patient needs to return for reexamination in

2 weeks. Contraception can be started the day of the procedure or during the patient's return visit in accordance with her needs and desires.

Problems Related to Menstruation

The normal menstrual cycle is discussed in Chapter 51. The hormonal changes related to the menstrual cycle are shown in Fig. 51-9. Menstruation may be irregular during the first few years after menarche and the years preceding menopause. Once established, a woman's menstrual cycles usually have a predictable pattern. However, considerable normal variation exists among women in cycle length, as well as in the duration, amount, and character of the menstrual flow (see Table 54-2).

PREMENSTRUAL SYNDROME

Premenstrual syndrome (PMS) is a common disorder in women in which a group of physical and psychologic symptoms occur during the last few days of the menstrual cycle and before the onset of menstruation. The symptoms can be severe enough to impair interpersonal relationships or interfere with usual activities. Because many symptoms are associated with PMS, it is difficult to concisely define it. However, PMS symptoms always occur cyclically during the luteal phase before the onset of menstruation and are not present at other times of the month.

Etiology and Pathophysiology

The etiology and pathophysiology are not well understood. PMS is thought to have a biologic trigger with compounding psychosocial factors. Neurotransmitters, such as serotonin, may also be involved. Some women may have a genetic predisposition to PMS. Other proposed causes of PMS include estrogen and progesterone imbalances and nutritional deficiencies of pyridoxine (vitamin B_6) or magnesium.[5] *Premenstrual dysphoric disorder* (PMD-D) is the term applied to a type of PMS. Women with PMD-D have a severe mood disorder in addition to PMS.

Clinical Manifestations

PMS is extremely variable in its clinical manifestation. Variation is common between women and, for an individual woman, from one cycle to another. Commonly occurring physical symptoms include breast discomfort, peripheral edema, abdominal bloating, sensation of weight gain, episodes of binge eating, and headache. Abdominal bloating and breast swelling are caused by fluid shifts because total body weight does not generally change. Symptoms of autonomic nervous system arousal (e.g., heart palpitations, dizziness) have been reported by women with PMS. Anxiety, depression, irritability, and mood swings are some of the emotional symptoms that women may experience.

Diagnostic Studies and Collaborative Care

PMS can be diagnosed only when other possible causes for the symptoms have been eliminated. A focused health history and physical examination are done to identify any underlying conditions such as thyroid dysfunction, uterine fibroids, or depression that may account for the symptoms. No definitive diagnostic test is available for PMS. When PMS or PMD-D is a possible diagnosis, a woman is given a symptom diary to record her symptoms prospectively for two or three menstrual cycles. Diagnosis is based on an evaluation of the woman's symptoms.

TABLE 54-4	*COLLABORATIVE CARE* Premenstrual Syndrome (PMS)

Diagnostic
History and physical examination
Symptom diary

Collaborative Therapy
Stress management and relaxation therapy
Nutritional therapy
- Avoid caffeine and alcohol
- Reduce refined carbohydrates
- Vitamin B$_6$
- Limit salt intake before menstruation
- Calcium and magnesium supplements
Aerobic exercise
Drug therapy
- Diuretics
- Prostaglandin inhibitors (e.g., ibuprofen [Advil, Motrin])
- buspirone (BuSpar)
- Tricyclic antidepressants (e.g., amitriptyline [Elavil])
- Selective serotonin reuptake inhibitors (e.g., sertraline [Zoloft])
- Combined oral contraceptives

Nonpharmacologic and pharmacologic strategies can relieve some PMS symptoms (Table 54-4). However, no single treatment is available. The goal of treatment is to reduce the severity of symptoms and enhance the woman's sense of control and quality of life.

Several conservative approaches to managing PMS symptoms are considered helpful, including stress management, diet changes, exercise, education, and counseling.[5] Techniques for stress reduction include yoga, meditation, imagery, and biofeedback training. To decrease autonomic nervous system arousal, women should avoid caffeine, reduce dietary intake of refined carbohydrates, exercise on a regular basis, and practice relaxation techniques. Eating complex carbohydrates with high fiber, foods rich in vitamin B$_6$, and sources of tryptophan (dairy and poultry) are thought to promote serotonin production, which improves the symptoms. Vitamin B$_6$ may be found in such foods as pork, milk, egg yolk, and legumes. Although no strongly supportive data exist, limiting salt intake before menstruation and increasing calcium intake have been proposed to alleviate fluid retention, weight gain, bloating, breast swelling, and tenderness.

Exercise results in a release of endorphins, leading to mood elevation. Aerobic exercise can also have a relaxing effect. Because fatigue tends to exaggerate the symptoms of PMS, adequate rest in the premenstrual period is a priority.

Explanations about PMS help the woman understand the complexity of the disorder and ways that she can regain a better sense of control. The patient needs to be assured that her symptoms are real, PMS exists, and she is not "crazy." Acknowledgment of having PMS can itself be therapeutic. Teaching the woman's partner about the nature of PMS assists the partner to better understand PMS and to provide support to the woman in making lifestyle changes to reduce the symptoms of PMS.

Drug Therapy. Drug therapy is considered when symptoms persist or interfere with daily functioning. Presently, no single drug can treat all the symptoms associated with PMS. One therapy may be tried for a time, and if no improvement is noted, another approach is tried. Many treatments are symptom specific. For fluid retention, diuretics such as spironolactone (Aldactone) are used. For reducing cramping pain, backache, and headache, prostaglandin inhibitors such as ibuprofen (Motrin, Advil) are used. To improve negative mood, vitamin B$_6$ supplementation (50 mg daily) may be used. Calcium and magnesium supplementation may also be effective in alleviating psychologic and physiologic symptoms. For anxiety, buspirone (BuSpar) taken during the luteal phase has helped some women. Women with PMD-D may benefit from antidepressants, including fluoxetine (Sarafem) and tricyclic antidepressants (e.g., amitriptyline [Elavil]).

Other pharmacologic treatments are directed at PMS in general. Selective serotonin reuptake inhibitors (SSRIs) (e.g., sertraline [Zoloft]) have provided significant relief to women with severe PMS.[6] Other general treatments include oral contraceptives containing estrogen and progesterone. Evening primrose oil, an herb, may help some women.

DYSMENORRHEA

Dysmenorrhea is abdominal cramping pain or discomfort associated with menstrual flow. The degree of pain and discomfort varies with the individual. The two types of dysmenorrhea are primary, when no pathology exists, and secondary, when pelvic disease is the underlying cause. Dysmenorrhea is one of the most common gynecologic problems, affecting approximately 50% of all women.[7]

Etiology and Pathophysiology

Primary dysmenorrhea is not a disease; it is caused by an excess of prostaglandin F$_2\alpha$ (PGF$_2\alpha$) and/or an increased sensitivity to it. The sequential stimulation of the endometrium by estrogen, followed by progesterone, results in a dramatic increase in prostaglandin production by the endometrium. With the onset of menses, degeneration of the endometrium releases prostaglandin. Locally, prostaglandins increase myometrial contractions and constriction of small endometrial blood vessels with consequent tissue ischemia and increased sensitization of the pain receptors, resulting in menstrual pain. Primary dysmenorrhea begins in the few years after menarche, typically with the onset of regular ovulatory cycles.

Secondary dysmenorrhea is usually acquired after adolescence, occurring most commonly at 30 to 40 years of age. Common pelvic conditions that cause secondary dysmenorrhea include endometriosis, chronic pelvic inflammatory disease, and uterine fibroids. Because secondary dysmenorrhea is caused by multiple conditions, symptoms vary. However, painful menses is present in all situations.[7]

Clinical Manifestations

Primary dysmenorrhea starts 12 to 24 hours before the onset of menses. The pain is most severe the first day of menses and rarely lasts more than 2 days. Characteristic manifestations include lower abdominal pain that is colicky in nature, frequently radiating to the lower back and upper thighs. The abdominal pain is often accompanied by nausea, diarrhea, loose stools, fatigue, headache, and light-headedness.

Secondary dysmenorrhea usually occurs after the woman has experienced problem-free periods for some time. The pain, which may be unilateral, is generally more constant in nature and usually continues longer than in primary dysmenorrhea. Depending on the cause, symptoms such as *dyspareunia* (painful intercourse), painful defecation, or irregular bleeding may occur at times other than menstruation.

Collaborative Care

Evaluation begins with distinguishing primary from secondary dysmenorrhea. A complete health history with special attention to menstrual and gynecologic history should be obtained. A pelvic examination is also performed. If the history reveals an onset shortly after menarche and symptoms only associated with menses in addition to normal pelvic examination findings, the probable diagnosis is primary dysmenorrhea. If any specific cause of dysmenorrhea is evident, the diagnosis is secondary dysmenorrhea.

Treatment for primary dysmenorrhea includes heat, exercise, and drug therapy. Heat is applied to the lower abdomen or back. Regular exercise is thought to be beneficial because it may reduce endometrial hyperplasia and subsequently reduce prostaglandin production. The primary drug therapy is nonsteroidal antiinflammatory drugs (NSAIDs) such as naproxen (Naprosyn), which has antiprostaglandin activity. NSAIDs should be started at the first sign of menses and continued every 4 to 8 hours to maintain a sufficient level of the drug to inhibit prostaglandin synthesis for the usual duration of discomfort. Oral contraceptives may also be used. They decrease dysmenorrhea by reducing endometrial hyperplasia.

Acupuncture and transcutaneous nerve stimulation also provide varying degrees of relief. (See Chapter 8 for a discussion of acupuncture.) These methods may be used for women who obtain inadequate relief from medications or who prefer not to take medications. Patients who are unresponsive to these treatments should be evaluated for chronic pelvic pain.

Treatment of secondary dysmenorrhea depends on the cause. Some individuals with secondary dysmenorrhea will be helped by the approaches used for primary dysmenorrhea. Depending on the underlying causes of dysmenorrhea, additional drug or surgical interventions are used.

NURSING MANAGEMENT
DYSMENORRHEA

One of the primary roles of the nurse is teaching. Women should be taught why dysmenorrhea occurs, as well as how to treat it. Teaching and supportive therapy can provide women with a foundation for coping with this common problem and increase feelings of control and self-reliance.

Women often ask the nurse what can be done for minor discomforts associated with menstrual cycles. Women should be advised that during acute pain, relief may be obtained by lying down for short periods, drinking hot beverages such as herbal teas, applying heat to the abdomen or back, taking warm tub baths, and taking NSAIDs for analgesia.[8] The nurse can also suggest noninvasive pain-relieving practices such as distraction and guided imagery.

Other health care measures can reduce the discomfort of dysmenorrhea. These include regular exercise and proper nutritional habits. Avoiding constipation, maintaining good body mechanics, and eliminating stress and fatigue, particularly during the time preceding menstrual periods, can also decrease discomfort. Staying active and interested in activities may also help.

ABNORMAL VAGINAL BLEEDING

Abnormal vaginal or uterine bleeding is a common gynecologic concern. Abnormalities include **oligomenorrhea** (long intervals between menses, generally greater than 35 days), **amenorrhea** (absence of menstruation), **menorrhagia** (excessive or prolonged

TABLE 54-5	Causes of Amenorrhea

Hypothalamic-Pituitary Axis
- Reversible CNS-mediated causes (e.g., emotional stress, anorexia nervosa or severe dieting, strenuous exercise, chronic or acute illness)
- Prolactinoma and other causes of hyperprolactinemia (e.g., drugs)
- Brainstem tumors
- Congenital conditions (e.g., isolated gonadotropin deficiency)*
- Trauma (e.g., head injury with hypothalamic contusion)
- Infiltrative processes (e.g., sarcoidosis)
- Vascular disease (e.g., hypothalamic vasculitis)
- Pituitary tumors

Ovaries
- Autoimmune disease (often involving thyroid, adrenal, and islet cells)
- Premature menopause
- Polycystic ovary disease
- Tumors
- Congenital or genetic conditions (e.g., Turner syndrome)*
- Infection (e.g., mumps oophoritis)
- Toxins (especially alkylating chemotherapeutic agents)
- Radiation
- Trauma, torsion (rare)

Hormonal Synthesis and Action
- Male pseudohermaphroditism (e.g., testicular feminization)*

CNS, Central nervous system.
*Usually manifests as primary amenorrhea.

menstrual bleeding), and **metrorrhagia** (irregular bleeding or bleeding between menses). The cause of abnormal bleeding may vary from anovulatory menstrual cycles to more serious causes such as ectopic pregnancy or endometrial cancer. The age of the woman provides direction for identifying the cause of bleeding. For example, a postmenopausal woman with abnormal bleeding must always be evaluated for endometrial cancer but does not need to be evaluated for possible pregnancy. For a 20-year-old woman with abnormal bleeding, the possibility of pregnancy must always be considered and the possibility of endometrial cancer would be unlikely. When bleeding is due to a disruption in the menstrual cycle (e.g., anovulation) it is called *dysfunctional uterine bleeding*.

Abnormal bleeding may be caused by dysfunction of the hypothalamic-pituitary-ovarian axis such as a pituitary adenoma. Another cause may be infection. Changes in lifestyle such as marriage, recent moves, a death in the family, financial stress, and other emotional crises can also cause irregular bleeding. Because psychologic factors can influence endocrine function, they should be considered when the patient is evaluated.

Types of Irregular Bleeding

Oligomenorrhea and Secondary Amenorrhea. Anovulation is the most common cause for missing menses once pregnancy has been ruled out. Additional causes of amenorrhea are listed in Table 54-5. *Primary amenorrhea* refers to the failure of menstrual cycles to begin by age 16 years or by age 14 years if secondary sex characteristics are present. *Secondary amenorrhea* refers to the cessation of menstrual cycles once they had been established.

Ovulation is often erratic for several years following menarche and before menopause. Thus oligomenorrhea due to anovulation is common for women at the beginning and end of menstruation.[9] In anovulatory cycles, the corpus luteum that produces progesterone does not form. This may result in a situation referred to as *unopposed estrogen.* When unopposed by progesterone, estrogen can cause excessive buildup of the endometrium. Persistent overgrowth of the endometrium increases a woman's risk for endometrial cancer. To reduce this risk, progesterone or oral contraceptives are prescribed to ensure that the patient's endometrial lining will be shed at least four to six times per year.

Menorrhagia. The excessive bleeding associated with menorrhagia can be characterized as an increased duration (more than 7 days), increased amount (more than 80 ml), or both. Anovulatory uterine bleeding is the most common cause of menorrhagia. An unopposed estrogen state continues to build up the endometrium until it becomes unstable, resulting in menorrhagia. For young women with excessive bleeding, clotting disorders must be considered. Uterine fibroids (also called *leiomyomas*) and endometrial polyps are common causes of menorrhagia for women in their 30s and 40s.

Metrorrhagia. Metrorrhagia, also referred to as *spotting* or *breakthrough bleeding,* is bleeding between menstrual periods. For all reproductive-age women, pregnancy complications such as spontaneous abortion or ectopic pregnancy must be considered as a possible cause. Other causes include cervical or endometrial polyps, infection, and carcinoma. Spotting is common during the first three cycles of oral contraceptives. If spotting continues past the woman's third cycle using oral contraceptives, a different pill formulation can be prescribed when other causes of metrorrhagia have been ruled out. Spotting with long-acting progestin therapy (e.g., Mirena IUD) or progestin-only pills (Depo-Provera) is also common. For postmenopausal women, endometrial cancer must be considered whenever spotting is experienced. In postmenopausal women, exogenous estrogen administration during hormone replacement therapy is a common cause of metrorrhagia. *Menometrorrhagia* is excessive bleeding that occurs at irregular intervals. It may be caused by endometrial cancer or uterine fibroids.

Diagnostic Studies and Collaborative Care

Because abnormal vaginal bleeding has multiple causes, the diagnostic and collaborative care varies. A health history and physical examination directed at the most likely causes of vaginal bleeding for the woman's age-group is the first step. These findings will provide the basis for selecting the necessary laboratory tests and diagnostic procedures. Treatment depends on the nature of the problem (e.g., menorrhagia, amenorrhea), degree of threat to the patient's health, and whether children are desired in the future.

Combined oral contraceptives may be prescribed for a woman with amenorrhea to ensure regular shedding of endometrium if she also wants contraception. If she wants to become pregnant, a fertility drug may be prescribed. If she does not need birth control, progesterone may be prescribed to ensure a shedding of the endometrial lining four to six times per year.

The treatment goal for women with menorrhagia is to minimize further blood loss. If menorrhagia is the result of anovulatory cycles, the endometrium must be stabilized by a combination of oral estrogen and progesterone.

Balloon thermotherapy is a technique for menorrhagia that involves the introduction of a soft, flexible balloon into the uterus; the balloon is then inflated with sterile fluid (Fig. 54-2). The fluid in the balloon is heated and maintained for 8 minutes, thus causing ablation (removal) of the uterine lining. When the treatment is com-

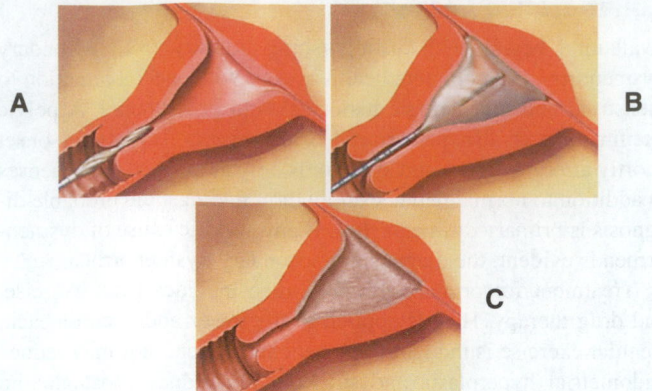

FIG. 54-2   Balloon thermotherapy for treatment of menorrhagia. **A,** Balloon-tipped catheter is inserted into the uterus through the vagina and cervix. **B,** The balloon is inflated with a sterile fluid that expands to fit the size and shape of the uterus. The fluid is heated to 188° F (87° C) and maintained for 8 minutes while the uterine lining is treated. **C,** Fluid is withdrawn from the balloon and the catheter is removed.

pleted, the fluid is withdrawn from the balloon and the catheter is removed from the uterus. The uterine lining sloughs off in the following 7 to 10 days. Uterine balloon thermotherapy is contraindicated for women who desire to maintain their fertility and for women with any suspected uterine abnormalities such as fibroids, suspected endometrial cancer, prior cesarean section, or myomectomy. With severe bleeding, hospitalization is indicated. All patients with menorrhagia should be evaluated for anemia and treated as indicated.

Surgical Therapy. Surgery may be indicated depending on the underlying cause of the abnormal vaginal bleeding. Dilation and curettage (D&C) was once a common therapy for excessive bleeding or for spotting in perimenopausal women. Now D&C is used only in extreme cases of bleeding or for older women when endometrial biopsy and ultrasonography have not provided the necessary diagnostic information. Endometrial ablation done by laser or electrosurgical technique has been successful with many patients with menorrhagia.[9] If menorrhagia is caused by uterine fibroids, a hysterectomy may be performed. A *myomectomy* (removal of fibroids without removal of the uterus) may be performed if the patient wants to preserve her uterus. The myomectomy is done via laparotomy, laparoscopy, or hysteroscopy. Hormonal regimens and embolization of the blood vessels supplying the fibroid tumor are other options.

NURSING MANAGEMENT
ABNORMAL VAGINAL BLEEDING

For some women, infrequent or no menses may or may not seem a desirable state. Teaching women about the characteristics of the menstrual cycle will assist them to identify normal variations.

Table 51-2 includes characteristics of the menstrual cycle and related patient teaching. This knowledge can diminish apprehension and dispel misconceptions about the menstrual cycle. If the patient's menstrual cycle pattern does not fall within the normal range, the nurse should urge her to visit her health care provider. Myths concerning activities allowed during menstruation are common. The nurse should be prepared to clarify the facts. The patient should be assured that bathing and hair washing are safe. A daily warm tub bath may help relieve pelvic discomfort. Women can swim, exercise, have intercourse, and basically continue their usual daily activities.

Frequent changing of tampons or pads meets comfort and hygiene needs during menstruation. The selection of internal or external sanitary protection is a matter of personal preference. Tampons are convenient and make menstrual hygiene easier, whereas pads may provide better protection. Using a combination of tampons and pads and avoiding prolonged use of superabsorbent tampons may decrease the risk of *toxic shock syndrome* (TSS). TSS is an acute life-threatening condition caused by a toxin from *Staphylococcus aureus*. TSS causes high fever, vomiting, diarrhea, weakness, myalgia, and a sunburn-like rash.[10]

Whenever excessive, the amount of the patient's vaginal bleeding should be assessed as accurately as possible. The number and size of pads or tampons used and the degree of saturation should be reported and recorded. The patient's fatigue level, along with variations in blood pressure and pulse, should be monitored because anemia and hypovolemia may be present. For the patient requiring a surgical procedure, the nurse should provide the appropriate preoperative and postoperative care.

ECTOPIC PREGNANCY

An **ectopic pregnancy** is the implantation of the fertilized ovum anywhere outside the uterine cavity (Fig. 54-3). Between 97% and 98% of ectopic pregnancies occur in the fallopian tube. The remaining 2% to 3% may be ovarian, abdominal, or cervical (Fig. 54-4). Ectopic pregnancy is a life-threatening condition. Earlier identification has contributed to a decrease in mortality rates. However, 40 to 50 deaths occur as a result of ectopic pregnancy each year in the United States. Ectopic pregnancy is the leading cause of pregnancy-related death.[11]

Etiology and Pathophysiology

Any blockage of the tube or reduction of tubal peristalsis that impedes or delays the zygote passing to the uterine cavity can result in tubal implantation. After implantation, the growth of the gestational sac expands the tubal wall. Eventually the tube ruptures, causing acute peritoneal symptoms. Less acute symptoms usually begin within 6 to 8 weeks after the last normal menstrual period and weeks before rupture would occur.

Risk factors for ectopic pregnancy include a history of pelvic inflammatory disease, prior ectopic pregnancy, current progestin-releasing intrauterine device (IUD), progestin-only birth control failure, and prior pelvic or tubal surgery. Additional risk factors for ectopic pregnancy include procedures used in infertility treatment, including in vitro fertilization procedures, embryo transfer, and ovulation induction.

Clinical Manifestations

The classic symptoms of ectopic pregnancy are abdominal or pelvic pain, missed menses, and irregular vaginal bleeding. Other symptoms include amenorrhea, morning sickness, breast tenderness, gastrointestinal disturbance, malaise, and syncope. Pain is almost always present and is caused by distention of the fallopian tube. It may start unilaterally and then spread to become bilateral. The character of the pain varies among women and can be colicky or vague. If tubal rupture occurs, the pain is intense and may be referred to the shoulder as a result of irritation of the diaphragm by blood released into the abdominal cavity. Symptom severity does not necessarily correlate with the extent of external bleeding pres-

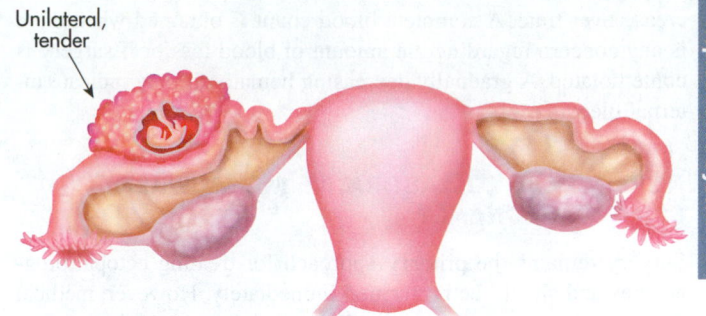

FIG. 54-3 Ectopic pregnancy occurring in the fallopian tube.

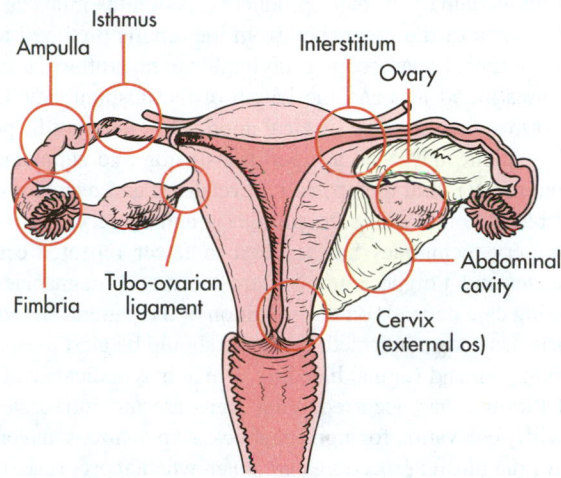

FIG. 54-4 Sites of implantation of ectopic pregnancies. Order of frequency of occurrence is ampulla, isthmus, interstitium, fimbria, tubo-ovarian ligament, ovary, abdominal cavity, and cervix (external os).

ent. With rupture, the risk of hemorrhage and hypovolemic shock is present. Suspected rupture is treated as an emergency.

The vaginal bleeding that may accompany ectopic pregnancy is usually described as spotting. However, it is also possible that bleeding may be heavier and can be confused with menses. The woman may also experience abnormal bleeding.

Diagnostic Studies

Because of the life-threatening nature of ectopic pregnancy, it should be considered whenever pregnancy is even remotely possible. Ectopic pregnancy can be a diagnostic challenge because of its similarity to other pelvic and abdominal disorders, such as salpingitis, spontaneous abortion, ruptured ovarian cyst, appendicitis, and peritonitis. A serum (radioimmunoassay) pregnancy test should be performed. If the test is negative, an ectopic pregnancy is not likely. If ectopic pregnancy cannot be excluded by the pregnancy test, further evaluation is warranted. If the patient is in a stable condition, a combination of serial β–human chorionic gonadotropin (β-hCG) and vaginal ultrasonography is used. β-hCG is expected to double about every 48 hours in a normal pregnancy. If the hCG level fails to double, the patient may have an ectopic pregnancy. Ultrasound can be used to confirm the presence of an intrauterine pregnancy once the β-hCG level has reached 1500 to 2000 mIU/ml.[12]

Absence of a normal intrauterine pregnancy means that the diagnosis is probably a spontaneous abortion or an ectopic pregnancy. With a spontaneous abortion, serial β-hCG levels will decrease over time. A complete blood count is obtained when there is any concern regarding the amount of blood loss or if surgery is contemplated. A gradually decreasing hematocrit may indicate internal bleeding.

NURSING *and* COLLABORATIVE MANAGEMENT
ECTOPIC PREGNANCY

Surgery remains the primary approach for treating ectopic pregnancies and should be performed immediately. However, medical management with methotrexate (Folex) is being used with increasing success with patients who are hemodynamically stable and have a mass less than 3 cm in size. A conservative surgical approach limits damage to the reproductive system as much as possible. Removal of the pregnancy from the tube is preferred to removing the tube. Laparoscopy is preferable to laparotomy, because it decreases blood loss and the length of the hospital stay. If the tube ruptures, conservative surgical approaches may not be possible. The patient may need a blood transfusion and supplemental intravenous (IV) fluid therapy to relieve shock and restore a satisfactory blood volume for safe anesthesia and surgery. The use of microsurgery techniques has resulted in fewer repeated ectopic pregnancies and a higher rate of future successful pregnancies.

Nursing care depends on the condition of the patient. Before the diagnosis has been confirmed, the nurse should be alert to signs of increasing pain and vaginal bleeding, which may indicate that rupture of the tube has occurred. Vital signs are monitored closely, along with observation for signs of shock. Explanations and preparation for diagnostic procedures are given when appropriate. Preparation of the patient for abdominal surgery may follow rapidly. The patient's emotional status should be assessed. Reassurance and support for the surgery should be given to the patient and her family. Postoperatively, the patient may express a fear of future ectopic pregnancies and have many questions about the impact of this experience on her future fertility.

PERIMENOPAUSE AND POSTMENOPAUSE

The **perimenopause** is a normal life transition that begins with the first signs of change in menstrual cycles and ends after cessation of menses. **Menopause** is the physiologic cessation of menses associated with declining ovarian function. It is usually considered complete after 1 year of *amenorrhea* (absence of menstruation). Menopause starts gradually and is usually associated with changes in menstruation, including menstrual flows that are increased, decreased, and/or irregular. Cessation of menses finally occurs. **Postmenopause** is a term that refers to the time in a woman's life after menopause.

The age at which menopause occurs ranges from 42 to 58 years, with the average being 51 years.[13] Menopause may occur earlier due to illness, surgical removal of the uterus or both ovaries, side effects of radiation therapy or chemotherapy, or drugs. The age at which menopause occurs is not affected by age at menarche, physical characteristics, number of pregnancies, date of last pregnancy, or oral contraceptive use. However, higher body mass index (BMI), cigarette smoking, racial/ethnic factors, and financial strain have been linked to an earlier age at menopause.[14]

Changes in the ovary start the cascade of events that finally result in menopause. The regression of the follicles within each ovary begins with puberty and accelerates after age 35. With age, fewer follicles remain that are responsive to follicle-stimulating hormone (FSH). FSH normally stimulates the dominant follicle to

TABLE 54-6	Clinical Manifestations of Perimenopause and Postmenopause

Perimenopause	Postmenopause
• Irregular menses	• Cessation of menses
• Vasomotor instability (hot flashes and night sweats)	• Occasional vasomotor symptoms
• Atrophy of genitourinary tissue (e.g., vaginal epithelium)	• Atrophy of genitourinary tissue with decreased support
• Stress and urge incontinence	• Stress and urge incontinence
• Breast tenderness	• Osteoporosis
• Mood changes	

TABLE 54-7	Signs and Symptoms of Estrogen Deficiency

Vasomotor
Hot flashes
Night sweats

Genitourinary
Atrophic vaginitis
Dyspareunia secondary to poor lubrication
Incontinence

Psychologic
Emotional lability
Change in sleep pattern
Decreased REM sleep

Skeletal
Increased fracture rate, particularly of vertebral bodies but also of humerus, distal radius, and upper femur

Cardiovascular
Decreased high-density lipoproteins (HDLs)
Increased low-density lipoproteins (LDLs)

Dermatologic
Diminished collagen content of skin
Breast tissue changes

REM, Rapid eye movement.

secrete estrogen. When the follicles can no longer respond to FSH, ovarian production of estrogen and progesterone declines. However, perimenopausal women can get pregnant until menopause has occurred. This is due to many women having long anovulatory cycles interspersed with shorter, ovulatory cycles.

With decreased ovarian function, decreased levels of estrogen cause a gradual increase in FSH and LH as a result of the negative feedback process. By the time menopause occurs, there is a 10-fold to 20-fold increase in FSH. The elevated FSH level may take several years to return to the premenopausal level. The reduced estrogen level also causes a decrease in the frequency of ovulation and results in changes in the reproductive organs and tissues (e.g., atrophy of vaginal tissue).

Clinical Manifestations

Clinical manifestations of perimenopause and postmenopause are presented in Table 54-6. The perimenopause is a time of erratic hormonal fluctuation. Irregular vaginal bleeding is common. With decreasing estrogen, hot flashes and other symptoms begin. The signs and symptoms of diminished estrogen are listed in Table 54-7. The loss of estrogen plays a significant role in the cause of age-related alterations. Changes most critical to a woman's well-being are the increased risks for coronary artery disease (CAD) and osteoporosis secondary to bone density loss. Other changes include a redistribution of fat, a tendency to gain weight more easily, muscle and joint pain, loss of skin elasticity, changes in hair amount and distribution, and atrophy of external genitalia and breast tissue.

Hallmarks of the perimenopause include *vasomotor instability* (hot flashes) and irregular menses. A hot flash is described as a sensation of warmth in the upper part of the chest, neck, and face followed by profuse perspiration.[15] These sensations last from several seconds to 5 minutes and occur most often at night, thereby disturbing sleep. The cause of hot flashes, or vasomotor instability, is not clearly understood. It has been theorized that temperature regulators in the brain are in proximity to the area where gonadotropin-releasing hormone (GnRH) is released. The lowered estrogen levels are correlated with dilation of cutaneous blood vessels resulting in hot flashes and increased sweating. The more sudden the withdrawal of estrogen (e.g., surgical removal of the ovaries), the more likely the symptoms will be severe if no hormone replacement is provided. These symptoms subside over time with or without hormone replacement therapy. Hot flashes can be triggered by situations that affect body temperature, such as eating a hot meal, hot weather, drinking an alcoholic beverage, stress, or warm clothing.

Atrophic vaginal changes secondary to decreased estrogen include thinning of the vaginal mucosa and disappearance of rugae. Vaginal secretions also decrease and become more alkaline. As a result of these changes, the vagina is easily traumatized and more susceptible to infection, including a higher risk for human immunodeficiency virus (HIV) transmission if exposed. *Dyspareunia* (painful intercourse) may also occur. This can lead to unnecessary and premature cessation of sexual activity. Dryness is a problem that can be easily corrected with water-soluble lubricants or, if needed, with hormonal creams or systemic hormone replacement therapy (see Evidence-Based Practice Box). In general, the extent and severity of the symptoms of menopause vary and are not easily predicted.

Atrophic changes in the lower urinary tract also occur with a decrease in estrogen. Bladder capacity decreases and the bladder and urethral tissue lose tone. These changes can cause symptoms that mimic a bladder infection (e.g., dysuria, urgency, frequency) when no infection is present.

Whether decreasing estrogen is responsible for the psychologic changes associated with perimenopause is unclear. The attributed depression, irritability, and cognitive problems could result from life stressors or sleep deprivation from hot flashes. Depressive symptoms appear to improve after menopause.[16]

Collaborative Care

The diagnosis of perimenopause should be made only after careful consideration of other possible causes for the woman's symptoms. Depression, thyroid dysfunction, anemia, or anxiety could be responsible for the same symptoms. Because of the hormonal fluctuations that occur before menopause, routine testing of the serum FSH level is not indicated. Levels of FSH in postmenopausal women are typically greater than 35 IU/L.[17]

Drug Therapy. Hormone replacement therapy (HRT) was standard therapy in the United States for treating menopausal symptoms until recently. HRT includes estrogen for women without ovaries or estrogen and progesterone for women with a uterus.

EVIDENCE-BASED PRACTICE

What Is the Effect of Localized Estrogen Preparations on Vaginal Atrophy?

Clinical Question

In women with vaginal atrophy (P), what is the effect of creams, pessaries, tablets, and vaginal rings (I) compared to no estrogen application (C) in relieving vaginal atrophy symptoms (O)?

Best Available Evidence

Systematic review of randomized controlled trials (RCTs)

Critical Appraisal and Synthesis of Evidence

- Meta-analysis of 16 RCTs (n = 2129) of postmenopausal women who administered intravaginal estrogen preparations for a duration of at least 3 months for symptom treatment of vaginal atrophy; 4 of the studies had a placebo control.

Conclusions

- Creams, pessaries, tablets, and the estradiol vaginal ring appeared to be equally effective in relieving symptoms of dyspareunia, pruritus, nocturia, urge incontinence, loss of libido, and dryness.
- Vaginal ring was the most acceptable.
- Long-term effect of localized estrogen on the endometrium is unknown.

Implications for Nursing Practice

- Instruct older women about the symptoms of vaginal atrophy and the beneficial effects of using localized estrogen.
- Include in patient education that lower doses of estrogen are used in the intravaginal preparations as compared with oral therapy.
- Optimum dose and frequency for best symptom relief is unknown.

Reference for Evidence

Suckling J, Lethaby A, Kennedy R: Local oestrogen for vaginal atrophy in postmenopausal women, *Cochrane Database of Systematic Reviews* 4, 2003.

PICO: P, Patient population of interest; *I*, intervention or area of interest; *C*, comparison of interest or comparison group; *O*, outcome(s) of interest (see p. 6).

Data from the Women's Health Initiative (WHI) studies changed this practice. The results of these studies showed that women who had taken estrogen plus progestin (Prempro) had an increased risk of breast cancer, stroke, heart disease, deep vein thrombosis, and pulmonary emboli. However, these women had fewer hip fractures and a lower risk of developing colorectal cancer.[18] In women who took only estrogen (Premarin), there was an increased risk for stroke and venous thrombosis (usually deep vein thrombosis). However, these women had neither an increased nor a decreased risk for heart disease, colorectal cancer, or breast cancer. Furthermore, they had fewer hip fractures. Neither estrogen plus progestin nor estrogen alone affected the risk of death.[18]

If women wish to consider taking HRT for the short-term treatment of menopausal symptoms, the risks and benefits (e.g., minimizes bone loss, hot flashes, vaginal atrophic changes) of therapy should be considered carefully. The decision to take HRT, and which ones to take, should be thoroughly discussed between the woman and her health care provider. If a woman chooses to use HRT, the lowest effective dose should be used.[19,20]

The side effects of estrogen include nausea, fluid retention, headache, and breast enlargement. Side effects of progesterone include increased appetite, weight gain, irritability, depression, spotting, and breast tenderness. A commonly used estrogen preparation is 0.625 mg of conjugated estrogen (Premarin) daily. For symptom relief, a higher dose may be needed. To receive the protective benefit of progesterone, 5 to 10 mg of medroxyprogesterone (Depo-Provera, Provera) is indicated for 12 days of each month on a cyclic regimen or 2.5 mg if on a continuous regimen. If the estrogen is to be increased for symptom relief, the progesterone should also be increased. Other forms of progesterone include norethindrone (Aygestin) and micronized progesterone creams, dermal patches, gels, and lotions; rings placed around the cervix; and subcutaneous pellets. Vaginal creams are especially useful for urogenital symptoms (e.g., dryness). Transdermal (skin patch) estrogen has the advantage of bypassing the liver, but has the disadvantage of causing skin irritation.

> **Drug Alert** - *Medroxyprogesterone (Depo-Provera, Provera)*
> • Report immediately the development of sudden loss of vision, severe headache, chest pain, hemoptysis, pain (especially with swelling, redness) in calves, numbness in arm/leg, abdominal pain/tenderness.

Antidepressants known as selective serotonin reuptake inhibitors (SSRIs), including paroxetine (Paxil), fluoxetine (Prozac), and venlafaxine (Effexor), are an effective alternative to HRT in reducing hot flashes. This effect is noted even if the user is not depressed.[15] The mechanism of action is unknown. Clonidine (Catapres), an antihypertensive drug, and gabapentin (Neurontin), an antiseizure drug, have also been shown to relieve hot flashes.

Selective estrogen receptor modulators (SERMs), such as raloxifene (Evista), are also used in treating menopausal problems. These drugs have some of the positive benefits of estrogen, such as preventing bone loss, without the negative effects such as endometrial hyperplasia. Raloxifene competes with estrogen for estrogen receptor sites. It decreases bone loss and serum cholesterol while having minimal effects on breast and uterine tissue. SERMs are also discussed in Chapter 64 with respect to their role in the management of osteoporosis.

Nonhormonal Therapy. Because of the associated risks with HRT, alternative therapies are receiving more attention for relieving menopausal symptoms. The frequency and severity of hot flashes can be reduced by promoting measures that support reduced heat production and increased heat loss. Keeping a cool environment and reducing caffeine and alcohol intake lowers heat production. Behavioral changes, such as relaxation techniques, also help. To promote heat loss at night when hot flashes can disrupt sleep, increasing air circulation in the room and avoiding bedding that traps the heat (e.g., heavy quilts) may help. Loose-fitting clothes do not retain body heat, whereas clothes with tight necks and wrists do. Cool cloths applied to flushed areas also aid in heat loss. A daily intake of vitamin E in doses up to 800 IU may also help reduce hot flashes.

Dry skin can be improved by the use of moisturizing soaps and body lotions. Kegel exercises may help decrease stress incontinence. Dyspareunia related to vaginal dryness can be managed with a water-soluble lubricant.

A focus on improving behaviors related to good nutrition with adequate amounts of exercise and sleep can help decrease anxiety and depression. Changing sleep patterns may be helped by avoiding alcohol and controlling hot flashes. Stress reduction techniques can promote a better night's sleep by decreasing anxiety. A regular moderate program (three to four times per week) of aerobic and weight-bearing exercises can slow the process of bone loss and a tendency toward weight gain. Exercise is important at menopause in modifying CAD risk factors, including stress, obesity, physical inactivity, and hypertension.

Nutritional Therapy. Good nutrition can decrease the risk of cardiovascular disease and osteoporosis in addition to assisting with vasomotor symptoms. A daily intake of about 30 kcal/kg of body weight is recommended. A decrease in metabolic rate and careless eating habits can cause the weight gain and fatigue often attributed to menopause. An adequate intake of calcium and vitamin D helps maintain healthy bones and counteracts loss of bone density. Postmenopausal women who are not receiving supplemental estrogen should have a daily calcium intake of at least 1500 mg; those who are taking estrogen replacement need at least 1000 mg per day. Calcium supplements are best absorbed when taken with meals. Either dietary calcium or calcium supplements may be used (see Chapter 64, Tables 64-15 and 64-16).

The diet should be high in complex carbohydrates and vitamin B complex, especially B_6. Research is inconclusive if phytoestrogens from plant sources can reduce menopausal symptoms. Examples of foods containing phytoestrogens include soy, tofu, chickpeas, and sunflower seeds. Herbal remedies, such as black cohosh, have become popular in treating menopausal symptoms (see Complementary and Alternative Therapies boxes on p. 1393). Consultation with an experienced herbal practitioner is recommended before initiating therapy. Many herbs can cause serious adverse effects.

CULTURALLY COMPETENT CARE
MENOPAUSE

Menopause is a universal phase in a woman's life, but the perception of this change varies by culture. Ethnic groups have their different traditions and beliefs regarding menopause. Nurses must be aware of the attitudes and beliefs regarding menopause among women from various ethnic backgrounds. In many cultures, menopause is considered a normal part of aging and little emphasis is placed on the physical and emotional symptoms that accompany the loss of fertility. A study of rural Irish women found that these women viewed menopause as a natural event and even looked forward to the end of childbearing.[21] In cultures where the elderly are revered, menopause is seen as a liberating transition to a state of being a "wise woman." In a study comparing women in the United States from different ethnic/racial groups, white women reported more psychosomatic menopausal symptoms (e.g., irritability, depression) than other ethnic groups. African American women reported more physical symptoms (e.g., hot flashes, vaginal dryness), and Asian women reported the fewest symptoms.[21] Australian women have a lower use of HRT and report more menopausal symptoms than British women.[22]

American culture generally has a negative attitude toward aging and places a high value on youth. Menopause is often considered a disorder that requires treatment. Menopausal symptoms are often viewed as troublesome, and there is a need to treat hot flashes and mood swings. Numerous substances, from HRT to herbal preparations, are used to treat menopausal symptoms.

Although menopause is experienced by all women, its meaning and symptoms vary. Menopause is a milestone in a woman's life that is embedded in her own personality and her culture. Nurses who approach the menopausal woman with this understanding can provide culturally competent care.

COMPLEMENTARY AND ALTERNATIVE THERAPIES
Herbs and Supplements for Menopause

Soy
Effects
Soy is used to decrease menopausal hot flashes.*

Nursing Implications
Women who have a history of breast, ovarian, or uterine cancer or endometriosis should consult with their health care provider before using soy or soy products. Soy may interact with warfarin. Patients taking warfarin should consult their health care provider before using soy or soy products.

Black Cohosh
Effects
Black cohosh is used to decrease menopausal symptoms.*

Nursing Implications
Black cohosh is generally safe when used for up to 6 months in otherwise healthy, nonpregnant women.

Ulbricht CE, Basch EM: Natural standard herb and supplement reference: evidence-based clinical reviews, St. Louis, 2005, Mosby. *www.naturalstandard.com.*
*Good scientific evidence exists for its use.

COMPLEMENTARY AND ALTERNATIVE THERAPIES
Valerian

Clinical Uses
- Insomnia*
- Anxiety disorder†
- Sedation‡

Effects
Appears to improve quality of sleep and to reduce time to fall asleep. Ongoing use may be more effective than single-dose uses, with increasing effects over 4 wk. Is nonsedating and appears to have little effect on concentration and coordination.

Nursing Implications
Generally safe in recommended dosages for up to 4-6 wk. Chronic use may result in insomnia. Liver toxicity has been reported in some multiple-herb preparations that include valerian. Contraindicated in pregnancy and lactation.

Ulbricht CE, Basch EM: Natural standard herb and supplement reference: evidence-based clinical reviews, St. Louis, 2005, Mosby. *www.naturalstandard.com.*
*Good scientific evidence exists for its use.
†Unclear scientific evidence exists for its use.
‡Fair scientific evidence exists against its use.

NURSING MANAGEMENT
PERIMENOPAUSE AND POSTMENOPAUSE

Nurses can play a key role in helping women to understand perimenopausal changes and options to minimize bothersome symptoms. Nurses can foster a positive image of perimenopause as a time of vitality and attractiveness. Perimenopause can provide women with a renewed incentive to enhance self-care and well-being.

Nurses need to provide teaching and reassurance to perimenopausal women who experience difficulty in managing their symptoms. They should be instructed that the symptoms are normal and often are temporary. Nonpharmacologic approaches to managing symptoms should be discussed. The nurse needs to address misconceptions about menopause to reduce unnecessary anxiety.

Sexual function can continue with little change in the vast majority of postmenopausal women. Cessation of menstruation and ability to bear children should not be equated with cessation of sexual capability; in fact it may be liberating. Femininity and libido do not disappear with menopause. Atrophic changes in vaginal epithelium associated with decreased estrogen may lead to dyspareunia. A water-soluble lubricant (e.g., Replens, Astroglide, K-Y jelly) is often effective in managing this problem. An active sex life helps increase lubrication and maintains the pliability of vaginal tissues. The patient should be given an opportunity to candidly discuss concerns related to sexual functioning.

CONDITIONS OF THE VULVA, VAGINA, AND CERVIX
Etiology and Pathophysiology

Infection and inflammation of the vagina, cervix, and vulva commonly occur when the natural defenses of the acid vaginal secretions (maintained by sufficient estrogen levels) and the presence of *Lactobacillus* are disrupted. The woman's resistance may also be decreased as a result of aging, poor nutrition, and the use of drugs (e.g., antibiotics, hormones) that alter the bacterial flora or mucosa. Organisms gain entrance to the areas through contaminated hands, clothing, and douche tips and during intercourse, surgery, and childbirth. Table 54-8 relates the specific etiologic factors, clinical manifestations and diagnostic methods, and collaborative care of common infections and inflammations.

Most lower genital tract infections are related to sexual intercourse. Intercourse can transmit organisms, injure tissues, and alter the acid-base balance of the vagina. Vulvar infections caused by viruses such as herpes and genital warts can be sexually transmitted when no lesions are apparent. Oral contraceptives, antibiotics, and corticosteroids may produce changes in the vaginal pH and trigger an overgrowth of the organisms present. For example, *Candida albicans* may be present in small numbers in the vagina. An overgrowth of this organism causes vulvovaginitis.

Clinical Manifestations

Abnormal vaginal discharge and reddened vulvar lesions are common clinical manifestations. In addition to a thick white curd-like discharge, women with vulvovaginal candidiasis (VVC) often experience intense itching and dysuria, which is the result of urine coming into contact with fissures and irritated areas on the vulva. The hallmark of bacterial vaginosis is the fishy odor of the discharge. Women with cervicitis may notice spotting after intercourse.

Common vulvar lesions include herpes infection and genital warts. Initial or primary herpes infections may be extremely painful. Herpes begins as a small vesicle followed by a superficial red ulcer. Most herpes lesions are painful. Dysuria is common when urine touches the lesion. Genital warts, caused by the human papillomavirus, vary in appearance. Irregularly shaped "cauliflower" lesions are common. Genital warts are painless unless traumatized. (Herpes infection and genital warts are discussed in Chapter 53.)

TABLE 54-8	Infections of the Lower Genital Tract	
Infection/Etiology	**Clinical Manifestations and Diagnostic Methods**	**Drug Therapy**
Vulvovaginal Candidiasis (VVC) (Monilial Vaginitis)		
Candida albicans (fungus)	Commonly found in mouth, gastrointestinal tract, and vagina; pruritus, thick white curdy discharge; KOH microscopic examination—pseudohyphae; pH 4.0-4.7	Antifungal agents (e.g., Monistat, Gyne-Lotrimin, Mycelex [available over the counter]) available in cream or suppository Fluconazole (Diflucan) 150 mg orally as single dose
Trichomonas Vaginitis		
Trichomonas vaginalis (protozoa)	Sexually transmitted; pruritus; frothy greenish or gray discharge; hemorrhagic spots on cervix or vaginal walls; saline microscopic examination—swimming trichomonads; pH >4.5	Metronidazole (Flagyl) 2 g orally in single dose or 500 mg orally twice a day for 7 days for patient and partner
Bacterial Vaginosis		
Gardnerella vaginalis *Corynebacterium vaginale*	Mode of transmission unclear; watery discharge with fishy odor; may or may not have other symptoms; saline microscopic examination—epithelial cells; pH >4.5	Metronidazole (Flagyl) 500 mg orally or clindamycin (Cleocin) 300 mg orally twice a day for 7 days or clindamycin (Clindesse) vaginal cream in single dose; examine and treat partner
Cervicitis		
Chlamydia trachomatis	Sexually transmitted; mucopurulent discharge with postcoital spotting from cervical inflammation; culture for chlamydia and gonorrhea	Azithromycin (Zithromax) 1 g orally as single dose or doxycycline 100 mg orally twice a day for 7 days; treat partner with same drugs
Severe Recurrent Vaginitis		
Candida albicans (most often)	May be indication of HIV infection; all women who are unresponsive to first-line treatment should be offered HIV testing	Drug appropriate to opportunistic organism

HIV, Human immunodeficiency virus; *KOH*, potassium hydroxide.

Postmenopausal older women may develop gynecologic problems such as *lichen sclerosis*.[23] This chronic inflammatory condition is associated with intense itching in the genital skin area (e.g., labia minora, clitoris). The lesions are white with a "tissue paper" appearance initially, although scratching produces changes in the appearance. The cause is unknown. High-potency topical corticosteroid ointment such as clobetasol (Temovate) helps relieve itching.

Collaborative Care

Genital problems are evaluated by taking a history, performing a physical examination, and obtaining the appropriate laboratory and diagnostic studies. Because many problems relate to sexual activity, a sexual history is essential. The nature of the problem directs specific aspects of the evaluation. Ulcerative lesions should be cultured for herpes. A blood test for syphilis may be done when ulcerative lesions are present. Genital warts are usually identified by their clinical appearance. Vulvar dystrophies may be examined via colposcopy, and a biopsy is taken for diagnosis.

Problems involving vaginal discharge are evaluated by microscopy and cultures. The most common vaginal conditions (i.e., bacterial vaginosis, VVC, and trichomoniasis) are diagnosed by a procedure called a *wet mount*. The findings characteristic of each condition are shown in Table 54-8. To assess for cervicitis, endocervical cultures are obtained for chlamydia and gonorrhea. If purulent discharge is observed coming from the cervix, a sample of endocervical cells may be taken to conduct a Gram stain. The Gram-stained slide is examined with a microscope to identify white blood cells and gram-negative diplococci (indicative of gonorrhea). (Sexually transmitted diseases [STDs] are discussed in Chapter 53.)

Drug therapy is based on the diagnosis and is shown in Table 54-8. Antibiotics taken as directed will cure bacterial infections. Antifungal preparations (in oral and cream preparations) are indicated for VVC. Women with vaginal conditions or cervical infection should abstain from intercourse for at least 1 week. Douching should be avoided. Douching disrupts the normal protective mechanisms within the vagina and may force the pathogens higher into the genital tract.[24] Sexual partners must be evaluated and treated if the patient is diagnosed with trichomoniasis, chlamydia, gonorrhea, syphilis, or HIV.

Treatment of vulvar dystrophies is symptomatic because no cures are available. Treatment involves controlling the itching and hence the scratching. Interrupting the "itch-scratch cycle" prevents further secondary damage to the skin.

NURSING MANAGEMENT
CONDITIONS OF THE VULVA, VAGINA, AND CERVIX

Nurses have the opportunity to teach women about common genital conditions and how to reduce their risks. Recognizing symptoms that indicate a problem helps women seek care in a timely manner. Discussing problems concerning one's genitals or sexual intercourse is frequently difficult. The nurse's nonjudgmental attitude makes women feel more comfortable and empowers them to ask questions seeking accurate information.

When a woman is diagnosed with a genital condition, the nurse should ensure that she fully understands the directions for treatment. Taking the full course of medication is especially important to decrease the chance of relapse. Because genitalia are such a private area, the use of graphs and models is especially helpful for patient teaching. When a woman will be using a vaginal medication for the first time, showing her the applicator and how to fill it is important. The woman should be taught where and how the applicator should be inserted using visual aids or models. Vaginal creams should be inserted before going to bed so that the medication will remain in the vagina for a long period of time. Women using vaginal creams or suppositories may wish to use panty liners during the day when the residual medication may drain out.

PELVIC INFLAMMATORY DISEASE

Pelvic inflammatory disease (PID) is an infectious condition of the pelvic cavity that may involve infection of the fallopian tubes (salpingitis), ovaries (oophoritis), and pelvic peritoneum (peritonitis). A tubo-ovarian abscess may also form. PID is referred to as "silent" when women do not perceive any symptoms. Other women with PID will be in acute distress. Pelvic pain may also be of a chronic nature.

Etiology and Pathophysiology

PID is often the result of untreated cervicitis. The organism infecting the cervix ascends higher into the uterus, fallopian tubes, ovaries, and peritoneal cavity (Fig. 54-5). *Chlamydia trachomatis* and *Neisseria gonorrhoeae* are the most common causative organisms of PID. These organisms, as well as anaerobes, mycoplasma, streptococci, and enteric gram-negative rods, gain entrance during sexual intercourse or after pregnancy termination, pelvic surgery, or childbirth. It is important to remember that not all cases of PID are the result of an STD.

Women at increased risk for chlamydial infections (younger than 24 years of age, have multiple sex partners, or have a new sex partner) should be routinely tested for chlamydia. Chlamydial infections can be asymptomatic and unknowingly transmitted during intercourse. Silent PID can cause damage that cannot be reversed. PID remains a major cause of female infertility.

Chronic pelvic pain is noncyclic pain greater than 6 months in duration, involving the pelvis, lower back, buttocks, and abdomen.[25] Up to one third of women have chronic pelvic pain after PID.[26] Factors also associated with chronic pelvic pain include interstitial cystitis, lower genital tract inflammation, irritable bowel syndrome, untreated uterine fibroids, endometriosis, and dysmenorrhea.

Clinical Manifestations

Women with PID usually go to a health care provider because they are experiencing lower abdominal pain. The pain typically starts gradually and is constant. The intensity may vary from mild to severe. Movement such as walking can increase the pain; pain is also frequently associated with intercourse. Spotting after intercourse and purulent cervical or vaginal discharge may also be noted. Fever and chills may also be present. Women with less acute symptoms notice increased cramping pain with menses, irregular bleeding, and some pain with intercourse. Women who have mild symptoms may go untreated either because they did not seek care or the health care provider misdiagnosed their complaints.

PID is a clinical diagnosis based on the patient's signs and symptoms. The diagnosis of PID is determined from data obtained during the bimanual portion of the pelvic examination. Women with PID have lower abdominal tenderness, adnexal tenderness, and positive cervical motion tenderness. Additional criteria useful for diagnosis may include fever and abnormal discharge (vaginal or cervical). Cultures for gonorrhea and chlamydia are also obtained, and a preg-

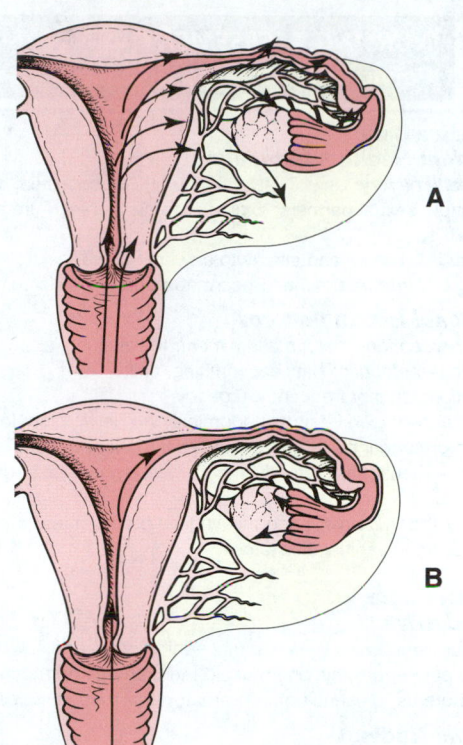

FIG. 54-5   Common routes of the spread of pelvic inflammatory disease. **A,** Direct spread of bacterial infection other than *Neisseria gonorrhoeae*. **B,** Direct spread of *N. gonorrhoeae*.

nancy test should be done to rule out ectopic pregnancy. Drug therapy begins when minimal diagnostic criteria are met, thus treatment is not delayed for culture results. When the patient's pain or obesity compromises the pelvic examination and a tubo-ovarian abscess may be present, a vaginal ultrasound is indicated.

Complications

Immediate complications of PID include septic shock and *Fitz-Hugh–Curtis syndrome,* which occurs when PID spreads to the liver and causes acute perihepatitis.[27] The patient will have symptoms of right upper quadrant pain, but liver function tests will be normal. Tubo-ovarian abscesses may "leak" or rupture, resulting in pelvic or generalized peritonitis. As the general circulation is flooded with bacterial endotoxins from the infected areas, septic shock may result. Embolisms may occur as the result of thrombophlebitis of the pelvic veins.

Long-term complications include ectopic pregnancy, infertility, and chronic pelvic pain. PID can cause adhesions and strictures to develop in the fallopian tubes. Ectopic pregnancy may result when a tube is partially obstructed because the sperm can pass through the stricture but the fertilized ovum cannot reach the uterus. After one episode of PID, the risk of having an ectopic pregnancy increases 10-fold. Further damage can obstruct the fallopian tubes and cause infertility.

Collaborative Care

PID is usually treated on an outpatient basis. The patient is given a combination of antibiotics such as cefoxitin (Mefoxin) and doxycycline (Vibramycin) to provide broad coverage against the causative organisms. With effective antibiotic therapy, the pain should subside. The patient must have no intercourse for 3 weeks. Her

TABLE 54-9	**NURSING ASSESSMENT** Pelvic Inflammatory Disease

Subjective Data

Important Health Information

Past health history: Use of IUD; previous PID, gonorrhea, or chlamydia; multiple sexual partners; exposure to partner with urethritis; infertility

Medications: Use of and allergy to any antibiotics

Surgery or other treatments: Recent abortion or pelvic surgery

Functional Health Patterns

Health perception–health management: Malaise

Nutritional-metabolic: Nausea, vomiting; chills, fever

Elimination: Urinary frequency, urgency

Cognitive-perceptual: Lower abdominal and pelvic pain; low back pain; pain on fundal palpation and cervical motion; onset of pain just after a menstrual cycle; dysmenorrhea, dyspareunia, dysuria, vulvar pruritus

Sexuality-reproductive: Abnormal vaginal bleeding and menstrual irregularity; vaginal discharge

Objective Data

Reproductive

Mucopurulent cervicitis, vulvar maceration, vaginal discharge (heavy and purulent to thin and mucoid), tenderness on motion of cervix and uterus; presence of inflammatory masses on palpation

Possible Findings

Leukocytosis; ↑ erythrocyte sedimentation rate; positive culture of secretions or endocervical fluid; pelvic inflammation and positive endometrial biopsy on laparoscopic examination; abscess or inflammation on ultrasonography

IUD, Intrauterine device; *PID,* pelvic inflammatory disease.

partner(s) must be examined and treated. An important part of care is physical rest and oral fluids. Reevaluation in 48 to 72 hours, even if symptoms are improving, is an essential part of outpatient care.

If outpatient treatment is unsuccessful or if the patient is acutely ill or in severe pain, admission to the hospital is indicated. If a tubo-ovarian abcess is present, hospitalization is also indicated. Maximum doses of parenteral antibiotics are given in the hospital. Some providers believe that the addition of corticosteroids to the antibiotic regimen reduces the inflammation, allowing for faster recovery and improvement in subsequent fertility. Application of heat to the lower abdomen or sitz baths may be used to improve circulation and decrease pain. Bed rest in the semi-Fowler position promotes drainage of the pelvic cavity by gravity and may prevent the development of abscesses high in the abdomen. Analgesics to relieve pain and IV fluids to prevent dehydration are also prescribed.

An indication for surgery is the presence of abscesses that fail to resolve with IV antibiotics. The abscess may be drained by laparoscopy or laparotomy. In extreme cases of infection or severe chronic pelvic pain, a hysterectomy may be performed. When surgery is necessary, the capacity for childbearing is preserved whenever possible.

Treatment for chronic pelvic pain should focus on the underlying disorder. If the source of the pain is unknown, treatment is directed at managing the symptoms.[25]

NURSING MANAGEMENT
PELVIC INFLAMMATORY DISEASE

Subjective and objective data that should be obtained from the woman with PID are presented in Table 54-9. Prevention, early recognition, and prompt treatment of vaginal and cervical infections can help prevent PID and its serious complications. Nurses

can provide accurate information about factors that place a woman at increased risk for PID. Nurses should urge women to seek medical attention for any unusual vaginal discharge or possible infection of their reproductive organs. Women should be helped to understand that not all discharge is indicative of infection, but that early diagnosis and treatment of an infection, if present, can prevent serious complications. Women should be informed of the methods to decrease the risk of getting STDs and to recognize the signs of infection in their partner(s).

The patient may have guilt feelings about having PID, especially if it was associated with an STD. She may also be concerned about the complications associated with PID, such as adhesions and strictures of the fallopian tubes, infertility, and the increased incidence of ectopic pregnancy. Discussion with the patient regarding her feelings and concerns can assist her to cope more effectively with them.

For patients requiring hospitalization, nurses have an important role in implementing drug therapy, monitoring the patient's health status, and providing symptom relief and patient teaching. Vital signs and the character, amount, color, and odor of the vaginal discharge should be recorded. Explanations about the need for limited activity, being in a semi-Fowler position, and increased fluid intake should increase patient cooperation. Assessing the degree of abdominal pain will provide information about the effectiveness of drug therapy.

ENDOMETRIOSIS

Endometriosis is the presence of normal endometrial tissue in sites outside the endometrial cavity. The most frequent sites are in or near the ovaries, the uterosacral ligaments, and the uterovesical peritoneum (Fig. 54-6). However, endometrial tissues can be in many other locations such as the stomach, lungs, intestines, and spleen. The tissue responds to the hormones of the ovarian cycle and undergoes a "mini–menstrual cycle" similar to the uterine endometrium.

Endometriosis is found equally among whites and African Americans, but is slightly more prevalent in Asian American women. The typical patient with endometriosis will be in her late twenties or early thirties, white, and never had a full-term pregnancy. Although it is not a life-threatening condition, endometriosis causes considerable pain and reduces a person's quality of life. Endometriosis is found in approximately 7% of women of reproductive age.[28]

Etiology and Pathophysiology

The etiology is not well understood, and many theories about the cause of endometriosis have been proposed. A widely held view is that retrograde menstrual flow passes through the fallopian tubes carrying viable endometrial tissues into the pelvis. The tissue attaches to various sites shown in Fig. 54-6. Another theory suggests that undifferentiated embryonic peritoneal cavity cells remain dormant in the pelvic tissue until the ovaries produce sufficient hormones to stimulate their growth. Other proposed causes include a genetic predisposition and altered immune function.

Clinical Manifestations

In patients with endometriosis a wide range of clinical manifestations and severity exists. The magnitude of a woman's symptoms does not necessarily correlate with the clinical extent of her endometriosis. Dysmenorrhea after years of relatively pain-free menses and infertility may serve as clues to the presence of endometriosis. The most common manifestations are secondary dysmenorrhea, infertility, pelvic pain, dyspareunia, and irregular bleeding. Less common manifes-

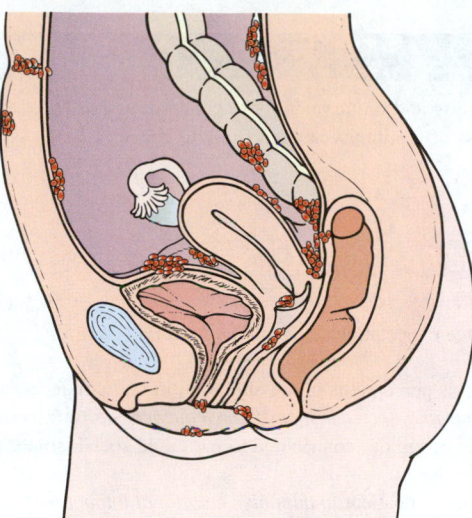

FIG. 54-6   Common sites of endometriosis.

TABLE 54-10	**COLLABORATIVE CARE** Endometriosis

Diagnostic
History and physical examination
Pelvic examination
Laparoscopy
Pelvic ultrasound
MRI

Collaborative Therapy
Conservative therapy (watch and wait)
Drug Therapy
* danazol (Danocrine)
* GnRH agonists (e.g., leuprolide [Lupron])
* Oral contraceptives
Surgical Therapy
* Laparotomy to remove implants and adhesions
* Total abdominal hysterectomy and bilateral salpingo-oophorectomy (TAH-BSO)

GnRH, Gonadotropin-releasing hormone; *MRI*, magnetic resonance imaging.

tations include backache, painful bowel movements, and dysuria. These symptoms may or may not correspond to the woman's menstrual cycles. With menopause, estrogen is no longer produced in the ovaries. This may lead to the disappearance of the symptoms.

When the ectopic endometrial tissues "menstruate," the blood collects in cystlike nodules that have a characteristic bluish black color. Nodules in the ovaries are sometimes called *chocolate cysts* because of the thick, chocolate-colored material they contain. When a cyst ruptures, the pain may be acute and the resulting irritation promotes the formation of adhesions, which fix the affected area to another pelvic structure. The adhesions may become severe enough to cause a bowel obstruction or painful micturition. Adhesions involving the uterus, tubes, or ovaries may result in infertility.[28]

Collaborative Care

Endometriosis may be suspected from a woman's history of the characteristic symptoms and the health care provider's palpation of firm nodular lumps in the adnexa on bimanual examination. However, laparoscopy is necessary for a definitive diagnosis. The treatment of endometriosis is influenced by the patient's age, desire for pregnancy, symptom severity, and extent and location of the disease. When symptoms are not disruptive, a "watch and wait" approach is used (Table 54-10). When endometriosis is identified as a probable cause of infertility, therapy proceeds more rapidly.

Drug Therapy. Drug therapy is used to reduce symptoms. Drugs are selected to inhibit estrogen production by the ovary so that the endometrial tissue will shrink. The various drugs used imitate a state of pregnancy or menopause. Continuous use (for 9 months) of combined oral contraceptives causes regression of endometrial tissue. Ovulation is suppressed and *pseudopregnancy* (hyperhormonal amenorrhea) is produced by progestin agents such as medroxyprogesterone (Depo-Provera). Another approach to hormonal treatment is danazol (Danocrine), a synthetic androgen that inhibits the anterior pituitary. This drug produces a *pseudomenopause* (ovarian suppression) with atrophy of ectopic endometrial tissue. Subjective relief of symptoms is noted within 6 weeks of danazol use. Side effects include weight gain, acne, hot flashes, and hirsutism. These side effects and the expense of this drug restrict its use.

Another class of drugs used is gonadotropin-releasing hormone (GnRH) agonists (e.g., leuprolide [Lupron], nafarelin [Synarel]). These drugs cause a hypoestrogenic state resulting in amenorrhea.

The side effects reported by patients are usually the same as menopause (hot flashes, vaginal dryness, and emotional lability). Loss of bone density has also been reported in women who remain on the therapy longer than 6 months. Endometriosis is controlled but not cured by hormonal therapy. Persistent lesions give rise to subsequent recurrences once the menstrual cycle is reestablished.

Drug Alert - *Leuprolide (Lupron)*
* *Assess patient for pregnancy before initiating therapy.*
* *Monitor patient for dysrhythmias, palpitations.*
* *Instruct patient to use contraceptive measures during therapy.*

Surgical Therapy. The only cure for endometriosis is surgical removal of all the endometrial implants. Surgical therapy may be conservative or definitive. Conservative surgery is done to confirm the diagnosis or to remove implants. It involves removal or destruction of endometrial implants and lysing or excision of adhesions by means of laparoscopic laser surgery or laparotomy. GnRH agonist therapy (e.g., leuprolide) can be administered for 4 to 6 months to reduce the size of the lesions before surgery. By reducing the extent of the surgery, this preoperative drug treatment helps reduce the development of adhesions that may further threaten fertility.

For women wishing to get pregnant, conservative surgical therapy is used to remove implants blocking the fallopian tube. Adhesions are removed from the tubes, ovaries, and pelvic structures. Efforts are made to conserve all tissues necessary to maintain fertility.

Definitive surgery involves removal of the uterus, tubes, ovaries, and as many endometrial implants as possible.[29] The individual woman should be actively involved in making the decision about preserving part or all of her ovaries, if surgically possible. Her feelings about maintaining her cyclic ovarian function need to be explored. The health care provider should assess the woman's risk for ovarian cancer and provide this information for her consideration.

NURSING MANAGEMENT
ENDOMETRIOSIS

Education of the patient and reassurance that a life-threatening situation does not exist may permit her to accept a conservative and progressive treatment. When the symptoms are less severe,

NURSING CARE PLAN 54-1

Patient with Abdominal Hysterectomy

NURSING DIAGNOSIS **Disturbed body image** *related to* perceived loss of femininity and future inability to conceive *as evidenced by* crying, weeping, depression; verbalization of perceived loss of femininity and/or ability to conceive

PATIENT GOALS 1. Verbalizes confidence in ability to adjust to postsurgical state
2. States acceptance of self and changes resulting from surgery

OUTCOMES (NOC)	**INTERVENTIONS (NIC) and *RATIONALES***
Sexual Identity	***Body Image Enhancement***
• Affirms self as a sexual being ____	• Determine patient's body image expectations *to establish need and plan for interventions.*
• Uses healthy coping behaviors to resolve sexual identity crisis ____	• Determine patient's and family's perceptions of the alteration in body image versus reality *to provide accurate facts and decrease fear of consequences of hysterectomy.*
• Reports healthy intimate relationships ____	• Determine if a change in body image has contributed to increased social isolation *to identify need for intervention.*
Measurement Scale	• Identify support groups available to patient *to minimize emotional impact of hysterectomy through open discussion.*
1 = Never demonstrated	• Assist the patient to discuss stressors affecting body image due to surgery (e.g., surgical menopause) *so patient is informed about possible treatment* (e.g., hormone replacement therapy).
2 = Rarely demonstrated	
3 = Sometimes demonstrated	
4 = Often demonstrated	
5 = Consistently demonstrated	

NURSING DIAGNOSES

Acute pain,* Ineffective breathing pattern,* Nausea,* Risk for imbalanced fluid volume,* Risk for infection*

COLLABORATIVE PROBLEMS

Hemorrhage,* Urinary retention,* Paralytic ileus*

*Postoperative care of the patient with an abdominal hysterectomy includes nursing diagnoses for the postoperative patient found in Nursing Care Plan 20-1: Postoperative Patient, p. 383 to 386.

teaching about nondrug comfort measures may be helpful. Nurses need to assist patients to understand the drugs that have been ordered to treat their condition. The action of the prescribed drug should be explained, as well as the possible side effects. Psychologic support may be needed for women experiencing severe disabling pain, sexual difficulties secondary to dyspareunia, and infertility.

If conservative surgery is the treatment selected, the nursing care is similar to the general preoperative and postoperative care of a patient undergoing laparotomy (see Chapter 43, pp. 1044 to 1045). If extensive surgery is planned, the nursing care is similar to the patient undergoing an abdominal **hysterectomy** (surgical removal of the uterus) (NCP 54-1). The nurse must know the extent of the procedure so that appropriate preoperative teaching can be done.

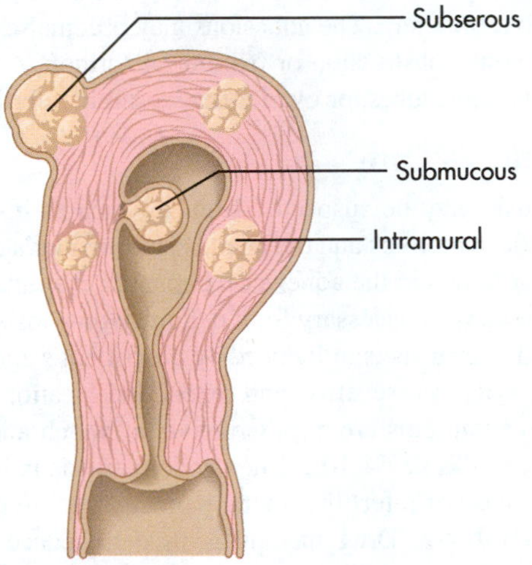

Benign Tumors of the Female Reproductive System

LEIOMYOMAS

Etiology and Pathophysiology

Leiomyomas (uterine fibroids) are benign smooth-muscle tumors that occur within the uterus. Leiomyomas are the most common benign tumors of the female genital tract (Fig. 54-7). By 30 years of age, 10% of white women and 30% of African American women have uterine leiomyomas. The cause of leiomyomas is unknown. They appear to depend on ovarian hormones because they grow slowly during the reproductive years and undergo atrophy after menopause.

FIG. 54-7 Leiomyomas. Uterine section showing whorl-like appearance and locations of leiomyomas, which are also called *uterine fibroids*.

Clinical Manifestations

The majority of women with leiomyomas do not have any symptoms. Of the women who develop symptoms, the most common include abnormal uterine bleeding, pain, and symptoms associated with pelvic pressure. Increased bleeding is thought to be associated with increased endometrial surface area that is associated with leiomyomas. Pain is thought to be associated with infection or twisting of the pedicle from which the tumor is growing. Devascularization and blood vessel compression are also thought to contribute to pain. Pressure on surrounding organs may result in rectal, bladder, and lower abdominal discomfort. Large tumors may cause a general enlargement of the lower abdomen. These tumors are sometimes associated with miscarriage and infertility.

Collaborative Care

Clinical diagnosis is based on the characteristic pelvic findings of an enlarged uterus distorted by nodular masses. Treatment depends on the symptoms, the age of the patient, her desire to bear children, and the location and size of the tumors. If the symptoms are minimal, the provider may elect to follow the patient closely for a time. If the woman is experiencing menorrhagia, the use of aspirin is discouraged because of its inhibitory effect on platelet aggregation.

Persistent heavy menstrual bleeding causing anemia and large or rapidly growing tumors are indications for surgery. The leiomyomas are removed by hysterectomy or myomectomy. A myomectomy is performed for women who wish to have children. In this case, only the fibroids are removed to preserve the uterus. Small tumors may be removed using a hysteroscope and laser resection instruments.

Uterine artery embolization is an increasingly used alternative treatment for uterine fibroids. In the procedure, embolic material (small plastic or gelatin beads) is injected into the uterine artery and carried to the fibroid branches.

Cryosurgery is another option. In cases of large leiomyomas, a GnRH agonist (e.g., leuprolide [Lupron]) may be used preoperatively to shrink the size of the tumor. However, the risks and benefits of this drug should be fully discussed, including the potential for irreversible loss of bone mass. The treatment should not be used on women planning to have children.

Another treatment option is the ExAblate 2000 system. It uses magnetic resonance imaging (MRI)–guided focused ultrasound to target and destroy uterine fibroids. Treatment requires repeated targeting and heating of the fibroid tissue while the patient lies inside the MRI machine. The procedure can last as long as 3 hours.

CERVICAL POLYPS

Cervical polyps are benign pedunculated lesions that generally arise from the endocervical mucosa and are seen protruding through the cervical os during a speculum examination. Polyps are a characteristic bright cherry-red and are soft and fragile in consistency. They are generally small, measuring less than 3 cm in length, and may be single or multiple. Their cause is unknown. Symptoms are usually not present, but metrorrhagia and bleeding after straining for a bowel movement and coitus can occur. Polyps are prone to infection. When the polyp is small, it can be excised in an outpatient procedure. If the point of attachment of the polyp cannot be identified and is not accessible to cautery, a polypectomy is performed in an operating room. All tissue removed is sent for pathologic review because polyps occasionally undergo malignant changes.

BENIGN OVARIAN TUMORS

There are many different types of benign tumors. The cause of most of them is unknown. They can be divided into cysts and neoplasms. *Cysts* are usually soft, are surrounded by a thin capsule, and may be detected during the reproductive years (Fig. 54-8). Follicle and corpus luteum cysts are common ovarian cysts. Multiple small ovarian follicles may occur in a condition called *polycystic ovary syndrome* (PCOS) (discussed in the next section). Epithelial ovarian neoplasms may be cystic or solid, or small or extremely large. Cystic teratomas, or dermoid cysts, originate from germ cells and can contain bits of any type of body tissue, such as hair or teeth.

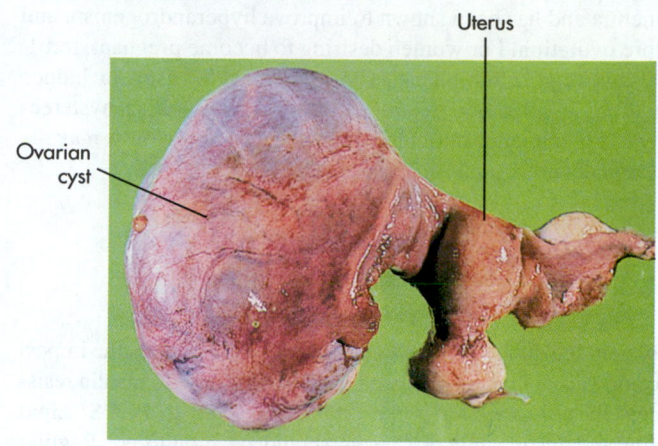

FIG. 54-8 Large ovarian cyst.

Ovarian masses are often asymptomatic until they are large enough to cause pressure in the pelvis. Constipation, menstrual irregularities, urinary frequency, a full feeling in the abdomen, anorexia, and peripheral edema may occur, depending on the size and location of the tumor. There may be an increase in abdominal girth. Pelvic pain may be present if the tumor is growing rapidly. Severe pain results when the cyst twists on its pedicle (ovarian torsion).

Pelvic examination reveals a mass or an enlarged ovary that demands further investigation. If the mass is cystic and smaller than 8 cm, the patient is asked to return for reexamination in 4 to 6 weeks. If the mass is cystic and greater than 8 cm or is solid, laparoscopic surgery or laparotomy is performed. Immediate surgery is necessary if ovarian torsion occurs, causing the ovary to rotate and cutting off circulation. Surgical techniques are used to save as much of the ovary as possible.

Polycystic Ovary Syndrome

Polycystic ovary syndrome (PCOS) is a chronic disorder in which many benign cysts form on the ovaries. It most commonly occurs in women under 30 years old. It affects about 5% of women of reproductive age. PCOS is caused by increased production of LH and decreased FSH. This imbalance prevents the ovaries from releasing an egg each month. The ovaries produce estrogen and excess testosterone but not progesterone. Small cysts develop in the ovaries related to chronic failure of the ovaries to release eggs. Research suggests a familial or genetic basis and a close association with obesity.[30]

Clinical manifestations include irregular menstrual periods (particularly long cycles), amenorrhea or oligomenorrhea, dysfunctional uterine bleeding, infertility, hirsutism, obesity, and acne. Many women start with normal menstrual periods and then after 1 to 2 years, the periods become irregular and then infrequent. If left untreated, cardiovascular disease, abnormal insulin resistance with type 2 diabetes mellitus, and ovarian and endometrial cancers may develop.[30-32]

Pelvic ultrasound will reveal enlarged ovaries with multiple small cysts. Successful management includes early diagnosis and treatment to improve quality of life and decrease the risk of complications. Oral contraceptives are useful in regulating menstrual cycles and controlling hirsutism. Hyperandrogenism can be treated with flutamide (Eulexin) and a GnRH agonist such as leuprolide (Lupron). Metformin (Glucophage) reduces hyperinsulinemia and has been shown to improve hyperandrogenism and restore ovulation. For women desiring to become pregnant, fertility drugs (e.g., clomiphene [Clomid]) may be used to induce ovulation. If all other treatments are unsuccessful, a hysterectomy with bilateral salpingectomy and oophorectomy may be performed.

> **Drug Alert** - *Clomiphene (Clomid)*
> • *Instruct patient to notify physician immediately if*
>   • *Lower abdominal pain occurs.*
>   • *Pregnancy is suspected.*

Patient teaching for the woman with PCOS includes the importance of weight management and exercise to decrease insulin resistance. Obesity exacerbates the problems related to PCOS. Lipid profile and fasting glucose levels should be monitored. Regular follow-up care is important to monitor the effectiveness of therapy and to detect any complications.

Cancers of the Female Reproductive System

CERVICAL CANCER

Approximately 10,370 women in the United States have invasive cervical cancer and 3700 women die from cervical cancer annually. Noninvasive cervical cancer is about four times more common than invasive cervical cancer. The mortality rate for cervical cancer in the United States is twice as high for African American women than for white women. Globally the annual incidence of cervical cancer is 471,000, with 80% of these cases occurring in underdeveloped countries.[33] The mortality rate in these countries is 50%. The increased incidence and mortality rates are attributed to a lack of screening and treatment programs.[34] An increased risk of cervical cancer is associated with low socioeconomic status, early sexual activity (before 17 years of age), multiple sexual partners, infection with human papillomavirus (HPV), immunosuppression, and smoking.

The number of deaths from cervical cancer in the United States has fallen steadily over the past 40 years. This is due to better and earlier diagnosis with the widespread use of the Papanicolaou (Pap) test. In addition to cancer, the Pap test screens for precancerous changes. By treating precancerous lesions, progression to cervical cancer can be prevented.

Etiology and Pathophysiology

The progression from normal cervical cells to dysplasia and then to invasive cervical cancer appears to be related to repeated injuries to the cervix. The progression occurs slowly over years rather than months. There is a strong relationship between sexual exposure of HPV and dysplasia.

Clinical Manifestations

Precancerous changes are asymptomatic. This highlights the importance of routine screening. The peak incidence of noninvasive cervical cancer is in women in their early 30s. The average age for women with invasive cervical cancer is 50 (Fig. 54-9). Early cervical cancer is generally asymptomatic, but leukorrhea and intermenstrual bleeding eventually occur. The discharge is usually thin and watery but becomes dark and foul smelling as the disease advances, suggesting the presence of an infection. The vaginal bleed-

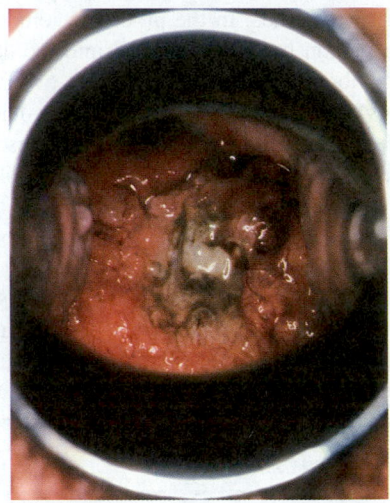

FIG. 54-9   Cervical cancer. View through a speculum inserted into the vagina.

ing is initially only spotting. As the tumor enlarges, it becomes heavier and more frequent. Pain is a late symptom and is followed by weight loss, anemia, and cachexia.

Diagnostic Studies

The American Cancer Society recommends that a Pap test be done at least once every 3 years, beginning 3 years after first sexual intercourse, but no later than age 21. Women ages 65 to 70 may decide with their health care provider after having no abnormal Pap tests in the last 10 years to stop having Pap tests.[35] Women who have had a total hysterectomy (uterus and cervix removed) do not need to be screened for cervical cancer, unless the surgery was done for cervical precancer or cancer.[36]

Pap tests are less than 100% accurate in screening for cervical cell abnormalities. There are problems with both false-positive and false-negative reports. ThinPrep, a newer liquid-based technique for Pap tests, has reduced the number of inaccurate Pap test results. Testing for HPV also identifies patients at risk for cervical cancer.

The finding of an abnormal Pap test indicates the need for follow-up. The type of follow-up depends on the findings. Women with minor changes may be followed with a repeated Pap test in 4 to 6 months for 2 years. Up to 80% may revert to normal spontaneously. Women with more prominent changes will receive additional procedures, such as colposcopy and biopsy, before a definitive diagnosis can be made. Colposcopy involves examination of the cervix with a binocular microscope with low levels of magnification (10× to 40×). The procedure helps in the identification of possible epithelial abnormalities and suggests areas for biopsy. The LUMA Cervical Imaging System may be used with colposcopy to identify these sites. Biopsies are sent to pathology for evaluation. Colposcopy and biopsy have improved diagnosis and allow more focused treatments to be selected.

The type and extent of the biopsy vary with the abnormality seen. A punch biopsy may be done on an outpatient basis with special punch biopsy forceps. The excision of a cone-shaped section of the cervix may be used for both diagnosis and treatment. Conization is accomplished using one of several techniques. The choice of procedure is determined by the health care provider's experience and the availability of equipment. *Cryotherapy* (freezing) and laser cone vaporization destroy the tissue. Laser cone excision and *loop electrosurgery excision procedure (LEEP)* remove the identified tissue and allow for histologic examination to ensure that all microinvasive tissue has been removed. These procedures can be performed as outpatient procedures with mild analgesics or sedation. Complications of these procedures include excessive bleeding and possible cervical stenosis after healing.

Collaborative Care

A vaccine is now available that reduces the incidence of both cervical-related neoplasia and cervical cancer due to infection from HPV types 16 and 18. It is approved for females aged 9 to 26. It requires three shots over six months.

The treatment of cervical cancer is guided by the stage of the tumor and the patient's age and general state of health (Table 54-11). There are four procedures in which fertility can be preserved. Conization may be the only type of therapy needed for noninvasive cervical cancer if analysis of removed tissue demonstrates that a wide area of normal tissue surrounds the excised tissue. Laser

treatments can be used in which a directed infrared beam is employed to destroy abnormal tissue. Cautery and cryosurgery may also be used.

Invasive cancer of the cervix is treated with surgery, radiation, and chemotherapy as single treatments or in combination. Surgical procedures include hysterectomy, radical hysterectomy (involving adjacent structures), and, rarely, pelvic exenterations. (Surgical therapy is discussed on pp. 1404 to 1407.) Radiation may be external (e.g., cobalt) or internal (e.g., cesium, radium). Standard radiation treatment is 4 to 6 weeks of external radiation followed by one or two treatments with internal implants. (Radiation therapy is discussed in Chapter 16.) Cisplatin-based chemotherapy regimens have shown benefit for patients with cancer spread beyond the cervix.[37]

ENDOMETRIAL CANCER

Cancer of the endometrium is the most common gynecologic malignancy, accounting for nearly 50% of female genital tract neoplasms in the United States. Approximately 41,000 newly diagnosed cases of endometrial cancer and 7300 deaths occur annually.[32] Endometrial cancer has a relatively low mortality rate, because most cases are diagnosed early. The survival rate is 94% if the cancer has not spread at the time of diagnosis.[38] About 25% of the cases of endometrial cancer are diagnosed before women reach menopause. The average age at the time of diagnosis is 61 years old.[38]

Etiology and Pathophysiology

The major risk factor for endometrial cancer is estrogen, especially unopposed estrogen. Additional risk factors include increasing age, nulliparity, late menopause, obesity, smoking, diabetes mellitus, and having a personal or family history of hereditary nonpolyposis colorectal cancer. Obesity is a risk factor because adipose cells store estrogen. Thus endogenous estrogen is increased. Pregnancy and oral contraceptives are protective factors.

Endometrial cancer arises from the lining of the endometrium. Most tumors are adenocarcinomas. The precursor may be a hyperplasic state that progresses to invasive carcinoma. Hyperplasia occurs when estrogen is not counteracted by progesterone. The cancer directly extends into the cervix and through the uterine serosa. As invasion of the myometrium occurs, regional lymph nodes, including the paravaginal and paraaortic, become involved. Hematogenous metastases develop concurrently. The usual sites of metastases are lung, bone, liver, and eventually the brain. Malignant cells can be found in the peritoneal cavity, probably having arrived by transport through the fallopian tubes.

Prognostic factors include histologic differentiation, uterine size at time of diagnosis, myometrial invasion, peritoneal cytology, lymph node and adnexal metastases, and tumor size. Endometrial cancer grows slowly, metastasizes late, and is amenable to therapy if diagnosed early.

Clinical Manifestations

The first sign of endometrial cancer is abnormal uterine bleeding, usually in postmenopausal women. Because perimenopausal women have sporadic periods for a time, it is important that this sign not be ignored or attributed to menopause. Pain occurs late in the disease process. Other manifestations that may arise are related to metastasis to other organs.

TABLE 54-11	**Staging and Treatment of Cervical Cancer**	
Stage	**Extent**	**Treatment**
Stage 0	In situ	Cervical conization, hysterectomy, cryosurgery, laser surgery
Stage I	Confinement to cervix	Radiation, radical hysterectomy
Stage II	Extension beyond cervix but not to pelvic wall, or the lower third of the vagina	Radiation, cisplatin-based chemotherapy, radical hysterectomy
Stage III	Extension to pelvic wall, no cancer-free space between tumor and pelvic wall on rectal examination, involvement of lower third of vagina, hydronephrosis or nonfunctioning kidney	Radiation, cisplatin-based chemotherapy
Stage IV	Extension beyond true pelvis or clinical involvement of the mucosa of bladder or rectum	Radiation, surgery (e.g., pelvic exenteration), cisplatin-based chemotherapy

Collaborative Care

Endometrial biopsy is the primary diagnostic test for endometrial cancer. Endometrial biopsy is done on an outpatient basis, and involves obtaining endometrial tissue from the uterus. Any occurrence of abnormal or unexpected bleeding in a postmenopausal woman mandates obtaining a tissue sample to exclude endometrial cancer. The American Cancer Society recommends that an endometrial biopsy be performed at menopause and then periodically in women who are at risk. The Pap test is not a reliable diagnostic tool for endometrial cancer, but it can rule out cervical cancer.

Treatment of endometrial cancer is a total hysterectomy and bilateral salpingo-oophorectomy with lymph node biopsies. Although they are not in widespread use, molecular markers help identify high-risk groups that could benefit from postoperative adjuvant therapy. These markers include p53 and p16 overexpression (tumor markers of high proliferative activity) and the expression of estrogen and/or progesterone receptors by the tumor cells. The absence of estrogen and progesterone receptors is a poor prognostic indicator.

Most cases of endometrial cancer are diagnosed at an early stage when surgery alone may result in cure. Surgery may be followed by radiation, either to the pelvis or abdomen externally or intravaginally, to decrease local recurrence.[37] Treatment of advanced or recurrent disease is difficult. Progesterone hormonal therapy (e.g., megestrol [Megace]) is the treatment of choice when the progesterone receptor status is positive and the tumor is well differentiated. Tamoxifen (Nolvadex), either alone or in combination with progesterone therapy, is also effective in women with advanced or recurrent endometrial cancer. Chemotherapy is considered when progesterone therapy is unsuccessful. Agents used include doxorubicin (Adriamycin), cisplatin (Platinol), 5-fluorouracil (5-FU), carboplatin (Paraplatin), and paclitaxel (Taxol).

OVARIAN CANCER

Ovarian cancer is a malignant neoplasm of the ovaries. About 25,500 new cases of ovarian cancer are diagnosed in the United States each year, and about 16,210 women die from the disease annually.[38] It is the fourth leading cause of cancer deaths in women in the United States. Most women with ovarian cancer have advanced disease at diagnosis. It occurs most frequently in women between 55 and 65 years of age. White women of North American or European descent are at greater risk for ovarian cancer as compared with African American women.

Etiology and Pathophysiology

The cause of ovarian cancer is not known. Women who have mutations of the BRCA genes have an increased susceptibility for ovarian cancer.[39] The BRCA genes are tumor suppressor genes that inhibit tumor growth when functioning normally. When they mutate, they lose their tumor suppressor ability. This results in an increased risk for women to develop ovarian or breast cancer (see the Genetics in Clinical Practice box).

The greatest risk factor for ovarian cancer is family history (one or more first-degree relatives). Having a family history of breast or colon cancer is also a risk factor. Other risk factors include a personal history of breast or colon cancer and hereditary nonpolyposis colorectal cancer. Women who have never been pregnant (nulliparity) are also at higher risk. Other risk factors include increasing age, high-fat diet, increased number of ovulatory cycles (usually

---

GENETICS IN CLINICAL PRACTICE
Ovarian Cancer

Genetic Basis
- Mutations in genes BRCA-1 and/or BRCA-2
- Autosomal dominant transmission
- Mutations can be passed down from either mother or father

Incidence
- About 10% of cases of ovarian cancer are related to hereditary factors.
- Women with BRCA-1 mutations have a 25% to 40% lifetime risk of developing ovarian cancer.
- Women with BRCA-2 mutations have a 10% to 20% lifetime risk of developing ovarian cancer.
- Family history of both breast and ovarian cancer increases the risk of having a BRCA mutation.
- BRCA mutations occur in 10% to 20% of patients with ovarian cancer who have no family history of breast or ovarian cancer.
- Family of genes associated with hereditary nonpolyposis colorectal cancer accounts for 10% of ovarian cancers.

Genetic Testing
- DNA testing is available for BRCA-1 and BRCA-2.

Clinical Implications
- Bilateral oophorectomy reduces the risk of ovarian cancer in women with BRCA-1 and BRCA-2 mutations.
- Genetic counseling and testing for BRCA mutations should be considered for women whose personal or family history puts them at high risk for a genetic predisposition to ovarian cancer.

---

associated with early menarche and late menopause), HRT, and possibly the use of infertility drugs. The use of oral contraceptives is associated with lower ovarian cancer risk.

Breastfeeding, multiple pregnancies, oral contraceptive use (greater than 5 years), and early age at first birth seem to reduce the risk of ovarian cancer. It is thought that these factors have a protective effect because they reduce the number of ovulatory cycles, and thus reduce the exposure to estrogen.

About 90% of ovarian cancers are epithelial carcinomas that arise from malignant transformation of the surface epithelial cells. Germ cell tumors account for another 10%. Histologic grading is an important prognostic determinant. Tumor cells are graded according to the level of differentiation. These include well differentiated (grade I), moderately well differentiated (grade II), and poorly differentiated (grade III). Grade III lesions carry a poorer prognosis than the other grades.

Ovarian cancer can metastasize directly by shedding malignant cells, which frequently implant on the uterus, bladder, bowel, and omentum. In addition, ovarian cancer can metastasize by lymphatic spread. Primary lymphatic drainage of the ovary is through the retroperitoneal lymph nodes, but drainage also can occur through the iliac and inguinal lymph nodes.

Clinical Manifestations

In the early stages, clinical manifestations are vague and may include a pattern of general abdominal discomfort (gas, indigestion, pressure, bloating, cramps), sense of pelvic heaviness, loss of appetite, feeling of fullness, and change in bowel habits.[40] Pain is not an early symptom. As the malignancy grows, a variety of manifestations can occur, including an increase in abdominal girth, bowel and bladder dysfunction, persistent pelvic or abdominal pain, menstrual irregularities, and ascites. An ovarian

TABLE 54-12	COLLABORATIVE CARE Ovarian Cancer

Diagnostic
History and physical examination
Pelvic examination
Abdominal and transvaginal ultrasound
CA-125 levels
Color Doppler imaging
Laparotomy for diagnostic staging

Collaborative Therapy
Surgery
- Abdominal hysterectomy and bilateral salpingo-oophorectomy with pelvic lymph node biopsies
- Debulking for advanced disease
Chemotherapy
- Adjuvant and palliative
Radiation therapy
- Adjuvant and palliative

malignancy should be considered when abnormal vaginal bleeding occurs.

Diagnostic Studies

Unlike the Pap test used to screen for cervical cancer, no screening test exists for ovarian cancer. Because early ovarian cancer has vague symptoms, yearly bimanual pelvic examinations should be performed to identify the presence of an ovarian mass (Table 54-12). Postmenopausal women should not have palpable ovaries, so a mass of any size should be suspected as possible ovarian cancer. An abdominal or a transvaginal ultrasound can be done to detect ovarian masses. An exploratory laparotomy may be used to establish the diagnosis and stage the disease.

For women with a high risk for ovarian cancer, screening using a combination of the tumor marker, CA-125, and ultrasound is often recommended in addition to a yearly pelvic examination. CA-125 is positive in 80% of women with epithelial ovarian cancer and is used to monitor the course of the disease. However, levels of CA-125 may be elevated with other nonovarian malignancies or with benign conditions such as fibroids or endometriosis (see Evidence-Based Practice Box).

Collaborative Care

Women identified as being at high risk based on family and health history may require counseling regarding options such as prophylactic oophorectomy and oral contraceptives. It is important to note that although oophorectomy will significantly reduce the risk of ovarian cancer, it will not completely eliminate the possibility of the disease.

If a diagnosis of ovarian cancer is made, staging is critical for guiding treatment decisions. Because of the numerous metastatic pathways for ovarian cancer, accurate staging usually involves multiple biopsies. Stage I describes disease limited to the ovaries; stage II, disease limited to the true pelvis; stage III, disease limited to the abdominal cavity; and stage IV, distant metastatic disease. The usual treatment for stage I malignancies is a total abdominal hysterectomy and bilateral salpingo-oophorectomy with removal of as much of the tumor as possible (i.e., tumor debulking). The remaining tissues in the abdomen and pelvis are carefully scrutinized. Ascitic fluid is submitted for cytologic study, and appropriate biopsies are performed to determine the stage of the disease.

EVIDENCE-BASED PRACTICE

Are Invasive Screening Methods for Ovarian Cancer Effective in Early Diagnosis?

Clinical Question
In asymptomatic women at risk for ovarian cancer (P), are routine gynecologic physical and history assessment screening (I) or invasive screening procedures such as transvaginal ultrasound and serum CA-125 (C) more effective in early diagnosis (O)?

Best Available Evidence
Evidence-based recommendations from U.S. Preventive Services Task Force (USPSTF) that address preventive health services for use in primary care clinical settings, including screening tests, counseling, and chemoprevention

Critical Appraisal and Synthesis of Evidence
- Earlier detection with invasive diagnostic tests might have a small effect, at best, on ovarian cancer mortality rates.
- Invasive screening such as transvaginal ultrasound and serum CA-125 has the potential for harm (e.g., unnecessary surgery) and should not be routinely used.

Conclusions
- All women should receive routine gynecologic assessment screening for ovarian cancer.
- The potential harm of invasive screening techniques outweighs potential benefits.
- In high-risk women with symptoms, invasive screening measures may be warranted.

Implications for Nursing Practice
- Assess ovarian cancer risk for women at their initial visit.
- Instruct all women about early signs and symptoms of ovarian cancer.
- Determine appropriate screening dependent on risk and symptoms.

Reference for Evidence
Calonge N: US Preventive Services Task Force screening for ovarian cancer: recommendation statement, *Am Fam Physician* 71:759, 2005.

PICO: P, Patient population of interest; *I*, intervention or area of interest; *C*, comparison of interest or comparison group; *O*, outcome(s) of interest (see p. 6).

The addition of chemotherapy or the instillation of intraperitoneal radioisotopes is usually suggested for stage I cancer that is poorly differentiated. The patient with stage II disease may receive external abdominal and pelvic radiation, intraperitoneal radiation, or systemic combined chemotherapy after tumor-reducing surgery. After completion of systemic chemotherapy in the patient who is clinically free of symptoms, a "second-look" surgical procedure is often performed to determine whether there is any evidence of disease. This option does not necessarily improve the outcome. If no disease is found, the patient is monitored for recurrent disease.

Chemotherapy (e.g., cisplatin [Platinol], carboplatin [Paraplatin]) is used for the treatment of stage III and stage IV diseases. Altretamine (Hexalen) is used for palliative treatment of persistent, recurrent ovarian cancer. Paclitaxel (Taxol) and topotecan (Hycamtin) are used to treat metastatic ovarian cancer. Surgical debulking is often done in conjunction with chemotherapy for advanced disease. Intraperitoneal chemotherapy, although associated with substantial side effects, is coming into wider use for the patient who has minimum residual disease after surgery. Gemcitabine (Gemzar) in combination with carboplatin (Paraplatin) is used to treat recurrent ovarian cancer.

The malignancy may have metastasized to the peritoneum, omentum, or bowel surface before discovery of the tumors. In these situations the prognosis is poor. Recurrent pleural effusion causing shortness of breath and discomfort may require frequent paracentesis. However, fluid accumulates again. Radiation and chemotherapy may be used to shrink the size of the tumor to relieve pressure and pain.

VAGINAL CANCER

Primary vaginal cancers are rare, with about 2140 new cases reported annually.[32] The peak incidence is between 50 and 70 years of age. Vaginal tumors are usually secondary sites or metastases of other cancers such as cervical or endometrial cancer. The most common type of vaginal cancer is squamous cell carcinoma. Intrauterine exposure to diethylstilbestrol (DES) places a woman at risk for clear cell adenocarcinoma of the vagina.

Treatment of vaginal cancer depends on the type of cells involved and the stage of the disease, the size of the tumor, and the location of the tumor. Squamous cell carcinomas can be treated with both surgery and radiation.

VULVAR CANCER

Cancer of the vulva is relatively rare, with about 3870 new cases reported annually.[32] Similar to cervical cancer, preinvasive lesions referred to as vulvar intraepithelial neoplasia (VIN) precede invasive vulvar cancer. The invasive form occurs mainly in women over 60 years of age, with the highest incidence being in women in their 70s. Patients with vulvar neoplasia may have symptoms of vulvar itching or burning, pain, bleeding, or discharge. Women who are immunosuppressed and/or have diabetes mellitus, hypertension, or chronic vulvar dystrophies are at a higher risk for developing vulvar cancers. Several subtypes of HPV have been identified in some but not all vulvar cancers.

Diagnosis of vulvar cancer is determined by the pathology report on the biopsy of the suspicious lesion. VIN is managed by eradicating the lesion medically with 5-fluorouracil (5-FU) or surgical excision. Larger lesions may require more extensive surgery and skin graft. The traditional treatment for vulvar cancer has been radical vulvectomy. However, the procedure results in extensive morbidity related to scarring and wound breakdown. For this reason, more conservative surgical techniques such as radical hemivulvectomy are being used. Cure rates are comparable between the radical vulvectomy and hemivulvectomy. Morbidity and loss of function have been significantly decreased with the hemivulvectomy.

SURGICAL PROCEDURES: FEMALE REPRODUCTIVE SYSTEM

A variety of surgical procedures are performed when benign or malignant tumors of the genital tract are found (Table 54-13). A *hysterectomy* (removal of the uterus) is the type of surgery performed for excision of cancerous tumors of the female reproductive system. A hysterectomy may be done either vaginally or abdominally. A vaginal route is often used when vaginal repair is to be done in addition to removal of the uterus. The abdominal route is used when large tumors are present and the pelvic cavity is to be explored or when the tubes and ovaries are to be removed at the same time (Fig. 54-10). The abdominal route can present more postoperative problems because it involves an incision and the opening of the abdominal cavity.

In both vaginal and abdominal hysterectomies, the ligaments that support the uterus are attached to the vaginal cuff so that nor-

TABLE 54-13	Surgical Procedures Involving the Female Reproductive System
Type of Surgery	**Description**
Hysterectomy	
Subtotal hysterectomy	Removal of uterus without cervix (rarely done today)
Total hysterectomy	Removal of uterus and cervix
Total abdominal hysterectomy and bilateral salpingo-oophorectomy (TAH-BSO)	Removal of uterus, cervix, fallopian tubes, and ovaries
Radical hysterectomy	Panhysterectomy, partial vaginectomy, and dissection of lymph nodes in pelvis
Laparoscopic-assisted vaginal hysterectomy (LAVH)	Vaginal removal of the uterus with laparoscopic assistance
Vulvectomy	
Simple vulvectomy	Excision of vulva and wide margin of skin
Radical vulvectomy	Excision of tissue from anus to few centimeters above symphysis pubis (skin, labia majora and minora, and clitoris) with superficial and deep lymph node dissection
Vaginectomy	Removal of vagina
Pelvic Exenteration	Radical hysterectomy, total vaginectomy, removal of bladder with diversion of urinary system and resection of bowel with colostomy
Anterior pelvic exenteration	Above operation without bowel resection
Posterior pelvic exenteration	Above operation without bladder removal

mal depth of the vagina is maintained. The cervix may or may not be removed depending on the findings.

A modified approach to a vaginal hysterectomy is laparoscopic-assisted vaginal hysterectomy (LAVH). LAVH utilizes a laparoscope to assist with the removal of the uterus. Another alternative is laparoscopic subtotal hysterectomy, which allows the cervix to remain. The advantage of these newer procedures is quicker recovery time and fewer complications.[40,41]

RADIATION THERAPY: CANCERS OF THE FEMALE REPRODUCTIVE SYSTEM

Radiation is used to cure, control, or act as a palliative measure for cancers of the female reproductive system either alone or in combination with other treatments. The goal of radiation therapy is to deliver a specific amount of high-energy (or ionizing) radiation to the cancer with minimal damage to the normal surrounding tissue. Radiation therapy may be external or internal (brachytherapy).

External Radiation Therapy

With external radiation therapy, a source outside of the body delivers electromagnetic radiation in the form of waves. (External radiation therapy is discussed in Chapter 16.)

Brachytherapy

Brachytherapy allows the radiation to be placed near or into the tumor. This method can deliver a high dose of radiation directly to the tumor. The dose decreases sharply the farther away from the

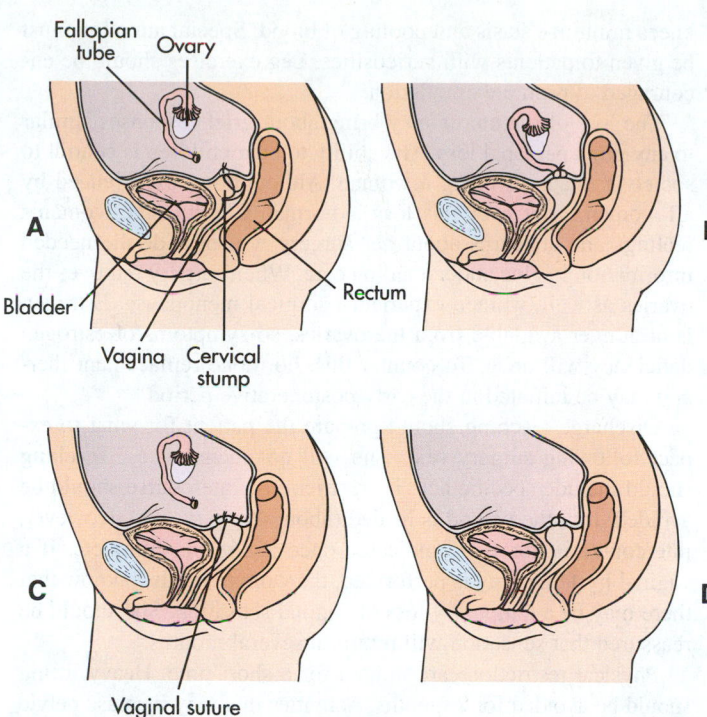

FIG. 54-10 **A,** Cross section of subtotal hysterectomy. Note that cervical stump, fallopian tubes, and ovaries remain. **B,** Cross section of total hysterectomy. Note that fallopian tubes and ovaries remain. **C,** Cross section of vaginal hysterectomy. Note that fallopian tubes and ovaries remain. **D,** Total hysterectomy, salpingectomy, and oophorectomy. Note that uterus, fallopian tubes, and ovaries are completely removed.

source, causing less damage to the surrounding normal tissue. A variety of forms are used to deliver brachytherapy, including wires, capsules, needles, tubes, and seeds. Brachytherapy is used in the management of cervical and endometrial cancer because of the accessibility of these body parts and the favorable results obtained. Radium and cesium are two commonly used isotopes. In preparation of the patient for the treatment, a cleansing enema is given to prevent straining at stool, which could cause displacement of the isotope. An indwelling catheter is inserted to prevent a distended bladder from coming into contact with the radioactive source.

A variety of applicators have been developed for intrauterine treatment. Applicators are inserted into the endometrial cavity and vagina of an anesthetized patient in the operating room. When the applicator contains the radioactive material, this is known as *preloading.* In *afterloading,* the applicator is implanted in the operating room but is not loaded with the radioactive material until its correct placement is verified and the patient has been returned to her room. Radiation exposure to the patient is precisely controlled. The radiation exposure to the physician and other personnel involved in the implantation is reduced when the afterload technique is used. The applicator is secured with vaginal packing and is left in place for 24 to 72 hours. The radiation oncologist determines the exact amount of radioactive substance to be used and the length of time it will be left in place so that destruction of cancer cells can occur with minimal damage to normal cells.

During the treatment the patient is placed in a lead-lined private room and is on absolute bed rest. She may be turned from side to side. The presence of an intrauterine applicator produces uterine contractions that may require analgesics. The destruction of cells results in a foul-smelling vaginal discharge, and a deodorizer is

helpful. Nausea, vomiting, diarrhea, and malaise may develop as a systemic reaction to the radiation.

At the end of the prescribed period of radiation, the radioactive material and the catheter are removed. The patient is allowed off bed rest and is discharged from the hospital when stable. Late complications that may arise after irradiation of the uterus include fistulas (vesicovaginal, ureterovaginal), cystitis, phlebitis, hemorrhage, and fibrosis. If fibrosis occurs, the vaginal wall becomes smaller in diameter and shorter. Dilation of the vagina through intercourse or the use of sequentially sized dilators may be indicated. The patient is urged to report any unusual symptoms or complaints to her physician. (Brachytherapy and related nursing care are discussed in Chapter 16.)

NURSING MANAGEMENT
CANCERS OF THE FEMALE REPRODUCTIVE SYSTEM

▪ *Nursing Assessment*

Malignant tumors of the female reproductive system can be found in the cervix, endometrium, ovaries, vagina, and vulva. The patient with any of these malignant tumors may experience a variety of clinical manifestations, including leukorrhea, irregular vaginal bleeding, vaginal discharge, increase in abdominal pain and pressure, bowel and bladder dysfunction, and vulvar itching and burning. Assessment for these signs and symptoms is an important nursing responsibility.

▪ *Nursing Diagnoses*

Nursing diagnoses for the female patient with cancer of the reproductive system include, but are not limited to, the following:

- Anxiety *related to* threat of a malignancy and lack of knowledge about the disease process and prognosis
- Acute pain *related to* pressure secondary to an enlarging tumor
- Disturbed body image *related to* loss of body part and loss of good health
- Ineffective sexuality pattern *related to* physiologic limitations and fatigue
- Ineffective breathing pattern *related to* presence of ascites and effusions
- Grieving *related to* poor prognosis of advanced disease

▪ *Planning*

The overall goals are that the patient with cancer of the female reproductive system will (1) actively participate in treatment decisions, (2) achieve satisfactory pain and symptom management, (3) recognize and report problems promptly, (4) maintain preferred lifestyle as long as possible, and (5) continue to practice cancer detection strategies.

▪ *Nursing Implementation*

Health Promotion. Through their contact with women in a variety of settings, nurses can teach women the importance of routine screening for cancers of the reproductive system. Cancer can be prevented when screening can reveal precancerous conditions of the vulva, cervix, endometrium, and, rarely, ovaries. Also, routine screening increases the chance that a cancer will be identified in its early stage. When cancer is identified earlier, treatment can be more conservative and the woman's prognosis improves. A yearly pelvic examination and Pap test will allow the health care provider to detect lesions on the vulva or any uterine or ovarian irregularities and screen for cervical cancer. Nurses can assist women to view routine cancer screening as an important self-care activity and can recommend vaccination against cervical cancer for those women at high risk.

Educating women about risk factors for cancers of the reproductive system is also important. Limiting sexual activity during adolescence, using condoms, having fewer sexual partners, and not smoking reduce the risk of cervical cancer. A high-fat diet increases risk for ovarian cancer. When high-risk behaviors are identified, nurses should assist women to modify their lifestyles to decrease risk.

Acute Intervention Related to Surgery. All patients experience a degree of anxiety when surgery is contemplated, but the prospect of major gynecologic surgery may heighten these concerns. Some women may fear a loss of femininity and worry about possible changes in their secondary sex characteristics. Others may experience feelings of guilt, anger, or embarrassment. Still others may focus on the effect the surgery will have on their reproductive and sexual functions. Some women view the whole process as annoying, whereas others are relieved by the thought of no longer having menstrual periods or becoming pregnant. Each patient must be understood in light of her fears and concerns and must be approached and evaluated individually. The nurse who exhibits interest and a willingness to listen can provide considerable psychologic support.

Preoperatively, the patient is prepared physically for surgery with the standard perineal or abdominal preparation. A vaginal douche and enemas may be given, according to the preference of the surgeon. The bladder should be emptied before the patient is sent to the operating room. An indwelling catheter is commonly inserted preoperatively.

Hysterectomy. Postoperatively, the patient who has had a hysterectomy will have an abdominal dressing (abdominal hysterectomy) or a sterile perineal pad (vaginal hysterectomy). (See NCP 54-1 for care of the patient after a total abdominal hysterectomy.) The dressing should be observed frequently for any sign of bleeding during the first 8 hours after surgery. A moderate amount of serosanguineous drainage on the perineal pad is expected following a vaginal hysterectomy.

The patient may experience urinary retention postoperatively because of temporary bladder atony resulting from edema or nerve trauma. This problem is more acute when a radical hysterectomy has been performed. At times an indwelling catheter is used for 1 to 2 days postoperatively to maintain constant drainage of the bladder and prevent strain on the suture line. If an indwelling catheter is not used, catheterization may be necessary if the patient has not urinated for 8 hours postoperatively. If residual urine is suspected after the removal of an indwelling catheter, catheterization is done to prevent bladder infection caused by pooling of urine. Accidental ligation of a ureter is a serious surgical complication. Any complaint of backache or decreased urine output should be reported to the surgeon.

Abdominal distention may develop from the sudden release of pressure on the intestines when a large tumor is removed or from paralytic ileus secondary to anesthesia and pressure on the bowel. Food and fluids may be restricted if the patient is nauseated. A rectal tube may be prescribed to relieve abdominal flatus, and ambulation is encouraged.

Special care must be taken to prevent the development of deep vein thrombosis (DVT). Frequent changes of position, avoidance of the high Fowler position, and avoidance of pressure under the knees minimize stasis and pooling of blood. Special attention must be given to patients with varicosities. Leg exercises should be encouraged to promote circulation.

The loss of the uterus may bring about grief responses similar to any great personal loss. The ability to bear children is central to society's image of being a woman. Although not experienced by all women, grief over this loss is normal. Eliciting the woman's feelings and concerns about her surgery will provide the needed information to give understanding care. When surgery removes the ovaries as well, women experience surgical menopause. Estrogen is no longer available from the ovaries, so symptoms of estrogen deficiency will arise. To counter this, hormone replacement therapy may be initiated in the early postoperative period.

Discharge teaching should prepare the patient for what to expect following surgery (e.g., she will not menstruate). Teaching should include specific activity restrictions. Intercourse should be avoided until the wound is healed (about 4 to 6 weeks). However, intercourse is not contraindicated once healing is complete. If a vaginal hysterectomy is performed, the woman needs to know that there may be a temporary loss of vaginal sensation. She should be reassured that sensation will return in several months.

Physical restrictions are limited for a short time. Heavy lifting should be avoided for 2 months. Activities that may increase pelvic congestion, such as dancing and walking swiftly, should be avoided for several months, whereas activities such as swimming may be both physically and mentally helpful. Wearing a girdle is allowed and may provide comfort. Once the patient has been assured that healing is complete, all previous activity can be resumed.

Salpingectomy and Oophorectomy. Postoperative care of the woman who has undergone removal of a fallopian tube (salpingectomy) or an ovary (oophorectomy) is similar to that for any patient having abdominal surgery. One exception is that if a large ovarian cyst is removed, there may be abdominal distention caused by the sudden release of pressure in the intestines. An abdominal binder may provide relief until the distention subsides.

When both ovaries are removed (bilateral oophorectomy), surgical menopause results. The symptoms are similar to those of regular menopause but may be more severe because of the sudden withdrawal of hormones. Attempts may be made to leave at least a portion of an ovary.

Vulvectomy. Although cancer of the vulva is relatively uncommon, it is important that the nurse recognize the extent of the vulvectomy and the significant effect it is likely to have on the patient's life. An honest, open attitude with the patient and her partner preoperatively can be most helpful in the postoperative period.

After a vulvectomy (see Table 54-13), the patient returns to the unit with a wound in the perineal area extending to the groin. The wound may be covered or left exposed and frequently has drains attached to portable suction (e.g., Hemovac). A heavy pressure dressing is often in place for the first 24 to 48 hours. The wound is cleaned with normal saline solution or an antiseptic twice daily. Solutions can be applied with an aseptic bulb syringe or a Water Pik machine. A heat lamp or a hair dryer is then used to dry the area. Wound care must be meticulous to prevent infection, which results in delayed healing.

Special attention to bowel and bladder care is needed. A low-residue diet and stool softeners prevent straining and wound contamination. An indwelling catheter is used to provide urinary drainage. Great care is taken not to dislodge the catheter because extensive edema makes its reinsertion difficult. Heavy, taut sutures are often used to close the wounds, resulting in severe discomfort for the patient. In other instances the wound may be allowed to heal by granulation. Analgesics may be required frequently to control pain. Careful positioning of the patient through the use of strategically placed pillows provides comfort. Ambulation is usually begun on the second postoperative day, but this varies with the preference of the surgeon. Anticoagulant therapy to prevent DVTs is common.

Because the surgery causes mutilation of the perineal area and the healing process is slow, the patient is likely to become discouraged. Opportunities for the patient to express her feelings and concerns about the operation should be provided. The patient needs specific instructions in self-care before she is discharged. She should be told to report any unusual odor, fresh bleeding, breakdown of incision, or perineal pain. Home care nursing can benefit the patient during her adjustment period. Sexual function is often retained. Whether clitoral sensation is retained may be critical to some women, particularly if it was a primary source of orgasmic satisfaction. A discussion of alternative methods of achieving sexual satisfaction may also be indicated.

Pelvic Exenteration. When other forms of therapy are ineffective in controlling the spread of cancer and no metastases have been found outside of the pelvis, pelvic exenteration may be performed. Although different types are done, this radical surgery usually involves removal of the uterus, ovaries, fallopian tubes, vagina, bladder, urethra, and pelvic lymph nodes (Fig. 54-11). In some situations, the descending colon, rectum, and anal canal may also be removed. Candidates for this procedure are selected on the basis of their likelihood of surviving the surgery and their ability to adjust to and accept the resulting limitations.

Postoperative care involves that of a patient who has had a radical hysterectomy, an abdominal perineal resection, and an ileostomy or a colostomy. The physical, emotional, and social adjustments to life on the part of the woman and her family are great. There are urinary or fecal diversions in the abdominal wall, a reconstructed vagina, and the onset of menopausal symptoms.

The patient's rehabilitative process should keep pace with her acceptance of the situation. Much understanding and support is needed from the nursing staff during a long recovery period. The patient should be gently encouraged to regain her independence. She needs to verbalize her feelings about her altered body structure. Inclusion of the family in the plan of care is important.

The patient will need to return to her health care provider at specified intervals. Early recurrence of the cancer may be identi-

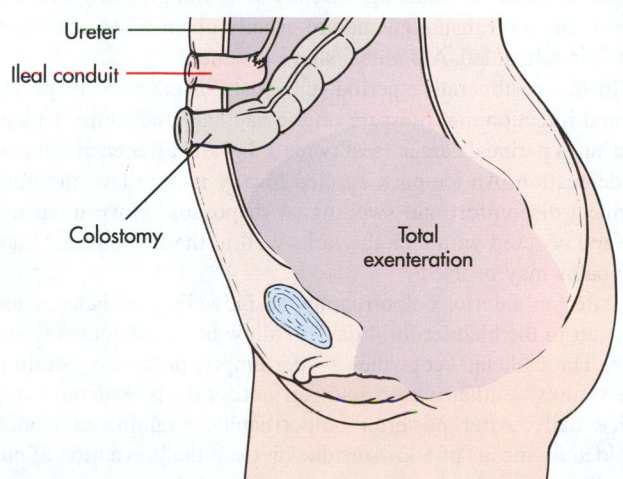

FIG. 54-11 Total exenteration is removal of all pelvic organs with creation of an ileal conduit and a colostomy.

fied and treated. At this time the patient's physical and emotional adjustment to the changes in body image produced by the surgery and her ability to carry out any treatment measures can also be assessed. Additional teaching and counseling can then be provided.

Acute Intervention with Radiation Therapy. Nursing management of the patient receiving brachytherapy requires special considerations. The nurse should not stay in the immediate area any longer than is necessary to give proper care and attention. No individual nurse should attend the patient for more than 30 minutes per day. The nurse should stay at the foot of the bed or at the entrance to the room to minimize radiation exposure. Visitors need to be told to stay 6 feet away from the bed and limit visits to less than 3 hours a day. Efficient organization of nursing care is essential so that the nurse does not stay in the immediate area of the patient any longer than is necessary. The reasons for these precautions must be explained fully to the patient and her visitors. (A more detailed discussion of nursing care of the patient receiving brachytherapy is given in Chapter 16.)

When the patient is to receive external radiation, she should be told to urinate immediately before the treatment to minimize radiation exposure to the bladder. She should be advised about radiation side effects, including enteritis and cystitis. These are natural reactions to radiation therapy and do not indicate an overdose. The patient should be fully informed of the possible side effects and measures to use to reduce their impact.

■ *Evaluation*

The expected outcomes are that the patient with cancer of the female reproductive system will
- actively participate in treatment decisions
- achieve satisfactory pain and symptom management
- recognize and report problems promptly
- maintain preferred lifestyle as long as possible
- continue to practice cancer detection strategies

Problems with Pelvic Support

The most commonly occurring problems with pelvic support are uterine prolapse, cystocele, and rectocele. Although vaginal birth increases the risk for these problems, these conditions can occur in women who have never experienced childbirth. Obesity, chronic coughing, and straining during bowel movements can increase the likelihood of these problems. The decreased estrogen that normally accompanies the perimenopause also reduces some connective tissue support.

UTERINE PROLAPSE

Uterine prolapse is the downward displacement of the uterus into the vaginal canal (Fig. 54-12). Prolapse is rated by degrees. In first-degree prolapse, the cervix rests in the lower part of the vagina. Second-degree prolapse means the cervix is at the vaginal opening. A third-degree prolapse means the uterus protrudes through the introitus. Symptoms vary with the degree of prolapse. The patient may describe a feeling of "something coming down." She may have dyspareunia, a dragging or heavy feeling in the pelvis, backache, and bowel or bladder problems if cystocele or rectocele is also present. Stress incontinence is a common and troubling problem. When third-degree uterine prolapse occurs, the protruding cervix and vaginal walls are subjected to constant irritation, and tissue changes may occur.

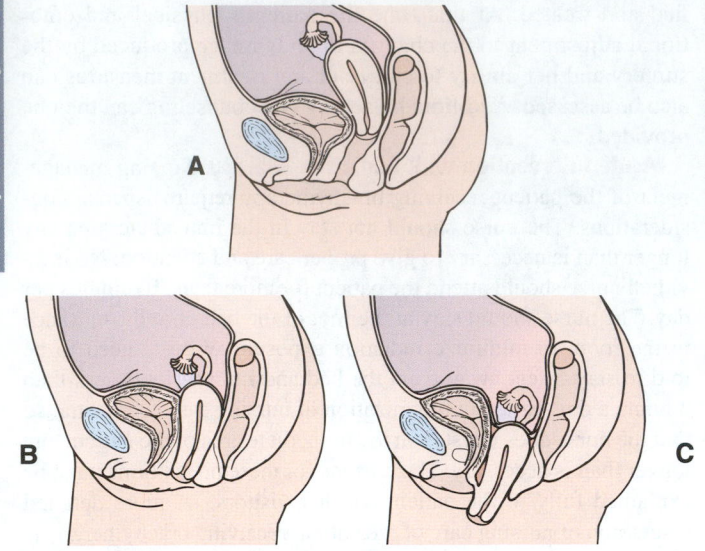

FIG. 54-12   Uterine prolapse. **A,** First-degree prolapse. **B,** Second-degree prolapse. **C,** Third-degree prolapse.

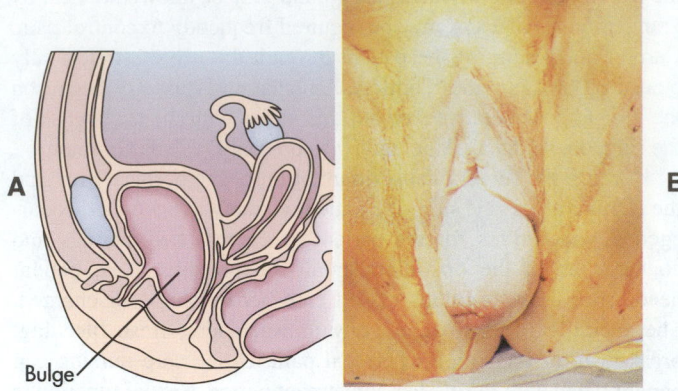

FIG. 54-13   **A,** Cystocele. **B,** Bladder has prolapsed into the vagina, causing a uterine prolapse.

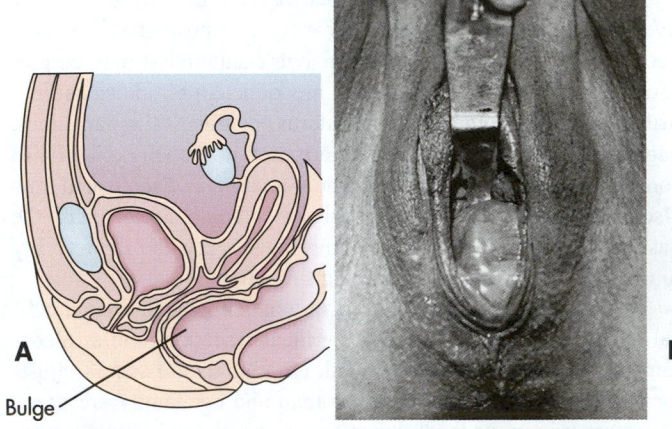

FIG. 54-14   **A,** Rectocele. **B,** Rectum has prolapsed into the vagina.

Therapy depends on the degree of prolapse and how much the woman's daily activities have been affected. Pelvic muscle strengthening exercises (Kegel exercises) may be effective for some women (see Table 46-20). If not, a pessary may be used. A *pessary* is a device that is placed in the vagina to help support the uterus.[41] A wide variety of shapes exist, including rings, arches, and balls. Most are made of plastic or wire coated with plastic. When a woman first receives a pessary, she needs instructions for its cleaning and follow-up. Pessaries that are left in place for long periods are associated with erosion, fistulas, and an increased incidence of vaginal carcinoma. If more conservative measures are not successful, surgery is indicated. Surgery generally involves a vaginal hysterectomy with anterior and posterior repair of the vagina and underlying fascia.

CYSTOCELE AND RECTOCELE

Cystocele occurs when support between the vagina and bladder is weakened (Fig. 54-13). Similarly, a **rectocele** results from weakening between the vagina and rectum (Fig. 54-14). These problems are common and asymptomatic in many women. With large cystoceles, complete emptying of the bladder can be difficult, predisposing women to bladder infections. A woman with a large rectocele may not be able to completely empty her rectum when defecating unless she helps push the stool out by putting her fingers in her vagina.

As with uterine prolapse, Kegel exercises (see Table 46-20) may be used to strengthen the weakened perineal muscles if the cystocele or rectocele is not too problematic. A pessary may be helpful for cystoceles. Surgery designed to tighten the vaginal wall is generally the method of treatment. A cystocele is corrected with a procedure called an anterior *colporrhaphy*, whereas a posterior colporrhaphy is done for a rectocele. If further surgery is needed to relieve stress incontinence, procedures to support the urethra and restore the proper angle between the urethra and the posterior bladder wall are used.

NURSING MANAGEMENT
PROBLEMS WITH PELVIC SUPPORT

Nurses can assist women to avoid or decrease problems with pelvic support by teaching them how to do Kegel exercises. Women of all ages may benefit from these exercises. Kegel exercises are especially important following childbirth or whenever women begin to have incontinence. To instruct a patient in this exercise, she should be told to pull in or contract her muscles as if she were trying to stop the flow of urine. She should hold the contraction for several seconds and then relax. Sets of 5 to 10 contractions each should be done several times daily.

If vaginal surgery is necessary, the preoperative preparation usually includes a cleansing douche the morning of surgery. A cathartic and a cleansing enema are usually given when a rectocele repair is scheduled. A perineal shave is done.

In the postoperative period, the goals of care are to prevent wound infection and pressure on the vaginal suture line. This necessitates perineal care at least twice a day and after each urination or defecation. An ice pack applied locally may relieve the initial perineal discomfort and swelling. A disposable glove filled with ice and covered with a cloth works well in these instances. Later, sitz baths may be used.

After an anterior colporrhaphy, an indwelling catheter is usually left in the bladder for 4 days to allow the local edema to subside. The catheter keeps the bladder empty, preventing strain on the sutures. Catheter care with an antiseptic is generally done twice daily. After posterior colporrhaphy, straining at stool is avoided by means of a low-residue diet and the prevention of constipation. A stool softener is usually given each night.

Discharge instructions should be reviewed before the patient leaves the hospital. They include the use of douches or a mild laxa-

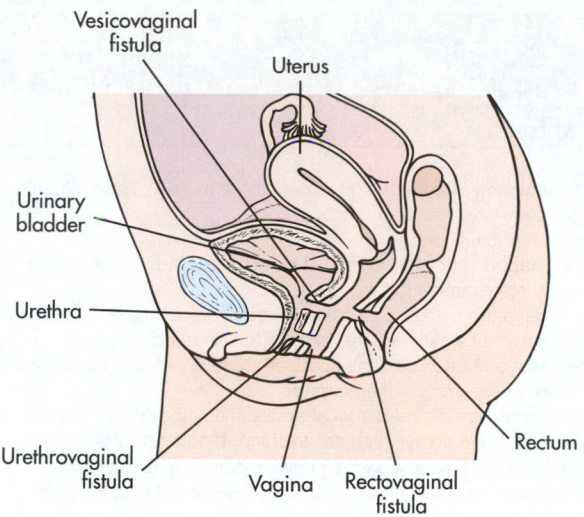

FIG. 54-15 Common fistulas involving the vagina.

tive as needed; restriction of heavy lifting and prolonged standing, walking, or sitting; and avoidance of intercourse until the physician gives permission. There may be a loss of vaginal sensation, which can last for several months. The patient needs to be reassured that this situation is temporary.

FISTULA

A *fistula* is an abnormal opening between internal organs or between an organ and the exterior of the body (Fig. 54-15). Gynecologic procedures cause the majority of urinary tract fistulas. Other causes include injury during childbirth and disease processes, such as carcinoma. They may develop between the vagina and the bladder, urethra, ureter, or rectum. When vesicovaginal fistulas (between the bladder and the vagina) develop, some urine leaks into the vagina, whereas with rectovaginal fistulas (between the rectum and the vagina), flatus and feces escape into the vagina. In both instances, excoriation and irritation of the vaginal and vulvar tissues occur and may lead to severe infections. In addition to wetness, offensive odors may develop, causing embarrassment and severely limiting socialization.

Because small fistulas may heal spontaneously within a matter of months, treatment may not be needed. If the fistula does not heal, surgical excision is required. Inflammation and tissue edema must be eliminated before surgery is attempted. This may involve a wait of up to 6 months for the surgery. The fistulectomy may result in the patient's having an ileal conduit or temporary colostomy.

NURSING MANAGEMENT
FISTULAS

Perineal hygiene is of great importance, both preoperatively and postoperatively. The perineum should be cleansed every 4 hours. Warm sitz baths should be taken three times daily if possible. Perineal pads should be changed frequently. The patient should be encouraged to maintain an adequate fluid intake. Encouragement and reassurance are needed in helping the patient cope with her problems.

Postoperatively, nursing care emphasis is on avoidance of stress on the repaired areas and prevention of infection. Care should be taken so that the indwelling catheter, usually in place for 7 to 10 days, is draining at all times. Oral fluids should be urged to provide

for internal catheter irrigation. Minimal pressure and strict asepsis are used if catheter irrigation becomes necessary. The first stool after bowel surgery may be purposely delayed to prevent contamination of the wound. Later, stool softeners or mild laxatives may be given. (See Chapter 46 for care of a patient with an ileal conduit and Chapter 43 for care of a patient with a colostomy.) Surgical repair of fistulas is not always effective, even in the best conditions. Therefore supportive nursing care for the patient and her significant others is especially important.

SEXUAL ASSAULT

Sexual assault is defined as the forcible perpetration of a sexual act on a person without his or her consent. It can include any of the following actions: sodomy, forced vaginal or anal intercourse, oral copulation, forced copulation of mouth or anus of another, assault with a foreign object, and serial battery. Sexual assault can dramatically disrupt the roles normally performed by the adult woman.

Clinical Manifestations

Physical. Of the women who seek help immediately after the assault, between one half and two thirds will not have any evidence of physical trauma. Evidence of trauma may be limited because women do not resist for fear of physical danger and injury. When present, physical injuries may include bruising and lacerations to the perineum, hymen, vulva, vagina, cervix, and anus. Fractures, subdural hematomas, cerebral concussions, and intraabdominal injuries have resulted in the need for hospitalization. Sexual assault also places women at risk for STDs and pregnancy.

Psychologic. Immediately after the assault, women may show shock, numbness, denial, or withdrawal. Some women may seem unnaturally calm; others may cry or express anger. Feelings of humiliation, degradation, embarrassment, anger, self-blame, and fear of another assault are commonly expressed. These symptoms usually decrease after 2 weeks, and victims may appear to have adjusted. Yet any time from 2 to 3 weeks to months to years after the assault, symptoms may return and become more severe. The rape-trauma syndrome is a classification of posttraumatic stress disorder. Flashbacks, intrusive recall, sleep disturbances, GI symptoms, and numbing of feelings are common initial symptoms. Women will feel embarrassment, self-blame, and powerlessness. Later symptoms include mood swings, irritability, and anger. Feelings of despair, shame, and hopelessness are often the cause of the anger. These feelings may be internalized and expressed as depression. Suicidal ideations may also occur.

Collaborative Care

In the acute care of an assault survivor, ensuring the woman's emotional and physical safety has the highest priority. Table 54-14 outlines the emergency management of the patient who has been sexually assaulted. Most emergency departments (EDs) have identified personnel who have received special training in order to work with women who have been assaulted. Many crime-fighting or victim advocate agencies within communities have implemented the position of the sexual assault nurse examiner (SANE).[42] Certification as a SANE is now being offered by nursing programs in institutions of higher education. The SANE is a registered nurse who is certified to provide care to victims of sexual assault, while ensuring evidence is safeguarded. Special procedures are followed in taking the history and conducting the examination in order to preserve all evidence in case of future prosecution.

Reproductive System

TABLE 54-14	*EMERGENCY MANAGEMENT* **Sexual Assault**

Etiology	Assessment Findings	Interventions
Sexual molestation Sodomy Assault involving genitalia (male or female) without consent	• Emotional or physical manifestations of shock • Hysteria • Crying • Anger • Silence • Decreased level of consciousness • Hyperventilation • Oral, vaginal, and rectal injuries • Extragenital injuries • Pain in genital area or extragenital area	**Initial** • Treat shock and other urgent medical problems (e.g., head injury, hemorrhage, wounds, fractures). • Assess emotional state. • Contact support person (i.e., social worker, rape advocate, sexual assault nurse examiner). • Do *not* clean the patient until all evidence is collected. Make sure the patient does not wash, douche, urinate, brush teeth, or gargle. • Place sheet on floor. Then have patient stand on sheet to remove clothing. Place sheet with clothing in paper bag. • Obtain forensic evidence per local protocol (i.e., body hair, nail scrapings, tissue, dried semen, vaginal washing, blood samples). • Maintain chain of evidence for all legal specimens. Clearly label evidence and keep in locked cabinet until given to law enforcement agency. • Obtain baseline HIV, syphilis, and other STD screening. • Determine method of contraception, date of last menstrual period, and date of last tetanus immunization. • Consider tetanus prophylaxis if lacerations contain soil/dirt. • Vaccinate with hepatitis B if not already done. **Ongoing Monitoring** • Monitor vital signs and emotional status. • Provide clothing as needed. • Counsel patient regarding confidential HIV and STD testing.

HIV, Human immunodeficiency virus; *STD,* sexually transmitted disease.

When the survivor of an assault is admitted to the ED or clinic, a specific chain of events occurs (Table 54-15). A signed informed consent is obtained from the woman before any data are collected. All materials gathered are well documented, labeled, and given to the appropriate person, such as the pathologist or a police officer. The materials are handled by as few people as possible, and signatures of all responsible for keeping and handling the data are obtained. Many items can be used as evidence if the victim chooses to file a complaint. Consequently, the integrity of the material must be maintained. The nurse's involvement in the medicolegal process depends on the policies of the individual institution and state law.

A gynecologic and sexual history and an account of the assault (who, what, when, and where), as well as a general physical and pelvic examination, add further information about the rape incident. Laboratory tests are done primarily to determine the presence of sperm in the vagina and to identify any existing STDs or pregnancy.

Follow-up physical and psychologic care is essential. Women should return weekly for the first month following the assault. This includes the time period when a woman's psychologic reactions may be the most severe. Providers should have the telephone numbers and names of contact persons for local resources for sexual assault survivors, including rape crisis centers, legal and law enforcement authorities, and human services.

NURSING MANAGEMENT
SEXUAL ASSAULT

Nurses can assist all women in becoming aware of prevention tactics (Table 54-16). They should also be encouraged to learn some basic techniques of self-defense. Local high schools and the YWCA usually have self-defense classes in which formal instruction is given.

Practicing the various techniques with a friend strengthens a woman's confidence in her ability to fight back. Learning self-defense can make the woman less vulnerable and more self-reliant.

When a sexual assault survivor is brought to the clinic or ED, a quiet, private area should be used for the initial assessment and the examinations that follow. The patient should not be left alone. Whenever possible, the same nurse should remain with her throughout her stay and provide needed emotional support. The patient's actions and words as she describes the incident may be inconsistent, confused, and inappropriate. The nurse should maintain a nonjudgmental attitude.

The patient usually has many feelings and thoughts about the assault and generally wants to talk about them to an interested listener. Talking may help the patient feel better and gain understanding of her reactions to the incident. When the nurse listens carefully, the patient feels that she is not alone and is better able to gain control over the situation.

The nurse should assess the patient's stress level before preparing her for the various procedures that will follow. The patient's coping mechanisms are supported when she knows what to expect and what is expected of her, as well as why the particular procedure must be done. Because the pelvic examination may trigger a flashback of the attack, the nurse should answer all related questions before the examination and be a supportive presence during the examination.

Following the examinations, the patient's physical comfort needs should be considered. She will need a change of clothing, because her original garments may be torn or soiled, or kept as evidence. Most women who have been sexually assaulted feel dirty and need a place to wash, as well as use a mouthwash, especially if oral sex was involved. Food and drink may also provide comfort to the victim.

TABLE 54-15	Evaluation of Alleged Sexual Assault

1. Medicolegal
- Valid written consent for examination, photographs, laboratory tests, release of information, and laboratory samples
- Appropriate "chain of evidence" documentation

2. History
- History of assault (who, what, when, where)
- Penetration, ejaculation, extragenital acts
- Activities since assault (e.g., changed clothes, bathed, douched)
- Inquire about safety
- Menstrual and contraceptive history
- Medical history
- Emotional status
- Current symptoms

3. General Physical Examination
- Vital signs and general appearance
- Extragenital trauma—mouth, breasts, neck
- Cuts, bruises, scratches (photographs taken)

4. Pelvic Examination
- Vulvar trauma, erythema; hymen, anal, and rectal status
- Matted hairs or free hairs
- Vaginal examination with unlubricated speculum for discharge, blood, lacerations
- Uterine size
- Adnexa, especially hematomas

5. Laboratory Samples
- Vaginal vault content sampling
- Vaginal smears—microscope evaluation for trichomonads and semen
- Oral or rectal swabs and smears, if indicated
- Blood samples—VDRL serology, pregnancy test; serologic testing for HIV and hepatitis B infection
- Freeze serum sample for later testing
- Cultures—cervix and other areas (if indicated) for gonorrhea and chlamydia
- Fingernail scrapings
- Pubic hair scrapings
- Clipping of matted pubic hairs

6. Treatment
- Care of injuries and emotional trauma
- Prophylaxis for STDs, tetanus, and hepatitis B (see appropriate chapters)
- Follow-up for pregnancy test in 2-3 wk (if appropriate)
- Testing for HIV, syphilis, and hepatitis B may be done at 6-8 wk
- Protection of legal rights
- Recommendation of continued follow-up and services of rape crisis center

HIV, Human immunodeficiency virus; *STDs,* sexually transmitted diseases; *VDRL,* Venereal Disease Research Laboratory.

Many sexual assault survivors are unaware of the availability of financial compensation (a law in most states) and appreciate information about the application process. This compensation is to assist them in paying for emergency services and for emotional injuries that may temporarily interfere with their ability to work.

When the patient is discharged, the nurse should make certain the patient has transportation home. If friends or family members are not available, the hospital or clinic should make arrangements with an appropriate community resource. The patient should not be sent home alone. The victim's partner and family have tremendous potential as both a negative and positive influence.

TABLE 54-16	*PATIENT AND FAMILY TEACHING GUIDE* Sexual Assault Prevention

1. Place and maintain lights at all entrances to your home.
2. Keep your doors locked and do not open them to a stranger; ask for identification if a service person comes to the door.
3. Do not advertise that you live alone; list only your initials with your last name in the telephone directory or on the mailbox; never reveal to a caller that you are home alone.
4. Avoid walking alone in deserted areas; walk to the parking lot with a friend; be sure you see each other leave.
5. Have your keys ready as you approach your car or home.
6. Keep all doors locked and the windows up when driving.
7. Never get on an elevator with a suspicious person; pretend you have forgotten something and get off.
8. Say what you mean in social situations; be sure your voice and body language reflect your response.
9. Proceed with caution in online correspondence.
10. Carry a loud whistle and use it when you think you are in danger.
11. Yell "Fire!" if you are attacked and run toward a lighted area.

Many communities today have crisis centers. These public service organizations have trained professional and nonprofessional volunteers who provide an emotional support system on request. Their programs provide advocacy to ensure dignified treatment throughout the medical and police procedures, short-term counseling for the woman and her family, and court assistance and public education on rape-related issues.

CRITICAL THINKING EXERCISE

CASE STUDY

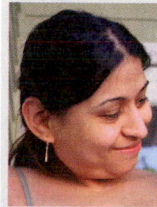

Case Study photo ©iStockphoto.com/ Brandon Clark.

Total Abdominal Hysterectomy

Patient Profile. Eva Torres, a 40-year-old Hispanic married woman with two children and type 2 diabetes, consulted her health care provider about experiencing menorrhagia and occasionally metrorrhagia for the past 5 months. She was diagnosed with leiomyomas and a total abdominal hysterectomy was recommended.

Subjective Data
- Was initially reluctant about surgery
- States her husband wants more children
- Concerned she may have uterine cancer

Objective Data

Physical Examination
- Has several large, firm masses in the body of the uterus
- Blood pressure (BP) is 160/100, pulse 110, respirations 20
- Moderate amount of dark red vaginal bleeding

Laboratory Studies
- Hemoglobin 10 g/dl (0.10 g/L)
- Hemoglobin A1C 9%

Postoperative Status
- Returned to room with indwelling urinary catheter in place
- Vaginal packing in place
- Legs wrapped in full-length elastic compression gradient stockings
- Patient-controlled analgesia (PCA) pump for pain management

Continued

CRITICAL THINKING EXERCISE—cont'd

Critical Thinking Questions

1. What are the common causes of menorrhagia and metrorrhagia?
2. Eva asks you about the effect of the surgery on getting pregnant. How would you respond?
3. What are priorities of care for Eva?
4. What possible complications (including their basis for development) can arise after abdominal hysterectomy?
5. What does Eva need to be taught before discharge related to her diabetes and hypertension?
6. Based on her assessment data, write one or more appropriate nursing diagnoses. Are there any collaborative problems?

NCLEX EXAMINATION REVIEW QUESTIONS

The number of the question corresponds to the same-numbered objective at the beginning of the chapter.

1. In telling a patient with infertility what she and her partner can expect, the nurse explains that
   a. ovulatory studies can help determine tube patency.
   b. a hysterosalpingogram is a common diagnostic study.
   c. the cause will remain unexplained for 40% of couples.
   d. if postcoital studies are normal, infection tests will be done.
2. A patient with a spontaneous abortion is more likely than a patient with an induced abortion to have
   a. a D&C.
   b. cramping and vaginal bleeding.
   c. complications such as infection and pelvic pain.
   d. emotional support from family members and friends.
3. An appropriate question to ask the patient with painful menstruation to differentiate primary from secondary dysmenorrhea is
   a. "Does your pain become worse with activity or overexertion?"
   b. "Have you had a recent personal crisis or change in your lifestyle?"
   c. "Is your pain relieved by nonsteroidal antiinflammatory medications?"
   d. "When in your menstrual history did the pain with your period begin?"
4. In caring for a patient after surgical treatment for an ectopic pregnancy, the nurse advises the patient that
   a. she has an increased risk for salpingitis.
   b. bed rest must be maintained for 12 hours to assist healing.
   c. having one ectopic pregnancy increases her risk for another.
   d. intrauterine devices and infertility treatments should be avoided.
5. To prevent or decrease age-related changes that occur after menopause in a patient who chooses not to take hormone therapy, the nurse teaches the patient that the most important self-care measure is
   a. maintaining usual sexual activity.
   b. increasing the intake of dairy products.
   c. performing regular aerobic, weight-bearing exercise.
   d. taking vitamin E and B-complex vitamin supplements.
6. The patient's history indicating thick, white, and curd-like vaginal discharge and vulvar pruritus is most consistent with
   a. trichomoniasis.
   b. monilial vaginitis.
   c. bacterial vaginosis.
   d. chlamydial cervicitis.
7. The nurse caring for a patient with pelvic inflammatory disease places her in semi-Fowler position. The rationale for this measure is to
   a. relieve pain.
   b. prevent the complication of sterility.
   c. promote drainage to prevent abscesses.
   d. improve circulation and promote healing.
8. In planning care for the patient receiving medical management of endometriosis, the nurse includes teaching regarding the side effects of
   a. estrogen usage.
   b. large doses of vitamins A and E.
   c. long-term treatment with NSAIDs.
   d. hormonal suppression of ovulation.
9. A 31-year-old woman who wishes to have children is diagnosed with leiomyoma. The nurse plans care for the patient based on the knowledge that
   a. a hysterectomy will be necessary to treat the tumor.
   b. a myomectomy may be performed to maintain fertility.
   c. aspirin and other NSAIDs used to control pain may cause fetal defects.
   d. hormonal therapy to shrink the tumor and increase fertility can be used.
10. Nursing responsibilities related to the patient receiving brachytherapy for endometrial cancer include
    a. maintaining absolute bed rest.
    b. allowing the patient bathroom privileges only.
    c. limiting an individual nurse's contact with the patient to 1 hour per day.
    d. allowing visitors to stay as long as desired if they stay 6 feet (2 meters) from the bed.
11. The nurse plans early and frequent ambulation for the patient who has undergone an abdominal hysterectomy in order to
    a. prevent urinary retention.
    b. promote pelvic circulation.
    c. relieve abdominal distention.
    d. maintain a sense of normalcy.
12. Preoperative and postoperative nursing care for the woman with a gynecologic fistula includes
    a. ambulation.
    b. bladder training.
    c. fluid restriction.
    d. perineal hygiene.
13. The first nursing intervention for the patient who has been sexually assaulted is to
    a. treat urgent medical problems.
    b. contact support person for the patient.
    c. provide supplies for the patient to cleanse self.
    d. document bruises and lacerations of the perineum and cervix.

REFERENCES

1. McKinney ES et al: *Maternal-child nursing,* ed 2, St Louis, 2005, Elsevier Saunders.
2. Speroff L, Fritz MA: Introduction of ovulation. In Speroff L, Fritz MA, editors: *Clinical gynecologic endocrinology and infertility,* ed 7, Philadelphia, 2005, Lippincott Williams & Wilkins.
3. Grewal M, Burkman RT: Contraception and family planning. In De Cheney AH, Nathan L, editors: *Current obstetric and gynecologic diagnosis and treatment,* ed 9, New York, 2003, Lange Medical Books/ McGraw-Hill.
4. U.S. Food and Drug Administration: FDA issues public health advisory for mifepristone, *FDA News.* Available at *www.fda.gov* (accessed December 28, 2005).
5. Shaughn O'Brien PM, Ismail K, Dimmock P: Premenstrual syndrome. In Shaw RW, Soutter WP, Stanton LS, editors: *Gynecology,* ed 3, Edinburgh, 2003, Churchill Livingstone.
6. Freeman E et al: Continuous or intermittent dosing with sertraline for patients with severe premenstrual syndrome or premenstrual dysphoric disorder, *Am J Psychiatry* 161:343, 2004.
7. Bader TJ, Allen RA: Premenstrual syndrome and dysmenorrhea. In Bader TJ, editor: *OB/GYN secrets,* ed 3, Philadelphia, 2005, Elsevier Mosby.
8. Skidmore-Roth L: *Mosby's handbook of herbs and natural supplements,* ed 2, St Louis, 2004, Mosby.

9. Ayers D, Lappin J, Liptok L: Abnormal vaginal bleeding, *Nursing* 35:51, 2005.

10. Centers for Disease Control and Prevention: *Toxic shock syndrome*, Atlanta, 2005, Division of Bacterial and Mycotic Diseases. Available at *www.cdc.gov* (accessed August 26, 2006).

11. Giustina D, Denny M: Ectopic pregnancy, *Emerg Med Clin North Am* 21:565, 2003.

12. Nelson AL, DeUgarte CM, Gambone JC: Ectopic pregnancy. In Hacker NF, Moore JG, Gambone JC, editors: *Essentials of obstetrics and gynecology*, ed 4, Philadelphia, 2004, Elsevier Saunders.

13. Smith P: Menopause assessment, treatment and patient education, *Nurs Pract* 30:32, 2005.

14. Santoro N, Chervenak J: The menopause transition, *Endocrinol Metab Clin North Am* 33:627, 2004.

15. Barton D, Loprinzi C: Making sense of the evidence regarding nonhormonal treatments for hot flashes, *Clin J Oncol Nurs* 8:39, 2004.

16. Gracia C, Freeman E: Acute consequences of the menopausal transition: the rise of common menopausal symptoms, *Endocrinol Metab Clin North Am* 33:675, 2004.

17. Laufer LR, Gambone JC: Climacteric. In Hacker NF, Moore JG, Gambone JC, editors: *Essentials of obstetrics and gynecology*, ed 4, Philadelphia, 2004, Elsevier Saunders.

18. Women's Health Initiative (WHI) Study: Findings from the WHI postmenopausal hormone therapy trials. Department of Health and Human Services. Available at *www.nhlbi.nih.gov/whi* (accessed August 26, 2006).

19. Women's Health Initiative Steering Committee: Effects of conjugated equine estrogen in postmenopausal women with hysterectomy, *JAMA* 291:1712, 2005.

20. Chlebowski R et al: Influence of estrogen plus progestin on breast cancer and mammography in healthy postmenopausal women: the Women's Health Initiative Randomized Trial, *JAMA* 289:3253, 2003.

21. Avis N, Stellato R, Crawford S: Is there a menopausal syndrome? Menopausal status and symptoms across racial/ethnic groups, *Soc Sci Med* 52:345, 2001.

22. Lee C, Mishra G, Kuh D: Country of birth, country of residence, and menopausal transitions and symptoms: British birth cohort and Australian Longitudinal Study on Women's Health, *Aust NZJ Public Health* 28:144, 2004.

23. Keehn C, Morgan M: Clinicopathologic attributes of common geriatric dermatologic entities, *Dermatol Clin* 22:115, 2004.

24. Iannacchione M: The vagina dialogues: do you douche? *Am J Nurs* 104:40, 2004.

25. Vega C: ACOG issues new guidelines for chronic pelvic pain, *Obstet Gynecol* 103:589, 2005.

26. Haggerty C, Peipert J, Weitzen S: Predictors of chronic pelvic pain in an urban population of women with symptoms and signs of pelvic inflammatory disease, *Sex Transm Dis* 32:293, 2005.

27. Beigi R, Wiesenfeld H: Pelvic inflammatory disease: new diagnostic criteria and treatment, *Obstet Gynecol Clin North Am* 30:777, 2003.

28. Adamson GD: Endometriosis. In Rakel R, Bope E, editors: *Conn's current therapy*, ed 57, St Louis, 2005, Saunders.

29. Fedele L et al: Tailoring radicality in demolitive surgery for deeply infiltrating endometriosis, *Am J Obstet Gynecol* 193:114, 2005.

30. Bulum S, Adashi E: Disorders of the female reproductive system. In Larsen P et al, editors: *Williams textbook of endocrinology*, ed 10, St Louis, 2003, Saunders.

31. Apridonidze T: Prevalence and characteristics of the metabolic syndrome in women with polycystic ovary syndrome, *J Clin Endocrinol Metab* 90:1929, 2005.

32. Jemal A et al: Cancer statistics 2005, *CA Cancer J Clin* 55:10, 2005.

33. Parkin DM: Global cancer statistics in the year 2000, *Lancet Oncol* 2:533, 2001.

34. Denny L et al: Screen-and-treat approaches for cervical cancer prevention in low-resource settings, *JAMA* 294:2173, 2005.

35. Saslow D et al: American Cancer Society guideline for the early detection of cervical dysplasia and cancer, *CA Cancer J Clin* 52:342, 2002. Available at *www.caonline.amcanersoc.org* (accessed August 26, 2006).

36. U.S. Preventive Services Task Force: *Screening for cervical cancer: recommendations and rationale*, Rockville, Md, 2003, Agency for Healthcare Research and Quality. Available at *www.ahrq.gov* (accessed August 26, 2006).

37. Russell A et al: Cancers of the cervix, vagina, and vulva. In Abeloff M et al, editors: *Clinical oncology*, ed 3, Edinburgh, 2004, Churchill Livingstone.

38. American Cancer Society: *Cancer facts and figures,* Atlanta, 2005, American Cancer Society.

39. Culler D et al: Cancer genetics in primary care, *Prim Care* 31:649, 2004.

*40. Koldjeski D et al: Ovarian cancer: early symptom patterns, *Oncol Nurs Forum* 30:927, 2003.

41. McIntosh L: The role of the nurse in the use of vaginal pessaries to treat organ prolapse and/or urinary incontinence, *Urol Nurs* 25:41, 2005.

42. Georgia Network to End Sexual Assault: Basic SANE training. Available at *www.gnesa.org* (accessed August 26, 2006).

*Nursing research–based reference.

RESOURCES

American Cancer Society
800-ACS-2345 or 404-320-3333
www.cancer.org

American College of Obstetricians and Gynecologists
202-863-2518
www.acog.org

American Urological Association
410-689-3700
www.auanet.org

Hysterectomy Educational Resources and Services (HERS) Foundation
888-750-HERS (4377)
610-667-7757
www.hersfoundation.com

National Women's Health Information Center
800-994-9662
www.4womam.org

North American Menopause Society
440-442-7550
www.menopause.org

Sexuality Information and Education Council of the United States (SIECUS)
212-819-9770
www.siecus.org

For additional Internet resources, see the website for this book at *http://evolve.elsevier.com/Lewis/medsurg.*

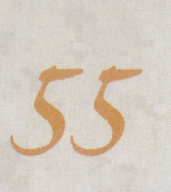

Health is the greatest gift, contentment the greatest wealth, faithfulness the best relationship.

The Buddha

55

Nursing Management
Male Reproductive Problems

Shannon Ruff Dirksen

LEARNING OBJECTIVES

1. Describe the pathophysiology, clinical manifestations, and collaborative care of benign prostatic hyperplasia.
2. Discuss the nursing management of benign prostatic hyperplasia.
3. Describe the pathophysiology, clinical manifestations, and collaborative care of prostate cancer.
4. Discuss the nursing management of prostate cancer.
5. Describe the pathophysiology, clinical manifestations, and collaborative and nursing management of problems of the penis, problems of the scrotum, and prostatitis.
6. Discuss the nursing management of problems related to male sexual functioning.
7. Identify the psychologic and emotional implications related to male reproductive problems.

KEY TERMS

andropause, p. 1437
benign prostatic hyperplasia, p. 1414
epididymitis, p. 1430
erectile dysfunction, p. 1434
prostate cancer, p. 1422
prostate-specific antigen, p. 1423
prostatitis, p. 1428
radical prostatectomy, p. 1424
transurethral resection of prostate,
   p. 1417
vasectomy, p. 1433

Electronic Resources

Supplemental content related to Chapter 55 can be found . . .

Companion CD
- Stress-Busting Kit for Nursing Students
- Interactive Case Study: Benign Prostatic Hyperplasia (BPH)
- NCLEX Examination Review Questions
- Comprehensive Glossary

Evolve Website *evolve*
http://evolve.elsevier.com/Lewis/medsurg
- Content Updates
- Key Points (Printable and CD/MP3 Download)
- Concept Map Creator
- Expanded Audio Glossary
- Key Term Flash Cards

- Customizable Nursing Care Plan: Prostate Surgery
- Patient Instruction Guide in English and Spanish: Testicular Self-Examination
- Electronic Calculators
- WebLinks

Problems of the male reproductive system can involve a variety of structures, including the prostate, penis, urethra, ejaculatory duct, scrotum, testes, epididymis, vas deferens, and rectum (Fig. 55-1).

Problems of the Prostate Gland

BENIGN PROSTATIC HYPERPLASIA

Benign prostatic hyperplasia (BPH) is an enlargement of the prostate gland resulting from an increase in the number of epithelial cells and stromal tissue. It is the most common urologic problem in male adults.[1] BPH occurs in about 50% of men over 50 years of age and in over 90% of men over 80 years of age. Approximately 25% of men require some form of treatment by the time they reach age 80. Prostate hyperplasia does not predispose the individual to the development of prostate cancer.

Etiology and Pathophysiology

Although the cause of BPH is not completely understood, it is thought that BPH results from endocrine changes associated with the aging process. Possible causes include excessive accumulation of dihydroxytestosterone (the principal intraprostatic

Reviewed by David Derrico, RN, MSN, Assistant Clinical Professor, University of Florida, Gainesville, Fla.

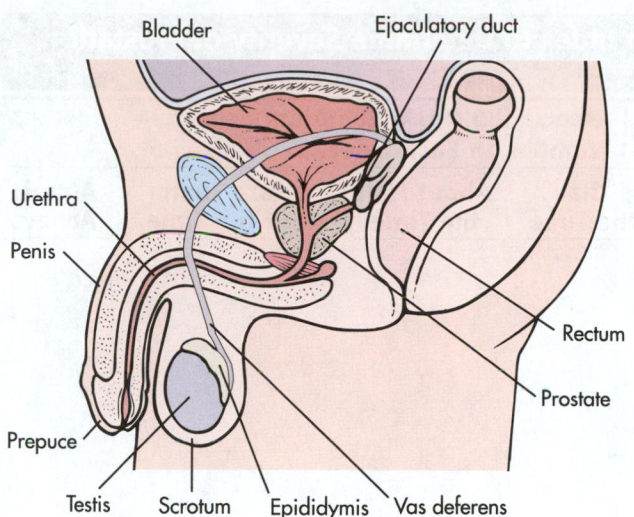

FIG. 55-1 Areas of the male reproductive system in which problems are likely to develop.

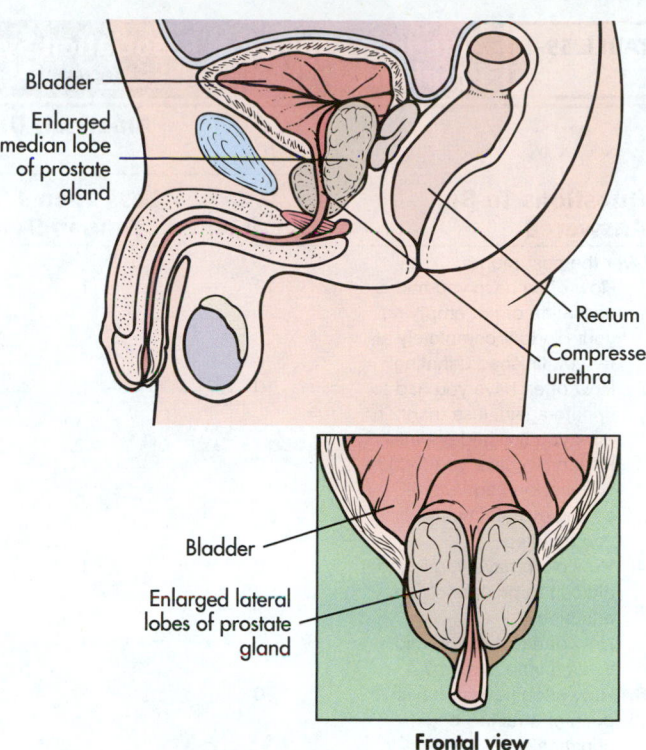

Frontal view

FIG. 55-2 Benign prostatic hyperplasia.

androgen), stimulation by estrogen, and local growth hormone action.

Typically BPH develops in the inner part of the prostate. (Prostate cancer is most likely to develop in the outer part.) This enlargement gradually compresses the urethra, eventually leading to partial or complete obstruction (Fig. 55-2). It is the compression of the urethra that ultimately leads to the development of clinical symptoms. There is no direct relationship between the size of the prostate and degree of obstruction. It is the location of the enlargement that is most significant in the development of obstructive symptoms. For example, it is possible for mild hyperplasia to cause severe obstruction; likewise, it is possible for extreme hyperplasia to cause few obstructive symptoms.

Risk factors for BPH include a family history (particularly involving first-degree relatives), environment, and diet. Although men from both Western and Eastern cultures develop BPH disease at about the same rates, men from Western cultures are much more likely to develop obstructive problems. Obesity, in particular increased waist circumference, appears to increase the risk for BPH.[2] A higher risk for BPH has also been found in association with a diet high in saturated fatty acids (e.g., butter, beef), whereas individuals who eat lots of fruits and vegetables are thought to have a lower risk for BPH. Physical activity and moderate alcohol consumption also have been found to decrease the risk of BPH.[2]

Clinical Manifestations

The symptoms of BPH experienced by the patient result from urinary obstruction. Symptoms are usually gradual in onset and may not be noticed until prostatic enlargement has been present for some time. Early symptoms are usually minimal because the bladder can compensate for a small amount of resistance to urine flow. The symptoms gradually worsen as the degree of urethral obstruction increases.

Symptoms fall into one of two groups: obstructive symptoms and irritative symptoms. *Obstructive symptoms* caused by prostate enlargement include a decrease in the caliber and force of the urinary stream, difficulty in initiating voiding, intermittency (stopping and starting stream several times while voiding), and dribbling at the end of urination. These symptoms are due to urinary retention. *Irritative symptoms,* which include urinary frequency,

urgency, dysuria, bladder pain, nocturia, and incontinence, are associated with inflammation or infection. The American Urological Association (AUA) Symptom Index for BPH (Table 55-1) is a tool used to assess voiding symptoms associated with obstruction.[3] Although this tool is not diagnostic, it is useful in determining the degree of symptoms.

Complications

The majority of complications that develop in BPH are related to urinary obstruction.[2] Acute urinary retention is a common complication and is an indication for surgical intervention in about 25% to 30% of patients. Another common complication is urinary tract infection (UTI) and potentially sepsis secondary to UTI. Incomplete bladder emptying (associated with partial obstruction) results in residual urine, which provides a favorable environment for bacterial growth. Calculi may develop in the bladder because of the alkalinization of the residual urine. Although bladder stones are eight times more common in men with BPH, the risk of renal calculi is not significantly increased. Other less common but potential complications include renal failure caused by *hydronephrosis* (distention of pelvis and calyces of kidney by urine that cannot flow through the ureter to the bladder), pyelonephritis, and bladder damage if treatment for acute urinary retention is delayed.

Diagnostic Studies

The primary methods used to diagnose BPH include a history and physical examination. The prostate can be palpated by digital rectal examination (DRE). Using DRE, the health care provider can estimate the size, symmetry, and consistency of the prostate gland. In BPH the prostate is symmetrically enlarged, firm, and smooth.

Additional diagnostic tests may be indicated, depending on the type and severity of symptoms and clinical findings. Diagnostic

TABLE 55-1	**American Urological Association Symptom Index to Determine Severity of Prostatic Problems**

American Urological Association (AUA) Symptom Score*
(Circle 1 Number on Each Line)

Questions To Be Answered	Not at All	Less Than 1 Time in 5	Less Than Half the Time	About Half the Time	More Than Half the Time	Almost Always
Over the past month,						
1. How often have you had a sensation of not emptying your bladder completely after you finished urinating?	0	1	2	3	4	5
2. How often have you had to urinate again, less than 2 hr after you finished urinating?	0	1	2	3	4	5
3. How often have you found you stopped and started again several times when you urinated?	0	1	2	3	4	5
4. How often have you found it difficult to postpone urination?	0	1	2	3	4	5
5. How often have you had a weak urinary stream?	0	1	2	3	4	5
6. How often have you had to push or strain to begin urination?	0	1	2	3	4	5
7. How many times did you most typically get up to urinate from the time you went to bed at night until the time you got up in the morning?	0 (None)	1 (1 time)	2 (2 times)	3 (3 times)	4 (4 times)	5 (5 times or more)
Sum of circled numbers (AUA Symptom Score): _____*						

From Barry B et al: The American Urological Association symptom index for benign prostatic hyperplasia, *J Urol* 148:1547, 1992. Used with permission.
*Score is interpreted as follows: 0-7, mild; 8-19, moderate; 20-35, severe.

tests are typically done to determine the presence of complications or for differential diagnosis. A urinalysis with culture is routinely done to determine the presence of infection. The presence of bacteria, white blood cells, or microscopic hematuria is an indication of infection or inflammation. The prostate-specific antigen (PSA) blood level is usually measured to rule out prostate cancer.[4] However, PSA levels may be slightly elevated in patients with BPH. Serum creatinine levels may be ordered to rule out renal insufficiency.

In patients with an abnormal DRE and elevated PSA, a *transrectal ultrasound* (TRUS) scan is typically indicated. This examination allows for accurate assessment of prostate size and is helpful in differentiating BPH from prostate cancer. Biopsies can be taken during the ultrasound procedure. *Uroflowmetry,* a study that measures the volume of urine expelled from the bladder per second, is helpful in determining the extent of urethral blockage and thus the type of treatment needed. Postvoid residual urine volume is often measured to determine the degree of urine flow obstruction. Cystourethroscopy, a procedure allowing internal visualization of the urethra and bladder, is performed if the diagnosis is uncertain and in patients who are scheduled for prostatectomy. Diagnostic studies are outlined in Table 55-2.

Collaborative Care

The goals of collaborative care are to restore bladder drainage, relieve the patient's symptoms, and prevent or treat the complications of BPH. Treatment is generally based on the degree to which the symptoms bother the patient or the presence of complications rather than the size of the prostate. Treatment for BPH has undergone major changes in recent years. Alternatives to surgical intervention for some patients now include drug therapy and minimally invasive procedures.[5]

The most conservative initial treatment for BPH is referred to as "watchful waiting." When there are no symptoms or only mild ones (AUA symptom scores 0 to 7), a wait-and-see approach is taken. Because symptoms may come and go, a conservative approach has value. Dietary changes (decreasing intake of caffeine and artificial sweeteners, limiting spicy or acidic foods), avoiding medications such as decongestants and anticholinergics, and restricting evening fluid intake may result in improvement of symptoms. A timed voiding schedule may reduce or eliminate symptoms, thus negating the need for further intervention. If the patient begins to have signs or symptoms that indicate an increase in obstruction, further treatment is indicated.

Drug Therapy. Drugs that have been used to treat BPH with variable degrees of success include 5-α-reductase inhibitors and α-adrenergic receptor blockers. Combination therapy using both types of these drugs has been shown to be more effective in reducing symptoms than using one drug alone.[6]

5-α-Reductase Inhibitors. These drugs work by reducing the size of the prostate gland. Finasteride (Proscar) blocks the enzyme 5-α-reductase, which is necessary for the conversion of testosterone to dihydroxytestosterone, the principal intraprostatic androgen. This drug results in regression of hyperplastic tissue through suppression of androgens. Finasteride is an appropriate treatment option for individuals who score between 12 and 26 on the AUA Symptom Index

TABLE 55-2	COLLABORATIVE CARE Benign Prostatic Hyperplasia

Diagnostic
History and physical examination
Digital rectal examination (DRE)
Urinalysis with culture
Serum creatinine
Prostate-specific antigen (PSA)
Postvoid residual
Uroflowmetry
Transrectal ultrasound (TRUS)
Cystourethroscopy

Collaborative Therapy
Conservative Therapy *("Watchful Waiting")*
Drug Therapy
• 5-α-Reductase inhibitors
• α-Adrenergic receptor blockers
• Saw palmetto

Invasive Therapy*
• Transurethral resection of the prostate (TURP)
• Transurethral incision of the prostate (TUIP)
• Open prostatectomy

Minimally Invasive Therapy
• Transurethral microwave thermotherapy (TUMT)
• Transurethral needle ablation (TUNA)
• Laser prostatectomy
• Transurethral electrovaporization of the prostate (TUVP)
• Intraprostatic urethral stents

*See Table 55-3.

COMPLEMENTARY AND ALTERNATIVE THERAPIES
Saw Palmetto

Clinical Uses
• Benign prostatic hyperplasia (BPH)*

Effects
Appears to be effective in managing symptoms of BPH. May alleviate nocturia, improve urinary flow, reduce postvoid residual bladder volume, and improve quality of life.

Nursing Implications
Generally well tolerated for up to 3 to 5 years. Most common side effects are gastrointestinal. Should be used with caution in patients with gastrointestinal disease. May increase risk of bleeding. Contraindicated in patients with bleeding disorders and those taking medications, herbs, or supplements that increase risk of bleeding. Contraindicated before surgical or dental procedures. May increase BP. Use with caution in patients with hypertension. Advise men to consult a physician for the correct diagnosis of BPH.

Ulbricht CE, Basch EM: *Natural standard herb and supplement reference: evidence-based clinical reviews,* St. Louis, 2005, Mosby. www.naturalstandard.com
*Strong scientific evidence exists for its use.

for BPH (see Table 55-1). Although 40% to 50% of those treated show symptom improvement, it takes between 3 and 6 months to be effective, and the medication must be taken on a continuous basis to maintain therapeutic results. Dutasteride (Avodart) has the same effect as finasteride and is a dual inhibitor of 5-α-reductase type 1 and 2 isoenzymes. (Finasteride inhibits only the type 2 isoenzyme.) Side effects of 5-α-reductase inhibitors include decreased libido, decreased volume of ejaculate, and erectile dysfunction.

Drug Alert - *Finasteride (Proscar)*
• *Patient should be aware of potential side effect of erectile dysfunction.*
• *Women who may be or are pregnant should not handle tablets.*

α-Adrenergic Receptor Blockers. Another drug treatment option for BPH is agents that block α$_1$-adrenergic receptors. Although this group of drugs is more commonly used for treatment of hypertension, these drugs promote smooth muscle relaxation in the prostate. α$_1$-Adrenergic receptors are abundant in the prostate and are increased in hyperplastic prostate tissue. Relaxation of the smooth muscle ultimately facilitates urinary flow through the urethra. Currently, the α-adrenergic blockers are the most widely prescribed drug for the patient with BPH who is experiencing moderate symptoms without the presence of other complications. These agents demonstrate a 50% to 60% efficacy in improvement of symptoms. Improvement of symptoms occurs within 2 to 3 weeks.

Several α-adrenergic blockers, including alfuzosin (UroXatral), doxazosin (Cardura), terazosin (Hytrin), and tamsulosin (Flomax), are currently being used. Side effects include orthostatic hypotension, dizziness, retrograde ejaculation, and nasal congestion. It should be noted that although these drugs offer symptomatic relief of BPH, they do not treat hyperplasia.

Herbal Therapy. Herbs extracted from plants have been used in the management of BPH. In particular, plant extracts, such as saw palmetto *(Serenoa repens),* have been used. Saw palmetto has been shown to improve urinary symptoms and urinary flow measures (see the Complementary and Alternative Therapies box).

Invasive Therapy. Invasive therapy is indicated when there is a decrease in urine flow sufficient to cause discomfort, persistent residual urine, acute urinary retention because of obstruction with no reversible precipitating cause, or hydronephrosis. Intermittent catheterization or insertion of an indwelling catheter can temporarily reduce symptoms and bypass the obstruction. However, long-term catheter use should be avoided because of the increased risk of infection.

Invasive treatment of symptomatic BPH primarily involves resection or ablation of the prostate. The choice of the treatment approach depends on the size and location of the prostatic enlargement, as well as patient factors such as age and surgical risk. Various invasive treatments are summarized in Table 55-3.

Transurethral Resection of the Prostate. Transurethral resection of the prostate (TURP) is a surgical procedure involving the removal of prostate tissue using a resectoscope inserted through the urethra. TURP has long been considered the "gold standard" surgical treatment for obstructing BPH. Although this procedure remains the most common operation performed, there has been a decrease in the number of TURP procedures done in recent years due to the development of less invasive technologies.[5]

The TURP is performed under a spinal or general anesthetic and requires a hospital stay. No external surgical incision is made. A resectoscope is inserted through the urethra to excise and cauterize obstructing prostatic tissue (Fig. 55-3). A large three-way indwelling catheter with a 30-ml balloon is inserted into the bladder after the procedure to provide hemostasis and to facilitate urinary drainage. The bladder is irrigated, either continuously or intermittently, usually for the first 24 hours to prevent obstruction from mucus and blood clots.

The outcome for 80% to 90% of patients is excellent, with marked improvements in symptoms and urinary flow rates. TURP

TABLE 55-3	Invasive Treatment Options for Benign Prostatic Hyperplasia		
Treatment	**Description**	**Advantages**	**Disadvantages**
Invasive			
Transurethral resection of the prostate (TURP)	Use of excision and cauterization to remove prostate tissue cystoscopically. Considered the most effective treatment of BPH.	Best long-term relief of prostatic obstruction Erectile dysfunction unlikely	Bleeding Retrograde ejaculation
Transurethral incision of the prostate (TUIP)	Involves making transurethral slits or incisions into prostatic tissue to relieve obstruction. Effective for men with relatively little prostatic enlargement.	Outpatient procedure Minimal complications No erectile dysfunction or retrograde ejaculation	Considered temporary solution to obstructive problem Urinary catheter needed after procedure
Open prostatectomy	Surgery of choice for men with large prostates. Involves external incision with three possible approaches (see Fig. 55-4).	Complete visualization of prostate and surrounding tissue Usually only indicated if prostate gland is very large	Erectile dysfunction Bleeding Postoperative pain Risk of infection
Minimally Invasive			
Transurethral microwave thermotherapy (TUMT)	Use of microwave radiating heat to produce coagulative necrosis of the prostate.	Outpatient procedure Erectile dysfunction and retrograde ejaculation are rare	Potential for damage to surrounding tissue Urinary catheter needed after procedure
Transurethral needle ablation (TUNA)	Low-wave radiofrequency used to heat the prostate, causing necrosis.	Outpatient procedure Erectile dysfunction and retrograde ejaculation are rare Precise delivery of heat to desired area Very little pain experienced	Urinary retention common Irritative voiding symptoms Hematuria
Laser prostatectomy	Procedure uses a laser beam to cut or destroy part of the prostate. Different techniques are available: Visual laser ablation of prostate (VLAP) Contact laser technique Interstitial laser coagulation (ILC)	Short procedure Minimal bleeding Fast recovery time Very effective	Postprocedure catheterization (up to 7 days) needed because of edema and urinary retention Delayed sloughing of tissue Takes several weeks to reach optimal effect Retrograde ejaculation
Transurethral electrovaporization of prostate (TUVP)	Electrosurgical vaporization and desiccation are used together to destroy prostatic tissue.	Minimal risks Minimal bleeding and sloughing	Retrograde ejaculation Intermittent hematuria
Intraprostatic urethral stents	Insertion of self-expandable metallic stent into the urethra where enlarged area of prostate occurs.	Safe and effective Low risk	Stent may move Long-term effect is unknown

BPH, Benign prostatic hyperplasia.

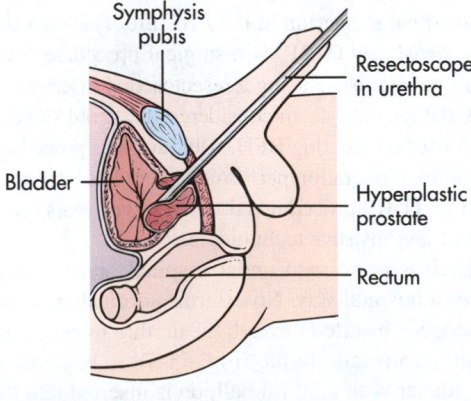

Symphysis pubis
Resectoscope in urethra
Bladder
Hyperplastic prostate
Rectum

FIG. 55-3 Transurethral resection of the prostate.

is a surgical procedure with relatively low risk. Some of the post-operative complications include bleeding, clot retention, and dilutional hyponatremia associated with irrigation. Because bleeding is a common complication, patients taking aspirin or warfarin (Coumadin) must discontinue these medications several days before surgery.

Transurethral Incision of the Prostate. Transurethral incision of the prostate (TUIP) is a surgical procedure done under local anesthesia. It is a surgical procedure indicated for men with moderate to severe symptoms and small prostates who are poor surgical candidates. Studies have shown that TUIP is as effective as TURP in relieving symptoms.[5]

Minimally Invasive Therapy. Minimally invasive nonsurgical therapies are an alternative to watchful waiting and surgical treatment. They generally do not require hospitalization or catheterization. The risk of complications is also reduced with these therapies.

Transurethral Microwave Thermotherapy. Transurethral microwave thermotherapy (TUMT) is an outpatient procedure that involves the delivery of microwaves directly to the prostate through a transurethral probe in order to raise the temperature of the prostate tissue to about 113° F (45° C). The heat causes death of tissue, thus relieving the obstruction.[7] A rectal temperature probe is used during the procedure to ensure that the rectal temperature is kept below 110° F (43.5° C) to prevent rectal tissue damage.

Postoperative urinary retention is a common complication. Thus the patient is generally sent home with an indwelling catheter for 2 to 7 days to maintain urinary flow and to facilitate the passing of small clots or necrotic tissue. Antibiotics, pain medication, and bladder antispasmodic medications are used to treat and prevent postprocedure problems. The procedure is not appropriate for men with rectal problems. Anticoagulant therapy should be stopped 10 days before treatment. Mild side effects include occasional problems of bladder spasm, hematuria, dysuria, and retention.

Transurethral Needle Ablation. Transurethral needle ablation (TUNA) is another procedure that increases the temperature of prostate tissue, thus causing localized necrosis. TUNA differs from TUMT in that low-wave radiofrequency is used to heat the prostate. Only prostate tissue in direct contact with the needle is affected, thus allowing greater precision in removal of the target tissue. The extent of tissue removed by this process is determined by the amount of tissue contact (needle length), amount of energy delivered, and duration of treatment. Seventy percent of patients undergoing TUNA report an improvement in symptoms, making this an attractive treatment option for men with BPH.

This procedure is performed in an outpatient unit or physician's office using local anesthesia and intravenous or oral sedation. The TUNA procedure typically lasts only 30 minutes. The patient typically experiences little pain and an early return to regular activities. Complications include urinary retention, urinary tract infection, and irritative voiding symptoms (e.g., frequency, urgency, dysuria). Some patients require a urinary catheter for a short duration. Patients typically have hematuria for up to a week.

Laser Prostatectomy. The use of laser therapy through visual or ultrasound guidance is an effective alternative to TURP in treating BPH.[8] The laser beam is delivered transurethrally through a fiber instrument and is used for cutting, coagulation, and vaporization of prostatic tissue. There are a variety of laser procedures using different sources, wavelengths, and delivery systems. A common laser procedure is laser coagulation of the prostate, which is often referred to as visual laser ablation of the prostate (VLAP). VLAP uses the laser beam to produce deep coagulation necrosis of the prostate. The affected prostate tissue gradually sloughs in the urinary stream. It takes several weeks before the patient reaches optimal results following this type of laser therapy. At the completion of VLAP, a urinary catheter is inserted to allow for drainage.

Contact laser techniques involve the direct contact of the laser to the prostate tissue. This produces an immediate vaporization of the prostate tissue. Blood vessels near the laser tip immediately are cauterized, thus bleeding during the procedure is rare. A three-way catheter with slow-drip irrigation is placed immediately after the procedure for a short time. Typically the catheter is removed within 6 to 8 hours after the procedure. Advantages of this procedure over TURP include minimal bleeding both during and after the procedure, faster recovery time, and ability to perform the surgery on patients taking anticoagulants.

Another approach to laser prostatectomy is interstitial laser coagulation (ILC).[9] The prostate is viewed through a cystoscope. A laser is used to quickly treat precise areas of the enlarged prostate by placement of interstitial light guides directly into the prostate tissue.

Intraprostatic Urethral Stents. Relief of symptoms from obstruction in patients who are poor surgical candidates can occur with intraprostatic urethral stents. Complications include chronic pain, infection, and encrustation. The long-term effects are not known.[10]

TABLE 55-4	**NURSING ASSESSMENT** Benign Prostatic Hyperplasia

Subjective Data
Important Health Information
Medications: Estrogen or testosterone supplementation
Surgery or other treatments: Previous treatment for BPH

Functional Health Patterns
Health perception–health management: Knowledge of the condition
Nutritional-metabolic: Voluntary fluid restriction
Elimination: Urinary urgency, diminution in caliber and force of urinary stream; hesitancy in initiating voiding; postvoiding dribbling; urinary retention; incontinence
Sleep: Nocturia
Cognitive-perceptual: Dysuria, sensation of incomplete voiding; bladder discomfort
Sexuality-reproductive: Anxiety about sexual dysfunction

Objective Data
General
Older adult male

Urinary
Distended bladder on palpation; smooth, firm, elastic enlargement of prostate on rectal examination

Possible Findings
Enlarged prostate on ultrasonography; vesicle neck obstruction on cystourethroscopy; residual urine with postvoiding catheterization; presence of white blood cells, bacteria, or microscopic hematuria with infection; ↑ serum creatinine levels with renal involvement

BPH, Benign prostatic hyperplasia.

NURSING MANAGEMENT
BENIGN PROSTATIC HYPERPLASIA

Because the nurse is most directly involved with care of patients with BPH having invasive procedures, the focus of nursing management in this section is on preoperative and postoperative care.

■ *Nursing Assessment*

Subjective and objective data that should be obtained from a patient with BPH are presented in Table 55-4.

■ *Nursing Diagnoses*

Nursing diagnoses for the patient with BPH preoperatively may include, but are not limited to, the following:

- Acute pain *related to* bladder distention secondary to enlarged prostate
- Risk for infection *related to* an indwelling catheter, urinary stasis, or environmental pathogens

Nursing diagnoses for the patient with BPH who has surgery may include, but are not limited to, those presented in NCP 55-1.

■ *Planning*

The overall preoperative goals for the patient having invasive procedures are to have (1) restoration of urinary drainage; (2) treatment of any urinary tract infection; and (3) understanding of the upcoming procedure, implications for sexual functioning, and urinary control. The overall postoperative goals are to have (1) no complications, (2) restoration of urinary control, (3) complete bladder emptying, and (4) satisfying sexual expression.

Reproductive System

NURSING CARE PLAN 55-1

Patient Having Prostate Surgery

NURSING DIAGNOSIS   **Acute pain** *related to* bladder irritability, irrigations, and distention; presence of catheter; and surgical trauma *as evidenced by* reports of pain; nonverbal signs of pain such as moaning, crying, legs drawn to abdomen

PATIENT GOAL   Patient reports satisfactory pain control

OUTCOMES (NOC)

Pain Control

- Reports pain controlled _____
- Uses analgesics appropriately _____
- Uses nonanalgesic relief measures _____
- Reports uncontrolled symptoms to health care professional _____

Measurement Scale

1 = Never demonstrated
2 = Rarely demonstrated
3 = Sometimes demonstrated
4 = Often demonstrated
5 = Consistently demonstrated

INTERVENTIONS (NIC) and *RATIONALES*

Patient-Controlled Analgesia (PCA) Assistance

- Teach patient and family to monitor pain intensity, quality, and duration.
- Teach patient and family members how to use the PCA device.
- Teach patient and family members the action and side effects of pain-relieving agents.

Pain Management

- Teach patient nonpharmacologic techniques (e.g., relaxation, guided imagery, distraction, and breathing exercises) before pain occurs or increases, and along with other pain-relief measures, *to alleviate pain through a variety of methods.*
- Explore with the patient factors that relieve/worsen pain.
- Evaluate the effectiveness of the pain control measures used through ongoing assessment of the pain experience.
- Institute and modify pain-control measures on the basis of the patient's response.

Tube Care: Urinary

- Maintain patency of urinary catheter system *because clots cause obstruction of urine flow resulting in painful bladder spasms.*

NURSING DIAGNOSIS   **Urge urinary incontinence** *related to* bladder irritation and poor sphincter control *as evidenced by* involuntary leakage of urine

PATIENT GOAL   Reports decrease in urine leakage between voidings

OUTCOMES (NOC)

Urinary Continence

- Urine leakage between voidings _____
- Starts and stops stream _____
- Empties bladder completely _____
- Responds to urge in timely manner _____

Measurement Scale

1 = Never demonstrated
2 = Rarely demonstrated
3 = Sometimes demonstrated
4 = Often demonstrated
5 = Consistently demonstrated

INTERVENTIONS (NIC) and *RATIONALES*

Urinary Elimination Management

- Identify factors that contribute to incontinence episodes *to plan appropriate interventions.*
- Instruct patient to respond immediately to urge to void *to prevent involuntary leakage.*

Urinary Incontinence Care

- Explain etiology of problem and rationale for actions *to help patient plan appropriate interventions.*
- Limit ingestion of bladder irritants (e.g., colas, coffee, tea, and chocolate) *to decrease urinary urgency.*
- Limit fluids for 2-3 hours before bedtime *to avoid nighttime urgency.*
- Assist to select appropriate incontinence garment/pad for short-term management while more definitive treatment is designed.

NURSING DIAGNOSIS   **Ineffective therapeutic regimen management** *related to* lack of knowledge regarding need for follow-up care and activity restriction postoperatively *as evidenced by* questioning or inaccurate comments about postoperative activity

PATIENT GOAL   Describes necessary follow-up care and activity restrictions

OUTCOMES (NOC)

Knowledge: Treatment Regimen

- Description of self-care responsibilities for ongoing treatment _____
- Description of prescribed activity _____
- Description of self-monitoring techniques _____

Measurement Scale

1 = None
2 = Limited
3 = Moderate
4 = Substantial
5 = Extensive

INTERVENTIONS (NIC) and *RATIONALES*

Discharge Planning

- Formulate a maintenance plan for postdischarge follow-up.
- Coordinate referrals relevant to linkages among health care providers.
- Assist patient/family/significant other in planning for supportive environment necessary *to provide for patient's posthospital care.*

Teaching: Disease Process

- Discuss lifestyle changes that may be required to prevent future complications and/or control disease process (e.g., avoid heavy lifting, straining during defecation, prolonged periods of travel, stair climbing, driving, and sexual activity—until surgeon approves such activity) *to prevent increases in intraabdominal pressure and the possibility of bleeding.*

▪ Nursing Implementation

Health Promotion. The cause of BPH is largely attributed to the aging process. The focus of health promotion is on early detection and treatment. The American Cancer Society, along with the AUA, recommends a yearly medical history and DRE for men over 50 years of age in an effort to provide early detection of prostate problems. When symptoms of prostatic hyperplasia become evident, further diagnostic screening may be necessary (see Table 55-2).

Some men find that the ingestion of alcohol and caffeine tends to increase prostatic symptoms because the diuretic effect of these substances increases bladder distention. Compounds found in common cough and cold remedies such as pseudoephedrine (in Sudafed) and phenylephrine (in Allerest and Coricidin preparations) often worsen the symptoms of BPH. These drugs are α-adrenergic agonists that cause smooth muscle contraction. If this happens, the patient should avoid these drugs.

The patient with obstructive symptoms should be advised to urinate every 2 to 3 hours and when first feeling the urge. This will minimize urinary stasis and acute urinary retention. Fluid intake should be maintained at a normal level to avoid dehydration or fluid overload. The patient may believe that if he restricts his fluid intake, symptoms will be less severe, but this only increases the chances of an infection. However, if the patient increases his intake too rapidly, bladder distention can develop because of the prostatic obstruction.

Acute Intervention. The following discussion focuses on preoperative and postoperative care for the patient undergoing a TURP.

Preoperative Care. Urinary drainage must be restored before surgery. Prostatic obstruction may result in acute retention or inability to void. A urethral catheter such as a Coudé (curved-tip) catheter may be needed to restore drainage. In many health care settings, 10 ml of sterile 2% lidocaine gel is injected into the urethra before insertion of the catheter. The lidocaine gel not only acts as a lubricant, but also provides local anesthesia and helps open the urethral lumen. If a sizable obstruction of the urethra exists, a urologist may insert a filiform catheter with sufficient rigidity to pass the obstruction. Aseptic technique is important at all times to avoid introducing bacteria into the bladder. (Urinary catheters are discussed in Chapter 46.)

Antibiotics are usually administered before any invasive procedure. Any infection of the urinary tract must be treated before surgery. Restoring urine drainage and encouraging a high fluid intake (2 to 3 L/day unless contraindicated) are also helpful in managing the infection.

The patient is often concerned about the impact of the impending surgery on his sexual functioning. Data gathered from the health history relating to sexual activities will identify possible problem areas. The nurse should provide an opportunity for the patient and partner to express their concerns. The patient needs to know how the surgery may affect sexual functioning. All types of prostatic surgery generally result in some degree of retrograde ejaculation. The patient should be informed that the ejaculate may be decreased in amount or totally absent. This may decrease orgasmic sensations felt during ejaculation. Retrograde ejaculation is not harmful because the semen is eliminated during the next urination.

Postoperative Care. The main complications following surgery are hemorrhage, bladder spasms, urinary incontinence, and infection. The plan of care should be adjusted to the type of surgery, the reasons for surgery, and the patient's response to surgery.

After surgery the patient will have a standard catheter or a triple-lumen catheter. Bladder irrigation is typically done to remove clotted blood from the bladder and ensure drainage of urine. The bladder is irrigated either manually on an intermittent basis or more commonly as a continuous bladder irrigation (CBI) with sterile normal saline solution or another prescribed solution. If the bladder is manually irrigated (if ordered), 50 ml of irrigating solution should be instilled and then withdrawn with a syringe to remove clots that may be in the bladder and catheter. Painful bladder spasms often occur as a result of manual irrigation. With CBI, irrigating solution is continuously infused and drained from the bladder. The rate of infusion is based on the color of drainage. Ideally the urine drainage should be light pink without clots. The inflow and outflow of irrigant must be continuously monitored. If outflow is less than inflow, the catheter patency should be assessed for kinks or clots. If the outflow is blocked and patency cannot be reestablished by manual irrigation, the CBI is stopped and the physician notified.

Careful aseptic technique should be used when irrigating the bladder because bacteria can easily be introduced into the urinary tract. Proper care of the catheter is important. To prevent urethral irritation and minimize the risk of bladder infection, the catheter must be secured to the leg with tape or a catheter strap. The catheter should be connected to a closed-drainage system and should not be disconnected unless it is being removed, changed, or irrigated. The secretions that accumulate around the meatus can be cleansed daily with soap and water.

Blood clots are expected after prostate surgery for the first 24 to 36 hours. However, large amounts of bright red blood in the urine can indicate hemorrhage. Postoperative hemorrhage may occur from displacement of the catheter, dislodging a large clot, or increases in abdominal pressure. Release or displacement of the catheter dislodges the balloon that provides counterpressure on the operative site. Traction on the catheter may be applied to provide counterpressure (tamponade) on the bleeding site in the prostate, thereby decreasing bleeding. Such traction can result in local necrosis if pressure is applied for too long. Pressure should therefore be relieved on a scheduled basis by qualified personnel. Activities that increase abdominal pressure, such as sitting or walking for prolonged periods and straining to have a bowel movement (Valsalva maneuver), should be avoided in the postoperative recovery period.

Bladder spasms are a distressing complication for the patient after transurethral procedures. They occur as a result of irritation of the bladder mucosa from the insertion of the resectoscope, presence of a catheter, or clots leading to obstruction of the catheter. The patient should be instructed not to urinate around the catheter because this increases the likelihood of spasm. If bladder spasms develop, the catheter should be checked for clots. If present, the clots should be removed by irrigation so that urine can flow freely. Belladonna and opium suppositories, or other antispasmodics (e.g., oxybutynin [Ditropan]) along with relaxation techniques, are used to relieve the pain and decrease spasm. The catheter is often removed 2 to 4 days after surgery. The patient should urinate within 6 hours after catheter removal. If he cannot, a catheter is reinserted for a day or two. If the problem continues, the nurse may need to instruct the patient in clean intermittent self-catheterization (see Chapter 46).

Sphincter tone may be poor immediately after catheter removal, resulting in urinary incontinence or dribbling. This is a common but distressing situation for the patient. Sphincter tone can be strengthened by having the patient practice Kegel exercises (pelvic floor muscle technique) 10 to 20 times per hour while awake. The patient should be encouraged to practice starting and stopping the stream several times during urination. This facilitates learning the pelvic floor exercises. It usually takes several weeks to achieve urinary continence. In some instances, control of urine may never be fully regained. Continence can improve for up to 12 months. If continence has not been achieved by that time, the patient may be referred to a continence clinic. A variety of methods, including biofeedback, have been used to achieve positive results. The patient can also be instructed to use a penile clamp, a condom catheter, or incontinence pads or briefs to avoid embarrassment from dribbling. In severe cases, an occlusive cuff that serves as an artificial sphincter can be surgically implanted to restore continence. The nurse should assist the patient in finding ways to manage the problem that will allow him to continue socializing and interacting with others.

The patient should be observed for signs of postoperative infection. If an external wound is present (from an open prostatectomy), the area should be observed for redness, heat, swelling, and purulent drainage. Special care must be taken if a perineal incision is present because of the proximity of the anus. Rectal procedures, such as taking rectal temperatures and administering enemas, should be avoided. The insertion of well-lubricated belladonna and opium suppositories is acceptable.

Dietary intervention and stool softeners are important in the postoperative period to prevent the patient from straining while having bowel movements. Straining increases the intraabdominal pressure, which can lead to bleeding at the operative site. A diet high in fiber facilitates the passage of stool.

Ambulatory and Home Care. Discharge planning and home care issues are important aspects of care after prostate surgery. Instructions include (1) caring for an indwelling catheter (if one is left in place); (2) managing urinary incontinence; (3) maintaining oral fluids between 2000 and 3000 ml per day; (4) observing for signs and symptoms of urinary tract and wound infection; (5) preventing constipation; (6) avoiding heavy lifting (more than 10 lb [4.5 kg]); and (7) refraining from driving or intercourse after surgery as directed by the physician.

The patient may experience a change in sexual functioning following surgery. Many men experience *retrograde ejaculation* because of trauma to the internal urethral sphincter. Semen is discharged into the bladder at orgasm and may produce cloudy urine when the patient urinates after orgasm. Physiologic erectile dysfunction (ED) may occur if the nerves are cut or damaged during surgery. The patient may experience anxiety over the change due to a perceived loss of his sex role, self-esteem, or quality of sexual interaction with his partner. The nurse should discuss these changes with the patient and his partner and allow them to ask questions and express their concerns. Sexual counseling and treatment options may be necessary if ED becomes a chronic or permanent problem. ED is discussed later in the chapter. It should be pointed out that although some patients experience concerns regarding change in sexual function, this is not a universal concern. Many men are comfortable with such changes and view them as appropriate for their age. If this is the case, nurses should be careful not to impose concern in their enthusiastic attempts to pursue such problems.

The bladder may take up to 2 months to return to its normal capacity. The patient should be instructed to drink at least 2 L of fluid per day and urinate every 2 to 3 hours to flush the urinary tract. Bladder irritants such as caffeine products, citrus juices, and alcohol should be avoided or limited to small amounts. Because the patient may be experiencing incontinence or dribbling, he may incorrectly believe that decreasing fluid intake will relieve this problem. Urethral strictures may result from instrumentation or catheterization. Treatment may include teaching the patient intermittent clean self-catheterization or having a urethral dilation.

The patient must be advised that he should continue to have a yearly DRE if he has had any procedure other than complete removal of the prostate. Hyperplasia or cancer can occur in the remaining prostatic tissue.

■ Evaluation

Expected outcomes for the patient with BPH who has surgery are presented in NCP 55-1.

PROSTATE CANCER

Prostate cancer is a malignant tumor of the prostate gland. It is estimated that 232,000 new cases of prostate cancer are diagnosed and 30,350 men die annually from the disease in the United States.[11] One of every five men will develop prostate cancer at some point during their lives. Prostate cancer is the most common cancer among men, excluding skin cancer. It is the second leading cause of cancer death in men (exceeded only by lung cancer). The majority (more than 75%) of cases occur in men over age 65. However, many cases occur in younger men who sometimes have a more aggressive type of cancer. There was a large increase in the incidence of newly diagnosed cases of prostate cancer between 1988 and 1992. This increase in number was attributed to the widespread use of prostate-specific antigen (PSA) as a screening procedure, allowing early detection of prostate cancer. The incidence of prostate cancer appears to have peaked and has now leveled off.[12]

Etiology and Pathophysiology

Prostate cancer is an androgen-dependent adenocarcinoma. The majority of tumors occur in the outer aspect of the prostate gland. Prostate cancer is usually slow growing. It can spread by three routes: direct extension, through the lymph system, or through the bloodstream. Spread by direct extension involves the seminal vesicles, urethral mucosa, bladder wall, and external sphincter. The cancer later spreads through the lymphatic system to the regional lymph nodes. The veins from the prostate seem to be the mode of spread to the pelvic bones, head of the femur, lower lumbar spine, liver, and lungs.

Age, ethnicity, and family history are three nonmodifiable risk factors for prostate cancer. The incidence of prostate cancer rises markedly after age 50, and more than 80% of men diagnosed are older than 65. The incidence of prostate cancer worldwide is higher in African Americans than in any other ethnic group. The reasons for the higher rate are unknown.[13] In addition, African American men are likely to have more aggressive tumors at diagnosis and have higher mortality rates from prostate cancer. A family history of prostate cancer, especially first-degree relatives (fathers, brothers), is also associated with an increased risk. Genetic mutations in certain genes may contribute to the risk of prostate cancer in susceptible men.

A high-fat diet is thought to be associated with an increased risk of prostate cancer.[14] Studies are examining the role of dietary carotenoids, such as lycopene, in reducing prostate cancer risk. Although occupational exposure to chemicals (e.g., cadmium) may be associated with higher prostate cancer risk, this possible risk continues to be studied.[15] A history of BPH is not a risk factor for prostate cancer.

Clinical Manifestations and Complications

Prostate cancer is usually asymptomatic in the early stages. Eventually the patient may have symptoms similar to those of BPH, including dysuria, hesitancy, dribbling, frequency, urgency, hematu-

TABLE 55-5	**Whitmore-Jewett Staging Classification of Prostate Cancer**
Stage A: Clinically Unrecognized	
A1	<5% of prostatic tissue neoplastic
A2	>5% of prostatic tissue neoplastic, all high-grade tumors
Stage B: Clinically Intracapsular	
B1	Nodule <2 cm and surrounded by palpably normal tissue
B2	Nodule >2 cm or multiple nodules
Stage C: Clinically Extracapsular, Localized to Periprostatic Area	
C1	Minimal extracapsular extension
C2	Large tumors involving seminal vesicles, adjacent structures, or both
Stage D: Metastatic Disease	
D1	Pelvic lymph node metastases or ureteral obstruction causing hydronephrosis
D2	Distant metastases to bone, viscera, or other soft tissue structures

Adapted from Schroeder F et al: TNM classification of prostate cancer, *Prostate* (suppl) 4:129, 1992; and American Joint Committee on Cancer, 1992.

ria, nocturia, retention, interruption of urinary stream, and inability to urinate. Pain in the lumbosacral area that radiates down to the hips or legs, when coupled with urinary symptoms, may indicate metastasis.

Early recognition and treatment is required to control growth, prevent metastasis, and preserve quality of life. The tumor can spread to pelvic lymph nodes, bones, bladder, lungs, and liver. Once the tumor has spread to distant sites, the major problem becomes the management of pain. As the cancer spreads to the bones (a common site of metastasis), pain can become severe, especially in the back and the legs because of compression of the spinal cord and destruction of bone.

Diagnostic Studies

Improved diagnostic techniques have greatly enhanced the detection of prostate cancer. The two primary screening tools are DRE and a blood test for **prostate-specific antigen** (PSA), a glycoprotein produced by the prostate. On DRE an abnormal prostate may feel hard, nodular, and asymmetric.

Elevated levels of PSA (normal level, 0 to 4 ng/ml [0 to 4 mcg/L]) indicate prostatic pathology, although not necessarily prostate cancer. Mild elevations in PSA may occur with aging, BPH, recent ejaculation, drugs (e.g., finasteride [Proscar]), herbs (e.g., saw palmetto), acute or chronic prostatitis, or after long bike rides. In addition, cystoscopy, indwelling urethral catheters, and prostate biopsies may also produce an elevation. When prostate cancer exists, serum PSA levels are a useful marker of tumor volume (i.e., the higher the PSA level, the greater the tumor mass).

There is controversy regarding the value of PSA testing in significantly reducing mortality rates of prostate cancer.[16] At the core of the controversy is that many people live and die *with* prostate cancer, but not *from* it. As screening has become more widespread, smaller cancers are being found in older men. Slow-growing cancers, in most cases, probably do not need to be diagnosed or treated.[17] However, early detection of aggressive cancers by PSA testing has saved lives. Some men with prostate cancer have normal PSA levels, which has led some health care providers to question if the upper limit of 4.0 ng/ml is too high.[18] This is another issue that currently is unresolved. Men are now being advised to discuss individually with their health care provider the need for and value of PSA testing.[19]

PSA is not only used to detect prostate cancer, but it is also used to monitor the success of treatment. When treatment has been successful in removing prostate cancer, PSA levels should fall to undetectable levels. Regular measurement of PSA levels following treatment is important to evaluate the effectiveness of treatment and possible recurrence of prostate cancer.

Elevated levels of prostatic isoenzyme of serum acid phosphatase (prostatic acid phosphatase [PAP]) is another indication of prostate cancer, especially if there is extracapsular spread. With advanced prostate cancer, serum alkaline phosphatase is increased as a result of bone metastasis. Investigation is now under way to locate a serum marker for prostate cancer similar to CA-125, which is a useful marker in ovarian cancer. (Ovarian cancer is discussed in Chapter 54.)

Neither PSA nor DRE is a definitive diagnostic test for prostate cancer. If PSA levels are elevated or if the DRE is abnormal, a biopsy of the prostate tissue is indicated. Biopsy of prostate tissue is necessary to confirm the diagnosis of prostate cancer. The biopsy is typically done using TRUS because it allows the physician to visualize the prostate and pinpoint abnormalities. When a suspicious area is located, a special biopsy needle is inserted into the prostate to obtain a tissue sample. A pathologic examination of the tissue specimen is done to assess for malignant changes. Other tests used to determine the location and extent of the spread of the cancer may include bone scan, computed tomography (CT), and magnetic resonance imaging (MRI) using an endorectal probe.

Collaborative Care

Early-stage prostate cancer is a curable disease in the majority of men. Based on findings from diagnostic studies, the prostate cancer is staged and graded. Two common classification systems used for staging prostate cancer are the Whitmore-Jewett and the tumor, node, metastasis (TNM) systems. They are both based on the size (volume) of the tumor and spread (Table 55-5). It is estimated that 80% of patients with prostate cancer are initially diagnosed when the cancer is in either a local or regional stage. The 5-year survival rate with an initial diagnosis at this stage is 100%.[12]

TABLE 55-6	**COLLABORATIVE CARE** **Prostate Cancer**

Diagnostic
History and physical examination
Digital rectal examination (DRE)
Prostate-specific antigen (PSA)
Prostatic acid phosphatase (PAP)
Transrectal ultrasound (TRUS)
Biopsy of prostate and lymph nodes
Computed tomography (CT), magnetic resonance imaging (MRI), bone scan (to evaluate for metastatic disease)

Collaborative Therapy
Stage A
Watchful waiting with annual PSA and DRE
Radical prostatectomy
Radiation therapy
- External beam
- Brachytherapy

Stage B
Radical prostatectomy
Radiation therapy

Stage C
Radical prostatectomy
Radiation therapy
Hormone therapy
Orchiectomy

Stage D
Hormone therapy
Orchiectomy
Chemotherapy
Radiation therapy to metastatic bone areas

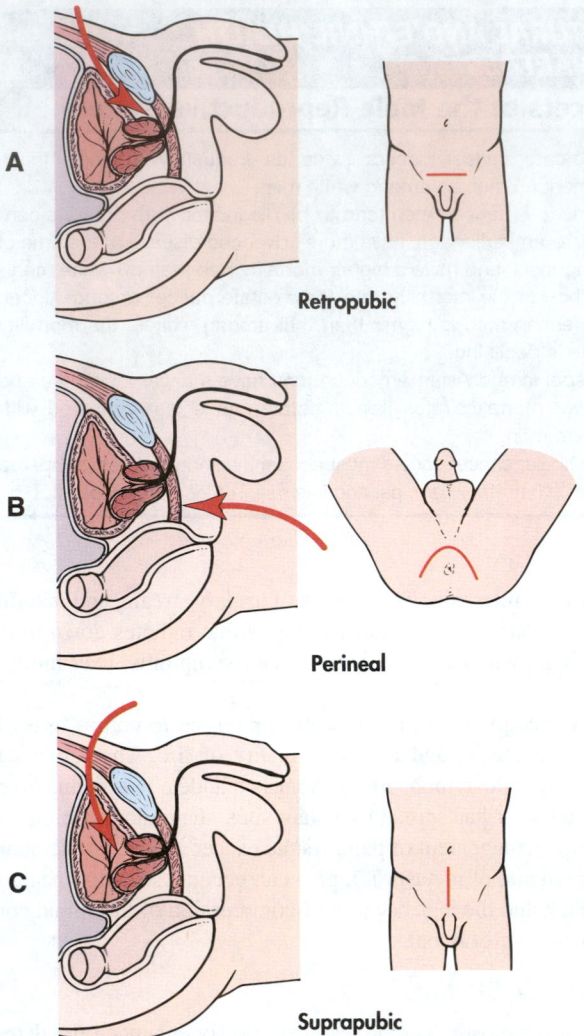

FIG. 55-4   Three approaches used to perform a prostatectomy. **A,** Retropubic approach involves a midline abdominal incision. **B,** Perineal approach involves an incision between the scrotum and anus. **C,** Suprapubic approach involves an abdominal incision.

Grading of the tumor is done based on tumor histology using the Gleason scale. With this scale, tumors are graded from 1 to 5 based on the degree of glandular differentiation. Grade 1 represents the most well differentiated (most like the original cells), and grade 5 represents the most poorly differentiated (undifferentiated). Gleason grades are given to the two most commonly occurring patterns of cells and added together. The Gleason score is a number from 2 to 10. This scale is used to predict how quickly the cancer will progress.

The collaborative care of the patient with prostate cancer depends on the stage of the cancer and the overall health of the patient. At all stages, there is more than one possible treatment option. The decision of which treatment course to pursue is made jointly by the patient, nurse, and the physician based on a careful analysis of the facts and the patient's preference.[20] Table 55-6 summarizes the various treatment options available.

Conservative Therapy. Prostate cancer is relatively slow growing. Therefore a conservative approach to management of prostate cancer is "watchful waiting" (also known as "deferred treatment"). The rationale behind this approach is that more men were dying *with* prostate cancer rather than dying *from* it.[21] The decision to adopt a strategy of watchful waiting is appropriate when there is (1) a life expectancy of less than 10 years, (2) presence of significant comorbid disease, and (3) presence of a low-grade, low-stage tumor. These patients are typically followed with frequent PSA measurements, along with DRE, to monitor the progress of the disease. Significant changes in either PSA, DRE, or the development of symptoms warrant a reevaluation of treatment options, whether they be definitive or palliative.

Surgical Therapy

Radical Prostatectomy. With **radical prostatectomy,** the entire prostate gland, seminal vesicles, and part of the bladder neck (ampulla) are removed.[20] The entire prostate is removed because the cancer tends to be in many different locations within the gland. In addition, a retroperitoneal lymph node dissection is usually done. A radical prostatectomy is the surgical procedure considered the most effective treatment for long-term survival. Thus it is the preferred treatment for men younger than 70 years of age who are in good health and with the cancer confined to the prostate (stages A and B). Surgery is usually not considered an option for stage D cancer (except to relieve symptoms associated with obstruction) because metastasis has already occurred. The two most common approaches for radical prostatectomy are retropubic and perineal resection (Fig. 55-4). With the more common *retropubic* approach, a low midline abdominal incision is made to access the prostate gland, and the pelvic lymph nodes can be dissected. With the *perineal* resection, an incision is made between the scrotum and anus. This procedure cannot remove lymph nodes. A laparoscopic approach to prostatectomy is being used in some settings. It has the potential to offer technologic improvement, less bleeding, less pain, and faster recovery compared with traditional approaches, but the long-term benefits are still being investigated.[18]

After surgery, the patient has a large indwelling catheter with a 30-ml balloon placed in the bladder via the urethra. This catheter is typically left in place for 1 to 2 weeks. A drain is left in the surgical site to aid in the removal of drainage from the area. This drain is typically removed after a couple of days. Because the perineal approach has a higher risk of postoperative infection (due to the location of the incision related to the anus), careful dressing changes and perineal care after each bowel movement are important for comfort and to prevent infection. The typical length of hospital stay postoperatively is 3 days.

The two major complications following a radical prostatectomy are erectile dysfunction and urinary incontinence. Because this procedure destroys the nerves needed for erection, erectile dysfunction occurs. The incidence of erectile dysfunction is dependent on the patient's age, preoperative sexual functioning, whether nerve-sparing surgery was performed, and the expertise of the surgeon. Problems with urinary control occur in nearly all men for the first few months following surgery because the bladder must be reattached to the urethra after the prostate is removed. Over time, the bladder adjusts and most men regain control. One study reported that only 8.7% were incontinent 24 months after surgery.[20] Other common complications associated with surgery include hemorrhage, urinary retention, infection, wound dehiscence, deep vein thrombosis, and pulmonary emboli.

Nerve-Sparing Procedure. Many men desire to retain sexual function following radical prostatectomy. In such cases a nerve-sparing procedure that spares the nerves responsible for erection may be possible. This procedure is the preferred choice for most men undergoing prostatectomy in the early stage of the disease. Nerve-sparing prostatectomy is indicated only for patients with cancer confined within the prostate gland. Although the risk of erectile dysfunction is significantly reduced with this procedure, there is no guarantee that potency will be maintained. Because the nerves lie directly beneath the prostate gland, the risk of damage is very high. The percent of success reported varies.[22]

Cryosurgery. Prostatic cryosurgery is a surgical technique that destroys cancer cells by freezing the tissue. It has been used both as an initial treatment and as a second-line treatment after radiation treatment failures. A transrectal ultrasound probe is inserted to visualize the prostate gland. Probes containing liquid nitrogen are then inserted into the prostate. Liquid nitrogen delivers freezing temperatures, destroying the tissue. The treatment takes about 2 hours under general or spinal anesthesia and does not involve an abdominal incision. Possible complications of prostatic cryosurgery include damage to the urethra and, in rare cases, a urethrorectal fistula (an opening between the urethra and the rectum) or a urethrocutaneous fistula (an opening between the urethra and the skin). Tissue sloughing, erectile dysfunction, urinary incontinence, prostatitis, and hemorrhage have also been reported.

Radiation Therapy. Radiation therapy is a common treatment option for prostate cancer, especially for men over 70, patients who are poor surgical risks, or those who wish to avoid surgery. The long-term outcome of radiation therapy is dependent on the stage of the cancer. Because many of the men choosing radiation therapy are older and perhaps not in as good health as those undergoing prostatectomy, comparisons are difficult.[21] Radiation therapy may be offered as the only treatment, or it may be offered in combination with surgery or with hormonal therapy.

PICO: P, Patient population of interest; *I*, intervention or area of interest; *C*, comparison of interest or comparison group; *O*, outcome(s) of interest (see p. 6).

Salvage radiation therapy is a new use of therapy in which radiation is given for cancer recurrence after radical prostatectomy. Early results have shown promise in reducing metastatic disease in some men.[23]

External Beam Radiation. External beam is the most widely used method of delivering radiation treatments for those with prostate cancer. This therapy can be used to treat patients with prostate cancer confined to the prostate and/or surrounding tissue (stages A, B, and C). Patients are treated on an outpatient basis 5 days a week for 6 to 8 weeks. Each treatment lasts only a few minutes. Side effects from radiation can be acute (occurring during treatment or within 90 days that follow) or delayed (occurring months or years after treatment). Common side effects involve the skin (dryness, redness, irritation, pain), gastrointestinal tract (diarrhea, abdominal cramping, bleeding), urinary tract (dysuria, frequency, hesitancy, urgency, nocturia), sexual functioning (erectile dysfunction), fatigue, and bone marrow suppression. These problems usually resolve 2 to 3 weeks after the completion of radiation therapy. In patients with clinically localized disease, cure rates with external beam radiation are comparable to those with radical prostatectomy.

Brachytherapy. *Brachytherapy* involves placing radioactive seed implants into the prostate gland, allowing higher radiation doses directly in the tissue while sparing the surrounding tissue

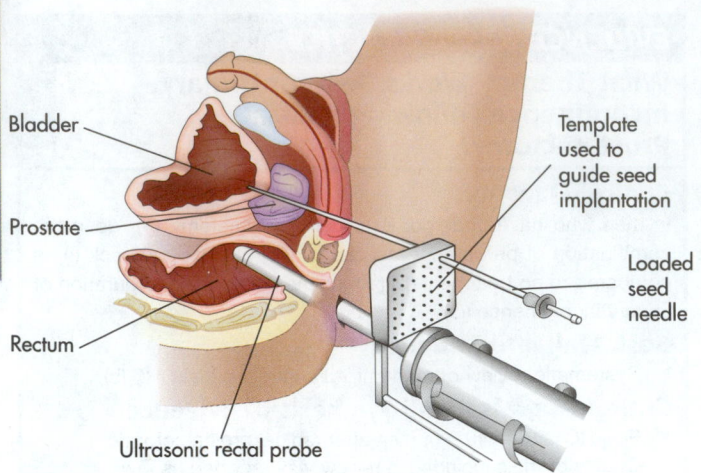

Bladder

Prostate

Rectum

Ultrasonic rectal probe

Template used to guide seed implantation

Loaded seed needle

FIG. 55-5   Prostate brachytherapy. Radioactive seeds are implanted with a needle guided by ultrasound and a template grid.

(rectum and bladder). The radioactive seeds are placed in the prostate gland with a needle through a grid template guided by transrectal ultrasound (Fig. 55-5). The grid template and ultrasound ensure accurate placement of the seeds. Because brachytherapy is a one-time outpatient procedure, many patients find this more convenient than external beam radiation treatment. Brachytherapy is best suited for patients with stage A or B prostate cancer. The most common side effect is the development of urinary irritative or obstructive problems. The AUA Symptom Index (see Table 55-1) can be used to measure urinary function for patients undergoing brachytherapy and can be incorporated into postoperative nursing management. For those with more advanced tumors, brachytherapy may be offered in combination with external beam radiation treatment.[20] (Brachytherapy is discussed further in Chapter 16.)

Drug Therapy.   The forms of drug therapy available for the treatment of prostate cancer are hormonal therapy, chemotherapy, or a combination of both.

Hormonal Therapy.   Prostate cancer growth is largely dependent on the presence of androgens. Therefore androgen deprivation is a primary therapeutic approach for some men with prostatic cancer. Hormone therapy is focused on reducing the levels of circulating androgens in order to reduce the tumor growth. Hormone or antiandrogen therapy can also be used as adjunct therapy before surgery or radiation therapy to reduce tumor size, and in men with locally advanced disease (stage C). One of the biggest challenges with hormonal therapy is that almost all tumors treated will become resistant to this therapy *(hormone refractory)* within a few years.[24] An elevated PSA level is often the first sign that hormonal therapy is no longer effective. Androgen ablation can be produced by interference with androgen production (e.g., luteinizing hormone–releasing hormone [LH-RH] agonists, orchiectomy) or androgen receptor blockers (Table 55-7).

Luteinizing Hormone–Releasing Hormone Agonists and Antagonists.   Luteinizing hormone–releasing hormone (LH-RH) is released from the hypothalamus to stimulate the anterior pituitary to produce luteinizing hormone (LH) and follicle-stimulating hormone (FSH). LH stimulates the testicular Leydig cells to produce testosterone. The LH-RH agonists superstimulate the pituitary. This ultimately results in downregulation of the LH-RH receptors, leading to a refractory condition in which the anterior pituitary is unresponsive to LH-RH. These drugs cause an initial transient increase in LH and

TABLE 55-7	**DRUG THERAPY** **Hormonal Therapy for Prostate Cancer**
Therapy	**Mechanism of Action**
LH-RH Agonists leuprolide (Lupron, Eligard, Viadur subcutaneous implant) goserelin (Zoladex) triptorelin (Trelstar) buserelin (Suprefact)	Reduce secretion of LH and FSH Decrease testosterone production
LH-RH Antagonist abarelix (Plenaxis)	Blocks LH receptors Immediate testosterone suppression
Androgen Receptor Blockers bicalutamide (Casodex) flutamide (Eulexin) nilutamide (Nilandron)	Block action of testosterone by competing with receptor sites
Estrogen diethylstilbestrol (DES)	Inhibits LH secretion Decreases testosterone production Blocks circulating testosterone
Orchiectomy Surgical removal of testicles	Removes 95% of testosterone source

FSH, Follicle-stimulating hormone; *LH,* luteinizing hormone; *LH-RH,* LH releasing hormone.

testosterone called a "flare." A worsening of symptoms may occur during this time. However, with continued administration, LH and testosterone levels are decreased. Current antiandrogen therapy includes leuprolide (Lupron, Eligard, Viadur), goserelin (Zoladex), and triptorelin (Trelstar). This therapy essentially produces a chemical castration similar to the effects of an orchiectomy. Antiandrogen medications are given by subcutaneous or intramuscular injections on a regular basis, and they must be taken indefinitely. Viadur is an implant that is placed subcutaneously and delivers leuprolide continuously for 1 year. Side effects of LH-RH agonists include hot flashes, gynecomastia, loss of libido, and erectile dysfunction.

Abarelix (Plenaxis) is an LH-RH antagonist that lowers testosterone levels. It is used for patients with advanced prostate cancer. Unlike the LH-RH agonists, abarelix does not cause a flare because it acts directly to block LH and FSH receptors. It is given as an intramuscular injection. Side effects include allergic reactions, hot flashes, gynecomastia, pain, and constipation.

Androgen Receptor Blockers.   Another classification of antiandrogens is drugs that compete with circulating androgens at the receptor sites. Flutamide (Eulexin), nilutamide (Nilandron), and bicalutamide (Casodex) are nonsteroidal androgen receptor blockers. They can be used in combination with goserelin or leuprolide. The combination has been found to be safe and well tolerated as a potency-sparing, androgen-ablative therapy. Adverse effects of androgen receptor blockers include loss of libido, erectile dysfunction, and hot flashes. Breast pain and gynecomastia may also occur in men treated with androgen receptor blockers. Combining an androgen receptor blocker with an LH-RH agonist is an often used treatment, which results in combined androgen blockade.[25]

Estrogen.   Estrogen (e.g., diethylstilbestrol [DES]) has been used as a form of androgen deprivation therapy. However, estrogen treatment is declining in popularity because of cardiovascular complications (e.g., myocardial infarction, deep vein thrombosis, cerebrovascular disease) and the development of more effective hormone therapies.

Orchiectomy. A bilateral orchiectomy is the surgical removal of the testes that may be done alone or in combination with prostatectomy. For advanced stages of prostate cancer (stage D) an orchiectomy is one treatment option for cancer control. Testosterone, produced by the testes, stimulates growth of the prostate cancer. An orchiectomy reduces the circulating testosterone levels by 90%. Another possible benefit of this procedure is the rapid relief of bone pain associated with advanced tumors. Orchiectomy may also induce sufficient shrinkage of the prostate to relieve urinary obstruction in later stages of disease when surgery is not an option.

Side effects of orchiectomy include hot flashes, erectile dysfunction, loss of sex drive, and irritability. Weight gain and loss of muscle mass, which are also common, can alter a man's physical appearance. Osteoporosis has also been reported as a consequence of orchiectomy. These physical changes can affect self-esteem, leading to grief and depression. Although this procedure is permanent and cost effective (compared with chemical hormone manipulation using LH-RH agonists), many men prefer drug therapy to orchiectomy.

Chemotherapy. The use of chemotherapeutic agents has primarily been limited to treatment for those with hormone-refractory prostate cancer (HRPC) in late-stage disease. In HRPC the cancer is progressing despite treatment. This occurs in patients who have taken an antiandrogen for a certain period of time. Historically, prostate cancer has been poorly responsive to chemotherapy and has not been shown to improve survival. Thus the goal of chemotherapy is palliation.[25] Some of the more commonly used chemotherapy drugs include mitoxantrone (Novantrone), cyclophosphamide (Cytoxan), idarubicin (Idamycin), epirubicin (Ellence), and estramustine (Emcyt).

The drug docetaxel (Taxotere) has recently been found to be the first drug to improve survival rates in men with advanced metastatic HRPC.[26] Docetaxel, when given in combination with prednisone, estramustine, or mitoxantrone (Novantrone), is being recognized as the new standard of care for HRPC.[24,25] Side effects of docetaxel include nausea, alopecia, and bone marrow suppression.

Clinical trials are now examining the effect of a vaccine (Provenge) on improving survival of patients with HRPC. The vaccine is designed to stimulate the patient's system against the cancer. The vaccine is currently being tested in men with metastatic prostate cancer.

CULTURALLY COMPETENT CARE
PROSTATE CANCER

Nurses must be aware of not only the epidemiologic differences that occur with prostate cancer, but also the differences that exist in health promotion practices. Demographic characteristics should be considered when providing information about the risk for prostate cancer and screening recommendations.

African American men suffer higher mortality rates than white men, in part because their prostate cancer often is more advanced at the time of diagnosis. Despite the availability of early screening measures (PSA and DRE), African American men and those in lower socioeconomic groups frequently do not use such services. This is partially related to actual and perceived knowledge levels

TABLE 55-8	**NURSING ASSESSMENT** Prostate Cancer

Subjective Data
Important Health Information
Medications: Testosterone supplements; use of any medications affecting urinary tract such as morphine, anticholinergics, monoamine oxidase inhibitors, and tricyclic antidepressants

Functional Health Patterns
Health perception–health management: Positive family history; increasing fatigue and malaise
Nutritional-metabolic: High-fat diet; anorexia, weight loss (possible indicators of metastasis)
Elimination: Hesitancy or straining to start stream, urinary urgency, frequency, retention with dribbling, weak stream, hematuria
Sleep: Nocturia
Cognitive-perceptual: Dysuria; low back pain radiating to legs or pelvis, bone pain (possible indicators of metastasis)
Self-perception–self-concept: Anxiety regarding self-concept

Objective Data
General
Older adult male; pelvic lymphadenopathy (late sign)

Urinary
Distended bladder on palpation; unilaterally hard, enlarged, fixed prostate on rectal examination

Musculoskeletal
Pathologic fractures (metastasis)

Possible Findings
↑ Serum PSA; ↑ serum PAP (metastasis); nodular and irregular prostate on ultrasonography, positive biopsy results; anemia

PAP, Prostatic acid phosphatase; *PSA,* prostate-specific antigen.

of prostate cancer. One study found that African American men did not participate in prostate cancer early detection screening activities because they felt disconnected from the health care system.[13] Although exposure to electronic and print media is successful in informing some men about prostate cancer, significant differences of effectiveness exist based on demographic variables such as ethnicity, age, education level, and socioeconomic level. Ideally, no man should be unaware of the risks associated with prostate cancer and screening methods available. The nurse must consider the best method to communicate this information to men of all cultures and ethnicities that will result in the greatest degree of understanding and participation in prostate cancer screening.

NURSING MANAGEMENT
PROSTATE CANCER

■ Nursing Assessment

Subjective and objective data that should be obtained from a patient with prostate cancer are presented in Table 55-8.

■ Nursing Diagnoses

Nursing diagnoses for the patient with prostate cancer depend on the stage of the cancer. General nursing diagnoses, which may or may not apply to every patient with cancer of the prostate, may include, but are not limited to, the following:

- Decisional conflict *related to* numerous alternative treatment options
- Acute pain *related to* surgery, prostatic enlargement, bone metastasis, and bladder spasms

- Urinary retention *related to* obstruction of urethra or bladder neck by the prostate, blood clots, and loss of bladder tone
- Impaired urinary elimination *related to* bladder neck sphincter damage
- Constipation or diarrhea *related to* treatment interventions
- Sexual dysfunction *related to* effects of treatment
- Anxiety *related to* uncertain outcome of disease process on life and lifestyle and effect of treatment on sexual functioning

■ Planning

The overall goals are that the patient with prostate cancer will (1) be an active participant in the treatment plan, (2) have satisfactory pain control, (3) follow the therapeutic plan, (4) understand the effect of the therapeutic plan on sexual function, and (5) find a satisfactory way to manage the impact on bladder or bowel function.

■ Nursing Implementation

Health Promotion. One of the most important roles for nurses in relation to prostate cancer is to encourage patients, in consultation with their health care providers, to have an annual prostate screening (PSA and DRE) starting at age 50 (or younger if risk factors are present). Because of their increased risk of prostate cancer, African American men and other men with a family history of prostate cancer should have an annual PSA and DRE beginning at age 45.[12]

Acute Intervention. Preoperative and postoperative phases of radical prostatectomy are similar to surgical procedures for BPH (see pp. 1424 to 1425). Nursing interventions for the patient who undergoes radiation therapy and chemotherapy are discussed in Chapter 16. An additional consideration is the psychologic response of the patient to a diagnosis of cancer. The nurse should provide sensitive, caring support for the patient and his family to help them cope with the diagnosis of cancer. Prostate support groups are available for men and their families to encourage them to be active, informed participants in their own care.

Ambulatory and Home Care. If the patient is discharged with an indwelling catheter in place, the nurse must teach appropriate catheter care. The patient should be instructed to clean the urethral meatus with soap and water once a day; maintain a high fluid intake; keep the collecting bag lower than the bladder at all times; keep the catheter securely anchored to the inner thigh or abdomen; and report any signs of bladder infection, such as bladder spasms, fever, or hematuria. If urinary incontinence is a problem, patients should be encouraged to practice pelvic floor muscle exercises (Kegel exercises) at every urination and throughout the day. Continuous practice during the 4- to 6-week healing process improves the success rate. Products used for incontinence specifically designed for men are available through home care product catalogs and many retail stores.

Although prostate cancer has a high cure rate if detected and treated early, prognosis for stage D prostate cancer is very unfavorable. Hospice care is often appropriate and beneficial to the patient and family. (Hospice care is discussed in Chapter 11.) Common problems experienced by the patient with advanced prostate cancer include fatigue, bladder outlet obstruction and ureteral obstruction (caused by compression of the urethra and/or ureters from tumor mass or lymph node metastasis), severe bone pain and fractures (caused by bone metastasis), spinal cord compression (from spinal metastasis), and leg edema (caused by lymphedema, deep vein thrombosis, and other medical conditions). Nursing interventions

must focus on all of these problems. However, management of pain is one of the most important aspects of nursing care for these patients. Pain control is managed through ongoing pain assessment, administration of prescribed medications (both opioid and nonopioid agents), and the use of nonpharmacologic methods of pain relief. (Pain management is discussed further in Chapter 10.)

■ Evaluation

Evaluation is based on expected outcomes. The outcomes are that the patient with prostate cancer will

- be an active participant in the treatment plan
- have satisfactory pain control
- follow the therapeutic plan
- understand the effect of the treatment on sexual function
- find a satisfactory way to manage the impact on bladder or bowel function

PROSTATITIS

Etiology and Pathophysiology

Prostatitis is a broad term that describes a group of inflammatory and noninflammatory conditions affecting the prostate gland. It is the most common urologic problem in men younger than 50 years of age. Nearly 2 million men are treated for prostatitis each year.[27] Historically, this condition has lacked a strong agreement regarding the cause, diagnosis, and optimal treatment. To bring greater consistency in approaching this common condition, the National Institutes of Health established consensus classifications of prostatitis syndromes. The consensus classifications include four categories: (1) acute bacterial prostatitis, (2) chronic bacterial prostatitis, (3) chronic prostatitis/chronic pelvic pain syndrome, and (4) asymptomatic inflammatory prostatitis.[28]

Both acute and chronic bacterial prostatitis generally result from organisms reaching the prostate gland by one of the following routes: ascending from the urethra, descending from the bladder, and invasion via the bloodstream or the lymphatic channels. Common causative organisms are *Escherichia coli, Klebsiella, Pseudomonas, Enterobacter, Proteus, Chlamydia trachomatis, Neisseria gonorrhoeae,* and group D streptococci. Chronic bacterial prostatitis differs from acute prostatitis in that it involves recurrent episodes of infection.[28]

Chronic prostatitis/chronic pelvic pain syndrome is a new term that describes a syndrome of prostate and urinary pain in the absence of an obvious infectious process. The etiology of chronic prostatitis/chronic pelvic pain syndrome is not known. It may occur after a viral illness, or it may be associated with sexually transmitted diseases (STDs), particularly in a younger adult. A culture reveals no causative organisms. However, leukocytes may be found in prostatic secretions.

Asymptomatic inflammatory prostatitis is usually diagnosed in individuals who have no symptoms, but are found to have an inflammatory process in the prostate. These patients are usually diagnosed during the evaluation of other genitourinary tract problems. Leukocytes are present in the seminal fluid from the prostate, but the cause of this process is unclear.

Clinical Manifestations and Complications

Common clinical manifestations of acute bacterial prostatitis include fever, chills, back pain, and perineal pain, along with acute urinary symptoms such as dysuria, urinary frequency, urgency, and cloudy urine.[29] The patient may also have acute urinary retention caused by prostatic swelling. With DRE, the prostate is extremely swollen, very tender, and firm. The complications of prostatitis are epididymitis and cystitis. Sexual functioning may be affected as manifested by postejaculation pain, libido problems, and erectile dysfunction. Prostatic abscess is also a potential, but uncommon, complication.

Chronic bacterial prostatitis and chronic prostatitis/pelvic pain syndrome manifest with similar symptoms that are generally milder than those associated with acute bacterial prostatitis. These include irritative voiding symptoms (frequency, urgency, dysuria), backache, perineal/pelvic pain, and ejaculatory pain. Obstructive symptoms are uncommon unless the patient has coexisting BPH. With DRE, the prostate feels enlarged and firm (often described as boggy) and is slightly tender with palpation. Chronic prostatitis can predispose the patient to recurrent urinary tract infections.

The clinical features of prostatitis can be mimicked by urinary tract infection. However, acute cystitis is not common in men.

Diagnostic Studies

Because patients with prostatitis have urinary symptoms, a urinalysis (UA) and urine culture are indicated. Often white blood cells (WBCs) and bacteria are present. If the patient has a fever, WBC count and blood cultures are also indicated. The PSA test may be done to rule out prostate cancer. However, PSA levels are often elevated with prostatic inflammation. Thus it is not considered diagnostic in itself.

Microscopic evaluation and culture of expressed prostate secretion is considered useful in the diagnosis of prostatitis. Expressed prostate secretion is obtained using a premassage and postmassage test. The patient is asked to void into a specimen cup just before and just after a vigorous prostate massage. Prostatic massage (for expressed prostate secretion) should be avoided if acute bacterial prostatitis is suspected, because compression is extremely painful and can increase the risk of bacterial spread. TRUS has not been particularly useful in the diagnosis of prostatitis. However, transabdominal ultrasound or MRI may be done to rule out an abscess on the prostate.

NURSING *and* COLLABORATIVE MANAGEMENT
PROSTATITIS

Antibiotics commonly used for acute and chronic bacterial prostatitis include trimethoprim/sulfamethoxazole (Bactrim), ciprofloxacin (Cipro), and ofloxacin (Floxin). Doxycycline (Vibramycin) or tetracycline may be prescribed for those patients with multiple sex partners. Antibiotics are usually given orally for up to 4 weeks for acute bacterial prostatitis. However, if the patient has high fever or other signs of impending sepsis, hospitalization and intravenous antibiotics are prescribed. Patients with chronic bacterial prostatitis are given oral antibiotic therapy for 4 to 16 weeks. A short course of oral antibiotics is usually prescribed for those with chronic prostatitis/chronic pelvic pain syndrome. However, antibiotic therapy often is ineffective for these patients.

Although patients with acute and chronic bacterial prostatitis tend to experience a great amount of discomfort, the pain resolves as the infection is treated. Pain management for patients with chronic prostatitis/chronic pelvic pain syndrome is more difficult because the pain persists for weeks to months. Antiinflammatory agents are the most common agents used for pain control in prostatitis, but these provide only moderate pain relief. Opioid pain

medications can be used, but because this pain is chronic in nature, the use of opioids should be approached cautiously. Thermal therapy, which may provide some relief, is being studied.[30]

Acute urinary retention can develop in acute prostatitis requiring bladder drainage with suprapubic catheterization. Passage of a catheter through an inflamed urethra is contraindicated in acute prostatitis. Repetitive prostatic massage is thought to be therapeutic for most types of prostatitis, but it is not an appropriate measure for acute bacterial prostatitis. This measure relieves congestion within the prostate by squeezing out excess prostatic secretions, thus providing pain relief. Prostatic massage is performed by using the index finger of a gloved hand and pressing down on the prostate, covering the entire gland's surface in longitudinal strokes. This is done two to three times a week for 6 weeks. Measures to stimulate ejaculation (masturbation and intercourse) help drain the prostate as well and are encouraged.

Because the prostate can serve as a source of bacteria, fluid intake should be kept at a high level for all patients experiencing prostatitis. Nursing interventions are aimed at encouraging the patient to drink plenty of fluids. This is especially important for those with acute bacterial prostatitis because of the increased fluid needs associated with fever and infection. Management of fever is also an important nursing intervention.

Problems of the Penis

Health problems of the penis are rare if STDs are excluded (see Chapter 53). Problems of the penis may be classified as congenital, problems of the prepuce, problems with the erectile mechanism, and cancer.

CONGENITAL PROBLEMS

Hypospadias is a urologic abnormality in which the urethral meatus is located on the ventral surface of the penis anywhere from the corona to the perineum. Hormonal influences in utero, environmental factors, and genetic factors are possible causes. Surgical repair of hypospadias may be necessary if it is associated with *chordee* (a painful downward curvature of the penis during erection) or if it prevents intercourse or normal urination. Surgery may also be done for cosmetic reasons or emotional well-being.

Epispadias, an opening of the urethra on the dorsal surface of the penis, is a complex birth defect that is usually associated with other genitourinary tract defects. Corrective surgery to place the urethra in a normal position in the penis is usually done in early childhood.

PROBLEMS OF THE PREPUCE

Problems of the prepuce in the United States are rare because circumcision has been a routine procedure for most male infants for many years. Circumcision, the surgical removal of the foreskin of the penis, is a procedure done to male infants for religious or cultural reasons. It is believed to prevent problems such as *phimosis* (tightness of the foreskin resulting in the inability to retract it), *paraphimosis* (tightness of the foreskin resulting in the inability to pull it forward from a retracted position), and cancer of the penis. A recent trend is that fewer parents are having their infants circumcised, which may result in an increased incidence of problems in the future.

Phimosis is a constriction of the uncircumcised foreskin around the head of the penis, making retraction difficult (Fig. 55-6, *A*). It is caused by edema or inflammation of the foreskin, usually associated with poor hygiene techniques that allow bacterial and yeast organisms to become trapped under the foreskin.

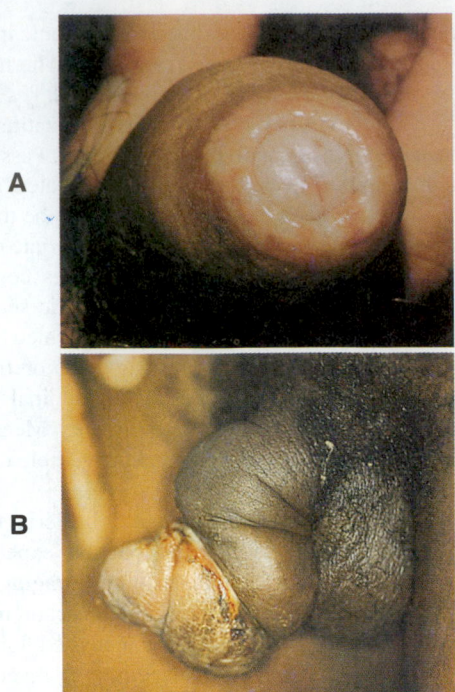

FIG. 55-6 **A,** Phimosis. Unable to retract the foreskin due to secondary lesions on the prepuce. **B,** Paraphimosis. Ulcer with edema from foreskin remaining contracted over the prepuce.

Paraphimosis is edema of the retracted uncircumcised foreskin, preventing normal return over the glans. An ulcer can develop if the foreskin remains contracted (see Fig. 55-6, *B*). This can occur when the foreskin is pulled back during bathing, use of urinary catheters, or intercourse and is not placed back in the forward position. Antibiotics, warm soaks, and sometimes circumcision or dorsal slit of the prepuce may be required. Careful cleaning followed by replacement of the foreskin generally prevents these problems.

PROBLEMS OF THE ERECTILE MECHANISM

Priapism is a painful erection lasting longer than 6 hours. The condition may constitute a medical emergency.[31] Causes of priapism include thrombosis of the corpus cavernosal veins, leukemia, sickle cell anemia, diabetes mellitus, degenerative lesions of the spine, neoplasms of the brain or spinal cord, prolonged foreplay, injection of vasoactive medications into the corpus cavernosa, and cocaine use. Treatment may include sedatives, injection of smooth muscle relaxants directly into the penis, aspiration and irrigation of the corpora cavernosa with a large-bore needle, or the surgical creation of a shunt to drain the corpora. Complications may include penile tissue necrosis caused by lack of blood flow or hydronephrosis from bladder distention. After an episode of priapism, the patient may be unable to achieve a normal erection.

Peyronie's disease, sometimes referred to as curved or crooked penis, is caused by plaque formation in one of the corpora cavernosa of the penis. The palpable, nontender, hard plaque formation is usually found on the posterior surface. It may result from trauma to the penile shaft or may occur spontaneously. The plaque prevents adequate blood flow into the spongy tissue, which results in a curvature during erection. The condition is not dangerous but can result in painful erections, erectile dysfunction, or embarrassment. If conservative measures do not correct the problem, surgery may be necessary.

CANCER OF THE PENIS

Cancer of the penis is rare. It occurs most commonly in men who have cancers associated with human papillomavirus (HPV) and in men who were not circumcised as infants. The tumor may appear as a superficial ulceration or a pimple-like nodule. The nontender warty lesion may be mistaken for a venereal wart. The majority of malignancies (95%) are well-differentiated squamous cell carcinomas. Treatment in the early stages is laser removal of the growth. A radical resection of the penis may be done if the cancer has spread. Surgery, radiation, or chemotherapy may be tried depending on the extent of the disease, lymph node involvement, or metastasis.

Problems of the Scrotum and Testes

INFLAMMATORY AND INFECTIOUS PROBLEMS

Skin Problems

The skin of the scrotum is susceptible to a number of common skin diseases. The most common conditions of the scrotal skin are fungal infections, dermatitis (neurodermatitis, contact dermatitis, seborrheic dermatitis), and parasitic infections (scabies, lice). These conditions involve discomfort for the patient but are associated with few, if any, severe complications (see Chapter 24).

Epididymitis

Epididymitis is an acute, painful inflammatory process of the epididymis (Fig. 55-7), usually secondary to an infectious process (sexually or nonsexually transmitted), trauma, or urinary reflux down the vas deferens. It is usually unilateral. Swelling may progress to the point that the epididymis and testis are indistinguishable. In men younger than 35 years of age, the most common cause is through sexual transmission of either gonorrhea or chlamydia.[27] The use of antibiotics is important for both partners if the transmission is through sexual contact. Patients should be encouraged to refrain from sexual intercourse during the acute phase. If they do engage in intercourse, a condom should be used. Conservative treatment consists of bed rest with elevation of the scrotum, use of ice packs, and analgesics. Ambulation places the scrotum in a dependent position and increases pain. Most tenderness subsides within 1 week, although swelling may last for weeks or months.

Orchitis

Orchitis refers to an acute inflammation of the testis. In orchitis, the testis is painful, tender, and swollen. It generally occurs after an episode of bacterial or viral infections such as mumps, pneumonia, tuberculosis, or syphilis. It can also be a side effect of epididymitis, prostatectomy, trauma, infectious mononucleosis, influenza, catheterization, or complicated urinary tract infection. Mumps orchitis is a condition contributing to infertility and could easily be avoided by childhood vaccination against mumps. Treatment involves the use of antibiotics (if the organism is known), pain medications, or bed rest with the scrotum elevated on an ice pack.

CONGENITAL PROBLEMS

Cryptorchidism (undescended testes) is failure of the testes to descend into the scrotal sac before birth. It is the most common congenital testicular condition. It may occur bilaterally or unilaterally and may be the cause of infertility if corrective surgery is

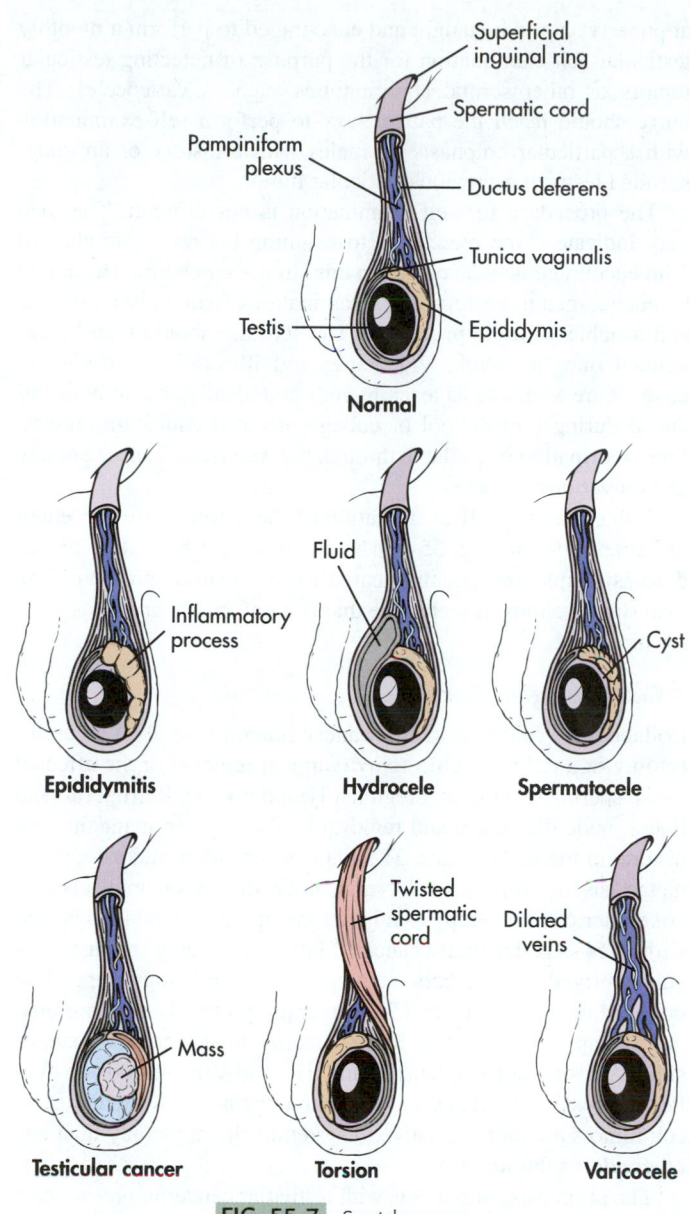

FIG. 55-7   Scrotal masses.

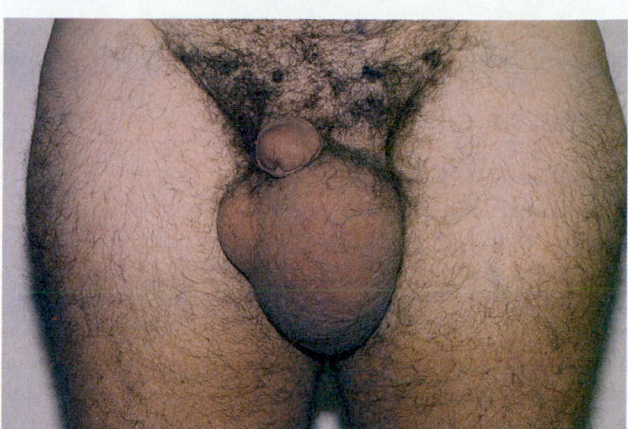

FIG. 55-8   Hydrocele.

Diagnosis is fairly simple because the mass can be seen by shining a flashlight through the scrotum (transillumination). No treatment is indicated unless the swelling becomes very large and uncomfortable, in which case aspiration or surgical drainage of the mass is performed.

Spermatocele

A **spermatocele** is a firm, sperm-containing, painless cyst of the epididymis that may be visible with transillumination (see Fig. 55-7). The cause is unknown, and surgical removal is the treatment. It is important for the patient to see his health care provider if he feels any scrotal lumps. He would be unable to distinguish this cyst from cancer when performing self-examination.

Varicocele

A **varicocele** is a dilation of the veins that drain the testes (see Fig. 55-7). The scrotum feels wormlike when palpated. The cause of the problem is unknown. The varicocele is usually located on the left side of the scrotum as a consequence of retrograde blood flow from the left renal vein. Surgery is indicated if the patient is infertile, because persistent varicoceles are associated with 40% to 50% of cases of infertility. Repair of the varicocele may be through injection of a sclerosing agent or by surgical ligation of the spermatic vein.

Testicular Torsion

Testicular torsion involves a twisting of the spermatic cord that supplies blood to the testes and epididymis (see Fig. 55-7). It is most commonly seen in males younger than age 20. The patient experiences severe scrotal pain, tenderness, swelling, nausea, and vomiting. Urinary symptoms, fever, and WBCs or bacteria in the urine are absent. The pain does not usually subside with rest or elevation of the scrotum. The cremasteric reflex is elicited by lightly stroking (with a reflex hammer or tongue blade) the inner aspect of the thigh in a downward direction. The normal response is a contraction of the cremaster muscle that pulls up the scrotum and testis on the side stroked. In testicular torsion this reflex is absent on the side of the swelling.

Nuclear technetium scan of the testes or Doppler ultrasound is typically performed to assess blood flow within the testicle. A decrease or absence in blood flow confirms the diagnosis. Unless it resolves spontaneously, surgery to untwist the cord and restore the blood supply must be performed immediately. Torsion constitutes a surgical emergency because if the blood supply to the affected

not done by 2 years of age. The incidence of testicular cancer is also higher if the condition is not corrected before puberty. Surgery is performed to locate and suture the testis or testes to the scrotum.

Absence of the vas deferens is a rare condition most often associated with cystic fibrosis. With the advent of advanced techniques to treat infertility, this defect can be circumvented by aspirating the sperm directly from the testis.

"DES sons" are the male children of women who took diethylstilbestrol (DES) during pregnancy. The effects of DES on males can include undescended or underdeveloped testes, small penis, varicocele, or epididymal cysts. These males also have an increased risk of infertility and testicular cancer.[32]

ACQUIRED PROBLEMS

Hydrocele

A **hydrocele** is a nontender, fluid-filled mass that results from interference with lymphatic drainage of the scrotum and swelling of the tunica vaginalis that surrounds the testis (Figs. 55-7 and 55-8).

testicle is not restored within 4 to 6 hours, ischemia to the testis will occur, leading to necrosis and the possible need for removal.

TESTICULAR CANCER

Etiology and Pathophysiology

Testicular cancer is relatively rare, accounting for less than 1% of all cancers found in males. However, testicular cancer is the most common type of cancer in young men between 15 and 34 years of age.[33] In the United States about 8000 new cases of and 400 deaths from testicular cancer occur annually.[11] The incidence of testicular cancer is four times higher in white males than in African American males, and it occurs more commonly in the right testicle than the left. Testicular tumors are also more common in males who have had undescended testes (cryptorchidism) or a family history of testicular cancer or anomalies. Other predisposing factors include orchitis, human immunodeficiency virus infection, maternal exposure to DES, and testicular cancer in the contralateral testis.

Most testicular cancers develop from embryonic germ cells. The two types of germ cell cancers are seminomas and nonseminomas. Although seminoma germ cell cancers are the most common, they are the least aggressive. Nonseminoma testicular germ cell tumors are rare, but are very aggressive. Non–germ cell tumors arise from other testicular tissue and include Leydig cell and Sertoli cell tumors. These account for less than 10% of testicular cancers.

Clinical Manifestations and Complications

Testicular cancer may have a slow or rapid onset depending on the type of tumor (see Fig. 55-7). The patient may notice a painless lump in his scrotum, as well as scrotal swelling and a feeling of heaviness. The scrotal mass usually is nontender and very firm. Some patients complain of a dull ache or heavy sensation in the lower abdomen, perianal area, or scrotum. Acute pain is the presenting symptom in about 10% of patients. Manifestations associated with metastasis to other systems are varied and include back pain, cough, dyspnea, hemoptysis, dysphagia (difficulty swallowing), alterations in vision or mental status, papilledema, and seizures.

Diagnostic Studies

Palpation of the scrotal contents is the first step in diagnosing testicular cancer. A cancerous mass is firm and does not transilluminate. Ultrasound of the testes is indicated whenever testicular cancer is suspected (e.g., palpable mass) or when persistent or painful testicular swelling is present. If a testicular neoplasm is suspected, blood is obtained to determine the serum levels of α-fetoprotein (AFP), lactate dehydrogenase (LDH), and human chorionic gonadotropin (hCG). (These tumor markers are discussed in Chapter 16.) A chest x-ray and CT scan of the abdomen and pelvis are done to detect metastasis. Anemia may be present and liver function may be elevated in metastatic disease.

NURSING *and* COLLABORATIVE MANAGEMENT
TESTICULAR CANCER

■ *Testicular Self-Examination*

As with many forms of cancer, the survival of the patient is closely associated with early diagnosis of the tumor. The scrotum is easily examined, and beginning tumors are usually palpable. Every male

at puberty should be taught and encouraged to perform a monthly testicular self-examination for the purpose of detecting testicular tumors or other scrotal abnormalities such as variceles. The nurse should teach the patient how to perform self-examination with a particular emphasis on males with a history of an undescended testis or a previous testicular tumor.

The procedure for self-examination is not difficult. The man may indicate some reluctance to examine his own genitals, but with encouragement he can learn this simple procedure. He should be encouraged to perform self-examinations frequently until he is comfortable with the procedure. The scrotum should then be examined once a month. Videotapes and illustrations on shower hangers are available as teaching aids and ideally should be introduced during high school or college physical education classes. Free information is available through the American Cancer Society and on various websites.

Guidelines for self-examination of the scrotum are presented in Table 55-9 and Fig. 55-9. The nurse should make this procedure as simple and uncomplicated for the man as possible. The man should choose a technique that is comfortable and consistent for him.

■ *Collaborative Care*

Collaborative care of testicular cancer generally involves an orchiectomy or a radical orchiectomy (surgical removal of the affected testis, spermatic cord, and regional lymph nodes). Retroperitoneal lymph node dissection and removal is also used in managing the disease in the early stages. These nodes are the primary route for metastasis. Retroperitoneal lymph node dissection may also be done after chemotherapy as adjunct therapy in patients diagnosed with later-stage testicular cancer.[34] Postorchiectomy treatment involves surveillance, radiation therapy, or chemotherapy, depending on the stage of the cancer. Chemotherapy protocols use combination therapy referred to as BEP—**b**leomycin (Blenoxane), **e**toposide (VePesid), and cisplatin (**P**latinol)—and VIP—etoposide (Ve-Pesid), **i**fosfamide (Ifex), and cisplatin (**P**latinol). (Testicular germ cell tumors are more sensitive to systemic chemotherapy than any other adult solid tumor.)

The prognosis for patients with testicular cancer in recent years has greatly improved, and 95% of the patients obtain complete remission if the disease is detected in the early stages. As a result of treatment successes, the majority of men with testicular cancer are long-term survivors and treatment-related toxicity is a significant issue. All patients with testicular cancer, regardless of pathology or stage, require meticulous follow-up and regular physical examinations, chest x-rays, CT scans, and assessment of hCG and AFP. The goal is to detect relapse when the tumor burden is minimal. Secondary malignancies that occur as a result of chemotherapy and radiation are described in Chapter 16.

Prior infertility or impaired fertility is often present at diagnosis. In treating testicular cancer, chemotherapy with cisplatin and/or pelvic irradiation often damages the testicular germ cells. Spermatogenesis can return, however, in some patients. Because of the high risk for infertility, the cryopreservation of sperm in a sperm bank before treatment begins should be discussed and recommended for the man with testicular cancer. Ejaculatory dysfunction may result from retroperitoneal lymph node dissection. These issues may be hard for the nurse to discuss with the newly diagnosed patient. Men may feel that the disease is a threat to their maleness and self-worth.[34]

TABLE 55-9	*PATIENT TEACHING GUIDE* **Testicular Self-Examination**

1. During a shower or bath is the easiest time to examine the testes. Warm temperatures make the testes hang lower in the scrotum (see Fig. 55-9).
2. Use both hands to feel each testis. Roll the testis between the thumb and first three fingers until the entire surface has been covered. Palpate each one separately.
3. Identify the structures. The testis should feel round and smooth, like a hard-boiled egg. Differentiate the testis from the epididymis. The epididymis is not as smooth as the egg-shaped testis. One testis may be larger than the other. Size is not as important as texture. Check for lumps, irregularities, pain in the testes, or a dragging sensation. Locate the spermatic cord, which is usually firm and smooth and goes up toward the groin.
4. Choose a consistent day of the month on which to examine the testes, such as a birth date, that is easy to remember. The examination can be performed more frequently if desired.
5. Notify the health care provider at once if any abnormalities are found.

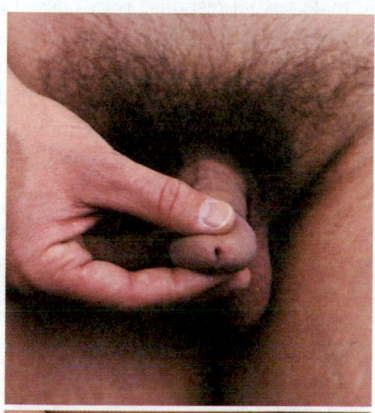
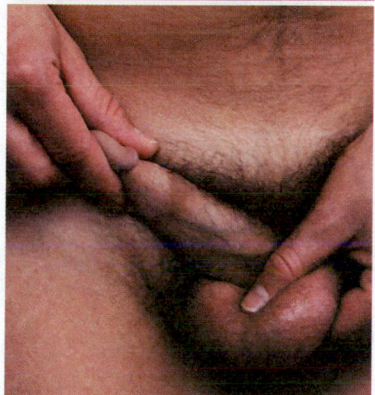

FIG. 55-9   Testicular self-examination.

Sexual Functioning

VASECTOMY

Vasectomy is the bilateral surgical ligation or resection of the vas deferens performed for the purpose of sterilization (Fig. 55-10). The procedure requires only 15 to 30 minutes and is usually performed with the patient under local anesthesia on an outpatient basis. Vasectomy is considered a permanent form of sterilization, although some successful reversals *(vasovasotomy)* have been reported.

ETHICAL DILEMMAS
Sterilization

Situation
A 43-year-old male patient is requesting a vasectomy and informs the nurse that he does not wish to discuss this with his wife. The physician's policy is to have the spouse or partner sign a form acknowledging the patient's desire to be sterilized. This patient explains that although his wife wants to have more children, the one they already have is all he wants.

Important Points for Consideration
• Patient autonomy suggests that matters of reproduction are left to the privacy and discretion of the individual. Competent adults may legally choose to be sterilized for medical reasons or convenience.
• To prevent possible future harm, this man should include his wife in the decision to permanently eliminate his ability to procreate.
• In most states, women can terminate a pregnancy without proof that their husbands are aware of their intentions. Sterilization, on the other hand, is a more permanent decision that has consequences for both parties in the relationship.
• This physician's standard is to have evidence of the spouse's or significant other's knowledge of the intent for sterilization. This is not a state requirement. The nurse should inform the man of the standard in this particular physician's practice and the benefits to the integrity of his marriage.
• If the patient is still unwilling to discuss the matter with his wife, either the nurse or physician should inform the man that they will not participate in deception and he is free to select another physician to perform the procedure.

Critical Thinking Questions
1. How would you approach this situation?
2. Should the nurse tell the wife of her husband's plans?
3. Are there ever circumstances in which deception of a patient or family would be justified?

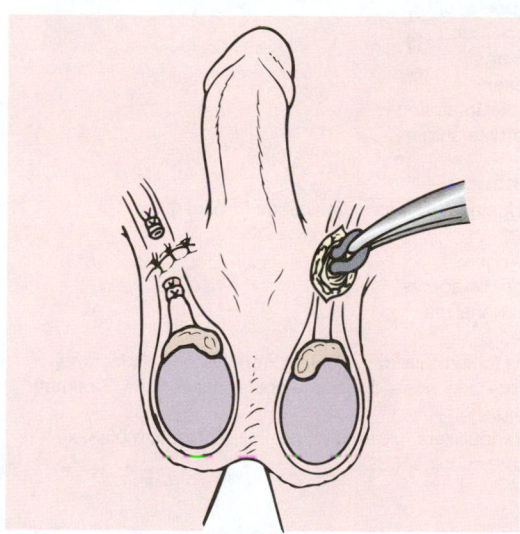

FIG. 55-10   Vasectomy procedure. The vas deferens is ligated or resected for the purpose of sterilization.

After vasectomy, the patient should not notice any difference in the look or feel of the ejaculate because its major component is seminal and prostatic fluid. The patient will need to use an alternative form of contraception until semen examination reveals no sperm. This usually requires at least 10 ejaculations or 6 weeks to evacuate sperm distal to the surgical site. Sperm cells continue to be produced by the testes but are absorbed by the body rather than being passed through the vas deferens. Occasionally postoperative hematoma and swelling of the scrotum occur.

Vasectomy does not affect the production of hormones, ability to ejaculate, or physiologic mechanisms related to erection or orgasm. Psychologic adjustment may be a problem after surgery. It may be difficult for the patient to separate vasectomy from castration at a subconscious level. Some men may develop erectile dysfunction or may feel the need to become much more sexually active than they were in the past to prove their masculinity. Careful discussion of the procedure and its outcome before the surgery can be helpful in detecting patients who may have problems with psychologic adjustment. Surgery should be delayed for these patients.

ERECTILE DYSFUNCTION

Erectile dysfunction (ED) is the inability to attain or maintain an erect penis that allows satisfactory sexual performance.[35] Although sexual function is a topic that many individuals are uncomfortable discussing, health care providers must be able and willing to address ED.

The effects of ED potentially interfere with a man's self-esteem, confidence, relationships, and overall sense of well-being. ED is a condition that is significant because of its prevalence; it is estimated that 20 million to 30 million men in the United States experience ED.[35] ED can occur at any age, although the incidence increases with age. In fact, it is estimated that about 50% of all men between ages 40 and 70 have at least some degree of ED. The problem is increasing in all segments of the sexually active male population and affects both the man and his partner. In younger men the increase is attributed to substance abuse, such as recreational drugs and alcohol. Middle-aged men are affected by medical conditions such as diabetes, hypertension, renal disease, organ transplants, coronary artery bypass surgeries, and cancer, or the therapy for these problems. Men are living longer, fuller lives and expect to remain sexually active, regardless of any existing medical conditions.

Etiology and Pathophysiology

ED can result from a number of factors in two general categories: physiologic (organic) and psychologic. *Physiologic ED* can result from a large number of etiologic factors (Table 55-10). Common causes include diabetes mellitus, vascular disease, side effects from medications, result of surgery (such as prostatectomy), trauma, chronic illness, and decreased gonadal hormone secretion. *Psychologic ED* can be caused by a number of issues but is most often associated with stress, difficulty in a relationship, depression, or low self-esteem. (The male sexual response is discussed in Chapter 51.)

Normal physiologic age-related changes are associated with changes in erectile function and may be an underlying cause of ED for some men.[36] Table 51-4 lists age-related changes in sexual function. Explanation of these age-related changes may be necessary to reassure an anxious older man regarding normal changes in his sexual abilities.

TABLE 55-10	Risk Factors for Erectile Dysfunction
Anatomic	**Genitourinary**
Congenital deformities of the penis (e.g., hypospadias)	Cystectomy
Peyronie's disease	Hydrocele
	Perineal or suprapubic prostatectomy
Cardiorespiratory	Phimosis
Angina pectoris	Post–kidney transplant
Atherosclerosis	Postpriapism
Emphysema	Prostatitis
Hypertension	Renal failure
Myocardial infarction	Varicocele
Post–cardiac surgery	
	Neurologic and Nerve Conduction
Drug Induced	Central nervous system disorders
5-α-Reductase inhibitors (finasteride [Proscar])	Electroshock therapy
Alcohol	Multiple sclerosis
Antiandrogens	Parkinson's disease
Antilipidemic agents	Peripheral neuropathic conditions
Antihypertensives	Spina bifida
Caffeine	Stroke
Diuretics (chlorothiazide [Diuril]; spironolactone [Aldactone])	Sympathectomy
Drugs for Parkinson's disease (carbidopa/levodopa [Sinemet])	Trauma to the spinal cord
Estrogens	Tumors or transection of spinal cord
Major tranquilizers (diazepam [Valium]; alprazolam [Xanax])	
Marijuana, cocaine, LSD	**Psychologic**
Nicotine	Depression
Opioids	Excessive stress in family, work, or interpersonal relationships
Tricyclic antidepressants (e.g., amitriptyline [Elavil])	Fatigue
	Fear of failure to perform
Endocrine	
Addison's disease	**Vascular**
Diabetes mellitus	Aortic aneurysm
Obesity	Aortofemoral bypass surgery
Pituitary tumor	Atherosclerosis of pelvic blood vessels
Prolactin (high levels)	
Testosterone deficiency	
Thyrotoxicosis	

Clinical Manifestations and Complications

A patient's self-report of problems associated with sexual performance is the typical symptom of ED. The patient usually describes an inability to attain or maintain an erection. The symptoms may occur only occasionally, or may be continual having had a gradual onset, or may occur with a sudden onset. A gradual onset of symptoms usually is associated with physiologic ED, whereas sudden or rapid onset of symptoms is typically associated with ED caused by psychologic issues.

The major complication of ED is that the man's inability to perform sexually can cause great distress in his interpersonal relationships and may interfere with his concept of himself as a man. Problems with ED can lead to a number of personal issues, including anger or depression.

Diagnostic Studies

The first step in diagnosis and management of ED begins with a thorough sexual, health, and psychosocial history. Self-administered assessment and treatment-related questionnaires have been developed and may prove useful as primary screening tools. For example, the International Index of Erectile Function (IIEF) identifies a man's response to five key areas of male sexual function: erectile function, orgasmic function, sexual desire, intercourse satisfaction, and overall satisfaction.[37] Second, a physical examination should be performed that focuses on secondary sexual characteristics, including pubic hair distribution, size and appearance of the penis and scrotum, and rectal examination. Assessment of blood pressure, palpation of peripheral pulses, and sensation of the genitalia should also be included.

Further examination or diagnostic testing is typically based on findings from the history and physical examination. A serum glucose and lipid profile is recommended to rule out diabetes mellitus. Hormonal levels for testosterone, prolactin, LH, and thyroid may help identify endocrine-related problems, and other blood chemistries and complete blood count may be helpful in identifying unrecognized systemic diseases.

Other diagnostic tests may be conducted to diagnose ED. Nocturnal penile tumescence and rigidity testing is a noninvasive method that involves the continuous measurement of penile circumference and axial rigidity during sleep. Such measurements are used to differentiate between physiologic or psychogenic causes of ED, as well as to evaluate the effectiveness of drug therapy. Vascular studies, including penile arteriography, penile blood flow study, and duplex Doppler ultrasound studies, are used to assess penile blood inflow and outflow. Such studies help assess vascular problems interfering with erection.

Collaborative Care

The goal of ED therapy is for the patient and his partner to achieve a satisfactory sexual relationship. The treatment for ED is based on the underlying cause.

A variety of treatment options are available[38] (Table 55-11). Patients should be advised that none of the options will restore ejaculation or tactile sensations if they were absent before treatment. The results of these interventions are usually most satisfactory when both partners are involved in the decision-making process and have realistic expectations of the treatment.

It is important to determine if ED is reversible before treatment is started. For example, if ED appears to be a side effect of prescribed drugs, alternative agents and/or treatments should be explored. When there is an established diagnosis of testicular failure

TABLE 55-11	*COLLABORATIVE CARE* **Erectile Dysfunction**

Diagnostic
History and physical examination
Sexual history
Serum glucose and lipid profile
Testosterone, prolactin, and thyroid hormone levels
Nocturnal penile tumescence and rigidity testing
Vascular studies

Collaborative Therapy
Modify reversible causes
Drug therapy
• sildenafil (Viagra)
• vardenafil (Levitra)
• tadalafil (Cialis)
Vacuum constriction device (VCD)
Intraurethral medication pellet
Intracavernosal self-injection
Penile implants
Sexual counseling

(hypogonadism), androgen replacement therapy may sometimes be effective in improving erectile function. For individuals who have ED that is psychologic in nature, counseling for the patient (and possibly his partner) is recommended.[38] This counseling should be carried out by a qualified therapist.

Oral Drug Therapy. Sildenafil (Viagra), tadalafil (Cialis), and vardenafil (Levitra) are erectogenic drugs. These drugs cause smooth muscle relaxation and increased blood flow into the corpus cavernosum, thus promoting penile erection. They are taken orally about 1 hour before sexual activity, but not more than once a day. These drugs have been found to be generally safe and effective for the treatment of most types of ED. A rare side effect of blindness due to a blockage of blood to the optic nerve may occur. Because these drugs may potentiate the hypotensive effect of nitrates, they are contraindicated for individuals taking nitrates (such as nitroglycerin).

Drug Alert - *Sildenafil (Viagra)*
• *Should not be used with nitrates (nitroglycerin) in any form.*
• *Can potentiate hypotensive effects of nitrates.*

Vacuum Constriction Devices. Vacuum constriction devices (VCDs) are suction devices that can be applied to the flaccid penis to produce an erection by pulling blood up into the corporeal bodies. A penile ring or constrictive band is placed around the base of the penis to retain venous blood, thereby preventing the erection from subsiding (Fig. 55-11). Special care must be taken in using these devices to prevent tissue bruising.

Intraurethral Devices. These interventions include the use of vasoactive drugs administered as topical gel, an injection into the penis (intracavernosal self-injection) (Fig. 55-12, *B*), or insertion of a medication pellet (alprostadil) into the urethra (intraurethral) using a medicated urethral system for erection (MUSE) device (Fig. 55-12, *A*). These vasoactive drugs enhance blood flow into the penile arteries. Current vasoactive medications include papaverine (topical gel or injection), alprostadil (Caverject) (topical gel, transurethral pellet, or injection), and phentolamine (Vasomax).

The vasoactive medication dose is regulated on an individual basis to prevent side effects. Side effects may include penile pain, priapism, corporal fibrosis, fibrotic nodules, and hypoten-

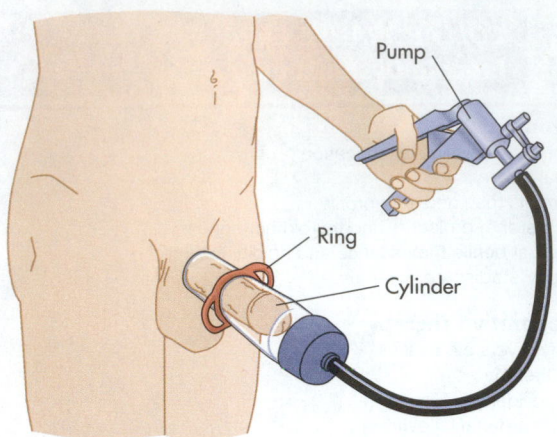

FIG. 55-11 Vacuum constriction device. With the vacuum device in place, blood can be drawn into the penis by means of a hand pump. This creates an erection. For intercourse, the ring is slipped to the base of the penis and the cylinder removed.

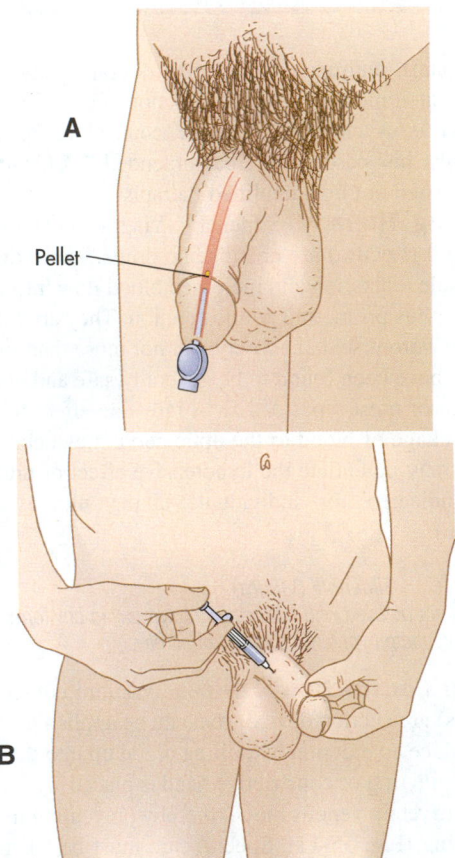

FIG. 55-12 **A,** Intraurethral insertion of medicated pellet (alprostadil) using a medicated urethral system for erection (MUSE) device. **B,** Intracavernosal self-injection. Self-injection therapy involves injecting a medication directly into the penis. This increases blood flow and causes an erection.

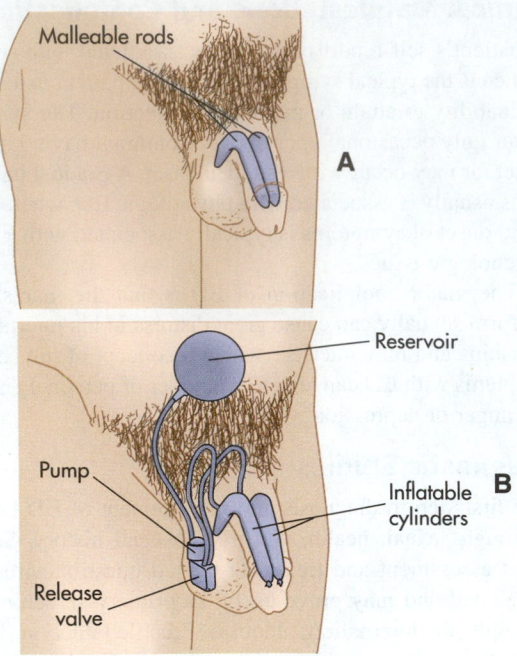

FIG. 55-13 Penile implants. **A,** Malleable implant is always erect but can be bent close to body for concealment. **B,** Inflatable implant consists of cylinders in the penis, a small pump in the scrotum, and a reservoir in the lower abdomen. When activated, the pump fills the cylinders with fluid from the reservoir. A small release valve permits the fluid to drain back into the reservoir after intercourse.

sion. It is important to instruct patients carefully on the specific administration techniques and precautions for any of the vasoactive medications.

Home injection therapy instruction is given to those men who are suitable candidates for the therapy. The injection is nearly painless and generally begins to work in 20 to 30 minutes. Success rates have been high when there is adequate patient teaching and follow-up. This treatment is not suitable for men with severe vas-

cular problems, intolerance for transient hypotension, severe psychiatric disease, poor manual dexterity, or poor vision or those receiving anticoagulant therapy. The man may discontinue treatment if he perceives a lack of spontaneity, has a needle phobia, or wants a more permanent treatment option.

Penile Implants. Surgical implants of semirigid or inflatable penile prostheses are shown in Fig. 55-13. These surgical procedures are highly invasive and associated with potential complications. Thus they are usually indicated for men with severe ED for which other interventions are ineffective.

The devices are implanted into the corporeal bodies to provide an erection firm enough for penetration. The semirigid malleable implant is displayed in Fig. 55-13, *A.* The inflatable implant consists of cylinders in the penis, a small pump in the scrotum, and a reservoir in the lower abdomen (Fig. 55-13, *B*). The main problems associated with penile prostheses are mechanical failure, infection, and erosions.

For healthy men the surgical procedure may be performed on an outpatient basis, with patients also being monitored on an outpatient basis. Complete recovery time varies from 4 to 6 weeks. Despite their high cost and invasiveness, penile implants are associated with high rates of personal satisfaction.

Sexual Counseling. Sexual counseling is often recommended before and after treatment. The ability to please both partners enhances satisfaction levels. Counseling should address psychologic or interpersonal factors that may enhance sexual expression, as well as other factors that are of concern. Counseling can be effective for the individual patient, but it is typically preferred to include his partner, particularly if he is involved in a long-term relationship. Counseling should begin before the start of medical treatment for ED.

TABLE 55-12	Clinical Manifestations of Andropause

- Loss of libido
- Fatigue and lethargy
- Erectile dysfunction
- Memory loss
- Depression and mood changes
- Sleep disturbances and irritability
- Infertility
- Increased body fat
- Decreased cognitive function
- Decreased bone density
- Loss of muscle mass and strength

NURSING MANAGEMENT
ERECTILE DYSFUNCTION

The man experiencing ED requires a great deal of emotional support for both himself and his partner. Men often do not feel comfortable discussing their problems with others because of society's expectations of a man's sexual abilities. The man may experience and demonstrate isolation from support systems, and he may also lose self-esteem.

The patient needs reassurance that confidentiality will be maintained. In conjunction with medical treatment, it often becomes necessary to provide counseling and therapy for the couple to establish realistic expectations and develop meaningful communication patterns. The majority of men delay seeking medical assistance. They are often highly motivated and expect immediate solutions to their problems. The health care team should provide a support system and accurate information as soon as possible.

Nurses are in a unique position of conducting routine health assessments on men seeking any form of medical treatment. It provides an opportunity to ask questions pertaining to general health, as well as sexual health and function. Given the opportunity, men will be less hesitant to answer these questions when they know that someone cares and can provide them with answers.

ANDROPAUSE

Andropause is a decline in androgen secretion that occurs in most men as they age. The slow and continuous loss of androgens (e.g., testosterone) has also been called *male menopause, late-onset hypogonadism,* and *aging male syndrome.*[39] Andropause can begin as early as age 40 with gradual decreases until the end of life. Factors that determine the rate of decline are not clearly known. Signs and symptoms associated with a lowered level of testosterone include loss of libido, fatigue, and erectile dysfunction (Table 55-12). Symptoms are often attributed to normal aging and are not frequently reported by the patient. Long-term effects can include osteoporosis and decreased muscle mass and strength.

A diagnosis of andropause is made after a complete physical examination with serum total testosterone levels obtained. Normal testosterone levels can range from 300 ng/dl to 1000 ng/dl. Replacement therapy may be considered once levels are below 250 ng/dl.[40] Testosterone replacement therapy (TRT) should not be started until the patient, in consultation with his health care provider, considers the risks and benefits of therapy. Symptoms may improve with TRT, but potential risks include lowered levels of high-density lipoprotein (HDL) cholesterol, increased hematocrit, and worsening sleep apnea. The effect of androgens on prostatic

tissue makes this therapy contraindicated in patients with BPH or prostate cancer. Before initiating treatment, a DRE and PSA test should be performed. Once TRT begins, patients should be closely monitored by their health care provider.

Replacement therapy is available in different forms. Oral TRT is not currently available in the United States due to concerns with liver damage. Intramuscular injections such as cypionate (Depo-Testosterone) and enanthate (Delatest) are available in varying dosages and are the least costly form of replacement. However, they create a cyclic rise and fall in serum testosterone levels. Side effects include mood swings with these fluctuations. Transdermal preparations include patches and gels (e.g., Androderm, Testim), which are more convenient but also more costly than injections. They are generally applied to the skin daily to various sites, including the back, arm, and abdomen. Skin irritation is the most common side effect. Triamcinolone creams (diacetate [Amcort], acetonide [Kenalog]) rubbed into the skin before application of the patch may decrease and prevent irritation. A newer form of sustained- and controlled-release TRT is by buccal administration.

INFERTILITY

Infertility in a couple is defined as the inability to achieve conception despite 1 year of frequent unprotected intercourse. Infertility is a disorder of a couple, not of one individual. For this reason, both partners must be involved in determining the cause of infertility. The primary cause of infertility is due to factors involving the man in about 33% of the cases. Male infertility can be caused by disorders of the hypothalamic-pituitary system, disorders of the testes, and abnormalities of the ejaculatory system.

The physical causes are generally divided into three categories: pretesticular, testicular, and posttesticular. The pretesticular or endocrine causes occur only in about 3% of the cases and can generally be treated with medication or surgery. Testicular problems make up 50% of the cases. The most common cause of male infertility is a varicocele.[41] Other factors that influence the testes include infection (e.g., mumps virus, STDs, bacterial infections), congenital anomalies, medications, radiation, substance abuse (alcohol, nicotine, drugs), and environmental hazards. Posttesticular causes account for approximately 5% to 7% of the cases, with obstruction, infection, or the result of a surgical procedure being the primary causes. The remaining 40% are classified as *idiopathic* or of unknown causes.

A careful health history and examination may reveal the cause of a patient's infertility. Thus the history is a starting point for determining cause and treatment. The history should include age; occupation; past injury, surgery, or infections to the genital tract; lifestyle issues such as hot tubs, weight training, or wearing tight undergarments; sexual practices; frequency of intercourse; and emotional factors such as stress levels and the desire for children. The use of drugs, such as chemotherapeutic agents, anabolic steroids (testosterone), sulfasalazine (Azulfidine), cimetidine (Tagamet), and recreational drugs, should be documented because these can reduce sperm count. A physical examination can disclose a varicocele, Peyronie's disease, or other physical abnormalities.

The first test in an infertility study is a semen analysis. The test determines the sperm concentration (count greater than 20 million/ml), forward progressive motility (at least 60% with a grade greater than 2), and morphology (at least 60% have normal oval head and long tail). Additional tests that may be helpful in determining the etiology include plasma testosterone and serum LH and FSH measurements. A test for sperm penetration abilities may also be done. The specific cause of infertility is often not determined.

The nurse should be concerned and tactful in dealing with the male patient undergoing infertility studies. For many men, fertility and masculinity are equated. The nurse must be sensitive to the problem of gender identity in the infertile man.

Treatment options for the man include medications, conservative lifestyle changes (e.g., avoidance of scrotal heat, substance abuse, high stress), in vitro fertilization techniques, and corrective surgery. Achievement of pregnancy varies from 8% to 60% and ranges in cost from several hundred to several thousand dollars. Infertility can seriously strain a marriage, and the couple may require counseling and discussion of alternatives if conception is not achieved. (Female infertility is discussed in Chapter 54.)

CRITICAL THINKING EXERCISE

CASE STUDY

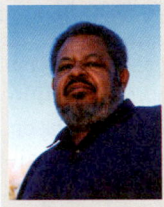

Benign Prostatic Hyperplasia

Patient Profile. Phillip Lockwood, a 66-year-old African American married man, comes to the primary health outpatient clinic because of an inability to void for the past 12 hours and pain in the lower abdomen.

Subjective Data
• Complains of the urge to void
• Is restless and agitated

Case Study photo ©iStockphoto.com/ Floyd Willis.

Objective Data
• Has prostate enlargement on digital rectal examination
• Has hematuria and WBCs in urine
• Has a tender and palpable bladder above the umbilicus
• PSA test: 6 ng/ml

Collaborative Care
• Indwelling catheter inserted by a urology resident
• Admitted to the hospital

Critical Thinking Questions

1. What risk factors for acute urinary retention and BPH are present in Phillip?
2. Explain the etiology of the objective symptoms Phillip exhibited.
3. Discuss the drug options available to Phillip.
4. Discuss the invasive options available to Phillip.
5. Phillip asks you about the effect of the various treatment options on his ability to have sex. How would you respond?
6. What is the priority nursing intervention for Phillip?
7. Write one or more appropriate nursing diagnoses based on the assessment data presented. Are there any collaborative problems?
8. On further assessment, you note that Phillip has a nursing diagnosis of decisional conflict. How would you help him resolve this conflict related to treatment options?

NCLEX EXAMINATION REVIEW QUESTIONS

The number of the question corresponds to the same-numbered objective at the beginning of the chapter.

1. An elderly male patient is experiencing difficulty in initiating voiding and a feeling of incomplete bladder emptying. These symptoms of BPH are primarily caused by
   a. obstruction of the urethra.
   b. decreased bladder compliance.
   c. prostate compression of the bladder.
   d. excessive accumulation of testosterone.

2. Postoperatively, a patient who has had a transurethral prostatectomy has continuous bladder irrigation with a three-way urinary catheter with a 30-ml balloon and traction applied. The patient complains of bladder spasms with the catheter in place. The nurse should
   a. deflate the catheter balloon to 10 ml to decrease bulk in the bladder.
   b. deflate the catheter balloon and then reinflate to ensure that it is patent.
   c. encourage the patient to try to have a bowel movement to relieve colon pressure.
   d. explain that this feeling is normal and that he should not try to urinate around the catheter.

3. In teaching health promotion related to early detection of prostate cancer, the nurse advises that beginning at middle age, men should have an annual
   a. urinalysis.
   b. prostatic ultrasound.
   c. digital rectal examination.
   d. prostatic acid phosphatase (PAP).

4. A patient scheduled for a prostatectomy for prostate cancer expresses the fear that he will have erectile dysfunction. In responding to the patient, the nurse must keep in mind that
   a. erectile dysfunction is a possibility even with a nerve-sparing procedure.
   b. the most common complication of this surgery is postoperative urinary retention.
   c. retrograde ejaculation occurs more frequently than erectile dysfunction in the long term.
   d. a penile implant is the best method to treat erectile dysfunction and should be considered after he has recovered from his surgery.

5. The nurse advises the patient with chronic prostatitis that management includes
   a. fluid restriction.
   b. an indwelling catheter.
   c. effective antibiotic therapy.
   d. sexual activities that result in ejaculation.

6. Discharge teaching for the patient who has had a vasectomy includes explaining that
   a. the procedure blocks the production of sperm.
   b. the ejaculate will be about half the volume it was before the procedure.
   c. an alternative form of contraception will be necessary for 6 to 8 weeks.
   d. erectile dysfunction is temporary and will return with continued sexual activity.

7. A nursing measure that can decrease the patient's discomfort over care involving his reproductive organs is
   a. relating his sexual concerns to his sexual partner.
   b. arranging to have only male nurses care for the patient.
   c. maintaining a nonjudgmental attitude toward his sexual practices.
   d. using only technical terminology when discussing reproductive function.

REFERENCES

1. Waldert M, Djavan B: Transurethral microwave therapy for treatment of benign prostatic hyperplasia, *J Men's Health Gender* 1:182, 2004.
2. Rohrmann S, Platz E, Giovannucci E: Lifestyle and benign prostatic hyperplasia in older men: what do we know? *J Men's Health Gender* 1:182, 2004.
3. Barry B et al: The American Urologic Association symptom index for benign prostatic hyperplasia, *J Urol* 148:1549, 1992.
4. National Kidney and Urologic Diseases Information Clearinghouse: Prostate enlargement: benign prostatic hyperplasia, National Institute of Diabetes and Digestive and Kidney Diseases, National Institutes of Health, February 2004. Available at *www.kidney.niddk.nih.gov* (accessed September 12, 2005).
5. Lam J, Cooper K, Kaplan S: Changing aspects in the evaluation and treatment of patients with benign prostatic hyperplasia, *Med Clin North Am* 88:281, 2004.
6. Barry M, Collins M: Benign prostatic hyperplasia and prostatitis. In Goldman L, editor: *Cecil textbook of medicine*, ed 22, St Louis, 2004, Saunders.
7. Atug F, Castle E, Thomas R: Office-based prostate procedures, *Urol Clin North Am* 32:327, 2005.
8. Hoffman R, MacDonald R, Wilt T: Laser prostatectomy for benign prostatic obstruction, *Cochrane Library* 3, 2005 (#CD001987).
9. Huynh P, Dickno A: Benign prostatic hyperplasia. In Rakel R, editor: *Conn's current therapy*, ed 57, St Louis, 2005, Elsevier.
10. Ogiste J, Cooper K, Kaplan S: Are stents a useful therapy for benign prostatic hyperplasia? *Curr Opin Urol* 13:51, 2003.
11. Jenal A et al: Cancer statistics 2005, *CA Cancer J Clin* 55:10, 2005.
12. American Cancer Society: *Cancer facts and figures 2005*, Atlanta, 2005, American Cancer Society. Available at *www.cancer.org*.
13. Woods et al: Culture, black men, and prostate cancer: what is reality? *Cancer Control* 11:388, 2004.
14. Calabrese D: Prostate cancer in older men, *Urol Nurs* 24:258, 2004.
15. Presti J: Neoplasms of the prostate gland. In Tanagho E, McAninch J, editors: *Smith's general urology*, ed 16, New York, 2004, McGraw-Hill.
16. Stoller M, Carroll P: Malignant genitourinary tract disorders. In Tierney L et al, editors: *Current medical diagnosis and treatment 2005,* ed 44, New York, 2005, McGraw-Hill.
17. Stamey T et al: The prostate specific antigen era in the United States is over for prostate cancer: what happened in the last 20 years? *J Urol* 172:1297, 2004.
18. Thompson I et al: Prevalence of prostate cancer among men with a prostate-specific antigen level ≤4.0 ng per milliliter, *N Engl J Med* 350:2239, 2004.
19. University of California, Berkeley, School of Public Health: *Wellness Letter* 21:2, 2005. Available at *www.WellnessLetter.com*.
20. Sweat G: Guiding prostate cancer treatment choices, *Postgrad Med* 117:45, 2005.
*21. Wallace M et al: The watchful waiting management option for older men with prostate cancer: state of the science, *Oncol Nurs Forum* 31:1057, 2004.
22. Talcott J, Manola J, Clark J: Time course and predictors of symptoms after primary prostate cancer therapy, *J Clin Oncol* 21:3979, 2003.
23. Stephenson A et al: Salvage radiotherapy for recurrent prostate cancer after radical prostatectomy, *JAMA* 291:1325, 2004.
24. McCarthy A: Advanced prostate cancer: a focus on therapies, *Cancer Updates, Research and Education (CURE)* 3:33, 2004. Available at *www.curetoday.com*.
25. Held-Warmkessel J: Prostate cancer. In Yarbro C et al, editors: *Cancer nursing principles and practice*, ed 6, Boston, 2005, Jones & Bartlett.
26. Diaz M, Patterson S: Management of androgen-independent prostate cancer, *Cancer Control* 11:364, 2004.
27. Naber K, Weidner W: Prostatitis, epididymitis and orchitis. In Cohen J, Powderly W, editors: *Infectious diseases*, ed 2, St Louis, 2004, Elsevier.
28. Krieger JN, Nyberg L, Nickel JC: NIH consensus definition and classification of prostatitis, *JAMA* 282:236, 1999.
29. Hua V, Schaeffer A: Acute and chronic prostatitis, *Med Clin North Am* 88:483, 2004.
30. McNaughton C, MacDonald W: Interventions for chronic abacterial prostatitis, *Cochrane Library* 3, 2005 (#CD002080).
31. Sadeghi N et al: Priapism, *Radiol Clin North Am* 42:427, 2004.
32. Schrager S: Diethylstilbestrol exposure, *Am Fam Physician* 69:2395, 2004.
33. Feder D: Testicular cancer, *Cancer Updates, Research and Education (CURE)* 3:50, 2004. Available at *www.curetoday.com*.
34. Stevenson T, McNeill J: Surgical management of testicular cancer, *Clin J Oncol Nurs* 8:355, 2004.
35. Lewis J, Rosen R, Goldstein I: Erectile dysfunction, *Nursing* 35:64, 2005.
36. Levy A, Freyberg Z: Sexual dysfunction and aging: building a bridge between genders, *Clin Geriatr* 12:36, 2004.
37. Rosen RC et al: The International Index of Erectile Function (IIEF): a multidimensional scale for assessment of erectile dysfunction, *Urology* 49:822, 1997.
38. Lewis J, Rosen R, Goldstein I: Erectile dysfunction: a panel's recommendation for management, *Am J Nurs* 103:48, 2003.
39. Charlton R: Aging male syndrome, andropause, androgen decline or mid-life crisis? *J Men's Health Gender* 1:55, 2004.
40. Liu P, Swerdloff R, Wong C: Relative testosterone deficiency in older men: clinical definition and presentation, *Endocrinol Metab Clin North Am* 34:957, 2005.
41. Brugh V: Male factor infertility: evaluation and management, *Med Clin North Am* 88:367, 2004.

RESOURCES

American Cancer Society
800-ACS-2345
www.cancer.org
American Urological Association
410-689-3933
www.auanet.org
Lance Armstrong Foundation
512-236-8820
www.livestrong.org
National Prostate Cancer Coalition
888-245-9455 or 202-463-9455
www.4npcc.org
Sexuality Information and Education Council of the United States
212-819-9770
www.siecus.org
Urologic Oncology Program
University of Michigan Comprehensive Cancer Center
Cancer Information Line: 800-865-1125
www.cancer.med.umich.edu/prostcan/prostcan.html
For additional Internet resources, see the website for this book at *http://evolve. elsevier.com/Lewis/medsurg*.

---

*Nursing research–based reference.

Problems Related to Movement and Coordination

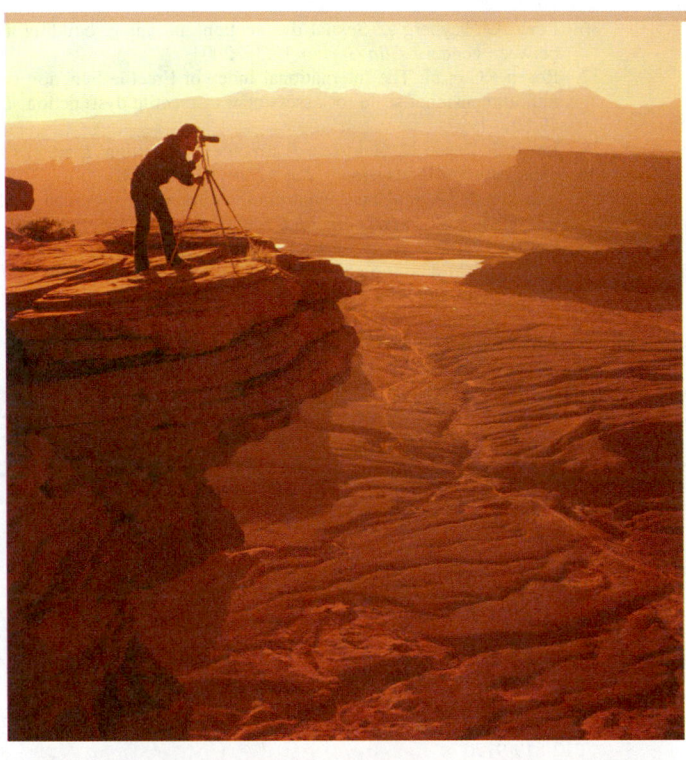

Section Outline

56 **Nursing Assessment**
Nervous System, p. 1441

57 **Nursing Management**
Acute Intracranial Problems, p. 1467

58 **Nursing Management**
Stroke, p. 1502

59 **Nursing Management**
Chronic Neurologic Problems, p. 1527

60 **Nursing Management**
Alzheimer's Disease and Dementia, p. 1561

61 **Nursing Management**
Peripheral Nerve and Spinal Cord Problems, p. 1580

62 **Nursing Assessment**
Musculoskeletal System, p. 1614

63 **Nursing Management**
Musculoskeletal Trauma and Orthopedic Surgery, p. 1629

64 **Nursing Management**
Musculoskeletal Problems, p. 1668

65 **Nursing Management**
Arthritis and Connective Tissue Diseases, p. 1693

It is nice to think how one can be recklessly lost in a daisy.

Anne Morrow Lindbergh

Nursing Assessment
Nervous System

56

Sherry Garrett Hendrickson

LEARNING OBJECTIVES

1. Describe the functions of neurons and neuroglia.
2. Explain the electrochemical aspects of nerve impulse transmission.
3. Explain the anatomic location and functions of the cerebrum, brainstem, cerebellum, spinal cord, peripheral nerves, and cerebrospinal fluid.
4. Identify the major arteries supplying the brain.
5. Describe the functions of the 12 cranial nerves.
6. Compare the functions of the two divisions of the autonomic nervous system.
7. Describe age-related changes in the neurologic system and differences in assessment findings.
8. Identify the significant subjective and objective data related to the nervous system that should be obtained from a patient.
9. Describe the techniques used in the physical assessment of the nervous system.
10. Differentiate normal from common abnormal findings of a physical assessment of the nervous system.
11. Describe the purpose, significance of results, and nursing responsibilities related to diagnostic studies of the nervous system.

KEY TERMS

autonomic nervous system, p. 1449
blood-brain barrier, p. 1452
central nervous system, p. 1442
cerebrospinal fluid, p. 1448
cranial nerves, p. 1448
dermatome, p. 1448
lower motor neurons, p. 1445
meninges, p. 1452
neuroglia, p. 1442
neuron, p. 1442
neurotransmitter, p. 1444
peripheral nervous system, p. 1442
reflex, p. 1445
synapse, p. 1443
upper motor neurons, p. 1445

Electronic Resources

Supplemental content related to Chapter 56 can be found . . .

Companion CD
- Stress-Busting Kit for Nursing Students
- NCLEX Examination Review Questions
- Animations:
  - Motor Pathways and Clinical Evaluation of the Central Nervous System
  - Reflex Arc
  - Sensory Pathways and Clinical Evaluation of the Central Nervous System
- Video Clips:
  - Evaluation: Smell, Cranial Nerve I—Olfactory Nerve
  - Evaluation: Central Vision and Visual Acuity, Cranial Nerve II—Optic Nerve
  - Evaluation: Pupil Responses, Direct and Accommodation, Cranial Nerves III, IV, and VI—Oculomotor, Trochlear, and Abducens Nerves

- Evaluation: Sensory, Light Touch; Face, Upper, and Lower Extremities, Cranial Nerve V—Trigeminal Nerve
- Inspection: Fine Motor Coordination, Upper Extremities
- Inspection: Fine Motor Coordination, Lower Extremities
- Evaluation: Sensory, Face, and Upper Extremities
- Evaluation: Deep Tendon Reflex, Patellar Tendon
- Comprehensive Glossary

Evolve Website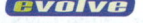
http://evolve.elsevier.com/Lewis/medsurg
- Content Updates
- Key Points (Printable and CD/MP3 Download)
- Concept Map Creator
- Expanded Audio Glossary
- Key Term Flash Cards
- Physical Examination Video Clips:
  - Head and Face; Eyes; Ears
  - Nose, Mouth, and Pharynx
  - Neck
  - Abdominal Reflexes, Abdominal Muscles, and Inguinal Area
  - Neurologic System: Sensory Function; Motor Function and Coordination; Gait and Balance
- Electronic Calculators
- WebLinks

Reviewed by Gayle H. Dasher, RN, PhD, CCRN, CNRN, Director of Clinical Practice and Standards, CHRISTUS Santa Rosa Health Care, San Antonio, Tex.

Nervous System

STRUCTURES AND FUNCTIONS OF THE NERVOUS SYSTEM

The human nervous system is a highly specialized system responsible for the control and integration of the body's many activities. The nervous system can be divided into the central nervous system (CNS) and the peripheral nervous system (PNS). The **central nervous system** consists of the brain and spinal cord. The **peripheral nervous system** consists of the cranial and spinal nerves and the peripheral components of the autonomic nervous system (ANS). Before considering higher order structures and their functions, cellular elements and nerve impulse transmission are discussed.

Cells of the Nervous System

The nervous system is made up of two types of cells: neurons and neuroglia. Although neuroglial cells are more numerous, they are mainly supportive to the **neuron** (the primary functional unit of the nervous system). Neurons are generally nonmitotic, not replicating or replacing themselves if irreversibly damaged. However, recent research demonstrates that neurogenesis from stem cells may occur in adult brains after cerebral injury.[1] Neuroglia are mitotic and can replicate. In general, when neurons are destroyed, the tissue is replaced by the proliferation of neuroglia cells.

Neurons. The neurons of the nervous system come in many different shapes and sizes, but they all share common characteristics: (1) *excitability,* or the ability to generate a nerve impulse; (2) *conductivity,* or the ability to transmit the impulse to other portions of the cell; and (3) the ability to influence other neurons, muscle cells, and glandular cells by transmitting nerve impulses to them.

A typical *neuron* consists of a cell body, an axon, and several dendrites (Fig. 56-1). The cell body containing the nucleus and cytoplasm is the metabolic center of the neuron. *Dendrites* are short processes extending from the cell body. They receive nerve impulses from the axons of other neurons and conduct impulses toward the cell body. The nerve *axon* projects varying distances from the cell body, ranging from several micrometers to more than a meter. Its function is to carry nerve impulses to other neurons or to end organs. The end organs are smooth and striated muscles and glands. Axons may be myelinated or unmyelinated. Many axons present in the CNS and the PNS are covered by a segmentally interrupted myelin sheath composed of a white, lipid substance that acts as an insulator for the conduction of impulses. Generally, the smaller fibers are unmyelinated.

Neuroglia. **Neuroglia,** or glial cells, provide support, nourishment, and protection to neurons. They constitute almost half the brain and spinal cord mass and are 5 to 10 times more numerous than neurons. Different types of glial cells, including oligodendrocytes, astrocytes, ependymal cells, and microglia, have specific functions. *Oligodendrocytes* are specialized cells that produce the myelin sheath of nerve fibers in the CNS (*Schwann cells* myelinate the nerve fibers in the periphery) and are primarily found in the white matter of the CNS.

Astrocytes provide structural support to neurons, and their delicate processes form the blood-brain barrier with the endothelium of the blood vessels, and play a role in synaptic transmission (conduction of impulses between neurons). They are found primarily in gray matter. When the brain is injured, astrocytes act as phagocytes for neuronal debris. They help restore the neurochemical milieu and provide support for repair. Proliferation of astrocytes contributes to the formation of scar tissue (gliosis) in the CNS. *Ependy-*

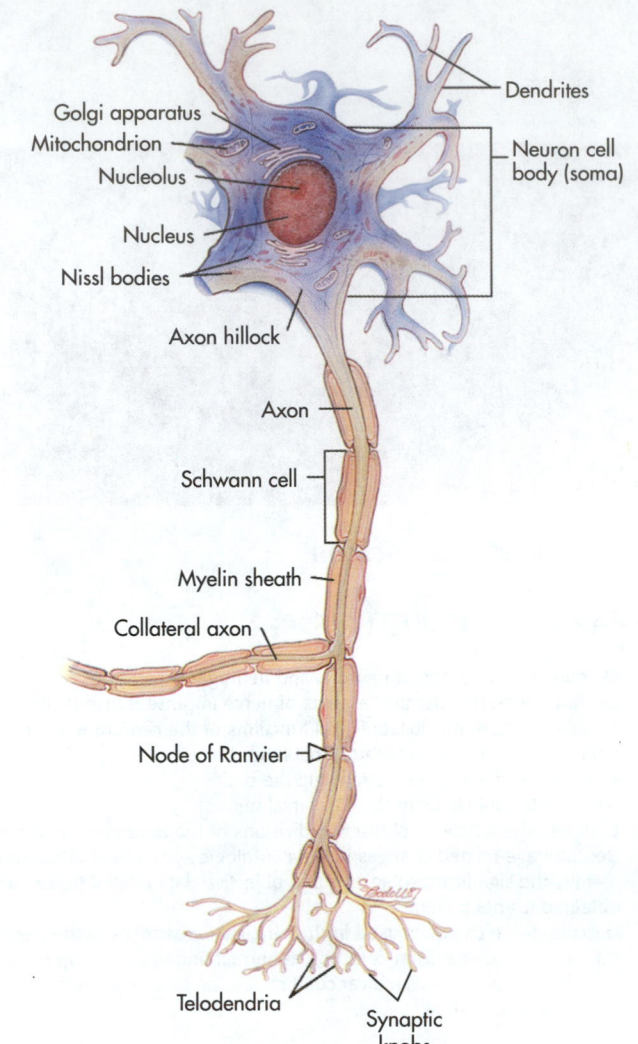

FIG. 56-1   Structural features of neurons: dendrites, cell body, and axons.

mal cells line the brain ventricles and aid in the secretion of cerebrospinal fluid (CSF). *Microglia,* a type of macrophage, are relatively rare in normal CNS tissue. They are phagocytes and are important in host defense.

Most primary CNS tumors involve neuroglia. Primary malignancies involving neurons are rare because these cells are not usually mitotic.

Nerve Regeneration

If the axon of the nerve cell is damaged, the cell attempts to repair itself. When damaged, all nerve cells attempt to grow back to their original destinations by sprouting many branches from the damaged ends of their axons. Unfortunately, axons in the CNS are less successful than peripheral axons in regenerating. Endogenous inhibitors such as neurite outgrowth inhibitor and myelin-associated glycoprotein reduce axon regeneration.[2]

In the PNS (outside the brain and the spinal cord), injured nerve fibers can regenerate by growing within the protective myelin sheath of the supporting Schwann cells if the cell body is intact. The final result of nerve regeneration depends on the number of axon sprouts that join with the appropriate Schwann cell columns and reinnervate appropriate end organs.

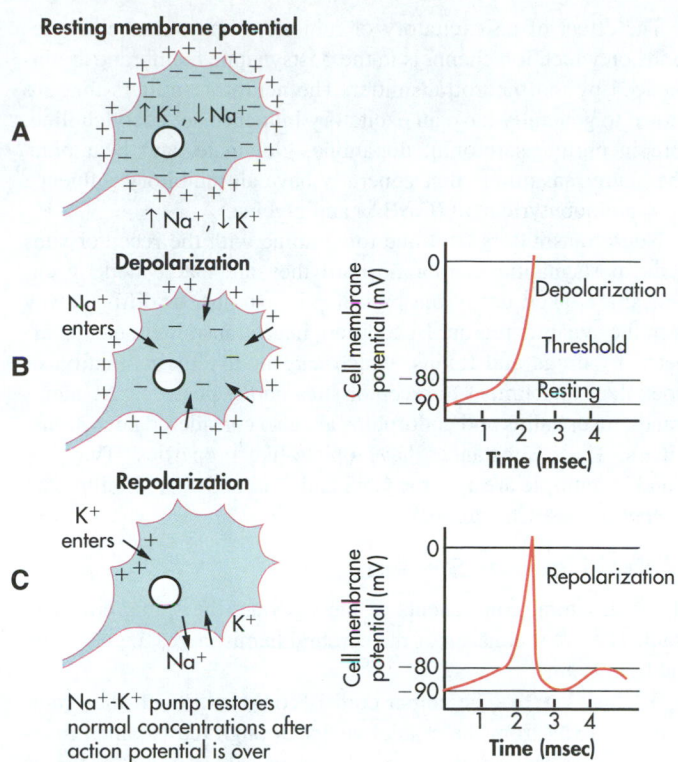

FIG. 56-2 A, Resting membrane potential. **B,** Depolarization. **C,** Repolarization.

Nerve Impulse

The purpose of a neuron is to initiate, receive, and process messages about events both within and outside the body. The initiation of a neuronal message (nerve impulse) involves the generation of an action potential. Once an action potential is initiated, a series of action potentials travel along the axon. When the impulse reaches the end of the nerve fiber, it is transmitted across the junction between nerve cells (synapse) by a chemical interaction involving neurotransmitters. This chemical interaction generates another set of action potentials in the next neuron. These events are repeated until the nerve impulse reaches its destination.

Action Potential. When nerve cells are in a resting (nonactive) state, the inside of the cell carries a negative electric charge relative to the outside of the cell. Sodium ions (Na^+) are in high concentration outside the cell, and potassium ions (K^+) are in high concentration inside the cell. The difference in electric charge across the cell membrane is termed the *resting membrane potential* (Fig. 56-2). An action potential occurs when a stimulus is of sufficient magnitude to alter the membrane potential.

Upon the initiation of the action potential, the cell membrane becomes more permeable to Na^+, allowing the Na^+ to move readily into the cell. The resulting change in the voltage across the cell membrane is called *depolarization*. The inside of the cell temporarily becomes positive relative to the outside. After rapid depolarization, *repolarization* (the inside of the cell becoming negative relative to the outside) is facilitated by a slower increase in K^+ permeability, which in turn is caused by the depolarization associated with entry of Na^+ into the cell. The process of depolarization and repolarization of the nerve cell membrane takes only 1 to 2 milliseconds. With repeated action potentials the cells accumulate Na^+. An active metabolic process within the cell is required to move Na^+ out of and K^+ back into the cell. This metabolic process

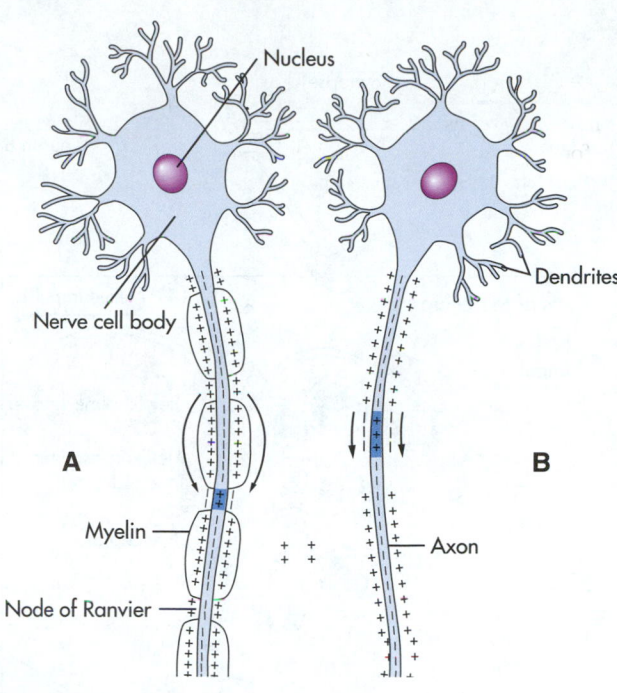

FIG. 56-3 A, Saltatory conduction in a myelinated nerve. **B,** Depolarization in an unmyelinated fiber.

is accomplished by the Na^+-K^+ pump, which requires energy from the breakdown of adenosine triphosphate (ATP).

The action potential has an all-or-none quality. Once the cell depolarizes enough to cause an action potential, the size of the action potential is independent of the strength of the stimulus. When an action potential is initiated at one point of a neuron, it is transmitted along the axon without losing its intensity.

Because of its insulating capacity, myelination of nerve axons facilitates the conduction of an action potential. Many peripheral nerve axons have gaps, termed *nodes of Ranvier,* at regular intervals in the myelin sheath surrounding them. An action potential traveling down one of these axons hops from node to node without traversing the insulated membrane segment between nodes, making the action potential travel much faster than it would otherwise. This is called *saltatory* (hopping) conduction. In an unmyelinated fiber the wave of depolarization traverses the entire length of the axon, with each portion of the membrane becoming depolarized in turn. Fig. 56-3 compares nerve impulse transmission of myelinated and unmyelinated fibers.

Synapse. A **synapse** is the structural and functional junction between two neurons. It is the point at which the nerve impulse is transmitted from one neuron to another or from neuron to glands or muscles. The essential structures of synaptic transmission are a presynaptic terminal, a synaptic cleft, and a receptor site on the postsynaptic cell (Fig. 56-4). There are two types of synapses: electrical and chemical. In an electrical synapse an action potential moves from neuron to neuron directly by allowing electric current to flow between neurons. In a chemical synapse an action potential reaches the end of the axon (presynaptic terminal); then it causes release of a chemical substance (neurotransmitter) from tiny vesicles within the axon terminal. This release depends on influx of calcium, initiated by depolarization of the nerve terminal. The neurotransmitter then crosses the microscopic space (synaptic cleft) between the two neurons and attaches to receptor

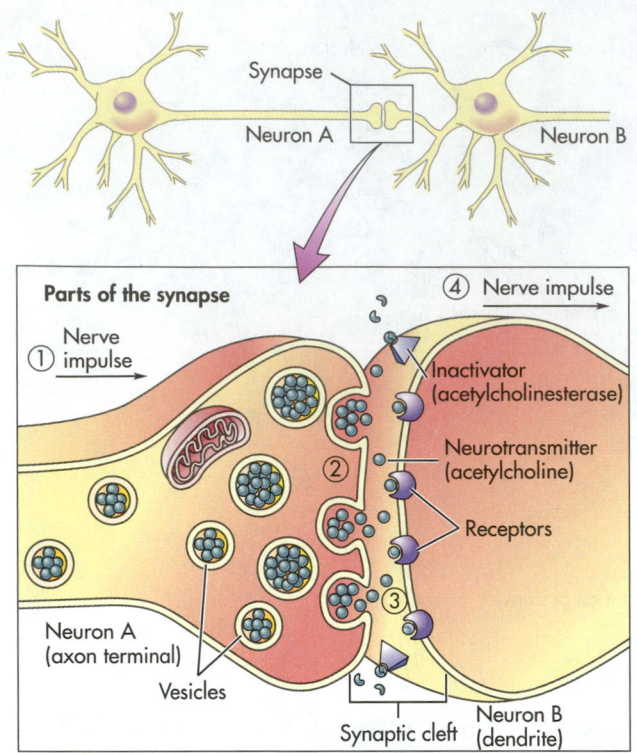

FIG. 56-4 The synapse is located in the space between neuron A and neuron B. Parts of the synapse include the neurotransmitters, inactivators, and receptors. The neurotransmitters are located in the vesicles of neuron A. The inactivators are located on the membrane of neuron B. The receptors are located on the membrane of neuron B.

sites of the receiving (postsynaptic) neuron. This causes a change in the permeability of the postsynaptic cell membrane to specific ions such as Na^+ and K^+ and a change in the electric potential of the membrane.

Neurotransmitters. A **neurotransmitter** is a chemical agent involved in the transmission of an impulse across the synaptic cleft. (Examples of neurotransmitters are presented in Table 56-1.) Some neurotransmitters are excitatory: they cause an increase in Na^+ permeability at the postsynaptic cell membrane, increasing the likelihood that an action potential will be generated. This type of synaptic input results in an excitatory postsynaptic potential. Other neurotransmitters are inhibitory: they cause an increase in permeability of K^+ and chloride (Cl^-) ions, decreasing the likelihood that an action potential will be generated. This type of synaptic input results in an inhibitory postsynaptic potential.

Each of the hundreds to thousands of synaptic connections of a single neuron has an influence on that neuron. The net effect of the input is sometimes excitatory and sometimes inhibitory. In general, the net effect depends on the number of presynaptic neurons that are releasing neurotransmitters on the postsynaptic cell. A presynaptic cell that releases an excitatory neurotransmitter does not always cause the postsynaptic cell to depolarize enough to generate an action potential. However, when many presynaptic cells release excitatory neurotransmitters on a single neuron, the sum of their input is enough to generate an action potential. The presynaptic input can be summed by the number of presynaptic cells firing (*spatial summation*) or by the frequency of firing of a single presynaptic cell (*temporal summation*). Summation usually occurs by both events.

The effect of an excitatory or inhibitory neurotransmitter depends on which ion channels in the postsynaptic membrane are influenced by that neurotransmitter. The neurotransmitters that are known to generally have an excitatory influence are acetylcholine, norepinephrine, serotonin, dopamine, glutamate, and histamine. The neurotransmitters that generally have an inhibitory influence are γ-aminobutyric acid (GABA) and glycine.

Neurotransmitters continue to combine with the receptor sites at the postsynaptic membrane until they are inactivated by enzymes, are taken up by the presynaptic endings, or diffuse away from the synaptic region. In addition, neurotransmitters can be affected by drugs and toxins, which can modify their function or block their attachment to receptor sites on the postsynaptic membrane. Enkephalins and endorphins are also considered neurotransmitters. These substances have opiate-like properties. They are found in multiple areas of the CNS and PNS and act to inhibit pain perception (see Chapter 10).

Central Nervous System

Major structural components of the CNS are the spinal cord and brain. The brain consists of the cerebral hemispheres, cerebellum, and brainstem.

Spinal Cord. The spinal cord is continuous with the brainstem and exits from the cranial cavity through the foramen magnum. A cross section of the spinal cord reveals gray matter that is centrally located in an H shape and is surrounded by white matter (Fig. 56-5). The gray matter contains the cell bodies of voluntary motor neurons and preganglionic autonomic motor neurons, as well as cell bodies of association neurons (interneurons). The white matter contains the axons of the ascending sensory and the descending (suprasegmental) motor fibers. The myelin surrounding these fibers gives them their white appearance. Specific ascending and descending pathways in the white matter can be identified. The spinal pathways or tracts are named for the point of origin and the point of destination (e.g., spinocerebellar tract [ascending], corticospinal tract [descending]). The major spinal pathways are presented in Fig. 56-5.

Ascending Tracts. In general, the ascending tracts carry specific sensory information to higher levels of the CNS. This information comes from special sensory endings (receptors) in the skin, muscles and joints, viscera, and blood vessels and enters the spinal cord by way of the dorsal roots of the spinal nerves. The fasciculus gracilis and the fasciculus cuneatus (commonly called the dorsal or posterior columns) carry information and transmit impulses concerned with touch, deep pressure, vibration, position sense, and kinesthesia (appreciation of movement, weight, and body parts). The *spinocerebellar tracts* carry subconscious information about muscle tension and body position to the cerebellum for coordination of movement. This information is not consciously perceived. The *spinothalamic tracts* carry pain and temperature sensations. Therefore the ascending tracts are organized by sensory modality, as well as by anatomy.

Although the functions of these pathways are generally accepted, other ascending tracts may also carry sensory modalities. The symptoms of various neurologic diseases suggest that additional pathways for touch, position sense, and vibration exist.

Descending Tracts. Descending tracts carry impulses that are responsible for muscle movement. Among the most important descending tracts are the corticobulbar and corticospinal tracts, collectively termed the *pyramidal tract*. These tracts carry volitional (vol-

TABLE 56-1	**Examples of Neurotransmitters**	
Substance	**Location***	**Clinical Example***
Acetylcholine	Many parts of the brain and spinal cord, neuromuscular junction of skeletal muscle, and many ANS synapses	A decrease in acetylcholine-secreting neurons is seen in Alzheimer's disease; myasthenia gravis results from a reduction in acetylcholine receptors.
Amines		
Epinephrine	Many areas of the brain	Acts as a hormone when secreted by the neurosecretory cells of the adrenal medulla.
Norepinephrine	Many areas of the brain; also in postganglionic neurons of sympathetic nervous system	Cocaine and amphetamines,[†] resulting in overstimulation of postsynaptic neurons.
Serotonin	Many areas of the brain and spinal cord	Involved with moods, emotions, and sleep; levels of serotonin elevated in schizophrenia.
Dopamine	Some areas of the brain	Involved in emotions and moods and regulating motor control. Parkinson's disease results from destructions of dopamine-secreting neurons.
Amino Acids		
γ-Aminobutyric acid (GABA)	Most neurons of the CNS	Drugs that increase GABA function have been used to treat seizure disorders.
Glycine	Spinal cord	Glycine receptors inhibited by strychnine.
Glutamate and aspartate	Widespread in the brain and spinal cord	Drugs that block glutamate or aspartate are under development; might prevent seizures and neural degeneration from overexcitation.
Neuropeptides		
Endorphins and enkephalins	Widely distributed in the CNS and PNS, retina, intestinal tract	The opiates morphine and heroin bind to endorphin and enkephalin receptors on presynaptic neurons and reduce pain by blocking the release of neurotransmitter.
Substance P	Spinal cord, brain, and sensory pathways associated with pain, GI tract	Neurotransmitter in pain transmission pathways; morphine blocks its release.

ANS, Autonomic nervous system; *CNS,* central nervous system; *GI,* gastrointestinal; *PNS,* peripheral nervous system.
*These are examples only; most of the neurotransmitters are also found in other locations and may have additional functions.
†Increase the release and block the reuptake of norepinephrine.

untary) impulses from the cortex to the cranial and peripheral nerves, respectively. Another group of descending motor tracts carries impulses from the extrapyramidal system, which includes all motor systems (except the pyramidal system) concerned with voluntary movement. It includes descending pathways originating in the brainstem, basal ganglia, and cerebellum. The motor output exits the spinal cord by way of the ventral roots of the spinal nerves.

Lower and Upper Motor Neurons. Lower motor neurons (LMNs) are the final common pathway through which descending motor tracts influence skeletal muscle, the effector organ for movement. The cell bodies of LMNs, which send axons to innervate the skeletal muscles of the arms, trunk, and legs, are located in the anterior horn of the corresponding segments of the spinal cord (e.g., cervical segments contain LMNs for the arms). LMNs for skeletal muscles of the eyes, face, mouth, and throat are located in the corresponding segments of the brainstem. These cell bodies and their axons make up the somatic motor components of the cranial nerves. LMN lesions generally cause weakness or paralysis, denervation atrophy, hyporeflexia or areflexia, and decreased muscle tone (flaccidity).

Upper motor neurons (UMNs) originate in the cerebral cortex and project downward. The corticobulbar tract ends in the brainstem, and the corticospinal tract descends into the spinal cord. These neurons influence skeletal muscle movement. UMN lesions generally cause weakness or paralysis, disuse atrophy, hyperreflexia, and increased muscle tone (spasticity).

Reflex Arc. A **reflex** is defined as an involuntary response to a stimulus. The components of a monosynaptic reflex arc (the simplest kind of reflex arc) are a receptor organ, an afferent neuron, an effector neuron, and an effector organ (e.g., skeletal muscle). The afferent neuron synapses with the efferent neuron in the gray matter of the spinal cord. A reflex arc is shown in Fig. 56-6. More complex reflex arcs have other neurons (interneurons) in addition to the afferent neuron influencing the effector neuron. In the spinal cord, reflex arcs play an important role in maintaining muscle tone, which is essential for body posture.

Brain. The brain can be divided into three major components: cerebrum, brainstem, and cerebellum.

Cerebrum. The *cerebrum* is composed of the right and left hemispheres. Both hemispheres can be further divided into four major lobes: frontal, temporal, parietal, and occipital (Fig. 56-7). The frontal lobe controls higher cognitive function, memory retention, voluntary eye movements, voluntary motor movement, and expressive speech in Broca's area. Behind the frontal lobe, the temporal lobe contains Wernicke's area, which is responsible for receptive speech and for integration of somatic, visual, and auditory data. The parietal lobe is composed of the sensory cortex, controlling and interpreting spatial information. Processing of sight takes place in the occipital lobe.

These divisions are useful to delineate portions of the neocortex (gray matter), which makes up the outer layer of the cerebral hemispheres. Neurons in specific parts of the neocortex are essential for various highly complex and sophisticated aspects of mental functioning, such as language, memory, and appreciation of visual-spatial relationships.

The functions of the cerebrum are multiple and complex. Specific areas of the cerebral cortex are associated with specific functions. Table 56-2 summarizes the location and function of the parts of the cerebrum.

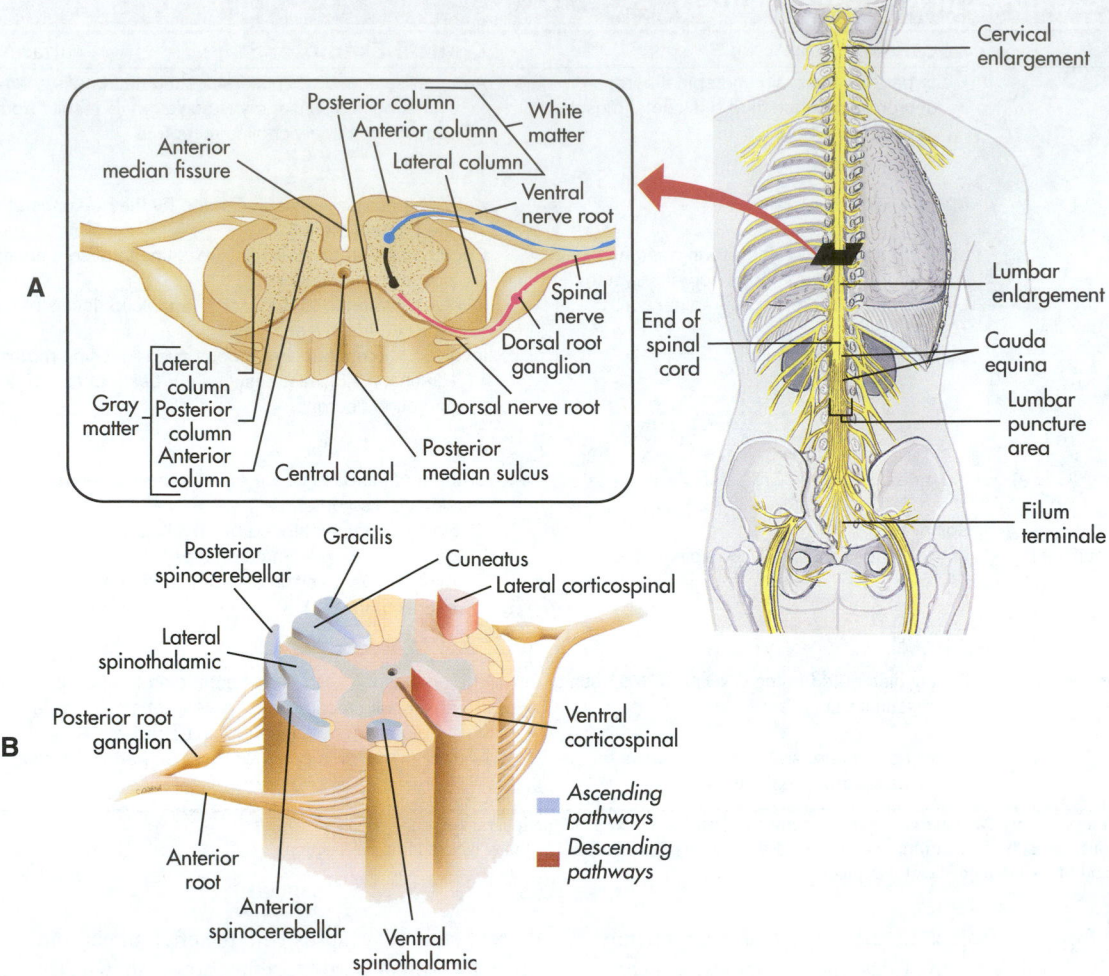

FIG. 56-5 Spinal cord. **A,** *Inset* illustrates a transverse section of the spinal cord shown in the broader view. **B,** Cross section of the spinal cord showing the horns, pathways (nerve tracts), and roots.

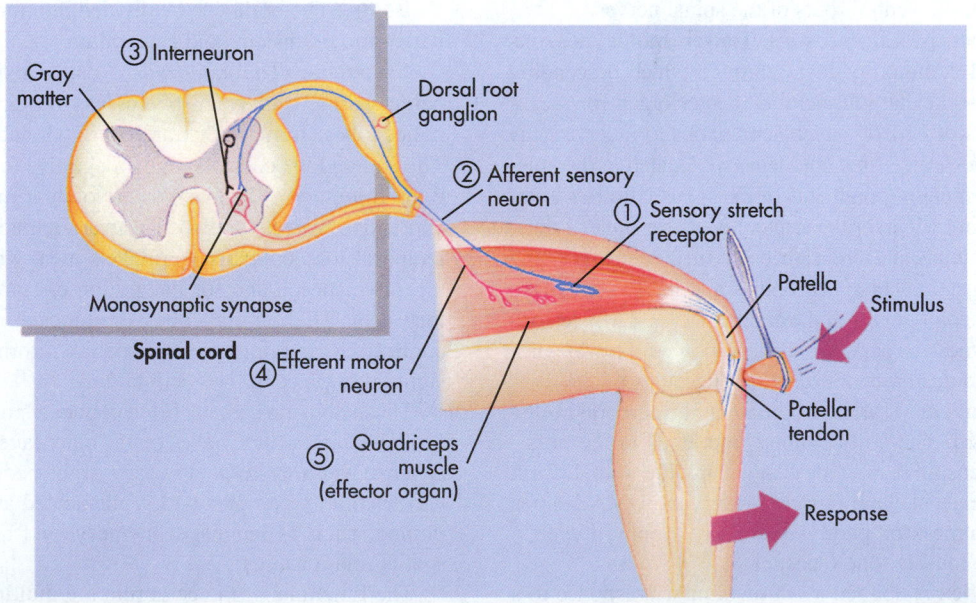

FIG. 56-6 Basic diagram of the patellar "knee jerk" reflex arc, including the *(1)* sensory stretch receptor, *(2)* afferent sensory neuron, *(3)* interneuron, *(4)* efferent motor neuron, and *(5)* quadriceps muscle (effector organ).

The basal ganglia, thalamus, hypothalamus, and limbic system are also located in the cerebrum. The basal ganglia are a group of paired structures located centrally in the cerebrum and midbrain; most of them are on both sides of the thalamus. The function of the basal ganglia is to modulate the initiation, execution, and completion of voluntary movements and automatic movements associated with skeletal muscle activity, such as swinging of the arms while walking, swallowing saliva, and blinking.

The thalamus (part of the diencephalon) lies directly above the brainstem (Fig. 56-8) and is the major relay center for sensory and other afferent (i.e., cerebellar) inputs to the cerebral cortex. The hypothalamus is located just inferior to the thalamus and slightly in front of the midbrain. It regulates the ANS and the endocrine system. The limbic system is, phylogenetically, an old part of the human cerebrum. It is located near the inner surfaces of the cerebral hemispheres (Fig. 56-9) and is concerned with emotion, aggression, feeding behavior, and sexual response.

Brainstem. The *brainstem* includes the midbrain, pons, and medulla (see Fig. 56-8). Ascending and descending fibers pass through the brainstem going to and from the cerebrum and cerebellum. The cell bodies, or nuclei, of cranial nerves III through XII are in the brainstem. Also located in the brainstem is the *reticular formation,* a diffusely arranged group of neurons and their axons that extends from the medulla to the thalamus and hypothalamus. The functions of the reticular formation include relaying sensory information, influencing excitatory and inhibitory control of spinal motor neurons, and controlling vasomotor and respiratory activity. The reticular activating system is part of the reticular formation and is the regulatory system for arousal, a component of consciousness.

The vital centers concerned with respiratory, vasomotor, and cardiac function are located in the medulla. The brainstem also contains the centers for sneezing, coughing, hiccupping, vomiting, sucking, and swallowing.

Cerebellum. The cerebellum is located in the posterior part of the cranial fossa, along with the brainstem, under the occipital lobe of the cerebrum. The function of the cerebellum is to coordinate voluntary movement and to maintain trunk stability and equilibrium. It influences motor activity through its axonal connections to the motor cortex, the brainstem nuclei, and their descending pathways. To perform these functions, the cerebellum receives information from the cerebral cortex, muscles, joints, and inner ear.

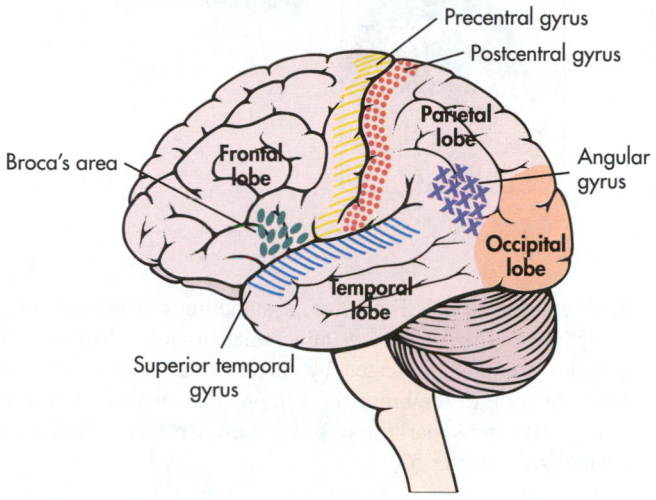

FIG. 56-7 Left hemisphere of cerebrum, lateral surface, showing major lobes and areas of the brain.

TABLE 56-2	Location and Function of the Parts of the Cerebrum	
Part	**Location**	**Function**
Cortical Areas		
Motor		
Primary	Precentral gyrus	Controls initiation of movement on opposite side of body
Supplemental	Anterior to precentral gyrus	Facilitates proximal muscle activity, including activity for stance and gait, and spontaneous movement and coordination
Sensory		
Somatic	Postcentral gyrus	Registers body sensations (e.g., temperature, touch, pressure, pain) from opposite side of body
Visual	Occipital lobe	Registers visual images
Auditory	Superior temporal gyrus	Registers auditory inputs
Association areas	Parietal lobe	Integrates somatic and special sensory inputs
	Posterior temporal lobe	Integrates visual and auditory inputs for language comprehension
	Anterior temporal lobe	Integrates past experiences
	Anterior frontal lobe	Controls higher order processes (e.g., judgment, insight, reasoning, problem solving, planning)
Language		
Comprehension	Wernicke's area	Integrates auditory language (understanding of spoken words)
Expression	Broca's area	Regulates verbal expression
Basal Ganglia	Near lateral ventricles of both cerebral hemispheres	Controls and facilitates learned and automatic movements
Thalamus	Below basal ganglia	Relays sensory and motor inputs to cortex and other parts of cerebrum
Hypothalamus	Below thalamus	Regulates endocrine and autonomic functions (e.g., feeding, sleeping, emotional and sexual responses)
Limbic System	Lateral to hypothalamus	Influences affective (emotional) behavior and basic drives such as feeding and sexual behavior

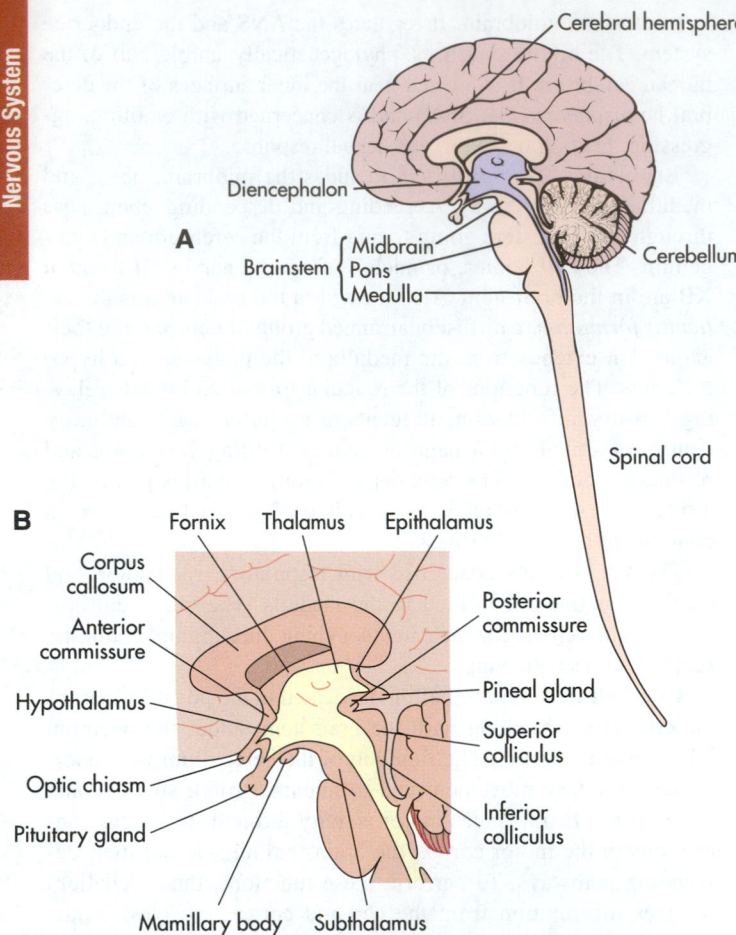

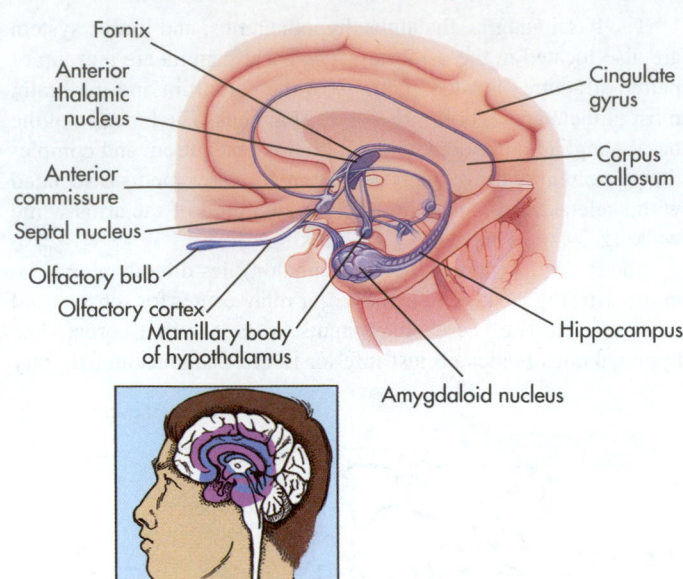

FIG. 56-9   Structures of the limbic system.

FIG. 56-8   **A,** Major divisions of the central nervous system (CNS). **B,** Diencephalon (thalamus and hypothalamus).

Ventricles and Cerebrospinal Fluid. Several supporting structures located within the CNS are important in regulating neuronal function and physical support of the brain. The ventricles are four fluid-filled cavities within the brain that connect with one another and with the spinal canal. The lower portion of the fourth ventricle becomes the central canal in the lower part of the brainstem. The spinal canal is located in the center and extends the full length of the spinal cord. Fig. 56-10 shows the ventricles and the flow of CSF in the CNS.

Cerebrospinal fluid circulates within the subarachnoid space that surrounds the brain, brainstem, and spinal cord. This fluid provides cushioning for the brain and spinal cord, allows fluid shifts from the cranial cavity to the spinal cavity, and carries nutrients. The formation of CSF in the choroid plexus in the ventricles involves both passive diffusion and active transport of substances. CSF resembles an ultrafiltrate of blood. Although CSF is continually being formed, many physiologic factors influence its rate of formation and absorption. The ventricles and central canal are normally filled with an average of 135 ml of CSF.

The CSF circulates throughout the ventricles and seeps into the subarachnoid space surrounding the brain and spinal cord. It is absorbed primarily through the *arachnoid villi* (tiny projections into the subarachnoid space), into the intradural venous sinuses, and eventually into the venous system. The analysis of CSF composition provides useful diagnostic information relating to certain ner-

vous system diseases. CSF pressure is sometimes measured in patients with actual or suspected intracranial diseases. Increases in intracranial pressure, indicated by increased CSF pressure, can lead to herniation of the brain and compression of vital brainstem structures. The signs marking this event are part of the herniation syndrome (see Chapter 57).

Peripheral Nervous System

The PNS includes all the neuronal structures that lie outside the CNS. It consists of the spinal and cranial nerves, their associated ganglia (groupings of cell bodies), and portions of the ANS.

Spinal Nerves. The spinal cord can be seen as a series of spinal segments, one on top of another. In addition to the cell bodies, each segment contains a pair of dorsal (afferent) sensory nerve fibers or roots and ventral (efferent) motor fibers or roots, which innervate a specific region of the neck, trunk, or limbs. This combined motor-sensory nerve is called a *spinal nerve* (Fig. 56-11). The cell bodies of the voluntary motor system are located in the anterior horn of the spinal cord gray matter. The cell bodies of the autonomic (involuntary) motor system are located in the anterolateral portion of spinal cord gray matter. The cell bodies of sensory fibers are located in the dorsal root ganglia just outside the spinal cord. On exiting the spinal column, each spinal nerve divides into ventral and dorsal rami, a collection of motor and sensory fibers that eventually goes to peripheral structures (e.g., skin, muscles, viscera). The sympathetic ganglia are attached to the ventral rami of the spinal nerves by gray and white rami communicantes.

A **dermatome** is the area of skin innervated by the sensory fibers of a single dorsal root of a spinal nerve. The dermatomes give a general picture of somatic sensory innervation by spinal segments. A *myotome* is a muscle group innervated by the primary motor neurons of a single ventral root. The dermatomes and myotomes of a given spinal segment overlap with those of adjacent segments because of the development of ascending and descending collateral branches of nerve fibers.

Cranial Nerves. The **cranial nerves** (CNs) are the 12 paired nerves composed of cell bodies with fibers that exit from the cranial

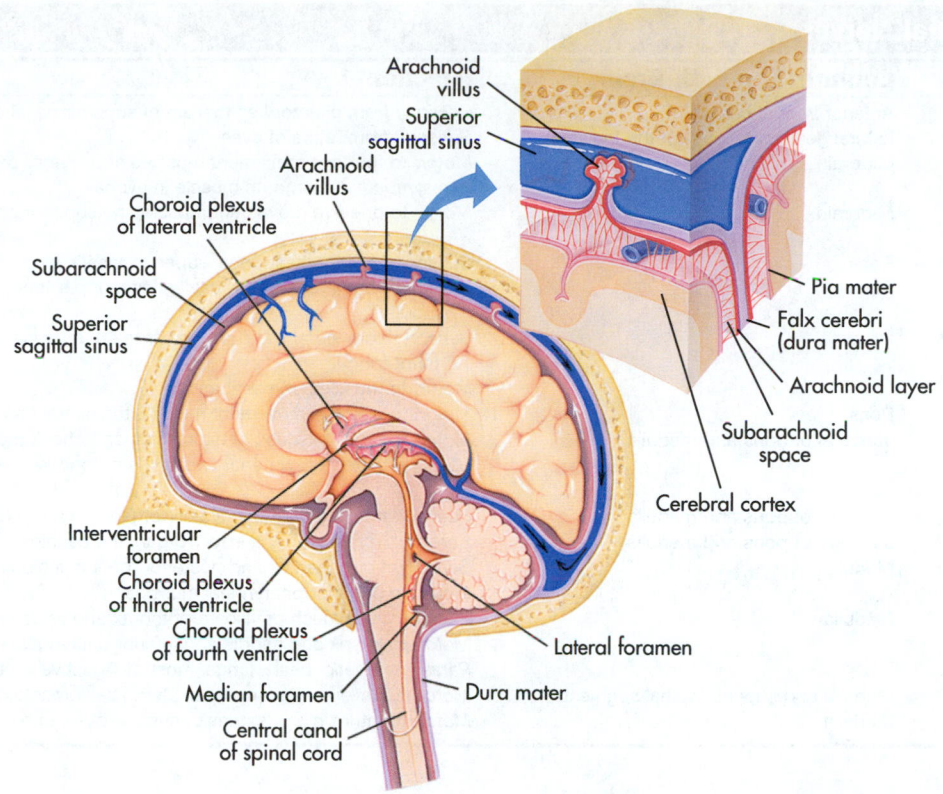

FIG. 56-10 Flow of cerebrospinal fluid (CSF). The fluid produced by filtration of blood by the choroid plexus of each ventricle flows inferiorly through the lateral ventricles, interventricular foramen, third ventricle, cerebral aqueduct, fourth ventricle, and subarachnoid space and to the blood.

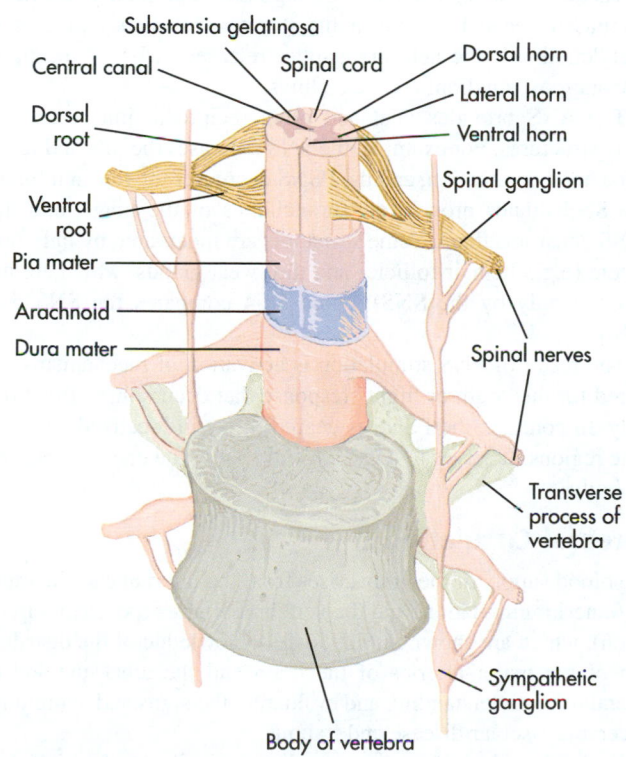

FIG. 56-11 Cross section of spinal cord showing attachments of spinal nerves and coverings of the spinal cord.

cavity. Unlike the spinal nerves, which always have both afferent sensory and efferent motor fibers, some CNs have only afferent and some only efferent fibers; others have both. Table 56-3 summarizes the motor and sensory components of the CNs. Fig. 56-12 shows the position of the CNs in relation to the brain and spinal cord. Just as the cell bodies of the spinal nerves are located in specific segments of the spinal cord, so are the cell bodies (nuclei) of the CNs located in specific segments of the brain. Exceptions are the nuclei of the olfactory and optic nerves. The primary cell bodies of the olfactory nerve are located in the nasal epithelium, and those of the optic nerve are in the retina. CN XI is a spinal nerve, and its efferent fibers migrate upward before exiting the neuroaxis at the level of the medulla.

Autonomic Nervous System. The **autonomic nervous system** (ANS) governs involuntary functions of cardiac muscle, smooth (involuntary) muscle, and glands.

The ANS is divided into two components, sympathetic and parasympathetic, which are anatomically and functionally different. These two systems function together to maintain a relatively balanced internal environment. The ANS is both an efferent and afferent system. It consists of preganglionic nerves and postganglionic nerves.

The preganglionic cell bodies of the *sympathetic nervous system* (SNS) are located in spinal segments T1 through L2. The sympathetic ganglia, which contain the cell bodies of the postganglionic neurons, lie close to the spinal column, along the vertebral bodies in the rami communicantes. These ganglia and the connecting nerves are called the paravertebral chain. The major neurotransmitter released by the postganglionic fibers of the SNS is

TABLE 56-3	**Cranial Nerves**

Nerve	Connnection with Brain	Function
I Olfactory	Anterior ventral cerebrum	*Sensory:* from olfactory epithelium of superior nasal cavity
II Optic	Lateral geniculate body of the thalamus	*Sensory:* from retina of eyes
III Oculomotor	Midbrain	*Motor:* to four eye movement muscles and levator palpebrae
		Parasympathetic: smooth muscle in eyeball
IV Trochlear	Midbrain	*Motor:* to one eye movement muscle, the superior oblique
V Trigeminal		
Ophthalmic branch	Pons	*Sensory:* from forehead, eye, superior nasal cavity
Maxillary branch	Pons	*Sensory:* from inferior nasal cavity, face, upper teeth, mucosa of superior mouth
Mandibular branch	Pons	*Sensory:* from surfaces of jaw, lower teeth, mucosa of lower mouth, and anterior tongue
		Motor: to muscles of mastication
VI Abducens	Pons	*Motor:* to one eye movement muscle, the lateral rectus
VII Facial	Junction of pons and medulla	*Motor:* to facial muscles of expression and cheek muscle, the buccinator
		Sensory: taste from anterior two thirds of tongue
VIII Vestibulocochlear		
Vestibular branch	Junction of pons and medulla	*Sensory:* from equilibrium sensory organ, the vestibular apparatus
Cochlear branch	Junction of pons and medulla	*Sensory:* from auditory sensory organ, the cochlea
IX Glossopharyngeal	Medulla	*Sensory:* from pharynx and posterior tongue, including taste
		Motor: to superior pharyngeal muscles
X Vagus	Medulla	*Sensory:* from much of viscera of thorax and abdomen
		Motor: to larynx and middle and inferior pharyngeal muscles
		Parasympathetic: heart, lungs, most of digestive system
XI Accessory	Medulla and superior spinal segments	*Motor:* to several neck muscles, sternocleidomastoid and trapezius
XII Hypoglossal	Medulla	*Motor:* to intrinsic and extrinsic muscles of tongue

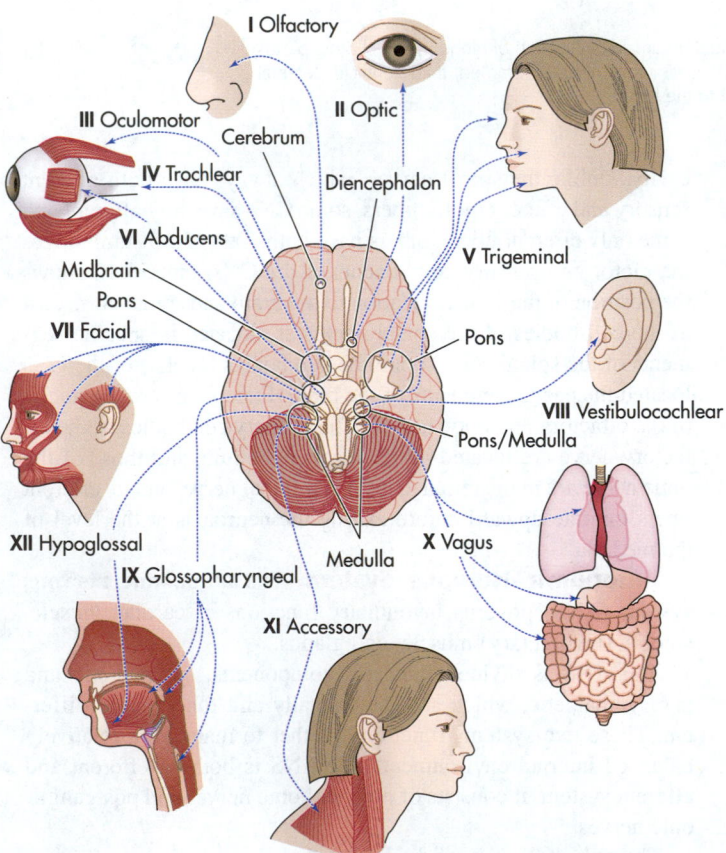

FIG. 56-12   The cranial nerves are numbered according to the order in which they leave the brain.

norepinephrine, and the neurotransmitter released by the preganglionic fibers is acetylcholine.

In contrast, the preganglionic cell bodies of the *parasympathetic nervous system* (PSNS) are located in the brainstem and in the sacral spinal segments (S2 through S4). The parasympathetic ganglia are located in or near the structures that they innervate. Acetylcholine is the neurotransmitter released at both preganglionic and postganglionic nerve endings.

The ANS provides dual and often reciprocal innervation to many structures. For example, the SNS increases the rate and force of the heart contraction, and the PSNS decreases the rate and force. The SNS dilates bronchi and bronchioles of the lungs, and the PSNS constricts them. Some structures are innervated by only one system (e.g., the hair follicles and the sweat glands, which are innervated only by the SNS). Table 56-4 compares the SNS and PSNS.

The result of SNS stimulation is activation of mechanisms required for the "fight or flight" response that occurs throughout the body. In contrast, the PSNS is geared to act in localized and discrete regions. It serves to conserve and restore the energy stores of the body.

Cerebral Circulation

The blood supply of the brain arises from the internal carotid arteries (anterior circulation) and the vertebral arteries (posterior circulation), which are shown in Fig. 56-13. Knowledge of the distribution of the major arteries of the brain and the area supplied is essential for understanding and evaluating the signs and symptoms of cerebrovascular disease and trauma.

Each internal carotid artery supplies the ipsilateral hemisphere, whereas the basilar artery, formed by the junction of the two vertebral arteries, supplies structures within the posterior fossa (cerebellum and brainstem). The *circle of Willis* arises from the basilar

TABLE 56-4 Effect of Sympathetic and Parasympathetic Nervous Systems

Visceral Effector	Effect of Sympathetic Nervous System*	Effect of Parasympathetic Nervous System†
Heart	↑ Rate and strength of heartbeat (β-receptors)	↓ Rate and strength of heartbeat
Smooth muscle of blood vessels		
Skin blood vessels	Constriction (α-receptors)	No effect
Skeletal muscle blood vessels	Dilation (β-receptors)	No effect
Coronary blood vessels	Dilation (β-receptors), constriction (α-receptors)	Dilation
Abdominal blood vessels	Constriction (α-receptors)	No effect
Blood vessels of external genitals	Ejaculation (contraction of smooth muscle in male ducts [e.g., epididymis, ductus deferens])	Dilation of blood vessels causing erection in male
Smooth muscle of hollow organs and sphincters		
Bronchi	Dilation (β-receptors)	Constriction
Digestive tract, except sphincters	↓ Peristalsis (β-receptors)	↑ Peristalsis
Sphincters of digestive tract	Contraction (α-receptors)	Relaxation
Urinary bladder	Relaxation (β-receptors)	Contraction
Urinary sphincters	Contraction (α-receptors)	Relaxation
Eye		
Iris	Contraction of radial muscle, dilation of pupil	Contraction of circular muscle, constriction of pupil
Cilia	Relaxation, accommodation for far vision	Contraction, accommodation for near vision
Hairs (pilomotor muscles)	Contraction producing goose pimples or piloerection (α-receptors)	No effect
Glands		
Sweat	↑ Sweat (neurotransmitter, acetylcholine)	No effect
Digestive (e.g., salivary, gastric)	↓ Secretion of saliva; not known for others	↑ Secretion of saliva and gastric HCl acid
Pancreas, including islets	↓ Secretion	↑ Secretion of pancreatic juice and insulin
Liver	↑ Glycogenolysis (β-receptors), increase in blood glucose level	No effect
Adrenal medulla‡	↑ Epinephrine secretion	No effect

Modified from Thibodeau GA, Patton KT: *Anatomy and physiology*, ed 6, St Louis, 2006, Mosby.
*Neurotransmitter is norepinephrine unless otherwise stated.
†Neurotransmitter is acetylcholine unless otherwise stated.
‡Sympathetic preganglionic axons terminate in contact with secreting cells of the adrenal medulla. Thus the adrenal medulla functions as a "giant sympathetic postganglionic neuron."

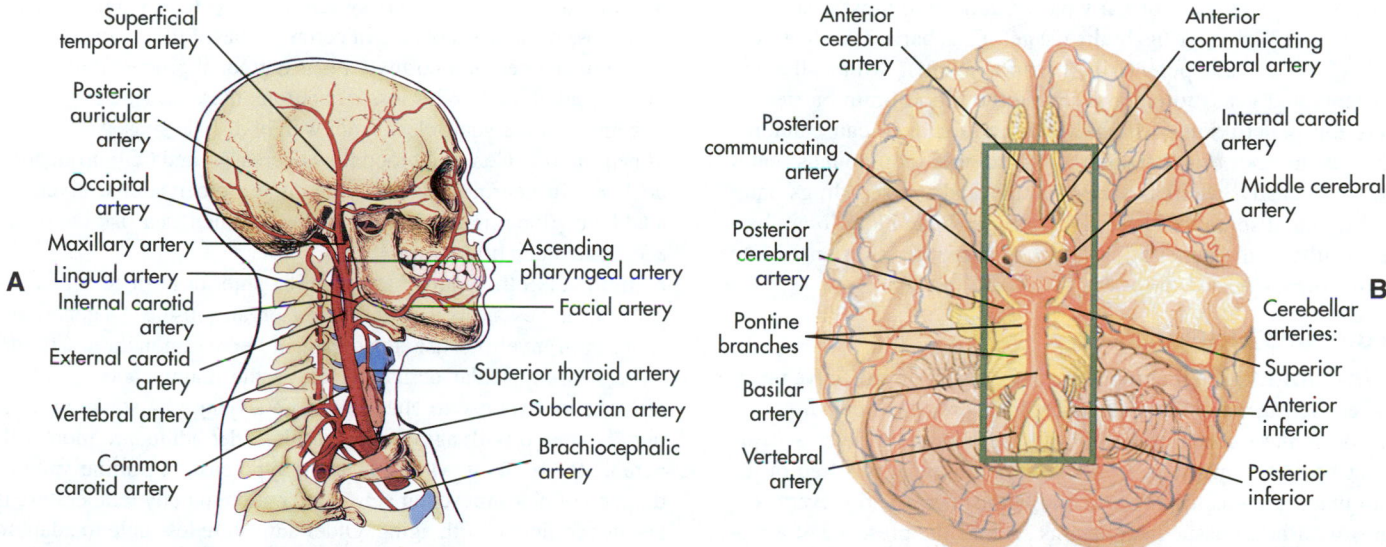

FIG. 56-13   Arteries of the head and neck. **A,** Brachiocephalic artery, right common carotid artery, right subclavian artery, and their branches. The major arteries to the head are the common carotid and vertebral arteries. **B,** Inferior view of the brain showing the vertebral, basilar, and internal carotid arteries and their branches.

Nervous System

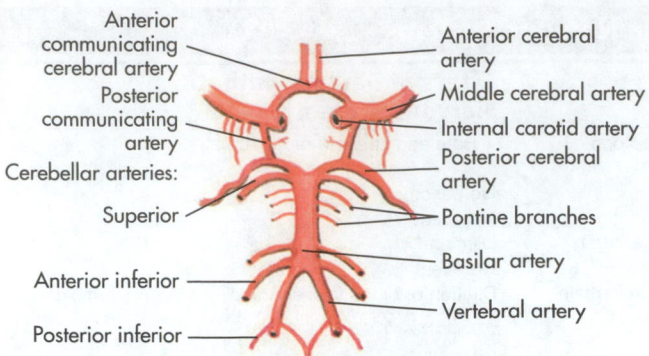

FIG. 56-14   Arteries at the base of the brain. The arteries that compose the circle of Willis are the two anterior cerebral arteries joined to each other by the anterior communicating cerebral artery and to the posterior cerebral arteries by the posterior communicating arteries.

artery and the two internal carotid arteries (Fig. 56-14). This vascular circle may act as a safety valve when differential pressures are present in these arteries. It also may function as an anastomotic pathway when occlusion of a major artery on one side of the brain occurs. In general, the two anterior cerebral arteries supply the medial and anterior portions of the frontal lobes. The two middle cerebral arteries supply the outer portions of the frontal, parietal, and superior temporal lobes. The two posterior cerebral arteries supply the medial portions of the occipital and inferior temporal lobes. Fig. 56-13 shows the major cerebral arteries. Venous blood drains from the brain through the dural sinuses, which form channels that drain into the two jugular veins.

Blood-Brain Barrier. The **blood-brain barrier** is a physiologic barrier between blood capillaries and brain tissue. The structure of brain capillaries differs from that of other capillaries. Some substances that normally pass readily into most tissues are prevented from entering brain tissue. This barrier protects the brain from certain potentially harmful agents, while allowing nutrients and gases to enter. Because the blood-brain barrier affects the penetration of drugs, only certain ones can enter the CNS from the bloodstream. Lipid-soluble compounds enter the brain easily, whereas water-soluble and ionized drugs enter the brain and spinal cord slowly. Damage to the blood-brain barrier results in the penetration of drugs and other substances into brain tissue.

Protective Structures

Meninges. The **meninges** are three layers of protective membranes that surround the brain and spinal cord. The thick *dura mater* forms the outermost layer, with the arachnoid layer and pia mater being the next two layers. The *falx cerebri* is a fold of the dura that separates the two cerebral hemispheres and prevents expansion of brain tissue in situations such as the presence of a rapidly growing tumor or acute hemorrhage. The expanding brain must squeeze under this structure, causing displacement toward the side opposite the lesion. The *tentorium cerebelli* is a fold of dura that separates the cerebral hemispheres from the posterior fossa (which contains the brainstem and cerebellum). Expansion of mass lesions in the cerebrum forces the brain to herniate through the opening created by the brainstem. This is termed *tentorial herniation* (see Chapter 57).

The *arachnoid* layer is a delicate, impermeable membrane that lies between the thick dura mater and the pia mater. The *subarach-*

noid space lies between the arachnoid layer and the pia mater. This space is filled with CSF. Structures passing to and from the brain and the skull or its foramina (holes through which blood vessels and nerves enter and exit the intracranial compartment) must pass through the subarachnoid space. Therefore all cerebral arteries and veins lie in this space, as do the CNs. A larger subarachnoid space is present in the region of the third and fourth lumbar vertebrae, which is the area penetrated to obtain CSF during a lumbar puncture. (The spinal cord itself ends between the first and second lumbar vertebrae.)

Skull. The bony skull protects the brain from external trauma. It is composed of 8 cranial bones and 14 facial bones. The structure of the skull cavity explains the pathophysiology of head injuries (see Chapter 57). Although the top and sides of the inside of the skull are relatively smooth, the bottom surface is uneven. It has many ridges, prominences, and foramina. The largest hole is the foramen magnum, through which the brainstem extends to the spinal cord. This foramen offers the only major space for the expansion of brain contents when increased intracranial pressure occurs.

Vertebral Column. The vertebral column protects the spinal cord, supports the head, and provides flexibility. The vertebral column is made up of 33 individual vertebrae: 7 cervical, 12 thoracic, 5 lumbar, 5 sacral (fused into one), and 4 coccygeal (fused into one). Each vertebra has a central opening through which the spinal cord passes. The vertebrae are held together by a series of ligaments. Intervertebral disks occupy the spaces between vertebrae. Fig. 56-15 shows the vertebral column in relation to the trunk.

GERONTOLOGIC CONSIDERATIONS
EFFECTS OF AGING ON THE NERVOUS SYSTEM

Several parts of the nervous system are affected by aging. In the CNS, loss of neurons occurs in certain areas of the brainstem, cerebellum, and cerebral cortex. This is a gradual process that begins in early adulthood. With loss of neurons there is widening or enlargement of the ventricles. Brain weight also decreases as a result of neuron loss. Cerebral blood flow decreases, and CSF production declines. In neurologically asymptomatic older adults, glycosylated hemoglobin (Hb A1C) has been identified as a risk factor for accelerated cerebral atropy.[3]

In the PNS there are changes in the anterior horn cells and peripheral nerves as well as the target organ muscle. Degenerative changes in myelin cause a decrease in nerve conduction. Coordinated neuromuscular activity, such as the maintenance of blood pressure in response to changing from a lying to a standing position, is altered with aging. As a result, older adults are more vulnerable to problems with orthostatic hypotension. Similarly, coordination of neuromuscular activity to maintain body temperature is also less efficient with aging. Older adults are less able to adapt to extremes in environmental temperature and are more vulnerable to both hypothermia and hyperthermia.

Additional relevant changes associated with aging include decreases in memory, vision, hearing, taste, smell, vibration and position sense, muscle strength, and reaction time.[4] Sensory changes, including decreases in taste and smell perception, may result in decreased dietary intake in the older adult. Reduced hearing and vision can result in perceptual confusion. Problems with balance and coordination can put the older adult at risk for falls and subsequent fractures.

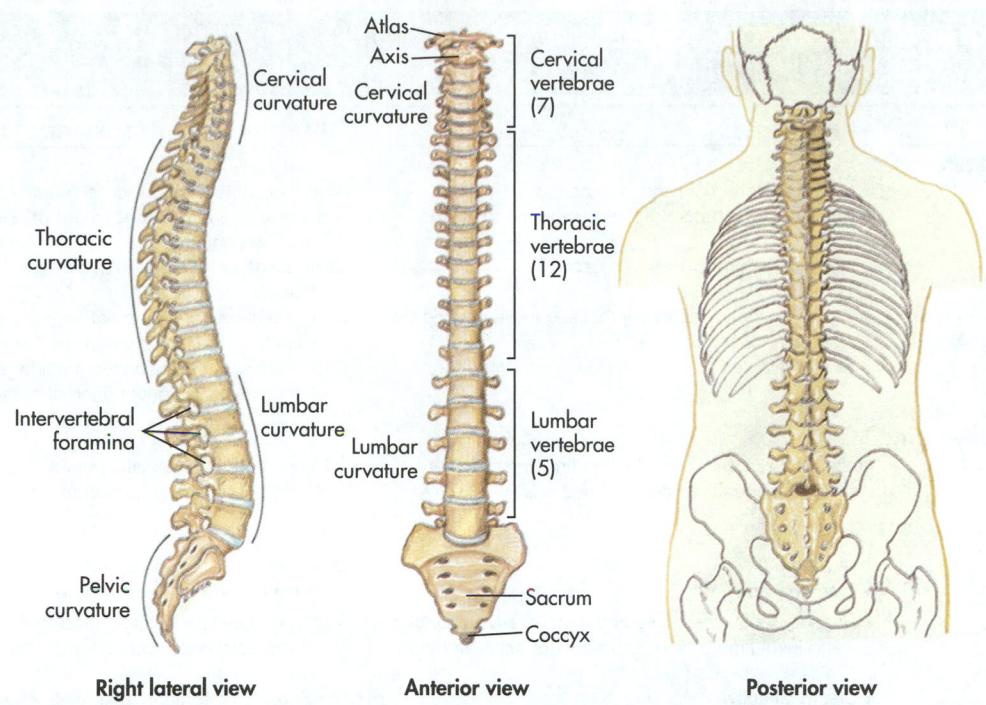

Right lateral view   **Anterior view**   **Posterior view**

FIG. 56-15   The vertebral column (three views).

Changes in assessment findings result from age-related alterations in the various components of the nervous system. Age-related changes in the nervous system and differences in assessment findings are presented in Table 56-5.

ASSESSMENT OF THE NERVOUS SYSTEM

Subjective Data

Important Health Information

Past Health History. Three points should be considered in taking the history of a patient with neurologic problems. First, avoid suggesting certain symptoms to the patient or asking leading questions such as, "Is your headache throbbing?" or "Are you weak on the right side?" It is better to ask open-ended questions such as, "What is your headache like?" or "Is there anything about your right side that bothers you?" Second, the mode of onset and the course of the illness are especially important aspects of the history. Often the nature of a neurologic disease process can be described by these facts alone. The nurse should obtain all pertinent data in the history of the present illness, especially data related to the characteristics and progression of the symptoms. Third, because many neurologic diseases affect a patient's mental functioning, the mental status must be accurately assessed before assuming that the history is factual. If the patient is not considered a reliable historian, obtain the history from a person who has firsthand knowledge of the patient's problems and complaints. Many times a health history cannot be obtained, and the nurse must proceed with only objective data.

The health history helps guide the approach for the neurologic examination, directing the health care provider toward the parts of the nervous system that need to be closely assessed. If the patient's primary complaint is dizziness, the examination may be focused on visual, vestibular, and cerebellar functions rather than on somatic motor and sensory functions.

Medications. Special attention should be given to obtaining a careful medication history, especially the use of sedatives, opioids, tranquilizers, and mood-elevating drugs. Many other drugs can also cause neurologic side effects.

Surgery or Other Treatments. The nurse should inquire about any surgery involving any part of the nervous system, such as the head, spine, or sensory organs. If a patient had surgery, the date, cause, procedure, recovery, and current status should be investigated.

The perinatal history may reveal exposure to toxic agents such as viruses, alcohol, tobacco, drugs, and radiation, which are known to adversely influence the development of the nervous system. The history may reveal a difficult labor and delivery, which can cause brain damage as a result of hypoxia, forceps delivery, or Rh incompatibility.

Growth and developmental history can be important in ascertaining whether nervous system dysfunction was present at an early age. The nurse should specifically inquire about major developmental tasks such as walking and talking. Successes at school or identified problems in an educational setting are other important developmental data to gather. Often this information is not available when the older patient is interviewed.

Functional Health Patterns. Key questions to ask a patient with a neurologic problem are presented in Table 56-6.

Health Perception–Health Management Pattern. The nurse should ask about the patient's health practices related to the nervous system, such as substance abuse and smoking, maintenance of adequate nutrition, safe participation in physical and recreational activities, use of seat belts and helmets, and control of hypertension. The nurse should ask about previous hospitalizations for neurologic problems. A careful family history may determine whether the neurologic problem has a hereditary or congenital background.

If the patient has an existing neurologic problem, the nurse should ask about how it affects daily living and the ability to carry

TABLE 56-5	*GERONTOLOGIC DIFFERENCES IN ASSESSMENT* Nervous System	

Component	Changes	Differences in Assessment Findings
Central Nervous System Brain	↓ Cerebral blood flow and metabolism ↓ Efficiency of temperature-regulating mechanism	Alterations in selected mental functioning ↓ Body temperature, impairment of ability to adapt to environmental temperature
	↓ Neurotransmitters, loss of neurons	Conduction of nerve impulses slowed, response time slowed
	↓ Oxygen supply, changes in basal ganglia caused by vascular changes Size of ventricles ↑	Changes in gait and ambulation (e.g., extrapyramidal, Parkinson-like gait); diminished kinesthetic sense Potential for altered balanced, vertigo, syncope; ↑ postural hypotension; proprioception diminished; ↓ sensory input
Peripheral Nervous System Cranial and spinal nerves	Loss of myelin and ↓ conduction time in some nerves Cellular degeneration, death of neurons	↓ Reaction time in specific nerves ↓ Speed and intensity of neuronal reflexes
Functional Divisions Motor	↓ Muscle bulk ↓ Electrical activity	Diminished strength and agility ↓ Reactions and movement time
Sensory*	↓ Sensory receptors caused by degenerative changes and involution of fine corpuscles of nerve endings	Diminished sense of touch; inability to localize stimuli; ↓ appreciation of touch, temperature, and peripheral vibrations
	↓ Electrical activity Atrophy of taste buds Degeneration and loss of fibers in olfactory bulb Degenerative changes in nerve cells in vestibular system of inner ear, cerebellum, and proprioceptive pathways in nervous system	Slowing of or alteration in sensory reception Signs of malnutrition, weight loss Diminished sense of smell Poor ability to maintain balance, widened gait
Reflexes	Possible ↓ deep tendon reflexes ↓ Sensory conduction velocity as result of myelin sheath degeneration	Below-average reflex score Sluggish reflexes, slowing of reaction time
Reticular Formation Reticular activating system	Modification of hypothalamic function, ↓ stage IV sleep	↑ Frequency of spontaneous awakening together with tiredness, interrupted sleep, insomnia
Autonomic Nervous System SNS and PSNS	Morphologic features of ganglia, slowing of ANS responses	Orthostatic hypotension, systolic hypertension
Sleep	Deep sleep ↑ Rapid eye movement (REM) ↓ in old-old adults	Difficulty falling asleep Period of wakefulness increased; sleep time averages 6 hr

ANS, Autonomic nervous system; *PSNS,* parasympathetic nervous system; *SNS,* sympathetic nervous system.
*Specific changes related to the eye are listed in Chapter 21, Table 21-1 and specific changes related to the ear are listed in Table 21-7.

out self-care. After a careful review of information, the nurse should ask someone who knows the patient well whether any mental or physical changes have been noticed in the patient. The patient with a neurologic problem may not be aware of it or may be a poor historian.[5]

Nutritional-Metabolic Pattern. Neurologic problems can result in problems of inadequate nutrition. Problems related to chewing, swallowing, facial nerve paralysis, and muscle coordination could make it difficult for the patient to ingest adequate nutrients. Also, certain vitamins such as thiamine (B_1), niacin, and pyridoxine (B_6) are essential for the maintenance and health of the CNS. Deficiencies in one or more of these vitamins could result in such nonspecific complaints as depression, apathy, neuritis, weakness, mental confusion, and irritability.[6] Cobalamin (vitamin B_{12}) deficiency is a risk for older adults as they tend to have problems with vitamin absorption from natural food sources such as meat, fish, and poultry. Untreated, the deficiency can cause mental function decline. It may not be diagnosed if there is a concurrent high folate intake, which prevents anemia but does not prevent neuron damage.[7]

Elimination Pattern. Bowel and bladder problems are often associated with neurologic problems, such as stroke, head injury, spinal cord injury, multiple sclerosis, and dementia. It is important to determine if the bowel or bladder problem was present before or after the neurologic event to plan appropriate interventions. Incontinence of urine and feces and urinary retention are the most common elimination problems associated with a neurologic problem. For example, nerve root compression (as occurs in cauda equina conditions) leads to a sudden onset of incontinence. Careful documentation of the details of the problem, such as number of episodes, accompanying sensations or lack of sensations, and measures to control the problem, is important.

Activity-Exercise Pattern. Many neurologic disorders can cause problems in the patient's mobility, strength, and coordination. These problems can result in changes in the patient's usual activity and exercise patterns. Falls can also result from such problems. Many aspects of daily living, such as getting out of a bed or chair, ambulating, preparing meals, and performing personal hygiene tasks, can be affected and should be assessed. The ability to

TABLE 56-6	**HEALTH HISTORY** Nervous System

Health Perception–Health Management Pattern
- What are your usual daily activities?
- Do you use any recreational drugs?*
- What safety practices do you perform in a car? On a motorcycle? On a bicycle?
- Do you have hypertension? If so, is it controlled?
- Have you ever been hospitalized for a neurologic problem?*
- How does it affect your daily living?

Nutritional-Metabolic Pattern
- Give a 24-hour dietary recall.
- Do you have any problems getting adequate nutrition because of chewing or swallowing difficulties, facial nerve paralysis, or poor muscle coordination?*
- Are you able to feed yourself?

Elimination Pattern
- Do you have incontinence of bowel or bladder? If yes, explain in detail the onset and pattern of the problem.
- What measures have you used to control the incontinence?
- Do you ever experience problems with hesitancy, urgency, retention?*
- Do you postpone defecation?*
- Does a neurologic problem make it difficult to reach a toilet when needed?
- Do you take any medication to manage neurologic problems? If so, what?

Activity-Exercise Pattern
- Describe any problems you experience with usual activities and exercise as a result of a neurologic problem.
- Do you have weakness or lack of coordination caused by a neurologic problem?*
- Does a neurologic problem keep you from performing your personal hygiene needs independently?*

Sleep-Rest Pattern
- Describe any problems you have with sleep.
- If you have trouble falling asleep, what do you do about it? (Ask specifically about use of sleep-inducing drugs.)

Cognitive-Perceptual Pattern
- Have you noticed any changes in your memory?*
- Do you experience vertigo, heat or cold sensitivity, numbness, or tingling?*
- Describe any pain you have experienced during the past 6 mo.
- Do you have any difficulty with verbal or written communication?*
- Have you noticed any changes in vision or hearing?*

Self-Perception–Self-Concept Pattern
- What effect has your neurologic problem had on how you feel about yourself? Your abilities? Your body?
- Describe your general emotional pattern.

Role-Relationship Pattern
- Have you experienced changes in roles such as spouse, parent, or breadwinner because of neurologic disease?*
- How do you feel about these changes?

Sexuality-Reproductive Pattern
- Are you satisfied with sexual functioning? Describe any problems you experience related to your sexuality and sexual functioning.
- Are problems related to sexual functioning causing tension in an important relationship?*
- Do you feel the need for professional counseling related to your sexual functioning?*
- Do you use alternative methods of achieving sexual satisfaction?

Coping–Stress Tolerance Pattern
- Describe your usual coping pattern.
- Do you think your present coping pattern is adequate to meet the stressors of your neurologic problem?*
- Is your support system adequate to meet your needs? If not, what needs are unmet?

Value-Belief Pattern
- Describe any culturally specific beliefs and attitudes that may influence the treatment of this neurologic problem.

*If yes, describe.

perform fine motor tasks may be affected, which increases the possibility of personal injury.

Sleep-Rest Pattern. Sleep can be disrupted by many neurologically related factors. Discomfort from pain and inability to move and change to a position of comfort because of muscle weakness and paralysis could interfere with sound sleep. Hallucinations resulting from dementia or drugs can also interrupt sleep. The nurse should carefully document the sleep problem and the patient's methods of dealing with the problem.

Cognitive-Perceptual Pattern. Because the nervous system controls cognition and sensory integration, many neurologic disorders affect these functions. The nurse should assess memory, language, calculation ability, problem-solving ability, insight, and judgment. Often a structured mental status questionnaire is used to evaluate these functions and provide baseline data.

Delirium (acute confusional state) is an acute disorder of cognition.[8] In elderly patients, delirium may be seen postoperatively. It is often an early indicator of various illnesses (see Chapter 60, Table 60-12). (Delirium is discussed in Chapter 60.)

Ability to both use and understand language is a cognitive function that the nurse should also assess. Appropriateness of responses is a useful indicator of cognitive and perceptual ability.

Pain is a common event associated with many health problems. It is often the reason a patient seeks health care. A careful assessment of the patient's pain should be carried out (see Chapter 10).

Neurologic problems and their treatment can be complex and confusing. The patient's understanding and ability to carry out necessary treatments should be determined. Neurologically related cognitive changes can interfere with the patient's understanding of the disease and compliance with related treatment. Frequently the patient's cognitive changes may not be adequately assessed by the health care team.[9]

Self-Perception–Self-Concept Pattern. Neurologic disease can drastically alter control over one's life and create dependency on others for daily needs. Also, the patient's physical appearance and emotional control can be affected. The nurse should ask about the patient's evaluation of self-worth, perception of abilities, body image, and general emotional pattern.

Role-Relationship Pattern. The patient should be asked if changes in roles, such as spouse, parent, or breadwinner, resulting from a neurologic problem have occurred. Physical impairments such as weakness and paralysis can alter or limit participation in usual roles and activities. Cognitive changes, however, can permanently change a person's ability to maintain previous roles. These changes can dramatically affect both the patient and significant others. Dependent relationships can develop.

Sexuality–Reproductive Pattern. The ability to participate in sexual activity should be assessed because many nervous system disorders can affect sexual response. Cerebral lesions may inhibit the desire phase or the reflex responses of the excitement phase. Brainstem and spinal cord lesions may partially or completely interrupt the connections between the brain and effector systems necessary for intercourse.

Neuropathies and spinal cord lesions that affect sensation, especially in the erotic zones, may decrease desire. Autonomic neuropathies and lesions of the sacral cord and cauda equina may prevent reflex activities of the sexual response. The nurse should determine if the patient and the spouse or significant other are satisfied with their sexual activity. The use of or need for alternative methods of achieving sexual satisfaction should be explored. Despite neurologically related changes in sexual functioning, many persons can achieve satisfying expression of intimacy and affection.

Coping–Stress Tolerance Pattern. The physical sequelae of a neurologic problem can seriously strain a patient's coping patterns. Often the problem is chronic and may require that the patient learn new coping skills. The nurse should assess the patient's usual coping pattern to determine if coping skills are adequate to meet the stress of a problem.

When the problem is a decrease in cognitive functioning, both the patient and the caregiver can be seriously stressed. The nurse should assess for the potential for suicide, abuse, and burnout. The presence of an adequate support system in this type of situation should be assessed.

Value–Belief Pattern. Many neurologic problems have serious, long-term, life-changing effects. These effects can strain the patient's belief system and should be assessed. The nurse should also determine if any religious or cultural beliefs could interfere with the planned treatment regimen.

Objective Data

Physical Examination. The standard neurologic examination helps determine the presence, location, and nature of disease of the nervous system. The examination assesses six categories of functions: mental status, function of CNs, motor function, cerebellar function, sensory function, and reflex function. The choice of particular parts of the examination depends on the purpose for which it is done. If a comprehensive baseline assessment of neurologic functioning is desired, all components of the examination are done. However, if a specific problem is to be evaluated, only certain components may be assessed. For example, if a patient's primary complaint is lack of sensation in the feet, the examination may be focused only on movement and sensation of the lower limbs.

With uncommunicative or comatose patients, data collection for the physical examination changes focus from the patient's subjective report to the nurse's objective findings. The 15-point Glasgow Coma Scale (GCS) (see Chapter 57, Table 57-5) is the classic tool used for patients who have deficits in eye opening, verbal ability, or motor function.[10]

Mental Status. Assessment of mental status (cerebral functioning) gives an indication of how the patient is functioning as a whole and how the patient is adapting to the environment. It involves determination of complex and high-level cerebral functions

that are governed by many areas of the cerebral cortex. Much of the area covered in this part of the examination is assessed during the history and therefore does not need to be evaluated further.[11] For example, language and memory can be assessed when the patient is asked for details of the illness and significant past events. The patient's cultural and educational background should be taken into account when evaluating mental status.

The components of the mental status examination are as follows:

- *General appearance and behavior.* This component includes motor activity, body posture, dress and hygiene, facial expression, and speech.
- *State of consciousness.* The patient must be conscious before other functions can be determined. The nurse should note orientation to time, place, person, and situation, as well as memory, general knowledge, insight, judgment, problem solving, and calculation. Common questions are "Who were the last three presidents?" "What does 'a stitch in time saves nine' mean?" "Subtract 7 from 100, and keep subtracting 7." The nurse should consider whether the patient's plans and goals match the physical and mental capabilities. Problems with memory may have implications for the ability to retain patient education.
- *Mood and affect.* The nurse should note agitation, anger, depression, or euphoria and the appropriateness of these states. Questions should be directed to bring out the feelings of the patient.
- *Thought content.* The nurse should note illusions, hallucinations, delusions, or paranoia.
- *Intellectual capacity.* The nurse should note retardation, dementia, and intelligence.

Cranial Nerves. Testing of each CN is an essential component of the neurologic examination (see Table 56-3).

Olfactory Nerve. After determining that both nostrils are patent, the olfactory nerve (CN I) is tested by asking the patient to close one nostril, close both eyes, and sniff from a bottle containing coffee, spice, soap, or some other readily recognized odor. The same is done for the other nostril. Generally, olfaction is not tested unless the patient has some disturbance with smell. Chronic rhinitis, sinusitis, and heavy smoking can often decrease the sense of smell. Disturbance in ability to smell may be associated with a tumor involving the olfactory bulb, or it may be the result of a basilar skull fracture that has damaged the olfactory fibers as they pass through the delicate cribriform plate of the skull.

Optic Nerve. Visual fields and visual acuity are assessed to test the function of the optic nerve (CN II). Peripheral visual fields are assessed by confrontation. The examiner, positioned directly opposite the patient, asks the patient to close one eye, look directly at the bridge of the examiner's nose, and indicate when an object (finger, pencil tip, head of pin) presented from the periphery of each of the four visual field quadrants is seen (Fig. 56-16). The same test is repeated for the other eye. The examiner is used as a control because both examiner and patient are sharing the same visual field. It is important to remember that the nasal side of the visual field is narrower because of the nasal bridge. Visual field defects may arise from lesions of the optic nerve, optic chiasm, or tracts that extend through the temporal, parietal, or occipital lobes. Visual field changes resulting from brain lesions are usually either a *hemianopsia* (one half of the visual field is affected), a *quadrantanopsia* (one fourth of the visual field is affected), or monocular.

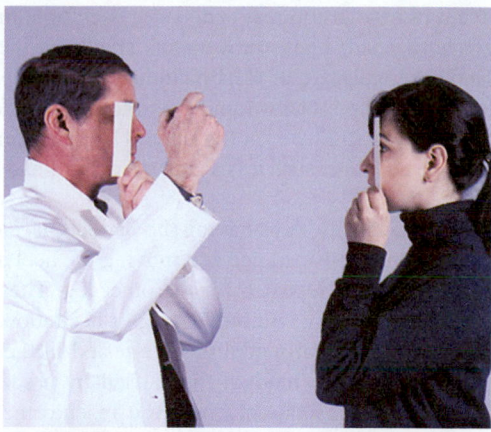

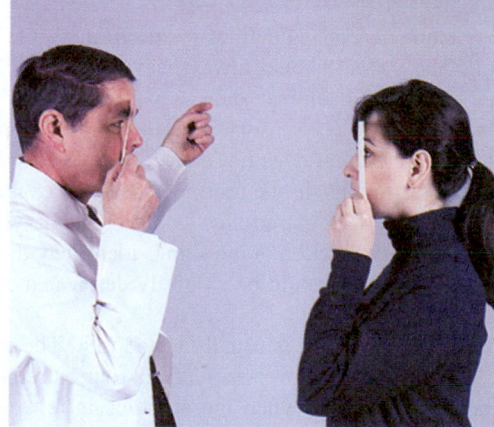

FIG. 56-16   Assessment of visual fields by gross confrontation.

Visual acuity is tested by asking the patient to read a Snellen chart from 20 feet away. The number on the lowest line that the patient can read with 50% accuracy is recorded. The patient who wears glasses should wear them during testing, unless they are used only for reading. The eyes should be tested individually and together. If a Snellen chart is not available, the patient should be asked to read newsprint for a gross assessment of acuity. The distance from the patient to the newsprint required for accurate reading should be recorded. Acuity may not be testable by these means if the patient does not read English or is aphasic.

Funduscopy reveals the physical condition of the optic disc (head of the optic nerve), as well as the retina and blood vessels. This procedure is routinely performed when the optic nerve is tested. Optic nerve atrophy and papilledema can be detected by this method.

Oculomotor, Trochlear, and Abducens Nerves. Because the oculomotor (CN III), trochlear (CN IV), and abducens (CN VI) nerves all help move the eye, they are tested together. The patient is asked to follow the examiner's finger as it moves horizontally and vertically (making a cross) and diagonally (making an X). If there is weakness or paralysis of one of the eye muscles, the eyes do not move together, and the patient has a *disconjugate gaze.* The presence and direction of *nystagmus* (fine, rapid jerking movements of the eyes) are observed at this time, even though this condition most often indicates vestibulocerebellar problems.

Other functions of the oculomotor nerve are tested by checking for pupillary constriction and for *convergence* (eyes turning inward) and *accommodation* (pupils constricting with near vision). To test pupillary constriction, the examiner shines a light into the pupil of one eye and looks for ipsilateral constriction of the same pupil and contralateral (consensual) constriction of the opposite eye. The size and shape of the pupils are also noted. The optic nerve must be intact for this reflex to occur. Testing for pupillary constriction is an important component of the neurologic assessment of patients at risk for herniation syndrome (see Chapter 57). Because the oculomotor nerve exits at the top of the brainstem at the tentorial notch, it can be easily compressed by expanding mass lesions in the cerebral hemispheres. The result is a pupil that does not constrict in response to light; it may become dilated because the sympathetic input to the pupil acts unopposed. Convergence and accommodation are tested by having the patient focus on the examiner's finger as it moves toward the patient's nose. Another function of the oculomotor nerve is to keep the eyelid open. Damage to the nerve can cause *ptosis* (drooping eyelid), pupillary abnormalities, and eye muscle weakness.

Trigeminal Nerve. The sensory component of the trigeminal nerve (CN V) is tested by having the patient identify light touch (cotton) and pinprick in each of the three divisions (ophthalmic, maxillary, and mandibular) of the nerve on both sides of the face. The patient's eyes should be closed during this part of the examination. The motor component is tested by asking the patient to clench the teeth and palpating the masseter muscles just above the mandibular angle. The corneal reflex test evaluates CN V and CN VII simultaneously. This reflex is not normally tested in patients who are awake and alert because other tests evaluate these two nerves. It involves applying a cotton wisp strand to the cornea. The sensory component of this reflex (corneal sensation) is innervated by the ophthalmic division of CN V. The motor component (eye blink) is innervated by the facial nerve (CN VII). For patients with a decreased level of consciousness, the corneal reflex test provides an evaluation of brainstem integrity at the level of the pons because the fibers of CN V and CN VII have connections in this area.

Facial Nerve. The facial nerve (CN VII) innervates the muscles of facial expression. Its function is tested by asking the patient to raise the eyebrows, close the eyes tightly, purse the lips, draw back the corners of the mouth in an exaggerated smile, and frown. The examiner should note any asymmetry in the facial movements because they can indicate damage to the facial nerve. Although taste discrimination of salt and sugar in the anterior two thirds of the tongue is a function of this nerve, it is not routinely tested unless a peripheral nerve lesion is suspected.

Acoustic Nerve. The cochlear portion of the acoustic (vestibulocochlear) nerve (CN VIII) is tested by having the patient close the eyes and indicate when a ticking watch or the rustling of the examiner's fingertips is heard as the stimulus is brought closer to the ear. Each ear is tested individually, and the distance from the patient's ear to the sound source when first heard is recorded. This test identifies only gross deficits in hearing. For more precise assessment of hearing, an audiometer is used (see Chapter 21). The vestibular portion of this nerve is not routinely tested unless the patient complains of dizziness, vertigo, or unsteadiness or has auditory dysfunction. If this is the case, caloric testing, which is beyond the scope of routine testing, may be done.

Glossopharyngeal and Vagus Nerves. The glossopharyngeal and vagus nerves are tested together because both innervate the pharynx. The glossopharyngeal nerve (CN IX) is primarily sensory. In the gag reflex (bilateral contraction of the palatal muscles initiated by stroking or touching either side of the posterior pharynx or soft palate with a tongue blade), the sensory component is mediated by CN IX and the major motor component by the vagus nerve (CN X). It is important to assess the gag reflex in patients who have a decreased level of consciousness, a brainstem lesion, or a disease involving the throat musculature. If the reflex is weak or absent, the patient is in danger of aspirating food or secretions. The strength and efficiency of swallowing are important to test in these patients for the same reason. Another test for the awake, cooperative patient is to have the patient phonate by saying "ah" and to note the bilateral symmetry of elevation of the soft palate. Any asymmetry can indicate weakness or paralysis. Swallowing is also assessed by lightly holding the examiner's hands on either side of the patient's throat and asking the patient to swallow. Any asymmetry is noted.

Spinal Accessory Nerve. The spinal accessory nerve (CN XI) is tested by asking the patient to shrug the shoulders against resistance and to turn the head to either side against resistance. There should be smooth contraction of the sternomastoid and trapezius muscles. Symmetry, atrophy, or fasciculation of the muscle should also be noted.

Hypoglossal Nerve. The hypoglossal nerve (CN XII) is tested by asking the patient to protrude the tongue. It should protrude in the midline. The patient should also be able to push the tongue to either side against the resistance of a tongue blade. Again, any asymmetry, atrophy, or fasciculation should be noted.

Motor System. The motor system examination includes assessment of bulk, tone, and power of the major muscle groups of the body, as well as assessment of balance and coordination. The examiner tests strength by asking the patient to push and pull against the resistance of the examiner's arm as it opposes flexion and extension of the patient's muscle. The patient should be asked to offer resistance at the shoulder, elbow, wrist, hips, knees, and ankles. The patient's grip strength can also be tested. Mild weakness of the upper extremities may be tested by having the patient extend both arms forward at shoulder height with palms up while the eyes are closed. Mild weakness of the arm is demonstrated by downward drifting of the arm or pronation of the palm (*pronator drift*). Any weakness or asymmetry of strength between the same muscle groups of the right and left side should be noted.[12]

Tone is tested by passively moving the limbs through their range of motion; there should be a slight resistance to these movements. Abnormal tone is described as *hypotonia* (flaccidity) or *hypertonia* (spasticity). Involuntary movements (e.g., tics, tremor, *myoclonus* [spasm of muscles], *athetosis* [slow, writhing, involuntary movements of extremities], *chorea* [involuntary, purposeless, rapid motions], *dystonia* [impairment of muscle tone]) should be noted.

Cerebellar function is tested by assessing balance and coordination. A good screening test for both balance and muscle strength is to observe the patient's stature (posture while standing) and gait. The examiner should note the pace and rhythm of the gait and observe the arm swing. (The arms should move symmetrically and in the opposite direction of the leg on the same side.) The patient's ability to ambulate is a key factor in determining the amount of nursing care that is needed and the risk of injury from falling. A patient with cerebellar disease may have an ataxic or staggering gait, in which the feet are placed wide apart and the steps are unsteady.

Coordination can be easily tested in several ways. The finger-to-nose test involves having the patient alternately touch the nose with the index finger, then touch the examiner's finger. The examiner repositions the finger while the patient is touching the nose so

that the patient must adjust to a new distance each time the examiner's finger is touched. These movements should be performed smoothly and accurately. Other tests include asking the patient to pronate and supinate both hands rapidly and to do a shallow knee bend, first on one leg and then on the other. Dysarthria or slurred speech should be noted because it is a sign of incoordination of the speech muscles.

The heel-to-shin test involves having the patient place one heel on the opposite shin below the knee and moving the heel down the shin to the ankle. This is repeated for the other leg. These movements should flow smoothly without jerking or hesitation.

Sensory System. Several modalities are tested in the somatic sensory examination. Each modality is carried by a specific ascending pathway in the spinal cord before it reaches the sensory cortex.

There are some general guidelines for performing the sensory examination. The patient should always have the eyes closed to avoid visual clues. The examiner should avoid giving verbal cues such as, "Is this sharp?" The sensory stimulus should be applied in such a way that the patient does not expect it, avoiding rhythmic application of the stimulus. In the routine neurologic examination, sensory testing of the four extremities is sufficient. However, if a disturbance in sensory function of the skin is identified, the boundaries of that dysfunction should be carefully delineated along the dermatome.

Light Touch. Light touch is usually tested first. The examiner gently strokes a cotton wisp over each of the four extremities and asks the patient to indicate when the stimulus is felt by saying "touch." (The sensory examination of the trigeminal nerve may be delayed until this time because the same material for testing sensation is used.)

Pain and Temperature. Pain is tested by touching the skin with the sharp end of a pin. This stimulus is irregularly alternated with a simple touch stimulus with the dull end of the pin to determine whether the patient can distinguish the two stimuli. Extinction or inhibition is assessed by simultaneously stimulating opposite sides of the body symmetrically with either a pain or a touch stimulus. Normally, the simultaneous stimuli are both perceived (sensed); perception of only one may indicate a parietal lobe lesion.

The sensation of temperature is tested by applying tubes of warm and cold water to the skin and asking the patient to identify the stimuli with the eyes closed. If pain sensation is intact, assessment of temperature sensation may be omitted because both sensations are carried by the same ascending pathways.

Vibration Sense. Vibration sense is assessed by applying a vibrating C128 tuning fork to the fingernails and the bony prominences of the hands, legs, and feet with the patient's eyes closed. The examiner asks the patient if the vibration or "buzz" is felt. The examiner then asks the patient to indicate when the vibration ceases. The examiner stops the vibration with the hand as desired.

Position Sense. Position sense is assessed by placing the thumb and forefinger on either side of the patient's forefinger or great toe and gently moving the finger up or down. The patient, with his or her eyes closed, is asked to indicate the direction in which the digit is moved.

Another test of position sense of the lower extremities is the Romberg test. The patient is asked to stand with the feet together and then close his or her eyes. If the patient is able to maintain balance with the eyes open but sways or falls with the eyes closed (i.e., a positive Romberg test), vestibulocochlear dysfunction or

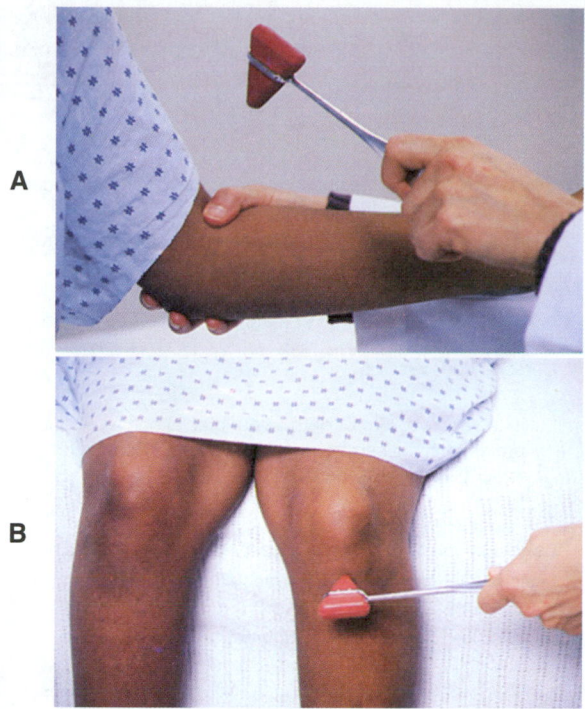

FIG. 56-17 The examiner strikes a swift blow over a stretched tendon to elicit a stretch reflex. **A,** Biceps reflex. **B,** Patellar reflex.

TABLE 56-7 | **Normal Physical Assessment of the Nervous System***

Mental Status
Alert and oriented, orderly thought processes, appropriate mood and affect

Cranial Nerves†
Smell intact to soap and coffee; visual fields full to confrontation; visual acuity 20/20 in both eyes; intact extraocular movements; no nystagmus; pupils equal, round, reactive to light and accommodation; intact facial sensation to touch and pinprick; facial movements full; intact gag and swallow reflexes; symmetric elevation of soft palate; full strength with head turning and shrugging of shoulders against resistance; midline protrusion of tongue

Motor System
Normal gait and station; normal tandem walk; negative Romberg test; normal and symmetric muscle bulk, tone, strength; smooth performance of finger-nose, heel-shin movements

Sensory System
Intact sensation to light touch, position sense, vibration, pinprick, heat and cold, two-point discrimination; intact stereognosis and graphesthesia

Reflexes‡
Biceps, triceps, brachioradialis, patellar, and Achilles tendon reflexes 2+ bilaterally; downgoing toes with plantar stimulation

*If some portion of the neurologic examination was not done, this should be indicated (e.g., "Smell not tested").
†May also be recorded as "CN I to XII intact."
‡May also be recorded as drawing of stick figure indicating reflex strength at appropriate sites.

disease in the posterior columns of the spinal cord may be indicated. It is important that the nurse be aware of patient safety during this test.

Cortical Sensory Functions. Several tests evaluate cortical integration of sensory perceptions (which occurs in the parietal lobes). Two-point discrimination is assessed by placing the two points of a calibrated compass on the tips of the fingers and toes. The minimum recognizable separation is 4 to 5 mm in the fingertips and a greater degree of separation elsewhere. This test is important in diagnosing diseases of the sensory cortex and peripheral nervous system.

Graphesthesia (ability to feel writing on skin) is tested by having the patient identify numbers traced on the palm of the hands while the eyes are closed. *Stereognosis* (ability to perceive the form and nature of objects) is tested by having the patient identify the size and shape of easily recognized objects (e.g., coins, keys, a safety pin) placed in the hands again with the eyes closed. Sensory extinction or inattention is evaluated by touching both sides of the body simultaneously. An abnormal response occurs when the patient perceives the stimulus only on one side. The other stimulus is "extinguished."

Reflexes. Tendons attached to skeletal muscles have receptors that are sensitive to stretch. A reflex contraction of the skeletal muscle occurs when the tendon is stretched. A simple muscle stretch reflex is initiated by briskly tapping the tendon of a stretched muscle, usually with a reflex hammer (Fig. 56-17). The response (muscle contraction of the corresponding muscle) is measured as follows: 0/5 = absent, 1/5 = weak response, 2/5 = normal response, 3/5 = exaggerated response, and 4/5 = hyperreflexia with clonus. *Clonus,* an abnormal response, is a continued rhythmic contraction of the muscle with continuous application of the stimulus.

In general, the biceps, triceps, brachioradialis, and patellar and Achilles tendon reflexes are tested. The examiner elicits the biceps reflex by placing the thumb over the biceps tendon in the antecubital space and striking the thumb with a hammer. The patient should have the arms partially flexed at the elbow with the palms up. The normal response is flexion of the arm at the elbow or contraction of the biceps muscle that can be felt by the examiner's thumb.

The triceps reflex is elicited by striking the triceps tendon above the elbow while the patient's arm is flexed. The normal response is extension of the arm or visible contraction of the triceps.

The brachioradialis reflex is elicited by striking the radius 3 to 5 cm above the wrist while the patient's arm is relaxed. The normal response is flexion and supination at the elbow or visible contraction of the brachioradialis muscle.

The patellar reflex is elicited by striking the patellar tendon just below the patella. The patient can be sitting or lying as long as the leg being tested hangs freely. The normal response is extension of the leg with contraction of the quadriceps.

The Achilles tendon reflex is elicited by striking the Achilles tendon while the patient's leg is flexed at the knee and the foot is dorsiflexed at the ankle. The normal response is plantar flexion at the ankle.

Table 56-7 is an example of a normal neurologic assessment. Common abnormal assessment findings of the neurologic system are presented in Table 56-8.

DIAGNOSTIC STUDIES OF THE NERVOUS SYSTEM

Diagnostic studies provide important information to the nurse in monitoring the patient's condition and planning appropriate interventions. These studies are considered to be objective data. Diagnostic studies used to assess the nervous system are presented in Table 56-9.

TABLE 56-8	**COMMON ASSESSMENT ABNORMALITIES** Nervous System	

Finding	Description	Possible Etiology and Significance
Mental Status		
Altered consciousness	Inability to speak, obey commands, open eyes appropriately with verbal or painful stimulus	Intracranial lesions, metabolic disorder, psychiatric disorders
Anosognosia	Inability to recognize bodily defect or disease	Lesions in right parietal cortex, common in right-brain stroke
Speech		
Aphasia	Loss of language faculty (comprehension, expression, or both)	Cerebral cortex lesion
Dysphasia	Impairment of or difficulty with use of language (comprehension, expression, or both)	Cerebral cortex lesion
Dysarthria	Lack of coordination in articulating speech	Lesions in cerebellum or pathway of cranial nerves (including brainstem); antiseizure drugs, sedatives, hypnotic drug toxicity (including alcohol)
Eyes		
Anisocoria	Inequality of pupil size	Lesion, injury, or intracranial pressure in area of midbrain
Diplopia	Double vision	Lesions affecting nerves of extraocular muscles, cerebellar damage
Homonymous hemianopsia	Loss of vision in one side of visual field	Injury or lesions in area of optic tract or its radiations to occipital cortex
Cranial Nerves		
Dysphagia	Difficulty in swallowing	Lesions involving motor pathways of CN IX, X (including lower brainstem)
Ophthalmoplegia	Paralysis of eye muscles	Lesions in brainstem or CN III, IV, VI
Papilledema	"Choked disc," swelling of optic nerve head	Increase in intracranial pressure on CN II
Motor System		
Apraxia	Inability to perform learned movements despite having desire and physical ability to perform them	Cerebral cortex lesion
Ataxia	Lack of coordination of movement	Lesions of sensory or motor pathways, cerebellum; antiseizure drugs, sedatives, hypnotic drug toxicity (including alcohol)
Dyskinesia	Impairment of power of voluntary movement, resulting in fragmentary or incomplete movements	Disorders of basal ganglia, idiosyncratic reaction to psychotropic drugs
Hemiplegia	Paralysis on one side	Stroke and other lesions involving motor cortex
Nystagmus	Jerking or bobbing of eyes as they track moving object	Lesions in cerebellum, brainstem, vestibular system; antiseizure drugs, sedatives, hypnotic toxicity (including alcohol)
Opisthotonus	Extreme arching of back with retraction of head	Meningitis, tonic phase of grand mal seizure
Sensory System		
Analgesia	Loss of pain sensation	Lesion in spinothalamic tract or thalamus, lack of or damage to sensory nerve endings
Anesthesia	Absence of sensation	Lesions in spinal cord, thalamus, sensory cortex, or peripheral sensory nerve
Hyperesthesia	Increase in sensation	
Hypoesthesia	Decrease in sensation	
Astereognosis	Inability to recognize form of object by touch	Lesions in parietal cortex
Reflexes		
Extensor plantar response (Babinski's sign)	Upgoing toes with plantar stimulation	Suprasegmental or upper motor neuron lesion
Brudzinski's sign (Fig. 56-18)	Neck lesion produces neck pain and results in reflex flexion of the hip and knee	Meningeal irritation
Kernig's sign (Fig. 56-19)	Reflex contraction and pain on extension of the leg from a position of 90-degree hip flexion while supine	Meningeal irritation

TABLE 56-8	COMMON ASSESSMENT ABNORMALITIES Nervous System—cont'd	

Finding	Description	Possible Etiology and Significance
Spinal Cord		
Bladder dysfunction		
Atonic (autonomous)	Absence of muscle tone and contractility, enlargement of capacity, no sensation of discomfort, overflow with large residual, inability to voluntarily empty or empty by reflex	Early stage of spinal cord injury
Hypotonic	More ability than atonic bladder but less than normal	Interruption of afferent pathways from bladder
Hypertonic	Increase in muscle tone, diminished capacity, reflex emptying, dribbling, incontinence	Lesions in pyramidal tracts (efferent pathways)
Paraplegia	Paralysis of lower extremities	Spinal cord transection or mass lesion (thoracolumbar region)
Tetraplegia (quadriplegia)	Paralysis of all extremities	Spinal cord transection or mass lesion (cervical region)

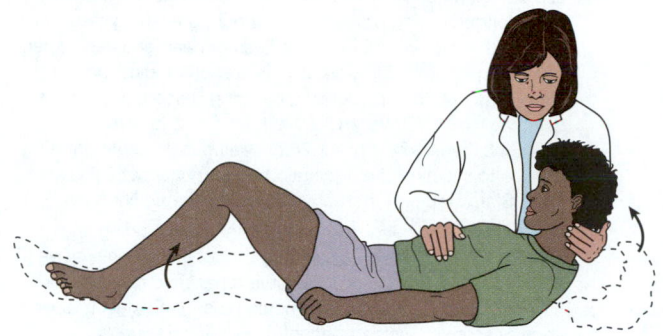

FIG. 56-18 Brudzinski's sign. Involuntary flexion of the hip and knees is a positive Brudzinski's sign for meningeal irritation.

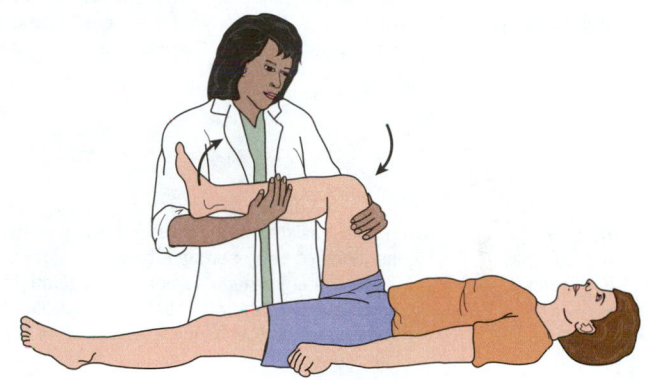

FIG. 56-19 Kernig's sign. Pain in the lower back and resistance to straightening the leg at the knee is a positive Kernig's sign, indicating meningeal irritation.

Cerebrospinal Fluid Analysis. CSF analysis provides information about a variety of CNS diseases. Normal CSF fluid is clear, colorless, and free of red blood cells and contains little protein. Normal CSF values are listed in Table 56-10.

Lumbar Puncture. Lumbar puncture is the most common method of obtaining CSF for analysis. It is contraindicated in the presence of increased intracranial pressure or infection at the site of puncture.

Nurses often assist in this procedure because it is usually performed in the patient's room. Before the procedure, the nurse should have the patient empty the bladder. The patient should lie in the lateral recumbent position, with the back as near as possible to the edge of the bed. The nurse should assist the patient to draw up the knees to the abdomen and flex the head to the chest. This helps separate the vertebrae so that the needle can be inserted more easily.

Using strict sterile technique, the physician inserts a long needle below the third lumbar vertebra. This may cause some local discomfort. There is no danger of injuring the spinal cord because the cord terminates between the first and second lumbar vertebrae. However, the patient may have some pain radiating down the leg or muscle twitching if the needle irritates the spinal root. The nurse can assure the patient that this is temporary and that the patient is not in danger of being paralyzed.

A manometer is attached to the needle, and CSF pressure is determined after the patient is asked to relax and extend the legs. If this is not done, the pressure appears abnormally high. CSF is withdrawn in a series of tubes and sent for analysis. Some examiners believe that the patient should be kept lying flat for at least a

few hours after the procedure to avoid a spinal headache, which is presumably the result of leakage of CSF at the puncture site. The prone position may be effective in preventing CSF leakage. Others do not believe that the lying position is necessary because headache seems to develop in some patients despite precautions. The headache intensity may also be reduced by increasing fluid intake. Meningeal irritation (*nuchal rigidity*) or signs and symptoms of local trauma (e.g., hematoma, pain) may develop in some patients.

Radiologic Studies

Cerebral Angiography. Cerebral angiography is indicated when vascular lesions or tumors are suspected. A catheter is inserted into the femoral (sometimes brachial) artery. It is then passed up the artery to the aortic arch and into the base of a carotid or a vertebral artery for injection of radiopaque contrast medium. A series of x-rays is taken in a timed sequence so that pictures of the arteries, smaller vessels, and veins can be obtained (Fig. 56-20). This study can help to localize and determine the presence of abscesses, aneurysms, hematomas, arteriovenous malformations, arterial spasm, and certain tumors.

Because this is an invasive procedure, adverse reactions may occur. The patient may have an allergic (anaphylactic) reaction to the contrast medium. This reaction usually occurs immediately after injection of the contrast medium and may require emergency resuscitation measures in the procedure room. The most common precaution for nurses to take in caring for the patient after the re-

TABLE 56-9	*DIAGNOSTIC STUDIES* Nervous System	

Study	Description and Purpose	Nursing Responsibility
Cerebrospinal Fluid Analysis		
Lumbar puncture	CSF is aspirated by needle insertion in L3-4 or L4-5 interspace to assess many CNS diseases (see Table 56-10).	Assure that patient has no cerebral tumor before start of procedure that could result in herniation with the removal of CSF. Patient assumes and maintains lateral recumbent position with knees flexed. Ensure maintenance of strict aseptic technique. Ensure labeling of CSF specimens in proper sequence. Keep patient flat for at least a few hours depending on physician preference. Encourage fluids. Monitor neurologic and VS. Administer analgesia as needed.
Radiology		
Skull and spine x-rays	Simple x-ray of skull and spinal column is done to detect fractures, bone erosion, calcifications, abnormal vascularity.	Explain that procedure is noninvasive. Explain positions to be assumed.
Cerebral angiography	Serial x-ray visualization of intracranial and extracranial blood vessels is performed to detect vascular lesions and tumors of brain. Contrast medium is used.	Assess patient for stroke risk prior to procedure as thrombi may be dislodged during procedure. Withhold preceding meal. Explain that patient will have hot flush of head and neck when contrast medium is injected. Administer premedication. Explain need to be absolutely still during procedure. Monitor neurologic and VS every 15-30 min for first 2 hr, every hour for next 6 hr, then every 2 hr for 24 hr. Maintain pressure dressing and ice to injection site. Maintain bed rest until patient is alert and VS are stable. Report any neurologic status changes.
Computed tomography (CT) scan	Computer-assisted x-ray of several levels or thin cross sections of body parts are done to detect problems such as hemorrhage, tumor, cyst, edema, infarction, brain atrophy, and other abnormalities. Contrast media may be used to enhance visualization of brain structures.	Assess for contraindications to contrast media, including shell fish/iodine/dye allergy. Explain that procedure is noninvasive (if no contrast medium used). Observe for allergic reaction and note puncture site (if contrast medium used). Explain appearance of scanner. Instruct patient to remain still during procedure.
Magnetic resonance imaging (MRI)	Imaging of brain, spinal cord, and spinal canal by means of magnetic energy (Fig. 56-21). Used in detection of strokes, multiple sclerosis, tumors, trauma, herniation, and seizures. No invasive procedures are required. Gadolinium contrast media may be used to enhance visualization. Has greater contrast in images of soft tissue structures than does CT scan.	Assess for contraindications, including heart pacemaker. Screen patient for metal parts and pacemaker in body. Instruct patient on need to lie very still for up to 1 hr. Sedation may be necessary if patient is claustrophobic.
Magnetic resonance angiography (MRA)	Uses differential signal characteristics of flowing blood to evaluate extracranial and intracranial blood vessels. Provides both anatomic and hemodynamic information. Can be used in conjunction with contrast media (contrast-enhanced MRA [cMRA]). Rapidly replacing cerebral angiography for use in diagnosing cerebrovascular diseases.	Similar to MRI (see above).
Magnetic resonance spectroscopy (MRS)	Provides information about chemical composition of tissue. Used to study brain diseases, including brain tumors, Alzheimer's disease, strokes, acquired immunodeficiency syndrome, seizure disorders, and multiple sclerosis. Markers of neuronal integrity (e.g., *N*-acetyl aspartate) used to determine loss of neurons.	Similar to MRI (see above).
Functional MRI (fMRI)	Use of MRI to detect changes in cerebral metabolism or blood flow, volume, or oxygenation in response to specific tasks, consisting of periods of activity and periods of rest. Can functionally map brain.	Similar to MRI (see above).
Myelography	X-ray of spinal cord and vertebral column after injection of contrast medium into subarachnoid space. Used to detect spinal lesions (e.g., herniated or ruptured disk, spinal tumor).	Administer preprocedure sedation as ordered. Instruct patient to empty bladder. Inform patient that test is performed with patient on tilting table that is moved during test. After procedure, patient should lie flat for a few hours. Encourage fluids. Monitor neurologic and VS. Headache, nausea, and vomiting may occur after procedure.
Positron emission tomography (PET)	Measures metabolic activity of brain to assess cell death or damage. Uses radioactive material that shows up as a bright spot on the image. Used for patients with stroke, Alzheimer's disease, seizure disorders, Parkinson's disease, and tumors.	Explain procedure to patient. Explain that two IV lines will be inserted. Instruct patient not to take sedatives or tranquilizers. Empty bladder before procedure. Assure glucose monitoring due to injected venous scan material. May be asked to perform different activities during test.

CSF, Cerebrospinal fluid; *CNS,* central nervous system; *IV,* intravenous; *VS,* vital signs.

TABLE 56-9	*DIAGNOSTIC STUDIES* Nervous System—cont'd	

Study	Description and Purpose	Nursing Responsibility
Radiology—cont'd		
Single-photon emission computed tomography (SPECT)	A method of scanning similar to PET, but it uses more stable substances and different detectors. Radiolabeled compounds are injected and their photon emissions can be detected. Images made are accumulation of labeled compound. Used to visualize blood flow or oxygen or glucose metabolism in the brain. Useful in diagnosing strokes, brain tumors, and seizure disorders.	Similar to PET (see above).
Electrographic Studies		
Electroencephalography (EEG)	Electrical activity of brain is recorded by scalp electrodes to evaluate seizure disorders, cerebral disease, CNS effects of systemic diseases, brain death.	Inform patient that procedure is painless and without danger of electric shock. Withhold stimulants. Determine whether any medications (e.g., tranquilizers, antiseizure drugs) should be withheld. Resume medications after test. Assist patient to wash electrode paste out of hair.
Magnetoencephalography (MEG)	Uses a sensitivity machine called a biomagnetometer, which detects very small magnetic fields generated by neural activity. It can accurately pinpoint the part of the brain involved in a stroke, seizure, or other disorder or injury. Measures extracranial magnetic fields as well as scalp electric field (EEG).	MEG, a passive sensor, does not make physical contact with patient. Explain procedure to patient.
Electromyography (EMG) and nerve conduction studies	Electrical activity associated with nerve and skeletal muscle is recorded by insertion of needle electrodes to detect muscle and peripheral nerve disease.	Inform patient of slight discomfort associated with insertion of needles.
Evoked potentials	Electrical activity associated with nerve conduction along sensory pathways is recorded by electrodes placed on skin and scalp. Stimulus generates the impulse. Procedure is used to diagnose disease, locate nerve damage, and monitor function intraoperatively.	Explain procedure to patient.
• Visual evoked potentials	Electrical activity in visual pathway is recorded with rapidly reversing checkerboard pattern on television screen. One eye is tested at a time.	Explain procedure to patient.
• Brainstem auditory evoked potentials	Electrical activity in auditory pathway is recorded with earphones that produce clicking sounds. One ear is tested at a time.	Explain procedure to patient.
• Somatosensory evoked potentials	Electrical activity in certain nerve pathways is recorded with mild electrical pulse (several per second).	Inform patient that stimulus may cause mild discomfort or muscle twitch.
Ultrasound		
Carotid duplex studies	Combined ultrasound and pulsed Doppler technology. Probe is placed over the carotid artery and slowly moved along the course of the common carotid to the bifurcation of the external and internal carotid arteries. Frequency of reflected ultrasound signal corresponds to the blood velocity. Increased blood flow velocity can indicate stenosis of a vessel. Duplex scanning is a noninvasive study that evaluates the degree of stenosis of the carotid and vertebral arteries.	Explain procedure to patient.
Transcranial Doppler	Same technology as carotid duplex, but evaluates blood flow velocities of the intracranial blood vessels. Probe is placed on the skin at various "windows" in the skull (areas in the skull that have only a thin bony covering) to register velocities of the blood vessels. Peak blood flow velocities and systolic/diastolic ratios can be calculated from this information. Noninvasive technique that is useful in assessing vasospasm associated with subarachnoid hemorrhage, altered intracranial blood flow dynamics associated with occlusive vascular disease, presence of emboli, and cerebral autoregulation.	Explain procedure to patient.

TABLE 56-10	Normal Cerebrospinal Fluid Values
Parameter	**Normal Value**
Specific gravity	1.007
pH	7.35
Appearance	Clear, colorless
RBCs	None
WBCs	0-8/μl (0-0.008/L)
Protein	
Lumbar	15-45 mg/dl (0.15-0.45 g/L)
Cisternal	15-25 mg/dl (0.15-0.25 g/L)
Ventricular	5-15 mg/dl (0.05-0.15 g/L)
Glucose	45-75 mg/dl (2.5-4.2 mmol/L)
Microorganisms	None
Opening pressure with lumbar puncture	60-150 mm H₂O

RBCs, Red blood cells; *WBCs,* white blood cells.

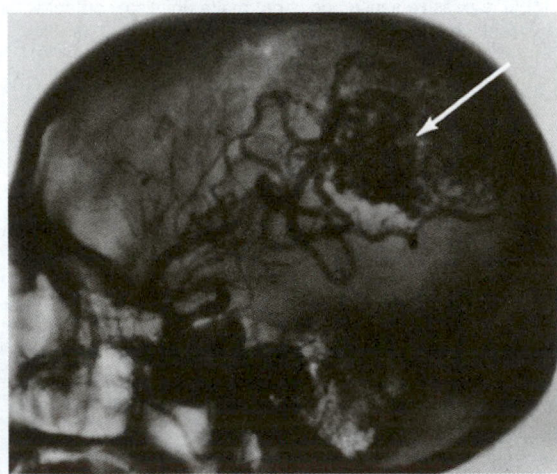

FIG. 56-20   Cerebral angiogram illustrating an arteriovenous malformation *(arrow).*

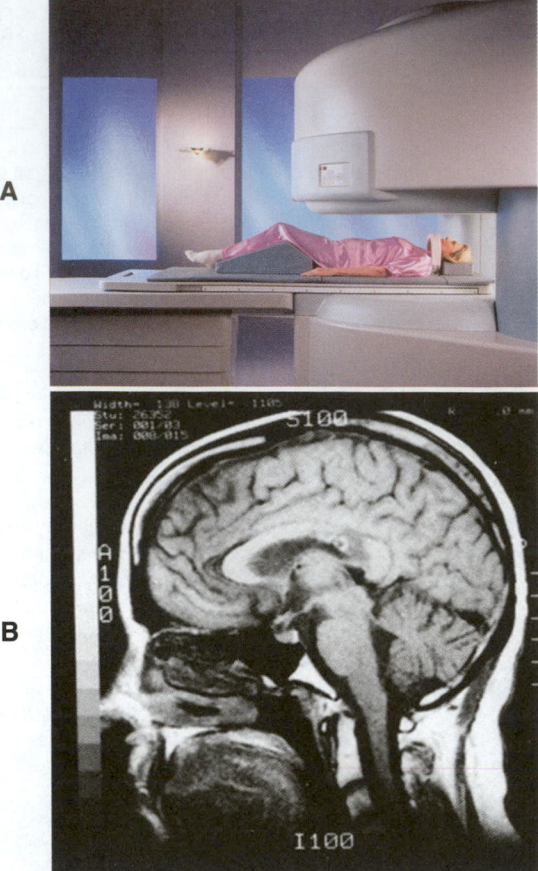

FIG. 56-21   **A,** Clinical setting for magnetic resonance imaging (MRI). **B,** Midline sagittal view of the brain using MRI.

turn to the room is observation for bleeding at the catheter puncture site (usually the groin). A pressure dressing and ice are usually placed on the site to promote hemostasis and prevent swelling.

Electrographic Studies

Electroencephalography. The technique of *electroencephalography (EEG)* involves the recording of the electrical activity of the surface cortical neurons of the brain by 8 to 16 electrodes placed on specific areas of the scalp. Specific tests may be done to evaluate the effects of bright lights and loud noises on the electrical activity. This test is done to evaluate not only cerebral disease but also the CNS effects of many metabolic and systemic diseases, and to determine brain death. Among the cerebral diseases assessed by EEG are seizure disorders, mass lesions (e.g., tumor, abscess, hematoma), cerebrovascular lesions, and brain injury (Fig. 56-22). The procedure is noninvasive. Patients sometimes have the misconception that the recording electrodes will give them an electric shock. They should be assured that this is not true and that the procedure is similar to electrocardiography.

Electromyography and Nerve Conduction Studies. *Electromyography (EMG)* is the recording of electrical activity as-

sociated with innervation of skeletal muscle. The recording is displayed on a computer screen and may be played on a loudspeaker for simultaneous analysis. Needle electrodes are inserted into the muscle to record specific motor units because recording from the skin is not sufficient. Normal muscle at rest shows no electrical activity. Typical electrical activity occurs when the muscle contracts. This activity may be altered in diseases of muscle itself (e.g., myopathic conditions) or in disorders of muscle innervation (e.g., segmental or LMN lesions, peripheral neuropathic conditions). Fibrillations are spontaneous, independent contractions of individual muscle fibers that can be detected only by EMG. They appear on EMG 1 to 3 weeks after a muscle has lost its nerve supply.

Nerve conduction studies involve application of a brief electrical stimulus to a distal portion of a sensory or mixed nerve and recording the resulting wave of depolarization at some point proximal to the stimulation. For example, a stimulus can be applied to the forefinger and a recording electrode placed over the median nerve at the wrist. The time between the onset of the stimulus and the initial wave of depolarization at the recording electrode is measured. This is termed *nerve conduction velocity*. Damaged nerves have slower conduction velocities.

Evoked Potentials. *Evoked potentials* are recordings of electrical activity associated with nerve conduction along sensory pathways. The activity is generated by a specific sensory stimulus related to the type of study (e.g., checkerboard patterns for visual evoked potentials, clicking sounds for auditory evoked

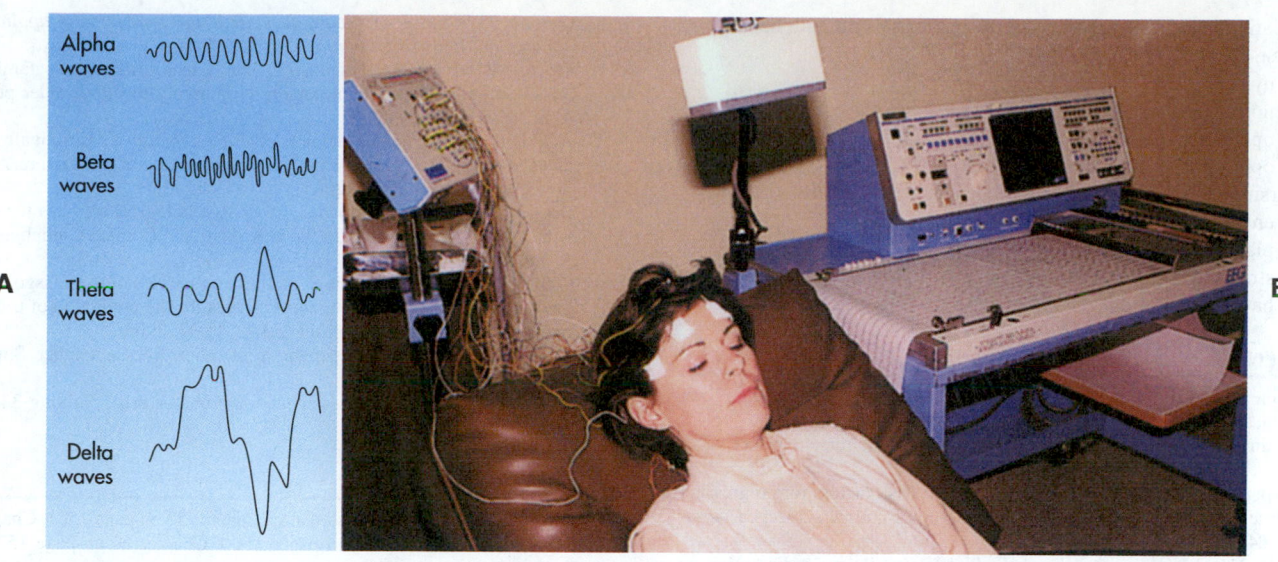

FIG. 56-22 Electroencephalogram (EEG). **A,** Examples of alpha, beta, theta, and delta waves seen on an EEG. **B,** Photograph showing a person undergoing an EEG test. Notice the scalp electrodes that detect voltage fluctuations within the cranium.

potentials, mild electrical pulses for somatosensory evoked potentials). Electrodes placed on specific areas of the skin and scalp record the electrical activity, which is stored and averaged by a computerized instrument. A wave pattern appears on a screen and is printed on paper. Peaks in the wave pattern correspond to conduction of the stimulus through certain points along the sensory pathway (e.g., peripheral nerve, brainstem, cortical areas). Increases in the normal time from stimulus onset to a given peak (latency) indicate slowed nerve conduction or nerve damage. This technique is useful in diagnosing abnormalities of the visual or auditory systems because it reveals whether a sensory impulse is reaching the appropriate part of the brain. Indications for these tests include evaluation of the optic nerve in conditions such as multiple sclerosis (optic neuritis) and of the vestibulocochlear nerve in acoustic neuroma.

NCLEX EXAMINATION REVIEW QUESTIONS

The number of the question corresponds to the same-numbered objective at the beginning of the chapter.

1. In a patient with a disease that affects the myelin sheath of nerves, such as multiple sclerosis, the glial cells that are affected are the
   a. microglia.
   b. astrocytes.
   c. ependymal cells.
   d. oligodendrocytes.
2. A state of hypoxia alters the repeated action potentials necessary for transmission of nerve impulses because energy is required for
   a. repolarization of the cell membrane.
   b. creation of cell membrane permeability.
   c. movement of sodium into the nerve cell.
   d. maintenance of the resting membrane potential.
3. Drugs or diseases that impair the function of the extrapyramidal system may cause loss of
   a. sensations of pain and temperature.
   b. regulation of the autonomic nervous system.

   c. integration of somatic and special sensory inputs.
   d. automatic movements associated with skeletal muscle activity.
4. An obstruction of the anterior cerebral arteries will affect functions of
   a. visual imaging.
   b. balance and coordination.
   c. judgment, insight, and reasoning.
   d. visual and auditory integration for language comprehension.
5. Paralysis of lateral gaze indicates a lesion of cranial nerve
   a. II.
   b. III.
   c. IV.
   d. VI.
6. A result of stimulation of the parasympathetic nervous system is
   a. dilation of skin blood vessels.
   b. increased secretion of insulin.
   c. increased blood glucose levels.
   d. relaxation of the urinary sphincters.
7. Assessment of muscle strength of older adults cannot be compared with that of younger adults because
   a. stroke is more common in older adults.
   b. nutritional status is better in young adults.
   c. most young people exercise more than older people.
   d. aging leads to a decrease in muscle bulk and strength.
8. Data regarding mobility, strength, coordination, and activity tolerance are important for the nurse to obtain because
   a. many neurologic diseases affect one or more of these areas.
   b. patients are less able to identify other neurologic impairments.
   c. these are the first functions to be affected by neurologic disease.
   d. aspects of movement are the most important functions of the nervous system.
9. During neurologic testing the patient is able to perceive pain elicited by pinprick. Based on this finding, the nurse may omit testing for
   a. position sense.
   b. patellar reflexes.
   c. temperature perception.
   d. heel-to-shin movements.

10. A patient's eyes jerk as they follow the nurse's moving finger. The nurse records this finding as
    a. nystagmus.
    b. normal tracking.
    c. ophthalmoplegia.
    d. ophthalmic dyskinesia.

11. Nursing responsibilities for lumbar puncture include
    a. ensuring the patient has a full bladder.
    b. placing the patient in the lateral recumbent position.
    c. straightening the patient's legs just before the puncture.
    d. having the patient cough when the needle has been inserted.

REFERENCES

1. Lichtenwalner RJ, Parent JM: Adult neurogenesis and the ischemic forebrain, *J Cereb Blood Flow Metab* 26:1, 2006.
2. Kastin AJ, Pan W: Targeting neurite growth inhibitors to induce CNS regeneration, *Curr Pharm Des* 11:1247, 2005.
3. Enzinger C, Fazekas F, Matthews PM, et al: Risk factors for progression of brain atrophy in aging: six-year follow-up of normal subjects, *Neurology* 64:1704, 2005.
4. Miller CA: *Nursing for wellness in older adults: theory and practice,* ed 4, Philadelphia, 2004, Lippincott, Williams & Wilkins.
5. Binder LM, Campbell KA: Medically unexplained symptoms and neuropsychological assessment, *J Clin Exp Neuropsychol* 26:369, 2004.
6. Grodner M, Long S, De Young S: *Foundations and clinical applications of nutrition: a nursing approach,* ed 3, St Louis, 2004, Mosby.
7. Morris MC, Evans DA, Bienias JL, et al: Dietary folate and vitamin B12 intake and cognitive decline among community-dwelling older persons, *Arch Neurol* 62:641, 2005.
8. Agnoletti V, Ansaloni L, Catena F, et al: Postoperative delirium after elective and emergency surgery: analysis and checking of risk factors. A study protocol, *BMC Surg* 5:12, 2005.
9. Bowen A, Knapp P, Hoffman A, et al: Psychological services for people with stroke: compliance with the U.K. National Clinical Guidelines, *Clin Rehabil* 19:323, 2005.
10. Gill M, Windemuth R, Steele R, et al: A comparison of the Glasgow Coma Scale score to simplified alternative scores for the prediction of traumatic brain injury outcomes, *Ann Emerg Med* 45:37, 2005.
11. Noah P: Neurological assessment: a refresher, *RN*, September, Suppl:18, 2004.
12. Pullen RL: Neurologic assessment for pronator drift, *Nursing* 34(3):22, 2004.

RESOURCES

Resources for this chapter are listed after Chapter 57 on page 1501, Chapter 58 on page 1526, Chapter 59 on pages 1560, Chapter 60 on page 1579, and Chapter 61 on page 1613.

For additional Internet resources, see the website for this book at *http://evolve. elsevier.com/Lewis/medsurg.*

You have not lived a perfect day unless you've done something for someone who will never be able to repay you.

Ruth Smeltzer

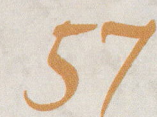

Nursing Management
Acute Intracranial Problems

57

Linda Laskowski-Jones

LEARNING OBJECTIVES

1. Identify the physiologic mechanisms that maintain normal intracranial pressure.
2. Identify the common etiologies, clinical manifestations, and collaborative care of the patient with increased intracranial pressure.
3. Describe the collaborative and nursing management of the patient with increased intracranial pressure.
4. Differentiate types of head injury by mechanism of injury and clinical manifestations.
5. Describe the collaborative care and nursing management of the patient with a head injury.
6. Compare the types, clinical manifestations, and collaborative care of patients with brain tumors.
7. Discuss the nursing management of the patient with a brain tumor.
8. Describe the nursing management of the patient undergoing cranial surgery.
9. Compare the primary causes, collaborative care, and nursing management of meningitis, encephalitis, and brain abscess.
10. Describe the etiology, clinical manifestations, and nursing and collaborative management of the patient with rabies.

KEY TERMS

cerebral edema, p. 1469
coma, p. 1469
concussion, p. 1482
contusion, p. 1482
encephalitis, p. 1497
epidural hematoma, p. 1483
Glasgow Coma Scale, p. 1476
intracerebral hematoma, p. 1484
intracranial pressure, p. 1468
meningitis, p. 1493
nuchal rigidity, p. 1494
subdural hematoma, p. 1483
unconsciousness, p. 1471

Electronic Resources

Supplemental content related to Chapter 57 can be found . . .

Companion CD
- Stress-Busting Kit for Nursing Students
- Interactive Case Studies:
  - Head Injury
  - Meningitis
- NCLEX Examination Review Questions
- Animation: Functional Areas of the Brain
- Comprehensive Glossary

Evolve Website *evolve*
http://evolve.elsevier.com/Lewis/medsurg
- Content Updates
- Key Points (Printable and CD/MP3 Download)
- Concept Map Creator
- Expanded Audio Glossary
- Key Term Flash Cards

- Customizable Nursing Care Plans:
  - Bacterial Meningitis
  - Increased Intracranial Pressure
- Patient and Family Instruction Guide in English and Spanish: Head Injury
- Electronic Calculators
- WebLinks

Acute intracranial problems include diseases and disorders that can increase intracranial pressure (ICP). This chapter discusses the mechanisms that maintain normal ICP, increased ICP, head injury, brain tumors, and cerebral inflammatory disorders.

INTRACRANIAL PRESSURE

Understanding the dynamics associated with ICP is important in caring for patients with many different neurologic problems. The skull is like a closed box with three essential volume components: brain tissue, blood, and cerebrospinal fluid (CSF) (Fig. 57-1). The intracellular and extracellular fluids of brain tissue make up ap-

proximately 78% of this volume. Blood in the arterial, venous, and capillary network makes up 12% of the volume, and the remaining 10% is the volume of the CSF. Under normal conditions, in which intracranial volume remains relatively constant, the balance among these components maintains the ICP. Factors that influence ICP under normal circumstances are changes in (1) arterial pressure, (2) venous pressure, (3) intraabdominal and intrathoracic pressure, (4) posture, (5) temperature, and (6) blood gases, particularly CO_2 levels. The degree to which these factors increase or decrease the ICP depends on the ability of the brain to accommodate to the changes.

Reviewed by Gayle H. Dasher, RN, PhD, CCRN, CNRN, Director of Clinical Practice and Standards, CHRISTUS Santa Rosa Health Care, San Antonio, Tex.

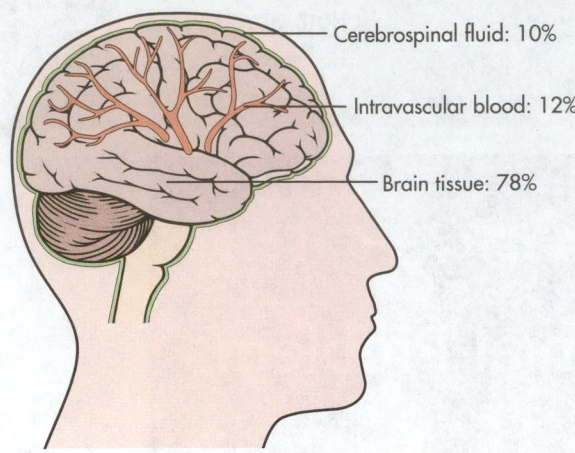

Cerebrospinal fluid: 10%

Intravascular blood: 12%

Brain tissue: 78%

FIG. 57-1   Components of the brain.

TABLE 57-1	Calculation of Cerebral Perfusion Pressure

CPP = MAP − ICP

$$MAP = DBP + \frac{1}{3}(SBP - DBP) \text{ or } \frac{SBP + 2(DBP)}{3}$$

Example: Systemic blood pressure = 122/84
                    MAP = 97
                    ICP = 12 mm Hg
                    CPP = 85 mm Hg

CPP, Cerebral perfusion pressure; *DBP,* diastolic blood pressure; *ICP,* intracranial pressure; *MAP,* mean arterial pressure; *SBP,* systolic blood pressure.

Regulation and Maintenance of Intracranial Pressure

Normal Intracranial Pressure. **Intracranial pressure** is the hydrostatic force measured in the brain CSF compartment. Normal ICP is the total pressure exerted by the three components within the skull: brain tissue, blood, and CSF. The modified Monro-Kellie doctrine describes the relatively constant volume of these three components within the rigid skull structure. If the volume of any one of the three components increases within the cranial vault and the volume from another component is displaced, the total intracranial volume will not change.[1] This hypothesis is only applicable in situations in which the skull is rigid (e.g., the hypothesis is not valid in neonates and in adults with displaced skull fractures).

Normal Compensatory Adaptations. In applying the modified Monro-Kellie doctrine, the body can adapt to volume changes within the skull to maintain a normal ICP. Initial compensatory mechanisms include changes in the CSF volume achieved by altering CSF absorption or production and by displacement of CSF into the spinal subarachnoid space. Alterations in intracranial blood volume occur through the collapse of cerebral veins and dural sinuses, regional cerebral vasoconstriction or dilation, and changes in venous outflow. Tissue brain volume compensates through distention of the dura or compression of brain tissue. Initially an increase in volume produces no increase in ICP as a result of these compensatory mechanisms. However, the ability to compensate to changes in volume is limited; as the volume increase continues, the ICP rises and decompensation ultimately occurs, resulting in compression and ischemia.[1]

Measuring ICP. ICP can be measured in the ventricles, subarachnoid space, subdural space, epidural space, or brain parenchymal tissue using a pressure transducer. Normal intracranial ICP ranges from 0 to 15 mm Hg. A sustained pressure above the upper limit is considered abnormal. ICP may rise due to head trauma, stroke, subarachnoid hemorrhage, brain tumor, inflammation, hydrocephalus, or brain tissue damage from other causes. Any patient who becomes acutely unconscious, regardless of the cause, is suspected of having increased ICP. Patients with conditions known to elevate ICP usually undergo ICP monitoring in an intensive care unit (ICU), except those with irreversible problems or advanced neurologic disease. Goals for nursing management of a patient with elevated ICP include preservation of cerebral oxygenation and perfusion, early identification of neurologic changes, and prevention of complications.

Cerebral Blood Flow

Cerebral blood flow (CBF) is the amount of blood in milliliters passing through 100 g of brain tissue in 1 minute. The global CBF is approximately 50 ml/min per 100 g of brain tissue. There is a difference in flow between the white and gray matter of the brain. The white matter has a slower blood flow, approximately 25 ml/min per 100 g, and the gray matter has a faster blood flow, approximately 75 ml/min per 100 g.[2] The maintenance of blood flow to the brain is critical because the brain requires a constant supply of oxygen and glucose. The brain uses 20% of the body's oxygen and 25% of its glucose.

Autoregulation of Cerebral Blood Flow. The brain has the ability to regulate its own blood flow in response to its metabolic needs despite wide fluctuations in systemic arterial pressure. *Autoregulation* is the automatic adjustment in the diameter of the cerebral blood vessels by the brain to maintain a constant blood flow during changes in arterial blood pressure (BP).[3] The purpose of autoregulation is to ensure a consistent CBF to provide for the metabolic needs of brain tissue and to maintain cerebral perfusion pressure within normal limits.

The lower limit of systemic arterial pressure at which autoregulation is effective in a normotensive person is a mean arterial pressure (MAP) of 50 mm Hg. Below this, CBF decreases, and symptoms of cerebral ischemia, such as syncope and blurred vision, occur. The upper limit of systemic arterial pressure at which autoregulation is effective is a MAP of 150 mm Hg.[2] When this pressure is exceeded, the vessels are maximally constricted, and further vasoconstrictor response is lost.

The *cerebral perfusion pressure* (CPP) is the pressure needed to ensure blood flow to the brain. CPP is equal to the MAP minus the ICP (CPP = MAP − ICP) (see example in Table 57-1). This formula is clinically useful, although it does not consider the effect of cerebral vascular resistance. Cerebral vascular resistance, generated by the arterioles within the cranium, links CPP and blood flow as follows:

$$CPP = Flow \times Resistance$$

When cerebral vascular resistance is high, blood flow to brain tissue is impaired. Transcranial Doppler is a noninvasive technique used in ICUs to monitor changes in cerebrovascular resistance.

As the CPP decreases, autoregulation fails and CBF decreases. Normal CPP is 60 to 100 mm Hg. CPP <50 mm Hg is associated with ischemia and neuronal death. A CPP below 30 mm Hg results in ischemia and is incompatible with life. Normally, autoregulation maintains an adequate CBF and perfusion pressure primarily by adjusting the diameter of cerebral blood vessels and metabolic factors that impact ICP. It is critical to maintain MAP when ICP is elevated. It is important to remember that CPP may not reflect perfusion pressure in all parts of the brain. There may be local areas of swelling and compression limiting regional perfusion pressure. Thus a higher CPP may be needed for these patients to prevent localized tissue damage.

Pressure Changes. The relationship of pressure to volume is depicted in the pressure-volume curve. The curve is affected by the brain's compliance.

Compliance is the expandability of the brain. It is represented as the volume increase for each unit increase in pressure. With low compliance, small changes in volume result in greater increases in pressure.

$$Compliance = Volume/Pressure$$

The concept of the pressure-volume curve can be used to represent the stages of increased ICP (Fig. 57-2). At stage 1 on the curve, there is high compliance. The brain is in total compensation, with accommodation and autoregulation intact. An increase in volume (in brain tissue, blood, or CSF) does not increase the ICP. At stage 2, the compliance is beginning to lessen, and an increase in volume places the patient at risk of increased ICP. At stage 3, there is significant reduction in compliance. Any small addition of volume causes a great increase in ICP. Compensatory mechanisms fail, there is a loss of autoregulation, and the patient will exhibit manifestations of increased ICP (e.g., headache, changes in level of consciousness or pupil responsiveness).

With a loss of autoregulation, there is a rise in systolic BP in an attempt to maintain cerebral perfusion through an elevation in systolic BP. However, decompensation is imminent. The patient's response is characterized by systolic hypertension with a widening pulse pressure, bradycardia with a full and bounding pulse, and altered respirations. This is known as *Cushing's triad*.

As the patient enters stage 4, the ICP rises to lethal levels with little increase in volume. *Herniation* occurs as the brain tissue is forcibly shifted from the compartment of greater pressure to a compartment of lesser pressure.

Factors Affecting Cerebral Blood Flow. Carbon dioxide, oxygen, and hydrogen ion concentration affect cerebral vessel tone. The partial pressure of carbon dioxide in arterial blood ($PaCO_2$) is a potent vasoactive agent. An increase in $PaCO_2$ relaxes smooth muscle, dilates cerebral vessels, decreases cerebrovascular resistance, and increases CBF. Alternately, a decrease in $PaCO_2$ constricts cerebral vessels, increases cerebrovascular resistance, and decreases CBF. Cerebral O_2 tension below 50 mm Hg results in cerebral vascular dilation. This dilation decreases cerebral vascular resistance, increases CBF, and raises O_2 tension. However, if O_2 tension is not raised, anaerobic metabolism begins, resulting in an accumulation of lactic acid. As lactic acid increases and hydrogen ions accumulate, the environment becomes more acidic. Within this acidic environment, further vasodilation occurs in a continued attempt to increase blood flow. The combination of a severely low partial pressure of oxygen in arterial blood (PaO_2) and an elevated hydrogen ion concentration (acidosis), which are both potent cerebral vasodilators, may produce a state wherein autoregulation is lost and compensatory mechanisms fail to meet tissue metabolic demands.[1]

CBF can be affected by cardiac or respiratory arrest, systemic hemorrhage, and other pathophysiologic states (e.g., diabetic

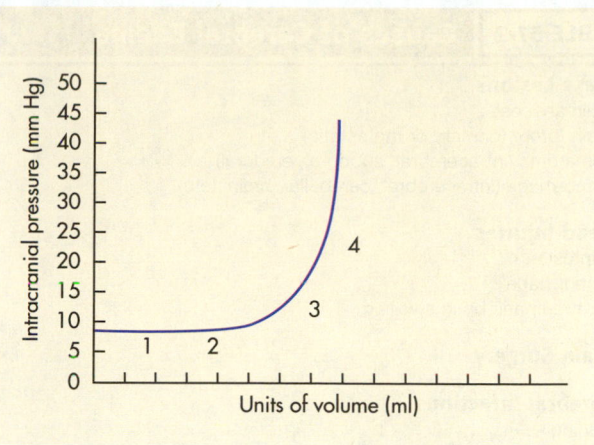

FIG. 57-2 Intracranial pressure-volume curve. (See text for descriptions of *1, 2, 3,* and *4.*)

coma, encephalopathies, infections, toxicities). Regional CBF can also be affected by trauma, tumors, cerebral hemorrhage, or stroke. When regional or global autoregulation is lost, CBF is no longer maintained at a constant level but is directly influenced by changes in systemic BP, hypoxia, or catecholamines.

INCREASED INTRACRANIAL PRESSURE

Increased ICP is a life-threatening situation that results from an increase in any or all of the three components (brain tissue, blood, CSF) within the skull. Cerebral edema is an important factor contributing to increased ICP.

Cerebral Edema

As shown in Table 57-2, there are a variety of causes of **cerebral edema** (increased accumulation of fluid in the extravascular spaces of brain tissue). Regardless of the cause, cerebral edema results in an increase in tissue volume that carries the potential for increased ICP. The extent and severity of the original insult are factors that determine the degree of cerebral edema.

There are three types of cerebral edema: vasogenic, cytotoxic, and interstitial. More than one type may occur in the same patient.

Vasogenic Cerebral Edema. *Vasogenic cerebral edema,* the most common type of edema, occurs mainly in the white matter and is attributed to changes in the endothelial lining of cerebral capillaries. These changes allow leakage of macromolecules from the capillaries into the surrounding extracellular space, resulting in an osmotic gradient that favors the flow of fluid from the intravascular to the extravascular space. A variety of insults, such as brain tumors, abscesses, and ingested toxins, may cause an increase in the permeability of the blood-brain barrier and produce an increase in the extracellular fluid volume. The speed and extent of the spread of the edema fluid are influenced by the systemic BP, the site of the brain injury, and the extent of the blood-brain barrier defect. This edema may produce a continuum of symptoms ranging from focal neurologic deficits to disturbances in consciousness, including **coma** (profound state of unconsciousness).

Cytotoxic Cerebral Edema. *Cytotoxic cerebral edema* results from local disruption of the functional or morphologic integrity of cell membranes and occurs most often in the gray matter. Cytotoxic cerebral edema develops from destructive lesions or trauma to brain tissue resulting in cerebral hypoxia or anoxia, so-

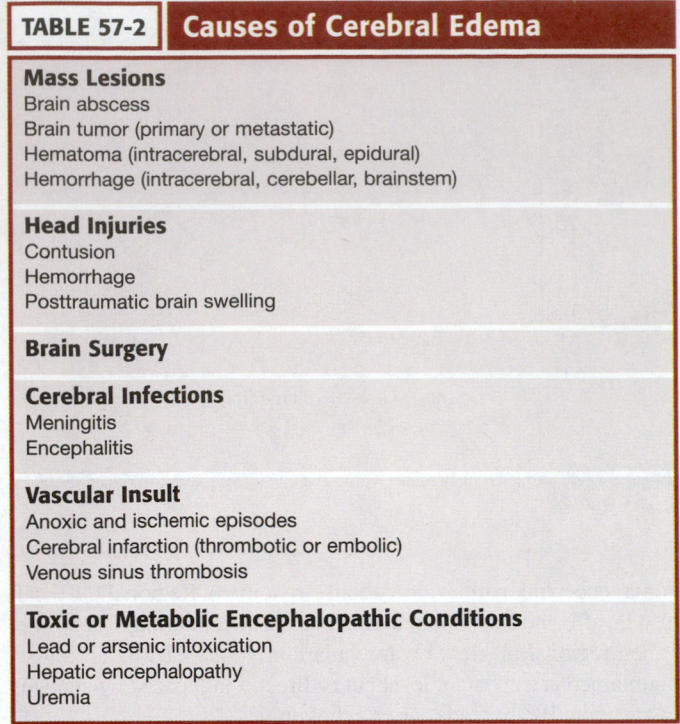

TABLE 57-2	Causes of Cerebral Edema

Mass Lesions
Brain abscess
Brain tumor (primary or metastatic)
Hematoma (intracerebral, subdural, epidural)
Hemorrhage (intracerebral, cerebellar, brainstem)

Head Injuries
Contusion
Hemorrhage
Posttraumatic brain swelling

Brain Surgery

Cerebral Infections
Meningitis
Encephalitis

Vascular Insult
Anoxic and ischemic episodes
Cerebral infarction (thrombotic or embolic)
Venous sinus thrombosis

Toxic or Metabolic Encephalopathic Conditions
Lead or arsenic intoxication
Hepatic encephalopathy
Uremia

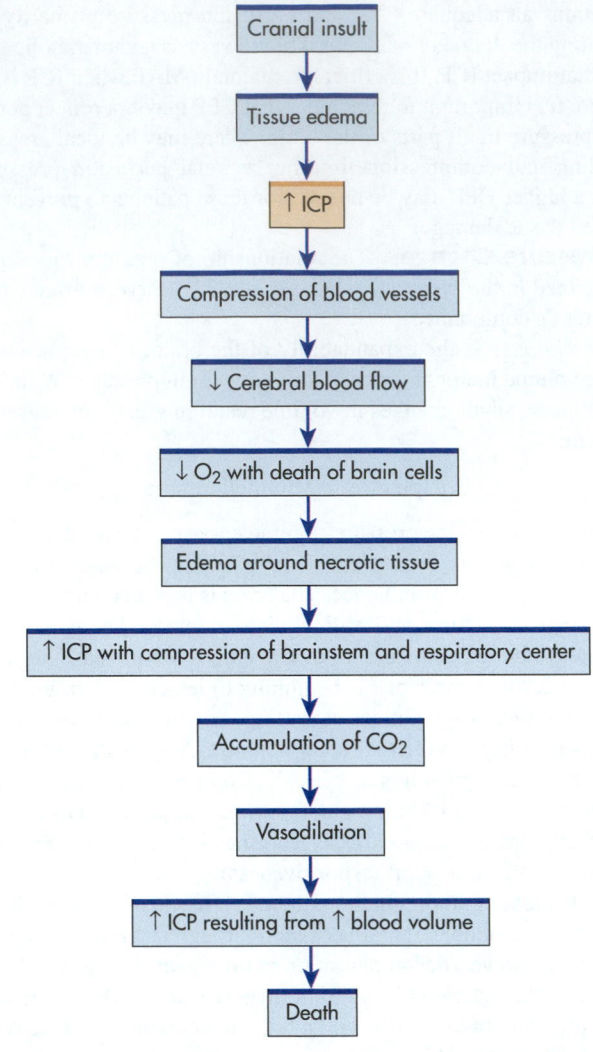

FIG. 57-3 Progression of increased intracranial pressure (ICP).

dium depletion, and syndrome of inappropriate antidiuretic hormone (SIADH) secretion. Cerebral edema results as fluid and protein shift from the extracellular space directly into the cells, with subsequent swelling and loss of cellular function.

Interstitial Cerebral Edema. *Interstitial cerebral edema* is the result of periventricular diffusion of ventricular CSF in a patient with uncontrolled hydrocephalus. It can also be caused by enlargement of the extracellular space as a result of systemic water excess (e.g., water intoxication, hyponatremia). Fluid moves into the cells to equilibrate with the hypoosmotic interstitial fluid. Regardless of the cause of cerebral edema, manifestations of increased ICP result, unless compensation is adequate.

Mechanisms of Increased Intracranial Pressure

Elevated ICP is clinically significant because it diminishes CPP, increases risks of brain ischemia and infarction, and is associated with a poor prognosis.[4] Increased ICP can be caused by several clinical problems, including a mass lesion (e.g., hematoma, contusion, abscess, tumor), cerebral edema (associated with brain tumors, hydrocephalus, head injury, or brain inflammation), or metabolic insult. These cerebral insults may result in hypercapnia, cerebral acidosis, impaired autoregulation, and systemic hypertension, which promote the formation and spread of cerebral edema. This edema distorts brain tissue, further increasing the ICP, which leads to even more tissue hypoxia and acidosis. Fig. 57-3 illustrates the progression of increased ICP.

Crucial to preservation of tissue is maintenance of CBF. Slowly developing increases in pressure or elevations that are more evenly distributed throughout the brain (e.g., an enlarging brain lesion) preserve blood flow better than a rapid increase, as in primary brain injury. Sustained increases in ICP result in brainstem compression and herniation of the brain from one compartment to another.

Displacement and herniation of brain tissue can cause a potentially reversible pathophysiologic process to become irreversible.

Ischemia and edema are further increased, compounding the preexisting problem. Compression of the brainstem and cranial nerves may be fatal. Fig. 57-4 illustrates the types of herniation. Herniations force the cerebellum and brainstem downward through the foramen magnum. If compression of the brainstem is unrelieved, respiratory arrest will occur due to compression of the respiratory control center in the medulla.

Clinical Manifestations

The clinical manifestations of increased ICP can take many forms, depending on the cause, location, and rate at which the pressure increase occurs (Fig. 57-5). The earlier the condition is recognized and treated, the better the patient outcome. The clinical manifestations of increased ICP are discussed below.

Change in Level of Consciousness. The *level of consciousness* (LOC) is the sensitive and reliable indicator of the patient's neurologic status. Changes in LOC are a result of impaired CBF, which deprives the cells of the cerebral cortex and the reticular activating system (RAS) of oxygen. The RAS is located in the brainstem, with neural connections to many parts of the nervous system. An intact RAS can maintain a state of wakefulness even in the absence of a functioning cerebral cortex. Interruptions of impulses from the RAS or alterations in functioning of the cerebral hemispheres can cause **unconsciousness** (abnormal state of complete or partial unawareness of self or environment).

The patient's state of consciousness is defined by both the behavior and the pattern of brain activity recorded by an electroencephalogram (EEG). The change in consciousness may be dramatic, as in coma, or subtle, such as a flattening of affect, change in orientation, or decrease in level of attention. In the deepest state of unconsciousness (i.e., coma), the patient does not respond to painful stimuli. Corneal and pupillary reflexes are absent. The pa-

tient cannot swallow or cough and is incontinent of urine and feces. The EEG pattern demonstrates decreased or absent neuronal activity.

Changes in Vital Signs. Changes in vital signs are caused by increasing pressure on the thalamus, hypothalamus, pons, and medulla. Manifestations such as Cushing's triad may be present but often do not appear until ICP has been increased for some time or is suddenly markedly increased (e.g., head trauma). A change in body temperature may also be noted because of increased ICP impacting the hypothalamus.

Ocular Signs. Compression of cranial nerve (CN) III, the oculomotor nerve, results in dilation of the pupil on the same side as or *ipsilateral* to the mass lesion, sluggish or no response to light, inability to move the eye upward, and ptosis of the eyelid. These signs can be the result of a shifting of the brain from the midline, compressing the trunk of CN III and paralyzing the muscles controlling pupillary size and shape. In this situation, a fixed, unilaterally dilated pupil is considered a neurologic emergency that indicates herniation of the brain. Other cranial nerves may also be affected, such as the optic (CN II), trochlear (CN IV), and abducens (CN VI) nerves. Signs of dysfunction of these cranial nerves include blurred vision, diplopia, and changes in extraocular eye movements. Central herniation may initially manifest as sluggish but equal pupil response. Uncal herniation may cause a dilated unilateral pupil. *Papilledema,* an edematous optic disc seen on retinal examination, is also noted and is a nonspecific sign associated with persistent increases in ICP.

Decrease in Motor Function. As the ICP continues to rise, the patient manifests changes in motor ability. A *contralateral* (opposite side of the mass lesion) hemiparesis or hemiplegia may develop, depending on the location of the source of the increased

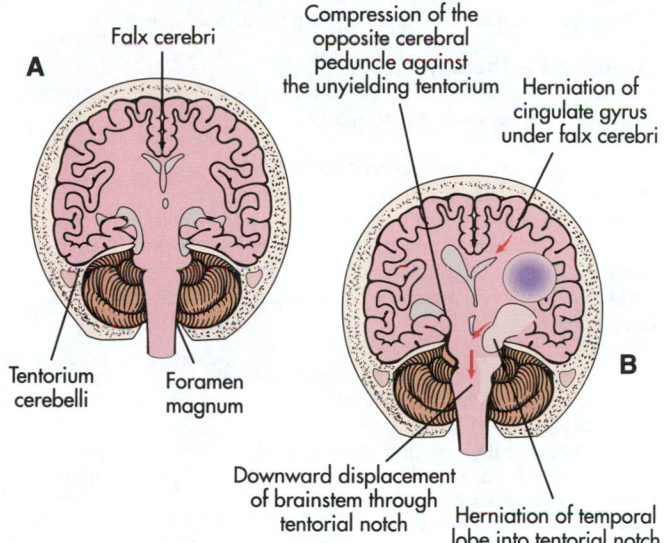

A

Falx cerebri

Compression of the opposite cerebral peduncle against the unyielding tentorium

Herniation of cingulate gyrus under falx cerebri

Tentorium cerebelli

Foramen magnum

B

Downward displacement of brainstem through tentorial notch

Herniation of temporal lobe into tentorial notch

FIG. 57-4 Herniation. **A,** Normal relationship of intracranial structures. **B,** Shift of intracranial structures.

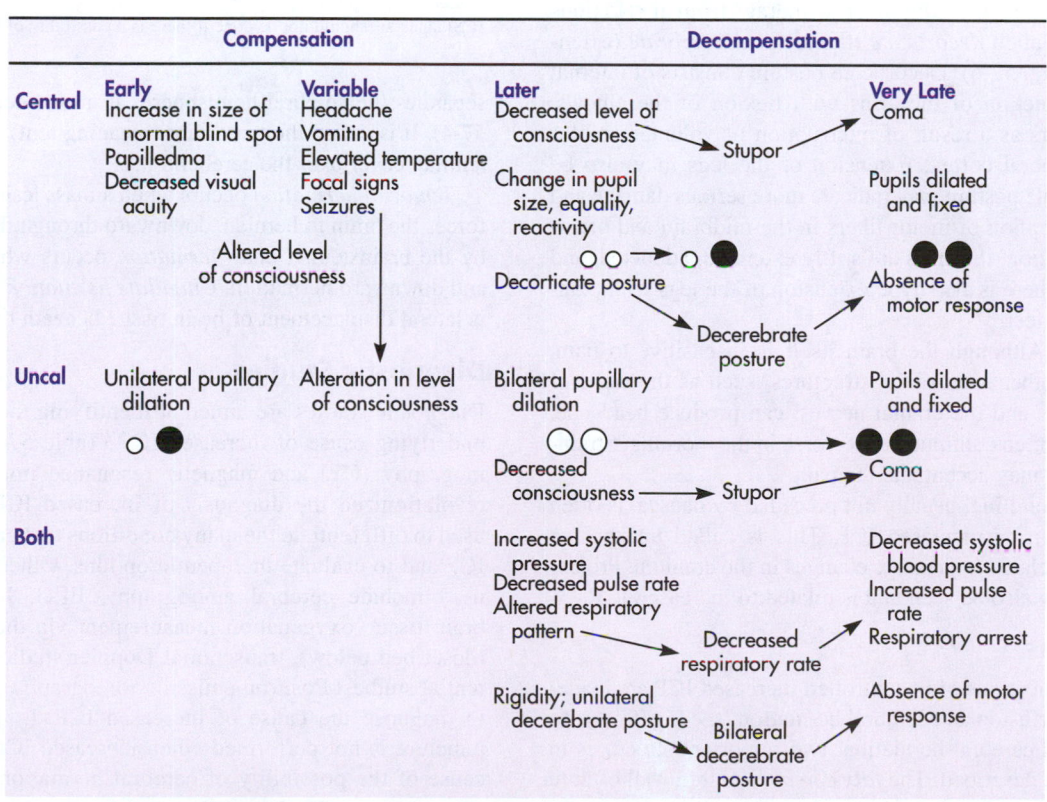

	Compensation		Decompensation	
Central	**Early** Increase in size of normal blind spot Papilledma Decreased visual acuity	**Variable** Headache Vomiting Elevated temperature Focal signs Seizures	**Later** Decreased level of consciousness → Stupor Change in pupil size, equality, reactivity ○ ○ → ○ ● Decorticate posture → Decerebrate posture	**Very Late** Coma Pupils dilated and fixed ● ● Absence of motor response
		Altered level of consciousness		
Uncal	Unilateral pupillary dilation ○ ●	Alteration in level of consciousness	Bilateral pupillary dilation ○ ○ → Decreased consciousness → Stupor	Pupils dilated and fixed ● ● Coma
Both			Increased systolic pressure Decreased pulse rate Altered respiratory pattern → Decreased respiratory rate Rigidity; unilateral decerebrate posture → Bilateral decerebrate posture	Decreased systolic blood pressure Increased pulse rate Respiratory arrest Absence of motor response

FIG. 57-5 Clinical manifestations of increased intracranial pressure.

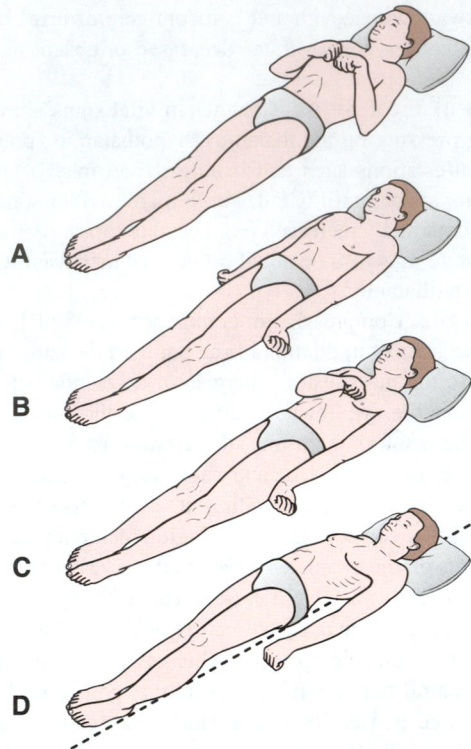

FIG. 57-6 Decorticate and decerebrate posturing. **A,** Decorticate response. Flexion of arms, wrists, and fingers with adduction in upper extremities. Extension, internal rotation, and plantar flexion in lower extremities. **B,** Decerebrate response. All four extremities in rigid extension, with hyperpronation of forearms and plantar flexion of feet. **C,** Decorticate response on right side of body and decerebrate response on left side of body. **D,** Opisthotonic posturing.

ICP. If painful stimuli are used to elicit a motor response, the patient may localize to the stimuli or withdraw from it. Noxious stimuli may also elicit *decorticate* (flexor) or *decerebrate* (extensor) posturing (Fig. 57-6). Decorticate posture consists of internal rotation and adduction of the arms with flexion of the elbows, wrists, and fingers as a result of interruption of voluntary motor tracts in the cerebral cortex. Extension of the legs may also be seen. A decerebrate posture may indicate more serious damage and results from disruption of motor fibers in the midbrain and brainstem. In this position, the arms are stiffly extended, adducted, and hyperpronated. There is also hyperextension of the legs with plantar flexion of the feet.

Headache. Although the brain itself is insensitive to pain, compression of other intracranial structures, such as the walls of arteries and veins and the cranial nerves, can produce headache. The headache is often continuous but worse in the morning. Straining or movement may accentuate the pain.

Vomiting. Vomiting, usually not preceded by nausea, is often a nonspecific sign of increased ICP. This is called unexpected vomiting and is related to pressure changes in the cranium. Projectile vomiting may also be seen and is related to increased ICP.

Complications

The major complications of uncontrolled increased ICP are inadequate cerebral perfusion and cerebral herniation (see Fig. 57-4). To better understand cerebral herniation, two important structures in the brain must be described. The *falx cerebri* is a thin wall of dura that folds down between the cortex, separating the two cerebral hemispheres. The *tentorium cerebelli* is a rigid fold of dura that

<table>
<tr><td>**TABLE 57-3**</td><td>*COLLABORATIVE CARE*
Increased Intracranial Pressure</td></tr>
</table>

Diagnostic

History and physical examination
Vital signs, neurologic assessments, ICP measurements
Skull, chest, and spinal x-ray studies
CT scan, MRI, PET, EEG, angiography
Transcranial Doppler studies
ECG
Laboratory studies, including CBC, coagulation profile, electrolytes, serum creatinine, ABGs, ammonia level, general drug and toxicology screen, CSF analysis for protein, cells, glucose*

Collaborative Therapy

Elevation of head of bed to 30 degrees with head in a neutral position
Intubation and mechanical ventilation
ICP monitoring
Cerebral oxygenation monitoring (LICOX, SjvO$_2$)
Maintenance of PaO$_2$ at 100 mm Hg or greater
Maintenance of fluid balance and assessment of osmolality
Maintenance of systolic arterial pressure between 100 and 160 mm Hg
Maintenance of CPP >60 mm Hg
Reduction of cerebral metabolism (e.g., high-dose barbiturates)
Drug therapy
- Osmotic diuretic (mannitol)
- Antiseizure drugs (e.g., phenytoin [Dilantin])
- Corticosteroids (dexamethasone [Decadron]) (for brain tumors, bacterial meningitis)
- Histamine (H$_2$)-receptor antagonist (e.g., cimetidine [Tagamet]) or proton pump inhibitor (e.g., pantoprazole [Protonix]) to prevent GI ulcers and bleeding

ABGs, Arterial blood gases; *CBC,* complete blood count; *CPP,* cerebral perfusion pressure; *CSF,* cerebrospinal fluid; *CT,* computed tomography; *ECG,* electrocardiogram; *EEG,* electroencephalogram; *GI,* gastrointestinal; *ICP,* intracranial pressure; *MRI,* magnetic resonance imaging; *PaO$_2$,* partial pressure of oxygen in arterial blood; *PET,* positron emission tomography; *SjvO$_2$,* jugular venous oxygen saturation.
*CSF analysis should not be done if there is a possibility of herniation.

separates the cerebral hemispheres from the cerebellum (see Fig. 57-4). It is called the tentorium (meaning tent) because it forms a tentlike cover over the cerebellum.

Tentorial herniation occurs when a mass lesion in the cerebrum forces the brain to herniate downward through the opening created by the brainstem. *Uncal herniation* occurs when there is lateral and downward herniation. *Cingulate herniation* occurs when there is lateral displacement of brain tissue beneath the falx cerebri.

Diagnostic Studies

Diagnostic studies are aimed at identifying the presence and the underlying cause of increased ICP (Table 57-3). Computed tomography (CT) and magnetic resonance imaging (MRI) have revolutionized the diagnosis of increased ICP. These tests are used to differentiate the many conditions that can cause increased ICP and to evaluate therapeutic options. Other tests that may be used include cerebral angiography, EEG, ICP measurement, brain tissue oxygenation measurement via the LICOX catheter (described below), transcranial Doppler studies, and evoked potential studies. Positron emission tomography (PET) is also used to diagnose the cause of increased ICP. In general, a lumbar puncture is not performed when increased ICP is suspected because of the possibility of cerebral herniation from the sudden release of the pressure in the skull from the area above the lumbar puncture.

Nervous System

Measurement of ICP

Indications for ICP Monitoring. ICP monitoring is used to guide clinical care when the patient is at risk for or has elevations in ICP. It may be used in patients with a variety of neurologic insults, including hemorrhage, stroke, tumor, infection, or traumatic brain injury. ICP should be monitored in patients admitted with a Glasgow Coma Scale (GCS) score of 8 or less and an abnormal CT scan or MRI (hematomas, contusion, edema, or compressed basal cisterns).[5] (The GCS is presented later in Table 57-5.)

Methods of Measuring ICP. Multiple methods and devices are available to monitor ICP (Fig. 57-7).

The "gold standard" for monitoring ICP is the ventriculostomy, in which a specialized catheter is inserted into the right lateral ventricle and coupled to an external transducer. This technique directly measures the pressure within the ventricles, facilitates removal and/or sampling of CSF, and allows for intraventricular drug administration. As with fluid-coupled BP monitoring systems, signals can be distorted by excessive tube length or bubbles in the line. In these systems, the transducer is external, and its position must remain constant with respect to the patient's head to produce comparable measures. An alternative technology, the fiberoptic catheter, uses a sensor transducer located within the catheter tip. The sensor tip is placed within the ventricle or the brain tissue and provides a direct measurement of brain pressure. Other methods of monitoring include the subarachnoid bolt and epidural wedge.

New technology is now available to measure cerebral oxygenation and cerebral ischemia. This technology offers an indirect assessment of cerebral oxygenation and perfusion. Two such devices are currently being used in ICU care settings: the *LICOX brain tissue oxygenation catheter* and the *jugular venous bulb catheter*. The LICOX catheter is placed in the frontal white matter of the brain and provides continuous monitoring of the pressure of oxygen in brain tissue ($PbtO_2$); the normal range for $PbtO_2$ is 20 to 40 mm Hg. A lower than normal $PbtO_2$ level is indicative of ischemia. The jugular venous bulb catheter is placed in the internal jugular vein and positioned so that the catheter tip is located in the jugular bulb; placement is verified by a lateral skull x-ray. This catheter provides a measurement of jugular venous oxygen saturation ($SjvO_2$), which indicates total venous brain tissue extraction of oxygen—a measure of cerebral oxygen supply and demand.[6] The normal $SjvO_2$ range is 55% to 75%. Values of <50% to 55% demonstrate impaired cerebral oxygenation. With the use of either device, inter-ventions can be specifically focused to improve brain tissue oxygen levels.

Infection is a serious consideration with ICP monitoring. Infection rates are highest in fluid-coupled systems. Prophylactic systemic antibiotics may be administered to reduce the chances of infection. Factors that contribute to the development of infection include ICP monitoring greater than 5 days, use of a ventriculostomy, the presence of a CSF leak, and a concurrent systemic infection. Routine care may include regular diagnostic testing for CSF organism growth.

ICP should be measured as a mean pressure at the end of expiration. If a CSF drainage device is in place, the drain must be closed for at least 6 minutes to ensure an accurate reading. The waveform strip should be recorded along with other pressure monitoring waveforms. The normal ICP waveform is shaped somewhat like an arterial pressure trace (Fig. 57-8), although the pressures are in a much lower range. This is because arterial pressure is transmitted to the choroid plexus and then to the CSF in the ventricular and subarachnoid spaces. When the waveform is monitored so that components in synchrony with the cardiac cycle can be visualized, the normal ICP waveform has three phases (Table 57-4).

It is important to monitor the ICP waveform, as well as mean CPP. When the height of P2 is higher than P1, the intracranial space may be noncompliant and the patient is at risk for development of elevated ICP (see Fig. 57-8). It is important to consider the rate at which changes occur and the patient's clinical condition. Neurologic deterioration might not occur until ICP elevation is pronounced and sustained. Any indication of ICP elevation, either as a mean increase in pressure or as an abnormal waveform configuration, should be reported to the health care provider immediately.

Inaccurate ICP readings can be caused by CSF leaks around the monitoring device, obstruction of the intraventricular catheter or bolt (from tissue or blood clot), difference between the height of the bolt and the transducer, kinks in the tubing, and incorrect height of the drainage system relative to the patient's reference point. In fluid-coupled systems, bubbles or air in the tubing also dampen the waveform.

CSF Drainage. With the ventricular catheter and certain fiberoptic systems, it is possible to control ICP by removing CSF. The level of the ICP at which to initiate drainage, amount of fluid to be drained, height of the system, and frequency of drainage are ordered by the physician. To remove CSF, a Y-connector is inserted in the line (Fig. 57-9). Using a closed system, elevations in ICP are controlled by removal of CSF by gravity drainage and by adjusting the height of the drip chamber and drainage bag relative to the patient's ventricular reference point. Typically a point 15 cm above the ear canal, which approximates the foramen of Monroe, is selected. Raising the system diminishes drainage, whereas lowering the system increases drainage volume. Careful monitoring of the volume of CSF drained is essential, keeping in mind that normal adult CSF production is about 20 to 30 ml/hr, with a total CSF volume of 90 to 150 ml within the ventricles and subarachnoid space. Prevention of infection by use of strict aseptic technique during dressing changes or sampling of CSF is imperative. The system must remain intact to ensure that the ICP readings are accurate because treatment is initiated on the basis of the pressures.

Complications of this type of drainage system include ventricular collapse, infection, and herniation or subdural hematoma formation from rapid decompression. Although it is generally recognized that CSF removal decreases ICP and improves CPP, guidelines for CSF

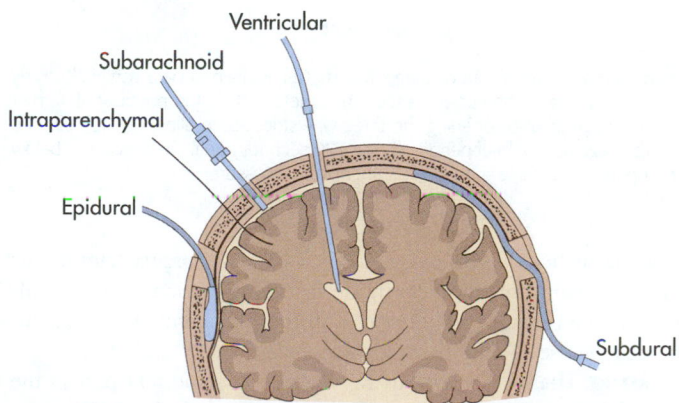

Ventricular

Subarachnoid

Intraparenchymal

Epidural

Subdural

FIG. 57-7 Coronal section of brain showing potential sites for placement of ICP monitoring devices.

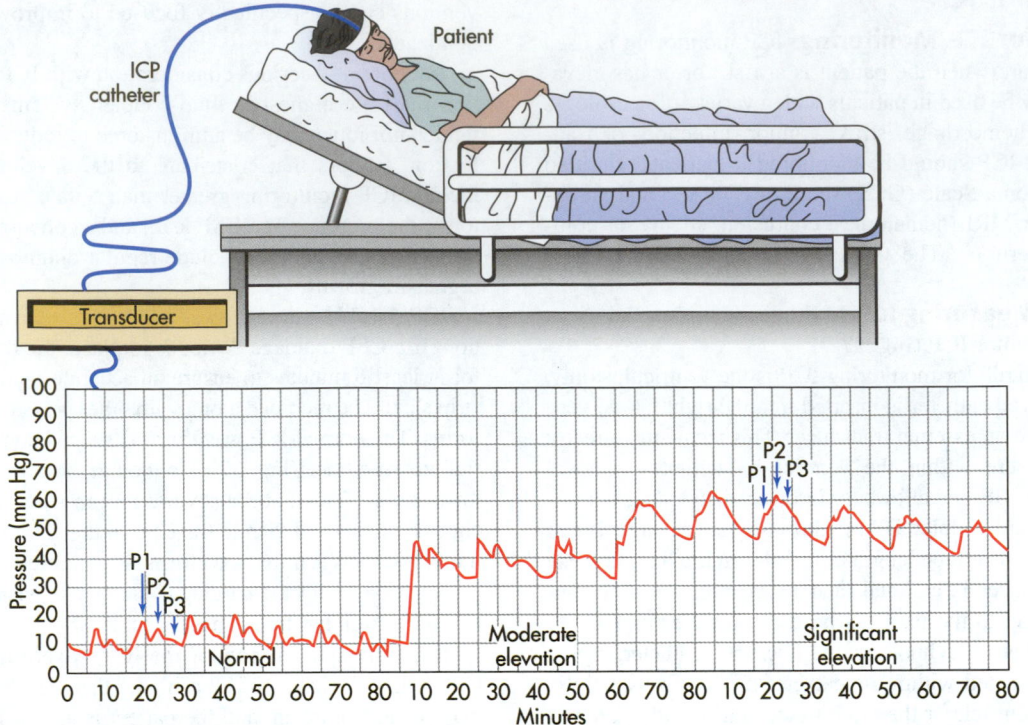

FIG. 57-8   Intracranial pressure monitoring can be used to continuously measure ICP. The ICP tracing shows normal, elevated, and plateau waves. At high ICP the P2 peak is higher than the P1 peak, and the peaks become less distinct and plateau.

TABLE 57-4	Normal ICP Waveforms*
Waveform	**Meaning**
P1 Percussion wave	Represents arterial pulsations; normally the highest of the three waveforms.
P2 Rebound wave or tidal wave	Reflects intracranial compliance or relative brain volume. When P2 is higher than P1, intracranial compliance is compromised.
P3 Dicrotic wave	Follows dicrotic notch; represents venous pulsations; normally the lowest waveform.

*See Fig. 57-8.

removal are not universally accepted but are typically based on institution or physician preference.[7]

Collaborative Care

The goals of collaborative care (see Table 57-3) are to identify and treat the underlying cause of increased ICP and to support brain function. A careful history is an important diagnostic aid that can direct the search for the underlying cause.

Ensuring adequate oxygenation to support brain function is the first step in the management of increased ICP. An endotracheal tube or tracheostomy may be necessary to maintain adequate ventilation. Arterial blood gas (ABG) analysis guides the oxygen therapy. The goal is to maintain the PaO_2 at 100 mm Hg or greater. It may be necessary to maintain the patient on a mechanical ventilator to ensure adequate oxygenation.

If the condition is caused by a mass lesion, such as a tumor or hematoma, surgical removal of the mass is the best management

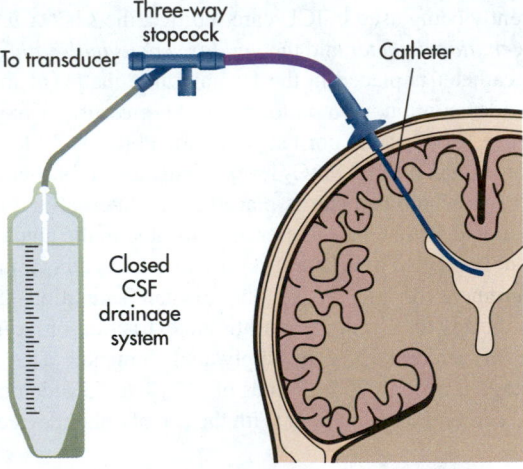

FIG. 57-9   Intermittent drainage system. CSF is drained via a ventriculostomy when ICP exceeds the upper pressure parameter set by the physician. Intermittent drainage involves opening the three-way stopcock to allow CSF to flow into the drainage bag for brief periods (30 to 120 seconds) until the pressure is below the upper pressure parameters. *ICP,* Intracranial pressure.

(see the sections on Brain Tumors and Cranial Surgery later in this chapter). Nonsurgical intervention for the reduction of tissue volume related to cerebral tissue swelling and cerebral edema includes the use of diuretics and corticosteroids.

Drug Therapy. Drug therapy plays an important part in the management of increased ICP. Mannitol (Osmitrol) (25%) is an osmotic diuretic and is given intravenously. Mannitol acts to decrease the ICP in two ways: plasma expansion and osmotic effect.

There is an immediate plasma-expanding effect that reduces the hematocrit and blood viscosity, thereby increasing CBF and cerebral oxygen delivery. A vascular osmotic gradient is created by mannitol. Thus fluid moves from the tissues into the blood vessels. Therefore the ICP is reduced by a decrease in the total brain fluid content. Fluid and electrolyte status must be monitored when osmotic diuretics are used. Mannitol may be contraindicated if renal disease is present and if serum osmolality is elevated.[7]

Corticosteroids (e.g., dexamethasone [Decadron]) are thought to control the vasogenic edema surrounding tumors and abscesses but are not recommended in the management of head-injured patients. The mode of action of corticosteroids is not completely known. It is theorized that they act by stabilizing the cell membrane and by inhibiting the synthesis of prostaglandins (see Chapter 13, Fig. 13-5), thus preventing the formation of proinflammatory mediators. Corticosteroids are also thought to improve neuronal function by improving CBF and restoring autoregulation.

Complications associated with the use of corticosteroids include hyperglycemia, increased incidence of infections, gastrointestinal (GI) bleeding, and hyponatremia. Fluid intake and sodium and glucose levels should be monitored regularly. Patients receiving corticosteroids should concurrently be given antacids or histamine (H_2)-receptor blockers (e.g., cimetidine [Tagamet], ranitidine [Zantac]) or proton pump inhibitors (e.g., omeprazole [Prilosec], pantoprazole [Protonix, Protonix I.V.]) to prevent GI ulcers and bleeding.

Drug therapy for reducing cerebral metabolism may be an effective strategy to control ICP. The reduction in the metabolic rate decreases the CBF and therefore the ICP. High-dose barbiturates (e.g., pentobarbital [Nembutal], thiopental [Pentothal]) are used in patients with increased ICP refractory to treatment. Barbiturates produce a decrease in cerebral metabolism and a subsequent decrease in ICP. A secondary effect is a reduction in cerebral edema and production of a more uniform blood supply to the brain.[7] Capabilities to monitor the patient's ICP, blood flow, EEG, and metabolism should be available when this treatment is used. Barbiturate dosing is typically based upon analysis of the bedside EEG tracing and the ICP. The physician orders the barbiturate infusion to be administered at a rate that achieves a desired level of brain wave suppression as a means to control ICP. Total *burst suppression,* recognized by the absence of spikes showing brain activity on the EEG monitor, indicates that maximal therapeutic effect has been achieved.[7] Antiseizure drugs such as phenytoin (Dilantin) also may be used because seizures can further increase ICP.

Hyperventilation Therapy. In the past, aggressive hyperventilation (PaCO$_2$ <25 mm Hg) had been a mainstay treatment of elevated ICP. The lowering of the PaCO$_2$ leads to constriction of the cerebral blood vessels, reducing CBF and thereby decreasing the ICP. More recent evidence suggests that aggressive hyperventilation increases the risk of focal cerebral ischemia and adversely affects outcomes.[7,8] Brief periods of less aggressive hyperventilation therapy (target PaCO$_2$ 30 to 35 mm Hg) may be useful for refractory intracranial hypertension. However, the effectiveness is time limited and transient. To prevent complications, it is important to maintain adequate intravascular volume and systemic blood pressure.

Nutritional Therapy. All patients must have their nutritional needs met, regardless of their state of consciousness or health. Early feeding following brain injury may improve outcomes.[9] The patient with increased ICP is in a hypermetabolic and hypercatabolic state that increases the need for glucose to provide the neces-

---

EVIDENCE-BASED PRACTICE

What Is the Best Time to Start Nutritional Support for Head-Injury Patients?

Clinical Question
In patients with head injuries (P), does early nutritional support (I) or delayed nutritional support (O) result in a better outcome (C)?

Best Available Evidence
Systematic review of randomized controlled trials (RCTs)

Critical Appraisal and Synthesis of Evidence
- 7 RCTs (*n* = 284) that compared the effect of early (within 48 hours of injury) versus delayed (usually 3 to 5 days after injury) feeding on survival and disability outcomes.
- 3 RCTS (*n* = 134) also examined route of administration.

Conclusions
- Early feeding showed a trend toward fewer infections and better outcomes.
- Timing of nutritional support was strongly influenced by the type of feeding used; parenteral feeding is usually begun earlier than enteral.
- Overall quality of trials was poor.

Implications for Nursing Practice
- There is currently not enough evidence to make a decision about the best time for nutritional support.
- Continued research on both the timing and route of nutritional support is needed to optimize patient outcomes.

Reference for Evidence
Yanagawa T, Bunn F, Roberts I, et al: Nutritional support for head-injured patients, Cochrane Injuries Group, *Cochrane Database Syst Rev* 4:CD001530, 2005.

PICO: P, Patient population of interest; *I,* intervention or area of interest; *C,* comparison of interest or comparison group; *O,* outcome(s) of interest (see p. 6).

---

sary fuel for metabolism of the injured brain. If the patient cannot maintain an adequate oral intake, other means of meeting the nutritional requirements, such as enteral feedings or parenteral nutrition, should be initiated. Nutritional replacements should begin within 3 days after injury to reach full nutritional replacement within 7 days after injury.[9] Because malnutrition promotes continued cerebral edema, maintenance of optimal nutrition is imperative. (Nutritional therapy is discussed in Chapter 40.) Feedings or supplements should be guided by the patient's fluid and electrolyte status, as well as the patient's metabolic needs.

It is controversial as to whether patients should be maintained in a state of moderate dehydration. Moderate dehydration is thought to be effective in reducing cerebral edema; in this case, fluids are restricted to 65% to 75% of normal requirements. However, the concern is that hypovolemia may result in a decrease in cardiac output and BP, which may decrease cerebral perfusion and the amount of oxygen delivered to the brain. There is additional concern that dehydrated patients do not respond well to vasoactive drugs. Because of this, the current therapy is directed at keeping patients normovolemic. The use of fluid restriction to reduce tissue volume should be evaluated on the basis of clinical factors such as urine output, insensible fluid loss, serum and urine osmolality, serum electrolytes, and the condition of the patient. Intravenous (IV) 0.9% sodium chloride is the preferred solution for administration of piggyback medications because a lowering of serum osmolarity and an increase in cerebral edema occur if 5% dextrose in water or 0.45% sodium chloride is used. Infusion of hypertonic saline

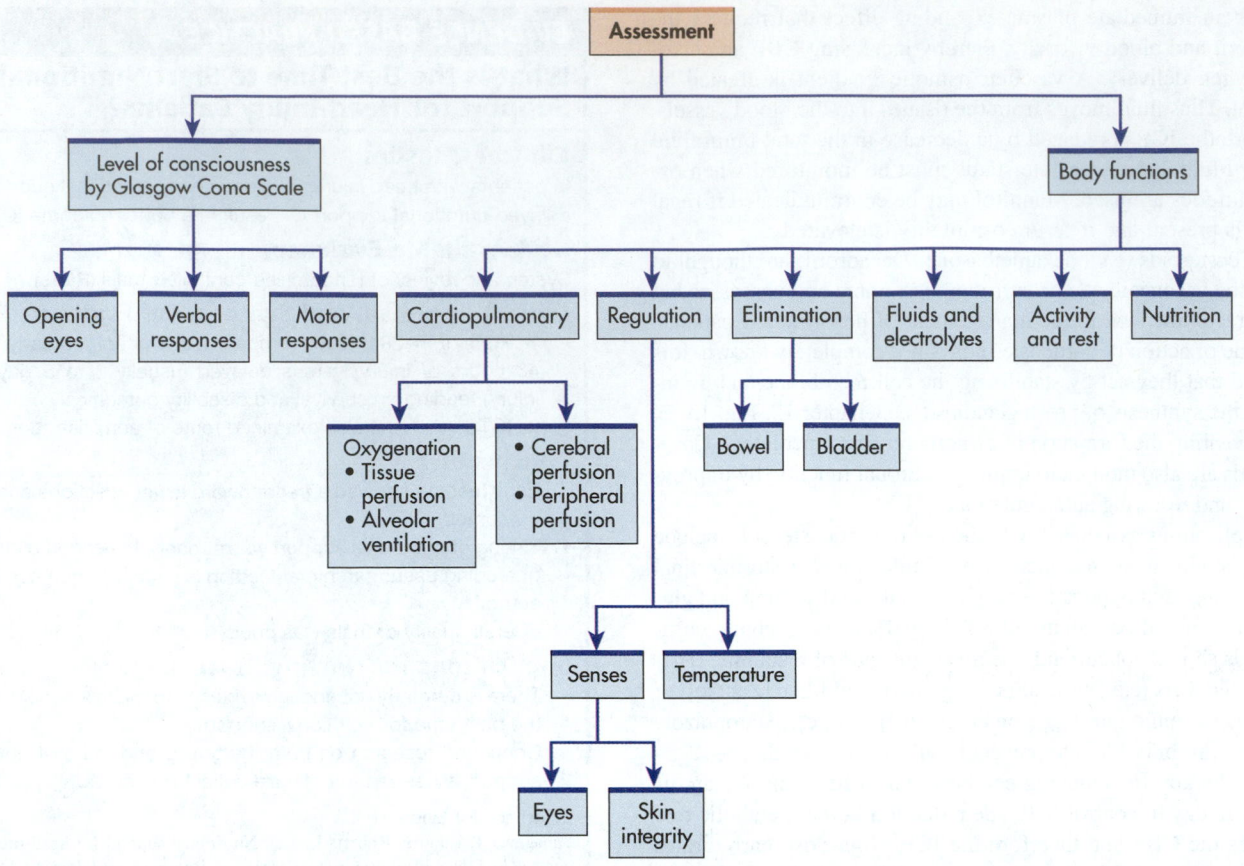

FIG. 57-10   Systematic approach to nursing assessment of the unconscious patient.

(2% to 7.5%) is another intervention currently used to acutely lower ICP and support intravascular volume. However, long-term patient outcome data are still being investigated.[7]

NURSING MANAGEMENT
INCREASED INTRACRANIAL PRESSURE

■ *Nursing Assessment*

Subjective data about the patient with increased ICP can be obtained from the patient or family members or other persons who are familiar with the patient. The nurse must learn appropriate neurologic assessment techniques and describe the LOC by noting the specific behaviors observed. When a deviation from the normal state of consciousness occurs, a more structured method of observation should be initiated. This type of systematic approach to nursing assessment is illustrated in Fig. 57-10 and consists of assessing the LOC by the Glasgow Coma Scale (Table 57-5) and by body functions. Adequate circulation and respiration are the most vital and should always be the first body functions assessed.

Glasgow Coma Scale. The **Glasgow Coma Scale** (GCS) is a quick, practical, and standardized system for assessing the degree of impaired consciousness. The three areas assessed in the GCS correspond to the definition of coma as the inability of a patient to speak, obey commands, or open the eyes when a verbal or painful stimulus is applied.[10] Specific assessments evaluate the patient's response to varying degrees of stimuli. Three indicators of response are evaluated: (1) opening of the eyes, (2) the best verbal response, and (3) the best motor response (see Table 57-5). Specific behaviors observed as responses to the testing stimulus in each of these three

areas are given a numeric value and can be plotted on a graph. The nurse's responsibility is to elicit the best response on each of the scales: the higher the scores, the higher the level of brain functioning. A graph can be used to determine whether the patient is stable, improving, or deteriorating. The subscale scores are particularly important if a patient is untestable in one area. For example, severe periorbital edema may make eye opening impossible. The total GCS score is the sum of the numeric values assigned to each of the three areas evaluated. The highest GCS score is 15 for a fully alert person, and the lowest possible score is 3. A GCS score of 8 or less is generally indicative of coma.[11]

The GCS offers several advantages in the assessment of the unconscious patient. It is specific and structured, allowing different health care professionals to arrive at the same conclusion regarding the patient's status. It saves time for the assessor because the ratings are done with numbers rather than with lengthy descriptions.

The GCS is also sensitive and specific enough to discriminate between different or changing states. The GCS is used to assess the arousal aspect of consciousness. Other components of the neurologic assessment include pupillary checks, extremity strength testing, and, if appropriate, corneal reflex testing.

Neurologic Assessment. The pupils are compared to one another for size, shape, movement, and reactivity (Fig. 57-11). If the oculomotor nerve [CN III] is compressed, the pupil on the affected side (ipsilateral) becomes larger until it fully dilates. If ICP continues to increase, both pupils dilate.

Pupillary reaction is tested with a penlight. The normal reaction is brisk constriction when the light is shone directly into the eye. A consensual response (a slight constriction in the opposite pupil)

TABLE 57-5	Glasgow Coma Scale		
Category of Response	**Appropriate Stimulus**	**Response**	**Score**
Eyes Open	• Approach to bedside • Verbal command • Pain	Spontaneous response	4
		Opening of eyes to name or command	3
		Lack of opening of eyes to previous stimuli but opening to pain	2
		Lack of opening of eyes to any stimulus	1
		Untestable	U
Best Verbal Response	• Verbal questioning with maximum arousal	Appropriate orientation, conversant; correct identification of self, place, year, and month	5
		Confusion; conversant, but disorientation in one or more spheres	4
		Inappropriate or disorganized use of words (e.g., cursing), lack of sustained conversation	3
		Incomprehensible words, sounds (e.g., moaning)	2
		Lack of sound, even with painful stimuli	1
		Untestable	U
Best Motor Response	• Verbal command (e.g., "raise your arm, hold up two fingers") • Pain (pressure on proximal nail bed)	Obedience of command	6
		Localization of pain, lack of obedience but presence of attempts to remove offending stimulus	5
		Flexion withdrawal,* flexion of arm in response to pain without abnormal flexion posture	4
		Abnormal flexion, flexing of arm at elbow and pronation, making a fist	3
		Abnormal extension, extension of arm at elbow usually with adduction and internal rotation of arm at shoulder	2
		Lack of response	1
		Untestable	U

*Added to the original scale by many centers.

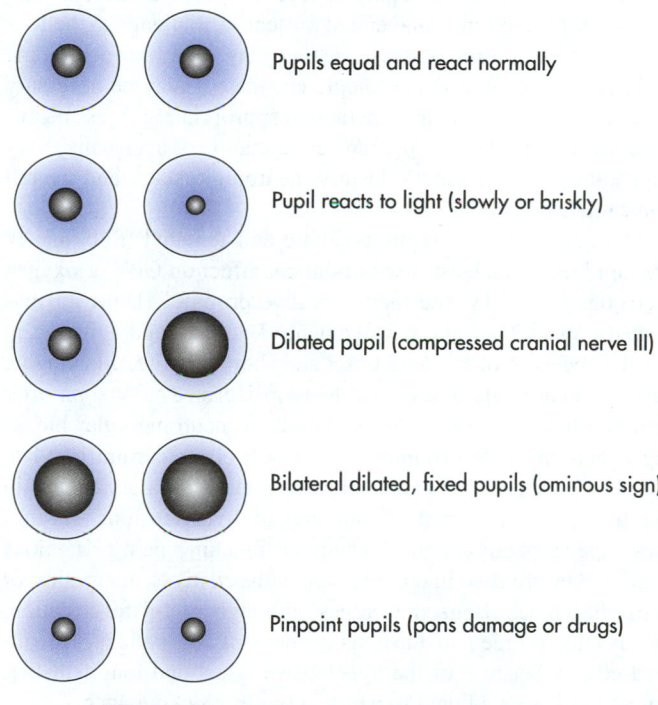

Pupils equal and react normally

Pupil reacts to light (slowly or briskly)

Dilated pupil (compressed cranial nerve III)

Bilateral dilated, fixed pupils (ominous sign)

Pinpoint pupils (pons damage or drugs)

FIG. 57-11 Pupillary check for size and response.

should also be noted at the same time. A sluggish reaction can indicate early pressure on CN III. A fixed pupil unresponsive to light stimulus usually indicates increased ICP. However, it is important to note that there are other causes of a fixed pupil, including direct injury to CN III (oculomotor nerve), previous eye surgery, and use of mydriatic eyedrops.

Evaluation of other cranial nerves can be included in the neurologic assessment. Eye movements controlled by cranial nerves III, IV, and VI can be examined in the patient who is awake and able to follow commands, and can be used to assess the function of the brainstem. In the unconscious patient, extraocular eye movements cannot be specifically tested. Testing the corneal reflex gives information on the functioning of cranial nerves V and VII. If this reflex is absent, routine eye care should be initiated to prevent corneal abrasion (see Chapters 21 and 22).

Eye movements of the uncooperative or unconscious patient can be elicited by reflex with the use of head movements (oculocephalic) and caloric stimulation (oculovestibular) (see Chapters 21 and 22). To test the oculocephalic reflex (doll's-eye reflex), the nurse turns the patient's head briskly to the left or right while holding the eyelids open. A normal response is movement of the eyes across the midline in the direction opposite that of the turning. Next, the nurse quickly flexes and then extends the neck. Eye movement should be opposite to the direction of head movement—up when the neck is flexed and down when it is extended. Abnormal responses can aid in locating the intracranial lesion. This test should not be attempted if a cervical spine problem is suspected. (The oculovestibular reflex is discussed in Chapter 21.)

Motor strength is tested by asking the awake patient to squeeze the nurse's hands to compare strength in the hands. The palmar drift test is an excellent measure of strength in the upper extremities. The patient raises the arms in front of the body with the palmar surface facing upward. If there is any weakness in the upper extremity, the palmar surface turns downward and the arm drifts downward. Asking the patient to raise the foot from the bed or to bend the knees up in bed is a good assessment of lower extremity strength. All four extremities should be tested for strength and evaluated for any asymmetry in strength or movement.

The motor response of the unconscious or uncooperative patient can be assessed by observation of spontaneous movement. If no spontaneous movement is possible, a pain stimulus should be applied to the patient, and the response should be noted. Resistance to movement during passive range-of-motion exercises is another measure of strength.

The vital signs, including BP, pulse, respiratory rate, and temperature, should also be systematically recorded. The nurse must be aware of Cushing's triad because this indicates severely increased ICP. Besides recording respiratory rate, the nurse should also note the respiratory pattern. Specific respiratory patterns are associated with severely increased ICP (Fig. 57-12).

■ Nursing Diagnoses

Nursing diagnoses for the patient with increased ICP include, but are not limited to, those presented in NCP 57-1.

■ Planning

The overall goals are that the patient with increased ICP will (1) maintain a patent airway, (2) have ICP within normal limits, (3) demonstrate normal fluid and electrolyte balance, and (4) have no complications secondary to immobility and decreased LOC.

■ Nursing Implementation

Acute Intervention

Respiratory Function. Maintenance of a patent airway is critical in the patient with increased ICP and is a primary nursing responsibility. As the LOC decreases, the patient is at increased risk of airway obstruction from the tongue dropping back and occluding the airway or from accumulation of secretions. Altered breathing patterns may become evident. Airway patency can be aided by keeping

the patient lying on one side, with frequent position changes. Snoring sounds indicate obstruction and require immediate intervention. Accumulated secretions are removed by suctioning as needed. An oral airway facilitates breathing and provides an easier suctioning route in the comatose patient. In general, any patient with an altered LOC who is unable to maintain a patent airway or effective ventilation needs intubation and mechanical ventilation.

The nurse must use measures to prevent hypoxia and hypercapnia. Proper positioning of the head is important. Elevation of the head of the bed to 30 degrees enhances respiratory exchange and aids in decreasing cerebral edema. Suctioning and coughing will cause transient decreases in the PaO_2 and increases in the ICP. Suctioning should be kept to a minimum and should be less than 10 seconds in duration, with administration of 100% oxygen before and after to prevent decreases in the PaO_2.[12] To avoid cumulative increases in the ICP with suctioning, it should be limited to two passes per suction procedure if possible. Patients with elevated ICP are at risk for lower CPP during suctioning. CPP must be maintained above 60 mm Hg to preserve cerebral perfusion.[13]

Abdominal distention can interfere with respiratory function and should be prevented. Insertion of a nasogastric tube to aspirate the stomach contents can prevent distention, vomiting, and possible aspiration. However, in patients with facial and skull fractures, a nasogastric tube is contraindicated, and oral insertion of a gastric tube is preferred.

Pain, anxiety, and fear from the initial injury, therapeutic procedures, or noxious stimuli can increase ICP and BP, thus complicating the management and recovery of the brain-injured patient. The appropriate choice or combination of sedatives, paralytics, and analgesics for symptom management presents a challenge to the ICU team. Administration of these agents may alter the neurologic state, thus masking true neurologic changes. It may be necessary to temporarily suspend drug therapy to appropriately assess neurologic status. The choice, dose, and combination of agents may vary depending on the patient's history, neurologic state, and overall clinical presentation.

Opioids, such as morphine sulfate and fentanyl (Sublimaze), are rapid-onset analgesics with minimal effect on CBF or oxygen metabolism. The IV anesthetic sedative propofol (Diprivan) has gained popularity in the management of anxiety and agitation in the ICU because of its rapid onset and short half-life, allowing an accurate neurologic assessment to be performed very soon after turning off the infusion.[7] Nondepolarizing neuromuscular blocking agents (e.g., vecuronium [Norcuron], cisatracurium besylate [Nimbex]) are useful for achieving complete ventilatory control in the treatment of refractory intracranial hypertension. Because these agents paralyze muscles without blocking pain or noxious stimuli, they are used in combination with sedatives, analgesics, or benzodiazepines. Benzodiazepines, although useful for sedation, are usually avoided in the management of the patient with increased ICP because of the hypotensive effect and long half-life, unless used as an adjunct to neuromuscular blocking agents.

ABGs should be measured and evaluated regularly (see Chapter 26). The nurse should frequently monitor the ABG values and take measures to maintain the levels within prescribed or acceptable parameters. The appropriate ventilatory support can be ordered on the basis of the PaO_2 and $PaCO_2$ values.

Fluid and Electrolyte Balance. Fluid and electrolyte disturbances can have an adverse effect on ICP. IV fluids should be closely monitored with the use of an accurate intravenous infusion control device or pump. Intake and output, with insensible losses

Pattern	Location of Lesion	Description
1. Cheyne-Stokes 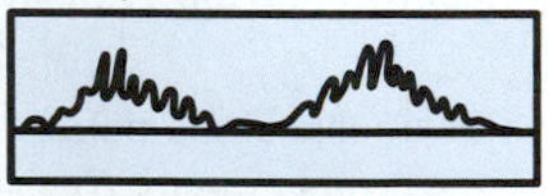	Bilateral hemispheric disease or metabolic brain dysfunction	Cycles of hyperventilation and apnea
2. Central neurogenic hyperventilation 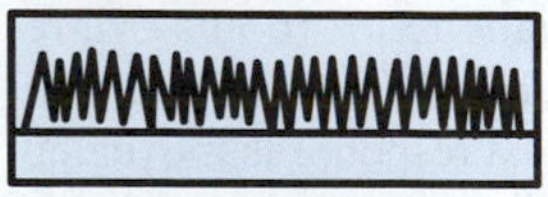	Brainstem between lower midbrain and upper pons	Sustained, regular rapid and deep breathing
3. Apneustic breathing 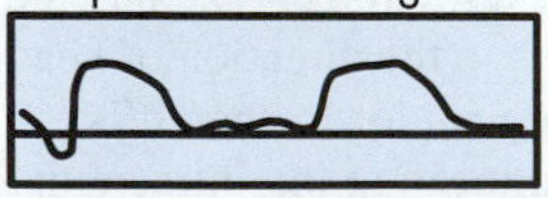	Mid or lower pons	Prolonged inspiratory phase or pauses alternating with expiratory pauses
4. Cluster breathing 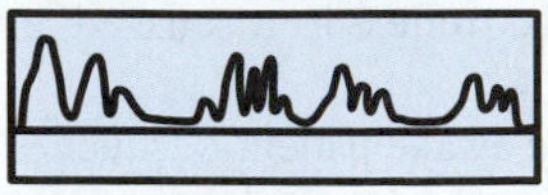	Medulla or lower pons	Clusters of breaths follow each other with irregular pauses between
5. Ataxic breathing 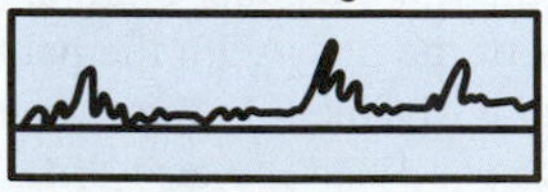	Reticular formation of the medulla	Completely irregular with some breaths deep and some shallow. Random, irregular pauses, slow rate

FIG. 57-12 Common abnormal respiratory patterns associated with coma.

NURSING CARE PLAN 57-1

Patient with Increased Intracranial Pressure

NURSING DIAGNOSIS   **Ineffective tissue perfusion (cerebral)** *related to* reduction of venous and/or arterial blood flow and cerebral edema *as evidenced by* CPP <60 mm Hg, Glasgow Coma Scale score <8, altered mental status, changes in motor response, behavioral changes

PATIENT GOAL   Maintains cerebral perfusion within normal parameters

OUTCOMES (NOC)	INTERVENTIONS (NIC) and *RATIONALES*
Tissue Perfusion: Cerebral	*Cerebral Perfusion Promotion*
• Neurologic function ____	• Consult with physician to determine hemodynamic parameters, and maintain hemodynamic parameters within this range.
• Intracranial pressure ____	• Induce hypertension with volume expansion or inotropic or vasoconstrictive agents, as ordered, *to maintain hemodynamic parameters and maintain/optimize cerebral perfusion*
• Systolic blood pressure ____	*pressure (CPP).*
• Diastolic blood pressure ____	• Monitor determinants of tissue oxygen delivery (e.g., PaCO₂, SaO₂, and hemoglobin levels and cardiac output), if available, *to ensure adequate oxygenation to support brain*
Measurement Scale	*function.*
1 = Severely compromised	• Calculate and monitor CPP *to evaluate adequacy of cerebral blood perfusion.*
2 = Substantially compromised	• Monitor neurologic status *to determine hemodynamic status.*
3 = Moderately compromised	• Monitor intake and output *to assess effects of diuretic and corticosteroid therapy.*
4 = Mildly compromised	
5 = Not compromised	

NURSING DIAGNOSIS   **Decreased intracranial adaptive capacity** *related to* decreased cerebral perfusion or sustained increase in ICP *as evidenced by* repeated increases of >10 mm Hg for more than 5 minutes following any of a variety of external stimuli, baseline ICP >20 mm Hg, elevated systolic blood pressure, bradycardia, and widened pulse pressure

PATIENT GOALS   1. Maintains intracranial pressure within normal parameters
2. Experiences no serious increases in intracranial pressure during or following care activities

OUTCOMES (NOC)	INTERVENTIONS (NIC) and *RATIONALES*
Neurologic Status	*Cerebral Edema Management*
• Cognitive ability ____	• Monitor vital signs and neurologic status closely and compare with baseline *to evaluate patient's response to treatment and enable immediate reporting and modification of treatment if necessary.*
• Cranial sensory/motor function ____	• Monitor respiratory status: rate, rhythm, depth of respirations; PaO₂, PaCO₂, pH, bicarbonate *because low PaO₂ and a high hydrogen ion concentration (acidosis) are potent cerebral blood vasodilators that increase cerebral blood flow and may increase ICP.*
• Intracranial pressure ____	
• Breathing pattern ____	• Analyze ICP waveform *to provide an accurate indicator of ICP.*
• Pulse pressure ____	• Monitor patient's ICP and neurologic responses to care activities.
• Blood pressure ____	• Position with head of bed up 30 degrees or greater *to promote venous drainage from head, reducing ICP.*
• Pulse rate ____	• Limit suction passes to <15 seconds *to prevent increased ICP.*
• Communication appropriate to situation ____	• Allow ICP to return to baseline between nursing activities *to prevent sustained increases in ICP.*
Measurement Scale	• Maintain normothermia *as elevated temperature increases cerebral metabolism and causes increased ICP.*
1 = Severely compromised	• Give sedation *to decrease agitation and hyperactivity that cause increased ICP.*
2 = Substantially compromised	• Decrease stimuli in patient's environment *to prevent increases in ICP.*
3 = Moderately compromised	
4 = Mildly compromised	
5 = Not compromised	

ICP, Intracranial pressure; *PaCO₂,* partial pressure of carbon dioxide in arterial blood; *PaO₂,* partial pressure of oxygen in arterial blood; *ROM,* range of motion; *SaO₂,* oxygen saturation of arterial blood.

Continued

and daily weights taken into account, are important parameters in the assessment of fluid balance.

Electrolyte determinations should be made daily, and any abnormal values should be discussed with the physician. It is especially important to monitor serum glucose, sodium, potassium, and osmolality. Urinary output is monitored to detect problems related to *diabetes insipidus* (e.g., increased urinary output related to a decrease in antidiuretic hormone secretion) and SIADH (syndrome of inappropriate antidiuretic hormone) secretion, which results in decreased urinary output. Besides urinary output, the serum sodium and osmolality are also used to diagnose diabetes insipidus

and SIADH. Diabetes insipidus may result in severe dehydration unless treated. The usual treatment is fluid replacement, vasopressin (Pitressin), or desmopressin acetate (DDAVP) (see Chapter 50). SIADH results in a dilutional hyponatremia that may produce cerebral edema, changes in LOC, seizures, and coma. (Treatment of SIADH is described in Chapter 50.)

Monitoring Intracranial Pressure. The measurement of ICP enhances clinical decision making by detecting early signs of intracranial hypertension and response to therapy. ICP monitoring is used in combination with other physiologic parameters to guide the care of the patient and assess the patient's response to routine

NURSING CARE PLAN 57-1

Patient with Increased Intracranial Pressure—cont'd

NURSING DIAGNOSIS   **Risk for disuse syndrome** *related to* altered level of consciousness, immobility, altered nutritional intake

PATIENT GOAL   Experiences no complications of immobility

OUTCOMES (NOC)	INTERVENTIONS (NIC) and *RATIONALES*
Immobility Consequences: Physiologic	***Airway Management***
• Lung congestion _____ • Pneumonia _____ • Pressure sore(s) _____ **Measurement Scale** 1 = Severe 2 = Substantial 3 = Moderate 4 = Mild 5 = None • Nutritional status _____ • Joint movement _____ • Muscle tone _____ **Measurement Scale** 1 = Severely compromised 2 = Substantially compromised 3 = Moderately compromised 4 = Mildly compromised 5 = Not compromised	• Position patient to maximize ventilation potential *to prevent aspiration and tongue from blocking airway.* • Remove secretions by encouraging coughing or by suctioning *to remove accumulated secretions, reduce risk of aspiration, and ensure patent airway.* • Perform chest physical therapy *to mobilize secretions and prevent pulmonary congestion.* ***Pressure Ulcer Prevention*** • Use an established risk assessment tool to monitor individual's risk factors (e.g., Braden scale [see Table 13-12]). • Inspect skin over bony prominences and other pressure points at least daily when repositioning *to identify potential or actual skin problems and initiate a plan of care.* • Turn every 1 to 2 hours as appropriate *as prolonged pressure decreases circulation and leads to tissue ischemia and necrosis.* • Turn with care (e.g., avoid shearing) *to prevent injury to fragile skin.* • Keep bed linen clean, dry, and wrinkle free *to protect skin.* • Use devices on bed (e.g., sheepskin) that protect the patient *to reduce pressure to bony prominences by distributing body weight evenly.* ***Nutrition Therapy*** • Complete a nutritional assessment *to determine current nutritional status and needs.* • Determine, in collaboration with the dietitian, the number of calories and type of nutrients needed to meet nutrition requirements. • Determine need for enteral tube feedings to meet nutritional needs *if patient unable to ingest foods and fluids.* ***Exercise Therapy: Joint Mobility*** • Perform passive or assisted ROM exercises *to maintain joint ROM and muscle strength.*

care. Valsalva maneuver, coughing, sneezing, hypoxemia, and arousal from sleep are factors that can increase ICP. Nurses should be alert to these factors and should attempt to minimize them. Nursing management of the patient with increased ICP is one of the most important aspects of the care provided for these patients.

Body Position. The patient with increased ICP should be maintained in the head-up position. The nurse must take care to prevent extreme neck flexion, which can cause venous obstruction and contribute to elevated ICP. The body position should be adjusted to decrease the ICP maximally and to improve the CPP. While traditional practice has been to elevate the head of the bed to 30 degrees unless otherwise contraindicated, research now suggests there is an inconsistent response of the ICP and the CPP to head elevation.[14] Elevation of the head of the bed reduces sagittal sinus pressure, promotes drainage from the head via the valveless venous system through the jugular veins, and decreases the vascular congestion that can produce cerebral edema. However, raising the head of the bed above 30 degrees may decrease the CPP by lowering systemic BP. Careful evaluation of the effects of elevation of the head of the bed on both the ICP and the CPP is required. The bed should be positioned so that it lowers the ICP while optimizing the CPP and other indices of cerebral oxygenation.

Care should be taken to turn the patient with slow, gentle movements because rapid changes in position may increase the ICP. Caution should be used to prevent discomfort in turning and positioning the patient because pain or agitation also increases pressure. Increased intrathoracic pressure contributes to increased ICP by im-

peding the venous return. Thus coughing, straining, and the Valsalva maneuver should be avoided. Extreme hip flexion should be avoided to decrease the risk of raising the intraabdominal pressure, which increases ICP. The patient should be turned at least every 2 hours.

Decorticate or decerebrate posturing is a reflex response in some patients with increased ICP. Turning, skin care, and even passive range of motion can elicit the posturing reflexes. Attempts should be made to provide needed physical care activities to minimize complications of immobility, such as atelectasis and contractures. In cases of severe posturing reflexes, these activities may have to be done less frequently because posturing can increase ICP.

Protection from Injury. The patient with increased ICP and a decreased LOC needs protection from self-injury. Confusion, agitation, and the possibility of seizures increase the risk for injury. Restraints should be used judiciously in the agitated patient. If restraints are absolutely necessary to keep the patient from removing tubes or falling out of bed, they should be secure enough to be effective, and the skin area under the restraints should be observed regularly for irritation. Agitation may increase with the use of restraints, which indicates the need for other measures to protect the patient from injury. Light sedation with agents such as haloperidol (Haldol) or lorazepam (Ativan) may be needed. Having a family member stay with the patient may have a calming effect. For the patient with seizures or the patient at risk for such activity, seizure precautions should be instituted. These include padded side rails, an airway at the bedside, suction readily available, accurate and timely administration of antiseizure drugs, and close observation.

The patient can benefit from a quiet, nonstimulating environment. The nurse should always use a calm, reassuring approach. Touching and talking to the patient, even one who is in a coma, is always appropriate. The nurse must create a balance between sensory deprivation and overload for the patient with increased ICP.

Psychologic Considerations. Besides the carefully planned physical care provided for patients with increased ICP, the nurse must also be aware of the psychologic well-being of patients and their families. Anxiety over the diagnosis and the prognosis can be distressing to the patient, the family, and the nursing staff. The nurse's competent and assured manner in performing care is reassuring to everyone involved. Short, simple explanations are appropriate and allow the patient and the family to acquire the amount of information they desire. There is a need for support, information, and education of both patients and families. The nurse should assess the family members' desire and need to assist in providing care for the patient and allow for their participation as appropriate.

■ Evaluation

The expected outcomes for the patient with ICP are addressed in NCP 57-1.

HEAD INJURY

Head injury includes any trauma to the scalp, skull, or brain. The term *head trauma* is used primarily to signify craniocerebral trauma, which includes an alteration in consciousness, no matter how brief.

Statistics regarding the occurrence of head injuries are incomplete because many victims die at the injury scene or because the condition is considered minor and health care services are not sought. In the United States, an estimated 1.1 million persons are treated and released with traumatic brain injury (TBI) in hospital emergency departments. Fifty thousand people die and 235,000 persons are hospitalized with TBI.[15] Of individuals hospitalized, 22% of the patients die.[15] It is estimated that there has been a 20% decline in fatalities related to head injury since 1980. In the past, motor vehicle collisions and falls were the most common causes of head injury in both Canada and the United States. More recently, in the United States, deaths from motor vehicle collisions and falls have decreased, whereas firearm-related head injury death rates have increased. Other causes of head injury include assaults, sports-related trauma, and recreational injuries. Males are twice as likely to sustain a traumatic brain injury as females.

Head trauma has a high potential for poor outcome.[16] Deaths from head trauma occur at three time points after injury: immediately after the injury, within 2 hours after injury, and approximately 3 weeks after injury. Factors that predict a poor outcome include the presence of an intracranial hematoma, increasing age of the patient, abnormal motor responses, impaired or absent eye movements or pupillary light reflexes, early sustained hypotension, hypoxemia or hypercapnia, and ICP levels higher than 20 mm Hg.[17] The majority of deaths after a head injury occur immediately after the injury, either from the direct head trauma or from massive hemorrhage and shock. Deaths occurring within a few hours of the trauma are caused by progressive worsening of the head injury or internal bleeding. Immediately recognizing changes in neurologic status and rapid surgical intervention are critical in the prevention of deaths at this point. Deaths occurring 3 weeks or more after injury result from multisystem failure. Expert nursing care in the weeks following the injury is crucial in decreasing mortality and in optimizing patient outcome.

TABLE 57-6	Types of Skull Fractures
Description	**Cause**
Linear Break in continuity of bone without alteration of relationship of parts	Low-velocity injuries
Depressed Inward indentation of skull	Powerful blow
Simple Linear or depressed skull fracture without fragmentation or communicating lacerations	Low to moderate impact
Comminuted Multiple linear fractures with fragmentation of bone into many pieces	Direct, high-momentum impact
Compound Depressed skull fracture and scalp laceration with communicating pathway to intracranial cavity	Severe head injury

Types of Head Injuries

Scalp Lacerations. *Scalp lacerations* are an easily recognized type of external head trauma. Because the scalp contains many blood vessels with poor constrictive abilities, most scalp lacerations are associated with profuse bleeding. Even relatively small wounds can bleed significantly. The major complications associated with scalp laceration are blood loss and infection.

Skull Fractures. *Skull fractures* frequently occur with head trauma. There are several ways to describe skull fractures: (1) linear or depressed; (2) simple, comminuted, or compound; and (3) closed or open (Table 57-6). Fractures may be closed or open, depending on the presence of a scalp laceration or extension of the fracture into the air sinuses or dura. The type and severity of a skull fracture depend on the velocity, the momentum, the direction of the injuring agent, and the site of impact.

The location of the fracture alters the presentation of the manifestations (Table 57-7). For example, a basilar skull fracture is a specialized type of linear fracture that occurs when the fracture involves the base of the skull. Manifestations can evolve over the course of several hours, vary with the location and severity of fracture, and may include cranial nerve deficits, Battle's sign (postauricular ecchymosis) (Fig. 57-13), and periorbital ecchymosis (raccoon eyes). This fracture generally is associated with a tear in the dura and subsequent leakage of CSF. *Rhinorrhea* (CSF leakage from the nose) or *otorrhea* (CSF leakage from the ear) generally confirms that the fracture has traversed the dura (Fig. 57-14). Rhinorrhea may also manifest as postnasal sinus drainage. The significance of rhinorrhea may be overlooked unless the patient is specifically assessed for this finding. The risk of meningitis is high with a CSF leak.

Two methods of testing can be used to determine whether the fluid leaking from the nose or ear is CSF. The first method is to test the leaking fluid with a Dextrostix or Tes-Tape strip to determine whether glucose is present. CSF gives a positive reading for glucose. If blood is present in the fluid, testing for the presence of glucose is unreliable because blood also contains glucose. In this event, the nurse should look for the *halo* or *ring* sign (see Fig. 57-14, *C*). To perform this test, the nurse allows the leaking fluid to drip onto a white pad (4 × 4) or towel and observes the drainage. Within a few minutes the blood coalesces into the center, and

TABLE 57-7	Clinical Manifestations of Different Types of Skull Fractures
Location	**Syndrome or Sequelae**
Frontal fracture	Exposure of brain to contaminants through frontal air sinus, possible association with air in forehead tissue, CSF rhinorrhea, or pneumocranium
Orbital fracture	Periorbital ecchymosis (raccoon eyes), optic nerve injury
Temporal fracture	Boggy temporal muscle because of extravasation of blood, oval-shaped bruise behind ear in mastoid region (Battle's sign), CSF otorrhea, middle meningeal artery disruption, epidural hematoma
Parietal fracture	Deafness, CSF or brain otorrhea, bulging of tympanic membrane caused by blood or CSF, facial paralysis, loss of taste, Battle's sign
Posterior fossa fracture	Occipital bruising resulting in cortical blindness, visual field defects; rare appearance of ataxia or other cerebellar signs
Basilar skull fracture	CSF or brain otorrhea, bulging of tympanic membrane caused by blood or CSF, Battle's sign, tinnitus or hearing difficulty, rhinorrhea, facial paralysis, conjugate deviation of gaze, vertigo

CSF, Cerebrospinal fluid.

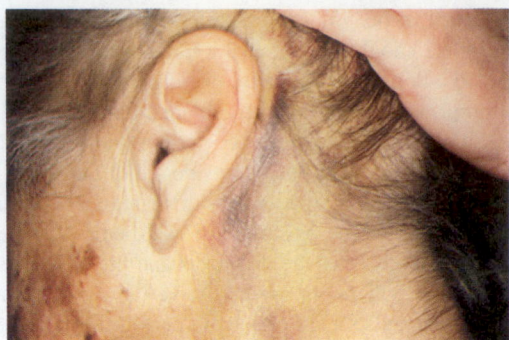

FIG. 57-13 Battle's sign.

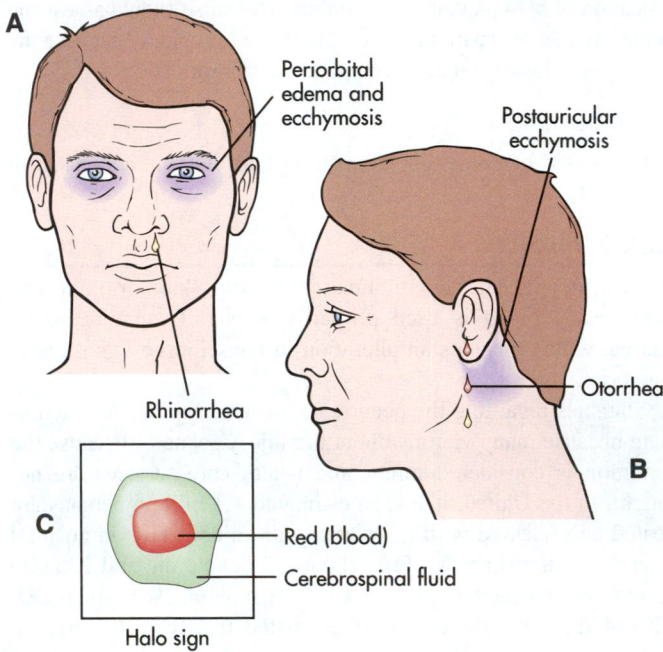

FIG. 57-14 **A,** Raccoon eyes and rhinorrhea. **B,** Battle's sign (postauricular ecchymosis) with otorrhea. **C,** Halo or ring sign (see text).

a yellowish ring encircles the blood if CSF is present. The color, appearance, and amount of leaking fluid must be noted because both tests can give false-positive results.

The major potential complications of skull fractures are intracranial infections and hematoma, as well as meningeal and brain tissue damage.

Minor Head Trauma. Brain injuries are categorized as being minor or major. **Concussion** (a sudden transient mechanical head injury with disruption of neural activity and a change in the LOC) is considered a minor head injury. The patient may or may not lose total consciousness with this injury.

Typical signs of concussion include a brief disruption in LOC, amnesia regarding the event (retrograde amnesia), and headache. The manifestations are generally of short duration. If the patient has not lost consciousness, or if the loss of consciousness lasts <5 minutes, the patient is usually discharged from the care facility with instructions to notify the health care provider if symptoms persist or if behavioral changes are noted.

Postconcussion syndrome may develop in some patients and is usually seen anywhere from 2 weeks to 2 months after the injury. Symptoms include persistent headache, lethargy, personality and behavioral changes, shortened attention span, decreased short-term memory, and changes in intellectual ability. This syndrome can significantly affect the patient's abilities to perform activities of daily living.

Although concussion is generally considered benign and usually resolves spontaneously, the symptoms may be the beginning of a more serious, progressive problem, especially in a patient with a history of prior concussion or head injury. At the time of discharge, it is important to give the patient and the family instructions for observation and accurate reporting of symptoms or changes in neurologic status.

Major Head Trauma. Major head trauma includes cerebral contusions and lacerations. Both injuries represent severe trauma to the brain.

A **contusion** is the bruising of the brain tissue within a focal area. It is usually associated with a closed head injury. A contusion may contain areas of hemorrhage, infarction, necrosis, and edema and frequently occurs at a fracture site. With contusion, the phenomenon of *coup-contrecoup injury* is often noted. Damage from coup-contrecoup injury occurs when the brain moves inside the skull due to high-energy or high-impact injury mechanisms. Contusions or lacerations occur both at the site of the direct impact of the brain on the skull *(coup)* and at a secondary area of damage on the opposite side away from injury *(contrecoup),* leading to multiple contused areas. Patient prognosis is dependent upon the amount of bleeding around the contusion site, which can range from minimal to severe. Contusions may continue to bleed or rebleed and appear to "blossom" on subsequent CT scans of the brain, which worsens neurologic outcome. Anticoagulant use and coagulopathy are associated with increased hemorrhage, more severe head injury, and a higher mortality rate.[18] Neurologic assessment may demonstrate focal as well as generalized findings, depending on the size and location of the contusion. Seizures are a common complication of brain contusion.

Lacerations involve actual tearing of the brain tissue and often occur in association with depressed and open fractures and penetrating injuries. Tissue damage is severe, and surgical repair of the laceration is impossible due to the nature of brain tissue. If bleeding is deep into the brain parenchyma, focal and generalized signs develop.

When major head trauma occurs, many delayed responses are seen, including hemorrhage, hematoma formation, seizures, and cerebral edema. Intracerebral hemorrhage is generally associated with cerebral laceration. This hemorrhage manifests as a space-occupying lesion accompanied by unconsciousness, hemiplegia on the contralateral side, and a dilated pupil on the ipsilateral side. As the hematoma expands, signs of increased ICP become more severe. Prognosis is generally poor for the patient with a large intracerebral hemorrhage. Subarachnoid hemorrhage and intraventricular hemorrhage can also occur secondary to head trauma.

Pathophysiology

Diffuse axonal injury (DAI) is widespread axonal damage occurring after a mild, moderate, or severe TBI. The damage occurs primarily around axons in subcortical white matter of the cerebral hemispheres, basal ganglia, thalamus, and brainstem.[19] Initially, DAI was believed to occur from the tensile forces of trauma that sheared axons, resulting in axonal disconnection. There is increasing evidence that axonal damage is not preceded by an immediate tearing of the axon from the traumatic impact, but rather the trauma changes the function of the axon, resulting in axon swelling and disconnection. This process takes approximately 12 to 24 hours to develop and may persist longer. The clinical signs include a decreased LOC, increased ICP, decortication or decerebration, and global cerebral edema. Approximately 90% of patients with DAI remain in a persistent vegetative state.[19]

Complications

Epidural Hematoma. An **epidural hematoma** results from bleeding between the dura and the inner surface of the skull (Fig. 57-15). An epidural hematoma is a neurologic emergency (Fig. 57-16) and is usually associated with a linear fracture crossing a major artery in the dura, causing a tear. It can have a venous or an arterial origin. Venous epidural hematomas are associated with a tear of the dural venous sinus and develop slowly. With arterial hematomas, the middle meningeal artery lying under the temporal bone is often torn. Hemorrhage occurs into the epidural space, which lies between the dura and the inner surface of the skull (see Fig. 57-15). Because this is an arterial hemorrhage, the hematoma develops rapidly and under high pressure. Classic signs typically include an initial period of unconsciousness at the scene, with a brief lucid interval followed by a decrease in LOC. Other manifestations may be a headache, nausea and vomiting, or focal findings. Rapid surgical intervention to evacuate the hematoma and prevent cerebral herniation can dramatically improve outcome.

Subdural Hematoma. A **subdural hematoma** occurs from bleeding between the dura mater and the arachnoid layer of the meninges (see Fig. 57-15). A subdural hematoma usually results from injury to the brain substance and its parenchymal vessels. The veins that drain from the surface of the brain into the sagittal sinus are the source of most subdural hematomas. Because a subdural hematoma is usually venous in origin, the hematoma may be slower to develop. However, a subdural hematoma may be caused by an arterial hemorrhage, in which case it develops more rapidly. Subdural hematomas may be acute, subacute, or chronic (Table 57-8). An *acute subdural hematoma* manifests signs within 48 hours of the injury. The signs and symptoms are similar to those associated with brain tissue compression in increased ICP and in-

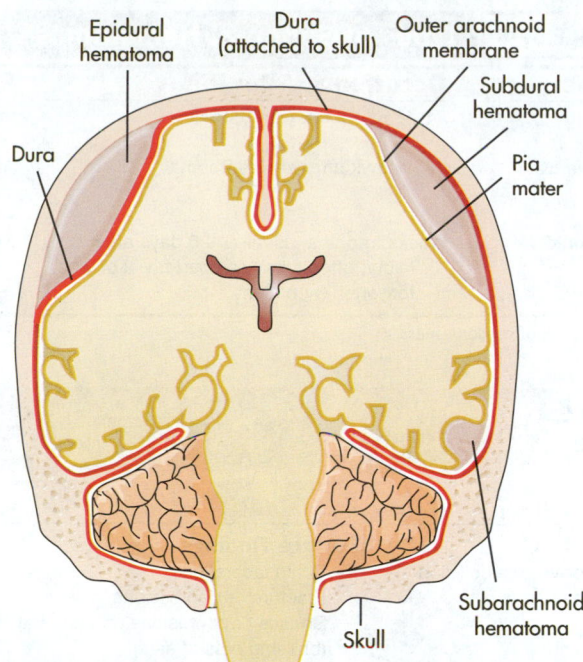

FIG. 57-15 Locations of epidural, subdural, and subarachnoid hematomas.

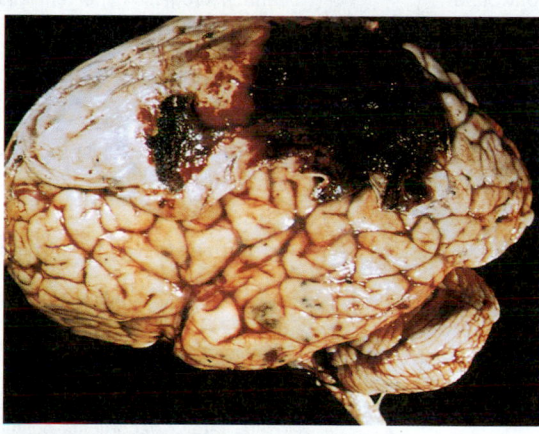

FIG. 57-16 Epidural hematoma covering a portion of the dura. Multiple small contusions are seen in the temporal lobe.

clude decreasing LOC and headache. The size of the hematoma determines the patient's clinical presentation as well as prognosis. The patient's appearance may range from drowsy and confused to unconscious. The ipsilateral pupil dilates and becomes fixed if ICP is significantly elevated. Blunt force injuries that produce acute subdural hematomas also may cause significant underlying brain injury with concomitant cerebral edema. The resulting increase in ICP from the cerebral edema can be the factor that causes increased morbidity and mortality despite surgical intervention to evacuate the hematoma. A *subacute subdural hematoma* usually occurs within 2 to 14 days of the injury. After the initial bleeding, a subdural hematoma may appear to enlarge over time as the breakdown products of the blood draw fluid into the subdural space to reach isotonicity.

A *chronic subdural hematoma* develops over weeks or months after a seemingly minor head injury. The peak incidence of chronic subdural hematoma is in the 50s and 60s when a potentially larger subdural space is available as a result of brain atrophy. With atrophy, the brain remains attached to the supportive structures, but

Nervous System

TABLE 57-8	**Types of Subdural Hematomas**		
Type	**Occurrence After Injury**	**Progression of Symptoms**	**Treatment**
Acute	24-48 hr after severe trauma	Immediate deterioration	Craniotomy, evacuation and decompression
Subacute	48 hr-2 wk after severe trauma	Alteration in mental status as hematoma develops; progression dependent on size and location of hematoma	Evacuation and decompression
Chronic	Weeks, months, usually >20 days after injury; often injury seemed trivial or was forgotten by patient	Nonspecific, nonlocalizing progression; progressive alteration in LOC	Evacuation and decompression, membranectomy

LOC, Level of consciousness.

TABLE 57-9	*EMERGENCY MANAGEMENT* **Head Injury**

Etiology	**Assessment Findings**	**Interventions**
Blunt	**Surface Findings**	**Initial**
Motor vehicle collision	• Scalp lacerations	• Ensure patent airway.
Pedestrian event	• Fracture or depressions in skull	• Stabilize cervical spine.
Fall	• Bruises or contusions on face, Battle's sign (bruising behind ears)	• Administer O_2 via non-rebreather mask.
Assault	• Raccoon eyes (dependent bruising around eyes)	• Establish IV access with two large-bore catheters to infuse normal saline or lactated Ringer's solution.
Sports injury		• Control external bleeding with sterile pressure dressing.
	Respiratory	• Assess for rhinorrhea, otorrhea, scalp wounds.
Penetrating	• Central neurogenic hyperventilation	• Remove patient's clothing.
Gunshot wound	• Cheyne-Stokes respirations	
Arrow	• Decreased O_2 saturation	**Ongoing Monitoring**
	• Pulmonary edema	• Maintain patient warmth using blankets, warm IV fluids, overhead warming lights, warm humidified O_2.
	Central Nervous System	• Monitor vital signs, level of consciousness, O_2 saturation, cardiac rhythm, Glasgow Coma Scale score, pupil size and reactivity.
	• Unequal or dilated pupils	• Anticipate need for intubation if gag reflex is impaired or absent.
	• Asymmetric facial movements	• Assume neck injury with head injury.
	• Garbled speech, abusive speech	• Administer fluids cautiously to prevent fluid overload and increasing ICP.
	• Confusion	
	• Decreased level of consciousness	
	• Combativeness	
	• Involuntary movements	
	• Seizures	
	• Bowel and bladder incontinence	
	• Flaccidity	
	• Depressed or hyperactive reflexes	
	• Decerebrate or decorticate posturing	
	• Glasgow Coma Scale score <12	
	• CSF leaking from ears or nose	

CSF, Cerebrospinal fluid; *ICP,* intracranial pressure; *IV,* intravenous.

tension is increased, and it is subject to tearing. The larger size of the subdural space also accounts for the presenting complaint often to be the focal symptoms, rather than the signs of increased ICP. Chronic alcoholics are also prone to cerebral atrophy and subsequent development of subdural hematoma due to an increased incidence of falls.

Delay in diagnosis of a subdural hematoma in the older adult can be attributed to symptoms that mimic other health problems in persons of this age-group, such as vascular disease and dementia. Somnolence, confusion, lethargy, and memory loss may be erroneously associated with health problems other than subdural hematoma.

Intracerebral Hematoma. **Intracerebral hematoma** occurs from bleeding within the parenchyma and occurs in approximately 16% of head injuries. It usually occurs within the frontal and temporal lobes, possibly from the rupture of intracerebral vessels at the time of injury. The size and location of the hematoma is a key determinant of patient outcome.

Diagnostic Studies and Collaborative Care

CT scan is considered the best diagnostic test to evaluate for craniocerebral trauma because it allows rapid diagnosis and intervention in the acute setting. MRI, PET, and evoked potential studies may also be used in the diagnosis and differentiation of head injuries. An MRI scan is more sensitive than the CT scan in detecting small DAI lesions. Transcranial Doppler studies allow for the measurement of CBF velocity. A cervical spine x-ray series or CT scan of the spine may also be indicated since cervical spine trauma often occurs concomitantly with head injury. In general, the diagnostic studies are similar to those used for a patient with increased ICP (see Table 57-3). The GCS can be used to classify head injury as mild (score of 13 to 15), moderate (score of 9 to 12), or severe (score of 3 to 8).

Emergency management of the patient with a head injury is presented in Table 57-9. In addition to measures to prevent secondary injury by treating cerebral edema and managing increased ICP, the principal treatment of head injuries is timely diagnosis and surgery if necessary. For the patient with concussion and contusion, observation and management of increased ICP are the primary management strategies.

The treatment of skull fractures is usually conservative. For depressed fractures and fractures with loose fragments, a craniotomy is necessary to elevate the depressed bone and remove the free fragments. If large amounts of bone are destroyed, the bone may be removed (craniectomy) and a cranioplasty will be needed at a later time (see the section on Cranial Surgery later in this chapter).

In cases of large acute subdural and epidural hematomas, or those associated with significant neurologic impairment, the blood must be removed through surgical evacuation. A craniotomy is generally performed to visualize and allow control of the bleeding vessels. Burr-hole openings may be used in an extreme emergency for a more rapid decompression, followed by a craniotomy. A drain is generally placed postoperatively for several days to prevent reaccumulation of blood.

NURSING MANAGEMENT
HEAD INJURY

■ Nursing Assessment

The patient with a head injury is always considered to have the potential for developing increased ICP. Increased ICP is associated with higher mortality rates and poorer functional outcomes.[4,6] The most important aspects of the objective data are noting the GCS score (see Table 57-5), assessing and monitoring the neurologic status (see Fig. 57-10), and determining whether a CSF leak has occurred. (Nursing assessment related to increased ICP is discussed on pp. 1476 to 1478.) Nursing assessment of the patient with a head injury is presented in Table 57-10.

■ Nursing Diagnoses

Nursing diagnoses and potential complication for the patient who has sustained a head injury may include, but are not limited to, the following:

- Ineffective tissue perfusion (cerebral) *related to* interruption of CBF associated with cerebral hemorrhage, hematoma, and edema
- Hyperthermia *related to* increased metabolism, infection, and loss of cerebral integrative function secondary to possible hypothalamic injury
- Acute pain (headache) *related to* trauma and cerebral edema
- Impaired physical mobility *related to* decreased LOC and treatment-imposed bed rest
- Anxiety *related to* abrupt change in health status, hospital environment, and uncertain future
- Potential complication: increased ICP *related to* cerebral edema and hemorrhage

■ Planning

The overall goals are that the patient with an acute head injury will (1) maintain adequate cerebral oxygenation and perfusion; (2) remain normothermic; (3) achieve control of pain and discomfort; (4) be free from infection; and (5) attain maximal cognitive, motor, and sensory function.

■ Nursing Implementation

Health Promotion. One of the best ways to prevent head injuries is to prevent car and motorcycle collisions. The nurse can be active in campaigns that promote driving safety and can speak to

ETHICAL DILEMMAS
Brain Death

Situation
The emergency nurse receives a radio call from emergency medical service (EMS) personnel about a young male who has been involved in a motorcycle crash. The patient was not wearing a helmet and has a large open skull fracture with obvious gray matter oozing from the area. Transport from the accident scene was delayed by 45 minutes as a result of a severe thunderstorm and traffic congestion. On the way to the hospital, the patient experiences fixed, dilated pupils and cardiac arrest. Estimated arrival at the hospital is still an additional 45 minutes as a result of the severe weather. EMS personnel request permission to stop resuscitation efforts.

Important Points for Consideration
- Death by neurologic criteria occurs when the cerebral cortex stops functioning or is irreversibly destroyed.
- Since technology has been developed that assists in supporting life, controversies have arisen related to an exact definition of death.
- Criteria for brain death include coma or unresponsiveness, absence of brainstem reflexes, and apnea (see Chapter 11). Specific assessments by a physician are required to validate each of the criteria.
- The patient's clinical manifestations indicate that brain death has occurred.
- Although there is a slight chance the patient's heart function could be resuscitated and supported with mechanical ventilation, there is no obligation to provide medically futile care for a patient with brain death.
- Brain death criteria do not address patients in a permanent vegetative state since the brainstem activity in these patients is adequate to maintain heart and lung function.

Critical Thinking Questions
1. What are your feelings about cessation of brain function versus cessation of heart and lung function as the criteria for death of a patient?
2. What are your state's laws or practices about stopping cardiopulmonary resuscitation (CPR) efforts by EMS personnel in the field?

driver education classes regarding the dangers of unsafe driving and of driving after drinking alcohol and using drugs. The use of seat belts in cars and the use of helmets for riding on motorcycles are the most effective measures for increasing survival after crashes. Increasingly, individual states are passing legislation requiring the use of automobile safety devices for both children and adults. The wearing of protective helmets by lumberjacks, construction workers, miners, horseback riders, bicycle riders, snowboarders, and skydivers is also recommended. The nurse should be familiar with data on outcomes with and without safety devices in working with groups who oppose safety legislation as an infringement of personal freedom.

Acute Intervention. Management at the injury scene can have a significant impact on the outcome of the head injury. Emergency management of head injury is presented in Table 57-9. The general goal of nursing management of the head-injured patient is to maintain cerebral oxygenation and perfusion and prevent secondary cerebral ischemia. Surveillance or monitoring for changes in neurologic status is critically important because the patient's condition may deteriorate rapidly, necessitating emergency surgery. Appropriate preoperative and postoperative nurs-

TABLE 57-10	**NURSING ASSESSMENT** **Head Injury**

Subjective Data

Important Health Information

Past health history: Motor vehicle collision, sports injury, industrial incident, assault, falls

Medications: Anticoagulant medication use

Functional Health Patterns

Health perception–health management: Use of alcohol or recreational drugs; risk-taking behaviors

Cognitive-perceptual: Headache, mood or behavioral change, mentation changes, aphasia, dysphasia, impaired judgment

Coping–stress tolerance: Fear, denial, anger, aggression, depression

Objective Data

General

Altered mental status

Integumentary

Lacerations, contusions, abrasions, hematoma, Battle's sign, periorbital edema and ecchymosis, otorrhea, exposed brain matter

Respiratory

Rhinorrhea, impaired gag reflex, inability to maintain a patent airway

Impending herniation: altered/irregular respiratory rate and pattern

Cardiovascular

Impending herniation: Cushing's response (systolic hypertension [widening pulse pressure], bradycardia [full and bounding pulse])

Gastrointestinal

Vomiting, projectile vomiting, bowel incontinence

Urinary

Bladder incontinence

Reproductive

Uninhibited sexual expression

Neurologic

Altered level of consciousness, seizure activity, pupil dysfunction, cranial nerve deficit(s)

Musculoskeletal

Motor deficit/impairment, weakness, palmar drift, paralysis, spasticity, decorticate or decerebrate posturing, muscular rigidity/increased tone, flaccidity, ataxia

Possible Findings

Location and type of hematoma, edema, skull fracture, and/or foreign body on CT scan and/or MRI; abnormal EEG; positive toxicology screen or alcohol level, ↓ or ↑ blood glucose level; ↑ ICP

CT, Computed tomography; *EEG,* electroencephalogram; *ICP,* intracranial pressure; *MRI,* magnetic resonance imaging.

TABLE 57-11	**PATIENT AND FAMILY TEACHING GUIDE** **Head Injury**

Teaching guidelines for the patient and family during the initial 2 to 3 days after a head injury include the following:

1. Notify your health care provider immediately if experiencing signs and symptoms that may indicate complications. These include:
   - Increased drowsiness (e.g., difficulty arousing, confusion)
   - Nausea and/or vomiting
   - Worsening headache or stiff neck
   - Seizures
   - Vision difficulties (e.g., blurring)
   - Behavioral changes (e.g., irritability, anger)
   - Motor problems (e.g., clumsiness, difficulty walking, slurred speech, weakness in arms or legs)
   - Sensory disturbances (e.g., numbness)
   - Slow heart rate
2. Have someone stay with you.
3. Abstain from alcohol.
4. Check with your health care provider before taking drugs that may increase drowsiness, including muscle relaxants, tranquilizers, and opioid pain medications.
5. Avoid driving, using heavy machinery, playing contact sports, and taking hot baths.

formation about the patient's diagnosis, the treatment plan, and the rationale for the interventions.[20] Other teaching points for the patient and family are presented in Table 57-11.

The nurse should perform neurologic assessments at intervals based on the patient's condition. The GCS is useful in assessing the level of consciousness (see Table 57-5). Indications of a deteriorating neurologic state, such as a decreasing LOC or a lessening of motor strength, should be reported to the health care provider, and the patient's condition should be closely monitored.

The major focus of nursing care for the brain-injured patient relates to increased ICP (see NCP 57-1). However, there may be specific problems that require nursing intervention.

Eye problems may include loss of the corneal reflex, periorbital ecchymosis and edema, and diplopia. Loss of the corneal reflex may necessitate administering lubricating eyedrops or taping the eyes shut to prevent abrasion. Periorbital ecchymosis and edema disappear spontaneously, but cold and, later, warm compresses provide comfort and hasten the process. Diplopia can be relieved by use of an eye patch.

Hyperthermia may occur from injury to or inflammation of the hypothalamus. Elevations in body temperature can result in increased CBF, cerebral blood volume, and ICP.[7] Increased metabolism secondary to hyperthermia increases metabolic waste, which in turn produces further cerebral vasodilation. The nurse should attempt to control hyperthermia and maintain normothermia in the head-injured patient.

If CSF rhinorrhea or otorrhea occurs, the nurse should inform the physician immediately. The head of the bed may be raised to decrease the CSF pressure so that a tear can seal. A loose collection pad may be placed under the nose or over the ear. No dressing should be placed into the nasal or ear cavities. The patient should be cautioned not to sneeze or blow the nose. NG tubes should not be used, and nasotracheal suctioning should not be performed on these patients due to the high risk of meningitis.

Nursing measures specific to the care of the immobilized patient, such as those related to bladder and bowel function, skin care, and infection, are also indicated. Nausea and vomiting may be a problem

ing interventions are initiated if surgery is anticipated. Because of the close association between hemodynamic status and cerebral perfusion, the nurse must be aware of any coexisting injuries or conditions. In the acute injury period, treating other life-threatening conditions (i.e., hemorrhage, hypoxia) will take initial priority in nursing care.

The nurse should explain the need for frequent neurologic assessments to both the patient and the family. Behavioral manifestations associated with head injury can result in a frightened, disoriented patient who is combative and resists help. The nurse's approach should be calm and gentle. A family member may be available to stay with the patient and thus prevent increasing anxiety and fear. Nursing research also validates that one of the most pressing needs for family members in the acute injury phase of care is desire for in-

and can be alleviated by antiemetic drugs. Headache can usually be controlled with acetaminophen or small doses of codeine.

If the patient's condition deteriorates, intracranial surgery may be necessary (see the section on Cranial Surgery later in this chapter). A burr-hole opening or craniotomy may be indicated, depending on the underlying injury that is causing the symptoms. The emergency nature of the surgery may hasten the usual careful preoperative preparation. The nurse should consult with the neurosurgeon to determine specific preoperative nursing measures.

The patient is often unconscious before surgery, making it necessary for a family member to sign the consent form for surgery. This is a difficult and frightening time for the patient's family and requires sensitive nursing management. The suddenness of the situation makes it especially difficult for the family to cope.

Ambulatory and Home Care. Once the condition has stabilized, the patient is usually transferred for acute rehabilitation management to prepare the patient for reentry into the community. As with any craniocerebral problem, there may be chronic problems related to motor and sensory deficits, communication, memory, and intellectual functioning. Many of the principles of nursing management of the patient with a stroke are appropriate (see Chapter 58). Conditions that may require nursing and collaborative management include poor nutritional status, bowel and bladder management, spasticity, dysphagia, neurogenic heterotopic ossification (overgrowth of bone), deep vein thrombosis, and hydrocephalus. The patient's outward appearance is not a good indicator of how well the patient will ultimately function in the home or work environment given recovery time and rehabilitation.

Seizure disorders are seen in approximately 5% of patients with a nonpenetrating head injury. The most vulnerable time for seizures to develop is during the first week after the head injury. Some patients may not develop a seizure disorder until years after the initial injury. Some health care providers recommend that antiseizure drugs be used prophylactically. Others may not institute treatment until a seizure is witnessed or an EEG demonstrates seizure activity. Phenytoin (Dilantin) is the typical antiseizure drug of choice to manage posttraumatic seizure activity.

The mental and emotional sequelae of brain trauma are often the most incapacitating problems. Many of the patients with head injuries who have been comatose for more than 6 hours undergo some personality change. They may suffer loss of concentration and memory and defective memory processing. Personal drive may decrease; apathy and apparent laziness may increase. Euphoria and mood swings, along with a seeming lack of awareness of the seriousness of the injury, may occur. The patient's behavior may indicate a loss of social restraint, judgment, tact, and emotional control.

Progressive recovery may continue for 6 months or more before a plateau is reached and a prognosis for recovery can be made. Specific nursing management in the posttraumatic phase depends on specific residual deficits.

In all cases the family must be given special consideration. They need to understand what is happening and be taught appropriate interaction patterns. The nurse must give guidance and referrals for financial aid, child care, and other personal needs and must assist the family in involving the patient in family activities whenever possible. Assisting the patient and family in developing and maintaining hope and keeping communication open are strategies perceived as supportive by families.[20,21]

The family often has unrealistic expectations of the patient as the coma begins to recede. The family expects full return to pretrauma

status. In reality, the patient experiences a reduced awareness and ability to interpret environmental stimuli. The nurse must prepare the family for the emergence of the patient from coma and must explain that the process of awakening often takes several weeks.

When the time for discharge planning arrives, the family and the patient may benefit from very specific posthospitalization instructions to avoid family-patient friction.[22] Special "no" policies that may be appropriately suggested by the neurosurgeon, neuropsychologist, and nurse include no drinking of alcoholic beverages, no driving, no use of firearms, no work with hazardous implements and machinery, and no unsupervised smoking. Family members, particularly spouses, go through role transition as the role changes from that of spouse to that of caregiver.

■ Evaluation

The expected outcomes are that the patient with a head injury will
- maintain normal cerebral perfusion pressure
- achieve maximal cognitive, motor, and sensory function
- experience no infection or hyperthermia
- achieve pain control

BRAIN TUMORS

The annual rate of newly diagnosed brain tumors in the United States is 18,500, with an estimated 12,760 deaths related to brain tumors.[23] The brain is also a frequent site for metastasis from other sites. The 5-year relative survival rate for brain tumors is approximately 33%.[23] Males have a slightly higher incidence of brain tumors than females.

Types

Brain tumors can occur in any part of the brain or spinal cord. Tumors of the brain may be *primary,* arising from tissues within the brain, or *secondary,* resulting from a metastasis from a malignant neoplasm elsewhere in the body. Secondary brain tumors are the most common type. Brain tumors are generally classified according to the tissue from which they arise. The most common primary brain tumors originate in astrocytes. These tumors are called gliomas (e.g., astrocytoma, glioblastoma multiforme) and account for 65% of primary brain tumors (Table 57-12). Glioblastoma multiforme is the most common primary brain tumor, followed by meningioma and astrocytoma. More than half of brain tumors are malignant; they infiltrate the brain parenchyma and are not amenable to complete surgical removal. Other tumors may be histologically benign but are located such that complete removal is not possible. Brain tumors are more commonly seen in middle-aged persons, but they may occur at any age.

TABLE 57-12	Types of Brain Tumors	
Type	**Tissue of Origin**	**Characteristics**
Gliomas		
• Astrocytoma	Supportive tissue, glial cells, and astrocytes	Can range from low-grade to moderate-grade malignancy
• Glioblastoma multiforme	Primitive stem cell (glioblast)	Highly malignant and invasive; among the most devastating of primary brain tumors
• Oligodendroglioma	Oligodendrocytes	Benign (encapsulation and calcification)
• Ependymoma	Ependymal epithelium	Range from benign to highly malignant; most are benign and encapsulated
• Medulloblastoma	Primitive neuroectodermal cell	Highly malignant and invasive; metastatic to spinal cord and remote areas of brain
Meningioma	Meninges	Can be benign or malignant; most are benign
Acoustic neuroma (Schwannoma)	Cells that form myelin sheath around nerves; commonly affects cranial nerve VIII	Many grow on both sides of the brain; usually benign or low-grade malignancy
Pituitary adenoma	Pituitary gland	Usually benign
Hemangioblastoma	Blood vessels of brain	Rare and benign; surgery is curative
Primary central nervous system lymphoma	Lymphocytes	Increased incidence in transplant recipients and acquired immunodeficiency syndrome (AIDS) patients
Metastatic tumors	Lungs, breast, kidney, thyroid, prostate	Malignant

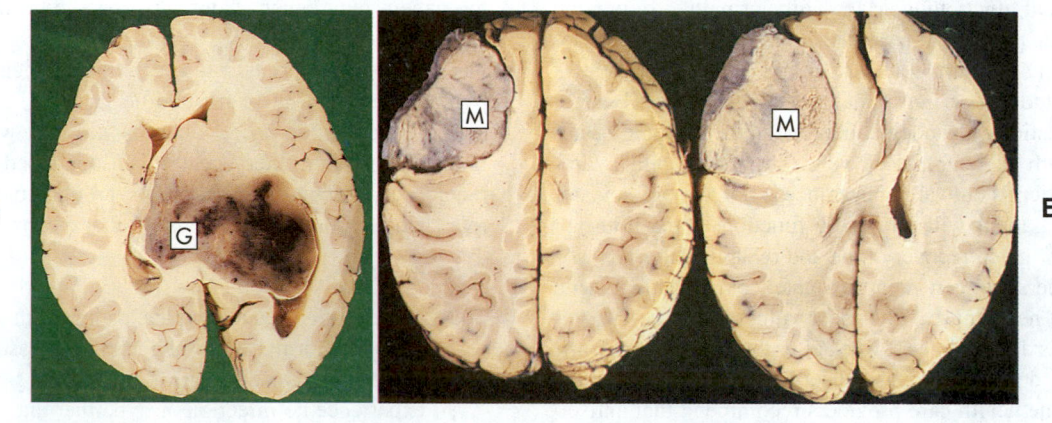

FIG. 57-17 **A,** Glioblastoma. A large glioblastoma *(G)* arises from one cerebral hemisphere and has grown to fill the ventricular system. **B,** Meningioma. These two different sections from different levels in the same brain show a meningioma *(M)* compressing the frontal lobe and distorting underlying brain.

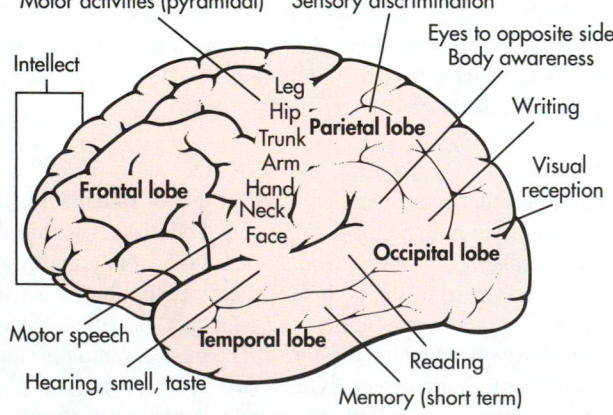

FIG. 57-18 Each area of the brain controls a particular activity.

Unless treated, all brain tumors eventually cause death from increasing tumor volume leading to increased ICP. Brain tumors rarely metastasize outside the central nervous system (CNS) because they are contained by structural (meninges) and physiologic (blood-brain) barriers. Table 57-12 compares the major brain tumors. A glioblastoma and meningioma are shown in Fig. 57-17.

Clinical Manifestations

The clinical manifestations of brain tumors depend mainly on the location and size of the tumor. The rate of growth and the appearance of manifestations depend on the location, size, and mitotic rate of the cells of the tissue of origin. Fig. 57-18 illustrates the functional areas of the cerebral cortex and can be used as a guide to correlate manifestations with the location of the tumor.

Wide ranges of possible clinical manifestations are associated with brain tumors. Headache is a common problem. Tumor-related headaches tend to be worse at night and may awaken the patient. The headaches are usually dull and constant but occasionally throbbing. Seizures are common in gliomas and brain metastases. Brain tumors can cause nausea and vomiting from increased ICP. Cognitive dysfunction, including memory problems and mood or personality changes, is another common manifestation, especially in patients with brain metastases. Muscle weakness, sensory losses, aphasia, and visuospatial dysfunction are also manifestations of brain tumors. As the brain tumor expands, it may also produce manifestations of increased ICP, cerebral edema, or obstruction of the CSF pathways. Manifestations may clearly indicate the location of the tumor by an alteration in the function controlled by the affected area (Table 57-13).

TABLE 57-13	Brain Tumor Locations and Presenting Manifestations
Tumor Location	**Presenting Manifestations**
Cerebral hemisphere	
• Frontal lobe (unilateral)	Unilateral hemiplegia, seizures, memory deficit, personality and judgment changes, visual disturbances
• Frontal lobe (bilateral)	Symptoms associated with unilateral frontal lobe tumors; ataxic gait
• Parietal lobe	Speech disturbance (if tumor is in the dominant hemisphere: inability to write, spatial disorders, unilateral neglect)
• Occipital lobe	Vision disturbances and seizures
• Temporal lobe	Few symptoms; seizures, dysphagia
Subcortical	Hemiplegia; other symptoms may depend on area of infiltration
Meningeal tumors	Symptoms are associated with compression of the brain and depend on tumor location
Metastatic tumors	Headache, nausea, or vomiting because of ↑ ICP; other symptoms depend on tumor location
Thalamus and sellar tumors	Headache, nausea, vision disturbances, papilledema, and nystagmus occur from ↑ ICP; diabetes insipidus may occur
Fourth ventricle and cerebellar tumors	Headache, nausea, and papilledema from ↑ ICP; ataxic gait and changes in coordination
Cerebellopontine tumors	Tinnitus and vertigo, deafness
Brainstem tumors	Headache on awakening, drowsiness, vomiting, ataxic gait, facial muscle weakness, hearing loss, dysphagia, dysarthria, "crossed eyes" or other visual changes, hemiparesis

ICP, Intracranial pressure.

Complications

If the tumor mass obstructs the ventricles or occludes the outlet, ventricular enlargement (hydrocephalus) can occur. Surgical treatment is necessary to relieve the pressure and involves placement of a ventriculoatrial or a ventriculoperitoneal shunt. A catheter with one-way valves is placed in the right lateral ventricle and then tunneled through the skin to drain CSF into the right atrium or the peritoneum. Rapid decompression of ICP can cause prostration and headache that may be prevented by gradually introducing the patient to the upright position. The patient should be instructed to avoid contact sports that may result in a blow to the valve or shearing of the catheter. Shunt malfunction is evidenced by signs of increased ICP, such as decreasing LOC, restlessness, headache, blurred vision, or vomiting. This may necessitate shunt revision or replacement. Signs of an infected shunt, such as high fever, persistent headache, and stiff neck, warrant investigation.

Diagnostic Studies

An extensive history and a comprehensive neurologic examination must be done in the workup of a patient with a suspected brain tumor. A careful history and physical examination may provide data with respect to location. A new-onset seizure disorder may be the first indication of a brain tumor. Diagnostic studies are similar to those used for a patient with increased ICP (see Table 57-3). The sensitivity of techniques such as MRI and PET allows for detection of very small tumors and may provide more reliable diagnostic information. CT and brain scanning are used to diagnose the location of the lesion. Other tests include magnetic resonance spectroscopy, functional MRI, PET scans, and single-photon emission computed tomography (SPECT). The EEG is useful but of less importance. A lumbar puncture is seldom diagnostic and carries with it the risk of cerebral herniation. Angiography can be used to determine blood flow to the tumor and further localize the tumor. Other studies are done to rule out a primary lesion elsewhere in the body. Endocrine studies are helpful when a pituitary adenoma is suspected (see Chapter 50).

The correct diagnosis of a brain tumor can be made by obtaining tissue for histologic study. In most patients, tissue is obtained at the time of surgery. Computer-guided stereotactic biopsy is also an option if complete resection is not possible or practical. A smear or frozen section can be performed in the operating room for a preliminary interpretation of the histologic type. With this information, the neurosurgeon can make a better decision about the extent of surgery. In some cases, immunohistochemical stains or electron microscopy may be necessary to ascertain the correct diagnosis. Determination of the MIB-1 index, a measure of mitotic rate, is often helpful in assessing the mitotic activity of a given tumor.

Collaborative Care

Treatment goals are aimed at (1) identifying the tumor type and location, (2) removing or decreasing tumor mass, and (3) preventing or managing increased ICP.

Surgical Therapy. Surgical removal is the preferred treatment for brain tumors (see the section on Cranial Surgery later in this chapter). Stereotactic surgical techniques are used with greater frequency to perform a biopsy and remove small brain tumors. The outcome of surgical therapy depends on the type, size, and location of the tumor. Meningiomas and oligodendrogliomas can usually be completely removed, whereas the more invasive gliomas and medulloblastomas can be only partially removed. Computer-guided stereotactic biopsy, ultrasound, functional MRI, and cortical mapping can be used to localize brain tumors intraoperatively. Complete surgical removal is not always possible because the tumor is not always accessible or it has involved vital parts of the brain. Surgery can reduce tumor mass, which decreases ICP and provides relief of symptoms with an extension of survival time. Tumors located in the deep central areas of the dominant hemisphere, the posterior corpus callosum, or the upper brainstem cause extensive neurologic damage and are considered probably inoperable.

Radiation Therapy and Radiosurgery. Radiation therapy is commonly used as a follow-up measure after surgery. Radiation seeds can also be implanted into the brain. Cerebral edema and rapidly increasing ICP may be a complication of radiation therapy, but they can be managed with high doses of corticosteroids (dexamethasone [Decadron], prednisone, or methylprednisolone [Solu-Medrol]). (Radiation therapy is discussed in Chapter 16.)

Stereotactic radiosurgery is a method of delivering a high concentrated dose of radiation precisely directed at a location within the brain. Stereotactic radiosurgery may be used when conventional surgery has failed or is not an option because of the tumor location. (Radiosurgery is discussed on pp. 1491 to 1492).

Chemotherapy. The effectiveness of chemotherapy has been limited by difficulty getting drugs across the blood-brain barrier, tumor cell heterogeneity, and tumor cell drug resistance. A group of chemotherapeutic drugs called the nitrosoureas (e.g., carmustine [BCNU], lomustine [CCNU]) are used to treat brain tumors. Normally the blood-brain barrier prohibits the entry of most drugs into the brain. The most malignant tumors cause a breakdown of the blood-brain barrier in the area of the tumor, allowing chemotherapeutic agents to be used to treat the malignancy. Chemotherapy-laden biodegradable wafers (e.g., Gliadel wafer [polifeprosan with carmustine implant]) implanted at the time of surgery can deliver chemotherapy directly to the tumor site. Other drugs being used include methotrexate and procarbazine (Matulane). One method used to deliver chemotherapeutic drugs directly to the CNS is intrathecal administration via an Ommaya reservoir.

Temozolomide (Temodar) is the first oral chemotherapeutic agent found to cross the blood-brain barrier. In contrast with many traditional chemotherapy drugs, which require metabolic activation to exert their effects, temozolomide has the ability to convert spontaneously to a reactive agent that directly interferes with tumor growth. It does not interact with other drugs commonly taken by patients with brain tumors, such as antiseizure medications, corticosteroids, and antiemetics.

> **Drug Alert** - *Temozolomide (Temodar)*
> * *Causes myelosuppression. Prior to giving dose, recommended that absolute neutrophil count be ≥1500/µl and platelet count ≥100,000/µl.*
> * *To reduce nausea and vomiting, take on empty stomach.*

Many techniques to control and treat brain tumors are currently under investigation. These include local hyperthermia and biologic therapy. Although progress in treatment has increased length and quality of survival of patients with gliomas, outcomes still remain poor.[24]

NURSING MANAGEMENT
BRAIN TUMORS

■ Nursing Assessment

The initial assessment should be structured to provide baseline data of the neurologic status and the information needed to design a realistic, individualized care plan. Areas to be assessed include the LOC and content of consciousness, motor abilities, sensory perception, integrated function (including bowel and bladder function), balance and proprioception, and the coping abilities of the patient and family. Watching a patient perform activities of daily living and listening to the patient's conversation are convenient ways to perform part of the neurologic assessment. Having the patient or the family explain the problem can be helpful in determining the patient's limitations and can also provide the nurse with information about the patient's insight into the problems. All initial data should be accurately recorded to provide a baseline for comparison to determine whether the patient's condition is improving or deteriorating.

Interview data are as important as the actual physical assessment. Questions concerning medical history, intellectual abilities and educational level, and history of nervous system infections and trauma should be asked. Determination of the presence of seizures, syncope, nausea and vomiting, and headaches or other pain is important in planning care for the patient.

■ Nursing Diagnoses

Nursing diagnoses for the patient with a brain tumor may include, but are not limited to, the following:

* Impaired tissue perfusion (cerebral) *related to* cerebral edema
* Acute pain (headache) *related to* cerebral edema and increased ICP
* Self-care deficits *related to* altered neuromuscular function secondary to tumor growth and cerebral edema
* Anxiety *related to* diagnosis and treatment
* Potential complication: seizures *related to* abnormal electrical activity of the brain
* Potential complication: increased ICP *related to* presence of tumor and failure of normal compensatory mechanisms

■ Planning

The overall goals are that the patient with a brain tumor will (1) maintain normal ICP, (2) maximize neurologic functioning, (3) achieve control of pain and discomfort, and (4) be aware of the long-term implications with respect to prognosis and cognitive and physical functioning.

■ Nursing Implementation

A primary or metastatic tumor of the frontal lobe can cause behavioral and personality changes. Loss of emotional control, confusion, disorientation, memory loss, and depression may be signs of a frontal lobe lesion. These behavioral changes are often not perceived by the patient but can be disturbing and even frightening to the family. These changes can also cause a distancing to occur between the family and the patient. Assisting the family in understanding what is happening to the patient and supporting the family through this diagnostic phase are important roles for the nurse.

The confused patient with behavioral instability can be a challenge. Protecting the patient from self-harm is an important part of nursing care.[25] At times when the patient manifests rage and aggression, the nurse must also be concerned about self-protection. Close supervision of activity, use of side rails, judicious use of restraints, appropriate sedative medications, padding of the rails and the area around the bed, and a calm, reassuring approach to care are all essential techniques in the care of these patients.

Perceptual problems associated with frontal lobe and parietal lobe tumors contribute to a patient's disorientation and confusion. Minimization of environmental stimuli, creation of a routine, and use of reality orientation can be incorporated into the care plan for the confused patient.

Seizures often occur with brain tumors. These are managed with antiseizure drugs. Seizure precautions should be instituted for the protection of the patient. Some behavioral changes seen in the patient with a brain tumor are a result of seizure disorders and can improve with adequate seizure control (see Chapter 59).

Motor and sensory dysfunctions are problems that interfere with the activities of daily living.[25] Alterations in mobility must be managed, and the patient should be encouraged to provide as much self-care as physically possible. Self-image often depends on the patient's ability to participate in care within the limitations of the physical deficits.

Language deficits can also occur in patients with brain tumors. Motor (expressive) or sensory (receptive) dysphasia may occur. The disturbance in communication can be frustrating for the patient and may interfere with the nurse's ability to meet the patient's

TABLE 57-14	Indications for Cranial Surgery		
Indication	**Cause**	**Manifestations**	**Procedure**
Intracranial infection	Bacteria	*Early findings:* stiff neck, headache, fever, weakness, seizures *Later findings:* seizures, hemiplegia, speech disturbances, ocular disturbances, decreased LOC	Excision or drainage of abscess
Hydrocephalus	Overproduction of CSF, obstruction to flow, defective reabsorption	*Early findings:* mental changes, disturbances in gait *Later findings:* memory impairment, urinary incontinence, increased tendon reflexes	Placement of ventriculoatrial or ventriculoperitoneal shunt
Brain tumors	Benign or malignant cell growth	Change in LOC, pupillary changes, sensory or motor deficit, papilledema, seizures, personality changes	Excision or partial resection of tumor
Intracranial bleeding	Rupture of cerebral vessels because of trauma or stroke	*Epidural:* momentary unconsciousness; lucid period, then rapid deterioration *Subdural:* headache, seizures, pupillary changes	Surgical evacuation through burr holes or craniotomy
Skull fractures	Trauma to skull	Headache, CSF leakage, cranial nerve deficit	Debridement of fragments and necrotic tissue, elevation and realignment of bone fragments
Arteriovenous (AV) malformation	Congenital tangle of arteries and veins (frequently in middle cerebral artery)	Headache, intracranial hemorrhage, seizures, mental deterioration	Excision of malformation
Aneurysm repair	Dilation of weak area in arterial wall (usually near anterior portion of circle of Willis)	*Before rupture:* headache, lethargy, visual disturbance *After rupture:* violent headache, decreased LOC, visual disturbances, motor deficit	Dissection and clipping or coiling of aneurysm

CSF, Cerebrospinal fluid; *LOC,* level of consciousness.

needs. Attempts should be made to establish a communication system that can be used by both the patient and the staff.

Nutritional intake may be decreased because of the patient's inability to eat, loss of appetite, or loss of desire to eat. Assessing the nutritional status of the patient and ensuring adequate nutritional intake are important aspects of care.[25] The patient may need encouragement to eat, or in some cases, may have to be fed orally by gastrostomy or nasogastric tube or by parenteral nutrition. The patient with a brain tumor who undergoes cranial surgery requires complex nursing care. This is discussed in the next section.

■ Evaluation

The expected outcomes are that the patient with a brain tumor will

- achieve control of pain, vomiting, and other discomforts
- maintain ICP within normal limits
- demonstrate maximal neurologic function (cognitive, motor, sensory) with regard to the location and extent of the tumor
- maintain optimal nutritional status
- accept the long-term consequences of the tumor and its treatment

CRANIAL SURGERY

The cause or indication for cranial surgery may be related to a brain tumor, CNS infection (e.g., abscess), vascular abnormalities, craniocerebral trauma, seizure disorder, or intractable pain (Table 57-14).

Types

Various types of cranial surgical procedures are presented in Table 57-15.

Stereotactic Surgery. Stereotactic surgery uses precision apparatus (often computer guided) to assist the surgeon to precisely target an area of the brain (Fig. 57-19). Stereotactic biopsy

TABLE 57-15	Types of Cranial Surgery
Type	**Description**
Burr hole	Opening into the cranium with a drill; used to remove localized fluid and blood beneath the dura
Craniotomy	Opening into the cranium with removal of a bone flap and opening the dura to remove a lesion, repair a damaged area, drain blood, or relieve ↑ ICP
Craniectomy	Excision into the cranium to cut away a bone flap
Cranioplasty	Repair of a cranial defect resulting from trauma, malformation, or previous surgical procedure; artificial material used to replace damaged or lost bone
Stereotaxis	Precision localization of a specific area of the brain using a frame or a frameless system based on 3-dimensional coordinates; procedure is used for biopsy, radiosurgery, or dissection
Shunt procedures	Alternate pathway to redirect cerebrospinal fluid from one area to another using a tube or implanted device; examples include ventriculoperitoneal shunt and Ommaya reservoir

ICP, Intracranial pressure.

can be performed to obtain tissue samples for histologic examination. CT scanning and MRI are used to image the targeted tissue. With the patient under general or local anesthesia, the surgeon drills a burr hole or creates a bone flap for an entry site and then introduces a probe and biopsy needle. Stereotactic procedures are used for removal of small brain tumors and abscesses, drainage of hematomas, ablative procedures for extrapyramidal diseases (e.g., Parkinson's disease), and repair of arteriovenous malformations. A major advantage of the stereotactic approach is a reduction in damage to surrounding tissue.

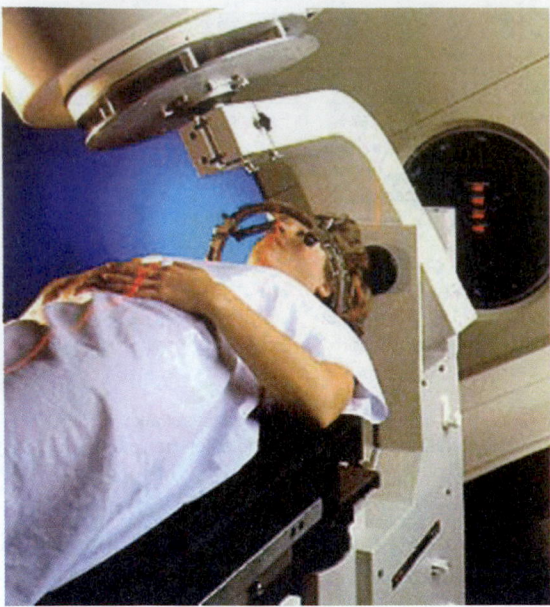

FIG. 57-19   Stereotactic frame.

Stereotactic radiosurgery is a procedure that involves closed-skull destruction of an intracranial target using ionizing radiation focused with the assistance of an intracranial guiding device. A sophisticated computer program is used while the patient's head is held still in a stereotactic frame. Radiosurgical techniques can use ionizing radiation generated by a linear accelerator or a gamma knife. In the gamma knife procedure, a high dose of cobalt radiation is delivered to precisely targeted tumor tissue. The dose of radiation can be delivered over a single 4- to 6-hour treatment time. In some situations, some tumors are treated over several weeks.

In combination with stereotactic procedures to identify and localize tumor sites, surgical lasers can be used to destroy tumors. Stereotactic procedures are used to identify the tumor site. Three surgical lasers currently used include the carbon dioxide, argon, and neodymium:yttrium-aluminum-garnet (Nd:YAG) lasers. All three work by creating thermal energy, which destroys the tissue on which it is focused. Laser therapy also provides the benefit of reducing damage to surrounding tissue.

Craniotomy. Depending on the location of the pathologic condition, a craniotomy may be frontal, parietal, occipital, temporal, or a combination of any of these. A set of burr holes is drilled, and a saw is used to connect the holes to remove the bone flap. Sometimes operating microscopes are used to magnify the site. After surgery the bone flap is wired or sutured. Sometimes drains are placed to remove fluid and blood. Patients are usually cared for in an ICU until stable.

NURSING MANAGEMENT
CRANIAL SURGERY

■ *Nursing Assessment*

The nursing assessment of the patient undergoing cranial surgery would be similar to that for the patient with increased ICP (see pp. 1476 to 1478).

ETHICAL DILEMMAS
Withholding Treatment

Situation
A 26-year-old patient in a permanent vegetative state is diagnosed with her fifteenth bladder infection. Her home care nurse must determine whether or not to seek antibiotics for this infection. The family members have expressed a concern that no heroic measures be used to extend the biologic life of their daughter and sister, but they have been unwilling to withdraw the existing treatment, which is enteral nutrition through a gastrostomy tube. Should antibiotics be withheld?

Important Points for Consideration
- Patients in a persistent vegetative state do not recover.
- Providing nutrition and hydration, even if by artificial means, can have significant cultural, religious, and psychologic meaning to patients and families.
- Clarification with the family about the goals of treatment and the patient's wishes, when she was competent and if they are known, is imperative. It is important to know whether treatment for an infection would be considered heroic based on the family's perspective of what the patient would want.
- The family's concerns about pain, suffering, and quality of life for the patient must be explored within the context of the overall plan of care.
- Withholding treatment is morally acceptable when a competent patient consents to it, if there is no medical benefit to the patient, if the treatment merely prolongs life, or if the burden of treatment outweighs the benefit to the patient.
- Surrogate decision making involving withholding or withdrawing treatment requires "clear and convincing evidence" of the patient's written or verbal wishes in most states.

Critical Thinking Questions
1. How would you approach the patient's family?
2. What are your feelings about providing nutrition, hydration, and treatments that will prolong life in a patient for whom there is no hope of recovery?

■ *Nursing Diagnoses*

Nursing diagnoses for the patient with cranial surgery are similar to those for the patient with increased ICP and may include, but are not limited to, those presented in NCP 57-1.

■ *Planning*

The overall goals are that the patient with cranial surgery will (1) return to normal consciousness, (2) achieve control of pain and discomfort, (3) maximize neuromuscular functioning, and (4) be rehabilitated to maximum ability.

■ *Nursing Implementation*

Acute Intervention. The general preoperative and postoperative nursing care for the patient undergoing cranial surgery is similar regardless of the cause. Nursing management is presented in NCP 57-1. The patient (if conscious and coherent) and the family will be gravely concerned about the potential physical and emotional problems that can result from surgery. The uncertainty regarding prognosis and outcome requires compassionate nursing care in the preoperative period.

Preoperative teaching is important in allaying the fears of the patient and the family and also in preparing them for the postoperative period. The patient and the family should be given general information concerning the type of operation that will be performed and what can be expected immediately after the operation. Explaining that some hair is shaved to allow for better exposure and prevention of contamination may prevent unnecessary concern over this task. The hair is usually removed in the operating room after induction of anesthesia. The family should also be informed that the patient will be taken to an ICU or to a special care unit after the operation.

The primary goal of care after cranial surgery is prevention of increased ICP. (Nursing management of the patient with increased ICP is presented on pp. 1478 to 1481.) Frequent assessment of the neurologic status of the patient is essential during the first 48 hours. In addition to the neurologic functions, fluid and electrolyte levels and serum osmolality are monitored closely to detect changes in sodium regulation, the onset of diabetes insipidus, or severe hypovolemia. The turning and positioning of the patient sometimes depend on the site of the operation. If the surgical approach is in the posterior fossa, the patient is generally kept flat or at a slight elevation (10 to 15 degrees). Lying on the back will be prevented as much as possible, and flexion of the neck will be avoided to protect the suture line. The maximum swelling in the operative area generally occurs within 24 to 48 hours after the surgery.

The surgical dressing is usually in place for 3 to 5 days. With an incision over the skull in the anterior or middle fossa, the patient will return from the operating room with the head elevated at an angle of 30 to 45 degrees. If a bone flap has been removed (craniectomy), care should be taken not to have the patient positioned on the operative side. The dressing should be observed for color, odor, and amount of drainage. The health care provider should be notified immediately of any excessive bleeding or clear drainage. Checking drains for placement and assessing the area around the dressing are also important. Scalp care should include meticulous care of the incision to prevent wound infection. The area should be cleansed and treated in accordance with hospital protocol or the health care provider's orders. Once the dressing is removed, use of an antiseptic soap for washing the scalp may also be beneficial. The psychologic impact of hair removal can be alleviated by the use of a wig, turban, scarves, or cap after the incision has completely healed. For the patient who is receiving radiation, use of a sunblock and head covering should be advocated if any exposure to the sun is anticipated.

Ambulatory and Home Care. The rehabilitative potential for a patient after cranial surgery depends on the reason for the surgery, the postoperative course, and the patient's general state of health. Nursing interventions must be based on a realistic appraisal of these factors. An overall goal for the nurse is to foster independence for as long as possible and to the highest degree possible.

Specific rehabilitation potential cannot be determined until cerebral edema and increased ICP subside postoperatively. Care must be taken to maintain as much function as possible through measures such as careful positioning, meticulous skin and mouth care, regular range-of-motion exercises, bowel and bladder care, and adequate nutrition.

Referrals may be made to other specialists on the health care team. For example, the speech therapist may be helpful to the patient who has a speech problem, or the physical therapist may provide an exercise plan to regain functional deficits. The needs and problems of each patient should be addressed individually because many variables affect the plan.

The mental and physical deterioration of the patient, including seizures, personality disorganization, apathy, and wasting, is difficult for both family and health professionals to endure. Cognitive and emotional residual deficits are often more difficult for the patient and the family to accept than are motor and sensory losses. Although progress is continually being made to help the patient with a brain tumor by means of chemotherapy, conventional and interstitial radiation, and biologic therapies, the prognosis remains grim for those with highly invasive tumors.[24] The nurse can provide much help and support during the adjustment phase and in long-range planning.

■ Evaluation

The expected outcomes are that the patient who has had cranial surgery will

- regain the maximal cognitive, motor, and sensory function possible
- be free of infection
- have pain and discomfort controlled
- be free of seizures
- have optimal nutritional intake

Inflammatory Conditions of the Brain

Meningitis, encephalitis, and brain abscesses are the most common inflammatory conditions of the brain and spinal cord. Inflammation can be caused by bacteria, viruses, fungi, and chemicals (e.g., contrast media used in diagnostic tests or blood in the subarachnoid space) (Table 57-16). CNS infections may occur via the bloodstream, by extension from a primary site, or along cranial and spinal nerves. The mortality rate is approximately 2% to 30% in the general population, with higher rates in elderly patients.[26,27] Up to 40% of those who recover can have long-term neurologic deficits, including hearing loss.[26]

BACTERIAL MENINGITIS

Etiology and Pathophysiology

Meningitis is an acute inflammation of the meningeal tissues surrounding the brain and the spinal cord. Meningitis specifically refers to infection of the arachnoid mater and the CSF. Bacterial meningitis is considered a medical emergency. Untreated bacterial meningitis has a mortality rate approaching 100%. The organisms usually gain entry to the CNS through the upper respiratory tract or the bloodstream, but they may enter by direct extension from penetrating wounds of the skull or through fractured sinuses in basal skull fractures.[27]

Meningitis usually occurs in the fall, winter, or early spring and is often secondary to viral respiratory disease. Older adults and persons who are debilitated are more often affected than is the general population. *Streptococcus pneumoniae* and *Neisseria meningitidis* are the leading causes of bacterial meningitis. *Haemophilus influenzae* was once the most common cause. However, the use of *H. influenzae* vaccine has resulted in a significant decrease in meningitis related to this organism.

Nervous System

TABLE 57-16	Comparison of Cerebral Inflammatory Conditions		
	Meningitis	**Encephalitis**	**Brain Abscess**
Causative Organisms	Bacteria (*Streptococcus pneumoniae, Neisseria meningitidis,* group B streptococcus, viruses, fungi)	Bacteria, fungi, parasites, herpes simplex virus (HSV), other viruses (e.g., West Nile virus)	Streptococci, staphylococci through bloodstream
CSF			
Pressure (normal, 60-150 mm H_2O)	↑	Normal to slight ↑	↑
WBC count (normal, 0-8/μl)	*Bacterial:* >1000/μl (mainly PMN) *Viral:* 25-500/μl (mainly lymphocytes)	500/μl, PMN (early), lymphocytes (later)	25-300/μl (PMN)
Protein (normal, 15-45 mg/dl [0.15-0.45 g/L])	*Bacterial:* >500 mg/dl *Viral:* 50-500 mg/dl	Slight ↑	Normal
Glucose (normal, 45-75 mg/dl [2.5-4.2 mmol/L])	*Bacterial:* ↓ *Viral:* normal or low	Normal	Low or absent
Appearance	*Bacterial:* turbid, cloudy *Viral:* clear or cloudy	Clear	Clear
Diagnostic Studies	CT scan, Gram stain, smear, culture, PCR*	CT scan, EEG, MRI, PET, PCR, IgM antibodies to virus in serum or CSF	CT scan
Treatment	Antibiotics, dexamethasone, supportive care, prevention of ↑ ICP	Supportive care, prevention of ↑ ICP, acyclovir (Zovirax) for HSV	Antibiotics, incision and drainage Supportive care

CSF, Cerebrospinal fluid; *CT,* computed tomography; *EEG,* electroencephalogram; *ICP,* intracranial pressure; *IgM,* immunoglobulin M; *MRI,* magnetic resonance imaging; *PCR,* polymerase chain reaction; *PET,* positron emission tomography; *PMN,* polymorphonuclear cells; *WBC,* white blood cell.
*PCR is used to detect viral RNA or DNA.

The inflammatory response to the infection tends to increase CSF production with a moderate increase in ICP. In bacterial meningitis the purulent secretions produced quickly spread to other areas of the brain through the CSF and cover the cranial nerves and other intracranial structures. If this process extends into the brain parenchyma or if concurrent encephalitis is present, cerebral edema and increased ICP become more of a problem. All patients with meningitis must be observed closely for manifestations of increased ICP, which is thought to be a result of swelling around the dura and increased CSF volume.

Clinical Manifestations

Fever, severe headache, nausea, vomiting, and **nuchal rigidity** (neck stiffness) are key signs of meningitis. A positive Kernig's sign (see Fig. 56-19), a positive Brudzinski's sign (see Fig. 56-18), photophobia, a decreased LOC, and signs of increased ICP may also be present. Coma is associated with a poor prognosis and occurs in 5% to 10% of patients with bacterial meningitis. Seizures occur in one third of all cases.[27] With meningitis the headache becomes progressively worse and may be accompanied by vomiting and irritability. If the infecting organism is a meningococcus, a skin rash is common and petechiae may be seen.

Complications

The most common acute complication of bacterial meningitis is increased ICP. Most patients will have increased ICP, and it is the major cause of an altered mental status. Another complication of bacterial meningitis is residual neurologic dysfunction. Cranial nerve dysfunction in bacterial meningitis often occurs with CN III, IV, VI, VII, or VIII. The dysfunction usually disappears within a few weeks. However, hearing loss may be permanent after bacterial meningitis.

Cranial nerve irritation can have serious sequelae. The optic nerve (CN II) is compressed by increased ICP. Papilledema is often present, and blindness may occur. When the oculomotor (CN III), trochlear (CN IV), and abducens (CN VI) nerves are irritated, ocular movements are affected. Ptosis, unequal pupils, and diplopia are common. Irritation of the trigeminal nerve (CN V) is evidenced by sensory losses and loss of the corneal reflex, and irritation of the facial nerve (CN VII) results in facial paresis. Irritation of the vestibulocochlear nerve (CN VIII) causes tinnitus, vertigo, and deafness.

Hemiparesis, dysphasia, and hemianopsia may also occur. These signs usually resolve over time. If resolution does not occur, a cerebral abscess, subdural empyema, subdural effusion, or persistent meningitis is suspected. Acute cerebral edema may occur with bacterial meningitis, causing seizures, CN III palsy, bradycardia, hypertensive coma, and death.

A noncommunicating hydrocephalus may occur if the exudate causes adhesions that prevent the normal flow of the CSF from the ventricles. CSF reabsorption by the arachnoid villi may also be obstructed by the exudate. In this situation surgical implantation of a shunt is the only treatment.

A complication of meningococcal meningitis is the *Waterhouse-Friderichsen syndrome.* The syndrome is manifested by petechiae, disseminated intravascular coagulation (DIC), adrenal hemorrhage, and circulatory collapse. DIC and shock are some of the most serious complications of meningitis and are associated with meningococcemia.[27] (DIC is discussed in Chapter 31.)

Diagnostic Studies

When a patient presents with manifestations suggestive of bacterial meningitis, a blood culture should be done. Diagnosis is usually verified by doing a lumbar puncture with analysis of the CSF.

TABLE 57-17	COLLABORATIVE CARE Bacterial Meningitis

Diagnostic
History and physical examination
Analysis of CSF for protein, glucose, WBC, Gram stain, and culture
CBC, coagulation profile, electrolyte levels, glucose, platelet count
Blood culture
CT scan, MRI, PET scan
Skull x-ray studies

Collaborative Therapy
Bed rest
IV fluids
Antibiotics IV
   ampicillin, penicillin
   cephalosporin (e.g., cefotaxime [Claforan], ceftriaxone [Rocephin])
codeine for headache
dexamethasone (Decadron)
acetaminophen or aspirin for temperature above 100.4° F (38° C)
Hypothermia
Clear liquids as desired or tolerated
phenytoin (Dilantin) IV
mannitol (Osmitrol) IV for diuresis

CBC, Complete blood count; *CSF*, cerebrospinal fluid; *CT*, computed tomography; *IV*, intravenous; *MRI*, magnetic resonance imaging; *PET*, positron emission tomography; *WBC*, white blood cells.

Variations in the CSF depend on the causative organism. Protein levels in the CSF are usually elevated and are higher in bacterial than in viral meningitis. CSF glucose concentration is commonly decreased in bacterial meningitis but may be normal in viral meningitis. The CSF is purulent and turbid in bacterial meningitis; it may be the same or clear in viral meningitis. The predominant white blood cell type in the CSF during bacterial meningitis is polymorphonuclear cells (see Table 57-16). Specimens of the CSF, sputum, and nasopharyngeal secretions are taken for culture before the start of antibiotic therapy to identify the causative organism. A Gram stain is done to detect bacteria.

X-rays of the skull may demonstrate infected sinuses. CT scans and MRI may be normal in uncomplicated meningitis. In other cases, CT scans may reveal evidence of increased ICP or hydrocephalus.

Collaborative Care

Bacterial meningitis is a medical emergency. Rapid diagnosis based on history and physical examination is crucial because the patient is usually in a critical state when health care is sought. When meningitis is suspected, antibiotic therapy is instituted after the collection of specimens for cultures, even before the diagnosis is confirmed (Table 57-17). The fundus of the eye should be examined via ophthalmoscope for papilledema before lumbar puncture for identification of possible increased ICP.

Ampicillin, penicillin, vancomycin, cefuroxime (Ceftin), cefotaxime (Claforan), ceftriaxone (Rocephin), ceftizoxime (Cefizox), and ceftazidime (Ceptaz) are commonly prescribed drugs of choice for treating bacterial meningitis. The corticosteroid dexamethasone may also be prescribed prior to or with the first dose of antibiotics. Although the data are limited, administration of dexamethasone appears to be associated with a lower mortality rate and a reduced incidence of hearing loss in patients with bacterial meningitis.[26]

NURSING MANAGEMENT
BACTERIAL MENINGITIS

■ *Nursing Assessment*

Initial assessment should include vital signs, neurologic evaluation, fluid intake and output, and evaluation of the lungs and skin (see Fig. 57-10).

■ *Nursing Diagnoses*

Nursing diagnoses for the patient with bacterial meningitis may include, but are not limited to, those presented in NCP 57-2.

■ *Planning*

The overall goals are that the patient with bacterial meningitis will have (1) return to maximal neurologic functioning, (2) resolution of infection, and (3) control of pain and discomfort.

■ *Nursing Implementation*

Health Promotion. Prevention of respiratory infections through vaccination programs for pneumococcal pneumonia and influenza should be supported by nurses.[27] A vaccine is available for protection against *Neisseria meningitides*. Routine vaccination is recommended for children ages 11 or 12, and catch-up vaccination for previously unvaccinated teens entering high school and for college freshmen.

Early and vigorous treatment of respiratory and ear infections is important. Persons who have close contact with anyone who has bacterial meningitis should be given prophylactic antibiotics.

Acute Intervention. The patient with bacterial meningitis is usually acutely ill. The fever is high, and head pain is severe. Irritation of the cerebral cortex may result in seizures. The changes in mental status and LOC depend on the degree of increased ICP. Assessment of vital signs, neurologic evaluation, fluid intake and output, and evaluation of lung fields and skin should be performed at regular intervals based on the patient's condition and recorded carefully.

Head pain and neck pain secondary to movement require attention. Codeine provides some pain relief without undue sedation for most patients. The patient should be assisted to a position of comfort, often curled up with the head slightly extended. The head of the bed should be slightly elevated, when permitted after lumbar puncture. A darkened room and a cool cloth over the eyes relieve the discomfort of photophobia.

For the delirious patient, additional low lighting may be necessary to decrease hallucinations. All patients suffer some degree of mental distortion and hypersensitivity and may be frightened and misinterpret the environment. Every attempt should be made to minimize environmental stimuli and prevent injury. Restraints should be avoided if possible. The presence of a familiar person at the bedside may have a calming effect. The nurse must be efficient with care but also should project an attitude of caring and of unhurried gentleness. The use of touch and a soothing voice to give simple explanations of activities is helpful. If seizures occur, appropriate observations should be made and protective measures should be taken. Antiseizure drugs such as phenytoin (Dilantin) are administered as ordered. Problems associated with increased ICP are also managed (see the section on Increased Intracranial Pressure earlier in this chapter).

Fever must be vigorously managed because it increases cerebral edema and the frequency of seizures. In addition, neurologic dam-

Nervous System

NURSING CARE PLAN 57-2

Patient with Bacterial Meningitis

NURSING DIAGNOSIS   Ineffective tissue perfusion (cerebral)*, Decreased intracranial adaptive capacity*

NURSING DIAGNOSIS   Disturbed sensory perception *related to* altered cognitive function *as evidenced by* inaccurate interpretation of environment, signs of fear or anxiety, disorientation, and restlessness

PATIENT GOALS   1. Demonstrates appropriate cognitive function
2. Is oriented to person, place, and time

OUTCOMES (NOC)	INTERVENTIONS (NIC) and *RATIONALES*
Cognition	**Delirium Management**
• Communicates clearly and appropriately for age and ability ____	• Monitor neurologic status on an ongoing basis *to determine extent of problem.*
• Comprehends the meaning of events and situations ____	• Administer PRN medications for anxiety or agitation *to reduce fear and anxiety.*
• Cognitive orientation ____	• Provide a low-stimulation environment for patient in whom disorientation is increased by overstimulation.
• Makes appropriate decisions ____	• Approach patient slowly and from the front *to avoid stimulating or frightening patient.*
Measurement Scale	• Provide appropriate level of supervision/surveillance to monitor patient and to allow for therapeutic actions.
1 = Severely compromised	• Reorient the patient to the health care provider with each contact *to assist with orientation and reduce anxiety.*
2 = Substantially compromised	
3 = Moderately compromised	
4 = Mildly compromised	
5 = Not compromised	

NURSING DIAGNOSIS   Acute pain *related to* headache and muscle aches *as evidenced by* general discomfort of head, joints, and muscles; apathy; grimacing on movements

PATIENT GOALS   1. Reports satisfaction with pain control
2. Demonstrates no effects of pain

OUTCOMES (NOC)	INTERVENTIONS (NIC) and *RATIONALES*
Pain Level	**Pain Management**
• Reported pain ____	• Provide patient optimal pain relief with prescribed analgesics *to relieve pain.*
• Facial expressions of pain ____	• Select and implement a variety of measures (e.g., pharmacologic, nonpharmacologic, interpersonal) to facilitate pain relief (e.g., massage, range of motion) *to promote comfort and show a caring attitude and to reduce joint stiffness and promote circulation.*
• Muscle tension ____	• Reduce or eliminate factors that precipitate or increase the pain experience (e.g., fear)
• Restlessness ____	• Control environmental factors that may influence the patient's response to discomfort (e.g., room temperature, lighting, noise) *as pain can be exhausting to the patient.*
Measurement Scale	
1 = Severe	
2 = Substantial	
3 = Moderate	
4 = Mild	
5 = None	

ICP, Intracranial pressure; *PRN,* as needed.

*Because cerebral edema and increased intracranial pressure may occur with bacterial meningitis, see the related nursing care plan, NCP 57-1, on page 1479 to 1480 for these nursing diagnoses.

age may result from an extremely high temperature over a prolonged time. Acetaminophen or aspirin may be used to reduce fever. However, if the fever is resistant to aspirin or acetaminophen, more vigorous means are necessary, such as an automatic cooling blanket. Care should be taken not to reduce the temperature too rapidly because shivering may result, causing a rebound effect and increasing the temperature. The extremities should be wrapped in soft towels, or a blanket covered with a sheet, to protect them from "frostbite." Care of the skin should be frequent to prevent breaks in the skin. If a cooling blanket is not available or desirable, tepid sponge baths with water may be effective in lowering the temperature. The skin must be protected from excessive drying and injury.

Because high fever greatly increases the metabolic rate and thus insensible fluid loss, the patient should be assessed for dehydration and adequacy of fluid intake. Diaphoresis further increases fluid losses, which should be taken into account on the output record. Replacement fluids should be calculated as 800 ml/day for respiratory losses and 100 ml for each degree of temperature above 100.4° F (38° C). Supplemental feeding to maintain adequate nutritional intake via tube or oral feedings may be necessary. The designated antibiotic schedule must be followed to maintain therapeutic blood levels. Observations should be made for side effects of the drugs used.

Meningitis generally requires respiratory isolation until the cultures are negative. Meningococcal meningitis is highly contagious, whereas other causes of meningitis may pose minimal to no infection risk with patient contact. However, standard precautions are essential to protect the patient and the nurse.

NURSING CARE PLAN 57-2

Patient with Bacterial Meningitis—cont'd

NURSING DIAGNOSIS **Hyperthermia** *related to* infection and abnormal temperature regulation by hypothalamus from increased ICP *as evidenced by* increased body temperature

PATIENT GOAL Experiences normal body temperature

OUTCOMES (NOC)

Thermoregulation
* Hyperthermia ____

Measurement Scale
1 = Severe
2 = Substantial
3 = Moderate
4 = Mild
5 = None

INTERVENTIONS (NIC) and *RATIONALES*

Fever Treatment
* Monitor temperature as frequently as appropriate.
* Monitor blood pressure, pulse, and respirations *to evaluate effects of hyperthermia.*
* Monitor intake and output *because increased body temperature increases the risk of fluid deficit.*
* Monitor for decreased levels of consciousness *because fever increases brain metabolism.*
* Encourage increased intake of oral fluids, as appropriate, *to replace fluids lost through increased metabolism and diaphoresis.*

COLLABORATIVE PROBLEM

NURSING GOALS

Potential Complication
* Monitor for seizure activity
* Carry out appropriate medical and nursing interventions
* Report and record any seizure activity

NURSING INTERVENTIONS and *RATIONALES*

Seizure activity *related to* cerebral irritation
* Monitor for seizure activity *so that interventions can be initiated immediately.*
* Keep side rails up and padded *to protect patient if a seizure occurs.*
* Administer sedative and antiseizure drugs as ordered *to control or prevent seizure activity.*
* Carry out interventions to treat underlying causes of inflammatory brain condition *to prevent seizure activity.*

Ambulatory and Home Care. After the acute period has passed, the patient requires several weeks of convalescence before normal activities can be resumed. In this period, adequate nutrition should be stressed, with an emphasis on a high-protein, high-calorie diet in small, frequent feedings.

Muscle rigidity may persist in the neck and the backs of the legs. Progressive range-of-motion exercises and warm baths are useful. Activity should be gradually increased as tolerated, but adequate rest and sleep should be encouraged.

Residual effects can result in sequelae such as dementia, seizures, deafness, hemiplegia, and hydrocephalus. Vision, hearing, cognitive skills, and motor and sensory abilities should be assessed after recovery, with appropriate referrals as indicated. Meningitis in infancy may have "silent" neurologic sequelae, which are manifested as learning and behavioral problems when the child reaches school age.

Throughout the acute and convalescent periods, the nurse should be aware of the anxiety and stress experienced by individuals close to the patient.

■ *Evaluation*

The expected outcomes for the patient with bacterial meningitis are addressed in NCP 57-2.

VIRAL MENINGITIS

The most common causes of viral meningitis are enteroviruses, arboviruses, human immunodeficiency virus, and herpes simplex virus (HSV). Enteroviruses are most often spread through direct contact with respiratory secretions. Viral meningitis usually presents as a headache, fever, photophobia, and stiff neck. The fever may be moderate or high. There are usually no symptoms of brain involvement.

The most important diagnostic test is examination of the CSF via lumbar puncture. The CSF can be clear or cloudy, and the typical finding is lymphocytosis (see Table 57-16). Organisms are not seen on Gram stain or acid-fast smears. Polymerase chain reaction (PCR) used to detect viral-specific DNA or RNA is a highly sensitive method for diagnosing CNS viral infections.[27]

Viral meningitis is managed symptomatically because the disease is self-limiting. Full recovery from viral meningitis is expected. Rare sequelae include persistent headaches, mild mental impairment, and incoordination.

ENCEPHALITIS

Encephalitis, an acute inflammation of the brain, is a serious, and sometimes fatal, disease. In the United States, encephalitis is responsible for about 20,000 cases and 1400 deaths annually.[28]

Etiology and Pathophysiology

Encephalitis is usually caused by a virus. Many different viruses have been implicated in encephalitis, some of them associated with certain seasons of the year and endemic to certain geographic areas. Ticks and mosquitoes transmit epidemic encephalitis. Examples include Eastern equine encephalitis, Japanese encephalitis (rarely seen in the United States at this time), La Crosse encephalitis, St. Louis encephalitis, West Nile encephalitis, and Western equine encephalitis. Nonepidemic encephalitis may occur as a complication of measles, chickenpox, or mumps. HSV encephalitis is the most common cause of acute nonepidemic viral encephalitis. Cytomegalovirus encephalitis is one of the common complications in patients with acquired immunodeficiency syndrome (AIDS).

The first outbreak of West Nile virus in North America occurred in New York City in the summer of 1999. Advanced age is the primary risk factor for encephalitis and mortality associated with this virus. The incubation period of West Nile virus is from 2 to 14 days. Most cases involve only mild flu-like symptoms. However, about 1 in 150 infections will result in severe neurologic disease, with encephalitis more commonly seen than meningitis.[29]

Clinical Manifestations and Diagnostic Studies

The onset of infection is typically nonspecific, with fever, headache, nausea, and vomiting. Encephalitis can be acute or subacute. Signs of encephalitis appear on day two or three and may vary from minimal alterations in mental status to coma. Virtually any CNS abnormality can occur, including hemiparesis, tremors, seizures, cranial nerve palsies, personality changes, memory impairment, amnesia, and dysphasia.

Early diagnosis and treatment of viral encephalitis are essential for favorable outcomes. Diagnostic findings related to viral encephalitis are shown in Table 57-16. Brain imaging techniques include CT, MRI, and PET. PCR tests allow for early detection of HSV and West Nile encephalitis. West Nile virus should be strongly considered in adults over 50 years old who develop encephalitis or meningitis in summer or early fall. The best diagnostic test for West Nile virus is a blood test that detects viral RNA. This test is also used in screening blood, organs, cells, and tissues that have been donated.[30]

NURSING *and* COLLABORATIVE MANAGEMENT
ENCEPHALITIS

To prevent encephalitis, mosquito control should be practiced, including cleaning rain gutters, removing old tires, draining bird baths, and removing water where mosquitoes can breed. In addition, insect repellant should be used during mosquito season.

Collaborative and nursing management of encephalitis, including West Nile virus infection, is symptomatic and supportive.[30] In the initial stages of encephalitis, many patients require intensive care.

Acyclovir (Zovirax) and vidarabine (Vira-A) are used to treat encephalitis caused by HSV infection. Acyclovir has fewer side effects than vidarabine and is often the preferred treatment. Use of these antiviral agents has been shown to reduce mortality rates, although neurologic complications may not be reduced. For maximal benefit, antiviral agents should be started before the onset of coma. Seizure disorders should be treated with antiseizure drugs. Prophylactic treatment with antiseizure drugs may be used in severe cases of encephalitis. Treatment of cytomegalovirus encephalitis in AIDS patients is discussed in Chapter 15.

RABIES

Rabies has been a threat to humans since ancient times. Between 30,000 and 70,000 people die each year from rabies worldwide, while only 1 to 3 people die annually in the United States.[31] Louis Pasteur developed the first rabies vaccine in 1885, which drastically reduced the risk of disease transmission from domestic animals to humans, particularly in developed countries where vaccine programs were effectively implemented. Despite the success of vaccines in domestic animals, rabies remains a serious public health concern due to the presence of the disease in wild animals.

Once a human contracts rabies and develops symptoms, the disease almost always ends in death.

Etiology and Pathophysiology

The etiology of rabies is an RNA virus that causes an acute, progressive viral encephalitis.[31,32] Although rabies is generally transmitted via saliva from the bite of an infected animal, it can also be spread by scratches, mucous membrane contact with infected secretions, and inhalation of aerosolized virus into the respiratory tract. Any warm-blooded mammal can carry rabies, including livestock. Throughout the world, rabid dogs are the most common disease vector. However, in developed countries, raccoons, skunks, bats, and foxes are the primary animal carriers. Even casual contact, such as being in proximity to an infected bat or petting the fur of an infected animal, is enough to potentially transmit rabies.

After introduction of the rabies virus into the human body, it spreads from the contact site through the central nervous system via peripheral nerve and possibly muscle fibers. The salivary glands and pharyngeal muscles are affected, leading to hypersalivation and pharyngeal spasm at the sight, taste, or sound of water.[31] This condition is termed *hydrophobia* and produces a characteristic frothing of the mouth. In its final stages, the nervous system fails and death ensues.

Clinical Manifestations

Two presentations of rabies include *encephalitic* rabies, which is the most common, and *paralytic* rabies, which only occurs in 15% to 20% of patients. The incubation period can last from 10 days to 1 year, with an average of 20 to 60 days.[31] The length of the incubation period is dependent upon the viral load transmitted and the location of the bite site. Bites that are closer to the brain progress more rapidly than distal extremity bites.[31]

After incubation, a prodromal period begins 2 to 10 days postexposure and lasts for up to 2 weeks. During this period, patients experience flu-like symptoms such as fever, headache, nausea, vomiting, and malaise. Typical findings include tingling, pain, paresthesias, or numbness at the bite site.[31] An acute neurologic syndrome then occurs 2 to 7 days later and is manifested by agitation, hypersalivation, hydrophobia, dysarthria, vertigo, diplopia, hallucinations, and other neurologic sequelae (e.g., hyperactive reflexes, nuchal rigidity, and a positive Babinski's sign). Coma develops within 7 to 10 days of the neurologic syndrome. Patients experience flaccid paralysis, apnea, hydrophobia, and seizures. Death ensues as a result of respiratory and cardiovascular collapse within a few days after the onset of coma.

Diagnostic Studies

The diagnosis of rabies is made based upon clinical examination as well as the presence of virus-specific fluorescent material in skin biopsies. In addition, the virus can be isolated in saliva. Antirabies antibodies also can be found in the blood and CSF. This is diagnostic if the patient has not been vaccinated against rabies in the past.

NURSING *and* COLLABORATIVE MANAGEMENT
RABIES

Because rabies is nearly always fatal, management efforts are directed at preventing the transmission and onset of the disease. Voluntary vaccination of domestic animals and strategies to avoid contact with wild animals, including bats, are the primary means of preventing rabies. Veterinary personnel, animal control officers, and laboratory staff who are at risk for contact with the rabies virus should be immunized with the rabies vaccine.[32] For all other individuals who have had contact with a potentially rabid animal but have not been vaccinated in advance against rabies, a specific postexposure prophylaxis regimen is indicated. Thorough wound cleansing with soap and water is the most important initial intervention to decrease the viral load and lower the risk of infection. The use of povidone iodine solutions or 70% isopropyl alcohol may serve to lower the risk of viral transmission.[32]

The next priority is to establish whether or not the animal is rabid. Domestic animals who are available after the contact may be observed for 10 days to determine whether or not signs of rabies develop. If the animal is healthy after 10 days, rabies treatment is not indicated. Rabies treatment is needed if clinical evidence of rabies occurs in the animal or if the domestic animal cannot be located after the bite. If possible, a wild animal that inflicts a bite should be humanely killed and transported to a lab that can analyze brain tissue for rabies infection. If the animal is not available for examination, then rabies postexposure prophylaxis should begin immediately. It is essential to begin the rabies postexposure prophylaxis regimen before clinical symptoms of rabies appear in the patient. At the point at which clinical manifestations develop, the rabies infection is ultimately fatal.

Rabies postexposure prophylaxis involves vaccines that confer passive immunity and active immunity to the disease in the patient. The first vaccine is rabies immune globulin (RIG), which confers passive immunity. RIG should be administered to the patient as soon as possible after contact with a rabid animal. Ideally the entire RIG dose is administered via infiltration in and around the bite wound. If the bite wound area is too small, such as a finger, or the contact with rabies occurred via mucous membrane or respiratory tract exposure, then the entire dose can be administered intramuscularly, generally in the posterior gluteal site.

Next, a vaccine series to induce active immunity is given. Antibodies take 7 to 10 days to develop. It is essential for the nurse to explain to the patient the need for strict compliance with the rabies vaccine regimen in order to prevent vaccine failure.

BRAIN ABSCESS

Brain abscess is an accumulation of pus within the brain tissue that can result from a local or a systemic infection. Direct extension from ear, tooth, mastoid, or sinus infection is the primary cause. Other causes for brain abscess formation include spread from a distant site (e.g., pulmonary infection, bacterial endocarditis), skull fracture, and prior brain trauma or surgery. Streptococci and *Staphylococcus aureus* are the primary infective organisms.

Manifestations are similar to those of meningitis and encephalitis and include headache, fever, and nausea and vomiting. Signs of increased ICP may include drowsiness, confusion, and seizures. Focal symptoms may be present and reflect the local area of the abscess. For example, visual field defects or psychomotor seizures are common with a temporal lobe abscess, whereas an occipital abscess may be accompanied by visual impairment and hallucinations. CT and MRI are used to diagnose a brain abscess.

Antimicrobial therapy is the primary treatment for brain abscess. Other manifestations are treated symptomatically. If drug therapy is not effective, the abscess may need to be drained, or removed if it is encapsulated. In untreated cases, the mortality rate approaches 100%. Nursing measures are similar to those for management of meningitis or increased ICP. If surgical drainage or removal is the treatment of choice, nursing care is similar to that described under cranial surgery.

Other infections of the brain include subdural empyema, osteomyelitis of the cranial bones, epidural abscess, and venous sinus thrombosis after periorbital cellulitis.

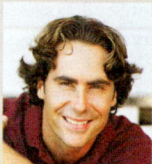

Head Injury

Patient Profile. T.J. is a 33-year-old white man who was the driver of a motorcycle that ran into an automobile broadside at a high rate of speed. He was sedated, paralyzed, and intubated by paramedics at the scene before transport by helicopter. He was brought to the emergency department (ED) with a prehospital report of multiple trauma and an open skull fracture. Paramedics also reported that he was not wearing a helmet.

Subjective Data
He was reportedly unresponsive at the scene, with a Glasgow Coma Scale score of 3, hypotension, tachycardia, and shallow irregular respirations.

Objective Data
At the Scene
- Unresponsive with obvious deformity to the left side of the skull and exposed brain matter
- Respirations were shallow and irregular
- O_2 saturations ranged from 88% to 90%
- Systolic BP ranged from 50 to 80 mm Hg
- Heart rate ranged from 100 to 130 beats/min

In the ED
- Right pupil, 5 mm nonreactive; left pupil, 3 mm nonreactive
- Glasgow Coma Scale score = 3
- Hypotension and tachycardia continued in spite of fluid resuscitation

Diagnostic Studies
- CT of the head was positive for an open left skull fracture, left subdural hematoma, bilateral intraventricular and subarachnoid hemorrhage, and cerebral edema
- CT of the abdomen/pelvis showed a lacerated liver, multiple infarcts to the right kidney, fluid around the duodenum and pancreas, and multiple left pelvic fractures.
- C-spine series was negative.
- Chest x-ray showed a right lung contusion and pneumomediastinum and subcutaneous emphysema.

Critical Thinking Questions

1. What could be the cause of T.J.'s hypoxia, hypotension, and tachycardia?
2. How could the injuries impact his neurologic condition?
3. What area of the brain do T.J.'s clinical manifestations suggest may be injured?
4. What nursing interventions should be implemented? What are the priorities?
5. Based on the assessment data presented, write one or more nursing diagnoses. Are there any collaborative problems?

NCLEX EXAMINATION REVIEW QUESTIONS

The number of the question corresponds to the same-numbered objective at the beginning of the chapter.

1. Vasogenic cerebral edema increases intracranial pressure by
   a. shifting fluid in the gray matter.
   b. altering the endothelial lining of cerebral capillaries.
   c. leaking molecules from the intracellular fluid to the capillaries.
   d. altering the osmotic gradient flow into the intravascular component.

2. A patient with intracranial pressure monitoring has pressure of 12 mm Hg. The nurse understands that this pressure reflects
   a. a severe decrease in cerebral perfusion pressure.
   b. an alteration in the production of cerebrospinal fluid.
   c. the loss of autoregulatory control of intracranial pressure.
   d. a normal balance between brain tissue, blood, and cerebrospinal fluid.

3. The nurse plans care for the patient with increased intracranial pressure with the knowledge that the best way to position the patient is to
   a. keep the head of the bed flat.
   b. elevate the head of the bed to 30 degrees.
   c. maintain patient on the left side with the head supported on a pillow.
   d. use a continuous-rotation bed to continuously change patient position.

4. The nurse is alerted to a possible acute subdural hematoma in the patient who
   a. has a linear skull fracture crossing a major artery.
   b. has focal symptoms of brain damage with no recollection of a head injury.
   c. develops decreased level of consciousness and a headache within 48 hours of a head injury.
   d. has an immediate loss of consciousness with a brief lucid interval followed by decreasing level of consciousness.

5. During admission of a patient with a severe head injury to the emergency department, the nurse places the highest priority on assessment for
   a. patency of airway.
   b. presence of a neck injury.
   c. neurologic status with the Glasgow Coma Scale.
   d. cerebrospinal fluid leakage from the ears or nose.

6. A patient is suspected of having a cranial tumor. The signs and symptoms include memory deficits, visual disturbances, weakness of right upper and lower extremities, and personality changes. The nurse recognizes that the tumor is most likely located in the
   a. frontal lobe.
   b. parietal lobe.
   c. occipital lobe.
   d. temporal lobe.

7. Nursing management of a patient with a brain tumor includes
   a. discussing with the patient methods to control inappropriate behavior.
   b. using diversion techniques to keep the patient stimulated and motivated.
   c. assisting and supporting the family in understanding any changes in behavior.
   d. limiting self-care activities until the patient has regained maximum physical functioning.

8. The primary goal of nursing care after a craniotomy is
   a. preventing infection.
   b. ensuring patient comfort.
   c. avoiding the need for secondary surgery.
   d. preventing increased intracranial pressure.

9. A nursing measure that is indicated to reduce the potential for seizures and increased intracranial pressure in the patient with bacterial meningitis is
   a. administering codeine for relief of head and neck pain.
   b. controlling fever with prescribed drugs and cooling techniques.
   c. keeping the room darkened and quiet to minimize environmental stimulation.
   d. maintaining the patient on strict bed rest with the head of the bed slightly elevated.

10. Which of the following best describes rabies?
    a. Bacterial infectious disease transmitted by mosquitoes
    b. Viral disease transmitted via saliva or bites from infected animal
    c. Bacterial disease transmitted via saliva or bites from infected animal
    d. Inflammatory reaction to previous viral infection of central nervous system

REFERENCES

1. Cushing H: *Studies in intracranial physiology and surgery,* London, 1925, Oxford University Press.
2. Cold GE: Measurement of cerebral blood flow and oxygen consumption, and the regulation of cerebral circulation, *Acta Neurochir Suppl* 49:1, 1990.
3. Arbour R: Intracranial hypertension: monitoring and nursing assessment, *Crit Care Nurs* 24(5):19, 2004.
4. Czosnyka M, Pickard JD: Monitoring and interpretation of intracranial pressure, *J Neurol Neurosurg Psychiatry* 75:813, 2004.
5. Bullock R, et al: The Brain Trauma Foundation. The American Association of Neurological Surgeons. The Joint Section on Neurotrauma and Critical Care. Recommendations for intracranial pressure monitoring technology, *J Neurotrauma* 17:497, 2000.
6. Stevens WJ: Multimodal monitoring: head injury management using SjvO$_2$ and LICOX, *J Neuroscience Nurs* 36:332, 2004.
7. Smith ER, Amin-Hanjani S: Evaluation and management of elevated intracranial pressure in adults—II. In Rose BD, editor: *Up to Date,* vol 13, p 1. Waltham, Mass., 2006. Available at *www.uptodate.com* (accessed August 28, 2006).
8. Robertson C: Every breath you take: hyperventilation and intracranial pressure, *Cleveland Clin J Med* 71(Suppl 1):S14, 2004.
9. Yanagawa T, Bunn F, Roberts I, et al: Nutritional support for head-injured patients, Cochrane Injuries Group, *Cochrane Database Syst Rev* 4:CD001530, 2005.
10. Jennett B, Teasdale G: Aspects of coma after severe head injury, *Lancet* 23:878, 1977.
11. Plum F, Posner J: *The diagnosis of stupor and coma,* ed 3, Philadelphia, 1980, FA Davis.
*12. Kerr ME, Rudy EB, Weber BB, et al: Effect of short-duration hyperventilation during endotracheal suctioning on intracranial pressure in severe head injured adults, *Nurs Res* 48:195, 1997.
13. The Brain Trauma Foundation: Update notice: guidelines for the management of severe traumatic brain injury: cerebral perfusion pressure, Approved by the American Association of Neurological Surgeons on March 14, 2003. Available at *www2.braintrauma.org* (accessed August 28, 2006).
*14. Fan JY: Effect of backrest position on intracranial pressure and cerebral perfusion pressure in individuals with brain injury: a systematic review, *J Neuroscience Nurs* 36:278, 2004.
15. Centers for Disease Control and Prevention: Traumatic brain injury in the United States: emergency department visits, hospitalizations and deaths. Available at *www.cdc.gov/ncipc/didop/tbi* (accessed August 28, 2006).
16. Centers for Disease Control and Prevention: Traumatic brain injury in the United States: a report to Congress. Available at *www.cdc.gov/doc.do/id/0900f3ec8001012b* (accessed August 28, 2006).
17. Marmarou A, et al: Impact of ICP instability and hypotension on outcome in patients with severe head trauma, *J Neurosurg* 75:S59, 1991.

*Nursing research–based reference.

18. Lavoie A, Ratte S, Clas D, et al: Preinjury warfarin use among elderly patients with closed head injuries in a trauma center, *J Trauma Injury Infect Crit Care* 56:802, 2004.

19. Wasserman JR: Diffuse axonal injury, *eMedicine Clinical Knowledge Base*, New York, 2006, eMedicine. Available at *www.emedicine.com* (accessed August 28, 2006).

*20. Bond AE, Draeger CRL, Mandleco B, et al: Needs of family members of patients with severe traumatic brain injury: implications for evidence-based practice, *Crit Care Nurs* 23(4):63, 2003.

21. Boyle GJ, Haines S: Severe traumatic brain injury: some effects on family caregivers, *Psychol Rep* 90:415, 2002.

22. Paterson B, Kieloch B, Gmiterek J: "They never told us anything": post-discharge instruction for families of persons with brain injuries, *Rehabil Nurs* 26:48, 2001.

23. Jemal A, et al: Cancer statistics, 2005, *CA Cancer J Clin* 55:10, 2005.

24. Remer S, Murphy ME: The challenges of long-term treatment outcomes in adults with malignant gliomas, *Clin J Oncol Nurs* 8:368, 2004.

25. Lovely MP: Symptom management of brain tumor patients, *Semin Oncol Nurs* 20:273, 2004.

26. van de Beek D, de Gans J, McIntyre P, et al: Corticosteroids in acute bacterial meningitis, *Cochrane Database Syst Rev* 1:CD004405, 2005.

27. Spiro CE, Spiro DM: Acute meningitis: focus on bacterial infection, *Clin Rev* 14(3):54, 2004.

28. Khetsuriani N, Holman RC, Anderson LJ: Burden of encephalitis-associated hospitalizations in the United States, 1988-1997, *Clin Infect Dis* 15:175, 2002.

29. Simmons C: West Nile virus versus meningitis: a challenging diagnosis, *Top Emerg Med* 26:237, 2004.

30. Watson JT, Pertel PE, Jones RC, et al: Clinical characteristics and functional outcomes of West Nile fever, *Ann Intern Med* 141:360, 2004.

31. Hankins DG, Rosenkrans JA: Overview, prevention, and treatment of rabies, *Mayo Clin Proc* 79:671, 2004.

32. Rupprecht CE, Gibbons RV: Prophylaxis against rabies, *N Engl J Med* 351:2626, 2004.

RESOURCES

American Association of Neuroscience Nurses
888-557-2266 or 847-375-4733
www.aann.org

American Brain Tumor Association
800-886-2282
www.abta.org

Brain Injury Association of America
800-444-6443 (family helpline) or 703-761-0750
www.biausa.org

Brain Trauma Foundation
212-772-0608
www2.braintrauma.org

Brain Tumor Center
617-724-8770
http://btc.mgh.harvard.edu

National Brain Tumor Foundation
800-934-CURE (2873) (Brian Tumor Information Line) or 415-834-9970
www.braintumor.org

For additional Internet resources, see the website for this book at *http://evolve.elsevier.com/Lewis/medsurg.*

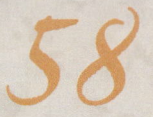

58

Nursing Management
Stroke

Julie T. Sanford

LEARNING OBJECTIVES

1. Describe the incidence of and risk factors for stroke.
2. Explain mechanisms that affect cerebral blood flow.
3. Compare and contrast the etiology and pathophysiology of ischemic and hemorrhagic strokes.
4. Correlate the clinical manifestations of stroke with the underlying pathophysiology.
5. Identify diagnostic studies performed for patients with strokes.
6. Describe the collaborative care, drug therapy, and nutritional therapy for a patient with a stroke.
7. Describe the acute nursing management of the patient with a stroke.
8. Describe the rehabilitative nursing management of the patient with a stroke.
9. Explain the psychosocial impact of a stroke on the patient and family.

KEY TERMS

aphasia, p. 1508
brain attack, p. 1502
embolic stroke, p. 1506
hemorrhagic strokes, p. 1506
intracerebral hemorrhage, p. 1506
ischemic stroke, p. 1505
stroke, p. 1502
subarachnoid hemorrhage, p. 1506
thrombotic stroke, p. 1505
transient ischemic attack, p. 1504

Electronic Resources

Supplemental content related to Chapter 58 can be found . . .

Companion CD
- Stress-Busting Kit for Nursing Students
- Interactive Case Study: Stroke
- NCLEX Examination Review Questions
- Comprehensive Glossary

Evolve Website *evolve*
http://evolve.elsevier.com/Lewis/medsurg
- Content Updates
- Key Points (Printable and CD/MP3 Download)
- Concept Map Creator
- Expanded Audio Glossary
- Key Term Flash Cards

- Customizable Nursing Care Plan: Stroke
- Patient and Family Instruction Guide in English and Spanish: Warning Signs of Stroke
- Electronic Calculators
- WebLinks

Stroke occurs when there is *ischemia* (inadequate blood flow) to a part of the brain or hemorrhage into the brain that results in death of brain cells. Functions such as movement, sensation, or emotions that were controlled by the affected area of the brain are lost or impaired. The severity of the loss of function varies according to the location and extent of the brain involved.

The term **brain attack** is increasingly being used to describe stroke. This term communicates the urgency of recognizing the clinical manifestations of a stroke and treating a medical emergency, similar to what would be done with a heart attack. Following the onset of a stroke, immediate medical attention is crucial to reduce disability and death.

Stroke is a major public health concern. An estimated 700,000 persons in the United States and 50,000 in Canada suffer a stroke annually.[1,2] Stroke is the third most common cause of death in the United States and Canada, behind cancer and heart disease.[1-3] Stroke is also a leading cause of serious, long-term disability. In the United States, there are an estimated 5.4 million individuals who have a history of stroke and up to 300,000 stroke survivors in Canada.[1,4] With an aging population, a further increase in stroke incidence can be expected.

In Canada about 16,000 die from stroke each year, while in the United States there are over 160,000 deaths from stroke.[4,5] After an initial stroke, 22% of men and 25% of women will die within

---

Reviewed by Mary Ciechanowski, RN, MSN, APRN-BC, CCRN, Trauma Advanced Practice Nurse, Christiana Care Health Systems, Newark, Del.

1 year.[1] The percentage is higher for people age 65 and older. Of those who survive, 50% to 70% will be functionally independent, and 15% to 30% will live with permanent disability. Twenty percent will require long-term care after 3 months.[1] Common long-term disabilities include hemiparesis, inability to walk, complete or partial dependence in activities of daily living (ADLs), aphasia, and depression.[1]

In addition to the physical, cognitive, and emotional impact of stroke on stroke survivors and their families, stroke also has an enormous financial impact. In 2005, the direct and indirect costs of strokes were estimated to be $56.8 billion per year in the United States and $2.7 billion per year in Canada.[1,4]

ETIOLOGY AND PATHOPHYSIOLOGY

Risk Factors for Stroke

The most effective way to decrease the burden of stroke is prevention. Awareness and control of modifiable risk factors can contribute to reducing the incidence and burden of stroke. Risk factors can be divided into nonmodifiable and modifiable. Stroke risk increases with multiple risk factors.

Nonmodifiable risk factors include age, gender, race, and family history/heredity. Stroke risk increases with age, doubling each decade after 55 years of age. Two thirds of all strokes occur in individuals over 65 years, but stroke can occur at any age. Strokes are more common in men, but more women die from stroke than men.[6,7] Because women tend to live longer than men, they have more opportunity to suffer a stroke. African Americans have a higher incidence of stroke as well as a higher death rate from stroke than whites.[1] This may be related in part to a higher incidence of hypertension, obesity, and diabetes mellitus in African Americans. African American men who are from the South are almost 4 times more likely to die from a stroke than Southern white men.[8] Hispanics, Native Americans/Alaska Natives, and Asian Americans also have higher death rates from intracerebral hemorrhage than whites. A family history of stroke, a prior transient ischemic attack, or a prior stroke also increases the risk of stroke.[1]

Modifiable risk factors are those that can potentially be altered through lifestyle changes and medical treatment, thus reducing the risk of stroke. Modifiable risk factors include hypertension, heart disease, smoking, excessive alcohol consumption, obesity, sleep apnea, metabolic syndrome, lack of physical exercise, poor diet, and drug abuse.

Hypertension is the single most important modifiable risk factor, but it is still often undetected and inadequately treated.[4] Increases in systolic and diastolic blood pressure (BP) independently increase the risk of stroke. Stroke risk can be reduced by up to 42% with appropriate treatment of hypertension.[1,7]

Heart disease, including atrial fibrillation, myocardial infarction, cardiomyopathy, cardiac valve abnormalities, and cardiac congenital defects, is also a risk factor for stroke. Of these, atrial fibrillation is the most important treatable cardiac-related risk factor.[1] The incidence of atrial fibrillation increases with age. Atrial fibrillation is responsible for about 15% to 20% of all strokes. Diabetes mellitus is a significant risk for stroke. The risk for stroke in people with diabetes mellitus is 4 to 5 times higher than in the general population.[1]

Increased serum cholesterol and smoking are risk factors for stroke.[1] In Canada, the use of tobacco is the major cause of preventable death.[7] Smoking nearly doubles the risk of stroke.[1] In the 2004 Health Consequences of Smoking report, the Surgeon General stated

that the risk associated with smoking decreases substantially over time after the smoker quits. After 5 to 10 years of no tobacco use, former smokers have the same chance of stroke as nonsmokers.[9]

The effect of alcohol on stroke risk appears to depend on the amount consumed. Women who drink more than one alcoholic drink per day and men who drink more than two alcoholic drinks per day are at higher risk for hypertension, which increases their chance of stroke.[10] Since 1991, the prevalence of obesity has increased 75%.

Abdominal obesity increases ischemic stroke risk in all ethnic groups. Individuals who are overweight or obese experience large decreases in life expectancy.[1] In addition, obesity is also associated with hypertension, high blood glucose, and elevated blood lipid levels, all of which increase the risk of stroke.

An association of physical inactivity and increased stroke risk is present in both men and women, regardless of ethnicity. Benefits of physical activity can occur with even light to moderate regular activity and may be in part related to the beneficial effect of exercise on other risk factors.[11] The effect of diet on stroke risk is not clear, although a diet high in saturated fat and low in fruits and vegetables may increase stroke risk. Illicit drug use, especially cocaine use, has been associated with stroke risk.[1]

The early forms of birth control pills that contained high levels of progestin and estrogen increased a woman's chance of experiencing a stroke, especially if they also smoked heavily. Newer, low-dose oral contraceptives have lower risks for stroke except in those individuals who are hypertensive and smoke.[12] Other conditions that may increase stroke risk include migraine headaches, inflammatory conditions, and hyperhomocystinemia. Sickle cell disease is another known risk factor for stroke.[1]

Pathophysiology

Anatomy of Cerebral Circulation. Blood is supplied to the brain by two major pairs of arteries: the internal carotid arteries (anterior circulation) and the vertebral arteries (posterior circulation). The carotid arteries branch to supply most of the frontal, parietal, and temporal lobes; the basal ganglia; and part of the diencephalon (thalamus and hypothalamus). The major branches of the carotid arteries are the middle cerebral and the anterior cerebral arteries. The vertebral arteries join to form the basilar artery, which branches to supply the middle and lower part of the temporal lobes, occipital lobes, cerebellum, brainstem, and part of the diencephalon. The main branch of the basilar artery is the posterior cerebral artery. The anterior and posterior cerebral circulation is connected at the circle of Willis by the anterior and posterior communicating arteries (Fig. 58-1). Anomalies in this area are common, and all connecting vessels may not be present.

Regulation of Cerebral Blood Flow. The brain requires a continuous supply of blood to provide the oxygen and glucose that neurons need to function. Blood flow must be maintained at 750 to 1000 ml/min (55 ml/100 g of brain tissue), or 20% of the cardiac output, for optimal brain functioning. If blood flow to the brain is totally interrupted (e.g., cardiac arrest), neurologic metabolism is altered in 30 seconds, metabolism stops in 2 minutes, and cellular death occurs in 5 minutes.

The brain is normally well protected from changes in mean systemic arterial BP over a range from 50 to 150 mm Hg by a mechanism known as *cerebral autoregulation.* This involves changes in the diameter of cerebral blood vessels in response to changes in pressure so that the blood flow to the brain stays constant. Cerebral autoregulation may be impaired following cerebral ischemia, and cerebral blood flow then changes directly in response to changes in BP. CO_2 is a potent cerebral vasodilator, and changes in arterial CO_2 levels have a dramatic effect on cerebral blood flow (increased CO_2 levels increase cerebral blood flow and vice versa). Very low arterial O_2 levels (partial pressure of arterial O_2 <50 mm Hg) or an increase in hydrogen ion concentration also increase cerebral blood flow.

Factors that affect blood flow to the brain include systemic BP, cardiac output, and blood viscosity. During normal activity, oxygen requirements vary considerably, but changes in cardiac output, vasomotor tone, and distribution of blood flow normally maintain adequate blood flow to the head. Cardiac output has to be reduced by one third before cerebral blood flow is reduced. Changes in blood viscosity affect cerebral blood flow, with decreased viscosity increasing flow.

Collateral circulation may develop to compensate for a decrease in cerebral blood flow. Because of the connections between arteries at the circle of Willis, an area of the brain can potentially receive blood supply from another blood vessel if its original blood supply is cut off (e.g., because of thrombosis). Individual differences in collateral circulation partly determine the degree of brain damage and functional loss when a stroke occurs.

Intracranial pressure (ICP) also influences cerebral blood flow (see Chapter 57). Increased ICP causes brain compression and reduced cerebral blood flow.

Atherosclerosis. *Atherosclerosis* (hardening and thickening of arteries) is a major cause of stroke. It can lead to thrombus formation and contribute to emboli. (The role of atherosclerosis in thrombosis and emboli development is discussed in Chapter 34 and shown in Fig. 34-2.) Initially there is abnormal infiltration of lipids in the intimal layer of the artery. This fatty streak further develops into a plaque. Plaques often develop in areas of increased turbulence of the blood, such as at the bifurcation of an artery or a tortuous area (Fig. 58-2). Calcified, brittle plaques may rupture or fissure, which leads to an inflammatory response. Platelets and fibrin are released and stick to the roughened plaque surface. Plaques lead to narrowing or occlusion of the artery. Also, parts of the plaque or thrombus can break off and travel to a narrower distal artery. Cerebral infarction occurs when a cerebral artery becomes blocked and blood supply to the brain beyond the blockage is cut off.

In response to ischemia, a series of metabolic events, termed the *ischemic cascade,* occur, including inadequate adenosine triphosphate (ATP) production, loss of ion homeostasis, release of excitatory amino acids (e.g., glutamate), free radical formation, and cell death. Around the core area of ischemia is a border zone of reduced blood flow called the *penumbra,* where ischemia is potentially reversible. If adequate blood flow can be restored early (e.g., within 3 hours) and the ischemic cascade can be interrupted, there may be less brain damage and less neurologic function lost. Research is ongoing to identify thrombolytic and neuroprotective therapies to reestablish blood flow and protect neurons from further ischemic damage.

Transient Ischemic Attack

A **transient ischemic attack** (TIA) is a temporary focal loss of neurologic function caused by ischemia of one of the vascular territories of the brain, lasting <24 hours and often lasting

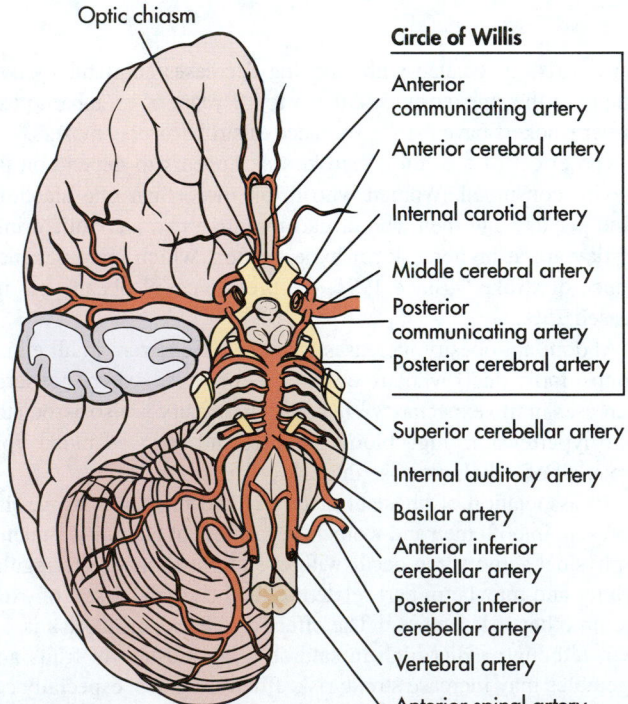

Optic chiasm

Circle of Willis

Anterior communicating artery

Anterior cerebral artery

Internal carotid artery

Middle cerebral artery

Posterior communicating artery

Posterior cerebral artery

Superior cerebellar artery

Internal auditory artery

Basilar artery

Anterior inferior cerebellar artery

Posterior inferior cerebellar artery

Vertebral artery

Anterior spinal artery

FIG. 58-1   Cerebral arteries and the circle of Willis. The tip of the temporal lobe has been removed to show the course of the middle cerebral artery.

<15 minutes. Most TIAs resolve within 3 hours. TIAs may be due to microemboli that temporarily block the blood flow. TIAs are a warning sign of progressive cerebrovascular disease. The signs and symptoms of a TIA depend on the blood vessel that is involved and the area of the brain that is ischemic. If the carotid system is involved, patients may have a temporary loss of vision in one eye *(amaurosis fugax)*, a transient hemiparesis, numbness or loss of sensation, or a sudden inability to speak. Signs of a TIA involving the vertebrobasilar system may include tinnitus, vertigo, darkened or blurred vision, diplopia, ptosis, dysarthria, dysphagia, ataxia, and unilateral or bilateral numbness or weakness.[13]

Evaluation must be done to confirm that the signs and symptoms of a TIA are not related to other brain lesions, such as a developing subdural hematoma or an increasing tumor mass. Computed tomography (CT) of the brain without contrast media is the most important initial diagnostic study. Cardiac monitoring and tests may reveal an underlying cardiac condition that is responsible for clot formation. Drugs that prevent platelet aggregation, such as aspirin, ticlopidine (Ticlid), clopidogrel (Plavix), dipyridamole (Persantine), combined dipyridamole and aspirin (Aggrenox), and anticoagulant drugs (e.g., oral warfarin [Coumadin]), may be prescribed for long-term therapy after a TIA.

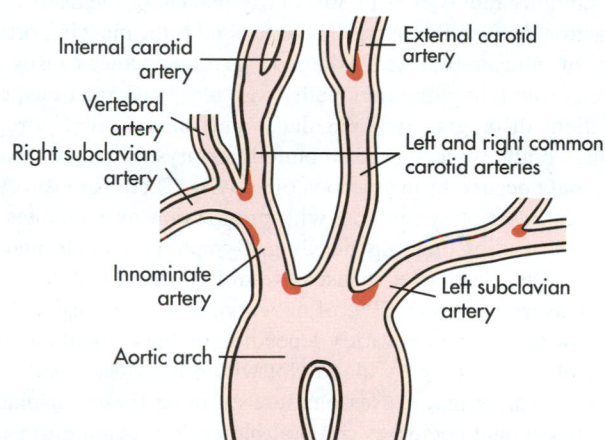

FIG. 58-2 Common sites for the development of atherosclerosis in extracranial and intracranial arteries. The main locations are just above the common carotid bifurcation (most common site) and the start of the branches from the aorta, innominate, and subclavian arteries.

Internal carotid artery
External carotid artery
Vertebral artery
Left and right common carotid arteries
Right subclavian artery
Innominate artery
Left subclavian artery
Aortic arch

 Drug Alert - *Ticlid (Ticlopidine) and Clopidogrel (Plavix)*
- *All health care providers and dentists must be informed that drug is being taken, especially before scheduling surgery or major dental procedures.*
- *Drug may need to be discontinued 10 to 14 days prior to surgery if antiplatelet effect is not desired.*

TYPES OF STROKE

Strokes are classified as ischemic or hemorrhagic based on the underlying pathophysiologic findings (Fig. 58-3 and Table 58-1).

Ischemic Stroke

An **ischemic stroke** results from inadequate blood flow to the brain from partial or complete occlusion of an artery; these account for approximately 80% of all strokes.[14] Ischemic strokes are further divided into thrombotic and embolic.

Thrombotic Stroke. A **thrombotic stroke** occurs from injury to a blood vessel wall and formation of a blood clot (Fig. 58-3, *A*). The lumen of the blood vessel becomes narrowed and, if it becomes occluded, infarction occurs. Thrombosis develops readily where atherosclerotic plaques have already narrowed blood vessels. Thrombotic stroke, which is the result of thrombosis or narrowing of the blood vessel, is the most common cause of stroke, accounting for about 60% of strokes.[15] Two thirds of thrombotic strokes are associated with hypertension or diabetes mellitus, both of which accelerate atherosclerosis. In 30% to 50% of individuals, thrombotic strokes have been preceded by a TIA.

The extent of the stroke depends on rapidity of onset, the size of the lesion, and the presence of collateral circulation. Most patients with ischemic stroke do not have a decreased level of consciousness in the first 24 hours, unless it is due to a brainstem stroke or other conditions such as seizures, increased ICP, or hemorrhage. Ischemic stroke symptoms may progress in the first 72 hours as infarction and cerebral edema increase.

A **lacunar stroke** refers to a stroke from occlusion of a small penetrating artery with development of a cavity in the place of the infarcted brain tissue. This most commonly occurs in the basal ganglia, thalamus, internal capsule, or pons. Although a large percentage of lacunar strokes are asymptomatic, when present, symptoms can cause considerable deficits. These include pure motor hemiplegia, pure sensory stroke (contralateral loss of all sensory modalities), contralateral leg and face weakness with arm and leg ataxia, and isolated motor or sensory stroke. Multiple small vessel

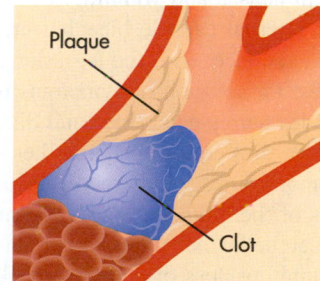

Thrombotic stroke. Cerebral thrombosis is a narrowing of the artery by fatty deposits called *plaque*. Plaque can cause a clot to form, which blocks the passage of blood through the artery.

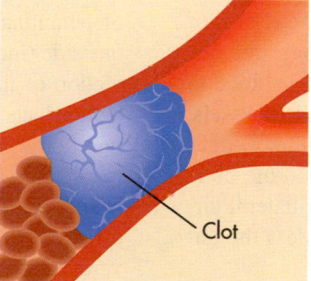

Embolic stroke. An embolus is a blood clot or other debris circulating in the blood. When it reaches an artery in the brain that is too narrow to pass through, it lodges there and blocks the flow of blood.

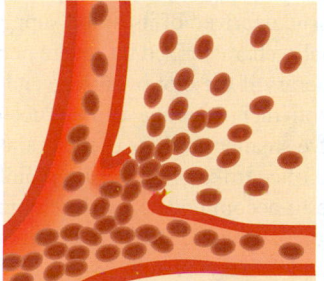

Hemorrhagic stroke. A burst blood vessel may allow blood to seep into and damage brain tissues until clotting shuts off the leak.

FIG. 58-3 Major types of stroke.

TABLE 58-1	Types of Stroke			
Type	**Gender/Age**	**Warning**	**Time of Onset**	**Course/Prognosis**
Ischemic				
Thrombotic	Men more than women, oldest median age	TIA (30%-50% of cases)	During or after sleep	Stepwise progression, signs and symptoms develop slowly, usually some improvement, recurrence in 20%-25% of survivors
Embolic	Men more than women	TIA (uncommon)	Lack of relationship to activity, sudden onset	Single event, signs and symptoms develop quickly, usually some improvement, recurrence common without aggressive treatment of underlying disease
Hemorrhagic				
Intracerebral	Slightly higher in women	Headache (25% of cases)	Activity (often)	Progression over 24 hr; poor prognosis, fatality more likely with presence of coma
Subarachnoid	Slightly higher in women, youngest median age	Headache (common)	Activity (often), sudden onset, most commonly related to head trauma	Usually single sudden event, fatality more likely with presence of coma

TIA, Transient ischemic attack.

infarcts may also result in a decrease in cognitive function (i.e., multiinfarct dementia)[16] (see Chapter 60).

Embolic Stroke. **Embolic stroke** occurs when an embolus lodges in and occludes a cerebral artery, resulting in infarction and edema of the area supplied by the involved vessel (Fig. 58-3, *B*). Embolism is the second most common cause of stroke, accounting for about 24% of strokes.[15] The majority of emboli originate in the endocardial (inside) layer of the heart, with plaque breaking off from the endocardium and entering the circulation. The embolus travels upward to the cerebral circulation and lodges where a vessel narrows or bifurcates. Heart conditions associated with emboli include atrial fibrillation, myocardial infarction, infective endocarditis, rheumatic heart disease, valvular prostheses, and atrial septal defects. Less common causes of emboli include air and fat from long bone (femur) fractures.

The patient with an embolic stroke commonly has a rapid occurrence of severe clinical symptoms. Embolic strokes can affect any age-group. Rheumatic heart disease is one cause of embolic stroke in young to middle-aged adults. An embolus arising from an atherosclerotic plaque is more common in older adults. Warning signs are less common with embolic than with thrombotic stroke. The onset of an embolic stroke is usually sudden and may or may not be related to activity. The patient usually remains conscious, although he or she may have a headache. Prognosis is related to the amount of brain tissue deprived of its blood supply. The effects of the emboli are initially characterized by severe neurologic deficits, which can be temporary if the clot breaks up and allows blood to flow. Smaller emboli then continue to obstruct smaller vessels, which in turn involve smaller portions of the brain with fewer deficits noted. The embolic stroke often occurs rapidly, and the body does not have time to accommodate by developing collateral circulation. Recurrence of embolic stroke is common unless the underlying cause is aggressively treated.

Hemorrhagic Stroke

Hemorrhagic strokes account for approximately 15% of all strokes and result from bleeding into the brain tissue itself (intracerebral or intraparenchymal hemorrhage) or into the subarachnoid space or ventricles (subarachnoid hemorrhage or intraventricular hemorrhage).[15]

Intracerebral Hemorrhage. **Intracerebral hemorrhage** is bleeding within the brain caused by a rupture of a vessel and accounts for about 10% of all strokes[17] (Fig. 58-3, *C*). The prognosis of patients with intracerebral hemorrhage is poor; the 30-day mortality rate is 40% to 80%. Fifty percent of the deaths occur within the first 48 hours.[18] Hypertension is the most important cause of intracerebral hemorrhage (Fig. 58-4). Other causes include cerebral amyloid angiopathy, vascular malformations, coagulation disorders, anticoagulant and thrombolytic drugs, trauma, brain tumors, and ruptured aneurysms. Hemorrhage commonly occurs during periods of activity. There is most often a sudden onset of symptoms, with progression over minutes to hours because of ongoing bleeding. Symptoms include neurologic deficits, headache, nausea, vomiting, decreased level of consciousness (in about 50% of patients), and hypertension. The extent of the symptoms varies depending on the amount and duration of the bleeding. A blood clot within the closed skull can result in a mass that causes pressure on brain tissue, displaces brain tissue, and decreases cerebral blood flow, leading to ischemia and infarction.[18]

Approximately half of intracerebral hemorrhages occur in the putamen and internal capsule, central white matter, thalamus, cerebellar hemispheres, and pons. Initially, patients experience a severe headache with nausea and vomiting. Clinical manifestations of putaminal and internal capsule bleeding include weakness of one side (including the face, arm, and leg), slurred speech, and deviation of the eyes. Progression of symptoms related to a severe hemorrhage includes hemiplegia, fixed and dilated pupils, abnormal body posturing, and coma. Thalamic hemorrhage results in hemiplegia with more sensory than motor loss. Bleeding into the subthalamic areas of the brain leads to problems with vision and eye movement. Cerebellar hemorrhages are characterized by severe headache, vomiting, loss of ability to walk, dysphagia, dysarthria, and eye movement disturbances. Hemorrhage in the pons is the most serious because basic life functions (e.g., respiration) are rapidly affected. Hemorrhage in the pons can be characterized by hemiplegia leading to complete paralysis, coma, abnormal body posturing, fixed pupils, hyperthermia, and death.[18]

Subarachnoid Hemorrhage. **Subarachnoid hemorrhage** occurs when there is intracranial bleeding into the cere-

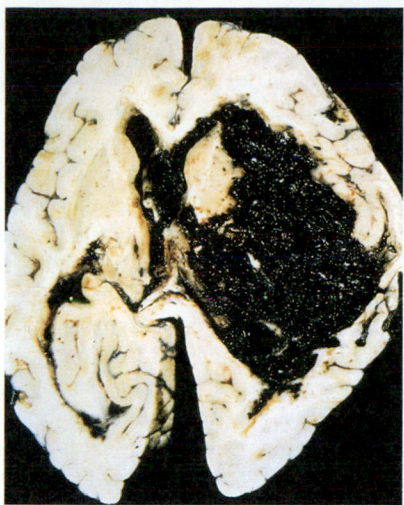

FIG. 58-4 Massive hypertensive hemorrhage rupturing into a lateral ventricle of the brain.

brospinal fluid–filled space between the arachnoid and pia mater membranes on the surface of the brain. Subarachnoid hemorrhage is commonly caused by rupture of a cerebral **aneurysm** (congenital or acquired weakness and ballooning of vessels). Aneurysms may be saccular or berry aneurysms, ranging from a few millimeters to 20 to 30 mm in size, or fusiform atherosclerotic aneurysms. The majority of aneurysms are in the circle of Willis. Other causes of subarachnoid hemorrhage include *arteriovenous malformations* (AVMs), trauma, and illicit drug (cocaine) abuse. About 35% of people who have a hemorrhagic stroke due to a ruptured aneurysm die during the first episode. Fifteen percent die from subsequent bleeding.[17] The annual incidence of subarachnoid hemorrhage caused by ruptured aneurysm is 6 to 25 per 100,000.[19] The incidence increases with age and is higher in women than men.

The patient may have warning symptoms if the ballooning artery applies pressure to brain tissue, or minor warning symptoms may result from leaking of an aneurysm before major rupture. The characteristic presentation of a ruptured aneurysm is the sudden onset of a severe headache that is different from a previous headache and typically the "worst headache of one's life." Loss of consciousness may or may not occur. The patient's level of consciousness may range from alert to comatose, depending on the severity of the bleed. Other symptoms include focal neurologic deficits (including cranial nerve deficits), nausea, vomiting, seizures, and stiff neck. Despite improvements in surgical techniques and management, many patients with subarachnoid hemorrhage die. Many are left with significant morbidity, including cognitive difficulties.[19]

Complications of aneurysmal subarachnoid hemorrhage include rebleeding before surgery or other therapy is initiated and cerebral vasospasm (narrowing of the large blood vessels at the base of the brain), which can result in cerebral infarction. Cerebral vasospasm is most likely due to an interaction between the metabolites of blood and the vascular smooth muscle. During the lysis of subarachnoid blood clots, metabolites are released. These metabolites can cause endothelial damage and vasoconstriction. In addition, release of endothelin (a potent vasoconstrictor) may play a major role in the induction of cerebral vasospasm after subarachnoid hemorrhage.

TABLE 58-2	Clinical Manifestations: Specific Cerebral Artery Involvement

Middle Cerebral Artery Involvement
Contralateral weakness (hemiparesis) or paralysis (hemiplegia)
Contralateral hemianesthesia; loss of proprioception, fine touch, localization
Dominant hemisphere: aphasia
Nondominant hemisphere: neglect of opposite side, anosognosia
Homonymous hemianopsia

Anterior Cerebral Artery Involvement
Occlusion of stem*
Occlusion distal to anterior communicating artery
• Contralateral sensory and motor deficits of foot and leg, greatest distally
• Contralateral weakness of proximal upper extremity
• Urinary incontinence (possibly unrecognized by patient)
• Sensory loss (discrimination, proprioception)
• Contralateral grasp and sucking reflexes may be present
• Apraxia
• Personality change: flat affect, loss of spontaneity, loss of interest in surroundings, distractibility, slowness in responding
• Possible cognitive impairment

Posterior Cerebral Artery and Vertebrobasilar Involvement†
Alert to comatose
Unilateral or bilateral sensory loss
Contralateral or bilateral weakness
Dysarthria
Dysphagia
Hoarseness
Ataxia
Horner's syndrome: miosis, ptosis, decreased sweating
Vertigo
Unilateral hearing loss
Nausea, vomiting
Visual disturbances (blindness, homonymous hemianopsia, nystagmus, diplopia)

*There is usually no problem if the stem is occluded near the anterior communicating artery because perfusion from the opposite side is maintained.
†The site of occlusion, the origin of the basilar arteries, and the arrangement of the circle of Willis are involved in the type of deficit seen. This can occur from a thrombus or embolus.

Clinical Manifestations

A stroke can have an effect on many body functions, including motor activity, bladder and bowel elimination, intellectual function, spatial-perceptual alterations, personality, affect, sensation, swallowing, and communication. The functions affected are directly related to the artery involved and area of the brain it supplies (Table 58-2). Manifestations related to right- and left-brain damage differ somewhat and are shown in Fig. 58-5.

Motor Function. Motor deficits are the most obvious effect of stroke. Motor deficits include impairment of (1) mobility, (2) respiratory function, (3) swallowing and speech, (4) gag reflex, and (5) self-care abilities. Symptoms are caused by the destruction of motor neurons in the pyramidal pathway (nerve fibers from the brain that pass through the spinal cord to the motor cells). The characteristic motor deficits include loss of skilled voluntary movement *(akinesia)*, impairment of integration of movements, alterations in muscle tone, and alterations in reflexes. The initial hyporeflexia (depressed reflexes) progresses to hyperreflexia (hyperactive reflexes) for most patients.

Motor deficits after a stroke follow certain specific patterns. Because the pyramidal pathway crosses at the level of the medulla,

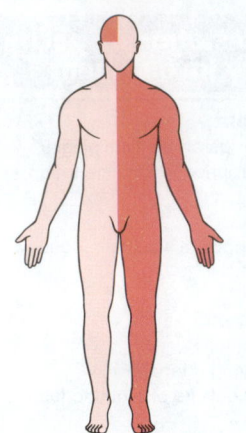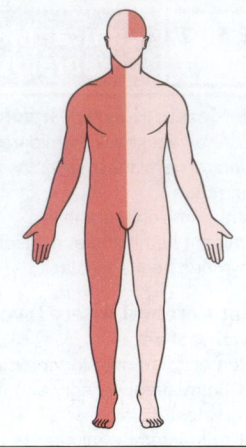

Right-brain damage (stroke on right side of the brain)	**Left-brain damage** (stroke on left side of the brain)
• Paralyzed left side: hemiplegia	• Paralyzed right side: hemiplegia
• Left-sided neglect	• Impaired speech/language aphasias
• Spatial-perceptual deficits	• Impaired right/left discrimination
• Tends to deny or minimize problems	• Slow performance, cautious
• Rapid performance, short attention span	• Aware of deficits: depression, anxiety
• Impulsive, safety problems	• Impaired comprehension related to language, math
• Impaired judgment	
• Impaired time concepts	

FIG. 58-5   Manifestations of right-brain and left-brain stroke.

a lesion on one side of the brain affects motor function on the opposite side of the brain (contralateral). The arms and legs of the affected side may be weakened or paralyzed to different degrees depending on which part of and to what extent the cerebral circulation was compromised. A stroke affecting the middle cerebral artery leads to a greater weakness in the upper extremity than the lower extremity. The affected shoulder tends to rotate internally, and the hip rotates externally. The affected foot is plantar flexed and inverted. An initial period of flaccidity may last from days to several weeks and is related to nerve damage. Spasticity of the muscles follows the flaccid stage and is related to interruption of upper motor neuron influence.

Communication. The left hemisphere is dominant for language skills in right-handed persons and in most left-handed persons. Language disorders involve expression and comprehension of written and spoken words. The patient may experience **aphasia** (total loss of comprehension and use of language) when a stroke damages the dominant hemisphere of the brain. **Dysphasia** refers to difficulty related to the comprehension or use of language and is due to partial disruption or loss. Patterns of dysphasia may differ as the stroke affects different portions of the brain. Dysphasias can be classified as *nonfluent* (minimal speech activity with slow speech that requires obvious effort) or *fluent* (speech is present but contains little meaningful communication). Most dysphasias are mixed, with impairment in both expression and understanding. A massive stroke may result in *global aphasia,* in which all communication and receptive function is lost.

Strokes affecting Wernicke's area of the brain exhibit symptoms of *receptive aphasia,* when neither the sounds of speech nor its meaning can be understood. This results in impairment of the patient's comprehension of both spoken and written language. Strokes affecting Broca's area of the brain cause *expressive aphasia* (difficulty in speaking and writing).

Many stroke patients also experience **dysarthria,** a disturbance in the muscular control of speech. Impairments may involve pronunciation, articulation, and phonation. Dysarthria does not affect the meaning of communication or the comprehension of language, but it does affect the mechanics of speech. Some patients experience a combination of aphasia and dysarthria.

Affect. Patients who have had a stroke may have difficulty controlling their emotions. Emotional responses may be exaggerated or unpredictable. Depression and feelings associated with changes in body image and loss of function can make this worse.[20] Patients may also be frustrated by mobility and communication problems. An example of unpredictable affect is as follows. A reserved professional engineer has returned home from the hospital following a stroke. During meals with his family, he becomes frustrated and begins to cry because of the difficulty getting food into his mouth and chewing, something that he was able to do easily before his stroke.

Intellectual Function. Both memory and judgment may be impaired as a result of stroke. These impairments can occur with strokes affecting either side of the brain. A left-brain stroke is more likely to result in memory problems related to language. Patients with a left-brain stroke often are very cautious in making judgments. The patient with a right-brain stroke tends to be impulsive and to move quickly. An example of behavior with right-brain stroke is the patient who tries to rise quickly from a wheelchair without locking the wheels or raising the footrests. The patient with a left-brain stroke would move slowly and cautiously from the wheelchair. Patients with either type of stroke may have difficulty making generalizations, which interferes with their ability to learn.

Spatial-Perceptual Alterations. A stroke on the right side of the brain is more likely to cause problems in spatial-perceptual orientation, although this can also occur with left-brain stroke. Spatial-perceptual problems may be divided into four categories. The first is related to the patient's incorrect perception of self and illness. This deficit follows damage to the parietal lobe. Patients may deny their illnesses or their own body parts. The second category concerns the patient's erroneous perception of self in space. The patient may neglect all input from the affected side. This may be worsened by *homonymous hemianopsia,* in which blindness occurs in the same half of the visual fields of both eyes. The patient also has difficulty with spatial orientation, such as judging distances. The third spatial-perceptual deficit is *agnosia,* the inability to recognize an object by sight, touch, or hearing. The fourth deficit is *apraxia,* the inability to carry out learned sequential movements on command. Patients may or may not be aware of their spatial-perceptual alterations.

Elimination. Most problems with urinary and bowel elimination occur initially and are temporary. When a stroke affects one hemisphere of the brain, the prognosis for normal bladder function is excellent. At least partial sensation for bladder filling remains, and voluntary urination is present. Initially, the patient may experience frequency, urgency, and incontinence. Although motor control of the bowel is usually not a problem, patients are frequently constipated. Constipation is associated with immobility, weak abdominal muscles, dehydration, and diminished response to the defecation reflex. Urinary and bowel elimination problems may also be related to inability to express needs and to manage clothing.

Diagnostic Studies

When manifestations of a stroke occur, diagnostic studies are done to (1) confirm that it is a stroke and not another brain lesion, such as a subdural hematoma, and (2) identify the likely cause of the stroke (Table 58-3). Tests also guide decisions about therapy to prevent a secondary stroke. The single most important diagnostic tool for patients who have experienced a stroke is the noncontrast CT scan.[21] The CT scan should optimally be obtained within 25 minutes and read within 45 minutes of arrival at the emergency department. The CT scan indicates the size and location of the lesion and differentiates between ischemic and hemorrhagic stroke. If the stroke is less than 3 hours old and is ischemic in nature, the CT will appear normal because the brain structures with or without blood flow appear the same in a noncontrast CT scan. For a patient to qualify for fibrinolytic therapy, the acute CT scan should appear normal with no sign of hemorrhage.[21] Computed tomographic angiography (CTA) provides visualization of vasculature and can be performed at the same time as the CT scan. CTA allows detection of intracranial or extracranial occlusive disease. Serial CT scans may be used to assess the effectiveness of treatment and to evaluate recovery.

Magnetic resonance imaging (MRI) is used to determine the extent of brain injury. MRI has greater specificity compared with CT. Diffusion-weighted MRI is a more sensitive MRI that better delineates ischemic brain injury early after a stroke when CT and standard MRI may appear normal. Use of MRI may be restricted in patients with claustrophobia or with devices such as pacemakers that would be affected by the magnetic field. Magnetic resonance angiography (MRA) is a noninvasive method of assessing vascular occlusive disease in the head or neck, similar to CTA.

Other tests used to diagnose stroke and assess the extent of tissue damage include positron emission tomography (PET), magnetic resonance spectroscopy (MRS), xenon CT, single-photon emission computed tomography (SPECT), and cerebral angiography. PET shows the metabolic activity of the brain and provides a depiction of the extent of tissue damage after a stroke. Less active or diseased tissue appears darker than healthy, active cells. MRS detects biochemical changes that may be present before physical changes are apparent.

Angiography is the "gold standard" for imaging the carotid arteries. Angiography can identify cervical and cerebrovascular occlusion, atherosclerotic plaques, and malformation of vessels. Intraarterial digital subtraction angiography (DSA) reduces the dose of contrast material, uses smaller catheters, and shortens the length of the procedure compared with conventional angiography. DSA involves the injection of a contrast agent to visualize blood vessels in the neck and the large vessels of the circle of Willis. It is considered safer than cerebral angiography because less vascular manipulation is required. Risks of angiography include dislodging an embolus, vasospasm, inducing further hemorrhage, and allergic reaction to contrast media.

Transcranial Doppler (TCD) ultrasonography is a noninvasive study that measures the velocity of blood flow in the major cerebral arteries. TCD has been shown to be effective in detecting microemboli and vasospasm. Other neurodiagnostic tests such as skull x-rays, brain scan, lumbar puncture, and electroencephalography (EEG) are currently used much less in the diagnosis of stroke. A skull x-ray result is usually normal after a stroke, but there may be a pineal gland shift with a massive infarction.

A lumbar puncture may be done to look for evidence of red blood cells in the cerebrospinal fluid if a subarachnoid hemorrhage

TABLE 58-3	**DIAGNOSTIC STUDIES** Stroke

Diagnosis of Stroke, Including Extent of Involvement
CT, CTA
MRI, MRA
SPECT
PET
MRS
Xenon CT
Electroencephalogram
Cerebral angiography
Cerebrospinal fluid analysis*

Cerebral Blood Flow Measures
Cerebral angiography
Digital subtraction angiography
Doppler ultrasonography
Transcranial Doppler
Carotid duplex
Carotid angiography

Cardiac Assessment
Electrocardiogram
Chest x-ray
Cardiac enzymes
Echocardiography (transthoracic, transesophageal)
Holter monitor (evaluation of dysrhythmias)

Additional Studies
Complete blood count
Platelets, prothrombin time, activated partial thromboplastin time
Electrolytes, blood glucose
Renal and hepatic studies
Lipid profile
Arterial blood gases (if hypoxia suspected)

CT, Computed tomography; *CTA,* computed tomographic angiography; *MRA,* magnetic resonance angiography; *MRI,* magnetic resonance imaging; *MRS,* magnetic resonance spectroscopy; *PET,* positron emission tomography; *SPECT,* single-photon emission computed tomography.
*A lumbar puncture to obtain cerebrospinal fluid is avoided if increased intracranial pressure is suspected.

is suspected but the CT does not show hemorrhage. A lumbar puncture is avoided if there are signs of increased ICP because of the danger of herniation of the brain downward, leading to pressure on cardiac and respiratory centers in the brainstem and potentially death. An EEG may show low-voltage, slow-wave activity suggestive of ischemic infarction. If the stroke is due to a hemorrhage, the EEG may show high-voltage slow waves. If the suspected cause of the stroke includes emboli from the heart, diagnostic cardiac tests should be done (see Table 58-3).

Blood tests are also done to help identify conditions contributing to stroke and to guide treatment (see Table 58-3).

Collaborative Preventive Care

Primary prevention is a priority for decreasing morbidity and mortality from stroke (Table 58-4). The goals of stroke prevention include health promotion for the well individual and education and management of modifiable risk factors to prevent a primary or secondary stroke. Health promotion focuses on (1) healthy diet, (2) weight control, (3) regular exercise, (4) no smoking, (5) limiting alcohol consumption, and (6) routine health assessments. Patients with known risk factors such as diabetes mellitus, hypertension, obesity, high serum lipids, or cardiac dysfunction require close management.

TABLE 58-4	COLLABORATIVE CARE Stroke

Diagnostic (see Table 58-3)
History and physical examination

Collaborative Therapy
Prevention
Control of hypertension
Control of diabetes mellitus
Treatment of underlying cardiac problem
Anticoagulation therapy for patients with atrial fibrillation
No smoking
Platelet inhibitors (e.g., aspirin)
Limiting alcohol intake
Surgical interventions for patients with aneurysms at risk of bleeding
Carotid endarterectomy
Stenting of carotid artery
Transluminal angioplasty
Extracranial-intracranial bypass

Acute Care
Maintenance of airway
Fluid therapy
Treatment of cerebral edema
Ischemic Stroke
Tissue plasminogen activator (tPA)
Merci retriever
Hemorrhagic Stroke
Surgical decompression if indicated
Clipping, wrapping, or coiling of aneurysm
Embolic Stroke
Treatment of underlying cause

Merci, Mechanical embolus retrieval in cerebral ischemia.

Drug Therapy. Measures to prevent the development of a thrombus or embolus are used in patients at risk for stroke. Antiplatelet drugs are usually the chosen treatment to prevent further stroke in patients who have had a TIA related to atherosclerosis.[22] Aspirin is the most frequently used antiplatelet agent, commonly at a dose of 81 to 325 mg/day. Other drugs include ticlopidine (Ticlid), clopidogrel (Plavix), dipyridamole (Persantine), and combined dipyridamole and aspirin (Aggrenox). Oral anticoagulation using warfarin is the treatment of choice for individuals with atrial fibrillation who have had a TIA.[22]

Surgical Therapy. Surgical interventions for the patient with TIAs from carotid disease include carotid endarterectomy, transluminal angioplasty, stenting, and extracranial-intracranial (EC-IC) bypass. In a carotid endarterectomy (CEA), the atheromatous lesion is removed from the carotid artery to improve blood flow[23,24] (Fig. 58-6).

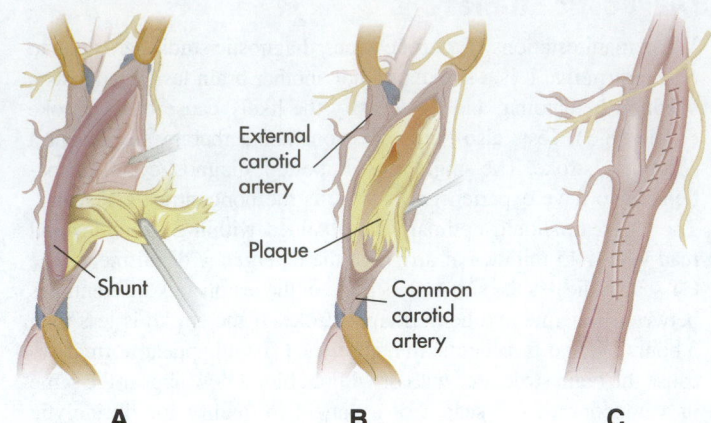

External carotid artery

Plaque

Shunt

Common carotid artery

A **B** **C**

FIG. 58-6 Carotid endarterectomy is performed to prevent impending cerebral infarction. **A,** A tube is inserted above and below the blockage to reroute the blood flow. **B,** Atherosclerotic plaque in the common carotid artery is removed. **C,** Once the artery is stitched closed, the tube can be removed. A surgeon may also perform the technique without rerouting the blood flow.

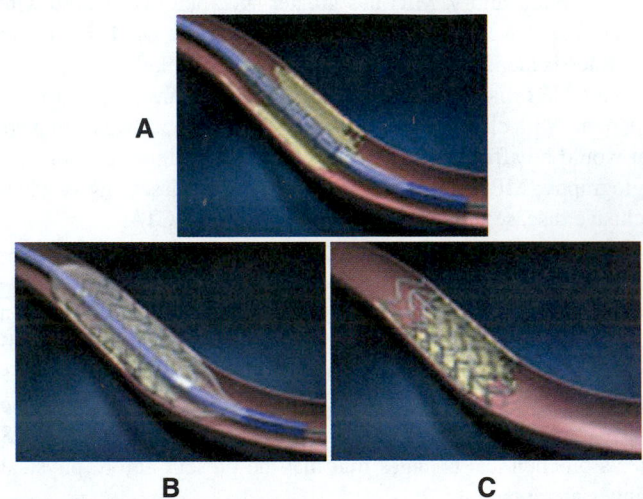

A

B **C**

FIG. 58-7 Brain stent used to treat blockages in cerebral blood flow. **A,** A balloon catheter is used to implant the stent into an artery of the brain. **B,** The balloon catheter is moved to the blocked area of the artery and then inflated. The stent expands due to the inflation of the balloon. **C,** The balloon is deflated and withdrawn, leaving the stent permanently in place holding the artery open and improving the flow of blood.

Transluminal angioplasty is the insertion of a balloon to open a stenosed artery and improve blood flow. The balloon is threaded up to the carotid artery via a catheter inserted in the femoral artery. Stenting involves intravascular placement of a stent in an attempt to maintain patency of the artery (Fig. 58-7). The stent can be inserted during an angioplasty. Once in place, the system can be used with a tiny filter that opens like an umbrella. The filter is used to catch and remove the debris that is stirred up during the stenting procedure before it floats to the brain, where it can trigger a stroke. Stenting is a less invasive strategy for revascularization in patients unable to withstand the CEA because of coexisting medical conditions. Initial research has shown the procedure to be as effective as the carotid endarterectomy.[24,25]

TABLE 58-5	*EMERGENCY MANAGEMENT* **Stroke**

Etiology	Assessment Findings	Interventions
• Sudden vascular compromise causing disruption of blood flow to the brain • Thrombosis • Trauma • Aneurysm • Embolism • Hemorrhage	• Altered level of consciousness • Weakness, numbness, or paralysis of portion of body • Speech or visual disturbances • Severe headache • Heart rate ↑ or ↓ • Respiratory distress • Unequal pupils • Hypertension • Facial drooping on affected side • Difficulty swallowing • Seizures • Bladder or bowel incontinence • Nausea and vomiting • Vertigo	**Initial** • Ensure patent airway. • Call a stroke code or the stroke team. • Remove dentures. • Perform pulse oximetry. • Maintain adequate oxygenation (SaO_2 >92%) with supplemental O_2, if necessary. • Establish IV access with normal saline. • Maintain BP according to guidelines (e.g., Cardiac Life Support).* • Remove clothing. • Obtain CT scan immediately. • Perform baseline laboratory tests (including blood glucose) immediately, and treat if hypoglycemic. • Position head midline. • Elevate head of bed 30 degrees if no symptoms of shock or injury. • Institute seizure precautions. • Anticipate thrombolytic therapy for ischemic stroke. **Ongoing Monitoring** • Monitor vital signs and neurologic status, including level of consciousness (Glasgow Coma Scale), motor and sensory function, pupil size and reactivity, SaO_2, and cardiac rhythm. • Reassure patient and family.

BP, Blood pressure; *CT*, computed tomography; *IV*, intravenous; *SaO₂*, arterial oxygen saturation.
*See Appendix A.

EC-IC bypass involves anastomosing (surgically connecting) a branch of an extracranial artery to an intracranial artery (most commonly, superficial temporal to middle cerebral artery) beyond an area of obstruction with the goal of increasing cerebral perfusion. This procedure is generally reserved for those patients who do not benefit from other forms of therapy.[26]

Collaborative Acute Care

The goals for collaborative care during the acute phase are preserving life, preventing further brain damage, and reducing disability. Treatment differs according to the type of stroke and changes as the patient progresses from the acute to the rehabilitation phase.

Table 58-5 outlines the emergency management of the patient with a stroke. Acute care begins with managing the airway, breathing, and circulation (the ABCs). Patients may have difficulty keeping an open and clear airway because of a decreased level of consciousness or decreased or absent gag and swallowing reflexes. Maintaining adequate oxygenation is important. Both hypoxia and hypercarbia are to be avoided because they can contribute to secondary neuronal injury. Oxygen administration, artificial airway insertion, intubation, and mechanical ventilation may be required. Baseline neurologic assessment is carried out, and patients are monitored closely for signs of increasing neurologic deficit. About 25% of patients will worsen in the first 24 to 48 hours. The American Heart Association recommends that acute care facilities have stroke teams in place. The stroke team generally consists of the registered nurse, neurologist, radiologist, and CT technician.[21,27]

Elevated BP is common immediately after a stroke and may be a protective response to maintain cerebral perfusion. Immediately following ischemic stroke, use of drugs to lower BP is recommended only if BP is markedly increased (mean arterial pressure >130 mm Hg or systolic pressure >220 mm Hg). Oral antihypertensive drugs are generally preferred. Although low BP immediately following a stroke is uncommon, hypotension and hypovolemia should be corrected if present. Hypervolemic hemodilution using crystalloids or colloids and drug-induced hypertension may be used in patients with ischemia caused by vasospasm following subarachnoid hemorrhage once the aneurysm has been successfully clipped or coiled (coils placed in aneurysm sac).

Fluid and electrolyte balance must be controlled carefully. The goal generally is to keep the patient adequately hydrated to promote perfusion and decrease further brain injury. Overhydration may compromise perfusion by increasing cerebral edema. Adequate fluid intake during acute care via oral, intravenous (IV), or tube feedings should be 1500 to 2000 ml/day. Urine output is monitored. If secretion of antidiuretic hormone (ADH) increases in response to the stroke, urine output decreases and fluid is retained. Low serum sodium (hyponatremia) may occur. IV solutions with glucose and water are avoided because they are hypotonic and may further increase cerebral edema and ICP. In addition, hyperglycemia may be associated with further brain damage and should be treated. In general, decisions regarding individualized fluid and electrolyte replacement therapy are based on the extent of intracranial edema, symptoms of increased ICP, central venous pressure levels, laboratory values for electrolytes, and intake and output.

Increased ICP is more likely to occur with hemorrhagic strokes but can occur with ischemic strokes. Increased ICP from cerebral edema usually peaks in 72 hours and may cause brain herniation. Management of increased ICP includes practices that improve venous drainage, such as elevating the head of the bed, maintaining head and neck in alignment, and avoiding hip flexion. Hyperthermia, which is seen commonly following stroke and may be associated with poorer outcome, needs to be avoided. Increased temperature contributes to increased cerebral metabolism. Other measures include pain management, avoidance of hypervolemia, and management of constipation. Cerebrospinal fluid drainage may be used in some patients to reduce ICP. Diuretic drugs, such as mannitol (Osmitrol) and furosemide (Lasix), may be used to decrease cerebral edema. The use of mannitol is being reexamined and compared to hypertonic saline and dextran solution infusions (HSD) for therapeutic treatment of increased ICP. Preliminary findings indicate that HSD is as effective as mannitol in lowering ICP.[28] As a last resort in the management of ICP, a bone flap may be removed to allow for cerebral edema without increases in ICP. The bone flap is frozen and replaced later.[29]

Drug Therapy. Recombinant tissue plasminogen activator (tPA) administered IV is used to reestablish blood flow through a blocked artery to prevent cell death in patients with the acute onset of ischemic stroke symptoms. Intraarterial infusion of tPA remains an option for a subgroup of patients with large vessel occlusions primarily in the middle cerebral artery. tPA produces localized fibrinolysis by binding to the fibrin in the thrombi. The fibrinolytic action of tPA occurs as the plasminogen is converted to plasmin, whose enzymatic action then digests fibrin and fibrinogen and thus lyses the clot. Other fibrinolytic agents cannot be substituted for tPA. (Fibrinolytic [thrombolytic] therapy is discussed in Chapter 34.)

tPA must be administered within 3 hours of the onset of clinical signs of ischemic stroke. Therefore the single most important factor is timing. Patients are screened carefully before tPA can be given. Screening includes a noncontrast CT or MRI scan to rule out hemorrhagic stroke, blood tests for coagulation disorders, and screening for recent history of gastrointestinal bleeding, stroke, or head trauma within the past 3 months, or major surgery within 14 days.[21]

During infusion of the drug, the patient's vital signs and neurologic status are monitored closely to assess for improvement or for potential deterioration related to intracerebral hemorrhage. Control of BP is critical during treatment and for 24 hours following.

The use of anticoagulants (e.g., heparin) in the emergency phase following an ischemic stroke is not indicated. However, the use of anticoagulants as an adjunct to tPA is still being investigated.[21]

Acetylsalicylic acid (aspirin) is used within 48 hours of the stroke. Complications of aspirin include gastrointestinal bleeding with higher doses. Aspirin administration should be done cautiously if the patient has a history of peptic ulcer disease.[30]

After the patient has stabilized and to prevent further clot formation, patients with strokes caused by thrombi and emboli may be treated with platelet inhibitors and anticoagulants (see discussion on prevention of stroke earlier in the chapter). Common anticoagulants include warfarin (Coumadin). Platelet inhibitors include aspirin, ticlopidine (Ticlid), clopidogrel (Plavix), and dipyridamole (Persantine).

Anticoagulants and platelet inhibitors are contraindicated in patients with hemorrhagic strokes. The calcium channel blocker nimodipine (Nimotop) is given to patients with subarachnoid hemorrhage to decrease the effects of vasospasm and minimize cerebral damage. Nimodipine restricts the influx of calcium ions into cells by reducing the number of open calcium channels. Although

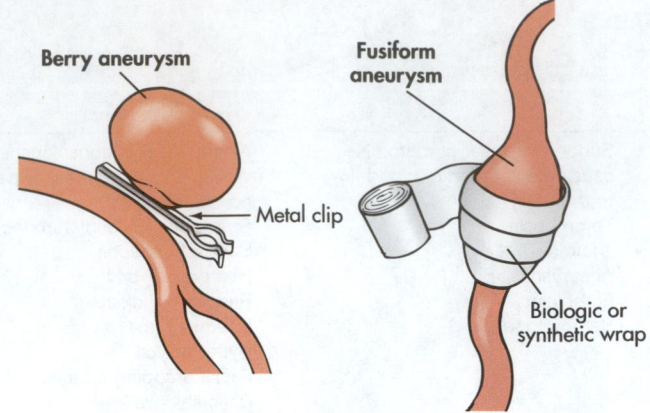

FIG. 58-8   Clipping and wrapping of aneurysms.

nimodipine is a calcium channel blocker, its exact mechanism of action in reducing vasospasm is not well understood.[31]

Drug Alert - *Nimodipine (Nimotop)*
- *Assess blood pressure and apical pulses prior to administration.*
- *If pulse is ≤60 beats/min or systolic BP <90 mm Hg, hold medication and contact physician.*

Drug therapies to treat hyperthermia include aspirin or acetaminophen (Tylenol). A temperature elevation of even 1° C can increase brain metabolism by 10% and contribute to further brain damage. Cooling blankets may be used cautiously to lower temperature. The nurse must closely monitor the patient's temperature. Hyperthermia prior to or during a stroke has been shown to result in negative outcomes. Aggressive management of temperature during the first 24 hours after a stroke is most effective in preventing detrimental outcomes.[32]

Seizures occur in 5% to 7% of stroke patients in the first 24 hours. An antiseizure drug, such as phenytoin (Dilantin), is given if a seizure occurs. The Stroke Council of the American Heart Association recommends uniform seizure prophylaxis in the acute period after intracerebral and subarachnoid hemorrhages.[33] In these patients, seizure activity may result in further neuronal injury and contribute to coma, although no clinical data support this recommendation. In other types of strokes, prophylactic use of antiseizure drugs is not recommended for patients who have not had a seizure.[33]

Surgical Therapy

Aneurysms and Hemorrhage. Surgical interventions for stroke include immediate evacuation of aneurysm-induced hematomas or cerebellar hematomas larger than 3 cm. Subarachnoid hemorrhage is usually caused by a ruptured aneurysm. Approximately 20% of patients will have multiple aneurysms. Treatment of an aneurysm involves clipping, wrapping, or coiling the aneurysm to prevent rebleeding (Figs. 58-8 and 58-9). A frequent surgical procedure used to prevent rebleeding is clipping of the aneurysm (see Fig. 58-8). Endovascular techniques may also be used. In the procedure known as *coiling,* a metal coil can be inserted into the lumen of the aneurysm via interventional neuroradiology (see Fig. 58-9). Guglielmi detachable coils (GDCs) provide immediate protection against hemorrhage by reducing the blood pulsations within the aneurysm. Eventually, a thrombus forms within the aneurysm and the aneurysm becomes sealed off from the parent vessel by the formation of an endothelialized layer of connective tissue. GDCs provide an alternative therapy to traditional surgical clipping of aneurysms.

Interventions to treat cerebral vasospasm either before or following aneurysm clipping or coiling include administration of the calcium channel blocker nimodipine (Nimotop). Following aneu-

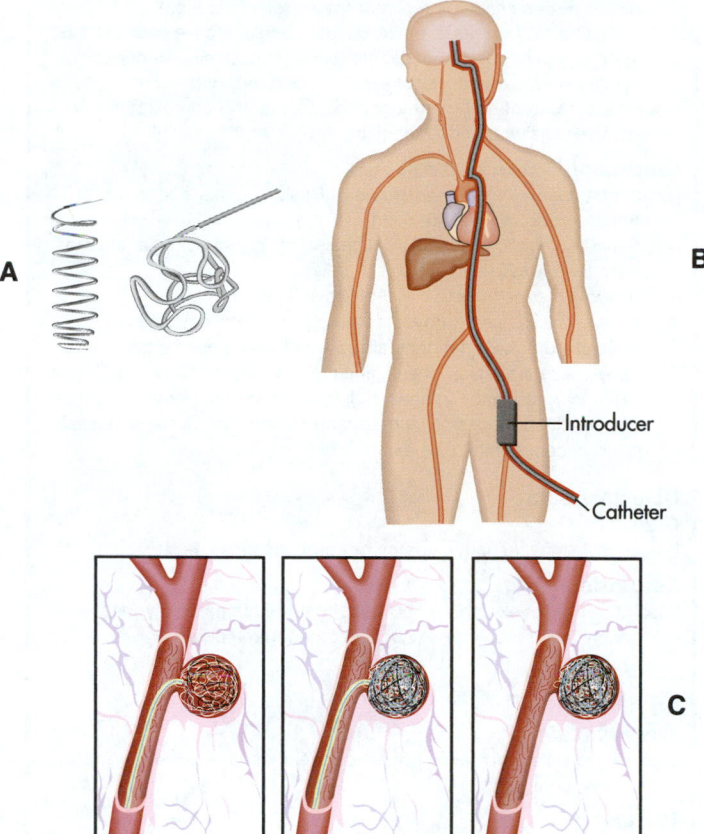

A

B

C

Introducer

Catheter

FIG. 58-9 GDC coil. **A,** A coil is used to occlude an aneurysm. Coils are made of soft, springlike platinum. The softness of the platinum allows the coil to assume the shape of irregularly shaped aneurysms while posing little threat of rupture of the aneurysm. **B,** A catheter is inserted through an introducer (small tube) in an artery in the leg. The catheter is threaded up to the cerebral blood vessels. **C,** Platinum coils attached to a thin wire are inserted into the catheter and then placed in the aneurysm until the aneurysm is filled with coils. Packing the aneurysm with coils prevents the blood from circulating through the aneurysm, reducing the risk of rupture.

rysmal occlusion, hyperdynamic therapy (hemodilution induced-hypertension using vasoconstricting agents such as phenylephrine or dopamine [Intropin] and hypervolemia) may be instituted in an effort to increase the mean arterial pressure and increase cerebral perfusion. Volume expansion is achieved via crystalloid or colloid solution.

The treatment of arteriovenous malformation (AVM) is surgical resection and/or radiosurgery (i.e., gamma knife). Both may be preceded by interventional neuroradiology to embolize the blood vessels that supply the AVM.

Subarachnoid and intracerebral hemorrhage can involve bleeding into the ventricles of the brain. This situation produces hydrocephalus, which further damages brain tissue from increased ICP. Insertion of a ventriculostomy for cerebrospinal fluid drainage can result in dramatic improvement in these situations.

Ischemic Stroke. The mechanical embolus retrieval in cerebral ischemia (Merci) retriever (Fig. 58-10) allows physicians to go inside the blocked artery of patients who are experiencing ischemic strokes. The retriever goes to the artery that is blocked, directly to the site of the problem, and pulls the clot out. The retriever is a tiny corkscrew device that uses a microcatheter inserted through a femoral artery balloon catheter. Once the corkscrew device reaches the clot in the brain, the device penetrates the clot, allowing it to be removed. Under x-ray guidance, the balloon catheter is maneuvered up to the carotid artery in the neck; a guidewire and the microcatheter are deployed through the balloon catheter and then placed just beyond the clot. The physician then deploys the Merci retriever device to engage and ensnare the clot. Once the clot is captured, the balloon catheter is inflated to temporarily arrest forward flow while the clot is being withdrawn. The clot is pulled into the balloon catheter and completely out of the body. The balloon is then deflated and blood flow is restored.

Collaborative Rehabilitation Care

After the stroke patient has stabilized for 12 to 24 hours, collaborative care shifts from preserving life to lessening disability and attaining optimal function. The patient may be evaluated by a physiatrist (a physician who specializes in physical medicine and rehabilitation). It is important to remember that some aspects of rehabilitation actually begin in the acute care phase as soon as the patient is stabilized. Depending on the patient's status, other medical conditions, rehabilitation potential, and available resources, the

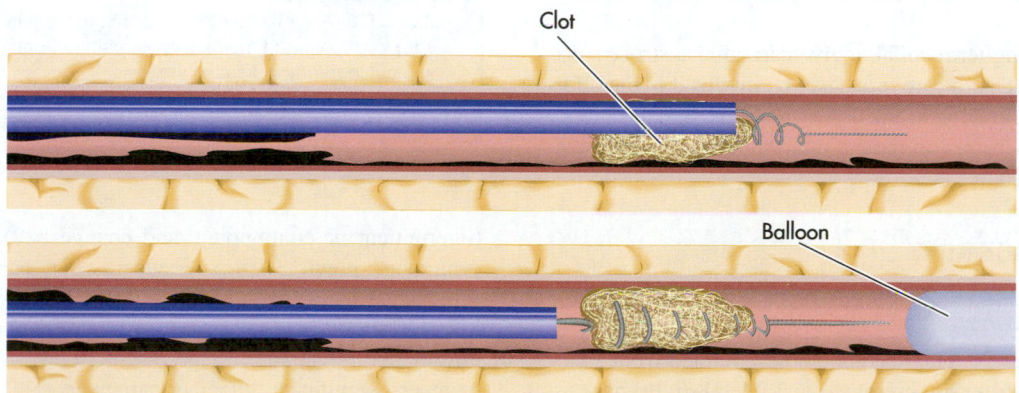

Clot

Balloon

FIG. 58-10 The Merci retriever removes blood clots in patients who are experiencing ischemic strokes. The retriever is a long, thin wire that is threaded through a catheter into the femoral artery. The wire is pushed through the end of the catheter up to the carotid artery. The wire reshapes itself into tiny loops that latch onto the clot and the clot can then be pulled out. To prevent the clot from breaking off, a balloon at the end of the catheter inflates to stop blood flow through the artery.

EVIDENCE-BASED PRACTICE

What Type of Exercise Program Is Most Effective for Stroke Patients?

Clinical Question

In older persons who have had a stroke (P), what is the effect of a weight lifting/stretching exercise program (I) as compared to an agility exercise program (C) on functional balance, mobility, postural reflexes, and falls (O)?

Best Available Evidence

Randomized controlled trial (RCT)

Critical Appraisal and Synthesis of Evidence

- RCT ($n = 61$) of community-dwelling older adults who have had a stroke.
- Participants randomly assigned to a weight lifting/stretching or agility exercise group. Both groups exercised three times per week for 10 weeks.
- Assessment occurred before, immediately after, and at 1 month postintervention. Falls were followed for up to 1 year later.

Conclusions

- Improvement was noted in both groups, with the agility group showing greater increases in step reaction time and postural reflexes and fewer induced falls.
- At 1 month, both groups had maintained improvement.
- In the agility group 1 year after the intervention, the number of people who had fallen was reduced by half in those with a prior history of falling.

Implications for Nursing Practice

- Instruct patient and family on importance of supervised balance training and agility to improve motor coordination.
- Emphasize the effect of exercise program on reducing risk of poststroke complications (e.g., falls) that can occur with sedentary lifestyle.
- Conduct more RCTs involving more subjects to support these findings.

Reference for Evidence

Marigold DS, Eng JJ, Dawson AS, et al: Exercise leads to faster postural reflexes, improved balance and mobility, and fewer falls in older persons with chronic stroke, *J Am Geriatr Soc* 53:416, 2005.

PICO: P, Patient population of interest; *I,* intervention or area of interest; *C,* comparison of interest or comparison group; *O,* outcome(s) of interest (see p. 6).

---

patient may be transferred to a rehabilitation unit. Other options for rehabilitation include outpatient therapy and home care–based rehabilitation.

As part of the long-term collaborative care after a stroke, various members of the health care team may be involved in the effort to promote optimal function of the patient and family. The composition of the team depends on patient and family needs and rehabilitation facility resources.

NURSING MANAGEMENT
STROKE

■ *Nursing Assessment*

Subjective and objective data that should be obtained from a person who has had a stroke are presented in Table 58-6. Primary assessment is focused on cardiac and respiratory status and neurologic assessment. If the patient is stable, the nursing history is obtained as follows: (1) description of the current illness with attention to initial symptoms, including onset and duration, nature

---

TABLE 58-6	NURSING ASSESSMENT Stroke

Subjective Data
Important Health Information
Past health history: Hypertension; previous stroke, TIA, aneurysm, cardiac disease (including recent myocardial infarction), dysrhythmias, heart failure, valvular disease, infective endocarditis; hyperlipidemia, polycythemia, diabetes, gout; family history of hypertension, diabetes, stroke, or coronary artery disease
Medications: Use of oral contraceptives; use of and compliance with antihypertensive and anticoagulant therapy

Functional Health Patterns
Health perception–health management: Positive family history of stroke; alcohol abuse, smoking
Nutritional-metabolic: Anorexia, nausea, vomiting; dysphagia, altered sensation of taste and smell
Elimination: Change in bowel and bladder patterns
Activity-exercise: Loss of movement and sensation; syncope; weakness on one side; generalized weakness, easy fatigability
Cognitive-perceptual: Numbness, tingling of one side of the body; loss of memory; alteration in speech, language, problem-solving ability; pain; headache, possibly sudden and severe (hemorrhage); visual disturbances; denial of illness

Objective Data
General
Emotional lability, lethargy, apathy or combativeness, fever

Respiratory
Loss of cough reflex, labored or irregular respirations, tachypnea, rhonchi (aspiration), airway occlusion (tongue), apnea

Cardiovascular
Hypertension, tachycardia, carotid bruit

Gastrointestinal
Loss of gag reflex, bowel incontinence, decreased or absent bowel sounds, constipation

Urinary
Frequency, urgency, incontinence

Neurologic
Contralateral motor and sensory deficits, including weakness, paresis, paralysis, anesthesia; unequal pupils, hand grasps; akinesia, aphasia (expressive, receptive, global), dysarthria (slurred speech), agnosias, apraxia, visual deficits, perceptual or spatial disturbances, altered level of consciousness (drowsiness to deep coma) and Babinski's sign, ↓ followed by ↑ deep tendon reflexes, flaccidity followed by spasticity, amnesia, ataxia, personality change, nuchal rigidity, seizures

Possible Findings
Positive CT, CTA, MRI, MRA, or other neuroimaging scans showing size, location, and type of lesion; positive Doppler ultrasonography and angiography indicating stenosis

CT, Computed tomography; *CTA,* computed tomographic angiography; *MRA,* magnetic resonance angiography; *MRI,* magnetic resonance imaging; *TIA,* transient ischemic attack.

(intermittent or continuous), and changes; (2) history of similar symptoms previously experienced; (3) current medications; (4) history of risk factors and other illnesses such as hypertension; and (5) family history of stroke or cardiovascular diseases. This information is gained through an interview of the patient, family members, significant others, or caregiver.

Secondary assessment should include a comprehensive neurologic examination of the patient. This includes (1) level of consciousness (Glasgow Coma Scale; see Table 57-5), (2) cognition, (3) motor abilities, (4) cranial nerve function, (5) sensation, (6)

TABLE 58-7	*PATIENT AND FAMILY TEACHING GUIDE* **Warning Signs of Stroke**

If someone is having one or more of these signs, do not ignore them. Call 911 and get medical help immediately.
- Sudden weakness, paralysis, or numbness of the face, arm, or leg, especially on one side of the body
- Sudden dimness or loss of vision in one or both eyes
- Sudden loss of speech, confusion, or difficulty speaking or understanding speech
- Unexplained sudden dizziness, unsteadiness, loss of balance or coordination
- Sudden severe headache

proprioception, (7) cerebellar function, and (8) deep tendon reflexes. Clear documentation of initial and ongoing neurologic examinations is essential to note changes in patient status.

▪ Nursing Diagnoses

Nursing diagnoses for the person with a stroke may include, but are not limited to, those presented in NCP 58-1.

▪ Planning

The patient, family, and nurse establish the goals of nursing care in a cooperative manner. Typical goals are that the patient will (1) maintain a stable or improved level of consciousness, (2) attain maximum physical functioning, (3) attain maximum self-care abilities and skills, (4) maintain stable body functions (e.g., bladder control), (5) maximize communication abilities, (6) maintain adequate nutrition, (7) avoid complications of stroke, and (8) maintain effective personal and family coping.

▪ Nursing Implementation

Health Promotion. In any health care setting and for the population as a whole, nurses can play a major role in the promotion of a healthy lifestyle. To reduce the incidence of stroke, the nurse should focus teaching efforts toward stroke prevention, particularly for persons with known risk factors. Nursing measures to reduce risk factors for stroke are similar to those for coronary artery disease (see Table 34-3) and are discussed on pp. 791 to 792. If a person is a diabetic, it is very important that the diabetes is well controlled. If an individual has atrial fibrillation, an anticoagulant such as warfarin (Coumadin) or aspirin may be used to treat the problem to prevent the risk of stroke. Because smoking is a major risk factor for stroke, the nurse needs to be actively involved in helping patients to stop smoking (see Chapter 12, Tables 12-4, 12-5, and 12-6).

Another very important aspect of health promotion is teaching patients and families about early symptoms associated with stroke or TIA. Table 58-7 presents information on when to seek health care for these symptoms.

Acute Intervention

Respiratory System. During the acute phase following a stroke, management of the respiratory system is a nursing priority. Stroke patients are particularly vulnerable to respiratory problems. Advancing age and immobility increase the risk for atelectasis and pneumonia. Risk for aspiration pneumonia may be high because of impaired consciousness or dysphagia. Airway obstruction can occur because of problems with chewing and swallowing, food pocketing (food remaining in the buccal cavity of the mouth), and the tongue falling back. Some stroke patients, especially those with

brainstem or hemorrhagic stroke, may require endotracheal intubation and mechanical ventilation, initially and/or with increasing cerebral edema and/or ICP. Enteral tube feedings also place the patient at risk for aspiration pneumonia.

Nursing interventions to support adequate respiratory function are individualized to meet the needs of the patient. An oropharyngeal airway may be used in comatose patients to prevent the tongue from falling back and obstructing the airway and to provide access for suctioning. Alternately, a nasopharyngeal airway may be used to provide airway protection and access. When an artificial airway will be required for a prolonged time, a tracheostomy may be performed. Nursing interventions include frequent assessment of airway patency and function, oxygenation, suctioning, patient mobility, positioning of the patient to prevent aspiration, and encouraging deep breathing. Patients who have an unclipped or uncoiled aneurysm may experience rebleeding and the possibility of further ICP increases with coughing exercises. Interventions related to maintenance of airway function are described in NCP 58-1.

Neurologic System. The patient's neurologic status must be monitored closely to detect changes suggesting extension of the stroke, increased ICP, vasospasm, or recovery from stroke symptoms. Neurologic assessment includes the Glasgow Coma Scale (a standardized assessment of level of consciousness), mental status, pupillary responses, and extremity movement and strength. (The Glasgow Coma Scale is shown in Table 57-5.) Vital signs are also closely monitored and documented. A decreasing level of consciousness may indicate increasing ICP. ICP and cerebral perfusion pressure may be monitored as well if the patient is in a critical care environment. Data from the nursing assessment are recorded on flow sheets to communicate evaluation of neurologic status to the interdisciplinary team.

Cardiovascular System. Nursing goals for the cardiovascular system are aimed at maintaining homeostasis. Many patients with stroke have decreased cardiac reserves secondary to cardiac disease. Cardiac efficiency may be further compromised by fluid retention, overhydration, dehydration, and/or blood pressure variations. Fluids are retained if there is increased production of ADH and aldosterone secondary to stress. Fluid retention plus overhydration can result in fluid overload. It can also increase cerebral edema and ICP. At the same time, dehydration can add to the morbidity and mortality associated with stroke, especially in the patient with cerebral vasospasm. IV therapy should be carefully regulated. The nurse should closely monitor intake and output. Central venous pressure, pulmonary artery pressure, or hemodynamic monitoring may be used as indicators of fluid balance or cardiac function in the critical care unit.

Nursing interventions include (1) monitoring vital signs frequently; (2) monitoring cardiac rhythms; (3) calculating intake and output, noting imbalances; (4) regulating IV infusions; (5) adjusting fluid intake to the individual needs of the patient; (6) monitoring lung sounds for crackles and rhonchi indicating pulmonary congestion; and (7) monitoring heart sounds for murmurs or for S_3 or S_4 heart sounds. Bedside monitors or telemetry may record cardiac rhythms. Hypertension is sometimes seen following a stroke as the body attempts to increase cerebral blood flow. It is important to monitor for orthostatic hypotension prior to ambulating the patient for the first time. Neurologic changes can occur with a sudden decrease in BP.

After a stroke, the patient is at risk for deep vein thrombosis, especially in the weak or paralyzed lower extremity. This is re-

Nervous System

NURSING CARE PLAN 58-1

Patient with Stroke

NURSING DIAGNOSIS   **Ineffective tissue perfusion (cerebral)** *related to* decreased cerebral blood flow secondary to thrombus, embolus, hemorrhage, or edema *as evidenced by* ICP >15 mm Hg for 15 to 30 seconds or longer, decreasing Glasgow Coma Scale (GCS) score, and altered respiratory pattern

PATIENT GOAL   Demonstrates signs of stable or improved cerebral perfusion

OUTCOMES (NOC)	INTERVENTIONS (NIC) and *RATIONALES*
Tissue Perfusion: Cerebral	**Cerebral Perfusion Promotion**

Tissue Perfusion: Cerebral

- Neurologic function _____
- Intracranial pressure _____
- Systolic blood pressure _____
- Diastolic blood pressure _____

Measurement Scale

1 = Severely compromised
2 = Substantially compromised
3 = Moderately compromised
4 = Mildly compromised
5 = Not compromised

Cerebral Perfusion Promotion

- Monitor neurologic status *to detect changes indicative of worsening or improving condition.*
- Monitor respiratory status (e.g., rate, rhythm, and depth of respirations; PaO_2, $PaCO_2$, pH, and bicarbonate levels) *to assess changes in neurologic status.*
- Monitor patient's ICP and neurologic responses to care activities *as ICP can increase with changes in positioning and movement.*
- Administer vasopressin, calcium channel blockers, anticoagulant medications, antiplatelet medications, thrombolytic medications (as ordered) *to increase tissue perfusion.*
- Administer volume expanders (as ordered) *to maintain hemodynamic parameters.*
- Avoid neck flexion or extreme hip/knee flexion *to avoid obstruction of arterial and venous blood flow.*

NURSING DIAGNOSIS   **Ineffective airway clearance** *related to* inability to raise secretions *as evidenced by* adventitious breath sounds, diminished breath sounds, and ineffective cough

PATIENT GOALS   1. Demonstrates effective coughing and increased air exchange
2. Maintains a clear airway

OUTCOMES (NOC)	INTERVENTIONS (NIC) and *RATIONALES*

Respiratory Status: Airway Patency

- Moves sputum out of airway _____
- Ease of breathing _____

Measurement Scale

1 = Severely compromised
2 = Substantially compromised
3 = Moderately compromised
4 = Mildly compromised
5 = Not compromised

Airway Management

- Auscultate breath sounds, noting areas of decreased/absent ventilation, and presence of adventitious sounds *to obtain ongoing data on patient's response to therapy.*
- Remove secretions by encouraging coughing or by suctioning *to clear airway.*

Cough Enhancement

- Assist patient to a sitting position with head slightly flexed, shoulders relaxed, and knees flexed *to provide optimal positioning for generating maximum intrathoracic pressure during cough.*
- Instruct patient to inhale deeply, bend forward slightly, and perform three or four huffs (against an open glottis) *to expel secretions.*
- Encourage use of incentive spirometry *to open collapsed alveoli, promote deep breathing, and prevent atelectasis.*

NURSING DIAGNOSIS   **Impaired physical mobility** *related to* neuromuscular and cognitive impairment and decreased muscle strength and control *as evidenced by* limited ability to perform gross and fine motor skills, limited range of motion, and difficulty turning

PATIENT GOALS   1. Demonstrates increased muscle strength and ability to move
2. Uses adaptive equipment to increase mobility

OUTCOMES (NOC)	INTERVENTIONS (NIC) and *RATIONALES*

Mobility

- Balance _____
- Muscle movement _____
- Joint movement _____
- Walking _____

Measurement Scale

1 = Severely compromised
2 = Substantially compromised
3 = Moderately compromised
4 = Mildly compromised
5 = Not compromised

Exercise Therapy: Muscle Control

- Collaborate with physical, occupational, and recreational therapists in developing and executing exercise program *to determine extent of problem and plan appropriate interventions.*
- Determine patient's readiness to engage in activity or exercise protocol *to assess expected level of participation.*
- Apply splints to achieve stability of proximal joints involved with fine motor skills *to prevent contractures.*
- Encourage patient to practice exercises independently *to promote patient's sense of control.*
- Provide restful environment for patient after periods of exercise *to facilitate recuperation.*

ICP, Intracranial pressure; *PaCO₂,* partial pressure of carbon dioxide in arterial blood; *PaO₂,* partial pressure of oxygen in arterial blood.

NURSING CARE PLAN 58-1

Patient wih Stroke—cont'd

NURSING DIAGNOSIS **Impaired verbal communication** *related to* residual aphasia *as evidenced by* refusal or inability to speak, word-finding problems, inappropriate verbalization, inability to follow verbal directions

PATIENT GOALS
1. Uses effective oral and written communication techniques
2. Demonstrates congruency of verbal and nonverbal communication

OUTCOMES (NOC)	INTERVENTIONS (NIC) and *RATIONALES*
Communication: Expressive	*Communication Enhancement: Speech Deficit*
• Use of spoken language: vocal ____	• Listen attentively *to convey the importance of patient's thoughts and to promote a positive environment for learning.*
• Use of written language ____	• Provide positive reinforcement and praise *to build self-esteem and confidence.*
• Directs messages appropriately ____	• Use simple words and short sentences *to avoid overwhelming patient with verbal stimuli.*
Measurement Scale	• Provide verbal prompts/reminders *to assist patient to express self.*
1 = Severely compromised	
2 = Substantially compromised	
3 = Moderately compromised	
4 = Mildly compromised	
5 = Not compromised	

NURSING DIAGNOSIS **Unilateral neglect** *related to* visual field cut and sensory loss on one side of body *as evidenced by* consistent inattention to stimuli on affected side

PATIENT GOALS
1. Cares for both sides of the body appropriately
2. Uses strategies to minimize unilateral neglect

OUTCOMES (NOC)	INTERVENTIONS (NIC) and *RATIONALES*
Body Image	*Unilateral Neglect Management*
• Description of affected body part ____	• Monitor for abnormal responses to three primary types of stimuli: sensory, visual, and auditory *to determine the presence of and degree to which unilateral neglect exists (i.e., inability to see objects on affected side, leaving food on a plate that corresponds to affected side, lack of sensation on affected side).*
• Willingness to touch affected body part ____	
• Adjustment to changes in body function ____	
• Willingness to use strategies to enhance function ____	• Instruct patient to scan from left to right to scan the entire environment.
Measurement Scale	• Rearrange the environment to use the right or left visual field; position personal items, television, or reading materials within view on unaffected side *to compensate for visual field deficits.*
1 = Never positive	
2 = Rarely positive	• Touch unaffected shoulder when initiating conversation *to attract patient's attention.*
3 = Sometimes positive	• Position bed in room so that individuals approach and care for patient on unaffected side.
4 = Often positive	• Gradually move personal items and activity to affected side, as patient demonstrates an ability to compensate for neglect.
5 = Consistently positive	• Include family in rehabilitation process to support the patient's efforts and assist with care *to promote reintegration with the whole body.*

NURSING DIAGNOSIS **Impaired urinary elimination** *related to* impaired impulse to void or inability to reach toilet or manage tasks of voiding *as evidenced by* incontinence and flow of urine at unpredictable times

PATIENT GOALS
1. Perceives impulse to void, removes clothing for toileting, and uses toilet
2. Demonstrates ability to urinate when the urge arises or with a timed schedule

OUTCOMES (NOC)	INTERVENTIONS (NIC) and *RATIONALES*
Urinary Continence	*Urinary Bladder Training*
• Recognizes urge to void ____	• Encourage patient to keep a voiding diary *to establish voiding pattern and plan appropriate interventions.*
• Maintains predictable pattern of voiding ____	• Establish interval of initial toileting schedule, based on voiding pattern *to initiate process of improving bladder functioning and increased muscle tone.*
Measurement Scale	• Toilet patient or remind patient to void at prescribed intervals *to assist patient in adapting to new toileting schedule.*
1 = Never demonstrated	• Teach patient to consciously hold urine until the scheduled toileting time *to improve muscle tone.*
2 = Rarely demonstrated	
3 = Sometimes demonstrated	• Discuss daily record of continence with patient *to provide reinforcement and to allow time to ask questions, make comments, or share concerns.*
4 = Often demonstrated	
5 = Consistently demonstrated	
5 = Never demonstrated	

Continued

NURSING CARE PLAN 58-1

Patient wih Stroke—cont'd

NURSING DIAGNOSIS   **Impaired swallowing** *related to* weakness or paralysis of affected muscles *as evidenced by* drooling, difficulty in swallowing, choking

PATIENT GOAL   Demonstrates effective swallowing without choking, coughing, or aspiration

OUTCOMES (NOC)	INTERVENTIONS (NIC) and *RATIONALES*
Swallowing Status	**Swallowing Therapy**

Swallowing Status

- Choking _____
- Coughing _____
- Gagging _____
- Discomfort with swallowing _____

Measurement Scale

1 = Severe
2 = Substantial
3 = Moderate
4 = Mild
5 = None

- Handles oral secretions _____
- Maintains food in mouth _____

Measurement Scale

1 = Severely compromised
2 = Substantially compromised
3 = Moderately compromised
4 = Mildly compromised
5 = Not compromised

Swallowing Therapy

- Collaborate with other members of health care team (i.e., occupational therapist, speech pathologist, and dietitian) *to provide continuity in patient's rehabilitative plan.*
- Assist patient to sit in an erect position (as close to 90 degrees as possible) for feeding/exercise *to provide optimal position for chewing and swallowing without aspirating.*
- Assist patient to position head in forward flexion in preparation for swallowing ("chin tuck").
- Assist patient to maintain sitting position for 30 minutes after completing meal *to prevent regurgitation of food.*
- Instruct patient/caregiver on emergency measures for choking *to prevent complications in the home setting.*
- Check mouth for pocketing of food after eating *to prevent collection and putrefaction of food and or aspiration.*
- Provide mouth care as needed *to promote comfort and oral health.*
- Monitor body weight *to determine adequacy of nutritional intake.*

NURSING DIAGNOSIS   **Situational low self-esteem** *related to* actual or perceived loss of function and altered body image *as evidenced by* refusal to touch or look at affected body parts, refusal to participate in self-care, and expressions of helplessness and uselessness

PATIENT GOALS   1. Expresses positive feelings of self-worth
2. Participates in self-care of affected body parts

OUTCOMES (NOC)	INTERVENTIONS (NIC) and *RATIONALES*
Self-Esteem	**Self-Esteem Enhancement**

Self-Esteem

- Maintenance of grooming/hygiene _____
- Acceptance of self-limitations _____
- Description of self _____
- Feelings about self-worth _____

Measurement Scale

1 = Never positive
2 = Rarely positive
3 = Sometimes positive
4 = Often positive
5 = Consistently positive

Self-Esteem Enhancement

- Monitor patient's statements of self-worth *to determine effect of stroke on self-esteem.*
- Encourage patient to identify strengths *to facilitate patient's recognition of intrinsic value.*
- Assist in setting realistic goals *to achieve higher self-esteem.*
- Reward or praise patient's progress toward reaching goals.
- Encourage increased responsibility for self *to promote sense of satisfaction, independence, and control, and to reduce frustrations.*
- Monitor levels of self-esteem over time *to determine stressors or situations that trigger low self-esteem and to teach coping mechanisms.*

Body Image Enhancement

- Monitor whether patient can look at the changed body part *to determine patient's level of acceptance of new image.*
- Help patient to determine the extent of actual changes in the body or its level of functioning *to prevent misperceptions concerning new level of physiologic functioning.*

---

lated to immobility, loss of venous tone, and decreased muscle pumping activity in the leg. The most effective prevention is to keep the patient moving. Active range-of-motion exercises should be taught if the patient has voluntary movement in the affected extremity. For the patient with hemiplegia, passive range-of-motion exercises should be done several times a day. Additional measures to prevent deep vein thrombosis include positioning to minimize the effects of dependent edema and the use of elastic compression gradient stockings or support hose. Intermittent pneumatic compression stockings may be ordered for bedridden patients. Deep vein thrombosis prophylaxis may include low-molecular-weight heparin (e.g., enoxaparin [Lovenox]). The nursing assessment for deep vein thrombosis includes measuring the calf and thigh daily, observing swelling of the lower extremities, noting unusual warmth of the leg, and asking the patient about pain in the calf.

Musculoskeletal System. The nursing goal for the musculoskeletal system is to maintain optimal function. This is accomplished by the prevention of joint contractures and muscular atrophy. In the acute phase, range-of-motion exercises and positioning are important nursing interventions. Passive range-of-motion exercise is begun on the first day of hospitalization. If the stroke is due to subarachnoid hemorrhage, the movement is limited to the extremities. The patient is taught to actively exercise as soon as possible. Muscle atrophy secondary to lack of innervation and activity can develop within 1 month following stroke.

The paralyzed or weak side needs special attention when the patient is positioned. Each joint should be positioned higher than the joint proximal to it to prevent dependent edema. Specific deformities on the weak or paralyzed side that may be present in patients with stroke include internal rotation of the shoulder; flexion contractures of the hand, wrist, and elbow; external rotation of the hip; and plantar flexion of the foot. Subluxation of the shoulder on the affected side is common. Careful positioning and moving of the affected arm may prevent the development of a painful shoulder condition. Immobilization of the affected upper extremity may precipitate a painful shoulder-hand syndrome.

Nursing interventions to optimize musculoskeletal function include (1) trochanter roll at the hip to prevent external rotation; (2) hand cones (not rolled washcloths) to prevent hand contractures; (3) arm supports with slings and lap boards to prevent shoulder displacement; (4) avoidance of pulling the patient by the arm to avoid shoulder displacement; (5) posterior leg splints, footboards or high-top tennis shoes to prevent footdrop; and (6) hand splints to reduce spasticity. Use of a footboard for the patient with spasticity is controversial. Rather than preventing plantar flexion (footdrop), the sensory stimulation of a footboard against the bottom of the foot increases plantar flexion. Likewise, there is disagreement on whether hand splints facilitate or diminish spasticity. The decision regarding the use of footboards or hand splints is made on an individual patient basis.

Integumentary System. The skin of the patient with stroke is particularly susceptible to breakdown related to loss of sensation, decreased circulation, and immobility. This is compounded by patient age, poor nutrition, dehydration, edema, and incontinence. The nursing plan for prevention of skin breakdown includes (1) pressure relief by position changes, special mattresses, or wheelchair cushions; (2) good skin hygiene; (3) emollients applied to dry skin; and (4) early mobility. The ideal position change schedule is side-back-side, with a maximum duration of 2 hours for any position. Nurses should position the patient on the weak or paralyzed side for only 30 minutes. If an area of redness develops and does not return to normal color within 15 minutes of pressure relief, the epidermis and dermis are damaged. The damaged area should not be massaged because this may cause additional damage. Control of pressure is the single most important factor in both the prevention and treatment of skin breakdown. Pillows can be used under lower extremities to reduce pressure on the heels. Vigilance and good nursing care are required to prevent pressure sores.

Gastrointestinal System. The stress of illness contributes to a catabolic state that can interfere with recovery. Neurologic, cardiac, and respiratory problems are considered priorities in the acute phase of stroke. However, gastrointestinal problems may hinder recovery. The most common bowel problem for the patient who has experienced a stroke is constipation. Patients may be prophylactically placed on stool softeners and/or fiber (psyllium [Metamucil]). If the patient does not have a daily or every-other-day bowel move-

ment, the patient should be checked for impaction. The patient who has liquid stools should also be checked for stool impaction. Depending on the patient's fluid balance status and swallowing ability, fluid intake should be at least 1800 to 2000 ml/day and fiber intake up to 25 g/day. Physical activity also promotes bowel function. Laxatives, suppositories, or additional stool softeners may be ordered if the patient does not respond to increased fluid and fiber. Similarly, enemas are used only if suppositories and digital stimulation are ineffective because they cause vagal stimulation and increase ICP.

Urinary System. In the acute stage of stroke, the primary urinary problem is poor bladder control, resulting in incontinence. Efforts should be made to promote normal bladder function and avoid the use of indwelling catheters. If an indwelling catheter must be used initially, it should be removed as soon as the patient is medically and neurologically stable. Long-term use of an indwelling catheter is associated with urinary tract infections and delayed bladder retraining. An intermittent catheterization program may be used for patients with urinary retention because of the lower incidence of urinary infections. An alternative to intermittent catheterizations is the external catheter for male patients with urinary incontinence. External catheters do not alleviate the problem of urine retention. Bladder overdistention should be avoided.

A bladder retraining program consists of (1) adequate fluid intake with the majority given between 8:00 AM and 7:00 PM; (2) scheduled toileting every 2 hours using bedpan, commode, or bathroom; and (3) noting signs of restlessness, which may indicate the need for urination.

Nutrition. The nutritional needs of the patient require quick assessment and treatment. The patient may initially receive IV infusions to maintain fluid and electrolyte balance, as well as for administration of drugs. Patients with severe impairment may require enteral or parenteral nutrition support. Depending on the severity of the stroke, individual assessment and planning for nutrition are necessary.

Speech therapists (if available) should perform a swallowing evaluation before patients are started on oral intake. The first oral feeding should be approached carefully because the gag reflex may be impaired due to dysphagia. Up to 64% of patients will experience dysphagia after a stroke.[34] Before initiation of feeding, the gag reflex should be assessed by gently stimulating the back of the throat with a tongue blade. If a gag reflex is present, the patient will gag spontaneously. If it is absent, feeding should be deferred and exercises to stimulate swallowing should be started. The speech therapist or occupational therapist is usually responsible for designing this program. However, the nurse may be called on to develop the program in some clinical settings.

To assess swallowing ability, the nurse should elevate the head of the bed to an upright position (unless contraindicated) and give the patient a small amount of crushed ice or ice water to swallow. If the gag reflex is present and the patient is able to swallow safely, the nurse may proceed with feeding.

After careful assessment of swallowing, chewing, gag reflex, and pocketing, oral feedings can be initiated. Mouth care before feeding helps stimulate sensory awareness and salivation and can facilitate swallowing. The patient should remain in a high Fowler's position, preferably in a chair with the head flexed forward, for the feeding and for 30 minutes following. Various dietary items may be recommended by the speech therapist. Foods should be easy to swallow and provide enough texture, temperature (warm or cold), and flavor to stimulate a swallow reflex. Crushed ice can be used

TABLE 58-8	Communication with a Patient with Aphasia

1. Decrease environmental stimuli that may be distracting and disrupting to communication efforts.
2. Treat the patient as an adult.
3. Present one thought or idea at a time.
4. Keep questions simple or ask questions that can be answered with "yes" or "no."
5. Let the person speak. Do not interrupt. Allow time for the individual to complete thoughts.
6. Make use of gestures or demonstration as an acceptable alternative form of communication. Encourage this by saying, "Show me . . ." or "Point to what you want."
7. Do not pretend to understand the person if you do not. Calmly say you do not understand and encourage the use of nonverbal communication, or ask the person to write out what he or she wants.
8. Speak with normal volume and tone.
9. Give the patient time to process information and generate a response before repeating a question or statement.
10. Allow body contact (e.g., the clasp of a hand, touching) as much as possible. Realize that touching may be the only way the patient can express feelings.
11. Organize the patient's day by preparing and following a schedule (the more familiar the routine, the easier it will be).
12. Do not push communication if the person is tired or upset. Aphasia worsens with fatigue and anxiety.

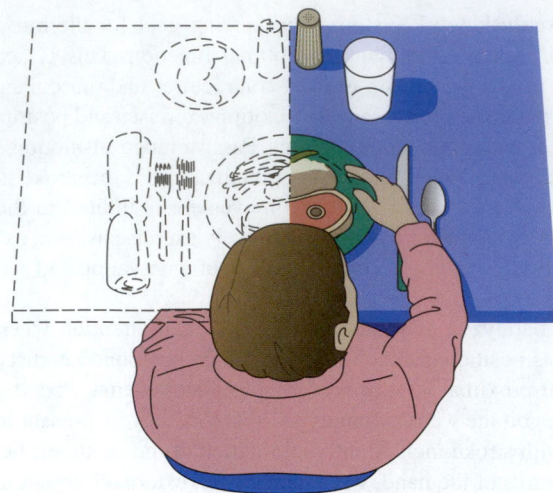

FIG. 58-11 Spatial and perceptual deficits in stroke. Perception of a patient with homonymous hemianopsia shows that food on the left side is not seen and thus is ignored.

as a stimulant. The patient is instructed to swallow and then swallow again. Pureed foods are not usually the best choice because they are often bland and too smooth. Thin liquids are often difficult to swallow and may promote coughing. Thin liquids can be thickened through the use of a commercially available thickening agent (Thick-It). Milk products should be avoided because they tend to increase the viscosity of mucus and increase salivation.

Food should be placed on the unaffected side of the mouth. The nurse should ensure an unrushed, nonstressful atmosphere. Feedings must be followed by scrupulous oral hygiene because food may collect on the affected side of the mouth.

Communication. During the acute stage of stroke, the nurse's role in meeting the psychologic needs of the patient is primarily supportive. An alert patient is usually anxious because of lack of understanding about what has happened and because of difficulty with, or inability to, communicate. The patient is assessed both for the ability to speak and the ability to understand. The patient's response to simple questions can give the nurse a guideline for structuring explanations and instructions. If the patient cannot understand words, gestures may be used to support verbal cues. It is helpful to speak slowly and calmly, using simple words or sentences to enhance communication. The nurse must give the patient extra time to comprehend and respond to communication. The stroke patient with aphasia may easily be overwhelmed by verbal stimuli. (Guidelines for communicating with a patient who has aphasia are presented in Table 58-8.) A picture board may be helpful for communicating with the stroke patient. Evaluation and treatment of language and communication deficits are often done by the speech pathologist once the patient has stabilized.

Sensory-Perceptual Alterations. *Homonymous hemianopsia* (blindness in the same half of each visual field) is a common problem after a stroke (Fig. 58-11). Persistent disregard of objects in part of the visual field should alert the nurse to this possibility. Initially, the nurse helps the patient to compensate by arranging the environment within the patient's perceptual field, such as arranging the food tray so that all foods are on the right side or the left

side to accommodate for field of vision (see Fig. 58-11). Later, the patient learns to compensate for the visual defect by consciously attending or by scanning the neglected side. The weak or paralyzed extremities are carefully checked for adequacy of dressing, for hygiene, and for trauma.

In the clinical situation it is often difficult to distinguish between a visual field cut and a neglect syndrome. Both problems may occur with strokes affecting either the right or the left side of the brain. A person may be unfortunate enough to have both homonymous hemianopsia and a neglect syndrome, which increases the inattention to the weak or paralyzed side. A neglect syndrome results in decreased safety awareness and places the patient at high risk for injury. Immediately after the stroke, the nurse must anticipate potential safety hazards and provide protection from injury. Safety measures can include close observation of the patient, elevating side rails, lowering the height of the bed, and video monitors. The use of restraints and soft vests is avoided because this may agitate the patient.

Other visual problems may include *diplopia* (double vision), loss of the corneal reflex, and *ptosis* (drooping eyelid), especially if the area of stroke is in the vertebrobasilar distribution. Diplopia is often treated with an eye patch. If the corneal reflex is absent, the patient is at risk for corneal abrasion and should be observed closely and protected against eye injuries. Corneal abrasion can be prevented with artificial tears or gel to keep the eyes moist and an eye shield (especially at night). Ptosis is generally not treated because it usually does not inhibit vision.

Coping. A stroke is usually a sudden, extremely stressful event for the patient, family members, and significant others. A stroke is often a family disease, affecting the family emotionally, socially, and financially, as well as changing roles and responsibilities within the family. An older couple may perceive the stroke as a very real threat to life and to accustomed lifestyle. Reactions to this threat vary considerably but may involve fear, apprehension, denial of the severity of stroke, depression, anger, and sorrow. During the acute phase of caring for the stroke patient and the family, nursing interventions designed to facilitate coping involve providing information and emotional support.

Explanations to the patient about what has happened and about diagnostic and therapeutic procedures should be clear and understandable. It is particularly challenging to keep the aphasic patient adequately informed. Tone, demeanor, and touch may also be used to convey support.

The patient's family should be given a careful, detailed explanation of what has happened to the patient. However, if the family is extremely anxious and upset during the acute phase, explanations may need to be repeated at a later time. Because family members usually have not had time to prepare for the illness, they may need assistance in arranging care for family members or pets and for transportation and finances. A social services referral is often helpful.

Ambulatory and Home Care. The patient is usually discharged from the acute care setting to home, an intermediate or long-term care facility, or a rehabilitation facility. Criteria for transfer to rehabilitation may include the patient's ability to participate in therapies for a minimum number of hours per day. Functional status scales such as the Barthel Index, Modified Rankin Scale, and Functional Independence Measure are used to evaluate the patient.[35] Ideally, discharge planning with the patient and family starts early in the hospitalization and promotes a smooth transition from one care setting to another. The interdisciplinary team provides the guidance for the appropriate care required after discharge. If the patient requires a short- or long-term health care facility, the team can make appropriate referrals that allow time for family selection and arrangement of care. A critical factor in discharge planning is the patient's level of independence in performing ADLs. If the patient is returning home, the team can make referrals for needed equipment and services in preparation for discharge.

Nurses have an excellent opportunity to prepare the patient and family for discharge through education, demonstration and return demonstration, practice, and evaluation of self-care skills before discharge. Total care is considered in discharge planning: medications, nutrition, mobility, exercises, hygiene, and toileting. Follow-up care is carefully planned to permit continuing nursing, physical, occupational, and speech therapy, as well as medical care. Community resources should be identified to provide recreational activities, group support, spiritual assistance, respite care, adult day care, and home assistance based on the individual patient's needs.

Rehabilitation is the process of maximizing the patient's capabilities and resources to promote optimal functioning related to physical, mental, and social well-being. The goals of rehabilitation are to prevent deformity and maintain and improve function. Regardless of the care setting, ongoing rehabilitation is essential to maximize the patient's abilities.

Rehabilitation requires a team approach so the patient and family can benefit from the combined, expert care of an interdisciplinary team. The team must communicate and coordinate care to achieve the patient's and family's goals. The nurse is in a good position to facilitate this process and is often key to successful rehabilitation efforts. The patient's and family's participation in decision making during rehabilitation is essential to goal achievement after a stroke. The interdisciplinary team is composed of many members, including nurses, physicians, psychiatrist, physical therapist, occupational therapist, speech therapist, registered dietitian, respiratory therapist, vocational therapist, recreational therapist, social worker, psychologist, pharmacist, and chaplain. Physical therapy focuses on mobility, progressive ambulation, transfer techniques, and equipment needed for mobility. Occupational therapy emphasizes retraining for skills of daily living such as eating, dressing, hygiene, and cooking. Occupational therapists are also skilled in cognitive and perceptual evaluation and training. Speech therapy focuses on speech, communication, cognition, and eating abilities.

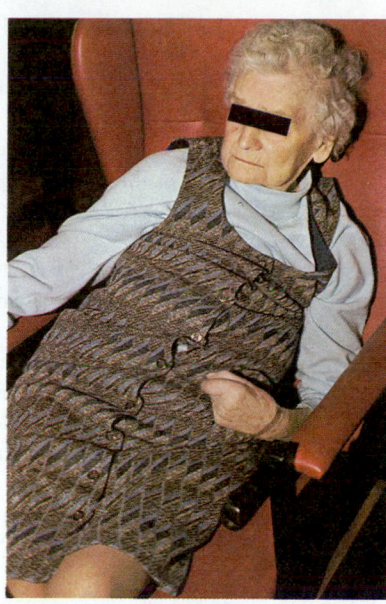

FIG. 58-12 Loss of postural stability is common after stroke. When the nondominant hemisphere is involved, walking apraxia and loss of postural control are usually apparent. The patient is unable to sit upright and tends to fall sideways. Appropriate support with pillows or cushions should be provided.

Many of the nursing interventions outlined in the nursing care plan for the patient with a stroke (see NCP 58-1) are initiated in the acute phase of care and continue throughout rehabilitation. Some of the interventions are independent nursing actions, whereas others involve the entire rehabilitation team.

The rehabilitation nurse assesses the patient and family with attention to (1) rehabilitation potential of the patient, (2) physical status of all body systems, (3) presence of complications caused by the stroke or other chronic conditions, (4) cognitive status of the patient, (5) family resources and support, and (6) expectations of the patient and family related to the rehabilitation program.

The goals for rehabilitation of the patient with stroke are mutually set by the patient, family, nurse, and other members of the rehabilitation team. The rehabilitation goals typically include the following:

- Learn techniques to self-monitor and maintain physical wellness
- Demonstrate self-care skills
- Exhibit problem-solving skills with self-care
- Avoid complications associated with stroke
- Establish and maintain a useful communication system
- Maintain nutritional and hydration status
- List community resources for equipment, supplies, and support
- Establish flexible role behaviors to promote family cohesiveness

Musculoskeletal Function. The nurse initially emphasizes the musculoskeletal functions of eating, toileting, and walking for the rehabilitation of the patient. Initial assessment consists of determining the stage of recovery of muscle function. If the muscles are still flaccid several weeks after the stroke, the prognosis for regaining function is poor and the focus of care is on preventing additional loss (Fig. 58-12). Most patients begin to show signs of spasticity with exaggerated reflexes within 48 hours following the stroke. Spasticity at this phase of stroke denotes progress toward recovery. As improvement continues, small voluntary movements of the hip or shoulder may be accompanied by involuntary movements in the rest of the extremity *(synergy)*. The final stage of recovery occurs when the patient has voluntary control of isolated muscle groups.

Interventions for the musculoskeletal system advance in a manner of progressive activity. Balance training is the initial step and begins with the patient sitting up in bed or dangling the lower extremities over the edge of the bed. The nurse evaluates tolerance by noting dizziness or syncope caused by vasomotor instability. The next step is transferring from bed to chair or wheelchair. The chair is placed beside the bed so that the patient can lead with the stronger arm and leg. The patient sits on the side of the bed, stands, places the strong hand on the far wheelchair arm, and sits down. The nurse may either supervise the transfer or provide minimal assistance by guiding the patient's strong hand to the wheelchair arm, standing in front of the patient blocking the patient's knees with the nurse's knees to prevent knee buckling, and guiding the patient into a sitting position.

In some rehabilitation units the Bobath method is used as an approach to mobility. The goal of this approach is to help the patient gain control over patterns of spasticity by inhibiting abnormal reflex patterns. Therapists and nurses use the Bobath approach to encourage normal muscle tone, normal movement, and promotion of bilateral function of the body. An example is to have the patient transfer into the wheelchair using the weak or paralyzed side and the stronger side to facilitate more bilateral functioning.

Another more recent approach to stroke rehabilitation is constraint-induced movement therapy (CIMT). CIMT encourages the patient to use the weakened extremity by restricting movement of the normal extremity. The ability of patients to comply with this approach is challenging and may limit its use.[36]

Supportive or assistive equipment, such as canes, walkers, and leg braces, may be needed on a short- or long-term basis for mobil-ity. The physical therapist usually selects the most appropriate supportive device(s) to meet individual needs and instructs the patient regarding use. The nurse should incorporate physical therapy activities into the patient's daily routine for additional practice and repetition of rehabilitation efforts.

Nutritional Therapy. After the acute phase, a dietitian can assist in determining the appropriate daily caloric intake based on the patient's size, weight, and activity level. If the patient is unable to take in an adequate oral diet, a percutaneous endoscopic gastrostomy (PEG) (see Chapter 40, Fig. 40-6) may be used for nutritional support if dysphagia persists. Most commercially prepared formulas provide about 1 calorie per milliliter. (Enteral feedings are described in Chapter 40.)

The nurse and speech therapist must assess the ability of the patient to swallow solids and fluids and adjust the diet appropriately. The dietitian plans the diet type, texture, calorie count, and fluids to meet the patient's nutritional needs. The occupational therapist and nurse must evaluate the patient's ability to feed himself or herself and recommend assistive devices to allow for independent eating. Nurses are involved in the daily planning, implementation, and evaluation of the nutritional status of the patient.

The inability to feed oneself can be frustrating and may result in malnutrition and dehydration. Interventions to promote self-feeding include using the unaffected upper extremity to eat; employing assistive devices such as rocker knives, plate guards, and nonslip pads for dishes (Fig. 58-13); removing unnecessary items from the tray or table, which can reduce spills; and providing a nondistracting environment to decrease sensory overload and distraction. The effectiveness of the dietary program is evaluated in terms of maintenance of weight, adequate hydration, and patient satisfaction.

Bowel Function. A bowel management program is implemented for problems with bowel control, constipation, or inconti-

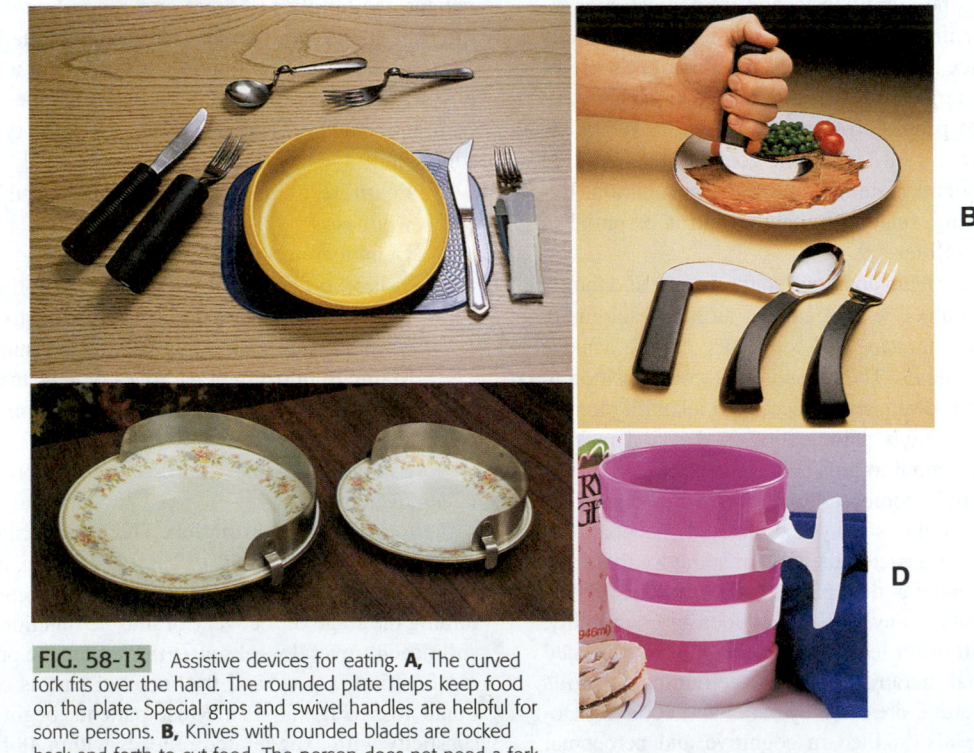

FIG. 58-13   Assistive devices for eating. **A,** The curved fork fits over the hand. The rounded plate helps keep food on the plate. Special grips and swivel handles are helpful for some persons. **B,** Knives with rounded blades are rocked back and forth to cut food. The person does not need a fork in one hand and a knife in the other. **C,** Plate guards help keep food on the plate. **D,** Cup with special handle.

nence. A high-fiber diet (see Chapter 43, Table 43-9) and adequate fluid intake (2500 to 3000 ml) are usually recommended. Patients with stroke frequently have constipation, which responds to the following dietary management:

- Fluid intake of 2500 to 3000 ml daily unless contraindicated
- Prune juice (120 ml) or stewed prunes daily
- Cooked fruit three times daily
- Cooked vegetables three times daily
- Whole-grain cereal or bread three to five times daily

The bowel management program for incontinence consists of placing the patient on the bedpan or bedside commode or taking the patient to the bathroom at a regular time daily to reestablish bowel regularity. A good time for the bowel program is 30 minutes after breakfast because eating stimulates the gastrocolic reflex and peristalsis. The time can be adjusted for individual bowel habits and preferred timing. Sitting on the commode or toilet promotes bowel elimination through both gravity and increased abdominal pressure. Stool softeners or suppositories may be ordered if the bowel program is ineffective in reestablishing bowel regularity. A glycerin suppository can be inserted 15 to 30 minutes before evacuation time to stimulate the anorectal reflex. The bisacodyl (Dulcolax) suppository is a chemical stimulant to the bowel and is used when other measures are ineffective. Ideally the suppository use is for short-term management.

Bladder Function. The nurse often assists the patient with urinary difficulties or incontinence that may follow a stroke. Often the patient with stroke has functional incontinence, which is associated with communication difficulties, mobility problems, and dressing or undressing difficulties. Nursing interventions focused on urinary continence include (1) assessment for bladder distention by palpation; (2) offering the bedpan, urinal, commode, or toilet every 2 hours during waking hours and every 3 to 4 hours at night; (3) focusing the patient on the need to urinate with direct command; (4) assistance with clothing and mobility; (5) scheduling the majority of fluid intake between 7:00 AM and 7:00 PM; and (6) encouraging the usual position for urinating (standing for men and sitting for women). Short-term interventions for urinary incontinence may include indwelling catheters, intermittent catheterization, external catheters for men, or incontinence briefs. These are not long-term solutions for urinary incontinence because complications such as urinary infections or skin irritation may occur. Assessment of postvoid residual volume is often completed by nurses using bladder ultrasound. The ultrasound measures how much urine is in the bladder following voiding. If urine remains in the bladder, incomplete emptying is a problem and may cause urinary tract infections. A coordinated program by the entire nursing staff is needed to achieve urinary continence.

Sensory-Perceptual Function. Patients who have had a stroke frequently have perceptual deficits. Patients with a stroke on the right side of the brain usually have difficulty in judging position, distance, and rate of movement. These patients are often impulsive and impatient and tend to deny problems related to strokes. They may fail to correlate spatial-perceptual problems with the inability to perform activities, such as guiding a wheelchair through the doorway. The patient with a right-brain stroke (left hemiplegia) is at higher risk for injury because of mobility difficulties. Directions for activities are best given verbally for comprehension. The task should be broken down to simple steps for ease of understanding. Environmental control, such as removing clutter and obstacles and using good lighting, aids in concentration and safer mobility. One-

sided neglect is common for people with right-brain stroke, so the nurse may assist or remind the patient to dress the weak or paralyzed side or shave the forgotten side of the face.

Patients with a left-brain stroke (right hemiplegia) commonly are slower in organization and performance of tasks. They tend to have impaired spatial discrimination. These patients usually admit to deficits and have a fearful, anxious response to a stroke. Their behaviors are slow and cautious. Nonverbal cues and instructions are helpful for comprehension with patients who have had a left-brain stroke.

Affect. Patients who have had strokes often exhibit emotional responses that are not appropriate or typical for the situation. Patients may appear apathetic, depressed, fearful, anxious, weepy, frustrated, and angry. Some patients exhibit exaggerated mood swings, especially those with a stroke on the left side of the brain (right hemiplegia). The patient may be unable to control emotions and may suddenly burst into tears or laughter. This behavior is out of context and often is unrelated to the underlying emotional state of the patient. Nursing interventions for atypical emotional response are to (1) distract the patient who suddenly becomes emotional, (2) explain to the patient and family that emotional outbursts may occur after a stroke, (3) maintain a calm environment, and (4) avoid shaming or scolding the patient during emotional outbursts.

Coping. The patient with a stroke may experience many losses, including sensory, intellectual, communicative, functional, role behavior, emotional, social, and vocational losses. The patient and family often go through the process of grief and mourning associated with the losses. Some patients experience long-term depression with symptoms such as anxiety, weight loss, fatigue, poor appetite, and sleep disturbances. In addition, the time and energy required to perform previously simple tasks can result in anger and frustration.

The patient and family need help with coping with the losses associated with stroke. The nurse may assist the coping by (1) supporting communication between the patient and family; (2) discussing lifestyle changes resulting from stroke deficits; (3) discussing changing roles and responsibilities within the family; (4) being an active listener to allow the expression of fear, frustration, and anxiety; (5) including the family and patient in short- and long-term goal planning and patient care; and (6) supporting family conferences. Maladjusted dependence with inadequate coping occurs when the patient does not maintain optimal functioning for self-care, family responsibilities, decision making, or socialization. This situation can cause resentment from both the patient and family with a negative cycle of interpersonal dependency and control. *Maladjusted independence* occurs when the patient overestimates personal cognitive or physical capabilities and energy levels. These patients are at risk for injury.

Family members must cope with three aspects of the patient's behavior: (1) recognition of behavioral changes resulting from neurologic deficits that are not changeable, (2) responses to multiple losses both by the patient and the family, and (3) behaviors that may have been reinforced during the early stages of stroke as continued dependency. The patient and family may express feelings of guilt over not living healthy lifestyles or not seeking professional help sooner. Family therapy is a helpful adjunct to rehabilitation. The patient and family need support and reassurance. Open communication, information regarding the total effects of stroke, education regarding stroke treatment, and therapy are helpful. Stroke support groups within rehabilitation facilities and in the community are helpful in terms of mutual sharing, education, coping, and understanding.

Sexual Function. A patient who has had a stroke may be concerned about the loss of sexual function. Many patients are comfortable talking about their anxieties and fears regarding sexual function if the nurse is comfortable and open to the topic. The nurse may initiate the topic with the patient and spouse or significant other. Common concerns regarding sexual activity involving the patient with a stroke are impotence and the occurrence of another stroke during sex. Nursing interventions for sexual activity include education on (1) optional positioning of partners, (2) timing for peak energy times, and (3) patient and partner counseling.

Communication. Speech, comprehension, and language deficits are the most difficult problems for the patient and family. Speech therapists can assess and formulate a plan of care to support communication. The nurse can be a role model for communication with the patient who has aphasia. Nursing interventions that support communication include (1) frequent, meaningful communication; (2) allowing time for the patient to comprehend and answer; (3) using simple, short sentences; (4) using visual cues; (5) structuring conversation so that it permits simple answers by the patient; and (6) praising the patient honestly for improvements with speech.

Community Integration. Traditionally, successful community integration following stroke has been difficult for the patient because of persistent problems with cognition, coping, physical deficits, and emotional lability that interfere with functioning. Older patients who have had a stroke often have more severe deficits and frequently experience multiple health problems. Failure to continue the rehabilitation regimen at home may result in deterioration and further complications. Advances in health care have resulted in an increased survival rate for patients with extensive stroke damage. Successful community integration can be redefined by the patient, family, and interdisciplinary health team as successful mobility, achievement of ADLs, and quality of life with family and friends.

Community resources can be an asset to patients and their families. The National Stroke Association provides information, resources, referral services, and quarterly newsletters on stroke. The American Stroke Association, a division of the American Heart Association, has information regarding stroke, hypertension, diet, exercise, and assistive devices. This association sponsors self-help groups in many areas. The Easter Seal Society provides wheelchairs and other assistive devices for stroke patients. Local groups can offer more daily assistance such as meals and transportation. These resources can be identified by nurse case managers, home health nurses, discharge planners, and clinical nurse specialists. (Resources are listed at the end of the chapter.)

GERONTOLOGIC CONSIDERATIONS
STROKE

Stroke is a significant cause of death and disability. The highest incidence of stroke occurs among older adults. Stroke can result in a profound disruption in the life of an older person. The magnitude of disability and changes in total function can leave patients wondering if they can ever return to their "old self," and loss of independence may be a major concern. The ability to perform ADLs may require many adaptive changes because of physical, emotional, perceptual, and cognitive deficits. Home management may be a particular challenge if the patient has an elderly spouse caregiver who also has health problems. There may be limited family

members (including adult children) living in close proximity to provide help.

The rehabilitative phase and assisting the older patient to deal with the residual deficits of stroke, as well as aging, can provide a challenging nursing experience. Patients may become fearful and depressed because they think they may have another attack or die. The fear can become immobilizing and interfere with effective rehabilitation.

Changes may occur in the patient-spouse relationship. The dependency resulting from a stroke may be threatening. The spouse may also have chronic medical problems that can affect the ability to take care of the stroke survivor. The patient may not want anyone other than the spouse to provide care, thus putting a significant burden on the spouse.

The nurse has the opportunity to assist the patient and family in the transition through acute hospitalization, rehabilitation, long-term care, and home care. The needs of the patient and family require ongoing nursing assessment and adaptation of interventions in response to changing needs to optimize quality of life for both the patient and family.

CRITICAL THINKING EXERCISE

CASE STUDY

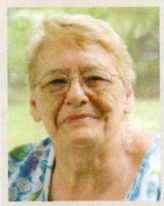

Case Study photo ©iStockphoto.com/ Roberta Osborne.

Stroke

Patient Profile. Suzanne, a 66-year-old white woman, awoke in the middle of the night and fell when she tried to get up and go to the bathroom. She fell because she was not able to control her left leg. Her husband took her to the hospital, where she was diagnosed with an acute ischemic stroke. Because she had awakened with symptoms, the actual time of onset was unknown and she was not a candidate for tPA.

Subjective Data
- Left arm and leg are weak and feel numb
- Feeling depressed and fearful
- Requires help with ADLs
- Concerned regarding having another stroke
- Says she has not taken her drugs for high cholesterol for many weeks
- History of a brief episode of left-sided weakness and tingling of the face, arm, and hand 3 months earlier, which totally resolved and for which she did not seek treatment

Objective Data
- BP 180/110
- Left-sided arm weakness (3/5) and leg weakness (4/5)
- Decreased sensation on the left side, particularly the hand
- Left homonymous hemianopsia
- Overweight
- Alert, oriented, and able to answer questions appropriately but mild slowness in responding

Critical Thinking Questions

1. How does Suzanne's prior health history put her at risk for a stroke?
2. How can the nurse address Suzanne's concerns regarding having another stroke?

3. How can Suzanne and her family address activity issues such as driving after the stroke?
4. What strategies might the home health nurse use to help Suzanne and her family cope with her feeling depressed?
5. What lifestyle changes should Suzanne make to reduce the likelihood of another stroke?
6. How will homonymous hemianopsia affect Suzanne's hygiene, eating, driving, and community activities?
7. What factors should the nurse assess for related to outpatient rehabilitation for Suzanne?
8. What are the priority nursing interventions for Suzanne?
9. Based on the assessment data provided, write one or more nursing diagnoses. Are there any collaborative problems?

NCLEX EXAMINATION REVIEW QUESTIONS

The number of the question corresponds to the same-numbered objective at the beginning of the chapter.

1. Of the following patients, the nurse recognizes that the one with the highest risk for a stroke is
   a. an obese 45-year-old Native American.
   b. a 35-year-old Asian American woman who smokes.
   c. a 32-year-old white woman taking oral contraceptives.
   d. a 65-year-old African American man with hypertension.
2. The factor related to cerebral blood flow that most often determines the extent of cerebral damage from a stroke is the
   a. amount of cardiac output.
   b. oxygen content of the blood.
   c. degree of collateral circulation.
   d. level of carbon dioxide in the blood.
3. Information provided by the patient that would help differentiate a hemorrhagic stroke from a thrombotic stroke includes
   a. sensory disturbance.
   b. a history of hypertension.
   c. presence of motor weakness.
   d. sudden onset of severe headache.
4. A patient with right-sided hemiplegia and aphasia resulting from a stroke most likely has involvement of the
   a. brainstem.
   b. vertebral artery.
   c. left middle cerebral artery.
   d. right middle cerebral artery.
5. The nurse explains to the patient with a stroke who is scheduled for angiography that this test is used to determine the
   a. presence of increased ICP.
   b. site and size of the infarction.
   c. patency of the cerebral blood vessels.
   d. presence of blood in the cerebrospinal fluid.
6. A patient experiencing TIAs is scheduled for a carotid endarterectomy. The nurse explains that this procedure is done to
   a. decrease cerebral edema.
   b. reduce the brain damage that occurs during a stroke in evolution.
   c. prevent a stroke by removing atherosclerotic plaques blocking cerebral blood flow.
   d. provide a circulatory bypass around thrombotic plaques obstructing cranial circulation.
7. Nursing management of the patient with hemiplegia during the acute phase of a stroke includes
   a. restricting active movement.
   b. positioning each joint higher than the proximal joint.

c. maintaining the patient in a recumbent, side-lying position.
d. performing passive range of motion on all limbs every 4 hours.
8. Bladder training in a male patient who has urinary incontinence after a stroke includes
   a. limiting fluid intake.
   b. keeping a urinal in place at all times.
   c. assisting the patient to stand to void.
   d. catheterizing the patient every 4 hours.
9. The most common response of the stroke patient to the change in body image is
   a. denial.
   b. depression.
   c. disassociation.
   d. intellectualization.

REFERENCES

1. American Heart Association. *Heart disease and stroke statistics: 2005 update,* Dallas, 2005, American Heart Association.
2. Heart and Stroke Foundation of Canada. Better blood pressure control dramatically reduces stroke. Available at *http://ww2.heartandstroke.bc.ca* (accessed August 30, 2006).
3. Canadian Statistics: Selected leading causes of death. Available at *www40.statcan.ca/l01/cst01/health36.htm?sdi=death* (accessed June 26, 2006).
4. Heart and Stroke Foundation of Canada. General info—stroke statistics. Available at *http://ww2.heartandstroke.bc.ca* (accessed August 30, 2006).
5. Centers for Disease Control and Prevention, National Center for Health Statistics: Stroke/cerebrovascular disease. Available at *www.cdc.gov/nchs/fastats/stroke.htm* (accessed August 30, 2006).
6. American Heart Association. Stroke risk factors. Available at *www.americanheart.org/presenter.jhtml?identifier=9217* (accessed August 30, 2006).
7. Heart and Stroke Foundation of Canada. The growing burden of heart disease and stroke. Available at *http://dsp-psd.pwgsc.gc.ca/Collection/H1-10-2003E.pdf* (accessed August 30, 2006).
8. Howard G, Felberg RA: *Regional differences in the increased stroke mortality of African Americans: the remarkable stroke burden of being a southern African American,* American Stroke Association's International Stroke Conference 2005, New Orleans, February 2-5, 2005.
9. Carmona R: The health consequences of smoking: a report of the Surgeon General. Available at *www.surgeongeneral.gov/library/smoking-consequences* (accessed August 30, 2006).
10. American Heart Association. Stroke risk factors. Available at *www.americanheart.org/presenter.jhtml?identifier=4716* (accessed August 30, 2006).
11. Gillum RF, Mussolino ME, Ingram DD: Physical activity and stroke incidence in women and men: the NHANES I epidemiologic follow-up study, *Am J Epidemiol* 143:9, 1996.
12. American Heart Association. Risk factors and coronary heart disease and stroke. Available at *www.americanheart.org/presenter.jhtml?identifier=539* (accessed August 30, 2006).
13. Weinberger J: Managing and preventing ischemic stroke: part 1—risk assessment and treatment of primary ischemic stroke, *Neurology* 12:48, 2004.
14. National Institute of Neurological Disorders and Stroke: Know Stroke. Know the Signs. Act in Time (last updated June 15, 2005). Available at *www.ninds.nih.gov/disorders/stroke/knowstroke.htm* (accessed August 30, 2006).
15. A.D.A.M. Healthcare Center: Stroke. Available at *http://adam.about.com/reports/000045.htm* (accessed August 30, 2006).
16. Gilroy J: *Basic neurology,* New York, 2000, McGraw-Hill.
17. The Merck Manual of Medical Information, hemorrhagic stroke. Available at *www.merck.com/mmhe/sec06/ch086/ch086d.html* (accessed August 30, 2006).
18. Nassisi D: Hemorrhagic stroke, New York, 2006, eMedicine. Available at *www.emedicine.com/EMERG/topic557.htm* (accessed August 30, 2006).
19. Kazzi AA, Ellis K: Subarachnoid hemorrhage, New York, 2006, eMedicine. Available at *www.emedicine.com/EMERG/topic559.htm* (accessed August 30, 2006).
20. Mathews M, Mathews M, Budut K, et al: Post-stroke depression, *Neuropsychiatry* 12:35, 2004.

21. Adams H, Adams R, Del Zoppo G, et al: Guidelines for the early management of patients with ischemic stroke, *Stroke* 36:916, 2005.

22. Cohen S: Preventing recurrent ischemic stroke: a 3-step plan, *J Family Pract* 54:412, 2005.

23. American Heart Association: What is carotid endarterectomy? Available at *www.americanheart.org/presenter.jhtml?identifier=3009563* (accessed August 30, 2006).

24. Yadav J, Wholey MH, Kuntz RE, et al: Protected carotid-artery stenting versus endarterectomy in high-risk patients, *N Engl J Med* 351:1493, 2004.

25. Society for Vascular Surgery: Final memo on carotid stent coverage Released by CMS. Available at *www.vascularweb.org/_CONTRIBUTION_PAGES/Government_Relations/Reimbursement/CMS_Coverage_Decision_on_Carotid_Stenting.html* (accessed November 30, 2005).

26. Hendrikse J, van der Zwan A, Ramos LM, et al: Hemodynamic compensation via an excimer laser-assisted, high-flow bypass before and after therapeutic occlusion of the internal carotid artery, *Neurosurgery* 53:858, 2003.

27. Miller J, Elmore S: Call a stroke code! *Nursing* 35(3):58, 2005.

28. Battison C, Andrews PJ, Graham C, et al: Randomized, controlled trial on the effect of a 20% mannitol solution and a 7.5% saline/6% dextran solution on increased intracranial pressure after brain injury, *Crit Care Med* 33:196, 2005.

29. Csokay A, Egyud L, Nagy L, et al: Vascular tunnel creation to improve the efficacy of decompressive craniotomy in post-traumatic cerebral edema and ischemic stroke, *Surg Neurol* 57:126, 2002.

30. Harvard Medical School: Aspirin study refocuses prevention message for women, *Harvard Women's Health Watch* 12:1, 2005.

31. López-Arrieta, Birks J: Nimodipine for primary degenerative, mixed and vascular dementia, *Cochrane Database Syst Rev* 1:CD000147, 2005.

32. Knies R: Research applied to clinical practice. Temperature management in acute stroke: Why does it matter? Available at *www.enw.org/Research-StrokeTemp.htm* (accessed August 30, 2006).

33. Arnold J: Stroke, ischemic (last updated March 24, 2005), New York, 2006, eMedicine. Available at *www.emedicine.com/EMERG/topic558.htm* (accessed August 30, 2006).

*34. Huhmann M, et al: Comparison of dysphagia screening by a registered dietitian in acute stroke patients to speech language pathologist's evaluation, *Top Clin Nutr* 19:239, 2004.

*35. Harris JE: Relationship of balance and mobility to fall incidence in people with chronic stroke, *Phys Ther* 85:150, 2005.

36. Barker E: New hope for stroke patients: a new therapy offers hope that movement will be restored to weakened limbs following a stroke, *RN* 68:38, 2005.

*Nursing research–based reference.

RESOURCES

American Association of Neuroscience Nurses (AANN)
888-557-2266 or 847-375-4733
www.aann.org

American Stroke Association
888-4-STROKE or 888-478-7653
www.strokeassociation.org

Association of Rehabilitation Nurses (ARN)
800-229-7530
www.rehabnurse.org

Canadian Association of Neuroscience Nurses (CANN)
www.cann.ca

Heart and Stroke Foundation of Canada
613-569-4361
www.heartandstroke.ca

National Institute of Neurological Disorders and Stroke
800-352-9424
www.ninds.nih.gov

National Stroke Association
800-STROKES (787-6537)
www.stroke.org

Society for Neuroscience
202-462-6688
www.sfn.org

For additional Internet resources, see the website for this book at *http://evolve.elsevier.com/Lewis/medsurg*.

Nursing Management
Chronic Neurologic Problems

59

Sherry Garrett Hendrickson, Stephanie A. Elms, and Virginia Shaw

LEARNING OBJECTIVES

1. Compare and contrast tension-type, migraine, and cluster headaches in terms of etiology, clinical manifestations, collaborative care, and nursing management.
2. Describe the etiology, clinical manifestations, diagnostic studies, collaborative care, and nursing management of seizure disorders, multiple sclerosis, Parkinson's disease, and myasthenia gravis.
3. Describe the clinical manifestations and nursing and collaborative management of restless legs syndrome, amyotrophic lateral sclerosis, and Huntington's disease.
4. Explain the potential impact of chronic neurologic disease on physical and psychologic well-being.
5. Outline the major goals of treatment for the patient with a chronic, progressive neurologic disease.

KEY TERMS

amyotrophic lateral sclerosis, p. 1558
epilepsy, p. 1533
headache, p. 1527
Huntington's disease, p. 1558
multiple sclerosis, p. 1542
myasthenia gravis, p. 1555
Parkinson's disease, p. 1547
restless legs syndrome, p. 1557
seizure, p. 1532

Electronic Resources

Supplemental content related to Chapter 59 can be found . . .

Companion CD
- Stress-Busting Kit for Nursing Students
- Interactive Case Studies:
  - Seizures
  - Parkinson's Disease and Hip Fracture
- NCLEX Examination Review Questions
- Comprehensive Glossary

Evolve Website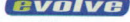
http://evolve.elsevier.com/Lewis/medsurg
- Content Updates
- Key Points (Printable and CD/MP3 Download)
- Concept Map Creator
- Expanded Audio Glossary
- Key Term Flash Cards

- Customizable Nursing Care Plans:
  - Headache
  - Multiple Sclerosis
  - Parkinson's Disease
  - Seizure Disorder or Epilepsy
- Patient and Family Instruction Guide in English and Spanish: Headache Management
- Electronic Calculators
- WebLinks

Headache

Headache is probably the most common type of pain experienced by humans. The majority of people have functional headaches, such as migraine or tension-type headaches; the remainder have organic headaches caused by intracranial or extracranial disease.

Not all tissues of the cranium are sensitive to pain. The pain-sensitive structures in the head include the venous sinuses, dura, cranial blood vessels, three divisions of the trigeminal nerve (cranial nerve [CN] V), facial nerve (CN VII), glossopharyngeal nerve (CN IX), vagus nerve (CN X), and the first three cervical nerves. Thus headache pain can arise from both intracranial and extracranial sources.

Headaches are classified using the International Headache Society (IHS) diagnostic criteria based on the characteristics of the headache. The primary classifications include tension-type, migraine, and cluster headaches. Characteristics of these headaches are shown in Table 59-1. A patient may have more than one type of headache. The history and neurologic examination are diagnostic keys to determining the type of headache.

TENSION-TYPE HEADACHE

Tension-type headache, the most common type of headache, is characterized by its bilateral location and pressing/tightening quality. Tension-type headaches are usually of mild or moderate inten-

Nervous System

TABLE 59-1	Comparison of Tension-Type, Migraine, and Cluster Headaches		
Pattern	**Tension-Type Headache**	**Migraine Headache**	**Cluster Headache**
Site	Bilateral, bandlike pressure at base of skull, in face, or in both	Unilateral (in 60%), may switch sides, commonly anterior	Unilateral, radiating up or down from one eye
Quality	Constant, squeezing tightness	Throbbing, synchronous with pulse	Severe, bone-crushing
Frequency	Cycles for several years	Periodic; cycles of several months to years	May have months or years between attacks; attacks occur in clusters: 1-3 times a day over a period of 4-8 wk
Duration	Intermittent for months or years	Continuous for hours or days	30-90 min
Time and mode of onset	Not related to time	May be preceded by prodrome; onset after awakening; gets better with sleep	Nocturnal; commonly awakens patient from sleep
Associated symptoms	Palpable neck and shoulder muscles, stiff neck, tenderness	Nausea or vomiting; edema; irritability; sweating; photophobia; phonophobia; prodrome of sensory, motor, or psychic phenomena; family history (in 65%)	Vasomotor symptoms such as facial flushing or pallor, unilateral lacrimation, ptosis, and rhinitis

GENDER DIFFERENCES
Headaches

Men
- Migraine headaches affect 6% of men.*
- Cluster headaches are more common in men.
- Exercise-induced headaches are more common in men.

Women
- Migraine headaches affect 18% of women.*

*From Lawrence EC: Diagnosis and management of migraine headaches, *South Med J* 97:1069, 2004.

sity and not aggravated by physical activity. Tension-type headaches are subcategorized as infrequent episodic, frequent episodic, or chronic.[1]

Etiology and Pathophysiology

It was originally thought that tension-type headache was the result of sustained and painful contraction of the muscles of the scalp and the neck. Recent evidence, however, does not support this mechanism in all patients with tension-type headaches. It is likely that neurovascular factors similar to those involved in migraine headaches play a role in the development of tension-type headaches.

Clinical Manifestations

There is no *prodrome* (early manifestation of impending disease) in tension-type headache. The headache does not involve nausea or vomiting but may involve sensitivity to light (*photophobia*) or sound (*phonophobia*). The headaches may occur intermittently for weeks, months, or even years. Many patients can have a combination of migraine and tension-type headaches, with features of both headaches occurring simultaneously. Patients with migraine headaches may experience tension-type headaches between migraine attacks.

Diagnostic Studies

Careful history taking is probably the most important tool for diagnosing tension-type headache. Electromyography (EMG) may be performed. This test may reveal sustained contraction of the neck, scalp, or facial muscles. However, many patients may not show increased muscle tension with this test, even when the test is done during the actual headache. Conversely, patients with diagnosed migraine headaches may show increased muscle tension on EMG. If tension-type headache is present during physical examination, increased resistance to passive movement of the head and tenderness of the head and neck may be present.

MIGRAINE HEADACHE

Migraine headache is a recurring headache characterized by unilateral or bilateral throbbing pain, a triggering event or factor, strong family history, and manifestations associated with neurologic and autonomic nervous system dysfunction. By puberty, migraine headaches are more common in girls, and by the late teens, females are about twice as likely to suffer from migraine headaches as males. The incidence of migraine headaches peaks for men and women between the ages of 25 to 55 years. In the United States the prevalence is higher in individuals of lower socioeconomic status.[2]

Etiology and Pathophysiology

Three different theories attempt to explain the etiology of migraine headaches. The vascular theory suggests that vasoconstriction followed by vasodilation with resulting changes in blood flow causes the throbbing pain. A second theory proposes that the pain is a result of muscular tension, and thus is related to tension-type headache. The third theory relates to biochemical changes, proposing that changes in the serotonin pathway result in the headache pain.[3] Serotonin, a neurotransmitter, is involved in mood, memory, sleep, temperature, and muscle function. During a migraine headache, the serotonin stored in platelets is released into the plasma and becomes inactive, thus altering the serotonin pathway.

In addition to the headache itself, migraines can be preceded by prodrome and aura. The prodrome may precede the headache phase by several hours or several days. The **aura** (sensation of light or warmth) of migraine is associated with "spreading depression," a wave of *oligemia* (diminished cerebral blood flow) beginning in the occipital lobe and spreading forward in the brain at a rate of 2 to 3 mm/min.

Migraine headaches, in many cases, have no known precipitating events. However, for other patients, the headache may be precipitated or triggered by foods, hormonal fluctuation, head trauma, physical exertion, fatigue, stress, and pharmacologic agents. Food triggers include chocolate, cheese, oranges, tomatoes, onions, monosodium glutamate, aspartame, red wine, and alcohol.[3]

Clinical Manifestations

Migraines are subdivided by the IHS into categories. The two most important are those without aura (formerly called common migraine) and those with aura (formerly called classic migraine). *Migraine without aura* is the most common type of migraine headache. *Migraine with aura* occurs in only 10% of migraine headache episodes. The sharply defined aura may last for 10 to 30 minutes before the start of the headache and may include sensory dysfunction (e.g., visual field defects, tingling or burning sensations, paresthesias), motor dysfunction (e.g., weakness, paralysis), dizziness, confusion, and even loss of consciousness.

Clinical manifestations that can occur in migraine are generalized edema, irritability, pallor, nausea and vomiting, and sweating. In migraine the prodrome is not sharply defined. The prodrome can include psychic disturbances, gastrointestinal upset, and changes in fluid balance.

During the headache phase, some patients with migraine may tend to "hibernate"; that is, they seek shelter from noise, light, odors, people, and problems. The headache is described as a steady, throbbing pain that is synchronous with the pulse. However, the presentation of migraine is varied in its severity. Not all migraine headaches are disabling, and many patients who have migraine headaches do not seek health care treatment for them. Although the headache is usually unilateral, it may switch to the opposite side in another episode. In some patients, the symptoms of the migraine headaches may become progressively worse over time.

Diagnostic Studies

There are no specific laboratory or radiologic tests for migraine headache. The diagnosis of migraine headache is usually made from the history. The neurologic and other diagnostic examinations are often normal.

The IHS criteria are used as the clinical basis for migraine diagnosis. If atypical features are present, secondary headaches must be ruled out. Neuroimaging techniques (e.g., head computed tomography [CT], with or without contrast, and magnetic resonance imaging [MRI]) are not recommended for routine evaluation of headache unless abnormal findings are found on the neurologic examination.

CLUSTER HEADACHE

Cluster headaches are a rare form of headache, affecting less than 0.1% of the population.[4] Cluster headaches involve repeated headaches that can occur for weeks to months at a time, followed by periods of remission.

Etiology and Pathophysiology

Neither the cause nor the pathophysiologic mechanism of cluster headache is fully known. The vasodilation that occurs in the affected part of the face is extracranial. The trigeminal nerve is implicated in the production of pain. Cluster headaches involve dysfunction of intracranial blood vessels, the sympathetic nervous system, and pain modulation systems. Due to the circadian rhythmicity of the headaches, the hypothalamus is believed to play a role. A genetic component has been noted in some families.[4] Smoking has been associated with cluster headache, but whether or not this association is causal remains unclear.[5] These headaches can also be triggered by alcohol ingestion.

Clinical Manifestations

The pain of cluster headache is described as sharp and stabbing, which is in contrast to the pulsing pain of the migraine headache. The cluster headache is one of the most severe forms of headache, with intense pain typically lasting about 1 hour. The pain is generally located around the eye, radiating to the temple, forehead, cheek, nose, or gums. Other manifestations may include swelling around the eye, lacrimation (tearing), facial flushing or pallor, rhinitis, and constriction of the pupil. During the headache, the patient is often agitated and restless, unable to sit still or relax. The headaches occur with regularity, usually occurring at the same time each day, during the same seasons of the year. Headaches typically last for 4 to 8 weeks, and then go into remission for months to years.

Diagnostic Studies

The diagnosis of cluster headache is primarily based on the history. Asking patients to keep a headache diary can be useful. However, CT scan, MRI, or magnetic resonance angiography (MRA) may be performed to rule out an aneurysm, tumor, or infection.

OTHER TYPES OF HEADACHES

Although tension, migraine, and cluster headaches are by far the most common types of headaches, other types of headaches can occur. These headaches may be the first symptom of a more serious illness. Headache can accompany subarachnoid hemorrhage; brain tumors; other intracranial masses; arteritis; vascular abnormalities; trigeminal neuralgia (tic douloureux); diseases of the eyes, nose, and teeth; and systemic illness (e.g., bacteremia, carbon monoxide poisoning, mountain sickness, polycythemia vera). The symptoms vary greatly. Because of the variety of causes of headache, clinical evaluation must be thorough. It should include an evaluation of personality, life adjustment, environment, and family situation, as well as a comprehensive evaluation of neurologic and physical status.

Collaborative Care for Headaches

If no systemic underlying disease is found, therapy is directed toward the functional type of headache. Table 59-2 outlines the general workup for a patient with headache to rule out any intracranial or extracranial disease. Table 59-3 summarizes the current therapies for prophylaxis and symptomatic relief of common headaches. These therapies include drugs, meditation,

TABLE 59-2	*DIAGNOSTIC STUDIES* **Headaches**

History and physical examination
Neurologic examination (often negative)
- Inspection for local infections
- Palpation for tenderness, bony swellings
- Auscultation for bruits over major arteries
Routine laboratory studies
- CBC
- Electrolytes
- Urinalysis
CT scan of sinuses
Special studies (e.g., CT scan, angiography, EMG, EEG, MRA, MRI)

CBC, Complete blood count; *CT,* computed tomography; *EEG,* electroencephalography; *EMG,* electromyography; *MRA,* magnetic resonance angiography; *MRI,* magnetic resonance imaging.

Nervous System

TABLE 59-3	*COLLABORATIVE CARE* Headaches		
	Tension-Type Headache	**Migraine Headache**	**Cluster Headache**
Diagnostic	History of neck and head tenderness, resistance to movement	History*	History
Collaborative Therapy			

Symptomatic	Nonopioid analgesics: aspirin, ibuprofen, acetaminophen
	Analgesic combinations:
	   butalbital and aspirin (Fiorinal)
	   butalbital and acetaminophen (Fioricet)
	   dichloralphenazone, acetaminophen, and isometheptene (Midrin)
	Muscle relaxants
		Nonopioid analgesics: aspirin, acetaminophen, ibuprofen
		Serotonin receptor agonists:
		   almotriptan (Axert)
		   eletriptan (Relpax)
		   frovatriptan (Frova)
		   naratriptan (Amerge)
		   rizatriptan (Maxalt)
		   sumatriptan (Imitrex)
		   zolmitriptan (Zomig)
		α-Adrenergic blockers: ergotamine tartrate (Ergomar), dihydroergotamine (D.H.E 45)
		Analgesic combination: acetaminophen, dichloralphenazone, and isometheptene (Midrin)
		Corticosteroids: dexamethasone (Decadron)
			α-Adrenergic blockers: ergotamine tartrate
			Vasoconstrictors
			Oxygen

Prophylactic	Tricyclic antidepressants:
	   doxepin (Sinequan)
	   amitriptyline (Elavil)
	β-Adrenergic blockers: propranolol (Inderal)
	Biofeedback
	Psychotherapy
	Muscle relaxation training
		β-Adrenergic blockers: propranolol (Inderal)
		Antidepressants:
		   amitriptyline (Elavil)
		   imipramine (Tofranil)
		Antiseizure:
		   valproate (Depakene)
		   topiramate (Topamax)
		Calcium channel blockers: verapamil (Isoptin)
		Serotonin antagonist:† methysergide (Sansert)
		Botox (BoNT-A)
		Biofeedback
		Relaxation therapy
		Cognitive-behavioral therapy
			α-Adrenergic blockers:
			   ergotamine tartrate
			Serotonin antagonist:
			   methysergide (Sansert)
			Corticosteroids: prednisone
			Calcium channel blockers:
			   verapamil (Isoptin)
			   lithium
			Biofeedback

*Magnetic resonance imaging (MRI) should be considered in nonacute headache patients with unexplained abnormal neurologic examination, atypical headache, headache features, or an additional risk factor such as immune deficiency.
†Only for patients suffering from one or more severe headaches per week.

yoga, biofeedback, cognitive-behavioral therapy, and relaxation training.

Biofeedback involves the use of physiologic monitoring equipment to give the patient information regarding muscle tension and peripheral blood flow (e.g., skin temperature of the fingers). The patient is trained to relax the muscles and raise the finger temperature, and is given reinforcement (operant conditioning) in accomplishing these changes.

Cognitive-behavioral therapy and relaxation therapy used alone or in conjunction with drug therapy may be beneficial to some patients. Acupuncture, acupressure, and hypnosis are also therapies that have worked well in some patients with headaches. These therapies are described further in Chapter 8.

Drug Therapy

Tension-Type Headache. Drug treatment for tension-type headache usually involves a nonopioid analgesic (e.g., aspirin, acetaminophen) used alone or in combination with a sedative, muscle relaxant, tranquilizer, or codeine. However, many of these drugs have serious side effects. The patient should be cautioned about the long-term use of aspirin and aspirin-containing drugs because they can cause upper gastrointestinal (GI) bleeding and coagulation abnormalities in susceptible patients. Long-term use

of Fiorinal should be avoided because, in addition to aspirin, it contains a barbiturate (butalbital), which may be habit forming. Drugs containing acetaminophen (Tylenol, Phenaphen, Midrin) can cause kidney damage with chronic use and liver damage when combined with alcohol.

Migraine Headache. Drug treatment of the acute migraine attack is aimed at terminating or decreasing the symptoms of the attack. Many people with mild or moderate migraine can obtain relief with aspirin or acetaminophen. For moderate to severe headaches, the triptans have become the first line of therapy. Triptans are drugs that affect selected serotonin receptors, and treat the primary cause of migraine. These drugs reduce the neurogenic inflammation of the cerebral blood vessels and produce vasoconstriction. They include sumatriptan (Imitrex), naratriptan (Amerge), rizatriptan (Maxalt), almotriptan (Axert), frovatriptan (Frova), zolmitriptan (Zomig), and eletriptan (Relpax). Some patients respond better to one triptan than to others, so health care providers need to be knowledgeable about all of them. Because these drugs cause constriction of coronary arteries, they need to be avoided in patients with heart disease. Triptans should be taken at the first symptom of migraine headache. When triptans are contraindicated, other drugs can be used (see Table 59-3).

EVIDENCE-BASED PRACTICE

Are Noninvasive Physical Treatments for Chronic Headaches Effective?

Clinical Question
In adults with chronic headaches (P), are noninvasive physical treatments (I) more effective than other treatments (C) in short- and long-term pain outcomes (O)?

Best Available Evidence
Systematic review of randomized controlled trials (RCTs)

Critical Appraisal and Synthesis of Evidence
- 22 RCTs ($n = 2628$) of individuals with five types of headaches: chronic or recurrent tension-type, cluster, cervicogenic,* migraine, and posttraumatic headaches.
- Nonphysical treatments included therapeutic heat/cold, traction, electrical stimulation, interferential therapy, electromagnetic therapy, microcurrent, ultrasound, laser, exercise, spinal manipulation, massage, reflexology, stretching, and trigger-point therapy.
- Treatments were compared either to placebo or to other available treatments.

Conclusions
- As a prophylactic treatment for migraine headache, spinal manipulation was more effective in the short term when compared to medication.
- As a prophylactic treatment for tension-type headache, many treatments with weak evidence of effectiveness were found.
- As a prophylactic treatment for cervicogenic headache, neck exercises and spinal manipulation were effective in the short and long term when compared to no treatment.

Implications for Nursing Practice
- Inform patients of the potential benefit and low risk of side effects with noninvasive treatments for chronic/recurrent headaches.
- Provide resource information about these treatments to patients.

Reference for Evidence
Bronfort G, Nilsson N, Haas M, et al: Non-invasive physical treatments for chronic/recurrent headache, Cochrane Pain, Palliative, and Supportive Care Group, *Cochrane Database Syst Rev* 4:CD001878, 2005.

PICO: P, Patient population of interest; *I,* intervention or area of interest; *C,* comparison of interest or comparison group; *O,* outcome(s) of interest (see p. 6).
*A condition in which headaches, particularly those classified as muscle tension headaches, involve referred pain and are the result of cervical subluxations.

Drug Alert - Sumatriptan (Imitrex)
- *Should not be given to patients with*
  - *history or manifestations of ischemic cardiac, cerebrovascular, or peripheral vascular problems.*
  - *uncontrolled hypertension as it may increase blood pressure.*
- *Excess dosage may produce tremor, decreased respirations.*

There is growing evidence for the role of preventive treatment in the management of migraine headaches.[6,7] The decision to initiate prophylactic treatment is individually determined based on frequency and severity of headaches as well as on any disability due to headaches. Topiramate (Topamax), taken daily, has been shown to be an effective therapy for migraine prevention in adults. Common side effects include hypoglycemia, paresthesia, weight loss, and cognitive changes. Usually these side effects are mild to moderate, and transient in nature. Topiramate must be used for 2 to 3 months to determine its effectiveness. Not all patients will become pain free on this medication. Health care providers must provide adequate teaching regarding topiramate in order to promote patient compliance.

Drug Alert - Topiramate (Topamax)
Instruct patient to
- *not abruptly discontinue as this may cause seizures.*
- *avoid tasks that require alertness until response to drug is established.*
- *take adequate fluid intake to decrease risk of renal stone development.*

Other preventive drugs for migraine headaches include β-adrenergic blockers (e.g., propranolol [Inderal], atenolol [Tenormin]), tricyclic antidepressants (e.g., amitriptyline [Elavil]), selective serotonin reuptake inhibitors (e.g., fluoxetine [Prozac]), calcium channel blockers (e.g., verapamil [Isoptin]), divalproex (Depakote), clonidine (Catapres), and thiazides. Another drug, methysergide (Sansert), competitively blocks serotonin receptors in the central and peripheral nervous systems. However, because of side effects, including retroperitoneal, pulmonary, and cardiac fibrosis, the patient taking methysergide requires regular follow-up. It is recommended that a patient taking methysergide have a break (drug holiday) every 4 to 6 months.

Botox [BoNT-A] is being successfully used in the prophylactic treatment of chronic daily headaches and migraines with minimal side effects. However, it is less likely to be effective in patients who have had migraine headaches with a duration greater than 30 years.[8,9]

Cluster Headache. Because cluster headaches occur suddenly, often at night, and are not long lasting, drug therapy is not as useful as it is for the other types of headaches. Prophylactic drugs may include verapamil, lithium, ergotamine, divalproex, or nonsteroidal antiinflammatory drugs (NSAIDs). Acute treatment of cluster headache is inhalation of 100% oxygen delivered at a rate of 7 to 9 L/min for 15 to 20 minutes, which may relieve headache by causing vasoconstriction. It can be repeated after a 5-minute rest. However, a drawback to this treatment is that the patient must have continuous access to the oxygen supply. Sumatriptan is also effective in treating acute cluster headache. Methysergide may be used prophylactically when the cluster headache recurs at a known time.

Other Headaches. Patients with frequent headaches may overuse analgesic drugs. Medication overuse headache (MOH), formerly referred to as analgesic rebound headache, is now an International Headache Society (IHS) classification. The dynamics of MOH probably involve factors beyond pain alone.[10] Drugs known to cause this problem are acetaminophen, aspirin, NSAIDs (e.g., ibuprofen), butalbital, sumatriptan, and opioids. Patients with daily headaches may complain of early awakening with decreased appetite, nausea, restlessness, decreased memory, and irritability. Treatment involves abrupt withdrawal of the offending drug (except for opioids, which need to be tapered) and initiation of alternative drugs such as amitriptyline.

NURSING MANAGEMENT
HEADACHES

■ Nursing Assessment
Subjective and objective data that should be obtained from a patient with headache are presented in Table 59-4. Because the history provides the key to assessment of headache, it should include specific details of the headache itself, such as the location and type of pain, onset, frequency, duration, relation to events (emotional, psychologic, physical), and time of day of the occurrence. Infor-

TABLE 59-4	*NURSING ASSESSMENT* **Headaches**

Subjective Data
Important Health Information
Past health history: Seizures, cancer, recent fall or trauma, cranial infection, stroke; asthma or allergies; mental illness; relationship of headache to overwork, stress, menstruation, exercise, food, sexual activity, travel, bright lights, or noxious environmental stimuli
Medications: Use of hydralazine (Apresoline), bromides, nitroglycerin, ergotamine (withdrawal), nonsteroidal antiinflammatory drugs (in high daily doses), estrogen preparations, oral contraceptives, over-the-counter or prescription remedies
Surgery or other treatments: Craniotomy, sinus surgery, facial surgery

Functional Health Patterns
Health perception–health management: Positive family history; malaise
Nutritional-metabolic: Ingestion of alcohol, caffeine, cheese, chocolate, monosodium glutamate, aspartame, lunch meats (nitrites in cured meats), sausage, hot dogs, onions, avocados; anorexia, nausea, vomiting (migraine prodrome); unilateral lacrimation (cluster)
Activity-exercise: Vertigo, fatigue, weakness, paralysis, fainting
Sleep-rest: Insomnia
Cognitive-perceptual:
- Migraine: Aura; unilateral, severe, throbbing (possible switching of side) headache; visual disturbances; photophobia; phonophobia; dizziness; tingling or burning sensations
- Cluster: Unilateral and severe, nocturnal headache; nasal stuffiness
- Tension-type: Bilateral, bandlike, dull and persistent, base-of-skull headache, neck tenderness

Self-perception–self-concept: Depression
Coping–stress tolerance: Stress, anxiety, irritability, withdrawal

Objective Data
General
Anxiety, apprehension

Integumentary
Cluster: Forehead diaphoresis, pallor, unilateral facial flushing with cheek edema, conjunctivitis
Migraine: Generalized edema (prodrome), pallor, diaphoresis

Neurologic
Horner's syndrome, restlessness (cluster), hemiparesis (migraine)

Musculoskeletal
Resistance of head and neck movement, nuchal rigidity (meningeal, tension-type), palpable neck and shoulder muscles (tension-type)

Possible Findings
Possible evidence of disease, deformity, or infection on brain imaging (CT, MRI, MRA), cerebral angiogram, lumbar puncture, EEG, EMG; nonspecific brain imaging or laboratory tests

CT, Computed tomography; *EEG,* electroencephalography; *EMG,* electromyography; *MRA,* magnetic resonance angiography; *MRI,* magnetic resonance imaging.

mation about previous illnesses, surgery, trauma, allergies, family history, and response to medication should also be obtained. The nurse can suggest that the patient keep a diary of headache episodes with specific details. This type of record can be of great help in determining the type of headache and the precipitating events. If the patient has a history of migraine, tension-type, or cluster headaches, it is important to determine if the character, intensity, or location of the headache has changed. This may be an important clue as to the cause of the headache.

■ *Nursing Diagnoses*

Nursing diagnoses for the patient with headache may include, but are not limited to, those presented in NCP 59-1.

■ *Planning*

The overall goals are that the patient with a headache will (1) have reduced or no pain, (2) experience increased comfort and decreased anxiety, (3) demonstrate understanding of triggering events and treatment strategies, (4) use positive coping strategies to deal with chronic pain, and (5) experience increased quality of life and decreased disability.

■ *Nursing Implementation*

Patients with chronic headache present a great challenge to health care providers. Headaches may be related to an inability to cope with daily stresses. The most effective therapy may be to help patients examine their lifestyle, recognize stressful situations, and learn to cope with them more appropriately. Precipitating factors can be identified, and ways of avoiding them can be developed. Daily exercise, relaxation periods, and socializing can be encouraged because each can help decrease the recurrence of headache. The nurse can suggest alternative ways of handling the pain of headache through techniques such as relaxation, meditation, yoga, and self-hypnosis.

In addition to using analgesics and analgesic combination drugs for the symptomatic relief of headache, the patient should be encouraged to use relaxation techniques because they are effective in relieving tension-type and migraine headaches. The migraine sufferer often needs a quiet, dimly lit environment. Massage and moist hot packs to the neck and head can help a patient with tension-type headaches. The patient should learn about the drugs prescribed for prophylactic and symptomatic treatment of headache and should be able to describe the purpose, action, dosage, and side effects of the drug. To prevent accidental overdose, the patient should make a written note of each dose of drug or headache remedy.

For the patient whose headaches are triggered by food, dietary counseling may be provided. The patient needs to be encouraged to eliminate foods that may provoke headaches, such as chocolate, cheese, oranges, tomatoes, onions, monosodium glutamate, aspartame, alcohol (particularly red wine), excessive caffeine, and fermented or marinated foods. Active challenge and provocative testing with specific foods may be necessary to determine the specific causative agents. However, food triggers may change over time. Patients should avoid smoking and exposure to triggers such as strong perfumes, volatile solvents, and gasoline fumes. Cluster headache attacks may occur at high altitudes with low oxygen levels during air travel. Ergotamine, taken before the plane takes off, may decrease the likelihood of these attacks. A teaching guide for the patient with a headache is presented in Table 59-5.

■ *Evaluation*

Expected outcomes for the patient with headache are addressed in NCP 59-1.

Chronic Neurologic Disorders

SEIZURE DISORDERS AND EPILEPSY

Seizure is a paroxysmal, uncontrolled electrical discharge of neurons in the brain that interrupts normal function. Seizures are often symptoms of an underlying illness. They may accompany a variety of disorders, or they may occur spontaneously without any apparent cause. Seizures resulting from systemic and metabolic disturbances are not considered epilepsy if the seizures cease when the underlying problem is corrected. In the adult, metabolic disturbances that

NURSING CARE PLAN 59-1

Patient with Headache

NURSING DIAGNOSIS **Acute pain** *related to* headache *as evidenced by* complaint of steady, throbbing, or severe crushing pain

PATIENT GOALS 1. Reports satisfaction with pain relief
2. Uses pharmacologic and nonpharmacologic measures appropriately to manage pain

OUTCOMES (NOC)	INTERVENTIONS (NIC) and *RATIONALES*
Pain Control	**Pain Management**
• Describes causal factors ____	• Perform a comprehensive assessment of pain to include location, characteristics, onset/duration, frequency, quality, intensity or severity of pain, and precipitating factors *to determine appropriate interventions.*
• Uses diary to monitor symptoms over time ____	• Utilize appropriate assessment method that allows for monitoring of change in pain and that will assist in identifying actual and potential precipitating factors (e.g., flowsheet, daily diary) *to provide patient some control in identifying and controlling factors that may precipitate headaches.*
• Uses preventive measures ____	
• Uses nonanalgesic relief measures ____	
• Uses analgesics appropriately ____	• Teach the use of nonpharmacologic techniques (e.g., biofeedback, relaxation, guided imagery, music therapy, distraction, and massage) before pain occurs or increases, and along with other pain-relief measures *to provide sense of control over pain.*
• Reports pain controlled ____	
Measurement Scale	• Provide the person optimal pain relief with prescribed analgesics *to reduce pain.*
1 = Never demonstrated	• Evaluate the effectiveness of the pain-control measures used through ongoing assessment of the pain experience *to assess efficacy and identify adverse drug effects.*
2 = Rarely demonstrated	
3 = Sometimes demonstrated	• Consider referrals for patient, family, and significant others to support groups and other resources *to reduce stress.*
4 = Often demonstrated	
5 = Consistently demonstrated	

TABLE 59-5	*PATIENT AND FAMILY TEACHING GUIDE* Headaches

1. Keep a diary or calendar of headaches and possible precipitating events.
2. Avoid factors that can trigger a headache:
   - Foods containing amines (cheese, chocolate), nitrites (meats such as hot dogs), vinegar, onions, monosodium glutamate
   - Fermented or marinated foods
   - Caffeine
   - Oranges
   - Tomatoes
   - Onions
   - Aspartame
   - Nicotine
   - Ice cream
   - Alcohol (particularly red wine)
   - Emotional stress
   - Fatigue
   - Drugs such as ergot-containing preparations and monoamine oxidase inhibitors
3. Describe the purpose, action, dosage, and side effects of drugs taken.
4. Be able to self-administer sumatriptan (Imitrex) subcutaneously if prescribed.
5. Use stress reduction techniques such as relaxation.
6. Participate in regular exercise.
7. Contact health care provider if the following occur:
   - Symptoms become more severe, last longer than usual, or are resistant to medication
   - Nausea and vomiting (if severe or not typical), change in vision, or fever occurs with the headache
   - Problems with drugs

Epilepsy is a condition in which a person has spontaneously recurring seizures caused by a chronic underlying condition. In the United States it is estimated that approximately 2.7 million people suffer from active epilepsy, with 200,000 new cases being diagnosed each year.[11] The prevalence of epilepsy in Canada is 5.2 to 5.6 per 1000 persons, and generally 5 to 10 per 1000 persons in other developed countries.[12,13] It is higher in underdeveloped countries. The incidence rates are high during the first year of life, decline through childhood and adolescence, plateau in middle age, and rise sharply again among the elderly. The population with the highest prevalence of new-onset epilepsy is those over the age of 60.[14]

Etiology and Pathophysiology

The most common causes of seizure disorder during the first 6 months of life are severe birth injury, congenital defects involving the central nervous system (CNS), infections, and inborn errors of metabolism. In patients between 2 and 20 years of age, the primary causative factors are birth injury, infection, trauma, and genetic factors. In individuals between 20 and 30 years of age, seizure disorder usually occurs as the result of structural lesions, such as trauma, brain tumors, or vascular disease. After 50 years of age the primary causes of seizure disorders are cerebrovascular lesions and metastatic brain tumors. Although many causes of seizure disorders have been identified, three fourths of all seizure disorder cases cannot be attributed to a specific cause and are considered *idiopathic.*

The role of heredity in the etiology of seizure disorders has been difficult to determine because of the problem of separating hereditary from environmental or acquired influences. In addition, some families carry a predisposition to seizure disorders in the form of an inherently low threshold to seizure-producing stimuli, such as trauma, disease, and high fever. The etiology of recurring seizures (epilepsy) has long been attributed to a group of abnormal neurons *(seizure focus)* that seem to undergo spontaneous firing. This firing spreads by physiologic pathways to involve adjacent or distant areas

cause seizures include acidosis, electrolyte imbalances, hypoglycemia, hypoxia, alcohol and barbiturate withdrawal, dehydration, and water intoxication. Extracranial disorders that can cause seizures are heart, lung, liver, or kidney diseases; systemic lupus erythematosus; diabetes mellitus; hypertension; and septicemia.

of the brain. If this activity spreads to involve the whole brain, a generalized seizure occurs. The factor that causes this abnormal firing is not clear. Any stimulus that causes the cell membrane of the neuron to depolarize induces a tendency to spontaneous firing. Often the area of the brain from which the epileptic activity arises is found to have scar tissue *(gliosis)*. The scarring is thought to interfere with the normal chemical and structural environment of the brain neurons, making them more likely to fire abnormally. Since epilepsy results from long-lasting changes in the brain, a vigorous attempt must be made to control recurring seizures.

Previously epilepsy research focused on neuronal causes. However, there is now evidence that astrocytes, or cerebral support cells, may play a key role in recurring seizures. Astrocytes release glutamate that triggers synchronous firing of neurons. Therefore drug therapy focused on suppressing astrocyte signaling or decreasing glutamate release may be a mechanism to achieve seizure control.[14]

Clinical Manifestations

The specific clinical manifestations of a seizure are determined by the site of the electrical disturbance. The preferred method of classifying recurring seizures is the International Classification System[15] (Table 59-6). This system is based on the clinical and electroencephalographic manifestations of seizures. In this system, seizures are divided into two major classes: *generalized* and *partial* (Fig. 59-1). Depending on the type, a seizure may progress through several phases, which include (1) the *prodromal phase,* with signs or activity which precede a seizure; (2) the *aural phase,* with a sensory warning; (3) the *ictal phase,* with full seizure; and (4) the *postictal phase,* which is the period of recovery after the seizure.

Generalized Seizures. **Generalized seizures** involve both sides of the brain and are characterized by bilateral synchronous epileptic discharges in the brain from the onset of the seizure. Because the entire brain is affected at the onset of the seizures, there is no warning or aura. In most cases, the patient loses consciousness for a few seconds to several minutes.

Tonic-Clonic Seizures. The most common generalized seizure is the generalized tonic-clonic (formerly known as *grand mal*) seizure. **Tonic-clonic seizure** is characterized by loss of consciousness and falling to the ground if the patient is upright, followed by stiffening of the body (tonic phase) for 10 to 20 seconds and subsequent jerking of the extremities (clonic phase) for another 30 to 40 seconds. Cyanosis, excessive salivation, tongue or cheek biting, and incontinence may accompany the seizure.

In the postictal phase the patient usually has muscle soreness, is very tired, and may sleep for several hours. Some patients may not feel normal for several hours or days after a seizure. The patient has no memory of the seizure.

Typical Absence Seizures. The **absence (petit mal) seizure** usually occurs only in children and rarely continues beyond adolescence. This type of seizure may cease altogether as the child matures, or it may evolve into another type of seizure. The typical clinical manifestation is a brief staring spell that lasts only a few

TABLE 59-6	International Classification of Seizure Disorders

Generalized Seizures (Nonfocal Origin)
Tonic-clonic seizures
Absence seizures
Myoclonic seizures
Tonic seizures
Atonic seizures
Clonic seizures

Partial Seizures (Focal Origin)
Simple partial seizures (no impairment of consciousness)
- With motor signs
- With sensory symptoms
- With autonomic symptoms
- With psychic symptoms
Complex partial seizures (impairment of consciousness)
- Simple partial onset followed by impaired consciousness
- Impairment of consciousness at onset
- With automatisms
Partial seizures evolving to secondary generalized seizures

Unclassified Epileptic Seizures

Adapted from Task Force on Epilepsy Classification and Treatment: Seizure types, International League Against Epilepsy, 2006. Available at *www.ilae-epilepsy.org/ Visitors/Centre/ctf/seizure_types.cfm.*

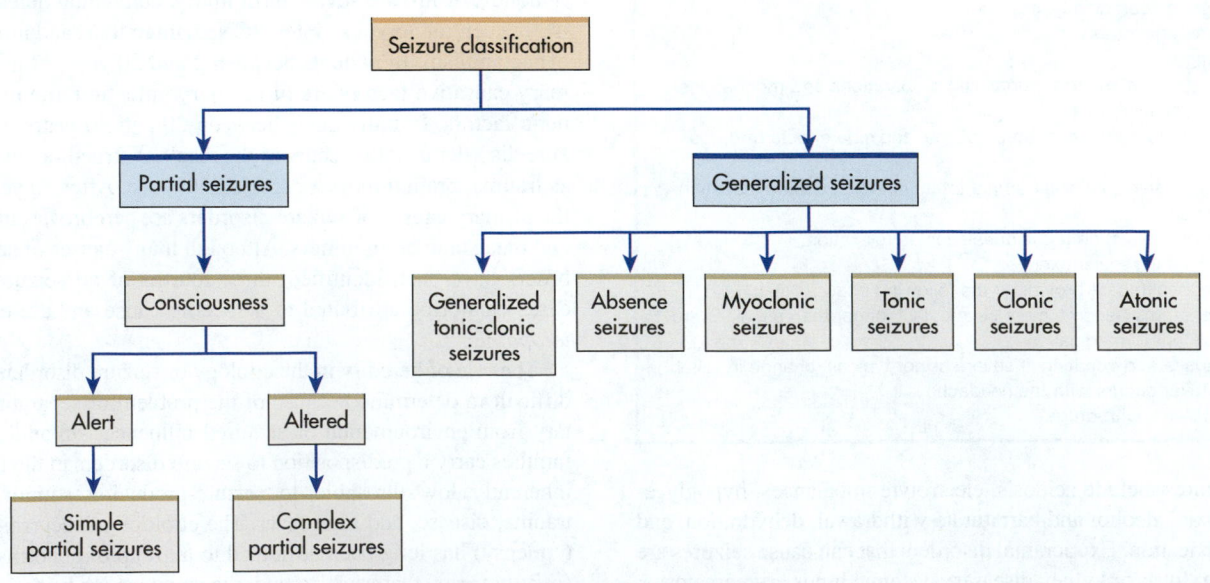

FIG. 59-1   Algorithm for classification of seizures.

seconds, so it often occurs unnoticed. There may be an extremely brief loss of consciousness. When untreated, the seizures may occur up to 100 times a day.

The electroencephalogram (EEG) demonstrates a 3-Hz (cycles per second) spike-and-wave pattern that is unique to this type of seizure. Absence seizures can often be precipitated by hyperventilation and flashing lights.

Atypical Absence Seizures. Another type of generalized seizure is **atypical absence seizure,** which is characterized by a staring spell accompanied by other signs and symptoms, including brief warnings, peculiar behavior during the seizure, or confusion after the seizure. The EEG demonstrates atypical spike-and-wave patterns, usually greater or less than 3 Hz.

Other Types of Generalized Seizures. Other generalized seizures are myoclonic, atonic, tonic, and clonic seizures. A *myoclonic seizure* is characterized by a sudden, excessive jerk of the body or extremities. The jerk may be forceful enough to hurl the person to the ground. These seizures are very brief and may occur in clusters.

An *atonic* ("drop attack") seizure involves either a tonic episode or a paroxysmal loss of muscle tone and begins suddenly with the person falling to the ground. Consciousness usually returns by the time the person hits the ground, and normal activity can be resumed immediately. Patients with this type of seizure are at a great risk of head injury and often have to wear protective helmets. A *tonic* seizure involves a sudden onset of maintained increased tone in the extensor muscles. These patients often fall. *Clonic* seizures begin with loss of consciousness and sudden loss of muscle tone, followed by limb jerking that may or may not be symmetric.

Partial Seizures. **Partial seizures** are the other major class of seizures in the International Classification System. They are also referred to as partial focal seizures. They are caused by focal irritations. They manifest with unilateral manifestations that arise from localized brain involvement. Partial seizures begin in a specific region of the cortex, as indicated by the EEG and usually by the clinical manifestations. For example, if the discharging focus is located in the medial aspect of the postcentral gyrus, the patient may experience paresthesias and tingling or numbness in the leg on the side opposite the focus. If the discharging focus is located in the part of the brain that governs a particular function, sensory, motor, cognitive, or emotional manifestations may occur.

Partial seizures may be confined to one side of the brain and remain partial or focal in nature, or they may spread to involve the entire brain, culminating in a generalized tonic-clonic seizure. Any tonic-clonic seizure that is preceded by an aura or warning is a partial seizure that generalizes secondarily. Many tonic-clonic seizures that appear to be generalized from the outset may actually be secondary generalized seizures, but the preceding partial component may be so brief that it is undetected by the patient, by the observer, or even on the EEG. Unlike the primary generalized tonic-clonic seizure, the secondary generalized seizure may result in a transient residual neurologic deficit postictally. This is called *Todd's paralysis* (focal weakness), which resolves after varying lengths of time.

Partial seizures are further divided into (1) simple partial seizures (those with simple motor or sensory phenomena) and (2) complex partial seizures (those with complex symptoms). *Simple partial seizures* with elementary symptoms do not involve loss of consciousness and rarely last longer than 1 minute. They may involve motor, sensory, or autonomic phenomena or a combination

of these. The terms *focal motor, focal sensory,* and *jacksonian* have been used to describe seizures of the simple partial type.

Complex partial seizures can involve a variety of behavioral, emotional, affective, and cognitive functions. The location of the discharging focus is usually in the temporal lobe, hence the term *temporal lobe seizure.* These seizures usually last longer than 1 minute and are frequently followed by a period of postictal confusion. Complex partial seizures are distinct from simple partial (focal motor, focal sensory) seizures in that they involve some alteration in consciousness. The sole manifestation of complex partial seizures may be clouding of consciousness or a confused state without any motor or sensory components. This type of attack is sometimes termed *temporal lobe absence.* There is rarely the complete loss of consciousness that is typical of the generalized absence attack, nor does the patient snap back to the preseizure state as does the patient who has had a generalized absence attack.

The most common complex partial seizure involves lip smacking and *automatisms* (repetitive movements that may not be appropriate). These are often called *psychomotor seizures.* The patient may continue an activity that was initiated before the seizure, such as counting out change or picking items from a grocery shelf, but after the seizure does not remember the activity performed during the seizure. Other automatisms are less organized, such as picking at clothing, fumbling with objects (real or imaginary), or simply walking away.

A variety of psychosensory symptoms may occur during a complex partial seizure, including distortions of visual or auditory sensations and vertigo. There may be alterations in memory, such as a feeling of having experienced an event before (*déjà vu*), or alterations in thought processes. Alterations in sexual functioning can vary from hyposexuality to hypersexuality. In addition, some antiseizure drugs can cause a decrease in sexual drive because of sedation. Others can cause erectile dysfunction.

 Drug Alert - *Antiseizure Drugs*
• *Abrupt withdrawal after long-term use may precipitate seizures.*

Complications

Physical. **Status epilepticus** is a state of continuous seizure activity or a condition in which seizures recur in rapid succession without return to consciousness between seizures. It is the most serious complication of epilepsy and is a neurologic emergency. Status epilepticus can occur due to any type of seizure. During repeated seizures the brain uses more energy than can be supplied. Neurons become exhausted and cease to function. Permanent brain damage may result. Tonic-clonic status epilepticus is the most dangerous because it can cause ventilatory insufficiency, hypoxemia, cardiac dysrhythmias, hyperthermia, and systemic acidosis, all of which can be fatal.

Another complication of seizures is severe injury and even death from trauma suffered during a seizure. Patients who lose consciousness during a seizure are at greatest risk. Seizures occurring throughout pregnancy or during delivery may also pose potential complications to a pregnant female and her baby.

Psychosocial. Perhaps the most common complication of seizure disorders is the effect it has on a patient's lifestyle. The patient may develop ineffective coping methods because of the psychosocial problems related to having a seizure disorder. Although attitudes have improved in recent years, epilepsy still carries a social stigma. The patient with epilepsy may experience discrimina-

Nervous System

TABLE 59-7	*COLLABORATIVE CARE* **Seizure Disorders and Epilepsy**

Diagnostic
History and Physical Examination
Birth and developmental history
Significant illnesses and injuries
Family history
Febrile seizures
Comprehensive neurologic assessment

Seizure History
Precipitating factors
Antecedent events
Seizure description (including onset, duration, frequency, postictal state)

Diagnostic Studies
CBC, urinalysis, electrolytes, creatinine, fasting blood glucose
Lumbar puncture for CSF analysis
CT, MRI, MRA, MRS, PET scan
Electroencephalography (EEG)

Collaborative Therapy
Antiseizure drugs (see Table 59-9)
Surgery (see Table 59-10)
Vagal nerve stimulation
Psychosocial counseling

CBC, Complete blood count; *CSF,* cerebrospinal fluid; *CT,* computed tomography; *MRA,* magnetic resonance angiography; *MRI,* magnetic resonance imaging; *MRS,* magnetic resonance spectroscopy; *PET,* position emission tomography.

tion in employment and educational opportunities. Transportation may be difficult because of legal sanctions against driving in most states and Canada.

Diagnostic Studies

A diagnosis of epilepsy or seizure disorder has many socioeconomic, physical, and psychologic consequences for the patient. Therefore an accurate diagnosis is crucial. The most useful diagnostic tools are an accurate and comprehensive description of the seizures and the patient's health history (Table 59-7). The EEG is a useful diagnostic adjuvant to the history but only if it shows abnormalities. Abnormal findings help determine the type of seizure and help pinpoint the seizure focus. Ideally, an EEG should be done within 24 hours of a suspected seizure.[16] Unfortunately, only a small percentage of patients with seizure disorders have abnormal findings on the EEG the first time the test is done. EEGs may need to be repeated often, or continuous EEG monitoring may be needed to detect abnormalities. Abnormal discharges may not occur during the 30 to 40 minutes of sampling during EEG, and the test may never indicate an abnormality. It is not a definitive test because some patients who do not have seizure disorders have abnormal patterns on their EEGs, whereas many patients with seizure disorders have normal EEGs between seizures. Magnetoencephalography may be done in conjunction with the EEG. This test has greater sensitivity in detecting small magnetic fields generated by neuronal activity.

A complete blood count, serum chemistries, studies of liver and kidney function, and urinalysis should be done to rule out metabolic disorders. A CT scan or MRI should be done in any new-onset seizure to rule out a structural lesion. Cerebral angiography, single-photon emission computed tomography (SPECT), magnetic resonance spectroscopy (MRS), magnetic resonance angiography (MRA), and positron emission tomography (PET) may be used in selected clinical situations.

If a patient is diagnosed with a seizure disorder, it is very important to classify the seizure type correctly (see Fig. 59-1 and Table 59-6). The choice of treatment depends on the classification of the type of seizure.

Collaborative Care

Most seizures do not require professional emergency medical care because they are self-limiting and rarely cause bodily injury. However, if status epilepticus occurs, if significant bodily harm occurs, or if the event is a first-time seizure, medical care should be sought immediately. Table 59-8 summarizes emergency care of the patient with a generalized tonic-clonic seizure, the seizure most likely to warrant professional emergency medical care. The diagnostic studies and collaborative care of seizure disorders are summarized in Table 59-7.

Drug Therapy. Seizure disorders are treated primarily with antiseizure drugs (Table 59-9). Therapy is aimed at preventing seizures because cure is not possible. Drugs generally act by stabilizing nerve cell membranes and preventing spread of the epileptic discharge. In about 70% of the patients, seizure disorders are controlled by medication. The primary goal of antiseizure drug therapy is to obtain maximum seizure control with a minimum of toxic side effects. The principle of drug therapy is to begin with a single drug based on patient age, weight, type, frequency, and cause of seizure and increase the dosage until seizures are controlled or toxic side effects occur.[13] Serum levels of the drug should be monitored if seizures continue to occur, if seizure frequency increases, or if drug compliance is questioned. The therapeutic range for each drug indicates the serum level above which most patients experience toxic side effects and below which most continue to have seizures. Therapeutic ranges are only guides for therapy. If the patient's seizures are well controlled with a subtherapeutic level, the drug dose need not be increased. Likewise, if a drug level is above the therapeutic range and the patient has good seizure control without toxic side effects, the drug dose need not be decreased. Many of the newer drugs do not require drug-level monitoring because the therapeutic range is very large. If seizure control is not achieved with a single drug, the drug dosage or timing of administration may be changed or a second drug may be added. About one third of patients require a combination regimen for adequate control.[16] Another consideration that is important when evaluating antiseizure medication is the various hormonal fluctuations in females during puberty, menses, pregnancy, and menopause.

For many years the primary drugs for treatment of generalized tonic-clonic and partial seizures were phenytoin (Dilantin), carbamazepine (Tegretol), phenobarbital, and divalproex (Depakote). For treatment of absence and myoclonic seizures the drugs include ethosuximide (Zarontin), divalproex (Depakote), and clonazepam (Klonopin).

> **Drug Alert** - *Carbamazepine (Tegretol)*
> • *Do not take with grapefruit juice.*
> • *Instruct patient to report visual abnormalities.*
> • *Instruct patient that abrupt withdrawal after long-term use may precipitate seizures.*

Other drugs that have become available include gabapentin (Neurontin), lamotrigine (Lamictal), topiramate (Topamax), tiagabine (Gabitril), levetiracetam (Keppra), and zonisamide (Zonegran). Vigabatrin (Sabril), another drug, is currently only available in Canada and Europe.[17] Some of these drugs are broad spectrum and appear to be effective for multiple seizure types.

TABLE 59-8	*EMERGENCY MANAGEMENT* **Tonic-Clonic Seizures**	
Etiology	**Assessment Findings**	**Interventions**

Etiology

Head Trauma
Epidural hematoma
Subdural hematoma
Intracranial hematoma
Cerebral contusion
Traumatic birth injury

Drug-Related Processes
Overdose
Withdrawal of alcohol, opioids, antiseizure drugs
Ingestion, inhalation

Infectious Processes
Meningitis
Septicemia
Encephalitis

Intracranial Events
Brain tumor
Subarachnoid hemorrhage
Stroke
Hypertensive crisis
Increased ICP secondary to clogged shunt

Metabolic Imbalances
Fluid and electrolyte imbalance
Hypoglycemia

Medical Disorders
Heart, liver, lung, or kidney disease
Systemic lupus erythematosus

Other
Cardiac arrest
Idiopathic
Psychiatric disorders
High fever

Assessment Findings
- Aura—peculiar sensations that precede seizure
- Loss of consciousness
- Bowel and bladder incontinence
- Tachycardia
- Diaphoresis
- Warm skin
- Pallor, flushing, or cyanosis
- *Tonic phase:* continuous muscle contractions
- *Hypertonic phase:* extreme muscular rigidity lasting 5-15 sec
- *Clonic phase:* rigidity and relaxation alternate in rapid succession
- *Postictal phase:* lethargy, altered level of consciousness
- Confusion and headache
- Repeated tonic-clonic seizures for several minutes

Interventions

Initial
- Ensure patent airway.
- Assist ventilations if patient does not breathe spontaneously after seizure. Anticipate need for intubation if gag reflex absent.
- Suction as needed.
- Stay with patient until seizure has passed.
- Protect patient from injury during seizure. *Do not restrain.* Pad side rails.
- Establish IV access.
- Anticipate administration of phenobarbital, phenytoin (Dilantin), or benzodiazepines (e.g., diazepam [Valium], midazolam [Versed], lorazepam [Ativan]) to control seizures.
- Remove or loosen tight clothing.

Ongoing Monitoring
- Monitor vital signs, level of consciousness, oxygen saturation, Glasgow Coma Scale results, pupil size and reactivity.
- Reassure and orient the patient after seizure.
- Never force an airway between a patient's clenched teeth.
- Give IV dextrose for hypoglycemia.

ICP, Intracranial pressure; *IV,* intravenous.

Felbamate (Felbatol) may be used to treat patients whose seizure disorders are refractory to other drugs. However, its use is limited because it can cause aplastic anemia and liver toxicity.

Treatment of status epilepticus requires initiation of a rapid-acting antiseizure drug that can be given intravenously. The drugs most commonly used are lorazepam (Ativan) and diazepam (Valium). Because these are short-acting drugs, they must be followed by administration of long-acting drugs such as phenytoin or phenobarbital.

Current drugs used in seizure management are shown in Table 59-9. Because many of these drugs (e.g., phenytoin, phenobarbital, ethosuximide, lamotrigine, topiramate) have a long half-life, they can be given in once- or twice-daily doses. This increases the patient's compliance with taking the drug by simplifying the drug regimen and avoiding the need to take it at work or school. Antiseizure drugs should not be discontinued abruptly because this can precipitate seizures. If weaning is to occur, the patient must be seizure free for a prolonged period of time (e.g., 2 to 5 years) and have a normal neurologic exam and EEG.[16]

Side effects of antiseizure drugs involve the CNS and include diplopia, drowsiness, ataxia, and mental slowing. Neurologic assessment for dose-related toxicity involves testing the eyes for nystagmus, hand and gait coordination, cognitive functioning, and general alertness.

Idiosyncratic side effects involve organs outside the CNS, including the skin (rashes), gingiva (hyperplasia), bone marrow (blood dyscrasias), liver, and kidneys. Nurses should be knowledgeable about these side effects so that patients can be informed and proper treatment can be instituted. A common side effect of phenytoin is gingival hyperplasia (excessive growth of gingival tissue), especially in young adults. This can be limited by good dental hygiene, including regular toothbrushing and flossing. If gingival hyperplasia is extensive, the hyperplastic tissue may have to be surgically removed (gingivectomy), and phenytoin may have to be replaced by another antiseizure drug. Phenytoin can also cause hirsutism in young people.

GERONTOLOGIC CONSIDERATIONS
DRUG THERAPY

The incidence of new-onset seizure disorders is high among the elderly. Special consideration needs to be given to the use of antiseizure medications with regard to normal changes that occur with aging. For example, phenytoin is widely used in the treatment of seizure disorders. However, because it is metabolized by the liver, taking phenytoin can be a problem for older patients with compromised liver function; enzyme changes in the liver that are age related decrease the ability of the liver to metabolize drugs in older adults. Phenobarbital and primidone (Mysoline) have been shown to have potential effects on cognitive function. Therefore their use may be less desirable for the older adult. Carbamazepine (Tegretol) has many significant drug interactions.[18]

Of the newer antiseizure medications available, several seem to offer greater treatment benefit to older adults. Gabapentin and levetiracetam seem to be safer, have fewer effects on cognitive function, and have fewer interactions with other drugs. Lamotrigine has also shown to be a relatively safe drug. Oxcarbazepine (Trileptal) has better tolerability than carbamazepine. Topiramate and zonisamide are also considered safe for the older patient.[18]

Surgical Therapy. A significant number of patients whose epilepsy cannot be controlled with drug therapy are candidates for surgical intervention to remove the epileptic focus or prevent spread of epileptic activity in the brain (Table 59-10). Surgical interventions include limbic resection, primarily anterior temporal lobe resection; amygdalohippocampectomy; neocortical resection, including extratemporal resection and lesionectomies; hemispherectomies; multilobar resections; and corpus collosum sections.[19]

The benefits of surgery include cessation or reduction in frequency of the seizures. However, not all types of epilepsy benefit from surgery. An extensive preoperative evaluation is important, including continuous EEG monitoring and other specific tests to ensure precise localization of the focal point. Before surgery is performed, three requirements must be met: (1) the diagnosis of epilepsy must be confirmed, (2) there must have been an adequate trial with drug therapy without satisfactory results, and (3) the electroclinical syndrome (type of seizure disorder) must be defined.

Other Therapies. Another treatment for seizure disorders is vagal nerve stimulation. An electrode is surgically placed around the left vagus nerve in the neck. It is connected to a battery placed beneath the skin in the upper chest. The device is programmed to deliver intermittent electrical stimulation to the brain to reduce the frequency and intensity of seizures. The exact mechanism of action is unknown, although the stimulation may interrupt synchronization of epileptic brain-wave activity. This method is currently used in only a small number of patients and can cause adverse effects such as coughing, hoarseness, dyspnea, and tingling in the neck. Battery replacement is required via surgery about every 5 years.[16]

Biofeedback to control seizures is aimed at teaching the patient to maintain a certain brain-wave frequency that is refractory to seizure activity. Further trials are needed to assess the effectiveness of biofeedback for seizure control.

NURSING MANAGEMENT
SEIZURE DISORDERS AND EPILEPSY

■ *Nursing Assessment*

Subjective and objective data that should be obtained from a patient with a seizure disorder are presented in Table 59-11. Data related to a specific seizure episode can be obtained from a witness.

■ *Nursing Diagnoses*

Nursing diagnoses for the patient with seizure disorders and epilepsy may include, but are not limited to, those presented in NCP 59-2.

■ *Planning*

The overall goals are that the patient with seizures will (1) be free from injury during a seizure, (2) have optimal mental and physical functioning while taking antiseizure drugs, and (3) have satisfactory psychosocial functioning.

■ *Nursing Implementation*

Health Promotion. Many cases of seizure disorders can be prevented by promotion of general safety measures, such as the wearing of helmets in situations involving risk of head injury. Im-

TABLE 59-9	*DRUG THERAPY* **Seizure Disorders and Epilepsy**

Generalized Tonic-Clonic and Partial Seizures
carbamazepine (Tegretol)
divalproex (Depakote)
felbamate (Felbatol)
gabapentin (Neurontin)
lamotrigine (Lamictal)
levetiracetam (Keppra)
oxcarbazepine (Trileptal)
phenobarbital
phenytoin (Dilantin)
primidone (Mysoline)
tiagabine (Gabitril)
topiramate (Topamax)
valproic acid (Depakene)
vigabatrin (Sabril)*
zonisamide (Zonegran)

Absence, Akinetic, and Myoclonic Seizures
clonazepam (Klonopin)
divalproex (Depakote)
ethosuximide (Zarontin)
phenobarbital
valproic acid (Depakene)

*Available for use in Europe and Canada only.

TABLE 59-10	**Surgical Procedures for Seizure Disorders and Epilepsy**		
Type of Seizure	**Surgical Procedure**	**Results**	
Complex partial seizure of temporal lobe origin	Resectioning of epileptogenic tissue	Absence of seizures 5 yr postoperatively in 55%-70% of patients	
Partial seizures of frontal lobe origin	Resectioning of epileptogenic tissue (if in resectable area)	Absence of seizures 5 yr postoperatively in 30%-50% of patients	
Generalized seizures (Lennox-Gastaut syndrome or drop attacks)	Sectioning of corpus callosum	Persistence of seizures; less violent, less frequent, less disabling events	
Intractable unilateral multifocal epilepsy associated with infantile hemiplegia	Hemispherectomy or callosotomy	Reduction in seizure frequency and type, improvement in behavior	

proved perinatal, labor, and delivery care have reduced fetal trauma and hypoxia and thereby have reduced brain damage leading to seizure disorders.

The patient with a seizure disorder should practice good general health habits (e.g., maintaining a proper diet, getting adequate rest, exercising). The patient should be helped to identify events or situations that precipitate the seizures and should be given suggestions for avoiding them or handling them better. Excessive alcohol intake, fatigue, and loss of sleep should be avoided, and the patient should be helped to handle stress constructively.

Acute Intervention. Nursing care for a hospitalized patient with a seizure disorder or a patient who has had seizures as a result of metabolic factors involves several responsibilities, including observation and treatment of the seizure, education, and psychosocial intervention.

When a seizure occurs, the nurse should carefully observe and record details of the event because the diagnosis and subsequent treatment often rest solely on the seizure description. All aspects of the seizure should be noted. What events preceded the seizure? When did the seizure occur? How long did each phase (aural [if any], ictal, postictal) last? What occurred during each phase?

Both subjective data (usually the only type of data in the aural phase) and objective data are important. Objective data should include the exact onset of the seizure (which body part was affected first and how); the course and nature of the seizure activity (loss of consciousness, tongue biting, automatisms, stiffening, jerking, total lack of muscle tone); the body parts involved and their sequence of involvement; and the presence of autonomic signs, such as dilated pupils, excessive salivation, altered breathing, cyanosis, flushing, diaphoresis, or incontinence. Assessment of the postictal period should include a detailed description of the level of consciousness, vital signs, memory loss, muscle soreness, speech disorders (aphasia, dysarthria), weakness or paralysis, sleep period, and the duration of each sign or symptom.

During the seizure it is important to maintain a patent airway. This may involve supporting and protecting the head, turning the patient to the side, loosening constrictive clothing, or easing the patient to the floor, if seated. The patient should not be restrained, and no objects should be placed in the mouth. After the seizure the patient may require suctioning, and oxygen may be needed.

A seizure can be a frightening experience for the patient and for others who may witness it. The nurse should assess the level of their understanding and provide information about how and why the event occurred. This is an excellent opportunity for the nurse to dispel many common misconceptions about seizures.

Ambulatory and Home Care. Prevention of recurring seizures is the major goal in the treatment of epilepsy. Because many seizure disorders cannot be cured, drugs must be taken regularly and continuously, often for a lifetime. The nurse should ensure that the patient knows this, as well as the specifics of the drug regimen and what to do if a dose is missed. Usually the dose should be made up if the omission is remembered within 24 hours. The patient should be cautioned not to adjust drug doses without professional guidance because this can increase seizure frequency and even cause status epilepticus. The patient should be encouraged to report any medication side effects and to keep regular appointments with the health care provider.

Nurses play an important role in teaching the patient and the family. Guidelines for teaching are shown in Table 59-12. Nurses should teach family members and significant others the emergency management of tonic-clonic seizures (see Table 59-8). They should be reminded that it is not necessary to call an ambulance or send a person to the hospital after a single seizure unless the seizure is prolonged, another seizure immediately follows, or extensive injury has occurred.

TABLE 59-11	**NURSING ASSESSMENT** **Seizure Disorders and Epilepsy**

Subjective Data

Important Health Information

Past health history: Previous seizures, birth defects or injuries, anoxic episodes; CNS trauma, tumors, or infections; stroke; metabolic disorders, alcoholism; exposure to metals and carbon monoxide; hepatic or renal failure; fever; pregnancy, systemic lupus erythematosus

Medications: Compliance with antiseizure medications; barbiturate or alcohol withdrawal; use and overdose of cocaine, amphetamines, lidocaine, theophylline, penicillin, lithium, phenothiazines, tricyclic antidepressants, benzodiazepines

Functional Health Patterns

Health perception–health management: Positive family history

Cognitive-perceptual: Headaches, aura, mood or behavioral changes before seizure; mentation changes; abdominal pain, muscle pain (postictal)

Self-perception–self-concept: Anxiety, depression; loss of self-esteem, social isolation

Sexuality-reproductive: Decreased sexual drive, erectile dysfunction; increased sexual drive (postictal)

Objective Data

General

Precipitating factors, including severe metabolic acidosis or alkalosis, hyperkalemia, hypoglycemia, dehydration, or water intoxication

Integumentary

Bitten tongue, soft tissue damage, cyanosis, diaphoresis (postictal)

Respiratory

Abnormal respiratory rate, rhythm, or depth; apnea (ictal); absent or abnormal breath sounds, possible airway occlusion

Cardiovascular

Hypertension, tachycardia or bradycardia (ictal)

Gastrointestinal

Bowel incontinence; excessive salivation

Urinary

Incontinence

Neurologic

Generalized

Tonic-clonic: Loss of consciousness, muscle tightening, then jerking; dilated pupils; hyperventilation, then apnea; postictal somnolence

Absence: Altered consciousness (5-30 sec), minor facial motor activity

Partial

Simple: Aura; consciousness; focal sensory, motor, cognitive, or emotional phenomena (focal motor); unilateral "marching" motor seizure (jacksonian)

Complex: Altered consciousness with inappropriate behaviors, automatisms, amnesia of event

Musculoskeletal

Weakness, paralysis, ataxia (postictal)

Possible Findings

Positive toxicology screen or alcohol level; altered serum electrolytes, acidosis or alkalosis, very low blood glucose level, ↑ blood urea nitrogen or serum creatinine, liver function tests, ammonia; abnormal CT scan or MRI of head, abnormal findings from lumbar puncture; abnormal discharges on EEG

CNS, Central nervous system; *CT,* computed tomography; *EEG,* electroencephalogram; *MRI,* magnetic resonance imaging.

Nervous System

NURSING CARE PLAN 59-2

Patient with Seizure Disorder or Epilepsy

NURSING DIAGNOSIS **Ineffective breathing pattern** *related to* neuromuscular impairment secondary to prolonged tonic phase of seizure or during postictal period *as evidenced by* abnormal respiratory rate, rhythm, and/or depth

PATIENT GOAL Experiences breathing pattern adequate to meet oxygen needs

OUTCOMES (NOC)

Respiratory Status: Ventilation

- Respiratory rate ____
- Respiratory rhythm ____
- Depth of inspiration ____

Measurement Scale

1 = Severely compromised
2 = Substantially compromised
3 = Moderately compromised
4 = Mildly compromised
5 = Not compromised

INTERVENTIONS (NIC) and *RATIONALES*

Airway Management

- Monitor respiratory and oxygenation status *to determine presence and extent of problem and to initiate appropriate interventions.*
- Position patient (side-lying) to maximize ventilation potential.
- Identify patient requiring actual/potential airway insertion *to facilitate intubation as necessary.*
- Perform endotracheal or nasotracheal suctioning *to maintain airway.*

Seizure Management

- Loosen clothing *to prevent restricted breathing.*
- Apply oxygen as appropriate *to maintain oxygenation and prevent hypoxia.*

NURSING DIAGNOSIS **Risk for injury** *related to* seizure activity and subsequent impaired physical mobility secondary to postictal weakness

PATIENT GOAL Experiences no seizure-related injury

OUTCOMES (NOC)

Seizure Control

- Describes precipitating seizure factors ____
- Avoids seizure triggers/risk factors ____
- Seeks medical attention immediately if seizure frequency increases ____
- Implements safety practices in home/work environment ____

Measurement Scale

1 = Never demonstrated
2 = Rarely demonstrated
3 = Sometimes demonstrated
4 = Often demonstrated
5 = Consistently demonstrated

INTERVENTIONS (NIC) and *RATIONALES*

Seizure Precautions

- Monitor compliance in taking antiseizure medications *to determine risk for seizures.*
- Remove potentially harmful objects from the environment.
- Keep suction, Ambu bag, oral or nasopharyngeal airway at bedside *to maintain airway and oxygenation if needed.*
- Use padded side rails *to prevent injury during a seizure.*

Seizure Management

- Remain with patient during seizure *to protect patient from injury.*
- Guide movements *to prevent injury during a seizure.*
- Record seizure characteristics: body parts involved, motor activity, and seizure progression.
- Monitor postictal period duration and characteristics *to plan appropriate interventions as needed.*

NURSING DIAGNOSIS **Ineffective coping** *related to* perceived loss of control and denial of diagnosis *as evidenced by* verbalizations about not having epilepsy, lack of truth-telling regarding seizure frequency, noncompliant behavior

PATIENT GOALS 1. Expresses acceptance of seizure disorder by admitting presence of epilepsy and maintaining compliant behavior
2. Maintains therapeutic levels of antiseizure medications

OUTCOMES (NOC)

Seizure Control

- Maintains positive attitude toward seizure disorder ____
- Maintains role performance ____
- Maintains social relationships ____

Acceptance: Health Status

- Recognizes reality of health situation ____
- Copes with health situation ____

Measurement Scale

1 = Never demonstrated
2 = Rarely demonstrated
3 = Sometimes demonstrated
4 = Often demonstrated
5 = Consistently demonstrated

INTERVENTIONS (NIC) and *RATIONALES*

Coping Enhancement

- Appraise patient's adjustment to changes in body image.
- Appraise impact of patient's life situation on roles and relationships *to determine extent of problem and to plan appropriate interventions.*
- Appraise and discuss alternative responses to situation.
- Provide factual information concerning diagnosis, treatment, and prognosis.
- Arrange situations that encourage patient's autonomy *to promote effective coping by providing correct information.*

Teaching: Disease Process

- Discuss lifestyle changes that may be required to prevent future complications and/or control the disease process.
- Describe possible chronic complications.
- Describe rationale behind management/treatment recommendations.

NURSING CARE PLAN 59-2

Patient with Seizure Disorder or Epilepsy—cont'd

NURSING DIAGNOSIS   **Ineffective therapeutic regimen management** *related to* lack of knowledge about management of seizure disorder *as evidenced by* verbalization of lack of knowledge, inaccurate perception of health status, noncompliance with prescribed health behavior

PATIENT GOALS
1. Describes factors involved in effective management of seizure disorder
2. Makes decisions about health and lifestyle modifications necessary for management of seizure disorder

OUTCOMES (NOC)	INTERVENTIONS (NIC) and *RATIONALES*
Knowledge: Disease Process	**Teaching: Disease Process**
• Description of specific disease process ____	• Discuss lifestyle changes (e.g., avoidance of precipitating factors, driving restrictions, wearing medical ID tags, moderation in drinking and eating, exposure to stress, and avoidance of hazardous activities) that may be required to prevent future complications and/or control the disease process.
• Description of measures to minimize disease progression ____	• Discuss therapy/treatment options and describe rationale behind management/treatment options *so patient and family can make lifestyle modifications to manage a chronic disease.*
• Description of precautions to prevent complications ____	
Measurement Scale	
1 = None	
2 = Limited	
3 = Moderate	
4 = Substantial	
5 = Extensive	

TABLE 59-12	*PATIENT AND FAMILY TEACHING GUIDE* — Seizure Disorders and Epilepsy

The patient should be taught the following:
1. Drugs must be taken as prescribed. Any and all side effects of drugs should be reported to the health care provider. When necessary, blood is drawn to ensure that therapeutic levels are maintained.
2. Use of nondrug techniques, such as relaxation therapy and biofeedback training, to potentially reduce the number of seizures.
3. Availability of resources in the community.
4. Need to wear a medical alert bracelet, necklace, and identification card.
5. Avoidance of excessive alcohol intake, fatigue, and loss of sleep.
6. Regular meals and snacks in between if feeling shaky, faint, or hungry.

Family members should be taught the following:
1. For first aid treatment of tonic-clonic seizure, it is not necessary to call an ambulance or send the patient to the hospital after a single seizure unless the seizure is prolonged, another seizure immediately follows, or extensive injury has occurred.
2. During an acute seizure, it is important to protect the patient from injury. This may involve supporting and protecting the head, turning the patient to the side, loosening constrictive clothing, and easing the patient to the floor, if seated.

Patients with a seizure disorder also experience concerns or fears related to recurrent seizures, incontinence, or loss of self-control. The nurse provides support for the patient through education and by helping to identify coping mechanisms.

Perhaps the greatest challenge that a seizure disorder presents to the patient is adjusting to the personal limitations imposed by the illness. Discrimination in employment is the most serious problem facing the person with a seizure disorder. For issues relating to job discrimination, patients can be referred to the state Human Rights Commission or the state Department of Vocational Rehabilitation.

A variety of other resources can be offered to the patient with a seizure disorder who has a specific problem. If the nurse believes that associating with others who have a seizure disorder would be beneficial, the patient can be referred to the local chapter of the Epilepsy Foundation (EF), a volunteer agency that offers a variety of services to patients with epilepsy. The patient who is an eligible veteran can be referred to a Department of Veterans Affairs medical center that provides comprehensive care.

Driving laws related to patients who have had a seizure vary from state to state. For example, some states require a 3-month seizure-free period before issuing or reissuing a driver's license, whereas others require up to 1 year. The EF provides current information on driving laws for each state.

The patient should be informed that medical alert bracelets, necklaces, and identification cards are available through the EF, local pharmacies, or companies specializing in identification devices (e.g., Medic Alert). However, the use of these medical identification tags is optional. Some patients have found them beneficial, but others have found them to be more a burden than a help because these individuals prefer not to be identified as having a seizure disorder.

Social workers and welfare agencies can help with financial problems and living arrangements. State services for individuals with developmental disabilities include assistance with job training and placement for patients whose seizures are not well controlled. Sheltered housing and funding for special needs, such as medical and psychologic evaluation and transportation, are also offered. State agencies specializing in vocational rehabilitation services can offer vocational assessment, counseling, funding for training, and assistance with job placement. They can also offer financial assistance for transportation and medical costs that are necessary for vocational rehabilitation or job maintenance. If intensive psychologic counseling is needed, the nurse can refer the patient to a community mental health center.

The patient should be encouraged to learn more about epilepsy through self-education materials. The EF provides several information pamphlets and may facilitate support groups. Many agencies that offer services to epileptic patients, as well as local chapters of EF, have these available as teaching aids.

▪ *Evaluation*

Expected outcomes for the patient with seizures are addressed in NCP 59-2.

MULTIPLE SCLEROSIS

Multiple sclerosis (MS) is a chronic, progressive, degenerative disorder of the CNS characterized by disseminated demyelination of nerve fibers of the brain and spinal cord. MS is considered a disease of young to middle-age adults, with the onset usually being between 15 and 50 years of age. Women are affected more often than men. High prevalence rates (over 30 per 100,000) occur in northern Europe, northern United States, southern Canada, and southern Australia and New Zealand. Low prevalence rates (<5 per 100,000) occur in southern Europe, Japan, China, and South America. MS is five times more prevalent in temperate climates (between 45 and 65 degrees of latitude), such as those found in the northern United States, Canada, and Europe, as compared with tropical regions. African American individuals have a prevalence rate that is 40% that of European Americans. Africans are thought to have a prevalence rate of approximately 1% that of European Americans. This suggests that the genetic susceptibility to MS may be related to ethnicity.[20]

Etiology and Pathophysiology

The cause of MS is unknown, although research findings suggest that MS is related to infectious (viral), immunologic, and genetic factors and is perpetuated as a result of intrinsic factors (e.g., faulty immunoregulation). The susceptibility to MS appears to be inherited. First-, second-, and third-degree relatives of patients with MS are at a slightly increased risk. Multiple genes confer susceptibility to MS.

The role of precipitating factors such as exposure to pathogenetic agents in the etiology of MS is controversial. It is possible that their association with MS is random and that there is no cause-and-effect relationship. Possible precipitating factors include infection, physical injury, emotional stress, excessive fatigue, pregnancy, and a poorer state of health.

MS is characterized by chronic inflammation, demyelination, and gliosis (scarring) in the CNS. The primary neuropathologic condition is an autoimmune disease orchestrated by autoreactive T cells (lymphocytes). This process may be initially triggered by a virus in genetically susceptible individuals. The activated T cells in the systemic circulation migrate to the CNS, causing blood-brain barrier disruption. This is likely the initial event in the development of MS. Subsequent antigen-antibody reaction within the CNS results in activation of the inflammatory response and, through multiple effector mechanisms, leads to demyelination of axons. The disease process consists of loss of myelin, disappearance of oligodendrocytes, and proliferation of astrocytes. These changes result in characteristic plaque formation, or sclerosis, with plaques scattered throughout multiple regions of the CNS.

Initially the myelin sheaths of the neurons in the brain and spinal cord are attacked (Fig. 59-2, *A* and *B*). Early in the disease the myelin sheath is damaged. However, the nerve fiber is not affected, and nerve impulses are still transmitted (Fig. 59-2, *C*). At this point the patient may complain of a noticeable impairment of function (e.g., weakness). However, the myelin can regenerate, and the symptoms will disappear. Therefore the patient experiences a remission.

In addition to myelin disruption, the axon also becomes involved (Fig. 59-2, *D*). Myelin is replaced by glial scar tissue,

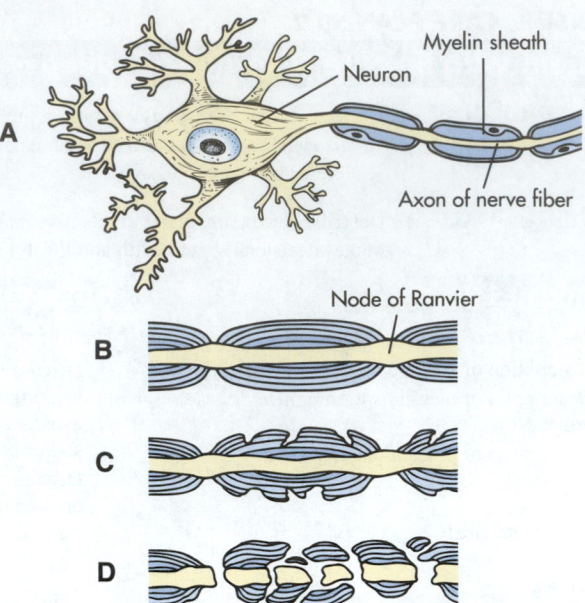

FIG. 59-2   Pathogenesis of multiple sclerosis. **A,** Normal nerve cell with myelin sheath. **B,** Normal axon. **C,** Myelin breakdown. **D,** Myelin totally disrupted; axon not functioning.

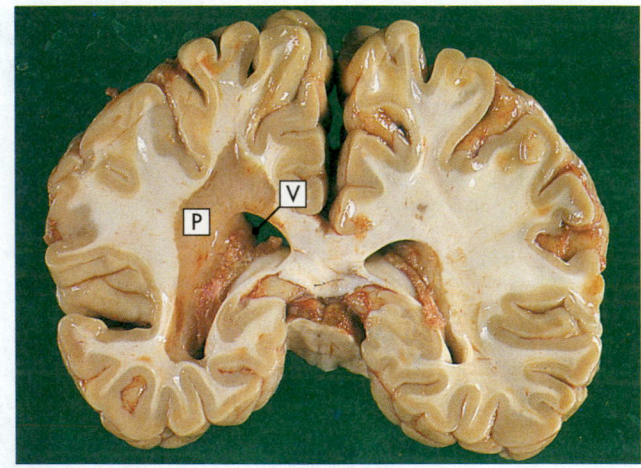

FIG. 59-3   Chronic multiple sclerosis. Demyelination plaque *(P)* at gray-white junction and adjacent partially remyelinated shadow plaque *(V)*.

which forms hard, sclerotic plaques in multiple regions of the CNS (Fig. 59-3). Without myelin, nerve impulses slow down. With destruction of nerve axons, impulses are totally blocked, resulting in permanent loss of function. In many chronic lesions, demyelination continues with progressive loss of nerve function.

Clinical Manifestations

The onset of the disease is often insidious and gradual, with vague symptoms occurring intermittently over months or years. Thus the disease may not be diagnosed until long after the onset of the first symptom. The disease process has a spotty distribution in the CNS, so the signs and symptoms vary over time. The disease is characterized by chronic, progressive deterioration in some persons and by remissions and exacerbations in others. With repeated exacerbations, however, progressive scarring of the myelin sheath occurs, and the overall trend is progressive deterioration in neurologic function.

The clinical manifestations vary according to the areas of the CNS involved. Some patients have severe, long-lasting symptoms

TABLE 59-13	Clinical Courses of Multiple Sclerosis
Category	**Characteristics**
Relapsing-remitting	Clearly defined relapses with full recovery or sequelae and residual deficit on recovery
Primary-progressive	Disease progression from onset with occasional plateaus and temporary minor improvements
Secondary-progressive	A relapsing-remitting initial course, followed by progression with or without occasional relapses, minor remissions, and plateaus
Progressive-relapsing	Progressive disease from onset, with clear acute relapses, with or without full recovery; periods between relapses are characterized by continuing progression

TABLE 59-14	*COLLABORATIVE CARE* **Multiple Sclerosis**

Diagnostic
History and physical examination
CSF analysis
Evoked response testing (also called evoked potential testing, e.g., somatosensory evoked potential [SSEP], auditory evoked potential [AEP], visual evoked potential [VEP])
CT scan
MRI, MRS

Collaborative Therapy
*Drug Therapy**
Corticosteroids
Immunomodulators
Immunosuppressants
Cholinergics
Anticholinergics
Muscle relaxants

Surgical Therapy
Thalamotomy (unmanageable tremor)
Neurectomy, rhizotomy, cordotomy (unmanageable spasticity)

CSF, Cerebrospinal fluid; *CT,* computed tomography; *MRI,* magnetic resonance imaging; *MRS,* magnetic resonance spectroscopy.
*See Table 59-15.

early in the course of the disease. Others may experience only occasional and mild symptoms for several years after onset. A classification scheme of MS by clinical course has been developed[21] (Table 59-13).

Common signs and symptoms of MS include motor, sensory, cerebellar, and emotional problems. Motor symptoms include weakness or paralysis of the limbs, trunk, or head; diplopia; scanning speech; and spasticity of the muscles that are chronically affected. Patients with MS experience a variety of sensory abnormalities, including numbness and tingling and other paresthesias, patchy blindness *(scotomas),* blurred vision, vertigo, tinnitus, decreased hearing, and chronic neuropathic pain. Radicular (nerve root) pains may be present, particularly in the low thoracic and abdominal regions. *Lhermitte's sign* is a transient sensory symptom described as an electric shock radiating down the spine or into the limbs with flexion of the neck. Cerebellar signs include nystagmus, ataxia, dysarthria, and dysphagia. Severe fatigue is present in many MS patients, and causes significant disability for some patients. The fatigue is usually associated with increased energy needs, deconditioning, depression, and medication side effects.[22]

Bowel and bladder function can be affected if the sclerotic plaque is located in areas of the CNS that control elimination. Problems with defecation usually involve constipation rather than fecal incontinence. Urinary problems are variable. A common problem in MS patients is a *spastic* (uninhibited) bladder. This indicates a lesion above the second sacral nerve, which cuts off suprasegmental inhibiting influences on bladder contractility. As a result, the bladder has a small capacity for urine, and its contractions are unchecked. This is accompanied by urinary urgency and frequency and results in dribbling or incontinence. A *flaccid* (hypotonic) bladder indicates a lesion in the reflex arc controlling bladder function. The bladder has a large capacity for urine because there is no sensation or desire to void, no pressure, and no pain. Generally, there is urinary retention, but urgency and frequency may also occur with this type of lesion. Another urinary problem is a combination of the previous two problems. Urinary problems cannot be adequately diagnosed and treated unless urodynamic studies are done.

Sexual dysfunction occurs in many persons with MS. Physiologic erectile dysfunction may result from spinal cord involvement in men. Women may experience decreased libido, difficulty with orgasmic response, painful intercourse, and decreased vaginal lubrication. Diminished sensation can prevent a normal sexual response in both sexes. The emotional effects of chronic illness and the loss of self-esteem also contribute to loss of sexual response.

MS has no apparent effect on the course of pregnancy, labor, delivery, or lactation. Some women with MS who become pregnant experience remission or an improvement in their symptoms during the gestation period. The hormonal changes associated with pregnancy appear to affect the immune system. However, during the postpartum period, women are at greater risk for exacerbation of the disease.

Although intellectual functioning generally remains intact, emotional stability may be affected. Cognitive sequelae can produce significant disability for some patients with MS. Persons may experience anger, depression, or euphoria. Signs and symptoms of MS are aggravated or triggered by physical and emotional trauma, fatigue, and infection.

The average life expectancy after the onset of symptoms is more than 25 years. Death usually occurs due to infective complications (e.g., pneumonia) of immobility or because of an unrelated disease.

Diagnostic Studies

Because there is no definitive diagnostic test for MS, diagnosis is based primarily on history, clinical manifestations, and the presence of multiple lesions over time as measured by MRI (Table 59-14). Certain laboratory tests are currently used as adjuncts to the clinical examination. In some patients, cerebrospinal fluid (CSF) analysis may show an increase in oligoclonal immunoglobulin G. The CSF also contains a high number of lymphocytes and monocytes. Evoked potential responses are often delayed in persons with MS because of decreased nerve conduction from the eye and the ear to the brain. MRI may be helpful because sclerotic plaques as small as 3 to 4 mm in diameter can be detected. Characteristic white-matter lesions scattered through the brain or spinal cord are evident on such a scan.[21]

Collaborative Care

Drug Therapy. Because there is currently no cure for MS, collaborative care is aimed at treating the disease process and providing symptomatic relief (see Table 59-14). The disease process is treated with drugs (Table 59-15). The symptoms are controlled with a variety of drugs and other forms of therapy. Adrenocorticotropic hormone (ACTH), methylprednisolone, and prednisone are helpful in treating acute exacerbations of the disease, probably by reducing edema and acute inflammation at the site of demyelination. Although the dose and route of administration may vary, these drugs are used in patients with all types of MS. However, these drugs do not affect the ultimate outcome or degree of residual neurologic impairment from the exacerbation.

Immunosuppressive drugs, such as azathioprine (Imuran), methotrexate, and cyclophosphamide (Cytoxan), have been shown to produce some beneficial effects in patients with progressive-relapsing, secondary-progressive, and primary-progressive MS. However, the potential benefits of these drugs in patients with MS must be counterbalanced against the potentially serious side effects.

Immunomodulator drugs modify the disease process. Interferon β-1b (Betaseron) is used for ambulatory patients with relapsing-remitting MS. Interferon β-1a (Avonex) is similar to interferon β-1b in efficacy and is used in similar patient groups with MS. Another formulation of interferon β-1a (Rebif) is administered subcutaneously three times weekly. Glatiramer acetate (Copaxone), formerly known as copolymer-1, is unrelated to interferon. It is given to patients with relapsing-remitting MS.

Drug Alert - *β-Interferon (Avonex, Betaseron, Rebif)*
- *Rotate injection sites with each dose.*
- *Assess for depression, suicidal ideation.*
- *Wear sunscreen and protective clothing while exposed to sun.*
- *Know that flu-like symptoms are common following initiation of therapy.*

Mitoxantrone (Novantrone) is a drug used for the treatment of primary-progressive and progressive-relapsing MS. It is an immunosuppressant drug that reduces both B and T lymphocytes and impairs antigen presentation. Unlike the other disease-modifying drugs, mitoxantrone has a lifetime dose limit because of cardiac toxicity.

Many other drugs are used to treat the symptoms of MS. Antispasmodics are used for spasticity. Amantadine (Symmetrel) and CNS stimulants (pemoline [Cylert], methylphenidate [Ritalin],

TABLE 59-15	**DRUG THERAPY** **Multiple Sclerosis**		
Drug	**Symptoms Relieved**	**Side Effects and Precautions**	**Patient Teaching**
Corticosteroids ACTH, prednisone, methylprednisolone	Exacerbations	Edema, mental changes (euphoria), weight gain, redistribution of body fat*; widespread effects on many metabolic processes; few adverse effects with use for <1 mo at a time	• Restrict salt intake. • Do not abruptly stop therapy. • Know drug interactions.
Immunomodulators β-interferon (Betaseron, Avonex, Rebif)	Exacerbations	Flu-like symptoms, local skin reactions, depression; monitor CBC, blood chemistries, and liver function tests every 3 mo	• Perform self-injection techniques. • Report side effects.
glatiramer acetate (Copaxone)	Exacerbations	Local skin reactions; chest pain, weakness; no laboratory monitoring required	• Perform self-injection techniques. • Report side effects.
Immunosuppressants mitoxantrone (Novantrone)	Exacerbations	Nausea, vomiting, diarrhea, mucositis, alopecia, hepatotoxicity, myelosuppression; cardiovascular disease; lifetime dose limit because of cardiotoxicity; monitor CBC and liver function every month	• Receive regular monitoring and follow-up. • Consult health care provider before getting immunizations. • Be aware that urine may turn a blue-green color initially. • Maintain adequate fluid intake.
Cholinergics bethanechol (Urecholine) neostigmine (Prostigmin)	Urinary retention (flaccid bladder)	Hypotension, diarrhea, diaphoresis, muscle weakness; history of cardiac dysfunction, hypotension, allergies, peptic ulcer disease, asthma	• Consult with health care provider before using other drugs, including over-the-counter drugs.
Anticholinergics propantheline (Pro-Banthine) oxybutynin (Ditropan)	Urinary frequency† and urgency (spastic bladder)	Dry mouth, blurred vision, constipation, hypertension, flushing, urinary retention (dose too high); contraindicated with history of glaucoma, benign prostatic hyperplasia, cardiac dysfunction, intestinal obstruction	• Consult health care provider before using other drugs, especially sleeping aids, antihistamines (possibly leading to potentiated effect).

ACTH, Adrenocorticotropic hormone; *CBC,* complete blood count; *CNS,* central nervous system; *MAO,* monoamine oxidase, *OTC,* over-the-counter; *SOB,* shortness of breath.
*See Chapter 50 for effects of long-term corticosteroid therapy.
†Urodynamic studies must be done before initiation of therapy because patients with MS have multiple lesions and type of bladder dysfunction cannot be diagnosed from symptoms alone.

and modafinil [Provigil]) are used for fatigue. Anticholinergics are used to treat bladder symptoms. Tricyclic antidepressants and antiseizure drugs are used for chronic pain syndromes.

Other Therapies. Spasticity is primarily treated with antispasmodic drugs. However, surgery (e.g., neurectomy, rhizotomy, cordotomy), dorsal-column electrical stimulation, or intrathecal baclofen (Lioresal) delivered by pump may be required. Tremors that become unmanageable with drugs are sometimes treated by thalamotomy or deep brain stimulation.

Neurologic dysfunction sometimes improves with physical and speech therapies. Exercise improves the daily functioning for patients with MS not experiencing an exacerbation. Exercise decreases spasticity, increases coordination, and retrains unaffected muscles to substitute for impaired ones.[23] An especially beneficial type of physical therapy is water exercise (Fig. 59-4). Water gives buoyancy to the body and allows the patient to perform activities that would normally be impossible because the patient has more control over the body.

TABLE 59-15	**DRUG THERAPY** Multiple Sclerosis—cont'd		

Drug	Symptoms Relieved	Side Effects and Precautions	Patient Teaching
Muscle Relaxants			
diazepam (Valium)	Spasticity	Drowsiness, ataxia, fatigue; contraindicated with history of narrow-angle glaucoma	• Avoid driving and similar activities because of CNS depressant effects. • Be aware of addictive potential. • Avoid long-term use. • Avoid concomitant use of barbiturates, MAO inhibitors, antidepressants.
baclofen (Lioresal)	Spasticity	Drowsiness, weakness; used cautiously with a history of hypersensitivity and renal damage; possible exacerbation of seizures in patients with seizure disorders	• Do not abruptly stop therapy (possibility of hallucinations). • Avoid driving and similar activities because of sedative effects. • Avoid use of other CNS depressants. • Take with food or milk.
dantrolene (Dantrium)	Spasticity	Drowsiness, dizziness, malaise, fatigue, diarrhea; used cautiously in patients with a history of respiratory or cardiac dysfunction; risk of hepatotoxicity	• Avoid driving when drug is used. • Avoid use with tranquilizers and alcohol (possibly causing photosensitivity). • Obtain baseline liver function tests.
tizanidine (Zanaflex)	Spasticity	Drowsiness, dry mouth, fatigue, nausea; used cautiously in patients with history of hypersensitivity, liver or renal disease, hypotension, bradycardia	• Avoid driving when drug is used. • Avoid use with tranquilizers and alcohol (possibly causing photosensitivity). • Eat small, frequent meals to reduce nausea. • Change position slowly when going from lying or sitting position to standing.
CNS Stimulants			
pemoline (Cylert)	Fatigue	Hyperactivity, insomnia, restlessness, tachycardia, nausea; used cautiously in pregnant or lactating patients, patients with a history of renal disease, drug abuse, or seizure disorders	• Decrease caffeine consumption (may increase stimulation). • Do not abruptly stop therapy. • Avoid use with alcohol. • Therapeutic effect may take 2-4 wk.
methylphenidate (Ritalin)	Fatigue	Hyperactivity, insomnia, restlessness, talkativeness, palpitations, tachycardia, nausea; used cautiously in pregnant or lactating patients, patient with a history of depression, seizures, or drug abuse	• Decrease caffeine consumption. • Do not break, crush, or chew time-released medication. • Do not abruptly stop therapy. • Avoid use with alcohol.
modafinil (Provigil)	Fatigue	Headache, nausea, nervousness, rhinitis, diarrhea, back pain, anxiety, insomnia, dizziness, dyspepsia; used cautiously in pregnant women and women using contraceptives	• Medication can alter the effectiveness of oral contraceptives. • Discuss the use of OTC vitamins and herbal supplements with your health care provider before taking with this medication. • Avoid use with alcohol. • Effects on fetus with use in pregnancy undetermined.
Antiviral/Antiparkinsonian			
symmetrel (Amantadine)	Fatigue	Dizziness, headache, irritability, loss of appetite, nausea, vomiting, nervousness, purplish red blotchy spots on skin, insomnia, constipation, dry mouth; more serious side effects include blurred vision, confusion, difficult urination, fainting, hallucinations, convulsions, unexplained SOB; undermined effects in pregnancy, passes into breast milk	• Side effects may go away as body adjusts. • Avoid use with alcohol (may increase side effects). • Notify health care provider if dry mouth lasts more than 2 wk. • Effects on fetus with use in pregnancy undetermined.

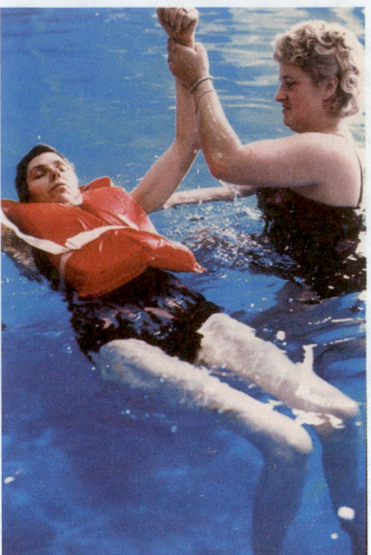

FIG. 59-4   Water therapy provides exercise and recreation for the patient with a chronic neurologic disease.

TABLE 59-16	*NURSING ASSESSMENT* **Multiple Sclerosis**

Subjective Data
Important Health Information
Past health history: Recent or past viral infections or vaccinations, other recent infections, residence in cold or temperate climates, recent physical or emotional stress, pregnancy, exposure to extremes of heat and cold
Medications: Use of and compliance in taking corticosteroids, immunomodulators, immunosuppressants, cholinergics, anticholinergics, antispasmodics

Functional Health Patterns
Health perception–health management: Positive family history; malaise
Nutritional-metabolic: Weight loss; difficulty in chewing, dysphagia
Elimination: Urinary frequency, urgency, dribbling or incontinence, retention; constipation
Activity-exercise: Generalized muscle weakness, muscle fatigue; tingling and numbness, ataxia (clumsiness)
Cognitive-perceptual: Eye, back, leg, joint pain; painful muscle spasms; vertigo; blurred or lost vision; diplopia; tinnitus
Sexuality-reproductive: Impotence, decreased libido
Coping–stress tolerance: Anger, depression, euphoria, social isolation

Objective Data
General
Apathy, inattentiveness

Integumentary
Pressure ulcers

Neurologic
Scanning speech, nystagmus, ataxia, tremor, spasticity, hyperreflexia, decreased hearing

Musculoskeletal
Muscular weakness, paresis, paralysis, spasms, foot dragging, dysarthria

Possible Findings
↓ T suppressor cells, demyelinating lesions on MRI or MRS scans, ↑ IgG or oligoclonal banding in cerebrospinal fluid, delayed evoked potential

IgG, Immunoglobulin G; *MRI,* magnetic resonance imaging; *MRS,* magnetic resonance spectroscopy.

Nutritional Therapy. Various nutritional measures have been used in the management of MS, including megavitamin therapy (cobalamin [vitamin B$_{12}$], vitamin C) and diets consisting of low-fat and gluten-free food and raw vegetables. Particular dietary measures are not widely used due to insufficient data for their effectiveness. Although not specific to MS patients, there is evidence that cranberry juice can prevent bacteria from sticking on the walls of the bladder, which may decrease the number of urinary infections, a common condition in patients with MS.[24]

A nutritious, well-balanced diet is essential. Although there is no standard prescribed diet, a high-protein diet with supplementary vitamins is often recommended. A diet high in roughage may help relieve the problem of constipation. Vitamins are merely supplemental and not curative.

NURSING MANAGEMENT
MULTIPLE SCLEROSIS

■ Nursing Assessment

Subjective and objective data that should be obtained from a patient with MS are presented in Table 59-16.

■ Nursing Diagnoses

Nursing diagnoses for the patient with MS may include, but are not limited to, those presented in NCP 59-3.

■ Planning

The overall goals are that the patient with MS will (1) maximize neuromuscular function, (2) maintain independence in activities of daily living for as long as possible, (3) manage disabling fatigue, (4) optimize psychosocial well-being, (5) adjust to the illness, and (6) reduce factors that precipitate exacerbations.

■ Nursing Implementation

The patient with MS should be aware of triggers that may cause exacerbations or worsening of the disease. Exacerbations of MS are triggered by infection (especially upper respiratory and urinary tract infections), trauma, immunization, delivery after pregnancy, stress, and change in climate. Each person responds differently to these triggers. The nurse should help the patient identify particular triggers and develop ways to avoid them or minimize their effects.

The most common reasons for hospitalization of the patient with MS are for a diagnostic workup and treatment of an acute exacerbation. During the diagnostic phase the patient needs reassurance that, even though there is a tentative diagnosis of MS, certain diagnostic studies must be done to rule out other neurologic disorders. The nurse should assist the patient in dealing with the anxiety caused by a diagnosis of a disabling illness. The patient with recently diagnosed MS may need assistance with the grieving process.

During an acute exacerbation the patient may be immobile and confined to bed. The focus of nursing intervention at this phase is to prevent major complications of immobility, such as respiratory and urinary tract infections and pressure ulcers.

Patient teaching should focus on building general resistance to illness, including avoiding fatigue, extremes of heat and cold, and exposure to infection. The last measure involves avoiding exposure to cold climates and to people who are sick, as well as vigorous

EVIDENCE-BASED PRACTICE

What Is the Effect of Exercise on Quality of Life in Patients with Multiple Sclerosis?

Clinical Question

In adults with multiple sclerosis (P), what is the effect of exercise (I) as compared to no exercise therapy (C) on activity limitations and quality of life (O)?

Best Available Evidence

Systematic review of randomized controlled trials (RCTs)

Critical Appraisal and Synthesis of Evidence

- 9 RCTs (*n* = 260) of persons with different types of multiple sclerosis (MS) presently without an exacerbation. Six studies compared exercise therapy versus no exercise therapy; three studies compared two interventions.

Conclusions

- Exercise strongly affects isometric strength, physical fitness, and mobility-related activities when compared to no exercise therapy.

- Exercise therapy also improves a person's mood (anxiety and depression).
- One type of exercise was not superior to another in improving activity or participation.

Implications for Nursing Practice

- Inform MS patients that daily functioning can be improved with exercise.
- Collaborate with the patient to determine the best "dose" and type of exercise to reach optimum beneficial effects.

Reference for Evidence

Rietberg MB, Brooks D, Uitdehaag BMJ, et al: Exercise therapy for multiple sclerosis, Cochrane Multiple Sclerosis Group, *Cochrane Database Syst Rev* 4, 2005.

PICO: P, Patient population of interest; *I,* intervention or area of interest; *C,* comparison of interest or comparison group; *O,* outcome(s) of interest (see p. 6).

NURSING CARE PLAN 59-3

Patient with Multiple Sclerosis

NURSING DIAGNOSIS   **Impaired physical mobility** *related to* muscle weakness or paralysis and muscle spasticity *as evidenced by* inability to ambulate, intermittent muscle spasms, pain associated with muscle spasms

PATIENT GOALS   1. Maintains or improves muscle strength and mobility
2. Uses assistive devices appropriately for ambulation and mobility

OUTCOMES (NOC)

Mobility

- Balance ____
- Coordination ____
- Muscle movement ____
- Joint movement ____
- Walking __

Measurement Scale

1 = Severely compromised
2 = Substantially compromised
3 = Moderately compromised
4 = Mildly compromised
5 = Not compromised

INTERVENTIONS (NIC) and RATIONALES

Exercise Therapy: Ambulation

- Apply/provide assistive device (e.g., cane, walker, or wheelchair) for ambulation if the patient is unsteady *to decrease fatigue and enhance independence, comfort, and safety.*
- Encourage independent ambulation within safe limits *to maintain mobility, promote independence, and provide for safety.*

Exercise Therapy: Joint Mobility

- Instruct patient/family how to systematically perform passive, assisted, or active ROM exercises, as indicated *to prevent contractures and minimize muscle atrophy.*

Exercise Promotion: Stretching

- Instruct patient to slowly extend muscle/joint to point of full stretch (or reasonable discomfort) and hold for specified time and slowly release the stretched muscles *to relieve spasms and contracted muscles.*

NURSING DIAGNOSIS   **Sexual dysfunction** *related to* neuromuscular deficits *as evidenced by* impotence, verbalization of problem, decreased libido

PATIENT GOAL   Verbalizes satisfaction with sexual expression

OUTCOMES (NOC)

Sexual Functioning

- Expresses comfort with sexual expression ____
- Adapts sexual technique as needed ____
- Communicates sexual needs with partner ____

Measurement Scale

1 = Never demonstrated
2 = Rarely demonstrated
3 = Sometimes demonstrated
4 = Often demonstrated
5 = Consistently demonstrated

INTERVENTIONS (NIC) and RATIONALES

Sexual Counseling

- Provide information about sexual functioning, as appropriate, *to give the patient permission to ask questions and discuss sexual problems.*
- Encourage patient to verbalize fears and to ask questions.
- Provide reassurance and permission to experiment with alternative forms of sexual expression *as intercourse may not be possible due to neuromuscular defects.*
- Include the spouse/sexual partner in the counseling as much as possible.
- Refer the patient to a sex therapist as appropriate *because complex sexual problems require the intervention of specialists.*

ROM, Range of motion.

Continued

Nervous System

NURSING CARE PLAN 59-3

Patient with Multiple Sclerosis—cont'd

NURSING DIAGNOSIS   **Impaired urinary elimination pattern** *related to* sensorimotor deficits *as evidenced by* posturination residual volume >50 ml, bladder distention, dribbling, urgency, frequency

PATIENT GOALS
1. Maintains urinary continence
2. Experiences posturination residual urine volume <50 ml
3. Uses intermittent catheterization to maintain urinary function if necessary

OUTCOMES (NOC)

Urinary Elimination

- Elimination pattern _____
- Empties bladder completely _____
- Adequate fluid intake _____
- Recognition of urge _____

Measurement Scale

1 = Severely compromised
2 = Substantially compromised
3 = Moderately compromised
4 = Mildly compromised
5 = Not compromised

- Urinary retention _____
- Urinary incontinence _____

Measurement Scale

1 = Severe
2 = Substantial
3 = Moderate
4 = Mild
5 = None

INTERVENTIONS (NIC) and *RATIONALES*

Urinary Elimination Management

- Teach patient to drink eight ounces of liquid with meals, between meals, and in early evening *to dilute urine and reduce risk of UTI.*
- Instruct patient to monitor for signs and symptoms of UTI *to ensure early identification and treatment.*
- Assist patient with development of toileting routine *to help ensure adequate bladder function.*

Urinary Retention Care

- Implement intermittent catheterization *to prevent distention or dribbling.*
- Provide Credé maneuver *as an alternative method of emptying the bladder.*
- Stimulate the reflex bladder by applying cold to the abdomen, stroking the inner thigh, or running water *to assist in emptying the bladder.*

NURSING DIAGNOSIS   **Interrupted family processes** *related to* changing family roles, potential financial problems, and fluctuating physical condition *as evidenced by* strained family relations, ineffective communication, verbalization of financial concerns

PATIENT GOALS
1. Maintains open communication within the family
2. Utilizes financial, social, and health services to maintain family processes

OUTCOMES (NOC)

Family Coping

- Confronts family problems _____
- Manages family problems _____
- Involves family members in decision making _____
- Expresses feelings and emotions freely among members _____
- Maintains financial stability _____
- Uses available social support _____

Measurement Scale

1 = Never demonstrated
2 = Rarely demonstrated
3 = Sometimes demonstrated
4 = Often demonstrated
5 = Consistently demonstrated

INTERVENTIONS (NIC) and *RATIONALES*

Family Process Maintenance

- Identify effects of role changes on family processes.
- Assist family members to implement normalizing strategies for their situation.
- Assist family members to use existing support mechanisms *to enable the family to handle the issues of long-term illness.*
- Design schedules of patient home care activities that minimize disruption of family routine.

Family Support

- Facilitate communication of concerns/feelings between patient and family or between family members.
- Provide assistance in meeting basic needs for family, such as shelter, food, and clothing, *to provide additional help in coping with a chronic debilitating disease.*
- Assist family to acquire necessary knowledge, skills, and equipment to sustain their decision about patient care *as lack of knowledge about multiple sclerosis affects ability to cope with its effects.*

UTI, urinary tract infection.

and early treatment of infection when it does occur. It is important to teach the patient to (1) achieve a good balance of exercise and rest, (2) eat nutritious and well-balanced meals, and (3) avoid the hazards of immobility (e.g., contractures, pressure ulcers). Patients should know their treatment regimens, the side effects of drugs and how to watch for them, and drug interactions with over-the-counter medications. The patient should consult a health care provider before taking nonprescription drugs.

Bladder control is a major problem for many patients with MS. Although anticholinergics may be beneficial for some patients to decrease spasticity, other patients may need to be taught self-catheterization (see Chapter 45). Bowel problems, particularly constipation, occur frequently in patients with MS. Increasing the dietary fiber intake may help some patients achieve regularity in bowel habits.

The patient with MS and the family must make many emotional adjustments because of the unpredictability of the disease, the need to change lifestyles, and the challenge of avoiding or decreasing precipitating factors. The National Multiple Sclerosis Society and its local chapters can offer a variety of services to meet the needs of patients with MS.

■ Evaluation

Expected outcomes for the patient with MS are addressed in NCP 59-3.

PARKINSON'S DISEASE

Parkinson's disease (PD) is a disease of the basal ganglia characterized by slowness in the initiation and execution of movement *(bradykinesia)*, increased muscle tone *(rigidity)*, tremor at rest, and impaired postural reflexes. It is the most common form of *parkinsonism* (a syndrome characterized by similar symptoms). PD is named after James Parkinson, who, in 1817, wrote a classic essay on "shaking palsy," a disease whose cause is still unknown.

Etiology and Pathophysiology

The prevalence of PD is about 160 per 100,000 and the incidence is about 20 per 100,000. The diagnosis of PD increases with age, with the peak onset in the 70s. To date, more than 10 autosomal dominant and recessive genes have been linked to familial PD. PD is more common in men by a ratio of 3:2.

There are many forms of parkinsonism other than PD. Encephalitis lethargica, or type A encephalitis, has been clearly associated with the onset of parkinsonism. However, the incidence of postencephalitic parkinsonism has dwindled since the 1920s, when there was a large outbreak of this infectious illness. Parkinsonism-like symptoms have occurred after intoxication with a variety of chemicals, including carbon monoxide and manganese (among copper miners) and the product of meperidine analog synthesis, MPTP. Drug-induced parkinsonism can follow reserpine (Serpasil), methyldopa (Aldomet), lithium, haloperidol (Haldol), and chlorpromazine (Thorazine) therapy. Parkinsonism can also be seen following the use of illicit drugs, including amphetamine and methamphetamine. Other causes of parkinsonism include hydrocephalus, hypoxia, infections, stroke, tumor, and trauma.[26]

The pathologic process of PD involves degeneration of the dopamine-producing neurons in the substantia nigra of the midbrain (Figs. 59-5 through 59-7), which in turn disrupts the normal balance between dopamine (DA) and acetylcholine (ACh) in the basal ganglia. DA is a neurotransmitter essential for normal func-

tioning of the extrapyramidal motor system, including control of posture, support, and voluntary motion. Symptoms of PD do not occur until 80% of neurons in the substantia nigra are lost.

Clinical Manifestations

The onset of PD is gradual and insidious, with a gradual progression and a prolonged course. It may involve only one side of the body initially. The classic manifestations of PD often include tremor, rigidity, and bradykinesia, which are often called the triad

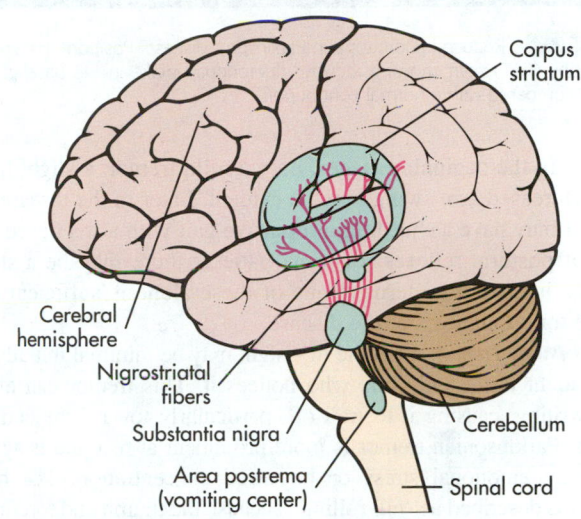

FIG. 59-5 Nigrostriatal disorders produce parkinsonism. Left-sided view of the human brain showing the substantia nigra and the corpus striatum *(shaded area)* lying deep within the cerebral hemisphere. Nerve fibers extend upward from the substantia nigra, divide into many branches, and carry dopamine to all regions of the corpus striatum.

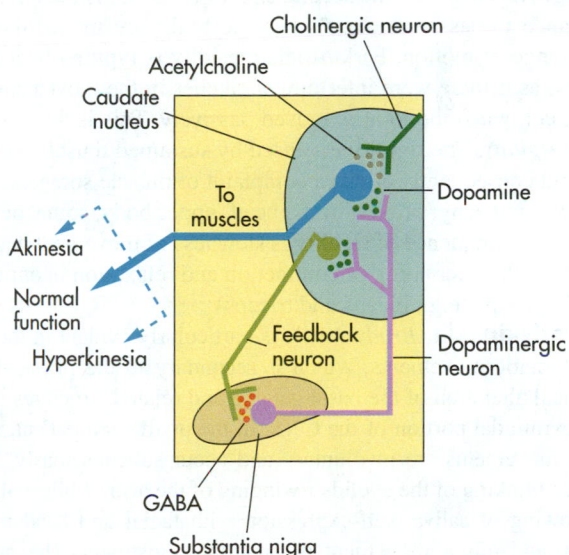

FIG. 59-6 Dopaminergic synaptic activity is mediated by dopamine. Cholinergic synaptic activity is mediated by acetylcholine. A balance between the two kinds of activity produces normal motor function. A relative excess of cholinergic activity produces akinesia and rigidity. A relative excess of dopaminergic activity produces involuntary movements. Neurons in the caudate nucleus contain γ-aminobutyric acid (GABA) and possibly control dopaminergic neurons in the substantia nigra through a feedback pathway.

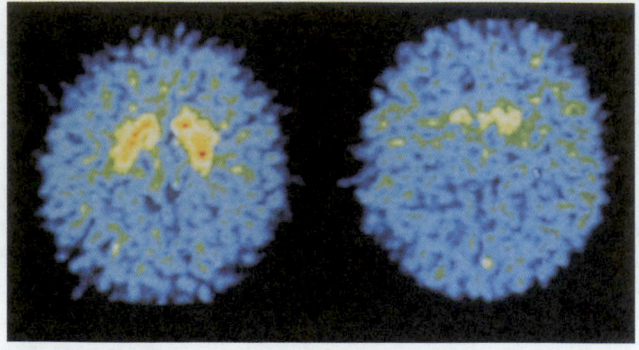

FIG. 59-7 Reduced fluorodopa in Parkinson's disease. Positron emission tomography (PET) scan showing reduced fluorodopa uptake in the basal ganglia *(right)* compared with a normal control *(left)*.

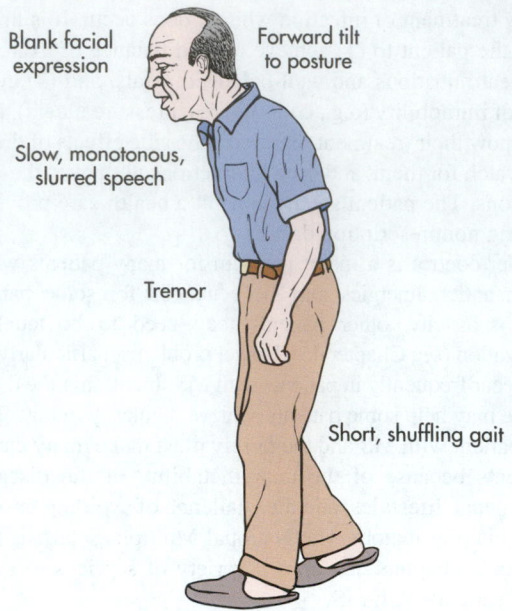

FIG. 59-8 Characteristic appearance of a patient with Parkinson's disease.

of PD. In the beginning stages, only a mild tremor, a slight limp, or a decreased arm swing may be evident. Later in the disease the patient may have a shuffling, propulsive gait with arms flexed and loss of postural reflexes. In some patients there may be a slight change in speech patterns. None of these alone is sufficient evidence for a diagnosis of the disease.

Tremor. *Tremor,* often the first sign, may be minimal initially, so the patient is the only one who notices it. This tremor can affect handwriting, causing it to trail off, particularly toward the ends of words. Parkinsonian tremor is more prominent at rest and is aggravated by emotional stress or increased concentration. The hand tremor is described as "pill rolling" because the thumb and forefinger appear to move in a rotary fashion as if rolling a pill, coin, or other small object. Tremor can involve the diaphragm, tongue, lips, and jaw but rarely causes shaking of the head. Unfortunately, in many people a benign essential tremor has mistakenly been diagnosed as PD. Essential tremor occurs during voluntary movement, has a more rapid frequency than parkinsonian tremor, and is often familial.

Rigidity. *Rigidity,* the second sign of the triad, is the increased resistance to passive motion when the limbs are moved through their range of motion. Parkinsonian rigidity is typified by a jerky quality, as if there were intermittent catches in the movement of a cogwheel, when the joint is moved passively. This is termed *cogwheel rigidity.* The rigidity is caused by sustained muscle contraction and consequently elicits a complaint of muscle soreness; feeling tired and achy; or pain in the head, upper body, spine, or legs. Another consequence of rigidity is slowness of movement because it inhibits the alternating of contraction and relaxation in opposing muscle groups (e.g., biceps and triceps).

Bradykinesia. *Bradykinesia* is particularly evident in the loss of automatic movements, which is secondary to the physical and chemical alteration of the basal ganglia and related structures in the extrapyramidal portion of the CNS. In the unaffected patient, automatic movements are involuntary and occur subconsciously. They include blinking of the eyelids, swinging of the arms while walking, swallowing of saliva, self-expression with facial and hand movements, and minor movement of postural adjustment. The patient with PD does not execute these movements, and there is a lack of spontaneous activity. This accounts for the stooped posture, masked face (deadpan expression), drooling of saliva, and shuffling gait (festination) that are characteristic of a person with this disease. The posture is that of a slowed "old man" image, with the head and trunk bent forward and the legs constantly flexed (Fig. 59-8).

Complications

In addition to the motor signs of PD, many nonmotor symptoms are common. They include depression, anxiety, apathy, fatigue, pain, constipation, impotence, and short-term memory impairment.[27] As the disease progresses, complications increase. These include motor symptoms (e.g., dyskinesias [spontaneous, involuntary movements], weakness, akinesia [total immobility]), neurologic problems (e.g., dementia), and neuropsychiatric problems (e.g., depression, hallucinations, psychosis). Dementia occurs in up to 40% of patients with PD.[28] As swallowing becomes more difficult (dysphagia), malnutrition or aspiration may result. General debilitation may lead to pneumonia, urinary tract infections, and skin breakdown. Orthostatic hypotension may occur in some patients and, along with loss of postural reflexes, may result in falls or other injury.

Sleep disorders in patients with PD are common, potentially severe, often underrecognized, and ineffectively treated.[29] Effective management of sleep disturbances can greatly improve the quality of life for patients with PD. It is important for the nurse to include an assessment of problems relating to sleep.

Diagnostic Studies

Because there is no specific diagnostic test for PD, the diagnosis is based solely on the history and the clinical features. A firm diagnosis can be made only when at least two of the three characteristic signs of the classic triad are present: tremor, rigidity, and bradykinesia. The ultimate confirmation of PD is a positive response to antiparkinsonian drugs. Research is ongoing using MRI to examine cognitive dysfunction in patients with PD.[30]

Collaborative Care

Because there is no cure for PD, collaborative management (Table 59-17) is aimed at relieving the symptoms.

Drug Therapy. Drug therapy for PD is aimed at correcting an imbalance of neurotransmitters within the CNS. Antiparkinsonian drugs either enhance the release or supply of DA (dopaminergic) or antagonize or block the effects of the overactive cholinergic neurons

TABLE 59-17	*COLLABORATIVE CARE* **Parkinson's Disease**

Diagnostic

History and physical examination
Tremor
Rigidity
Bradykinesia
Positive response to antiparkinsonian drugs*
MRI
Rule out side effects of phenothiazines, reserpine, benzodiazepines, haloperidol

Collaborative Therapy

Antiparkinsonian drugs*
Surgical destruction or deep brain stimulation of ventrolateral nucleus of the thalamus or posteroventral globus pallidus

MRI, Magnetic resonance imaging.
*See Table 59-18.

in the striatum (anticholinergic). Levodopa with carbidopa (Sinemet) is often the first drug to be used. Levodopa is a chemical precursor of DA and can cross the blood-brain barrier. It is converted to DA in the basal ganglia. Sinemet is the preferred drug because it also contains carbidopa, an agent that inhibits the enzyme dopa-decarboxylase in the peripheral tissues. Dopa-decarboxylase breaks down levodopa before it reaches the brain. The net result of the combination of levodopa and carbidopa is that more levodopa reaches the brain, and therefore less drug is needed. Carbidopa/levodopa is also available as Paracopa, which is a tablet that rapidly dissolves in the mouth. It can be given with or without water.

 Drug Alert - *Carbidopa/Levodopa (Sinemet)*
- *Monitor for signs of dyskinesia.*
- *Effects may be delayed for several weeks to months.*
- *Instruct patient or family member to report any uncontrolled movement of face, eyelids, mouth, tongue, arms, hands, legs; mental changes; palpitations; severe nausea/vomiting; difficulty urinating.*

Many patients are given Sinemet early in the disease course. However, some health care providers believe that, after a few years of therapy, the effectiveness of Sinemet wears off. Therefore they prefer to initiate therapy with a DA receptor agonist instead. These drugs include bromocriptine (Parlodel), pergolide (Permax), ropinirole (Requip), and pramipexole (Mirapex). These drugs directly stimulate DA receptors. When more moderate to severe symptoms are present, levodopa with carbidopa (Sinemet) is added to the drug regimen.

Drug Alert - *Bromocriptine (Parlodel)*
- *Patient may become dizzy or faint due to orthostatic hypotension, especially following the first dose.*
- *Notify physician immediately if a severe headache develops that does not let up or continues to get worse.*

Anticholinergic drugs are also used to manage PD. These drugs act by decreasing the activity of acetylcholine, thus providing balance between cholinergic and dopaminergic actions. Antihistamines (e.g., diphenhydramine [Benadryl]) with anticholinergic properties or a β-adrenergic blocker (e.g., propranolol [Inderal]) are used to manage tremors. The antiviral agent amantadine (Symmetrel) is also an effective antiparkinsonian drug. Although its ex-

act mechanism of action is not known, amantadine promotes the release of DA from neurons.

Selegiline (Eldepryl) is a monoamine oxidase (MAO) inhibitor that is sometimes used in combination with Sinemet. By inhibiting MAO, the degradative enzyme for DA, the levels of DA are increased. Rasagiline (Azilect), a type B MAO inhibitor, is a new drug used in the treatment of Parkinson's disease. It is used as an initial drug therapy in early Parkinson's disease and as an addition to levodopa in patients with more advanced disease.

Entacapone (Comtan) and tolcapone (Tasmar) block the enzyme catechol-o-methyl transferase (COMT), which breaks down levodopa in the peripheral circulation, thus prolonging the effect of Sinemet. These drugs are used only as adjuncts to levopoda.[31,32]

Table 59-18 summarizes the drugs commonly used in PD, the symptoms they relieve, and their common side effects. The use of only one drug is preferred because there are fewer side effects and the drug dosage is easier to adjust than when several drugs are used. However, as the disease progresses, combination therapy is often required. Excessive amounts of dopaminergic drugs can lead to *paradoxic intoxication* (aggravation rather than relief of symptoms).

The most commonly prescribed medication for PD is levodopa, and this drug has many side effects and drug interactions. Prolonged use often results in dyskinesias and "off-on" periods when the medication will unpredictably start or stop working.

Within 3 to 5 years of treatment with standard Parkinson's drug treatments, many patients experience episodes of hypomobility (e.g., inability to rise from chair, to speak, or to walk). The episodes can occur toward the end of a dosing interval with standard medications (so-called end-of-dose wearing off) or at unpredictable times (spontaneous "on/off").

Apomorphine (Apokyn) can be used for treating Parkinson's patients during these episodes of "hypomobility," or "off periods" in which the patient becomes immobile or unable to perform activities of daily living. Apomorphine, which is given by a subcutaneous injection, needs to be taken with an antiemetic drug (e.g., trimethobenzamide [Tigan]) because, when taken alone, it causes severe nausea and vomiting. It must not be taken with the antiemetics in the serotonin (5-HT$_3$) receptor antagonist class (e.g., ondansetron [Zofran]), because the combination of apomorphine and these drugs can lead to very low blood pressure and loss of consciousness.

Rivastigmine (Exelon) or donezepil (Aricept) is used to treat mild to moderate Parkinson's dementia. Amitriptyline (Elavil) may be used to treat depression.

Surgical Therapy. Surgical procedures are aimed at relieving symptoms of PD and are usually used in patients who are unresponsive to drug therapy or who have developed severe motor complications. Surgical procedures fall into three categories: ablation (destruction), deep brain stimulation (DBS), and transplantation. *Ablation surgery* involves stereotactic ablation of areas in the thalamus *(thalamotomy),* globus pallidus *(pallidotomy),* and subthalamic nucleus *(subthalamic nucleotomy).* Ablative procedures have been used for PD for over 50 years, but they have been replaced recently by DBS. DBS involves placing an electrode in either the thalamus, globus pallidus, or subthalamic nucleus and connecting it to a generator placed in the upper chest (like a pacemaker). The device is programmed to deliver a specific current to the targeted brain location. Unlike ablation procedures, DBS can be adjusted to control symptoms better and is reversible (the de-

| TABLE 59-18 | *DRUG THERAPY* **Parkinson's Disease** | | |

Drug	Mechanism of Action	Symptoms Relieved	Side Effects and Precautions
Dopaminergics			
levodopa (L-dopa)	Converted to dopamine in basal ganglia	Bradykinesia, tremor, rigidity	Nausea, dyskinesia, hypotension, palpitations, dysrhythmias; agitation, hallucinations, confusion (in older patient); avoidance of foods high in vitamin B_6 (reversal of effect of levodopa); contraindicated in narrow-angle glaucoma
levodopa-carbidopa (Sinemet, Paracopa [orally dissolving tablet])	Same as above	Same as above	Less nausea but greater chance of dyskinesia, confusion, hallucinations; periodic check of BUN, AST, WBCs, Hct; contraindicated in melanoma, narrow-angle glaucoma, combination with reserpine, methyldopa, guanethidine, antipsychotics
bromocriptine mesylate (Parlodel)	Same as above	Same as above	Orthostatic hypotension, nausea, vomiting, toxic psychosis, limb edema, phlebitis, dizziness, headache, insomnia
pergolide (Permax)	Same as above	Same as above	Same as above
pramipexole (Mirapex)		Same as above	Same as above
ropinirole (Requip)	Same as above	Same as above	Same as above
amantadine (Symmetrel)	Blocks reuptake of dopamine into presynaptic neurons	Rigidity, akinesia	Nervousness, insomnia, confusion, hallucinations, dry mouth, nausea, edema, orthostatic hypotension
apomorphine (Apokyn)	Stimulates postsynaptic dopamine receptors	Hypomobility, including difficulty starting movements, muscle stiffness, slow movements	Causes severe nausea and vomiting; needs to be taken with antiemetic drug; dyskinesia, sleepiness, dizziness, runny nose, chest pain, increased sweating, flushing
Anticholinergics			
trihexyphenidyl (Artane) benztropine (Cogentin) biperiden (Akineton)	Block cholinergic receptors, thus helping to balance cholinergic and dopaminergic activity	Tremor	Dry mouth, blurred vision, constipation, delirium, anxiety, agitation, hallucinations; avoidance of drugs with similar actions, including over-the-counter drugs containing scopolamine or antihistamines (e.g., Sominex), antispasmodics (e.g., Donnatal), tricyclic antidepressants (e.g., imipramine [Tofranil], amitriptyline [Elavil])
Antihistamine			
diphenhydramine (Benadryl)	Has anticholinergic effect	Tremor, rigidity	Sedation, same precautions as for anticholinergic drugs
Monoamine Oxidase Inhibitors			
selegiline (Eldepryl, Carbex) rasagiline (Azilect)	Block breakdown of dopamine	Bradykinesia, rigidity, tremor	Similar to dopaminergic drugs
Catechol-O-Methyl Transferase (COMT) Inhibitors			
entacapone (Comtan) tolcapone (Tasmar)		Block COMT and slow the breakdown of levodopa, thus prolonging the action of levodopa	Similar to dopaminergic drugs; these drugs are used in combination with levodopa Tolcapone requires additional monitoring for liver function

AST, Aspartate aminotransferase; *BUN,* blood urea nitrogen; *Hct,* hematocrit; *MAO,* monoamine oxidase; *WBCs,* white blood cells.

vice can be removed). These ablative and DBS procedures work by reducing the increased neuronal activity produced by DA depletion. DBS has been shown to improve motor function and reduce dyskinesia and medication usage.[33]

Transplantation of fetal neural tissue into the basal ganglia is designed to provide DA-producing cells in the brains of patients with PD. This form of therapy is still in the experimental stages.

Nutritional Therapy. Diet is of major importance to the patient with PD because malnutrition and constipation can be serious consequences of inadequate nutrition. Patients who have dysphagia and bradykinesia need appetizing foods that are easily chewed and swallowed. The diet should contain adequate roughage and fruit to avoid constipation. Food should be cut into bite-sized pieces before it is served, and it should be served on a warmed plate to preserve its appeal. Eating six small meals a day may be less exhausting than eating three large meals a day. Ample time should be planned for eating to avoid frustration and encourage independence. In addition, absorption of levodopa can be impaired by protein ingestion and vitamin B_6. Some patients are advised to limit their protein intake to the evening meal to decrease this problem, and to consult with their health care provider regarding vitamin B_6 in their multivitamins and fortified cereals.

NURSING MANAGEMENT
PARKINSON'S DISEASE

■ *Nursing Assessment*

Subjective and objective data that should be obtained from a patient with PD are presented in Table 59-19.

■ *Nursing Diagnoses*

Nursing diagnoses for the patient with PD may include, but are not limited to, those presented in NCP 59-4.

■ *Planning*

The overall goals are that the patient with PD will (1) maximize neurologic function, (2) maintain independence in activities of daily living for as long as possible, and (3) optimize psychosocial well-being.

■ *Nursing Implementation*

Promotion of physical exercise and a well-balanced diet are major concerns for nursing care. Exercise can limit the consequences of decreased mobility, such as muscle atrophy, contractures, and constipation. The American Parkinson Disease Association (see Resources at the end of this chapter) publishes a series of booklets and videotapes that are helpful in terms of exercise that can be used by family members and health care professionals.

A physical therapist may be consulted to design a personal exercise program aimed at strengthening and stretching specific muscles. Overall muscle tone, as well as specific exercises to strengthen the muscles involved with speaking and swallowing, should be included. Although exercise will not halt the progress of the disease, it will enhance the patient's functional ability. An occupational therapist can also assist the patient with strategies to increase self-care measures, including eating and dressing.

Because PD is a chronic degenerative disorder with no acute exacerbations, nurses should note that teaching and nursing care are directed toward maintenance of good health, encouragement of independence, and avoidance of complications such as contractures.

Problems secondary to bradykinesia can be alleviated by relatively simple measures. The following are helpful hints for patients who tend to "freeze" while walking: consciously think about stepping over imaginary or real lines on the floor, drop rice kernels and step over them, rock from side to side, lift the toes when stepping, or take one step backward and two steps forward. The patient should be assessed for the possibility of levodopa overdose because it is a common cause of akinesic "freezing." A brief period of dyskinesia, usually *athetosis* (slow, writhing, continuous, and involuntary movement) of the neck, should alert the nurse to this possibility.

Getting out of a chair can be facilitated by using an upright chair with arms and placing the back legs on small (2-inch) blocks. Other aspects of the environment can be altered. Rugs and excess furniture can be removed to avoid stumbling. An ottoman can be used to elevate the legs and avoid dependent ankle edema. Clothing can be simplified by the use of slip-on shoes and Velcro hook-and-loop fasteners or zippers on clothing, instead of buttons and hooks. An elevated toilet seat can facilitate getting on and off the toilet. The nurse should work closely with the patient's family in exploring creative adaptations that allow maximum independence and self-care.

In the early stages of PD many patients experience depression and anxiety. Patients may need to make adjustments in their life-

TABLE 59-19	*NURSING ASSESSMENT* **Parkinson's Disease**

Subjective Data
Important Health Information
Past health history: CNS trauma, cerebrovascular disorders, exposure to metals and carbon monoxide, encephalitis
Medications: Use of major tranquilizers, especially haloperidol (Haldol), and phenothiazines, reserpine, methyldopa, amphetamines

Functional Health Patterns
Health perception–health management: Fatigue
Nutritional-metabolic: Excessive salivation, dysphagia; weight loss
Elimination: Constipation, incontinence; excessive sweating
Activity-exercise: Difficulty in initiating movements; frequent falls; loss of dexterity; micrographia (handwriting deterioration)
Sleep-rest: Insomnia
Cognitive-perceptual: Diffuse pain in head, shoulders, neck, back, legs, and hips; muscle soreness and cramping
Self-perception–self-concept: Depression; mood swings, hallucinations

Objective Data
General
Blank (masked) facies, slow and monotonous speech, infrequent blinking

Integumentary
Seborrhea, dandruff; ankle edema

Cardiovascular
Postural hypotension

Gastrointestinal
Drooling

Neurologic
Tremor at rest, first in hands (pill rolling), later in legs, arms, face, and tongue; aggravation of tremor with anxiety, absence in sleep; poor coordination; subtle dementia, impaired postural reflexes

Musculoskeletal
Cogwheel rigidity, dysarthria, bradykinesia, contractures, stooped posture, shuffling gait

Possible Findings
Lack of specific tests; diagnosis on basis of history and physical findings and ruling out of other diseases

CNS, Central nervous system.

style, including work and role responsibilities. As the disease progresses, the impact on the psychologic well-being of the patient also increases. The nurse can assist the patient through listening, providing education, challenging distorted thoughts, and encouraging social interactions.

In the early stage of the disease there are also subtle changes in cognitive function that can progress to dementia. This results in increased caregiver burden and the potential for long-term care placement. Information on care of the patient with dementia is provided in Chapter 60.

The majority of patients with PD are cared for by family caregivers (e.g., spouse, children). As the disease progresses, the burden of caregiving increases. The burden of caregiving has been associated with decreases in physical and mental health of the caregiver. Strategies to reduce caregiver burden are described in Chapter 60. Other interventions for the patient with dementia are presented in NCP 59-4.

■ *Evaluation*

Expected outcomes for the patient with PD are addressed in NCP 59-4.

NURSING CARE PLAN 59-4

Patient with Parkinson's Disease

NURSING DIAGNOSIS　**Impaired physical mobility** *related to* rigidity, bradykinesia, and akinesia *as evidenced by* difficulty in initiation of purposeful movements, deterioration of spontaneity of movement

PATIENT GOALS　1. Uses physical exercise appropriately to deter muscle atrophy and joint contractures
2. Uses assistive devices appropriately for ambulation and mobility

OUTCOMES (NOC)	INTERVENTIONS (NIC) and *RATIONALES*
Mobility	*Exercise Therapy: Ambulation*
• Gait _____ • Walking _____	• Assist patient with initial ambulation *to determine degree of impairment and prevent injury.* • Consult physical therapist about ambulation plan *to facilitate activities of daily living and safe ambulation.* • Apply/provide assistive device (cane, walker, or wheelchair) for ambulation, if the patient is unsteady.
Coordinated Movement	
• Smooth movement _____ • Balanced movement _____ • Steadiness of movement _____	*Exercise Therapy: Balance* • Assist patient to stand (or sit) and rock body from side to side *to stimulate balance mechanisms and decrease akinesia.* • Encourage patient to maintain wide base of support *to prevent shuffling gait and loss of balance.*
Measurement Scale 1 = Severely compromised 2 = Substantially compromised 3 = Moderately compromised 4 = Mildly compromised 5 = Not compromised	

NURSING DIAGNOSIS　**Impaired verbal communication** *related to* dysarthia, tremor, and bradykinesia *as evidenced by* decreased amount of communication, slow and slurred speech, inability to move facial muscles, decreased tongue mobility, and micrographia

PATIENT GOAL　Develops methods of communication that meet needs for interaction with others

OUTCOMES (NOC)	INTERVENTIONS (NIC) and *RATIONALES*
Communication: Expressive	*Communication Enhancement: Speech Deficit*
• Use of spoken language: vocal _____ • Clarity of speech _____ • Use of pictures and drawings to communicate _____ • Use of nonverbal language _____	• Listen attentively *to reduce patient's frustration.* • Reinforce need for follow-up with speech therapist after discharge *to provide specialized guidance in care of the patient.* • Use picture board *because muscle involvement has impaired writing and speaking ability.* • Encourage patient to repeat words *to provide exercise and enhance understanding of words.*
Measurement Scale 1 = Severely compromised 2 = Substantially compromised 3 = Moderately compromised 4 = Mildly compromised 5 = Not compromised	

NURSING DIAGNOSIS　**Deficient diversional activity** *related to* inability to perform usual leisure activities *as evidenced by* boredom, lack of participation, restlessness, depression

PATIENT GOAL　Engages in satisfying diversional activities

OUTCOMES (NOC)	INTERVENTIONS (NIC) and *RATIONALES*
Leisure Participation	*Activity Therapy*
• Participates in low physical demand leisure activities _____ • Selects leisure activities of interest _____ • Expresses satisfaction with leisure activities _____ • Enjoys leisure activities _____	• Determine patient's commitment to increasing frequency and/or range of activity *to determine need for motivational interventions.* • Assist to focus on what patient can do, rather than on deficits. • Assist patient to identify meaningful activities *to meet individual needs.* • Assist patient to schedule specific periods for diversional activity into daily routine. • Assist patient to choose activities consistent with physical, psychologic, and social capabilities *so individual needs are considered.* • Monitor emotional, physical, social, and spiritual responses to activity *to evaluate effectiveness of interventions.*
Measurement Scale 1 = Never demonstrated 2 = Rarely demonstrated 3 = Sometimes demonstrated 4 = Often demonstrated 5 = Consistently demonstrated	*Emotional Support* • Assist patient in recognizing feelings such as anxiety, anger, or sadness *to promote problem solving and substitution of new activities for those no longer able to perform.*

NURSING CARE PLAN 59-4

Patient with Parkinson's Disease—cont'd

NURSING DIAGNOSIS **Imbalanced nutrition: less than body requirements** *related to* dysphagia *as evidenced by* difficulty swallowing and chewing, drooling, decreased gag reflex, weight loss

PATIENT GOALS 1. Maintains nutritional intake adequate for metabolic needs
2. Maintains body weight within normal parameters

OUTCOMES (NOC)

Nutritional Status
- Food intake ____
- Fluid intake ____
- Weight/height ratio ____

Measurement Scale

1 = Severe deviation from normal range
2 = Substantial deviation from normal range
3 = Moderate deviation from normal range
4 = Mild deviation from normal range
5 = No deviation from normal range

Swallowing Status
- Handles oral secretions ____
- Timely swallow reflex ____
- Swallow study findings ____

Measurement Scale

1 = Severely compromised
2 = Substantially compromised
3 = Moderately compromised
4 = Mildly compromised
5 = Not compromised

INTERVENTIONS (NIC) and *RATIONALES*

Nutritional Therapy
- Provide needed nourishment within limits of prescribed diet.
- Ensure that diet includes foods high in fiber content *to prevent constipation.*
- Assist patient to a sitting position before eating or feeding *to promote swallowing and reduce risk of aspiration.*

Swallowing Therapy
- Monitor for signs and symptoms of aspiration.
- Monitor patient's tongue movements while eating *to evaluate patient's level of impairment and minimize risk of aspiration.*
- Collaborate with other members of health care team (i.e., occupational therapist, speech pathologist, and dietitian) to provide continuity in patient's rehabilitative plan *as they can provide specific plans to improve swallowing.*

Aspiration Precautions
- Keep suction setup available *to remove pooled secretions and prevent choking and aspiration.*
- Offer foods or liquids that can be formed into a bolus before swallowing *as this consistency is more easily swallowed.*

MYASTHENIA GRAVIS

Myasthenia gravis (MG) is an autoimmune disease of the neuro-muscular junction characterized by the fluctuating weakness of certain skeletal muscle groups. MG occurs in either gender and in persons of any ethnicity. The prevalence rate is 14 per 100,000 in the United States. MG can occur at any age but most commonly occurs between the ages of 10 and 65. The peak age at onset in women is 20 to 30 years. MG is three times more common in women, but at older ages both sexes are equally affected. MG is considered infrequent over age 70.[34]

Etiology and Pathophysiology

MG is caused by an autoimmune process in which antibodies attack acetylcholine (ACh) receptors, resulting in a decreased number of ACh receptor (AChR) sites at the neuromuscular junction. This pre-vents ACh molecules from attaching and stimulating muscle con-traction. Anti-AChR antibodies are detectable in the serum of 85% to 90% of patients with generalized MG and in 50% to 60% of pa-tients with ocular myasthenia. The explanation for muscular weak-ness in the 10% to 15% of patients who lack autoantibodies to AChR may be related to autoantibodies to muscle-specific receptor tyro-sine kinase.[35] Thymic tumors are found in about 15% of patients, and abnormal thymus tissue is found in most others.

Clinical Manifestations and Complications

The primary feature of MG is fluctuating weakness of skeletal muscle. Strength is usually restored after a period of rest. The muscles most often involved are those used for moving the eyes and eyelids, chewing, swallowing, speaking, and breathing. These muscles are generally the strongest in the morning and become exhausted with continued activity. Consequently, by the end of the day, muscle weakness is prominent.

In 90% of cases, the eyelid muscles or extraocular muscles are involved. Facial mobility and expression can be impaired. There may be difficulty in chewing and swallowing food. Speech is af-fected, and the voice often fades after a long conversation. The muscles of the trunk and limbs are less often affected. Of these, the proximal muscles of the neck, shoulder, and hip are more often af-fected than the distal muscles. No other signs of neural disorder accompany MG. There is no sensory loss, reflexes are normal, and muscle atrophy is rare.

The course of this disease is highly variable. Some patients may have short-term remissions, others may stabilize, and others may have severe, progressive involvement. Restricted ocular myasthe-nia, usually seen only in men, has a good prognosis. Exacerbations of MG can be precipitated by emotional stress, pregnancy, menses, secondary illness, trauma, temperature extremes, and hypokale-mia. Ingestion of drugs, including aminoglycoside antibiotics, β-adrenergic blockers, procainamide, quinidine, and phenytoin, can aggravate MG. Psychotropic drugs (e.g., lithium carbonate, phenothiazines, benzodiazepines, tricyclic antidepressants) have also been associated with worsening of myasthenia, as have neu-romuscular blocking agents (tubocurarine chloride, pancuronium, succinylcholine [Anectine]).

Myasthenic crisis is an acute exacerbation of muscle weakness triggered by infection, surgery, emotional distress, drug overdose, or inadequate drugs. The major complications of MG result from muscle weakness in areas that affect swallowing and breathing.

TABLE 59-20	COLLABORATIVE CARE Myasthenia Gravis	
Diagnostic	**Collaborative Therapy**	
History and physical examination	Drugs	
Fatigability with prolonged upward gaze (2-3 min)	• Anticholinesterase agents	
Muscle weakness	• Corticosteroids	
EMG	• Immunosuppressive agents	
Tensilon test	Surgery (thymectomy)	
Acetylcholine receptor antibodies	Plasmapheresis	

EMG, Electromyography.

This results in aspiration, respiratory insufficiency, and respiratory infection.

Diagnostic Studies

The diagnosis of MG can be made on the basis of history and physical examination. However, other tests may be used if the diagnosis is still in doubt. EMG may show a decrementing response to repeated stimulation of the hand muscles, indicative of muscle fatigue. Use of drugs may also aid in the diagnosis. The Tensilon test in a patient with MG reveals improved muscle contractility after intravenous injection of the anticholinesterase agent edrophonium chloride (Tensilon). (Anticholinesterase blocks the enzyme acetylcholinesterase.) This test also aids in the diagnosis of cholinergic crisis (secondary to overdose of anticholinesterase drug), which occurs when there is too much cholinesterase inhibition. Clinical features include muscle fasciculation, sweating, excessive salivation, and constricted pupils. In this condition, Tensilon does not improve muscle weakness but may actually increase it. Atropine, a cholinergic antagonist, should be readily available to counteract the effects of Tensilon when it is used diagnostically.

Collaborative Care

Drug Therapy. Drug therapy for MG includes anticholinesterase drugs, alternate-day corticosteroids, and immunosuppressants (Table 59-20). Anticholinesterase drugs are aimed at enhancing function of the neuromuscular junction. Acetylcholinesterase is the enzyme that breaks down ACh. Thus inhibition of this enzyme by an anticholinesterase inhibitor will prolong the action of ACh and facilitate transmission of impulses at the neuromuscular junction. Neostigmine (Prostigmin) and pyridostigmine (Mestinon) are the most successful drugs of this group in treating MG. Tailoring the dose to avoid a myasthenic or cholinergic crisis often presents a clinical challenge. Corticosteroids (specifically prednisone) are used to suppress the immune response. Drugs such as azathioprine (Imuran) and cyclophosphamide (Cytoxan) may also be used for immunosuppression.

Many drugs are contraindicated or must be used with caution in patients with MG. Classes of drug that should be cautiously evaluated before use include anesthetics, antidysrhythmics, antibiotics, quinine, antipsychotics, barbiturates and sedative-hypnotics, cathartics, diuretics, opioids, muscle relaxants, thyroid preparations, and tranquilizers.

Surgical Therapy. Because the presence of the thymus gland in the patient with MG appears to enhance the production of AChR antibodies, removal of the thymus gland results in improvement in a majority of patients. Thymectomy is indicated for almost all patients with thymoma, for patients with generalized MG between the ages of puberty and about 65 years, and for patients with purely ocular MG.

Other Therapies. Plasmapheresis can yield a short-term improvement in symptoms and is indicated for patients in crisis or in preparation for surgery when corticosteroids must be avoided. (Plasmapheresis is discussed in Chapter 14.) Intravenous (IV) immunoglobulin G has been used with some success and is recommended as a second-line treatment for MG. However, there is insufficient evidence that intravenous immunoglobulin is better than plasmapheresis for treating exacerbations or for moderately severe MG.[36]

NURSING MANAGEMENT
MYASTHENIA GRAVIS

■ Nursing Assessment

The nurse can assess the severity of MG by asking the patient about fatigability, what body parts are affected, and how severely they are affected. The patient's coping abilities and understanding of the disorder should also be assessed. Some patients become so fatigued that they are no longer able to work or even ambulate.

Objective data should include respiratory rate and depth, oxygen saturation, arterial blood gas analyses, pulmonary function tests, and evidence of respiratory distress in patients with acute myasthenic crisis. Muscle strength of all face and limb muscles should be assessed, as should swallowing, speech (volume and clarity), and cough and gag reflexes.

■ Nursing Diagnoses

Nursing diagnoses for the patient with MG may include, but are not limited to, the following:

- Ineffective breathing pattern *related to* intercostal muscle weakness
- Ineffective airway clearance *related to* intercostal muscle weakness and impaired cough and gag reflex
- Impaired verbal communication *related to* weakness of the larynx, lips, mouth, pharynx, and jaw
- Imbalanced nutrition: less than body requirements *related to* impaired swallowing
- Disturbed sensory perception (visual) *related to* ptosis, decreased eye movements, and disconjugate gaze
- Activity intolerance *related to* muscle weakness and fatigability
- Disturbed body image *related to* inability to maintain usual lifestyle and role responsibilities

■ Planning

The overall goals are that the patient with MG will (1) have a return of normal muscle endurance, (2) manage fatigue, (3) avoid complications, and (4) maintain a quality of life appropriate to disease course.

■ Nursing Implementation

The patient with MG who is admitted to the hospital usually has a respiratory tract infection or is in an acute myasthenic crisis. Nursing care is aimed at maintaining adequate ventilation, continuing drug therapy, and watching for side effects of therapy. The nurse must be able to distinguish cholinergic from myasthenic crisis (Table 59-21) because the causes and treatment of the two conditions differ greatly.

TABLE 59-21	Comparison of Myasthenic Crisis and Cholinergic Crisis	
Myasthenic Crisis		**Cholinergic Crisis**
Causes		
Exacerbation of myasthenia following precipitating factors or failure to take drug as prescribed or drug dose too low		Overdose of anticholinesterase drugs resulting in increased ACh at the receptor sites, remission (spontaneous or after thymectomy)
Differential Diagnosis		
Improved strength after IV administration of anticholinesterase drugs; increased weakness of skeletal muscles manifesting as ptosis, bulbar signs (e.g., difficulty in swallowing, difficulty in articulating words), or dyspnea		Weakness within 1 hr after ingestion of anticholinesterase; increased weakness of skeletal muscles manifesting as ptosis, bulbar signs, dyspnea; effects on smooth muscle include pupillary miosis, salivation, diarrhea, nausea or vomiting, abdominal cramps, increased bronchial secretions, sweating, or lacrimation

ACh, Acetylcholine; *IV,* intravenous.

As with other chronic illnesses, care focuses on the neurologic deficits and their impact on daily living. A balanced diet with food that can be chewed and swallowed easily should be prescribed. Semisolid foods may be easier to eat than solids or liquids. Scheduling doses of drugs so that peak action is reached at mealtime may make eating less difficult. Diversional activities that require little physical effort and match the interests of the patient should be arranged. Teaching should focus on the importance of following the medical regimen, potential adverse reactions to specific drugs, planning activities of daily living to avoid fatigue, the availability of community resources, and the complications of the disease and therapy (crisis conditions) and what to do about them. Contact with the Myasthenia Gravis Foundation or an MG support group may be helpful and should be explored.

■ *Evaluation*

The overall expected outcomes are that the patient with MG will
- maintain optimal muscle function
- be free from side effects of drugs
- not experience complications, in particular myasthenic or cholinergic crises, from the disease
- maintain a quality of life appropriate to the disease course

RESTLESS LEGS SYNDROME

Etiology and Pathophysiology

Restless legs syndrome (RLS) is characterized by unpleasant sensory (paresthesias) and motor abnormalities of one or both legs. Prevalence rates vary from 3% to 15%. However, the numbers may be higher because the condition is underdiagnosed. Although the exact cause of RLS is not known, probably more than half of all cases are transmitted in an autosomal dominant pattern.[37] There are two distinct types of RLS, primary (idiopathic) and secondary. The majority of cases are primary, and many patients with this type of RLS report a positive family history. Secondary RLS can be seen in metabolic abnormalities associated with iron deficiency, renal failure, polyneuropathy associated with diabetes mellitus, rheumatic disorders (e.g., rheumatoid arthritis), or pregnancy. Anemia, deficient iron condition, and certain medications can cause or worsen symptoms.

The pathophysiology of primary RLS is related to abnormal iron metabolism and functional alterations in central dopaminergic neurotransmitter systems.[37] Although primary RLS may be related to nervous system dysfunction, the exact cause remains to be determined. Several theories include (1) an alteration in dopaminergic transmission in the basal ganglia, (2) axonal neuropathy, or (3) a brainstem disinhibition phenomenon resulting in motor and sensory disturbances.

Clinical Manifestations

The severity of RLS sensory symptoms ranges from infrequent minor discomfort (paresthesias, including numbness, tingling, and "pins and needles" sensation) to severe pain. Sensory symptoms often appear first and are manifested as an annoying and uncomfortable (but usually not painful) sensation in the legs. The sensation is often compared with the sensation of bugs creeping or crawling on the legs. The leg pain is localized within the calf muscles. Patients can also experience pain in the upper extremities and trunk. The discomfort occurs when the patient is sedentary and is most common in the evening or at night.

The pain at night can produce sleep disruptions and is often relieved by physical activity such as walking, stretching, rocking, or kicking. In the most severe cases, patients sleep only a few hours at night, resulting in daytime fatigue and disruption of the daily routine. The motor abnormalities associated with RLS consist of voluntary restlessness and stereotyped, periodic, involuntary movements. The involuntary movements usually occur during sleep. Symptoms are aggravated by fatigue. Over time, RLS advances to more frequent and severe episodes.

Diagnostic Studies

RLS is a clinical diagnosis and is based in large part on the patient's history or the report of the bed partner related to nighttime activities. The International Restless Legs Study Group has proposed four minimum diagnostic criteria.[37] They are (1) desire to move the limbs, (2) motor restlessness, (3) symptoms that are worse or exclusively present at rest with at least partial and temporary relief by activity, and (4) symptoms that are worse in the evening or night.

Polysomnography studies during sleep may be performed for the patient with RLS to distinguish the problem from other clinical conditions (e.g., sleep apnea) that can disturb sleep. However, periodic leg movements in sleep are a common feature in RLS patients. The patient's history of diabetes mellitus and its management may provide information to determine whether paresthesias are caused by peripheral neuropathy or RLS.

NURSING *and* COLLABORATIVE MANAGEMENT
RESTLESS LEGS SYNDROME

The goal of collaborative management is to reduce patient discomfort and distress and to improve sleep quality. When RLS is secondary to renal failure or iron deficiency, correction of these conditions will decrease symptoms. Nonpharmacologic approaches to RLS management include establishing regular sleep habits, encouraging exercise, avoiding activities that cause symptoms, and eliminating aggravating factors such as alcohol, caffeine, and certain drugs (neuroleptics, lithium, antihistamines, and antidepressants).

If nonpharmacologic measures fail to provide symptom relief, drug therapy may be started. The main drugs used in RLS are dopaminergic agents, opioids, and benzodiazepines. Dopaminergic agents such as carbidopa/levodopa (Sinemet) and DA agonists (pergolide [Permax], bromocriptine [Parlodel], pramipexole [Mirapex]) are the drugs of choice in treating RLS. Ropinirole (Requip), a drug used to treat PD, is used to treat moderate to severe RLS.[38] These agents are effective in managing sensory and motor symptoms. Dopaminergic agents have a number of side effects, including hypotension and gastric irritation.

Other agents that may be used include antiseizure drugs such as gabapentin (Neurontin), divalproex (Depakote), lamotrigine (Lamictal), and carbamazepine (Tegretol). Clonidine (Catapres) and propranolol (Inderal) are also effective in some patients. Opioids (e.g., oxycodone) are usually reserved for those patients with severe symptoms who fail to respond to other drug therapies. When used, opioids given in low doses have also been found to be effective in reducing the symptoms associated with RLS. The main side effect of opioids is constipation, so the patient may need to take a stool softener or laxative.

AMYOTROPHIC LATERAL SCLEROSIS

Amyotrophic lateral sclerosis (ALS) is a rare progressive neurologic disorder characterized by loss of motor neurons. ALS usually leads to death within 2 to 6 years after diagnosis. This disease became known as Lou Gehrig's disease when the famous baseball player was stricken with it in the early 1940s. The onset is usually between 40 and 70 years of age. ALS is more common in men than women by a ratio of 2:1.

For unknown reasons, motor neurons in the brainstem and spinal cord gradually degenerate in ALS (Fig. 59-9). Dead motor neurons cannot produce or transport vital signals to muscles. Consequently, electrical and chemical messages originating in the brain do not reach the muscles to activate them.

The typical symptoms are weakness of the upper extremities, dysarthria, and dysphagia. However, weakness may begin in the legs. Muscle wasting and fasciculations result from the denervation of the muscles and lack of stimulation and use. Death usually results from respiratory infection secondary to compromised respiratory function. Unfortunately, there is no cure for ALS. Riluzole (Rilutek) slows the progression of ALS.[39] This drug works to decrease the amount of glutamate (an excitatory neurotransmitter) in the brain. In clinical trials, riluzole has been shown to delay the need for tracheostomy and death by a few months.[39]

The illness trajectory for ALS is devastating because the patient remains cognitively intact while wasting away. The challenge of nursing care is to guide the patient in use of moderate intensity, endurance-type exercises for the trunk and limbs, as this may help to reduce ALS spasticity.[40] Additionally, the nurse needs to support the patient's cognitive and emotional functions. Nursing interventions may include (1) facilitating communication, (2) reducing risk of aspiration, (3) decreasing pain secondary to muscle weakness, (4) decreasing risk of injury related to falls, (5) providing diversional activities such as reading and human companionship, and (6) helping the patient and family manage the disease process, to include grieving related to loss of motor function and ultimately death.

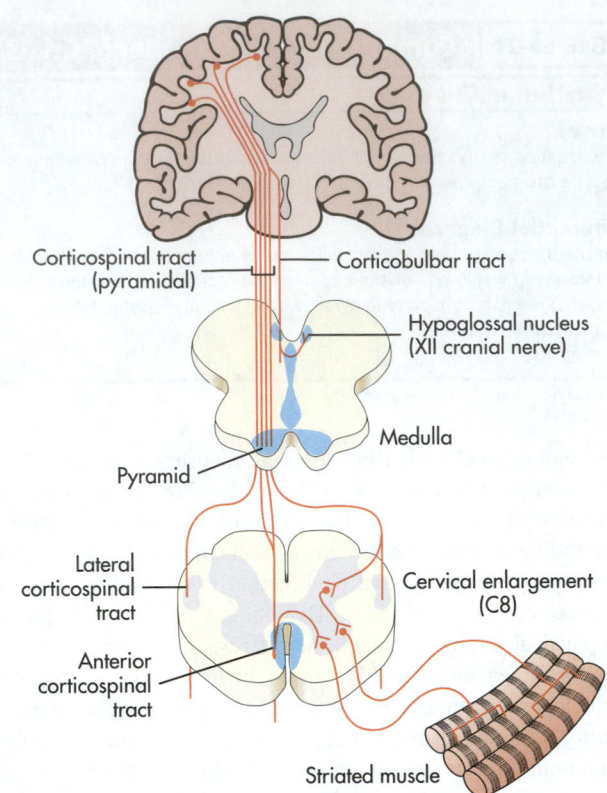

FIG. 59-9   Pathogenesis of amyotrophic lateral sclerosis. This disease is characterized by degeneration of the pyramidal tract and the motor cells in the anterior gray horns. In cases with corticobulbar involvement, the motor nuclei of cranial nerves V, VII, IX, X, XI, and XII also undergo degeneration.

HUNTINGTON'S DISEASE

Huntington's disease (HD) is a genetically transmitted, autosomal dominant disorder that affects both men and women of all races. The offspring of a person with this disease have a 50% risk of inheriting it (see Genetics in Clinical Practice box on p. 1559). The onset of HD is usually between 30 and 50 years of age. Often the diagnosis is made after the affected individual has had children. In the United States the incidence of HD is 1 in 10,000, and the incidence is fairly uniform throughout the world.[41] Diagnosis in the past was based on family history and clinical symptoms. However, since the gene for HD has been discovered, one now can be tested for the presence of the gene. People who are asymptomatic but who have a positive family history of HD face the dilemma of whether or not to get tested. If the test is positive, the person will develop HD, but when and to what extent the disease develops cannot be determined.

Like PD, the pathologic process of HD involves the basal ganglia and the extrapyramidal motor system. However, instead of a deficiency of DA, HD involves a deficiency of the neurotransmitters ACh and γ-aminobutyric acid (GABA). The net effect is an excess of DA, which leads to symptoms that are the opposite of those of parkinsonism. The clinical manifestations are characterized by abnormal and excessive involuntary movements (*chorea*). These are writhing, twisting movements of the face, limbs, and body. The movements get worse as the disease progresses. Facial movements involving speech, chewing, and swallowing are affected and may cause aspiration and malnutrition. The gait deteriorates, and ambulation eventually becomes impossible. Perhaps the most devastating deterioration is in mental functions, which include intellectual decline, emotional lability, and psychotic behavior. Death usually occurs 10 to 20 years after the onset of

GENETICS IN CLINICAL PRACTICE
Huntington's Disease

Genetic Basis
- Autosomal dominant disorder
- Caused by mutation of single gene located on chromosome 4
- Expression similar in homozygotes and heterozygotes

Incidence
- 1 in 10,000
- Higher incidence in people of European ancestry
- With each pregnancy an affected parent has a 50% chance of having a child with Huntington's disease (HD)

Genetic Testing
- DNA testing is available
- DNA testing can be done on fetal cells obtained by amniocentesis or chorionic biopsy
- Genetic testing can determine whether a person is a carrier
- No test is available to predict when symptoms will develop

Clinical Implications
- Onset of disease usually occurs at 30 to 50 years of age
- HD is a progressive, degenerative brain disorder
- No cure is available
- Drugs are available to control movements and behavioral problems
- Genetic counseling may be considered if there is a family history of HD

symptoms and occurs due to medical problems associated with the effects of HD, such as infection, choking, or pneumonia.

Because there is no cure, collaborative care is palliative. Antipsychotic (e.g., haloperidol [Haldol]), antidepressant (fluoxetine [Prozac], sertraline [Zoloft], nortriptyline [Aventyl]), and antichorea (clonazepam [Klonopin]) drugs are prescribed and have some benefit. However, they do not alter the course of the disease. Transplantation of fetal striatal neural tissues into the striatum (caudate and putamen) of the brain is an experimental treatment that may be effective.[42] HD presents a great challenge to health care professionals. The goal of nursing management is to provide the most comfortable environment possible for the patient and the family by maintaining physical safety, treating the physical symptoms, and providing emotional and psychologic support. Because of the choreic movements, caloric requirements are high. Patients may require as many as 4000 to 5000 calories per day to maintain body weight. As the disease progresses, meeting caloric needs becomes a greater challenge when the patient has difficulty swallowing and holding the head still. Depression and mental deterioration can also compromise nutritional intake.

CRITICAL THINKING EXERCISE

CASE STUDY

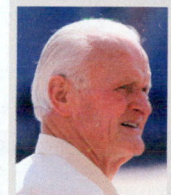

Parkinson's Disease
Patient Profile. Mr. Porter is a 79-year-old white man who was diagnosed with Parkinson's disease 2 years ago when he presented with mild hand tremors and complaints of "muscle aches." He was placed on Sinemet and reports it has been effective. Recently he and his wife have noticed new symptoms that are of concern to them. Mr. Porter reports that his hand tremors

Case Study photo ©iStockphoto.com/ Bernrd Klumpp.

are a "bit worse" and he feels achy more often than before. He also is embarrassed because he is drooling occasionally. His wife adds that she has noticed his facial expressions to be very blank and feels he may be showing signs of early dementia.

Objective Data
- Alert and oriented to person
- Mild dandruff
- Slightly slurred speech
- Rigidity with passive range of motion
- Bilateral hand tremors at rest
- Increased oral secretions but no drooling at present
- Stiff gait

Subjective Data
- Feels anxious about the future
- Worried about ability to care for his wife

Critical Thinking Questions

1. What is parkinsonism?
2. What is the pathophysiology of Parkinson's disease?
3. What is the likely explanation of the progression of his disease?
4. What is a priority nursing intervention for Mr. Porter?
5. What teaching plan regarding the course of the disease should be developed for Mr. Porter and his wife?
6. What additional medications might be added to Mr. Porter's regimen?
7. Write one or more appropriate nursing diagnoses based on the assessment data presented.

NCLEX EXAMINATION REVIEW QUESTIONS

The number of the question corresponds to the same-numbered objective at the beginning of the chapter.

1. The nurse plans care for the patient with a migraine headache based on the knowledge that, during a migraine, the patient is most likely to
   a. withdraw from stimuli.
   b. act out with bizarre behavior.
   c. seek out the company of others.
   d. experience painful facial spasms and tearing.
2. The triad of symptoms the nurse would expect to find during assessment of the patient with Parkinson's disease is
   a. spasticity, diplopia, tremor.
   b. tremor, rigidity, bradykinesia.
   c. ataxia, drowsiness, dysarthria.
   d. diplopia, tremor, bradykinesia.
3. During assessment of the patient with ALS the nurse would expect to find
   a. emotional lability.
   b. mental deterioration.
   c. muscle weakness and wasting.
   d. sensory loss in the extremities.
4. The emotional response of the patient with a chronic neurologic disease is often
   a. symptoms of intellectual deterioration.
   b. absent in patients with cognitive impairment.
   c. a result of physical disability and changes in body image.
   d. reduced in patients who have family members to care for them.

5. A major goal of treatment for the patient with a chronic, progressive neurologic disease is
   a. reversal of pathophysiology.
   b. total remission of the disease.
   c. continuation of usual lifestyle.
   d. adaptation by patient and family to the disease.

REFERENCES

1. Lipton RB, Bigal ME, Steiner RJ, et al: Classification of primary headaches, *Neurology* 63:427, 2005.
2. Lipton RB, Bigal ME: Migraine: epidemiology, impact, and risk factors for progression, *Headache* 45 (Suppl) 1:S3, 2005.
3. O'Malley P: "Oh! My aching head"—safety managing migraine headaches: update for the clinical nurse specialist, *Clin Nurse Specialist* 19:187, 2005.
4. May A: Cluster headache: pathogenesis, diagnosis, and management, *Lancet* 366:843, 2005.
5. Black DF, Swanson JW, Stang PE: Decreasing incidence of cluster headache: a population-based study in Olmsted County, Minnesota, *Headache* 45:220, 2005.
6. Loder E, Biondi D: General principles of migraine management: the changing role of prevention, *Headache* 45 (Suppl 1):S33, 2005.
7. Brandes JL: Practical use of topiramate for migraine prevention, *Headache* 45 (Suppl 1):S66, 2005.
8. Mathew NT, Frishberg BM, Gawel M, et al; BOTOX CDH Study Group: Botulinum toxin type A (BOTOX) for the prophylactic treatment of chronic daily headache: a randomized, double-blind, placebo-controlled trial, *Headache* 45:293, 2005.
9. Eross EJ, Gladstone JP, Lewis S, et al: Duration of migraine is a predictor for response to botulinum toxin type A, *Headache* 45:308, 2005.
10. Saper JR, Dodick D, Gladstone JP: Management of chronic daily headache: challenges in clinical practice, *Headache* 45 (Suppl 1):S74, 2005.
11. Epilepsy Foundation. *Epilepsy and seizure statistics*. Available at *www.epilepsyfoundation.org/answerplace/statistics.cfm* (accessed August 31, 2006).
12. Tellez-Zenteno JF, Pondal-Sordo M, Matijevic S, et al: 2004 national and regional prevalence of self-reported epilepsy in Canada, *Epilepsia* 45:1623, 2004.
13. Sander JW: The use of antiepileptic drugs, *Principles and Practice* 45:28, 2005.
14. Tian GF, Azmi H, Takano T, et al: An astrocytic basis of epilepsy, *Nat Med* 11:973, 2005.
15. Task Force on Epilepsy Classification and Terminology: Seizure types, International League Against Epilepsy, 2006. Available at *www.ilae-epilepsy.org/Visitors/Centre/ctf/seizure_types.cfm*.
16. Gambrell M, Flynn N: Seizures 101, *Nursing* 34(8):36, 2004.
17. Cole A: Initial individualized selection of long-term anticonvulsant drugs by neurologists, *Neurology* 63(10 Suppl 4):S1, 2004.
18. Bergey G: Initial treatment of epilepsy: special issues in treating the elderly, *Neurology* 63(10 Suppl 4):S40, 2004.
19. Chilcott J, Howell S, Kemeny A, et al: The effectiveness of surgery in the management of epilepsy, Cochrane Centre for Reviews and Dissemination, *Database of Abstracts of Reviews of Effects* 3:DARE-20008004, 2005.
20. Hafler DA, Salvik JM, Anderson DE, et al: Multiple sclerosis, *Immunol Rev* 204:208, 2005.
21. Lubin FD, Reingold SC: Defining the clinical course of multiple sclerosis: results of an international survey, *Neurology* 46:907, 1996.
22. Holland N, Madonna M: Nursing grand rounds, *J Neurosci Nurs* 37:15, 2005.
23. Rietberg MB, Brooks D, Uitdehaag BMJ, et al: Exercise therapy for multiple sclerosis, *Cochrane Database Syst Rev* 3:CD003980, 2005.
24. Jepson RG, Mihaljevic L, Craig J: Cranberries for preventing urinary tract infections, *Cochrane Database Syst Rev* 3:CD001321, 2005.
25. Nutt JG, Wooten GF: Diagnosis and initial management of Parkinson's disease, *N Engl J Med* 353:1021, 2005.
26. Zhang L, Dawson VL, Dawson TM: Role of nitric oxide in Parkinson's disease, *Pharmacol Ther* 109:33, 2006.
27. Frucht SJ: Parkinson disease: an update, *Neurologist* 10:185, 2004.
28. Ghazi-Noori S, Chung TH, Deane KHO, et al: Therapies for depression in Parkinson's disease, *Cochrane Database Syst Rev* 3:CD003465, 2005.
29. Adler CH: Sleep issues in Parkinson's disease, *Neurology* 64(12 Suppl 3):S12, 2005.
30. Nagano-Saito A, Washimi Y, Arahata Y, et al: Cerebral atrophy and its relation to cognitive impairment in Parkinson disease, *Neurology* 64:224, 2005.
31. Deane KHO, Spieker S, Clarke CE: Catechol-O-methyltransferase inhibitors for levodopa-induced complications in Parkinson's disease, *Cochrane Database Syst Rev* 3:CD004554, 2005.
32. Goetz CG, Poewe W, Rascol O, et al: Evidence-based medical review update: pharmacological and surgical treatments of Parkinson's disease: 2001-2004, *Mov Disord* 20:523, 2005.
33. Olanow CW, Watts RL, Koller WC: An algorithm (decision tree) for the management of Parkinson's disease (2001): treatment guidelines, *Neurology* 56:1, 2001.
34. Aragones JM, Bolibar I, Bonfill X, et al: Myasthenia gravis: a higher than expected incidence in the elderly, *Neurology* 60:1024, 2003.
35. Vincent AC, McConville J, Newsom-Davis J, et al: Is "seronegative" MG explained by autoantibodies to MuSK? *Neurology* 64:399, 2005.
36. Gajdos P, Chevret S, Toyka K: Intravenous immunoglobulin for myasthenia gravis, *Cochrane Database Syst Rev* 3:CD002277, 2005.
37. Thorpy MJ: New paradigms in the treatment of restless legs syndrome, *Neurology* 64:S28, 2005.
38. FDA Talk Paper: FDA approves Requip for restless legs syndrome, May 5, 2005. Available at *www.fda.gov/bbs/topics/ANSWERS/2005/ANS01356.html* (accessed August 31, 2006).
39. Miller RG, Mitchell JD, Lyon M, et al: Riluzole for amyotrophic lateral sclerosis (ALS)/motor neuron disease (MND), *Cochrane Database Syst Rev* 3:CD001447, 2005.
40. Ashworth NL, Satkunam LE, Deforge D: Treatment for spasticity in amyotrophic lateral sclerosis/motor neuron disease, *Cochrane Database Syst Rev* 3:CD004156, 2005.
41. Ekestern E, Lebhart G: Long-term monitoring of the mortality trend of Huntington's disease in Austria, *Eur J Epidemiol* 20:169, 2005.
42. Kim SU: Human neural stem cells genetically modified for brain repair in neurological disorders, *Neuropathology* 24:159, 2004.

RESOURCES

ALS Association (ALSA)
 800-782-4747 or 818-880-9007
 www.alsa.org
American Association of Neuroscience Nurses (AANN)
 888-557-2266 or 847-375-4733
 www.aann.org
American Council for Headache Education (ACHE)
 856-423-0258
 www.achenet.org
American Parkinson Disease Association
 800-223-2732 or 718-981-8001
 www.apdaparkinson.org
Association of Rehabilitation Nurses (ARN)
 800-229-7530 or 847-375-4710
 www.rehabnurse.org
Epilepsy Foundation
 800-332-1000
 www.efa.org
Huntington's Disease Society of America
 800-345-HDSA or 212-242-1968
 www.hdsa.org
Myasthenia Gravis Foundation of America
 800-541-5454 or 651-917-6256
 www.myasthenia.org
National Headache Foundation
 888-NHF-5552
 www.headaches.org
National Institute of Neurological Disorders and Stroke
 800-352-9424 or 301-496-5751
 www.ninds.nih.gov
National Multiple Sclerosis Society
 800-FIGHT-MS
 www.nmss.org
Restless Legs Syndrome Foundation
 877-463-6757 or 507-287-6465
 www.rls.org
For additional Internet resources, see the website for this book at *http://evolve.elsevier.com/Lewis/medsurg.*

Nursing Management
Alzheimer's Disease and Dementia

60

Virginia Shaw and Sharon L. Lewis

LEARNING OBJECTIVES

1. Define dementia and describe its impact on society.
2. Compare and contrast different etiologies of dementia.
3. Describe the clinical manifestations, diagnostic studies, and collaborative management of dementia.
4. Describe the clinical manifestations of mild cognitive impairment.
5. Describe the clinical manifestations, diagnostic studies, and collaborative management of Alzheimer's disease.
6. Describe the nursing management of the patient with Alzheimer's disease.
7. Describe other neurodegenerative disorders associated with dementia, including Lewy body dementia, Pick's disease, Creutzfeldt-Jakob disease, and normal pressure hydrocephalus.
8. Describe the etiology, pathophysiology, clinical manifestations, diagnostic studies, and collaborative management of delirium.

KEY TERMS

Alzheimer's disease, p. 1564
Creutzfeldt-Jakob disease, p. 1575
delirium, p. 1576
dementia, p. 1561
frontotemporal dementia, p. 1576
Lewy body dementia, p. 1575
mild cognitive impairment, p. 1564
neurofibrillary tangles, p. 1565
Pick's disease, p. 1576
sundowning, p. 1573
vascular dementia, p. 1562

Electronic Resources

Supplemental content related to Chapter 60 can be found . . .

Companion CD
- Stress-Busting Kit for Nursing Students
- Interactive Case Study: Alzheimer's Disease
- NCLEX Examination Review Questions
- Comprehensive Glossary

Evolve Website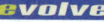
http://evolve.elsevier.com/Lewis/medsurg
- Content Updates
- Key Points (Printable and CD/MP3 Download)
- Concept Map Creator
- Expanded Audio Glossary
- Key Term Flash Cards
- Customizable Nursing Care Plans:
  - Alzheimer's Disease
  - Caregiver of the Patient with Alzheimer's Disease

- Audio Lecture: Alzheimer's Disease
- Patient and Family Instruction Guides in English and Spanish:
  - Early Warning Signs of Alzheimer's Disease
  - Managing Alzheimer's Disease
- Electronic Calculators
- WebLinks

The three most common cognitive problems in adults are dementia, delirium (acute confusion), and depression. Table 60-1 provides an overview of these conditions. Although this chapter focuses on dementia and delirium, the nurse needs to recognize that depression is often associated with these conditions.

DEMENTIA

Dementia is a syndrome characterized by dysfunction or loss of memory, orientation, attention, language, judgment, and reasoning. Personality changes and behavioral problems such as agita-tion, delusions, and hallucinations may result.[1] Ultimately these problems result in alterations in the individual's ability to work, to fulfill social and family responsibilities, and to perform activities of daily living. Physicians usually diagnose dementia when two or more brain functions, such as memory loss or language skills, are significantly impaired.

Dementia is not a normal part of aging, although it occurs most often in older adults. Fifteen percent of older Americans have dementia. As the average life span of humans increases, the number of those affected with dementia is growing. It is now a major inter-

---

Reviewed by Judith L. Roy, RN, BSN, BC (Gerontological Nursing), Staff Developmental Coordinator and Infection Control Officer, Maine Veterans' Home, Scarborough, Maine.

TABLE 60-1	Comparison of the Clinical Features of Delirium, Dementia, and Depression		
Feature	**Dementia**	**Delirium**	**Depression**
Onset	Usually insidious	Rapid, often at night	Coincides with life changes; often abrupt
Course	Long; symptoms progressive yet relatively stable over time	Fluctuates, worse at night; lucid intervals	Diurnal effects, typically worse in the morning; situational fluctuations
Progression	Slow but even	Abrupt	Variable, rapid to slow but uneven
Duration	Months to years	Hours to <1 mo	At least 2 wk, but can be several months to years
Awareness	Clear	Reduced	Clear
Alertness	Generally normal	Fluctuates, lethargic or hypervigilant	Normal
Orientation	Progressive impairment	Fluctuates in severity, generally impaired	Selective disorientation resulting from impaired concentration and attention span, which may manifest as memory deficit
Thinking	Difficulty with abstraction, thoughts impoverished, judgment impaired, words difficult to find	Disorganized, distorted, fragmented; slow or accelerated incoherent speech	Intact but with apathy, fatigue; may not want to live; may be at risk for suicide
Perception	Misperceptions often present; delusions, illusions, and hallucinations	Distorted; illusions, delusions, and hallucinations	May deny depression
Psychomotor behavior	Apraxia	Variable; hypokinetic, hyperkinetic, or mixed	Variable; psychomotor retardation or agitation
Sleep-wake cycle	Frequent awakenings	Disturbed, cycle reversed	Disturbed, often early morning awakening
Mental status testing	Frequent "near miss" answers, struggles with test, great effort to find an appropriate reply; consistently poor performances	Distracted from task; poor performance; improves when patient recovers	Frequent "don't know" answers, little effort, frequently gives up, indifferent

national public health concern. There are about 100 causes of dementia, with 60% to 80% of the patients with dementia having the diagnosis of Alzheimer's disease (AD).[2] In the United States, half of all patients in long-term care facilities have AD or a related dementia. In Canada, approximately 60,000 new cases of dementia are identified each year.[3]

Etiology and Pathophysiology

Dementia is due to both treatable and nontreatable conditions (Table 60-2). The two most common causes of dementia are neurodegenerative conditions (e.g., AD) and vascular disorders. Neurodegenerative conditions account for 60% to 80% of all dementias. Advanced age and family history are important risk factors for dementia. Infectious conditions such as bacterial meningitis and viral encephalitis can result in both vascular and neurodegenerative changes that may ultimately result in dementia.

Dementia is sometimes caused by treatable conditions that are potentially reversible (see Table 60-2). Initially these conditions may be reversible. However, with prolonged exposure or disease, irreversible changes may occur.

Vascular causes are the second most common cause of dementia. **Vascular dementia,** also called multiinfarct dementia, is the loss of cognitive function resulting from ischemic, ischemic-hypoxic, or hemorrhagic brain lesions caused by cardiovascular disease. This type of dementia is the result of decreased blood supply from narrowing and blocking of arteries that supply the brain. Vascular dementia may be caused by a single stroke (infarct) or by multiple strokes.

A history of smoking, cardiac dysrhythmias (e.g., atrial fibrillation), hypertension, hypercholesterolemia, diabetes mellitus, and coronary artery disease predispose to vascular dementia. Patients with metabolic syndrome have an increased risk of dementia and Alzheimer's disease.[4]

Clinical Manifestations

Depending on the cause of the dementia, the onset of symptoms may be insidious and gradual or more abrupt. Often dementia associated with neurologic degeneration is gradual and progressive over time. Causes of vascular dementia often result in more abrupt symptoms or symptoms that progress in a more stepwise pattern. However, it is difficult to distinguish the etiology of dementia (vascular versus neurodegenerative) based on symptom progression alone. An acute (days to weeks) or subacute (weeks to months) pattern of change may be indicative of an infectious or metabolic cause, including encephalitis, meningitis, hypothyroidism, or drug-related dementia.

Clinical manifestations of dementia are classified as mild, moderate, and severe (Table 60-3). Regardless of the cause of dementia, the initial symptoms are related to changes in cognitive functioning. Patients may have complaints of memory loss, mild disorientation, and/or trouble with words and numbers. Often it is a family member, in particular the spouse, who reports to the health care provider about the patient's declining memory. Almost all adults experience some changes with memory related to aging. Normal age-related memory decline is characterized as mild changes that do not impact activities of daily living. In dementia the memory loss initially relates to recent events, with remote memories still intact. With time and progression of the dementia, memory loss includes both recent and remote memory and ultimately affects the ability to perform self-care.

Diagnostic Studies

The diagnosis of dementia is focused on determining the cause (e.g., reversible versus nonreversible factors). An important first step is a thorough medical, neurologic, and psychologic history. A thorough physical examination is performed to rule out other potential medical conditions. Screening for cobalamin (vitamin B_{12})

TABLE 60-2	**Causes of Dementia**		
Neurodegenerative disorders	Alzheimer's disease Lewy body dementia Frontal lobe dementia Frontal-temporal dementia (e.g., Pick's disease) Down syndrome Amyotrophic lateral sclerosis (ALS) Parkinson's disease Huntington's disease	**Immunologic diseases or infections**	Multiple sclerosis Chronic fatigue syndrome Infections (e.g., Creutzfeldt-Jakob disease) Acquired immunodeficiency syndrome (AIDS) Meningitis* Encephalitis* Neurosyphilis*
Vascular diseases	Vascular (multiinfarct) dementia Cardiac disease causing emboli or decreased perfusion Binswanger's disease Subarachnoid hemorrhage* Chronic subdural hematoma*	**Systemic diseases** **Trauma** **Tumors**	Systemic lupus erythematosus* Uremic encephalopathy* Dialysis dementia* Hepatic encephalopathy* Wilson's disease Head injury* Brain tumors (primary)* Metastatic tumors*
Toxic or metabolic diseases	Alcoholism Thiamine (vitamin B_1) deficiency* Cobalamin (vitamin B_{12}) deficiency* Folate deficiency* Hyperthyroidism* Hypothyroidism* Hypoglycemia* Hypercalcemia*	**Ventricular disorders** **Seizure disorders** **Drugs†**	Hydrocephalus* Epilepsy Diuretics digoxin Anticholinergics Opioids Hypnotics Antihypertensives Antiparkinsonian drugs Antihistamines

*Potentially reversible.

†These are examples of drugs that may cause cognitive impairment that is potentially reversible.

TABLE 60-3	**Clinical Manifestations of Dementia**	
Early (Mild)	**Middle (Moderate)**	**Late (Severe)**
• Forgetfulness beyond what is seen in a normal person • Short-term memory impairment, especially for new learning • Difficulty recognizing what numbers mean • Loss of initiative and interests • Decreased judgment • Geographic disorientation	• Impaired ability to recognize close family or friends • Agitation • Wandering, getting lost • Loss of remote memory • Confusion • Impaired comprehension • Forgets how to do simple tasks • Apraxia • Receptive aphasia • Expressive aphasia • Insomnia • Delusions • Illusions, hallucinations • Behavioral problems	• Little memory, unable to process new information • Cannot understand words • Difficulty eating, swallowing • Repetitious words or sounds • Unable to perform self-care activities • Immobility • Incontinence

deficiency and hypothyroidism are often performed. Based on patient history, testing for neurosyphilis (see Chapter 59) may be performed. The American Academy of Neurology recommends cognitive evaluation and ongoing clinical monitoring of persons with mild cognitive impairment (MCI) because of their increased risk of developing dementia.[5] (MCI is described later in this chapter.)

Mental status testing is an important component of the patient evaluation. Patients with mild dementia may be able to compensate, making it difficult to evaluate cognitive function through conversation. Cognitive testing is focused on evaluating memory, ability to calculate, language, visuospatial skills, and degree of alertness. The Mini-Mental State Examination (Table 60-4) is the most commonly used tool to assess cognitive functioning.

Depression is often mistaken for dementia in older adults, and, conversely, dementia for depression. Manifestations of depression (especially in the older adult) include sadness, difficulty thinking and concentrating, fatigue, apathy, feelings of despair, and inactivity. When the depression is severe, poor concentration and attention may result, causing memory and functional impairment. When dementia and depression occur together (which may occur in up to 40% of patients with dementia), the intellectual deterioration can be more extreme. Depression, alone or in combination with dementia, is treatable. The challenge is to make an accurate and early assessment and diagnosis.

Diagnosis of dementia related to vascular causes is based on the presence of cognitive loss, the presence of vascular brain lesions demonstrated by neuroimaging techniques, and the exclusion of other causes of dementia (e.g., AD). The American Academy of Neurology guidelines include the use of structural neuroimaging with computed tomography (CT) or magnetic resonance imaging (MRI) in the evaluation of patients with dementia.[6] Although both single-photon emission computed tomography (SPECT) and positron emission tomography (PET) scanning techniques can be used

TABLE 60-4	Mini-Mental State Examination (MMSE)

MMSE Sample Items

Orientation to Time
"What is the date?"

Registration
"Listen carefully, I am going to say three words. You say them back after I stop. Ready? Here they are . . . HOUSE (pause), CAR (pause), LAKE (pause). Now repeat those words back to me." (Repeat up to five times, but score only the first trial.)

Naming
"What is this?" (Point to a pencil or pen.)

Reading
"Please read this and do what it says." (Show examinee the words CLOSE YOUR EYES on the stimulus form.)

Reproduced by special permission of the Publisher, Psychological Assessment Resource, Inc., 16204 North Florida Avenue, Lutz, Florida 33549, from the Mini Mental State Examination, by Marshal Folstein and Susan Folstein, Copyright 1975, 1998, 2001 by Mini-Mental, LLC, Inc. Published 2001 by Psychological Assessment Resources, Inc. Further reproduction is prohibited without permission from PAR, Inc. The MMSE can be purchased from PAR, Inc., by calling (813) 968-3003.

to characterize central nervous system (CNS) changes in dementia, these tools are not routinely used in the initial diagnosis of dementia. There are no genetic markers or cerebrospinal fluid (CSF) markers that are currently recommended for routine evaluation of patients with dementia.

NURSING and COLLABORATIVE MANAGEMENT
DEMENTIA

In many ways, management of the patient with dementia is similar to management of the patient with AD (described later in this chapter). One form of dementia, vascular dementia, can often be prevented. Preventive measures include treatment of risk factors such as hypertension, diabetes, smoking, hyperfibrinogenemia, hyperhomocystinemia, orthostatic hypotension, and cardiac dysrhythmias. (Stroke is discussed in Chapter 58.) Cholinesterase inhibitors (e.g., donepezil [Aricept]) that are used for patients with AD are also useful in patients with vascular dementia.

MILD COGNITIVE IMPAIRMENT

Mild cognitive impairment (MCI) is a state of cognitive functioning that is below defined norms, yet does not meet the criteria for dementia (Table 60-5). Criteria for MCI as established by the American Academy of Neurology include: (1) memory complaint, preferably confirmed by another person, (2) measurable memory impairment as detected with standard assessment tests, (3) normal overall thinking and cognitive function, and (4) ability to perform activities of daily living.[5]

Causes of MCI may include stress, anxiety, depression, or physical illness. Subgroups of MCI are based on the cause (e.g., degenerative, vascular, psychiatric, or medical) and on which aspects of cognition are affected. The subgroup with memory impairment as the predominant deficit (often called MCI with memory loss or amnestic MCI) is the group most likely to develop AD. The percentage of patients with MCI who develop AD remains unknown. Controversy exists as to whether MCI is a precursor to AD, a multifaceted condition in which AD is one of several potential causes, or a separate clinical condition.

TABLE 60-5	Mild Cognitive Impairment (MCI)
Description	• MCI refers to a state of cognition and functional ability below defined norms that does not meet criteria for dementia.
	• Individuals are memory impaired but otherwise functionally normal.
	• Subtypes of MCI are based on cause and which type of cognition is affected.
	• Subtype that features memory impairment is called MCI with memory loss or amnestic MCI.
Characteristics	• Memory complaint
	• Abnormal memory for age
	• Intact activities of daily living
	• Normal general cognitive functioning
Significance	• It is important to identify and treat patients with MCI.
	• Treatment strategies must be developed to stop or reverse the decline in cognitive function.

More research is needed to better understand and treat the patient with MCI. Presently there is no widely accepted guideline for treatment. There is insufficient evidence to recommend a standard approach. Research is being conducted to determine whether these patients benefit from the medications used in AD (e.g., acetylcholinesterase inhibitors). Until research determines the risk and benefits of administering AD medications, the primary treatment consists of ongoing monitoring.

The nurse caring for the patient with MCI must recognize the importance of monitoring the patient for changes in memory and thinking skills that would indicate a worsening of symptoms or a progression to dementia. It is critical that the nurse understand the 10 early warning signs of AD (see Table 60-6 later in this chapter).

ALZHEIMER'S DISEASE

Alzheimer's disease is a chronic, progressive, degenerative disease of the brain. It is the most common form of dementia, accounting for approximately 60% to 80% of all cases of dementia. AD is named after Alois Alzheimer, a German physician who in 1906 described changes in the brain tissue of a 51-year-old woman who had died of an unusual mental illness.

Approximately 4.5 million Americans suffer from AD. It is estimated that 5% of people ages 65 to 74, and nearly 50% of those over age 85, have AD.[7] Most patients live 8 to 10 years after being diagnosed, although some patients live for 20 years. The economic cost of caring for persons in the United States with AD is at least $100 billion annually.[8] The burden on the patient, family, caregivers, and society as a whole is staggering.

The incidence of AD is slightly higher in African Americans and Hispanic Americans. AD has been associated with lower socioeconomic status and education level and poor access to health care. Therefore additional research is needed to determine whether ethnic differences are related to genetic or environmental risk factors. Women are more likely than men to develop AD, primarily because they live longer (see the Gender Differences box).

Etiology and Pathophysiology

The exact etiology of AD is unknown. Similar to other forms of dementia, age is the most important risk factor for developing AD. However, AD is a disease that destroys brain cells, which is not a normal part of aging. Only a small percentage of people younger than 60 years old will develop AD. When AD develops in someone less than the age of 60, it is referred to as *early-onset AD*. AD that becomes evident in individuals after the age of 60 is called *late-onset AD* (see the Genetics in Clinical Practice box).

Persons in whom a clear pattern of inheritance within a family is established are said to have **familial Alzheimer's disease** (FAD). Other cases in persons in whom no familial connection can be made are termed *sporadic*. FAD is associated with earlier onset (before 60 years of age) and more rapid disease course. In both FAD and sporadic AD, the pathogenesis of AD is similar.

Characteristic findings of AD relate to changes in the brain's structure and function: (1) amyloid plaques, (3) neurofibrillary tangles, and (3) loss of connections between cells and cell death.[9] Fig. 60-1 shows the pathologic changes in AD disease.

As part of aging, people develop some plaques in their brain tissue, but in AD there are more plaques in certain parts of the brain. These plaques consist of clusters of insoluble deposits of a protein called *β-amyloid*, other proteins, remnants of neurons, non-nerve cells such as microglia (cells that surround and digest damaged cells or foreign substances), and other cells, such as astrocytes. β-Amyloid is cleaved from amyloid precursor protein (APP), which is associated with the cell membrane (Fig. 60-2). The normal function of APP is unknown. In AD, plaques develop first in areas of the brain used for memory and cognitive function, including the hippocampus (a structure that is important in forming and storing short-term memories). Eventually AD attacks the cerebral cortex, especially the areas responsible for language and reasoning.

Neurofibrillary tangles are abnormal collections of twisted protein threads inside nerve cells. The main component of these structures is a protein called *tau*. Tau proteins in the CNS are involved in providing support for intracellular structure through their support of microtubules. Tau proteins hold the microtubules together like railroad ties hold railroad tracks together. In AD the tau protein is altered, and as a result, the microtubules twist together in a helical fashion (see Fig. 60-2). This ultimately forms the neurofibrillary tangles observed in the neurons of persons with AD.

Plaques and neurofibrillary tangles are not unique to patients with AD or dementia. They are also found in the brains of individuals without evidence of cognitive impairment. However, they are more plentiful in the brains of individuals with AD.

The third feature of AD is the gradual loss of connections between neurons. This process leads to damage and then death of the neurons. Affected parts of the brain begin to shrink in a process called brain atrophy. By the final state of AD, brain tissue has shrunk significantly (Fig. 60-3).

Genetic Factors. Genetic factors may play a critical role in how the brain processes the β-amyloid protein.[9] Overproduction of β-amyloid appears to be an important risk factor for AD. Abnormally high levels of β-amyloid are thought to produce cell damage either directly or through eliciting an inflammatory response and ultimately neuron death. Understanding why neurons produce β-amyloid led researchers to examine the enzymes (and their genes) that are responsible for both the synthesis and processing of APP.

In patients with early-onset AD, three genes have been identified as important in the etiology of AD (see Genetics in Clinical Practice box above). When the presenilin-1 and presenilin-2 genes are mutated, they cause brain cells to overproduce β-amyloid.

The first gene associated with AD was the epsilon (E)-4 allele of the apolipoprotein E (ApoE) gene on chromosome 19.[9] ApoE comes in several different forms or alleles, but three occur most commonly. People inherit one allele (i.e., ApoE-2, ApoE-3, ApoE-4) from each parent. ApoE may play a role in clearing amyloid plaques. Mutations in this gene result in greater amyloid deposition. The presence of ApoE-4 increases the risk of a person developing late-onset AD. However, the presence of the gene alone is not adequate to account for AD as many people with ApoE-4 do not develop AD.

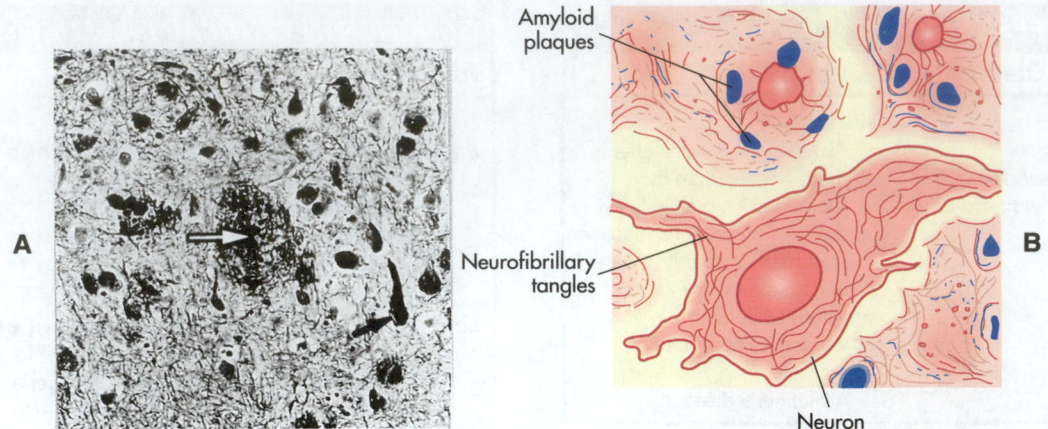

FIG. 60-1 Pathologic changes in Alzheimer's disease. **A,** Plaque with central amyloid core *(white arrow)* next to a neurofibrillary tangle *(black arrow)* on the histologic specimen from a brain autopsy. **B,** Schematic representation of amyloid plaque and neurofibrillary tangle.

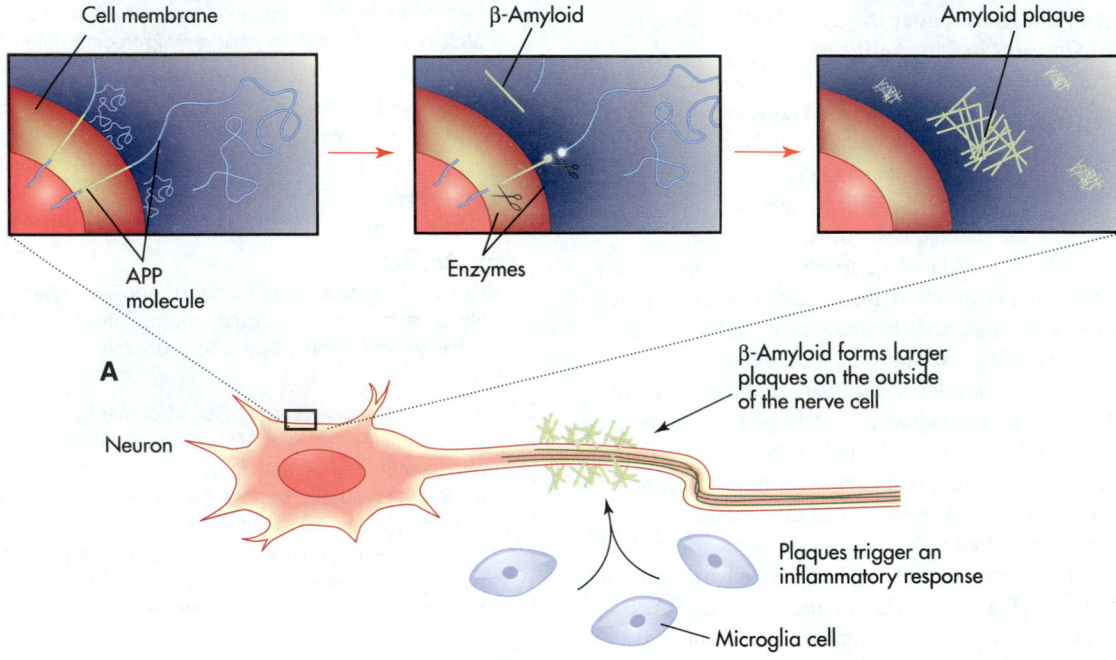

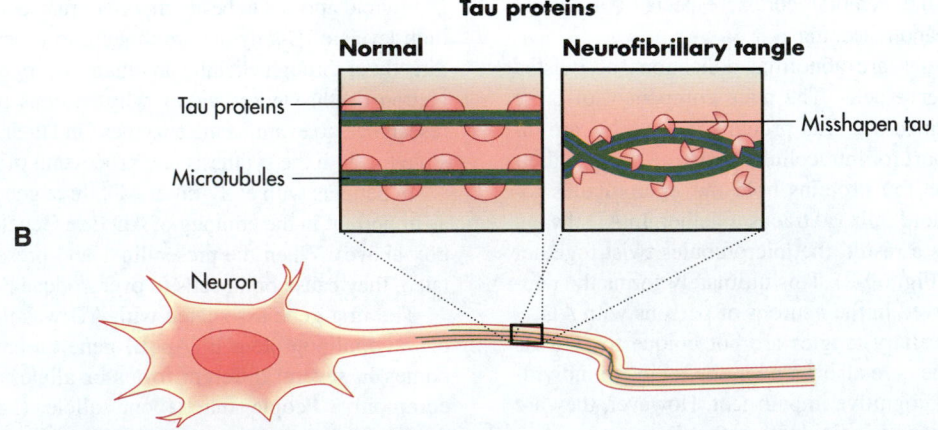

FIG. 60-2 Current etiologic theories for the development of Alzheimer's disease. **A,** Abnormal amounts of β-amyloid are cleaved from the amyloid precursor protein (APP) and released into the circulation. The β-amyloid fragments come together in clumps to form plaques that attach to the neuron. Microglia react to the plaque and an inflammatory response results. **B,** Tau proteins provide structural support for the neuron microtubules. Chemical changes in the neuron produce structural changes in tau proteins. This results in twisting and tangling (neurofibrillary tangles).

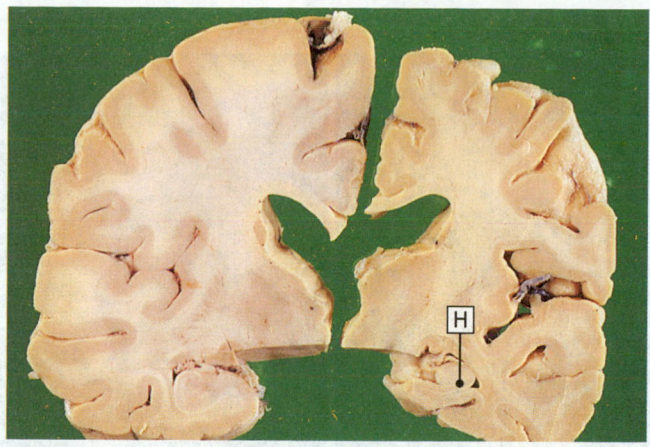

FIG. 60-3 Effects of Alzheimer's disease on the brain. This figure shows slices from two brains. On the left is a normal brain from a 70-year-old; on the right is the same region from a 70-year-old with Alzheimer's disease. The diseased brain is atrophic with loss of cortex and white matter, most marked in the hippocampal region (H).

Cellular and Other Factors.

Researchers are very interested in the possible link between inflammation and the development of AD. One theory links aging and inflammation. The theory of aging suggests that, over time, formation of free radicals (by-products of normal cell metabolism) damages neurons, thus resulting in loss of function. This oxidative damage leads to inflammation, which may be a factor in the development of AD.[9]

Another area of research focuses on the link between cardiovascular disease and AD. Studies have shown that common risk factors for heart disease (e.g., hypertension, obesity, smoking, atherosclerosis, elevated cholesterol levels, and elevated homocysteine [an amino acid] levels) are also associated with an increased risk of AD. Clinical trials are underway to determine if dietary supplements and vitamins that may help to control free radicals (e.g., folic acid, vitamins C and E) and that reduce homocysteine levels (e.g., vitamins B_6 and B_{12}) reduce the risk for AD.[9]

Epidemiologic Factors.

Epidemiologic studies focus on groups of people, thus hoping to learn more about the causes of AD. Early findings have shown that individuals who engage in activities that involve information processing (e.g., reading, doing crossword puzzles, learning a new language) have a lower risk of developing AD. Lifestyle factors that may relate to AD risk include dietary patterns, physical activity, leisure activities, and educational attainment.[9]

Clinical Manifestations

Pathologic changes often precede clinical manifestations of dementia by anywhere from 5 to 20 years. The Alzheimer's Association has developed a list of warning signs that include common manifestations of AD (Table 60-6). The manifestations of AD can be categorized similarly to those for dementia as mild, moderate, and late (see Table 60-3). The rate of progression from mild to late is highly variable from individual to individual and ranges from 3 to 20 years.

An initial sign of AD is a subtle deterioration in memory. Inevitably this progresses to more profound memory loss that interferes with the patient's ability to function. As the disease progresses, manifestations are more easily noticed and become serious enough to cause people with AD or their family members to seek medical help. Recent events and new information cannot be recalled. Personal hygiene deteriorates, as does the ability to concentrate and

TABLE 60-6	**PATIENT AND FAMILY TEACHING GUIDE** **Early Warning Signs of Alzheimer's Disease (AD)**

1. **Memory loss that affects job skills**
   - Frequent forgetfulness or unexplainable confusion at home or in the workplace may signal that something is wrong.
   - This type of memory loss goes beyond forgetting an assignment, colleague's name, deadline, or phone number.
2. **Difficulty performing familiar tasks**
   - It is not abnormal for most people to become distracted and to forget something (e.g., leave something on the stove too long).
   - People with AD may cook a meal but then forget not only to serve it but also that they made it.
3. **Problems with language**
   - Most people have trouble with finding the "right" word from time to time.
   - Persons with AD may forget simple words or substitute inappropriate words, making their speech difficult to understand.
4. **Disorientation to time and place**
   - While most individuals occasionally forget the day of the week or what they need from the store, people with AD can become lost on their own street, not knowing where they are, how they got there, or how to get back home.
5. **Poor or decreased judgment**
   - Many individuals from time to time may choose not to dress appropriately for the weather (e.g., not bringing a coat or sweater on a cold evening).
   - Person with AD may dress inappropriately in more noticeable ways, such as wearing a bathrobe to the store or a sweater on a hot day.
6. **Problems with abstract thinking**
   - For the person with AD, this goes beyond challenges such as balancing a checkbook.
   - Person with AD may have difficulty recognizing numbers or doing even basic calculations.
7. **Misplacing things**
   - For many individuals, temporarily misplacing keys, purses, or wallets is a normal albeit frustrating event.
   - Person with AD may put items in inappropriate places (e.g., eating utensils in clothing drawers) but have no memory of how they got there.
8. **Changes in mood or behavior**
   - Most individuals experience mood changes.
   - Person with AD tends to exhibit more rapid mood swings for no apparent reason.
9. **Changes in personality**
   - As most individuals age, they may demonstrate some change in personality (e.g., become less tolerant).
   - Person with AD can change dramatically, either suddenly or over time.
   - For example, someone who is generally easygoing may become angry, suspicious, or fearful.
10. **Loss of initiative**
    - Person with AD may become and remain uninterested and uninvolved in many or all of his or her usual pursuits.

Adapted from Alzheimer's Association: *Early warning signs,* Chicago, Alzheimer's Association.

maintain attention. Ongoing loss of neurons in AD can cause a person to act in altered or unpredictable ways. Behavioral manifestations of AD (e.g., agitation) result from changes that take place within the brain. They are neither intentional nor controllable by the individual with the disease. Some patients develop psychotic manifestations (e.g., delusions, illusions, hallucinations).

With progression of AD, additional cognitive impairments are noted. These include *dysphasia* (difficulty comprehending language

TABLE 60-7	*COLLABORATIVE CARE* **Alzheimer's Disease**

Diagnostic

History and physical examination, including psychologic evaluation

Neuropsychologic testing, including Mini-Mental State Examination (see Table 60-4)

Brain imaging tests: CT, MRI, MRS, SPECT, PET

Complete blood count

Electrocardiogram

Serum glucose, creatinine, BUN

Serum levels of vitamins B_1, B_6, B_{12}

Thyroid function tests

Liver function tests

Screening for depression

Collaborative Therapy

Drug therapy for cognitive problems (see Table 60-8)

Drug therapy for behavioral problems (see Table 60-8)

Behavioral modification

Moderate exercise

Assistance with functional independence

Music, particularly with meals and bathing

Assistance and support for caregiver

BUN, Blood urea nitrogen; *CT,* computed tomography; *MRI,* magnetic resonance imaging; *MRS,* magnetic resonance spectroscopy; *PET,* positron emission tomography; *SPECT,* single-photon emission computed tomography.

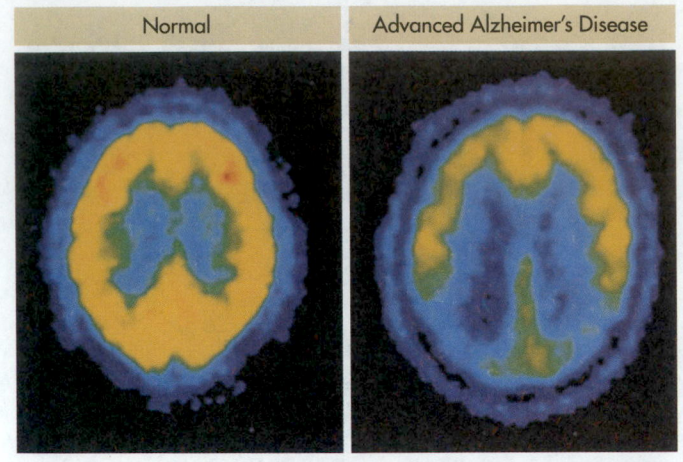

Normal	Advanced Alzheimer's Disease
A	B

FIG. 60-4 Positron emission tomography (PET) scan can be used to assist in the diagnosis of Alzheimer's disease (AD). Radioactive fluorine is applied to glucose (fluorodeoxyglucose), and the yellow areas indicate metabolically active cells. **A,** A normal brain. **B,** Advanced AD is recognized by hypometabolism in many areas of the brain.

and oral communication), *apraxia* (inability to manipulate objects or perform purposeful acts), *visual agnosia* (inability to recognize objects by sight), and *dysgraphia* (difficulty communicating via writing). Eventually long-term memories cannot be recalled, and patients lose the ability to recognize family members and friends. Other problems include aggression and a tendency to wander.

Later in the disease, the ability to communicate and to perform activities of daily living is lost. In the late or final stages of AD, the patient is unresponsive and incontinent and requires total care.

Diagnostic Studies

The diagnosis of AD is primarily a diagnosis of exclusion. No single clinical test can be used to diagnose AD. In patients with cognitive impairment, there is increased emphasis on early and careful evaluation of the patient. As indicated earlier in this chapter, many conditions can cause manifestations of dementia, some of which are treatable or "reversible" (see Table 60-2).

When all other possible conditions that can cause cognitive impairment have been ruled out, a clinical diagnosis of AD can be made. A comprehensive patient evaluation includes a complete health history, physical examination, neurologic and mental status assessments, and laboratory tests (Table 60-7). Brain imaging tests include CT or MRI. A CT or an MRI scan may show brain atrophy and enlarged ventricles in the later stages of the disease, although this finding occurs in other diseases and can also be seen in persons without cognitive impairment. Newer techniques include SPECT, magnetic resonance spectroscopy (MRS), and PET (Fig. 60-4). These techniques allow for detection of changes early in the disease as well as monitoring of treatment response. Research is ongoing to develop diagnostic tests to detect and quantify AD, and most involve some form of brain imaging technique. Although many different tests (neuroimaging, neuropsychologic testing, examination of genetic markers) may provide a diagnosis of possible or probable AD, a definitive diagnosis requires examination of brain tissue and the presence of neurofibrillary tangles and neuritic plaques at autopsy.

Neuropsychologic testing with tools such as the Mini-Mental State Examination (see Table 60-4) can help document the degree of cognitive impairment. Neuropsychologic testing is important not only for diagnostic purposes but also to determine a baseline from which changes over time can be evaluated.

Collaborative Care

At this time there is no cure for AD. The collaborative management of AD is aimed at (1) improving or controlling decline in cognition and (2) controlling the undesirable behavioral manifestations that the patient may exhibit (see the Table 60-7).

Drug Therapy. Drug therapy for AD is listed in Table 60-8. Cholinesterase inhibitors are used in the treatment of mild and moderate dementia.[10-12] They block cholinesterase, the enzyme responsible for the breakdown of acetylcholine in the synaptic cleft (Fig. 60-5). Cholinesterase inhibitors include donepezil (Aricept), rivastigmine (Exelon), and galantamine (Razadyne). These drugs have been shown to either improve or stabilize cognitive decline in some people with AD. As a result, they can enhance the patient's functional abilities. However, these drugs do not cure or reverse the progression of the disease. It is not known whether the long-term administration of these drugs will actually delay the progression of the neurologic damage.

Memantine (Namenda) is used for the treatment of the middle to late stages of AD. Memantine appears to protect the brain's nerve cells against excess amounts of glutamate, which is released in large amounts by cells damaged by AD. The attachment of glutamate to *N*-methyl-D-aspartate (NMDA) receptors permits calcium to flow freely into the cell, which in turn may lead to cell degeneration. Memantine may prevent this destructive sequence by blocking the action of glutamate.

Drug therapy is often used for the management of behavioral problems that occur in patients with AD. Conventional antipsychotic drugs (e.g., haloperidol [Haldol]) can be used to manage acute episodes of agitation, aggressive behavior, and psychosis. However, these antipsychotics are often associated with side effects, including extrapyramidal symptoms and anticholinergic activity, especially in older adults. Therefore atypical antipsychotics are being used more commonly for behavioral management in AD. These include risperidone (Risperdal), olanzapine (Zyprexa), and

Problem	Drugs
Decreased memory and cognition	Cholinesterase inhibitors • donepezil (Aricept) • rivastigmine (Exelon) • galantamine (Razadyne) *N*-methyl-D-aspartate (NMDA) receptor antagonist • memantine (Namenda)
Depression	Selective serotonin reuptake inhibitors (SSRIs) • sertraline (Zoloft) • fluvoxamine (Luvox) • citalopram (Celexa) • fluoxetine (Prozac) Tricyclic antidepressants • nortriptyline (Aventyl, Pamelor) • amitriptyline (Elavil) • imipramine (Tofranil) • doxepin (Sinequan) Atypical antidepressant • trazodone (Desyrel)
Behavioral problems (e.g., agitation, disinhibition)	Conventional antipsychotics (neuroleptics) • loxapine (Loxitane) • haloperidol (Haldol) Atypical antipsychotics (neuroleptics) • risperidone (Risperdal) • olanzapine (Zyprexa) • quetiapine (Seroquel) Benzodiazepines • lorazepam (Ativan) • temazepam (Restoril) • oxazepam (Serax)
Sleep disturbances	zolpidem (Ambien)

TABLE 60-8

DRUG THERAPY
Alzheimer's Disease

COMPLEMENTARY AND ALTERNATIVE THERAPIES
Ginkgo biloba

Clinical Uses
• Dementia treatment (multiinfarct and Alzheimer's disease), claudication (peripheral vascular disease)*
• Cerebral insufficiency†

Effects
Appears to benefit patients in the early stage of Alzheimer's disease and multiinfarct dementia. May improve blood flow to the brain, but additional research is needed. May result in small improvements of symptoms due to claudication.

Nursing Implications
Generally well tolerated in recommended dosages for up to 6 months. May increase risk of bleeding. Use with caution in patients with bleeding disorders and those taking medications, herbs, or supplements that increase risk of bleeding. Contraindicated prior to surgical or dental procedures. May affect blood glucose. Caution is advised in patients with diabetes or those taking medications, herbs, or supplements that affect blood glucose levels. Advise these patients to have close monitoring of blood glucose by a health care professional. May lower BP, although studies are inconclusive. Contraindicated in pregnancy or lactation. High doses may reduce fertility. Due to possible monoamine oxidase inhibitor properties, high doses may result in elevated BP when taken with tyramine-containing foods (e.g., anchovies, avocados, pickled herring, raisins).

Adapted from Ulbricht CE, Basch EM: *Natural standard herb and supplement reference: evidence-based clinical reviews,* St Louis, 2005, Mosby. Available at *www.naturalstandard.com.*
BP, Blood pressure.
*Strong scientific evidence for its use.
†Good scientific evidence for its use.

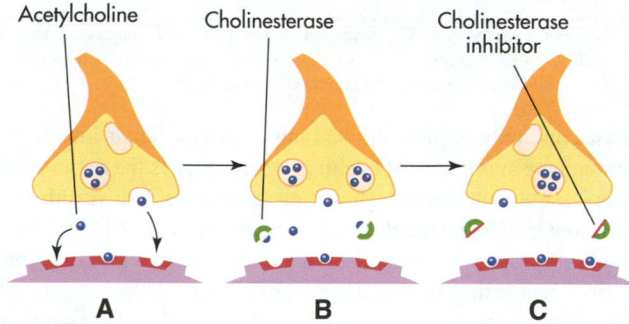

FIG. 60-5 Mechanism of action of cholinesterase inhibitors. **A,** Acetylcholine is released from the nerve synapses and carries a message across the synapse. **B,** Cholinesterase breaks down acetylcholine. **C,** Cholinesterase inhibitors block cholinesterase, thus giving acetylcholine more time to transmit the message.

quetiapine (Seroquel). However, recent evidence shows that their clinical benefits are uncertain and adverse side effects may limit their effectiveness.[13]

Treating the depression that is often associated with AD may improve cognitive ability. Depression is often treated with selective serotonin reuptake inhibitors, including fluoxetine (Prozac), sertraline (Zoloft), fluvoxamine (Luvox), and citalopram (Celexa). The antidepressant trazodone (Desyrel) may help with problems related to sleep. However, this agent may result in hypotension. Antiseizure drugs (neuroleptics), including valproic acid (Depakene) and carbamazepine (Tegretol), are also used to

manage behavioral problems. These drugs tend to act as mood stabilizers.

There has been some debate about the ability of certain hormones and herbs (e.g., ginkgo biloba) to prevent or treat AD. Ginkgo biloba (see the Complementary and Alternative Therapies box above) can be used in patients with AD. Observational and longitudinal studies suggest that hormone replacement therapy (HRT) may attenuate age-associated cognitive impairment or decrease AD, but this has not been confirmed by randomized clinical trials. A critical window of time may exist around the menopause when HRT may delay or decrease cognitive changes. However, hormone therapy initiated in the late postmenopause does not improve global cognition and may increase dementia risk.[14]

Preliminary results from studies investigating the incidence and onset of AD in patients with arthritis who have taken nonsteroidal antiinflammatory drugs (NSAIDs) suggest that NSAIDs may have a protective effect. Although NSAIDs have been shown through epidemiologic studies to be associated with a reduced risk of AD, controlled clinical trials in patients with AD have not demonstrated a clear benefit.[12] When NSAIDs are used in older adults at high doses, there are concerns related to increased potential for upper gastrointestinal bleeding.

Scientists are studying other possible treatments for AD, which include cholesterol-lowering drugs (statins), antioxidants (e.g., vitamins C and E), folic acid, substances that prevent formation of β-amyloid plaques, and nerve growth factor to keep neurons healthy. A number of ongoing clinical drug trials are attempting to find drugs that can limit or decrease the rate of disease progression, as well as manage the signs and symptoms of AD.

NURSING MANAGEMENT
ALZHEIMER'S DISEASE

■ Nursing Assessment

Subjective and objective data that should be obtained from a person with AD are presented in Table 60-9. Useful questions for the patient and informant are, "When did you first notice the memory loss?" and "How has the memory loss progressed since then?"

■ Nursing Diagnoses

Nursing diagnoses for AD may include, but are not limited to, those presented in NCP 60-1.

■ Planning

The overall goals are that the patient with AD will (1) maintain functional ability for as long as possible, (2) be maintained in a safe environment with a minimum of injuries, (3) have personal care needs met, and (4) have dignity maintained. The overall goals for the caregiver of a patient with AD are to (1) reduce caregiver stress; (2) maintain personal, emotional, and physical health; and (3) cope with the long-term effects of caregiving.

■ Nursing Implementation

Health Promotion. At this time there is no known method of reducing the risk of AD. Ongoing studies suggest that antioxidants may be beneficial. However, additional data are clearly needed. Because traumatic brain injury may be a risk factor for developing AD, the nurse should promote safety in physical activities and driving. Depression should be recognized and treated early. At this time genetic testing for AD is not performed on a regular basis.

Early recognition and treatment of AD are important. The nurse has a responsibility in terms of informing patients and their families regarding the early signs of AD. The warning signs of AD developed by the Alzheimer's Association are shown in Table 60-6.

Acute Intervention. The diagnosis of AD is traumatic for both the patient and the family. It is not unusual for the patient to respond with depression, denial, anxiety and fear, isolation, and feelings of loss. The nurse is in an important position to assess for depression and suicidal ideation. Antidepressant drugs and counseling may be indicated. Family members may also be in denial and may not seek medical attention early in the disease. Along with patient assessment, the nurse must assess family members and their ability to accept and cope with the diagnosis.

Although there is no current treatment for reversing AD, there is a need for ongoing monitoring of both the patient with AD and the patient's caregiver. An important nursing responsibility is to work collaboratively with the patient's caregiver to manage clinical manifestations effectively as they change over time. The nurse is often responsible for teaching the caregiver to perform the many tasks that are required to manage the patient's care. The nurse must consider both the patient with AD and the caregiver as patients with overlapping but unique problems. To aid in identifying the many problems of the caregiver, a nursing care plan for the caregiver of a person with AD is presented on the website at *http://evolve.elsevier.com/Lewis/medsurg*.

Patients with AD may be hospitalized for other health care problems. Patients with AD are subject to acute and other chronic

TABLE 60-9	**NURSING ASSESSMENT** **Alzheimer's Disease**

Subjective Data
Important Health Information
Past health history: Repeated head trauma, stroke, exposure to metals (e.g., mercury, aluminum), previous CNS infection, family history of dementia
Medications: Use of any drug to decrease symptoms (e.g., tranquilizers, hypnotics, antidepressants, antipsychotics)

Functional Health Patterns
Health perception–health management: Positive family history; emotional lability
Nutritional-metabolic: Anorexia, malnutrition, weight loss
Elimination: Incontinence
Activity-exercise: Poor personal hygiene; gait instability, weakness; inability to perform activities of daily living
Sleep-rest: Frequent nighttime awakening, daytime napping
Cognitive-perceptual: Forgetfulness, inability to cope with complex situations, difficulty with problem solving (early signs); depression, withdrawal, suicidal ideation (early)

Objective Data
General
Disheveled appearance, agitation

Neurologic
Early: Loss of recent memory; disorientation to date and time; flat affect; lack of spontaneity; impaired abstraction, cognition, and judgment
Middle: Agitation; impaired ability to recognize close family and friends; loss of remote memory; confusion, apraxia, agnosia, alexia (inability to understand written language); aphasia; inability to do simple tasks
Late: Inability to do self-care; incontinence; immobility; limb rigidity; flexor posturing

Possible Findings
Diagnosis by exclusion, cerebral cortical atrophy on CT scan, poor scores on mental status tests, hippocampal atrophy on MRI scan, abnormal changes on PET, SPECT, and MRS

CNS, Central nervous system; *CT,* computed tomography; *MRI,* magnetic resonance imaging; *MRS,* magnetic resonance spectroscopy; *PET,* position emission tomography; *SPECT,* single-photon emission computed tomography.

illnesses and may require surgical interventions. Their inability to communicate symptoms of health problems places the responsibility for assessment and diagnosis on caregivers and health care professionals. Hospitalization of the patient with AD can be a traumatic event for both the patient and the caregiver and can precipitate a worsening of the disease or delirium. Patients with AD hospitalized in the acute care setting will need to be observed more closely because of concerns for safety, frequently oriented to place and time, and given reassurance. The use of consistent nurses may be helpful in reducing anxiety or disruptive behavior.

Ambulatory and Home Care. Currently, family members and friends care for the majority of individuals with AD in their homes. Others with AD reside in various facilities, including long-term care and assisted living facilities. A facility that is good for one person may not be suitable for another. Also, what is helpful for a person at one point in the disease process may be completely different from what is best when the disease progresses.[15]

Patients with AD progress through the stages at variable rates. The nursing care required by the patient with AD changes as the disease progresses, emphasizing the need for regular assessment and support. Regardless of the setting, the severity of the problems and the amount of nursing care intensify over time. The specific manifestations of the disease will depend on the area of the brain

NURSING CARE PLAN 60-1

Patient with Alzheimer's Disease

NURSING DIAGNOSIS   **Disturbed thought processes** *related to* effects of dementia *as evidenced by* loss of memory and other cognitive deficits

PATIENT GOAL   Functions at highest level of cognitive ability

OUTCOMES (NOC)

Cognition

- Communicates clearly and appropriately for age and ability ____
- Comprehends the meaning of events and situations ____
- Attentiveness ____
- Cognitive orientation ____
- Demonstrates immediate memory ____
- Demonstrates recent memory ____
- Demonstrates remote memory ____
- Processes information ____
- Makes appropriate decisions ____

Measurement Scale

1 = Severely compromised
2 = Substantially compromised
3 = Moderately compromised
4 = Mildly compromised
5 = Not compromised

INTERVENTIONS (NIC) and *RATIONALES*

Dementia Management

- Determine type and extent of cognitive deficit(s), using standardized assessment tool, *to establish baseline function.*
- Include family members in planning, providing, and evaluating care to the extent desired *to plan appropriate and consistent interventions.*
- Discuss with family members and friends how best to interact with patient *to maintain consistency.*
- Identify usual patterns of behavior for such activities as sleep, medication use, elimination, food intake, and self-care *to maintain familiar routines.*
- Give one simple direction at a time *to decrease confusion and frustration.*
- Use distraction, rather than confrontation, to manage behavior, *which will decrease anxiety.*
- Provide cues—such as current events, seasons, location, and names—to assist orientation *to promote memory and reduce confusion.*
- Limit number of choices patient has to make, *so as not to cause anxiety.*

Reality Orientation

- Stimulate memory by repeating patient's last expressed thought.
- Inform patient of person, place, and time *to promote memory and reduce confusion.*
- Avoid frustrating patient by quizzing with orientation questions that cannot be answered.
- Use environmental cues (e.g., signs, pictures, clocks, calendars, and color coding of environment) *to stimulate memory, reorient, and promote appropriate behavior.*

NURSING DIAGNOSIS   **Self-care deficit (bathing, dressing, toileting)** *related to* memory deficit and neuromuscular impairment *as evidenced by* inability to independently and appropriately bathe, dress, or toilet

PATIENT GOAL   Performs self-care bathing, dressing, and toileting with assistance as needed

OUTCOMES (NOC)

Self-Care: Bathing

- Gets in and out of bathroom ____
- Regulates water temperature ____
- Washes face ____
- Washes upper body ____
- Washes lower body ____
- Cleans perineal area ____
- Dries body ____

Self-Care: Dressing

- Puts clothing on upper body ____
- Puts clothing on lower body ____
- Uses zippers ____
- Buttons clothing ____
- Ties shoes ____

Self-Care: Toileting

- Gets to and from toilet ____
- Removes clothing ____
- Empties bladder ____
- Empties bowel ____
- Wipes self after urinating ____
- Wipes self after bowel movement ____

Measurement Scale

1 = Severely compromised
2 = Substantially compromised
3 = Moderately compromised
4 = Mildly compromised
5 = Not compromised

INTERVENTIONS (NIC) and *RATIONALES*

Self-Care Assistance

- Monitor patient's ability for independent self-care *to plan appropriate interventions specific to patient's unique problems.*
- Use consistent repetition of health routines as a means of establishing them *as memory loss impairs patient's ability to plan and complete specific sequential activities.*
- Assist patient in accepting dependency needs *to ensure all needs are met.*
- Teach patient/family to encourage independence, to intervene only when patient is unable to perform *to promote independence.*

Self-Care Assistance: Bathing/Hygiene

- Provide desired personal articles (e.g., deodorant, toothbrush, and bath soap) *to enhance memory and provide care.*
- Facilitate patient's bathing self *to facilitate independence and provide appropriate help in hygiene.*

Self-Care Assistance: Dressing/Grooming

- Provide patient's clothes in accessible area (e.g., at bedside) *to enhance memory and provide care.*
- Be available for assistance in dressing *to facilitate independence and provide appropriate help in dressing.*

Self-Care Assistance: Toileting

- Assist patient to toilet/commode/bedpan/fracture pan/urinal at specified intervals *to promote regularity.*
- Facilitate toilet hygiene after completion of elimination *to prevent discomfort and skin excoriation.*

Continued

NURSING CARE PLAN 60-1

Patient with Alzheimer's Disease—cont'd

NURSING DIAGNOSIS **Risk for injury** *related to* impaired judgment, possible gait instability, muscle weakness, and sensory/perceptual alteration

PATIENT GOALS 1. Experiences no injury
2. Uses assistive devices appropriately for ambulation support

OUTCOMES (NOC)	INTERVENTIONS (NIC) and *RATIONALES*
Fall Prevention Behavior	**Fall Prevention**
• Uses assistive devices correctly ____	• Identify cognitive or physical deficits of the patient that may increase potential falls in a particular environment *to decrease or prevent occurrence of injury.*
• Controls agitation and restlessness ____	• Provide assistive devices (e.g., walker) *to steady gait and provide ambulation support.*
• Uses well-fitting tied shoes ____	• Ensure that patient wears shoes that fit properly, fasten securely, and have nonskid soles *to provide support during ambulation.*
• Uses vision-correcting devices ____	• Instruct patient to wear prescription glasses when out of bed *to allow for proper vision.*
Measurement Scale	
1 = Never demonstrated	
2 = Rarely demonstrated	
3 = Sometimes demonstrated	
4 = Often demonstrated	
5 = Consistently demonstrated	

NURSING DIAGNOSIS **Wandering** *related to* disease process *as evidenced by* getting lost numerous times a day and patient's statement of "I don't know where I am"

PATIENT GOAL Remains in restricted area during ambulation and activity

OUTCOMES (NOC)	INTERVENTIONS (NIC) and *RATIONALES*
Fall Prevention Behavior (Caregiver)	**Fall Prevention**
• Places barriers to prevent falls ____	• Use a bed alarm *to alert caregiver that individual is getting out of bed.*
• Controls agitation and restlessness ____	**Dementia Management**
• Provides assistance with mobility ____	• Provide space for safe pacing and wandering *to prevent injury and getting lost.*
Measurement Scale	• Use symbols, other than written signs, to assist patient to locate room, bathroom, or other area *to orient patient to environment.*
1 = Never demonstrated	**Surveillance: Safety**
2 = Rarely demonstrated	• Monitor environment for potential safety hazards *to prevent injury to patient.*
3 = Sometimes demonstrated	• Monitor patient for alterations in physical or cognitive function that might lead to unsafe behavior *to assess any changes that may occur.*
4 = Often demonstrated	• Provide appropriate level of supervision/surveillance *to monitor patient and to allow for therapeutic actions.*
5 = Consistently demonstrated	

involved. Nursing care is focused on decreasing clinical manifestations, preventing harm, and supporting the patient and caregiver throughout the disease process.

In the early stages of AD, memory aids (e.g., calendars) may be beneficial. Patients often develop depression during this phase. Depression may be related to the diagnosis of an incurable disorder, as well as the impact of the disease on activities of daily living (e.g., driving, socializing with friends, participating in hobbies or recreational activities). Drug therapy with cholinesterase inhibitors appears to be most effective during the early stages of AD. However, not all patients will show improvement. The drugs must be taken on a regular basis. Because memory is one of the key functions to be altered in AD, drug compliance may be challenging.

Following the initial diagnosis, patients need to be aware that the progression of the disease is variable. Effective management of the disease can slow the progress of the disease and decrease the burden on the patient, caregiver, and family. However, decisions related to care should be made with the patient, family members, and health care team early in the disease. The nurse has a role in advising the patient and the caregiver to initiate health care deci-

sions, including advance directives, while the patient has the capacity to do so. This can ease the burden for the caregiver as the disease progresses.

Adult day care is one of the options available to the person with AD. Although programs vary in size, structure, physical environment, and degree of experience of staff, the common goals of all day care programs are to provide respite for the family and a protective environment for the patient. During the early and middle stages of AD, the person can still benefit from stimulating activities that encourage independence and decision making in a protective environment. The patient returns home tired, content, less frustrated, and ready to be with the family. The respite from the demands of care allows the caregiver to be more responsive to the patient's needs.

As the disease progresses, the demands on the caregiver eventually exceed the resources, and the person with AD may need to be placed in a long-term care facility. Special units to care for persons with AD are becoming increasingly common in long-term care settings. The Alzheimer's unit is designed with an emphasis on safety. For example, many facilities have designated areas that allow the patient to walk freely within the unit, while the unit is secured so that the patient cannot wander outside of it.

As the patient with AD progresses to the late stages (severe impairment) of AD, there is increased difficulty with the most basic functions, including walking and talking. Total care is required.

Specific problems relate to the care of the patient with AD across the phases of the disease. These problems are described below.

Behavioral Problems. Behavioral problems occur in about 90% of patients with AD. These problems include repetitiveness (asking the same question repeatedly), delusions (false beliefs), illusions, hallucinations, agitation, aggression, altered sleeping patterns, wandering, and resisting care. Many times these behaviors are unpredictable and may challenge caregivers. Caregivers need to be aware that these behaviors are not intentional and are often difficult to control. Behavioral symptoms often lead to the placement of patients in institutional care settings.

These behaviors are often the patient's way of responding to a precipitating factor (e.g., pain, frustration, temperature extremes, anxiety). When these behaviors become problematic, the nurse must plan interventions carefully. Initially the nurse must assess the patient's physical status. The patient is checked for changes in vital signs, urinary and bowel patterns, and pain that could account for behavioral problems. The environment is then assessed to identify those factors that may trigger behavior disruptions. Extremes in temperature, as well as excessive noise, may result in behavior changes. When the patient is agitated by the environment, either the patient or the stimulus should be moved. The patient can be assisted to call family members if this is reassuring. When a patient resists or pulls tubes or dressings, these items can be covered with stretch tube gauze or removed from the visual field. The patient should be reassured that the nurse is present to keep him or her safe. Reality orientation can be used to orient to time, place, and person. The confused or agitated patient should not be asked challenging "why" questions. If the patient cannot verbalize distress, his or her mood should be validated. The patient's statement can be rephrased to validate its meaning. The patient's emotional state should be closely observed.

Nursing strategies that address difficult behavior include redirection, distraction, and reassurance. For the patient who is restless or agitated, redirecting involves a change in the patient's focus (e.g., having the patient perform activities such as sweeping, raking, or dusting). Ways to distract the agitated patient may include providing snacks, taking a car ride, sitting on a porch swing or rocker, listening to favorite music, watching videotapes, looking at family photographs, or walking. Reassurance involves communicating to the patient that he or she will be protected from danger, harm, or embarrassment. Use of repetitive activities, songs, poems, music, massage, aromas, or a favorite object can be soothing to patients.

When dealing with the difficult patient, the nurse's frustration should be acknowledged. The nurse should not threaten to restrain the patient or threaten to call the physician. A calming family member can be requested to stay with the patient until the patient becomes calmer. The patient should be monitored frequently, and all interventions should be documented. The use of positive nurse actions can reduce the use of physical and chemical (drug therapy) restraints.

When nonpharmacologic therapies are ineffective or there is concern about self-injury, disruptive behavior may be treated by medications (see Table 60-8). However, many of these drugs have adverse side effects that can be distressing for the patient and caregiver. The side effects of the drugs must be weighed against the distress of and potential safety concerns for the patient. As verbal skills decline, the caregiver and nurse may need to rely more on the patient's body language to communicate care needs.

A specific type of agitation is termed **sundowning,** in which the patient becomes more confused and agitated in the late afternoon or evening. Behaviors commonly exhibited include agitation, aggressiveness, wandering, resistance to redirection, and increased verbal activity such as yelling. The cause of sundowning is unclear, but several theories propose it is due to a disruption of circadian rhythms. Other possible causes include fatigue, unfamiliar environment, and noise (especially in an acute care setting), medications, reduced lighting, and sleep fragmentation. The nurse must remain calm and avoid confrontation. She must assess the situation for possible causes of the agitation. Nursing interventions that may be helpful include: (1) creating a quiet calm environment, (2) maximizing exposure to daylight (open blinds and turn on lights during the day), (3) evaluating medications to determine if any could cause sleep disturbance, (4) limiting naps and caffeine, and (5) consulting with the health care provider regarding drug therapy. Management of sundowning can be challenging for the nurse, the patient, and the family. The nurse must place emphasis on patient safety while planning and providing nursing care.

Safety. The person with AD is at risk for problems related to personal safety. These risks include injury from falls, injury from ingesting dangerous substances, wandering, injury to others and self with sharp objects, fire or burns, and inability to respond to crisis situations. These concerns require careful attention to the home environment to minimize risk, as well as the need for supervision. As the patient's cognitive function declines over time, the patient may have difficulty navigating physical spaces and interpreting environmental cues. Stairwells must be well lit. Handrails should be graspable, with the end of the rail shaped differently to alert the patient that it is the end of the stairway. Carpet edges should be tacked down, and throw rugs should be removed. Polished floor surfaces and linoleum can predispose to falls. Extension cords should be removed as the patient may trip over them. In the bathroom, nonskid mats should be used in the tub or shower, and handrails should be installed in the bath and commode. The nurse can assist the caregiver in assessing the home environment for safety risks.

Wandering is a major concern for caregivers. Wandering may be related to loss of memory or to side effects of drugs, or it may be an expression of a physical or emotional need, restlessness, curiosity, or stimuli that trigger memories of earlier routines. As with other behaviors, the nurse should observe for factors or events that may precipitate wandering. For example, the patient may be sensitive to stress and tension in the environment. In such cases, wandering may reflect an attempt to leave the environment. AD patients who tend to wander can be registered with Safe Return, a federally supported program operated through the Alzheimer's Association. The Safe Return program includes identification products (e.g., wallet cards), a national photo/information database, a 24-hour toll-free emergency crisis line, local chapter support, and wandering behavior education and training for caregivers and families.[16]

Pain Management. Because of difficulties with oral and written language associated with AD, patients may have difficulty expressing physical complaints, including pain. The nurse must rely on other clues, including the patient's behavior. Pain can result in alterations in the patient's behavior, such as increased vocalization, agitation, withdrawal, and changes in function. Pain should be recognized and treated promptly and the patient's response monitored.

Eating and Swallowing Difficulties. Undernutrition is a problem in the middle and late stages of AD, with patients in long-term facilities having the highest incidence of undernutrition.[17] Loss of interest in food and decreased ability to self-feed (*feeding apraxia*), as well as comorbid conditions, can result in significant nutritional deficiencies in the patient with AD. In long-term care facilities, inadequate assistance with feeding may add to the problem.

Pureed foods, thickened liquids, and nutritional supplements can be used when chewing and swallowing become problematic for the patient. Patients may need reminders to chew their food and to swallow. Patients need a quiet and unhurried environment for eating. Distractions at mealtimes, including the television, should be avoided. Low lighting, music, and simulated nature sounds may improve eating behaviors. Easy-grip eating utensils and finger foods may allow the patient to self-feed. Liquids should be offered frequently.

When oral feeding is not possible, alternative routes may be explored. Nasogastric (NG) feeding may be used for short periods. However, for the long term the NG tube is uncomfortable and may add to the patient's agitation. A percutaneous endoscopic gastrostomy (PEG) tube provides another option (see Fig. 40-6). However, PEG tubes can be problematic as patients with AD are particularly vulnerable to aspiration of feeding formula and tube dislodgment. The potential positive outcomes to be gained from nutritional therapies are considered in light of overall outcome goals and potential adverse effects of the specific therapy. Nutritional support therapies are described in Chapter 40.

Oral Care. In the late stages of AD, the patient will be unable to perform oral self-care. With decreased toothbrushing and flossing, dental problems are likely to occur. Because of swallowing difficulties, patients may pocket food in the mouth, adding to the potential for tooth decay. Dental caries and tooth abscess can add to patient discomfort or pain and subsequently may increase agitation. The mouth should be inspected regularly and mouth care provided to those patients unable to do self-care.

Infection Prevention. Urinary tract infection and pneumonia are the most common infections to occur in patients with AD. Such infections are ultimately the cause of death in many patients with AD. Because of feeding and swallowing problems, the patient with AD is at risk for aspiration pneumonia. Immobility can also predispose to pneumonia. Reduced fluid intake, prostate hyperplasia in men, poor hygiene, and urinary drainage devices (e.g., catheter) can predispose to bladder infection. Any manifestations of infection, such as a change in behavior, fever, cough (pneumonia), or pain on urination (bladder), need prompt evaluation and treatment.

Skin Care. It is important to monitor the patient's skin over time. Rashes, areas of redness, and skin breakdown should be noted and treated as appropriate. In the late stages, incontinence along with immobility and undernutrition can place the patient at risk for skin breakdown. The skin should be kept dry and clean and the patient's position changed regularly to avoid areas of pressure over bony prominences.

Elimination Problems. During the middle and late stages of AD, urinary and fecal incontinence lead to increased need for nursing care. When possible, habit or behavioral retraining of bladder and bowel function (e.g., scheduled toileting) may help decrease episodes of incontinence. Drug therapy (e.g., oxybutynin [Ditropan]) may decrease bladder excitability and improve control. For women, estrogen cream may be helpful if atrophic vaginitis is present.

Another common elimination problem is constipation. Causes may relate to immobility, dietary intake (e.g., reduced fiber intake), and decreased fluid intake. Increasing dietary fiber, fiber supple-

---

TABLE 60-10   **FAMILY AND CAREGIVER TEACHING GUIDE**
Alzheimer's Disease

Mild Stage
1. Confirm the diagnosis. Many treatable (and potentially reversible) conditions can mimic Alzheimer's disease (see Table 60-2).
2. Get the person to stop driving. Confusion and poor judgment can impair driving skills and potentially put others at risk.
3. Encourage activities such as visiting with friends and family, listening to music, participating in hobbies, and exercising.
4. Provide cues in the home, establish a routine, and determine specific location where essential items (e.g., glasses) need to be kept.
5. Do not correct misstatements or faulty memory.
6. Register with Safe Return, a program established by the Alzheimer's Association to locate individuals who may wander from their homes.
7. Make plans for the future in terms of care options, financial concerns, and personal preference for care.

Moderate Stage
1. Install door locks for patient safety.
2. Provide protective wear for urinary and fecal incontinence.
3. Ensure that the home has good lighting, install handrails in stairways and bathroom, and remove area rugs or ensure that they are tacked down.
4. Label drawers and faucets (hot and cold) to ensure safety.
5. Develop strategies such as distraction and diversion to cope with behavioral problems. Identify and reduce potential triggers (e.g., reduce stress, extremes in temperature) for disruptive behavior.
6. Provide memory triggers, such as pictures of family and friends.

Late Stage
1. Provide a regular schedule for toileting to reduce incontinence.
2. Provide care to meet needs, including oral care and skin care.
3. Monitor diet and fluid intake to ensure their adequacy.
4. Continue communication through talking and touching.
5. Consider placement in a long-term care facility when providing total care becomes too difficult.

---

ments, and stool softeners are the first lines of management. The combination of aging, other health problems, and swallowing difficulties may increase the risk of complications associated with the use of mineral oil, stimulants, osmotic agents, and enemas. Management of constipation is discussed in Chapter 43.

Caregiver Support. AD is a disease that disrupts all aspects of personal and family life. Persons caring for the person with AD describe it as very stressful. These caregivers also exhibit adverse consequences relating to their employment and to their emotional and physical health, which then result in family conflict and caregiver strain. Caregivers with a history of depression may have greater difficulty in adjusting to the demands placed on them. Suggested caregiver needs based on the disease stages are provided in Table 60-10. Other tips for caregivers are listed in Table 60-11.

As the disease progresses, the relationship of the caregiver to the patient changes. Family roles may be altered or reversed (e.g., son caring for father). Decisions must be made including when to tell the patient about the diagnosis, when to have the patient stop driving or doing activities that might be dangerous, when to ask for assistance, and when to place the patient in adult day care or a long-term care facility. With early-onset AD, the patient is affected during his or her most productive years in terms of career and family. The consequences can be devastating for the patient and the family.

Sexual relations for couples are also seriously affected by AD. As the disease progresses, sexual interest may decline for both the patient and the partner. A number of reasons account for this, in-

TABLE 60-11	Guidelines for Dealing with Patients with Dementia

Do	Do Not
Treat them as adults, with respect and dignity, even when their behavior is childlike.	Criticize, correct, or argue.
Use gentle touch and direct eye contact.	Rush or hurry the patient.
Remain patient, flexible, and understanding.	Talk about the patient as if he or she were not there.
Anticipate challenging behaviors as the patient's ability to think logically has been affected.	Take challenging behaviors personally. These behaviors are due to the patient's disease.
Simplify tasks.	Use condescending terms, such as "honey" or "sweetie."
Give directions using gestures or pictures.	
Focus on one thing at a time.	
Avoid questions or topics that require extensive thought, memory, or words.	
Be flexible. If one approach does not work, try another.	
Use distraction, changing the subject, redirecting to another activity.	
Provide reassurance.	

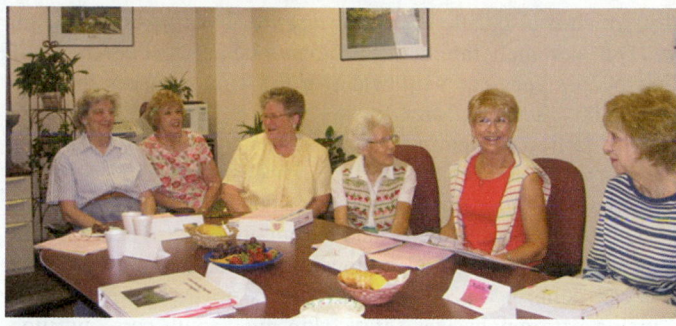

FIG. 60-6 Support groups are an effective way to help caregivers cope.

The Alzheimer's Association has many educational and support systems available to help family caregivers. This organization can provide help in many different ways to caregivers. (See resources at the end of the chapter.)

■ Evaluation

Expected outcomes for the patient with AD are addressed in NCP 60-1.

OTHER NEURODEGENERATIVE DISEASES

Parkinson's disease and Huntington's disease are both neurodegenerative diseases (see Chapter 59). Both diseases are chronic, progressive, and incurable. Despite differences in the etiology and pathophysiology of these diseases, both are associated with the development of dementia in the later stages of disease.

Lewy body dementia (LBD) is a condition characterized by the presence of Lewy bodies (intraneural cytoplasmic inclusions) in the brainstem and cortex. A common cause of dementia, it is often unrecognized by health care providers. Patients typically present with symptoms of parkinsonism, hallucinations, short-term memory loss, unpredictable cognitive shifts, and sleep disturbances. Dementia plus two of the following symptoms indicates a possible diagnosis of LBD: (1) extrapyramidal signs such as bradykinesia, rigidity, and postural instability, but not always a tremor; (2) fluctuating cognitive ability; and (3) hallucinations.[18] This disease has features of both AD and Parkinson's disease, and it is imperative that a correct diagnosis be reached.

Medications for LBD are determined on an individual basis, as a standardized treatment plan has not been determined. Medications may include levodopa/carbidopa and acetylcholinesterase inhibitors. Nursing care for these patients relates to management of the dementia, as well as problems due to dysphagia and immobility. Swallowing problems can lead to impaired nutrition. These patients are at risk for falls due to impaired mobility and balance. Pneumonia is a common complication. The diagnostic criteria for LBD is based on clinical signs and symptoms and confirmed at autopsy by histologic examination of brain tissue.

Creutzfeldt-Jakob disease (CJD) is a rare and fatal brain disorder thought to be caused by a prion protein. A *prion* is a small infectious pathogen containing protein but lacking nucleic acids. Worldwide, sporadic CJD affects 1 in 1 million individuals each year.

There are three types of CJD: sporadic CJD, familial CJD, and acquired CJD.[19] A variant form of CJD (vCJD) was identified in 1996. The source of this infection appeared to be beef obtained from animals contaminated with bovine spongiform encephalopa-

cluding fatigue, as well as memory impairment and episodes of incontinence in the patient with AD. It is also possible for the patient to become very sexually driven as the disease progresses and the patient becomes more uninhibited.

The nurse should work with the caregiver to assess stressors and to identify coping strategies to reduce the burden of caregiving. For example, the nurse should ask which behaviors are most disruptive to family life at a given time, while remembering that this is likely to change over time as the disease progresses. Determining what the caregiver views as most disruptive or distressful can help to establish priorities for care. Risk to the safety of the patient and caregiver is given high priority. It is also important to assess what the caregiver's expectations are regarding the patient's behavior. Are the expectations reasonable given the progression of the disease? Working with the caregiver to identify risk factors for complications, including behavioral problems, is an important responsibility of the nurse.

Caregivers, most of whom are women, may be older adults themselves. Caregiving stress or burden can have adverse outcomes for their health, especially for those who have chronic health problems. Adult children are often caregivers. The impact of the caregiving role can be overwhelming for adult children caregivers. They may need to relocate their family or their parent(s), juggle employment and family responsibilities, face financial strain, and realize the "loss" of their own lives.

Support groups for caregivers and family members (Fig. 60-6) have been formed throughout the United States and other countries to provide an atmosphere of understanding and to give current information about the disease itself and related topics such as safety, legal, ethical, and financial issues. Nurses often receive personal and professional satisfaction in participating in such support groups. Strategies related to stress management are discussed in Chapter 9.

thy, which is also called *mad cow disease.* The risk of contracting vCJD is extremely rare. It affects about one person in every 1 million people per year worldwide; in the United States there are about 200 cases per year.[20]

The earliest symptom of the disease may be memory impairment and behavior changes. The disease progresses rapidly with mental deterioration, involuntary movements (muscle jerks), weakness in the limbs, blindness, and eventually coma. There is no diagnostic test for CJD. Only autopsy and examination of brain tissue can confirm the diagnosis. There is no treatment for CJD. Nursing care emphasizes safety, skin and mouth care, nutrition, and comfort.[20]

Pick's disease, a type of **frontotemporal dementia,** is a rare brain disorder characterized by disturbances in behavior, sleep, personality, and eventually memory. The major distinguishing characteristic between these disorders and AD is marked symmetric lobar atrophy of the temporal and/or frontal lobes. The disease is relentless in its progression, which may ultimately include language impairment, erratic behavior, and dementia. Because of the strange behavior associated with Pick's disease and frontotemporal dementia, psychiatrists often see these patients first. There is no specific treatment. The diagnosis can be confirmed at autopsy.

Normal pressure hydrocephalus is an uncommon disorder characterized by an obstruction in the flow of CSF, which causes a buildup of this fluid in the brain. Symptoms of the condition include dementia, urinary incontinence, and difficulty in walking. Meningitis, encephalitis, or head injury may cause the condition. If diagnosed early in the disease, normal pressure hydrocephalus is treatable by surgery in which a shunt is inserted to divert the fluid away from the brain.

DELIRIUM

Delirium, a state of temporary but acute mental confusion, is a common, life-threatening, and possibly preventable syndrome in older adults. Incidence of delirium is highest in hospitalized older adults, with delirium accounting for more than 49% of all hospital days. In the hospital setting, 15% to 53% of older adults experience delirium postoperatively, and 70% to 87% experience delirium in the intensive care setting.[21]

Etiology and Pathophysiology

The pathophysiologic mechanism of delirium is poorly understood. Cholinergic deficiency, excess release of dopamine, and both increased and decreased serotonergic activity may contribute to delirium.[21,22] Cytokines, including interleukin-1, interleukin-2, interleukin-6, tumor necrosis factor-α, and interferon, appear to play a role.[21] Chronic stress has also been linked to the onset of delirium.

Clinically, delirium is rarely caused by a single factor. It is often the result of the interaction of the patient's underlying condition with a precipitating event. Delirium can occur following a relatively minor insult in a vulnerable patient. For example, the patient with underlying health problems such as heart failure, cancer, cognitive impairment, or sensory limitations may develop delirium in response to a relatively minor change (e.g., use of a sleeping medication). In other nonvulnerable patients, it may take a combination of factors (e.g., anesthesia, major surgery, infection, prolonged sleep deprivation) to precipitate delirium.[22] Delirium can also be a symptom of a serious medical illness such as bacterial meningitis.

Understanding factors that can lead to delirium can help in determining effective interventions. Several factors that can precipitate delirium are listed in Table 60-12. Many of these factors are more

TABLE 60-12	Factors That Can Precipitate Delirium
Demographic Characteristics Age of 65 years or older Male gender	**Drugs** Sedative-hypnotics Opioids Anticholinergic drugs Treatment with multiple drugs Alcohol or drug withdrawal
Cognitive Status Dementia Cognitive impairment History of delirium Depression	**Coexisting Medical Conditions** Severe acute illness Chronic renal or hepatic disease History of stroke Neurologic disease Infection/sepsis Fracture or trauma Terminal illness Infection with human immunodeficiency virus
Environmental Admission to an intensive care unit Use of physical restraints Pain (especially untreated) Emotional stress Prolonged sleep deprivation	
Functional Status Functional dependence Immobility History of falls	**Surgery** Orthopedic surgery Cardiac surgery Prolonged cardiopulmonary bypass Noncardiac surgery
Sensory Sensory deprivation Sensory overload	
Decreased Oral Intake Dehydration Malnutrition	

Adapted from Inoye SK: Delirium in older persons, *N Engl J Med* 354:1157, 2006.

common is older patients. In addition, older patients have limited compensatory mechanisms to deal with physiologic insults such as hypoxia, hypoglycemia, and dehydration. Older adults are more susceptible to drug-induced delirium, in part because of their increased use of multiple drugs. Many medications, including sedative-hypnotics, opioids (especially meperidine [Demerol]), benzodiazepines, and drugs with anticholinergic properties, can cause or contribute to delirium, especially in older or vulnerable patients. An important risk factor for delirium is preexisting dementia.

Clinical Manifestations

Patients with delirium can present with a variety of manifestations ranging from hypoactivity and lethargy to hyperactivity, including agitation and hallucinations. Patients can also have mixed delirium, manifesting both hypoactive and hyperactive symptoms. In most patients, delirium usually develops over a 2- to 3-day period. The early manifestations often include inability to concentrate, irritability, insomnia, loss of appetite, restlessness, and confusion. Later the manifestations may include agitation, misperception, misinterpretation, and hallucinations.

Acute delirium occurs frequently in hospitalized older adults. This transient condition is characterized by disorganized thinking, difficulty concentrating, and sensory misperceptions that last from 1 to 7 days. However, some delirium manifestations may persist up to and after discharge. Delirium is one of the most frequent consequences following unscheduled surgery on the older adult, especially when the patient has not been stabilized physically or prepared emotionally. Often this patient will experience a decline in ability to perform activities of daily living as well as an increase in risk for falls.

Manifestations of delirium are sometimes confused with dementia. A key distinction between delirium and dementia is that the person who exhibits sudden cognitive impairment, disorientation, or clouded sensorium is more likely to have delirium rather than dementia. (A comparison of delirium and dementia is presented in Table 60-1.)

Diagnostic Studies

A careful medical and psychologic history and physical examination are the first steps in the diagnosis of delirium. This includes careful attention to medications, both prescription and over-the-counter drugs. A variety of cognitive measures can be used, including the Mini-Mental State Examination (see Table 60-4). The information may have to be obtained from a reliable informant if the patient is unable to provide the information. It is important to distinguish whether the delirium is part of an underlying problem of dementia.

Once delirium has been diagnosed, potential causes of the delirium are explored. These include a careful review of the patient's health history and medication record. Laboratory tests include complete blood count, serum electrolytes, blood urea nitrogen, and creatinine levels; electrocardiogram; urinalysis; liver and thyroid function tests; and oxygen saturation level. Drug and alcohol levels may be obtained. If unexplained fever or nuchal rigidity is present and meningitis or encephalitis is suspected, a lumbar puncture may be performed. CSF is examined for glucose and protein and the presence of bacteria. If the patient's history includes head injury, appropriate x-rays or scans may be ordered. In general, brain imaging studies such as CT and MRI are used only in those situations in which head injury is known or suspected.

NURSING and COLLABORATIVE MANAGEMENT
DELIRIUM

In caring for the patient with delirium, the roles of the nurse include prevention, early recognition, and treatment.[23] Prevention of delirium involves recognition of high-risk patients. Patient groups at risk include those with neurologic disorders (e.g., stroke, dementia, CNS infection, Parkinson's disease), sensory impairment, and advanced age. Other risk factors include hospitalization in an intensive care unit, lack of a watch or calendar, and absence of reading glasses. Untreated pain may also precipitate delirium.

Care of the patient with delirium is focused on eliminating precipitating factors. If it is drug induced, medications are discontinued. It is important to keep in mind that delirium can also accompany drug and alcohol withdrawal. Depending on patient history, drug screening may be performed. Fluid and electrolyte imbalances and nutritional deficiencies (e.g., thiamine) are corrected if appropriate. If the problem is related to environmental conditions (e.g., an overstimulating or understimulating environment), changes should be made. If delirium is secondary to infection, appropriate antibiotic therapy is started. Similarly, if delirium is secondary to chronic illness such as chronic kidney disease or heart failure, treatment is focused on these conditions.

Care of the patient experiencing delirium includes protecting the patient from harm. Priority is given to creating a calm and safe environment. This may include encouraging family members to stay at the bedside, providing familiar objects, transferring the patient to a private room or one closer to the nurses' station, and planning for consistency of nursing staff if possible. Reorientation and behavioral interventions should be used in all patients with

EVIDENCE-BASED PRACTICE
What Is the Effect of Music on Confusion and Delirium in Surgical Patients?

Clinical Question
In elderly patients having orthopedic surgery (P), does music therapy (I) as compared to no music intervention (C) decrease acute confusion and delirium postoperatively (O)?

Best Available Evidence
One RCT (randomized controlled trial)

Critical Appraisal and Synthesis of Evidence
- RCT (n = 66) persons 65 years and older who were having elective hip or knee surgery.
- Subjects randomly assigned to either listen to music or not during the postoperative recovery period.
- Music therapy consisted of a bedside compact disc (CD) player with various musical choices to be in use for at least 1 hour, three times per day.
- Data were collected on episodes of acute confusion and delirium and ability to ambulate.

Conclusions
- Patients who listened to music had significantly fewer episodes of confusion and delirium. This group also showed a significant and greater readiness to ambulate the day of surgery.
- Music was reported to have an additional calming effect on family members and nurses in rooms where music was played.

Implications for Nursing Practice
- Surgical patients should be given an opportunity to choose and listen to music during their hospitalization.
- Further examination of music therapy and its effect on improving patient outcomes in hospitalized patients is warranted.

Reference for Evidence
McCaffrey R, Locsin R: The effect of music listening on acute confusion and delirium in elders undergoing elective hip and knee surgery, *J Clin Nurs* 13:91, 2004.

PICO: *P*, Patient population of interest; *I*, intervention or area of interest; *C*, comparison of interest or comparison group; *O*, outcome(s) of interest (see p. 6).

delirium. The patient is provided with reassurance and reorienting information as to place, time, and procedures. Clocks, calendars, and listing the patient's scheduled activities are also useful in reducing confusion. Environmental stimuli, including noise and light levels, often need to be reduced.

Personal contact through touch and verbal communication can be an important reorienting strategy. If the patient uses eyeglasses or a hearing aid, it should be made readily available because sensory deprivation can precipitate delirium. The use of restraints should be avoided. Other interventions, including relaxation techniques, music therapy, and massage, may also be appropriate for some patients with delirium.

Comprehensive, multicomponent interventions to prevent delirium are the most effective and should be implemented through institution-based programs that are interdisciplinary.[23] These interdisciplinary teams may also address issues related to polypharmacy, pain, nutritional status, and potential for incontinence. The patient experiencing delirium is also at risk for the adverse consequences of immobility, including skin breakdown. Attention is given to increasing physical activity or providing range-of-motion exercises, when appropriate, and maintaining skin integrity.

The nurse should also focus on supporting the family and caregivers during episodes of delirium. Family members need to understand factors that may have precipitated the delirium, as well as the potential outcomes.

Drug Therapy. Drug therapy is reserved for those patients with severe agitation, especially those whose agitation interferes with needed medical therapy (e.g., fluid replacement, intubation, dialysis). Agitation can put the patient at risk for falls and injury. Drug therapy is used cautiously because many of the drugs used to manage agitation have psychoactive properties.

Patients are often treated with low-dose antipsychotics (neuroleptics) such as haloperidol (Haldol). Haloperidol can be administered intravenously, intramuscularly, or orally and will produce sedation. In addition to sedation, other side effects include hypotension; extrapyramidal side effects, including *tardive dyskinesia* (involuntary muscle movements of the face, trunk, and arms) and *athetosis* (involuntary writhing movements of the limbs); muscle tone changes; and anticholinergic effects. Older patients receiving antipsychotic agents need to be carefully monitored. Newer antipsychotics, including risperidone (Risperdal), olanzapine (Zyprexa), and quetiapine (Seroquel), may be used to manage agitated behavior in older adults. Although these drugs have fewer side effects compared with haloperidol, they also have significant side effects.

Short-acting benzodiazepines (e.g., lorazepam [Ativan]) can be used to treat delirium associated with sedative and alcohol withdrawal or in conjunction with antipsychotics to reduce extrapyramidal side effects. However, these drugs may worsen delirium caused by other factors and must be used cautiously.

CRITICAL THINKING EXERCISE

CASE STUDY

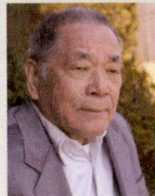

Case Study photo ©iStockphoto.com/ Nancy Louie.

Alzheimer's Disease

Patient Profile. Mr. Y., an 80-year-old Asian American man, was diagnosed with AD 3 years ago. Today his 78-year-old wife brings him to the emergency department because he wandered from his home, fell, and injured his left hip.

Subjective Data
• Can state his name
• Confused as to place and time
• Denies memory of wandering or falling
• Agitated, trying to get up
• Denies pain

Objective Data

Physical Examination
• Left leg shorter than right leg
• Tense and anxious

Diagnostic Studies
• X-ray of left hip indicates a fracture
• Mini-Mental State Examination shows cognitive impairment

Critical Thinking Questions

1. What is the pathogenesis of AD?
2. What precipitating factors may have resulted in Mr. Y.'s fall?
3. What precautions need to be taken regarding the inpatient care of Mr. Y.?
4. What is the priority nursing intervention for Mr. Y.?

5. What teaching plan should be developed for Mr. Y. and his wife?
6. Surgery is planned to repair his fractured hip. Why is he at risk for delirium?
7. Write one or more appropriate nursing diagnoses based on the assessment data presented. Are there any collaborative problems?

NCLEX EXAMINATION REVIEW QUESTIONS

The number of the question corresponds to the same-numbered objective at the beginning of the chapter.

1. Dementia is defined as a
   a. syndrome that results only in memory loss.
   b. disease associated with abrupt changes in behavior.
   c. disease that is always due to reduced blood flow to the brain.
   d. syndrome characterized by cognitive dysfunction and loss of memory.

2. Vascular dementia is associated with
   a. transient ischemic attacks.
   b. bacterial or viral infection of neuronal tissue.
   c. cognitive changes secondary to cerebral ischemia.
   d. abrupt changes in cognitive function that are irreversible.

3. The clinical diagnosis of dementia is based on
   a. CT or MRS.
   b. brain biopsy.
   c. electroencephalogram.
   d. patient history and cognitive assessment.

4. Which of the following statements accurately describes mild cognitive impairment?
   a. Always progresses to AD
   b. Caused by variety of factors and may progress to AD
   c. Should be aggressively treated with acetylcholinesterase drugs
   d. Caused by vascular infarcts that, if treated, will delay progression to AD

5. The early stage of AD is characterized by
   a. no noticeable change in behavior.
   b. memory problems and mild confusion.
   c. increased time spent sleeping or in bed.
   d. incontinence, agitation, and wandering behavior.

6. A major goal of treatment for the patient with AD is to
   a. maintain patient safety.
   b. maintain or increase body weight.
   c. return to a higher level of self-care.
   d. enhance functional ability over time.

7. Creutzfeldt-Jakob disease is characterized by
   a. remissions and exacerbations over many years.
   b. memory impairment, muscle jerks, and blindness.
   c. parkinsonian symptoms including muscle rigidity and tremors at rest.
   d. increased intracranial pressure secondary to decreased CSF drainage.

8. Which of the following patients is most at risk for developing delirium?
   a. A 50-year-old woman with cholecystitis
   b. A 19-year-old man with a fractured femur
   c. A 42-year-old woman having an elective hysterectomy
   d. A 78-year-old man admitted to the medical unit with complications related to heart failure

Nervous System

REFERENCES

1. National Institute of Neurological Disorders and Stroke: Dementia information page. Available at *www.ninds.nih.gov/disorders/dementias.htm* (accessed March 24, 2006).
2. American Psychiatric Association: Healthy minds, healthy lives, mental health of the elderly. Available at *http://healthyminds.org/mentalhealthofelderly.cfm* (accessed March 24, 2006).
3. Alzheimer Society: Alzheimer's disease statistics. Available at *www.alzheimer.ca/english/disease/stats-people.htm*.
4. Morris JC: Dementia update 2005, *Alzheimer Dis Assoc Disord* 19:100, 2005.
5. Feldman HH, Jacova C: Mild cognitive impairment, *Am J Geriatr Psychiatry* 13:645, 2005.
6. Desai AK, Grossberg GT: Diagnosis and treatment of Alzheimer's disease, *Neurology* 64(Suppl):S34, 2005.
7. Alzheimer's Disease Education and Referral Center: General information. Available at *www.alzheimers.org/generalinfo.htm* (accessed August 31, 2006).
8. Alzheimer's Association: Alzheimer's disease fact sheet. Available at *www.alz.org* (accessed August 31, 2006).
9. National Institute on Aging: 2004-2005 progress report on Alzheimer's disease. Available at *www.nia.nih.gov/Alzhemiers/PublicationsADProgress 2004_2005* (accessed August 31, 2006).
10. Desai AK, Grossberg GT: Diagnosis and treatment of Alzheimer's disease, *Neurology* 64(Suppl):S34, 2005.
11. Sink KM, Holden KF, Yaffe K: Pharmacological treatment of neuropsychiatric symptoms of dementia, *JAMA* 293:596, 2005.
12. Potyk D: Treatments for Alzheimer disease, *South Med Assoc* 98:628, 2005.
13. Schneider LS, Tariot PN, Dagerman KS, et al: Effectiveness of atypical antipsychotic drugs in patients with Alzheimer's disease, *NEJM* 355(15):1525, 2006.
14. Pinkerton JV, Henderson VW: Estrogen and cognition, with a focus on Alzheimer's disease, *Semin Reprod Med* 23:172, 2005.
15. Nair M: Nursing management of the patient with Alzheimer's disease, *Br J Nurs* 15:258, 2006.
16. Alzheimer's Association Safe Return. Available at *www.alz.org/services/safereturn* (accessed August 31, 2006).
17. Furman EF: Undernutrition in older adults across the continuum of care, *J Gerontol Nurs* 32(1):22, 2006.
18. Keiser J: Lewy body dementia, Lewy Body Dementia Association. Available at *www.lewybodydementia.org/AR0507LBD1.shtml* (accessed February 25, 2006).
19. Hilton DA: Pathogenesis and prevalence of variant Creutzfeldt-Jakob disease, *J Pathol* 208:134, 2006.
20. Sheff B: Mad cow disease and vCJD: understanding the risks, *Nursing* 35(2):74, 2005.
21. Inouye SK: Delirium in older adults, *N Engl J Med* 354:1157, 2006.
22. Leentjens AFG, van der Mast RC: Delirium in elderly people: an update, *Curr Opin Psychiatry* 18:325, 2005.
23. Milisen K, Lemiengre J, Braes T, et al: Multicomponent intervention strategies for managing delirium in hospitalized older people: systematic review, *J Adv Nurs* 52:79, 2005.

RESOURCES

Administration on Aging (AoA)
202-619-0724
www.aoa.dhhs.gov
Alzheimer's Association
800-272-3900 or 312-335-8700
www.alz.org
Alzheimer's Disease Education and Referral Center
800-438-4380
www.alzheimers.org
American Association for Geriatric Psychiatry
301-654-7850
www.aagponline.org
American Association of Retired Persons
800-687-2277
www.aarp.org
Lewy Body Dementia Association
800-539-9767
www.lewybodydementia.org
National Alliance for Caregiving
www.caregiving.org
National Council on the Aging (NCOA)
800-373-4906
www.ncoa.org
National Family Caregivers Association (NFCA)
800-896-3650
www.nfcacares.org
National Institute on Aging
800-222-2225 or 301-496-1752
www.nia.nih.gov
National Institute of Mental Health (NIMH)
800-421-4211 or 301-443-4513
www.nimh.nih.gov
National Institute of Neurological Disorders and Strokes
800-352-9424
www.ninds.nih.gov
National Mental Health Association
Alexandria, VA 22311
800-969-NMHA (6642) or 703-684-7722
www.nmha.org

For additional Internet resources, see the website for this book at *http://evolve. elsevier.com/Lewis/medsurg*.

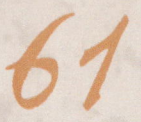

Character cannot be developed in ease and quiet. Only through experience of trial and suffering can the soul be strengthened, ambition inspired, and success achieved.

Helen Keller

61

Nursing Management
Peripheral Nerve and Spinal Cord Problems

Linda Laskowski-Jones

LEARNING OBJECTIVES

1. Explain the etiology, clinical manifestations, collaborative care, and nursing management of trigeminal neuralgia and Bell's palsy.
2. Explain the etiology, clinical manifestations, collaborative care, and nursing management of Guillain-Barré syndrome, botulism, tetanus, and neurosyphilis.
3. Describe the classification of spinal cord injuries and associated clinical manifestations.
4. Describe the clinical manifestations, collaborative care, and nursing management of spinal cord shock.
5. Correlate the clinical manifestations of spinal cord injury with the level of disruption and rehabilitation potential.
6. Describe the nursing management of the major physical and psychologic problems of the patient with a spinal cord injury.
7. Describe the effects of spinal cord injury on the older adult population.
8. Explain the types, clinical manifestations, collaborative care, and nursing management of spinal cord tumors.
9. Describe the pathophysiology, clinical manifestations, and nursing and collaborative management of postpolio syndrome.

KEY TERMS

autonomic dysreflexia, p. 1603
Bell's palsy, p. 1584
botulism, p. 1587
Brown-Séquard syndrome, p. 1591
Guillain-Barré syndrome, p. 1585
neurogenic bladder, p. 1604
neurogenic shock, p. 1590
neurosyphilis, p. 1589
paraplegia, p. 1590
postpolio syndrome, p. 1610
spinal shock, p. 1590
tetanus, p. 1588
tetraplegia, p. 1589
trigeminal neuralgia, p. 1581

Electronic Resources

Supplemental content related to Chapter 61 can be found . . .

Companion CD
- Stress-Busting Kit for Nursing Students
- Interactive Case Study: Spinal Cord Injury
- NCLEX Examination Review Questions
- Comprehensive Glossary

Evolve Website *evolve*
http://evolve.elsevier.com/Lewis/medsurg
- Content Updates
- Key Points (Printable and CD/MP3 Download)
- Concept Map Creator
- Expanded Audio Glossary
- Key Term Flash Cards

- Customizable Nursing Care Plan: Spinal Cord Injury
- Patient and Family Instruction Guides in English and Spanish:
  - Autonomic Dysreflexia
  - Bowel Management After Spinal Cord Injury
  - Skin Care for Patient with Spinal Cord Injuries
- Electronic Calculators
- WebLinks

Reviewed by Gayle H. Dasher, RN, PhD, CCRN, CNRN, Director of Clinical Practice and Standards, CHRISTUS Santa Rosa Health Care, San Antonio, Tex.

Cranial Nerve Disorders

Cranial nerve disorders are commonly classified as peripheral neuropathies. The 12 pairs of cranial nerves are considered the peripheral nerves of the brain. The disorders usually involve the motor or sensory (or both) branches of a single nerve (*mononeuropathies*). Causes of cranial nerve problems include tumors, trauma, infections, inflammatory processes, and idiopathic (unknown) causes. Two cranial nerve disorders are trigeminal neuralgia (tic douloureux) and acute peripheral facial paralysis (Bell's palsy).

TRIGEMINAL NEURALGIA

Etiology and Pathophysiology

Trigeminal neuralgia (*tic douloureux*) is a relatively uncommon cranial nerve disorder diagnosed in approximately 15,000 Americans each year. However, it is the most commonly diagnosed neuralgic condition. It is seen approximately twice as often in women as in men. The majority of cases (over 90%) are diagnosed in individuals over the age of 40.[1] The trigeminal nerve is the fifth cranial nerve (CN V) and has both motor and sensory branches. In trigeminal neuralgia the sensory or afferent branches, primarily the maxillary and mandibular branches, are involved (Fig. 61-1).

The pathophysiology of trigeminal neuralgia is not fully understood. One theory is that compression of blood vessels, especially the superior cerebellar artery, occurs. This results in chronic irritation of the trigeminal nerve at the root entry zone. This irritation leads to increased firing of the afferent or sensory fibers. Other factors that may result in neuralgia include herpesvirus infection, infection of the teeth and jaw, and a brainstem infarct. The effectiveness of antiseizure drug therapy in reducing pain may be related to the ability of these drugs to stabilize the neuronal membrane and decrease paroxysmal afferent impulses of the nerve.[1]

Clinical Manifestations

The classic feature of trigeminal neuralgia is an abrupt onset of paroxysms of excruciating pain described as a burning, knifelike, or lightning-like shock in the lips, upper or lower gums, cheek, forehead, or side of the nose. Intense pain, twitching, grimacing, and frequent blinking and tearing of the eye occur during the acute attack (giving rise to the term *tic*). Some patients may also experience facial sensory loss. The attacks are usually brief, lasting only seconds to 2 or 3 minutes, and are generally unilateral. Recurrences are unpredictable; they may occur several times a day or weeks or months apart. After the refractory (pain-free) period, a phenomenon known as *clustering* can occur. Clustering is characterized by a cycle of pain and refractoriness that continues for hours.

The painful episodes are usually initiated by a triggering mechanism of light cutaneous stimulation at a specific point (*trigger zone*) along the distribution of the nerve branches. Precipitating stimuli include chewing, toothbrushing, a hot or cold blast of air on the face, washing the face, yawning, or even talking. Touch and tickle seem to predominate as causative triggers, rather than pain or changes in temperature. As a result, the patient may eat improperly, neglect hygienic practices, wear a cloth over the face, and withdraw from interaction with other individuals. The patient may sleep excessively as a means of coping with the pain.

Although this condition is considered benign, the severity of the pain and the disruption of lifestyle can result in almost total physical and psychologic dysfunction or even suicide.

Diagnostic Studies

It is important to rule out other problems with similar manifestations, such as other forms of facial and cephalic neuralgias and pain arising from the sinuses, teeth, and jaws. In young adults with bilateral facial pain, a computed tomography (CT) scan is performed to rule out any lesions or vascular abnormalities, and a lumbar puncture and magnetic resonance imaging (MRI) are done to rule out multiple sclerosis. A complete neurologic assessment is done, including audiologic evaluation, although results are usually normal. Additional tests used to rule out other pathologic conditions include electromyography (EMG), cerebrospinal fluid (CSF) analysis, arteriography, and myelography. Once the diagnosis is made, the goal of treatment is relief of pain either medically or surgically (Tables 61-1 and 61-2).

Collaborative Care

Drug Therapy. The majority of patients obtain adequate relief through antiseizure drugs such as carbamazepine (Tegretol), phenytoin (Dilantin), and valproate (Depakene). Carbamazepine is consid-

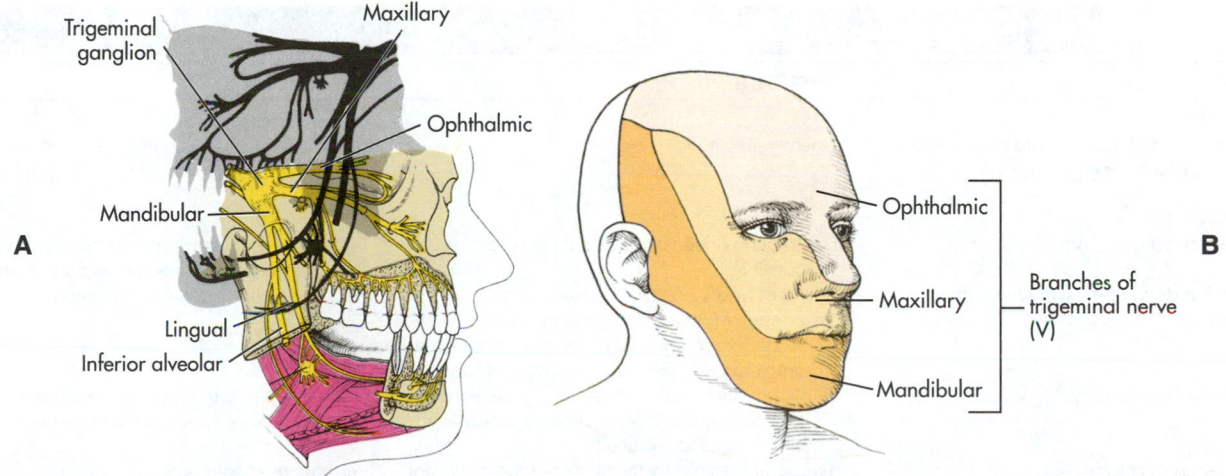

FIG. 61-1 A, Trigeminal (fifth cranial) nerve and its three main divisions—the ophthalmic, maxillary, and mandibular nerves. **B,** Cutaneous innervation of the head.

ered the first-line therapy for trigeminal neuralgia. By acting on sodium channels, carbamazepine and other antiseizure drugs lengthen the time needed for neuron repolarization, resulting in decreased neuron firing. Side effects of carbamazepine may include bone marrow suppression leading to blood abnormalities. Therefore routine complete blood cell (CBC) counts are required. Newer antiseizure drugs used in the management of trigeminal neuralgia include oxcarbazepine (Trileptal), gabapentin (Neurontin), lamotrigine (Lamictal), and topiramate (Topamax). These antiseizure drugs may prevent an acute attack or promote a remission of symptoms. Because drug therapy may not provide permanent pain relief, some patients may seek continued help by numerous visits to otolaryngologists or from therapies such as acupuncture and megavitamins.

Conservative Therapy. Nerve blocking with local anesthetics is another treatment option. Local nerve blocking results in complete anesthesia of the area supplied by the injected branches. Relief of pain is temporary, lasting from 6 to 18 months. This treatment is usually tolerated well by older adults.

Biofeedback is another strategy that may be helpful for some patients. In addition to controlling the pain, the patient may experience a strong sense of personal control by mastering the technique and altering certain body functions. (Biofeedback is discussed in Chapter 8.)

Surgical Therapy. If a conservative approach including drug therapy is not effective, surgical therapy is available (see Table 61-2). *Glycerol rhizotomy* is a percutaneous procedure that consists of an injection of glycerol through the foramen ovale into the trigeminal cistern (Fig. 61-2). It is a more benign procedure with less sensory loss and fewer sensory aberrations than radiofrequency rhizotomy and with comparable or better pain relief. However, for some patients the pain will return over time.[2,3]

Percutaneous radiofrequency rhizotomy (electrocoagulation) and microvascular decompression afford the greatest relief of pain. *Percutaneous radiofrequency rhizotomy* consists of placing a needle into the trigeminal rootlets that are adjacent to the pons and destroying the area by means of a radiofrequency current. This can result in facial numbness (although some degree of sensation may be retained), corneal anesthesia, and trigeminal motor weakness. This procedure is easily performed with minimal risk to the patient and is based on the exchange of pain for numbness. The procedure is usually performed on an outpatient basis with few complications. It is tolerated well by older adults and avoids a major operative procedure in the high-risk patient.[2]

Microvascular decompression of the trigeminal nerve is another commonly used procedure for neuralgia. It is accomplished by displacing and repositioning blood vessels that appear to be compressing the nerve at the root entry zone where it exits the pons. This procedure relieves pain without residual sensory loss, but it is potentially dangerous, as is any surgery near the brainstem. Microvascular decompression has a long-term success rate equal to or superior to percutaneous procedures without the higher rate of permanent neurologic outcomes such as numbness. It is a safe procedure with an almost negligible mortality and low morbidity when performed in younger adults by a skilled surgeon.[2]

Gamma knife radiosurgery is another surgical treatment that is used for trigeminal neuralgia. Radiosurgery using the gamma knife provides precise radiation of the proximal trigeminal nerve identified on high-resolution imaging. This image-guided approach has been useful both for patients with persistent pain after other surgeries and as a primary surgical option.[3] Two other intra-

TABLE 61-1	**COLLABORATIVE CARE** **Trigeminal Neuralgia**

Diagnostic
History and physical examination
Audiologic evaluation
CT scan
MRI
EMG
CSF analysis
Arteriography
Posterior myelography

Collaborative Therapy
Drug therapy (e.g., phenytoin [Dilantin], carbamazepine [Tegretol], valproate [Depakene], oxcarbazepine [Trileptal], gabapentin [Neurontin], lamotrigine [Lamictal], topiramate [Topamax])
Local nerve blocking
Biofeedback
Surgical intervention (see Table 61-2)

CSF, Cerebrospinal fluid; *CT,* computed tomography; *EMG,* electromyography; *MRI,* magnetic resonance imaging.

TABLE 61-2	**Surgical Interventions for Trigeminal Neuralgia**

Procedure	**Technique**	**Benefit**
Peripheral		
Glycerol rhizotomy (injection into one or more branches of the trigeminal nerve)	Chemical ablation	Total pain relief with sparing of touch and corneal reflex
Intracranial		
Percutaneous radiofrequency rhizotomy	Destruction of sensory fibers by low-voltage current	Total pain relief, sparing of touch and corneal reflex (increased risk for sensory changes)
Microvascular decompression (Jannetta procedure)	Lifting of artery pressing on nerve root in posterior fossa with wedge of sponge, leading to removal of pressure at nerve-root entry zone or removing the involved vessel	Pain relief without loss of sensation
Gamma knife radiosurgery	Technique that uses high doses of radiation focused on the trigeminal nerve root using stereotactic localization	Pain relief 1 day to 4 mo posttreatment; noninvasive; no loss of sensation
Retrogasserian rhizotomy	Temporal craniotomy (sectioning of sensory root in middle cranial fossa)	Permanent anesthesia
Suboccipital craniotomy	Sectioning of sensory root of posterior fossa	Permanent anesthesia

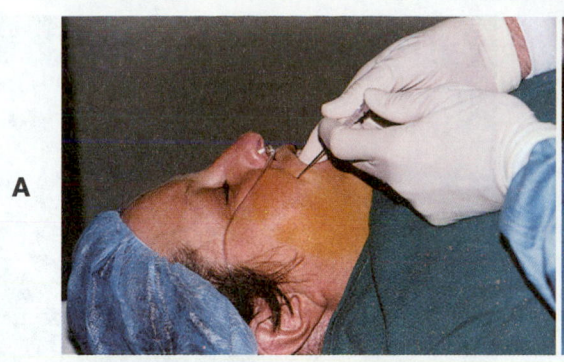 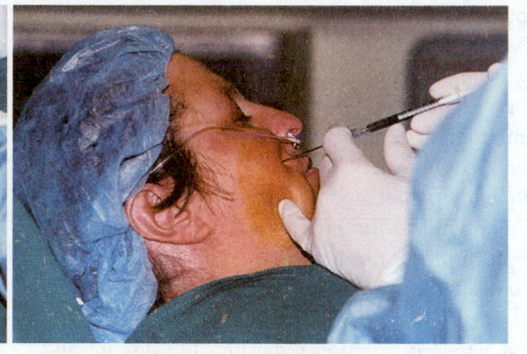

FIG. 61-2 A, Patient with trigeminal neuralgia having needle placed. **B,** Physician injecting glycerol.

cranial procedures include the retrogasserian rhizotomy and sub-occipital craniotomy (see Table 61-2).

NURSING MANAGEMENT
TRIGEMINAL NEURALGIA

■ Nursing Assessment

Assessment of the attacks, including the triggering factors, characteristics, frequency, and pain management techniques, helps the nurse plan for patient care. The nursing assessment should include the patient's nutritional status, hygiene (especially oral), and behavior (including withdrawal). Evaluation of the degree of pain and its effects on the patient's lifestyle, drug history, emotional state, and suicidal tendencies are other important factors.

■ Nursing Diagnoses

Nursing diagnoses for the patient with trigeminal neuralgia include, but are not limited to, the following:

- Acute pain *related to* inflammation or compression of the trigeminal nerve
- Imbalanced nutrition: less than body requirements *related to* fear of triggering pain by eating or chewing
- Anxiety *related to* uncertainty of timing and initiating event of pain and uncertainty regarding effectiveness of pain-relieving treatments
- Impaired oral mucous membrane *related to* unwillingness to practice oral hygiene measures secondary to potential for initiating pain
- Social isolation *related to* anxiety over pain attacks and desire to maintain nonstimulating environment

■ Planning

The overall goals are that the patient with trigeminal neuralgia will (1) be free of pain, (2) maintain adequate nutritional and oral hygiene status, (3) have minimal to no anxiety, and (4) return to normal or previous socialization and occupational activities.

■ Nursing Implementation

Health Promotion. Because the etiology of trigeminal neuralgia remains unknown, health promotion is directed at reducing recurrent episodes in those who have trigeminal neuralgia. Awareness and reduction of triggering events may be possible in some patients.

Acute Intervention. Patients with trigeminal neuralgia are treated primarily on an outpatient basis. Pain relief is primarily obtained by the administration of the recommended drug therapy.

The nurse monitors the patient's response to therapy and notes any side effects. Strong opioids such as morphine should be used cautiously because of the potential for addiction over time. Alternative pain-relief measures, such as biofeedback, should be explored for the patient who is not a surgical candidate and whose pain is not controlled by other therapeutic measures. Careful assessment of pain, including history, pain relief, and drug dependency, can assist in selecting appropriate interventions.

Environmental management is essential during an acute period to lessen triggering stimuli. The room should be kept at an even, moderate temperature and free of drafts. A private room is preferred during an acute period. The nurse must use care to avoid touching the patient's face or jarring the bed. Many patients prefer to carry out their own care, fearing that someone else will inadvertently injure them.

The nurse must teach the patient about the importance of nutrition, hygiene, and oral care and convey understanding if previous oral neglect is apparent. The nurse should provide lukewarm water and soft cloths or cotton saturated with solutions not requiring rinsing for cleansing the face. A small, soft-bristled toothbrush or a warm mouthwash assists in promoting oral care. Hygiene activities are best carried out when analgesia is at its peak.

The patient will probably not engage in extensive conversation during the acute period. Alternative communication methods such as paper and pencil should be provided.

Food should be high in protein and calories and easy to chew. It should be served lukewarm and offered frequently. The diet should be individualized according to personal, cultural, and religious preferences. When oral intake is sharply reduced and the patient's nutritional status is compromised, a nasogastric tube can be inserted on the unaffected side for enteral feedings.

The nurse is responsible for instruction related to diagnostic studies to rule out other problems, such as multiple sclerosis, dental or sinus problems, and neoplasms, and for preoperative teaching if surgery is planned. The nurse may also need to reinforce the surgeon's instructions related to postoperative expectations. Appropriate teaching related to postoperative activities depends on the type of procedure planned (e.g., percutaneous, intracranial). The patient needs to know that he or she will be awake during local procedures so that he or she can cooperate when corneal and ciliary reflexes and facial sensations are checked. Patients are informed about the potential risk of postoperative facial numbness.

After the procedure the patient's pain is compared with the preoperative level. The corneal reflex, extraocular muscles, hearing, sensation, and facial nerve function are evaluated frequently (see Chapter 56). If there is impairment of the corneal reflex, special attention must be paid to eye protection. This includes the use of artificial tears or eye shields. General postoperative nursing care after a craniotomy is appropriate if intracranial surgery is performed. (Nursing care related to craniotomy is discussed in Chapter 57.) Diet and ambulation should be increased according to the patient's progress or specific orders.

After a radiofrequency percutaneous electrocoagulation procedure, an ice pack is applied to the jaw on the operative side for 3 to 5 hours. To avoid injuring the mouth, the patient should not chew on the operative side until sensation has returned.

Ambulatory and Home Care. Regular follow-up care should be planned. The patient needs instruction regarding the dosage and side effects of medications. Although relief of pain may be complete, the patient should be encouraged to keep environmental stimuli to a moderate level and to use stress-reduction methods. The patient may have developed protective practices to prevent pain and may need counseling or psychiatric assistance in the readjustment, especially in reestablishing personal relationships. Herpes simplex infection (cold sores) can occur from manipulation of the gasserian ganglion. Treatment consists of antiviral agents such as acyclovir (Zovirax) (see Chapter 24).

Long-term management after surgical intervention depends on the residual effects of the type of procedure. If anesthesia is present or the corneal reflex is altered, the patient should be taught to (1) chew on the unaffected side; (2) avoid hot foods or beverages, which can burn the mucous membranes; (3) check the oral cavity after meals to remove food particles; (4) practice meticulous oral hygiene and continue with semiannual dental visits; (5) protect the face against extremes of temperature; (6) use an electric razor; and (7) wear a protective eye shield.

■ Evaluation

The expected outcomes are that the patient with trigeminal neuralgia will

- have decreased or relief from pain
- appear more comfortable and less anxious
- have normal facial sensation
- return to previous socialization and occupational activities

BELL'S PALSY

Etiology and Pathophysiology

Bell's palsy (peripheral facial paralysis, acute benign cranial polyneuritis) is a disorder characterized by a disruption of the motor branches of the facial nerve (CN VII) on one side of the face in the absence of any other disease such as a stroke. Bell's palsy is an acute, peripheral facial paresis of unknown cause. Each year approximately 20 per 100,000 individuals will be diagnosed with Bell's palsy. It can affect any age group, but it is more commonly seen in the 20- to 60-year-old age range. Despite its good prognosis, Bell's palsy leaves more than 8000 people a year in the United States with permanent, potentially disfiguring facial weakness.[4]

Although the exact etiology is not known, there is evidence that reactivated herpes simplex virus (HSV) may be involved in some cases. The reactivation of the HSV causes inflammation, edema, ischemia, and eventual demyelination of the nerve, creating pain and alterations in motor and sensory function.

Bell's palsy is considered benign, with full recovery after 6 months in most patients, especially if treatment is instituted im-

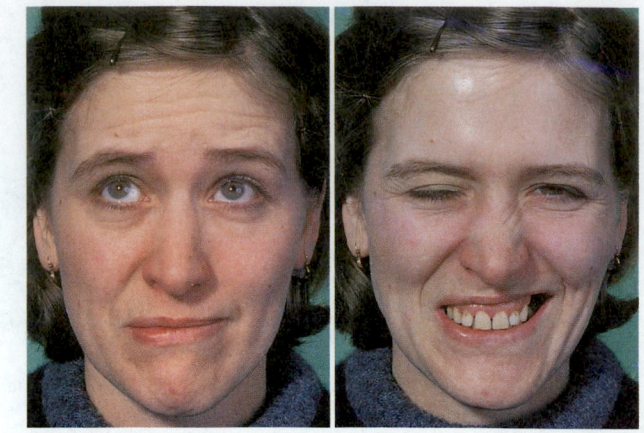

FIG. 61-3 Facial characteristics of Bell's palsy. **A,** At rest the face may look almost normal, but the patient is not able to wrinkle her forehead on the affected side and the right corner of the mouth droops. **B,** When she is asked to close her eyes and show her teeth, the differences between the affected and unaffected sides become more obvious.

mediately. The remaining patients continue to be bothered by weakness and asymmetric movement of facial muscles.[4]

Clinical Manifestations

The onset of Bell's palsy is often accompanied by an outbreak of herpes vesicles in or around the ear. Patients may complain of pain around and behind the ear. In addition, manifestations may include fever, tinnitus, and hearing deficit. The paralysis of the motor branches of the facial nerve typically results in a flaccidity of the affected side of the face, with drooping of the mouth accompanied by drooling (Fig. 61-3). An inability to close the eyelid, with an upward movement of the eyeball when closure is attempted, is also evident. A widened *palpebral fissure* (the opening between the eyelids); flattening of the nasolabial fold; and inability to smile, frown, or whistle are also common. Unilateral loss of taste is common. Decreased muscle movement may alter chewing ability, and although some patients may experience a loss of tearing, many patients complain of excessive tearing. The muscle weakness causes the lower lid to turn out, allowing overflow of normal tear production. Pain may be present behind the ear on the affected side, especially before the onset of paralysis.

Complications can include psychologic withdrawal because of changes in appearance, malnutrition, dehydration, mucous membrane trauma, corneal abrasions, muscle stretching, and facial spasms and contractures.

Diagnostic Studies

The diagnosis of Bell's palsy is one of exclusion. There is no definitive test. The diagnosis and prognosis are indicated by observation of the typical pattern of onset and signs and the testing of percutaneous nerve excitability by EMG.

Collaborative Care

Methods of treatment for Bell's palsy include moist heat, gentle massage, and electrical stimulation of the nerve and prescribed exercises. Stimulation may maintain muscle tone and prevent atrophy. Care is primarily focused on relief of symptoms, prevention of complications, and protection of the eye on the affected side.

Drug Therapy. Corticosteroids, especially prednisone, are started immediately, and the best results appear to be obtained if corticosteroids are initiated before paralysis is complete. When the patient improves to the point that the corticosteroids are no longer necessary, they should be tapered off over a 2-week period. Usually, the corticosteroid treatment decreases the edema and pain, but mild analgesics can be used if necessary. Because the HSV is implicated in approximately 70% of cases of Bell's palsy, treatment with acyclovir (Zovirax), alone or in conjunction with prednisone, may be used.[4] Additional antiviral agents, including valacyclovir (Valtrex) and famciclovir (Famvir), have also been used in the management of Bell's palsy.

NURSING MANAGEMENT
BELL'S PALSY

■ Nursing Assessment

Early recognition of the possibility of Bell's palsy is important. Because HSV is a possible etiologic factor, any person who is prone to herpes simplex should be alerted to seek health care if pain occurs in or around the ear. Assessment of facial muscles for any signs of weakness should also be done. Careful recording of assessment data provides information related to the progress of the syndrome.

■ Nursing Diagnoses

The nursing diagnoses for the patient with Bell's palsy may include, but are not limited to, the following:

- Acute pain *related to* the inflammation of CN VII (facial nerve)
- Imbalanced nutrition: less than body requirements *related to* inability to chew secondary to muscle weakness
- Risk for injury (corneal abrasion) *related to* inability to blink
- Disturbed body image *related to* change in facial appearance secondary to facial muscle weakness

■ Planning

The overall goals are that the patient with Bell's palsy will (1) be pain free or have pain controlled, (2) maintain adequate nutritional status, (3) maintain appropriate oral hygiene, (4) not experience injury to the eye, (5) return to normal or previous perception of body image, and (6) be optimistic about disease outcome.

■ Nursing Implementation

The patient with Bell's palsy is treated on an outpatient basis. The following interventions are used throughout the course of the disease. Mild analgesics can relieve pain. Hot wet packs can reduce the discomfort of herpetic lesions, aid circulation, and relieve pain. The face should be protected from cold and drafts because trigeminal *hyperesthesia* (extreme sensitivity to pain or touch) may accompany the syndrome. Maintenance of good nutrition is important. The patient should be taught to chew on the unaffected side of the mouth to avoid trapping food and to enjoy the taste of food. Thorough oral hygiene must be carried out after each meal to prevent the development of parotitis, caries, and periodontal disease from accumulated residual food.

Dark glasses may be worn for protective and cosmetic reasons. Artificial tears (methylcellulose) should be instilled frequently during the day to prevent drying of the cornea. The eye should be inspected for the presence of eyelashes. Ointment and an impermeable eye shield can be used at night to retain moisture. In some patients, taping the lids closed at night may be necessary to provide protection. The patient is taught to report ocular pain, drainage, or discharge.

A facial sling may be helpful to support affected muscles, improve lip alignment, and facilitate eating. The facial sling is usually made and fitted by a physical or occupational therapist. Vigorous massage can break down tissues, but gentle upward massage has psychologic benefits even if physical effects other than the maintenance of circulation are questionable. When function begins to return, active facial exercises are performed several times a day.

The change in physical appearance as a result of Bell's palsy can be devastating. The patient must be reassured that a stroke did not occur and that chances for a full recovery are good. The patient's need for privacy should be respected, especially during meals, but the nurse's assistance in the patient's adjustment to the physical changes should not be delayed. Enlisting support from family and friends is important. It is important to share with the patient that most patients recover within about 6 weeks of the onset of symptoms.

■ Evaluation

The expected outcomes are that the patient with Bell's palsy will

- be free of pain
- not experience any complications
- maintain appropriate nutritional intake
- experience minimal side effects associated with corticosteroid treatment
- return to previous perception of body image

Polyneuropathies

GUILLAIN-BARRÉ SYNDROME

Etiology and Pathophysiology

Guillain-Barré syndrome (Landry–Guillain-Barré–Strohl syndrome, postinfectious polyneuropathy, ascending polyneuropathic paralysis) is an acute, rapidly progressing, and potentially fatal form of polyneuritis. It affects the peripheral nervous system and results in loss of myelin (a segmental demyelination) and edema and inflammation of the affected nerves, causing a loss of neurotransmission to the periphery. The syndrome affects males 1.5 times more frequently than females and is typically seen in adults, although it is observed in all age groups. Worldwide the incidence has varied from 0.4 to 1.7 cases per 100,000 persons per year. Because the management of the disease is often prolonged, Guillain-Barré syndrome has an estimated annual cost of $2 to $3 billion dollars in the United States. With adequate supportive care, 85% to 95% of patients recover completely from this disorder.

The etiology of this disorder is unknown, but it is believed to be a cell-mediated immunologic reaction directed at the peripheral nerves. The syndrome is often preceded by immune system stimulation from a viral infection, trauma, surgery, viral immunizations, or human immunodeficiency virus (HIV).[5] *Campylobacter jejuni* is the most recognized organism associated with Guillain-Barré syndrome.[6] *C. jejuni* gastroenteritis is thought to precede Guillain-Barré syndrome in approximately 30% of cases. Other potential pathogens include *Mycoplasma pneumoniae,* cytomegalovirus, Epstein-Barr virus, varicella-zoster virus, and vaccines (rabies, swine influenza). These stimuli are thought to cause an alteration in the immune system, resulting in sensitization of T lymphocytes to the patient's myelin and, ultimately, myelin damage. Demyelination occurs, and the transmission of nerve impulses is stopped or slowed down. The muscles innervated by the damaged peripheral nerves undergo denervation and atrophy. In the recovery phase, remyelination occurs slowly, and neurologic function returns in a proximal-to-distal pattern.

Clinical Manifestations

Guillain-Barré syndrome is a heterogeneous condition with symptoms ranging from mild to severe. Symptoms of Guillain-Barré syndrome usually develop 1 to 3 weeks after an upper respiratory or gastrointestinal (GI) infection. Weakness of the lower extremities (evolving more or less symmetrically) occurs over hours to days to weeks, usually peaking about the fourteenth day. Distal muscles are more severely affected. *Paresthesia* (numbness and tingling) is frequent, and paralysis usually follows in the extremities. *Hypotonia* (reduced muscle tone) and *areflexia* (lack of reflexes) are common, persistent symptoms. Objective sensory loss is variable, with deep sensitivity more affected than superficial sensations.

Miller Fisher syndrome is a clinical variant of Guillain-Barré syndrome, accounting for 5% to 10% of cases. It is characterized by a triad of symptoms including ataxia, areflexia, and *ophthalmoplegia* (paralysis of motor nerves of the eye). Other subtypes include acute inflammatory demyelinating polyneuropathy, acute motor axonal neuropathy, and acute motor and sensory axonal neuropathy.

In Guillain-Barré syndrome, autonomic nervous system dysfunction results from alterations in both the sympathetic and parasympathetic nervous systems. Autonomic disturbances are usually seen in patients with severe muscle involvement and respiratory muscle paralysis. The most dangerous autonomic dysfunctions include orthostatic hypotension, hypertension, and abnormal vagal responses (bradycardia, heart block, asystole). Other autonomic dysfunctions include bowel and bladder dysfunction, facial flushing, and diaphoresis. Patients may also have syndrome of inappropriate antidiuretic hormone (SIADH) secretion. SIADH is discussed in Chapter 50. Progression of Guillain-Barré syndrome to include the lower brainstem involves the facial, abducens, oculomotor, hypoglossal, trigeminal, and vagus nerves (CNs VII, VI, III, XII, V, and X, respectively). This involvement manifests itself through facial weakness, extraocular eye movement difficulties, dysphagia, and paresthesia of the face.

Pain is a common symptom in the patient with Guillain-Barré syndrome. The pain can be categorized as paresthesias, muscular aches and cramps, and hyperesthesias. Pain appears to be worse at night. Opioids may be indicated for those experiencing severe pain. Pain may lead to a decrease in appetite and may interfere with sleep.

Complications. The most serious complication of this syndrome is respiratory failure, which occurs as the paralysis progresses to the nerves that innervate the thoracic area. Constant monitoring of the respiratory system by checking respiratory rate and depth, forced vital capacity, and negative inspiratory force provides information about the need for immediate intervention, including intubation and mechanical ventilation. Respiratory or urinary tract infections (UTIs) may occur. Fever is generally the first sign of infection, and treatment is directed at the infecting organism. Immobility from the paralysis can cause problems such as paralytic ileus, muscle atrophy, deep vein thrombosis, pulmonary emboli, skin breakdown, orthostatic hypotension, and nutritional deficiencies.

Diagnostic Studies

Diagnosis is based primarily on the patient's history and clinical signs. CSF is normal or has a low protein content initially, but after 7 to 10 days it shows an elevated protein level to 700 mg/dl (7 g/L) (normal protein is 15 to 45 mg/dl [0.15 to 0.45 g/L]) with a normal cell count. Results of EMG and nerve conduction studies are markedly abnormal (reduced nerve conduction velocity) in the affected extremities.

Collaborative Care

Management is aimed at supportive care, particularly ventilatory support, during the acute phase. Plasmapheresis is used in the first 2 weeks of Guillain-Barré syndrome. In patients with severe disease who are treated within 2 weeks of onset, there is a distinct reduction in the length of hospital stay, length of time on a ventilator, and time required to resume walking. Intravenous (IV) administration of high-dose immunoglobulin (Sandoglobulin) has also been shown to be as effective as plasma exchange and has the advantage of immediate availability and greater safety. However, patients receiving high-dose immunoglobulin need to be well hydrated and have adequate renal function. (Plasmapheresis is discussed in Chapter 14.) Beyond 3 weeks after disease onset, plasma exchange and immunoglobulin therapies have little value. Corticosteroids appear to have little effect on the prognosis or duration of the disease.[7]

Nutritional Therapy. Nutritional intake is compromised in the patient with Guillain-Barré syndrome. During the acute phase, the patient may experience difficulty swallowing because of cranial nerve involvement. Mild dysphagia can be managed by placing the patient in an upright position and flexing the head forward during feeding. For more severe dysphagia, tube feedings may be required. Patients who experience paralytic ileus or intestinal obstruction may require parenteral nutrition. Later in the course of the disease, motor paralysis or weakness continues to affect the ability to self-feed. The patient's nutritional status, including body weight, serum albumin levels, and calorie counts, must be evaluated at regular intervals.

NURSING MANAGEMENT
GUILLAIN-BARRÉ SYNDROME

■ *Nursing Assessment*

Assessment of the patient is the most important aspect of nursing care during the acute phase. During the routine assessment the nurse must monitor the ascending paralysis; assess respiratory function; monitor arterial blood gases (ABGs); and assess the gag, corneal, and swallowing reflexes. Reflexes are usually decreased or absent.

Monitoring blood pressure and cardiac rate and rhythm is also important during the acute phase because transient cardiac dysrhythmias have been reported. Autonomic dysfunction is common and usually takes the form of bradycardia and dysrhythmias. Orthostatic hypotension secondary to muscle atony may occur in severe cases. Vasopressor agents and volume expanders may be needed to treat the low blood pressure. However, the presence of SIADH may require fluid restriction.

■ *Nursing Diagnoses*

Nursing diagnoses for the patient with Guillain-Barré syndrome may include, but are not limited to, the following:

- Impaired spontaneous ventilation *related to* progression of disease process resulting in respiratory muscle paralysis
- Risk for aspiration *related to* dysphagia

- Acute pain *related to* paresthesias, muscle aches and cramps, and hyperesthesias
- Impaired verbal communication *related to* intubation or paralysis of the muscles of speech
- Fear *related to* uncertain outcome and seriousness of the disease
- Self-care deficits *related to* inability to use muscles to accomplish activities of daily living (ADLs)

■ *Planning*

The overall goals are that the patient with Guillain-Barré syndrome will (1) maintain adequate ventilation, (2) be free from aspiration, (3) be pain free or have pain controlled, (4) maintain an acceptable method of communication, (5) maintain adequate nutritional intake, and (6) return to usual physical functioning.

■ *Nursing Implementation*

The objective of therapy is to support body systems until the patient recovers. Respiratory failure and infection are serious threats. Monitoring the vital capacity and ABGs is essential. If the vital capacity drops to less than 800 ml (15 ml/kg or two thirds of the patient's normal vital capacity) or the ABGs deteriorate, endotracheal intubation or tracheostomy may be done so that the patient can be mechanically ventilated (see Chapter 68). Meticulous suctioning technique is needed to prevent infection whether the patient has an endotracheal tube or tracheostomy. Thorough bronchial hygiene and chest physiotherapy help clear secretions and prevent respiratory deterioration. If fever develops, sputum cultures should be obtained to identify the pathogen. Appropriate antibiotic therapy is then initiated.

A communication system must be established based upon the patient's abilities. This is extremely difficult if the disease progresses to involvement of the cranial nerves. At the peak of a severe episode the patient may be incapable of communicating. The nurse must explain all procedures before doing them and reassure the patient that muscle function will return.

Urinary retention is common for a few days. Intermittent catheterization is preferred to an indwelling catheter to avoid urinary tract infections. However, for the acutely ill patient receiving a large volume of fluids (>2.5 L/day), indwelling catheterization may be safer to reduce overdistention of a temporarily flaccid bladder and to prevent vesicoureteral reflux. Physical therapy is indicated early to help prevent problems related to immobility. Range-of-motion exercises and attention to body position help maintain function and prevent contractures. Patients who develop facial paralysis must receive meticulous eye care to avoid corneal irritation or damage *(exposure keratitis).* Artificial tears should be instilled frequently during the day to prevent drying of the cornea. The eyes should be inspected for the presence of eyelashes. Ointment and an impermeable eye shield can be used at night to retain moisture.

Nutritional needs must be met in spite of possible problems associated with delayed gastric emptying, paralytic ileus, and potential for aspiration if the gag reflex is lost. In addition to checking for the gag reflex, nurses should note drooling and other difficulties with secretions, which may be more indicative of an inadequate gag reflex. Initially, tube feedings or parenteral nutrition may be used to ensure adequate caloric intake. Because of delayed gastric emptying, residual volumes of the feedings should be assessed at regular intervals or before feedings (see Chapter 40). Fluid and

electrolyte therapy must be monitored carefully to prevent electrolyte imbalances. A bowel program should be initiated because constipation is a common problem related to diet changes, immobility, and decreased GI motility.

Throughout the course of the illness, the nurse needs to provide support and encouragement to the family and patient. Because residual problems and relapses are uncommon except in the chronic form of the disease, complete recovery can be anticipated, although it is generally a slow process that takes months or years if axonal degeneration occurs.

■ *Evaluation*

The expected outcomes are that the patient with Guillain-Barré syndrome will

- return to usual level of physical functioning
- be free from pain and discomfort
- maintain nutritional status

BOTULISM

Etiology and Pathophysiology

Botulism is the most serious type of food poisoning. It is caused by GI absorption of the neurotoxin produced by *Clostridium botulinum.* This organism is found in the soil, and the spores are difficult to destroy. It can grow in any food contaminated with the spores. Improper home canning of foods is often the cause. In 2001, 169 cases of botulism were reported to the Centers for Disease Control and Prevention (CDC).[8] It is thought that the neurotoxin destroys or inhibits the neurotransmission of acetylcholine at the myoneural junction, resulting in disturbed muscle innervation.

Clinical Manifestations

Symptoms consist of nausea, vomiting, diarrhea, and abdominal cramping pain, generally within 12 to 36 hours after consumption of the contaminated food. Neurologic manifestations can develop rapidly or evolve over several days. They include development of a descending flaccid paralysis with intact sensation, photophobia, ptosis, paralysis of extraocular muscles, blurred vision, diplopia, dry mouth, sore throat, and difficulty in swallowing. Other manifestations include paralytic ileus, seizures, and respiratory muscle weakness that can rapidly deteriorate to respiratory arrest and/or cardiac arrest. The course of the disease depends on the amount of toxin absorbed from the gut. If only a small amount is absorbed, symptoms are mild and recovery is complete. When large amounts are absorbed, death may occur from circulatory failure, respiratory paralysis, or development of pulmonary complications. Approximately 5% of patients with botulism die.[8] Because botulism is a reportable disease, local, state, and federal health agencies, particularly the CDC in Atlanta, must be notified. Botulism can also be contracted through infected wounds or nasal inhalation, as well as oral ingestion. It has been highlighted as a potential bioterrorism agent and is discussed further in Chapter 69.

Diagnostic Studies and Collaborative Care

Blood and CSF are obtained for studies to rule out other diseases. In the patient with botulism the blood and CSF results are normal.

Drug Therapy. The initial treatment of botulism is IV administration of botulinum antitoxin. Before administration of the antitoxin, an intradermal test dose for sensitivity to horse serum is given. If there are no reactions, the test dose is followed by the therapeutic dose of botulism antitoxin, which may be repeated in 2 to 4 hours if symptoms persist, and again at 12- to 24-hour intervals if required.

The GI tract is purged by non–magnesium-containing laxatives, high colonic enemas, and gastric lavage to decrease the absorption of the toxin. Magnesium is contraindicated because it worsens toxin-induced neuromuscular blockade.

NURSING MANAGEMENT
BOTULISM

Primary prevention is the goal of nursing management by educating consumers to be alert to situations that may result in botulism. Particular attention should be given to foods with a low acid content, which support germination and the production of botulin, a deadly poison. These foods include fish, vichyssoise, and peppers. Although bacteria and the botulism toxin can be destroyed by boiling for 10 minutes, spores are extremely heat resistant and can survive in boiling water for 3 to 5 hours. High-temperature pressure cooking is the only safe method of home canning. Specific suggestions related to the preparation, storage, and use of food include the following:

- In home canning, the equipment manufacturer's directions should be followed. Only fresh fruits and vegetables (with all questionable spots removed) should be used. All containers and utensils must be cleansed, and the seal on the can or jar must be airtight. Canned foods should be stored properly in a cool, dry place.
- A can with a swollen end should never be used; the swelling may be caused by gases from *C. botulinum*.
- If the food is forcefully expelled when a container is opened, it should be discarded immediately and the contents should not be tasted.
- If the contents of a can look or smell bad after opening, the can should be discarded without tasting the contents. Materials may be flushed down the toilet or disposed of in the garbage disposal if a large amount of water is used.

Nursing care during the acute illness is similar to that for Guillain-Barré syndrome. Supportive nursing interventions include rest, activities to maintain respiratory function, adequate nutrition, and prevention of loss of muscle mass. Because the recovery process is slow, the patient may develop problems related to a feeling of helplessness, boredom, and low morale.

TETANUS

Etiology and Pathophysiology

Tetanus (lockjaw) is an extremely severe polyradiculitis and polyneuritis affecting spinal and cranial nerves. It results from the effects of a potent neurotoxin released by the anaerobic bacillus *Clostridium tetani*. The toxin interferes with the function of the reflex arc by blocking inhibitory transmitters at the presynaptic sites in the spinal cord and brainstem. The spores of the bacillus are present in soil, garden mold, and manure. Thus *C. tetani* enters the body through a traumatic or suppurative wound that provides an appropriate low-oxygen environment for the organisms to mature and produce toxin. Other possible sources include dental infection, chronic otitis media, injections of heroin, human and animal bites, burns, frostbite, open fractures, and gunshot wounds. The incubation period is usually 7 days but can range from 3 to

21 days, with symptoms frequently appearing after the original wound is healed. In general, the longer the incubation period, the milder the illness and the better the prognosis.

Worldwide the number of cases per year is estimated to be 1 million. In the United States about 50 to 70 cases occur each year and are typically due to infection of deep, penetrating wounds or IV drug use.[9] Of the reported cases, the majority of patients are over the age of 40 years.[10] However, the number of individuals under the age of 40 with tetanus is increasing, which is most likely related to IV drug use. Mortality rates vary according to age, with infants and persons over 50 years of age most seriously affected. Overall mortality rates are declining and are at about 10% in the United States.[10]

Clinical Manifestations

Initial manifestations of generalized tetanus include stiffness in the jaw *(trismus)* and neck, fever, and other symptoms of general infection. Generalized tonic spasms occur because of the lack of reciprocal innervation. As the disease progresses, the neck muscles, back, abdomen, and extremities become progressively rigid. In severe forms, continuous tonic convulsions may occur with *opisthotonos* (extreme arching of the back and retraction of the head). Laryngeal and respiratory spasms cause apnea and anoxia. Additional effects are manifested by overstimulation of the sympathetic nervous system, including profuse diaphoresis, labile hypertension, episodic tachycardia, hyperthermia, and dysrhythmias. The slightest noise, jarring motion, or bright light can set off the seizure. These seizures are agonizingly painful. Mortality is almost 100% in the severe form. Death is usually attributable to asphyxia or heart failure, the result of constantly recurring spasms. Residual injury, such as vertebral fracture, muscle contracture, and brain damage secondary to hypoxia, may be long-term consequences.

Collaborative Care

Serum electrolytes, CBC count, albumin, clotting factors, glucose, and ABGs are monitored. Cardiac function is monitored by electrocardiogram and auscultation. As increasing numbers of nerve cells become involved, their inhibitory control over muscle activity decreases and symptoms develop.

Drug Therapy. The management of tetanus includes administration of a tetanus and diphtheria toxoid (Td) booster and tetanus immune globulin (TIG) in different sites before the onset of symptoms to neutralize circulating toxins (see Table 69-6). A much larger dose of TIG is administered to patients with manifestations of clinical tetanus. Control of spasms is essential and is managed by deep sedation and skeletal muscle relaxation, usually with diazepam (Valium), barbiturates and, in severe cases, neuromuscular blocking agents such as vecuronium that act to paralyze skeletal muscles. Opioid analgesics such as morphine or fentanyl are also indicated for pain management. A 10- to 14-day course of penicillin, metronidazole, tetracycline, or doxycycline is recommended to inhibit further growth of *C. tetani*.

Because of laryngospasm and the potential need for neuromuscular blocking drugs, a tracheostomy is usually performed early and the patient is maintained on mechanical ventilation. Sedative agents and opioid analgesics are given concomitantly to all patients who are pharmacologically paralyzed. Any recognized wound should be debrided or an abscess drained. Antibiotics may be given to prevent secondary infections.

Nutrition is maintained through parenteral nutrition or nasogastric feeding. The mortality rate associated with tetanus is declining. However, for those who recover, there is a long convalescence that includes extensive physical therapy.

NURSING MANAGEMENT
TETANUS

Health teaching is aimed at ensuring tetanus prophylaxis, which is the most important factor influencing the incidence of this disease. Tetanus prevention and immunization protocols are summarized in Table 69-6. Adults should receive a tetanus and diphtheria toxoid booster every 10 years. The patient should be taught that immediate, thorough cleansing of all wounds with soap and water is important in the prevention of tetanus. If an open wound occurs and the patient has not been immunized within 5 years, the health care provider should be contacted so that a tetanus booster can be given.

If equine tetanus antitoxin is to be used, the patient should be tested for sensitivity. Administration of equine antitoxin is not recommended if sensitivity occurs; anaphylactic shock is potentially life threatening, and desensitization is ineffective. The side effects of routine administration of the antitoxin are mild and include a sore arm, swelling at the site, and itching. Serious side effects rarely occur. Routine administration of a booster shot to an adequately immunized patient can cause arm swelling and lymphadenopathy.

Every patient should receive a written record of immunizations and be encouraged to complete the active immunization schedule. The patient's immunization history should be accurately recorded to protect the patient and health care providers.

The acute nursing management of the patient with tetanus is aimed at supportive care based on the treatment of clinical manifestations. The patient should be placed in a quiet, darkened room that is insulated against noise. Judicious sedation should be given. Nursing care should be administered with the utmost caution to avoid triggering spasms. For example, the nurse should avoid unnecessary touching, use firm touching when necessary, and maintain a slightly higher than normal ambient temperature to minimize the use of linens to cover the patient. Nursing care related to tracheostomy and mechanical ventilation is given as appropriate. An indwelling urinary catheter may be used to prevent bladder distention and urinary reflux in the presence of spasms in the muscles of the pelvic floor. Attention is also given to skin care. The patient needs emotional support during the acute phase because the fear of death is real. The family also needs support and education.

NEUROSYPHILIS

Neurosyphilis (tertiary syphilis) is an infection of any part of the nervous system by the organism *Treponema pallidum*. It is the result of untreated or inadequately treated syphilis (see Chapter 53). The organism can invade the central nervous system within a few months of the original infection. Except for causing some changes in the CSF, including increased white blood cells (WBCs) and protein and positive serologic reaction, the organism lies dormant for years. Untreated neurosyphilis, although not contagious, can be fatal. Penicillin therapy is effective for syphilitic meningitis, but the neurologic deficits remain.

Late neurosyphilis results from degenerative changes in the spinal cord (tabes dorsalis) and brainstem (general paresis). *Tabes dorsalis* (progressive locomotor ataxia) is characterized by vague, sharp pains in the legs; ataxia; "slapping" gait; loss of proprioception and deep tendon reflexes; and zones of hyperesthesia. *Charcot's joints,* which are characterized by enlargement, bone destruc-

tion, and hypermobility, also occur as a result of joint effusion and edema. Other manifestations of neurosyphilis include seizures and vision and hearing problems.

Neurologic symptoms associated with neurosyphilis are numerous and many times nonspecific. Neurosyphilis is a differential diagnosis for patients with neurologic and psychiatric symptoms. *Dementia paralytica* is an ongoing spirochetal meningoencephalitis that causes a general dissolution of mental and physical capabilities. It may mimic a number of major or minor psychoses. Management includes treatment with penicillin, symptomatic care, and protection from physical injury.

Spinal Cord Problems

SPINAL CORD INJURY

Before World War II, the life expectancy for a person with a spinal cord injury ranged from months to 10 years from the onset of injury. The leading causes of death were renal failure and sepsis. Today, with improved treatment strategies, even the very young patient with a spinal cord injury can anticipate a long life. The prognosis for life is generally only about 5 years less than for persons of the same age without spinal cord injury. The cause of premature death in the patient with **tetraplegia** (paralysis of both arms and legs), which was formerly called quadriplegia, is usually related to compromised respiratory function.

The potential for disruption of individual growth and development, altered family dynamics, economic loss in terms of absence from work, and the high cost of rehabilitation and long-term health care make spinal cord trauma a major problem. According to estimates from the Centers for Diseases Control and Prevention (CDC), 11,000 Americans suffer spinal cord injuries each year.[11] The number of persons with spinal cord injuries living in the United States at any one time ranges from 222,000 to 285,000.[12] The cost of spinal cord injury care can be high. The average cost of care for a person with a high cervical injury is $682,957 in the first year and $122,334 in each subsequent year.[12] Although many people with spinal cord injuries can care for themselves independently, those with the highest level of injury may require round-the-clock care at home or in a long-term care facility. Today almost 90% of patients with spinal cord injury are discharged from the hospital to home or another noninstitutional residence.[12] The remaining 10% are discharged to nursing homes, chronic care facilities, or group homes.

Etiology and Pathophysiology

The segment of the population with the greatest risk for spinal cord injury is young adult men between the ages of 16 and 30 years. Seventy-eight percent of people with spinal cord injury are male, and the most common age at injury is 19.

Causes of spinal cord injury include many types of trauma. Motor vehicle crashes account for 50%; falls, 24%; violence, 11%; sports injuries, 9%; and other miscellaneous causes, 6%. In large urban areas, gunshot wounds may surpass falls as a cause of spinal cord injuries.[12]

There has also been an increase in the number of older adults with spinal cord injuries. People who were at least 61 years of age when injured increased from 4.7% of patients with spinal cord injury in the 1970s to 11% currently. Besides having greater mortality, older adults with traumatic injuries experience more complications than younger ones, and they are hospitalized longer. This trend toward older age at time of injury explains the overall increase in mean age of people with spinal cord injury from 28 years in the 1970s to 38 years at this time.[12]

Initial Injury. The spinal cord is wrapped in tough layers of dura and is rarely torn or transected by direct trauma. Spinal cord injury can be due to cord compression by bone displacement, interruption of blood supply to the cord, or traction resulting from pulling on the cord. Penetrating trauma, such as gunshot and stab wounds, can result in tearing and transection. The initial mechanical disruption of axons as a result of stretch or laceration is referred to as the *primary injury. Secondary injury* refers to the ongoing, progressive damage that occurs after the initial injury.[13]

There are several theories on what causes this ongoing damage at the molecular and cellular levels. These include free radical formation, uncontrolled calcium influx, ischemia, and lipid peroxidation. At the molecular level, *apoptosis* (cell death) occurs and may continue sometimes for weeks or months after the initial injury. Thus the complete cord damage (previously thought to be transection) in severe trauma is related to autodestruction of the cord. This is confirmed by observations that, shortly after the injury, petechial hemorrhages are noted in the central gray matter of the cord. Hemorrhagic areas in the center of the spinal cord appear within 1 hour, and by 4 hours there may be infarction in the gray matter.[13] This ongoing destructive process makes it critical that the initial care and management of the patient with a spinal cord injury limit further activation of these processes.

Fig. 61-4 illustrates the cascade of events causing secondary injury following traumatic spinal cord injury. The resulting hypoxia reduces the oxygen tension below the level that meets the metabolic needs of the spinal cord. Lactate metabolites and an increase in vasoactive substances, including norepinephrine, serotonin, and dopamine, are noted. At high levels, these vasoactive substances cause vasospasms and hypoxia, leading to subsequent necrosis. Unfortunately, the spinal cord has minimal ability to adapt to vasospasm.

By 24 hours or less, permanent damage may occur because of the development of edema. Edema secondary to the inflammatory response is particularly harmful because of lack of space for tissue expansion. Therefore resultant compression of the cord and extension of edema above and below the injury increase the ischemic damage.

The extent of the neurologic damage caused by a spinal cord injury results from primary injury damage (actual physical disruption of axons) and secondary injury damage (ischemia, hypoxia, microhemorrhage, and edema).[13] Because secondary injury processes occur over time, the extent of injury and prognosis for recovery are most accurately determined at least 72 hours or more after injury.[14]

Spinal and Neurogenic Shock. About 50% of people with acute spinal cord injury experience a temporary neurologic syndrome known as **spinal shock** that is characterized by decreased reflexes, loss of sensation, and flaccid paralysis below the level of the injury.[15] This syndrome lasts days to months and may mask postinjury neurologic function. Active rehabilitation may begin in the presence of spinal shock. **Neurogenic shock,** in contrast, is due to the loss of vasomotor tone caused by injury and is characterized by hypotension and bradycardia, which are important clinical clues. Loss of sympathetic nervous system innervation causes peripheral vasodilation, venous pooling, and a decreased cardiac output. These effects are generally associated with a cervical or high thoracic injury.

Classification of Spinal Cord Injury. Spinal cord injuries are classified by the mechanism of injury, skeletal and neurologic level of injury, and completeness or degree of injury.

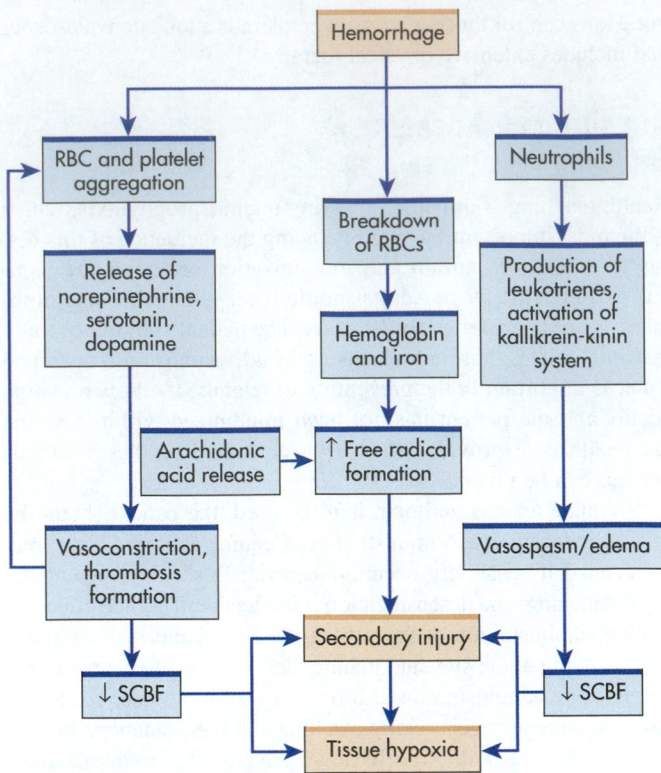

FIG. 61-4 Cascade of metabolic and cellular events that leads to spinal cord ischemia and hypoxia of secondary injury. *RBCs,* red blood cells; *SCBF,* spinal cord blood flow. *(Redrawn from Marciano F et al: BNI Quarterly 11:6, 1995.)*

Mechanisms of Injury. The major mechanisms of injury are flexion, hyperextension, flexion-rotation, extension-rotation, and compression (Fig. 61-5). The flexion-rotation injury is the most unstable of all injuries because the ligamentous structures that stabilize the spine are torn. This injury is most often implicated in severe neurologic deficits.

Level of Injury. *Skeletal level* of injury is the vertebral level where there is the most damage to vertebral bones and ligaments. *Neurologic level* is the lowest segment of the spinal cord with normal sensory and motor function on both sides of the body. The level of injury may be cervical, thoracic, or lumbar. Cervical and lumbar injuries are most common because these levels are associated with the greatest flexibility and movement. If the cervical cord is involved, paralysis of all four extremities occurs, resulting in tetraplegia. However, when the damage is high in the cervical cord, the arms are rarely completely paralyzed. If the thoracic or lumbar cord is damaged, the result is **paraplegia** (paralysis and loss of sensation in the legs). Fig. 61-6 shows affected structures and functions at different levels of cord injury.

Degree of Injury. The degree of spinal cord involvement may be either complete or incomplete (partial). *Complete cord involvement* results in total loss of sensory and motor function below the level of the lesion (injury). *Incomplete cord involvement* results in a mixed loss of voluntary motor activity and sensation and leaves some tracts intact. The degree of sensory and motor loss varies depending on the level of the lesion and reflects the specific nerve tracts damaged and those spared. Six syndromes are associated with incomplete lesions: central cord syndrome, anterior cord syndrome, Brown-Séquard syndrome, posterior cord syndrome, cauda equina syndrome, and conus medullaris syndrome.

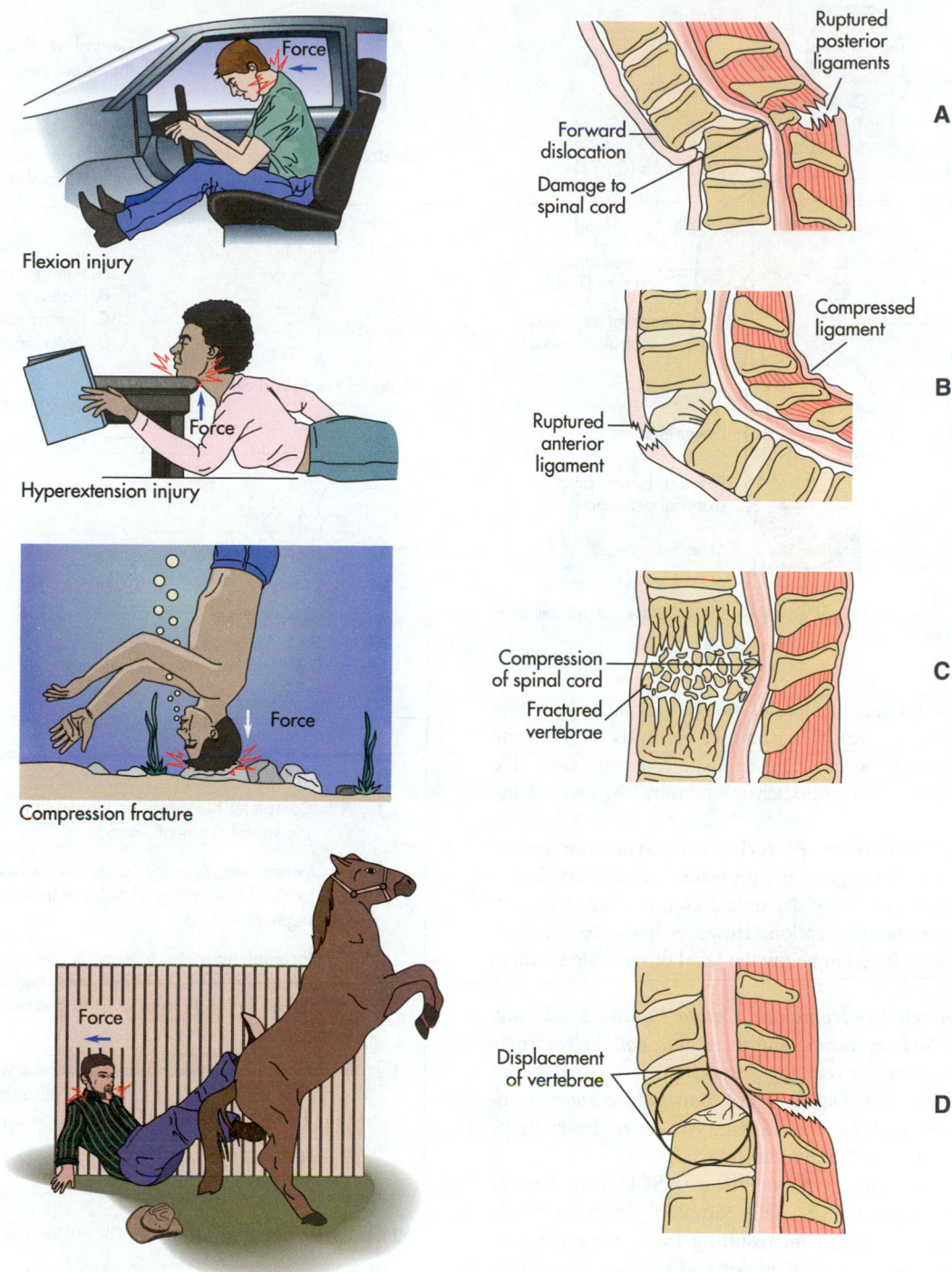

FIG. 61-5   Mechanisms of spinal cord injury. Many situations may produce these injuries. This only shows some examples. **A,** Flexion injury of the cervical spine ruptures the posterior ligaments. **B,** Hyperextension injury of the cervical spine ruptures the anterior ligaments. **C,** Compression fractures crush the vertebrae and force bony fragments into the spinal canal. **D,** Flexion-rotation injury of the cervical spine often results in tearing of ligamentous structures that normally stabilize the spine.

Central Cord Syndrome. Damage to the central spinal cord is termed **central cord syndrome** (Fig. 61-7). It occurs most commonly in the cervical cord region and is more common in older adults. Motor weakness and sensory loss are present in both the upper and lower extremities, but the upper extremities are affected more than the lower ones.

Anterior Cord Syndrome. **Anterior cord syndrome** is caused by damage to the anterior spinal artery. This results in compromised

blood flow to the anterior spinal cord. It typically results from injury causing acute compression of the anterior portion of the spinal cord, often a flexion injury (see Fig. 61-7). Manifestations include motor paralysis and loss of pain and temperature sensation below the level of injury. Because the posterior cord tracts are not injured, sensations of touch, position, vibration, and motion remain intact.

Brown-Séquard Syndrome. **Brown-Séquard syndrome** is a result of damage to one half of the spinal cord (see Fig. 61-7). This

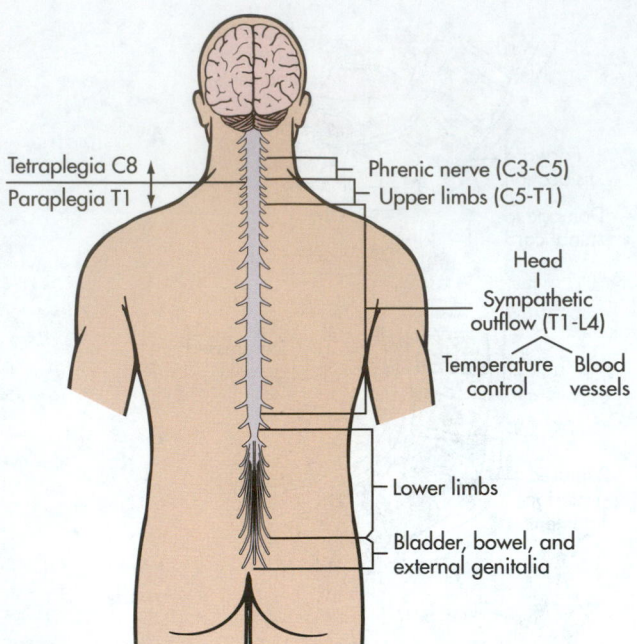

FIG. 61-6 Symptoms, degree of paralysis, and potential for rehabilitation depend on the level of the lesion.

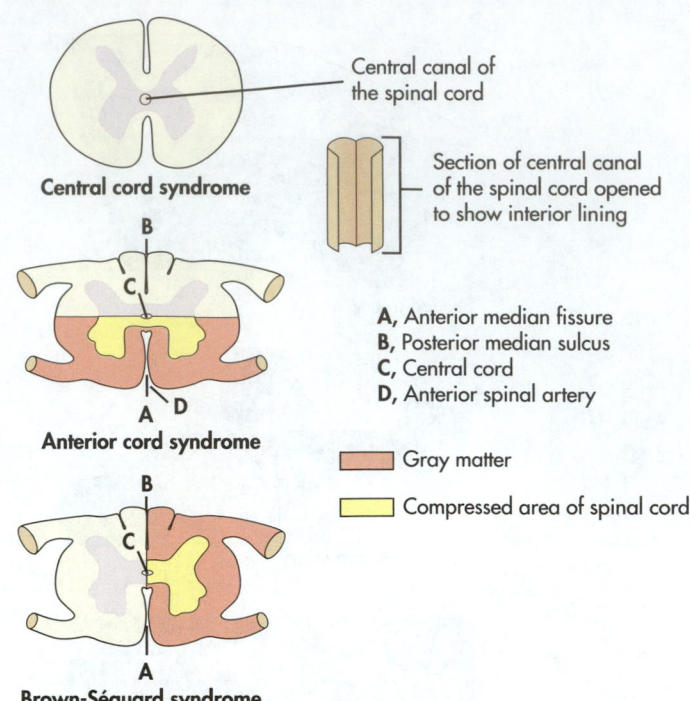

FIG. 61-7 Syndromes associated with incomplete cord lesions.

syndrome is characterized by a loss of motor function and position and vibratory sense, as well as vasomotor paralysis on the same side *(ipsilateral)* as the lesion. The opposite *(contralateral)* side has loss of pain and temperature sensation below the level of the lesion.

Posterior Cord Syndrome. **Posterior cord syndrome** results from compression or damage to the posterior spinal artery. It is a very rare condition. Generally the dorsal columns are damaged, resulting in loss of proprioception. However, pain, temperature sensation, and motor function below the level of the lesion remain intact.

Conus Medullaris Syndrome and Cauda Equina Syndrome. The *conus medullaris syndrome* and the *cauda equina syndrome* result from damage to the very lowest portion of the spinal cord *(conus)* and the lumbar and sacral nerve roots *(cauda equina)*. Injury to these areas produces flaccid paralysis of the lower limbs and areflexic (flaccid) bladder and bowel.

American Spinal Injury Association (ASIA) Impairment Scale. The ASIA Impairment Scale is commonly used for classifying the severity of impairment resulting from spinal cord injury. It combines assessments of motor and sensory function to determine neurologic level and completeness of injury[16] (Figs. 61-8 and 61-9). This scale is useful for recording changes in neurologic status and identifying appropriate functional goals for rehabilitation.

Clinical Manifestations

The manifestations of spinal cord injury are generally the direct result of trauma that causes cord compression, ischemia, edema, and possible cord transection. Manifestations of spinal cord injury are related to the level and degree of injury. The patient with an incomplete lesion may demonstrate a mixture of symptoms. The higher the injury, the more serious the sequelae because of the proximity of the cervical cord to the medulla and brainstem. Movement and rehabilitation potential related to specific locations

American Spinal Injury Association (ASIA) Impairment Scale

☐ **A = Complete:** No motor or sensory function is preserved in the sacral segments S4-S5.

☐ **B = Incomplete:** Sensory but not motor function is preserved below the neurologic level and includes the sacral segments S4-S5.

☐ **C = Incomplete:** Motor function is preserved below the neurologic level, and more than half of key muscles below the neurologic level have a muscle grade less than 3.

☐ **D = Incomplete:** Motor function is preserved below the neurologic level, and at least half of key muscles below the neurologic level have a muscle grade of 3 or more.

☐ **E = Normal:** Motor and sensory function are normal.

FIG. 61-8 The American Spinal Injury Association Impairment Scale.

of the spinal cord injury are described in Table 61-3. In general, sensory function closely parallels motor function at all levels.

Immediate postinjury problems include maintaining a patent airway, adequate ventilation, and adequate circulating blood volume and preventing extension of cord damage (secondary damage).

Respiratory System. Respiratory complications closely correspond to the level of the injury.[15] Cervical injury above the level of C4 presents special problems because of the total loss of respiratory muscle function. Mechanical ventilation is required to keep the patient alive. At one time the majority of these patients died at the scene of the injury, but with improved emergency medical services, more of these patients are surviving the initial events of their spinal cord injury. Injury or fracture below the level of C4 results in diaphragmatic breathing if the phrenic nerve is function-

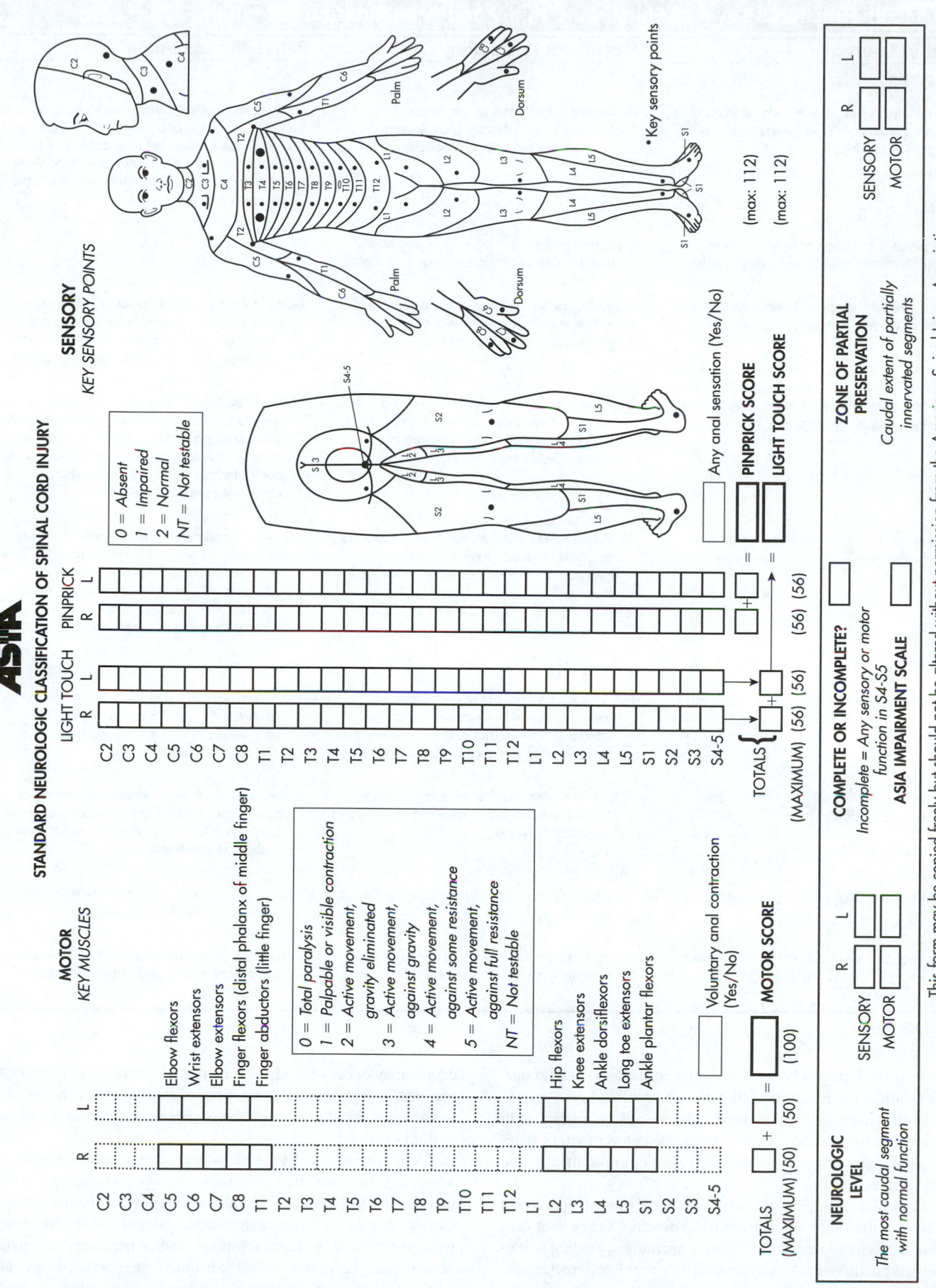

FIG. 61-9   Standard neurologic classification of spinal cord injury.

TABLE 61-3	Functional Level of Spinal Cord Injury and Rehabilitation Potential	
Level of Injury	**Movement Remaining**	**Rehabilitation Potential**
Tetraplegia		
C1-3 Often fatal injury; vagus nerve domination of heart, respiration, blood vessels, and all organs below injury	Movement in neck and above, loss of innervation to diaphragm, absence of independent respiratory function	Ability to drive electric wheelchair equipped with portable ventilator by using chin control or mouth stick, headrest to stabilize head; computer use with mouth stick, head wand, or noise control; 24-hr attendant care, able to instruct others
C4 Vagus nerve domination of heart, respirations, and all vessels and organs below injury	Sensation and movement in neck and above; may be able to breathe without a ventilator	Same as C1-C3
C5 Vagus nerve domination of heart, respirations, and all vessels and organs below injury	Full neck, partial shoulder, back, biceps; gross elbow, inability to roll over or use hands; decreased respiratory reserve	Ability to drive electric wheelchair with mobile hand supports; indoor mobility in manual wheelchair; able to feed self with setup and adaptive equipment; attendant care 10 hr/day
C6 Vagus nerve domination of heart, respirations, and all vessels and organs below injury	Shoulder and upper back abduction and rotation at shoulder, full biceps to elbow flexion, wrist extension, weak grasp of thumb, decreased respiratory reserve	Ability to assist with transfer and perform some self-care; feed self with hand devices; push wheelchair on smooth, flat surface; drive adapted van from wheelchair; independent computer use with adaptive equipment; attendant care 6 hr/day
C7-8 Vagus nerve domination of heart, respirations, and all vessels and organs below injury	All triceps to elbow extension, finger extensors and flexors, good grasp with some decreased strength, decreased respiratory reserve	Ability to transfer self to wheelchair; roll over and sit up in bed; push self on most surfaces; perform most self-care; independent use of wheelchair; ability to drive car with powered hand controls (in some patients); attendant care 0-6 hr/day
Paraplegia		
T1-6 Sympathetic innervation to heart, vagus nerve domination of all vessels and organs below injury	Full innervation of upper extremities; back, essential intrinsic muscles of hand; full strength and dexterity of grasp; decreased trunk stability, decreased respiratory reserve	Full independence in self-care and in wheelchair; ability to drive car with hand controls (in most patients); independent standing in standing frame
T6-12 Vagus nerve domination only of leg vessels, GI and genitourinary organs	Full, stable thoracic muscles and upper back; functional intercostals, resulting in increased respiratory reserve	Full independent use of wheelchair; ability to stand erect with full leg brace, ambulate on crutches with swing (although gait difficult); inability to climb stairs
L1-2 Vagus nerve domination of leg vessels	Varying control of legs and pelvis, instability of lower back	Good sitting balance; full use of wheelchair; ambulation with long leg braces
L3-4 Partial vagus nerve domination of leg vessels, GI and genitourinary organs	Quadriceps and hip flexors, absence of hamstring function, flail ankles	Completely independent ambulation with short leg braces and canes; inability to stand for long periods

GI, Gastrointestinal.

ing. Even if the injury is below C4, spinal cord edema and hemorrhage can affect the function of the phrenic nerve and cause respiratory insufficiency. Hypoventilation almost always occurs with diaphragmatic respirations because of the decrease in vital capacity and tidal volume, which occurs as a result of impairment of the intercostal muscles.

Cervical and thoracic injuries cause paralysis of abdominal muscles and often intercostal muscles. Therefore the patient cannot cough effectively enough to remove secretions, leading to atelectasis and pneumonia. An artificial airway provides direct access for pathogens, making bronchial hygiene and chest physiotherapy extremely important to reduce infection. Neurogenic pulmonary edema may occur secondary to a dramatic increase in sympathetic nervous system activity at the time of injury, which shunts blood to the lungs. In addition, pulmonary edema may occur in response to fluid overload.

Cardiovascular System. Any cord injury above the level of T6 greatly decreases the influence of the sympathetic nervous system. Bradycardia occurs. Peripheral vasodilation results in hypotension. A relative hypovolemia exists because of the increase in venous capacitance. Cardiac monitoring is necessary. In marked bradycardia (heart rate <40 beats/min), appropriate drugs (atropine) to increase the heart rate and prevent hypoxemia are necessary.[15] The peripheral vasodilation reduces the venous return of blood to the heart and subsequently decreases cardiac output, resulting in hypotension. IV fluids or vasopressor drugs may be required to support blood pressure.

Urinary System. Urinary retention is a common development in acute spinal cord injuries and spinal shock. While the patient is in spinal shock, the bladder is atonic and becomes overdistended. An indwelling catheter is inserted to drain the bladder. In the postacute phase the bladder may become hyperirritable, with a loss of inhibition from the brain resulting in reflex emptying. Chronic indwelling catheterization increases the risk of infection. Once the patient is medically stable and large quantities of IV fluids are no longer required, the indwelling catheter should be removed and intermittent catheterization should begin as early as possible. This helps to maintain bladder tone and decrease risk of infection. (Intermittent catheterization is discussed in Chapter 46.)

Gastrointestinal System. If the cord injury has occurred above the level of T5, the primary GI problems are related to hypomotility. Decreased GI motor activity contributes to the development of paralytic ileus and gastric distention. A nasogastric tube for intermittent suctioning may relieve the gastric distention. Metoclopramide (Reglan) may be used to treat delayed gastric emptying. The development of stress ulcers is common because of excessive release of hydrochloric acid in the stomach. Histamine H_2 receptor blockers, such as ranitidine (Zantac) and famotidine (Pepcid), and proton pump inhibitors (e.g., pantoprazole [Protonix IV], omeprazole [Prilosec], lansoprazole [Prevacid]) are frequently used to prevent the occurrence of ulcers during the initial phase. Intraabdominal bleeding may occur and is difficult to diagnose because no subjective signs such as pain, tenderness, and guarding are observed. Continued hypotension in spite of vigorous treatment and decreased hemoglobin and hematocrit may be indications of bleeding. Expanding girth of the abdomen may also be noted.

Less voluntary neurologic control over the bowel results in a *neurogenic bowel*. In the early period after injury when spinal shock is present and for patients with an injury level of T12 or below, the bowel is areflexic and sphincter tone is decreased. As reflexes return, the bowel becomes reflexic, sphincter tone is enhanced, and reflex emptying occurs. Both types of neurogenic bowel can be managed successfully with a regular bowel program coordinated with the gastrocolic reflex to minimize untimely incontinence.

Integumentary System. A major consequence of lack of movement is the potential for skin breakdown over bony prominences in areas of decreased or absent sensation. Pressure ulcers can occur quickly and can lead to major infection or sepsis.

Thermoregulation. Poikilothermism is the adjustment of the body temperature to the room temperature. This occurs in spinal cord injuries because the interruption of the sympathetic nervous system prevents peripheral temperature sensations from reaching the hypothalamus. With spinal cord disruption there is also decreased ability to sweat or shiver below the level of the lesion, which also affects the ability to regulate body temperature. The degree of poikilothermism depends on the level of injury. Patients with high cervical injuries have a greater loss of the ability to regulate temperature than do those with thoracic or lumbar injuries.

Metabolic Needs. Nasogastric suctioning may lead to metabolic alkalosis, and decreased tissue perfusion may lead to acidosis. Electrolyte levels, including sodium and potassium, can be altered by gastric suctioning and must be monitored until suctioning is discontinued and a normal diet is resumed. Loss of body weight (10% or more) is common, with nitrogen excretion mirroring weight loss.[15] Nutritional needs are much greater than what would be expected for an immobilized person. A positive nitrogen balance and a high-protein diet help to prevent skin breakdown and infections and decrease the rate of muscle atrophy.

Peripheral Vascular Problems. Deep vein thrombosis (DVT) is a common problem accompanying spinal cord injury during the first 3 months. It is more difficult to detect a DVT in a person with a spinal cord injury because the usual signs and symptoms, such as pain and tenderness, will not be present.[17] Pulmonary embolism is one of the leading causes of death in patients with spinal cord injury. Techniques for assessment of DVT include Doppler examination, impedance plethysmography, and measurement of leg and thigh girth.

Diagnostic Studies

Complete spine films are performed to assess for vertebral fracture. X-rays visualizing C1 through T1 are done to document the presence of vertebral injury. A CT scan may be used to assess the stability of the injury, location and degree of bony injury, and degree of spinal canal compromise.[15] MRI is used to assess for soft tissue and neural changes and when there is unexplained neurologic deficit or worsening of neurologic status. A comprehensive neurologic examination is performed along with assessment of head, chest, and abdomen for additional injuries or trauma. Patients with cervical injuries who demonstrate altered mental status may also need vertebral angiography to rule out vertebral artery damage.

Collaborative Care

The initial goals for the patient with a spinal cord injury are to sustain life and prevent further cord damage. Table 61-4 outlines the emergency management of the patient with a spinal cord injury. Systemic and neurogenic shock must be treated to maintain blood pressure. For injury at the cervical level, all body systems must be maintained until the full extent of the damage can be evaluated.

Collaborative care during the acute phase for a patient with a cervical injury is described in Table 61-5. The systemic support required by the patient is less intense for spinal cord injuries of the thoracic and lumbar vertebrae. Respiratory compromise is not as severe, and bradycardia is not a problem. Specific problems are treated symptomatically. After stabilization at the injury scene, the person is transferred to a medical facility. A thorough assessment is done to specifically evaluate the degree of deficit and to establish the level and degree of injury. A history is obtained, with emphasis on how the incident occurred and the extent of injury as perceived by the patient immediately after the event. Assessment involves testing muscle groups rather than individual muscles. Muscle groups should be tested with and against gravity, alone and against resistance, and on both sides of the body. Spontaneous movement should be noted. The patient should be asked to move legs and then hands, spread fingers, extend wrists, and shrug shoulders. After assessment of motor status, a sensory examination including touch and pain as tested by pinprick should be carried out, starting at the toes and working upward. If time and conditions permit, position sense and vibration can also be assessed.

The types of injury mechanisms that cause spinal cord trauma, especially those involving the cervical cord, may also result in brain injury. The patient should therefore be assessed for history of unconsciousness, signs of concussion, and increased intracranial pressure (see Chapter 57). In addition, a careful assessment for musculoskeletal injuries and trauma to internal organs should be

TABLE 61-4	*EMERGENCY MANAGEMENT* Spinal Cord Injury	
Etiology	**Assessment Findings**	**Interventions**

Etiology

Blunt

Compression, flexion, extension, or rotational injuries to spinal column
Motor vehicle collisions
Pedestrian incidents
Falls
Diving

Penetrating

Stretched, torn, crushed, or lacerated spinal cord
Gunshot wounds
Stab wounds

Assessment Findings

- Pain, tenderness, deformities, or muscle spasms adjacent to vertebral column
- Numbness, paresthesias
- Alterations in sensation: temperature, light touch, deep pressure, proprioception
- Weakness or heaviness in limbs
- Weakness, paralysis, or flaccidity of muscles
- Spinal shock
- Cuts; bruises; open wounds over head, face, neck, or back
- Neurogenic shock: hypotension; bradycardia; dry, flushed skin
- Bowel and bladder incontinence
- Urinary retention
- Difficulty breathing
- Priapism
- Diminished rectal sphincter tone

Interventions

Initial

- Ensure patent airway.
- Stabilize cervical spine.
- Administer oxygen via nasal cannula or non-rebreather mask.
- Establish IV access with two large-bore catheters to infuse normal saline or lactated Ringer's solution as appropriate.
- Assess for other injuries.
- Control external bleeding.
- Obtain cervical spine x-rays, CT scan, or MRI.
- Prepare for stabilization with cranial tongs and traction.
- Administer high-dose methylprednisolone if ordered.

Ongoing Monitoring

- Monitor vital signs, level of consciousness, oxygen saturation, cardiac rhythm, urine output.
- Keep warm.
- Monitor for urinary retention, hypertension.
- Anticipate need for intubation if gag reflex absent.

CT, Computed tomography; *IV,* intravenous; *MRI,* magnetic resonance imaging.

---

performed. Because there are no muscle, bone, or visceral sensations, the only clue to internal trauma with hemorrhage may be a rapidly falling hematocrit level. Urinary output is examined for hematuria, which is also indicative of internal injuries.

The patient must be moved in alignment as a unit or "logrolled" during transfers and when repositioning to prevent further injury. Respiratory, cardiac, urinary, and GI functions should be monitored closely. The patient may go directly to surgery following initial immobilization and stabilization or to the intensive care unit (ICU) for monitoring and management.

Nonoperative Stabilization. Nonoperative treatments are focused on stabilization of the injured spinal segment and decompression, either through traction or realignment. Stabilization methods eliminate damaging motion at the injury site. They are intended to prevent secondary spinal cord damage caused by repeated contusion or compression.[15]

Surgical Therapy. The decision to perform surgery on a patient with a spinal cord injury often depends on the preference of a particular physician. When cord compression is certain or the neurologic disorder progresses, benefit may be seen following immediate surgery. Surgery stabilizes the spinal column. There is some evidence to suggest that early cord decompression results in reduced secondary injury to the spinal cord and therefore improved outcomes.[18] Other criteria used in the decision for early surgery include (1) evidence of cord compression, (2) progressive neurologic deficit, (3) compound fracture of the vertebrae, (4) bony fragments (may dislodge and penetrate the cord), and (5) penetrating wounds of the spinal cord or surrounding structures.

The more common surgical procedures include decompression laminectomy by anterior cervical and thoracic approaches with fusion, posterior laminectomy with the use of acrylic wire mesh and fusion, and insertion of stabilizing rods (e.g., Harrington rods for the correction and stabilization of thoracic deformities). (Specific surgical and nursing interventions for these techniques are discussed in Chapter 63.)

Drug Therapy. The National Acute Spinal Cord Injury Study II (NASCIS II, 1990) and NASCIS III (1997) reported that methylprednisolone (MP), when administered early and in a large dose, resulted in greater recovery of neurologic function.[19] Based on these studies, MP was adopted as a standard of care for acute spinal cord injury management. However, further studies showed that deleterious effects could result from the use of MP, including higher risk of complications, higher acute care costs, and longer hospital stays.

Currently MP (Solu-Medrol) is considered a treatment option.[20] The physician needs to consider whether the potential benefits outweigh the risks. If ordered, MP is to be given within 8 hours of injury. When the loading dose of 30 mg/kg is given within 3 hours of injury, this is followed by 24 hours of 5.4 mg/kg/hr IV drip. If this loading dose is given between 3 and 8 hours postinjury, the IV drip is maintained for 48 hours. There is no reported benefit from MP if it is given more than 8 hours postinjury.[21] MP, a blocker of lipid peroxidation by-products, is thought to improve blood flow and reduce edema in the spinal cord. Side effects of MP include immunosuppression, increased frequency of upper GI bleeding, and increased risk of infection. Other neuroprotective drugs are being tested, and more treatment options may be available soon.[22]

Vasopressor agents such as dopamine (Intropin) are used in the acute phase as adjuvants to treatment. These agents are used to maintain the mean arterial pressure at a level greater than 80 to 90 mm Hg so that perfusion to the spinal cord is improved.

Pharmacologic properties and drug metabolism are altered in spinal cord injury. Therefore drug interactions may occur. The differences in drug metabolism correlate with level and completeness of injury, with greater change apparent in people with cervical injury than in those with injury of lower spinal levels.[23]

TABLE 61-5	COLLABORATIVE CARE

Cervical Cord Injury

Diagnostic
History and physical examination, including complete neurologic examination
ABGs
Serial bedside PFTs
Electrolytes, glucose level, coagulation profile, hemoglobin and hematocrit levels
Urinalysis
Anteroposterior, lateral, and odontoid spinal x-ray studies
CT scan, MRI
X-rays of spine
Myelography
EMG to measure evoked potentials
Venous duplex studies

Collaborative Therapy
Acute Care
Immobilization of vertebral column by skeletal traction
Maintenance of heart rate (e.g., atropine) and blood pressure (e.g., dopamine [Intropin])
Methylprednisolone high-dose therapy (if ordered)
Insertion of nasogastric tube and attachment to suction
Intubation (if indicated by ABGs and PFTs)
O_2 by high-humidity mask
Indwelling urinary catheter
Administration of IV fluids
Stress ulcer prophylaxis
Deep vein thrombosis prophylaxis
Bowel and bladder training

Rehabilitation and Home Care
Physical therapy
 • Range-of-motion exercises
 • Mobility training
 • Muscle strengthening
Occupational therapy (splints, activities of daily living training)
Bowel and bladder training
Autonomic dysreflexia prevention
Pressure ulcer prevention
Recreational therapy
Patient and family education

ABGs, Arterial blood gases; *CT,* computed tomography; *EMG,* electromyography; *IV,* intravenous; *MRI,* magnetic resonance imaging; *PFTs,* pulmonary function tests.

TABLE 61-6	NURSING ASSESSMENT

Spinal Cord Injury

Subjective Data
Important Health Information
Past health history: Motor vehicle crash, sports injury, industrial incident, gunshot or stabbing injury, falls

Functional Health Patterns
Health perception–health management: Use of alcohol or recreational drugs; risk-taking behaviors
Activity-exercise: Loss of strength, movement, and sensation below level of injury; dyspnea, inability to breathe adequately ("air hunger")
Cognitive-perceptual: Presence of tenderness, pain at or above level of injury; numbness, tingling, burning, twitching of extremities
Coping–stress tolerance: Fear, denial, anger, depression

Objective Data
General
Poikilothermism (unable to regulate body heat)

Integumentary
Warm, dry skin below level of injury (neurogenic shock)

Respiratory
Lesions at C1-C3: apnea, inability to cough; lesions at C4: poor cough, diaphragmatic breathing, hypoventilation; lesions at C5-T6: decreased respiratory reserve

Cardiovascular
Lesions above T5: bradycardia, hypotension, postural hypotension, absence of vasomotor tone

Gastrointestinal
↓ or absent bowel sounds (paralytic ileus in lesions above T5), abdominal distention, constipation, fecal incontinence, fecal impaction

Urinary
Retention (for lesions between T1 and L2); flaccid bladder (acute stages); spasticity with reflex bladder emptying (later stages)

Reproductive
Priapism, loss of sexual function

Neurologic
Complete: Flaccid paralysis and anesthesia below level of injury resulting in tetraplegia (for lesions above C8) or paraplegia (for lesions below C8), hyperactive deep tendon reflexes, bilaterally positive Babinski test (after resolution of spinal shock)
Incomplete: Mixed loss of voluntary motor activity and sensation

Musculoskeletal
Muscle atony (in flaccid state), contractures (in spastic state)

Possible Findings
Location of level and type of bony involvement on spinal x-ray: lesion, edema, compression on CT scan and MRI; positive finding on myelogram

CT, Computed tomography; *MRI,* magnetic resonance imaging.

Pharmacologic agents are used to treat specific autonomic dysfunctions such as GI hypoactivity, bradycardia, orthostatic hypotension, inadequate emptying of the bladder, and autonomic dysreflexia. The nurse must know the intended effects of such agents, observe responses, and provide specific interventions when adverse reactions are seen.

NURSING MANAGEMENT
SPINAL CORD INJURY

■ Nursing Assessment

Subjective and objective data that should be obtained from a patient with a recent spinal cord injury are presented in Table 61-6.

■ Nursing Diagnoses

Nursing diagnoses for the patient with a spinal cord injury depend on the severity of the injury and the level of dysfunction. The nursing diagnoses for a patient with a spinal cord injury may include, but are not limited to, those presented in NCP 61-1. The care plan presented is for a patient with a complete cervical cord injury.

■ Planning

The overall goals are that the patient with a spinal cord injury will (1) maintain an optimal level of neurologic functioning; (2) have minimal or no complications of immobility; (3) learn new skills, gain new knowledge, and acquire new behaviors to be able to care for self or successfully direct others to do so; and (4) return to home and the community at an optimal level of functioning.

■ Nursing Implementation

Health Promotion. Nursing interventions for injury prevention include identification of high-risk populations, counseling, and education. Support of legislation related to seat belt use in cars, helmets for motorcyclists and bicyclists, child safety seats, and

NURSING CARE PLAN 61-1

Patient with a Spinal Cord Injury

NURSING DIAGNOSIS   **Impaired gas exchange** *related to* intercostal muscle and diaphragmatic fatigue or paralysis and retained secretions *as evidenced by* decreased PaO_2, increased $PaCO_2$, decreased tidal volume, fatigue, diminished breath sounds

PATIENT GOALS
1. Maintains adequate gas exchange
2. Demonstrates no signs of respiratory distress

OUTCOMES (NOC)	INTERVENTIONS (NIC) and *RATIONALES*
Respiratory Status: Gas Exchange	**Respiratory Monitoring**
• Cognitive status _____	• Monitor rate, rhythm, depth, and effort of respirations *to note baseline and changes in status.*
• PaO_2 _____	• Monitor for diaphragmatic muscle fatigue (paradoxical motion).
• $PaCO_2$ _____	• Auscultate breath sounds, noting areas of decreased/absent ventilation and presence of adventitious sounds.
• Oxygen saturation __	• Note changes in SaO_2, SvO_2, end-tidal CO_2, and ABG values.
Respiratory Status: Ventilation	• Monitor PFT values, particularly vital capacity, maximal inspiratory force, and forced expiratory volume, *to identify hypoventilation requiring mechanical ventilation.*
• Respiratory rate _____	• Monitor patient's ability to cough effectively *to identify need for suctioning.*
• Tidal volume _____	**Airway Management**
• Auscultated breath sounds _____	• Identify patient requiring actual/potential airway insertion *to ensure timely intervention.*
Measurement Scale	• Perform endotracheal or nasotracheal suctioning *to stimulate coughing and to clear respiratory secretions.*
1 = Severely compromised	
2 = Substantially compromised	
3 = Moderately compromised	
4 = Mildly compromised	
5 = Not compromised	

NURSING DIAGNOSIS   **Impaired skin integrity** *related to* skull tong placement, immobility, and poor tissue perfusion *as evidenced by* reddened skin over bony prominences and open tong sites

PATIENT GOALS
1. Demonstrates no signs of infection at skull tong sites
2. Maintains intact skin over bony prominences

OUTCOMES (NOC)	INTERVENTIONS (NIC) and *RATIONALES*
Tissue Integrity: Skin and Mucous Membranes	**Infection Protection**
	• Inspect condition of any surgical incision/wound *to detect early signs of infection.*
• Skin lesions _____	**Infection Control**
• Erythema _____	• Ensure appropriate wound care technique *to prevent bacterial colonization at tong sites.*
• Necrosis _____	**Pressure Management**
• Induration and blanching _____	• Monitor skin for areas of redness and breakdown *so that interventions can be initiated promptly if a problem develops.*
Measurement Scale	• Facilitate small shifts of body weight *to relieve pressure without disrupting traction.*
1 = Severe	• Monitor the patient's nutritional status *to maintain healthy skin resistant to breakdown.*
2 = Substantial	
3 = Moderate	
4 = Mild	
5 = None	

ABG, Arterial blood gases; *$PaCO_2$,* partial pressure of carbon dioxide in arterial blood; *PaO_2,* partial pressure of oxygen in arterial blood; *PFT,* pulmonary function tests; *SaO_2,* arterial oxygen saturation; *SvO_2,* venous oxygen saturation.

tougher penalties for drunk-driving offenses is a professional responsibility.

It is important that the nurse emphasize the importance of other health promotion and health screening in addition to spinal cord injury care. After injury, health-promoting behaviors can have a significant impact on the health and well-being of the individual with a spinal cord injury. Nursing interventions include education, counseling, and referral to programs such as smoking cessation classes, recreation and exercise programs, and alcohol treatment programs, and maintaining routine physical examinations for non-neurologic problems. Outpatient health care requires that screening and prevention programs be accessible to people with spinal cord injury. Nurses in these settings should facilitate wheelchair-accessible examination rooms, adjustable-height examination tables, and scheduling that allows extra time if needed.

Acute Intervention. High cervical injury caused by flexion-rotation is the most complex spinal cord injury and is discussed in this section. Interventions for this type of injury can be modified for patients with less severe problems.

Immobilization. Proper immobilization of the neck involves the maintenance of a neutral position. A blanket or towel roll, a hard cervical collar, and a backboard can be used to stabilize the neck to prevent lateral rotation of the cervical spine. The body should always be correctly aligned, and turning should be performed so that the patient is moved as a unit (e.g., logrolling) to prevent movement of the spine. For cervical injuries, skeletal trac-

NURSING CARE PLAN 61-1

Patient with a Spinal Cord Injury—cont'd

NURSING DIAGNOSIS **Constipation** *related to* neurogenic bowel, inadequate fluid intake, diet low in roughage, and immobility *as evidenced by* lack of bowel movement for more than 2 days, decreased bowel sounds, palpable impaction, hard stool, or stool incontinence

PATIENT GOALS 1. Establishes a bowel management program based on neurologic function and personal preference
2. Maintains a bowel movement every other day

OUTCOMES (NOC)	**INTERVENTIONS (NIC) and *RATIONALES***
Bowel Elimination	***Bowel Management***

OUTCOMES (NOC)

Bowel Elimination

- Elimination pattern _____
- Control of bowel movements _____
- Stool soft and formed _____
- Ease of stool passage _____
- Muscle tone to evacuate stool _____

Measurement Scale

1 = Severely compromised
2 = Substantially compromised
3 = Moderately compromised
4 = Mildly compromised
5 = Not compromised

INTERVENTIONS (NIC) and *RATIONALES*

Bowel Management

- Monitor bowel movements, including frequency, consistency, shape, volume, and color, *to establish baseline function.*
- Monitor bowel sounds *to determine if peristalsis is present.*
- Instruct patient on foods high in fiber *because bulk and fiber are necessary to the success of a bowel program.*
- Initiate a bowel training program *to establish a bowel routine as quickly as possible.*

NURSING DIAGNOSIS **Impaired urinary elimination** *related to* spinal injury and limited fluid intake *as evidenced by* urinary retention, bladder distention, involuntary emptying of bladder (after spinal shock)

PATIENT GOAL Establishes a bladder management program based on neurologic function, caregiver status, and lifestyle choices

OUTCOMES (NOC)

Urinary Elimination

- Urinary retention _____
- Urinary incontinence _____

Measurement Scale

1 = Severe
2 = Substantial
3 = Moderate
4 = Mild
5 = None

INTERVENTIONS (NIC) and *RATIONALES*

Urinary Retention Care

- Monitor intake and output *to evaluate fluid balance.*
- Monitor degree of bladder distention by palpation and percussion *because loss of autonomic and reflex control of bladder and sphincter can cause distention.*
- Insert urinary catheter *to relieve urinary retention in spinal shock.*
- Implement intermittent catheterization *in postacute phase of spinal cord injury to maintain bladder tone and avoid infection associated with long-term use of indwelling catheter.*
- Refer to urinary continence specialists *to establish long-term bladder management program.*

NURSING DIAGNOSIS **Ineffective protection** *related to* spinal cord injury, vertebral column instability, or forced immobilization by traction *as evidenced by* inability to move purposefully, limited muscle strength, impaired perception of position or presence of body parts

PATIENT GOAL Develops no complications of immobility

OUTCOMES (NOC)

Immobility Consequences: Physiologic

- Contracted joints _____
- Urinary calculi _____
- Venous thrombosis _____
- Lung congestion _____
- Stool impaction _____
- Hypoactive bowel _____
- Urinary tract infection _____

Measurement Scale

1 = Severe
2 = Substantial
3 = Moderate
4 = Mild
5 = None

INTERVENTIONS (NIC) and *RATIONALES*

Bed Rest Care

- Place on an appropriate therapeutic mattress/bed *to allow for frequent turning without disrupting cervical traction and spinal alignment.*
- Apply appliances to prevent footdrop.
- Turn the immobilized patient at least every 2 hours, according to specific schedule, with use of turning frames or beds *to prevent prolonged pressure.*
- Perform passive and/or active range-of-motion exercises *to promote circulation, prevent thrombosis, and prevent contractures.*
- Apply pneumatic compression devices and/or antiembolism stockings *to promote circulation and prevent thrombosis.*
- Monitor pulmonary status *because pulmonary complications are a common sequela of immobility.*
- Monitor for urinary function *because bed rest contributes to urinary stasis and calculi formation.*

Continued

Nervous System

NURSING CARE PLAN 61-1

Patient with a Spinal Cord Injury—cont'd

NURSING DIAGNOSIS **Risk for autonomic dysreflexia** *related to* reflex stimulation of sympathetic nervous system after spinal shock resolves

PATIENT GOALS 1. Experiences no episodes of dysreflexia
2. Describes causes, prevention, symptoms, and management of dysreflexia

OUTCOMES (NOC)

Neurologic Status: Autonomic

- Apical heart rate _____
- Systolic blood pressure _____
- Diastolic blood pressure _____
- Bowel elimination pattern _____
- Urinary elimination pattern _____
- Thermoregulation _____

Measurement Scale

1 = Severely compromised
2 = Substantially compromised
3 = Moderately compromised
4 = Mildly compromised
5 = Not compromised

- Headaches _____
- Dysreflexia _____

Measurement Scale

1 = Severe
2 = Substantial
3 = Moderate
4 = Mild
5 = None

INTERVENTIONS (NIC) and *RATIONALES*

Dysreflexia Management

- Identify and minimize stimuli that may precipitate dysreflexia: bladder distention, renal calculi, infection, fecal impaction, rectal examination, suppository insertion, skin breakdown, and constrictive clothing or bed linen.
- Monitor for signs and symptoms of autonomic dysreflexia: paroxysmal hypertension, bradycardia, tachycardia, diaphoresis above the level of injury, facial flushing, pallor below the level of injury, headache, nasal congestion, engorgement of temporal and neck vessels, conjunctival congestion, chills without fever, pilomotor erection, and chest pain.
- Investigate and treat or remove offending cause (e.g., distended bladder, fecal impaction, skin lesions, and constricting bed clothes).
- Place head of bed in upright position if hyperreflexia occurs *to reduce blood pressure by allowing blood to pool in the lower extremities.*
- Stay with patient and monitor status every 3 to 5 minutes if hyperreflexia occurs.
- Administer antihypertensive agents intravenously as ordered *to reduce blood pressure.*
- Instruct patient and family about causes, symptoms, treatment, and prevention of dysreflexia *to reverse occurrence and prevent occurrence of status epilepticus, stroke, and possible death.*

NURSING DIAGNOSIS **Ineffective coping** *related to* loss of control over bodily functions and altered lifestyle secondary to paralysis *as evidenced by* verbalization of inability to cope, expression of anger or other negative feelings, refusal to discuss changes in function and participate in social contacts

PATIENT GOALS 1. Reports ability to cope with effects of spinal cord injury
2. Expresses feelings of grief in adapting to losses related to chronic condition

OUTCOMES (NOC)

Coping

- Identifies effective coping patterns _____
- Identifies ineffective coping patterns _____
- Verbalizes sense of control _____
- Verbalizes acceptance of situation _____
- Seeks information concerning illness and treatment _____
- Modifies lifestyle as needed _____
- Uses available social support _____
- Reports decrease in negative feelings _____

Measurement Scale

1 = Never demonstrated
2 = Rarely demonstrated
3 = Sometimes demonstrated
4 = Often demonstrated
5 = Consistently demonstrated

INTERVENTIONS (NIC) and *RATIONALES*

Coping Enhancement

- Appraise patient's adjustment to changes in body image.
- Appraise impact of patient's life situation on roles and relationships.
- Provide an atmosphere of acceptance.
- Encourage verbalization of feelings, perceptions, and fears *to aid patient in clarifying feelings.*
- Provide factual information concerning diagnosis, treatment, and prognosis *because knowledge of expectations can help patient cope with the future.*
- Provide patient with realistic choices about certain aspects of care.
- Support use of appropriate defense mechanisms.
- Assist patient to identify positive strategies to deal with limitations and manage needed lifestyle or role changes *to prevent patient from practicing ineffective behaviors such as smoking, drinking, or angry outbursts.*
- Encourage family involvement *to enhance patient's sense of worth and value as a person.*
- Assist patient to grieve and work through the losses of chronic illness and/or disability *because spinal cord injury results in a real loss, which requires adjustment through grieving.*

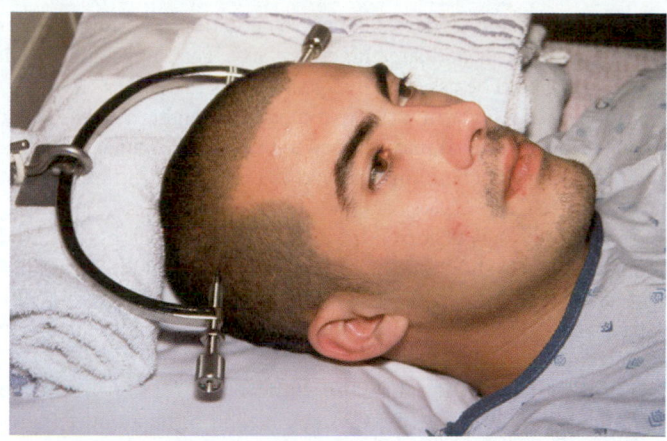

FIG. 61-10 Cervical traction is attached to tongs inserted in the skull.

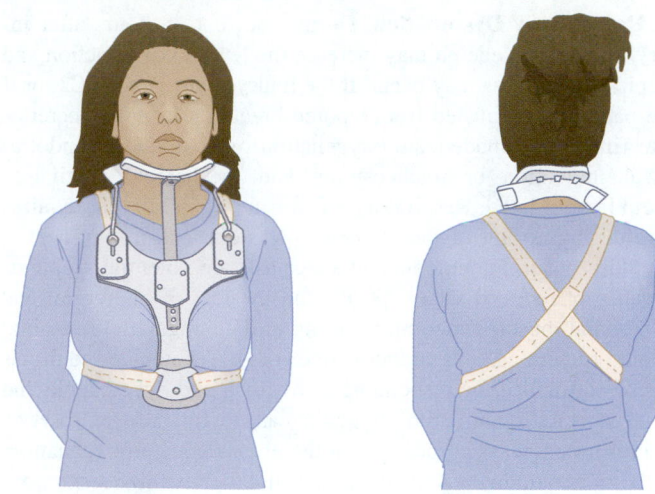

FIG. 61-11 Sternal-occipital-mandibular immobilizer (SOMI) brace.

tion is used less frequently with the development of better surgical stabilization. When skeletal traction is used, realignment or reduction of the injury is targeted. Crutchfield (Fig. 61-10), Vinke, or Gardner-Wells tongs or other types of devices are used to provide this type of traction. Traction is provided by a rope that is extended from the center of the tongs over a pulley and has weights attached at the end. Traction must be maintained at all times. Depending on the type of injury and the goal of treatment, the tongs and traction may be removed 1 to 4 weeks after the injury. One disadvantage of skull tongs is that the skull pins can be displaced. If this occurs, the head should be held in a neutral position and help should be summoned. The nurse should stabilize the head while the physician reinserts the tongs.

Infection at the sites of tong insertion is another potential problem. Preventive care includes cleansing the sites twice a day with normal saline solution and applying an antibiotic ointment, which acts as a mechanical barrier to the entrance of bacteria. The preventive care of insertion sites may vary depending on individual hospital standards of care.

Special beds are often used in the management of the patient with a spinal cord injury. Kinetic therapy uses a continual side-to-side slow rotation laterally with the patient in constant motion. The bed allows a frequency of turns greater than 200 times per day. The bed is used to decrease the likelihood of pressure sores and cardiopulmonary complications. However, in some patients the turning can induce motion sickness and fear of falling out of bed when turned to the extremes. (Motion sickness is unlikely when automatic rather than manual turning is used.)

After cervical fusion or other stabilization surgery, a hard cervical collar or sternal-occipital-mandibular immobilizer brace can be worn until the fusion becomes solid[24] (Fig. 61-11).

In a stable injury for which surgery is not done, a halo fixation apparatus may be applied. The halo is the most frequently used method of stabilizing cervical injuries. The halo apparatus can be used to apply cervical traction by means of a jacket-like arrangement (Fig. 61-12). Hanging weights, such as those used with tongs, can be incorporated with the halo. In addition, the apparatus can be attached to a body vest, stabilizing the injured area and allowing ambulation if the patient is neurologically intact. Another alternative is to use the halo after the patient has had traction removed. It allows the patient to be more mobile and to begin active rehabilitation.

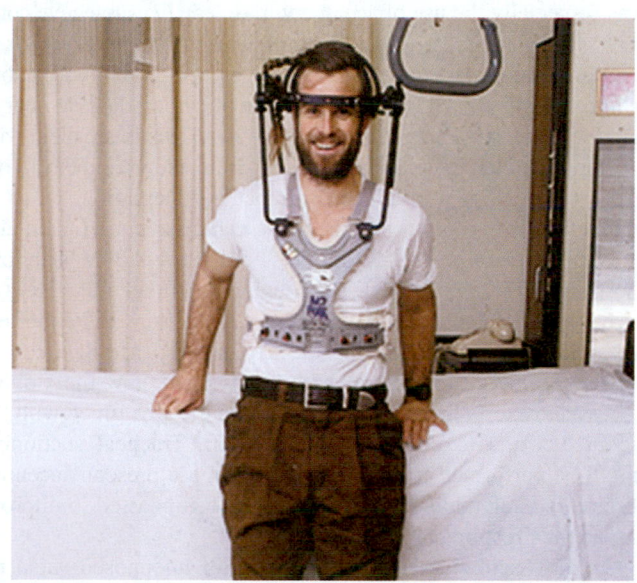

FIG. 61-12 Halo vest, Ace manufacturing design. Note the rigid shoulder straps and encompassing vest. Various vest sizes are available prefabricated. The halo ring, superstructure, and vest are MRI compatible.

Patients with thoracic or lumbar spine injuries are immobilized with a custom thoracolumbar orthosis ("body jacket"), which inhibits spinal flexion, extension, and rotation, or with a Jewett brace, which restricts forward flexion.

Immobilization of the neck of the patient with a spinal cord injury prevents further injury, but the effects of immobility are profound. Meticulous skin care is critical because decreased sensation and circulation make the patient particularly susceptible to skin breakdown. Patients should be removed from backboards as soon as possible, and cervical collars should be properly fitted or replaced with other forms of immobilization to prevent coccygeal and occipital area skin breakdown. It is important that areas under the halo vest or jacket or under braces or orthoses be inspected to assess skin condition.

Respiratory Dysfunction. During the first 48 hours after injury, spinal cord edema may increase the level of dysfunction and respiratory distress may occur. If the injury is at or above C3, or if the patient is exhausted from labored breathing or ABGs deteriorate (indicating inadequate oxygenation or ventilation), endotracheal intubation or tracheostomy and mechanical ventilation should be initiated. Respiratory arrest is a possibility that requires careful monitoring of the respiratory system and prompt action, should it occur. Pneumonia and atelectasis are potential problems because of reduced vital capacity and the loss of intercostal and abdominal muscle function, resulting in diaphragmatic breathing, pooled secretions, and an ineffective cough.[25] The older adult has a more difficult time responding to hypoxia and hypercapnia and is extremely intolerant of hypoxia caused by lack of reserve. Therefore aggressive chest physiotherapy, adequate oxygenation, and proper pain management are essential to maximize respiratory function and gas exchange. Other problems include nasal stuffiness and bronchospasms.

The nurse needs to regularly assess (1) breath sounds, (2) ABGs, (3) tidal volume, (4) vital capacity, (5) skin color, (6) breathing patterns (especially the use of accessory muscles), (7) subjective comments about the ability to breathe, and (8) the amount and color of sputum. A PaO_2 (partial pressure of oxygen in arterial blood) above 60 mm Hg and a $PaCO_2$ (partial pressure of carbon dioxide in arterial blood) below 45 mm Hg are acceptable values in a patient with uncomplicated tetraplegia. A patient who is unable to count to 10 out loud without taking a breath needs immediate attention.

In addition to monitoring, the nurse can intervene in maintaining ventilation. Oxygen is administered until ABGs stabilize. Chest physiotherapy and assisted coughing facilitate the raising of secretions. Assisted coughing simulates the action of the ineffective abdominal muscles during the expiratory phase of a cough. The nurse places the heels of both hands just below the xiphoid process and exerts firm upward pressure to the area timed with the patient's efforts to cough (see Fig. 68-6). Tracheal suctioning should be performed if crackles or rhonchi are present. Incentive spirometry is an additional technique that can be used to improve the patient's respiratory status.

Cardiovascular Instability. Because of unopposed vagal response, the heart rate is slowed, often to below 60 beats/min. Any increase in vagal stimulation, such as turning or suctioning, can result in cardiac arrest. Loss of sympathetic tone in peripheral vessels results in chronic low blood pressure with potential postural hypotension. Lack of muscle tone to aid venous return can result in sluggish blood flow and predispose the patient to DVT.

Vital signs should be assessed frequently. If bradycardia is symptomatic, an anticholinergic drug such as atropine is administered. A temporary or permanent pacemaker may be inserted in some instances. Hypotension is managed with a vasopressor agent, such as dopamine or norepinephrine, and fluid replacement.

In the older adult, the prevalence of cardiovascular disease must be considered. The cardiovascular system becomes less able to handle the stress of traumatic injury because heart contractions weaken, and cardiac output is reduced. Maximum heart rate is also reduced.

Compression gradient stockings can be used to prevent thromboemboli and to promote venous return. The stockings must be removed every 8 hours for skin care. The use of pneumatic compression devices for the calves is advocated, and they must be applied as soon as possible after admission and maintained throughout the hospitalization. Venous duplex studies may be performed before applying compression devices. The nurse should also perform range-of-motion exercises and stretching regularly. The thighs and calves of the legs should be assessed every shift for signs of DVT.

Prophylactic heparin or low-molecular-weight heparin (e.g., enoxaparin [Lovenox]) may be used to prevent DVT unless contraindicated. Contraindications include internal bleeding and recent surgery.

If blood loss has occurred from other injuries, hemoglobin and hematocrit levels should be monitored and blood should be administered according to protocol. The nurse also should monitor the patient for indications of hypovolemic shock secondary to hemorrhage.

Fluid and Nutritional Maintenance. During the first 48 to 72 hours after the injury, the GI tract may stop functioning (paralytic ileus) and a nasogastric tube must be inserted. Because the patient cannot have oral intake, fluid and electrolyte needs must be carefully monitored. Specific solutions and additives are ordered based on individual requirements. Once bowel sounds are present or flatus is passed, oral food and fluids can gradually be introduced. Because of severe catabolism, a high-protein, high-calorie diet is necessary for energy and tissue repair. In patients with high cervical cord injuries, swallowing must be evaluated before starting oral feedings. If the patient is unable to resume eating, total parenteral nutrition may be started to provide nutritional support.

Some patients experience anorexia, which can be due to psychologic depression, boredom with institutional food, or discomfort at being fed (often by a hurried nurse). Some patients have a normally small appetite. Occasionally, refusal to eat is used as a means of maintaining control over the environment because of diminished or absent body control. If the patient is not eating adequately, the cause should be thoroughly assessed. On the basis of this assessment, a contract may be made with the patient using mutual goal setting regarding the diet. This gives the patient increased control of the situation and often results in improved nutritional intake. General measures such as providing a pleasant eating environment, allowing adequate time to eat (including any self-feeding the patient can achieve), encouraging the family to bring in special foods, and planning social rewards for eating may be useful. A calorie count should be kept, and the patient's daily weight recorded as a means of evaluating progress. If feasible, the patient should participate in recording calorie intake. Dietary supplements may be necessary to meet nutritional needs. Increased dietary fiber should be included to promote bowel function. The nurse should avoid allowing the patient's nutritional intake to become a basis for a power struggle.

Bladder and Bowel Management. Immediately after injury, urine is retained because of the loss of autonomic and reflex control of the bladder and sphincter. Because there is no sensation of fullness, overdistention of the bladder can result in reflux into the kidney with eventual renal failure. Bladder overdistention may even result in rupture of the bladder. Consequently, an indwelling catheter is usually inserted as soon as possible after injury. Its patency must be ensured by frequent inspection and irrigation if necessary. In some institutions a physician's order is required for this procedure. Strict aseptic technique for catheter care is essential to avoid introducing infection.

After the patient is stabilized, the best means of managing long-term urinary function is assessed. Usually the patient is started on an intermittent catheterization program. The patient is often maintained on a fluid restriction of 1800 to 2000 ml/day to facilitate a bladder training program. Urinary output is monitored closely.

UTIs are a common problem. The best method for preventing UTIs is regular and complete bladder drainage. During the period of indwelling catheterization, a large fluid intake is required. The catheter should be checked frequently to prevent kinking and ensure free flow of urine. During intermittent catheterization, fluid intake should be moderate and regular (200 to 300 ml every 2 to 3 hours). Catheterization should be done every 3 to 4 hours to prevent bacterial overgrowth resulting from urinary stasis. Cranberry juice and/or cranberry extract tablets may be helpful for UTI prevention because there is some evidence that they may prevent bacteria from adhering to the bladder wall. If the appearance or odor of the urine is suspicious or if the patient develops symptoms of a UTI (e.g., chills, fever, malaise), a specimen is sent for culture.

Age-related changes in renal function should be considered. The older adult is more likely to develop renal calculi, and older men may have prostatic hyperplasia, which may interfere with urinary flow and complicate management of urinary problems.

Constipation is generally a problem during spinal shock because no voluntary or involuntary (reflex) evacuation of the bowels occurs. A bowel program should be started during acute care. This consists of choosing a rectal stimulant (suppository or mini-enema) to be inserted daily at a regular time of day followed by gentle digital stimulation or manual evacuation done by the nurse until evacuation is complete. Initially the program may be done in bed in the side-lying position, but as soon as the patient has resumed sitting, it should be done in the upright position on a padded bedside commode chair.

Temperature Control. Because there is no vasoconstriction, piloerection, or heat loss through perspiration below the level of injury, temperature control is largely external to the patient. Therefore the nurse must monitor the environment closely to maintain an appropriate temperature. Body temperature should be monitored regularly. The patient should not be overloaded with covers or unduly exposed (such as during bathing). If an infection with high fever develops, more extensive means of temperature control, such as a cooling blanket, may be necessary.

Stress Ulcers. Stress ulcers are a problem for the patient with a spinal cord injury because of the physiologic response to severe trauma, psychologic stress, and high-dose corticosteroids. Peak incidence of stress ulcers is 6 to 14 days after injury. Stool and gastric contents are tested daily for blood, and the hematocrit is observed for a slow drop. When corticosteroids are given, they should be accompanied by antacids or food. Histamine H_2-receptor blockers, such as ranitidine (Zantac) and famotidine (Pepcid), or proton pump inhibitors, such as pantoprazole sodium (Protonix I.V.) or omeprazole (Prilosec), may be given prophylactically to decrease the secretion of hydrochloric acid.

Sensory Deprivation. The nurse must compensate for the patient's absent sensations to prevent sensory deprivation. This is done by stimulating the patient above the level of injury. Conversation, music, strong aromas, and interesting flavors should be a part of the nursing care plan. Prism glasses are provided so that the patient can read and watch television. Every effort should be made to prevent the patient from withdrawing from the environment.

Patients with spinal cord injury often report altered sensorium and vivid dreams during the acute phase of their treatment. Whether this is due to drugs used to manage pain and anxiety is not known. Patients may also experience disrupted sleep patterns as a result of the hospital environment or posttraumatic stress disorder.

Reflexes. Once spinal cord shock is resolved, the return of reflexes may complicate rehabilitation. Lacking control from the higher brain centers, reflexes are often hyperactive and produce exaggerated responses. Penile erections can occur from a variety of stimuli, causing embarrassment and discomfort. Spasms ranging from mild twitches to convulsive movements below the level of the lesion may also occur. This reflex activity may be interpreted by the patient or family as a return of function, and the nurse must tactfully explain the reason for the activity. The patient may be informed of the positive use of these reflexes in sexual, bowel, and bladder retraining. Spasms may be controlled with the use of antispasmodic drugs. Most commonly prescribed are baclofen (Lioresal), dantrolene (Dantrium), and tizanidine (Zanaflex). Botulism toxin injections may also be given to treat severe spasticity.

Autonomic Dysreflexia. The return of reflexes after the resolution of spinal shock means that patients with an injury level at T6 or higher may develop autonomic dysreflexia. **Autonomic dysreflexia** (also known as autonomic hyperreflexia) is a massive uncompensated cardiovascular reaction mediated by the sympathetic nervous system. It occurs in response to visceral stimulation once spinal shock is resolved in patients with spinal cord lesions. The condition is a life-threatening situation that requires immediate resolution. If resolution does not occur, this condition can lead to status epilepticus, stroke, myocardial infarction, and even death.

The most common precipitating cause is a distended bladder or rectum, although any sensory stimulation may cause autonomic dysreflexia. Contraction of the bladder or rectum, stimulation of the skin, or stimulation of the pain receptors may also cause autonomic dysreflexia. Manifestations include hypertension (up to 300 mm Hg systolic), throbbing headache, marked diaphoresis above the level of the lesion, bradycardia (30 to 40 beats/min), *piloerection* (erection of body hair) as a result of pilomotor spasm, flushing of the skin above the level of the lesion, blurred vision or spots in the visual fields, nasal congestion, anxiety, and nausea. It is important to measure blood pressure when a patient with a spinal cord injury complains of a headache.[26]

The pathology of autonomic dysreflexia involves the stimulation of sensory receptors below the level of the cord lesion. The intact autonomic nervous system below the level of the lesion responds to the stimulation with a reflex arteriolar vasoconstriction that increases blood pressure. Baroreceptors in the carotid sinus and the aorta sense the hypertension and stimulate the parasympathetic system. This results in a decrease in heart rate, but the visceral and peripheral vessels do not dilate because efferent impulses cannot pass through the cord lesion.

Nursing interventions in this serious emergency are elevation of the head of the bed 45 degrees or sitting the patient upright, notification of the physician, and assessment to determine the cause. The most common cause is bladder irritation. Immediate catheterization to relieve bladder distention may be necessary. Lidocaine jelly should be instilled in the urethra before catheterization. If a catheter is already in place, it should be checked for kinks or folds. If plugged, small-volume irrigation should be performed slowly and gently to open a plugged catheter, or a new catheter may be inserted. Stool impaction can also result in autonomic dysreflexia. A digital rectal examination should be performed only after application of an anesthetic ointment to decrease rectal stimulation and to prevent an increase of symptoms. The nurse should remove all skin stimuli, such as constrictive clothing and tight shoes. Blood pressure should be monitored frequently during the episode. If symptoms persist after the source has been relieved, an α-adrenergic blocker or an arteriolar vasodilator (e.g., nifedipine [Procardia]) is administered. Careful monitoring must continue until the vital signs stabilize.

TABLE 61-7	**PATIENT AND FAMILY TEACHING GUIDE** Autonomic Dysreflexia

Patient and family members must know the signs and symptoms of autonomic dysreflexia so that timely intervention can occur. These include the following:
- Sudden onset of acute headache
- Elevation in blood pressure and/or reduction in pulse rate
- Flushed face and upper chest (above the level of the lesion) and pale extremities (below the level of the lesion)
- Sweating above the level of the lesion
- Nasal congestion
- Feeling of apprehension

Immediate interventions include the following:
- Raise the person to a sitting position.
- Remove the noxious stimulus (fecal impaction, kinked urinary catheter, tight clothing).
- Call the health care provider if above actions do not relieve the signs and symptoms.

Efforts to decrease the likelihood of autonomic dysreflexia include the following:
- Maintain regular bowel function.
- If manual rectal stimulation is used, local anesthetics may reduce stimulation of autonomic dysreflexia.
- Monitor urine output.
- Wear a Medic Alert bracelet indicating a history of autonomic dysreflexia.

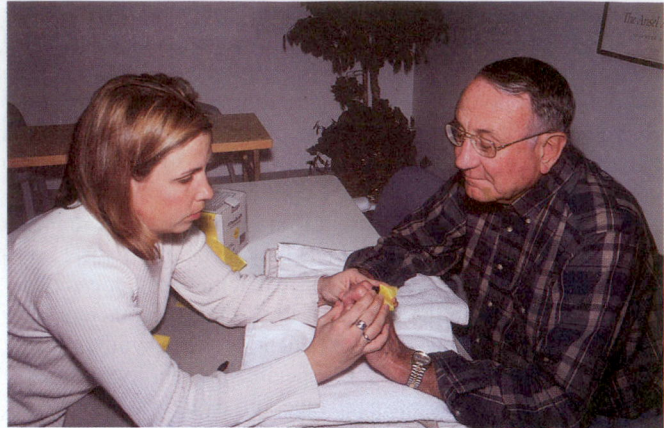

FIG. 61-13 Patient participating in occupational therapy.

The patient and family should be taught to recognize the causes and symptoms of autonomic dysreflexia (Table 61-7). They must understand the life-threatening nature of this dysfunction and must know how to relieve the cause.

Rehabilitation and Home Care. The physiologic and psychologic rehabilitation of the person with spinal cord injury is complex and involved. With physical and psychologic care and intensive and specialized rehabilitation, the patient with a spinal cord injury learns to function at the highest level of wellness. It is recommended that all patients with a new spinal cord injury receive comprehensive inpatient rehabilitation in a rehabilitation unit or center that specializes in spinal cord rehabilitation.

Many of the problems identified in the acute period become chronic and continue throughout life. Rehabilitation focuses on refined retraining of physiologic processes and extensive patient and family teaching about how to manage the physiologic and life changes resulting from injury (Fig. 61-13).

Rehabilitation is a multidisciplinary endeavor carried out through a team approach. Team members include rehabilitation nurses, physicians, physical therapists, occupational therapists, speech therapists, vocational counselors, psychologists, therapeutic recreation specialists, prosthetists, orthotists, and dietitians. Rehabilitation care is organized around the individual patient's goals and needs. During rehabilitation, patients are expected to be involved in therapies and learn self-care for several hours each day. Such intensive work at a time when the patient is dealing with the sudden change in health and functional status can be very stressful. Progress may be slow, and frequent encouragement may be required. The rehabilitation nurse has a pivotal role in providing encouragement, specialized nursing care, and patient and family teaching, and helping to coordinate the efforts of the rehabilitation team.

Respiratory Rehabilitation. The patient with high cervical spinal cord injury may have greatly increased mobility with phrenic nerve stimulators or electronic diaphragmatic pacemakers. These devices are not appropriate for all ventilator-dependent patients but may be helpful for those with an intact phrenic nerve. Today, ventila-

tors are also reasonably portable, and ventilator-dependent tetraplegic patients can be mobile and somewhat independent. Patients and family members should be taught all aspects of home ventilator care, and referrals should be made to appropriate community agencies. Patients with cervical-level injuries who are not ventilator dependent should be taught assisted coughing and regular use of incentive spirometry or deep-breathing exercises.

Neurogenic Bladder. A **neurogenic bladder** is any type of bladder dysfunction related to abnormal or absent bladder innervation. After spinal cord shock resolves, depending on the completeness of the spinal cord injury, patients usually have some degree of neurogenic bladder. Normal voiding requires nervous system coordination of urethral and pelvic floor relaxation with simultaneous contraction of the detrusor muscle. Depending on the lesion, a neurogenic bladder may have no reflex detrusor contractions (areflexic, flaccid), may have hyperactive reflex detrusor contractions (hyperreflexic, spastic), or may have lack of coordination between detrusor contraction and urethral relaxation *(dyssynergia)*. Common problems with a neurogenic bladder include urgency, frequency, incontinence, inability to void, and high bladder pressures resulting in reflux of urine into the kidneys.

Neurogenic bladder can be classified according to reflex detrusor activity, intravesical filling pressure, and continence function. Types of neurogenic bladder are outlined in Table 61-8. Diagnostic and collaborative care of neurogenic bladder is described in Table 61-9. The patient with a spinal cord injury and a neurogenic bladder requires a comprehensive program to manage bladder function.

After the patient's overall condition is stable and there is evidence of neurologic reflexes, urodynamic testing and a urine culture are done. The method used for urinary drainage depends on the type of neurogenic bladder dysfunction, the preference of the patient, and availability of a family caregiver, the physician, and the nursing staff. Numerous drainage methods are possible, including bladder reflex retraining if partial voiding control remains, indwelling catheter, intermittent catheterization, and external catheter (condom catheter). Surgical options include sphincterotomy, implantation of a functional electrical stimulation device, and urinary diversion.

Many factors are considered when selecting a bladder management strategy. These include upper extremity function, caregiver burden, and lifestyle choices. The type of bladder dysfunction also defines treatment goals and management options. A reflexic bladder with detrusor and sphincter dyssynergia requires interventions to provide low-pressure storage, low-pressure voiding, and adequate emptying. Anticholinergic drugs (oxybutynin [Ditropan],

TABLE 61-8	Types of Neurogenic Bladder		
Type	**Characteristics**	**Causes**	**Clinical Manifestations**
Reflexic (spastic, uninhibited, upper motor neuron)	No inhibitions influence time and place of voiding; bladder empties in response to stretching of bladder wall	Corticospinal tract lesion; observed in spinal cord injury, stroke, multiple sclerosis, brain tumor, brain trauma	Incontinence, frequency, urgency; voiding is unpredictable and incomplete
Areflexic (autonomous, flaccid, lower motor neuron)	Bladder acts as if there were paralysis of all motor functions, fills without emptying	Lower motor neuron lesion caused by trauma involving S2-S4; lesions of cauda equina, pelvic nerves	If sensory function intact, feels bladder distention and hesitancy; no control of micturition, resulting in overdistention of bladder and overflow incontinence
Sensory	Lack of sensation of need to urinate	Damage to sensory limb of bladder spinal reflex arc; seen in multiple sclerosis, diabetes mellitus	Poor bladder sensation, infrequent voiding of large residual volume

tolterodine [Detrol]) may be used to suppress bladder contraction. α-Adrenergic blockers (e.g., terazosin [Hytrin], doxazosin [Cardura]) may be used to decrease outflow resistance at the bladder neck, and antispasmodic drugs (e.g., baclofen [Lioresal]) may be used to decrease spasticity of pelvic floor muscles.

Drainage options include intermittent catheterization, external catheter, or indwelling catheter. A reflexic bladder with detrusor hyperreflexia may be treated with anticholinergic drugs, intravesical capsaicin, or botulinum A toxin. An areflexic bladder is usually managed with intermittent catheterization or an indwelling catheter.

The long-term use of an indwelling catheter should be carefully evaluated because of the associated high incidence of UTI, fistula formation, and diverticula. However, there may be patients for whom this is the best option. Adequate fluid intake and patency of the catheter should be ensured. The frequency of routine catheter changes ranges from 1 week to 1 month, depending on the type of catheter used and agency policy.

Intermittent catheterization is the most commonly recommended method of bladder management (see Chapter 46). Nursing assessment is important in selecting the time interval between catheterizations. Initially, catheterization is done every 4 hours. Bladder volume can be assessed before catheterization using the portable bladder ultrasound machine. If less than 200 ml of urine is measured, the time interval may be extended. If 500 ml or more of urine is measured, the time interval is shortened. An overdistended bladder can cause ischemia of the bladder wall, which may predispose tissues to bacterial invasion and infection. Patients often experience diuresis at a regular time during a 24-hour period. The number of intermittent catheterizations per day is usually five or six.

Urinary diversion surgery may be necessary if the patient has repeated UTIs with renal involvement or repeated stones or if therapeutic intervention has been unsuccessful (see Chapter 46). Surgical treatment of neurogenic bladder includes bladder neck revision (sphincterotomy), bladder augmentation (augmentation cystoplasty), penile prosthesis, artificial sphincter, perineal ureterostomy, cystotomy, vesicotomy, and anterior urethral transplantation.

No matter which bladder management strategy is selected, the nurse must teach the patient and the family or caregivers about how to accomplish successful self-management. Management techniques, how to obtain necessary supplies, care of supplies and equipment, and when to seek health care must be taught. Resources and referrals for supplies and ongoing care must be arranged.

Neurogenic Bowel. Careful management of bowel evacuation is necessary in the patient with a spinal cord injury because volun-

TABLE 61-9	COLLABORATIVE CARE — Neurogenic Bladder

Diagnostic
History and physical examination, including neurologic examination
Urodynamic testing
IV pyelogram
Urine culture

Collaborative Therapy
Drug therapy
- Suppress bladder contractions (anticholinergics)
- Relaxation of urethral sphincter (α-adrenergic blockers)
- Suppress pelvic floor spasticity (baclofen [Lioresal])
Fluid intake of 1800-2000 ml/day
Urine drainage
- Voluntary or reflex voiding
- Intermittent catheterization
- Indwelling catheter
Surgery
- Sphincterotomy
- Electrical stimulation
- Urinary diversion

IV, Intravenous.

tary control of this function may be lost as a result of a condition called **neurogenic bowel.** The usual measures for preventing constipation include a high-fiber diet and adequate fluid intake (see Table 43-9). Patient and family teaching guidelines related to bowel management are presented in Table 61-10. However, these measures by themselves may not be adequate to stimulate evacuation. In addition, suppositories (bisacodyl [Dulcolax] or glycerin) or small-volume enemas and digital stimulation by the nurse or patient may be necessary. In the patient with an upper motor neuron lesion, digital stimulation is necessary to relax the external sphincter to promote defecation. A stool softener such as docusate sodium (Colace) can be used to regulate stool consistency. Oral stimulant laxatives should be used only if absolutely necessary for a day or two and not on a regular basis.

Valsalva maneuver and manual stimulation are useful in patients with lower motor neuron lesions. The Valsalva maneuver requires intact abdominal muscles, so it is used in those patients with injuries below T12. In general, a bowel movement every other day is considered adequate. However, preinjury patterns should be considered. Incontinence can result from too much stool softener or a fecal impaction.

TABLE 61-10	PATIENT AND FAMILY TEACHING GUIDE Bowel Management After Spinal Cord Injury

The following are teaching guidelines for a patient with a spinal cord injury:

1. Optimal nutritional intake includes:
   - Three well-balanced meals each day
   - Two servings from the milk group
   - Two or more servings from the meat group, including beef, pork, poultry, eggs, fish
   - Four or more servings from the vegetable and fruit groups
   - Four or more servings from the bread and cereal group
2. Fiber intake should be approximately 20 to 30 g/day. The amount of fiber eaten should be increased gradually over 1 to 2 weeks.
3. Two to three quarts of fluid per day should be consumed unless contraindicated. Water or fruit juices should be used, and caffeinated beverages such as coffee, tea, and cola should be limited. Fluid softens hard stools; caffeine stimulates fluid loss through urination.
4. Foods that produce gas (e.g., beans) or upper GI upset (spicy foods) should be avoided.
5. *Timing:* A regular schedule for bowel evacuation should be established. A good time is 30 minutes after the first meal of the day.
6. *Position:* If possible, an upright position with feet flat on the floor or on a stepstool enhances bowel evacuation. Staying on the toilet, commode, or bedpan for longer than 20 to 30 minutes may cause skin breakdown. Based on stability, someone may need to stay with the patient.
7. *Activity:* Exercise is important for bowel function. In addition to improving muscle tone, it also increases GI transit time and increases appetite. Muscles should be exercised. This includes stretching, range-of-motion, position changing, and functional movement.
8. *Drug treatment:* Suppositories may be necessary to stimulate a bowel movement. Manual stimulation of the rectum may also be helpful in initiating defecation. Stool softeners should be used as needed to regulate stool consistency. Oral laxatives should be used only if necessary.

GI, Gastrointestinal.

Careful recording of bowel movements, including amount, time, and consistency, is important to the overall success of the program. Timing of defecation may also be an important factor. If bowel evacuation is planned for 30 to 60 minutes following the first meal of the day, this may enhance success by taking advantage of the gastrocolic reflex induced by eating. Again, patient and family education is required to promote successful independent bowel management.

Neurogenic Skin. Prevention of pressure ulcers and other types of injury to insensitive skin are essential for every patient with spinal cord injury. Nurses in rehabilitation are responsible for teaching these skills and providing information about daily skin care. A comprehensive visual and tactile examination of the skin should be done twice daily, with special attention given to areas over bony prominences. The areas most vulnerable to breakdown include the ischia, trochanters, heels, and sacrum. Careful positioning and repositioning should be done initially every 2 hours, with gradual increases in the times between turns if there is no redness over bony prominences at the time of turning. Pressure-relieving cushions must be used in wheelchairs, and special mattresses may also be needed. Movement during turns and transfers should be done carefully to avoid stretching and folding of soft tissues (shear), as well as friction or abrasion.[27]

Nutritional status should be assessed regularly. Both body weight loss and weight gain can contribute to skin breakdown.

TABLE 61-11	PATIENT AND FAMILY TEACHING GUIDE Skin Care for Patient with Spinal Cord Injury

Skin breakdown is a potential problem after spinal cord injury. The following measures are used to decrease this possibility:

Change Position Frequently
- If in a wheelchair, lift self up and shift weight every 15 to 30 minutes.
- If in bed, a regular turning schedule (at least every 2 hours) that includes sides, back, and abdomen is encouraged to change position.
- Use special mattresses and wheelchair cushions.
- Use pillows to protect bony prominences when in bed.

Monitor Skin Condition
- Inspect skin frequently for areas of redness, swelling, and breakdown.
- Keep fingernails trimmed to avoid scratches and abrasions.
- If a wound develops, follow standard wound care management procedures.

TABLE 61-12	PATIENT AND FAMILY TEACHING GUIDE Halo Vest Care

The following are teaching guidelines for a patient with a halo vest:

1. Inspect the pins on the halo traction ring. Report to health care provider if pins are loose or if there are signs of infection, including redness, tenderness, swelling, or drainage at the insertion sites.
2. Clean around pin sites carefully with hydrogen peroxide, water, or alcohol on a cotton swab as directed.
3. Apply antibiotic ointment as prescribed.
4. To provide skin care, have the patient lie down on a bed with his or her head resting on a pillow to reduce pressure on the brace. Loosen one side of the vest. Gently wash the skin under the vest with soap and water, rinse it, and then dry it thoroughly. At the same time, check the skin for pressure points, redness, swelling, bruising, or chafing. Close the open side and repeat the procedure on the opposite side.
5. If the vest becomes wet or damp, it can be carefully dried with a blow dryer.
6. An assistive device (e.g., cane, walker) may be used to provide greater balance. Flat shoes should be worn.
7. Turn the entire body, not just the head and neck, when trying to view sideways.
8. In case of an emergency, keep a set of wrenches close to the halo vest at all times.
9. Mark the vest strap such that consistent buckling and fit can be maintained.
10. Avoid grabbing bars or vest to assist patient.
11. Keep sheepskin pad under vest. Change and wash at least weekly.
12. If perspiration or itching is a problem, a cotton T-shirt can be worn under sheepskin. The T-shirt can be modified with a Velcro seam closure on one side.

Adequate intake of protein is essential for skin health. Measurement of prealbumin, total protein, and albumin can help identify inadequate protein intake. The importance of nutrition to skin health should be stressed to the patient and family.

Protection of the skin also requires avoidance of thermal injury. Burns can be caused by hot food or liquids, bath or shower water that is too warm, radiators, heating pads, and uninsulated plumbing. Thermal injury also can result from extreme cold (frostbite). Injuries may not be noticed until severe damage is done. Anticipatory guidance about potential risks is essential. Patient and family education related to skin is provided in Tables 61-11 and 61-12.

TABLE 61-13	Potential for Sexual Function in Men with Spinal Cord Injury		
Erection	**Ejaculation**	**Orgasm**	
Upper Motor Neuron			
Complete			
Frequent (92%), reflexogenic only	Rare (4%)	Rare	
Incomplete			
Most frequent (99%), including reflexogenic (80%) and psychogenic (19%)	Less frequent (32%), after reflexogenic erection (74%), after psychogenic erection (26%)	Present (if ejaculation occurs)	
Lower Motor Neuron			
Complete			
Infrequent (26%)	Infrequent (18%)	Present (if ejaculation occurs)	
Incomplete			
Psychogenic and reflexogenic	Frequent (70%), after psychogenic and reflexogenic erections	Present (if ejaculation occurs)	

Sexuality. Knowledge of the level and completeness of injury is needed to understand the male patient's potential for orgasm, erection, and fertility and the patient's capacity for sexual satisfaction (Table 61-13). Sexuality is an important issue regardless of the patient's age or gender. To provide accurate and sensitive counseling and education about sexuality, the nurse must have an awareness and an acceptance of personal sexuality, as well as knowledge of human sexual responses. When discussing sexual potential, the nurse should use scientific terminology rather than slang whenever possible.

Reflex sexual function capability is possible if the patient has an upper motor neuron lesion. The presence of tone in the external rectal sphincter indicates an upper motor lesion. The absence of external rectal sphincter tone, bulbocavernosus reflex, or both indicates that the patient has lower motor neuron involvement and may be capable of psychogenic erection but not reflex erection. If ejaculation occurs, it may be retrograde into the bladder.

The type of lesion determines the physical sexual response. Men with upper motor neuron lesions may have reflexogenic erections that are produced by reflex activity or external stimuli or that occur spontaneously. These spontaneous erections are often short lived and uncontrolled and cannot be maintained or summoned at the time of coitus. Orgasm and ejaculation are usually not possible for men with a complete upper motor neuron lesion.

Most patients with a complete lower motor neuron lesion are unable to have either psychogenic or reflexogenic erections. Patients with incomplete lower motor neuron lesions have the highest possibility of successful psychogenic erection with ejaculation, and up to 10% of these patients are fertile.

Treatments for erectile dysfunction include drugs, vacuum devices, and surgical procedures. Sildenafil (Viagra) has become the treatment of choice since several studies have documented its effectiveness in men with spinal cord injury. Penile injection of vasoactive substances (papaverine, prostaglandin E) is another medical treatment. Risks include *priapism* (prolonged penile erection) and scarring, so these substances are often considered only after failure of sildenafil. Vacuum suction devices use negative pressure to encourage blood flow into the penis. Erection is maintained by a constriction band placed at the base of the penis. The main surgical option is implantation of a penile prosthesis. (Erectile dysfunction is discussed in Chapter 55.)

Male fertility is affected by spinal cord injury causing poor sperm quality and ejaculatory dysfunction. Recent advances in methods of retrieving sperm (penile vibratory stimulation and electroejaculation) combined with ovulation induction and intra-

EVIDENCE-BASED PRACTICE
Sexuality Following Spinal Cord Injury

Clinical Question
What is the impact of spinal cord injury on sexuality and reproductive health?

Best Available Evidence
Meta-analysis of descriptive exploratory studies

Critical Appraisal and Synthesis of Evidence
- 122 studies ($n = 6668$) explored the sexual function and fertility of patients with spinal cord injuries ranging in age from 16 to 81 years old.
- The overwhelming majority of study participants were male.
- Ejaculation rates were studied using vibration and/or electrode stimulation.
- Sexual function was studied with sildenafil [Viagra], vacuum devices, and penile injections.
- The sample size of women was too small to reach any conclusions.

Conclusions
- Using vibration and electroejaculation, most males (95%) can produce semen for fertility purposes.
- Vibration should be tried first for those with upper motor neuron injuries, with electroejaculation reserved for those in whom vibration failed or for those with lower motor neuron injuries.
- Sildenafil, vacuum devices, and penile injections can help most men with short-term erectile function problems.

Implications for Nursing Practice
- Provide information to patients about the effects of spinal cord injury on sexual health and options for fertility and improving sexual function.
- Long-term sexual adjustment and activity has not been studied in patients with spinal cord injuries.

Reference for Evidence
DeForge D, Blackmer J, Moher D, et al: Sexuality and reproductive health following spinal cord injury, *Evidence Report/Technology Assessment No 109* (AHRQ Publication No 05-E003-2), Rockville, Md, 2004, Agency for Healthcare Research and Quality. Available at *www.ncbi.nlm.nih.gov/books/bv.fcgi?rid =hstat1a.chapter.76018.*

uterine insemination of the female partner have changed the prognosis for men with spinal cord injury to father children from unlikely to a reasonable possibility of successful outcomes.[28]

The effect of spinal cord injury on female sexual response is less clear. Lubrication is similar to erections in males, with reflex and psychogenic components. Women with upper motor neuron injuries may retain the capacity for reflex lubrication, whereas psychogenic lubrication depends on the completeness of injury. Orgasm is reported by about 50% of women with spinal cord injury.[28]

The woman of childbearing age with a spinal cord injury usually remains fertile. The injury does not affect the ability to become pregnant or to deliver normally through the birth canal. Menses may cease for as long as 6 months after injury. If sexual activity is resumed, protection against an unplanned pregnancy is necessary. A normal pregnancy may be complicated by UTIs, anemia, and autonomic dysreflexia. Because uterine contractions are not felt, a precipitous delivery is always a danger.

Sexual rehabilitation for both men and women should begin informally after the acute phase of the injury has passed. Questions such as, "Have you had an erection since your injury?" and "Have your menstrual periods continued since the injury?" are nonthreatening ways to introduce the topic of sexual functioning. The male patient may pose a question such as, "Can I ever be a man again?"

Open discussion with the patient is essential. This important aspect of rehabilitation should be handled by someone specially trained in sexual counseling. A nurse or other rehabilitation professional with such expertise works with the patient and partner to provide support, with the emphasis on open communication. The nurse's educational role requires respect for every couple's personal standards of religious and cultural beliefs. Alternative methods of obtaining sexual satisfaction, such as oral-genital sex (cunnilingus and fellatio), may be suggested. Explicit films may also be used, such as a film demonstrating the sexual activities of a patient with paraplegia and a nondisabled partner. Graphics should be used cautiously because they may be too limiting or focus too much on the mechanics of sex rather than on the relationship.

Sexual activities may require more planning and be less spontaneous than before the injury. For example, an attendant may have to undress the patient and remove equipment. A relaxed atmosphere with music and perfume creates an attractive environment. Ample time for caressing, fondling, and kissing is essential. The partners should be encouraged to explore each other's erogenous areas, such as the lips, neck, and ears, which can arouse psychogenic erection or orgasm. Few demands should be made initially.

Care should be taken not to dislodge an indwelling catheter during sexual activity. If an external catheter is used, it should be removed before sexual activity and the patient should refrain from fluids. The bowel program should include evacuation the morning of sexual activity. The partner should be informed that incontinence is always possible. The woman may need a water-soluble lubricant to supplement diminished vaginal secretions and facilitate vaginal penetration.

Grief and Depression. Patients with spinal cord injuries may feel an overwhelming sense of loss. They may temporarily lose control over everyday life activities and must depend on others for ADLs and for life-sustaining measures. Patients may believe that they are useless and burdens to their families. At a stage when independence is often of the greatest importance, they may be totally dependent on others.

The patient's response and recovery differ in some important aspects from those of patients experiencing loss from amputation or terminal illness. First, regression can and does occur at different stages. Working through grief is a difficult, lifelong process with which the patient needs support and encouragement. With recent advances in rehabilitation, it is usual for the patient to be independent

TABLE 61-14	**Mourning Process and Nursing Interventions in Spinal Cord Injury**	
Patient Behavior	**Nursing Intervention**
Shock and Denial Struggle for survival, complete dependence, excessive sleep, withdrawal, fantasies, unrealistic expectations	• Employ meticulous nursing care. • Provide honest information. • Use simple diagrams to explain injury. • Encourage patient to begin road to recovery. • Establish agreement to use and improve all current abilities while not denying the possibility of future improvement.
Anger Refusal to discuss paralysis, decreased self-esteem, manipulation, hostile and abusive language	• Coordinate care with patient and encourage self-care. • Support family members; prevent alleviation of guilt by supporting dependency. • Use humor liberally. • Allow patient outbursts. • Do not allow fixation on injury.
Depression Sadness, pessimism, anorexia, nightmares, insomnia, agitation, psychomotor retardation, "blues," suicidal preoccupation, refusal to participate in any self-care activities	• Encourage family involvement and resources. • Plan graded steps in rehabilitation to give success with minimal opportunity for frustration. • Give cheerful and willing assistance with activities of daily living. • Avoid sympathy. • Use firm kindness.
Adjustment Planning for future, active participation in therapy, finding of personal meaning in experience and continuation of growth, return to premorbid personality	• Remember that patients have individual personalities. • Balance support systems to encourage independence. • Set goals with patient input. • Emphasize potentials.

dent physically and discharged from the rehabilitation center before completion of the grief process. The goal of recovery is related more to adjustment than to acceptance. Adjustment implies the ability to go on with living with certain limitations. Although the patient who is cooperative and accepting is easier to treat, the nurse should expect a wide fluctuation of emotions from a patient with a spinal cord injury. Depression may not be a component of the recovery process. Societal norms allow depression after severe loss and almost impose it on those confronted with death or radical lifestyle changes. However, every patient may not experience depression.

The nurse's role in grief work is to allow mourning as a component of the rehabilitation process. Table 61-14 summarizes the mourning process and appropriate nursing interventions. Maintaining hope is an important strategy during the grieving process and should not be interpreted as denial.[29] During the shock and denial stage, the nurse reassures the patient and stresses the expertise of the entire health care team. During the anger stage, the nurse assists the patient in achievement of control over the environment, particularly by allowing the patient's input into the plan of care. The nurse should not respond to anger or manipulation or become involved in a power struggle with the patient. As self-care abilities increase, the patient's independence increases.

The patient's family also requires counseling to avoid promoting dependency in the patient through guilt or misplaced sympathy. The family is also experiencing an intense grieving process. A support group of family members and friends of patients with spinal cord injury can help increase family members' knowledge of and participation in the grieving process, physical difficulties, the rehabilitation plan, and the meaning of the disability in society.[30]

During the stage of depression, the nurse must be patient and persistent and maintain a sense of humor. Sympathy is not helpful. The patient should be treated in an adult manner and be involved in decision making about care, but the nurse must insist that the care be performed. A primary nurse relationship is helpful. Staff planning and sessions in which staff members can express their feelings are helpful in providing consistency of care. To achieve the stage of adjustment, the patient needs continual support throughout the rehabilitation process in the forms of acceptance, affection, and caring. The nurse must be attentive when the patient needs to talk and sensitive to needs at the various stages of the grief process.[29]

Although the stage of depression during the grief process usually lasts days to weeks, there are some individuals who may become clinically depressed and require treatment for depression. Evaluation by a psychiatric nurse or psychiatrist is recommended. Treatment may include drugs and psychotherapy.

▪ Evaluation

Expected outcomes for the patient with a spinal cord injury are presented in NCP 61-1.

GERONTOLOGIC CONSIDERATIONS
SPINAL CORD INJURY

The demographics of patients living with spinal cord injury are changing. The fact that persons with spinal cord injury now have longer life spans has contributed to the increasing number of older adults living with a spinal cord injury. Aging is also associated with an increased occurrence of other chronic illnesses in the person with a spinal cord injury. This can have a serious impact on these older adults. As patients with spinal cord injury age, both individual aging changes and length of time since injury can impact functional ability. For example, bowel and bladder dysfunction can increase with the duration and severity of spinal cord injury.

Health promotion and screening are important for the older patient with a spinal cord injury. Daily skin inspections, UTI prevention measures, and monthly breast examinations for women and regular prostate cancer screening for men are recommended. Cardiovascular disease is the most common cause of morbidity and mortality among spinal cord–injured persons. The lack of sensation, including chest pain, in those with high-level injuries may mask acute myocardial ischemia. Altered autonomic nervous system function and decreases in physical activity can place the patient at risk for cardiovascular problems, including hypertension.

At the same time, because of increased work and recreational activities of older adults, more older adults are experiencing spinal cord

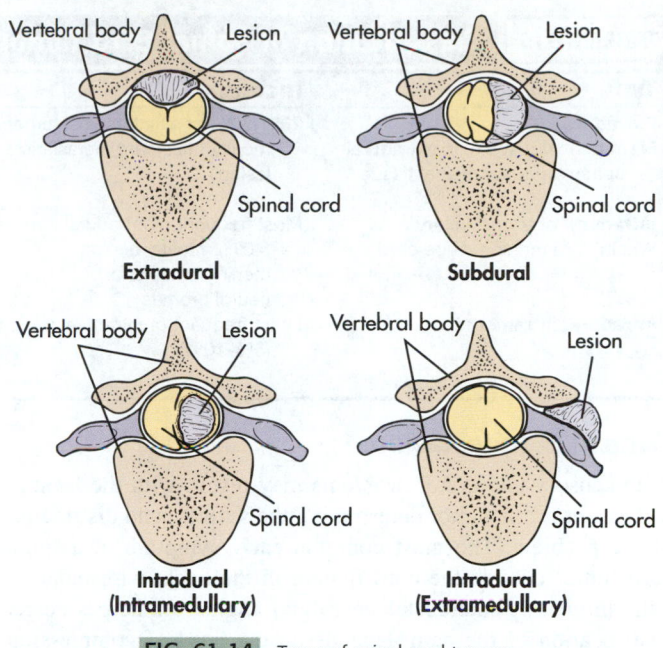

FIG. 61-14 Types of spinal cord tumors.

injury. Health promotion to decrease the risk of injuries includes fall prevention strategies (e.g., using a stepstool or a grab bar to reach high shelves, handrails on stairs). Rehabilitation for the older person who has undergone a spinal cord injury may take longer because of other preexisting conditions and poorer health status at the time of the initial injury. An interdisciplinary team approach to rehabilitation is essential in preventing secondary complications associated with spinal cord injury, especially in older adults.[31]

SPINAL CORD TUMORS

Etiology and Pathophysiology

Tumors that affect the spinal cord account for 0.5% to 1% of all neoplasms. These tumors are classified as primary (arising from some component of cord, dura, nerves, or vessels) or secondary (from primary growths in the breast, thyroid, lung, kidney, and other sites). Spinal cord tumors are further classified as extradural (outside the spinal cord), intradural extramedullary (within the dura but outside the actual spinal cord), and intradural intramedullary (within the spinal cord itself). These latter tumors are usually astrocytomas or ependymomas (Fig. 61-14, Table 61-15). Approximately 90% of all spinal tumors are extradural. Extradural tumors are usually metastatic and most often arise in the vertebral bodies. These metastatic lesions can invade intradurally and compress the spinal cord. Spinal intradural-extramedullary tumors account for two thirds of all intraspinal neoplasms and mainly consist of meningiomas and schwannomas.

Because many of these tumors are slow growing, their symptoms stem from the mechanical effects of slow compression and irritation of nerve roots, displacement of the cord, or gradual obstruction of the vascular supply. The slowness of growth does not cause autodestruction (secondary injury) as in traumatic lesions. Therefore complete functional restoration may be possible when the tumor is removed, except with the intradural-intramedullary tumors.

Most metastatic tumors are extradural lesions. Tumors that commonly metastasize to the spinal epidural space are those that spread to bone, such as carcinomas of the breast, lung, prostate, and kidney.

TABLE 61-15	**Classification of Spinal Cord Tumors**		
Type	**Incidence**	**Treatment**	**Prognosis**
Extradural From bones of spine, in extradural space, or in paraspinal tissue	20%-50% of all intraspinal tumors, mostly malignant metastatic lesions	Relief of cord pressure by surgical laminectomy, radiation, chemotherapy, or combination approach	Poor
Intradural extramedullary Within dura mater outside cord	Most frequent of intradural tumors (40%), mostly benign meningiomas and neurofibromas	Complete surgical removal of tumor (if possible), partial removal followed by radiation	Usually very good if lack of damage to cord from compression
Intradural intramedullary	Least frequent of intradural tumors (5%-10%)	Partial surgical removal, radiation therapy (resulting in only temporary improvement)	Very poor

Clinical Manifestations

Both sensory and motor problems may result, with the location and extent of the tumor determining the severity and distribution of the problem. The most common early symptom of a spinal cord tumor outside the cord is pain in the back, with radicular pain simulating intercostal neuralgia, angina, or herpes zoster. The location of the pain depends on the level of compression. The pain worsens with activity, coughing, straining, and lying down. Sensory disruption is later manifested by coldness, numbness, and tingling in an extremity or in several extremities, slowly progressing upward until it reaches the level of the lesion. Impaired sensation of pain, temperature, and light touch precedes a deficit in vibration and position sense that may progress to complete anesthesia. Motor weakness accompanies the sensory disturbances and consists of slowly increasing clumsiness, weakness, and spasticity. The sensory and motor disturbances are ipsilateral to the lesion. Bladder disturbances are marked by urgency with difficulty in starting the flow and progressing to retention with overflow incontinence.

Manifestations of intradural spinal tumor develop as progressive damage to the long spinal tracts, producing paralysis, sensory loss, and bladder dysfunction. Pain can be severe as a result of compression of spinal roots or vertebrae.

NURSING and COLLABORATIVE MANAGEMENT
SPINAL CORD TUMORS

Extradural tumors are seen early on routine spinal x-rays, whereas intradural and intramedullary tumors require MRI or CT scans for detection. CSF analysis may reveal tumor cells. The cord is decompressed after removal of the tumor by a laminectomy. More than 85% of primary neoplasms are benign and can be completely resected; 90% of patients recover without residual problems.

Compression of the spinal cord is an emergency. Relief of the ischemia related to the compression is the goal of therapy. Corticosteroids are generally prescribed immediately to relieve tumor-related edema. Dexamethasone (Decadron) is also usually used to treat edema, and often in large doses.

Treatment for nearly all spinal cord tumors is surgical removal. The exception is the metastatic tumor that is sensitive to radiation and that has caused only minimal neurologic deficits in the patient. In general, tumors of the extradural or intradural-extramedullary groups can be completely removed surgically. Intradural-intramedullary tumors have a less favorable prognosis. However, exploration and removal are usually attempted.

Radiation therapy after the operation is fairly effective. Maximum permissible tissue dose is given over 6 to 8 weeks. Chemotherapy has also been used in conjunction with radiation therapy.

Relief of pain and return of function are the ultimate goals of treatment. Nurses must be aware of the neurologic status of the patient before and after treatment. Ensuring that the patient receives pain medication as needed is an important nursing responsibility. Depending on the amount of neurologic dysfunction exhibited, the patient may need to be cared for as though recovering from a spinal cord injury. Rehabilitation of patients with spinal cord tumors is similar to spinal cord injury rehabilitation.[31]

POSTPOLIO SYNDROME

Polio, also known as *poliomyelitis,* is an infectious viral disease transmitted through the oral route by ingestion of contaminated water or food, or contact with infected sources such as unwashed hands. The virus is shed in the feces of infected individuals for as long as 6 weeks. The disease produces a range of presentations from flu-like symptoms (abortive poliomyelitis) that resolve in 24 to 36 hours (nonparalytic) to paralytic poliomyelitis that attacks the motor neurons in the anterior horn of the spinal cord and/or brainstem. Polio once ravaged American communities in postwar epidemics during the 1940s and 1950s. Approximately 1.6 million people currently living in the United States were afflicted. More than 600,000 of these individuals suffered paralytic poliomyelitis and subsequently recovered motor function.

Polio was effectively eradicated in the United States by the development of the Salk injectable polio vaccine in 1955 and the Sabin oral polio vaccine in 1961. It is still a threat in developing countries due to lack of effective immunization programs. Polio survivors who recovered from the disease decades ago, notably those who had paralytic poliomyelitis, are now experiencing a recurrence of neuromuscular symptoms as they age. These late effects of polio are collectively referred to as **postpolio syndrome.**

Etiology and Pathophysiology

The etiology of postpolio syndrome is not completely clear. The most commonly accepted theory is that enlarged distal motor neurons that had recovered after polio degenerate and subsequently begin to fail.[32] It appears that cellular damage caused by the effects of the polio virus may lead to exhaustion and premature failure of the motor neurons. The result is slowly progressive muscle weakness and fatigue. Factors thought to contribute to postpolio syndrome include age-related motor neuron loss, musculoskeletal overuse and disuse, weight gain, pain, and other neuromuscular or systemic illnesses. There is no evidence to support the theory that postpolio syndrome is caused by reactivation of the original polio virus.

Clinical Manifestations and Diagnostic Studies

Postpolio syndrome is manifested by a new onset of joint and muscle weakness, easy fatigability, generalized fatigue, and pain. Uncommonly, individuals may also exhibit speech, swallowing, and respiratory difficulties. Postpolio syndrome is diagnosed by exclusion. There is no definitive test that identifies this disorder. Patients should undergo thorough diagnostic testing to rule out other medical conditions that may produce similar symptoms. Criteria used to establish the diagnosis of postpolio syndrome include a history of polio in the abortive, nonparalytic, or paralytic forms; recovery from polio; a lengthy period of stability of at least 10 to 20 years' duration; and clinical manifestations of postpolio syndrome that are not associated with other medical disorders. Although the disabilities caused by postpolio syndrome are not necessarily obvious, they can have a significant impact on the patient's quality of life.

NURSING *and* COLLABORATIVE MANAGEMENT POSTPOLIO SYNDROME

There is no specific treatment for postpolio syndrome. Management approaches are targeted at controlling symptoms, particularly fatigue, weakness, and pain. An interdisciplinary team approach is essential to manage the patient. The cornerstone of management is lifestyle modification to conserve energy and support performance of activities of daily living.

During the polio epidemic, polio victims were subjected to rigorous therapy to regain muscle function. A particular challenge may be helping the patient to understand that aggressive or strenuous therapy to strengthen muscles is now considered to be counterproductive in treating postpolio symptoms. Overexertion can worsen fatigue and weakness. Instead, it is important to promote pacing of activities to avoid feelings of fatigue. Planning to include rest periods as well as utilizing assistive devices such as scooters, canes, and wheelchairs may be beneficial. Adaptive equipment can be helpful to patients who experience difficulty with self-care. Other strategies include arranging for a handicapped license plate or sticker to facilitate parking close to shops and public buildings, shopping on the Internet to avoid walking, and enlisting the support of family and friends to perform necessary tasks. Physical therapy can be ordered to support mobility and fitness in light of the patient's limitations. Weight loss interventions should be considered for the individual who is overweight.

Effective pain management through both pharmacologic and nonpharmacologic approaches can enable an individual to remain active and achieve a greater sense of well-being. Nonpharmacologic measures include massage, relaxation strategies, and guided imagery (see Chapter 9). Protection from the cold can also aid in pain relief; the individual with postpolio syndrome may be especially sensitive to a cold environment. It is important to collaborate with the health care provider or pain management team to derive an effective plan that meets individual patient needs.

For the individual with speech, swallowing, or respiratory difficulties, it is important to take measures to prevent aspiration, maintain airway patency, and promote optimal nutrition. Nursing interventions for these problems are similar to those described for patients with Guillain-Barré syndrome and spinal cord injury.

Experiencing the reemergence of symptoms related to polio can have a devastating impact on the patient's psychosocial well-being.

Memories of paralysis and the challenges of recovery can lead to fear in a patient diagnosed with postpolio syndrome. Anxiety and depression as well as difficulties with coping can occur. The nurse can assist the individual by actively listening to concerns, providing information about postpolio syndrome and available resources, and referring the patient to support groups or counseling when necessary. Gaining a sense of control through active participation in lifestyle modifications and therapy may improve the patient's ability to better cope with postpolio syndrome.

CRITICAL THINKING EXERCISE

CASE STUDY

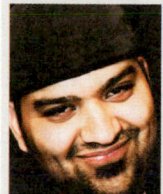

Case Study photo
©iStockphoto.com/
Kevin Russ.

Spinal Cord Injury

Patient Profile. Bruce V., a 24-year-old white man, is admitted to the emergency department with the diagnosis of a cervical spinal cord injury. Bruce was swimming at a neighbor's backyard pool. He dove into the shallow end, striking his head on the bottom of the pool. His friends noticed that he did not resurface. They rescued him and brought him to the side of the pool. They maintained neck immobilization until the rescue crews arrived.

Subjective Data
- Is awake and alert
- Has complaints of neck pain
- Is anxious and asking why he cannot move his legs
- Is asking to see his family

Objective Data

Physical Examination
- Weak biceps movement
- No triceps movement
- Gross elbow movement present
- Decreased sensation from the shoulders down
- No bladder or bowel control
- BP 90/56; pulse 56; respirations 32 and labored

Diagnostic Studies
- X-rays revealed C5 fracture dislocation

Collaborative Care
- Intubated in the emergency department
- Started on mechanical ventilation
- Placed in tongs and traction in the emergency department
- Admitted to ICU

Critical Thinking Questions

1. What nursing activities would be a priority on Bruce V.'s arrival in the ICU?
2. What physiologic problems are causing Bruce V. to have hypotension and bradycardia?
3. What would be the first line of treatment for Bruce V.'s hypotension and bradycardia?
4. What signs and symptoms would indicate respiratory distress and what physiologic problem would cause respiratory distress in Bruce V.'s injury state?
5. What can the nurse do to decrease Bruce V.'s anxiety?
6. Based on the assessment data provided, write one or more nursing diagnoses. Are there any collaborative problems?

NCLEX EXAMINATION REVIEW QUESTIONS

The number of the question corresponds to the same-numbered objective at the beginning of the chapter.

1. During assessment of the patient with trigeminal neuralgia, the nurse should
   a. inspect all aspects of the mouth and teeth.
   b. lightly palpate the affected side of the face for edema.
   c. test for temperature and sensation perception on the face.
   d. ask the patient to describe factors that initiate an episode.

2. During routine assessment of a patient with Guillain-Barré syndrome, the nurse finds the patient to be short of breath. The patient's respiratory distress is caused by
   a. elevated protein levels in the CSF.
   b. immobility resulting from ascending paralysis.
   c. degeneration of motor neurons in the brainstem and spinal cord.
   d. paralysis ascending to the nerves that stimulate the thoracic area.

3. A patient is admitted to the ICU with a C7 spinal cord injury and diagnosed with Brown-Séquard syndrome. On physical examination, the nurse would most likely find
   a. upper extremity weakness only.
   b. complete motor and sensory loss below C7.
   c. loss of position sense and vibration in both lower extremities.
   d. ipsilateral motor loss and contralateral sensory loss below C7.

4. A patient is admitted to the hospital with a spinal cord injury following an automobile collision. The nurse recognizes that the pathophysiology of secondary spinal cord injury involves
   a. initial infarction of the white matter of the cord.
   b. mechanical transection of the cord by the trauma.
   c. necrotic destruction of the cord from hemorrhage and edema.
   d. release of epinephrine leading to massive vasodilation of spinal cord vessels.

5. A rehabilitation goal for the patient with an injury at the C5 level includes
   a. feeding self with hand devices.
   b. driving an electric wheelchair.
   c. assisting with transfer activities.
   d. controlling bowel and bladder functions.

6. A patient with a C7 spinal cord injury undergoing rehabilitation tells the nurse he must have the flu because he has a bad headache and nausea. The initial action of the nurse is to
   a. call the physician.
   b. check the patient's temperature.
   c. take the patient's blood pressure.
   d. elevate the head of the bed to 90 degrees.

7. For a 65-year-old female patient who has lived with a T1 spinal cord injury for 20 years, the nurse would emphasize the following health teaching information:
   a. A mammogram is needed every year.
   b. Bladder function tends to improve with age.
   c. Heart disease is not common in persons with spinal cord injury.
   d. As a person ages, the need to change body position is less important.

8. The most common early symptom of a spinal cord tumor is
   a. urinary incontinence.
   b. back pain that worsens with activity.
   c. paralysis below the level of involvement.
   d. impaired sensation of pain, temperature, and light touch.

9. Which of the following descriptions best describes postpolio syndrome?
   a. Autoimmune disease of motor neurons triggered by polio virus
   b. Reactivation of poliomyelitis resulting in acute musculoskeletal disease
   c. Degeneration of enlarged motor neurons many years following poliomyelitis
   d. Disorder characterized by active viral destruction of the upper motor neurons

REFERENCES

1. Cheshire WP: Trigeminal neuralgia: diagnosis and treatment, *Curr Neurol Neurosci Rep* 5:79, 2005.
2. Lopez BC, Hamlyn PJ, Zakrzewska JM: Systematic review of ablative neurosurgical techniques for the treatment of trigeminal neuralgia, *Neurosurgery* 54:973, 2004.
3. Liu JK, Apfelbaum RI: Treatment of trigeminal neuralgia, *Neurosurg Clin N Am* 15:319, 2004.
4. Gilden DH: Bell's palsy, *N Engl J Med* 351:1323, 2004.
5. Yamamoto L, Texas V: Guillain-Barré syndrome versus electrolyte imbalances: comorbidities that complicate the neurologic examination, *Top Emerg Med* 26:186, 2004.
6. Hughes R: *Campylobacter jejuni* in Guillain-Barré syndrome, *Lancet Neurol* 3:644, 2004.
7. Kuwabara S: Guillain-Barré syndrome: epidemiology, pathophysiology, and management, *Drugs* 64:597, 2004.
8. Centers for Disease Control and Prevention: Botulism. Available at *www.cdc.gov/ncidod/dbmd/diseaseinfo/botulism* (accessed November 25, 2005).
9. Goonetilleke A, Harris JB: Clostridial neurotoxins, *J Neurol Neurosurg Psychiatry* 75(Suppl III):35, 2004.
10. Centers for Disease Control and Prevention: Tetanus. Available at *www.cdc.gov/nip/publications/pink/tetanus* (accessed November 25, 2005).
11. Centers for Disease Control and Prevention, National Center for Injury Prevention and Control: Spinal cord injury (SCI): fact sheet. Available at *www.cdc.gov/ncipc/factsheets/scifacts.htm* (accessed November 25, 2005).
12. Spinal Cord Injury Information Network: Facts and figures at a glance—August 2004. Available at *www.spinalcord.uab.edu* (accessed November 25, 2005).
13. Norenberg MD, Smith J, Marcillo A: The pathology of human spinal cord injury: defining the problems, *J Neurotrauma* 21:429, 2004.
14. Ditunno JF, Little JW, Tessler A, et al: Spinal shock revisited: a four-phase model, *Spinal Cord* 42:383, 2004.
15. Royster RA, Barboi C, Peruzzi WT: Critical care in the acute cervical spinal cord injury, *Top Spinal Cord Injury Rehabil* 9:11, 2004.
16. American Spinal Injury Association/International Medical Society of Paraplegia (ASIA/IMSOP): *International standards for neurological functional classification of spinal cord injury patients* (revised), Chicago, 2002, American Spinal Injury Association.
17. Burns SP, Nelson AL, Bosshart HT, et al: Implementation of clinical practice guidelines for prevention of thromboembolism in spinal cord injury, *J Spinal Cord Med* 28:33, 2005.
18. Kishan S, Vives MJ, Reiter MF: Timing of surgery following spinal cord injury, *J Spinal Cord Med* 28:11, 2005.
19. Bracken MB, Holford TR: Neurological and functional status 1 year after acute spinal cord injury: estimates of functional recovery in National Acute Spinal Cord Injury Study II from results modeled in National Acute Spinal Cord Injury Study III, *J Neurosurg* 96:259, 2002.
20. Bracken MB: Steroids for acute spinal cord injury, Cochrane Injuries Group, *Cochrane Database Syst Rev* 4:CD001046, 2005.
21. McCutcheon EP, Selassie AW, Gu JK, et al: Acute traumatic spinal cord injury, 1993–2000. A population-based assessment of methylprednisolone administration and hospitalization, *J Trauma Injury Infect Crit Care* 56:1076, 2004.
22. Dobkin BH, Havton LA: Basic advances and new avenues in therapy of spinal cord injury, *Ann Rev Med* 55:255, 2004.
23. Bravo G, Guizar-Sahagun G, Ibarra A, et al: Cardiovascular alterations after spinal cord injury: an overview, *Curr Medicinal Chem Cardiovasc Hematol Agents* 2:133, 2004.
24. Patel RV, DeLong W, Vresilovic EJ: Evaluation and treatment of spinal injuries in the patient with polytrauma, *Clin Orthop Rel Res* 422:43, 2004.
25. March A: A review of respiratory management in spinal cord injury, *J Orthop Nurs* 9:19, 2005.
26. Krassioukov A: Autonomic dysreflexia in acute spinal cord injury: incidence, mechanisms, and management, *Sci Nurs* 21:215, 2004.
27. Holloway NM: *Medical-surgical care planning,* ed 4, Philadelphia, 2004, Lippincott Williams & Wilkins.

28. DeForge D, Blackmer J, Moher D, et al: Sexuality and reproductive health following spinal cord injury, *Evidence Report/Technology Assessment No 109* (AHRQ Publication No 05-E003-2), Rockville, Md, 2004, Agency for Healthcare Research and Quality. Available at *www.ncbi.nlm.nih.gov/ books/bv.fcgi?rid=hstat1a.chapter.76018.*

29. Lohne V, Severinsson E: Patients' experiences of hope and suffering during the first year following acute spinal cord injury, *J Clin Nurs* 14:285, 2005.

30. Meade MA, Taylor A, Kreutzer JS, et al: A preliminary study of acute family needs after spinal cord injury: analysis and implications, *Rehabil Psychol* 49:150, 2004.

31. Gittler MS: Acute rehabilitation in cervical spinal cord injury, *Top Spinal Cord Injury Rehabil* 9:60, 2004.

32. Trojan DA, Cashman NR: Post-poliomyelitis syndrome, *Muscle Nerve* 31:6, 2005.

RESOURCES

American Association of Spinal Cord Injury Nurses (AASCIN)
718-803-3782
www.aascin.org

American Paraplegia Society
718-803-3782
www.apssci.org

Canadian Paraplegic Association
800-720-4933 or 613-723-1033
Fax: 613-723-1060
www.canparaplegic.org

Christopher Reeve Paralysis Foundation
800-225-0292
www.christopherreeve.org

Guillain-Barré Syndrome Foundation International
www.guillain-barre.com

National Institute of Neurological Disorders and Stroke (NINDS)
800-352-9424 or 301-496-5751
www.ninds.nih.gov

National Rehabilitation Information Center (NARIC)
800-346-2742 or 301-459-5900
www.naric.com

National Spinal Cord Injury Association
800-962-9629 or 301-214-4006
www.spinalcord.org

Paralyzed Veterans of America
800-424-8200
www.pva.org

Spinal Cord Society
218-739-5252 or 218-739-5261
http://members.aol.com/scsweb

For additional Internet resources, see the website for this book at *http://evolve. elsevier.com/Lewis/medsurg.*

62

Nursing Assessment
Musculoskeletal System

Dottie Roberts

LEARNING OBJECTIVES

1. Describe the gross anatomic and microscopic composition of bone.
2. Explain the classification system of joints and movements at synovial joints.
3. Describe the types and structure of muscle tissue.
4. Describe the functions of cartilage, muscles, ligaments, tendons, fascia, and bursae.
5. Describe age-related changes in the musculoskeletal system and differences in assessment findings.
6. Identify the significant subjective and objective data related to the musculoskeletal system that should be obtained from a patient.
7. Describe the appropriate techniques used in the physical assessment of the musculoskeletal system.
8. Differentiate normal from abnormal findings of a physical assessment of the musculoskeletal system.
9. Describe the purpose, significance of results, and nursing responsibilities related to diagnostic studies of the musculoskeletal system.

KEY TERMS

ankylosis,* p. 1623
arthrocentesis, p. 1627
arthroscopy, p. 1624
atrophy,* p. 1623
contracture,* p. 1623
crepitation,* p. 1623
isometric contractions, p. 1618
isotonic contractions, p. 1618
kyphosis,* p. 1623
lordosis,* p. 1623

*See Table 62-6 on pp. 1623-1624.

Electronic Resources

Supplemental content related to Chapter 62 can be found . . .

Companion CD
- Stress-Busting Kit for Nursing Students
- NCLEX Examination Review Questions
- Animations:
  - Classification of Joints: Condyloid Joint
  - Classification of Joints: Gliding Joint—Hand
  - Classification of Joints: Hinge Joint
- Video Clips:
  - Inspection: Gait in Older Adult
  - Inspection: General Muscular Strength
  - Inspection and Palpation: Muscular Development
- Comprehensive Glossary

Evolve Website *evolve*
http://evolve.elsevier.com/Lewis/medsurg
- Content Updates
- Key Points (Printable and CD/MP3 Download)
- Concept Map Creator
- Expanded Audio Glossary
- Key Term Flash Cards
- Electronic Calculators
- Physical Examination Video Clips:
  - Neck
  - Upper Extremities

- Back and Posterior Chest
- Anterior Chest, Lungs, and Heart
- Abdominal Reflexes, Abdominal Muscles, and Inguinal Area
- Feet, Legs, and Hips
- Musculoskeletal Function
- Spine
- WebLinks

The unique structures of the musculoskeletal system allow human beings to complete complex movements in their interactions with the environment. The dexterity of the upper extremities enables an individual to perform complicated technical tasks, while stronger lower extremities allow mobility for varied activities. The musculoskeletal system is composed of voluntary muscle and five types of connective tissue: bones, cartilage, ligaments, tendons, and fascia.[1]

Resilient bone and cartilage absorb energy from any impact, minimizing the risk of injury to other body structures. However, this characteristic ability makes the musculoskeletal system itself particularly vulnerable to injury from external forces. Any damage to bone and related soft tissues can cause functional disruption for an individual. Deformity, alteration in body image and mobility, self-care deficit, pain, or permanent disability may result from musculoskeletal injury.

Reviewed by Jan Foecke, RN, MS, ONC, Orthopedic Operations and Clinical Resource Specialist, Providence Medical Center, Kansas City, Kan.

STRUCTURES AND FUNCTIONS OF THE MUSCULOSKELETAL SYSTEM

Bone

Function. The main functions of bone are support, protection of internal organs, voluntary movement, blood cell production, and mineral storage.[2] Bones provide the supporting framework that keeps the body from collapsing and also allow the body to bear weight. Bones also protect underlying vital organs and tissues. For example, the skull encloses the brain, the vertebrae surround the spinal cord, and the rib cage contains the lungs and heart. Bones serve as a point of attachment for muscles, which are connected to bones by tendons. Bones act as a lever for muscles, and movement occurs as a result of muscle contractions applied to these levers. Bones contain hematopoietic tissue for the production of red and white blood cells. Bones also serve as a site for storage of inorganic minerals such as calcium and phosphorus.

Bone was previously considered to be a static, inert substance. In reality, it is a dynamic tissue that continually changes form and composition. It contains both organic material (collagen) and inorganic material (calcium, phosphate). The internal and external growth and remodeling of bone are ongoing processes. Bone is classified according to structure as *cortical* (compact and dense) or *cancellous* (spongy).

Microscopic Structure. Cylinder-shaped structural units (*haversian* systems) fit closely together in compact bone, creating a dense bone structure (Fig. 62-1, *A*). Within the systems, the haversian canals run parallel to the bone's long axis and contain the blood vessels that travel to the bone's interior from the periosteum.

Surrounding the haversian canals are concentric rings known as *lamellae,* which characterize mature bone. Smaller canals (*canaliculi*) extend from the haversian canals to the *lacunae,* where mature bone cells are embedded. Cancellous bone lacks the organized structure of cortical (compact) bone. The lamellae are not arranged in concentric rings but rather along the lines of maximum stress placed on the bone. Networks of bone tissue are filled with red or yellow marrow, and blood reaches the bone cells by passing through spaces in the marrow.

The three types of bone cells are osteoblasts, osteocytes, and osteoclasts. *Osteoblasts* synthesize organic bone matrix (collagen) and are the basic bone-forming cells. *Osteocytes* are the mature bone cells. *Osteoclasts* participate in bone remodeling by assisting in the breakdown of bone tissue. *Bone remodeling* is the removal of old bone by osteoclasts (*resorption*) and the deposition of new bone by osteoblasts (*ossification*). The inner layer of bone is primarily made up of osteoblasts with a few osteoclasts.

Gross Structure. The anatomic structure of bone is best represented by a typical long bone such as the humerus (see Fig. 62-1, *B*). Each long bone consists of the epiphysis, the diaphysis, and the metaphysis. The *epiphysis,* the widened area found at each end of a long bone, is composed primarily of cancellous bone. The wide epiphysis allows for greater weight distribution and provides stability for the joint. The epiphysis is also the location of muscle attachment. Articular cartilage covers the ends of the epiphysis to provide a smooth surface for joint movement. The *diaphysis* is the main shaft of the bone. It provides structural support and is composed of compact bone. The tubular structure of the diaphysis allows it to more easily withstand bending and

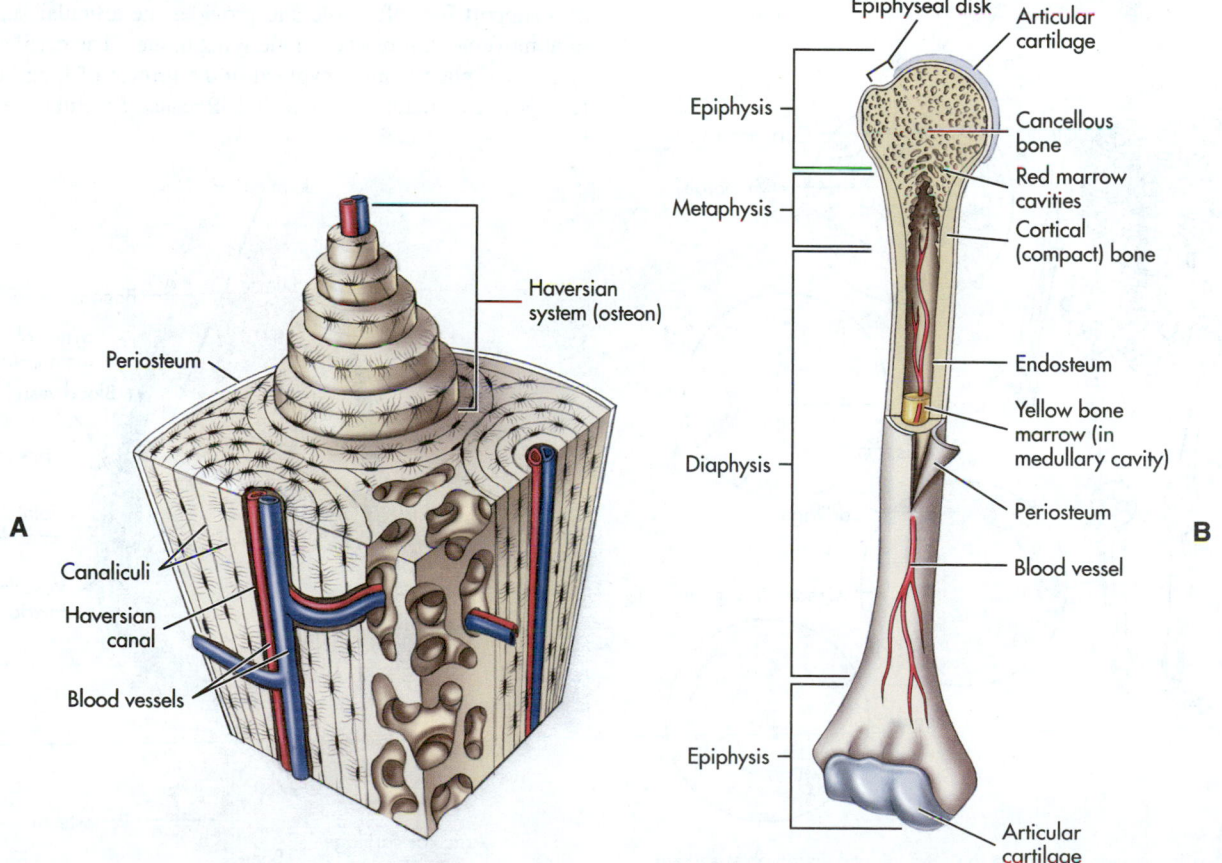

FIG. 62-1 Bone structure. **A,** Cortical (compact) bone showing haversian system. **B,** Anatomy of a long bone (humerus).

twisting forces. The *metaphysis* is the flared area between the epiphysis and the diaphysis. Like the epiphysis, it is composed of cancellous bone. The *epiphyseal plate,* or growth zone, is the cartilaginous area between the epiphysis and metaphysis. It actively produces bone to allow longitudinal growth in children. Injury to the epiphyseal plate in a growing child can lead to a shorter extremity that can cause significant functional problems. In the adult, the metaphysis and epiphysis become joined as this plate hardens to mature bone.

The *periosteum* is composed of fibrous connective tissue that covers the bone. Tiny blood vessels penetrate the periosteum to provide nutrition to underlying bone. Musculotendinous fibers anchor to the outer layer of the periosteum. The inner layer of the periosteum is attached to the bone by bundles of collagen. No periosteum exists on the articular surfaces of long bones. These bone ends are covered by articular cartilage.

The medullary (marrow) cavity is in the center of the diaphysis and contains either red or yellow bone marrow.[3] In the growing child, red bone marrow is actively involved in blood cell production (hematopoiesis). In the adult, the medullary cavity of long bones contains yellow bone marrow, which is mainly adipose tissue. Yellow marrow will only be involved in hematopoiesis in times of great blood cell need. Blood cell production in the adult normally occurs in the red bone marrow of the skull, ribs, sternum, pelvis, vertebrae, and shoulder bones.

Types. The skeleton consists of 206 bones, which are classified according to shape as long, short, flat, or irregular.

Long bones are characterized by a central shaft (diaphysis) and two widened ends (epiphyses) (see Fig. 62-1, *B*). Examples include the femur, humerus, and radius. Short bones are composed of cancellous bone covered by a thin layer of compact bone. Examples include the carpals in the hand and the tarsals in the foot.

Flat bones have two layers of compact bone separated by a layer of cancellous bone. Examples include the ribs, skull, scapula, and sternum. The spaces in the cancellous bone contain bone marrow. Irregular bones appear in a variety of shapes and sizes. Examples include the vertebrae, sacrum, and mandible.

Joints

A *joint* (articulation) is a place where the ends of two bones are in proximity and move in relation to each other. Joints are classified according to the degree of movement that they allow (Fig. 62-2).

The most common joint is the freely movable *diarthrodial* (synovial) type. Each joint is enclosed in a capsule of fibrous connective tissue, which joins the two bones together to form a cavity (Fig. 62-3). The capsule is lined by a synovial membrane, which secretes a thick synovial fluid to lubricate the joint, reduce friction, and allow for sliding of opposing surfaces. The end of each bone is covered with articular (hyaline) cartilage. Supporting structures (e.g., ligaments, tendons) reinforce the joint capsule and provide limits and stability to joint movement.[4] Types of diarthrodial joints are shown in Fig. 62-4.

Cartilage

Cartilage is a rigid connective tissue in synovial joints that serves as a support for soft tissue and provides the articular surface for joint movement. It protects underlying tissues. The cartilage in the epiphyseal plate is also involved in the growth of long bones before physical maturity is reached. Because articular cartilage is

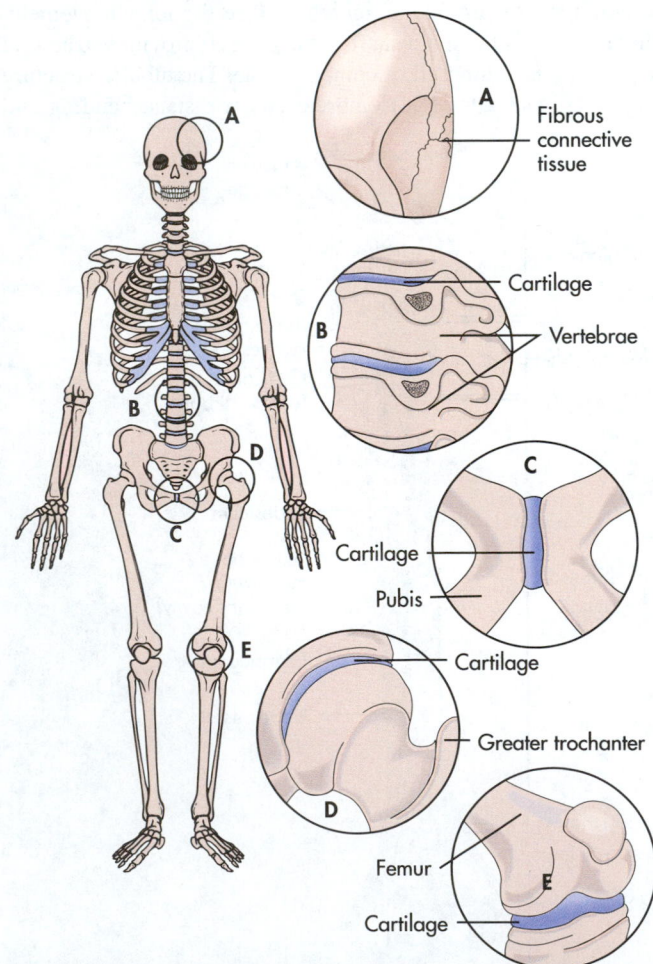

FIG. 62-2   Classification of joints. **A** to **C,** Synarthrotic (immovable) and amphiarthrotic (slightly movable) joints. **D** and **E,** Diarthrodial (freely movable) joints.

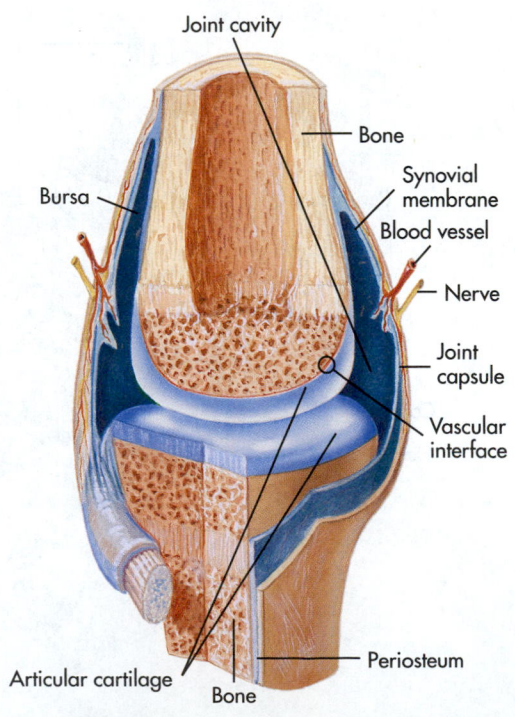

FIG. 62-3   Structure of synovial joint.

Joint	Movement	Examples	Illustration
Hinge joint	Flexion, extension	Elbow joint (shown), interphalangeal joints, knee joint	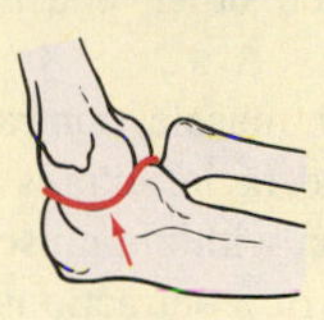
Ball and socket (spheroidal)	Flexion, extension; adduction, abduction; circumduction	Shoulder (shown), hip	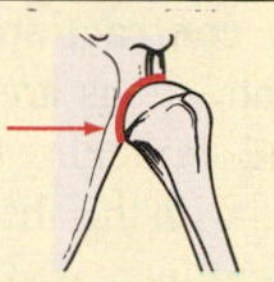
Pivot (rotary)	Rotation	Atlas-axis, proximal radioulnar joint (shown)	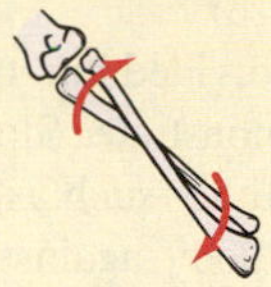
Condyloid	Flexion, extension; abduction, adduction; circumduction	Wrist joint (between radial and carpals) (shown)	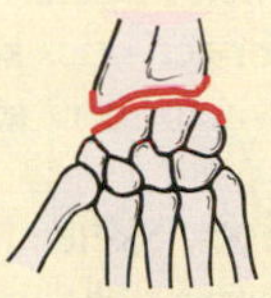
Saddle	Flexion, extension; abduction, adduction; circumduction, thumb-finger opposition	Carpometacarpal joint of thumb	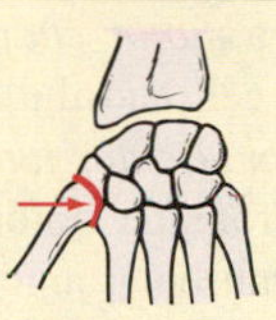
Gliding	One surface moves over another surface	Between tarsal bones, sacroiliac joint, between articular processes of vertebrae, between carpal bones (shown)	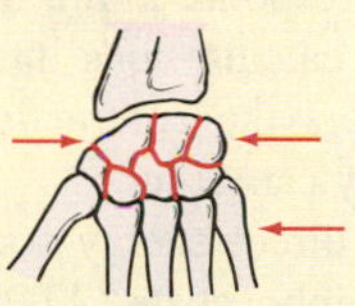

FIG. 62-4   Types of diarthrodial (synovial) joints.

relatively avascular, it must receive nourishment by the diffusion of material from the synovial fluid. The lack of a direct blood supply contributes to the slow metabolism of cartilage cells and explains why cartilage tissue heals slowly.

The three types of cartilage tissue are hyaline, elastic, and fibrous. *Hyaline cartilage,* the most common, contains a moderate amount of collagen fibers. It is found in the trachea, bronchi, nose, epiphyseal plate, and articular surfaces of bones. *Elastic cartilage,* which contains both collagen and elastic fibers, is more flexible than hyaline cartilage. It is found in the ear, epiglottis, and larynx. *Fibrous cartilage* (fibrocartilage) consists mostly of collagen fibers and is a tough tissue that often functions as a shock absorber. It is found between the vertebral disks and also forms a protective cushion between the bones of the pelvic girdle, knee, and shoulder.

Muscle

Types. The three types of muscle tissue are *cardiac* (striated, involuntary), *smooth* (nonstriated, involuntary), and *skeletal* (striated, voluntary) muscle. Cardiac muscle is found in the heart. Its spontaneous contractions propel blood through the circulatory system. Smooth muscle occurs in the walls of hollow structures such as airways, arteries, gastrointestinal (GI) tract, urinary bladder, and uterus. Smooth muscle contraction is modulated by neuronal and hormonal influences. Skeletal muscle, which requires neuronal stimulation for contraction, accounts for about half of a human being's body weight. It is the focus of the following discussion.

Structure. The entire muscle is enclosed by the *epimysium,* a continuous layer of deep fascia. The epimysium helps muscles to slide over nearby structures. Connective tissue surrounding and extending into the muscle can be subdivided into fiber bundles or *fasciculi.* These bundles are covered by *perimysium* and an innermost connective tissue layer called the *endomysium* that surrounds each fiber.

The structural unit of muscle is the muscle cell or muscle fiber, which is highly specialized for contraction. Skeletal muscle fibers are long, multinucleated cylinders that contain many mitochondria to support their high metabolic activity. Muscle fibers are composed of myofibrils, which in turn are made up of contractile filaments (protein). The *sarcomere* is the contractile unit of the myofibrils.[5] Each sarcomere consists of myosin (thick) filaments and actin (thin) filaments. The arrangement of the thin and thick filaments accounts for the characteristic banding of muscle when it is seen under a microscope. Muscle contraction occurs as thick and thin filaments slide past each other, causing the sarcomeres to shorten.

Contractions. Skeletal muscle contractions allow posture maintenance, movement, and facial expressions. **Isometric contractions** increase the tension within a muscle but do not produce movement. Repeated isometric contractions make muscles grow larger and stronger. **Isotonic contractions** shorten a muscle to produce movement. Most contractions are a combination of tension generation (isometric) and shortening (isotonic). Muscular atrophy (decrease in size) occurs with the absence of contraction that results from immobility, whereas increased muscular activity leads to *hypertrophy* (increase in size).

Skeletal muscle fibers are divided into two groups based on the type of activity that they demonstrate. Slow-twitch muscle fibers support prolonged muscle activity such as marathon running. Because they also support the body against gravity, they assist in posture maintenance. Fast-twitch muscle fibers are used for rapid muscle contraction required for activities such as blinking the eye, jumping, or sprinting. Fast-twitch fibers tend to tire more readily than slow-twitch fibers.

Neuromuscular Junction. Skeletal muscle fibers require a nerve impulse to contract. A nerve fiber and the skeletal muscle fibers it stimulates are called a *motor endplate*. The junction between the axon of the nerve cell and the adjacent muscle cell is called the *myoneural* or *neuromuscular junction* (Fig. 62-5).

Acetylcholine is released from the motor endplate of the neuron and diffuses across the neuromuscular junction to bind with receptors on the muscle fiber. In response to this stimulation, the sarcoplasmic reticulum releases calcium ions into the cytoplasm. The presence of calcium triggers the contraction in the myofibrils. When calcium is low, tetany can occur.

Energy Source. The direct energy source for muscle fiber contractions is adenosine triphosphate (ATP). ATP is synthesized by cellular oxidative metabolism in numerous mitochondria located close to the myofibrils. It is rapidly depleted through conversion to adenosine diphosphate (ADP) and must be rephosphorylated. Phosphocreatine provides a rapid source for the resynthesis of ATP, but it is in turn converted to creatine and must be recharged. Glycolysis can serve as a source of ATP when the oxygen supply is inadequate for the metabolic needs of the muscle tissue.

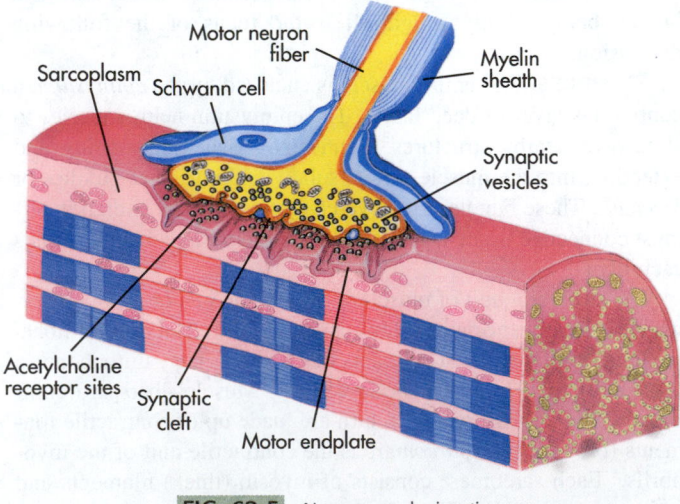

FIG. 62-5   Neuromuscular junction.

Motor neuron fiber
Sarcoplasm
Schwann cell
Myelin sheath
Synaptic vesicles
Acetylcholine receptor sites
Synaptic cleft
Motor endplate

Glucose is broken down to pyruvic acid, which can be further converted to lactic acid to make more oxygen available. An accumulation of lactic acid in tissues leads to fatigue and pain.

Ligaments and Tendons

Ligaments and tendons are both composed of dense, fibrous connective tissue that contains bundles of closely packed collagen fibers arranged in the same plane for additional strength. Tendons attach muscles to bones as an extension of the muscle sheath that adheres to the periosteum. Ligaments connect bones to bones (e.g., tibia to femur at knee joint). They have a higher elastic content than tendons.[6] Ligaments provide stability while permitting controlled movement at the joint.

Ligaments and tendons have a relatively poor blood supply, usually making tissue repair a slow process after injury. For example, the stretching or tearing of ligaments that occurs with a sprain may require a long time to mend.

Fascia

Fascia refers to layers of connective tissue with intermeshed fibers that can withstand limited stretching. Superficial fascia lies immediately under the skin. Deep fascia is a dense, fibrous tissue that surrounds the muscle bundles, nerves, and blood vessels. It also encloses individual muscles, allowing them to act independently and to glide over each other during contraction. In addition, fascia provides strength to muscle tissues.

Bursae

Bursae are small sacs of connective tissue lined with synovial membrane and containing synovial fluid. They are typically located at bony prominences or joints to relieve pressure and prevent friction between moving parts. For example, bursae are found between the patella and the skin (prepatellar bursa), between the olecranon process of the elbow and the skin (olecranon bursa), between the head of the humerus and the acromion process of the scapula (subacromial bursa), and between the greater trochanter of the proximal femur and the skin (trochanteric bursa). *Bursitis* is an inflammation of a bursa sac. The inflammation may be acute or chronic.

GERONTOLOGIC CONSIDERATIONS
EFFECTS OF AGING ON THE MUSCULOSKELETAL SYSTEM

Many of the functional problems experienced by the aging adult are related to changes of the musculoskeletal system. Although some changes begin in early adulthood, obvious signs of musculoskeletal impairment may not appear until later adult years. Alterations may affect the older adult's ability to complete self-care tasks and pursue other customary activities. Effects of musculoskeletal changes may range from mild discomfort and decreased ability to perform activities of daily living to severe, chronic pain and immobility. The risk for falls also increases in the older adult.

The bone remodeling process is altered in the aging adult. Increased bone resorption and decreased bone formation cause a loss of bone density, contributing to development of osteopenia and osteoporosis (see Chapter 64). Muscle mass and strength also decrease with aging. Almost 30% of muscle mass is lost by the 70s. A loss of motor neurons can cause additional problems

TABLE 62-1	*GERONTOLOGIC DIFFERENCES IN ASSESSMENT* Musculoskeletal System	

Changes	Differences in Assessment Findings
Muscle	
Decreased number and diameter of muscle cells; replacement of muscle cells by fibrous connective tissue	Decreased muscle strength and bulk; abdominal protrusion; flabby muscle Increased rigidity in neck, shoulders, hips, and knees
Loss of elasticity in ligaments and cartilage	Decreased fine motor dexterity, decreased agility
Reduced ability to store glycogen; decreased ability to release glycogen as quick energy during stress	Slowed reaction times and reflexes as a result of slowing of impulse conduction along motor units; earlier fatigue with activity
Joints	
Increased risk for cartilage erosion that contributes to direct contact between bone ends and overgrowth of bone around joint margins	Joint stiffness, decreased mobility, limited ROM, possible crepitation on movement; pain with motion and/or weight bearing
Loss of water from disks between vertebrae; narrowing of intervertebral spaces	Loss of height from disk compression; posture change
Bone	
Decrease in bone density	Loss of height from vertebral compression, back pain; deformity such as dowager's hump (kyphosis) caused by vertebral compression

ROM, Range of motion.

with skeletal muscle movement. Tendons and ligaments become less flexible, and movement becomes more rigid. Joints in the aging adult are also more likely to be affected by osteoarthritis (see Chapter 65).

In addition to the usual musculoskeletal assessment with a particular emphasis on exercise practices, the nurse should determine the impact of age-related changes of the musculoskeletal system on the functional status of the older patient. The nurse should identify any musculoskeletal changes that increase the patient's risk for falls, and discuss fall prevention strategies.[7] Functional limitations that are accepted by older adults as a normal part of aging can often be halted or reversed with appropriate preventive strategies (see Chapter 63, Table 63-1).

Diseases such as osteoarthritis and osteoporosis are not the normal consequences of growing old. The nurse should carefully differentiate between expected changes and the effects of disease in the aging adult. Symptoms of disease can be treated in many cases, helping the older adult to return to a higher functional level. Age-related changes in the musculoskeletal system and differences in assessment findings are presented in Table 62-1.

ASSESSMENT OF THE MUSCULOSKELETAL SYSTEM

Correct diagnosis of any complaint depends on a complete patient history and thorough physical examination. Musculoskeletal assessment can focus on a specific body part, or it can be done as part of a general physical examination or as an examination in itself. The nurse uses the patient's complaint as a guide in selecting all or part of the components of the musculoskeletal history and physical examination. For example, accidents may result in multisystem trauma. Because serious or life-threatening injuries do not usually involve the musculoskeletal system, critical information about the patient's condition is obtained to support immediate treatment. A complete assessment of the musculoskeletal system may be deferred for the secondary survey.

The most common symptoms of musculoskeletal impairment include pain, weakness, deformity, limitation of movement, stiffness, and joint crepitation. Information should also be sought about changes in sensation or in the size of a muscle.

Subjective Data

Important Health Information. Appropriate questions to ask during a musculoskeletal assessment are included in Table 62-2.

Past Health History. Because certain illnesses are known to affect the musculoskeletal system either directly or indirectly, the nurse should carefully question the patient about past medical problems. These include tuberculosis, poliomyelitis, diabetes mellitus, parathyroid problems, hemophilia, rickets, scurvy, soft tissue infection, and neuromuscular disabilities. In addition, past or developing musculoskeletal problems can affect the patient's overall health. Trauma to the musculoskeletal system is a common reason for seeking medical evaluation. Questions should also focus on symptoms of arthritic and connective tissue diseases (e.g., gout, psoriatic arthritis, systemic lupus erythematosus), osteomalacia, osteomyelitis, and fungal infection of the bones or joints. The patient should also be asked about possible sources of a secondary bacterial infection, such as the ears, tonsils, teeth, sinuses, lungs, or genitourinary tract. These infections can enter the bones, resulting in osteomyelitis. A detailed account of the course and treatment of any of these problems should be obtained.

Medications. The nurse should carefully question the patient regarding prescription and over-the-counter drugs and herbal products and nutritional supplements (see the Complementary and Alternative Therapies box in Chapter 4 on p. 44). Detailed information should be obtained about each treatment, including its name, the dose and frequency, length of time it was taken, its effects, and any possible side effects. Specific inquiry should be made about skeletal muscle relaxants, opioids, nonsteroidal antiinflammatory drugs, and systemic and topical corticosteroids. The patient who has taken antiinflammatory drugs should be questioned about GI distress or signs of bleeding.

In addition to drugs taken for treatment of a musculoskeletal problem, the patient should be questioned about drugs that can have detrimental effects on this system. These drugs and their potential side effects include antiseizure drugs (osteomalacia), phenothiazines (gait disturbances), corticosteroids (avascular necrosis, decreased bone and muscle mass), and potassium-depleting diuretics (muscle cramps and weakness). Women should be questioned

TABLE 62-2	*HEALTH HISTORY* **Musculoskeletal System**

Health Perception–Health Management Pattern
- Describe your usual daily activities.
- Do you experience any difficulties performing these activities?* Describe what you do if you experience difficulty in dressing, preparing meals and feeding yourself, performing basic hygiene, or maintaining your home.
- Do you use any mechanical assistive devices?*
- Do you have to lift heavy objects? Describe any specialized equipment you use or wear when you work or exercise that helps protect you from injury.
- What other safety precautions do you take?
- Do you take any drugs or herbal products to manage your musculoskeletal problem? If so, what are their names and what are the expected effects?
- When did you have your last tetanus and polio immunizations? When were you last tested for tuberculosis?

Nutritional-Metabolic Pattern
- Give a 24-hr diet recall.
- What dietary supplements do you take? (Ask specifically about calcium, vitamin D supplements, and herbal products.)
- What is your weight? Describe any recent weight loss or gain. Were your musculoskeletal symptoms affected by the change in your weight?*

Elimination Pattern
- Does your musculoskeletal problem make it difficult for you to reach the toilet in time?*
- Do you need any assistive devices or equipment to achieve satisfactory toileting?*
- Do you experience constipation related to decreased mobility or to drugs taken for your musculoskeletal problem?*

Activity-Exercise Pattern
- Do you require assistance in completing your usual daily activities because of a musculoskeletal problem?*
- Describe your usual exercise pattern. Do you experience musculoskeletal symptoms before, during, or after exercising?*
- Are you able to move all your joints comfortably through full range of motion? Describe any limitations in mobility.
- Do you use any prosthetic or orthotic devices?*

Sleep-Rest Pattern
- Do you experience any difficulty sleeping because of a musculoskeletal problem?* Do you require frequent position changes at night?*
- Do you wake up at night because of musculoskeletal pain?*

Cognitive-Perceptual Pattern
- Describe any musculoskeletal pain you experience. How do you manage your pain? (Ask specifically about adjunctive therapies such as heat and cold or alternative therapies such as acupuncture.)

Self-Perception–Self-Concept Pattern
- Describe how changes in your musculoskeletal system (posture, walking, muscle strength) and decreased ability to do certain things have affected how you feel about yourself. How have these changes affected your lifestyle?

Role-Relationship Pattern
- Do you live alone?
- Describe how family members or others assist you with your musculoskeletal problem.
- Describe the effect of your musculoskeletal problem on your work and on your social relationships.

Sexuality-Reproductive Pattern
- Describe any sexual concerns related to your musculoskeletal problem.

Coping–Stress Tolerance Pattern
- Describe how you deal with problems such as pain or immobility that have resulted from your musculoskeletal problem.

Value-Belief Pattern
- Describe any cultural practices or religious beliefs that may influence the treatment of your musculoskeletal problem.

*If yes, describe.

---

about their menstrual history. Episodes of amenorrhea can contribute to early development of osteoporosis. Questions about the use of hormone replacement therapy are important for postmenopausal women. Calcium and vitamin D supplements should be inquired about for both women and men.

Surgery or Other Treatments. Information should be obtained about past hospitalizations from a musculoskeletal problem. The nurse should carefully document the reason for hospitalization, the date and duration, and the treatment, including ongoing rehabilitation. Details of emergency treatment for musculoskeletal injuries should also be sought. Specific information should also be obtained regarding any surgical procedure, postoperative course, and complications. If the patient experienced a period of prolonged immobilization, the development of osteoporosis and muscle atrophy should be considered.

Functional Health Patterns. The use of functional health patterns assists the nurse in organizing the assessment data and formulating diagnoses based on information collected about the musculoskeletal system. Table 62-2 summarizes specific questions to ask in relation to functional health patterns.

Health Perception–Health Management Pattern. The nurse should ask about the patient's health practices related to the musculoskeletal system, such as maintenance of a normal body weight, avoidance of excessive stress on muscles and joints, and the use of proper body mechanics when lifting objects.[8]

The patient should be specifically questioned about tetanus and polio immunizations. The most current date and reaction to a tuberculin skin test should also be obtained.

Food or contact allergies have little direct relation to musculoskeletal problems, but the general malaise often associated with allergic reactions may manifest in musculoskeletal stiffness and lethargy. Allergic reactions to drugs used to treat musculoskeletal problems can be significant if they interfere with therapy.

The patient who is a good historian can recount numerous minor and major injuries of the musculoskeletal system. Information should be recorded chronologically and should include the following:

1. Mechanism of the injury (e.g., twist, crush, stretch)
2. Circumstances related to the injury
3. Diagnostic evaluations
4. Methods of treatment

5. Duration of treatment
6. Current status related to the injury
7. Need for assistive devices
8. Interference with activities of daily living

A family history should be obtained related to rheumatoid arthritis, systemic lupus erythematosus, osteoarthritis, gout, osteoporosis, and scoliosis because a patient may have genetic predisposition to these or other musculoskeletal disorders.

Safety practices can affect the patient's predisposition for certain injuries and illnesses. Therefore the nurse should ask the patient about safety practices as they relate to work environment, home life, recreation, and exercise. For example, if the patient is a computer programmer, the nurse should ask about ergonomic adaptations in the office that decrease the risk of carpal tunnel syndrome or low back pain. Identification of problems in this area will direct the plan for patient teaching.

Nutritional-Metabolic Pattern. The patient's description of a typical day's diet provides clues to areas of nutritional concern that can affect the musculoskeletal system. Adequate amounts of vitamins C and D, calcium, and protein are essential for a healthy, intact musculoskeletal system. Abnormal nutritional patterns can predispose individuals to problems such as osteomalacia and osteoporosis. In addition, maintenance of normal weight is an important nutritional goal. Obesity places additional stress on weight-bearing joints such as the knees, hips, and spine, and it predisposes individuals to ligamentous instability.

Elimination Pattern. Questions about the patient's mobility may reveal difficulty with ambulating to the toilet. The patient should be asked if an assistive device such as an elevated toilet seat or a grab bar is necessary to accomplish toileting. Decreased mobility secondary to a musculoskeletal problem can lead to constipation. In addition, musculoskeletal problems can contribute to bowel or bladder incontinence.

Activity-Exercise Pattern. The nurse should obtain a detailed account of the type, duration, and frequency of exercise and recreational activities. Daily, weekend, and seasonal patterns should be compared because occasional or sporadic exercise can be more problematic than regular exercise. Many musculoskeletal problems can affect the patient's activity-exercise pattern. The nurse should question the patient about limitations in movement, pain, weakness, clumsiness, crepitus, or any change in the bones or joints that interferes with daily activities.

Extremes of activity related to occupation can also affect the musculoskeletal system. A sedentary occupation can negatively impact muscle flexibility and strength. Jobs that require extreme effort through heavy lifting or pushing can lead to damage of joints and supporting structures. The nurse should specifically question the patient about work-related injuries to the musculoskeletal system, including treatment and time lost from work.

Sleep-Rest Pattern. The discomfort caused by musculoskeletal disorders can interfere with a normal sleep pattern. The patient should be questioned about possible alterations in sleep patterns. If the patient describes sleep interference related to a musculoskeletal problem, the nurse should inquire further about the type of bedding and pillows used, bedtime routine, sleeping partner, and sleeping positions.

Cognitive-Perceptual Pattern. Any pain experienced by the patient as a result of a musculoskeletal problem should be fully explored and documented. To provide a baseline for later reassessment, the patient should be asked to describe the intensity of the pain on a scale from 1 to 10 (0 = no pain, 10 = most severe pain imaginable). Reassessments over time will assist in determining the effectiveness of any treatment plan. The patient should also be questioned about measures used at home for pain management and about related problems such as joint swelling or muscle weakness. (Pain is discussed in Chapter 10.)

Self-Perception–Self-Concept Pattern. Many chronic musculoskeletal problems lead to deformities and a reduction in activities that can have a serious negative impact on the patient's body image and sense of personal worth. The nurse should address the patient's feelings about each of these changes.

Role-Relationship Pattern. Impaired mobility and chronic pain from musculoskeletal problems can negatively affect the patient's ability to perform in roles of spouse, parent, or employee. The ability to pursue and maintain meaningful social and personal relationships can also be affected by musculoskeletal problems. The nurse should carefully question the patient about role performance and relationships.

If the patient lives alone, the current musculoskeletal problem and its rehabilitation may make it difficult or impossible to continue this arrangement. The degree of assistance available from family, friends, and organized caregivers should be determined.

Sexuality-Reproductive Pattern. The pain of musculoskeletal problems can greatly affect the patient's ability to obtain sexual satisfaction. The nurse should sensitively explore this area, helping the patient feel comfortable in discussing any sexual problems related to pain, movement, and positioning.

Coping–Stress Tolerance Pattern. Mobility limitations and pain, whether acute or chronic, are serious potential stressors that challenge the patient's coping resources. The nurse must recognize the potential for ineffective coping in the patient and family or significant other. Additional questioning will help determine if a musculoskeletal problem is causing coping difficulties.

Value-Belief Pattern. The patient should be questioned about cultural or religious beliefs that might influence a patient's acceptance of care for the musculoskeletal problem.

Objective Data

Physical Examination. Examination involves observation, palpation, motion, and muscular assessment. Although a general overview will be conducted, data obtained in a careful health history will guide the nurse in choosing areas on which to concentrate the local examination. Specific measurements may be taken as indicated by the local examination.

Inspection. A systematic inspection is performed starting at the head and neck and proceeding to the upper extremities, the lower extremities, and the trunk. A specific order is not required, but the regular use of a systematic approach is important to avoid missing important aspects of the examination. The skin is inspected for general color, scars, or other overt signs of previous injury or surgery. Certain cutaneous lesions require additional investigation because they can represent underlying disorders. For example, café-au-lait spots are characteristic markers of neurofibromatosis. General body build, muscle configuration, and symmetry of joints are noted. The nurse observes any swelling, deformity, nodules or masses, and discrepancies in limb length or muscle size. The patient's opposite body part is used for comparison when an abnormality is suspected.

Palpation. Any area that has aroused concern because of a subjective complaint or appears abnormal on inspection should be carefully palpated. As with inspection, palpation usually proceeds cephalopedally (head to toe) to examine the neck, shoulders, elbows, wrists, hands, back, hips, knees, ankles, and feet. Both superficial and deep palpation are usually performed consecutively.

The nurse's hands should be warm to prevent muscle spasm, which can interfere with identification of essential landmarks or soft tissue structures. Palpation of both muscles and joints allows for evaluation of skin temperature, local tenderness, swelling, and crepitation. The nurse must establish the relationship of adjacent structures and evaluate the general contour, abnormal prominences, and local landmarks.

Motion. When assessing the patient's joint mobility, the nurse must carefully evaluate both passive and active **range of motion;** measurements should be similar for both maneuvers. *Active range of motion* means the patient takes his or her own joints through all movements without assistance. *Passive range of motion* occurs when someone else moves the patient's joints without his or her participation. The nurse should be cautious in performing passive range of motion because of the risk of injury to underlying structures. Manipulation must cease immediately if pain or resistance is encountered. If deficits in active or passive range of motion are noted, the nurse must also assess functional range of motion to determine if performance of activities of daily living has been affected by joint changes. This is done by asking the patient if activities such as eating and bathing must be performed with assistance or cannot be done at all.

Range of motion is most accurately assessed with a goniometer, which measures the angle of the joint (Fig. 62-6). Specific degrees of range of motion of all joints are usually not measured unless a musculoskeletal problem has been identified. A less exact but valuable assessment method is to compare the range of motion of one extremity with the range of motion on the opposite side. Common movements that occur at the synovial joints, including *abduction, adduction, flexion,* and *extension,* are described in Table 62-3.

Muscle-Strength Testing. The nurse grades the strength of individual muscles or groups of muscles during contraction (Table 62-4). Normal muscle strength should be graded as a "5" bilaterally, with full resistance to opposition. The patient should be instructed to apply resistance to the force exerted by the nurse. For example, the examiner tries to pull the bent arm down while the patient tries to raise it. Muscle strength should also be compared with the strength of the opposite extremity. Subtle variations in muscle strength may be noted when comparing the patient's dominant side with the nondominant side. Variations in strength also exist between individuals.

Measurement. When length discrepancies or subjective problems are noted, the nurse will often obtain limb length and circumferential muscle mass measurements. For example, leg length should be measured when gait disorders are observed. The affected limb is measured between the anterior-superior iliac crest and the bottom of the medial malleolus. It is then compared with the similar measurement of the opposite extremity. Muscle mass is measured circumferentially at the largest area of the muscle. When re-

TABLE 62-3	Movement at Synovial Joints
Movement	**Description**
Abduction	Movement of part away from midline of body
Adduction	Movement of part toward midline of body
Circumduction	Combination of flexion, extension, abduction, and adduction resulting in circular motion of a body part
Dorsiflexion	Flexion of the ankle and toes toward the shin
Eversion	Turning of sole outward away from midline of body
Extension	Straightening of joint that increases angle between two bones
External rotation	Movement along longitudinal axis away from midline of body
Flexion	Bending of joint as a result of muscle contraction that results in decreased angle between two bones
Hyperextension	Extension in which angle exceeds 180 degrees
Internal rotation	Movement along longitudinal axis toward midline of body
Inversion	Turning of sole inward toward midline of body
Opposition	Moving the first and fifth metacarpals anteriorly from a flattened palm ("cupping position"); makes it possible to hold objects between the thumb and fingers
Plantar flexion	Flexion of the ankle and toes toward the plantar surface of the foot ("toes pointed")
Pronation	Turning of palm downward
Supination	Turning of palm upward

TABLE 62-4	Muscle Strength Scale
0	No detection of muscular contraction
1	A barely detectable flicker or trace of contraction with observation or palpation
2	Active movement of body part with elimination of gravity
3	Active movement against gravity only and not against resistance
4	Active movement against gravity and some resistance
5	Active movement against full resistance without evident fatigue (normal muscle strength)

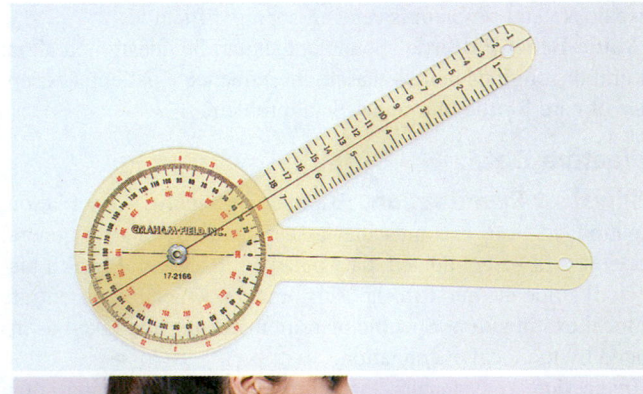
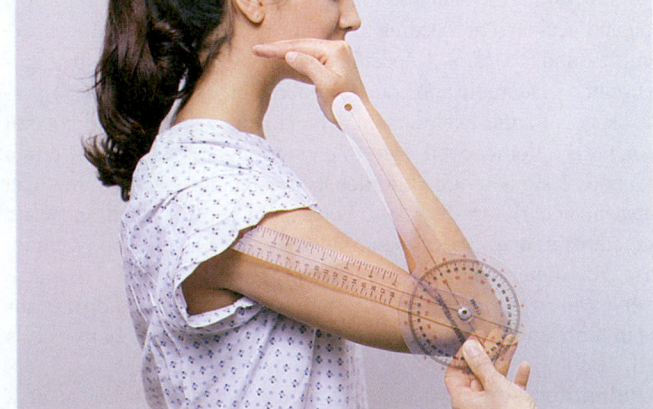

A

B

FIG. 62-6   A, Goniometer. **B,** Measurement of joint motion with a goniometer.

cording measurements, the nurse should document the exact location at which the measurements were obtained (e.g., the quadriceps muscle is measured 15 cm above the patella). This informs the next examiner of the exact area to be measured and ensures consistency during reassessment.

Other. The patient's use of an assistive device such as a walker or cane should be noted. If the patient is able to move independently, the nurse should assess posture and gait by watching the patient walk, stand, and sit.[9] Musculoskeletal and neurologic problems can result in abnormal gait patterns. Assessment of reflexes is discussed in Chapter 56. Neurovascular assessment is discussed in Chapter 63. Table 62-5 is an example of how to record a normal physical assessment of the musculoskeletal system. Common abnormal assessment findings of the musculoskeletal system are presented in Table 62-6.

Scoliosis is a lateral S-shaped curvature of the thoracic and lumbar spine.[8] Unequal shoulder and scapula height is usually noted when the patient is observed from the back (Fig. 62-7). The patient also should be asked to place fingertips together as if diving into a swimming pool and slowly bend forward, allowing the nurse

---

TABLE 62-5	Normal Physical Assessment of the Musculoskeletal System

- Normal spinal curvatures
- No muscle atrophy or asymmetry
- No joint swelling, deformity, or crepitation
- No tenderness on palpation of spine
- Full range of motion of all joints without pain or laxity
- Muscle strength of 5

TABLE 62-6	COMMON ASSESSMENT ABNORMALITIES Musculoskeletal System

Finding	Description	Possible Etiology and Significance
Achilles tendonitis	Pain in posterior leg when running or walking initially; can progress to pain at rest	Cumulative stress on Achilles tendon resulting in inflammation
Ankylosis	Stiffness and fixation of a joint	Chronic joint inflammation (e.g., rheumatoid arthritis)
Antalgic gait	Shortened stride with as little weight bearing as possible on the affected side	Pain or discomfort in the lower extremity on weight bearing; can be related to trauma or other disorders
Ataxic gait	Staggering, uncoordinated gait often with sway	Neurogenic disorders (e.g., spinal cord lesion)
Atrophy	Flabby appearance of muscle leading to decreased function and tone	Muscle denervation, contracture, prolonged disuse as a result of immobilization
Boutonnière deformity	Finger abnormality, flexion of proximal interphalangeal (PIP) joint and hyperextension of the distal interphalangeal (DIP) joint of the fingers (see Fig. 65-4)	Typical deformity of rheumatoid and psoriatic arthritis caused by rupture of extensor tendons over the fingers
Contracture	Resistance of movement of muscle or joint as a result of fibrosis of supporting soft tissues	Shortening of muscle or ligaments, tightness of soft tissue, incorrect positioning of immobilized extremity
Crepitation (crepitus)	Audible crackling sound with palpable grating that accompanies movement	Fracture, dislocation, temporomandibular joint dysfunction, osteoarthritis
Dislocation	Bone is displaced from its normal joint	Trauma, disorders of surrounding soft tissues
Festinating gait	While walking, the neck, trunk, and knees flex while the body is rigid; delayed start with short, quick, shuffling steps; speed may increase as if patient is unable to stop (festination)	Neurogenic disorders (e.g., Parkinson's disease)
Ganglion cyst	Small fluid-filled bump or mass over a tendon sheath or joint, usually on dorsal surface of wrist or foot	Inflammation of tissues around a joint, can increase in size or disappear
Kyphosis (dowager's hump)	Forward bending of thoracic spine, slight flexion of knees; exaggerated thoracic curvature	Poor posture, tuberculosis, arthritis, osteoporosis, growth disturbance of vertebral epiphyses
Lateral epicondylitis (tennis elbow)	Dull ache along outer aspect of elbow, worsens with twisting and grasping motions	Partial tearing of tendon at its insertion on epicondyle
Limited range of motion (ROM)	Joint does not achieve the expected degrees of motion	Injury, inflammation, contracture
Lordosis (swayback)	Asymmetric scapulae and shoulders, exaggerated lumbar curvature	Secondary to other spinal deformities, muscular dystrophy, obesity, flexion contracture of hip, congenital dislocation of hip
Muscle spasticity	Increased muscle tone (rigidity) with sustained muscle contractions (spasms); stiffness or tightness may interfere with gait, movement, speech	Neuromuscular disorders such as multiple sclerosis (MS) or cerebral palsy
Myalgia	General muscle tenderness and pain	Chronic rheumatic syndromes (e.g., fibromyalgia)
Paresthesia	Numbness and tingling, often described as a "pins and needles" sensation	Compromised sensory nerves, often due to edema in a closed space such as a cast or bulky dressing
Pes planus (flat foot)	Abnormal flatness of the sole and arch of the foot	Hereditary, muscle paralysis, mild cerebral palsy, early muscular dystrophy, injury to posterior tibial tendon
Plantar fasciitis	Burning, sharp pain on sole of foot; worse in the morning	Chronic degenerative/reparative cycle resulting in inflammation

Continued

TABLE 62-6	*COMMON ASSESSMENT ABNORMALITIES* Musculoskeletal System—cont'd	

Finding	Description	Possible Etiology and Significance
Scoliosis	Asymmetric elevation of shoulders, scapulae, and iliac crests (see Fig. 62-7)	Idiopathic or congenital condition, fracture or dislocation, osteomalacia
Short-leg gait	A limp, unless corrective footwear used	Leg length discrepancy of 1 inch or more, generally of structural origin (arthritis, fracture)
Spastic gait	Short steps with dragging of foot; jerky, uncoordinated, cross-knee (scissor) movement	Neurogenic (e.g., cerebral palsy, hemiplegia)
Steppage gait	Increased hip and knee flexion in order to clear the foot from the floor; footdrop is evident, foot slaps down and along walking surface	Neurogenic disorders (e.g., peroneal nerve injury, paralyzed dorsiflexor muscles)
Subluxation	Partial dislocation of joint	Instability of joint capsule and supporting ligaments (e.g., trauma, arthritis)
Swan neck deformity	Hyperextension of the PIP joint with flexion of the metacarpophalangeal (MCP) and DIP joints of the fingers (see Fig. 65-4)	Typical deformity of rheumatoid and psoriatic arthritis caused by contracture of muscles and tendons
Swelling	Enlargement, often of a joint due to fluid collection; generally leads to pain, stiffness	Trauma or inflammation
Tenosynovitis	Superficial swelling, pain, and tenderness along a tendon sheath	Inflammation that often occurs with repetitive motion (e.g., carpal tunnel syndrome)
Torticollis (wryneck)	Neck is twisted in unusual position to one side	Prolonged contraction of neck muscles, congenital or acquired
Ulnar deviation (ulnar drift)	Fingers drift to ulnar side of forearm (see Fig. 65-4)	Typical deformity of rheumatoid arthritis due to tendon contracture
Valgum deformity (knock-knees)	When knees are together and there is more than 1 inch (2.5 cm) between the medial malleoli	Poliomyelitis, congenital deformity, arthritis
Varum deformity (bowlegs)	When knees are apart and the medial malleoli are together, a space of more than 1 inch (2.5 cm) exists	Arthritis, congenital deformity

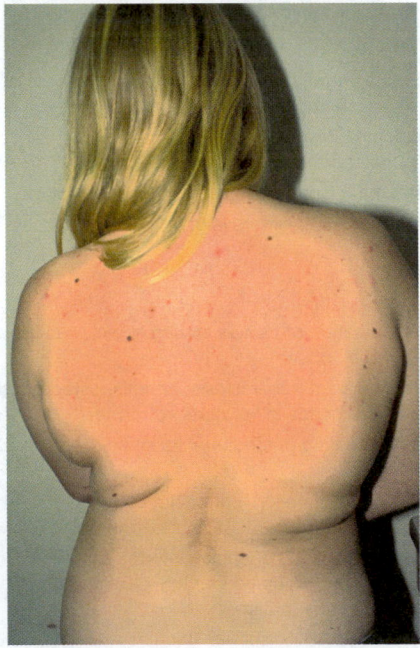

FIG. 62-7 Scoliosis in a standing erect posture.

to assess for thoracic rib prominence or paravertebral muscle prominence in the lumbar spine.[1] If the deformity is greater than 45 degrees, lung and cardiac function is generally impaired.

The *straight-leg-raising test* is performed by the nurse on the supine patient who complains of sciatica or leg pain. The patient's leg is passively raised 60 degrees or less. The test is positive if the patient complains of pain along the distribution of the sciatic nerve. A positive test indicates nerve root irritation from intervertebral disk prolapse and herniation, particularly at the level of L4-5 or L5-S1.

DIAGNOSTIC STUDIES OF THE MUSCULOSKELETAL SYSTEM

Diagnostic studies provide important objective data that aid the nurse in monitoring the patient's condition and planning appropriate interventions. Table 62-7 contains diagnostic studies common to the musculoskeletal system. The use of studies such as x-rays, magnetic resonance imaging (MRI), and bone scans has greatly improved orthopedic care. Tests must be carefully chosen to enhance or clarify information gained from the patient's history and physical examination.

The **x-ray,** or roentgenogram, is the most common diagnostic study used to assess musculoskeletal problems and to monitor the effectiveness of treatment. Because bones are denser than other tissues, x-rays do not penetrate them. Dense areas show as white on the standard x-ray. X-rays provide information about bone deformity, joint congruity, bone density, and calcification in soft tissue. Fracture diagnosis and management are the primary indications for x-ray, but it is also useful in the evaluation of hereditary, developmental, infectious, inflammatory, neoplastic, metabolic, and degenerative disorders.

A small fiberoptic tube called an arthroscope is used to directly examine the interior of a joint cavity in a procedure known as **arthroscopy.** After anesthesia has been administered, a large-bore needle is inserted into the joint, and the joint is distended with

TABLE 62-7	*DIAGNOSTIC STUDIES* **Musculoskeletal System**	

Study	Description and Purpose	Nursing Responsibility
Radiologic Studies		
Standard x-ray	An x-ray is taken to determine density of bone. Study evaluates structural or functional changes of bones and joints. In anteroposterior view, x-ray beam passes from front to back, allowing one-dimensional view; lateral position provides two-dimensional view.	Avoid excessive exposure of patient and self. Before procedure, remove any radiopaque objects that can interfere with results. Explain procedure to patient. Verify patient is not pregnant.
Diskogram	An x-ray of cervical or lumbar intervertebral disk is done after injection of contrast dye into nucleus pulposus. Study permits visualization of intervertebral disk abnormalities.	Assess patient for possible allergy to contrast medium. Explain procedure.
Computed tomography (CT) scan	An x-ray beam is used with a computer to provide a three-dimensional picture. It is used to identify soft tissue abnormalities, bony abnormalities, and various musculoskeletal trauma.	Inform patient that procedure is painless. Inform patient of importance of remaining still during procedure. If contrast medium is being used, verify that patient does not have shellfish allergy.
Myelogram with or without CT	A myelogram involves injecting a radiographic opaque dye (dye that is picked up by x-ray) into the sac around the nerve roots. CT scan may follow to show how the bone is affecting the nerve roots. Very sensitive test for nerve impingement and can pick up even very subtle lesions and injuries.	Main risk is the potential for spinal headache. Inform patient that headache should resolve in 1-2 days with rest and fluids, but should be reported to health care provider.
Magnetic resonance imaging (MRI)	Radio waves and magnetic field are used to view soft tissue. Study is especially useful in the diagnosis of avascular necrosis, disk disease, tumors, osteomyelitis, ligament tears, and cartilage tears. Patient is placed inside scanning chamber. Gadolinium may be injected into a vein to enhance visualization of the structures. Open MRI does not require the patient to be placed inside a chamber.	Inform patient that procedure is painless. Be aware that it is contraindicated in patient with aneurysm clips, metallic implants, pacemakers, electronic devices, hearing aids, and shrapnel. Ensure that patient has no metal on clothing (e.g., snaps, zippers, jewelry, credit cards). Inform patient of importance of remaining still throughout examination. Inform patients who are claustrophobic that they may experience symptoms during examination. Administer antianxiety agent if indicated and ordered. Open MRI may be indicated for obese patient or patient with large chest and abdominal girth or severe claustrophobia. Open MRI may not be available at all facilities.
Bone Mineral Density (BMD) Measurements		
Dual-energy x-ray absorptiometry (DEXA)	Technique measures bone mass of spine, femur, forearm, and total body. Allows assessment of bone density with minimal radiation exposure; used to diagnose metabolic bone disease and to monitor changes in bone density with treatment.	Inform patient that procedure is painless.
Quantitative ultrasound (QUS)	Evaluates density, elasticity, and strength of patella and calcaneus using ultrasound rather than radiation.	Inform patient that procedure is painless.
Radioisotope Studies		
Bone scan	Technique involves injection of radioisotope (usually technetium-99m [^{99m}Tc]) that is taken up by bone. A uniform uptake of the isotope is normal. Increased uptake is seen in osteomyelitis, osteoporosis, primary and metastatic malignant lesions of bone, and certain fractures. Decreased uptake is seen in areas of avascular necrosis.	Explain that technician gives a calculated dose of radioisotope 2 hr before procedure. Ensure that bladder is emptied before scan. Inform patient that procedure requires 1 hr while patient lies supine and that no pain or harm will result from isotopes. Explain that no follow-up scans are required. Increase fluids after the examination.
Endoscopy		
Arthroscopy	Study involves insertion of arthroscope into joint (usually knee) for visualization of structure and contents. It can be used for exploratory surgery (removal of loose bodies and biopsy) and for diagnosis of abnormalities of meniscus, articular cartilage, ligaments, or joint capsule. Other structures that can be visualized through the arthroscope include the shoulder, elbow, wrist, jaw, hip, and ankle.	Inform patient that procedure can be performed in outpatient setting with strict asepsis and that either local or general anesthesia is used. After procedure, cover wound with sterile dressing.

Continued

TABLE 62-7	*DIAGNOSTIC STUDIES* Musculoskeletal System—cont'd	
Study	**Description and Purpose**	**Nursing Responsibility**
Mineral Metabolism		
Alkaline phosphatase	This enzyme, produced by osteoblasts of bone, is needed for mineralization of organic bone matrix. Elevated levels are found in healing fractures, bone cancers, osteoporosis, osteomalacia, and Paget's disease. *Normal:* 30-120 U/L (0.5-2.0 μkat/L).	Obtain blood samples by venipuncture. Observe venipuncture site for bleeding or hematoma formation. Inform patient that procedure does not require fasting.
Calcium	Bone is primary organ for calcium storage. Calcium provides bone with rigid consistency. Decreased serum level is found in osteomalacia, renal disease, and hypoparathyroidism; increased level is found in hyperparathyroidism, some bone tumors. *Normal:* 9-11 mg/dl (4.5-5.5 mEq/L, 2.25-2.74 mmol/L)	Same as above.
Phosphorus	Amount present is indirectly related to calcium metabolism. Decreased level is found in osteomalacia; increased level is found in chronic renal disease, healing fractures, osteolytic metastatic tumor. *Normal:* 2.8-4.5 mg/dl (0.9-1.45 mmol/L).	Same as above.
Serologic Studies		
Rheumatoid factor (RF)	Study assesses presence of autoantibody (rheumatoid factor) in serum. Factor is not specific for rheumatoid arthritis and is seen in other connective tissue diseases, as well as in a small percentage of normal population. *Normal:* Negative or titer <1:20.	Same as above.
Erythrocyte sedimentation rate (ESR)	Study is nonspecific index of inflammation. Study measures rapidity with which red blood cells settle out of unclotted blood in 1 hr. Results are influenced by physiologic factors, as well as diseases. Elevated levels are seen with any inflammatory process (especially rheumatoid arthritis, rheumatic fever, osteomyelitis, and respiratory infections). *Normal:* <20 mm/hr. Some gender and age variation.	Same as above.
Antinuclear antibody (ANA)	Study assesses presence of antibodies capable of destroying nucleus of body's cells. Finding is positive in 95% of patients with SLE and may also be positive in individuals with systemic sclerosis (scleroderma) or rheumatoid arthritis and in a small percentage of normal population. *Normal:* Negative or titer <1:10.	Same as above.
Anti-DNA antibody	Study detects serum antibodies that react with DNA. It is the most specific test for SLE. *Normal:* Negative or titer <1:10.	Same as above.
Complement	Complement, a normal body protein, is essential to both immune and inflammatory reactions. Complement components used up in these reactions are depleted. Complement depletions may be found in patients with rheumatoid arthritis or SLE.	Same as above.
Uric acid	End product of purine metabolism is normally excreted in urine. Although not specific, levels are usually elevated in gout. *Normal:* Men, 4.5-6.5 mg/dl (268-387 μmol/L); women, 2.5-5.5 mg/dl (149-327 μmol/L).	Obtain blood samples by venipuncture. Observe venipuncture site for bleeding or hematoma formation. Inform patient that procedure does not require fasting.
C-reactive protein (CRP)	Study is used to diagnose inflammatory diseases, infections, and active widespread malignancy. CRP is synthesized by the liver and is present in large amounts in serum 18-24 hr after onset of tissue damage. *Normal:* Negative.	Same as above.
Human leukocyte antigen (HLA)-B27	Antigen present in disorders such as ankylosing spondylitis and rheumatoid arthritis.	Same as above.

SLE, Systemic lupus erythematosis.

TABLE 62-7	*DIAGNOSTIC STUDIES* Musculoskeletal System—cont'd	
Study	**Description and Purpose**	**Nursing Responsibility**
Markers of Muscle Injury		
Creatine kinase (CK)	Highest concentration is found in skeletal muscle. Increased values are found in progressive muscular dystrophy, polymyositis, and traumatic injuries. *Normal:* Men, 15-105 U/L (0.26-1.79 μkat/L); women, 10-80 U/L (0.17-1.36 μkat/L).	Same as above.
Serum potassium	Increased values are found in muscle trauma as cell destruction releases this electrolyte into the serum. *Normal:* 3.5-5 mEq/L.	Monitor trauma patients for cardiac dysrhythmias related to hyperkalemia.
Aldolase	Study is useful in monitoring muscular dystrophy and dermatomyositis. *Normal:* 1-7.5 U/L (0.02-0.13 μkat/L).	Same as above.
Invasive Procedures		
Arthrocentesis	Incision or puncture of joint capsule is done to obtain samples of synovial fluid from within joint cavity or to remove excess fluid. Local anesthesia and aseptic preparation are used before needle is inserted into joint and fluid aspirated. Study is useful in diagnosis of joint inflammation, infection, and subtle fractures.	Inform patient that procedure is usually done at bedside or in examination room. Send samples of synovial fluid to laboratory for examination (if indicated). After procedure, apply compression dressing. Observe for leakage of blood or fluid on dressing.
Electromyogram (EMG)	Study evaluates electrical potential associated with skeletal muscle contraction. Small-gauge needles are inserted into certain muscles. Needle probes are attached to leads that feed information to EMG machine. Recordings of electrical activity of muscle are traced on audiotransmitter, as well as on oscilloscope and recording paper. Study is useful in providing information related to lower motor neuron dysfunction and primary muscle disease.	Inform patient that procedure is usually done in electromyogram laboratory while patient lies supine on special table. Keep patient awake to cooperate with voluntary movement. Inform patient that procedure involves some discomfort from needle insertion. Avoid administration of stimulants, including caffeine and sedatives, 24 hr before procedure.
Miscellaneous		
Duplex venous Doppler	Ultrasound of the veins, usually of the lower extremities, to detect blood flow abnormalities that could indicate deep vein thrombosis.	Inform patient that procedure is painless and noninvasive.
Thermography	Technique uses infrared detector that measures degree of heat radiating from skin surface. Study is useful in investigation of cause of inflamed joint and in following up patient's response to antiinflammatory drug therapy.	Inform patient that procedure is painless and noninvasive.
Plethysmography	Study records variations in volume and pressure of blood passing through tissues. Test is nonspecific.	Inform patient that procedure is painless and noninvasive.
Somatosensory evoked potential (SSEP)	Study evaluates evoked potential of muscle contractions. Electrodes are placed on skin and provide recordings of electrical activity of muscle. Study is useful in identifying subtle dysfunction of lower motor neuron and primary muscle disease. SSEP measures nerve conduction along pathways not accessible by EMG. Transcutaneous or percutaneous electrodes are applied to the skin and help identify neuropathy and myopathy. Test is often used during spinal surgery for scoliosis to detect neurologic compromise when the patient is under anesthesia.	Inform patient that procedure is similar to EMG but does not involve needles. Electrodes are applied to the skin.

fluid or air (Fig. 62-8). When the arthroscope is inserted, the surgeon is able to perform extensive, accurate visualization of the joint cavity.[10] Photographs or videotapes can be made through the scope, and a biopsy of the synovium or cartilage can be obtained. Torn tissue can be repaired through arthroscopic surgery, eliminating the need for a larger incision and greatly decreasing the recovery time.

An **arthrocentesis** or joint aspiration is usually performed for a synovial fluid analysis. It may also be used to instill medications for the patient with septic arthritis or to remove fluid from joints to relieve pain. After the skin has been cleaned, a local anesthetic is instilled. An 18-gauge or larger needle is inserted into the joint, and fluid is withdrawn. The appropriate sterile container should be readily available to receive the aspirated fluid, which must be transported immediately to the laboratory.

The fluid will be examined grossly for volume, color, clarity, viscosity, and mucin clot formation. Normal synovial fluid is transparent and colorless or straw-colored. It should be scant in amount

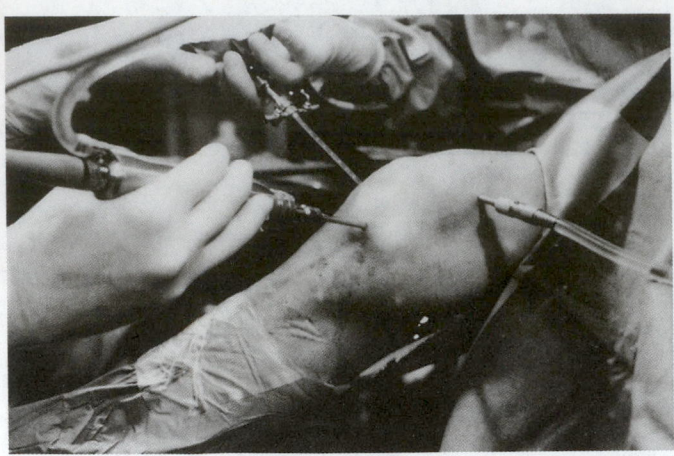

FIG. 62-8 Arthroscopy of a knee.

and of low viscosity. Fluid from an infected joint may be purulent and thick or gray and thin. In gout the fluid may be whitish yellow. Blood may be aspirated if there is hemarthrosis because of injury or a bleeding disorder. The mucin clot test indicates the character of the protein portion of the synovial fluid. Normally a white, rope-like mucin clot is formed. In the presence of an inflammatory process, the clot breaks apart easily and fragments. The fluid is examined grossly for floating fat globules, which indicate bone injury. Protein content is elevated and glucose is considerably decreased in septic arthritis. Presence of uric acid crystals suggests a diagnosis of gout. A Gram stain and culture may also be done of the aspirated fluid.

NCLEX EXAMINATION REVIEW QUESTIONS

The number of the question corresponds to the same-numbered objective at the beginning of the chapter.

1. The bone cells that function in the forming of bone tissue are called
   a. osteoids.
   b. osteocytes.
   c. osteoclasts.
   d. osteoblasts.
2. While performing passive range of motion for a patient, the nurse puts a synovial joint through the movements of
   a. rotation.
   b. flexion and extension.
   c. flexion, extension, abduction, and adduction.
   d. flexion, extension, abduction, adduction, and circumduction.
3. The nurse teaches a patient with a leg immobilized in traction to prevent muscle atrophy in the affected leg by performing
   a. flexion contractions.
   b. tetanic contractions.
   c. isotonic contractions.
   d. isometric contractions.
4. A patient with bursitis of the shoulder asks the nurse what the bursa does. The nurse's response is based on the knowledge that bursae
   a. connect bone to bone.
   b. separate muscle from muscle.
   c. lubricate joints with synovial fluid.
   d. relieve friction between moving parts.

5. The decreased agility found during assessment of the older adult is caused by the age-related change of
   a. decrease in bone mass.
   b. erosion of articular cartilage.
   c. loss of elasticity in ligaments and cartilage.
   d. decrease in number and diameter of muscle cells.
6. While obtaining subjective assessment data related to the musculoskeletal system, it is particularly important for the nurse to ask about family history in the patient with
   a. osteomyelitis.
   b. osteomalacia.
   c. low back pain.
   d. rheumatoid arthritis.
7. When grading muscle strength, the nurse records a score of 2, indicating
   a. active movement against gravity.
   b. a barely detectable flicker of contraction.
   c. active movement with elimination of gravity.
   d. active movement against full resistance without evident fatigue.
8. A normal assessment finding of the musculoskeletal system is
   a. ulnar deviation.
   b. muscle strength of 4.
   c. angulation of bone toward midline.
   d. no tenderness with spine palpation.
9. A patient is scheduled for an electromyogram. The nurse explains that this diagnostic test involves
   a. placement of thin needles into the muscles.
   b. placement of electrodes on the skin to record electrical activity of muscles.
   c. measurement of the heat of muscle contractions radiating from the skin surface.
   d. administration of a calculated dose of radioisotope 2 hours before the procedure.

REFERENCES

1. Maher AB, Salmond SW, Pellino TA, editors: *Orthopaedic nursing,* ed 3, Philadelphia, 2002, Saunders.
2. National Association of Orthopaedic Nurses: *An introduction to orthopaedic nursing,* ed 3, Chicago, 2002, National Association of Orthopaedic Nurses.
3. Thibodeau GA, Patton KT: *The human body in health and disease,* ed 4, St Louis, 2005, Mosby.
4. Taggert H: NAON *core curriculum for orthopaedic nursing,* ed 5, Boston, 2006, Pearson Custom Publishers.
5. McCance KL, Huether SE: *Pathophysiology: the biologic basis for disease in adults and children,* ed 3, St Louis, 2006, Mosby.
6. Herlihy B, Maebius NK: *The human body in health and illness,* ed 3, Philadelphia, 2007, Elsevier Saunders.
7. Meiner S: Safety. In Meiner S, Lueckenotte A, editors: *Gerontologic nursing,* ed 3, St Louis, 2006, Elsevier Mosby.
8. Jarvis C: *Physical examination and health assessment,* ed 4, Philadelphia, 2004, Saunders.
9. Rubenstein L, Trueblood P: Gait and balance assessment in older persons, *Ann Long-term Care* 12:39, 2004.
10. Chernecky C, Berger B: *Laboratory tests and diagnostic procedures,* ed 4, St Louis, 2004, Saunders.

RESOURCES

Resources for this chapter are listed after Chapter 63 on p. 1667, Chapter 64 on p. 1692, and Chapter 65 on p. 1731.

Nursing Management
Musculoskeletal Trauma and Orthopedic Surgery

63

Sharon G. Childs

LEARNING OBJECTIVES

1. Explain the etiology, pathophysiology, clinical manifestations, and collaborative care of soft tissue injuries, including strains, sprains, dislocations, subluxations, bursitis, repetitive strain injury, carpal tunnel syndrome, rotator cuff injury, meniscus injury, and muscle spasms.
2. Describe the sequential events involved in fracture healing.
3. Differentiate among closed reduction, cast immobilization, open reduction, and traction regarding purpose, complications, and nursing management.
4. Describe the neurovascular assessment of an injured extremity.
5. Explain common complications associated with a fracture and fracture healing.
6. Describe the collaborative care and nursing management of patients with specific fractures.
7. Describe the indications for and the collaborative care and nursing management of the patient with an amputation.
8. Describe the types of joint replacement surgery associated with arthritis and connective tissue diseases.
9. Identify the preoperative and postoperative management of the patient having joint replacement surgery.

KEY TERMS

arthroplasty, p. 1662
bursitis, p. 1635
carpal tunnel syndrome, p. 1633
compartment syndrome, p. 1650
dislocation, p. 1632
fat embolism syndrome, p. 1651
fracture, p. 1635
phantom limb sensation, p. 1660
repetitive strain injury, p. 1633
sprain, p. 1630
strain, p. 1630
subluxation, p. 1632
synovectomy, p. 1662
traction, p. 1638

Electronic Resources

Supplemental content related to Chapter 63 can be found . . .

Companion CD
- Stress-Busting Kit for Nursing Students
- Interactive Case Study: Musculoskeletal Trauma
- NCLEX Examination Review Questions
- Comprehensive Glossary

Evolve Website *evolve*
http://evolve.elsevier.com/Lewis/medsurg
- Content Updates
- Key Points (Printable and CD/MP3 Download)
- Concept Map Creator
- Expanded Audio Glossary
- Key Term Flash Cards
- Customizable Nursing Care Plans:
  - Fracture
  - Orthopedic Surgery

- Patient and Family Instruction Guides in English and Spanish:
  - Care After a Femoral Head Prosthesis
  - Care Following an Amputation
  - Prevention of Musculoskeletal Problems in the Older Adult
- Electronic Calculators
- WebLinks

The most common cause of musculoskeletal injuries is a traumatic event resulting in fracture, dislocation, and associated soft tissue injuries. Although most of these injuries are not fatal, the cost in terms of pain, disability, medical expense, and lost wages is enormous. For all ages, accidents are exceeded only by heart disease, cancer, and strokes as a cause of death. Accidental injuries (e.g., motor vehicle crashes, drowning, burns) are the leading cause of death in children and young adults in the United States.[1]

The nurse has an important role in educating the public about the basic principles of safety and accident prevention. The morbidity associated with accidents can be significantly reduced if people are aware of environmental hazards, use appropriate safety equip-

---

Reviewed by Kathleen Rourke, RN, BSN, ANP, ONC, Orthopedic Nurse Practitioner, Harvard Vanguard Medical Associates, Boston, Mass.

ment, and apply safety and traffic rules. In the occupational and industrial setting, the nurse should teach employees and employers about the use of proper safety equipment and avoidance of hazardous working situations.

In the home environment, falls account for many musculoskeletal injuries. Preventive education should be directed toward the importance of wearing shoes with functional and stable soles and heels, avoidance of wet or slippery surfaces, careful placement of throw rugs, and removal of obstacles from the pathway of high-risk individuals such as persons with gait instability or visual or cognitive impairment. Ways to prevent common musculoskeletal problems in the older adult are listed in Table 63-1.

TABLE 63-1	*PATIENT AND FAMILY TEACHING GUIDE* **Prevention of Musculoskeletal Problems in the Older Adult**

1. Use ramps in buildings and at street corners instead of steps to prevent falls.
2. Eliminate scatter rugs in the home.
3. Treat pain and discomfort from osteoarthritis.
   - Rest in positions that decrease discomfort.
   - Use plain or enteric-coated aspirin or nonsteroidal antiinflammatory drugs to decrease inflammation of joints and reduce pain.
4. Use a walker or cane to help with walking to prevent falls.
5. Eat the amount and kind of foods to prevent excess weight gain because obesity adds stress to joints, which may predispose to osteoarthritis.
6. Get regular and frequent exercise.
   - Activities of daily living provide range-of-motion exercises.
   - Hobbies (e.g., jigsaw puzzles, needlework, model building) exercise finger joints and prevent stiffness.
   - Performing weight-bearing exercise daily (e.g., walking) is essential and should be done 2 or 3 times daily.
7. Use shoes with good support to provide for safety and promote comfort.
8. Gradually initiate activities to promote optimal coordination. Rise slowly to a standing position to prevent dizziness, falls, and fractures.
9. Avoid walking on uneven surfaces and wet floors.

Soft Tissue Injuries

Soft tissue injuries include sprains, strains, dislocations, and subluxations. These common injuries are usually caused by trauma. The increase in the number of people who have committed themselves to a fitness program or participating in sports has contributed to the increased incidence of soft tissue injuries. Common sports-related injuries are summarized in Table 63-2. Most sport injuries result from direct trauma, contusion, or indirect sprain/strain injury.[2]

SPRAINS AND STRAINS

Sprains and strains are the two most common types of injury affecting the musculoskeletal system. These injuries are usually associated with abnormal stretching or twisting forces that may occur during vigorous activities. These injuries tend to occur around joints and in the spinal musculature.

A **sprain** is an injury to tendinoligamentous structures surrounding a joint, usually caused by a wrenching or twisting motion. A sprain is classified according to the amount of ligament fibers torn. A *first-degree (mild) sprain* involves tears of only a few fibers resulting in mild tenderness and minimal swelling. A *second-degree (moderate) sprain* is partial disruption of the involved tissue with more swelling and tenderness. A *third-degree (severe) sprain* is a complete tearing of the ligament in association with moderate to severe swelling. A gap in the muscle may be apparent or palpated through the skin if the muscle is torn. Because areas around joints are rich in nerve endings, the injury can be extremely painful. The most common areas of sprains occur in the ankle and wrist.

A **strain** is an excessive stretching of a muscle and its fascial sheath. It often involves the tendon. Strains may also be classified as first degree (mild or slightly pulled muscle), second degree (moderate or moderately torn muscle), and third degree (severely ruptured or torn muscle).[3] The clinical manifestations of sprains and strains are similar and include pain, edema, decrease in function, and contusion. Pain aggravated by continued use is common. Edema develops in the injured area because of tiny hemorrhages within the disrupted tissues and the ensuing local inflammatory response. Usually the patient will recount a history of traumatic in-

TABLE 63-2	Common Sports-Related Injuries	
Injury	**Definition**	**Treatment**
Impingement syndrome	Entrapment of soft tissue structures under coracoacromial arch of the shoulder	NSAIDs; rest until symptoms decrease and then gradual ROM and strengthening exercises
Rotator cuff tear	Tear within muscle or tendinoligamentous structures about the shoulder	If minor tear, rest shoulder, NSAIDs, and gradual mobilization with ROM and strengthening exercises If major tear, surgical repair
Shin splints	Inflammation along anterior aspect of calf from periostitis caused by improper shoes, overuse, or running on hard pavement	Rest, ice, NSAIDs, proper shoes; gradual increase in activity; if pain persists, x-ray should be done to rule out stress fracture of tibia
Tendinitis	Inflammation of tendon as a result of overuse or incorrect use	Rest, ice, NSAIDs; gradual return to sport activity; protective brace (orthosis) may be necessary if symptoms recur
Ligament injury	Tearing or stretching of ligament; usually occurs as a result of inversion, eversion, shearing, or torque applied to a joint; characterized by sudden pain, swelling, and instability	Rest, ice, NSAIDs; protection of affected extremity by use of brace; if symptoms persist, surgical repair may be necessary
Meniscal injury	Injury to fibrocartilage of the knee characterized by popping, clicking, or tearing sensation, effusion, and swelling	Rest, ice, NSAIDs; gradual return to regular activities; if symptoms persist, surgical arthroscopy to diagnose and repair meniscal injury may be necessary

NSAIDs, Nonsteroidal antiinflammatory drugs; *ROM,* range of motion.

jury, possibly of an inversion or twisting nature, or recent exercise activity.

Mild sprains and strains are usually self-limiting, with full function returning within 3 to 6 weeks. A severe sprain can result in a concomitant *avulsion fracture,* in which the ligament pulls loose a fragment of bone. Alternatively, the joint structure may become unstable and result in subluxation or dislocation. At the time of injury, *hemarthrosis* (bleeding into a joint space or cavity) or disruption of the synovial lining may occur. An acute strain may involve partial or complete rupture of a muscle. Severe strains may require surgical suturing of the muscle and surrounding fascia.

X-rays of the affected part may be taken to rule out a fracture or widening of the joint structure. However, some health care providers utilize an assessment protocol called the "Ottawa rules or guidelines" for the examination of an injured ankle or knee before ordering x-rays.[4] These rules specify x-rays for a patient based on age, capability of flexion, location of tenderness, and ability to bear weight immediately after the injury or when examined. Surgical repair may be necessary if the injury is significant enough to produce complete or severe disruption of ligamentous or muscle structures, fracture, or dislocation.

NURSING MANAGEMENT
SPRAINS AND STRAINS

■ *Nursing Implementation*

Health Promotion. Stretching and warm-up prior to exercising and before vigorous activity significantly reduce sprains and strains. Preconditioning exercise protects an inherently weak joint because tissues tolerate slow stretching better than quick stretching. Warm-up exercises "prelengthen" potentially strained tissues by avoiding the quick stretch often encountered in sports. Warm-up exercises also increase the temperature of muscle tissue, increase oxygen utilization within muscle, and increase cell metabolism and nerve impulse transmission. Stretching improves balance, coordination, flexibility, and kinesthetic awareness, thus lessening the chance of injury to muscle or joints.

Strengthening, balancing, and endurance exercises are also important. Strengthening exercises involve lifting or pushing weights. These exercises build up muscle strength and bone density. Balance exercises, which may overlap with some strengthening exercises, help to prevent falling. Endurance exercises should start at a low level of effort and progress gradually to moderate activities (e.g., swimming, gardening, walking briskly). They should be done for 30 minutes.[5] Exercise instructions for these types of physical activity are available at *www.weboflife.ksc.nasa.gov/exerciseandaging.*

The use of elastic support bandages or adhesive tape wrapping before beginning a vigorous activity is thought to reduce the occurrence of sprains and is often used to support an injured joint postinjury while the athlete is competing and training. However, some health care providers do not believe in using elastic bandages or preventive wrapping or taping because it may predispose the athlete to injury.

Acute Intervention. If an injury occurs, the immediate care focuses on (1) stopping the activity and limitation of movement, (2) applying ice compresses to the injured area, (3) compressing the involved extremity, (4) elevating the extremity, and (5) providing analgesia as necessary (Table 63-3). RICE (rest, ice, compression, elevation) has been found to decrease local inflammation and pain for most musculoskeletal injuries.[6] Movement should be re-

stricted and the extremity rested as soon as pain is felt. Unless the injury is severe, prolonged rest is usually not necessary. Cold *(cryotherapy)* in several forms can be used to produce hypothermia to the involved part. Physiologic changes that occur in soft tissue as a result of the use of cold include vasoconstriction and a reduction in the transmission and perception of nerve pain impulses. These changes result in analgesia and anesthesia, reduction of muscle spasm without changes in muscular strength or endurance, reduction of local edema and inflammation, and reduction of local metabolic requirements. Cold is most useful when applied immediately after the injury has occurred. Ice applications should not exceed 20 to 30 minutes per application, allowing a "warm-up" time of 10 to 15 minutes between applications.

Compression also helps limit swelling, which, if left uncontrolled, could lengthen healing time. An elastic compression bandage can be wrapped around the injured part. The bandage is too tight if numbness is felt below the area of compression or there is additional pain or swelling beyond the edge of the bandage. The bandage can be left in place for 30 minutes and then removed for 15 minutes. However, some elastic wraps are left on during training, athletic, and occupational activities.

The injured part should be elevated above the heart level to help mobilize excess fluid from the area and prevent further edema. The injured part should be elevated even during sleep. Mild analgesics and nonsteroidal antiinflammatory drugs (NSAIDs) may be necessary to manage patient discomfort.

After the acute phase (usually lasting 24 to 48 hours), warm, moist heat may be applied to the affected part to reduce swelling and provide comfort. Heat applications should not exceed 20 to 30 minutes, allowing a "cool-down" time between applications. NSAIDs may be recommended to decrease edema and pain. The patient is encouraged to use the limb, provided that the joint is protected by means of casting, bracing, taping, or splinting. Movement of the joint maintains nutrition to the cartilage, and muscle contraction improves circulation and resolution of the contusion and swelling.

Ambulatory and Home Care. With the exception of treatment in the hospital emergency department following the injury, sprains and strains are treated in the outpatient setting. The patient should be instructed in the use of ice and elevation for 24 to 48 hours after the injury to reduce edema. The use of mild analgesics to promote comfort should be encouraged. Use of an elastic wrap may provide additional support during activity. The patient should learn proper measures of strengthening and conditioning to prevent reinjury.

TABLE 63-3	**EMERGENCY MANAGEMENT** **Acute Soft Tissue Injury**	
Etiology	**Assessment Findings**	**Interventions**
Falls Direct blows Crush injury Motor vehicle collisions Sports injuries	• Edema • Ecchymosis/contusion • Pain, tenderness • Decreased sensation with severe edema • Decreased pulse, coolness, and capillary refill greater than 2 sec • Decreased movement • Pallor • Shortening or rotation of extremity • Inability to bear weight when lower extremity involved • Limited or decreased function with upper extremity involvement • Muscle spasms	**Initial** • Ensure airway, breathing, and circulation. • Assess neurovascular status of involved limb. • Elevate involved limb. • Apply compression bandage unless dislocation present. • Apply ice packs to affected area. • Immobilize affected extremity in the position found. Do *not* attempt to realign or reinsert protruding bones. • Anticipate x-rays of injured extremity. • Give analgesia as necessary. • Administer tetanus and diphtheria prophylaxis if skin integrity breached or open fracture. • Administer antibiotic prophylaxis for open fracture, large tissue defects, or mangled extremity injury. **Ongoing Monitoring** • Monitor for changes in neurovascular status. • Eliminate weight bearing when lower extremity involved. • Anticipate compartment pressure monitoring if neurovascular status changes and compartment syndrome suspected. • Monitor the patient for signs of infection/sepsis.

The physical therapist may help in providing pain relief by means of modalities such as ultrasound. The therapist may also teach the patient exercises to perform for flexibility and strength.

DISLOCATION AND SUBLUXATION

A **dislocation** is a severe injury of the ligamentous structures that surround a joint. Dislocation results in the complete displacement or separation of the articular surfaces of the joint. A **subluxation** is a partial or incomplete displacement of the joint surface. The clinical manifestations of a subluxation are similar to those of a dislocation but are less severe. Treatment of subluxation is similar to that of a dislocation, but subluxation may require less healing time.

Dislocations characteristically result from forces transmitted to the joint that cause a disruption of the soft tissue support structures surrounding the joint. The joints most frequently dislocated in the upper extremity include the thumb, elbow, and shoulder. In the lower extremity, the hip is vulnerable to dislocation occurring as a result of severe trauma, often associated with motor vehicle collisions (Fig. 63-1). The patella may dislocate because of instability of the tendons, ligaments, and muscles surrounding the knee or a severe twisting blow. Dislocations may also be the result of a congenital anomaly or be of pathologic origin. Patellar dislocation has an increased incidence in females because the quadriceps muscles, particularly the vastus medialis, are not as toned and strong as in males. Overtraining and poor training techniques also contribute to injury.

The most obvious clinical manifestation of a dislocation is deformity. For example, if a hip is dislocated, the limb is shorter and often found externally rotated on the affected side. Additional manifestations include local pain, tenderness, loss of function of the injured part, and swelling of the soft tissues in the region of the joint. The major complications of a dislocated joint are open joint injuries, intraarticular fractures, fracture-dislocation, *avascular necrosis* (bone cell death as a result of inadequate blood supply),

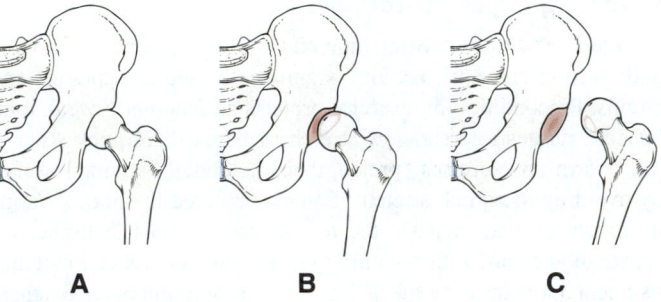

FIG. 63-1   Soft tissue injury of the hip. **A,** Normal. **B,** Subluxation (partial dislocation). **C,** Dislocation.

and damage to adjacent neurovascular tissue. Neurovascular assessment is critical (see pp. 1642 to 1643).

X-ray studies are performed to determine the extent of displacement of the involved structures. The joint may also be aspirated to determine the presence of hemarthrosis or fat cells. Fat cells in the aspirate indicate a probable intraarticular fracture.

NURSING *and* COLLABORATIVE MANAGEMENT
DISLOCATION

A dislocation requires prompt attention and is considered an orthopedic emergency. The longer the joint remains unreduced, the greater the possibility of avascular necrosis. Compartment syndrome may also occur after dislocation and is associated with significant vascular injury. The hip joint is particularly susceptible to avascular necrosis. The first goal of management is to realign the dislocated portion of the joint in its original anatomic position. This can be accomplished by a closed reduction, which may be performed under local or general anesthesia or intravenous (IV) conscious sedation. Anesthesia is often necessary to produce muscle relaxation so that the bones can be manipulated. In some situations, surgical open reduction may be necessary. After reduction, the extremity is usually immobilized by bracing, splinting, taping, or using a sling to allow the torn ligaments and capsular tissue time to heal.

Nursing management of subluxation or dislocation is directed toward relief of pain and support and protection of the injured joint. After the joint has been reduced and immobilized, motion is usually restricted. A carefully regulated rehabilitation program can prevent fracture instability and joint dysfunction. Gentle range of motion (ROM) may be started if the joint is stable and well supported. An exercise program slowly restores the joint to its original ROM without causing another dislocation. The patient should gradually return to normal activities.

A patient who has dislocated a joint may be at greater risk for repeated dislocations because shortened ligaments and scar tissue have weakened the joint. Activity restrictions of the affected joint may be imposed to decrease the risk of repeatedly dislocating the joint.

REPETITIVE STRAIN INJURY

Repetitive strain injury (RSI) is a cumulative traumatic disorder resulting from prolonged, forceful, or awkward movements. RSI is also reported as repetitive trauma disorder, nontraumatic musculoskeletal injury, overuse syndrome (sports medicine), regional musculoskeletal disorder, work-related musculoskeletal disorder, and "nintendinitis" (from playing Nintendo games).[7] Repeated movements strain the tendons, ligaments, and muscles, causing tiny tears that become inflamed. If the tissues are not given time to heal properly, scarring can occur. Blood vessels of the arms and hands may become constricted, depriving tissues of vital nutrients and causing an accumulation of lactic acid. Without intervention, tendons and muscles can deteriorate and nerves can become hypersensitive. At this point even the slightest movement can cause pain.

In addition to the repetitive movements, other factors related to RSI include poor posture and positioning, poor work space ergonomics, a badly designed keyboard, and repetitive lifting of heavy workloads without sufficient muscle rest. The result may be inflammation, swelling, and pain in the muscles, tendons, and nerves of the neck, spine, shoulder, forearm, and hand. Symptoms of RSI include pain, weakness, numbness, or impairment of motor function. Persons who may be affected by RSI include musicians, dancers, butchers, grocery clerks, vibratory tool workers, and those with frequent use of a computer mouse and keyboard.

Competitive athletes and poorly trained athletes may also develop RSI. Swimming, overhead throwing (e.g., baseball), weight lifting, gymnastics, dancing, tennis, skiing, kicking sports (e.g., soccer), and horseback riding require repetitive motion, and overtraining compounds the effects of RSI.

RSI can be prevented through education and ergonomics (consideration of the interaction of humans and their work environment). A few ergonomic considerations include keeping the hips and knees flexed to 90 degrees with the feet flat, keeping the wrist straight to type, having the top of the computer monitor even with the forehead, and taking at least hourly stretch breaks. Once diagnosed, the treatment of RSI consists of identifying the precipitating activity, modification of equipment or activity, pain management including heat/cold application, NSAIDs, rest, physical therapy for strengthening and conditioning exercises, and lifestyle changes.

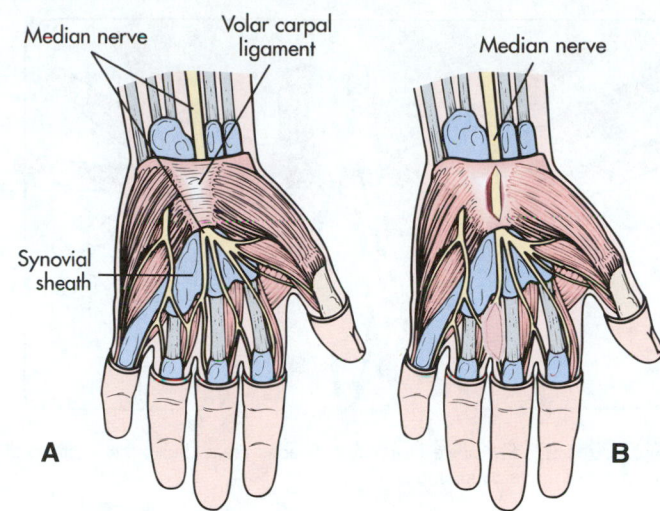

FIG. 63-2 **A,** Wrist structures involved in carpal tunnel syndrome. **B,** Decompression of median nerve by incision through the transverse carpal ligament.

CARPAL TUNNEL SYNDROME

Carpal tunnel syndrome (CTS) is a condition caused by compression of the median nerve, which enters the hand through the narrow confines of the carpal tunnel (Fig. 63-2). The carpal tunnel is formed by ligaments and bones. CTS is the most common compression neuropathy in the upper extremity. This condition often is caused by pressure from trauma or edema caused by inflammation of a tendon (tenosynovitis), neoplasm, rheumatoid arthritis, or soft tissue masses such as ganglia. Symptoms of CTS are often seen during the premenstrual period, pregnancy, and menopause, suggesting hormones may be involved. Persons with diabetes mellitus and hypothyroidism also have a higher incidence of symptoms.[7,8] This syndrome is associated with hobbies or occupations that require continuous wrist movement (e.g., butchers, seamstresses, musicians, painters, carpenters, computer operators, bowlers, knitters). Women are more likely than men to develop CTS, possibly due to a smaller carpal tunnel.[8]

The clinical manifestations of CTS are weakness (especially of the thumb), burning pain (causalagia) and numbness, or impaired sensation in the distribution of the median nerve and clumsiness in performing fine hand movements. Numbness and tingling may be present that awaken the patient at night. Holding the wrists for 60 seconds produces tingling and numbness over the distribution of the median nerve: the palmar surface of the thumb, index finger, middle finger, and part of the ring finger (Fig. 63-3). This is known as a positive *Phalen's test.* Tapping gently over the volar aspect of the wrist (area of the inflamed median nerve) may reproduce paresthesia. This is known as a positive *Tinel's sign.* In late stages there is atrophy of the thenar muscles around the base of the thumb, resulting in recurrent pain and eventual dysfunction of the hand.

NURSING *and* COLLABORATIVE MANAGEMENT CARPAL TUNNEL SYNDROME

Prevention of CTS involves educating employees and employers to identify risk factors. Adaptive devices such as wrist splints may be worn to hold the wrist in a slight extension to relieve pressure on the median nerve. Special keyboard pads and mouses that help prevent repetitive pressure on the median nerve are available for

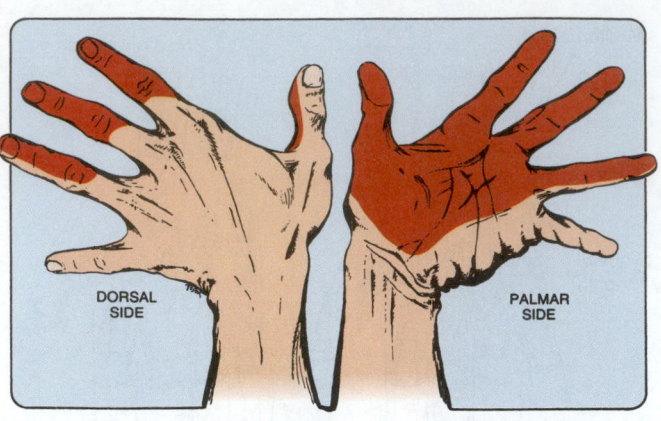

FIG. 63-3   Median nerve distribution. Shaded areas depict the locations of pain in carpal tunnel syndrome.

computer users. Other ergonomic changes include workstation modifications, change in body positions, and frequent breaks from work-related activities.

Collaborative care of the patient with CTS is directed toward relieving the underlying cause of the nerve compression. The early symptoms associated with CTS can usually be relieved by stopping the aggravating movement and by placing the hand and wrist at rest by immobilizing them in a hand splint. Injection of a corticosteroid drug directly into the carpal tunnel may provide short-term relief. As CTS may result in impaired sensation, the patient should be instructed to avoid hazards such as extremes of heat and cold because of the risk of thermal injury. The patient may be required to consider temporary occupational changes because of discomfort and sensory and functional changes.

If the problem continues, the median nerve may need to be surgically decompressed by longitudinal division of the transverse carpal ligament under local, regional, or general anesthesia (see Fig. 63-2, *B*). This surgery is done on an outpatient basis. After surgery, the neurovascular status of the hand should be evaluated before discharge, and the patient should be instructed in the appropriate assessments to perform at home. Endoscopic carpal tunnel release is a surgical procedure in which the decompression is performed through a small incision puncture site with the patient under local anesthesia. Modified open carpal tunnel release procedure is another alternative surgical intervention. Rehabilitation can last up to 7 weeks.[8]

ROTATOR CUFF INJURY

The rotator cuff is a complex of four muscles in the shoulder: the supraspinatus, infraspinatus, teres minor, and subscapularis muscles. These muscles act to stabilize the humeral head in the glenoid fossa while assisting with the ROM of the shoulder joint and rotation of the humerus. Degenerative changes of the rotator cuff may be associated with normal aging.

A tear in the rotator cuff may occur as a gradual, degenerative process resulting from aging, repetitive stress (especially overhead arm motions), or injury to the shoulder while falling.[9] The rotator cuff can tear as a result of sudden adduction forces applied to the cuff while the arm is held in abduction. In sports, repetitive overhead motions, such as in swimming, racquet sports (tennis, racquetball), and baseball (especially pitching), are often activities that initiate injury. A fall onto an outstretched arm and hand or a blow to the upper arm, heavy lifting, or repetitive work motions are also causative factors.

Manifestations of a rotator cuff injury include shoulder weakness and pain and decreased ROM. The patient usually experiences severe pain when the arm is abducted between 60 and 120 degrees (the painful arc). The *drop arm test,* in which the arm falls suddenly after the patient is asked to slowly lower the arm to the side after it has been abducted 90 degrees, is another sign of rotator cuff injury. An x-ray alone is usually not beneficial in the diagnosis of a rotator cuff injury. A tear can be confirmed by arthrogram or magnetic resonance imaging (MRI).

The goal of treatment emphasizes maintaining passive ROM and the return of abduction strength. The patient with a partial tear or cuff inflammation may be treated conservatively with rest, ice and heat, NSAIDs, corticosteroid injections into the joint, and physical therapy. If the patient does not respond to conservative treatment or if a complete tear is present, a surgical repair may be necessary.[10] Surgical repair may be performed through an arthroscope. If an extensive tear is present, *acromioplasty* (surgical removal of part of the acromion to relieve compression of rotator cuff during movement) may be necessary. An immobilization device such as a sling or, more commonly, a shoulder immobilizer may be used immediately after surgery. However, the shoulder should not be immobilized for too long a period because "frozen" shoulder or arthrofibrosis may occur. Pendulum exercises and physical therapy begin the first postoperative day.

MENISCUS INJURY

The menisci are crescent-shaped pieces of fibrocartilage in the knee. Menisci also line other joints. Meniscus injuries are closely associated with ligament sprains commonly occurring in athletes engaged in sports such as basketball, rugby, football, soccer, and hockey. These activities produce rotational stress when the knee is in varying degrees of flexion and the foot is planted or fixed. A blow to the knee can cause the meniscus to be sheared between the femoral condyles and the tibial plateau, resulting in a torn meniscus. (The knee joint is shown in Fig. 63-4.) Persons who work in occupations that require squatting or kneeling may be at higher risk for meniscus injuries.

Meniscus injuries alone do not usually cause significant edema because most of the cartilage is avascular. However, an acutely torn meniscus may be suspected when localized tenderness, pain, and effusion are noted (Fig. 63-5). Pain is elicited by flexion, internal rotation, and then extension of the knee (called the McMurray's test). The usual clinical picture is a feeling by the patient that the knee is unstable and a report that the knee may "click, pop, lock, or give way."[11] Quadriceps atrophy may be evident if the injury has been present for some time. Traumatic arthritis may occur from repeated meniscus injury and chronic inflammation.

An arthrogram, arthroscopy, or both can diagnose knee problems. MRI is beneficial in confirming the diagnosis before arthroscopy is used. MRI has eliminated the use of an arthrogram as a diagnostic tool in many cases. Surgery may be indicated for a torn meniscus. The degree of knee pain and dysfunction, occupation, sport activities, and age may affect the patient's decision to have or postpone surgery.

NURSING *and* COLLABORATIVE MANAGEMENT
MENISCUS INJURY

Because meniscal injuries are commonly caused by sports-related activity, athletes should be taught to do warm-up activities. Proper stretching may make the patient less prone to meniscal injury

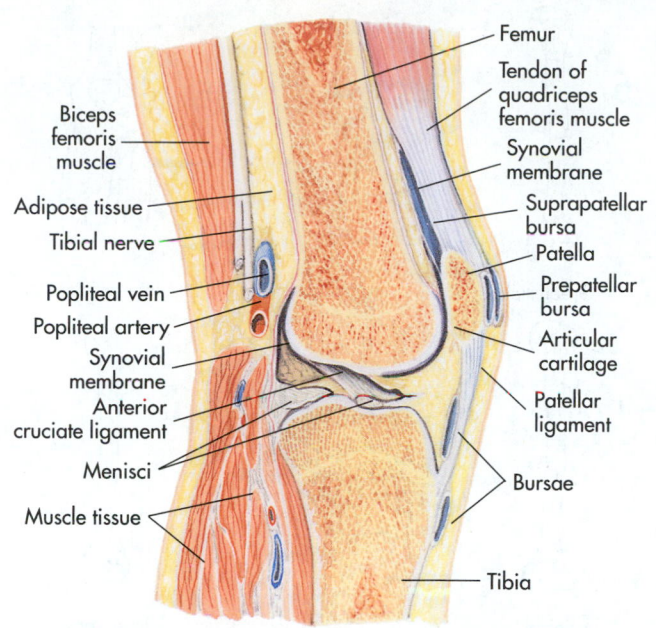

FIG. 63-4 Sagittal section through knee joint.

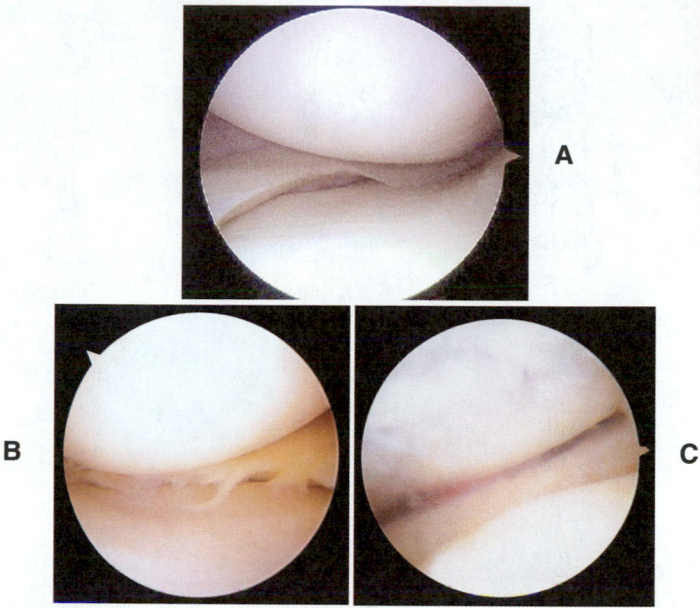

FIG. 63-5 Arthroscopic views of the meniscus. **A,** Normal meniscus. **B,** Torn meniscus. **C,** Surgically repaired meniscus.

when a fall or twisting occurs. Examination of the acutely injured knee should occur within 24 hours of injury. Initial care of this type of injury involves application of ice, immobilization, and partial weight bearing with crutches. Most meniscal injuries are treated in an outpatient setting. The patient should be allowed to ambulate as tolerated. Crutches may be necessary. Use of a knee brace or immobilizer during the first few days after the injury protects the knee and offers some pain relief.

After acute pain has decreased, physical therapy can help with gradual increases in flexion and muscle strengthening to assist the patient to reach full functioning. Surgical repair or excision of part of the meniscus (meniscectomy) may be necessary (see Fig. 63-5). Meniscal surgery is performed by arthroscopy. Pain relief may include NSAIDs or other analgesics. Rehabilitation starts soon after surgery, including quadriceps and hamstring strengthening exercises and ROM. When the patient's strength is back to its preinjury level, normal activities may be resumed.

BURSITIS

Bursae are closed sacs that are lined with synovial membrane and contain a small amount of synovial fluid. They are located at sites of friction, such as between tendons and bones and near the joints. **Bursitis** (inflammation of the bursa) results from repeated or excessive trauma or friction, gout, rheumatoid arthritis, or infection. The primary clinical manifestations of bursitis are warmth, pain, swelling, and limited ROM in the affected part. Sites at which bursitis commonly occurs include the hand, knee, greater trochanter of the hip, shoulder, and elbow. Improper body mechanics, repetitive kneeling (carpet layers, coal miners, and gardeners), jogging in worn-out shoes, and prolonged sitting with crossed legs are common precipitating factors of injury.

Attempts are made to determine and correct the cause of the bursitis. Rest is often the only treatment needed. Icing the area will decrease pain and may reduce local inflammation. The affected part may be immobilized in a compression dressing or splint. NSAIDs may be used to reduce inflammation and pain. Aspiration of the bursal fluid and intraarticular injection of a corticosteroid

may be necessary.[11] If the bursal wall has become thickened and continues to interfere with normal joint function, surgical excision (bursectomy) may be necessary. Septic bursae usually require surgical incision and drainage.

MUSCLE SPASMS

Local muscle spasms are a common condition often associated with sports and excessive everyday activities. Injury to a muscle results in inflammation and edema, which irritates nerve endings, resulting in muscle spasm. The spasms produce additional pain, creating a repetitive cycle. The clinical manifestations of muscle spasm include pain; palpable, tense, firm muscle mass; diminished ROM if a joint is involved; and limitation of daily or occupational activities.

A careful history and physical examination should be performed to rule out central nervous system (CNS) problems. Muscle spasms may be managed with drug therapy, physical therapy, or both. Drugs used for treatment of local muscle spasms include mild analgesics, NSAIDs, and skeletal muscle relaxants. A physical therapy program might include the use of heat or ice, supervised exercise, massage, hydrotherapy, local heat-producing applications (oil of wintergreen), ultrasound (deep heat), manipulation, and bracing.

Fractures

Classification

A **fracture** is a disruption or break in the continuity of the structure of bone. Traumatic injuries account for the majority of fractures, although some fractures are secondary to a disease process (pathologic fractures from cancer or osteoporosis). Fractures are described and classified according to (1) type (Fig. 63-6), (2) communication or noncommunication with the external environment (Fig. 63-7), and (3) anatomic location of fracture on the involved bone (Fig. 63-8). Fractures are also described as stable or unstable. A *stable fracture* occurs when a piece of the periosteum is intact across the fracture and either external or internal fixation has ren-

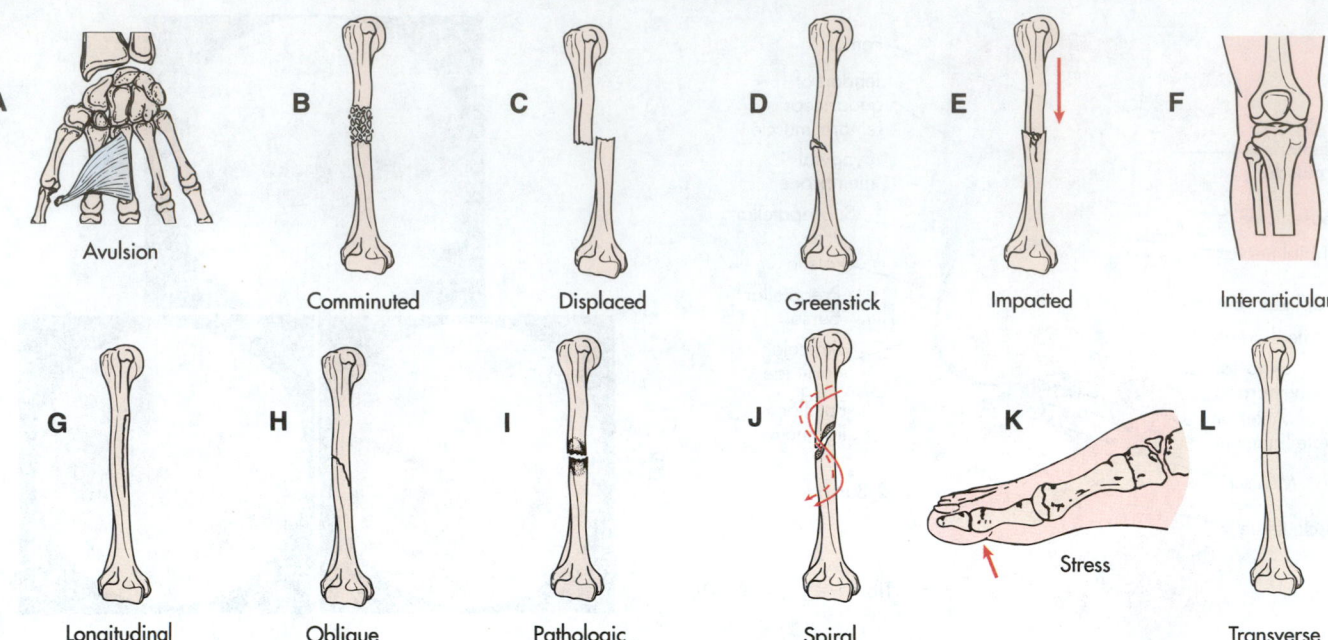

FIG. 63-6   Types of fractures. **A,** Avulsion is a fracture of bone resulting from the strong pulling effect of tendons or ligaments at the bone attachment. **B,** Comminuted fracture is a fracture with more than two fragments. The smaller fragments appear to be floating. **C,** Displaced (overriding) fracture involves a displaced fracture fragment that is overriding the other bone fragment. The periosteum is disrupted on both sides. **D,** Greenstick fracture is an incomplete fracture with one side splintered and the other side bent. **E,** Impacted fracture is a comminuted fracture in which more than two fragments are driven into each other. **F,** Interarticular fracture is a fracture extending to the articular (joint) surface of the bone. **G,** Longitudinal fracture is an incomplete fracture in which the fracture line runs along the longitudinal axis of the bone. The periosteum is not torn away from the bone. **H,** Oblique fracture is a fracture in which the line of the fracture extends in an oblique direction. **I,** Pathologic fracture is a spontaneous fracture at the site of a bone disease. **J,** Spiral fracture is a fracture in which the line of the fracture extends in a spiral direction along the shaft of the bone. **K,** Stress fracture is a fracture that occurs in normal or abnormal bone that is subject to repeated stress, such as from jogging or running. **L,** Transverse fracture is a fracture in which the line of the fracture extends across the bone shaft at a right angle to the longitudinal axis.

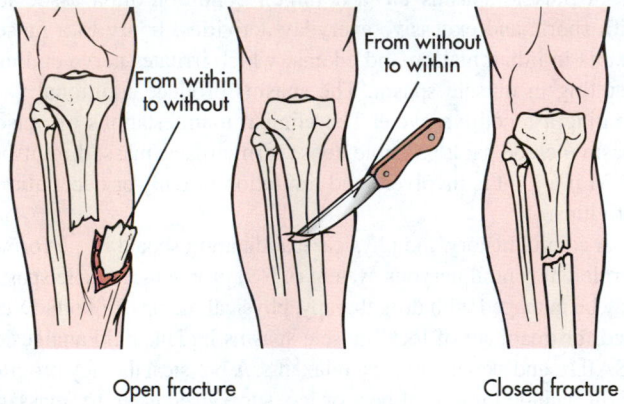

FIG. 63-7   Fracture classification according to communication with the external environment.

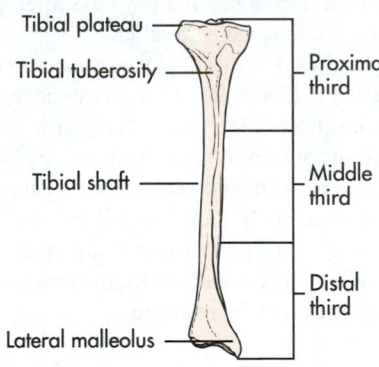

FIG. 63-8   Fracture classification according to location.

dered the fragments stationary. Stable fractures are usually transverse, spiral, or greenstick. An *unstable fracture* is grossly displaced during injury and is a site of poor fixation. Unstable fractures are usually comminuted or oblique.

A fracture can also be classified as closed (simple) or open. An *open fracture* (formerly called compound fracture) involves communication of the fracture through the skin with the external environment (see Fig. 63-7).

Clinical Manifestations

The patient's history indicates a mechanism of injury associated with numerous signs and symptoms, including immediate localized pain, decreased function, and inability to bear weight on or use the affected part (Table 63-4). The patient guards and protects the extremity against movement. The fracture may not be accompanied by obvious bone deformity. If a fracture is suspected, the extremity is immobilized in the position in which it is found. Unnecessary movement increases soft tissue damage and may convert a closed fracture to an open fracture or create further injury to adjacent neurovascular structures.

Fracture Healing

It is important to understand the principles of fracture healing (Fig. 63-9) to provide appropriate therapeutic interventions. Bone goes through a remarkable reparative process of self-healing (termed *union*) that occurs in the following stages:

1. *Fracture hematoma.* When a fracture occurs, bleeding creates a hematoma, which surrounds the ends of the fragments. The hematoma is extravasated blood that changes from a liquid to a semisolid clot. This occurs in the initial 72 hours after injury.

TABLE 63-4	Clinical Manifestations of Fracture
Manifestation	**Significance**
Edema and Swelling Disruption and penetration of bone through skin or soft tissues, or bleeding into surrounding tissues	Unchecked bleeding, swelling, and edema in closed space can occlude circulation and damage nerves (e.g., there is a risk of compartment syndrome).
Pain and Tenderness Muscle spasm as a result of involuntary reflex action of muscle, direct tissue trauma, increased pressure on nerves, movement of fracture parts	Pain and tenderness encourage splinting of musculature around the fracture with reduction in motion of injured area.
Muscle Spasm Irritation of tissues and protective response to injury and fracture	Muscle spasms may displace nondisplaced fracture or prevent it from reducing spontaneously.
Deformity Abnormal position of extremity/part as result of original forces of injury and action of muscles pulling fragment into abnormal position; seen as a loss of normal bony contours	Deformity is cardinal sign of fracture; if uncorrected, it may result in problems with bony union and restoration of function of injured part.
Ecchymosis/Contusion Discoloration of skin as a result of extravasation of blood in subcutaneous tissues	Ecchymosis may appear immediately after injury and may appear distal to injury. The nurse should reassure patient that process is normal and discoloration will eventually leave.
Loss of Function Disruption of bone or joint, preventing functional use of limb or part	Fracture must be managed properly to ensure restoration of function to limb/part.
Crepitation Grating or crunching together of bony fragments, producing palpable or audible crunching or popping sensation	Crepitation may increase chance for nonunion if bone ends are allowed to move excessively. Micromovement of bone-end fragments (postfracture) assists in osteogenesis (new bone growth).

2. *Granulation tissue.* During this stage, active phagocytosis absorbs the products of local necrosis. The hematoma converts to granulation tissue. Granulation tissue (consisting of new blood vessels, fibroblasts, and osteoblasts) produces the basis for new bone substance called *osteoid* during days 3 to 14 postinjury.

3. *Callus formation.* As minerals (calcium, phosphorus, and magnesium) and new bone matrix are deposited in the osteoid, an unorganized network of bone is formed that is woven about the fracture parts. Callus is primarily composed of cartilage, osteoblasts, calcium, and phosphorus. It usually appears by the end of the second week after injury. Evidence of callus formation can be verified by x-ray.

4. *Ossification.* Ossification of the callus occurs from 3 weeks to 6 months after the fracture and continues until the fracture has healed. Callus ossification is sufficient to prevent movement at the fracture site when the bones are gently stressed. However, the fracture is still evident on x-ray. During this stage of *clinical union* the patient may be allowed limited mobility or the cast may be removed.

5. *Consolidation.* As callus continues to develop, the distance between bone fragments diminishes and eventually closes. This stage is called consolidation, and ossification continues. It can be equated with radiologic union.

6. *Remodeling.* Excess bone tissue is reabsorbed in the final stage of bone healing, and union is completed. Gradual return of the injured bone to its preinjury structural strength and shape occurs. Bone remodels in response to physical loading stress or Wolf's law.[12] Initially, stress is provided

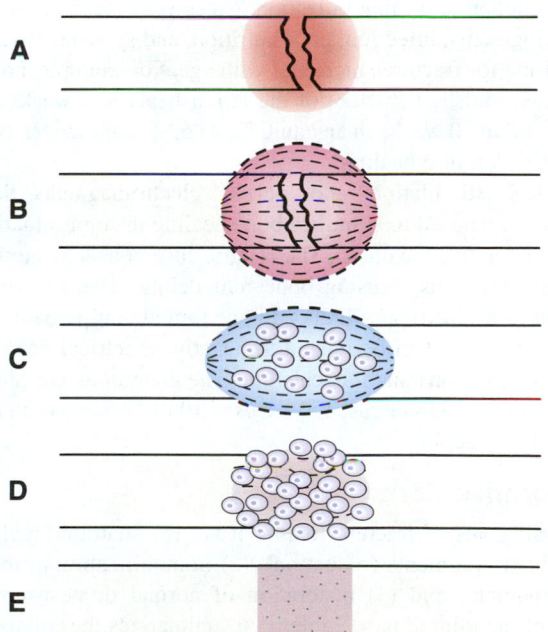

FIG. 63-9 Bone healing (schematic representation). **A,** Bleeding at fractured ends of the bone with subsequent hematoma formation. **B,** Organization of hematoma into fibrous network. **C,** Invasion of osteoblasts, lengthening of collagen strands, and deposition of calcium. **D,** Callus formation: new bone is built up as osteoclasts destroy dead bone. **E,** Remodeling is accomplished as excess callus is reabsorbed and trabecular bone is laid down.

TABLE 63-5	Complications of Fracture Healing
Problem	**Description**
Delayed union	Fracture healing progresses more slowly than expected; healing eventually occurs.
Nonunion	Fracture fails to heal properly despite treatment, resulting in fibrous union or pseudoarthrosis.
Malunion	Fracture heals in expected time but in unsatisfactory position, possibly resulting in deformity or dysfunction.
Angulation	Fracture heals in abnormal position in relation to midline of structure (type of malunion).
Pseudoarthrosis	Type of nonunion occurring at fracture site in which false joint is formed on shaft of long bones. It is a fracture site that failed to fuse. Each bone end is covered with fibrous scar tissue.
Refracture	New fracture occurs at original fracture site.
Myositis ossificans	Deposition of calcium in muscle tissue at the site of significant blunt muscle trauma or repeated muscle injury.

TABLE 63-6	COLLABORATIVE CARE Fractures

Diagnostic
History and physical examination
X-ray
CT scan, MRI

Collaborative Therapy
Fracture Reduction
Manipulation
Closed reduction
Traction devices
Skin traction
Skeletal traction
Open reduction/internal fixation

Fracture Immobilization
Casting or splinting
Traction
External fixation
Internal fixation

Open Fractures
Surgical debridement and irrigation
Tetanus and diphtheria immunization
Prophylactic antibiotic therapy
Immobilization

CT, Computed tomography; *MRI,* magnetic resonance imaging.

through exercise. Weight bearing is gradually introduced. New bone is deposited in sites subjected to stress and resorbed at areas where there is little stress. *Radiologic union* occurs when there is x-ray evidence of complete bony union. This phase can occur up to a year following injury.

Many factors, such as age, initial displacement of the fracture, site of the fracture, blood supply to the area, immobilization, implants, infection, and hormones, influence the time required for fracture healing to be complete. Fracture healing may not occur in the expected time *(delayed union)* or may not occur at all *(nonunion)*. The ossification process is arrested by causes such as inadequate reduction and immobilization, excessive movement of the fracture fragments, infection, poor nutrition, and systemic disease. Healing time for fractures increases with age. For example, an uncomplicated midshaft fracture of the femur heals in 3 weeks in a newborn and in 20 weeks in an adult. Table 63-5 summarizes complications of fracture healing.

Electrical stimulation and pulsed electromagnetic fields (PEMFs) can be used to stimulate bone healing in some situations of nonunion or delayed union. The electric current acts by modifying cell mechanisms, causing bone remodeling. The underlying mechanism for electrically induced bone remodeling remains unknown. It is thought to be related to negative electrical fields attracting positive ions such as calcium. The electrodes are placed over the patient's skin or cast and are used 10 to 12 hours each day, usually while sleeping.

Collaborative Care

The overall goals of fracture treatment are (1) anatomic realignment of bone fragments (reduction), (2) immobilization to maintain realignment, and (3) restoration of normal or near-normal function of the injured part. Table 63-6 summarizes the collaborative care of fractures.

Fracture Reduction

Closed Reduction. *Closed reduction* is a nonsurgical, manual realignment of bone fragments to their previous anatomic position. Traction and countertraction are manually applied to the bone fragments to restore position, length, and alignment. Closed reduction is usually performed while the patient is under local or general anesthesia. After reduction, traction, casting, external fixation, splints, or orthoses (braces) immobilize the injured part to maintain alignment until healing occurs.

Open Reduction. *Open reduction* is the correction of bone alignment through a surgical incision. It usually includes internal fixation of the fracture with the use of wires, screws, pins, plates, intramedullary rods, or nails. The type and location of the fracture, age of patient, and presence of concurrent disease, as well as the result of attempted closed reduction by means of traction, may influence the decision to use open reduction. The chief disadvantages of this form of fracture management are the possibility of infection, the complications associated with anesthesia, and the effects of premorbid medical conditions (e.g., diabetes) in the patient.

If open reduction with internal fixation (ORIF) is used for intraarticular fractures (involving joint surfaces), early initiation of ROM of the joint is indicated. Machines that provide continuous passive motion (CPM) to various joints (e.g., knee, shoulder) are now available. Use of these machines can help prevent extraarticular and intraarticular adhesions and result in faster reconstruction of the subchondral (beneath cartilage) bone plate, more rapid healing of the articular cartilage, and possibly decreased incidence of later posttraumatic arthritis. ORIF facilitates early ambulation, which decreases the risk of complications related to prolonged immobility, and promotes fracture healing with gradually increasing increments of stress placed upon the affected joint and soft tissue structures.

Traction. Traction is the application of a pulling force to an injured or diseased part of the body or an extremity while counter traction pulls in the opposite direction. The purpose of any traction is to (1) prevent or reduce muscle spasm, (2) immobilize a joint or part of the body, (3) reduce a fracture or dislocation, and (4) treat a pathologic joint condition. Traction is also indicated to (1) provide immobilization to prevent soft tissue damage, (2) reduce muscle spasm associated with low back pain or cervical whiplash,

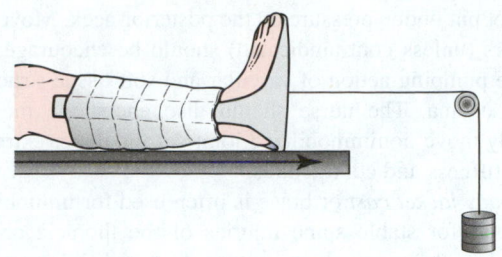

FIG. 63-10 Buck's traction. Commonly used for fractures of the hip, femur, knee, or back.

(3) expand a joint space during arthroscopic procedures, and (4) expand a joint space before major joint reconstruction.

Traction devices apply a pulling force on a fractured extremity to attain realignment while countertraction pulls in the opposite direction. The two most common types of traction are skin traction and skeletal traction. *Skin traction* is generally used for short-term treatment (48 to 72 hours) until skeletal traction or surgery is possible. Tape, boots, or splints are applied directly to the skin to maintain alignment, assist in reduction, and help diminish muscle spasms in the injured extremity. The traction weights are usually limited to 5 to 10 lb (2.3 to 4.5 kg). Pelvic or cervical skin traction may require heavier weights applied intermittently.

Skeletal traction, generally in place for longer periods than skin traction, is used to align injured bones and joints or to treat joint contractures and congenital hip dysplasia. It provides a long-term pull that keeps the injured bones and joints aligned. To apply skeletal traction, the physician inserts a pin or wire into the bone, either partially or completely, to align and immobilize the injured body part. Weight for skeletal traction ranges from 5 to 45 lb (2.3 to 20.4 kg). The use of too much weight can result in delayed union or nonunion. The major disadvantages of skeletal traction are infection in the area of the bone where the skeletal pin has been inserted and the consequences of prolonged immobility.

When traction is used to treat fractures, the forces are usually exerted on the distal fragment to obtain alignment with the proximal fragment. Several types of traction can be used for this purpose. One of the more common types is Buck's traction (Fig. 63-10). Fracture alignment depends on the correct positioning and alignment of the patient while the traction forces remain constant. For extremity traction to be effective, forces must be pulling in the opposite direction (countertraction) to prevent the patient from sliding to the end or side of the bed. Countertraction is commonly supplied by the patient's body weight or may be augmented by elevating the end of the bed. It is imperative that the nurse maintains the traction constantly and does not interrupt the weight applied to the traction.

Fracture Immobilization

Casts. A cast is a temporary circumferential immobilization device. Casting is a common treatment following closed reduction. It allows the patient to perform many normal activities of daily living while providing sufficient immobilization to ensure stability. Cast materials are natural (plaster of paris), synthetic acrylic, fiberglass free, latex-free polymer, or a hybrid of materials. Application of a cast generally incorporates the joints above and below a fracture. Immobilization above and below a joint restricts tendinoligamentous movement, therefore assisting with joint stabilization while the fracture heals.

After immersion in water, plaster of paris is wrapped and molded around the affected part after the bony prominences have

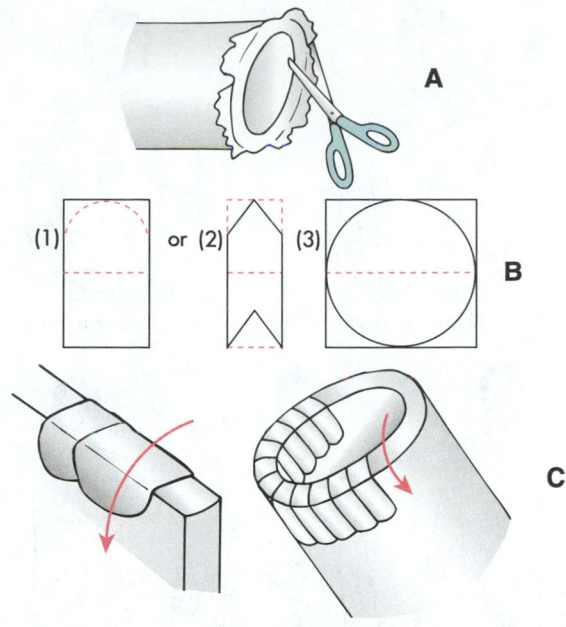

FIG. 63-11 Petaling edges of cast with waterproof adhesive strips. **A,** Cast must be thoroughly dry. The health care provider trims the excess sheet wadding and stretches the stockinette over the cast edge (when possible). **B,** Several strips (petals) of waterproof adhesive tape (2-inch-wide strips for wide areas and 1-inch-wide strips for small areas, each 1 inch long) are made in advance. **C,** Uncut end of the tape is placed beneath the cast edge. Each succeeding petal overlaps the previous one by one half inch, ensuring a smooth cast edge.

been padded. The number of layers of plaster bandage and the technique of application determine the strength of the cast. After the cast is completely dry, it is strong and firm and can withstand stresses. The plaster sets within 15 minutes, so the patient may move around without difficulty. However, it is not strong enough for weight bearing until about 24 to 72 hours.

A fresh plaster cast should never be covered with a blanket because air cannot circulate and heat builds up in the cast. During the drying period the cast should be kept dry and clean, and direct pressure should be avoided. Once the cast is thoroughly dry, the edges may need to be petaled to avoid skin irritation from rough edges and to prevent plaster of paris debris from falling into the cast and causing irritation or pressure necrosis (Fig. 63-11).

Synthetic casting materials (thermolabile plastic, thermoplastic resins, polyurethane, and fiberglass) are molded to fit the torso or extremity after being activated by submersion in cool or tepid water. Casts made of synthetic materials are being used more than plaster because they are lightweight and relatively waterproof and provide for immediate mobilization.

Types of Casts. Immobilization of an acute fracture or soft tissue injury of the upper extremity is often accomplished by use of (1) the sugar-tong splint, (2) the posterior splint, (3) the short arm cast, and (4) the long arm cast (Fig. 63-12). The sugar-tong splint is typically used for acute wrist injuries or injuries that may result in significant swelling. Plaster splints are applied over a well-padded forearm, beginning at the phalangeal joints of the hand, extending up the dorsal aspect of the forearm around the distal humerus, and then extending down the volar aspect of the forearm to the distal palmar crease. The splinting material is wrapped with either elastic bandage or bias stockinette. The sugar-tong posterior splint accommodates for swelling in the fractured extremity that occurs postinjury.

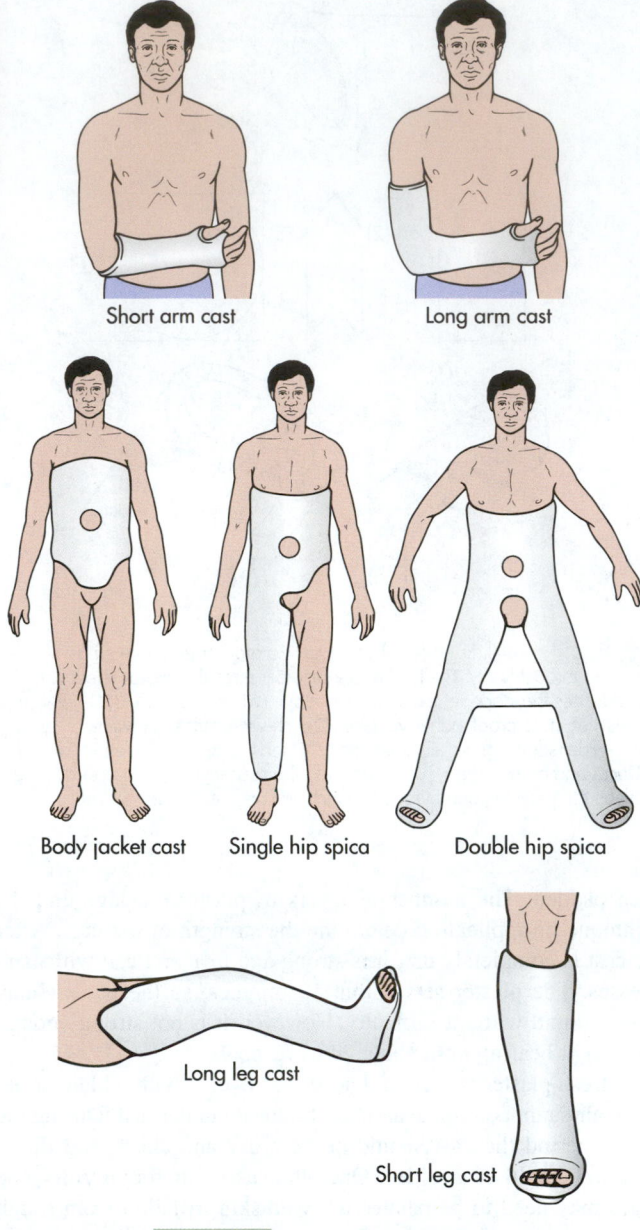

FIG. 63-12 Common types of casts.

The *short arm cast* is often used for the treatment of stable wrist or metacarpal fractures. An aluminum finger splint can be fabricated into the short arm cast for concurrent treatment of phalangeal injuries. The *short arm cast* is a circular cast extending from the distal palmar area to the proximal forearm. This cast provides wrist immobilization and permits unrestricted elbow motion.

The *long arm cast* is commonly used for stable forearm or elbow fractures and unstable wrist fractures. It is similar to the short arm cast but extends to the proximal humerus, restricting motion in the wrist and elbow. Nursing measures should be directed toward supporting the extremity and reducing the effects of edema by maintaining extremity elevation with a sling. However, when a hanging arm cast is used for a proximal humerus fracture, elevation or a supportive sling is contraindicated because hanging provides traction and promotes fracture healing.

When a sling is used, the nurse must ensure that the axillary area is well padded to prevent skin excoriation and maceration associated with direct skin-to-skin contact. Placement of the sling should not put undue pressure on the posterior neck. Movement of the fingers (unless contraindicated) should be encouraged to enhance the pumping action of vascular and soft tissue structures to decrease edema. The nurse should also encourage the patient to actively move nonimmobilized joints of the upper extremity to prevent stiffness and contractures.

The *body jacket cast* or brace is often used for immobilization and support for stable spine injuries of the thoracic or lumbar spine. This cast is applied around the chest and abdomen and extends from above the nipple line to the pubis. After application of the cast, the nurse must assess the patient for the development of *cast syndrome.* This condition occurs if the body cast is applied too tightly and the cast compresses the superior mesenteric artery against the duodenum. The patient generally complains of abdominal pain, abdominal pressure, nausea, and vomiting. The abdomen should be assessed for decreased bowel sounds (a window may be left over the umbilicus). Treatment includes gastric decompression with a nasogastric (NG) tube and suction. The cast may need to be removed or split. Nursing assessment also includes observation of respiratory status, bowel and bladder function, and areas of pressure over the bony prominences, especially the iliac crest. During the time required for the cast to dry, the nurse should reposition the patient every 2 to 3 hours to promote even cast drying and to relieve pressure and discomfort.

The *hip spica cast* is used for treatment of femoral fractures. The purpose of the hip spica cast is to immobilize the affected extremity and the trunk securely. It includes two casts joined together: (1) the body jacket cast and (2) the long leg cast. The location of the femoral fracture will determine whether the thigh of the unaffected extremity will have to be immobilized to restrict rotation of the pelvis and possible hip motion on the side of the femur fracture. The hip spica cast extends from above the nipple line to the base of the foot (single spica) and may include the opposite extremity up to an area above the knee (spica and a half) or both extremities (double spica).

The nurse should assess the patient with a hip spica cast for the same problems that are associated with the body jacket cast. During the initial drying stage the patient should not be placed in the prone position because the cast may break. The patient should be turned to an oblique side position and supported with pillows. When the patient is repositioned, the support bar joining the thighs must never be used to assist in moving because the bar can break and cause cast disruption. After the cast has dried, the nurse (with assistance) can turn the patient to the prone position and provide pillow support under the chest and immobilized extremity. Skin care around the cast edges (petaling) and the areas not encompassed by plaster is important to prevent any pressure sores. The nurse should instruct the patient in the positioning activities required to get on and off the bedpan. A fracture bedpan may be used to provide comfort and ease the movement of getting on and off the bedpan. After the hip spica cast has dried sufficiently, the patient may be instructed in ambulation techniques by the physical therapist.

Injuries to the Lower Extremity. Injuries to the lower extremity are often immobilized by a long leg cast, short leg cast, cylinder cast, a Jones dressing, or a prefabricated splint or immobilizer. The usual indications for applying a long leg cast are an unstable ankle fracture, soft tissue injuries, a fractured tibia, and knee injuries. The cast usually extends from the base of the toes to the groin and gluteal crease. The short leg cast can be used for a variety of conditions

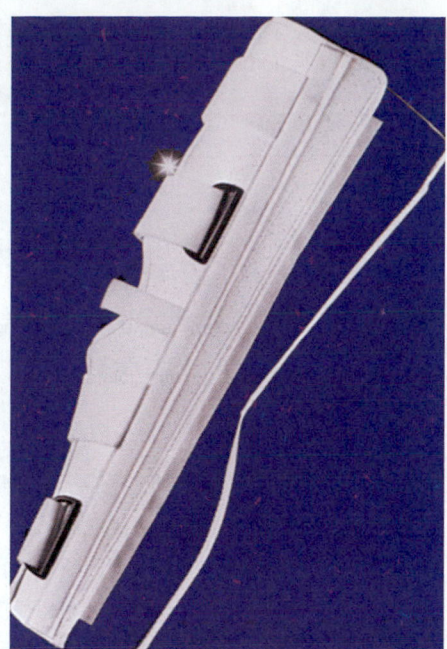

FIG. 63-13 Knee immobilizer.

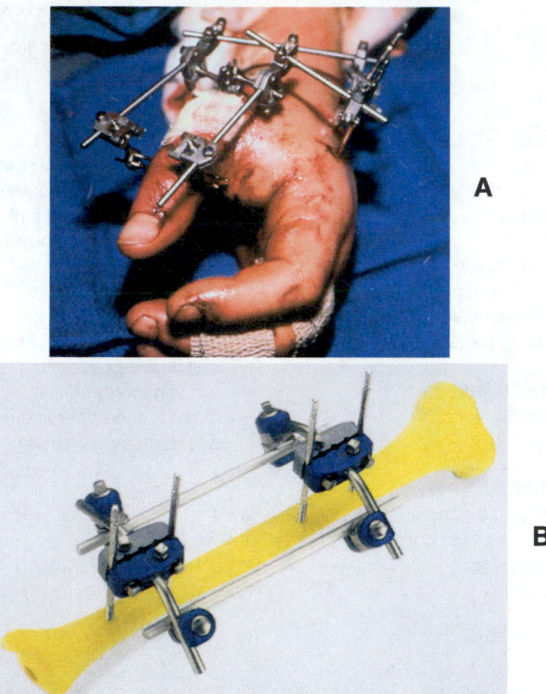

FIG. 63-14 External fixators. **A,** Mini-Hoffman system in use on hand. **B,** Hoffman II on the tibia (standard system).

but is primarily used for stable ankle and foot injuries. A cylinder cast is used for knee injuries or fractures. The cast extends from the groin to the malleoli of the ankle. A Jones dressing is composed of bulky padding materials (absorption dressing and cotton sheet wadding), splints, and an elastic wrap or bias-cut stockinette. After the application of a lower extremity cast or dressing, the extremity should be elevated onto pillows above the heart level for the first 24 hours. After the initial phase, the casted extremity should not be placed in a dependent position because of the possibility of excessive edema. Following cast application, the nurse should observe for signs of pressure, especially in the regions of the heel, anterior tibial border, fibular head, and malleoli.

Prefabricated knee and ankle splints and immobilizers are being used in many settings. This type of immobilization is easy to apply and remove, which permits close observation of the affected joint for signs of swelling and skin breakdown (Fig. 63-13). Depending on the injury, removal of the splint or immobilizer facilitates ROM of the affected joint and a faster return to function.

External Fixation. An external fixator is a metallic device composed of metal pins that are inserted into the bone and attached to external rods to stabilize the fracture while it heals. It can be used to apply traction or to compress fracture fragments and to immobilize reduced fragments when the use of a cast or other traction is not appropriate. The external device holds fracture fragments in place similar to a surgically implanted internal device. The external fixator is attached directly to the bones by percutaneous transfixing pins or wires (Fig. 63-14). External fixation is indicated in simple fractures (either open or closed), complex fractures with extensive soft tissue damage, correction of bony defects (congenital), pseudoarthrosis, and nonunion or malunion and for limb lengthening.

External fixation has many advantages over other fracture management strategies and is often employed in an attempt to salvage extremities that otherwise might require amputation. Because the use of an external device is a long-term process, ongoing assessment for pin loosening and infection is critical. Infection signaled by exudate, erythema, tenderness, and pain may require removal of the device.

The nurse should instruct the patient and family about meticulous pin care. Although each physician has a protocol for pin care cleaning, half-strength hydrogen peroxide with normal saline is often used.

Internal Fixation. Internal fixation devices (pins, plates, intramedullary rods, and metal and bioabsorbable screws) are surgically inserted at the time of realignment. Biologically inert metal devices such as stainless steel, Vitallium, or titanium are used to realign and maintain bony fragments. Proper alignment is evaluated by x-ray studies at regular intervals.

Drug Therapy. Patients with fractures experience varying degrees of pain associated with muscle spasms. Involuntary reflexes that result from edema and nerve injury following muscle injury cause these spasms. Central and peripheral muscle relaxants, such as carisoprodol (Soma), cyclobenzaprine (Flexeril), or methocarbamol (Robaxin) may be prescribed for relief of pain associated with muscle spasms.

Common side effects associated with muscle relaxants are drowsiness, lassitude, headache, weakness, fatigue, blurred vision, ataxia, and gastrointestinal upset.[13] Hypersensitivity reactions may include skin rash or pruritus. Ingestion of large doses of muscle relaxants may cause hypotension, tachycardia, or respiratory depression. The possible habituating effects associated with long-term use and the potential for abuse must be carefully considered.

In an open fracture the threat of tetanus can be reduced with tetanus and diphtheria toxoid or tetanus immunoglobulin for the patient who has not been previously immunized. Bone-penetrating antibiotics, such as a cephalosporin (e.g., cefazolin [Kefzol, Ancef]), are used prophylactically.

Nutritional Therapy. Proper nutrition is an essential component of the reparative process in injured tissue. An adequate energy source is needed to promote muscle strength and tone, build endurance, and provide energy for ambulation and gait-training skills. The patient's dietary requirements must include ample protein

TABLE 63-7	*EMERGENCY MANAGEMENT* **Fractured Extremity**

Etiology	Assessment Findings	Interventions

Blunt
Motor vehicle collision
Pedestrian event
Falls
Direct blows
Forced flexion or
    hyperextension
Twisting forces
 	
Penetrating
Gunshot
Blast
 	
Other
Pathologic conditions
Violent muscle contractions
    (seizures)
Crush injury
	• Deformity (loss of normal
	  bony contours) or unnatural
	  position of affected limb
	• Edema and ecchymosis
	• Muscle spasm
	• Tenderness and pain
	• Loss of function
	• Numbness, tingling, loss of
	  distal pulses
	• Grating (crepitus)
	• Open wound over injured
	  site, exposure of bone
		Initial
		• Treat life-threatening injuries first.
		• Ensure airway, breathing, and circulation.
		• Control external bleeding with direct pressure or sterile pressure dressing and
		  elevation of the extremity.
		• Splint joints above and below fracture site.
		• Check neurovascular status distal to injury before and after splinting.
		• Elevate injured limb if possible.
		• Do *not* attempt to straighten fractured or dislocated joints.
		• Do *not* manipulate protruding bone ends.
		• Apply ice packs to affected area.
		• Obtain x-rays of affected limb.
		• Administer tetanus and diphtheria prophylaxis if skin integrity is compromised.
		• Mark location of pulses to facilitate repeat assessment.
		• Splint fracture site, including joints above and below fracture site.
		
		Ongoing Monitoring
		• Monitor vital signs, level of consciousness, oxygen saturation, neurovascular
		  status, and pain.
		• Monitor for compartment syndrome characterized by excessive pain, pain
		  with passive stretch of the affected extremity muscles, pallor, paresthesia,
		  paralysis, and pulselessness.
		• Monitor for fat embolism (dyspnea, chest pain, temperature elevation).

(e.g., 1 g/kg of body weight), vitamins (especially B, C, and D), and calcium, phosphorus, and magnesium to ensure optimal soft tissue and bone healing. Low serum protein levels and vitamin C deficiencies interfere with tissue healing. Immobility and callus formation increase calcium needs. Three well-balanced meals a day will usually provide the necessary nutrients. The well-balanced meal should be supplemented by a fluid intake of 2000 to 3000 ml/day to promote optimal bladder and bowel function. Adequate fluid and a high-fiber diet with fruits and vegetables will prevent constipation. If immobilized in bed with skeletal traction or in a body jacket or hip spica cast, the patient should be instructed to eat six small meals so as not to overeat and thus avoid abdominal pressure and cramping.

NURSING MANAGEMENT
FRACTURES

▪ *Nursing Assessment*

A brief history of the traumatic episode, mechanism of injury, and the position in which the victim was found can be obtained from the patient or witnesses. As soon as possible, the patient should be transported to an emergency department where a thorough assessment and treatment can be initiated (Table 63-7). Subjective and objective data that should be obtained from an individual with a fracture are presented in Table 63-8.

Special emphasis must be placed on the region distal to the site of injury. Clinical findings must be documented before fracture treatment is initiated to avoid doubts about whether a problem discovered later was missed during the original examination or was caused by the treatment.

Neurovascular Assessment. Musculoskeletal injuries have the potential for causing changes in the neurovascular status of an injured extremity. With musculoskeletal trauma, application of a cast or constrictive dressing, poor positioning, and the physiologic responses to the traumatic injury can cause nerve or vascular damage, usually distal to the injury. A thorough neurovascular assessment consists of a peripheral vascular assessment (color, temperature, capillary refill, peripheral pulses, and edema) and a peripheral neurologic assessment (sensation, motor function, and pain). Throughout the neurovascular assessment, both extremities are compared to obtain an accurate assessment.

An extremity's color (pink, pale, cyanotic) and temperature (hot, warm, cool, cold) in the area of the affected extremity are assessed. Pallor or a cool/cold extremity below the injury could indicate arterial insufficiency. A warm, cyanotic extremity could indicate poor venous return. Capillary refill (blanching of the nail bed) is assessed next. The standard for a compressed nail bed to return to its original color is within 2 seconds. Accurate documentation and ongoing neurovascular assessments are the cornerstones of nursing care for the individual with a musculoskeletal injury.

Pulses on both the unaffected and injured extremity are compared to identify differences in rate or quality. Pulses are described as strong, diminished, audible by Doppler, or absent. A diminished or absent pulse distal to the injury can indicate vascular dysfunction and insufficiency. However, some adults do not have specific pulses, including an absent dorsalis pedis (17% of adults) and an absent posterior tibial (9% of African Americans).[12] Peripheral edema is also assessed; pitting edema may be present with severe injury.

Evaluating the ulnar, median, and radial nerves assesses sensation and motor innervation in the upper extremity. Neurovascular status can be assessed by abduction and adduction of the fingers,

TABLE 63-8	**NURSING ASSESSMENT** Fracture

Subjective Data
Important Health Information
Past health history: Traumatic injury; long-term repetitive forces (stress fracture); bone or systemic diseases, prolonged immobility, osteopenia, osteoporosis
Medications: Use of corticosteroids (osteoporotic fractures); analgesics
Surgery or other treatments: First aid treatment of fracture, previous musculoskeletal surgeries

Functional Health Patterns
Health perception–health management: Estrogen replacement therapy, calcium supplementation
Activity-exercise: Loss of motion or weakness of affected part; muscle spasms
Cognitive-perceptual: Sudden and severe pain in affected area; numbness, tingling, loss of sensation distal to injury; chronic pain that increases with activity (stress fracture)

Objective Data
General
Apprehension, guarding of injured site

Integumentary
Skin lacerations, pallor and cool skin or bluish and warm skin distal to injury; ecchymosis, hematoma, edema at site of fracture

Cardiovascular
Reduced or absent pulse distal to injury, ↓ skin temperature, delayed capillary refill

Neurovascular
Paresthesias, absent or ↓ sensation, hypersensation

Musculoskeletal
Restricted or lost function of affected part; local bony deformities, abnormal angulation; shortening, rotation, or crepitation of affected part; muscle weakness

Possible Findings
Localization and extent of fractures on x-ray, bone scans, CT scan, or MRI

CT, Computed tomography; *MRI,* magnetic resonance imaging.

opposition of the fingers, and supination and pronation of the hand. In the lower extremity, dorsiflexion and plantar flexion assess motor function of the peroneal and tibial nerves. Sensory innervation is evaluated for the peroneal nerve on the dorsal part of the foot between the web space of the great and second toes. Tibial nerve assessment is performed by stroking the plantar surface (sole) of the foot. Contralateral evaluation is critical. Paresthesia (abnormal sensation [e.g., numbness, tingling]), decreased sensation, hypersensation/hyperesthesia, or partial or full loss of sensation (paresis/paralysis) may be reported by the patient. Reduced motion or strength in an injured extremity alerts the nurse to potential limb-threatening complications or disability.

Pain is the final element of the neurovascular assessment. The nurse must carefully assess the location, quality, and intensity of the pain (see Chapter 10). Current nursing practice is to evaluate the patient's level of pain on a scale of 1 to 10. Pain unrelieved by drugs and out of proportion to the level of injury is an indication of compartment syndrome.

Patients should be instructed to report any changes in their neurovascular status. Patients must verbalize and demonstrate a thorough understanding of all elements before discharge from the treatment setting.

■ Nursing Diagnoses

Nursing diagnoses for the patient with a fracture may include, but are not limited to, those presented in NCP 63-1.

■ Planning

The overall goals are that the patient with a fracture will (1) have physiologic healing with no associated complications, (2) obtain satisfactory pain relief, and (3) achieve maximal rehabilitation potential.

■ Nursing Implementation

Health Promotion. The public should be taught to take appropriate safety precautions to prevent injuries while at home, at work, when driving, or when participating in sports. Nurses should be staunch advocates for personal actions known to reduce injuries, such as the regular use of seat belts, driving within posted speed limits, stretching and warming up muscles prior to exercise, use of protective athletic equipment (helmets and knee, wrist, and elbow pads), use of safety equipment at work, and not combining drinking and driving.

Individuals (especially older adults) should be encouraged to participate in moderate exercise to aid in the maintenance of muscle strength and balance. To reduce falls, living environments should be examined so that scatter rugs are removed, adequate footwear and lighting are maintained, and paths to the bathroom cleared for nighttime use. The nurse should also stress the importance of adequate calcium and vitamin D intake.

Acute Intervention. Patients with fractures may be treated in an emergency department or a physician's office and released to home care, or they may require hospitalization for varying amounts of time. Specific nursing measures depend on the type of treatment used and the setting in which patients are placed.

Preoperative Management. If surgical intervention is required to treat a fracture, patients will need preoperative preparation. In addition to the usual preoperative nursing measures (see Chapter 18), the nurse should inform patients of the type of immobilization and assistive devices that will be used and the expected activity limitations after surgery. Patients must be assured that their needs will be met by the nursing staff until they can again meet their own needs. Assurance that pain medication will be available if needed is often beneficial.

Proper skin preparation is an important part of preoperative preparation. The protocol for skin preparation varies among agencies and may be the responsibility of the nurse. The aim of skin preparation is to assist in the cleansing of the skin and remove debris and hair to reduce the possibility of infection. Careful attention to this preoperative treatment can influence the postoperative course.

Postoperative Management. In general, postoperative nursing care and management are directed toward monitoring vital signs and applying the general principles of postoperative nursing care (see Chapter 20). Frequent neurovascular assessments of the affected extremity are necessary to detect early and subtle neurovascular changes. Any limitations of movement or activity related to turning, positioning, and extremity support should be monitored closely. Pain and discomfort can be minimized through proper alignment and positioning. Dressings or casts should be carefully observed for any overt signs of bleeding or drainage. A significant increase in size of the drainage area should be reported. If a wound drainage system is in place, the patency of the system and the

NURSING CARE PLAN 63-1

Patient with a Fracture

NURSING DIAGNOSIS **Impaired physical mobility** *related to* loss of integrity of bone structures, movement of bone fragments, soft tissue injury, and prescribed movement restrictions *as evidenced by* limited joint range of motion, inability to purposefully move, and inability to bear weight

PATIENT GOALS
1. Experiences uncomplicated bone healing and return of skeletal function
2. Uses assistive devices as necessary to increase physical mobility
3. Experiences no complications of immobility

OUTCOMES (NOC)

Bone Healing
- Intact peripheral circulation ____
- Return of skeletal function ____

Measurement Scale

1 = None
2 = Limited
3 = Moderate
4 = Substantial
5 = Extensive

- Hematoma ____
- Pain ____
- Edema ____
- Infection in surrounding tissue ____
- Infection in bone ____

Measurement Scale

1 = Extensive
2 = Substantial
3 = Moderate
4 = Limited
5 = None

Mobility
- Balance ____
- Coordination ____
- Joint movement ____
- Moves with ease ____

Measurement Scale

1 = Severely compromised
2 = Substantially compromised
3 = Moderately compromised
4 = Mildly compromised
5 = Not compromised

INTERVENTIONS (NIC) and *RATIONALES*

Splinting
- Support the affected body part *to avoid fracture displacement and soft tissue injury.*
- Move the injured extremity as little as possible *to avoid additional injury.*
- Monitor for bleeding at injury site *to plan appropriate intervention.*

Traction/Immobilization Care
- Position in proper body alignment *to enhance traction and skeletal function.*
- Maintain traction at all times *to prevent misalignment of bone fragments.*
- Monitor circulation, movement, and sensation of affected extremity *to detect complications of peripheral vascular function.*
- Provide trapeze for movement in bed *to reduce complications of immobility.*
- Monitor skin and body prominences for signs of skin breakdown.
- Administer appropriate skin care at friction points *to prevent skin breakdown.*

Cast Care: Wet
- Expose drying cast to air *to promote even drying.*
- Support cast with pillows during the drying period *to prevent denting and flattening of the cast.*
- Apply plastic to cast if close to groin *to prevent soiling of cast.*
- Mark the circumference of any drainage *as a gauge for future assessments.*

Cast Care: Maintenance
- Instruct patient not to scratch skin under the cast with any objects *to prevent skin injury and infection.*
- Position cast on pillows *to lessen strain on other body parts.*
- Pad rough cast edges and traction connections *to prevent skin irritation and breakdown of cast.*

NURSING DIAGNOSIS **Ineffective therapeutic regimen management** *related to* lack of knowledge regarding muscle atrophy, exercise program, and care of casts or external immobilizers *as evidenced by* questions about long-term effect of immobilization, devices, activity restrictions

PATIENT GOALS
1. Describes the prescribed activity and its rationale
2. Demonstrates appropriate care of cast or immobilizer

OUTCOMES (NOC)

Knowledge: Prescribed Activity
- Description of prescribed activity ____
- Description of purpose of activity ____
- Description of strategies for gradual activity increase ____

Measurement Scale

1 = None
2 = Limited
3 = Moderate
4 = Substantial
5 = Extensive

INTERVENTIONS (NIC) and *RATIONALES*

Teaching: Prescribed Activity/Exercise
- Inform patient of the purpose for, and the benefits of, the prescribed activity/exercise *so patient will exercise involved extremity when immobilization is no longer necessary.*
- Instruct the patient how to perform prescribed activity/exercise.
- Observe the patient perform the prescribed activity/exercise.

Teaching: Psychomotor Skill
- Demonstrate the skill for the patient.
- Provide written information/diagrams.
- Provide frequent feedback to patient on what he/she is doing correctly and incorrectly *so that bad habits are not formed.*

NURSING CARE PLAN 63-1

Patient with a Fracture—cont'd

NURSING DIAGNOSIS   **Risk for peripheral neurovascular dysfunction** *related to* vascular insufficiency and nerve compression secondary to edema and application of traction, splints, or casts

PATIENT GOAL   Experiences no peripheral neurovascular dysfunction

OUTCOMES (NOC)	INTERVENTIONS (NIC) and *RATIONALES*
Tissue Perfusion: Peripheral	**Circulatory Precautions**

Tissue Perfusion: Peripheral

- Capillary refill fingers _____
- Capillary refill toes _____
- Extremity skin temperature _____
- Sensation _____
- Skin color _____
- Muscle function _____
- Skin integrity _____

Measurement Scale

1 = Severely compromised
2 = Substantially compromised
3 = Moderately compromised
4 = Mildly compromised
5 = Not compromised

- Localized extremity pain _____
- Peripheral edema _____

Circulatory Precautions

- Perform a comprehensive appraisal of peripheral circulation (e.g., check peripheral pulses, edema, capillary refill, color, temperature of extremity) *to monitor for diminished tissue perfusion and plan appropriate intervention.*
- Prevent infection in wounds *to prevent further edema and inflammation, which may contribute further to vascular insufficiency and nerve compression.*
- Maintain adequate hydration *to prevent increased blood viscosity.*

Positioning

- Immobilize or support affected body part *to prevent pressure and injury.*
- Maintain position and integrity of traction *to prevent compression of blood vessels and nerves.*
- Elevate affected limb 20 degrees or greater above the level of the heart *to reduce edema by promoting venous return.* (*Note:* if compartment syndrome is suspected, elevate extremity no higher than heart level.)

Peripheral Sensation Management

- Monitor for paresthesia: numbness, tingling, hyperesthesia, and hypoesthesia.
- Monitor sharp/dull and/or hot/cold discrimination *to assure early recognition of and intervention for compromised circulation or nerve compression.*

NURSING DIAGNOSIS   **Acute pain** *related to* edema, movement of bone fragments, and muscle spasm *as evidenced by* pain descriptors, guarding, crying

PATIENT GOAL   Reports satisfaction with pain-relief measures

OUTCOMES (NOC)	INTERVENTIONS (NIC) and *RATIONALES*

Pain Control

- Uses preventive measures _____
- Uses nonanalgesic relief measures _____
- Uses analgesics appropriately _____
- Reports uncontrolled symptoms to health care professional _____
- Reports pain controlled _____

Measurement Scale

1 = Never demonstrated
2 = Rarely demonstrated
3 = Sometimes demonstrated
4 = Often demonstrated
5 = Consistently demonstrated

Pain Management

- Perform a comprehensive assessment of pain to include location, characteristics, onset/duration, intensity or severity of pain, and precipitating factors *to plan appropriate interventions.*
- Provide patient optimal pain-relief with prescribed analgesics *to relieve pain and promote muscle relaxation.*
- Notify physician if measures are unsuccessful or if current complaint is a significant change from patient's past experience of pain *since this may indicate an impending compartment syndrome.*
- Teach the use of nonpharmacologic techniques (e.g., relaxation, guided imagery, hot/cold application, and massage) before, after, and, if possible, during painful activities; before pain occurs or increases; and along with other pain-relief measures *to reduce edema and promote comfort.*

volume of drainage should be regularly measured and assessed. Whenever the contents of a drainage system are measured or emptied, the nurse should use sterile technique to avoid contamination. Additional nursing responsibilities depend on the type of immobilization used. A blood salvage and reinfusion system that allows for recovery and reinfusion of the patient's own blood may be used. The blood is retrieved from a joint space or cavity, and the patient receives this blood in the form of an autotransfusion. (Autotransfusion is discussed in Chapter 31.) NCP 63-2 is for the patient who has had orthopedic surgery.

Other Measures. Patients often have reduced mobility as a result of the fracture. The nurse must plan care to prevent the many complications associated with immobility. Constipation can be prevented by increased activity and maintenance of a high fluid intake (more than 2500 ml/day unless contraindicated by the patient's health status) and a diet high in bulk and roughage (fresh fruits and vegetables). If these measures are not effective in maintaining the patient's normal bowel pattern, warm fluids, stool softeners, laxatives, or suppositories may be necessary. Maintaining a regular time for elimination aids in promoting regularity.

Renal calculi can develop as a result of bone demineralization. The hypercalcemia from demineralization causes a rise in urine pH and stone formation resulting from the precipitation of calcium. Unless contraindicated, a fluid intake of 2500 ml/day is recommended.

EVIDENCE-BASED PRACTICE

Are Interventions to Reduce the Incidence of Falls Effective?

Clinical Question

In elderly persons (P), are interventions to reduce risk factors for falls (I) more effective than the usual care (C) in reducing the incidence of falls (O)?

Best Available Evidence

Systematic review of randomized controlled trials (RCTs)

Critical Appraisal and Synthesis of Evidence

- 62 RCTs (*n* = 21,668) comparing exercise/physical therapy programs, cognitive/behavioral programs, medication withdrawal, home hazard modification, cardiac pacing, and nutrition and hormonal supplementation.
- Participants were at risk for or had a history of falling, and lived in a community or institutional care facility. Most participants were over age 80, with the majority being female.

Conclusions

- Interventions found to be beneficial included muscle strengthening and balance retraining, Tai Chi exercise, psychotropic medication withdrawal, home hazard assessment and modification, and cardiac pacemaker insertion for persons with cardioinhibitory carotid sinus hypersensitivity.
- Interventions delivered by a health care professional that are individually focused are more effective than standard or group-delivered programs.

Implications for Nursing Practice

- Instruct patients at risk for falling on the value of interventions that are likely to be effective.
- Locate programs and resources that can assist persons in decreasing their risk of falling.
- Further study is needed to determine if interventions that are effective in reducing falls also help in reducing fall severity (e.g., fractures).

Reference for Evidence

Gillespie LD, Gillespie WJ, Robertson MC, et al: Interventions for preventing falls in elderly people, Cochrane Bone, Joint and Muscle Trauma Group, *Cochrane Database Syst Rev* 4:CD000340, 2005.

PICO: P, Patient population of interest; *I,* intervention or area of interest; *C,* comparison of interest or comparison group; *O,* outcome(s) of interest (see p. 6).

TABLE 63-9	PATIENT AND FAMILY TEACHING GUIDE Cast Care

Do Not

- Get plaster cast wet.
- Remove any padding.
- Insert any objects inside cast.
- Bear weight on new cast for 48 hr (not all casts are made for weight bearing; check with health care provider when unsure).
- Cover cast with plastic for prolonged periods.

Do

- Apply ice directly over fracture site for first 24 hr (avoid getting cast wet by keeping ice in plastic bag and protecting cast with cloth).
- Check with health care provider before getting fiberglass cast wet.
- Dry cast thoroughly after exposure to water.
  - Blot dry with towel.
  - Use hair dryer on low setting until cast is thoroughly dry.
- Elevate extremity above level of heart for first 48 hr.
- Move joints above and below cast regularly.
- Report signs of possible problems to health care provider.
  - Increasing pain.
  - Swelling associated with pain and discoloration of toes or fingers.
  - Pain during movement.
  - Burning or tingling under cast.
  - Sores or foul odor under the cast.
- Keep appointment to have fracture and cast checked.

---

regular removal of exudate with half-strength hydrogen peroxide, rinsing pin sites with sterile saline, and drying of the area with sterile gauze.[14]

External rotation of the hip can occur when skin traction is used on the lower extremity. The nurse can correct this position by placing a pillow, sandbag, or rolled-up draw sheet along the greater trochanteric region of the femur. Generally, the patient should be in the center of the bed in a supine position. Incorrect alignment can result in increased pain and nonunion or malunion.

To offset some of the problems associated with prolonged immobility, the nurse should discuss specific patient activity with the health care provider. If exercise is permitted, the nurse should encourage participation by the patient in a simple exercise regimen based on activity restrictions. Activities that the patient should participate in include frequent position changes, ROM exercises of unaffected joints, deep breathing exercises, isometric exercises, and use of the trapeze bar (if permitted) to raise oneself off the bed for linen changes and use of the bedpan. These activities should be performed several times each day.

If allowed, active exercises that move uninvolved joints through the ROM are the preferred activity. Frequent exercise of the trunk and extremities is an excellent stimulus to deep breathing. Active, resistive exercise (isotonic) of uninvolved extremities helps reduce deconditioning from prolonged immobility.

Ambulatory and Home Care

Cast Care. Because many fractures are casted in an outpatient setting, the patient often requires only a short hospitalization or none at all. Regardless of the type of cast material, a cast can interfere with circulation and nerve function from being applied too tightly or because of excessive edema that occurs after application. Thus frequent neurovascular assessments of the immobilized extremity are critical. The patient must be taught about signs of cast complications so that they can be reported promptly. Elevation of the extremity above the level of the heart to promote venous return and applications of ice to control or prevent edema are mea-

Cranberry juice or ascorbic acid (500 to 1500 mg/day) may be recommended to acidify the urine and prevent calcium precipitation in the urine. (Renal calculi are discussed in Chapter 46.)

Rapid deconditioning of the cardiopulmonary system can occur as a result of prolonged bed rest, resulting in orthostatic hypotension and decreased lung capacity. Unless contraindicated, these effects can be diminished by permitting the patient to sit on the side of the bed, allowing the patient's lower limbs to dangle over the bedside, and having the patient perform standing transfers. When the patient is allowed to increase activity, careful evaluation should be made to assess for orthostatic hypotension. Patients must also be assessed for deep vein thrombosis (DVT) and pulmonary emboli. (DVT is discussed in Chapter 38.)

Traction. When slings are used with traction, the nurse should inspect exposed skin areas regularly. Pressure over a bony prominence created by the wrinkling of sheets or bedclothes may cause pressure necrosis. Persistent skin pressure may impair blood flow and cause injury to the peripheral neurovascular structures. Skeletal traction pin sites must be observed for signs of infection. Pin site care varies but usually includes

NURSING CARE PLAN 63-2

Patient Having Orthopedic Surgery*

NURSING DIAGNOSIS **Acute pain** *related to* tissue trauma, disruption of skin integrity, and edema *as evidenced by* reluctance to move, guarding of affected area, persistent score of >8 on 10-point pain scale, and facial grimacing

PATIENT GOAL Reports satisfactory relief of pain

OUTCOMES (NOC)	INTERVENTIONS (NIC) and *RATIONALES*
Pain Control	**Pain Management**
• Uses nonanalgesic relief measures ____ • Uses analgesics appropriately ____ • Reports uncontrolled symptoms to health care professional ____ • Reports pain controlled ____	• Encourage patient to monitor own pain and to intervene appropriately *to increase patient's control over pain management.* • Implement use of patient-controlled analgesia (PCA) *to give patient control.* • Medicate prior to an activity *to increase participation but evaluate hazard of sedation.* • Evaluate effectiveness of pain-control measures used through ongoing assessment of pain experience *so that pain relief is in accordance with healing process.*
Measurement Scale 1 = Never demonstrated 2 = Rarely demonstrated 3 = Sometimes demonstrated 4 = Often demonstrated 5 = Consistently demonstrated	**Positioning** • Position in proper body alignment *to reduce pressure on nerves and tissues.*

NURSING DIAGNOSIS **Impaired physical mobility** *related to* pain, stiffness, and surgical procedure *as evidenced by* limited joint movement, difficulty ambulating, inability to participate in physical rehabilitation, guarded movement

PATIENT GOALS 1. Participates in exercise therapy to increase joint mobility
2. Demonstrates ability to transfer, walk with assistive devices, and move with ease

OUTCOMES (NOC)	INTERVENTIONS (NIC) and *RATIONALES*
Mobility	**Exercise Therapy: Joint Mobility**
• Joint movement ____ • Transfer performance ____ • Moves with ease ____	• Determine limitations of joint movement and effect on function *to plan appropriate interventions.* • Assist patient to optimal body position for passive/active joint movement *to prevent dislocation or other complications.* • Initiate pain-control measures before beginning joint exercise *to decrease discomfort from exercise and increase patient participation.* • Perform passive or assisted ROM exercises. • Collaborate with physical therapy in developing and executing an exercise program *to increase patient compliance and promote continuity of exercise.*
Ambulation • Bears weight ____ • Walks with effective gait ____ • Walks at slow pace ____ • Walks at moderate pace ____	
Measurement Scale 1 = Severely compromised 2 = Substantially compromised 3 = Moderately compromised 4 = Mildly compromised 5 = Not compromised	**Exercise Therapy: Ambulation** • Assist patient to sit on side of bed *to facilitate postural adjustments.* • Apply/provide assistive device (cane, walker, or wheelchair) for ambulation, if the patient is unsteady, *to prevent falls.* • Assist patient with initial ambulation *to promote mobility according to patient's abilities.* • Consult physical therapist about ambulation plan *to reinforce plan and to provide unified approach to patient.*

*This NCP is appropriate for a patient with an open reduction with internal fixation (ORIF) or joint replacement surgery.   *Continued*
ROM, Range of motion.

---

sures frequently used during the initial phase. The nurse should instruct the patient to exercise joints above and below the cast. Pulling out cast padding and scratching or placing foreign objects inside the cast is forbidden because it predisposes the patient to skin breakdown and infection.

Patient and family teaching is an important nursing responsibility to prevent complications. In addition to specific instructions for cast care and recognition of complications, the nurse should encourage the patient to contact the clinic or care provider should questions arise. Table 63-9 summarizes patient and family instructions for cast care. The nurse should validate the patient's and family's understanding of these instructions before discharge from the inpatient and ambulatory settings. A follow-up phone contact

is appropriate, and home care nursing visits are warranted, especially with body or spica casts.

Cast removal is done in the outpatient setting. Patients often fear being cut by the oscillating blade of the cast saw. The nurse should reassure the patient. More importantly, the nurse should educate the patient as to the possible alteration in the appearance of the skin that has been beneath the cast. Anxiety will also be present related to weight bearing and continued follow-up care.

Psychosocial Problems. Short-term rehabilitative goals are directed toward the transition from dependence to independence in performing simple activities of daily living and preservation or increasing strength and endurance. Long-term rehabilitative goals are aimed at preventing problems associated with musculoskeletal

NURSING CARE PLAN 63-2

Patient Having Orthopedic Surgery—cont'd

NURSING DIAGNOSIS   **Risk for peripheral neurovascular dysfunction** *related to* edema, circulatory stasis, dislocated prosthesis or fixation devices*

NURSING DIAGNOSIS   **Deficient knowledge** *related to* lack of exposure to information and resources for follow-up care *as evidenced by* expression of concern with ability to care for self after discharge, frequent questioning about follow-up care, lack of plan for follow-up care

PATIENT GOALS   1. Describes activities related to treatments, activities of daily living, and obtaining assistance if needed
           2. Verbalizes confidence in ability to follow prescribed discharge plan

OUTCOMES (NOC)

Discharge Readiness: Independent Living

- Seeks assistance appropriately ____
- Uses available social support ____
- Describes prescribed treatments ____
- Describes risks for complications ____
- Manages own medications ____
- Performs activities of daily living (ADLs) independently ____

Measurement Scale

1 = Never demonstrated
2 = Rarely demonstrated
3 = Sometimes demonstrated
4 = Often demonstrated
5 = Consistently demonstrated

INTERVENTIONS (NIC) and *RATIONALES*

Discharge Planning

- Communicate patient's discharge plans (e.g., activity limitations, medications, follow-up visit, signs of infection, dislocation) *to prepare for self-care and decision making.*
- Assist patient/family/significant others in planning for the supportive environment necessary to provide patient's posthospital care *so appropriate changes can be made.*
- Coordinate referrals relevant to linkages among health care providers *to monitor long-term rehabilitation program at home.*

*See NCP 63-1 on pp. 1644 to 1645 for outcomes and interventions.

injury (Table 63-10). An important part of nursing care during the rehabilitative phase is assisting the patient to adjust to any problems caused by the injury (e.g., separation from family, financial impact of medical care, loss of income from inability to work, potential for lifetime disability). The nurse must exhibit gentleness, support, and encouragement and should actively listen to the patient's and family's fears.

Ambulation. The nurse must know the overall goals of physical therapy in relation to the patient's abilities, needs, and tolerance. Mobility training and instruction in the use of assistive aids (cane, crutches, walker) constitute major areas of responsibility of the physical therapist. The nurse should reinforce these instructions to the patient. The patient with lower extremity dysfunction usually starts mobility training when able to sit in bed and dangle the feet over the side. This activity should be done two or three times for 10 to 15 minutes, with the nurse assisting as necessary. Collaboration of the nurse and physical therapist to coordinate pain management prior to a physical therapy session will assist in patient participation at therapy sessions. As endurance increases, the patient is instructed in the techniques of transferring from bed to chair. Progressive ambulation is usually started with parallel bars and progresses to ambulatory assistive devices. When the patient begins to ambulate, the nurse must know the patient's weight-bearing status and the correct technique if the patient is using an assistive device. There are different degrees of weight-bearing ambulation: (1) non–weight-bearing (no weight borne) ambulation, (2) touch-down/toe-touch weight-bearing ambulation (contact with floor but no weight borne), (3) partial–weight-bearing ambulation (25% to 50% of patient's weight borne),

(4) weight bearing as tolerated (dictated by patient's pain and tolerance), and (5) full–weight-bearing ambulation (no limitations).

Assistive Devices. Devices for ambulation range from a cane, which can relieve up to 40% of the weight normally borne by a lower limb, to a walker or crutches, which may allow for complete non–weight-bearing ambulation. The decision about which device is appropriate for a patient is made by the health care provider and involves balancing the need for maximum stability and safety versus maneuverability (this is required in small spaces such as bathrooms and buses). Discussing with patients the requirements of their lifestyles and determining the device with which each patient feels most secure and independent is essential.

The technique for using assistive devices varies. The involved limb is usually advanced at the same time or immediately after the advance of the device. The uninvolved limb is advanced last. In almost all cases, canes are held in the hand opposite the involved extremity.

The common gait patterns with assistive devices are the two-point gait, the four-point gait, the swing-to gait, and the swing-through gait:

- *Two-point gait:* Crutch on one side advances simultaneously with the opposite foot; this gait is also used with cane ambulation.
- *Four-point gait:* A slower version of the two-point gait in which each "point" is advanced separately.
- *Swing-to gait:* Both crutches are advanced together, followed by the lifting of both lower limbs to the same place; this gait is also used with walkers.
- *Swing-through gait:* This gait is similar to the swing-to gait,

TABLE 63-10	Problems Associated with Injury of the Musculoskeletal System	
Problem	**Description**	**Nursing Considerations**
Muscle atrophy	Decreased muscle mass normally occurs as a result of disuse following prolonged immobilization. Loss of nerve innervation can precipitate muscle atrophy.	An isometric muscle-strengthening exercise regimen within the confines of the immobilization device assists in reducing the amount of atrophy. Muscle atrophy interferes with and prolongs the rehabilitation process.
Contracture	Abnormal condition of joint characterized by flexion and fixation. Caused by atrophy and shortening of muscle fibers or by loss of normal elasticity of skin over a joint.	Can be prevented by frequent position change, correct body alignment, and active-passive range-of-motion exercises several times a day. Intervention requires gradual and progressive stretching of the muscles or ligaments in the region of the joint.
Footdrop	Plantar-flexed position of the foot (footdrop) occurs when the Achilles tendon in the ankle shortens because it has been allowed to assume an unsupported position. Peroneal nerve palsy (a compression neuropathy) also causes footdrop.	Nursing management of the patient with long-term injuries must include preventive measures by supporting the foot in a neutral position. Once footdrop has developed, ambulation and gait training may be significantly hindered. The patient may require a splint to keep foot/feet in a neutral position.
Pain	Frequently associated with fractures, edema, and muscle spasm; pain varies in intensity from mild to severe and is usually described as aching, dull, burning, throbbing, sharp, or deep.	Causes of pain include incorrect positioning and alignment of the extremity, incorrect support of the extremity, sudden movement of the extremity, and immobilization device that is applied too tightly or in an incorrect position, constrictive dressings, and motion occurring at the fracture site. Causes of pain should be determined so that corrective nursing action can be taken.
Muscle spasms	Caused by involuntary muscle contraction after fracture, muscle strain, or nerve injury and may last as long as several weeks. Pain associated with muscle spasms is often intense and can last from several seconds to several minutes.	Nursing measures to reduce the intensity of the muscle spasms are similar to the corrective actions for pain control. Muscle spasms should not be massaged because massaging stimulates muscle tissue contraction that increases spasm and pain. Thermotherapy, especially heat, may reduce muscle spasm.

but the patient swings the body past the crutches. An alternate four-point sweep-through gait for patients with concurrent visual and neuromuscular disability provides exploration of upcoming terrain by the crutches before they are placed in the traditional position.

A transfer belt should be placed around the patient's waist to provide stability during the learning stages. The nurse should discourage the patient from reaching for furniture or relying on another person for support. When there is inadequate upper limb strength or poorly fitted crutches, the patient bears weight at the axilla rather than at the hands, endangering the neurovascular bundle that passes across the axilla. If verbal coaching does not correct the problem, the patient should be instructed in another form of ambulation until strength is adequate (e.g., platform crutches, walker).

Patients who must ambulate without weight bearing require sufficient upper limb strength to lift their own weight at each step. Because the muscles of the shoulder girdle are not accustomed to this work, they require vigorous and diligent training in preparation for this task. Push-ups, pull-ups using the overhead trapeze bar, and lifting weights develop the triceps and biceps. Straight-leg raises and quadriceps-setting exercises strengthen the quadriceps.

Counseling and Referrals. During the rehabilitative process the patient's family assumes an important role in the provision and follow-through of long-term care plans. The family must be instructed in the techniques of strength and endurance exercises, assistance with mobility training, and promoting activities that enhance the quality of daily living. Sexual counseling should be included in discharge planning. Unless nurses have specific preparation for sexual health counseling, they should remember that wrong answers might be more harmful than no answers. For referral purposes, nurses must know whether weight-bearing status will affect sexual activity and whether any immobilization or support devices are necessary.

Patients also need to be evaluated for posttraumatic stress disorder. This is especially important if significant injury to others or fatalities were associated with the patient's injuries.

■ Evaluation

The expected outcomes for a patient with a fracture are presented in NCP 63-1 and NCP 63-2.

COMPLICATIONS OF FRACTURES

The majority of fractures heal without complications. If death occurs after a fracture, it is usually the result of damage to underlying organs and vascular structures or from complications of the fracture or immobility. Complications of fractures may be either direct or indirect. Direct complications include problems with bone infection, bone union, and avascular necrosis. Indirect complications of fractures are associated with blood vessel and nerve damage resulting in conditions such as compartment syndrome, venous thrombosis, fat embolism, and traumatic or hypovolemic shock.[12] Although most musculoskeletal injuries are not life threatening, open fractures or fractures accompanied by severe blood loss and fractures that damage vital organs (such as the lung, heart, or bladder) are medical emergencies requiring immediate attention.

Infection

Open fractures and soft tissue injuries have a high incidence of infection. An open fracture usually results from the impact of severe external forces. Massive or blunt soft tissue injury often has more serious consequences than the fracture. Devitalized and contaminated tissue is an ideal medium for many common pathogens, including gas-forming (anaerobic) bacilli. Treatment of infection is costly in terms of extended nursing and medical care, time for treatment, and loss of patient income. Osteomyelitis can become chronic (see Chapter 64).

Collaborative Care. Open fractures require aggressive surgical debridement.[15] The wound is initially cleansed by jet-pulsed lavage in the operating room. Gross contaminants are irrigated and mechanically removed. Contused, contaminated, and devitalized tissue such as muscle, subcutaneous fat, skin, and fragments of bone are surgically excised *(debridement)*. The extent of the soft tissue damage determines whether the wound will be closed at the time of surgery, whether closed suction drainage may be necessary, and whether skin grafting will be needed. Depending on the location and extent of the fracture, reduction may be maintained by external fixation or traction. During surgery the open wound may be irrigated with antibiotic solution. Antibiotic-impregnated beads may also be placed in the surgical site. During the postoperative phase the patient will have antibiotics administered intravenously for 3 to 7 days. Antibiotics, in conjunction with aggressive surgical management, have greatly reduced the occurrence of infection.

Compartment Syndrome

Compartment syndrome is a condition in which elevated intracompartmental pressure within a confined myofascial compartment compromises the neurovascular function of tissues within that space. Compartment syndrome causes capillary perfusion to be reduced below a level necessary for tissue viability and is classified as acute, chronic/exertional, or crush syndrome. Thirty-eight compartments are located in the upper and lower extremities. Two basic types of compartment syndrome include (1) decreased compartment size resulting from restrictive dressings, splints, casts, excessive traction, or premature closure of fascia; and (2) increased compartment content related to bleeding, edema, chemical response to snakebite, or IV infiltration. Depending on the patient's age and body mass index, the expected range of intracompartmental pressure readings is 0 to 15 mm Hg. Readings of 30 to 50 mm Hg indicate compartment syndrome.[16]

Edema can create sufficient pressure to obstruct circulation and cause venous occlusion, which further increases edema. Eventually arterial flow is compromised, resulting in ischemia to the extremity. As ischemia continues, muscle and nerve cells are destroyed over time, and fibrotic tissue replaces the healthy tissue. Contracture, disability, and loss of function can occur. Delay in diagnosis and treatment can result in irreversible muscle and nerve ischemia, resulting in a functionally useless or severely impaired extremity.

Compartment syndrome is associated with trauma, fractures, extensive soft tissue damage, crush injury, reperfusion syndrome, severe burns, and venomous snakebite, or occurs following knee or leg surgery. Prolonged pressure on a muscle compartment may occur when someone is trapped under a heavy object or a person's limb is trapped beneath the body because of an obtunded state such as drug or alcohol overdose. It has even been known to occur as a result of a massive infiltration of IV fluids. Exertional compartment syndrome may occur after intensive exercise.[17] The upper arm and lower leg are the most common sites of compartment syndrome. Fractures of the distal humerus and proximal tibia are the most common fractures associated with compartment syndrome. In the upper extremity this condition is referred to as *Volkmann's ischemic contracture* (Fig. 63-15) and in the lower extremity as anterior tibial compartment syndrome, although the underlying pathophysiologic mechanism is similar.

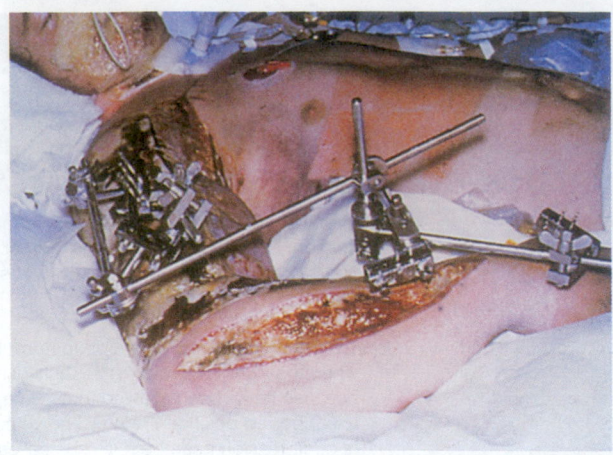

FIG. 63-15   Volkmann's ischemic contracture of the forearm following acute compartment syndrome secondary to a supracondylar fracture of the humerus. Note the incision line of an unsuccessful fasciotomy.

Clinical Manifestations. Early recognition and treatment of compartment syndrome are essential to avoid permanent damage to muscles and nerves. Ischemia can occur within 4 to 12 hours after onset. Regular neurovascular assessments should be performed and documented on all patients with fractures, but especially those with injury of the distal humerus or proximal tibia or soft tissue disruption in these areas. Compartment syndrome may occur initially from the physiologic response of the body or may be delayed for several days from the original insult/injury.

The six Ps are characteristic of an impending compartment syndrome: (1) *paresthesia* (numbness and tingling); (2) *pain* distal to the injury that is not relieved by opioid analgesics and pain on passive stretch of muscle traveling through the compartment; (3) *pressure* increases in the compartment; (4) *pallor,* coolness, and loss of normal color of the extremity; (5) *paralysis* or loss of function; and (6) *pulselessness* or diminished/absent peripheral pulses. The patient may present with one or all of the six Ps. Absence of a peripheral pulse and paralysis are late and ominous signs that indicate a severe disturbance of neurovascular status.[18] The health care provider should be notified immediately of a patient's changing condition.

Because of the possibility of muscle damage, urine output must be assessed. Myoglobin released from damaged muscle cells precipitates as a gel-like substance, causing obstruction in renal tubules because of its high molecular weight. Large amounts of myoglobinemia may result in acute tubular necrosis, which causes acute renal failure. Common signs of myoglobinuria are (1) dark reddish brown urine and (2) clinical manifestations associated with acute renal failure (see Chapter 47).

Collaborative Care. Prompt, accurate diagnosis of compartment syndrome is critical. Prevention or early recognition is the key. Elevation of the extremity may raise venous pressure and slow arterial perfusion, thus the extremity should not be elevated above heart level. Similarly, the application of cold compresses may result in vasoconstriction and exacerbate compartment syndrome. Elevation and ice should not be used in patients with suspected compartment syndrome. It may also be necessary to remove or loosen the bandage and bivalve the cast. A reduction in traction weight may also decrease external circumferential pressures.

Surgical decompression (e.g., fasciotomy) of the involved compartment may be necessary.[17] The fasciotomy site is left open for several days to ensure adequate soft tissue decompression. Infection resulting from delayed wound closure is a potential problem following a fasciotomy. Severe compartment syndrome may require amputation to decrease myoglobinemia or to replace a functionally useless extremity with a prosthesis.

Venous Thrombosis

The veins of the lower extremities and pelvis are highly susceptible to thrombus formation after fracture, especially hip fracture. Precipitating factors are venous stasis caused by incorrectly applied casts or traction, local pressure on a vein, or immobility. Venous stasis is aggravated by inactivity of the muscles that normally assist in the pumping action of venous blood returning to the extremities. In addition to wearing compression gradient stockings (antiembolism hose) and using sequential compression devices, the patient should be instructed to move (dorsiflex/plantar flex) the fingers or toes of the affected extremity against resistance and to perform ROM exercises on the unaffected lower extremities.

Because of the high risk of venous thrombosis in the patient with limited mobility, prophylactic anticoagulant drugs such as aspirin, warfarin, or heparin may be ordered. Low-molecular-weight heparin (LMWH) (e.g., enoxaparin [Lovenox]) is frequently used to prevent venous thrombosis. Because LMWH has a predictable dose response, monitoring of prothrombin time is not necessary. A newer class of antithrombotic drugs (e.g., fondaparinux [Arixtra]) works by inhibiting factor Xa, a key blood-clotting component. (Assessment and management of venous thrombosis are discussed in Chapter 38.)

Fat Embolism Syndrome

Fat embolism syndrome (FES) is characterized by the presence of systemic fat globules from fractures that are distributed into tissues and organs after a traumatic skeletal injury.[19] FES is a contributory factor in many deaths associated with fractures. The fractures that most often cause FES are those of the long bones, ribs, tibia, and pelvis. FES has also been known to occur following total joint replacement, spinal fusion, liposuction, crush injuries, and bone marrow transplantation. Two theories related to the origin of fat emboli include the mechanical theory and the biochemical theory. The *mechanical theory* suggests that fat is released from the marrow of injured bone. It is driven out by an increase in intramedullary pressure and enters the circulation through draining veins traveling to pulmonary capillaries, where it lodges. The fat droplets traverse the capillary bed to enter the systemic circulation, where they then embolize to other organs such as the brain. The *biochemical theory* postulates that catecholamines released at the time of trauma mobilize free fatty acids from the adipose tissue, causing the loss of chylomicron emulsion stability. The chylomicrons form large fat globules that eventually lodge in the lungs. This biochemical change initiated by injury sets up an inflammatory response secondary to destabilization of free fatty acids, which causes a biochemical injury to the lung parenchyma. The tissues of the lungs, brain, heart, kidneys, and skin are most often affected.

Clinical Manifestations. Early recognition of FES is crucial in preventing a potentially lethal course. Initial manifestations usually occur 12 to 72 hours after injury.[20] Severe forms have occurred within hours of injury. The fat globules transported to the lungs cause a hemorrhagic interstitial pneumonitis that produces signs and symptoms of acute respiratory distress syndrome (ARDS), such as chest pain, tachypnea, cyanosis, dyspnea, apprehension, tachycardia, and decreased partial pressure of arterial oxygen (PaO_2). All of these symptoms are caused by poor oxygen exchange. Because they are frequently the presenting symptoms, changes in mental status as a result of hypoxemia are important to recognize. Memory loss, restlessness, confusion, elevated temperature, and headache should prompt further investigation so that CNS involvement is not mistaken for alcohol withdrawal or acute head injury. The continued change in level of consciousness and petechiae located around the neck, anterior chest wall, axilla, buccal membrane, and conjunctiva of the eye helps distinguish fat emboli from other problems. Petechiae result from intravascular thromboses caused by decreased oxygenation.

The clinical course of a fat embolus may be rapid and acute. Frequently the patient expresses a feeling of impending disaster. In a short time, skin color changes from pallor to cyanosis, and the patient may become comatose. No specific laboratory examinations are available to aid in the diagnosis. However, certain diagnostic abnormalities may be present. These include fat cells in the blood, urine, or sputum; a decrease of the PaO_2 to less than 60 mm Hg; ST segment changes on electrocardiogram; a decrease in the platelet count and hematocrit levels; and a prolonged prothrombin time resulting from hemorrhaging into the lungs. A chest x-ray may reveal areas of pulmonary infiltrate or multiple areas of consolidation. This is sometimes referred to as the white-out effect.

Collaborative Care. Treatment for fat embolism is directed at prevention.[20] Careful immobilization of a long bone fracture is probably the most important factor in the prevention of fat embolism. Management of FES is essentially symptom related and supportive, and fluid resuscitation is given to prevent hypovolemic shock, correction of acidosis, and replacement of blood loss. Coughing and deep breathing should be encouraged. The patient should be repositioned as little as possible before fracture immobilization or stabilization because of the danger of dislodging more fat droplets into the general circulation. Use of corticosteroids to prevent or treat fat embolism is controversial. Oxygen is administered to treat hypoxia. Intubation or intermittent positive pressure ventilation may be considered if a satisfactory PaO_2 cannot be obtained with supplemental oxygen alone. Some patients may develop pulmonary edema, ARDS, or both, leading to an increased mortality rate. Most persons survive FES with few sequelae.

Types of Fractures

COLLES' FRACTURE

A *Colles' fracture* is a fracture of the distal radius and is one of the most common fractures in adults. The styloid process of the ulna may be involved as well. The injury usually occurs when the patient attempts to break a fall with an outstretched arm and hand. This type of fracture most often occurs in women over age 50 whose bones are osteoporotic. The clinical manifestations of Colles' fracture are pain in the immediate area of injury, pronounced swelling, and dorsal displacement of the distal fragment (dinner-fork deformity). This will appear as an obvious deformity of the wrist. The major complication associated with a Colles' fracture is vascular insufficiency as a result of edema. Carpel tunnel syndrome can be a later complication.

A Colles' fracture is usually managed by closed manipulation of the fracture and immobilization by either a splint or a cast or, if displaced, by internal or external fixation. The elbow must be immobilized to prevent wrist supination and pronation. Nursing

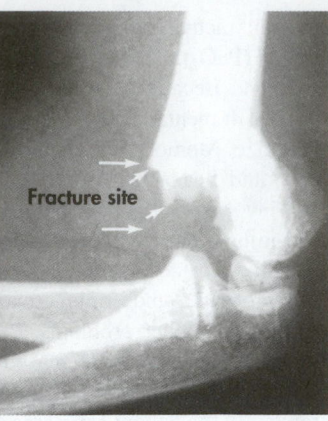

A

B

FIG. 63-16 **A,** Supracondylar fracture of the humerus. This type of injury results in the formation of a large hematoma. **B,** Fracture of distal shaft of humerus.

management should include measures to prevent or reduce edema and frequent neurovascular assessments. Support and protection of the extremity should be provided, along with encouragement of active movement of the thumb and fingers. This type of movement helps reduce edema and increases venous return. The patient should be instructed to perform active movements of the shoulder to prevent stiffness or contracture.

FRACTURE OF THE HUMERUS

Fractures involving the shaft of the humerus are a common injury among young and middle-aged adults. The prominent clinical manifestations are an obvious displacement of the humerus shaft, shortened extremity, abnormal mobility, and pain (Fig. 63-16). The major complications associated with fracture of the humerus are radial nerve injury and vascular injury to the brachial artery as a result of laceration, transection, or muscle spasm.

The treatment for a fracture of the humerus depends on the location and displacement of the fracture. Nonoperative treatment may include a hanging arm cast, a shoulder immobilizer, or the sling and swathe, which is a type of immobilization that prevents glenohumeral movement. The swathe encircles the trunk and humerus as an additional binder. It is often used for surgical repairs and shoulder dislocation.

When these devices are used, the head of the bed should be elevated to assist gravity in reducing the fracture. The arm should be allowed to hang freely when the patient is sitting and standing. Nursing care should include measures to protect the axilla and prevent skin maceration by placing lightly powdered absorbable dressing pads in the axilla and changing them twice daily or as needed. Skin or skeletal traction may be used for purposes of reduction and immobilization.

During the rehabilitative phase, an exercise program geared toward improving strength and motion of the injured extremity is extremely important. This should include assisted motion of the hand and fingers. The shoulder can also be exercised if the fracture is stable. This helps to prevent stiffness secondary to frozen shoulder or arthrofibrosis.

FRACTURE OF THE PELVIS

Pelvic fractures range from benign to life threatening depending on the mechanism of injury and associated vascular insult. High-speed vehicular or motorcycle crashes or skiing accidents can result in open book (anterior-posterior compression) fractures result-

ing in hemorrhagic life-threatening situations. An *open book fracture* is sustained when the external force pulls the pelvis apart, such as when struck or crushed from the front. A *closed book fracture* is sustained from lateral force compression, whereas a vertical shear injury is the result of a fall. Although only a small percentage of all fractures are pelvic fractures, this type of injury is associated with the highest mortality rate.[21] Preoccupation with associated injuries at the time of a traumatic event may result in an oversight of pelvic injuries. Pelvic fractures may cause serious intraabdominal injury such as paralytic ileus, hemorrhage, and laceration of the urethra, bladder, or colon. Patients may survive the initial pelvic injury, only to die from sepsis, FES, or DVT complications.

Physical examination demonstrates local swelling, tenderness, deformity, unusual pelvic movement, and ecchymosis on the abdomen. The neurovascular status of the lower extremities and manifestations of associated injuries should be assessed. Pelvic fractures are diagnosed by x-ray and computed tomography (CT) scan.

Treatment of a pelvic fracture depends on the severity of the injury. Stable, nondisplaced fractures such as those sustained in a fall require limited intervention and early mobilization. Bed rest for stable pelvic fractures is maintained from a few days to 6 weeks. More complex fractures may be treated with pelvic sling traction, skeletal traction, hip spica casts, external fixation, open reduction, or a combination of these methods. Open reduction and internal fixation of a pelvic fracture may be necessary if the fracture is displaced.[22] Extreme care in handling or moving the patient is important to prevent serious injury from a displaced fracture fragment. Because a pelvic fracture can damage other organs, assessment of bowel and urinary tract function and distal neurovascular status are important nursing measures.

The patient should be turned only when specifically ordered by the health care provider. Back care is provided while the patient is raised from the bed either by independent use of the trapeze or with adequate assistance. Weight bearing on the affected side should be avoided until healing is complete. If the pelvic fracture is nondisplaced, the patient is usually allowed to ambulate using a walker or crutches to distribute the weight bearing between the upper and lower extremities.

FRACTURE OF THE HIP

Hip fractures are common in older adults. More than 200,000 hip fractures occur annually. It is estimated that, by the age of 90, 33% of all women and 17% of all men will have sustained a hip fracture.[23] In adults over age 65, hip fracture occurs more frequently in women than in men because of osteoporosis. It is estimated that 10% to 20% of patients who experience a hip fracture will die within 1 year of injury because of medical complications caused by the fracture or resulting immobility. Many older adults with a hip fracture develop disabilities necessitating long-term care.[24]

A fracture of the hip (Fig. 63-17) refers to a fracture of the proximal third of the femur, which extends up to 5 cm below the lesser trochanter. Fractures that occur within the hip joint capsule are called *intracapsular fractures.* Intracapsular fractures (femoral neck) are further identified by a name derived from specific locations: (1) capital (fracture of the head of the femur), (2) subcapital (fracture just below the head of the femur), and (3) transcervical (fracture of the neck of the femur). These fractures are often associated with osteoporosis and minor trauma. Extracapsular fractures occur outside the joint capsule and are termed (1) intertrochanteric if they occur in a region between the greater and lesser trochanter or (2) subtrochanteric if they occur in the region below the lesser trochanter. Extracapsular fractures are usually caused by severe direct trauma or a fall.

Clinical Manifestations

The clinical manifestations of hip fractures are external rotation, muscle spasm, shortening of the affected extremity, and severe pain and tenderness in the region of the fracture site. Displaced femoral neck fractures cause serious disruption of the blood supply to the femoral head, which can result in avascular necrosis of the femoral head.

Collaborative Care

Surgical repair is the preferred method of managing intracapsular and extracapsular hip fractures. Surgical treatment permits early mobilization of the patient and decreases the risk of major complications. Initially the affected extremity may be temporarily immobilized by Buck's traction (see Fig. 63-10) until the patient's physi-

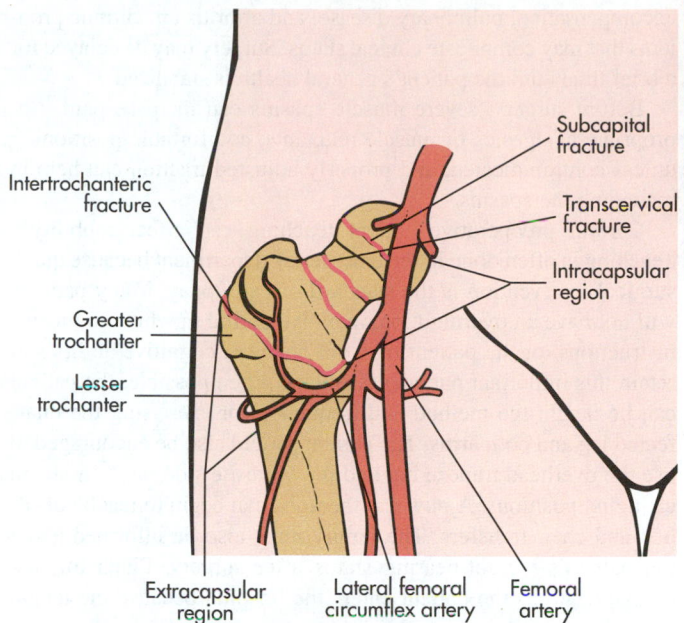

FIG. 63-17 Femur with location of various types of fracture.

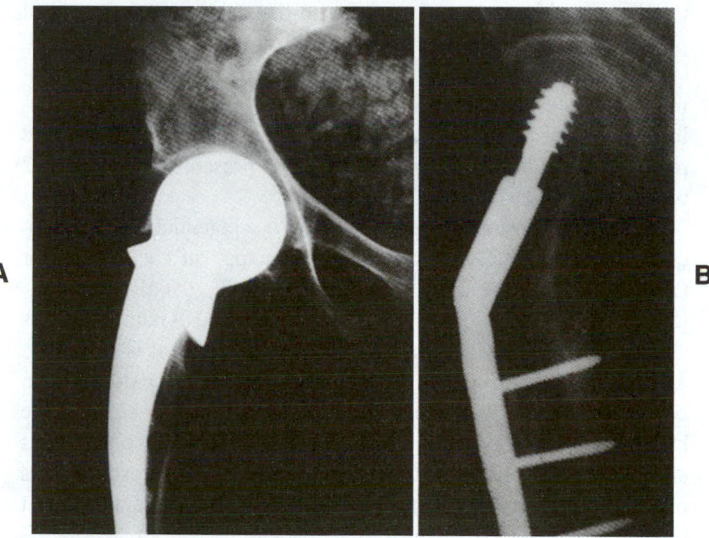

FIG. 63-18 Types of internal fixation for a hip fracture. **A,** Femoral head endoprosthesis. **B,** Type of hip compression screw with side plate.

cal condition is stabilized and surgery can be performed. Buck's traction relieves painful muscle spasms and is used for 24 to 48 hours maximum.

Intracapsular (femoral neck) fractures are usually repaired with the use of an endoprosthesis to replace the femoral head (hemiarthroplasty) (Fig. 63-18, *A*). Extracapsular fractures are repaired using fixed nail plates, sliding nail plates, intramedullary devices, and replacement prostheses (Fig. 63-18, *B*). The principles of patient care for these procedures are similar.

NURSING MANAGEMENT
HIP FRACTURE

■ *Nursing Implementation*

Preoperative Management. Because older adults are most prone to hip fractures, chronic health problems must often be considered when planning treatment. Diabetes mellitus, hypertension, cardiac decompensation, pulmonary disease, and arthritis are chronic problems that may complicate clinical status. Surgery may be delayed for a brief time until the patient's general health is stabilized.

Before surgery, severe muscle spasms can increase pain. Appropriate analgesics or muscle relaxants, comfortable positioning unless contraindicated, and properly adjusted traction can help in managing the spasms.

Careful preoperative patient teaching can affect mobility.[25] Teaching is often done in the emergency department because quick surgical intervention is the standard of care today. Many patients will not have an overnight preoperative period in which to receive instructions, or the patient may not have the cognitive abilities to retain this important patient education. When possible, the patient can be taught the method and frequency for exercising the unaffected leg and both arms. The patient should also be encouraged to use the overhead trapeze bar and the opposite side rail to assist in changing positions. A physical therapist can begin to teach out-of-bed and chair transfers. The family must also be informed about the patient's weight-bearing status after surgery. Plans for discharge begin as the patient enters the hospital because the length of stay postoperatively will be only a few days.

Postoperative Management. The initial postoperative management of a patient following open reduction with internal fixation (ORIF) of a hip fracture is similar to that for any older surgical patient. The nurse must monitor vital signs, intake, and output; supervise respiratory activities, such as deep breathing and coughing; administer pain medication cautiously; and observe the dressing and incision for signs of bleeding and infection. A nursing care plan for the orthopedic surgical patient is presented in NCP 63-2 on pp. 1647 to 1648.

In the early postoperative period there is a potential for neurovascular impairment. The nurse assesses the patient's extremity for (1) color, (2) temperature, (3) capillary refill, (4) distal pulses, (5) edema, (6) sensation, (7) motor function, and (8) pain. Edema is alleviated by elevation of the leg whenever the patient is in a chair. The pain resulting from poor alignment of the affected extremity can be reduced by keeping pillows (or an abductor splint) between the knees when the patient is turning to either side. Sandbags and pillows are also used to prevent external rotation. If an endoprosthesis was placed, the patient is at risk for hip dislocation. Hip precautions must be demonstrated and explained to the patient.

The physical therapist usually supervises active-assistance exercises for the affected extremity and ambulation when the surgeon permits it. Ambulation usually begins on the first or second postoperative day. The nurse in collaboration with the physical therapist monitors the patient's ambulation status for proper crutch walking or use of the walker. For the patient to be discharged home, the patient must be able to safely demonstrate use of crutches or a walker, the ability to transfer into and from a chair and bed, and the ability to ascend and descend stairs.

Complications associated with femoral neck fracture include non-union, avascular necrosis, dislocation, and degenerative arthritis. As a result of an intertrochanteric fracture, the affected leg may be shortened. A cane or built-up shoe may be required for safe ambulation.

If the hip fracture has been treated by insertion of a femoral head prosthesis, measures to prevent dislocation must always be used (Table 63-11). The patient and family must be fully aware of positions and activities that predispose the patient to dislocation (greater than 90 degrees of flexion, adduction, or internal

---

TABLE 63-11   PATIENT AND FAMILY TEACHING GUIDE
Femoral Head Prosthesis

Do Not
- Force hip into greater than 90 degrees of flexion (e.g., sitting in low chairs or toilet seats)
- Force hip into adduction
- Force hip into internal rotation
- Cross legs
- Put on own shoes or stockings until 8 weeks after surgery without adaptive device (e.g., long-handled shoehorn or stocking-helper)
- Sit on chairs without arms to aid rising to a standing position

Do
- Use toilet elevator on toilet seat
- Place chair inside shower or tub and remain seated while washing
- Use pillow between legs for first 8 weeks after surgery when lying on "good" side or when supine
- Keep hip in neutral, straight position when sitting, walking, or lying
- Notify surgeon if severe pain, deformity, or loss of function occurs
- Inform dentist of presence of prosthesis before dental work so that prophylactic antibiotics can be given

---

rotation). Many daily activities may reproduce these positions, including putting on shoes and socks, crossing the legs or feet while seated, assuming the side-lying position incorrectly, standing up or sitting down while the body is flexed greater than 90 degrees relative to the chair, and sitting on low seats, especially low toilet seats. Until the soft tissue capsule surrounding the hip has healed sufficiently to stabilize the prosthesis, these activities must be avoided, usually for at least 6 weeks. Sudden severe pain, a lump in the buttock, limb shortening, and external rotation indicate prosthesis dislocation. This requires a closed reduction with conscious sedation or open reduction to realign the femoral head in the acetabulum.

In addition to teaching the patient and family how to prevent prosthesis dislocation, the nurse should (1) place a large pillow between the patient's legs when turning, (2) avoid extreme hip flexion, and (3) avoid turning the patient on the affected side until approved by the surgeon. In addition, some health care providers prefer that the patient keep leg abductor splints on except when bathing.

The patient is out of bed on the first postoperative day. Weight bearing on the involved extremity varies. Weight bearing of especially fragile fractures may be restricted until x-ray examination indicates adequate healing, usually 6 to 12 weeks.

The nurse assists both the patient and the family in adjusting to the restrictions and dependence imposed by the hip fracture. Anxiety and depression can easily occur, but creative nursing care and awareness of the problem can do much to prevent it. The patient and family may need to be informed about community referral services that can assist in the postdischarge rehabilitation phase. Hospitalization averages 3 or 4 days. Patients frequently require care in a subacute unit, at a skilled nursing facility, or in a rehabilitation facility for a few weeks before returning home. Regular follow-up care after discharge, including home health nursing, should be arranged.

■ Evaluation

The expected outcomes for the patient with fracture of the hip are presented in NCP 63-2.

GERONTOLOGIC CONSIDERATIONS
HIP FRACTURE

Factors that contribute to the occurrence of a hip fracture in older adults include a propensity to fall, inability to correct a postural imbalance, orientation of the fall, inadequacy of local tissue shock absorbers (e.g., fat, muscle bulk), and underlying skeletal strength. Several factors have been identified in older persons that increase their risk of falling. These include gait and balance problems, decreased vision and hearing, decreased reflexes, orthostatic hypotension, and medication use. Leading hazards of falls are loose rugs and slippery or uneven surfaces. Many falls are associated with getting in or out of a chair or bed. Falls to the side, the most common type in the frail elderly, are more likely to result in a hip fracture than a forward fall. External hip protectors have not been shown to be effective in reducing hip fractures in the elderly after a fall.[26] A low level of patient compliance in wearing hip protectors, which are plastic shields or foam pads held in place with specially designed underwear, may be one reason for these results.

Two important factors influencing the amount of force imposed on the hip are the presence of energy-absorbing soft tissue over the greater trochanter and the state of leg muscle contraction at the time of the fall. Because many elderly persons have poor muscle tone, these are important factors in the severity of a fall. Elderly women often have osteoporosis and accompanying low bone density, which increases the risk of hip fracture and other types of fractures.[27]

Targeted interventions to reduce hip fractures in the elderly include a variety of strategies. Calcium and vitamin D supplementation, estrogen replacement, and bisphosphonate drug therapy have been shown to decrease bone loss or increase bone density and decrease the likelihood of fracture. (Osteoporosis is discussed in Chapter 64.) Nurses must be vigilant in planning interventions for the elderly that are known to reduce the incidence of hip fracture.

FEMORAL SHAFT FRACTURE

Femoral shaft fracture is a common injury occurring particularly in young adults. Severe direct force is required to produce this injury because the femur can bend slightly before actual fracture occurs. The force exerted to cause the fracture often causes damage to the adjacent soft tissue structures. These injuries may be more serious than the bone injury. Displacement of the fracture fragments often results in open fracture and increased soft tissue damage. This can result in considerable blood loss (1 to 1.5 L).

The clinical manifestations of a fracture of the femoral shaft are usually obvious. They include marked deformity and angulation, shortening of the extremity, inability to move either the hip or knee, and pain. The common complications associated with fracture of the femoral shaft include fat embolism, nerve and vascular injury, and problems associated with bone union, open fracture, and soft tissue damage.

Initial management is directed toward stabilization of the patient and immobilization of the fracture. Treatment may consist of skeletal traction via a femoral or tibial pin and balanced suspension traction for 8 to 12 weeks. The nurse must encourage the patient to perform exercises and ROM activities for the uninvolved extremities and joints to discourage deconditioning. The physician determines when active exercise can be instituted on the affected

---

EVIDENCE-BASED PRACTICE
Should Hip Fracture Patients Use Weight-Bearing Exercises?

Clinical Question

In patients who have suffered a hip fracture (P), is weight-bearing (I) or non–weight-bearing (C) exercise more effective in recovery (O)?

Best Available Evidence

Randomized controlled trial (RCT)

Critical Analysis and Synthesis of Evidence

- RCT (n = 120) of older patients who had received the usual care for a hip fracture.
- The study design involved three groups: a weight-bearing home exercise group, a non–weight-bearing home exercise group, and a control group.
- Participants were tested on strength, balance, gait, and functional performance as well as a self-report.
- A follow-up retest was performed at 1 and 4 months.

Conclusions

- The weight-bearing group showed the most improvement in balance and functional ability.
- More people in the weight-bearing group at the 4-month follow-up were walking unaided.
- No significant differences were found between the two exercise groups in regard to strength or gait.
- Weight-bearing exercise was found to have no adverse effects on falls or pain.

Implications for Nursing Practice

- Encourage patients to exercise in the home after a hip fracture.
- Educate patients about the benefits of using weight-bearing exercises and the importance of safety measures at home.

Reference for Evidence

Sherrington C, Lord SR, Herbert RD: A randomized controlled trial of weight-bearing versus non-weight-bearing exercise for improving physical ability after usual care for hip fracture, *Arch Phys Med Rehabil* 84:710, 2004.

PICO: P, Patient population of interest; *I,* intervention or area of interest; *C,* comparison of interest or comparison group; *O,* outcome(s) of interest (see p. 6).

---

extremity. When there is sufficient clinical evidence of bone union, a hip spica or long leg cast may be applied. Use of prolonged traction is uncommon as the current standard of care.

ORIF has become the preferred method to manage a femoral fracture. It is carried out with an intramedullary rod, compression plate, and screws or side plate with an intercondylar nail. Internal fixation is often the preferred treatment because it reduces hospital stay and the complications associated with prolonged bed rest. Other indications for internal fixation are failure to obtain satisfactory reduction by nonsurgical methods and multiple associated injuries. In some instances the surgically repaired femur may be supported by suspension traction for 3 to 4 days to prevent excessive movement of the extremity and to control rotation; non–weight-bearing gait training is then begun. Fractures associated with extensive soft tissue injury may be treated with external fixation.

Promotion and maintenance of strength in the affected extremity usually include gluteal and quadriceps isometric exercises. It is important to ensure performance of ROM and strengthening exercises for all uninvolved extremities in preparation for ambulation.

The patient may be immobilized in a hip spica cast and gradually progress to an articulating cast brace or may be allowed to begin non–weight-bearing activities with an ambulatory assistive device. Full weight bearing is usually restricted until there is x-ray evidence of union of the fracture fragments.

FRACTURE OF THE TIBIA

Although the tibia is vulnerable to injury because it lacks a covering of anterior muscle, strong force is required to produce a fractured tibia. As a result, soft tissue damage, devascularization, and open fracture are frequent. The tibia is one of the more common sites of a stress fracture. Complications associated with tibial fractures are compartment syndrome, fat embolism, problems associated with bony union, and possible infection associated with open fracture. Amputation, although rare, may be required if adequate muscle and tissue coverage is not achieved following muscle and flap grafts.

The recommended management for closed tibial fracture is closed reduction followed by immobilization in a long leg cast. ORIF with intramedullary rods or compression plate or external fixation is indicated for complex fractures and those with extensive soft tissue damage. With either method of reduction, emphasis is placed on maintaining the strength of the quadriceps.

The neurovascular status of the affected extremity must be assessed at least every 2 hours during the first 48 hours. Patients are instructed to perform active ROM exercises with all uninvolved extremities, as well as exercises for the upper extremities, to build the strength required for crutch walking. When the health care provider has determined that the patient is ready for gait training, the patient is instructed in the principles of crutch walking. The patient may be on non–weight-bearing status for 6 to 12 weeks depending on healing. Patients with external fixation must be taught pin care and dressing changes if extensive tissue has been debrided. Home nursing visits can be initiated to augment outpatient appointments and monitor the patient's progress.

STABLE VERTEBRAL FRACTURES

Stable fractures of the vertebral column are usually caused by motor vehicle collisions, falls, diving, or athletic injuries. A stable fracture is one in which the fracture or the fragment is not likely to move or cause spinal cord damage. This type of injury is frequently confined to the anterior element (vertebral body) of the spinal column in the lumbar region, and involves the cervical and thoracic regions less frequently. The vertebral bodies are usually protected from displacement by the intact spinal ligaments.

Most patients with spinal fractures have stable fractures and experience only brief periods of disability. However, if the ligamentous structures are significantly disrupted, dislocation of the vertebral structures may occur, resulting in instability and injury to the spinal cord (unstable fracture). These injuries generally require surgery. The most serious complication of vertebral fractures is fracture displacement, which can cause damage to the spinal cord (see Chapter 61). Although stable vertebral fractures are not associated with abnormal spinal cord pathologic conditions, all spinal injuries should initially be considered unstable and potentially serious until diagnostic tests are performed and the fracture is determined to be stable.

The most common injury to the vertebral body is the compression type of fracture caused by excessive vertical axial loading, such as a severe fall on the buttocks from a height, or injury resulting from sudden flexion that forces the spine beyond its normal ROM.

The patient usually complains of pain and tenderness in the affected region of the spine. Sudden loss of function below the level of fracture indicates severe fracture with spinal cord impingement and paraplegia. Stable compression fractures are associated with a kyphotic deformity (flexion angulation of several vertebrae). This deformity may be noted during the physical examination. In patients with osteoporosis, several vertebral levels may be involved as evidenced by a "dowager's hump" (abnormal curvature of thoracic spine). The cervical spine may also be involved. Bowel and bladder dysfunction may be an indication of an interruption of the autonomic nervous system nerves or injury to the spinal cord.

The overall goal in management of stable vertebral fractures is to keep the spine in good alignment until union has been accomplished. Many nursing interventions are aimed at assessing for the possibility of spinal cord trauma. Vital signs and bowel and bladder function should be evaluated regularly, as should the motor and sensory status of the peripheral nerves distal to the injured region. Any deterioration in the patient's neurovascular status should be promptly reported.

Treatment includes support, heat, and traction. The patient is usually placed in a standard hospital bed with firm support from the mattress or a bedboard. The aim is to support the spinal column, relax muscles, decrease edema, and release potential compression on nerve roots. Heat and traction may be used to relieve muscle spasms resulting from the fracture. Traction may also be used to reduce and immobilize fracture fragments. A trapeze is not usually allowed because its use increases intrathoracic pressure. Both an upright position and turning of the torso are prohibited. When turning, the patient should be taught to keep the spine straight by turning the shoulders and pelvis together. Nursing assistance is necessary for the patient to learn the technique of "logrolling."[28] Several days after the initial injury, the health care provider may apply a specially constructed orthotic device (e.g., Milwaukee, Jewett, or Taylor brace), a jacket cast, or a removable corset if there is no evidence of neurologic deficit.

Vertebral compression fractures, which are often due to osteoporosis, can be treated with two newer outpatient procedures, vertebroplasty and kyphoplasty. *Vertebroplasty* uses guided imaging to inject bone cement into the fractured area. The cement (when hardened) serves to stabilize and prevent further vertebral deterioration. *Kyphoplasty* initially involves inserting an inflated balloon to lift apart the injured vertebrae. The surgeon then fills the cavity with bone cement after the balloon has been deflated. Kyphoplasty results in a lower leakage of bone cement when compared to vertebroplasty. Many patients experience marked pain relief and improved function following these procedures.[29,30]

If the fracture is in the cervical spine, the patient may wear a cervical collar. Some cervical fractures are immobilized by use of a halo vest (see Fig. 61-12). This consists of a plastic jacket or cast fitted about the chest and attached to a halo that is held in place by skeletal pins inserted into the cranium. These devices immobilize the spine in the fracture area but allow the patient to ambulate. The patient is discharged after (1) regaining ambulation skills, (2) learning care of the cast or orthotic device, and (3) learning how to cope with interferences in safety and security imposed by injury and treatment.

FACIAL FRACTURES

Any bone of the face can be fractured as a result of trauma. Fractures can occur as a result of collision with another person or object, fighting, or blunt trauma. The primary concern after facial in-

TABLE 63-12	Clinical Manifestations of Facial Fractures
Fracture	**Clinical Manifestation**
Frontal bone	Rapid edema that may mask underlying fractures
Periorbital bone	Possible frontal sinus involvement, entrapment of ocular muscles
Nasal bone	Displacement of nasal bones, epistaxis
Zygomatic arch	Depression of zygomatic arch and entrapment of ocular muscles
Maxilla	Segmental motion of maxilla and alveolar fracture of teeth
Mandible	Tooth fractures, bleeding, limited motion of mandible

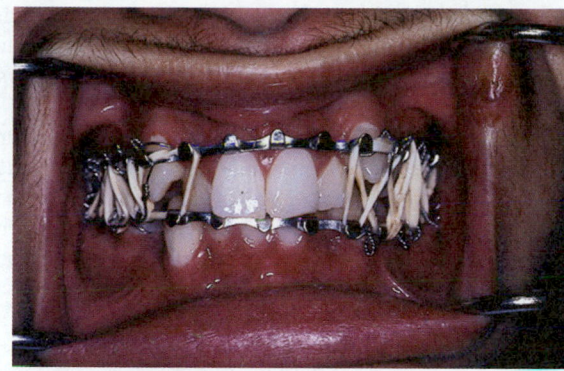

FIG. 63-19 Intermaxillary fixation.

jury is to establish and maintain a patent airway and to provide adequate ventilation by removal of foreign material and blood. Suctioning may be necessary. An alternative airway (tracheostomy) may be needed if a patent airway cannot be maintained. Pressure packing controls hemorrhage. Cervical spine injuries are common. All patients with facial injuries should be treated as though they have a cervical injury until proven otherwise by examination and imaging studies (e.g., CT scan, x-ray). Table 63-12 describes the clinical manifestations of common facial fractures.

Concurrent soft tissue injury often makes assessment of a facial injury difficult. Oral and facial examinations should be performed after the patient has been stabilized and any life-threatening situations have been treated. Careful assessment is made of the ocular muscles and cranial nerve involvement (cranial nerves III, IV, and VI). An x-ray documents the extent of the injury. CT scanning helps differentiate between bone and soft tissue and gives a more specific view of the fracture.

Injury to the eye must be suspected when a facial injury occurs, particularly if the injury is near the orbit. If an eye-globe rupture is suspected, the examination is stopped and a protective shield is placed over the eye. Signs of globe rupture include the extrusion of vitreous humor, or brown tissue (iris or ciliary body) on the surface of the globe or penetrating through a laceration with an eccentric or teardrop-shaped pupil. Specific treatment of a facial fracture depends on the site and extent of the fracture and the associated soft tissue injury. Immobilization or surgical stabilization may be necessary.

The patient who sustains a facial fracture requires sensitive nursing care because an alteration in appearance after the trauma may be drastic. Edema and discoloration subside with time, but concurrent soft tissue injuries may result in permanent scarring. Attention to maintenance of a patent airway and adequate nutrition are ongoing concerns of the nurse throughout the recovery period. Suction should always be available to maintain a patent airway for facial trauma patients.

Mandible Fracture

A fracture of the mandible may result from trauma to the face or jaws. Maxillary fractures may also occur, but they are less common than mandibular fractures. The fracture may be simple, with no bone displacement, or it may involve loss of tissue and bone. The fracture may require immediate and sometimes long-term treatment to ensure survival and restore satisfactory appearance and function. Mandibular fracture may also be therapeutically performed to correct an underlying malocclusion problem that cannot be corrected by orthodontic procedures alone. In these conditions,

the mandible is resected during surgery and manipulated forward or backward depending on the occlusion problem. For this patient, the procedure is performed on an elective basis.

Surgery consists of immobilization, usually by wiring the jaws *(intermaxillary fixation)*. Internal fixation may be accomplished with screws and plates. In a simple fracture with no loss of teeth, the lower jaw is wired to the upper jaw. Wires are placed around the teeth, and then cross-wires or rubber bands are used to hold the lower jaw tight against the upper jaw (Fig. 63-19). Arch bars may be placed on the maxillary and mandibular arches of the teeth. Vertical wires are placed between the arch bars holding the jaws together. When teeth are missing or if there is bone displacement, other forms of fixation such as metal arch bars in the mouth or insertion of a pin in the bone may be needed. Bone grafting may also be required. Immobilization is usually necessary for only 4 to 6 weeks because the fractures generally heal rapidly.

NURSING MANAGEMENT
MANDIBULAR FRACTURE

■ *Nursing Implementation*

Preoperative Management. The patient should be informed preoperatively about the surgical procedure, including what it involves, how the face will look afterward, and alterations caused by the surgery. The patient must be reassured about the ability to breathe normally, speak, and swallow liquids. Hospitalization for respiratory monitoring is brief unless there are other injuries or problems.

Postoperative Management. Postoperative care should focus on a patent airway, oral hygiene, communication, pain management, and adequate nutrition. Two major potential problems in the immediate postoperative period are airway obstruction and aspiration of vomitus. Because the patient cannot open the jaws, measures to ensure an airway are essential. The nurse must observe for signs of respiratory distress (e.g., dyspnea; alterations in rate, quality, and depth of respirations). The patient should be placed on the side with the head slightly elevated immediately after surgery. A wire cutter or scissors (for rubber bands) must be taped to the head of the bed and sent with the patient on all appointments and examinations away from the bedside. These may be used to cut the wires or elastic bands in case of an emergency. The wires should be cut only as a last resort. Once the patient is awake, the wires should be cut only in case of cardiac arrest or respiratory distress requiring access to the pharynx or lungs.

The surgeon should explain, by using a picture, the appropriate wire or wires to cut, and this should be included in the care plan.

In some cases, cutting the wires may cause the entire facial and upper jaw structure to shift or collapse and worsen the problem. A tracheostomy tray or an endotracheal tray should always be available.

If the patient begins to vomit or choke, the nurse should try to clear the mouth and airway. Suctioning may be necessary and may be done by the nasopharyngeal or oral route, depending on the extent of injury and the type of repair. An NG tube may be used for decompression to remove fluids and gas from the stomach to help prevent aspiration. It also helps prevent vomiting. Antiemetics may also be used. The NG tube can later be used as a feeding tube. The nurse should teach the patient to clear secretions and vomitus.

Oral hygiene is an extremely important part of the nursing care. The mouth should be rinsed frequently, particularly after meals and snacks, to remove food debris. Warm normal saline solution, water, or alkaline mouthwashes may be used. A soft rubber catheter or a Water Pik is effective for a thorough oral cleansing. The nurse should inspect the mouth several times a day to see that it is clean. A flashlight is necessary, and a tongue depressor is used to retract the cheeks. The lips and corners of the mouth should be kept moist as well as the buccal mucosa.

Communication may be a problem, particularly in the early postoperative period. An effective way of communication must be established preoperatively (e.g., use of picture board, pad and pencil, small chalkboard). Usually the patient can speak well enough to be understood, especially after the first few postoperative days.

Ingestion of sufficient nutrients poses a challenge because the diet must be liquid. The patient easily tires of sucking through a straw or laboriously using a spoon. The diet must be planned to include adequate calories, protein, and fluids. Liquid protein supplements may be helpful for improving the nutritional status. The nurse works with the dietitian and the patient to ensure adequate nutrition. The low-bulk, high-carbohydrate diet and the intake of air through the straw create a problem with constipation and flatus. Ambulation, prune juice, and bulk-forming laxatives may help relieve these problems.

The patient is usually discharged with the wires in place. The nurse should encourage the patient to verbalize feelings about the altered appearance. Discharge teaching should include oral care, techniques of handling secretions, diet, how and when to use wire cutters, and when to notify the health care provider for concerns and problems.

AMPUTATION

During the past 20 years, major advances have been made in surgical amputation techniques, prosthetic design, and rehabilitation programs. These advances are enabling amputees to return to productive and satisfying social roles. There are an estimated 1.6 million people in the United States living with limb loss.[31] The middle and older age-groups have the highest incidence of amputation because of the effects of peripheral vascular disease, atherosclerosis, and vascular changes related to diabetes mellitus. Amputation in the young is usually secondary to trauma (e.g., motor vehicle collisions, land mines, farm-related injury).

Clinical Indications

The clinical indications for an amputation depend on the underlying disease or trauma. Amputation is required more often in persons engaged in hazardous occupations, with a greater incidence in men. Common indications for amputation include circulatory im-

TABLE 63-13	COLLABORATIVE CARE Amputation

Diagnostic
History and physical examination
Physical appearance of soft tissues
Skin temperature
Sensory function
Presence of peripheral pulses
Arteriography
Venography
Plethysmography
Transcutaneous ultrasonic Doppler recordings

Collaborative Therapy
Medical
Appropriate management of underlying disease
Stabilization of trauma victim

Surgical
Selective type of amputation
Residual limb management
Immediate prosthetic fitting
Delayed prosthetic fitting

Rehabilitation
Coordination of prosthesis-fitting and gait-training activities
Coordination of muscle-strengthening and physical therapy regimens

pairment resulting from a peripheral vascular disorder, traumatic and thermal injuries, malignant tumors, uncontrolled or widespread infection of the extremity (e.g., gas gangrene, osteomyelitis), and congenital disorders. These conditions may manifest as loss of sensation, inadequate circulation, pallor, and local or systemic manifestations of sepsis. Although pain is often present, it is not usually the primary reason for an amputation. The underlying problem dictates whether the amputation is performed as elective or emergency surgery. Consideration must also be given to the patient's ability to successfully use a prosthetic device.

Diagnostic Studies

The types of diagnostic studies performed depend on the underlying problem that makes the amputation necessary (Table 63-13). An elevated white blood cell (WBC) count with differential may indicate infection. Vascular tests such as arteriography, Doppler studies, and venography provide information about the circulatory status of the extremity.

Collaborative Care

The potential for revascularization surgery rather than amputation can be assessed on the basis of vascular studies. If amputation is to be considered "elective," the patient's general health is carefully assessed. Chronic illnesses and the presence of infection are monitored closely. The patient and family should be assisted to understand the need for the amputation and be assured that rehabilitation can result in an active, useful life. If the amputation is performed on an emergency basis as a result of trauma, management of the patient is physically and emotionally more complicated.

The goal of amputation surgery is to preserve extremity length and function while removing all infected, pathologic, or ischemic tissue. This improves the possibility of good prosthetic, cosmetic, and functional satisfaction. (Levels of amputation of upper and

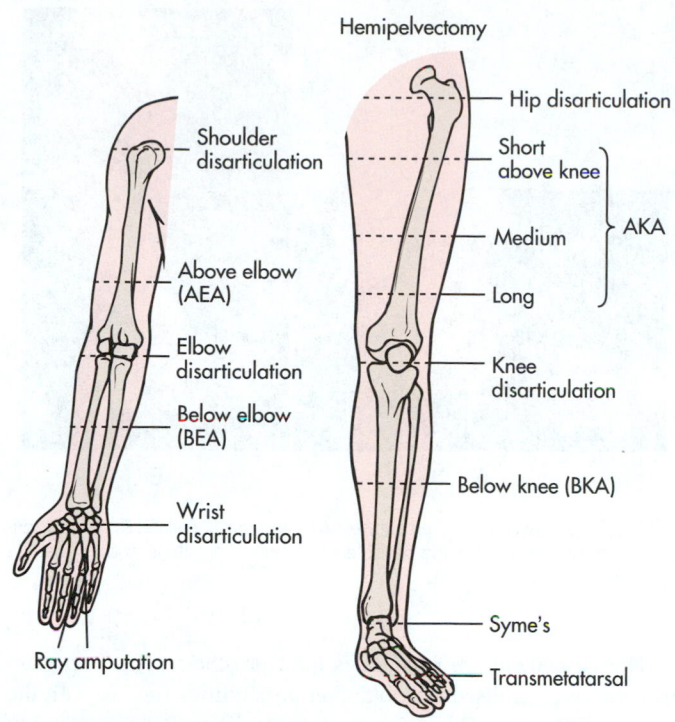

Hemipelvectomy

Hip disarticulation

Short above knee

Medium } AKA

Long

Knee disarticulation

Below knee (BKA)

Syme's

Transmetatarsal

Shoulder disarticulation

Above elbow (AEA)

Elbow disarticulation

Below elbow (BEA)

Wrist disarticulation

Ray amputation

FIG. 63-20 Location and description of amputation sites of the upper and lower extremities. *AKA,* Above-the-knee amputation.

lower extremities are illustrated in Fig. 63-20.) The type of amputation depends on the reason for the surgery. A closed amputation is performed to create a weight-bearing residual limb (or stump). An anterior skin flap with dissected soft tissue padding covers the bony part of the residual limb. The skin flap is sutured posteriorly so that it will not be positioned in a weight-bearing area. Special care is necessary to prevent the accumulation of drainage, which can produce pressure and harbor bacteria that may cause infection. Disarticulation is an amputation performed through a joint. A *Syme's amputation* is a form of disarticulation at the ankle. An open amputation leaves a surface on the residual limb that is not covered with skin. This type of surgery is generally indicated for control of actual or potential infection. The wound is usually closed later by a second surgical procedure or closed by skin traction surrounding the residual limb. This type of amputation is often called a "guillotine amputation."

NURSING MANAGEMENT
AMPUTATION

■ Nursing Assessment

Preexisting illnesses must be adequately assessed because most amputations are performed as a result of vascular problems. Assessment of the vascular and neurologic status is an important part of the assessment process (see Chapters 32 and 56).

■ Nursing Diagnoses

Nursing diagnoses for the patient with an amputation may include, but are not limited to, the following:

- Disturbed body image *related to* amputation and impaired mobility
- Impaired skin integrity *related to* immobility and improperly fitted prosthesis

- Chronic pain *related to* phantom limb sensation
- Impaired physical mobility *related to* amputation of lower limb

■ Planning

The overall goals are that the patient with an amputation will (1) have adequate relief from the underlying health problem, (2) have satisfactory pain control, (3) reach maximum rehabilitation potential with the use of a prosthesis (if indicated), (4) cope with the body image changes, and (5) make satisfying lifestyle adjustments.

■ Nursing Implementation

Health Promotion. Most lower limb amputations result from peripheral vascular disease, and most upper limb amputations result from severe trauma. Knowing this, the nurse directs patient education toward prevention of amputation. Control of causative illnesses such as peripheral vascular disease, diabetes mellitus, chronic osteomyelitis, and pressure ulcers can eliminate or delay the need for amputation. Patients with these problems should be taught to carefully examine their lower extremities daily for signs of potential problems. If the patient cannot assume this responsibility, a family member should be instructed in the procedure. Patients and their families should be instructed to report problems such as change in skin color or skin temperature, decrease or absence of sensation in the feet and/or toes, tingling, burning pain, or the presence of a lesion to the health care provider.

Instruction in proper safety precautions in recreational activities and in the performance of potentially hazardous work is an important nursing responsibility, especially for occupational health nurses. A mangled extremity with subsequent amputation is a serious consequence of trauma that can be avoided.

Acute Intervention. The nurse must recognize the tremendous psychologic and social implications of an amputation for the patient. The disruption in body image caused by an amputation often causes a patient to go through the psychologic stages of the grieving process. Allowing the patient to go through the grieving process and recognizing it as a normal consequence may do much to aid the patient's acceptance of the amputation. The patient's family must also be helped to work through the transitional process to arrive at a realistic and positive attitude about the future. The reasons for an amputation and the rehabilitation potential depend on age, diagnosis, occupation, personality, resources, and support systems. Understanding and meeting the special needs of day laborers, such as farmers and their families, is also important for the nurse and staff.[32]

Preoperative Management. Before surgery, the nurse should reinforce information that the patient and family have received about the reasons for the amputation, the proposed prosthesis, and the mobility-training program. In addition to the usual preoperative instructions, the patient undergoing an amputation has special educational needs. To meet these needs, the nurse must know the level of amputation, the type of postsurgical dressings to be applied, and the type of prosthesis to be utilized. The patient should receive instruction in the performance of upper extremity exercises such as push-ups in bed or the wheelchair to promote arm strength. This instruction is essential later for crutch walking and gait training. General postoperative nursing care should be discussed, including positioning, support, and residual limb care. If a compression bandage is to be used after surgery, the patient should be instructed about its purpose and how it will be applied. If an immediate prosthesis is planned, the general ambulation expectations and program should be discussed.

The patient should be warned that it might feel as if the amputated limb is still present after surgery. This phenomenon, termed **phantom limb sensation,** occurs in 80% of amputees and may cause patients grave concern unless they are forewarned. If pain was present in the affected limb preoperatively, the patient may also experience phantom limb pain postoperatively. The patient may complain of feelings of coldness and heaviness, cramping, shooting, burning, or crushing pain. Often, the patient may be extremely anxious about this pain because the patient knows the limb is gone but still perceives pain in it. As recovery and ambulation progress, phantom limb sensation and pain usually subside, although the pain may become chronic.[33,34]

Postoperative Management. General postoperative care for the patient who has had an amputation depends largely on the patient's general state of health, the reason for the amputation, and the patient's age. Nursing care must be individualized on the basis of these factors. For example, an older adult patient needs careful monitoring of respiratory status. A victim of a motor vehicle collision may need careful neurologic monitoring. Individuals who undergo amputation as a result of a traumatic injury need to be monitored for posttraumatic stress disorder because they have had no time to prepare or perhaps even participate in the decision to have a limb amputated.

Prevention and detection of complications are important nursing responsibilities during the postoperative period. Careful monitoring of the patient's vital signs and dressings can alert the nurse to hemorrhage in the operative area. Careful attention to sterile technique during dressing changes reduces the potential for wound infection.

If an immediate postoperative prosthesis has been applied, the nurse must monitor vital signs. Careful surveillance of the surgical site is also required. A surgical tourniquet must always be available for emergency use. If excessive bleeding occurs, the surgeon should be notified immediately. Efforts to maintain hemostasis and to control the hemorrhage should begin at once.

The orthopedic surgeon will decide the type of prosthetic fitting that will be used after surgery. An immediate prosthetic fitting may be performed in the operating room after the amputation. For example, for a lower extremity amputation, a rigid, castlike bandage is applied around the closed residual limb with a prosthetic pylon and an ankle-foot assembly. While the patient is still anesthetized, the prosthetic pylon and ankle-foot assembly are aligned and adjusted to provide a smooth gait and to avoid excessive pressure on the residual limb area. A strap is placed on the proximal anterior surface of the rigid plaster bandage and attached to a waistband to prevent slippage. The main advantages of this device are reduction of edema and the psychologic benefit of early ambulation. A disadvantage in the application of an immediate postoperative device is the inability to directly visualize the surgical site.

The delayed prosthetic fitting may be the best choice for certain patients. Patients who have had amputations above the knee or below the elbow, older adults, debilitated individuals, and those with infection usually have delayed prosthetic fittings (Fig. 63-21). The appropriate time for use of a prosthesis depends on satisfactory healing of the residual limb, as well as on the general condition of the patient. A temporary prosthesis may be used for partial weight bearing once the sutures are removed. Barring any problems, patients can bear full weight on permanent prostheses approximately 3 months after amputation.

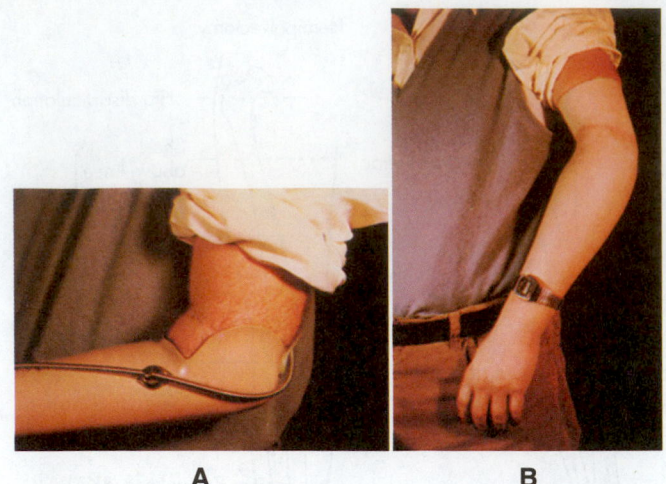

FIG. 63-21 Two types of prostheses. **A,** Traditional fiberglass. **B,** New materials and techniques have made possible fabrication of prosthetic sockets that are light, soft, flexible, and secure.

Not all patients are candidates for a prosthesis. It is important that the surgeon discuss ambulation possibilities frankly with the patient and family. The seriously ill or debilitated patient may not have the upper body strength and energy required to use a lower extremity prosthesis. Mobility with a wheelchair may be the most realistic goal for patients who are not candidates for prostheses.

Collaborative care also includes the direction and coordination of the rehabilitation program for the amputee. Success depends on the physical and emotional health of the patient. Chronic illness and deconditioning complicate aggressive rehabilitation efforts. Both physical and occupational therapy must be an integral component of the patient's overall plan of care.

Flexion contractures may delay the rehabilitation process. The most common and debilitating contracture is hip flexion. Hip adduction contracture is rare. Patients should avoid sitting in a chair for more than 1 hour with hips flexed or having pillows under the surgical extremity to prevent flexion contractures. Unless specifically contraindicated, patients should lie on their abdomen for 30 minutes three or four times each day and position the hip in extension while prone.

Proper residual limb bandaging fosters shaping and molding for eventual prosthesis fitting (Fig. 63-22). The physician usually orders a compression bandage to be applied immediately after surgery to support the soft tissues, reduce edema, hasten healing, minimize pain, and promote residual limb shrinkage and maturation. This bandage may be an elastic roll applied to the residual limb or a residual limb shrinker, which is an elastic stocking that fits tightly over the residual limb and lower trunk area.[35]

The compression bandage is initially worn at all times except during physical therapy and bathing. The bandage is taken off and reapplied several times daily, and care is taken so that it is applied snugly but not so tight as to interfere with circulation. Shrinker bandages should be washed and changed daily. It is recommended that the patient have two residual limb shrinker bandages so that one can be worn while the other is being washed. After healing has occurred, the residual limb is bandaged only when the patient is not wearing the prosthesis. The patient should be instructed to avoid dangling the residual limb over the bedside to minimize edema formation.

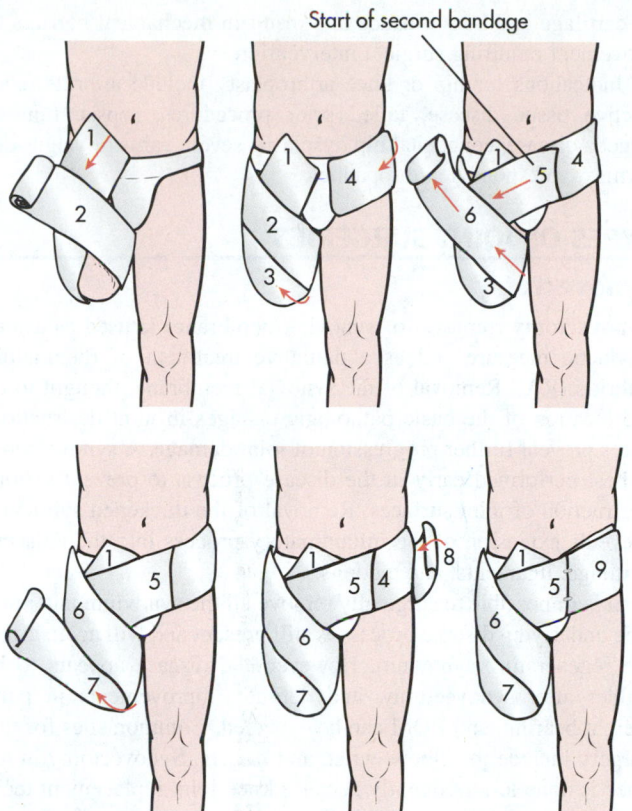

Start of second bandage

FIG. 63-22 Bandaging for the above-the-knee amputation residual limb. Figure-eight style covers progressive areas of the residual limb. Two elastic wraps are required.

TABLE 63-14	*PATIENT AND FAMILY TEACHING GUIDE* **Following an Amputation**

1. Inspect the residual limb daily for signs of skin irritation, especially erythema, excoriation, and odor. Pay particular attention to areas prone to pressure.
2. Discontinue use of the prosthesis if an irritation develops. Have the area checked before resuming use of the prosthesis.
3. Wash residual limb thoroughly each night with warm water and a bacteriostatic soap. Rinse thoroughly and dry gently. Expose the residual limb to air for 20 min.
4. Do not use any substance such as lotions, alcohol, powders, or oil unless prescribed by the health care provider.
5. Wear only a residual limb sock that is in good condition and supplied by the prosthetist.
6. Change residual limb sock daily. Launder in a mild soap, squeeze, and lay flat to dry.
7. Use prescribed pain-management techniques.
8. Perform ROM to all joints daily. Perform general strengthening exercises including the upper extremities daily.
9. Do not elevate the residual limb on a pillow.
10. Lay prone with hip extension for 30 min three or four times daily.

ROM, Range of motion.

As the patient's overall condition improves, the nurse begins instruction in the principles and techniques of transferring from bed to chair and back. Active exercises and conditioning are essential in developing ambulation skills. The exercise regimen is normally started under the supervision of the health care provider and the physical therapist. The nurse must have a clear understanding of the exercise regimen to reinforce it and ensure that the exercises are performed correctly. Active ROM exercises of all joints should be started as soon after surgery as the patient's pain level and medical status permit. In preparation for mobility, the patient should increase triceps and shoulder strength and lower limb support and learn balance of the altered body. The loss of the weight of an amputated limb requires adaptation of the patient's proprioceptive and coordination mechanisms to prevent falls and injury.

Crutch walking is started as soon as patients are physically able. If they have had immediate postsurgical fitting, orders related to weight bearing must be carefully followed to avoid disruption of the skin flap and delay of the tissue healing process. Initial periods of ambulation should not exceed 5 minutes to prevent dependent edema.

Before discharge, the patient and family need careful instruction related to residual limb care, ambulation, prevention of contractures, recognition of complications, exercise, and follow-up care. Table 63-14 outlines patient and family teaching following an amputation.

Ambulatory and Home Care. When the healing has occurred satisfactorily and the residual limb is well molded, the patient is ready for fitting of the prosthesis. Walking with a below-the-knee prosthesis requires 40% additional energy, and an above-the-knee

prosthesis requires 60% more energy. Matching a patient with a suitable prosthesis involves many factors, including age, general health, intelligence, motivation, occupation, and finances. After the physician makes the recommendation, the patient is referred to a prosthetist, who initially makes a mold of the residual limb and measures landmarks for the fabrication of the prosthesis. The molded limb socket allows the residual limb to fit snugly into the prosthesis. The limb is covered with a residual limb stocking to ensure good fit and prevent skin breakdown. The residual limb may continue to shrink, causing a loose fit, in which case a new socket has to be fabricated. The patient may need to have the prosthesis adjusted to prevent rubbing and friction between the residual limb and the socket. Excessive movement of a loose prosthesis can cause severe skin irritation and breakdown.

The prosthesis is fitted by the prosthetist, who may also train the amputee to use it. It is important for the nurse to be familiar with the training program to encourage and assist the patient. Most often this learning occurs after the patient has been discharged from the inpatient setting. Learning to use a prosthesis is frustrating, and the patient may easily become discouraged. The nurse must continually offer support until the patient is able to manage alone.

Artificial limbs become an integral part of the patient's changed body image. Proper care ensures their long life and useful functioning. The patient should be instructed to clean the prosthesis socket daily with a mild soap and rinse thoroughly to remove irritants. The leather and metal parts of the prosthesis should not get wet. The patient should be encouraged to have regular maintenance of the prosthesis. Consideration of the condition of the shoe is also necessary. A badly worn shoe alters the gait and may cause damage to the prosthesis.

Referral to a community health nurse can foster optimal physical and emotional adjustment. The family should be instructed on ambulation and transfer techniques and proper residual limb care.

Special Considerations in Upper Limb Amputation. The emotional implications of an upper limb amputation are often more devastating than those for lower limb amputation. The enforced dependency brought about by one-handedness is both frustrating and humiliating to many patients. Because most upper extremity amputations result from trauma, the patient has not had the opportunity to adjust psychologically to an amputation or to participate in the decision-making process about amputation.

Both immediate and delayed prosthetic fittings are possible for the below-the-elbow amputee. Prosthetic fitting is delayed for the above-the-elbow amputee. The usual functional prosthesis is the arm and hook. A cosmetic hand is available but has limited functional value. As with the lower limb prosthesis, patient motivation and endurance are major factors contributing to a satisfactory outcome.

■ Evaluation

The expected outcomes are that the patient with an amputation will:

- accept changed body image and integrate changes into lifestyle
- have no evidence of skin breakdown
- have reduction or absence of pain
- become mobile within limitations imposed by amputation

GERONTOLOGIC CONSIDERATIONS
AMPUTATION

If a lower limb amputation has been performed on an older adult, the patient's previous ability to ambulate may affect the extent of recovery. Use of a prosthesis requires significant strength and energy for ambulation. Older adults whose general health is altered and weakened by disorders such as cardiac or pulmonary dysfunction may not be candidates for prosthesis use. The patient's ability to ambulate may be limited. If possible, this should be discussed with the patient and family before surgery so that realistic expectations can be set.

Common Joint Surgical Procedures

Surgery plays an important role in the treatment and rehabilitation of patients with various forms of arthritis, conditions related to trauma, and other painful conditions resulting in functional disability. Joint replacement surgery is the most common orthopedic operation performed on older adults. Significant advances in the field of reconstructive surgery have resulted in improvements in prosthetic design, materials, and surgical techniques that provide significant relief of pain and deformity and improve function and joint motion.

Indications for Joint Surgery

Surgery is aimed at relieving pain, improving joint motion, correcting deformity and malalignment, and removing intraarticular causes of erosion. Debilitating joint pain is one of the primary reasons for arthroplasty. In addition to the effects of chronic pain on the physical and emotional health of the patient, any movement of the painful joint is often avoided. If this decreased functional ability is not corrected, contraction with permanent limitation of motion often occurs. Limitation of motion at any joint can be demonstrated on physical examination and by joint-space narrowing on radiologic examination.

There may also be a slow loss of cartilage in affected joints, which may be related to loss of motion. Synovitis can cause tendon damage, resulting in rupture or subluxation of the joint and subsequent loss of function. Continuing disease activity may cause loss

of cartilage and bony surface and result in mechanical barriers to movement requiring surgical intervention.

Indications for hip or knee arthroplasty include arthritis, connective tissue disease, failed prior procedures, sepsis, tumors, Paget's disease, congenital hip dysplasia, severe varus or valgus deformity, and spondyloarthropathies.

TYPES OF JOINT SURGERIES

Synovectomy

Synovectomy (removal of synovial membrane) is used as a prophylactic measure and as a palliative treatment of rheumatoid arthritis (RA). Removal of the synovial membrane, thought to be the location of the basic pathologic changes in joint destruction, helps prevent further progression of joint damage. A synovectomy is best performed early in the disease process to prevent serious destruction of joint surfaces. Removal of the thickened synovium prevents extension of the inflammatory process into the adjacent cartilage, ligaments, and tendons.

It is impossible to surgically remove all the synovium in a joint. The underlying disease process is still present and will again affect the regenerating synovium. However, the disease appears to be milder after synovectomy, and definite improvements in pain, weight bearing, and ROM can be expected. Common sites for this surgery include the elbow, wrist, and fingers. Synovectomy in the knee is done less frequently because knee joint replacement techniques are usually used.

Osteotomy

An **osteotomy** is performed by removing or adding a wedge or slice of bone to change alignment (joint and vertebral) and to shift weight bearing, thereby correcting deformity and relieving pain. Cervical osteotomy may be used to correct deformity in some patients with ankylosing spondylitis. A halo and body jacket is worn until fusion occurs (3 to 4 months). Subtrochanteric or femoral osteotomy may provide some relief of pain and improve motion in selected patients with hip osteoarthritis. Osteotomy has proven ineffective in patients with inflammatory joint disease. Osteotomy of the knee (tibia) provides relief of pain in selected patients, but advanced joint destruction is usually corrected by joint replacement surgery. The postoperative care is similar to the treatment of an internal fixation of a fracture at a comparable site (see pp. 1643 to 1646). Internal wires, screws and plates, bone grafts, or an external fixator usually fix the bone in place.

Debridement

Debridement is the removal of degenerative debris such as loose bodies, osteophytes, joint debris, and degenerated menisci from a joint. This procedure is usually performed on the knee or the shoulder using a fiberoptic arthroscope. The procedure is usually done on an outpatient basis. A compression dressing is applied postoperatively. Weight bearing is permitted following knee arthroscopy. Patient education includes monitoring for signs of infection, managing pain, and restricting excessive activity for 24 to 48 hours.

Arthroplasty

Arthroplasty is the reconstruction or replacement of a joint. This surgical procedure is performed to relieve pain, improve or maintain ROM, and correct deformity. The most common uses of arthroplasty are for patients with osteoarthritis (OA), RA, avascular necrosis, congenital deformities or dislocations, and other sys-

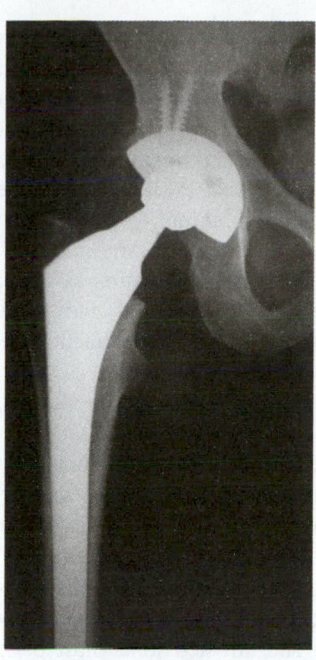

FIG. 63-23 Total hip arthroplasty. Porous coated, noncemented femoral prosthesis of metal alloy with a cemented high-density plastic acetabular socket.

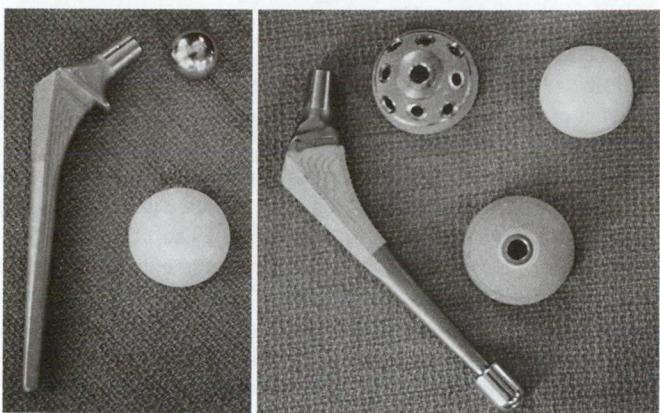

FIG. 63-24 Total hip replacements. **A,** Coated cemented components. **B,** Porous cementless components.

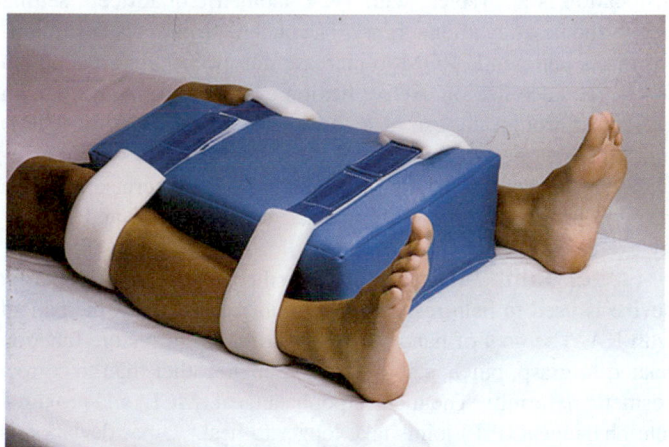

FIG. 63-25 Maintaining postoperative abduction following total hip replacement.

temic problems. There are several types of arthroplasty, including replacement of part of a joint (hemiarthroplasty), surgical reshaping of the bones of the joints, and total joint replacement. Replacement arthroplasty is available for the elbow, shoulder, phalangeal joints of the fingers, wrist, hip, knee, ankle, and foot.

Hip Arthroplasty. Total hip arthroplasty (THA) provides significant relief of pain and improvement of function for patients with OA and RA. Implants are often "cemented" in place with polymethylmethacrylate, which bonds to the bone. With time, a significant number of femoral components loosen and require revision surgery. Because of this risk, cemented THAs are recommended for less active, older adults with compromised bone density. Younger individuals receive "cementless" arthroplasties in an effort to prolong the lifetime of the prosthesis. Cementless THAs provide long-term implant stability by facilitating biologic ingrowth of new bone tissue into the porous surface coating of the prosthesis (Fig. 63-23). A patient with a high activity potential and a life expectancy of 25 years or more is an excellent candidate for a cementless prosthesis. Total hip replacements are shown in Fig. 63-24.

In both types of arthroplasties, extremes of internal rotation, adduction, and 90-degree flexion of the hip must be avoided for 4 to 6 weeks postoperatively. A foam abduction pillow is sometimes placed between the legs to prevent dislocation of the new joint (Fig. 63-25). Following surgery, flexion of the hip past 90 degrees is contraindicated and elevated toilet seats and chair alterations at home are necessary. Tub baths and driving a car are not allowed for 4 to 6 weeks. An occupational therapist may teach the patient to use assistive devices, such as reach bars ("reachers") to avoid bending over to pick something off the floor, long-handled shoehorns, or sock pullers. The knees must be kept apart; the patient must never cross the legs or twist to reach behind. Physical therapy is initiated the first postoperative day, with ambulation and weight bearing with a walker for patients with a cemented prosthesis and weight bearing on the operative side for those with an uncemented prosthesis.

Exercises designed to restore strength and muscle tone in the quadriceps and muscles about the hip are essential to improved

function and ROM. These include quadriceps setting (e.g., tightening the kneecap), gluteal muscle setting (e.g., tightening the buttocks), leg raises in supine and prone positions, and abduction exercises (e.g., swinging the leg out but never crossing midline) from the supine and standing positions. The patient will continue these exercises for many months after discharge, and the family should be well acquainted with the exercise program to offer encouragement at home.

Home care considerations include ongoing assessment of pain management, monitoring for infection, and prevention of DVT. Not all patients will qualify for home nursing visits. The incision may be closed with metal staples, which are removed at the surgeon's office. Because of the high risk for DVT, prothrombin times will be determined weekly and anticoagulation adjusted accordingly if warfarin is used. Enoxaparin (Lovenox), a low-molecular-weight heparin (LMWH), is administered subcutaneously and can be given at home by the patient or family member. An advantage of enoxaparin is that it does not require monitoring of the patient's coagulation status. The patient should be instructed to obtain prophylactic antibiotics prior to dental appointments and surgical procedures that might put the patient at risk for bacteremia.

A physical therapist will assess ROM, ambulation, and compliance with the exercise regimen. The patient will gradually increase the number of repetitions of exercises, add weights to ankles, and swim, and may eventually use a stationary bicycle to tone quadriceps and improve cardiovascular fitness. High-impact exercises and sports, such as jogging and tennis, may loosen the implant and should be avoided. The elderly adult may require rehabilitation at a subacute or extended care facility until able to function independently.[36]

Knee Arthroplasty.

Unremitting pain and instability as a result of severe destructive deterioration of the knee joint is the main indication for total knee arthroplasty (TKA). The presence of osteoporosis may necessitate bone grafting to augment defects and to correct bone deficiencies. Either part of or the entire knee joint may be replaced with a metal and plastic prosthetic device. A compression dressing is used to immobilize the knee in extension immediately after the operation. This is removed before discharge and may be replaced with a knee immobilizer or posterior plastic shell, which maintains extension during ambulation and at rest for about 4 weeks.

Great emphasis is placed on postoperative physical therapy, and dislocation is not typical with TKA. Isometric quadriceps setting begins the first day after surgery. The patient progresses to straight-leg raises and gentle ROM to increase muscle strength and obtain 90-degree knee flexion. Active flexion exercises or passive flexion exercises through the use of a continuous passive motion (CPM) machine postoperatively promote joint mobility. Full weight bearing is begun before discharge. An active home exercise program involves progressive ROM with muscle strengthening, and flexibility exercises.

Finger Joint Arthroplasty.

A silicone rubber arthroplastic device is used to help restore function in the fingers of the patient with RA. The goal of hand surgery is primarily to restore function related to grasp, pinch, stability, and strength rather than to correct cosmetic deformity. The metacarpophalangeal (MCP) and proximal interphalangeal (PIP) joints take longer to heal.[6] Ulnar deviation is often present, which results in severe functional limitations of the hand. Before surgery the patient is instructed in hand exercises, including flexion, extension, abduction, and adduction of the fingers. Postoperatively, the hand is kept elevated with a bulky dressing in place. Neurovascular assessment is conducted postoperatively, and the nurse assesses for signs of infection. The success of the surgery depends largely on the postoperative treatment plan, which is often carried out under the direction of an occupational therapist. Once the dressing is removed, a guided splinting program is initiated. The patient is discharged with splints to use while sleeping and hand exercises to perform for 10 to 12 weeks at least three or four times a day. The patient is also instructed to avoid lifting heavy objects.

Elbow and Shoulder Arthroplasty.

Although available, total replacement of elbow and shoulder joints is not as common as other forms of arthroplasty. Shoulder replacements are performed in patients with severe pain because of RA, OA, avascular necrosis, or an old trauma. The shoulder replacement is usually considered if the patient has adequate surrounding muscle strength and bone stock. If joint replacement is necessary for both elbow and shoulder, the elbow is usually done first because a severely painful elbow interferes with the shoulder rehabilitation program.

Significant pain relief has been achieved following arthroplasty, with 90% of patients having no pain at rest or minimal pain with activity. Functional improvements have resulted in better hygiene and increased ability to perform activities of daily living in most patients. Rehabilitation is longer and more difficult than with other joint surgeries.

Ankle Arthroplasty.

Total ankle arthroplasty (TAA) is indicated for RA, OA, trauma, and avascular necrosis. Ankle fusion is often selected over arthroplasty because the result is more durable. However, the patient is left with a stiff foot and the inability to change heel height. TAA is advantageous because a more normal gait pattern can be achieved. Postoperatively, the patient may not bear weight for 6 weeks and must elevate the extremity to reduce and prevent edema, be extremely careful to prevent postoperative infection, and maintain immobilization as directed by the physician. Although the use of TAA is not widespread, it is becoming a viable alternative to fusion for the treatment of severe ankle arthritis in selected patients.

Arthrodesis

Arthrodesis is the surgical fusion of a joint. This procedure is indicated only if articular surfaces are too severely damaged or infected to allow joint replacement or for reconstructive surgery failures. Arthrodesis relieves pain and provides a stable but immobile joint. The fusion is usually accomplished by removal of the articular hyaline cartilage and the addition of bone grafts across the joint surface. The affected joint must be immobilized until bone healing has occurred. Common areas of fusion are the wrist, ankle, cervical spine, lumbar spine, and metatarsophalangeal (MTP) joint of the great toe.

Complications of Joint Surgery

Infection is a serious complication of joint surgery, particularly joint replacement surgery. The most common causative organisms are gram-positive aerobic streptococci and staphylococci. Infection almost always leads to pain and loosening of the prosthesis, generally requiring extensive surgery. Efforts to reduce the incidence of infection include the use of specially designed self-contained operating suites, operating rooms with laminar airflow, and prophylactic antibiotic administration.

DVT is another potentially serious complication after joint surgeries, particularly those involving the lower extremities. Prophylactic measures such as aspirin, warfarin, LMWH, and pneumatic compression of the legs are usually instituted. Patients may be followed postoperatively with venous Doppler ultrasound to detect DVT, the source of most pulmonary emboli. Fat embolism syndrome (FES) may also occur after total hip arthroplasty.

Collaborative Care

Preoperative Management.

As surgical techniques and care improve, more patients with chronic diseases such as RA are being considered as surgical candidates. The primary goal of preoperative assessment is to identify risk factors associated with postoperative complications so that nursing strategies can be implemented to promote optimal positive outcomes. A careful history will include previous medical diagnoses and complications such as diabetes and thrombophlebitis, pain tolerance and management preferences, current functional status and expectations following surgery, and level of social support and home care needs after discharge. The patient should be free from infection and acute joint inflammation.

If lower extremity surgery is planned, upper extremity muscle strength and joint function are assessed to determine the type of assistive devices needed postoperatively for ambulation and activities of daily living. Preoperative teaching informs the patient and family of the expected hospital course and postoperative management at home. In addition, it prepares them to maximize the usefulness and longevity of the prosthesis. Research has shown that preoperative education alone is not sufficient to ensure successful joint replacement; the patient must have a sense of self-efficacy for an optimal outcome to be achieved.[37] Patients also need to realize that recovery is "not going to happen overnight." Both patients and their families or significant others need to speak with individuals who have had a total joint arthroplasty to better understand the reality of dealing with a joint replacement.

Postoperative Management. Postoperatively, neurovascular assessment is performed to assess nerve function and circulatory status. Anticoagulation therapy, analgesia, and parenteral antibiotics are administered. In general, the affected joint is exercised, and ambulation is encouraged as early as possible to prevent complications of immobility. Specific protocols vary according to patient, type of prosthesis, and surgeon preference. Pain management techniques used postoperatively may include epidural analgesia, patient-controlled analgesia, IV injections, oral opioids or NSAIDs, and the On-Q pump. The On-Q pump administers analgesics locally to an operative area.[37]

The hospital stay after arthroplasty is 3 to 5 days depending on the patient's course and need for physical therapy. Physical therapy and ambulation enhance mobility, build muscle strength, and reduce the risk of thrombus formation. If the patient is taking warfarin, therapy starts on the day of surgery and continues for 3 weeks, with a prothrombin time measured on a regular basis. For those taking LMWH (e.g., enoxaparin), therapy starts 24 to 36 hours after surgery and continues for 2 weeks postoperatively. Daily monitoring of the patient's coagulation status is not necessary when the patient is taking LMWH. The decision to use warfarin or LMWH depends on many factors, including the patient's age and overall state of health.

NURSING MANAGEMENT
JOINT SURGERY

The nursing management of the patient undergoing joint surgery begins with preoperative teaching and realistic goal setting. It is important that the patient understands and accepts the limitations of the proposed surgery and realizes that it will not remove the underlying disease or inflammatory process. Postoperative procedures such as turning, deep breathing, use of bedpan and bedside commode, and use of abductor pillows should be explained and opportunities for practice provided. The patient should be reassured that pain relief will be available. Patient-controlled analgesia can be helpful. A preoperative visit from a physical therapist allows practice of postoperative exercises and measurement for crutches or other assistive devices.

Discharge planning begins immediately. The duration of the hospital stay and the expected postoperative events should be discussed because the patient and family must prepare ahead. The home environment must be assessed for safety (e.g., presence of scatter rugs and electrical cords) and accessibility. Are the bathroom and bedroom on the first floor? Are door frames wide enough to accommodate a walker? Social support must also be assessed. Is a friend or family member available to assist the patient in the home? Will the patient require homemaker or meal services? The

elderly patient may need the rehabilitation services of a subacute or extended care facility for a few weeks postoperatively to progressively develop independent living skills. Specific nursing interventions related to surgery for the patient having orthopedic surgery are summarized in NCP 63-2.

Patient teaching includes instructions on reporting complications, including infection (e.g., fever, increased pain, drainage) and dislocation of the prosthesis (e.g., pain, loss of function, shortening or malalignment of an extremity). The home care nurse acts as the liaison between the patient and the surgeon, monitoring for postoperative complications, assessing comfort and ROM, and facilitating improvements in functional performance.

CRITICAL THINKING EXERCISE

CASE STUDY

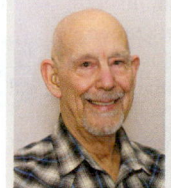

Hip Fracture

Patient Profile. Gene Wells is an 82-year-old white male admitted to the hospital through the emergency department. He fell on an icy patch outside his home. It appears he may have sustained a fracture to his right hip. He has a history of type 2 diabetes mellitus and has a 60 pack-year smoking history that is now complicated by chronic obstructive pulmonary disease.

Case Study photo
©iStockphoto.com.

Subjective Data
- Complains of excruciating pain and tenderness in right hip

Objective Data

Physical Examination
- Blood pressure: 166/94
- Diaphoretic and pale skin
- Respiratory rate 36; crackles, expiratory wheeze
- Pain not relieved with morphine

Diagnostic Studies
- X-ray of right hip reveals extracapsular fracture
- Hematocrit 30%; hemoglobin 15 g/dl; WBC 15,000/μl (15×10^9/L)

Collaborative Care
- Right hip repair with compression plate and bone screws
- Cefazolin (Ancef) 1 g IV every 8 hours
- Intake and output for 48 hours postoperatively
- Morphine sulfate per patient-controlled analgesia pump

Critical Thinking Questions

1. How do preexisting medical conditions predispose Gene to postoperative complications?
2. What are the most likely postoperative complications to develop for Gene?
3. What pre- and postoperative nursing interventions will be essential while taking care of this patient?
4. What are the priority nursing interventions?
5. Based on the data presented, write one or more appropriate nursing diagnoses.
6. What are the collaborative care concerns for the elderly patient with a hip fracture?

NCLEX EXAMINATION REVIEW QUESTIONS

The number of the question corresponds to the same-numbered objective at the beginning of the chapter.

1. The nurse suspects an ankle sprain when a patient at the urgent care center
   a. was hit by another soccer player on the field.
   b. has ankle pain after running a 10-mile race.
   c. dropped a 10-lb weight on his lower leg at the health club.
   d. had an inversion or twisting injury while running bases during a baseball game.

2. The nurse explains to a patient with a distal tibial fracture returning for a 3-week checkup that healing is indicated by
   a. callus formation.
   b. complete union of bone.
   c. presence of granulation tissue.
   d. formation of a hematoma at the fracture site.

3. A patient with a comminuted fracture of the femur is to have an open reduction with internal fixation (ORIF) of the fracture. The nurse explains that ORIF is indicated when
   a. a cast would be too large to provide normal mobility.
   b. the patient is able to tolerate long-term immobilization.
   c. the patient cannot tolerate the discomfort of a closed reduction.
   d. adequate alignment cannot be obtained by other nonsurgical methods.

4. An indication of a neurovascular problem noted during assessment of the patient with a fracture is
   a. exaggeration of extremity movement.
   b. petechiae on the head and upper thorax.
   c. decreased sensation distal to the fracture site.
   d. purulent drainage at the site of an open fracture.

5. A patient with a stable, closed fracture of the humerus caused by trauma to the arm has a temporary splint with bulky padding applied with an elastic bandage. The nurse suspects compartment syndrome and notifies the physician when the patient experiences
   a. pain at the fracture site.
   b. increasing edema of the limb.
   c. muscle spasms of the lower arm.
   d. pain when the nurse passively extends the fingers.

6. A patient with symphysis pubis and pelvic rami fractures should be monitored for
   a. sudden thirst.
   b. changes in urinary output.
   c. a palpable lump in the buttock.
   d. sudden decrease in blood pressure.

7. During the postoperative period, the patient with an above-the-knee amputation should be instructed that the residual limb should not be routinely elevated because
   a. the flexed position can promote hip flexion contracture.
   b. this position reduces the development of phantom limb sensation.
   c. this position promotes clot formation at the incision site and thigh.
   d. unnecessary movement of the extremity can cause wound dehiscence.

8. A patient with rheumatoid arthritis is scheduled for an arthroplasty. The nurse explains that the purpose of this procedure is to
   a. fuse a joint and reduce pain.
   b. prevent further joint damage.
   c. assess and remove degenerative debris.
   d. replace the joint and improve function.

9. The nurse teaches a patient scheduled for a total hip replacement that it is important after surgery to avoid
   a. sleeping on the abdomen.
   b. sitting with the legs crossed.
   c. abduction exercises of the affected leg.
   d. bearing weight on the affected leg for 4 to 6 weeks.

REFERENCES

1. National Center for Injury Prevention and Control: *Fatal injuries: leading causes of death reports,* Atlanta, 2002, Centers for Disease Control and Prevention. Available at *www.webapp.cdc.gov* (accessed August 31, 2006).
2. Centers for Disease Control and Prevention: Nonfatal sports and recreation-related injuries treated in emergency departments—United States, *MMWR Morb Mortal Wkly Rep* 51:736, 2002. Available at *www.cdc.gov/mmwr* (accessed July 31, 2006).
3. Maher A: Trauma. In Taggart HM: *NAON core curriculum for orthopedic nursing,* ed 5, Boston, 2006, Pearson Custom Publishing.
4. Derksen RJ: Diagnostic accuracy and reproducibility in the interpretation of Ottawa ankle and foot rules by specialized emergency nurses, *Am J Emerg Med* 23:725, 2005.
5. National Institute of Aging and the National Aeronautics and Space Administration: *Exercise: guide from the National Institute of Aging,* Available at *www.weboflife.ksc.nasa.gov/exerciseandaging* (accessed August 31, 2006).
6. Childs S: Hand and wrist problems. In Taggart HM: *NAON core curriculum for orthopaedic nursing,* ed 5, Boston, 2006, Pearson Custom Publishing.
7. Bagwell-Crum C: The shoulder. In Taggart HM: *NAON core curriculum for orthopaedic nursing,* ed 5, Boston, 2006, Pearson Custom Publishing.
8. John Hopkins Medical Letter: Relief is at hand for carpel tunnel syndrome, *Johns Hopkins Health After 50 Newsletter* 16:3, 2006.
9. Browning DG: Rotator cuff injuries and treatment, *Prim Care* 31:807, 2004.
10. Childs S: Athletic performance and injury. In Maher AB, Salmond SW, Pellino TA, editors: *Orthopaedic nursing,* ed 3, St Louis, 2002, Mosby.
11. Deu R, Carek P: Common sport injuries: upper extremity injuries, *Clin Fam Pract* 7:249, 2005.
12. Childs SG, Holmes SB: *Guidelines for orthopaedic nursing,* Pitman, NJ, 1998, Jannetti.
13. *Saunders nursing drug handbook,* St Louis, 2005, Saunders.
14. Holmes SB, Brown SJ: Skeletal pin site care: National Association of Orthopaedic Nursing guidelines. *Orthop Nurs* 24:99, 2005.
15. Zalavras CG, Patzakis MJ, Holtom PD, et al: Management of open fractures, *Infect Dis Clin North Am* 19:915, 2005.
16. Malinoski D, Slater M, Mullins R: Crush injury and rhabdomyolysis, *Crit Care Clin* 20:171, 2004.
17. Glazer J, Hosey R: Soft-tissue injuries of the lower extremity, *Prim Care* 31:1005, 2004.
18. Kostler W, Strohm PC, Sudkamp NP: Acute compartment syndrome of the limb, *Injury* 35:1221, 2004.
19. Harris H: Fat embolism, *Nursing* 43(6):96, 2004.
20. Mirza A, Ellis T: Initial management of pelvic and femoral fractures in the multiply injured patient, *Crit Care Clin* 20:159, 2004.
21. Whyte J: Stress fractures of the pelvis and lower extremities: diagnosis and management, *Adv Nurs Pract* 13(7):55, 2005.

22. Friese G, La May G: Emergency stabilization of unstable pelvic fractures, *Emerg Med Serv* 34:67, 2005.
23. Bischoff-Ferrari HA, Willett WC, Wong JB, et al: Fracture prevention with vitamin D supplementation: a meta-analysis of randomized controlled trials, *JAMA* 293:2257, 2005.
*24. Archibald G: Patients' experiences of hip fracture, *J Adv Nurs* 44:385, 2003.
*25. Hayes KS, Steinke E, Heilman A: Case study of hip fracture in an older person, *J Am Acad Nurs Pract* 15:450, 2003.
26. Parker MJ, Gillespie WJ, Gillespie LD: Hip protectors for preventing hip fractures in older people, *Cochrane Database Syst Rev* 3:CD001255, 2005.
*27. Martin JT, Coviak CP, Gendler P, et al: Female adolescents' knowledge of bone health promotion behaviors and osteoporosis risk factors, *Orthop Nurs* 23:235, 2004.
28. Pullen RL: Logrolling a patient, *Nursing* 34(2):22, 2004.
29. Ledlie J, Renfro M: Kyphoplasty treatment of vertebral fractures: 2 year outcomes show sustained benefits, *Spine* 1:57, 2006.
30. Hochmuth K: Percutaneous vertebroplasty in the therapy of osteoporotic vertebral compression fractures: a critical review, *Eur Radiol* 5:1, 2006.
31. Amputee Coalition of America: Amputation statistics by cause: limb loss in the United States, *National Limb Loss Information Center Fact Sheet*. Available at *www.amputee-coalition.org* (accessed August 31, 2006).
*32. Reed D: Understanding and meeting the needs of farmers with amputations, *Orthop Nurs* 23:397, 2004.
33. Siddle L: The challenge and management of phantom limb pain with amputation, *Br J Nurs* 13:664, 2004.
34. Woodhouse A: Phantom limb sensation, *Clin Exp Pharmacol Physiol* 32:132, 2005.
35. Hayes D: How to wrap an above-the-knee amputation stump, *Nursing* 33(1):70, 2003.
36. Oldmeadow LB, McBurney H, Robertson VJ, et al: Targeted postoperative care improves discharge outcome after hip or knee arthroplasty, *Arch Phys Med Rehabil* 85:1424, 2004.
37. Altizer L: Patient education for total hip and knee replacement, *Orthop Nurs* 23:283, 2004.

*Nursing research–based reference.

RESOURCES

American Academy of Orthopedic Surgeons (AAOS)
847-823-7186
www.aaos.org
American Association of Hand Surgery
312-236-3307
www.handsurgery.org
Amputee Coalition of America
888-267-5669
www.amputee-coalition.org
American College of Sports Medicine (ACSM)
317-637-9200
www.acsm.org
Easter Seals Disability Services
312-726-6200
www.easterseals.com
National Amputation Foundation
516-887-3600
www.nationalamputation.org
National Arthritis/Musculoskeletal and Skin Diseases Information Clearinghouse
301-495-4484
www.nih.gov/niams
National Association of Orthopaedic Nurses, Inc. (NAON)
800-289-NAON (6266) or 856-256-2310
www.orthonurse.org
National Center on Physical Activity and Disability (NCPAD)
800-900-8086
www.ncpad.org
Older Women's League
800-825-3695
www.owl-national.org

For additional Internet resources, see the website for this book at *http://evolve. elsevier.com/Lewis/medsurg.*

It is health that is real wealth and not pieces of gold and silver.

Mahatma Gandhi

64

Nursing Management
Musculoskeletal Problems

Colleen R. Walsh

LEARNING OBJECTIVES

1. Describe the pathophysiology, clinical manifestations, collaborative care, and nursing management of osteomyelitis.
2. Describe the types, pathophysiology, clinical manifestations, and collaborative care of bone cancer.
3. Differentiate between the causes and characteristics of acute and chronic low back pain.
4. Describe the conservative and surgical therapy of intervertebral disk damage.
5. Describe the postoperative nursing management of a patient who has undergone spinal surgery.
6. Explain the etiology and nursing management of common foot disorders.
7. Describe the etiology, pathophysiology, clinical manifestations, and collaborative and nursing management of osteomalacia, osteoporosis, and Paget's disease.

KEY TERMS

degenerative disk disease, p. 1680
herniated intervertebral disk, p. 1680
muscular dystrophy, p. 1675
osteochondroma, p. 1673
osteogenic sarcoma, p. 1674
osteomalacia, p. 1686
osteomyelitis, p. 1668
osteoporosis, p. 1686
Paget's disease, p. 1690

Electronic Resources

Supplemental content related to Chapter 64 can be found . . .

Companion CD
- Stress-Busting Kit for Nursing Students
- Interactive Case Study: Osteoporosis
- NCLEX Examination Review Questions
- Comprehensive Glossary

Evolve Website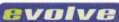
http://evolve.elsevier.com/Lewis/medsurg
- Content Updates
- Key Points (Printable and CD/MP3 Download)
- Concept Map Creator
- Expanded Audio Glossary
- Key Term Flash Cards
- Customizable Nursing Care Plans:
  - Osteomyelitis
  - Low Back Pain

- Patient and Family Instruction Guides in English and Spanish:
  - Back Exercises
  - Low Back Problems
- Electronic Calculators
- WebLinks

OSTEOMYELITIS

Etiology and Pathophysiology

Osteomyelitis is a severe infection of the bone, bone marrow, and surrounding soft tissue. The most common infecting microorganism is *Staphylococcus aureus*. A variety of microorganisms can cause osteomyelitis[1] (Table 64-1). Aerobic gram-negative bacteria alone or mixed with gram-positive organisms are often found. The widespread use of antibiotics in conjunction with surgical treatment has significantly reduced the mortality rate and complications associated with osteomyelitis.

The infecting microorganisms can invade by indirect or direct entry. The *indirect entry* (hematogenous) of microorganisms in osteomyelitis most frequently affects growing bone in boys less than 12 years old, and is associated with their higher incidence of blunt trauma. The most common sites of indirect entry in children are the distal femur, proximal tibia, humerus, and radius.[2] Adults with vascular insufficiency disorders (e.g., diabetes mellitus) and genitourinary and respiratory infections are at higher risk for a primary infection to spread via the blood to the bone. The pelvis, tibia, and vertebrae, which are vascular-rich sites of bone, are the most common sites of infection.

Reviewed by Jan Foecke, RN, MS, ONC, Orthopedic Operations and Clinical Resource Specialist, Providence Medical Center, Kansas City, Kan.

TABLE 64-1	Causative Organisms in Osteomyelitis
Organism	**Possible Predisposing Problem**
Staphylococcus aureus	Pressure ulcer, penetrating wound, open fracture, orthopedic surgery, vascular insufficiency disorders (e.g., diabetes, atherosclerosis)
Staphylococcus epidermidis	Indwelling prosthetic devices (e.g., joint replacements, fracture fixation devices)
Streptococcus viridans	Abscessed tooth, gingival disease
Escherichia coli	Urinary tract infection
Mycobacterium tuberculosis	Tuberculosis
Neisseria gonorrhoeae	Gonorrhea
Pseudomonas	Puncture wounds, intravenous drug use
Salmonella	Sickle cell disease
Fungi, mycobacteria	Immunocompromised host

Direct entry osteomyelitis can occur at any age when there is an open wound (e.g., penetrating wounds, fractures) and microorganisms gain entry to the body. Osteomyelitis may also occur in the presence of a foreign body such as an implant or an orthopedic prosthetic device (e.g., plate, total joint prosthesis). After gaining entrance to the bone by way of the blood, the microorganisms then lodge in an area of bone in which circulation slows, usually the metaphysis. The microorganisms grow, resulting in an increase in pressure because of the nonexpanding nature of most bone. This increasing pressure eventually leads to ischemia and vascular compromise of the periosteum. Eventually the infection passes through the bone cortex and marrow cavity, ultimately resulting in cortical devascularization and necrosis. Once ischemia occurs, the bone dies. The area of devitalized bone eventually separates from the surrounding living bone, forming *sequestra*. The part of the periosteum that continues to have a blood supply forms new bone called *involucrum* (Fig. 64-1).

Once formed, a sequestrum continues to be an infected island of bone, surrounded by pus. It is difficult for blood-borne antibiotics or white blood cells (WBCs) to reach the sequestrum. A sequestrum may enlarge and serve as a site for microorganisms that spread to other sites, including the lungs and brain. The sequestrum can move out of the bone and into the soft tissue. Once outside the bone, the sequestrum may revascularize and then undergo removal by normal immune processes. Another possibility is that the sequestrum can be surgically removed through debridement of the necrotic bone. If the necrotic sequestrum is not resolved naturally or surgically, it may develop a sinus tract, resulting in chronic, purulent cutaneous drainage.

Chronic osteomyelitis is either a continuous, persistent problem (a result of inadequate acute treatment) or a process of exacerbations and remissions (Fig. 64-2). Over time, granulation tissue turns to scar tissue. This avascular scar tissue provides an ideal site for continued microorganism growth and is impenetrable by antibiotics.

Clinical Manifestations

Acute osteomyelitis refers to the initial infection or an infection of less than 1 month in duration. The clinical manifestations of acute osteomyelitis are both systemic and local. Systemic manifestations include fever, night sweats, chills, restlessness, nausea, and malaise. Local manifestations include constant bone pain that is unrelieved by rest and worsens with activity; swelling, tenderness, and

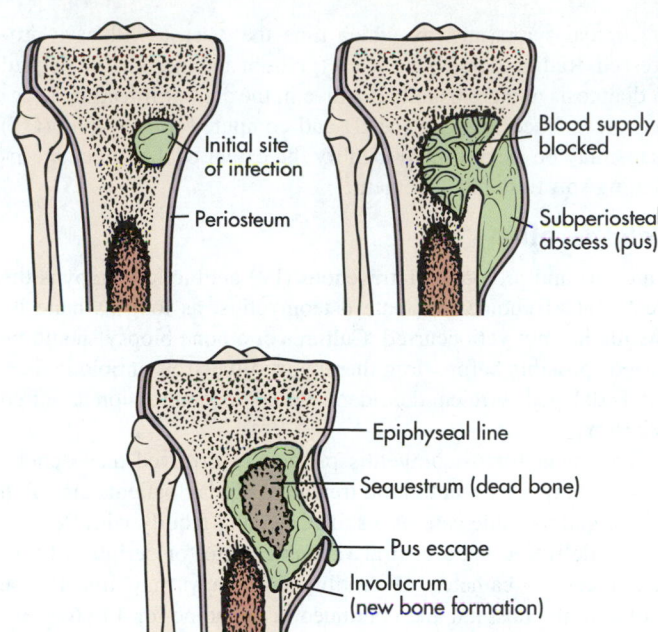

FIG. 64-1 Development of osteomyelitis infection with involucrum and sequestrum.

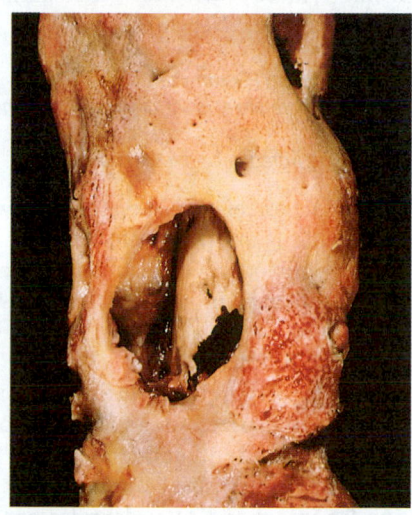

FIG. 64-2 Chronic osteomyelitis of the femur.

warmth at the infection site; and restricted movement of the affected part. Later signs include drainage from sinus tracts to the skin and/or the fracture site.

Chronic osteomyelitis refers to a bone infection that persists for longer than 1 month or an infection that has failed to respond to the initial course of antibiotic therapy. Systemic signs may be diminished, with local signs of infection more common, including constant bone pain and swelling, tenderness, and warmth at the infection site.

Diagnostic Studies

A bone or soft tissue biopsy is the definitive way to determine the causative microorganism. The patient's blood and/or wound cultures are frequently positive for the presence of microorganisms. An elevated WBC count and erythrocyte sedimentation rate (ESR) may also be found. Radiologic signs suggestive of osteomyelitis usually do not appear until 10 days to weeks after the appearance of clinical symptoms, by which time the disease will have progressed. Radionuclide bone scans (gallium and indium) are helpful in diagnosis and are usually positive in the area of infection. Magnetic resonance imaging (MRI) and computed tomography (CT) scans may be used to help identify the extent of the infection, including soft tissue involvement.[3]

Collaborative Care

Vigorous and prolonged intravenous (IV) antibiotic therapy is the treatment of choice for acute osteomyelitis, as long as bone ischemia has not yet occurred. Cultures or a bone biopsy should be done if possible before drug therapy is initiated. If antibiotic therapy is delayed, surgical debridement and decompression are often necessary.

Treatment for osteomyelitis previously involved an extended hospital stay for IV antibiotic treatment. Today patients are often discharged to home care or a skilled nursing facility with IV antibiotics delivered via a central venous catheter or peripherally inserted central catheter. IV antibiotic therapy may initially be started in the hospital and continued in the home for 4 to 6 weeks or as long as 3 to 6 months. A variety of antibiotics may be prescribed depending on the microorganism. These drugs include penicillin, nafcillin (Nafcil), neomycin, vancomycin, cephalexin (Keflex), cefazolin (Ancef), cefoxitin (Mefoxin), gentamicin (Garamycin), and tobramycin (Nebcin).

> **Drug Alert** - *Gentamicin (Garamycin)*
> • *Instruct patient to notify physician if any visual, hearing, or urinary problems develop.*
> • *Assess patient for dehydration before starting therapy.*

In adults with chronic osteomyelitis, oral therapy with a fluoroquinolone (ciprofloxacin [Cipro]) for 6 to 8 weeks may be prescribed instead of IV antibiotics. Oral antibiotic therapy may also be given after acute IV therapy is complete to ensure resolution of the infection. The patient's response to drug therapy is monitored through bone scans and ESR tests.

Surgical treatment for chronic osteomyelitis includes removal of the poorly vascularized tissue and dead bone and the extended use of antibiotics. Antibiotic-impregnated polymethylmethacrylate bead chains may also be implanted at this time to aid in combating the infection.[4] After debridement of the devitalized and infected tissue, the wound may be closed, and a suction irrigation system is inserted. Intermittent or constant irrigation of the affected bone with antibiotics may also be initiated. Protection of the limb or surgical site with casts or braces is frequently done. Negative pressure (Wound VAC) over the site of the infection may be used to draw the wound together (see Chapter 13).

Hyperbaric oxygen therapy with 100% oxygen may be administered as an adjunct therapy in refractory cases of chronic osteomyelitis. This therapy is thought to stimulate circulation and healing in the infected tissue (see Chapter 13). Orthopedic prosthetic devices, if a source of chronic infection, must be removed. Muscle flaps or skin grafting provide wound coverage over the dead space (cavity) in the bone. Bone grafts may help to restore blood flow. Amputation of the extremity may be indicated when there is extensive bone destruction and amputation is necessary to preserve the person's life and/or improve quality of life.

Long-term and mostly rare complications of osteomyelitis include septicemia, septic arthritis, pathologic fractures, and amyloidosis.

NURSING MANAGEMENT
OSTEOMYELITIS

■ *Nursing Assessment*

Subjective and objective data that should be obtained from an individual with osteomyelitis are presented in Table 64-2.

■ *Nursing Diagnoses*

Nursing diagnoses for the patient with osteomyelitis may include, but are not limited to, those presented in NCP 64-1.

■ *Planning*

The overall goals are that the patient with osteomyelitis will (1) have satisfactory pain and fever control, (2) not experience any complications associated with osteomyelitis, (3) cooperate with the treatment plan, and (4) maintain a positive outlook on the outcome of the disease.

■ *Nursing Implementation*

Health Promotion. The control of infections already in the body (e.g., urinary, respiratory tract) is important in preventing osteomyelitis. Adults who are immunocompromised, have orthopedic prosthetic devices, and/or have vascular insufficiencies are especially susceptible. These patients should be instructed regarding the local and systemic manifestations of osteomyelitis. Family members should also be aware of their role in monitoring the patient's health. Symptoms of bone pain, fever, swelling, and restricted limb movement should be reported immediately to the health care provider.

TABLE 64-2	*NURSING ASSESSMENT* **Osteomyelitis**

Subjective Data
Important Health Information
Past health history: Bone trauma, open fracture, open or puncture wounds, other infections (e.g., streptococcal sore throat, bacterial pneumonia, sinusitis, skin or tooth infection, chronic urinary tract infection)
Medications: Use of analgesics or antibiotics
Surgery or other treatments: Bone surgery

Functional Health Patterns
Health perception–health management: IV drug abuse; malaise
Nutritional-metabolic: Anorexia, weight loss; chills
Activity-exercise: Weakness, paralysis, muscle spasms around affected bone
Cognitive-perceptual: Local tenderness over affected area, increase in pain with movement of affected bone
Coping–stress tolerance: Irritability, withdrawal, dependency, anger

Objective Data
General
Restlessness; high, spiking temperature; night sweats

Integumentary
Diaphoresis; erythema, warmth, edema at infected bone

Musculoskeletal
Restricted movement; wound drainage; spontaneous fractures

Possible Findings
Leukocytosis, positive blood and/or wound cultures, ↑ erythrocyte sedimentation rate; presence of sequestrum and involucrum on x-rays, radionuclide bone scans, CT, and MRI

CT, Computed tomography; *IV,* intravenous; *MRI,* magnetic resonance imaging.

Musculoskeletal System

NURSING CARE PLAN 64-1

Patient with Osteomyelitis

NURSING DIAGNOSIS **Acute pain** *related to* inflammatory process secondary to infection *as evidenced by* guarding, moaning, crying, restlessness, altered muscle tone, decreased activity, rated pain as >4 on 10-point rating scale

PATIENT GOALS 1. Reports satisfactory pain relief with pain <4 on 10-point scale
2. Uses analgesics and nonpharmacologic measures effectively to control pain

OUTCOMES (NOC)

Pain Control

- Uses nonanalgesic relief measures _____
- Uses analgesics appropriately _____
- Reports uncontrolled symptoms to health care professional _____
- Reports pain controlled _____

Measurement Scale

1 = Never demonstrated
2 = Rarely demonstrated
3 = Sometimes demonstrated
4 = Often demonstrated
5 = Consistently demonstrated

INTERVENTIONS (NIC) and *RATIONALES*

Pain Management

- Perform a comprehensive assessment of pain to include location, characteristics, onset/duration, frequency, quality, intensity or severity of pain, and precipitating factors *to plan appropriate interventions.*
- Evaluate effectiveness of pain-control measures used through ongoing assessment of pain experience.
- Provide patient optimal pain relief with prescribed analgesics *to relieve pain.*
- Use pain-control measures before pain becomes severe.
- Teach the use of nonpharmacologic techniques (e.g., relaxation, guided imagery, distraction) *to augment or reduce the need for analgesics.*

Positioning

- Immobilize or support affected body part *to reduce pain and prevent pathologic fractures.*
- Position in proper body alignment *to prevent unusual position or muscle stretching from increasing pain.*
- Elevate affected body part *to reduce swelling and provide comfort.*

NURSING DIAGNOSIS **Ineffective therapeutic regimen management** *related to* lack of knowledge regarding long-term management of osteomyelitis *as evidenced by* verbalization of concern and uncertainty about procedures and skills needed for home care

PATIENT GOALS 1. Describes treatment regimen and verbalizes confidence in ability to implement it at home
2. Demonstrates wound care, aseptic technique, care of intravenous (IV) access, and administration of antibiotics correctly

OUTCOMES (NOC)

Treatment Behavior: Illness or Injury

- Follows recommended treatment regimen _____
- Uses treatment devices correctly _____
- Follows medication regimen _____
- Performs self-care consistent with ability _____
- Monitors treatment's effects _____
- Monitors changes in disease status _____
- Seeks advice from health care professional as needed _____

Measurement Scale

1 = Never demonstrated
2 = Rarely demonstrated
3 = Sometimes demonstrated
4 = Often demonstrated
5 = Consistently demonstrated

INTERVENTIONS (NIC) and *RATIONALES*

Teaching: Psychomotor Skill

- Demonstrate skills (e.g., wound care, aseptic technique, antibiotic administration) for the patient.
- Instruct patient to perform skills one step at a time.
- Observe patient return demonstrate skills *to evaluate patient's knowledge and performance.*
- Provide written information/diagrams *for future reference.*

Teaching: Prescribed Medication

- Inform patient of both generic and brand names of each medication.
- Instruct patient on purpose and action of each medication.
- Instruct patient on dosage, route, and duration of each medication.
- Evaluate patient's ability to self-administer medications.
- Instruct patient on possible adverse effects of each medication.
- Inform patient of consequences of not taking or abruptly discontinuing medication(s) *as long-term antibiotic therapy is required.*
- Provide patient with written information about action, purpose, and side effects of medications.

Continued

Acute Intervention. Some immobilization of the affected limb (e.g., splint, traction) is usually indicated to decrease pain. The involved limb should be handled carefully to avoid excessive manipulation, which increases pain and may cause pathologic fracture. An important nursing responsibility is to assess the patient's pain. Minor to severe pain may be experienced with muscle spasms. Nonsteroidal antiinflammatory drugs (NSAIDs), opioid analgesics, and muscle relaxants may be prescribed to provide patient comfort. Nonpharmacologic (e.g., guided imagery, hypnosis) approaches to pain should be encouraged by the nurse (see Chapters 9 and 10).

Dressings are used to absorb the exudate from draining wounds and to debride devitalized tissue from the wound site when removed. Types of dressings used include dry, sterile dressings; dressings saturated in saline or antibiotic solution; and wet-to-dry dressings. Soiled dressings should be handled carefully to prevent

NURSING CARE PLAN 64-1

Patient with Osteomyelitis—cont'd

NURSING DIAGNOSIS   **Impaired physical mobility** *related to* pain, immobilization devices, and weight-bearing limitations *as evidenced by* inability or unwillingness to change bed positions and ambulate with assistive devices

PATIENT GOALS   1. Demonstrates a consistent increase in mobility and range of motion, turning in bed, and performing range-of-motion exercises
       2. Ambulates with assistive devices to prevent weight bearing on limb

OUTCOMES (NOC)

Mobility

- Muscle movement _____
- Joint movement _____
- Walking _____
- Moves with ease _____

Measurement Scale

1 = Severely compromised
2 = Substantially compromised
3 = Moderately compromised
4 = Mildly compromised
5 = Not compromised

INTERVENTIONS (NIC) and *RATIONALES*

Exercise Therapy: Ambulation

- Assist patient to stand and ambulate specified distance and with specified number of staff *to reduce patient's frustration with impaired mobility and prevent injury.*
- Encourage patient to be "up ad lib" *to maintain muscle function and strength.*
- Apply/provide assistive device (e.g., cane, walker, wheelchair) for ambulation.
- Monitor patient's use of crutches or other walking aids *to prevent pathologic fracture, pain, and increased stress on bone.*

---

cross-contamination of the wound or spread of the infection to other patients. When the dressing is changed, sterile technique is essential.

The patient is frequently on bed rest in the early stages of the acute infection.[5] Good body alignment and frequent position changes prevent complications associated with immobility and promote comfort. Flexion contracture, especially of the hip or knee, is a common sequela of osteomyelitis of the lower extremity because the patient frequently positions the affected extremity in a flexed position to promote comfort. The contracture may then progress to a deformity. Footdrop can develop quickly in the lower extremity if the foot is not correctly supported in a neutral position by a splint or if there is excessive pressure from a splint, which can injure the peroneal nerve. The patient should be instructed to avoid any activities such as exercise or heat application that increase circulation and swelling and serve as stimuli to the spread of infection. Uninvolved joints and muscles should continue to be exercised.

The patient should also be taught the potential adverse and toxic reactions associated with prolonged and high-dose antibiotic therapy. These reactions include hearing deficit, fluid retention, and neurotoxicity, which can occur with the aminoglycosides (e.g., tobramycin, neomycin), jaundice, colitis, and photosensitivity from the extended use of the cephalosporins (e.g., cefazolin). Peak and trough blood levels of most antibiotics must be carefully monitored throughout the course of therapy to avoid these adverse effects. Lengthy antibiotic therapy can also result in an overgrowth of *Candida albicans* in the genitourinary and oral cavities, especially in immunosuppressed and older patients. The nurse should instruct the patient to report any whitish, yellow, curdlike lesions to the health care provider.

The patient and family are often frightened and discouraged because of the serious nature of the disease, the uncertainty of the outcome, and the cost and lengthy course of treatment. Continued psychologic and emotional support is an integral part of nursing management.

Ambulatory and Home Care. With the introduction of various intermittent venous access devices, IV antibiotics can be administered to the patient in a skilled nursing facility or home setting. If at home, the patient and family must be instructed on the proper care and management of the venous access device. They must also be taught how to administer the antibiotic when scheduled and the need for follow-up laboratory testing. The importance of continuing to take antibiotics after the symptoms have subsided should be stressed. Periodic home nursing visits provide the family with support, which helps to reduce anxiety. If there is an open wound, dressing changes are often necessary. The patient and family may require supplies and instruction in the technique. Family members also need to understand that the infection is not contagious.

If the osteomyelitis becomes chronic, patients need physical and psychologic support for a prolonged period. They may become suspicious and angry toward the health care providers when treatment plans do not result in a cure. Well-informed patients are better able to participate in decisions and cooperate in treatment plans.

■ Evaluation

The expected outcomes for the patient with osteomyelitis are presented in NCP 64-1.

Bone Tumors

Primary bone tumors, both benign and malignant, are relatively rare in adults. Metastatic bone cancer in which the cancer has spread from another site is a more common problem. The name given to the tumor is based on the area of the bone and surrounding tissue that is affected, and on the type of cells forming the tumor. The main types of benign tumors include osteochondroma, osteoclastoma, and endochroma (Table 64-3). These types of tumors are often cured by surgery and are more common than primary malignant tumors.

Primary bone cancer is called **sarcoma.** Sarcomas can also develop in cartilage, muscle fibers, fatty tissue, and nerve tissue.[6] The more common types of bone cancer are osteogenic sarcoma, chondrosarcoma, Ewing's sarcoma, and chordoma (see Table 64-3). Annually about 2700 new cases of bone (and joint) cancer occur in the United States, with an estimated 1200 deaths.[7] Primary malignant tumors occur most often during childhood through young

TABLE 64-3	Types of Primary Bone Tumors
Types	**Description**
Benign	
Osteochondroma	Most common benign bone tumor; frequently located in metaphyseal portion of long bones, particularly the leg, pelvis, or scapula; occurs most often in persons ages 10-25; malignant transformation may occur (chondrosarcoma).
Osteoclastoma	A tumor that arises in the cancellous ends of the arm and leg bones; about 10% of all osteoclastomas (giant cell tumor) are locally aggressive and may spread to the lungs; high rate of local recurrence after surgery and chemotherapy (Fig. 64-3).
Endochroma	An intramedullary cartilage tumor usually found in the cavity of a single hand or foot bone; rare malignant transformation can occur; if tumor becomes painful, a surgical resection is done; peak incidence in persons ages 10-20.
Malignant	
Osteogenic sarcoma	Most common primary bone cancer (osteosarcoma); occurs mostly in young males between ages 10 and 25; most often in bones of the arms, legs, or pelvis (Fig. 64-4).
Chondrosarcoma	Occurs in cartilage cells most commonly in the arm, leg, and pelvic bones of older adults ages 50-70; can also arise from benign bone tumors (osteochondromas); wide surgical resection is mostly done as tumor rarely responds to radiation and chemotherapy; survival rate depends on stage, size, and grade of tumor (Fig. 64-5).
Ewing's sarcoma	Develops in medullary cavity of long bones, especially the femur, humerus, pelvis, and tibia; usually occurs in children and teenagers; use of wide surgical resection, radiation, and chemotherapy has greatly improved the 5-yr survival rate to 60%; occurs most often in white people.
Chordoma	Rare tumor that occurs in base of the skull and vertebral bones of older adults ages 50-70; wide surgical resection and radiation are difficult because the spinal cord and nerves may also be involved; chemotherapy may be used for late-stage disease; tumor may recur 10 or more yr after treatment.

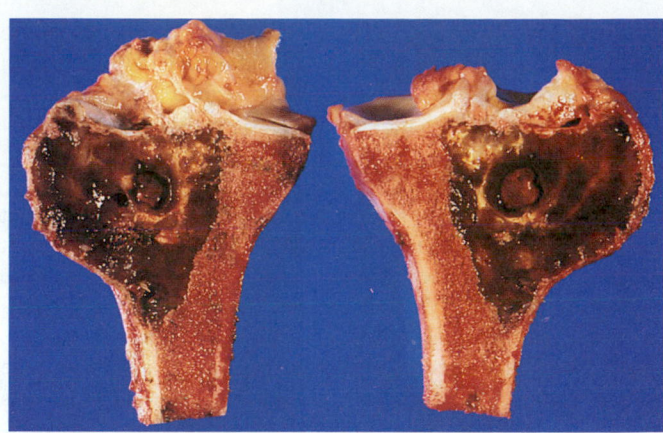

FIG. 64-3 Osteoclastoma (giant cell tumor) in a long bone.

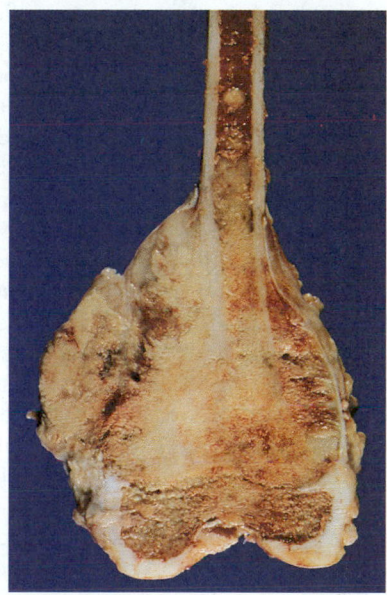

FIG. 64-4 Osteogenic sarcoma in the femur. Bone cortex has been destroyed.

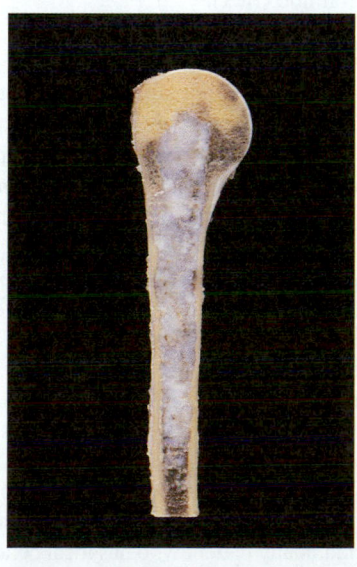

FIG. 64-5 Chondrosarcoma of proximal humerus. Note shiny appearance of the hyaline cartilage tumor in the medullary cavity.

adulthood. They are characterized by their rapid metastasis and bone destruction.

OSTEOCHONDROMA

Osteochondroma is a primary benign bone tumor that is characterized by an overgrowth of cartilage and bone near the end of the bone at the growth plate. Osteochondromas can occur in any bone where cartilage assists in forming bone. It is more commonly found in the long bones of the leg, pelvis, or scapula. One form of the disease is hereditary, with multiple tumors forming before age 10.

Clinical manifestations include a painless, hard, and immobile mass, lower-than-normal-height for age, soreness of muscles in close proximity to the tumor, one leg or arm longer than the other, and pressure or irritation with exercise. Patients may also have no symptoms. Diagnosis is confirmed from x-ray, CT scan, and MRI.

No treatment is necessary for asymptomatic osteochondroma. If the tumor is causing pain or neurologic symptoms due to compression, surgical resection is usually done. As long as the entire cartilage cap is removed, the tumor should not recur. Patients with many large osteochondromas should have regular screening examinations to detect malignant transformation early.

OSTEOGENIC SARCOMA

Osteogenic sarcoma (osteosarcoma) is a primary bone tumor that is extremely aggressive and rapidly metastasizes to distant sites. It usually occurs in the metaphyseal region of the long bones of the extremities, particularly in the regions of the distal femur, proximal tibia, and proximal humerus, as well as the pelvis (see Fig. 64-4). Osteogenic sarcoma is the most common malignant bone tumor affecting children and young adults; the highest incidence is in males in the 10- to 25-year-old age-group. Secondary osteosarcoma is known to occur in adults over age 60 and is most commonly associated with Paget's disease.[8]

Clinical manifestations of osteogenic sarcoma are usually associated with the gradual onset of pain and swelling, especially around the knee. A minor injury does not cause the neoplasm but may bring the preexisting condition to medical attention. The neoplasm can restrict joint motion if the tumor is close to a joint structure. The diagnosis is confirmed from biopsied tissue specimens; elevation of serum alkaline phosphatase and calcium levels; and findings on x-ray, CT or positron emission tomogram (PET) scans, and MRI. Metastasis is present in 10% to 20% of individuals on diagnosis, with the lung being the most frequent site.

Major advances continue to be made in the treatment of osteosarcoma. Preoperative chemotherapy is used to decrease tumor size. As a result, limb salvage procedures, including a wide surgical resection of the tumor, are being used more often. Limb salvage procedures are considered when there is a clear 6- to 7-cm margin surrounding the lesion. Limb salvage is contraindicated if there is major neurovascular involvement, pathologic fracture, infection, skeletal immaturity, or extensive muscle involvement.[9] Quality-of-life considerations also factor in the decision of limb salvage compared with amputation. Current use of adjunct chemotherapy following amputation has increased the projected 5-year survival rate to 60%.[10] Chemotherapeutic agents include methotrexate, doxorubicin (Adriamycin), cisplatin (Platinol), cyclophosphamide (Cytoxan), bleomycin (Blenoxane), dactinomycin (Cosmegen), and ifosfamide (Ifex).

METASTATIC BONE CANCER

The most common type of malignant bone tumor occurs as a result of metastasis from a primary tumor. Common sites for the primary tumor include the breast, prostate, gastrointestinal (GI) tract, lungs, kidney, ovary, and thyroid.[11] Metastatic cancer cells travel from the primary tumor to the bone via the lymph and blood supply. The metastatic bone lesion is commonly found in the vertebrae, pelvis, femur, humerus, or ribs. Pathologic fractures at the site of metastasis are common because of a weakening of the involved bone. High serum calcium levels result as calcium is released from damaged bones.

Once a primary lesion has been identified, radionuclide bone scans are often done to detect the presence of metastatic lesions before they are visible on x-ray. It is important to note that metastatic bone lesions may occur at any time (even years later) following diagnosis and treatment of the primary tumor. Metastasis to the bone should be suspected in any patient who has local bone pain and a past history of cancer. Treatment may be palliative and consists of radiation and pain management (see Chapter 10). Surgical stabilization of the fracture may be indicated if there is a fracture or pending fracture. Prognosis depends on the extent of metastasis and location.

■ Nursing Assessment

The patient with bone cancer should be assessed for the location and severity of pain. Weakness caused by anemia and decreased mobility may also be noted. Swelling at the involved site and decreased joint function, depending on the tumor site, should also be monitored.

■ Nursing Diagnoses

Nursing diagnoses for the patient with bone cancer may include, but are not limited to, the following:
- Acute pain *related to* the disease process or inadequate pain medication or comfort measures
- Impaired physical mobility *related to* disease process, pain, weakness, and debility
- Disturbed body image *related to* possible amputation, deformity, swelling, and effects of chemotherapy
- Grieving *related to* poor prognosis of the disease
- Risk for injury *related to* disease process, possible pathologic fracture, or inadequate handling or positioning of affected body part
- Impaired home maintenance *related to* lack of knowledge about care needed at home or how to perform the necessary skills

■ Planning

The overall goals are that the patient with bone cancer will (1) have satisfactory pain relief; (2) maintain preferred activities as long as possible; (3) demonstrate acceptance of body image changes resulting from chemotherapy, radiation, and surgery; (4) be free from injury; and (5) verbalize a realistic idea of disease progression and prognosis.

■ Nursing Implementation

Health Promotion. The nurse should teach the public to recognize the warning signs of bone cancer, including swelling, bone pain of unexplained origin, limitation of joint function, and changes in skin temperature. As with all forms of cancer, health promotion should stress the importance of periodic screening and health examinations.

Acute Intervention. Nursing care of the patient with a malignant bone neoplasm does not differ significantly from the care given to the patient with a malignant disease of any other body system (see Chapter 16). However, special attention is required to reduce the complications associated with prolonged bed rest and to prevent falls and pathologic fractures. Careful handling and support of the affected extremity and logrolling for those on bed rest is important to prevent pathologic fractures.[12] The patient is often reluctant to participate in therapeutic activities because of weakness from the disease and treatment and fear of pain. Regular rest periods should be provided between activities.

Ambulatory and Home Care. The nurse must be able to assist the patient and family in accepting the guarded prognosis associated with bone neoplasms. Inability to accomplish age-specific developmental tasks can increase the frustrations with this condition. General principles related to cancer nursing are applicable (see Chapter 16). Special attention is necessary for the problems of

TABLE 64-4	Types of Muscular Dystrophy	
Type	**Genetic Basis**	**Clinical Manifestations**
Duchenne (pseudohypertrophic)	X-linked Mutation of dystrophin gene	Onset before age 5; progressive weakness of pelvic and shoulder muscles; unable to walk after age 12; cardiomyopathy; respiratory failure in teens or 20s; mental impairment
Becker (benign pseudo-hypertrophic)	X-linked Mutation of dystrophin gene	Onset between 5 and 15 yr; slower course of pelvic and shoulder muscle wasting than Duchenne; cardiomyopathy; respiratory failure; may survive into 30s or 40s
Landouzy-Déjérine (facioscapulohumeral)	Autosomal dominant Deletion of chromosome 4q35	Onset before age 20; slowly progressive weakness of face, shoulder muscles, and foot dorsiflexion; deafness
Erb (limb-girdle)	Autosomal recessive or autosomal dominant	Onset ranges from early childhood to early adulthood; slow progressive weakness of shoulder and hip muscles

pain and disability, chemotherapy, and specific surgery such as spinal cord decompression or amputation.

■ Evaluation

The expected outcomes are that the patient with bone cancer will
- have minimal pain
- have no falls
- accept changes in body image
- retain dignity and active participation in treatment decisions
- have maximal functional ability

MUSCULAR DYSTROPHY

Muscular dystrophy (MD) is a group of genetically transmitted diseases characterized by progressive symmetric wasting of skeletal muscle without evidence of neurologic involvement. In all forms of MD an insidious loss of strength occurs with increasing disability and deformity. The types of MD differ in the groups of muscles affected, age of onset, rate of progression, and mode of genetic inheritance.[13] Types of MD are presented in Table 64-4.

Duchenne and Becker MD are sex-linked recessive disorders usually seen only in males. In these disorders there is a genetic mutation of the dystrophin gene. Dystrophin in normal muscle cells helps to attach skeletal muscle fibers to the basement membrane. Abnormalities in dystrophin can lead to defects in the plasma membrane of muscle fiber with subsequent muscle fiber degeneration.

Diagnostic studies for MD include muscle serum enzymes (especially creatine kinase), electromyogram (EMG) testing, muscle fiber biopsy, electrocardiogram abnormalities reflective of cardiomyopathy, and genetic pedigree (see Chapter 14). Muscle biopsy confirms the diagnosis with classic findings of fat and connective tissue deposits, degeneration and necrosis of muscle fibers, and a deficiency of the muscle protein dystrophin.

Presently, no definitive therapy is available to stop the progressive wasting of MD. Corticosteroid therapy may significantly halt the disease progression for up to 3 years.[14] The goal of treatment is to preserve mobility and independence through exercise, physical therapy, and orthopedic appliances. The nurse should encourage communication among family members (and parents) to cope with the emotional and physical strains of MD.[15] An emphasis should be placed on teaching the patient and family range-of-motion exercises, nutrition, and signs of progression. Genetic testing and counseling may be recommended for individuals with a family history of MD.

Nursing care should focus on keeping the patient active as long as possible. Prolonged bed rest should be avoided because immobility can lead to further muscle wasting. As the disease progresses, the focus will shift to teaching the patient to limit sedentary peri-

GENETICS IN CLINICAL PRACTICE
Duchenne Muscular Dystrophy (MD)

Genetic Basis
- Sex-linked recessive disorder

Incidence
- About 30 in 100,000 males

Genetic Testing
- DNA testing for mutation in dystrophin gene

Clinical Implications
- Duchenne MD is present at birth but does not usually become clinically apparent until at least age 3.
- Very few individuals with the disease live to adulthood.
- Genetic testing and counseling should be considered in individuals with a family history of Duchenne MD.
- Because there are many types of MD with different genetic bases, establishing the type of MD is important to determine treatment and possible genetic counseling recommendations.

ods when skin integrity or respiratory complications could develop. Ongoing medical and nursing care will be required throughout the individual's lifetime.

Low Back Pain

Etiology and Pathophysiology

Low back pain is common and has probably affected about 80% of adults in the United States at least once during their lifetime.[16] Backache is second only to headache as the most common pain complaint. In persons under age 45, low back pain is responsible for more lost working hours than any other medical condition and represents one of the nation's most costly health problems.[17] Low back pain is a common problem because the lumbar region (1) bears most of the weight of the body, (2) is the most flexible region of the spinal column, (3) contains nerve roots that are vulnerable to injury or disease, and (4) has an inherently poor biomechanical structure.

Several risk factors are associated with low back pain, including lack of muscle tone and excess body weight, poor posture, cigarette smoking, and stress. Jobs that require repetitive heavy lifting, vibration (such as a jackhammer operator), and prolonged periods of sitting are also associated with low back pain. **Low back pain** is most often due to a musculoskeletal problem. The causes of low back pain of musculoskeletal origin include (1) acute lumbosacral strain, (2) instability of the lumbosacral bony mechanism, (3) osteoarthritis

Musculoskeletal System

of the lumbosacral vertebrae, (4) degenerative disk disease, and (5) herniation of an intervertebral disk.

ACUTE LOW BACK PAIN

Acute low back pain lasts 4 weeks or less. Acute low back pain is usually associated with some type of activity that causes undue stress (often hyperflexion) on the tissues of the lower back. Often symptoms do not appear at the time of injury but develop later because of a gradual increase in paravertebral muscle spasms. Few definitive diagnostic abnormalities are present with paravertebral muscle strain. One test is the straight-leg raise. This test is positive for disk herniation when radicular pain occurs. MRI and CT scans are generally not done unless trauma or systemic disease (e.g., cancer, spinal infection) is suspected.

Collaborative Care

If the acute muscle spasms and accompanying pain are not severe and debilitating, the patient may be treated on an outpatient basis with a combination of the following: (1) analgesics, such as NSAIDs; (2) muscle relaxants (e.g., cyclobenzaprine [Flexeril]); (3) massage and back manipulation; and (4) the alternating use of heat and cold compresses. Severe pain may require a brief course of opioid analgesics.

A brief period (1 to 2 days) of rest at home may be necessary for some persons, with most persons doing better with a continuation of their regular activities.[18] Invasive treatments, such as epidural corticosteroid injections and implanted devices that deliver pain medication, are reserved for patients with chronic back pain who are refractory to the usual therapeutic options.[19] All patients during this time should avoid activities that aggravate the pain, including lifting, bending, twisting, and prolonged sitting. Most cases improve within 2 weeks.

NURSING MANAGEMENT
ACUTE LOW BACK PAIN

■ Nursing Assessment

Subjective and objective data that should be obtained from the patient with low back pain are summarized in Table 64-5.

■ Nursing Diagnoses

Nursing diagnoses for the patient with low back pain may include, but are not limited to, those presented in NCP 64-2.

■ Planning

The overall goals are that the patient with low back pain will (1) have satisfactory pain relief, (2) avoid constipation secondary to medication and immobility, (3) learn back-sparing practices, and (4) return to previous level of activity within prescribed restrictions.

■ Nursing Implementation

Health Promotion. The nurse is a significant role model and teacher for patients with low back problems. As a role model, the nurse should use proper body mechanics at all times. This should be a primary consideration when teaching patients and health care providers transfer and turning techniques. The nurse should assess the patient's use of body mechanics and offer advice when activities that could produce back strain are used (Table 64-6).

Some health care providers refer patients with back pain to a program called "Back School." It is a formal program usually taught by health professionals such as physicians, nurses, and

TABLE 64-5	*NURSING ASSESSMENT* **Low Back Pain**

Subjective Data
Important Health Information
Past health history: Acute or chronic lumbosacral strain/trauma, osteoarthritis, degenerative disk disease, obesity
Medications: Use of opioid and nonopioid analgesics, muscle relaxants, nonsteroidal antiinflammatory drugs, corticosteroids, over-the-counter remedies including herbal products and nutritional supplements
Surgery or other treatments: Previous back surgery, epidural corticosteroid injections

Functional Health Patterns
Health perception–health management: Smoking, lack of exercise
Nutritional-metabolic: Obesity
Activity-exercise: Poor posture, muscle spasms; activity intolerance
Elimination: Constipation
Sleep-rest: Interrupted sleep
Cognitive-perceptual: Pain in back, buttocks, or leg associated with walking, turning, straining, coughing, leg raising; numbness or tingling of legs, feet, toes
Role-relationship: In occupations requiring heavy lifting, vibrations, or extended driving, change in role within family structure due to inability to work and provide income

Objective Data
General
Guarded movement

Neurologic
Depressed or absent Achilles tendon reflex or patellar tendon reflex; positive straight-leg-raising test, positive crossover straight-leg-raising test, positive Trendelenburg test

Musculoskeletal
Tense, tight paravertebral muscles on palpation, ↓ range of motion of spine

Possible Findings
Localization of site of lesion or disorder on myelogram, CT scan, or MRI; determination of nerve root impingement on electromyography

CT, Computed tomography; *MRI,* magnetic resonance imaging.

physical therapists. It is designed to teach the patient how to minimize back pain and avoid repeat episodes of low back pain. Tips for prevention of back injury are listed in Table 64-6. Exercises to strengthen the back are presented in Table 64-7.

Patients are also advised to maintain appropriate body weight. Excess body weight places extra stress on the lower back and weakens the abdominal muscles that support the lower back. Flat shoes and/or shoes with low heels and shock-absorbing shoe inserts are recommended for women.

The position assumed while sleeping is also important in preventing low back pain. Sleeping in a prone position should be avoided because it produces excessive lumbar lordosis, placing excessive stress on the lower back. A firm mattress is recommended. The patient should sleep in either a supine or side-lying position with the knees and hips flexed to prevent unnecessary pressure on support muscles, ligamentous structures, and lumbosacral joints. Patients should be educated about the necessity to avoid or cease smoking. Nicotine has been shown to decrease circulation to the vertebral disks, and a causal relationship exists between smoking and some types of low back pain.

Acute Intervention. The primary nursing responsibilities in acute low back pain are to assist the patient to maintain activity

HEALTHY PEOPLE
Prevention of Low Back Pain

- Maintain healthy weight
- Do not sleep in a prone position
- Avoid cigarette smoking and tobacco products
- Obtain regular physical activity, including strength and endurance training
- Use proper body mechanics to avoid low back strain (e.g., when lifting heavy objects, bend at the knees, not at the waist, and stand up slowly while holding object close to your body)
- Sleep on side with knees flexed and a pillow between the knees

---

TABLE 64-6
PATIENT AND FAMILY TEACHING GUIDE
Low Back Problems

Do Not
- Lean forward without bending knees.
- Lift anything above level of elbows.
- Stand in one position for prolonged time.
- Sleep on abdomen or on back or side with legs out straight.
- Exercise without consulting health care provider if having severe pain.
- Exceed prescribed amount and type of exercises without consulting health care provider.

Do
- Prevent lower back from straining forward by placing a foot on a step or stool during prolonged standing.
- Sleep in a side-lying position with knees and hips bent.
- Sleep on back with a lift under knees and legs or on back with 10-inch-high pillow under knees to flex hips and knees.
- Exercise 15 min in the morning and in the evening regularly; begin exercises with a 2- or 3-min warm-up period by moving arms and legs, by alternately relaxing and tightening muscles; exercise slowly with smooth movements.
- Maintain appropriate body weight.
- Use local heat and cold application.
- Use a lumbar roll or pillow for sitting.

TABLE 64-7
PATIENT AND FAMILY TEACHING GUIDE
Back Exercises

Knee-to-Chest Lift (to stretch hip, buttocks, lower back muscles)
- Lie on back on the floor with knees bent and feet flat on floor.
- Draw both knees up to chest.
- Place both hands around knees and pull them firmly against chest. Hold for 30 seconds.
- Lower legs and return to starting position.
- Repeat 5 to 10 times.

Simple Leg Lift
- Lie flat on back on floor with left knee bent and left foot flat on floor.
- Raise right leg as high as comfortably possible.
- Hold for count of 5.
- Slowly return leg to floor.
- Bend right knee and put right foot flat on floor.
- Raise left leg and hold for count of 5.
- Repeat 5 to 10 times for each leg.

Double Leg Lift
- Lie flat on back.
- Slowly lift legs until feet are 12 inches from the floor.
- Keep legs straight and hold this position for count of 10.
- Lower legs to floor.
- Repeat 5 times.

Pelvic Tilt
- Lie flat on back on floor with knees bent and feet flat on the floor.
- Firmly tighten buttock muscles.
- Hold for count of 5.
- Relax buttocks.
- Repeat 5 to 10 times.
- Be sure to keep lower back flat against floor.

Half Sit-Ups (to strengthen abdominal muscles)
- Lie flat on floor on back with knees bent, feet flat on floor, and hands on chest.
- Slowly raise head and neck to top of chest.
- Reach both hands forward and place them on knees.
- Hold for count of 5.
- Return to starting position.
- Repeat 5 to 10 times.

Elbow Props (to extend lower back)
- Lie face down with arms beside body and head turned to one side.
- Stay in this position for 2 to 5 minutes, making sure that you relax completely.
- Remain face down and prop yourself on your elbows.
- Hold this position for 2 to 3 minutes.
- Return to starting position and relax for 1 minute.
- Repeat 5 to 10 times.

Hip Tilts
- Lie flat on back with knees bent.
- Slowly bend legs and hips to one side as far as possible.
- Bend to other side.
- Repeat 5 times.

Toe Touches
- Stand straight and relaxed.
- Lower head and body and try to touch floor with fingertips.
- Keep knees straight.
- Do not jerk or lunge toward floor.
- Bend only as far as you can.
- Repeat 5 times.

From Canobbio MM: *Mosby's handbook of patient teaching,* ed 3, St Louis, 2006, Mosby.

---

limitations, promote comfort, and educate the patient about the health problem and appropriate exercises. Other nursing interventions are summarized in NCP 64-2. The use of analgesics, NSAIDs, muscle relaxants, and thermotherapy (ice and heat) while avoiding continued bed rest is incorporated into the plan of care.

Muscle stretching and strengthening exercises may be part of the management plan. Although the actual exercises are often taught by the physical therapist, it is the nurse's responsibility to ensure that the patient understands the type and frequency of exercise prescribed, as well as the rationale for the program.

Ambulatory and Home Care. The goal of management is to make an episode of acute low back pain an isolated incident. If the lumbosacral mechanism is unstable, repeated episodes can be anticipated. The lumbosacral spine may be unable to meet the demands placed on it without strain because of factors such as obesity, poor posture, poor muscular support, advancing age, or local trauma. Intervention is aimed at strengthening the supporting muscles by exercise. A corset limits extremes of movement and may increase the risk of back pain if used for prolonged periods.[20]

Persistent use of poor body mechanics may also result in repeated episodes of low back pain. If the strain is work related, occupational counseling may be necessary. The frustration, pain, and

NURSING CARE PLAN 64-2

Patient with Low Back Pain

ACUTE MANAGEMENT

NURSING DIAGNOSIS   **Acute pain** *related to* muscle spasm and ineffective comfort measures *as evidenced by* verbalization of back pain on movement, guarded movements, palpable muscle spasm, decreased physical activity, rating pain as >4 on 10-point pain scale

PATIENT GOAL   Reports satisfactory pain relief with pain <4 on 10-point scale

OUTCOMES (NOC)

Pain Level

- Reported pain _____
- Muscle tension _____
- Narrowed focus _____

Pain: Disruptive Effects

- Impaired physical mobility _____

Measurement Scale

1 = Severe
2 = Substantial
3 = Moderate
4 = Mild
5 = None

Pain Control

- Uses nonanalgesic relief measures _____
- Uses analgesics appropriately _____
- Reports pain controlled _____

Measurement Scale

1 = Never demonstrated
2 = Rarely demonstrated
3 = Sometimes demonstrated
4 = Often demonstrated
5 = Consistently demonstrated

INTERVENTIONS (NIC) and RATIONALES

Pain Management

- Perform a comprehensive assessment of pain to include location, characteristics, onset/duration, frequency, quality, intensity or severity of pain, and precipitating factors, *to plan appropriate interventions.*
- Evaluate effectiveness of pain-control measures used through ongoing assessment of pain experience.
- Ensure that patient receives attentive analgesic care *to promote comfort and evaluate effectiveness.*
- Promote adequate rest/sleep *to facilitate pain relief and to reduce paravertebral muscle spasm and resulting pain.*
- Teach the use of nonpharmacologic techniques (e.g., relaxation, distraction, hot/cold application, and massage) before pain occurs or increases, and along with other pain-relief measures *to promote muscle relaxation and decrease tension.*
- Provide patient with optimal pain relief with prescribed analgesics *to help decrease pain and inflammation.*

Positioning

- Place in the designated therapeutic position (e.g., keep head of bed elevated 20 degrees and knee of bed flexed) *to promote comfort by reducing stress on lower back muscles.*

NURSING DIAGNOSIS   **Impaired physical mobility** *related to* pain *as evidenced by* limited range of motion (ROM), movement restrictions, muscle spasms

PATIENT GOALS   1. Demonstrates return to prior level of mobility within prescribed restrictions
2. Demonstrates correct performance of exercises

OUTCOMES (NOC)

Mobility

- Gait _____
- Muscle movement _____
- Coordination _____
- Joint movement _____
- Body positioning performance _____
- Moves with ease _____

Measurement Scale

1 = Severely compromised
2 = Substantially compromised
3 = Moderately compromised
4 = Mildly compromised
5 = Not compromised

INTERVENTIONS (NIC) and RATIONALES

Exercise Therapy: Joint Mobility

- Determine limitations of joint movement and effect on function.
- Initiate pain-control measures before beginning joint exercises *to assist in completion of exercises and ROM.*
- Encourage active range-of-motion (ROM) exercises, according to regular, planned schedule, *to maintain all joints in normal ROM.*
- Encourage ambulation *to promote gradual and progressive return to previous mobility level.*
- Provide written discharge instructions for exercise.

NURSING CARE PLAN 64-2

Patient with Low Back Pain—cont'd

CHRONIC MANAGEMENT

NURSING DIAGNOSIS **Chronic pain** *related to* progressive degenerative changes of the muscles and skeletal structures of the back *as evidenced by* verbal report of back pain over more than 6 months, fatigue, and protective and guarding behaviors

PATIENT GOAL Reports ability to control pain at an acceptable level with the use of preventive and nonpharmacologic measures

OUTCOMES (NOC)	INTERVENTIONS (NIC) and *RATIONALES*
Pain Control	**Pain Management**
• Uses preventive measures ____	• Evaluate effectiveness of pain-control measures used through ongoing assessment of pain experience.
• Uses nonanalgesic relief measures ____	• Select and implement a variety of measures (e.g., pharmacologic, nonpharmacologic) *to facilitate pain relief.*
• Uses analgesics appropriately ____	
• Uses available resources ____	• Collaborate with patient, significant other, and other health professionals to select and implement nonpharmacologic pain-relief measures (e.g., use of heat, transcutaneous electrical nerve stimulation) *to provide information about supplementary methods of pain management.*
• Reports pain controlled ____	
Measurement Scale	
1 = Never demonstrated	
2 = Rarely demonstrated	• Explore with patient factors that relieve/worsen pain *to make adjustments in lifestyle so that pain is reduced.*
3 = Sometimes demonstrated	• Use therapeutic communication strategies *to acknowledge pain experience and convey acceptance of patient's response to pain.*
4 = Often demonstrated	
5 = Consistently demonstrated	• Inform other health care professionals/family members of nonpharmacologic strategies being used by patient *to encourage preventive approaches to pain management.*

NURSING DIAGNOSIS **Ineffective coping** *related to* effects of chronic pain *as evidenced by* verbalization of hopelessness and inability to cope, irritability, inability to meet role expectations, ineffective or inappropriate use of coping behaviors

PATIENT GOALS 1. Uses coping behaviors effectively to adapt to effects of chronic pain
2. Reports a positive sense of control and hope
3. Reports satisfaction with lifestyle

OUTCOMES (NOC)	INTERVENTIONS (NIC) and *RATIONALES*
Pain: Disruptive Effects	**Coping Enhancement**
• Leisure activities ____	• Appraise and discuss alternative responses to situation.
• Life enjoyment ____	• Assist patient in developing an objective appraisal of the event.
• Sense of control ____	• Seek to understand patient's perception of a stressful situation.
• Sense of hope ____	• Support use of appropriate defense mechanisms.
Measurement Scale	• Arrange situations that encourage patient's autonomy *to foster effective coping behaviors and adjustments to chronic pain.*
1 = Severely compromised	• Foster constructive outlets for anger and hostility.
2 = Substantially compromised	• Assist patient to identify positive strategies to deal with limitations and manage needed lifestyle or role changes.
3 = Moderately compromised	
4 = Mildly compromised	
5 = Not compromised	
Coping	**Hope Instillation**
• Verbalizes sense of control ____	• Encourage therapeutic relationships with significant others *to increase hope through a connection with others.*
• Verbalizes acceptance of situation ____	
• Modifies lifestyle as needed ____	• Teach family about the positive aspects of hope (e.g., develop meaningful conversational themes that reflect love and need for patient) *to promote hopeful state.*
• Uses effective coping strategies ____	
• Reports decrease in negative feelings ____	• Develop plan of care that involves degree of goal attainment, moving from simple to more complex goals *to promote hope for the future.*
Measurement Scale	
1 = Never demonstrated	
2 = Rarely demonstrated	
3 = Sometimes demonstrated	
4 = Often demonstrated	
5 = Consistently demonstrated	

Continued

NURSING CARE PLAN 64-2

Patient with Low Back Pain—cont'd

NURSING DIAGNOSIS **Ineffective therapeutic regimen management** *related to* knowledge deficit, complexity of therapeutic regimen, or lack of perceived benefits regarding posture, exercises, and body mechanics *as evidenced by* verbalization that action has not been taken to reduce risk factors for progression of illness and to include treatment regimens in daily routines

PATIENT GOALS Integrates a program of appropriate posture, body mechanics, exercises, and weight management into daily routine

OUTCOMES (NOC)

Knowledge: Body Mechanics

- Description of the proper standing posture _____
- Description of proper sitting posture _____
- Description of proper lying posture _____
- Description of proper lifting techniques _____
- Description of exercises to increase muscle strength _____
- Description of exercises to strengthen lower abdominal muscles _____

Measurement Scale

1 = None
2 = Limited
3 = Moderate
4 = Substantial
5 = Extensive

INTERVENTIONS (NIC) and *RATIONALES*

Teaching: Prescribed Activity/Exercise

- Observe patient perform prescribed activity/exercise *to identify incorrect techniques and intervene appropriately.*
- Instruct patient on good posture and body mechanics *to reduce risk of reinjury, provide back support, and maintain proper body alignment.*
- Assist patient to incorporate activity/exercise regimen into daily routine/lifestyle *to make desired behaviors a habit.*
- Refer patient to physical therapist/occupational therapist/exercise physiologist *to develop abdominal and paravertebral muscle strength exercises and to provide increased support.*

Weight Management

- Discuss risks associated with being over- and underweight *as increased abdominal weight alters posture and puts strain on low back.*
- Develop with patient a method to keep a daily record of intake, exercise sessions, and/or changes in body weight *to evaluate management of therapeutic regimen.*

---

disability imposed on the patient with low back pain require emotional support and understanding care by the nurse.

■ Evaluation

The expected outcomes for the patient with low back pain are presented in NCP 64-2.

CHRONIC LOW BACK PAIN

Chronic back pain lasts more than 3 months or is a repeated incapacitating episode. The causes of chronic low back pain include degenerative disk disease, lack of physical exercise, prior injury, obesity, structural and postural abnormalities, and systemic disease. Osteoarthritis (OA) of the lumbar spine is found in patients over 50, whereas chronic back pain in younger patients with OA usually involves the thoracic or lumbar spine. Discomfort is increased following periods of inactivity, particularly on awakening or after long periods of sitting.

Spinal stenosis is a narrowing of the vertebral canal or nerve root canals caused by encroachment of bone on the space. The stenosis may be congenital or, more typically, it is acquired through degenerative or traumatic changes to the spine. When it occurs in the lumbar area of the spine, it is a common cause of chronic or recurrent low back pain. Compression of the nerve roots can result, with subsequent disk herniation. The pain associated with lumbar spinal stenosis often starts in the low back and then radiates to the buttock and leg.[21] It worsens with walking and, in particular, standing without walking.

Treatment regimens for chronic back pain are much the same as for acute low back pain. These include a reduction in the pain associated with daily activities, a formal back pain program, and ongoing medical care. Cold, damp weather aggravates the back pain, but this can be relieved with rest and local heat application.

Relief of pain and stiffness by the use of mild analgesics, such as NSAIDs, is integral to the daily comfort of the individual with chronic low back pain. Weight reduction, sufficient rest periods, local heat or cold application, and exercise and activity throughout the day help to keep the muscles and joints mobilized. Tricyclic antidepressants (e.g., amitriptyline [Elavil]) and selective serotonin reuptake inhibitors (e.g., sertraline [Zoloft]) have been shown to improve the chronic symptoms of low back pain.[22]

Surgical intervention may be indicated in patients with severe chronic low back pain who do not respond to conservative care and/or have continued neurologic deficits. (Surgery for low back pain is discussed on pp. 1681 to 1683.)

INTERVERTEBRAL LUMBAR DISK DAMAGE

Etiology and Pathophysiology

An intervertebral disk is interposed between the vertebrae from the cervical axis to the sacrum. Structural degeneration of the lumbar disk is often caused by **degenerative disk disease** (DDD) (Fig. 64-6). This progressive degeneration is a normal process of aging, and results in the intervertebral disks losing their elasticity, flexibility, and shock-absorbing capabilities. Thinning of the disks occurs as the nucleus pulposus (gelatinous center of the disk) starts to dry out and shrink.[23] Most persons by age 60 have some degree of DDD. Compression of the nerve roots and cord may then occur. Damage to the spine by DDD contributes to osteoarthritis of the spine by the formation of osteophytes (bone spurs).

An acute **herniated intervertebral disk** (slipped disk) can be the result of natural degeneration with age or repeated stress and trauma to the spine. The nucleus pulposus may first bulge and then it can herniate, placing pressure on nearby nerves. The most

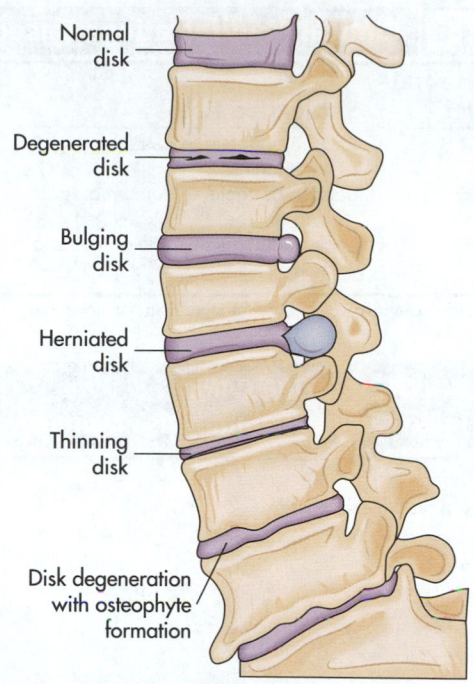

FIG. 64-6 Common causes of degenerative disk damage.

Labels: Normal disk; Degenerated disk; Bulging disk; Herniated disk; Thinning disk; Disk degeneration with osteophyte formation

common sites of rupture are the lumbosacral disks, specifically L4-5 and L5-S1. Disk herniation may also occur at C5-6 and C6-7. Disk herniation may be the result of spinal stenosis, in which narrowing of the spinal canal creates a bulging of the intervertebral disk.

Clinical Manifestations

The most common feature of lumbar disk damage is low back pain. Radicular pain that radiates down the buttock and below the knee, along the distribution of the sciatic nerve, generally indicates disk herniation. (Specific manifestations for lumbar disk herniation are summarized in Table 64-8.) The straight-leg-raising test may be positive, indicating nerve root irritation. Back or leg pain may be reproduced by raising the leg and flexing the foot at 90 degrees. Low back pain from other causes may not be accompanied by leg pain. Reflexes may be depressed or absent, depending on the spinal nerve root involved. Paresthesia or muscle weakness in the legs, feet, or toes may be reported by the patient. Multiple nerve root (*cauda equina*) compression may be manifested as bowel and bladder incontinence or impotence.

Diagnostic Studies

X-rays are done to note any structural defects. A myelogram, MRI, or CT scan is helpful in localizing the damaged site. An epidural venogram or diskogram may be necessary if other methods of diagnosis are unsuccessful. An EMG of the extremities can be per-

formed to determine the severity of nerve irritation, or to rule out other pathologic conditions such as peripheral neuropathy.

Collaborative Care

The patient with suspected disk damage is usually managed first with at least 4 weeks of conservative therapy (Table 64-9). This includes limitation of extremes of spinal movement (brace, corset, or belt), local heat or ice, ultrasound and massage, traction, and transcutaneous electrical nerve stimulation (TENS). Drug therapy includes NSAIDs, short-term opioids, and muscle relaxants. Epidural corticosteroid injections may be effective in reducing inflammation and relieving acute pain. If the underlying cause remains, the pain tends to recur. Conservative treatment can result in a healing over of the damaged area if not due to DDD, with a concomitant decrease in pain. Once the symptoms subside, back strengthening exercises are begun twice a day and are encouraged for a lifetime. The patient should be taught the principles of good body mechanics. Extremes of flexion and torsion are strongly discouraged.

Most patients initially recover with a conservative treatment plan. However, if conservative treatment is unsuccessful, *radiculopathy* (nerve root pain) becomes progressively worse, or loss of bowel or bladder control (cauda equina) is documented, surgery may then be indicated.

Surgical Therapy. Surgery for a damaged disk is generally indicated when diagnostic tests indicate that the problem is not responding to conservative treatment and the patient is in consistent pain and/or has a persistent neurologic deficit. Surgery should be carefully considered as some patients, for unknown reasons, do not improve and symptoms may actually worsen after surgery.[24]

An *intradiscal electrothermoplasty* (IDET) is a minimally invasive outpatient procedure that may help in treating back and sciatica pain.[25] The procedure involves the insertion of a needle into the affected disk with the guidance of an x-ray. A wire is then threaded down through the needle and into the disk. The wire is then heated, which denervates the small nerve fibers that have grown into the

TABLE 64-8 | **Clinical Manifestations Based on Level of Disk Herniation***

Intervertebral Level	Subjective Pain	Affected Reflex	Motor Function	Sensation
L3-4	Back to buttocks to posterior thigh to inner calf	Patellar	Quadriceps, anterior tibialis	Inner aspect of lower leg, anterior part of thigh
L4-5	Back to buttocks to dorsum of foot and big toe	None	Anterior tibialis, extensor hallucis longus, gluteus medius	Dorsum of foot and big toe
L5-S1	Back to buttocks to sole of foot and heel	Achilles	Gastrocnemius, hamstring, gluteus maximus	Heel and lateral foot

*A disk herniation can involve pressure on more than one nerve root.

TABLE 64-9 | *COLLABORATIVE CARE*
Intervertebral Lumbar Disk Damage

Diagnostic
History and physical examination
X-ray
CT scan
MRI
Myelogram
Diskogram
EMG

Collaborative Therapy
Conservative
Restricted activity for several days, limit total bed rest
Medication
Analgesics
Nonsteroidal antiinflammatory drugs
Muscle relaxants (e.g., cyclobenzaprine [Flexeril])
Local ice or heat
Physical therapy
Epidural corticosteroid injections

Surgical
Intradiscal electrothermoplasy (IDET)
Radiofrequency discal nucleoplasty
Interspinous process decompression system (X Stop)
Laminectomy with or without spinal fusion
Diskectomy
Percutaneous laser diskectomy
Artificial disc replacement (Charité disk)
Spinal fusion with (e.g., plates, screws) or without instrumentation

CT, Computed tomography; *EMG,* electromyogram; *MRI,* magnetic resonance imaging.

COMPLEMENTARY AND ALTERNATIVE THERAPIES

Acupuncture

Acupuncture is a traditional Chinese medical practice of inserting very fine needles into the skin to stimulate specific anatomic points in the body (called acupoints) for therapeutic purposes. Acupuncture is used to regulate the flow of Qi (life force or energy). The acupuncture needles unblock the obstruction of Qi through the meridians (see Chapter 8).

Clinical Uses
Pain management
Postoperative and chemotherapy-associated nausea and vomiting
Addiction, asthma, menstrual cramps, menopausal symptoms, and stroke rehabilitation
Table 8-8 lists other conditions that may benefit from acupuncture

Effects
Release of endorphins, activation of the hypothalamus and pituitary gland, and alterations in the levels of neurotransmitters.

Nursing Implications
Acupuncture is a safe therapy when the practitioner has been appropriately trained. Advise patients to ensure that their practitioner has appropriate education and licensure.

cracks and have invaded the degenerating disk. The heat also partially melts the annulus, which triggers the body to generate new reinforcing proteins in the fibers of the annulus. Although some patients have reported a large reduction in pain with IDET, long-term studies are still needed.[25]

Another outpatient technique is *radiofrequency discal nucleoplasty* (coblation nucleoplasty). A needle is inserted into the disk similar to IDET. Instead of a heating wire, a special radiofrequency probe is used. The probe generates energy that breaks up the molecular bonds of the gel in the nucleus. The result is that up to 20% of the nucleus is removed, which decompresses the disk and reduces the pressure on both the disk and the surrounding nerve roots. Relief from pain varies among patients. Additional study is needed to determine the effectiveness of this procedure.

A third procedure is the use of an *interspinous process decompression system* (X Stop). This device is made of titanium and fits onto a mount that is placed on vertebrae in the lower back. The

X Stop is indicated for use in patients with pain due to lumbar spinal stenosis. The device works by pushing open the spinal cord by pressing against parts of either side of the vertebrae. The effect is similar to and less invasive than a laminectomy.[26]

A traditional and most common surgical procedure for lumbar disk disease is a *laminectomy.* It involves the surgical excision of part of the posterior arch of the vertebra (referred to as the lamina) to gain access to part of or the entire protruding disk to remove it. A minimal hospital stay is usually required after the procedure.

A *diskectomy* is another common type of surgical procedure that may be performed to decompress the nerve root. Microsurgical diskectomy is a version of the standard diskectomy in which the surgeon uses a microscope to allow better visualization of the disk and disk space during surgery to aid in the removal of the damaged portion. This helps maintain the bony stability of the spine.

A *percutaneous laser diskectomy* is an outpatient surgical procedure using a tube that is passed through the retroperitoneal soft tissues to the lateral border of the disk with local anesthesia and the aid of fluoroscopy. A laser is then used on the damaged portion of the disk. Small stab wounds are used, and minimal blood loss occurs during the procedure. The procedure is effective and safe and decreases rehabilitation time.

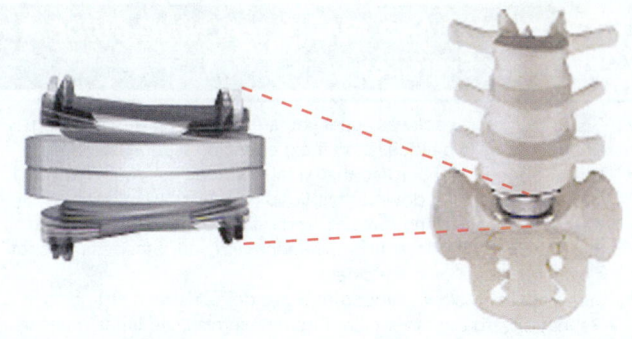

FIG. 64-7 The Charité artificial disk, used in degenerative disk disease to replace a damaged intervertebral disk. The Charité artificial disk consists of two cobalt-chromium alloy endplates sandwiched around a movable high-density plastic core. The design of the disk helps align the spine and preserve its natural ability to move.

The *Charité disk* is used in patients with disk damage associated with DDD.[27] This artificial disk is made up of a high-density core sandwiched between two cobalt-chromium endplates (Fig. 64-7). This device is surgically placed in the spine through a small incision below the umbilicus after the damaged disk is removed. The disk allows for movement at the level of the implant.

A *spinal fusion* may be performed if an unstable bony mechanism is present. The spine is stabilized by creating an ankylosis (fusion) of contiguous vertebrae with a bone graft from the patient's fibula or iliac crest or from a donated cadaver bone. Metal fixation with rods, plates, or screws may be implanted at the time of spinal surgery to provide more stability and decrease vertebral motion. A posterior lumbar interbody fusion may be performed in patients to provide extra support for bone grafting or a prosthetic device. A more recent device, the InFuse Bone Graft/LT-CAGE, is being used to eliminate the need to use bone from the patient in grafting. The device contains genetically engineered protein that stimulates the body to grow new bone at the spinal fusion site.[28]

NURSING MANAGEMENT
SPINAL SURGERY

Postoperative nursing interventions focus on maintaining proper alignment of the spine at all times until healing has occurred. Depending on the extent and type of surgery, bed rest may be maintained for 1 to 2 days. Logrolling patients when turning is essential to maintain proper body alignment. Pillows can be used under the thighs of each leg when supine and between the legs when in the side-lying position to provide comfort and ensure alignment. The patient often fears turning or any movement that increases pain by straining the surgical area. The nurse must offer reassurance to the patient that the proper technique is being used to maintain body alignment. Sufficient staff should be available to move the patient without undue pain or strain on staff members or the patient. Depending on the type and extent of surgery and the surgeon's preference, the patient may be able to dangle the legs at the side of the bed, stand, or even ambulate the first day after surgery.

Postoperatively, most patients will require opioids such as morphine IV for 24 to 48 hours. Patient-controlled analgesia allows for optimal analgesic levels and is the preferred method of continued pain management during this time. Once fluids are being taken, the patient may be switched to oral drugs such as acetaminophen with codeine, hydrocodone (Vicodin), or oxycodone (Percocet). Diazepam (Valium) may be prescribed for muscle relaxation. The nurse should monitor and document pain management and its effectiveness after surgery.

Because the spinal canal may be entered during surgery, there is potential for cerebrospinal fluid (CSF) leakage. Severe headache or leakage of CSF on the dressing should be reported immediately. CSF appears as clear or slightly yellow drainage on the dressing. It has a high glucose concentration and will be positive for glucose when a dipstick test is done. The amount, color, and characteristics of drainage should be noted.

Frequent monitoring of peripheral neurologic signs of the extremities is a routine postoperative nursing responsibility after spinal surgery. Movement of the arms and legs and assessment of sensation should be unchanged when compared with the preoperative status. These assessments are repeated every 2 to 4 hours during the first 48 hours after surgery, and findings are compared with the preoperative assessment. Paresthesias, such as numbness and tingling, may not be relieved immediately after surgery. Any new muscle weakness or paresthesias should be documented and reported to the surgeon immediately. Extremity circulation should be assessed by temperature, capillary refill, and pulses.

Paralytic ileus and interference with bowel function may occur for several days and may manifest as nausea, abdominal distention, and constipation. The nurse should assess whether the patient is passing flatus, has bowel sounds in all quadrants, and has a flat, soft abdomen. Stool softeners (e.g., docusate [Colace]) may aid in relieving and preventing constipation.

Adequate bladder emptying may be altered because of activity restrictions, opioids, or anesthesia. If allowed by the surgeon, men should be encouraged to dangle the legs over the side of the bed or stand to urinate. Patients should use the commode or ambulate to the bathroom when allowed to promote adequate emptying of the bladder. The nurse should ensure that privacy is maintained. It is necessary to clarify whether the patient can be allowed up to ambulate to the bathroom without the corset or brace. Intermittent catheterization or an indwelling catheter may be necessary for patients who have difficulty urinating.

Loss of sphincter tone or bladder tone may indicate nerve damage. Incontinence or difficulty evacuating the bowel or bladder must be monitored closely and reported to the surgeon.

Activity prescriptions vary with surgeons, but the patient who has had spinal surgery usually ambulates early in the postoperative period. It is a nursing responsibility to know the specific orders related to activity for any patient.

In addition to the nursing care appropriate for a patient who has had a laminectomy, there are other nursing responsibilities if the patient has also had a spinal fusion. Because a bone graft is usually involved, the postoperative healing time is prolonged compared with that of a laminectomy. Immobilization over an extended time may be necessary. A rigid orthosis (thoracic-lumbar-sacral orthosis or chairback brace) is often used during the period of immobilization. Some surgeons require that the patient be taught to put it on and take it off by logrolling in bed, whereas others allow their patients to apply the brace in a sitting or standing position. The nurse should verify the preferred method before initiating this activity. The extended immobilization required by a spinal fusion carries with it all the potential problems related to immobility.

In addition to the primary surgical site, the donor site for the bone graft must be regularly assessed. The posterior iliac crest is the most commonly used donor site, although the fibula may also

TABLE 64-10	Causes of Neck Pain

- Poor posture
- Strain or sprain
- Degenerative disk disease, including herniation
- Trauma (e.g., fractures and subluxation)
- Spondylosis
- Rheumatoid arthritis
- Tumor
- Osteoporosis
- Osteomyelitis
- Meningitis
- Paget's disease
- Psychiatric chronic syndromes
- Referred from visceral pain

TABLE 64-11	PATIENT AND FAMILY TEACHING GUIDE
	Neck Exercises

- Bend your head backward until you are looking up at the ceiling. Repeat slowly five times. Stop if experiencing dizziness.
- Bring your head forward so that your chin touches your chest and your face is looking down at the floor. Repeat slowly five times.
- Keep your head facing forward, and bend your ear down toward one shoulder. Alternate this movement with your other ear. Repeat slowly five times on each side.
- Turn your head slowly around to one side as far as it will go. Repeat toward the other side. Repeat exercise five times on each side.

be used. The donor site usually causes greater postoperative pain than the fused area. The donor site is bandaged with a pressure dressing to prevent excessive bleeding. If the donor site is the fibula, neurovascular assessments of the extremity are a postoperative nursing responsibility.

As the bone graft heals, the patient must adjust to the permanent immobility at the graft or fusion site. Instruction in proper body mechanics is essential and should be evaluated during the hospital stay.

The patient should be instructed to avoid sitting or standing for prolonged periods. Activities that should be encouraged include walking, lying down, and shifting weight from one foot to the other when standing. The patient should learn to mentally think through an activity before starting any potentially injurious task such as bending, lifting, or stooping. Any twisting movement of the spine is contraindicated. The thighs and knees, rather than the back, should be used to absorb the shock of activity and movement. A firm mattress or bedboard is essential.

NECK PAIN

Neck pain may occur almost as frequently as low back pain, affecting up to 90% of adults at some point in their life.[29] Neck pain may be the result of many conditions, both benign (e.g., poor posture) and serious (e.g., traumatic injury) (Table 64-10).

Cervical neck sprains and strains occur from hyperflexion and hyperextension injury. Patients have symptoms of stiffness and neck pain and possible pain radiating into the arm and hand. Pain may also radiate into the head, anterior chest, thoracic spine region, and shoulders. Cervical nerve root compression from stenosis, degenerative disk disease, or herniation may be indicated by weakness or paresthesia of the arm and hand. Diagnosing the cause of neck pain is done by history, physical examination, x-ray, MRI, CT scan, and myelogram. An EMG of the upper extremities is done to diagnose cervical radiculopathy.

Conservative treatment for neck pain that can commonly occur in patients without an underlying disorder includes head support via soft cervical collars, heat and ice applications, massage, rest until symptoms subside, physical therapy, ultrasound, and NSAIDs. Most neck pain resolves without surgical intervention. Indications for cervical spine surgery are similar to those for the lower back. Types of surgery are also similar, including a diskectomy, laminectomy, and spinal fusion. If surgery is done on the cervical spine, the nurse must be alert for symptoms of spinal cord edema such as respiratory distress and a worsening neurologic status of the upper extremities. An orthosis or halo may be

necessary after surgery depending on the degree of spine stabilization. After surgery, the patient's neck is immobilized in either a soft or hard cervical collar.

Preventing benign neck pain that occurs due to everyday activities such as prolonged sitting at a computer or television, sleeping in nonalignment spinal positions, or jarring movements during exercise is important. Preventive strategies can begin by practicing good posture and maintaining neck flexibility (Table 64-11).

FOOT DISORDERS

The foot is the platform that provides support for the weight of the body and absorbs considerable shock in ambulation. It is a complicated structure composed of bony structures, muscles, tendons, and ligaments. It can be affected by (1) congenital conditions, (2) structural weakness, (3) traumatic injuries, and (4) systemic conditions such as diabetes mellitus and rheumatoid arthritis. Abnormalities of the foot affect over 80 million persons in the United States. Much of the pain, deformity, and disability associated with foot disorders can be directly attributed to or accentuated by improperly fitting shoes, which cause crowding and angulation of the toes and inhibition of the normal movement of foot muscles.

The purposes of footwear are to (1) provide support, foot stability, protection, shock absorption, and a foundation for orthoses; (2) increase friction with the walking surface; and (3) treat foot abnormalities. (Table 64-12 summarizes common foot disorders.) One of the most common forefoot disorders is a bunion (Fig. 64-8). A lateral deviation of the great toe, termed *hallux valgus*, occurs with a bunion.[30]

NURSING MANAGEMENT
FOOT DISORDERS

■ **Nursing Implementation**

Health Promotion. Well-constructed and properly fitted shoes are essential for healthy, pain-free feet. Instead of considerations of comfort and support, fashion styles, especially for women, often influence selection of footwear. Patient teaching should stress the importance of having a shoe that conforms to the foot rather than to current fashion trends. The shoe must be long enough and wide enough to prevent crowding of the toes and forcing of the great toe into a position of hallux valgus. At the metatarsal head, the width of the shoe should be sufficient to allow free movement of the foot muscles and permit bending of the toes. The shank (narrow part of sole under the instep) of the shoe should be rigid enough to give optimal support. The height of the heel should be realistic in relation to the purpose for which the shoe is worn. Ideally, the heel of

TABLE 64-12	Common Foot Disorders	
Disorder	**Description**	**Treatment**
Forefoot		
Hallux valgus (bunion)	Painful deformity of great toe consisting of lateral angulation of great toe toward second toe, bony enlargement of medial side of first metatarsal head, and formation of bursa or callus over bony enlargement (Fig. 64-8)	Conservative treatment includes wearing shoes with wide forefoot or "bunion pocket" and use of bunion pads to relieve pressure on bursal sac. Surgical treatment is removal of bursal sac and bony enlargement and correction of lateral angulation of great toe; may include temporary or permanent internal fixation.
Hallux rigidus	Painful stiffness of first MTP joint caused by osteoarthritis or local trauma	Conservative treatment includes intraarticular corticosteroids and passive manual stretching of first MTP joint. A shoe with a stiff sole decreases pain in the joint during walking. Surgical treatment is joint fusion or arthroplasty with silicone rubber implant.
Hammer toe	Deformity of the second through fifth toes, including flexion deformity of PIP and DIP joints, hyperextension of MTP joint, flexion deformity of DIP joint alone (mallet toe); callus formation and flexion of PIP and DIP joint hyperextension (claw toe) (Fig. 64-9); complaints related to hammer toe include burning on bottom of foot, and pain and difficulty in walking when wearing shoes	Conservative treatment consists of passive manual stretching of PIP joint and use of metatarsal arch support. Surgical correction consists of resection of base of middle phalanx and head of proximal phalanx and bringing raw bone ends together. Kirschner wire maintains straight position.
Morton's neuroma (Morton's toe or plantar neuroma)	Neuroma in web space between third and fourth metatarsal heads, causing sharp, sudden attacks of pain and burning sensations	Surgical excision is the usual treatment.
Midfoot		
Pes planus (flatfoot)	Loss of metatarsal arch causing pain in foot or leg	Symptoms are relieved by use of resilient longitudinal arch supports. Surgical treatment consists of triple arthrodesis or fusion of subtalar joint.
Pes cavus	Elevation of longitudinal arch of foot resulting from contracture of plantar fascia or bony deformity of arch	Treatment is manipulation and casting (in patients <6 yr of age); surgical correction is necessary if it interferes with ambulation (in patients >6 yr of age).
Hindfoot		
Painful heels	Complaint of heel pain with weight bearing; common cause of plantar bursitis, plantar fasciitis, or bone spur in adult	Corticosteroids are injected locally into inflamed bursa and sponge-rubber heel cushion is used; surgical excision of bursa or spur is performed; stretching exercises and shock-wave therapy, along with NSAIDs and corticosteroids, are used for plantar fasciitis.
Local Problems		
Corn	Localized thickening of skin caused by continual pressure over bony prominences, especially metatarsal head, frequently causing localized pain	Corn is softened with warm water or preparations containing salicylic acid and trimmed with razor blade or scalpel. Pressure on bony prominences caused by shoes is relieved.
Soft corn	Painful lesion caused by bony prominence of one toe pressing against adjacent toe; usual location in web space between toes; softness caused by secretions keeping web space relatively moist	Pain is relieved by placing cotton between toes to separate them. Surgical treatment is excision of projecting bone spur (if present).
Callus	Similar formation to corn but covering of wider area and usual location on weight-bearing part of foot	Same as for corn.
Plantar wart	Painful papillomatous growth caused by virus that may occur on any part of skin on sole of foot; they tend to cluster on pressure points	Remedies containing salicyclic acid (e.g., Compound W); excision with electrocoagulation or surgical removal; laser treatments may also be used; many disappear without treatment.

DIP, Distal interphalangeal; *MTP,* metatarsophalangeal; *NSAIDs,* nonsteroidal antiinflammatory drugs; *PIP,* proximal interphalangeal.

the shoe should not rise more than 1 inch higher than the forefoot support.

Acute Intervention. Many foot problems require referral to a podiatrist. Depending on the problem, conservative therapies are usually tried first (see Table 64-12). These therapies include NSAIDs, shock-wave therapy, icing, physical therapy, alterations in footwear, stretching, warm soaks, orthotics, ultrasound, and corticosteroid injections. If these methods do not offer relief, surgery may then be recommended.

When surgery is performed, the foot is usually immobilized by a bulky dressing, short leg cast, slipper (plaster) cast, or a platform "shoe" that fits over the dressing and has a rigid sole (known as a

bunion boot). The foot should be elevated with the heel off the bed to help reduce discomfort and prevent edema. Neurovascular status should be assessed frequently during the immediate postoperative period. Depending on the type of surgery, pins or wires may extend through the toes, or a protective splint that extends over the end of the foot may be in place. Care must be taken not to jar these devices and cause pain. The devices may interfere with or preclude assessment for movement. The nurse should be aware that sensation may be difficult to evaluate because postoperative pain can interfere with the patient's ability to differentiate pain caused by the surgical procedure from pain resulting from nerve pressure or circulatory impairment.

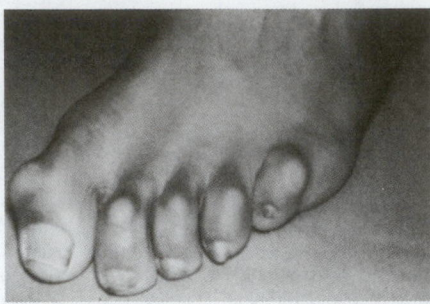

FIG. 64-8   Hallux valgus with bunion of the great toe.

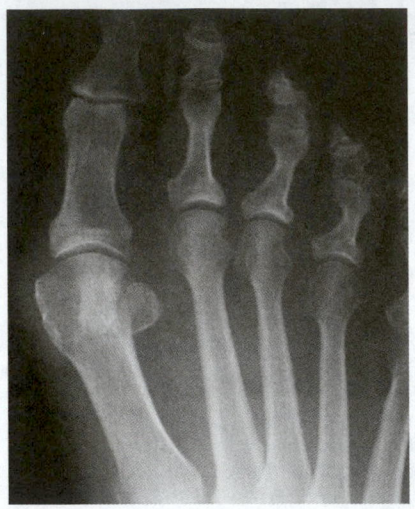

FIG. 64-9   Claw-toe deformity. A type of hammer toe caused by chronic irritation from poorly fitting shoes.

The type and extent of surgery determine the degree of ambulation allowed. Crutches, a walker, or a cane may be necessary. The patient may experience pain or a throbbing sensation when starting ambulation. The nurse should reinforce instructions given by the physical therapist and ensure that the patient does not develop a faulty gait pattern such as walking on the heels in an attempt to avoid excessive pain or pressure. The nurse must reinforce the importance of walking with an erect posture and with proper weight distribution. Dysfunction of gait or continued pain should be reported to the physician. The nurse should instruct the patient on the importance of frequent rest periods with the foot elevated.

Ambulatory and Home Care. Foot care should include daily hygienic care and the wearing of clean stockings. Stockings should be long enough to avoid wrinkling and the development of pressure areas. Trimming toenails straight across helps prevent ingrown toenails and reduces the possibility of infection. Persons with impaired circulation or diabetes mellitus require detailed instruction to prevent serious complications associated with blisters, pressure areas, and infections. (See Table 49-22 for guidelines for foot care.)

GERONTOLOGIC CONSIDERATIONS
FOOT PROBLEMS

The older adult is prone to developing foot problems because of poor circulation, atherosclerosis, and decreased sensation in the lower extremities. This is especially a problem for older patients with diabetes mellitus. A patient may develop an open wound but not feel it because of altered sensation.[31] This may be the result of peripheral vascular disease or diabetic neuropathy. Older adults should be instructed to inspect their feet daily and report any open wounds or breaks in the skin to their health care provider. If left untreated, wounds may become infected, lead to osteomyelitis, and require surgical debridement. If the infection becomes widespread, lower limb amputation may be necessary.

Metabolic Bone Diseases

Normal bone metabolism is affected by hormones, nutrition, and hereditary factors. When there is dysfunction in any of these factors, a generalized reduction in bone mass and strength may result. Metabolic bone diseases include osteomalacia, osteoporosis, and Paget's disease.

OSTEOMALACIA

Osteomalacia is a rare condition of adult bone associated with vitamin D deficiency, resulting in decalcification and softening of bone. This disease is the same as rickets in children except that the epiphyseal growth plates are closed in the adult. Vitamin D, with its complex actions and method of synthesis, is required for the absorption of calcium from the intestine. Insufficient vitamin D intake can interfere with the normal mineralization of bone, causing failure or insufficient calcification of bone, which results in bone softening. Etiologic factors in the development of osteomalacia include lack of exposure to ultraviolet rays (which is needed for vitamin D synthesis), GI malabsorption, extensive burns, chronic diarrhea, pregnancy, kidney disease, and drugs such as phenytoin (Dilantin).

The most common clinical features of osteomalacia are localized bone pain, difficulty rising from a chair, and difficulty walking.[32] Other clinical manifestations include low back and bone pain; progressive muscular weakness, especially in the pelvic girdle; weight loss; and progressive deformities of the spine (kyphosis) or extremities. Fractures are common and demonstrate delayed healing when they occur. Mineralization may take 2 to 3 months as opposed to the normal 6 to 10 days.

Laboratory findings commonly associated with osteomalacia are decreased serum calcium or phosphorus levels, decreased serum 25-hydroxyvitamin D, and elevated serum alkaline phosphatase. X-rays may demonstrate the effects of generalized bone demineralization, especially loss of calcium in the bones of the pelvis and the presence of associated bone deformity. *Looser's transformation zones* (ribbons of decalcification in bone found on x-ray) are diagnostic of osteomalacia. However, significant osteomalacia may exist without changes noted on x-ray.

Collaborative care of osteomalacia is directed toward correction of the vitamin D deficiency. Vitamin D_3 (cholecalciferol) and vitamin D_2 (ergocalciferol) can be supplemented, and the patient often shows a dramatic response. Calcium salts or phosphorus supplements may also be prescribed. Dietary ingestion of eggs, low-fat milk, fish, and vegetables is encouraged. Exposure to sunlight (and ultraviolet rays) is also valuable, along with weight-bearing exercise.

OSTEOPOROSIS

Osteoporosis, or porous bone (fragile bone disease), is a chronic, progressive metabolic bone disease characterized by low bone mass and structural deterioration of bone tissue, leading to in-

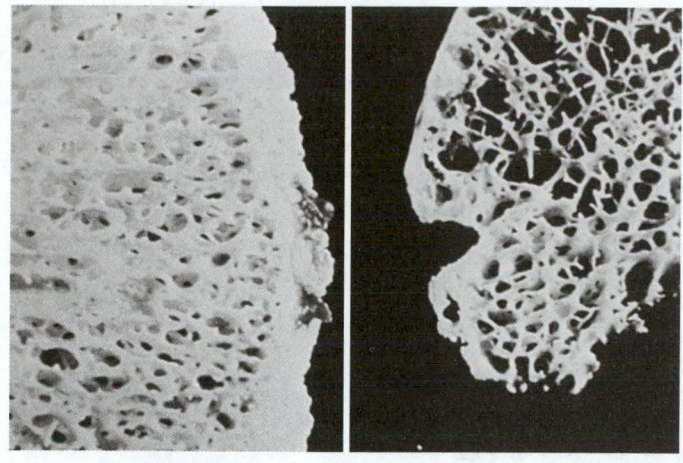

FIG. 64-10 **A,** Normal bone. **B,** Osteoporotic bone.

TABLE 64-13	Risk Factors for Osteoporosis

- Advanced age
- Female gender
- Thin, small framed
- Family history of osteoporosis
- Diet low in calcium
- White or Asian ethnicity
- Excessive use of alcohol
- Cigarette smoking
- Inactive lifestyle
- Long-term use of corticosteroids, thyroid replacements, heparin, long-acting sedatives, or antiseizure medications
- Postmenopausal, including early or surgically induced menopause
- History of anorexia nervosa or bulimia, chronic liver disease, or malabsorption syndromes
- Excess caffeine use
- Low testosterone levels (hypogonadism in men)

CULTURAL AND ETHNIC HEALTH DISPARITIES
Osteoporosis

- White and Asian American women have a higher incidence of osteoporosis than African American women.
- African American women have 10% more bone mass than non–African American women.
- Hispanic women have a lower incidence of osteoporosis than white women.
- Postmenopausal women are at the highest risk for osteoporosis regardless of ethnic group.

GENDER DIFFERENCES
Osteoporosis

Men	Women
• Men are underdiagnosed and undertreated for osteoporosis as compared to women. • One in eight men over the age of 50 will have an osteoporosis-related fracture in their lifetime.	• Osteoporosis is 8 times more common in women than in men. • One in two women over the age of 50 will have an osteoporosis-related fracture in their lifetime.

creased bone fragility (Fig. 64-10). At least 10 million persons in the United States (80% of them women) have osteoporosis, and with the projected increase in life expectancy, this number is expected to grow. One in two women and one in eight men over the age of 50 will sustain an osteoporosis-related fracture during their lifetime. In the United States, the total cost of osteoporosis in terms of medical care, nursing home fees, and loss of income is estimated to exceed $13 billion. Osteoporosis is known as the "silent thief" because it slowly and insidiously over many years robs the skeleton of its banked resources. Bones can eventually become so fragile that they cannot withstand normal mechanical stress.[33]

Osteoporosis is 8 times more common in women than in men for several reasons: (1) women tend to have lower calcium intake than men throughout their lives (men between 15 and 50 years of age consume twice as much calcium as women); (2) women have less bone mass because of their generally smaller frame; (3) bone resorption begins at an earlier age in women and is accelerated at menopause; (4) pregnancy and breastfeeding deplete a woman's skeletal reserve unless calcium intake is adequate; and (5) longevity increases the likelihood of osteoporosis. Although osteoporosis is more common in women than men, it is important to realize that men can also develop osteoporosis.

Women age 65 and older should be routinely screened for osteoporosis. Screening should begin by age 60 for women at increased risk of osteoporotic fractures (Table 64-13). No general recommendations for screening have been made for women who are younger than age 60, or for women age 60 to 64 who are not at increased risk for osteoporosis.[34]

Etiology and Pathophysiology

Risk factors for osteoporosis are female gender, increasing age, family history of osteoporosis, white (European descent) or Asian race, small stature, early menopause, history of anorexia or oophorectomy, sedentary lifestyle, and insufficient dietary calcium. Increased risk is associated with cigarette smoking and alcoholism. Decreased risk is associated with regular weight-bearing exercise and fluoride and vitamin D ingestion.[35] Risk factors for osteoporosis are listed in Table 64-13. Low testosterone levels are a major risk factor in men.

Peak bone mass (maximum bone tissue) is mainly achieved before age 20. It is determined by a combination of four major factors: hereditary, nutrition, exercise, and hormone function. Hered-

ity may be responsible for up to 70% of a person's peak bone mass. Bone loss from midlife (age 35 to 40 years) onward is inevitable, but the rate of loss varies. At menopause, women experience rapid bone loss when the decline in estrogen production is the sharpest. This rate of loss then slows, and eventually matches the rate of bone lost by men 65 to 70 years old.

Bone is continually being deposited by osteoblasts and resorbed by osteoclasts, a process called *remodeling*. Normally the rates of bone deposition and resorption are equal to each other so that the total bone mass remains constant. In osteoporosis, bone resorption exceeds bone deposition. Although resorption affects the entire skeletal system, osteoporosis occurs most commonly in the bones of the spine, hips, and wrists. Over time, wedging and fractures of the vertebrae produce gradual loss of height and a humped back known as "*dowager's hump*," or *kyphosis*. The usual first signs are back pain or spontaneous fractures. The loss of bone substance causes the bone to become mechanically weakened and prone to either spontaneous fractures or fractures from minimal trauma. A person who has one spinal vertebral fracture due to osteoporosis has a 25% chance of having a second vertebral fracture within 1 year.[35]

Specific diseases associated with osteoporosis include intestinal malabsorption, kidney disease, rheumatoid arthritis, hyperthyroidism, chronic alcoholism, cirrhosis of the liver, hypogonadism, and diabetes mellitus.

Many drugs can interfere with bone metabolism, including corticosteroids, antiseizure drugs (e.g., valproate [Depakote], phenytoin [Dilantin]), aluminum-containing antacids, heparin, certain cancer treatments, and excessive thyroid hormones.[36] At the time a drug is prescribed, the patient should be informed of this possible side effect. Long-term corticosteroid use is a major contributor to osteoporosis. When a corticosteroid is taken, there is a loss of bone and inhibition of new bone formation.[37]

Clinical Manifestations

Osteoporosis is often called the "silent disease" because bone loss occurs without symptoms. People may not know they have osteoporosis until their bones become so weak that a sudden strain, bump, or fall causes a hip, vertebral, or wrist fracture. Collapsed vertebrae may initially be manifested as back pain, loss of height, or spinal deformities such as kyphosis or severely stooped posture.

Diagnostic Studies

Osteoporosis often goes unnoticed because it cannot be detected by conventional x-ray until more than 25% to 40% of calcium in the bone is lost. Serum calcium, phosphorus, and alkaline phosphatase levels usually are normal, although alkaline phosphatase may be elevated after a fracture. Bone mineral density (BMD) measurements are typically used to measure bone density. BMD assesses the mass of bone per unit volume, or how tightly the bone is packed. (BMD measurements are presented in Chapter 62, Table 62-7.) Quantitative ultrasound (QUS) measures bone density with sound waves in the heel, kneecap, or shin.[37] One of the most common BMD studies is dual-energy x-ray absorptiometry (DEXA), which measures bone density in the spine, hips, and forearm (the most common sites of fractures resulting from osteoporosis). DEXA studies are also useful to evaluate changes in bone density over time and to assess the effectiveness of treatment. DEXA results are frequently reported as T-scores.

Osteoporosis is quantitatively defined as a BMD of at least 2.5 standard deviations below the mean BMD of young adults. *Osteopenia* is defined as bone loss that is more than normal (a T-score less than or equal to a range of 1 to 2.5), but not yet at the level for a diagnosis of osteoporosis. Over 14 million women over age 50 have osteopenia.[34] Bone biopsy is also used to differentiate the diagnosis of osteoporosis from osteomalacia.

NURSING *and* COLLABORATIVE MANAGEMENT
OSTEOPOROSIS

Collaborative care of osteoporosis focuses on proper nutrition, calcium supplementation, exercise, prevention of fractures, and medications (Table 64-14). The National Osteoporosis Foundation (*www.nof.org*) recommends treatment for osteoporosis for postmenopausal women who have (1) a T-score of less than or equal to −2, (2) a T-score less than or equal to −1.5 with additional risk

TABLE 64-14	COLLABORATIVE CARE Osteoporosis

Diagnostic
History and physical examination
Serum calcium, phosphorus, alkaline phosphatase, and vitamin D levels
Bone mineral densitometry
Dual-energy x-ray absorptiometry (DEXA)
Quantitative ultrasound

Collaborative Therapy
Diet high in calcium (see Table 64-15)
Calcium supplements (see Table 64-16)
Vitamin D supplements
Exercise program
Estrogen replacement therapy
calcitonin (Calcimar)
Bisphosphonates
- alendronate (Fosamax)
- clodronate (Bonefos)
- etidronate (Didronel)
- ibandronate (Boniva)
- pamidronate (Aredia)
- risedronate (Actonel)
- tiludronate (Skelid)
Selective estrogen receptor modulator
- raloxifene (Evista)
- teriparatide (Forteo)

factors (see Table 64-13), or (3) prior history of a hip or vertebral fracture.[34]

Prevention and treatment of osteoporosis focuses on adequate calcium intake (1000 mg/day in premenopausal women and postmenopausal women taking estrogen and 1500 mg/day in postmenopausal women who are not receiving supplemental estrogen). If dietary intake of calcium is inadequate, supplemental calcium may be recommended. Foods that are high in calcium content include whole and skim milk, yogurt, turnip greens, cottage cheese, ice cream, sardines, and spinach (Table 64-15). The amount of elemental calcium varies in different calcium preparations (Table 64-16). Calcium supplementation inhibits age-related bone loss; however, no new bone is formed.

Vitamin D is important in calcium absorption and function and may have a role in bone formation. Most people get enough vitamin D from the diet or naturally through synthesis in the skin from exposure to sunlight. Being in the sun more than 20 min/day is generally enough. However, supplemental vitamin D (400 to 800 IU) may be recommended for older adults, those who are homebound, and those who get minimal sun exposure.

Moderate amounts of exercise are important to build up and maintain bone mass. Exercise also increases muscle strength, coordination, and balance. The best exercises are weight-bearing exercises that force an individual to work against gravity. These exercises include walking, hiking, weight training, stair climbing, tennis, and dancing. Walking is preferred to high-impact aerobics or running, both of which may put too much stress on the bones resulting in stress fractures. Walking 30 minutes, three times a week, is recommended.

Cigarette smoking and excess alcohol intake are risk factors for osteoporosis. Regular consumption of 2 to 3 ounces of alcohol a day may increase the degree of osteoporosis, even in young men and women. Patients should be instructed to quit smoking

TABLE 64-15	NUTRITIONAL THERAPY Sources of Calcium

Food	Calcium (mg)
1 cup milk	
Buttermilk	285
Whole	291
Skim	302
Half and half	254
Evaporated, canned	657
Eggnog	330
1 oz cheese	
American	174
Blue	150
Brie	52
Cheddar	130
Cottage	130
Parmesan	390
8 oz yogurt	415
1 cup ice cream	176
Soft serve	272
3 oz seafood	
Salmon	167
Sardines with bones	372
Oysters	113
1 medium stalk cooked broccoli	158
1 cup cooked spinach	200
1 cup turnip greens	252
1 cup bok choy	250
1 cup kale	206
Bonus Sources	
1 cup almonds	304
1 cup hazelnuts	240
1 tbs blackstrap molasses	137
Poor Sources	
Egg	28
1 cup cabbage	44
1 oz cream cheese	23
3 oz beef, pork, poultry	10
Apple, banana	10
1/2 grapefruit	20
1 med potato	14
1 med carrot	14
1/4 head lettuce	27

TABLE 64-16	Elemental Calcium Content of Various Oral Calcium Preparations

Calcium Preparation	Elemental Calcium Content
Calcium carbonate (Tums 500)	500 mg/tablet
Calcium carbonate + 5 mcg vitamin D_2 (Os-Cal 250)	250 mg/tablet
Calcium gluconate	40 mg/500 mg
Calcium carbonate	400 mg/g
Calcium lactate	80 mg/600 mg
Calcium citrate	40 mg/300 mg

therapy is most effective when combined with calcium (see Table 64-16). The greatest benefit of estrogen is probably in the first 10 years after menopause. Transdermal estrogen treatment (e.g., Menostar) given once a week in a very low dose has been shown to be effective in the prevention of osteoporosis in postmenopausal women by increasing bone density by 3%. Data from the Women's Health Initiative Study has indicated an increased risk for breast cancer and coronary events in women who took hormone replacement therapy (HRT).[38,39] Until further information is known, patients should discuss with their health care provider the potential risks and benefits of using HRT for osteoporosis prevention. (See Chapter 54 for further discussion of estrogen replacement therapy.)

Calcitonin is secreted by the thyroid gland and inhibits osteoclastic bone resorption by directly interacting with active osteoclasts. Salmon calcitonin (Calcimar) is available in intramuscular, subcutaneous, and intranasal forms. The nasal form is easy to administer, and patients should be taught to alternate nostrils daily. Nasal dryness and irritation are the most frequent side effects. Administration of the intramuscular or subcutaneous form of the drug at night has been shown to decrease the side effects of nausea and facial flushing. Nausea does not occur with the nasal spray. When calcitonin is used, calcium supplementation is necessary to prevent secondary hyperparathyroidism.[40]

Bisphosphonates inhibit osteoclast-mediated bone resorption, thereby increasing BMD and total bone mass. This group of drugs has been shown to increase BMD by 5%. These drugs include etidronate (Didronel), alendronate (Fosamax), pamidronate (Aredia), risedronate (Actonel), clodronate (Bonefos), tiludronate (Skelid), and ibandronate (Boniva). Common side effects are anorexia, weight loss, and gastritis. Patients should be instructed on the proper administration of a bisphosphonate to aid in its absorption (see Drug Alert). These precautions have been shown to decrease gastrointestinal side effects (especially esophageal irritation) and increase absorption. Alendronate is available as a once-per-week oral tablet and ibandronate is available as a once-per-month oral tablet. An injectable version of ibandronate that would last for 3 months is under development.

Drug Alert - Bisphosphonates
Instruct patient to:
• Take with full glass of water.
• Take 30 min before food or other medications.
• Remain upright for at least 30 min after taking.

Another type of drug used in treating osteoporosis is selective estrogen receptor modulators, such as raloxifene (Evista). These drugs mimic the effect of estrogen on bone by reducing bone re-

and cut down on alcohol intake to decrease the likelihood of losing bone mass.

Although loss of bone cannot be significantly reversed, further loss can be prevented if the patient follows a regimen of calcium and vitamin D supplementation, exercise, estrogen replacement, and alendronate (Fosamax) or raloxifene (Evista), if indicated. Efforts should be made to keep patients with osteoporosis ambulatory to prevent further loss of bone substance as a result of immobility. Treatment also involves the use of a gait aid as needed, and protecting areas of potential pathologic fractures. For example, a corset can be used to prevent vertebral collapse. (Fractures are discussed in Chapter 63.)

■ **Drug Therapy**

Estrogen replacement therapy after menopause may be used to prevent osteoporosis. Although the exact mechanism for the protective function of estrogen is not known, it is believed that estrogen inhibits osteoclast activity, leading to decreased bone resorption and preventing both cortical and trabecular bone loss. Estrogen replacement sorption without stimulating the tissues of the breast or uterus. Raloxifene in postmenopausal women significantly increases BMD. The most commonly reported side effects are leg cramps and hot flashes.

Teriparatide (Forteo) is used for the treatment of osteoporosis in men and postmenopausal women who are at high risk for having a fracture. Teriparatide is a portion of human parathyroid hormone (PTH) and works by increasing the action of osteoblasts. Teriparatide is the first drug approved for the treatment of osteoporosis that stimulates new bone formation. Most drugs used to treat osteoporosis prevent further bone loss. Teriparatide is administered by subcutaneous injection once a day.[41] Side effects can include leg cramps and dizziness. This drug is expensive, and long-term use (>2 years) may increase the risk for osteosarcoma.

Medical management of patients receiving corticosteroids includes prescribing the lowest possible dose of the drug. In addition, calcium and vitamin D supplementation is needed. If osteopenia is evident on bone densitometry, treatment with bisphosphonate agents, such as alendronate (Fosamax), should be considered.

PAGET'S DISEASE

Paget's disease *(osteitis deformans)* is a skeletal bone disorder in which there is excessive bone resorption followed by replacement of normal marrow by vascular, fibrous connective tissue. The new bone is larger, disorganized, and structurally weaker. The regions of the skeleton commonly affected are the pelvis, long bones, spine, ribs, sternum, and cranium. The etiology of Paget's disease is unknown, although a viral cause has been proposed. Up to 40% of all patients with Paget's disease have at least one relative with the disorder. Men are affected 2:1 over women, and Paget's disease is rarely seen in persons under 40 years of age.[42]

In milder forms of Paget's disease, patients may remain free of symptoms, and the disease may be discovered incidentally on x-ray or serum chemistry. The initial clinical manifestations are usually insidious development of bone pain (which may progress to severe intractable pain), complaints of fatigue, and progressive development of a waddling gait. Patients may complain that they are becoming shorter or that their heads are becoming larger. Headaches, dementia, visual deficits, and loss of hearing can result with an enlarged, thickened skull. Increased bone volume in the spine can cause spinal cord or nerve root compression. Pathologic fracture is the most common complication of Paget's disease and may be the first indication of the disease. Other complications include osteosarcoma, fibrosarcoma, and osteoclastoma (giant cell) tumors.

Serum alkaline phosphatase levels are markedly elevated (indicating high bone turnover) in advanced forms of the disease. X-rays may demonstrate that the normal contour of the affected bone is curved and the bone cortex is thickened and irregular, especially the weight-bearing bones and cranium. Bone scans using a radiolabeled bisphosphate demonstrate increased uptake in the skeletal areas affected.

Collaborative care of Paget's disease is usually limited to symptomatic and supportive care and correction of secondary deformities by either surgical intervention or braces. Bone resorption, relief of acute symptoms, and lowering the serum alkaline phosphatase levels may be significantly influenced by the administration of human calcitonin (Cibacalcin), which inhibits osteoclastic activity. It is available as a subcutaneous injection. Salmon calcitonin (Calcimar) can also be used as a subcutaneous or IM injection for treat-

ing Paget's disease. Salmon calcitonin has a longer half-life and greater milligram potency than human calcitonin. Response to calcitonin therapy is not permanent and often stops when therapy is discontinued. Bisphosphonate drugs, including risedronate (Actonel), etidronate (Didronel), pamidronate (Aredia), ibandronate (Boniva), tiludronate (Skelid), and alendronate (Fosamax), are also used to retard bone resorption. Calcium and vitamin D are often given to decrease hypocalcemia, a common side effect with these drugs. Drug effectiveness may be monitored by serum alkaline phosphatase levels. Calcitonin therapy is recommended for patients who cannot tolerate bisphosphonate drugs. Pain is usually managed by NSAIDs. Orthopedic surgery for fractures, hip and knee replacements, and knee realignment may be necessary.

A firm mattress should be used to provide back support and to relieve pain. The patient may be required to wear a corset or light brace to relieve back pain and provide support when in the upright position. The patient should be proficient in the correct application of such devices and know how to regularly examine areas of the skin for friction damage. Activities such as lifting and twisting should be discouraged. Physical therapy may increase muscle strength. Good body mechanics are essential. A properly balanced nutrition program is important in the management of metabolic disorders of bone, especially pertaining to vitamin D, calcium, and protein, which are necessary to ensure the availability of the components for bone formation. Prevention measures such as patient education, use of an assistive device, and environmental changes should be actively pursued to prevent falls and subsequent fractures.[43]

GERONTOLOGIC CONSIDERATIONS
METABOLIC BONE DISEASES

Osteoporosis and Paget's disease are common in older adults. Patients should be instructed in proper nutritional management to prevent further bone loss such as that occurring from osteoporosis.

Because metabolic bone disorders increase the possibility of pathologic fractures, the nurse must use extreme caution when the patient is turned or moved. It is important to keep the patient as active as possible to retard demineralization of bone resulting from disuse or extended immobilization. A supervised exercise program is an essential part of the treatment program. If the patient's condition permits, ambulation without causing fatigue must be encouraged.

CRITICAL THINKING EXERCISE

CASE STUDY

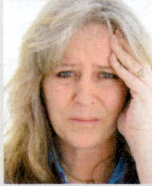

Case Study photo ©iStockphoto.com/ Roberta Osborne.

Osteoporosis

Patient Profile. Alice Lang is a 58-year-old white librarian who had a total hysterectomy and salpingo-oophorectomy for removal of a benign ovarian cyst 4 years ago. She also has a history of a seizure disorder since childhood and Addison's disease.

Subjective Data
• Experiences chronic, mild lumbar pain and tenderness that radiates to her right hip and the lateral thigh
• Regular walking offers some relief
• Had a stress fracture in wrist 6 months ago

- Reports no noticeable loss of height
- Has maternal history of osteoporosis
- Has been taking corticosteroids and mineralocorticoids for past 6 years for Addison's disease
- Has been taking phenytoin (Dilantin) every evening
- Drinks socially—two alcoholic beverages per day
- Dislikes dairy products

Objective Data
- 5 feet 6 inches tall, 116 lb

Diagnostic Studies
- Bone mass/density tests show decreased bone mineral density at spine and hip
- Lumbar spine radiographs reveal a nondisplaced L4 compression fracture
- Laboratory tests reveal normal serum calcium, phosphorus, and alkaline phosphatase levels

Collaborative Care
- Premarin 0.625 mg PO daily
- alendronate (Fosamax) 70 mg PO once/wk
- Calcium supplements 1500 mg PO daily
- High-calcium diet
- Reduce alcohol intake
- Maintain regular low-impact weight-bearing exercise program

Critical Thinking Questions

1. What risk factors made Alice prone to develop osteoporosis?
2. Why does regular exercise help Alice's symptoms?
3. What is the purpose of prescribing estrogen replacement for Alice?
4. What is the priority nursing intervention for Alice?
5. What teaching should the nurse provide to Alice regarding alendronate?
6. How might the nurse assist Alice in increasing her intake of calcium?
7. Based on the assessment data presented, write one or more nursing diagnoses. Are there any collaborative problems?

NCLEX EXAMINATION REVIEW QUESTIONS

The number of the question corresponds to the same-numbered objective at the beginning of the chapter.

1. A patient with osteomyelitis is treated with surgical debridement followed by continuous irrigation of the affected bone with antibiotics. In responding to the patient who asks why oral or IV antibiotics cannot be used alone, the nurse explains that
   a. the irrigation is necessary to wash out dead tissue and pus from the infected area.
   b. there are no effective oral or IV antibiotics to treat *S. aureus*, the most common cause of osteomyelitis.
   c. an irrigation can penetrate involucrum created by the infection and prevent bacterial spreading to other tissue.
   d. the ischemia and bone death associated with osteomyelitis are frequently impenetrable to most blood-borne antibiotics.

2. A patient with metastatic bone cancer has a nursing diagnosis of risk for injury (pathologic fracture) related to bone tissue changes. The nursing management of this patient is primarily directed toward
   a. preventing pain.
   b. relieving edema.
   c. increasing physical mobility.
   d. supporting and positioning the leg.

3. In identifying people at risk for back injuries, the nurse recognizes that the person at greatest risk for low back pain is a(n)
   a. long-distance truck driver.
   b. 62-year-old widow who walks daily.
   c. aerobics instructor who weighs 100 lb.
   d. 25-year-old nurse who works in a newborn nursery.

4. The primary nursing responsibility in caring for a patient with a suspected disk herniation who presents with severe pain and muscle spasms is
   a. teaching exercises such as straight-leg raises to decrease pain.
   b. positioning the patient on the abdomen with the legs extended.
   c. providing pain medication to promote an early return to exercise and ambulation.
   d. assisting the patient to maintain activity restrictions with a gradual increase in activity.

5. In caring for the patient after a spinal fusion, the nurse recognizes that interventions for this surgery differ from a simple laminectomy in that
   a. body alignment is maintained by the fusion procedure.
   b. earlier ambulation is permitted because the spine is more stabilized.
   c. the donor site for the bone graft may be more painful than the spinal incision.
   d. teaching regarding body mechanics and prevention of future back injuries is not as critical.

6. Before discharge from the same-day surgery unit, the nurse instructs the patient who has had a surgical correction of bilateral hallux valgus to
   a. rest frequently with the feet elevated.
   b. soak the feet in warm water several times a day.
   c. walk primarily on the heels to relieve pressure on the toes.
   d. expect the feet to be numb for several days postoperatively.

7. The nurse advises the patient with early osteoporosis (osteopenia) to
   a. lose weight.
   b. stop smoking.
   c. eat a high-protein diet.
   d. start swimming for exercise.

REFERENCES

1. Crowley LV: *An introduction to human disease: pathology and pathophysiology considerations,* Sudbury, Mass., 2004, Jones & Bartlett.
2. Zvulunov G, Segev Z: Acute hematogenous osteomyelitis of the pelvis in childhood: diagnostic clues and pitfalls, *Pediatric Emergency Care* 19:29, 2003.
3. Weinstein MA, Eismont FJ: Infections of the spine in patients with human immunodeficiency virus, *J Bone Joint Surg* 87:604, 2005.
4. Bosse MJ, Gruber HE, Ramp WK: Internalization of bacteria by osteoblasts in a patient with recurrent, long term osteomyelitis, *J Bone Joint Surg Am* 87:1343, 2005.
5. Salmond S, Fine C: Infections of the musculoskeletal system. In Maher AB, Salmond SW, Pellino TA, editors: *Orthopaedic nursing,* ed 3, St Louis, 2002, Saunders.
6. Sumner J: Bone and soft-tissue sarcomas. In Yarbro C, Frogge M, Goodman M, editors: *Cancer nursing,* ed 6, Sudbury, Mass., 2005, Jones & Bartlett.
7. Jemal A, Murray T, Ward E, et al: Cancer statistics, 2005, *CA Cancer J Clin* 55:10, 2005.
8. Maylivahanan N, Bose JC, Paraskumar M, et al: Paget's sarcoma: limb salvage by custom mega prostheses, *J Orthop Surg (Hong Kong)* 12:243, 2004.
9. Davidson AW, Hong A, McCarthy SW, et al: En-bloc resection, extracorporeal irradiation, and reimplantation in limb salvage for bony malignancies, *J Bone Joint Surg Br* 87:851, 2005.
10. St. Jude's Children's Research Hospital: Osteogenic sarcoma. Available at *www.stjude.org/disease-summaries* (accessed August 31, 2006).
11. American Cancer Society: Detailed guide: bone metastasis. Available at *www.cancer.org* (accessed August 31, 2006).

12. Walsh CR: Tumors of the musculoskeletal system. In Taggert H, editor: *NAON: core curriculum for orthopaedic nursing,* ed 5, Boston, 2006, Pearson Custom Publishing.

13. Porth CM, Curtis R: Alterations in neuromuscular function. In Porth CM, editor: *Essentials of pathophysiology: concepts of altered health states,* ed 7, Philadelphia, 2004, Lippincott Williams & Wilkins.

14. Beenakker EA, Foch JM, Van Tol MJ, et al: Intermittent prednisone therapy in Duchenne muscular dystrophy: a randomized controlled study, *Arch Neurol* 62:128, 2005.

15. Bostrom K, Ahlstrom G: Quality of life in patients with muscular dystrophy and their next of kin, *Int J Rehabil Res* 28:103, 2005.

16. Blue C, Levin P: Ergonomics. In Maher AB, Salmond SW, Pellino TA, editors: *Orthopaedic nursing,* ed 3, St Louis, 2002, Saunders.

17. Landers SJ: Aching backs and shoulders taking a toll, *Am Med News* 48:33, 2005.

18. Shekelle PG, Delitto AM: Treating low back pain, *Lancet* 365:1987, 2005.

19. Deyo RA: Treatments for back pain: can we get past trivial effects? *Ann Intern Med* 141:958, 2004.

20. Anonymous: Primary care interventions to prevent low back pain in adults: recommendation statement, *Am Fam Physician* 71:2337, 2005.

21. Petropoulos P: Spinal stenosis lumbar. In Ferri FR, editor: *Ferri's clinical advisor: instant diagnosis and treatment,* St Louis, 2006, Mosby.

22. Hainline B: Chronic pain: physiological, diagnostic, and management considerations, *Psychiatric Clin North Am* 28:713, 2005.

23. Roh J, Teng AL, Yoo JU, el al: Degenerative disorders of the lumbar and cervical spine, *Orthop Clin North Am* 36:255, 2005.

24. Johns Hopkins University: Back pain: the evidence points to "heal thyself", *Health After 50 Newsletter* 17:4, 2004.

25. Bezyack M: Getting back at back pain: emerging techniques in spinal surgery. Available at *www.nurseweek.com* (accessed August 31, 2006).

26. U.S. Food and Drug Administration: PMA final decisions rendered for November 2005: X STOP Interspinous Process Decompression System, Available at *www.fda.gov/cdrh/pdf4/p040001.html* (accessed August 31, 2006).

27. U.S. Food and Drug Administration: FDA Talk Paper: FDA approves artificial disc; another alternative to treat low back pain. Available at *www.fda.gov/bbs/topics/ANSWERS/2004/ANS01320.html* (accessed August 31, 2006).

28. Author. Surgical technology: transforaminal lumbar interbody fusion with minimal access study released, *Pain Central Nervous System Week* 217, 2005. Available at *www.newsrx.com/newsletters* (accessed September 2, 2006).

29. Cleveland Clinic: Neck pain: what causes it, how to treat it, *Arthritis Advisor* 5:1, 2006. Available at *www.arthritis-advisor.com.*

30. Oh IS, Kim MK, Lee SH: New modified technique of osteotomy for hallux valgus, *J Orthop Surg (Hong Kong)* 12:235, 2004.

31. Boulton AJ, Kirsner RS, Vileikyte L: Clinical practice: neuropathic diabetic foot ulcers, *N Engl J Med* 351:48, 2004.

32. Lyman D: Undiagnosed vitamin D deficiency in the hospitalized patient, *Am Fam Physician* 71:299, 2005.

33. Burke SM: Osteoporosis: a neglected but treatable disease, *Ann Long-Term Care* 12:20, 2004.

34. U.S. Preventive Services Task Force: Screening for osteoporosis in postmenopausal women: rationale and recommendations, *Am J Nurs* 103:73, 2003. Available at *www.preventiveservices.ahrg.gov.*

35. South-Paul J: Nonvertebral fractures due to post menopausal osteoporosis: evaluation of effective preventive interventions, *Clin Geriatr* 13:30, 2005.

36. Hetzell C: New help for old bones, *Nursing* 35(5):20, 2005.

37. Satoshi S, et al: Glucocorticoid-induced osteoporosis: skeletal manifestations of glucocorticoid use and 2004 Japanese Society for Bone and Mineral Research-proposed guidelines for its management, *Mod Rheumatol* 15:163, 2005.

38. National Institutes of Health: Postmenopausal hormone therapy. Available at *www.nhibi.nih.gov/health/women* (accessed August 31, 2006).

39. Barrett-Connor E, Grady D, Stefanick ML: The rise and fall of menopausal hormone therapy, *Annu Rev Public Health* 126:115, 2005.

40. Kuehn BM: Longer lasting osteoporosis drugs sought, *JAMA* 293:2458, 2005.

41. Zizic T: Pharmacological prevention of osteoporotic fractures, *Am Fam Physician* 70:1293, 2004.

42. Roodman GD, Windle JJ: Paget disease of bone, *J Clin Invest* 115:200, 2005.

*43. McCarter-Bayer A, Bayer F, Hall K: Fall prevention in acute care: an innovative approach, *J Gerontol Nurs* 31(3):25, 2005.

RESOURCES

American Academy of Orthopedic Surgeons (AAOS)
800-346-AAOS or 847-823-7186
www.aaos.org

American Cancer Society
800-ACS-2345
www.cancer.org

American College of Foot and Ankle Surgeons (ACFAS)
773-693-9304
www.acfas.org

American College of Sports Medicine
317-637-9200
www.acsm.org/

American Podiatric Medical Association
800-FOOT-CARE
www.apma.org

Cancer Survivors Network
800-333-HOPE (4673)
www.acscsn.org

International Osteoporosis Foundation
www.osteofound.org

Muscular Dystrophy Association
800-344-4683
www.mdausa.org

National Association of Orthopaedic Nurses (NAON)
856-256-6266
www.orthonurse.org

National Institute of Arthritis and Musculoskeletal and Skin Disorders Information Clearinghouse, National Institutes of Health
877-22-NIAMS or 301-495-4484
www.nih.gov/niams

National Osteoporosis Foundation
800-223-9994
www.nof.org

NIH Osteoporosis and Related Bone Diseases—National Resource Center
www.niams.gov/bone

Older Women's League
800-825-3695
www.owl-national.org

The Paget Foundation for Paget Disease of Bone and Related Disorders
212-509-5335
www.paget.org

For additional Internet resources, see the website for this book at *http://evolve.elsevier.com/Lewis/medsurg.*

*Nursing research–based reference.

Nursing Management
Arthritis and Connective Tissue Diseases

65

Dottie Roberts

LEARNING OBJECTIVES

1. Compare and contrast the sequence of events leading to joint destruction in osteoarthritis and rheumatoid arthritis.
2. Describe the clinical manifestations, collaborative care, and nursing management of osteoarthritis and rheumatoid arthritis.
3. Compare and contrast the pathophysiology, clinical manifestations, collaborative care, and nursing management of ankylosing spondylitis, psoriatic arthritis, and reactive arthritis.
4. Describe the pathophysiology, clinical manifestations, and collaborative care of septic arthritis, Lyme disease, and gout.
5. Describe the pathophysiology, clinical manifestations, collaborative care, and nursing management of systemic lupus erythematosus, polymyositis, dermatomyositis, and Sjögren's syndrome.
6. Describe the drug therapy and related nursing management associated with arthritis and connective tissue diseases.
7. Compare and contrast the possible etiologies, clinical manifestations, and collaborative and nursing management of myofascial pain syndrome, fibromyalgia syndrome, and chronic fatigue syndrome.

KEY TERMS

ankylosing spondylitis, p. 1711
arthritis, p. 1693
chronic fatigue syndrome, p. 1728
dermatomyositis, p. 1725
fibromyalgia syndrome, p. 1727
gout, p. 1715
Lyme disease, p. 1714
myofascial pain syndrome, p. 1726
osteoarthritis, p. 1693
polymyositis, p. 1725
Raynaud's phenomenon, p. 1723
rheumatoid arthritis, p. 1702
Sjögren's syndrome, p. 1726
systemic lupus erythematosus, p. 1716
systemic sclerosis, p. 1723

Electronic Resources

Supplemental content related to Chapter 65 can be found . . .

Companion CD
- Stress-Busting Kit for Nursing Students
- Interactive Case Studies:
  - Rheumatoid Arthritis
  - Systemic Lupus Erythematosus
- NCLEX Examination Review Questions
- Comprehensive Glossary

Evolve Website *evolve*
http://evolve.elsevier.com/Lewis/medsurg
- Content Updates
- Key Points (Printable and CD/MP3 Download)
- Concept Map Creator
- Expanded Audio Glossary
- Key Term Flash Cards
- Customizable Nursing Care Plans:
  - Rheumatoid Arthritis
  - Systemic Lupus Erythematosus

- Patient and Family Instruction Guides in English and Spanish:
  - Joint Protection and Energy Conservation
  - Protection of Small Joints
- Electronic Calculators
- WebLinks

Arthritis

Arthritis refers to the inflammation of a joint, while *rheumatic disease* involves the bones and muscles as well as the joints.[1] Over 100 different types of arthritis and rheumatic disorders exist. It is estimated that, by the year 2030, 65 million Americans will be affected by arthritis.[2] Arthritis affects women twice as much as men, and the economic cost to the United States is estimated at $83 bil-

lion.[1] The most prevalent types of arthritis are osteoarthritis, rheumatoid arthritis, and gout.

OSTEOARTHRITIS

Osteoarthritis (OA), the most common form of joint (articular) disease in North America, is a slowly progressive noninflammatory disorder of the diarthrodial (synovial) joints. Currently 20 million Americans are affected by OA, with the numbers ex-

Reviewed by Geri B. Neuberger, RN, EdD, Professor, School of Nursing, University of Kansas, Kansas City, Kan.

pected to greatly increase as the population ages. Previously identified as *degenerative joint disease* or degenerative arthritis, it is now known to involve the formation of new joint tissue in response to cartilage destruction.[3]

Etiology and Pathophysiology

OA is no longer considered to be a normal part of the aging process, but growing older continues to be consistently identified as one risk factor for disease development.[4] Cartilage destruction can actually begin between ages 20 and 30, and the majority of adults are affected by age 40. Few patients experience symptoms until after age 50 or 60, but more than half of those over 65 years of age have x-ray evidence of the disease in at least one joint.[5] Before the age of 50, men are more often affected than women. However, the incidence of OA after age 50 is higher in women than men.

OA may occur as an idiopathic (formerly primary) or secondary disorder. The cause of idiopathic OA is unknown. Secondary OA, on the other hand, is caused by a known event or condition that directly damages cartilage or causes joint instability (Table 65-1).

Researchers have been unable to identify a single cause for OA, but a number of factors have been linked to disease development. The increased incidence of OA in aging women is believed to be due to estrogen reduction at menopause. Genetic factors also appear to play a significant role in the occurrence of OA. Modifiable risk factors have been identified, including obesity, which contributes to hip and knee OA. Regular moderate exercise, which also helps with weight control, has been shown to decrease the likelihood of disease development and progression. Overuse of knees by strenuous exercise with quick stops and pivoting as in football and soccer has been linked to an increased risk of knee OA.[6] Occupations that require frequent kneeling and stooping are also linked to a higher risk of knee OA.

OA results from cartilage damage that triggers a metabolic response at the level of the chondrocytes (Fig. 65-1). Progression of OA causes the normally smooth, white, translucent articular cartilage to become dull, yellow, and granular. Affected cartilage gradually becomes softer, less elastic, and less able to resist wear with heavy use. The body's attempts at cartilage repair cannot keep up with the destruction that is occurring. Continued changes in the collagen structure of the cartilage lead to fissuring and erosion of the articular surfaces. As the central cartilage becomes thinner, cartilage and bony growth (osteophytes) increase at the joint margins. The resulting incongruity in joint surfaces creates an uneven distribution of stress across the joint and contributes to a reduction in motion.

While inflammation is not characteristic of OA, a secondary synovitis may result when phagocytic cells try to rid the joint of small pieces of cartilage torn from the joint surface. These inflammatory changes contribute to the early pain and stiffness of OA. The pain of later disease results from contact between exposed bony joint surfaces after the articular cartilage has completely deteriorated.

Clinical Manifestations

Systemic. Systemic manifestations, such as fatigue, fever, and organ involvement, are not present in OA. This is an important distinction between OA and inflammatory joint disorders such as rheumatoid arthritis.

Joints. Manifestations of OA range from mild discomfort to significant disability. Joint pain is the predominant symptom of OA and the typical reason that the patient seeks medical attention. Pain generally worsens with joint use. In the early stages of OA, joint pain is relieved by rest. In advanced disease, however, the patient may complain of pain with rest or experience sleep disruptions caused by increasing joint discomfort. Pain may also become worse as the barometric pressure falls before inclement weather. As OA progresses, increasing pain can contribute significantly to disability and loss of function. The pain of OA may be referred to the groin, buttock, or medial side of the thigh or knee. Sitting down becomes difficult, as does rising from a chair when the hips are lower than the knees. As OA develops in the intervertebral (apophyseal) joints of the spine, localized pain and stiffness are common.

Unlike pain, which is typically provoked by activity, joint stiffness occurs after periods of rest or static position. Early morning stiffness is common but generally resolves within 30 minutes, a factor distinguishing OA from inflammatory arthritic disorders. Overactivity can cause a mild joint effusion that temporarily increases stiffness. *Crepitation,* a grating sensation caused by loose particles of cartilage in the joint cavity, can also contribute to stiffness. Crepitation indicates the loss of cartilage integrity and is present in more than 90% of patients with knee OA.

TABLE 65-1	**Causes of Secondary Osteoarthritis**
Cause	**Effects on Joint Cartilage**
Trauma	Dislocations or fractures may lead to avascular necrosis or uneven stress on cartilage.
Mechanical stress	Repetitive physical activities (e.g., sports activities) cause cartilage deterioration.
Inflammation	Release of enzymes in response to local inflammation can affect cartilage integrity.
Joint instability	Damage to supporting structures causes instability, placing uneven stress on articular cartilage.
Neurologic disorders	Pain and loss of reflexes from neurologic disorders, such as diabetic neuropathy, and Charcot joint cause abnormal movements that contribute to cartilage deterioration.
Skeletal deformities	Congenital or acquired conditions such as Legg-Calvé-Perthes disease or dislocated hip contribute to cartilage deterioration.
Hematologic/endocrine disorders	Chronic hemarthrosis (e.g., hemophilia) can contribute to cartilage deterioration.
Use of selected drugs	Drugs such as indomethacin (Indocin), colchicine, and corticosteroids can stimulate collagen-digesting enzymes in joint synovium.

GENDER DIFFERENCES

Osteoarthritis

Men	**Women**
• Men are more often affected than women before the age of 50.	• Women are affected twice as often as men after the age of 50.
• Hip OA is more common in men after the age of 55.	• OA in interphalangeal joints and thumb base is more common in women after the age of 55.
• Knee OA is more common in men before the age of 45.	• Knee OA is more common in women after the age of 45.

OA, Osteoarthritis.

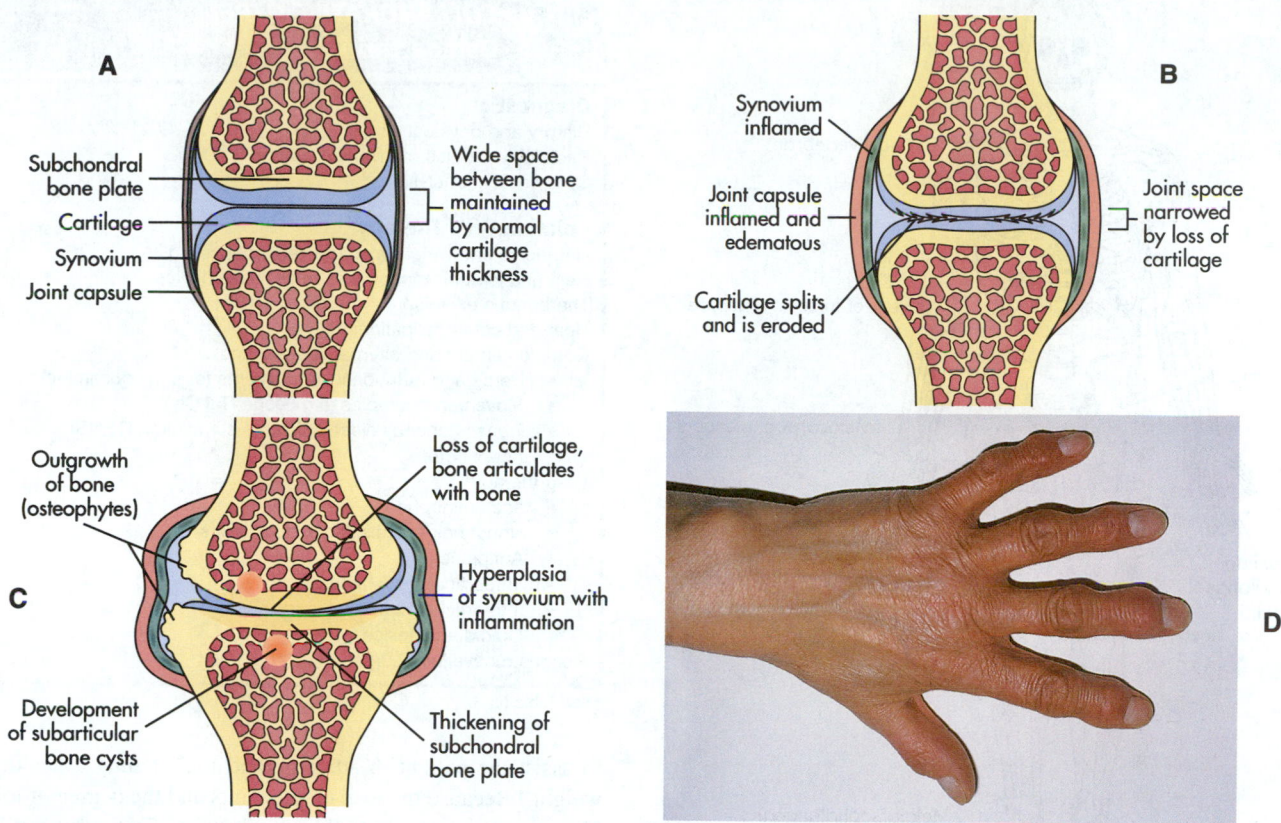

FIG. 65-1 Pathologic changes in osteoarthritis. **A,** Normal synovial joint. **B,** Early change in osteoarthritis is destruction of articular cartilage and narrowing of the joint space. There is inflammation and thickening of the joint capsule and synovium. **C,** With time, there is thickening of subarticular bone caused by constant friction of the two bone surfaces. Osteophytes form around the periphery of the joint by irregular overgrowths of bone. **D,** In osteoarthritis of the hands, osteophytes on the distal interphalangeal joints of the fingers are termed Heberden's nodes and appear as small nodules.

OA usually affect joints asymmetrically. The most commonly involved joints are the distal interphalangeal (DIP) and proximal interphalangeal (PIP) joints of the fingers, the metacarpophalangeal (MCP) joint of the thumb, weight-bearing joints (hips, knees), the metatarsophalangeal (MTP) joint of the foot, and the cervical and lower lumbar vertebrae (Fig. 65-2).

Deformity. Deformity or instability associated with OA is specific to the involved joint. For example, *Heberden's nodes* occur on the DIP joints as an indication of osteophyte formation and loss of joint space (see Fig. 65-1, *D*). They can appear in the OA patient as early as age 40 and tend to be seen in family members. *Bouchard's nodes* on the PIP joints indicate similar disease involvement. Heberden's and Bouchard's nodes are often red, swollen, and tender. Although these bony enlargements do not usually cause significant loss of function, the patient may be distressed by the visible disfigurement.

Knee OA often leads to joint malalignment as a result of cartilage loss in the medial compartment. The patient has a characteristic bowlegged appearance and may develop an altered gait in response to the obvious deformity. In advanced hip OA, one of the patient's legs may become shorter from a loss of joint space.

Diagnostic Studies

A bone scan, computed tomography (CT) scan, or magnetic resonance imaging (MRI) may be useful in early OA because of the sensitivity of these tests to detect joint changes. X-rays are helpful in confirming disease and staging the progression of joint damage.

As OA progresses, x-rays typically show joint space narrowing, bony sclerosis, and osteophyte formation. However, these changes do not always correlate with the degree of pain experienced by the patient. Despite significant radiologic indications of disease, the patient may be relatively free of symptoms. Conversely, another patient may have severe pain with only minimal x-ray changes.

No laboratory abnormalities or biomarkers have been identified that are specific diagnostic indicators of OA. The erythrocyte sedimentation rate (ESR) is normal except in instances of acute synovitis, when minimal elevations may be noted. Other routine blood tests (e.g., complete blood count [CBC], renal and liver function tests) are useful only in screening for related conditions or for establishing baseline values before the initiation of therapy. Synovial fluid analysis allows differentiation between OA and other forms of inflammatory arthritis. In the presence of OA, the fluid remains clear yellow with little or no sign of inflammation.

Collaborative Care

Because there is no cure for OA, collaborative care focuses on managing pain and inflammation, preventing disability, and maintaining and improving joint function (Table 65-2). Nonpharmacologic interventions are the foundation for OA management and should be maintained throughout the patient's treatment period. Drug therapy serves as an adjunct to nonpharmacologic treatments. Symptoms of disease are often managed conservatively for many years, but the patient's loss of joint function, unrelieved pain, and diminished ability to independently perform self-care may

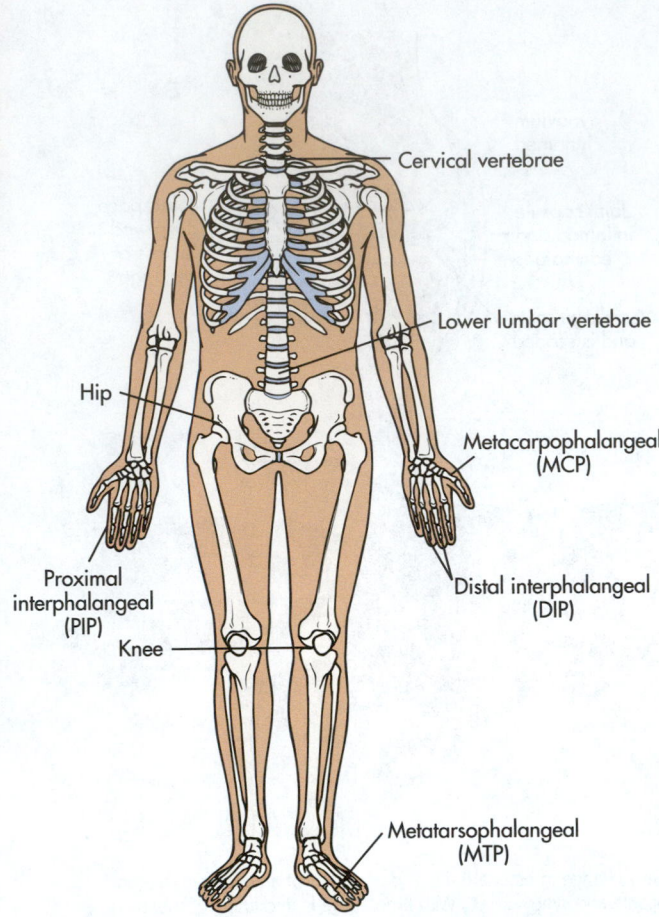

Cervical vertebrae

Lower lumbar vertebrae

Hip

Metacarpophalangeal
(MCP)

Proximal
interphalangeal
(PIP)

Distal interphalangeal
(DIP)

Knee

Metatarsophalangeal
(MTP)

FIG. 65-2 Joints most frequently involved in osteoarthritis.

TABLE 65-2	*COLLABORATIVE CARE* **Osteoarthritis**

Diagnostic
History and physical examination
Radiologic studies of involved joints
Synovial fluid analysis

Collaborative Therapy
Nutritional and weight management counseling
Rest and joint protection, use of assistive devices
Therapeutic exercise
Heat and cold applications
Complementary and alternative therapies
- Herbs and nutritional supplements (e.g., glucosamine)
- Movement therapies (e.g., yoga, Tai Chi)
- Transcutaneous electrical nerve stimulation (TENS)
- Acupuncture
Drug therapy*
- acetaminophen
- Nonsteroidal antiinflammatory drugs
- Antibiotics
- Intraarticular hyaluronic acid
- Intraarticular corticosteroids
- Opioid analgesics
Reconstructive joint surgery

*See Table 65-3.

prompt a recommendation for surgery. Reconstructive surgical procedures are discussed in Chapter 63. In general, arthroscopic surgery for debridement is usually not recommended for OA. However, arthroscopic surgery to repair cartilage or ligament tears or remove bone bits or cartilage is effective in reducing pain and improving function.[7]

Rest and Joint Protection. The OA patient must understand the importance of a balance of rest and activity. The affected joint should be rested during any periods of acute inflammation and maintained in a functional position with splints or braces if necessary. However, immobilization should not exceed 1 week because of the risk of joint stiffness with inactivity. The patient may need to modify his or her usual activities to decrease stress on affected joints. For example, the patient with knee OA should avoid prolonged periods of standing, kneeling, or squatting. Using an assistive device such as a cane, walker, or crutches can also help decrease stress on arthritic joints.

Heat and Cold Applications. Applications of heat and cold may help reduce complaints of pain and stiffness. Although ice is not used as often as heat in the treatment of OA, it can be appropriate if the patient experiences acute inflammation. Heat therapy is especially helpful for stiffness, including hot packs, whirlpool baths, ultrasound, and paraffin wax baths.

Nutritional Therapy and Exercise. If the patient is overweight, a weight-reduction program is a critical part of the total treatment plan. The nurse should help the patient evaluate the current diet to make appropriate changes. (Chapter 41 discusses ways

to assist the patient in attaining and maintaining a healthy body weight.) Because the load on the joints and the degree of joint mobilization are essential to the preservation of articular cartilage integrity, the American College of Rheumatology has identified exercise as a fundamental part of OA management.[8] Aerobic conditioning and specific programs for muscle strengthening have led to a modest reduction in pain and disability for some patients with knee OA.

Complementary and Alternative Therapies. Complementary and alternative therapies for symptom management of arthritis have become increasingly popular with patients who have failed to find relief through traditional medical care. Acupuncture, for example, has been found to be a safe and effective method for arthritis pain management.[9] Other therapies include the use of yoga, massage, guided imagery, and therapeutic touch (see Chapter 8). In particular, the use of nutritional supplements such as glucosamine and chondroitin sulfate for relieving moderate to severe arthritis pain in the knees and improving joint mobility has shown promising results. These promising results were not noted in patients with mild OA[10] (see the Complementary and Alternative Therapies box).

Drug Therapy. Drug therapy is based on the severity of the patient's symptoms (Table 65-3). The patient with mild to moderate joint pain may receive relief from acetaminophen (Tylenol). The patient may receive up to 1000 mg every 6 hours, with the daily dose not to exceed 4 g. A topical agent such as capsaicin cream (Zostrix) may also be beneficial, either alone or in conjunction with acetaminophen. It blocks pain by locally interfering with substance P, which is responsible for the transmission of pain impulses. A concentrated product is available by prescription, but creams of 0.025% to 0.075% capsaicin are sold over the counter (OTC). Additional OTC products that contain camphor, eucalyptus oil, and menthol (e.g., BenGay, ArthriCare) may also provide temporary pain relief. Topical salicylates (e.g., Aspercreme) that can be absorbed into the blood are another alternative for patients who are able to take aspirin-containing medication.

For the patient who fails to obtain adequate pain management with acetaminophen or for the patient with moderate to severe OA pain, a nonsteroidal antiinflammatory drug (NSAID) may provide greater relief. NSAID therapy is typically initiated in low-dose OTC strengths (ibuprofen [Motrin] 200 mg up to four times daily), with the dose increased as patient symptoms indicate. If the patient is at risk for or experiences gastrointestinal (GI) side effects with a conventional NSAID, supplemental treatment with a protective agent such as misoprostol (Cytotec) may be indicated. Arthrotec, a combination of misoprostol and the NSAID diclofenac (Voltaren), is also available.

Because traditional NSAIDs block the production of prostaglandins from arachidonic acid by inhibiting the production of cyclooxygenase-1 (COX-1) and cyclooxygenase-2 (COX-2) (see Fig. 13-5), the risk for GI erosion and bleeding is increased. Traditional NSAIDs affect platelet aggregation, leading to a prolonged bleeding time. Patients on both warfarin (Coumadin) and an NSAID are at high risk for bleeding. Concerns have also been raised regarding the possible negative effects of long-term NSAID treatment on cartilage metabolism, particularly in older patients who may already have diminished cartilage integrity. As an alternative to traditional NSAIDs, treatment with the COX-2 inhibitor celecoxib (Celebrex) may be considered in selected patients.[11] Two other COX-2 inhibitors (valdecoxib [Bextra], rofecoxib [Vioxx]) were withdrawn from the market after several large studies indicated increased cardiovascular risks for patients after 18 months of treatment. Additional studies are underway for further evaluation of this class of drugs.[11]

When given in equivalent antiinflammatory dosages, all NSAIDs are considered comparable in efficacy but vary widely in cost. Individual responses to the NSAIDs are also variable. Aspirin is still preferred by some patients, but it is no longer a common treatment, and it should not be used in combination with NSAIDs because both inhibit platelet function and prolong bleeding time.

Antibiotics may also be useful in the treatment of OA. Doxycycline (Vibramycin) has been shown to decrease the loss of carti-

lage in persons with knee OA.[12] Its action may be due to a disruption in the production of cartilage-degrading enzymes. Intraarticular injections of corticosteroids may be appropriate for the elderly patient with local inflammation and effusion. Four or more injections without relief should suggest the need for additional intervention. Systemic use of corticosteroids is not indicated and can actually accelerate the disease process.

Another treatment for mild to moderate OA is hyaluronic acid (HA), a type of viscosupplementation. HA is found in normal joint fluid and articular cartilage. It contributes to both the viscosity and elasticity of synovial fluid, and its degradation can result in joint damage. Synthetic and naturally occurring HA derivatives (Orthovisc, Synvisc, Supartz, Nuflexxa, and Hyalgan) are administered in three weekly injections directly into the knee. Pain relief can occur for some people for up to 1 year.[1] HA may also be added to oral

Musculoskeletal System

| TABLE 65-3 | DRUG THERAPY — Arthritis and Connective Tissue Disorders | | |

Drug	Mechanism of Action	Side Effects	Nursing Considerations
Salicylates aspirin, salsalate (Disalcid, Asaphen) choline salicylate (Arthropan) choline magnesium trisalicylate (Trilisate)	Antiinflammatory Analgesic Antipyretic Act by inhibiting synthesis of prostaglandins	GI irritation (dyspepsia, nausea, ulcer, hemorrhage) Prolonged bleeding time Exacerbation of asthma (aspirin-sensitive asthma) Tinnitus, dizziness with repeated large doses	Administer drug with food, milk, antacids as prescribed, or full glass of water; may use enteric-coated aspirin. Report signs of bleeding (e.g., tarry stools, bruising, petechiae, nosebleeds).
Nonsteroidal Antiinflammatory Drugs (NSAIDs) ibuprofen (Motrin, Advil, Novoprofen) naproxen (Naprosyn, Anaprox, Aleve) ketoprofen (Orudis, Actron) piroxicam (Feldene, Novopirocam) indomethacin (Indocin, Indocid) sulindac (Clinoril, Apo-Sulin, NovoSundac) tolmetin (Tolectin) diclofenac (Voltaren, Apo-Diclo SR) meclofenamate (Meclomen) nabumetone (Relafen) oxaprozin (Daypro) meloxicam (Mobic) celecoxib (Celebrex)	Antiinflammatory Analgesic Antipyretic Act by inhibiting synthesis of prostaglandins	GI irritation (dyspepsia, nausea, ulcer, hemorrhage) Prolonged bleeding time Headache, tinnitus Rash Acute renal insufficiency and other renal medullary changes Exacerbation of asthma (cross-reactivity with aspirin)	Administer drug with food, milk, or antacids as prescribed. Report signs of bleeding (e.g., tarry stools, bruising, petechiae, nosebleeds), edema, skin rashes, persistent headaches, visual disturbances. Monitor BP for elevations related to fluid retention. Needs to be used regularly for maximal effect.
Antibiotics doxycycline (Vibramycin) minocycline (Minocin)	Decreases action of enzymes on cartilage degradation Antirheumatic effect possibly related to immunomodulatory/antiinflammatory properties	Monilial vaginitis, sun sensitivity, nonspecific GI irritation GI effects (nausea/vomiting, diarrhea, stomach cramps) Dizziness Photosensitivity (severe)	May be reasonable alternative with mild disease
Topical Analgesics capsaicin cream (Zostrix, Capzasin)	Depletes substance P from nerve endings, interrupting pain signals to the brain	Rash, urticaria Localized burning sensation, erythema	Must be used regularly over time for maximal effect. Aloe vera cream may moderate burning sensation. Advise patient not to use cream with external heat source (heating pad) because of risk of burns. Available in OTC and prescriptive strengths.
Corticosteroids *Intraarticular Injections* methylprednisolone acetate (Depo-Medrol) triamcinolone (Aristospan)	Antiinflammatory Analgesic Act by inhibiting synthesis and/or release of mediators of inflammation	Local osteoporosis, tendon rupture, neuropathic arthropathy from frequent injection Dermal/subdermal changes leading to depression at injection site Possibility of local infection	Use strict aseptic technique for joint fluid aspiration or corticosteroid injection. Inform patient that joint may feel worse immediately after injection. Inform patient that improvement lasts weeks to months after injection. Advise patient to avoid overusing affected joint after injection.

BP, Blood pressure; *GI*, gastrointestinal; *OTC*, over-the-counter.

TABLE 65-3	**DRUG THERAPY** Arthritis and Connective Tissue Disorders—cont'd

Drug	Mechanism of Action	Side Effects	Nursing Considerations
Corticosteroids—cont'd *Systemic* hydrocortisone sodium succinate (Solu-Cortef) methylprednisolone sodium succinate (Solu-Medrol) dexamethasone (Decadron) prednisone triamcinolone (Aristocort)	Antiinflammatory Analgesic Act by inhibiting synthesis and/or release of mediators of inflammation	Cushing syndrome (including fluid retention), GI irritation, osteoporosis, insomnia, hypertension, steroid psychosis, diabetes mellitus, acne, menstrual irregularities, hirsutism, risk of antibiotic-resistant infection, bruising	Use only in life-threatening exacerbation or when symptoms persist after treatment with less potent antiinflammatory drugs. Administer for limited time only, tapering dose slowly. Be aware that exacerbation of symptoms occurs with abrupt withdrawal of drug. Monitor BP, weight, CBC, and potassium level. Limit sodium intake. Report signs of infection. Instruct patient to report corticosteroid use to surgeon or dentist to avoid postoperative adrenal insufficiency.
Disease-Modifying Antirheumatic Drugs (DMARDs)			
methotrexate (Rheumatrex, Trexall)	Antimetabolite Inhibits DNA, RNA, protein synthesis	Hepatotoxicity occurs more often with frequent small doses than with large intermittent doses Smaller dose and different administration schedule for RA make it less likely that patient will develop symptoms related to drug's antineoplastic activity (e.g., GI and skin toxicity, bone marrow depression, nephropathy)	Monitor CBC and hepatic and renal function. Advise patient to report signs of anemia (fatigue, weakness). Keep patient well hydrated. Teratogenic potential cautions against use for women of childbearing age. Inform patient that contraception should be used during and 3 mo after treatment.
sulfasalazine (Azulfidine, Salazopyrin)	Sulfonamide Antiinflammatory Blocks prostaglandin synthesis	GI effects (anorexia, nausea/vomiting) Bleeding, bruising, jaundice Headache Rash, urticaria, pruritus	Advise patient that drug may cause orange-yellow discoloration of urine or skin. Space doses evenly around the clock, taking drug after food with 8 oz water. Treatment may be continued even after symptoms are relieved. Monitor CBC.
leflunomide (Arava)	Antiinflammatory Immunomodulatory agent that inhibits proliferation of lymphocytes	Hepatotoxicity (especially if also taking methotrexate or prior alcohol abuse) Nausea, or ongoing diarrhea Respiratory tract infection Alopecia Rash	Monitor hepatic function. Evaluate for relief of pain, swelling, stiffness; increase in joint mobility. Advise women of childbearing age to avoid pregnancy.
penicillamine (Cuprimine, Depen)	Antiinflammatory Exact mechanism of action in RA unknown but may suppress cell-mediated immune response	GI irritation (nausea/vomiting, anorexia, diarrhea), reduced/altered taste Rash Proteinuria, hematuria Iron deficiency (especially in menstruating women)	Monitor WBC count, platelets, urinalysis. Advise patient to take medication 1 hr before or 2 hr after meals or at least 1 hr from any other drug, food, or milk.
Gold Compounds Parenteral (gold sodium thiomalate [Myochrysine], aurothioglucose [Solganal]) Oral (auranofin [Ridaura])	Alters immune responses, suppressing synovitis of active RA Antirheumatic	Decreased hemoglobin, leukopenia, thrombocytopenia Proteinuria, hematuria Stomatitis	Rule out pregnancy before beginning treatment. Monitor CBC, urinalysis, and hepatic and renal function. Advise patient that therapeutic response may not occur for 3-6 mo. Advise patient to immediately report pruritus, rash, sore mouth, indigestion, or metallic taste.

BP, Blood pressure; *CBC,* complete blood count; *GI,* gastrointestinal; *RA,* rheumatoid arthritis; *TNF,* tumor necrosis factor; *WBC,* white blood cell.

Continued

TABLE 65-3	*DRUG THERAPY* Arthritis and Connective Tissue Disorders—cont'd		
Drug	**Mechanism of Action**	**Side Effects**	**Nursing Considerations**
Antimalarials hydroxychloroquine (Plaquenil)	Antirheumatic action unknown but may suppress formation of antigens	Ocular toxicity (retinopathy); may progress even after drug is discontinued Ototoxicity Peripheral neuritis, neuromyopathy, hypotension, electrocardiogram changes with prolonged therapy	Monitor CBC and hepatic function. Advise patient that therapeutic response may not occur for up to 6 mo. Advise patient to immediately report visual difficulties, muscular weakness, and decreased hearing/tinnitus.
Immunosuppressants azathioprine (Imuran) cyclophosphamide (Cytoxan)	Inhibit DNA, RNA, protein synthesis	GI irritation (nausea/vomiting; anorexia with large doses) Rash	Evaluate for relief of pain, swelling, stiffness; increase in joint mobility. Advise patient to immediately report unusual bleeding or bruising. Advise patient that therapeutic response may take up to 12 wk. Advise women of childbearing age to avoid pregnancy.
Biologic/Targeted Therapy etanercept (Enbrel)	Binds TNF, blocking its interaction with cell surface receptors to decrease inflammatory and immune responses	Injection site reaction including erythema, pain, itching, swelling Abdominal pain, vomiting Dizziness, headache Rhinitis, pharyngitis, cough	Evaluate for relief of pain, swelling, stiffness; increase in joint mobility. Advise patient that injection site reaction generally occurs in first month of treatment and decreases with continued therapy. Advise patient to not receive live virus vaccines during treatment.
infliximab (Remicade) adalimumab (Humira)	Monoclonal antibodies that bind to TNF; reduce infiltration of inflammatory cells	Abdominal pain, nausea/vomiting, dizziness, headache, rhinitis, cough, sinusitis, pharyngitis	Evaluate for relief of pain, swelling, stiffness; increase in joint mobility.
anakinra (Kineret)	Blocks the action of interleukin-1, thus decreases the inflammatory response	Injection site reaction, leukopenia, headache, abdominal pain, rash	Evaluate for relief of pain, swelling, stiffness; increase in joint mobility. Advise patient that injection site reaction generally occurs in first month of treatment and decreases with continued therapy. Evaluate renal function. Monitor for infection. Do not take drug with other TNF inhibitors.
abatacept (Orencia)	Modulates T-cell activation; suppresses immune response	Headache, upper respiratory infection, nausea, sore throat, injection site reaction	Not recommended for concomitant use with TNF inhibitors. Evaluate for relief of pain, swelling, stiffness; increase in joint mobility.
rituximab (Rituxan)	Monoclonal antibody that targets B cells	Dizziness, palpitations, fever, itching, difficulty breathing, sore throat	Given in combination with methotrexate. Monitor for infection and bleeding. Advise patient to not receive live virus vaccines with treatment. Monitor for low BP if also taking BP medication.

TABLE 65-4 | **PATIENT AND FAMILY TEACHING GUIDE**
Joint Protection and Energy Conservation

- Lose or maintain weight.
- Use assistive devices, if indicated.
- Avoid forceful repetitive movements.
- Avoid positions of joint deviation and stress.
- Use good posture and proper body mechanics.
- Seek assistance with necessary tasks that may cause pain.
- Develop organizing and pacing techniques for routine tasks.
- Modify home and work environment to create less stressful ways to perform tasks.

supplements of glucosamine and chondroitin. Few side effects have been reported.

NURSING MANAGEMENT
OSTEOARTHRITIS

▪ Nursing Assessment

The nurse should carefully assess and document the type, location, severity, frequency, and duration of the patient's joint pain and stiffness. The patient should also be questioned about the extent to which these symptoms affect his or her ability to perform activities of daily living. Pain-relieving practices should be noted, and the patient should be questioned about the duration and success of treatment for each intervention. Physical examination of the affected joint or joints includes assessment of tenderness, swelling, limitation of movement, and crepitation. An involved joint should be compared with the contralateral joint if it is not affected.

▪ Nursing Diagnoses

Nursing diagnoses for the patient with OA may include, but are not limited to, the following:

- Acute and chronic pain *related to* physical activity and lack of knowledge of pain self-management techniques
- Insomnia *related to* pain
- Impaired physical mobility *related to* weakness, stiffness, or pain on ambulation
- Self-care deficits *related to* joint deformity and pain with activity
- Imbalanced nutrition: more than body requirements *related to* intake in excess of energy output
- Chronic low self-esteem *related to* changing physical appearance and social and work roles

▪ Planning

The overall goals are that the patient with OA will (1) maintain or improve joint function through a balance of rest and activity, (2) use joint protection measures (Table 65-4) to improve activity tolerance, (3) achieve independence in self-care and maintain optimal role function, and (4) use pharmacologic and nonpharmacologic strategies to manage pain satisfactorily.

▪ Nursing Implementation

Health Promotion. Prevention of primary OA is not possible. However, community education should focus on the alteration of modifiable risk factors through weight loss and the reduction of occupational and recreational hazards. Athletic instruction and physical fitness programs should include safety measures that protect and reduce trauma to the joint structures. Congenital conditions, such as Legg-Calvé-Perthes disease, that are known to predispose a patient to the development of OA should be treated promptly.

Acute Intervention. The person with OA most often complains of pain, stiffness, limitation of function, and the frustration of coping with these physical difficulties on a daily basis. The older adult may believe that OA is an inevitable part of aging and that nothing can be done to ease the discomfort and related disability.

The patient with OA is usually treated on an outpatient basis, often by an interdisciplinary team of health care providers that includes a rheumatologist, a nurse, an occupational therapist, and a physical therapist. Health assessment questionnaires are often used to pinpoint areas of difficulty for the patient with arthritis. Questionnaires are updated at regular intervals to document disease and treatment progression. Treatment goals can be developed based on data from the questionnaires and the physical examination, with specific interventions to target identified problems. The patient is usually hospitalized only if joint surgery is planned (see Chapter 63).

Drugs are administered for the relief of pain and inflammation. Nonpharmacologic pain management strategies may include massage, the application of heat (thermal packs) or cold (ice packs), relaxation, and guided imagery. Splints may be prescribed to rest and stabilize painful or inflamed joints. Once an acute flare has subsided, a physical therapist can provide valuable assistance in planning an exercise program. Therapists may often recommend Tai Chi as a low-impact form of exercise. Tai Chi can be performed by patients of all ages and may be done in a wheelchair. The nurse should emphasize the importance of warming up before practice to prevent stretch injuries.

Patient and family teaching related to OA is an important nursing responsibility in any care setting and is the foundation of successful disease management. Teaching should include information about the nature and treatment of the disease, pain management, correct posture and body mechanics, correct use of assistive devices such as a cane or walker, principles of joint protection and energy conservation (see Table 65-4), nutritional choices, weight and stress management, and a therapeutic exercise program. The patient should be assured that OA is a localized disease and that severe deforming arthritis is not the usual course. The patient can also gain support and understanding of the disease process through community resources such as the Arthritis Foundation's Self-Help Course (*www.arthritis.org*).

Ambulatory and Home Care. Chronic pain and a loss of function of the affected joints continue to be primary concerns. Home management goals must be individualized to meet the patient's needs, and family members or significant others should be included in goal setting and teaching. Home and work environment modification is essential for patient safety.[13] Measures include removing scatter rugs, providing rails at the stairs and bathtub, using night-lights, and wearing well-fitting supportive shoes. Assistive devices such as canes, walkers, elevated toilet seats, and grab bars also reduce the load on an affected joint and promote safety. The nurse should urge the patient to continue all prescribed therapies at home and also be open to the discussion of new approaches to symptom management.

Sexual counseling may help the patient and significant other to enjoy physical closeness by introducing the idea of alternate positions and timing for intercourse. Discussion also increases awareness of each partner's needs. The nurse should encourage the patient to take analgesics or a warm bath to decrease joint stiffness before sexual activity.

▪ Evaluation

The expected outcomes are that the patient with OA will
- experience adequate amounts of rest and activity
- achieve satisfactory pain management
- maintain joint flexibility and muscle strength through joint protection and therapeutic exercise
- verbalize acceptance of OA as a chronic disease, collaborating with health care providers in disease management

RHEUMATOID ARTHRITIS

Rheumatoid arthritis (RA) is a chronic, systemic autoimmune disease characterized by inflammation of connective tissue in the diarthrodial (synovial) joints, typically with periods of remission and exacerbation. RA is frequently accompanied by extraarticular manifestations.

RA occurs globally, affecting all ethnic groups. It can occur at any time of life, but the incidence increases with age, peaking between the 30s and 50s. Nearly 2.1 million Americans are affected by RA, with women having an incidence three times higher than men.

Etiology and Pathophysiology

The cause of RA is unknown. Despite past theories, no infectious agent has been cultured from blood and synovial tissue or fluid with enough reproducibility to suggest an infectious cause for the disease. An autoimmune etiology is currently the most widely accepted.

1. *Autoimmunity.* The autoimmune theory suggests that changes associated with RA begin when a susceptible host experiences an initial immune response to an antigen. The antigen, which is probably not the same in all patients, triggers the formation of an abnormal immunoglobulin G (IgG). RA is characterized by the presence of autoantibodies against this abnormal IgG. The autoantibodies are known as rheumatoid factor (RF), and they combine with IgG to form immune complexes that initially deposit on synovial membranes or superficial articular cartilage in the joints. Immune complex formation leads to the activation of complement, and an inflammatory response results. (Complement activation is discussed in Chapter 13, and immune complex formation is discussed in Chapter 14.) Neutrophils are attracted to the site of inflammation, where they release proteolytic enzymes that can damage articular cartilage and cause the synovial lining to thicken (Fig. 65-3). Other inflammatory cells include

T helper (CD4) cells, which are the primary orchestrators of cell-mediated immune responses. Activated CD4 cells stimulate monocytes, macrophages, and synovial fibroblasts to secrete the proinflammatory cytokines interleukin-1 (IL-1), interleukin-6 (IL-6), and tumor necrosis factor (TNF). These cytokines are the primary factors that drive the inflammatory response in RA.

Joint changes from chronic inflammation begin when the hypertrophied synovial membrane invades the surrounding cartilage, ligaments, tendons, and joint capsule. *Pannus* (highly vascular granulation tissue) forms within the joint. It eventually covers and erodes the entire surface of the articular cartilage. The production of inflammatory cytokines at the pannus-cartilage junction further contributes to cartilage destruction. The pannus also scars and shortens supporting structures such as tendons and ligaments, ultimately causing joint laxity, subluxation, and contracture.

2. *Genetic factors.* Genetic predisposition appears to be important in the development of RA. For example, a higher occurrence of the disease has been noted in identical than in fraternal twins. The strongest evidence for a familial influence is the increased occurrence of a human leukocyte antigen (HLA) known as HLA-DR4 in white RA patients. Other HLA variants have also been identified in patients from other ethnic groups. (HLA is discussed in Chapter 14.) Smoking significantly increases the risk of RA in both men and women who are genetically predisposed to the disease.[14]

The pathogenesis of RA is more clearly understood than its etiology. If unarrested, the disease progresses through four stages, which are identified in Table 65-5.

Clinical Manifestations

Joints. The onset of RA is typically insidious. Nonspecific manifestations such as fatigue, anorexia, weight loss, and generalized stiffness may precede the onset of arthritic complaints. The stiffness becomes more localized in the following weeks to months. Some patients report a history of a precipitating stressful event such as infection, work stress, physical exertion, childbirth, surgery, or emotional upset. However, research has been unable to correlate such events directly with the onset of RA.

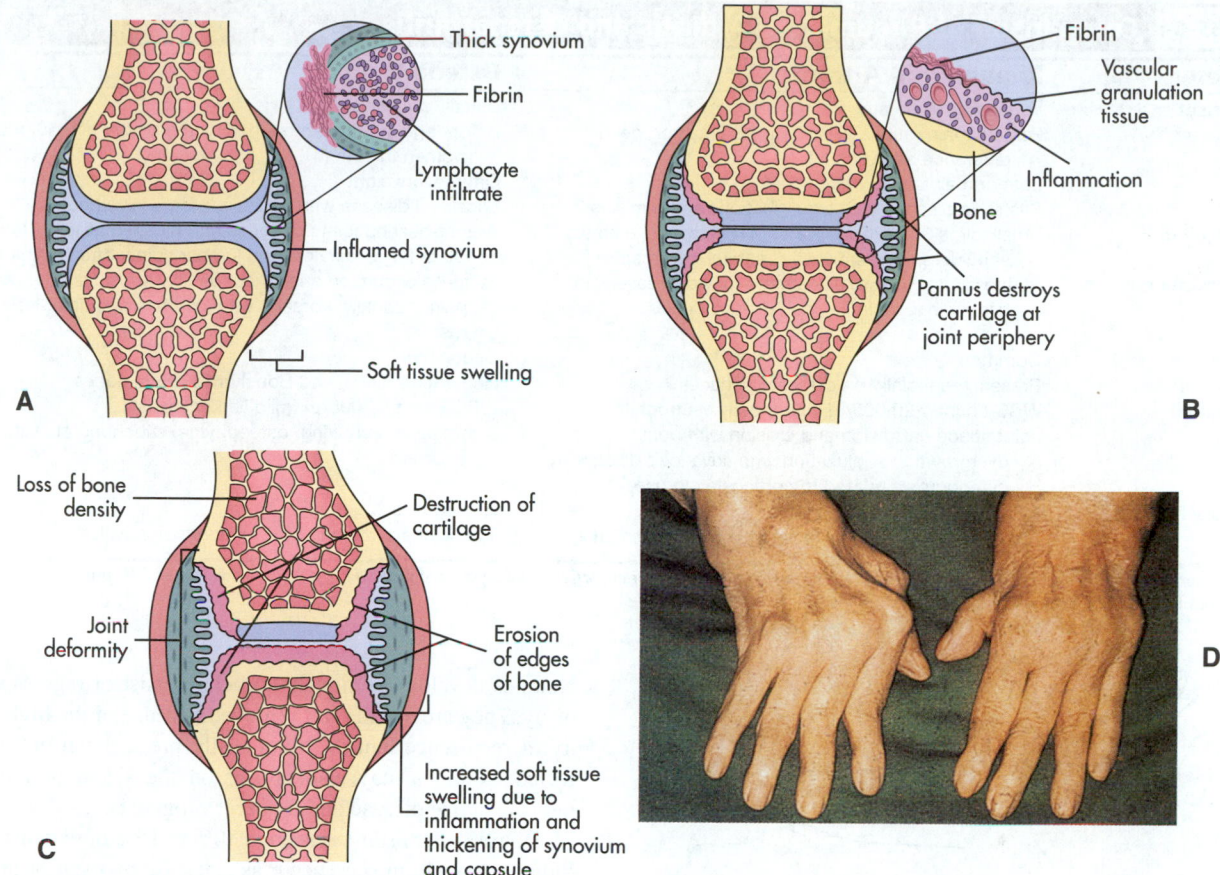

FIG. 65-3 Rheumatoid arthritis. **A,** Early pathologic change in rheumatoid arthritis is rheumatoid synovitis. The synovium is inflamed. There is a great increase in lymphocytes and plasma cells. **B,** With time, there is articular cartilage destruction; vascular granulation tissue grows across the surface of the cartilage (pannus) from the edges of the joint, and the articular surface shows loss of cartilage beneath the extending pannus, most marked at the joint margins. **C,** Inflammatory pannus causes focal destruction of bone. At the edges of the joint there is osteolytic destruction of bone, responsible for erosions seen on x-rays. This phase is associated with joint deformity. **D,** Characteristic deformity and soft tissue swelling associated with long-standing rheumatoid disease of the hands.

TABLE 65-5	**Anatomic Stages of Rheumatoid Arthritis**

Stage I: Early
No destructive changes on x-ray, possible x-ray evidence of osteoporosis

Stage II: Moderate
X-ray evidence of osteoporosis, with or without slight bone or cartilage destruction; no joint deformities (although possibly limited joint mobility); adjacent muscle atrophy; possible presence of extraarticular soft tissue lesions (e.g., nodules, tenosynovitis)

Stage III: Severe
X-ray evidence of cartilage and bone destruction in addition to osteoporosis; joint deformity, such as subluxation, ulnar deviation, or hyperextension, without fibrous or bony ankylosis; extensive muscle atrophy; possible presence of extraarticular soft tissue lesions (e.g., nodules, tenosynovitis)

Stage IV: Terminal
Fibrous or bony ankylosis, stage III criteria

Data from American College of Rheumatology: Classification criteria for determining progression of rheumatoid arthritis. Available at *www.hopkins-arthritis.som.jhmi.edu* (accessed April 30, 2006).

Specific articular involvement is manifested clinically by pain, stiffness, limitation of motion, and signs of inflammation (e.g., heat, swelling, tenderness).[15] Joint symptoms occur symmetrically and frequently affect the small joints of the hands (PIP and MCP) and feet (MTP). Larger peripheral joints such as the wrists, elbows, shoulders, knees, hips, ankles, and jaw may also be involved. The cervical spine may be affected, but the axial spine is generally spared. Table 65-6 compares the manifestations of RA and OA.

The patient characteristically experiences joint stiffness after periods of inactivity. Morning stiffness may last from 60 minutes to several hours or more, depending on disease activity. MCP and PIP joints are typically swollen. In early disease, the fingers may become spindle shaped from synovial hypertrophy and thickening of the joint capsule (see Fig. 65-3, *D*). Joints become tender, painful, and warm to the touch. Joint pain increases with motion, varies in intensity, and may not be proportional to the degree of inflammation. Tenosynovitis frequently affects the extensor and flexor tendons around the wrists, producing manifestations of carpal tunnel syndrome and making it difficult for the patient to grasp objects.

As disease activity progresses, inflammation and fibrosis of the joint capsule and supporting structures may lead to deformity and disability. Atrophy of muscles and destruction of tendons around the joint cause one articular surface to slip past the other *(sublux-*

TABLE 65-6	Comparison of Rheumatoid Arthritis and Osteoarthritis	
Parameter	**Rheumatoid Arthritis**	**Osteoarthritis**
Age at onset	Young to middle age	Usually >40 yr of age
Gender	Female/male ratio is 2:1 or 3:1; less marked gender difference after age 60	Before age 50, more men than women; after age 50, more women than men
Weight	Lost or maintained weight	Often overweight
Disease	Systemic disease with exacerbations and remissions	Localized disease with variable, progressive course
Affected joints	Small joints first (PIPs, MCPs, MTPs), wrists, elbows, shoulders, knees; usually bilateral, symmetric	Weight-bearing joints of knees and hips, small joints (MCPs, DIPs, PIPs), cervical and lumbar spine; often asymmetric
Pain characteristics	Stiffness lasts 1 hr to all day and may decrease with use, pain is variable, may disrupt sleep	Stiffness occurs on arising but usually subsides after 30 min, pain gradually worsens with joint use and time, lessens with rest
Effusions	Common	Uncommon
Nodules	Present, especially on extensor surfaces	Heberden's (DIPs) and Bouchard's (PIPs) nodes
Synovial fluid	WBC count >20,000/μl with mostly neutrophils	WBC count <2000/μl (mild leukocytosis)
X-rays	Joint space narrowing and erosion with bony overgrowths, subluxation with advanced disease; osteoporosis related to corticosteroid use	Joint space narrowing, osteophytes, subchondral cysts, sclerosis
Laboratory findings	RF positive in 80% of patients	RF negative
	Elevated ESR, CRP indicative of active inflammation	Transient elevation in ESR related to synovitis

CRP, C-reactive protein; *DIP,* distal interphalangeal; *ESR,* erythrocyte sedimentation rate; *MCP,* metacarpophalangeal; *MTP,* metatarsophalangeal; *PIP,* proximal interphalangeal; *RF,* rheumatoid factor; *WBC,* white blood cell.

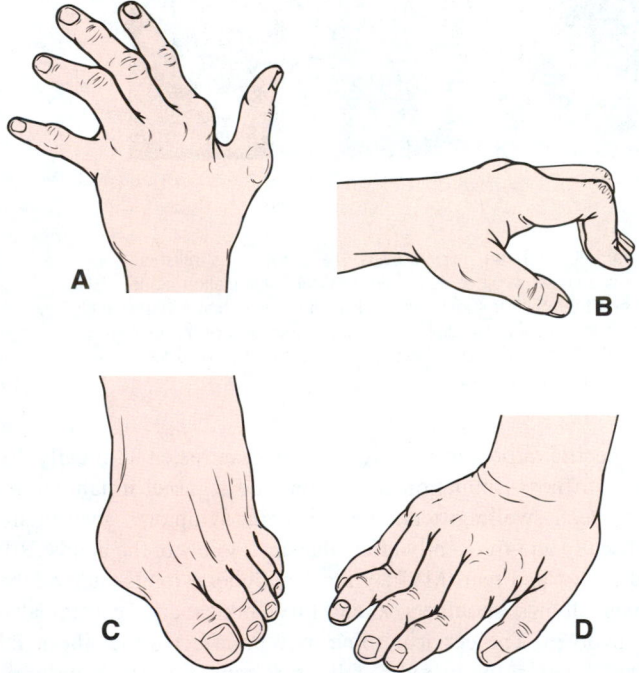

FIG. 65-4 Typical deformities of rheumatoid arthritis. **A,** Ulnar drift. **B,** Boutonnière deformity. **C,** Hallux valgus. **D,** Swan neck deformity.

ation). Typical distortions of the hand include ulnar drift ("zig-zag deformity"), swan neck, and boutonnière deformities (Fig. 65-4). Metatarsal head subluxation and hallux valgus (bunion) in the feet may cause pain and walking disability.

Extraarticular Manifestations. RA can affect nearly every system in the body. Extraarticular manifestations of RA are depicted in Fig. 65-5. The three most common are rheumatoid nodules, Sjögren's syndrome, and Felty syndrome.

Rheumatoid nodules develop in up to 25% of all patients with RA. Those affected with nodules usually have high titers of RF. Rheumatoid nodules appear subcutaneously as firm, nontender, granuloma-type masses and are usually located over the extensor surfaces of joints such as fingers and elbows. Nodules at the base of the spine and back of the head are common in older adults.

Nodules develop insidiously and can persist or regress spontaneously. They are usually not removed because of the high probability of recurrence, but they can easily break down or become infected. Nodules may also appear on the sclera or lungs; these indicate active disease and a poorer prognosis.

Sjögren's syndrome is seen in 10% to 15% of patients with RA. Sjögren's syndrome can occur as a disease by itself or in conjunction with other arthritic disorders such as RA and systemic lupus erythematosus (SLE). Affected patients have diminished lacrimal and salivary gland secretion, leading to complaints of burning, gritty, itchy eyes. They experience decreased tearing and photosensitivity. (Sjögren's syndrome is discussed later in this chapter.)

Felty syndrome occurs most commonly in patients with severe, nodule-forming RA. It is characterized by inflammatory eye disorders, splenomegaly, lymphadenopathy, pulmonary disease, and blood dyscrasias (anemia, thrombocytopenia, granulocytopenia).

Complications

Without treatment, joint destruction begins as early as the first year of the disease. Flexion contractures and hand deformities cause diminished grasp strength and affect the patient's ability to perform self-care tasks. Nodular myositis and muscle fiber degeneration can lead to pain similar to that of vascular insufficiency. Cataract development and loss of vision can result from scleral nodules. Complications can also result from rheumatoid nodules. On the skin, these nodules can ulcerate, similar to pressure ulcers. Nodules on the vocal cords lead to progressive hoarseness, and nodules in the vertebral bodies can cause bone destruction. In later disease, cardiopulmonary effects may occur. These may include pleurisy, pleural effusion, pericarditis, pericardial effusion, and cardiomyopathy. Carpal tunnel syndrome can result from swelling of the synovial membrane.

Diagnostic Studies

An accurate diagnosis is essential to the initiation of appropriate treatment and the prevention of unnecessary disability. A diagnosis is often made based on history and physical findings, but some laboratory tests are useful for confirmation and to monitor disease progression (see Table 65-6). Positive RF occurs in approximately 80% of patients, and titers rise during active disease. ESR and C-reactive

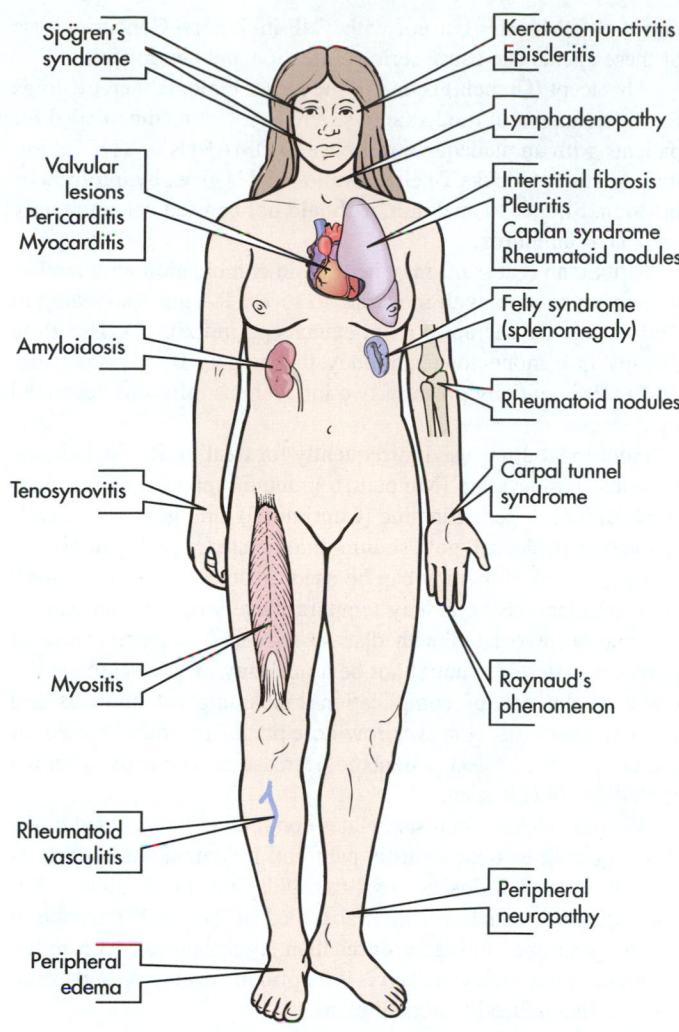

FIG. 65-5 Extraarticular manifestations of rheumatoid arthritis.

Sjögren's syndrome

Keratoconjunctivitis Episcleritis

Lymphadenopathy

Valvular lesions Pericarditis Myocarditis

Interstitial fibrosis Pleuritis Caplan syndrome Rheumatoid nodules

Felty syndrome (splenomegaly)

Amyloidosis

Rheumatoid nodules

Tenosynovitis

Carpal tunnel syndrome

Myositis

Raynaud's phenomenon

Rheumatoid vasculitis

Peripheral neuropathy

Peripheral edema

TABLE 65-7	American Rheumatism Association Classification

Criteria for Rheumatoid Arthritis
Rheumatoid arthritis is defined as having at least 4 of 7 of the following criteria:

- Morning stiffness that lasts ≥1 hr*
- Swelling in three or more joints*
- Swelling in hand joints*
- Symmetric joint swelling*
- Erosions or decalcification seen on hand x-rays
- Rheumatoid nodules
- Presence of serum RF

From Arnett FC, Edworthy SM, Bloch DA, et al: The American Rheumatism Association 1987 revised criteria for the classification of rheumatoid arthritis, *Arthritis Rheum* 31:315, 1988. Available at *www.rheumatology.org.*
RF, Rheumatoid factor.
*Must be present for at least 6 weeks.

protein (CRP) are general indicators of active inflammation. Antinuclear antibody (ANA) titers are also seen in some RA patients.

Synovial fluid analysis in early disease often shows a straw-colored fluid with many fibrin flecks. The white blood cell (WBC) count of synovial fluid is elevated (up to 25,000/µl). Inflammatory changes in the synovium can be confirmed by tissue biopsy.

X-rays are not specifically diagnostic of RA. They may be inconclusive during early stages of the disease, revealing only soft tissue swelling and possible bone demineralization. In later disease, narrowing of the joint space, destruction of articular cartilage, erosion, subluxation, and deformity are seen. Malalignment and ankylosis are often evident in advanced disease. Baseline films may be useful in monitoring disease progression and treatment effectiveness. Bone scans are more useful in detecting early joint changes and confirming a diagnosis so that RA treatment can be initiated. Criteria for the diagnosis of RA are described in Table 65-7.

Collaborative Care

Care of the patient with RA begins with a comprehensive program of education and drug therapy. Education regarding drug therapy includes correct administration, reporting of side effects, and frequent medical and laboratory follow-up visits. The patient and family are educated about the disease process and home management strategies. NSAIDs are prescribed to promote physical comfort. Physical therapy helps the patient maintain joint motion and

muscle strength. Occupational therapy develops upper extremity function and encourages joint protection through the use of splints or other assistive devices and strategies for activity pacing.

An individualized treatment plan considers the nature of the disease activity, joint function, age, gender, family and social roles, and response to previous treatment (Table 65-8). A caring, long-term relationship with an arthritis health care team can promote the patient's self-esteem and positive coping.

Drug Therapy. Drugs remain the cornerstone of RA treatment (see Table 65-3). Instead of maintaining the patient on high doses of aspirin or NSAIDs until x-rays show clear evidence of the disease, health care providers now aggressively prescribe disease-modifying antirheumatic drugs (DMARDs) with the knowledge that irreversible joint changes can occur as early as the first year of RA. These drugs have the potential to lessen the permanent effects of RA, such as joint erosion and deformity. The choice of drug is based on disease activity, the patient's level of function, and lifestyle considerations, such as the desire to bear children. Many of the drugs used to treat RA are expensive.

Usually methotrexate (Rheumatrex) is the drug of first choice. The rapid antiinflammatory effect of methotrexate reduces clinical symptoms in days to weeks. It also is inexpensive and has a lower toxicity compared to other drugs. Side effects include bone marrow suppression and hepatotoxicity. Methotrexate therapy requires frequent laboratory monitoring, including CBC and chemistry panel. Sulfasalazine (Azulfidine) and the antimalarial drug hydroxychloroquine (Plaquenil) may be effective DMARDs for mild to moderate disease. They are rapidly absorbed, relatively safe, and well-tolerated medications. A newer synthetic DMARD is leflunomide (Arava), which blocks immune cell overproduction. Efficacy is similar to methotrexate and sulfasalazine, with side effects including liver toxicity, diarrhea, and teratogenesis.[16]

Drug Alert - *Hydroxychloroquine (Plaquenil)*
- *Retinopathy may occur and progress even after drug is discontinued.*
- *Report any visual disturbances immediately.*

The use of combination therapy, in which the patient takes two or more drugs simultaneously, can slow symptoms and joint damage while improving function. Drug combinations are individualized to the patient and often include a DMARD, an NSAID, and a corticosteroid.

Biologic/targeted drug therapies are also used to slow disease progression in RA.[17] These drugs include etanercept (Enbrel), in-

Musculoskeletal System

TABLE 65-8	COLLABORATIVE CARE Rheumatoid Arthritis

Diagnostic

History and physical examination
Laboratory studies
- Complete blood cell count (CBC)
- Erythrocyte sedimentation rate (ESR)
- Rheumatoid factor (RF)
- Antinuclear antibody (ANA)
- C-reactive protein (CRP)

Radiologic studies of involved joints
Synovial fluid analysis

Collaborative Therapy

Nutritional and weight management counseling
Therapeutic exercise
Rest and joint protection, use of assistive devices
Heat and cold applications
Complementary and alternative therapies
- Herbal products
- Movement therapies

Drug therapy*
- Disease-modifying antirheumatic drugs (DMARDs)
- Intraarticular or systemic corticosteroids
- Nonsteroidal antiinflammatory drugs (NSAIDs)
- Biologic/targeted therapy

Reconstructive surgery
Implants
Arthroplasty

*See Table 65-3.

fliximab (Remicade), adalimumab (Humira), anakinra (Kineret), and abatacept (Orencia). They can be used to treat patients with moderate to severe disease who have not responded to DMARDs, or in combination therapy with an established DMARD such as methotrexate.

Etanercept is a biologically engineered copy (using recombinant DNA technology) of the TNF cell receptor. This soluble TNF receptor binds to TNF in circulation before TNF can bind to the cell surface receptor. By inhibiting binding of TNF, etanercept inhibits the inflammatory response. This drug is given in 25-mg doses twice per week, or as a 50-mg dose once weekly in a subcutaneous injection.

Drug Alert - *Etanercept (Enbrel)*
- *Increased risk of serious infection and heart failure is a concern.*
- *Report persistent fever, bruising, bleeding, or other signs of infection.*

Infliximab and adalimumab are monoclonal antibodies against TNF. They bind to TNF, thus preventing it from binding to TNF receptors on cells. Infliximab is given intravenously (IV) as an initial dose, followed by additional dosing at 2 and 6 weeks, and then every 8 weeks thereafter. It should be given in combination with methotrexate. Adalimumab is given subcutaneously every other week. If the response is inadequate, dosing can be increased to weekly.

Drug Alert - *Infliximab (Remicade)*
- *Administer tuberculin test and chest x-ray before initiation of therapy.*
- *Monitor for signs of infection and stop drug if acute infection develops.*

Anakinra is a recombinant version of IL-1 receptor antagonist (IL-1Ra). It blocks the biologic activity of IL-1 by competitively inhibiting IL-1 binding to the IL-1 receptor. It is given as a subcutaneous injection. Anakinra is used to reduce the pain and swelling associated with moderate to severe RA. It can be used in combination with DMARDs but not with TNF inhibitors. Concurrent use of these agents can cause serious infection and neutropenia.

Abatacept (Orencia) is one of the newer biologic therapy drugs for the treatment of moderate to severe RA. It is recommended for patients with an inadequate response to DMARDs or TNF inhibitors. Abatacept blocks T-cell activation and is given by intravenous infusion. Similar to anakinra, it should not be used concomitantly with TNF inhibitors.

Rituximab (Rituxan) may be used in combination with methotrexate for patients with moderate to severe RA not responding to TNF antagonist therapies (e.g., etanercept, infliximab). This drug therapy is a monoclonal antibody that targets B cells (see Fig. 16-21). It is initially given in two intravenous infusions separated by 2 weeks.

Additional drugs used infrequently for treating RA include antibiotics (minocycline [Minocin]), immunosuppressants (azathioprine [Imuran], penicillamine [Cuprimine]), and gold compounds (auranofin [Ridaura], gold sodium thiomalate [Myochrysine]).

Corticosteroid therapy can be used to aid in symptom control. Intraarticular injections may temporarily relieve the pain and inflammation associated with disease flare-ups. Long-term use of oral corticosteroids should not be a mainstay of RA treatment because of the risk of complications, including osteoporosis and avascular necrosis. However, low-dose prednisone may be used for a limited time in select patients to decrease disease activity until a DMARD effect is seen.

Various NSAIDs and salicylates continue to be included in the drug regimen to treat arthritis pain and inflammation. Aspirin is often used in high dosages of 4 to 6 g/day (10 to 18 tablets). Because enteric-coated aspirin is absorbed in the small intestine, it can be prescribed in higher doses than regular tablets. The ability to obtain serum salicylate levels is helpful in developing and evaluating individualized treatment plans.

NSAIDs have antiinflammatory, analgesic, and antipyretic properties. Although many NSAIDs are potent inhibitors of inflammation, they do not appear to alter the natural history of RA. Some relief may be noted within days of the start of treatment with NSAIDs, but full effectiveness may take 2 to 3 weeks. NSAIDs may be used when the patient cannot tolerate high doses of aspirin. Those antiinflammatory drugs that are taken only once or twice a day may improve the patient's ability to follow the treatment regimen (see Table 65-3). A newer generation of NSAIDs, the COX-2 inhibitors, are effective in RA as well as OA. Celecoxib (Celebrex) is currently the only available COX-2 inhibitor.

Apheresis. A blood filtration device used in apheresis called the Prosorba column is infrequently used to treat moderate to severe RA in patients who have failed to respond or are intolerant to DMARDs. RF is removed from the patient's blood as it passes through the column. Patients are treated once a week for 12 weeks. Limited data have shown a decrease in RA signs and symptoms for some patients.[18] (Apheresis is discussed in Chapter 14.)

Nutritional Therapy. Although there is no special diet for RA, balanced nutrition is important. Fatigue, pain, depression, limited endurance, and mobility deficits often accompany RA and may cause a loss of appetite or interfere with the patient's ability to shop for and prepare food. Weight loss may result. The occupational therapist may help the patient to modify the home environment and to use assistive devices to make food preparation easier.

Corticosteroid therapy or immobility secondary to pain may result in unwanted weight gain. A sensible weight loss program consisting of balanced nutrition and exercise reduces stress on affected joints. Corticosteroids also increase the appetite, resulting in a higher caloric intake. In addition, the patient may become distressed as signs and symptoms of Cushing syndrome, including moon face and the redistribution of fatty tissue to the trunk, change the physical appearance. The patient must be encouraged to continue a balanced diet and not to alter the corticosteroid dose or stop therapy abruptly. Weight slowly adjusts to normal several months after cessation of therapy.

NURSING MANAGEMENT
RHEUMATOID ARTHRITIS

■ Nursing Assessment

Subjective and objective data that should be obtained from the patient with RA are presented in Table 65-9.

■ Nursing Diagnoses

Nursing diagnoses for the patient with RA may include, but are not limited to, those presented in NCP 65-1.

■ Planning

The overall goals are that the patient with RA will (1) have satisfactory pain relief, (2) have minimal loss of functional ability of the affected joints, (3) participate in planning and carrying out the therapeutic regimen, (4) maintain a positive self-image, and (5) perform self-care to the maximum amount possible.

■ Nursing Implementation

Health Promotion. Prevention of RA is not possible at this time. However, community education programs should focus on symptom recognition to promote early diagnosis and treatment of RA. The Arthritis Foundation offers many publications, classes, and support activities to assist people (see Resources at end of this chapter).

Acute Intervention. The primary goals in the management of RA are the reduction of inflammation, management of pain, maintenance of joint function, and prevention or correction of joint deformity. Goals may be met through a comprehensive program of drug therapy, rest, joint protection, heat and cold applications, exercise, and patient and family teaching. The nurse is an integral member of the health team, working closely with the health care provider, physical and occupational therapists, and social worker to restore function and to help the patient make appropriate lifestyle adjustments to chronic illness.

The newly diagnosed RA patient is usually treated on an outpatient basis, although hospitalization may be necessary for patients with extraarticular complications or advancing disease requiring reconstructive surgery for disabling deformities. Nursing intervention begins with a careful physical assessment (e.g., joint pain, swelling, range of motion [ROM], and general health status). The nurse must also evaluate psychosocial needs (e.g., family support, sexual satisfaction, emotional stress, financial constraints, vocation and career limitations) and environmental concerns (e.g., transportation, home or work modifications). After problem identification, a carefully planned program for rehabilitation and education can be coordinated by the nurse for the interdisciplinary health care team.

Suppression of inflammation may be effectively achieved through the administration of NSAIDs, DMARDs, and biologic therapies. Careful attention to timing is critical to sustain a thera-

TABLE 65-9	**NURSING ASSESSMENT** **Rheumatoid Arthritis**

Subjective Data
Important Health Information
Past health history: Recent infections; presence of precipitating factors such as emotional upset, infections, overwork, childbirth, surgery; pattern of remissions and exacerbations
Medications: Use of aspirin, NSAIDs, corticosteroids, DMARDs
Surgery or other treatments: Any joint surgery

Health Patterns
Health perception–health management: Positive family history for rheumatoid arthritis or other autoimmune disorders; malaise, ability to participate in therapeutic regimen
Nutritional-metabolic: Anorexia, weight loss; dry mucous membranes of mouth and pharynx
Activity-exercise: Stiffness and joint swelling, muscle weakness, difficulty walking, fatigue
Cognitive-perceptual: Paresthesias of hands and feet; numbness, tingling, loss of sensation; symmetric joint pain and aching that increases with motion or stress on joint

Objective Data
General
Lymphadenopathy, fever

Integumentary
Keratoconjunctivitis; subcutaneous rheumatoid nodules on forearm, elbows; skin ulcers; shiny, taut skin over involved joints; peripheral edema

Cardiovascular
Symmetric pallor and cyanosis of fingers (Raynaud's phenomenon); distant heart sounds, murmurs, dysrhythmias

Respiratory
Chronic bronchitis, tuberculosis, histoplasmosis, fibrosing alveolitis

Gastrointestinal
Splenomegaly (Felty syndrome)

Musculoskeletal
Symmetric joint involvement with swelling, erythema, heat, tenderness, and deformities; enlargement of proximal phalangeal and metacarpophalangeal joints; limitation of joint movement; muscle contractures, muscle atrophy

Possible Findings
Positive rheumatoid factor, ↑ ESR, anemia; ↑ WBC in synovial fluid; evidence of joint space narrowing, and bony erosion and deformity on x-ray (osteoporosis with advanced disease)

DMARDs, Disease-modifying antirheumatic drugs; *ESR,* erythrocyte sedimentation rate; *NSAIDs,* nonsteroidal antiinflammatory drugs; *WBC,* white blood cells.

peutic drug level and reduce early morning stiffness. The nurse should discuss the action and side effects of each prescribed drug and the importance of necessary laboratory monitoring. Many patients with RA will take several different drugs, and the nurse must make the drug regimen as understandable as possible.

Nonpharmacologic relief of pain may include the use of therapeutic heat and cold, rest, relaxation techniques, joint protection (see Tables 65-4 and 65-10), biofeedback (see Chapter 8), transcutaneous electrical nerve stimulation (see Chapter 10), and hypnosis. Assessment for individual differences and preference allows the nurse to help the patient and family choose therapies that promote optimal comfort within the parameters of their lifestyle.

Lightweight splints may be prescribed to rest an inflamed joint and prevent deformity from muscle spasms and contractures. The occupational therapist may help to identify additional self-help devices that can assist in activities of daily living. Splints should be removed at regular intervals to give skin care and perform ROM

NURSING CARE PLAN 65-1

Patient with Rheumatoid Arthritis

NURSING DIAGNOSIS   **Chronic pain** *related to* joint inflammation, overuse of joints, and ineffective pain and/or comfort measures *as evidenced by* communication of pain descriptors, guarding behavior, and limited joint function; hot, swollen, painful joints

PATIENT GOALS
1. Effectively uses analgesics and nonanalgesic relief measures
2. Verbalizes satisfactory pain control

OUTCOMES (NOC)	INTERVENTIONS (NIC) and *RATIONALES*
Pain Control	**Pain Management**
• Uses preventive measures ____	• Perform a comprehensive assessment of pain to include location, characteristics, onset/duration, frequency, quality, intensity or severity of pain, and precipitating factors *to establish a pattern and baseline assessment and to plan appropriate interventions.*
• Uses nonanalgesic relief measures ____	• Evaluate, with patient and health care team, effectiveness of past pain-control measures that have been used *to determine what has helped and not helped in the past.*
• Uses analgesics appropriately ____	• Reduce or eliminate factors that precipitate or increase the pain experience (e.g., fear, fatigue, and lack of knowledge) *to minimize negative stimuli that may increase pain.*
• Reports uncontrolled symptoms to health care professional ____	• Teach use of nonpharmacologic techniques (e.g., relaxation, distraction, hot/cold applications, and massage) before pain occurs or increases, and along with other pain relief measures, *to promote muscle relaxation and decrease tension.*
• Reports pain controlled ____	• Provide the person with optimal pain relief with prescribed analgesics *to help decrease pain and inflammation.*
Measurement Scale	
1 = Never demonstrated	
2 = Rarely demonstrated	
3 = Sometimes demonstrated	
4 = Often demonstrated	
5 = Consistently demonstrated	

NURSING DIAGNOSIS   **Impaired physical mobility** *related to* joint pain, stiffness, and deformity *as evidenced by* limitation of joint motion, strength, and endurance; inability to perform routine activities of daily living

PATIENT GOALS
1. Performs prescribed joint exercises to maintain and improve joint function
2. Uses joint protection measures to prevent increased joint inflammation

OUTCOMES (NOC)	INTERVENTIONS (NIC) and *RATIONALES*
Mobility	**Exercise Therapy: Joint Mobility**
• Joint movement ____	• Determine limitations of joint movement and effect on function *to establish baseline for plan of care.*
• Muscle movement ____	• Collaborate with physical therapy in developing and executing an exercise program *to maintain and improve joint function.*
• Moves with ease ____	• Explain to patient/family the purpose and plan for joint exercises *to provide information and support for the patient.*
Endurance	• Initiate pain-control measures before beginning joint exercise (e.g., hot packs, warm shower) *to relieve stiffness and increase mobility.*
• Performance of usual routine ____	• Assist patient to optimal body position for passive/active joint movement (e.g., with correct application of resting splints, selection of properly fitting footwear, and selection and use of assistive devices) *to prevent or limit joint deformity.*
• Muscle endurance ____	
• Activity ____	
Measurement Scale	
1 = Severely compromised	
2 = Substantially compromised	
3 = Moderately compromised	
4 = Mildly compromised	
5 = Not compromised	

exercises. After assessment has been completed and supportive care has been given, the splints should be reapplied as prescribed.

Morning care and procedures should be planned around the patient's morning stiffness. Sitting or standing in a warm shower, sitting in a tub with warm towels around the shoulders, or simply soaking the hands in a basin of warm water may help relieve joint stiffness and allow the patient to more comfortably perform activities of daily living. Gentle skin care should be offered, with assistance particularly needed by the patient who is confined to bed.

Ambulatory and Home Care

Rest. Alternating scheduled rest periods with activity throughout the day helps relieve fatigue and pain. The amount of rest needed varies according to the severity of the disease and the patient's limitations. The patient should rest before becoming exhausted. Total bed rest is rarely necessary and should be avoided to prevent stiffness and immobility. However, even a patient with mild disease may require daytime rest in addition to 8 to 10 hours of sleep at night. The nurse should help the patient identify ways to modify daily activities to avoid overexertion that can lead to fatigue and an exacerbation of disease activity. For example, the patient may tolerate meal preparation more easily while sitting on a high stool in front of the sink. The nurse should assist the patient to pace activities and set priorities on the basis of realistic goals.

Good body alignment while resting can be maintained through use of a firm mattress or bedboard. Positions of extension should be encouraged, and positions of flexion should be avoided. Splints and casts may be helpful in maintaining proper alignment and

NURSING CARE PLAN 65-1

Patient with Rheumatoid Arthritis—cont'd

NURSING DIAGNOSIS   **Disturbed body image** *related to* chronic disease activity, long-term treatment, deformities, stiffness, and inability to perform usual activities *as evidenced by* social withdrawal, flat affect, altered self-concept, and reduced sexual interest

PATIENT GOALS   1. Discusses feelings about and the meaning of changes in physical appearance
2. Verbalizes acceptance of body appearance and function
3. Identifies community resources for sexual counseling for self and partner

OUTCOMES (NOC)	INTERVENTIONS (NIC) and *RATIONALES*
Body Image • Internal picture of self ____ • Congruence between body reality, body ideal, and body presentation ____ • Description of affected body part ____ • Adjustment to changes in physical appearance ____ • Adjustment to changes in body function ____ **Measurement Scale** 1 = Never positive 2 = Rarely positive 3 = Sometimes positive 4 = Often positive 5 = Consistently positive	**Body Image Enhancement** • Identify effects of patient's culture, religion, race, sex, and age in terms of body image *to determine extent of problems and plan appropriate interventions.* • Assist patient to discuss changes caused by illness or surgery *to identify problems and plan appropriate interventions.* • Assist patient to separate physical appearance from feelings of personal worth *so a positive body image is fostered in spite of physical manifestations.* • Facilitate contact with individuals with similar changes in body image *to promote sharing and socialization for patient.* **Sexual Counseling** • Refer patient to sex therapist *as sexual problems and concerns can have a serious impact on body image.* • Include spouse/sexual partner in counseling as much as possible *to encourage communication.*

NURSING DIAGNOSIS   **Ineffective therapeutic regimen management** *related to* complexity of chronic health problem, sense of powerlessness, pain, and decisional conflicts *as evidenced by* questioning management plan, self-doubt about ability to manage disease, ability to perform activities for only short periods

PATIENT GOALS   1. Participates in planning and carrying out therapeutic regimen
2. Expresses confidence in ability to make treatment decisions

OUTCOMES (NOC)	INTERVENTIONS (NIC) and *RATIONALES*
Motivation • Self-initiates goal directed behavior ____ • Expresses belief in ability to perform action ____ • Expresses that performance will lead to desired outcome ____ **Treatment Behavior: Illness or Injury** • Follows recommended treatment regimen ____ • Performs self-care consistent with ability ____ • Avoids behaviors that potentiate pathology ____ • Monitors changes in disease status ____ • Balances treatment, exercise, work, leisure, rest, and nutrition ____ **Measurement Scale** 1 = Never demonstrated 2 = Rarely demonstrated 3 = Sometimes demonstrated 4 = Often demonstrated 5 = Consistently demonstrated	**Anticipatory Guidance** • Determine patient's usual method of problem solving *to identify where interventions need to focus.* • Provide information on realistic expectations related to patient's behavior *to ensure correct understanding of disease management.* • Refer patient to community agencies (e.g., Meals on Wheels, Arthritis Foundation) *to allow the patient to meet desired outcomes.* • Include family/significant others *to increase their sense of control and to increase patient's sense of support.* **Pain Management** • Determine impact of pain experience on quality of life (e.g., sleep, appetite, activity, cognition, mood, relationships, performance of job, and role responsibilities) *because these are major deterrents to successful disease management and must be addressed.*

Continued

promoting rest, especially when joint inflammation is present. Lying prone for half an hour twice daily is also recommended. To decrease the risk of joint contracture, pillows should never be placed under the knees. A small, flat pillow may be used under the head and shoulders.

Joint Protection. Protecting joints from stress is important. The nurse can help the patient to identify ways to modify tasks to put less stress on joints during routine activities (see Table 65-10). Energy conservation requires careful planning. The emphasis is on work simplification techniques. Work should be done in short periods with scheduled rest breaks to avoid fatigue (pacing). Work should be spread throughout the week rather than attempted at one time (e.g., all cleaning should not be done on the weekend). Activities should be carefully organized to avoid going up and down

NURSING CARE PLAN 65-1

Patient with Rheumatoid Arthritis—cont'd

NURSING DIAGNOSIS **Self-care deficit (total)** *related to* disease progression, weakness, and contracture *as evidenced by* inability to perform activities of daily living

PATIENT GOALS 1. Performs activities of daily living to the maximum amount possible
2. Determines when assistance is needed for performance of activities of daily living

OUTCOMES (NOC)	INTERVENTIONS (NIC) and *RATIONALES*
Self-Care: Activities of Daily Living (ADLs)	**Self-Care Assistance**
• Eating _____ • Dressing _____ • Toileting _____ • Bathing _____ • Grooming _____ **Measurement Scale** 1 = Severely compromised 2 = Substantially compromised 3 = Moderately compromised 4 = Mildly compromised 5 = Not compromised	• Monitor patient's ability for independent self-care *to plan appropriate interventions.* • Monitor patient's need for adaptive devices for personal hygiene, dressing, grooming, toileting, and eating *to compensate for contractures and weakness so patient can perform as many self-care activities as possible.* • Establish a routine for self-care activities *to foster maximum independence.* • Assist patient in accepting dependency needs *to ensure all needs are met.* • Teach family to encourage independence, and to intervene only when patient is unable to perform *to promote independence.*

TABLE 65-10	*PATIENT AND FAMILY TEACHING GUIDE* **Protection of Small Joints**

1. Maintain joint in neutral position to minimize deformity.
    - Press water from a sponge instead of wringing.
2. Use strongest joint available for any task.
    - When rising from chair, push with palms rather than fingers.
    - Carry laundry basket in both arms rather than with fingers.
3. Distribute weight over many joints instead of stressing a few.
    - Slide objects instead of lifting them.
    - Hold packages close to body for support.
4. Change positions frequently.
    - Do not hold book or grip steering wheel for long periods without resting.
    - Avoid grasping pencil or cutting vegetables with knife for extended periods.
5. Avoid repetitive movements.
    - Do not knit for long periods.
    - Rest between rooms when vacuuming.
    - Modify home environment to include faucets and doorknobs that are pushed rather than turned.
6. Modify chores to avoid stress on joints.
    - Avoid heavy tasks.
    - Sit on stool instead of standing during meal preparation.

stairs repeatedly. Carts should be used to carry supplies, or materials that are used often can be stored in a convenient, easily reached area. Time-saving joint protective devices (e.g., electric can opener) should be used whenever possible. Tasks can also be delegated to other family members.

Patient independence may be increased by occupational therapy training with assistive devices that help simplify tasks, such as built-up utensils, buttonhooks, modified drawer handles, lightweight plastic dishes, and raised toilet seats. Wearing shoes with Velcro fasteners and clothing with buttons or a zipper down the front instead of the back makes dressing easier. A cane or a walker offers support and relief of pain when walking. A platform-wheeled walker further minimizes strain on the small joints of the hands and wrists.

Heat and Cold Therapy and Exercise. Heat and cold applications can help relieve stiffness, pain, and muscle spasm. Application of ice is especially beneficial during periods of disease exacerbation, whereas moist heat appears to offer better relief of chronic stiffness. The treatment modality should be selected according to disease severity, ease of application, and cost. Superficial heat sources such as heating pads, moist hot packs, paraffin baths, whirlpool baths, and warm baths or showers can relieve stiffness to allow participation in therapeutic exercises. Plastic bags of frozen vegetables (peas or corn), which can easily mold around the shoulder, wrists, or knees, are an easy home treatment. The patient can also use ice cubes or small paper cups of frozen water to massage proximal or distal to a painful joint. Heat and cold can be used as often as desired; however, the heat application should not exceed 20 minutes at one time, and the cold application should not exceed 10 to 15 minutes at one time. The nurse should alert the patient to the possibility of a burn, and to avoid the use of a heat-producing cream (e.g., capsaicin) with another external heat device.

Individualized exercise is an integral part of the treatment plan.[19] A therapeutic exercise program is usually developed by a physical therapist and includes exercises that improve the flexibility and strength of the affected joints, and the patient's overall endurance. The nurse should reinforce program participation and ensure that the exercises are being done correctly. Inadequate joint movement can result in progressive joint immobility and muscle weakness, and overaggressive exercise can result in increased pain, inflammation, and joint damage. The nurse should emphasize that participating in a recreational exercise program (e.g., walking or swimming) or performing usual daily activities does not eliminate the patient's need for therapeutic exercise to maintain adequate joint motion.

Gentle ROM exercises are usually done daily to keep the joints functional. The patient should have the opportunity to practice the exercises with supervision. Careful adherence to the prescribed exercise program should be a prime goal of the teaching program. Aquatic exercises in warm water (78° to 86° F [25° to 30° C]) allow easier joint movement because of the buoyancy of the water.

At the same time, although movement seems easier, water provides two-way resistance that makes muscles work harder than they would on land. Aerobic conditioning programs have been shown to improve the physical fitness levels of patients with RA. During acute inflammation, exercise should be limited to one or two repetitions.

Psychologic Support. Self-management and adherence to an individualized home treatment program can only be accomplished if the patient has a thorough understanding of RA, the nature and course of the disease, and the goals of therapy. In addition, the patient's value system and perception of the disease must be considered. The patient is constantly challenged by problems of limited function and fatigue, loss of self-esteem, altered body image, and fear of disability and deformity. Alterations in sexuality should be discussed. Chronic pain or loss of function may make the patient vulnerable to unproven or even dangerous remedies through the claims of false advertising. The nurse can help the patient recognize fears and concerns that are faced by all people who live with chronic illness.

Evaluation of the family support system is important. Financial planning may be necessary. Community resources such as a home care nurse, homemaker services, and vocational rehabilitation may be considered. Self-help groups are beneficial for some patients.

GERONTOLOGIC CONSIDERATIONS
ARTHRITIS

The prevalence of arthritis in older adults is high, and the disease is accompanied by problems unique to this age-group. The most problematic areas related to connective tissue disease in older adults include the following:

1. The high incidence of OA expected in older adults often keeps the health care provider from considering the presence of other types of arthritis.
2. Age alone causes changes in serologic profiles, making interpretation of laboratory values such as RF and ESR more difficult.
3. Polypharmacy in the older adult can result in iatrogenic arthritis.
4. Nonorganic musculoskeletal pain syndromes and weakness may be related to depression and physical inactivity.
5. Diseases such as SLE, which commonly occurs in younger adults, can develop in a milder form in older adults.

Aging brings many physical and metabolic changes that may increase the older patient's sensitivity to both the therapeutic and toxic effects of some drugs. The use of NSAIDs with a shorter half-life may require more frequent dosing but may also produce fewer side effects in the older patient with altered drug metabolism. The older adult who takes NSAIDs has an increased risk for side effects, particularly GI bleeding and renal toxicity. The common occurrence of polypharmacy makes the use of additional drugs in RA treatment particularly problematic in the older adult because of the increased likelihood of untoward drug interactions. The drug regimen should be simplified as much as possible to increase compliance in the older adult (e.g., limited number of drugs with decreased frequency of administration), particularly for the patient without regular assistance.

A major concern of treatment in the older patient relates to the use of corticosteroid therapy. Corticosteroid-induced osteopenia can add to the problem of decreased bone density related to age and inactivity. It can also increase the occurrence of pathologic fractures, especially compression fractures of vertebrae. Corticosteroid-induced myopathy can be minimized or prevented by an age-appropriate exercise program. Although important for all age-groups, an adequate support system for the older adult is a critical factor in the ability to follow a treatment regimen that includes nutritional planning, exercise, general health maintenance, and appropriate pharmacotherapy.

Spondyloarthropathies

The **spondyloarthropathies** are a group of interrelated multisystem inflammatory disorders that affect the spine, peripheral joints, and periarticular structures. These disorders are all negative for RF, thus they are often referred to as seronegative arthropathies. Inheritance of HLA-B27 is strongly associated with occurrence of these diseases. Both genetic and environmental factors play a role in the development of this group of diseases, which includes ankylosing spondylitis, psoriatic arthritis, and reactive arthritis. (HLAs and their relationship to autoimmune diseases are discussed in Chapter 14.) The spondyloarthropathies share clinical and laboratory characteristics that make it difficult to distinguish among them in early disease. According to the European Spondyloarthropathy Study Group criteria, a diagnosis is made when inflammatory spinal pain or asymmetric synovitis is accompanied by one or more of the following: (1) episodes of alternating buttock pain; (2) radiographic evidence of sacroiliitis; (3) heel enthesopathy (e.g., plantar fasciitis, Achilles tendinitis); (4) positive family history of spondyloarthropathy in a first-degree relative; (5) current or documented history of psoriasis; (6) current or documented history of inflammatory bowel disease; and (7) urethritis, cervicitis, or acute diarrhea that occurred within the month preceding onset of arthritic symptoms.[20]

ANKYLOSING SPONDYLITIS

Ankylosing spondylitis (AS) is a chronic inflammatory disease that primarily affects the axial skeleton, including the sacroiliac joints, intervertebral disk spaces, and costovertebral articulations. The HLA-B27 antigen is found in approximately 90% of whites and 50% of African Americans with AS. The prevalence of HLA-B27 is high in the Eskimo population (25% to 40%) and extremely low in Japan (0.006%).[20] Although the usual age of onset is 15 to 35 years of age, the highest incidence of the disease is in persons 25 to 34 years of age. Men are three to five times more likely to develop AS than women.[3] The disease may go undetected in women because of a milder course and because the disease is not often considered in a differential diagnosis for women.

Etiology and Pathophysiology

The cause of AS is unknown. Genetic predisposition appears to play an important role in the disease pathogenesis, but the precise mechanisms are unknown. Aseptic synovial inflammation in joints and adjacent tissue causes the formation of granulation tissue (pannus) and the development of dense fibrous scars that lead to fusion of articular tissues. Extraarticular inflammation can affect the eyes, lungs, heart, kidneys, and peripheral nervous system.

Clinical Manifestations and Complications

AS is characterized by symmetric sacroiliitis and progressive inflammatory arthritis of the axial skeleton. Symptoms of inflammatory spine pain are the first clues to a diagnosis of AS. The patient typically complains of low back pain, stiffness, and limitation of

GENETICS IN CLINICAL PRACTICE
Ankylosing Spondylitis

Genetic Basis
- Inheritance of human leukocyte antigen HLA-B27

Incidence
- More than 90% of white patients with ankylosing spondylitis (AS) have HLA-B27 antigen.
- Only 2% of people with HLA-B27 have clinically detectable disease.
- AS is three to five times more common in men than women.
- It occurs more often in whites than other ethnic groups.
- It affects 7 in 100,000 people.

Genetic Testing
- Testing for HLA-B27 antigen

Clinical Implications
- AS usually occurs in the teens and 20s.
- It is a systemic disease often affecting the eyes and heart.
- Genetic and environmental factors play a role in pathogenesis of disease.
- AS is present in about 3% to 10% of patients with inflammatory bowel disease (IBD).
- About 50% to 70% of patients with both AS and IBD are HLA-B27 positive.

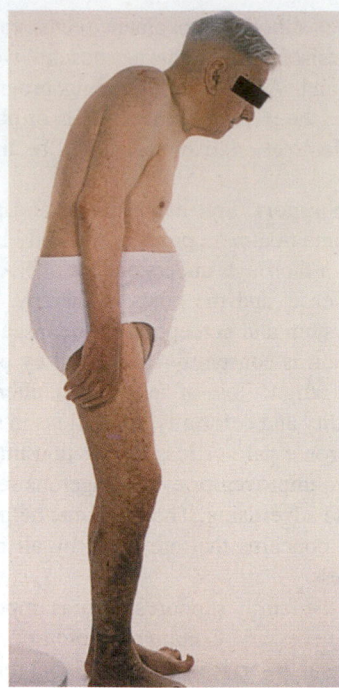

FIG. 65-6   Advanced ankylosing spondylitis. Eventually the neck remains fixed with rigid lumbar and thoracic kyphosis.

motion that is worse during the night and in the morning but improves with mild activity. In women, early symptoms of disease may present as pain and stiffness in the neck rather than the lower back. General symptoms such as fever, fatigue, anorexia, and weight loss are rarely present. *Uveitis* (intraocular inflammation) is the most common nonskeletal symptom. It can appear as an initial presentation of the disease years before arthritic symptoms develop. AS patients may also experience chest pain and sternal/costal cartilage tenderness that can be distressing.

Severe postural abnormalities and deformity can lead to significant disability for the patient with AS (Fig. 65-6). Impaired spinal ROM and fixed kyphosis contribute to altered visual function, raising concerns about safe ambulation. Aortic insufficiency and pulmonary fibrosis are frequent complications. Cauda equina syndrome can also result, contributing to lower extremity weakness and bladder dysfunction. In addition, the patient is at risk for spinal fracture because of osteoporosis.

Diagnostic Studies

X-rays are essential for the diagnosis of AS. However, spinal x-rays are seldom useful in initial diagnosis. Instead, pelvic x-rays demonstrate characteristic changes of sacroiliitis that range from subtle erosion to completely fused joints in which the joint spaces have been obliterated. Changes on later spinal films include the appearance of "bamboo spine," which is due to calcifications *(syndesmophytes)* that bridge from one vertebra to another. Laboratory testing is not specific, but an elevated ESR and mild anemia may be seen. When the suspicion of AS is high, the presence of the HLA-B27 antigen improves the likelihood of this diagnosis.

Collaborative Care

Prevention of AS is not possible. However, families with other diagnosed HLA-B27–positive rheumatic diseases (e.g., acute anterior uveitis, juvenile spondyloarthritis) should be alert to signs of low back pain for early identification and treatment of AS.

Care of the AS patient is aimed at maintaining maximal skeletal mobility while decreasing pain and inflammation. Heat applications can help in the relief of local symptoms. NSAIDs and salicylates are commonly prescribed. DMARDs such as sulfasalazine (Azulfidine) or methotrexate have little effect on spinal disease but may be helpful with peripheral joint disease. Local corticosteroid injections may be beneficial in relieving symptoms. Etanercept (Enbrel), a type of biologic therapy, binds TNF and inhibits its action. TNF, which promotes inflammation, is found in elevated levels in the blood and certain tissues of patients with AS. Etanercept has been shown to reduce disease activity and improve patient functioning.[21] Additional anti-TNF biologic agents (infliximab [Remicade], adalimumab [Humira]) may also be effective.

Once pain and stiffness are managed, exercise is essential. Postural control is important to minimize spinal deformity. The exercise regimen should include back, neck, and chest stretches. Hydrotherapy has also been shown to decrease pain and facilitate spinal extension. Surgery may be indicated for severe deformity and mobility impairment. Spinal osteotomy and total joint replacement are the most commonly performed procedures (see Chapter 63).

NURSING MANAGEMENT
ANKYLOSING SPONDYLITIS

The key nursing responsibility for the patient with AS is education about the disease and principles of therapy. The home management program should include regular exercise and attention to posture, local moist heat applications, and knowledgeable use of drugs.

Baseline ROM assessment by the nurse should include chest expansion (using breathing exercises). Smoking cessation should be encouraged to decrease the risk for lung complications in those with reduced chest expansion. Ongoing physical therapy should include gentle, graded stretching and strengthening exercises to preserve ROM and improve thoracolumbar flexion and extension.

Excessive physical exertion during periods of active flare-up of the disease should be discouraged. Proper positioning at rest is essential. The mattress should be firm, and the patient should sleep on the back with a flat pillow, avoiding positions that encourage flexion deformity. Postural training emphasizes avoiding spinal flexion (e.g., leaning over a desk); heavy lifting; and prolonged walking, standing, or sitting. Sports that facilitate natural stretching, such as swimming and racquet games, should be encouraged. Family counseling and vocational rehabilitation are important.

PSORIATIC ARTHRITIS

Psoriasis is a common benign, inflammatory skin disorder that appears to have a genetic predisposition (see Chapter 24). Approximately 10% of the 3 million people with psoriasis develop psoriatic arthritis (PsA). PsA is now recognized as a progressive inflammatory disease that can cause significant disability. The exact cause of PsA is unknown, but a combination of immune, genetic, and environmental factors is suspected. PsA can occur in five forms:

- Arthritis involving primarily the small joints of the hands and feet
- Asymmetric arthritis involving joints of the extremities
- Symmetric polyarthritis resembling RA
- Arthritis of the sacroiliac joints and spine (psoriatic spondylitis)
- Arthritis mutilans, a rare but very deforming and destructive disease[22]

On x-ray, the cartilage loss and erosion resemble that of RA. Advanced cases of PsA often reveal widened joint spaces, and a "pencil in cup" deformity is common at the DIP joints as a result of osteolysis. Elevated ESR, mild anemia, and elevated blood uric acid levels can be seen in some patients; gout must be excluded. Treatment includes splinting, joint protection, and physical therapy. Intramuscular gold therapy has been used to treat PsA in the past with some success but now has been replaced by newer DMARDs such as methotrexate, which are effective for both articular and cutaneous manifestations. Sulfasalazine (Azulfidine) and cyclosporine have also have been used with some success in the treatment of PsA. Biologic therapy drugs, including etanercept (Enbrel) and infliximab (Remicade), are also being used for treating PsA.

REACTIVE ARTHRITIS

Reactive arthritis (*Reiter's syndrome*) occurs more commonly in young men as compared to young women. It is associated with a symptom complex that includes urethritis, conjunctivitis, and mucocutaneous lesions.[23] In women, symptoms include cervicitis. Although the exact etiology is unknown, reactive arthritis appears to occur after a genitourinary or GI tract infection.[21] *Chlamydia trachomatis* is most often implicated in sexually transmitted reactive arthritis. Men and women appear to have equal risk for developing dysenteric reactive arthritis, which typically occurs within days or weeks after infection with *Shigella, Salmonella, Campylobacter,* or *Yersinia.* Individuals with inherited HLA-B27 are at increased risk of developing reactive arthritis after sexual contact or exposure to certain enteric pathogens, supporting the likelihood of a genetic predisposition.

Urethritis develops within 1 to 2 weeks after sexual contact or dysentery. Low-grade fever, conjunctivitis, and arthritis may occur over the next several weeks. This type of arthritis tends to be asymmetric, frequently involving the large joints of the lower extremities and the toes. Lower back pain may occur with severe disease. Mucocutaneous lesions commonly occur as small, painless, superficial ulcerations on the tongue, oral mucosa, and glans penis. Soft tissue manifestations commonly include enthesopathies such as Achilles tendinitis or plantar fasciitis. Few laboratory abnormalities occur, although the ESR may be elevated.

Prognosis is favorable, with most patients recovering after 2 to 16 weeks. Because reactive arthritis is often associated with *C. trachomatis* infection, treatment of patients and their sexual partners with doxycycline (Vibramycin) 100 mg twice daily for up to 3 months is widely recommended. Conjunctivitis and lesions require no treatment, but topical ophthalmic corticosteroids are typically prescribed for treatment of uveitis. Physical therapy may be helpful during disease recovery.

Joints heal completely, and many patients have complete remission with full joint function. Up to 50% may develop chronic or recurring disease, which can result in major disability. X-ray changes in chronic disease closely resemble those of AS. Treatment of chronic reactive arthritis is symptomatic.

SEPTIC ARTHRITIS

Septic arthritis (infectious or bacterial arthritis) is caused by an invasion of the joint cavity with microorganisms. Bacteria can travel through the bloodstream from another site of active infection, resulting in hematogenous seeding of the joint. Organisms can also be introduced directly through trauma or surgical incision. Any bacteria can cause the infection. In the immunocompromised patient, even nonpathogenic bacteria can be responsible for development of septic arthritis. *Staphylococcus aureus* is the most common causative organism. *Streptococcus hemolyticus* is also seen. *Neisseria gonorrhoeae* is the most common cause in sexually active young adults. Factors that increase the risk of infection include diseases in which there is decreased host resistance, such as leukemia and diabetes mellitus; treatment with corticosteroids or immunosuppressive drugs; and debilitating chronic illness.

In septic arthritis, large joints such as the knee and hip are most frequently involved. Inflammation of the joint cavity causes severe pain, erythema, and swelling. Because infection has often spread from a primary site elsewhere in the body, fever or shaking chills often accompany articular manifestations. A diagnosis may be made by aspiration of the joint (arthrocentesis) and culture of the synovial fluid. Blood cultures for aerobic and anaerobic organisms should also be obtained.[24]

Septic arthritis requires prompt treatment to prevent joint destruction. Broad-spectrum antibiotics against gram-negative organisms, pneumococci, and staphylococci are often started before cultures identify the causative organism. Once the organism is determined, the treatment can be narrowed. Infections may respond to treatment within 2 weeks or may take as long as 4 to 8 weeks, depending on the causative organism. Local aspiration and surgical drainage may be required. If diagnosis and treatment are delayed, destruction of articular cartilage can occur, followed by loss of joint function. Chronic infection can also develop. Septic arthritis of the hip can contribute to development of avascular necrosis.

Nursing intervention includes assessment and monitoring of joint inflammation, pain, and fever. Immobilization of affected joints to control pain can be achieved by use of resting splints or traction. Local hot compresses can also help relieve pain. Gentle ROM exercises should be initiated as soon as tolerated to prevent muscle atrophy and joint contractures. The nurse should explain the need for antibiotics and the importance of their continued use until the infection is resolved. Support should be offered to the patient who requires arthrocentesis or operative drainage. Strict aseptic technique should be used during assistance with joint aspiration procedures.

LYME DISEASE

Lyme disease is a spirochetal infection caused by *Borrelia burgdorferi* and transmitted by the bite of an infected deer tick. It was first identified in 1975 in Lyme, Connecticut, after an unusual clustering of arthritis in children and is now the most common vector-borne disease in the United States. The tick typically feeds on mice, dogs, cats, cows, horses, deer, and humans. Wild animals do not exhibit the illness, but clinical Lyme disease does occur in domestic animals. Person-to-person transmission does not occur. The peak season for human infection is during the summer months. Most U.S. cases occur in three endemic areas: along the northeastern coast from Maryland to Massachusetts; in the midwestern states of Wisconsin and Minnesota; and along the northwestern coast of California and Oregon. Over 23,000 cases were reported in the United States in 2002.[25]

Lyme disease symptoms can mimic other diseases such as multiple sclerosis, mononucleosis, and meningitis. The most characteristic clinical symptom of early localized disease is erythema migrans (EM), a skin lesion that occurs at the site of the tick bite within 2 to 30 days after exposure (Fig. 65-7). The lesion begins as a red macule or papule that slowly expands to form a large round lesion with a bright red border and central clearing. The EM lesion is often accompanied by acute viral-like symptoms, such as fever, chills, headache, stiff neck, fatigue, swollen lymph nodes, and migratory joint and muscle pain. Symptoms usually occur in a week but may be delayed for up to 30 days.

If not treated, symptoms of Lyme disease can progress within several weeks or months to include nervous system problems such as severe headaches, temporary facial paralysis (e.g., Bell's palsy), or poor motor coordination. In late disease, which can occur from months to years after the initial infection, arthritis pain and swelling may occur in large joints. Arthritic symptoms are often temporary, but about 10% of people with Lyme disease will develop chronic Lyme arthritis if untreated. Neurologic disorders can also occur at this stage, including one condition known as tertiary neuroborreliosis that results in confusion and forgetfulness.

A diagnosis of Lyme disease is often based on clinical manifestations, in particular the EM lesion, and a history of exposure in an endemic area. CBC and ESR results are usually normal. Lyme serology tests for antibodies may be falsely negative in early disease but are reliable for diagnosis in later disease.[26] Cerebrospinal fluid should be examined in individuals with neurologic involvement.

Active lesions can be treated with oral antibiotic therapy. Doxycycline (Vibramycin), cefuroxime (Ceftin), and amoxicillin are often effective in early-stage infection and in prevention of later stages of the disease. Doxycycline has also shown to be effective in preventing Lyme disease when given within 3 days after the bite of a deer tick. Short-term therapy of 2 to 3 weeks is usually effective for solitary EM, but long-standing infection may require extended parenteral antibiotic therapy. Intravenous ceftriaxone (Rocephin) is prescribed for severe cardiac or neurologic problems. Reducing exposure to ticks is the best way to prevent Lyme disease. Patient and family teaching for those in endemic areas is outlined in Table 65-11. A vaccine for Lyme disease is no longer available.

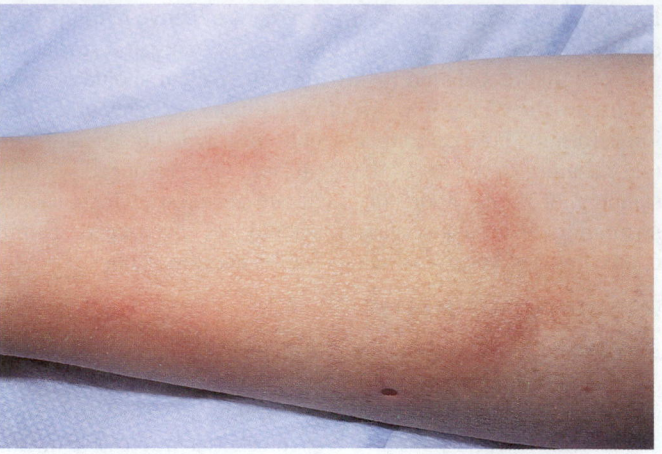

FIG. 65-7   Erythema migrans. Early skin lesion in Lyme disease.

TABLE 65-11	***PATIENT AND FAMILY TEACHING GUIDE*** **Prevention of Lyme Disease (Endemic Areas)**

- Avoid walking through tall grasses and low brush, and sitting on logs.
- Mow grass and remove brush around paths, buildings, and campsites.
- Move woodpiles and bird feeders away from house.
- Wear long pants or nylon tights of tightly woven, light-colored fabric so that ticks can be easily seen.
- Tuck pants into boots or long socks, tuck long-sleeved shirts into pants, and wear closed shoes when hiking.
- Check often for ticks crawling from pantlegs to open skin.
- Thoroughly inspect and wash clothes.
- Spray insect repellent containing DEET on skin or permethrin on clothes, especially on lower extremities.
- Have pets wear tick collars, inspect them often, and do not allow pets on furniture or beds.
- Remove attached ticks with tweezers (not fingers). Grasp tick's mouth parts as close to skin as possible and gently pull straight out. Do not twist or jerk.
- Save the tick in a bottle of alcohol, if you need later for identification.
- Wash bitten area with soap and water and apply antiseptic. Wash hands.
- See a doctor immediately if flu-like symptoms or a bulls-eye rash appears within 2 to 30 days after removal of tick.

DEET, N,N-diethyl-M-toluamide.

HUMAN IMMUNODEFICIENCY VIRUS–ASSOCIATED RHEUMATIC DISEASE

A variety of rheumatic disorders can develop in the course of human immunodeficiency virus (HIV) infection.[27] The cause of these disorders in HIV-infected persons is not clearly known. However, an autoimmune process and an inflammatory response may be occurring at the same time in the patient who is immunosuppressed. Up to 70% of HIV-infected patients may develop a rheumatic disease in the later stages of HIV infection. Rheumatic diseases associated with HLA-B27 appear to be more severe in HIV-infected patients. Conditions typically associated with HIV infection include SLE, reactive arthritis, PsA, Sjögren's syndrome, polymyositis, and fibromyalgia syndrome. The knees and ankles are generally the most affected joints. Most patients improve with conventional arthritis treatments such as NSAIDs, but patients with reactive arthritis or PsA may not respond

TABLE 65-12	Conditions That Can Cause Hyperuricemia

- Acidosis or ketosis
- Alcoholism
- Atherosclerosis
- Chemotherapeutic drugs
- Diabetes mellitus
- Drug-induced renal impairment
- Hyperlipidemia
- Hypertension
- Malignant disease
- Myeloproliferative disorders
- Obesity or starvation
- Renal disease
- Sickle cell anemia
- Use of certain common drugs (salicylates, diuretics)

GENDER DIFFERENCES
Gout

Men
- Occurs more commonly in men than in women.
- Occurs predominantly in middle-aged men.

Women
- Almost no occurrence of gout in premenopausal women.

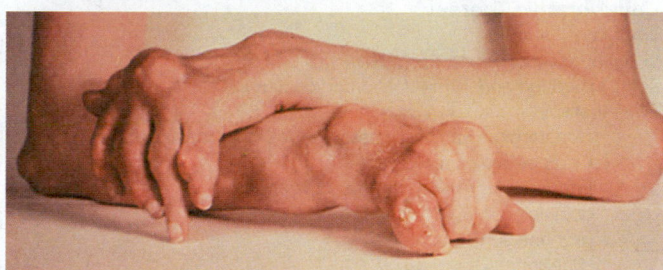

FIG. 65-8   Tophaceous gout.

as well and develop progressive deformities. As with other patients, appropriate physical therapy is recommended.

GOUT

Gout is caused by an increase in uric acid production, underexcretion of uric acid by the kidneys, or increased intake of foods containing purines, which are metabolized to uric acid by the body. Characteristic deposits of sodium urate crystals occur in articular, periarticular, and subcutaneous tissues. Joint involvement includes recurrent attacks of acute arthritis. Over 2 million Americans are affected by gout.

Gout may be classified as primary or secondary.[28] In *primary gout,* a hereditary error of purine metabolism leads to the overproduction or retention of uric acid. *Secondary gout* may be related to another acquired disorder (Table 65-12) or may be the result of drugs known to inhibit uric acid excretion. Secondary gout may also be caused by drugs that increase the rate of cell death, such as the chemotherapeutic agents used in treating leukemia. Primary gout, which accounts for 90% of cases, occurs predominantly in middle-aged men, with almost no incidence in premenopausal women. Hyperuricemia may also develop in patients taking thiazide diuretics, in postmenopausal women, and in organ transplant recipients who are receiving immunosuppressive agents.

Obesity in men has been shown to increase the risk of gout.[29] Hypertension, diuretic use, and excessive alcohol consumption are additional risk factors. A diet high in purine-rich foods (e.g., shellfish such as crab and shrimp; vegetables such as lentils, asparagus, and spinach; meats such as beef, chicken, and pork) will not cause gout but can trigger an acute attack if a person is susceptible to gout.

Etiology and Pathophysiology

Uric acid is the major end product of purine catabolism and is primarily excreted by the kidneys. Hyperuricemia may be the result of increased purine synthesis, decreased renal excretion, or both. A high dietary intake of purine alone has relatively little effect on uric acid levels. Hyperuricemia may result from prolonged fasting or excessive alcohol drinking because of the increased production of keto acids, which then inhibit uric acid excretion.

Clinical Manifestations and Complications

In the acute phase, gouty arthritis may occur in one or more joints but usually less than four. Affected joints may appear dusky or cyanotic and are extremely tender. Inflammation of the great toe (*podagra*) is the most common initial problem. Other affected joints may include the midtarsal area of the foot, ankle, knee, and wrist.

Olecranon bursae may also be involved. Acute gouty arthritis is usually precipitated by trigger events such as trauma, surgery, alcohol ingestion, or systemic infection. The onset of symptoms typically occurs at night with sudden swelling and excruciating pain peaking within several hours, often accompanied by low-grade fever. Individual attacks usually subside, treated or untreated, in 2 to 10 days. The affected joint returns entirely to normal, and patients are often free of symptoms between attacks.

Chronic gout is characterized by multiple joint involvement and visible deposits of sodium urate crystals called *tophi.* These are typically noted in the synovium, subchondral bone, olecranon bursae, and vertebrae; along tendons; and in the skin and cartilage (Fig. 65-8). Tophi are rarely present at the time of the initial attack and are generally noted only many years after the onset of disease.

The severity of gouty arthritis is variable. The clinical course may consist of infrequent mild attacks or multiple severe episodes (up to 12/yr) associated with a slowly progressive disability. In general, the higher the serum uric acid level, the earlier the appearance of tophi and the greater the tendency toward more frequent, severe episodes of acute gout. Chronic inflammation may result in joint deformity, and cartilage destruction may predispose the joint to secondary OA. Large and unsightly tophaceous deposits may perforate overlying skin, producing draining sinuses that often become secondarily infected. Excessive uric acid excretion may lead to kidney or urinary tract stone formation. Pyelonephritis associated with intrarenal sodium urate deposits and obstruction may contribute to renal disease.

Diagnostic Studies

Serum uric acid levels are usually elevated above 6 mg/dl. However, hyperuricemia is not specifically diagnostic of gout because increased levels may be related to a variety of drugs or may exist as a totally asymptomatic abnormality in the general population. Specimens for 24-hour urine uric acid levels may be obtained to determine if the disease is caused by decreased renal excretion or overproduction of uric acid.

Synovial fluid aspiration is a controversial part of patient evaluation because an accurate diagnosis of gout is possible in 80% of patients based on clinical symptoms alone. However, aspiration

TABLE 65-13	COLLABORATIVE CARE Gout

Diagnostic
History and physical examination
Family history of gout
Presence of sodium urate crystals in synovial fluid
Elevated serum uric acid levels
Elevated 24-hr urine for uric acid levels
X-ray

Collaborative Therapy
Joint immobilization
Local application of heat or cold
Joint aspiration and intraarticular corticosteroids
Drug therapy
- Nonsteroidal antiinflammatory drugs (e.g., naproxen [Naprosyn])
- Corticosteroids (prednisone)
- Intraarticular (methylprednisolone acetate)
- colchicine
- probenecid (Benemid)
- allopurinol (Zyloprim)
- Adrenocorticotropic hormone (ACTH)
Dietary avoidance of food/fluids with high purine content (e.g., anchovies, liver, wine/beer)

may have therapeutic value by decompressing a swollen joint capsule. Joint aspiration is also the only reliable method to distinguish gout from septic arthritis and *pseudogout* (calcium phosphate crystals are formed). Affected fluid characteristically contains needle-like crystals of sodium urate. X-rays appear normal in the early stages of gout, with tophi, an indicator of chronic disease, appearing as eroded areas in the bone.

Collaborative Care

Goals for care of the patient with gout (Table 65-13) include termination of an acute attack through use of an antiinflammatory agent such as colchicine, with NSAIDs prescribed adjunctively for pain management. Future attacks are prevented by a maintenance dose of allopurinol (Zyloprim, Alloprim) in combination with weight reduction, as needed, and possible avoidance of alcohol and food high in purine (red and organ meats). Treatment is also aimed at preventing the formation of uric acid kidney stones and the development of associated conditions such as hypertriglyceridemia and hypertension.

Drug Therapy. Acute gouty arthritis is treated with colchicine and NSAIDs. Colchicine has known antiinflammatory effects but no analgesic properties, so an NSAID is added to the treatment regimen primarily for pain management. Oral administration of colchicine generally produces dramatic pain relief within 24 to 48 hours. Colchicine also has diagnostic merit in that a good response to this drug gives further evidence for the diagnosis of gout. Recurrent gout may be prevented by combining colchicines with a xanthine oxidase inhibitor such as allopurinol or a uricosuric drug such as probenecid (Benemid). Corticosteroids either orally or by intraarticular injection can be helpful in treating acute attacks. Systemic corticosteroids may be used only if routine therapies are contraindicated or ineffective. Adrenocorticotropic hormone (ACTH) may also be used for treating acute gout.

For many years the standard therapy for hyperuricemia caused by urate underexcretion has been uricosuric drugs such as probenecid, which inhibit renal tubular reabsorption of urates. However, this class of drugs is ineffective when creatinine clearance is reduced, as

can occur in patients over the age of 60. Aspirin inactivates the effect of uricosurics, resulting in urate retention, and should be avoided while patients are taking uricosuric drugs. Acetaminophen can be used safely if analgesia is required.

Adequate urine volume with normal renal function (2 to 3 L/day) must be maintained to prevent precipitation of uric acid in the renal tubules. Allopurinol, which blocks the production of uric acid, is particularly useful in patients with uric acid stones or renal impairment, in whom uricosuric drugs may be ineffective or dangerous. For patients who cannot tolerate allopurinol because of side effects, oxypurinol can be prescribed. Oxypurinol is the active metabolite of allopurinol. The angiotensin II receptor antagonist losartan (Cozaar) may be especially useful for treatment of elderly patients with both gout and hypertension. Losartan given 50 mg daily will promote urate diuresis and may normalize serum urate levels. Combination therapy with losartan and allopurinol may also be given. Regardless of which drugs are prescribed, serum uric acid levels must be checked regularly to monitor treatment effectiveness.

Febuxostat, a selective inhibitor of xanthine oxidase, has recently been shown in clinical trials to reduce serum uric acid in persons with chronic gout.[30] This is the first drug developed in 40 years to treat gout.

Nutritional Therapy. Traditional dietary restrictions include limiting the use of alcohol and the consumption of foods high in purine (see Table 46-13). However, drugs can often control gout without necessitating these changes. Obese patients should be instructed in a carefully planned weight-reduction program.

NURSING MANAGEMENT
GOUT

Nursing interventions for the patient with acute gouty arthritis include supportive care of the inflamed joints. Special care is taken to avoid causing pain to an inflamed joint by careless handling. Bed rest may be appropriate with affected joints properly immobilized. Involvement of a lower extremity may require use of a cradle or footboard to protect the painful area from the weight of bed clothes. The limitation of motion and degree of pain should be assessed, and treatment effectiveness should be documented.

The nurse should help the patient and the family to understand that hyperuricemia and gouty arthritis are chronic problems that can be controlled with careful adherence to a treatment program. Thorough explanations should be given concerning the importance of drug therapy and the need for periodic determination of serum uric acid levels. The patient should be able to demonstrate knowledge of precipitating factors that may cause an attack, including excessive caloric intake or overindulgence in purine-containing foods and alcohol; starvation (fasting); drug use (e.g., niacin, aspirin, diuretics); and major medical events (e.g., surgery, myocardial infarction).

SYSTEMIC LUPUS ERYTHEMATOSUS

Systemic lupus erythematosus (SLE) is a multisystem inflammatory disease of autoimmune origin. It is a complex disorder of multifactorial origin resulting from interactions among genetic, hormonal, environmental, and immunologic factors. SLE typically affects the skin, joints, and serous membranes (pleura, pericardium), along with the renal, hematologic, and neurologic systems.

The overall incidence of SLE in the United States is 2 to 8 per 100,000. Most cases of SLE occur in women in their childbearing years. Women are 10 times more likely to develop SLE than men. African Americans (especially), Asian Americans, Hispanics, and Native Americans are more likely than whites to develop the disease.[31] SLE is characterized by variability within and among persons. Its chronic unpredictable course is marked by alternating periods of exacerbations and remissions.

Etiology and Pathophysiology

The etiology of the abnormal immune response in SLE is unknown.[32] Based on the high prevalence of SLE among family members, a genetic influence has long been suspected. Multiple susceptibility genes from the HLA complex show associations with SLE, including HLA-DR3. Hormones are also known to play a role in the etiology of SLE. Onset or exacerbation of disease symptoms sometimes occurs after the onset of menarche, with the use of oral contraceptives, and during and after pregnancy. The disease tends to worsen in the immediate postpartum period.

Environmental factors are believed to contribute to the occurrence of SLE, with sun exposure and sunburns as the most significant environmental triggers. Infectious agents may serve as a stimulus for immune hyperactivity. SLE may also be precipitated or aggravated by certain drugs such as procainamide (Pronestyl), hydralazine (Apresoline), and a number of antiseizure drugs.

SLE is characterized by the production of a large variety of autoantibodies against nucleic acids (e.g., single- and double-stranded DNA), erythrocytes, coagulation proteins, lymphocytes, platelets, and many other self proteins. Most characteristically the autoimmune reactions are directed against constituents of the cell nucleus (antinuclear antibodies [ANAs]), particularly DNA.

Circulating immune complexes containing antibody against DNA are deposited in the basement membranes of capillaries in the kidneys, heart, skin, brain, and joints. Complement is activated and inflammation occurs. The overaggressive antibody response is also related to activation of B and T cells. The specific manifestations of SLE depend on which cell types or organs are involved. (SLE is a type III hypersensitivity response [see Chapter 14].)

Clinical Manifestations and Complications

SLE is extremely variable in its severity, ranging from a relatively mild disorder to a rapidly progressive one affecting many body systems (Fig. 65-9). No characteristic pattern occurs in the progressive involvement of SLE. Any organ can be affected by an accumulation of circulating immune complexes. The most commonly affected tissues are the skin and muscle, the lining of the lungs, the heart, nervous tissue, and the kidneys. Generalized com-

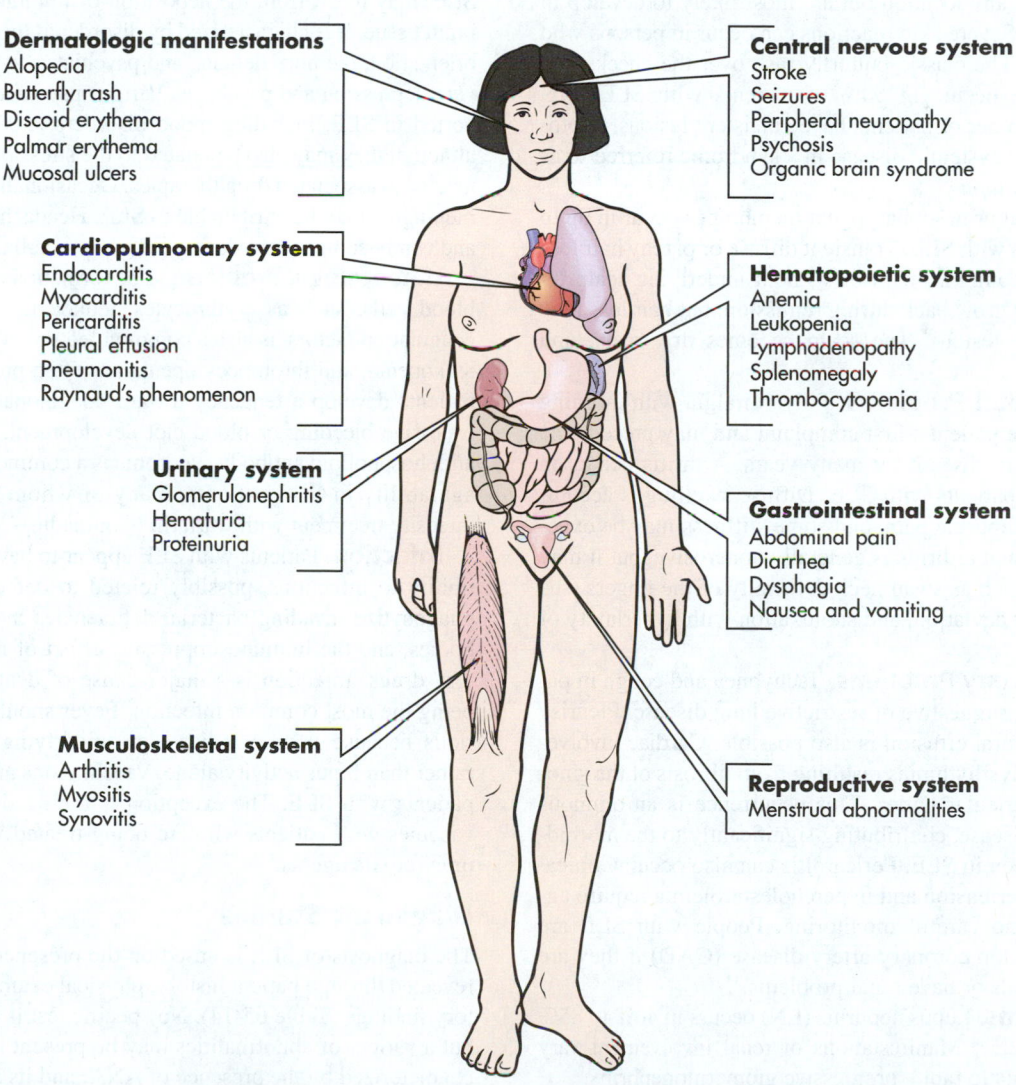

Dermatologic manifestations
Alopecia
Butterfly rash
Discoid erythema
Palmar erythema
Mucosal ulcers

Cardiopulmonary system
Endocarditis
Myocarditis
Pericarditis
Pleural effusion
Pneumonitis
Raynaud's phenomenon

Urinary system
Glomerulonephritis
Hematuria
Proteinuria

Musculoskeletal system
Arthritis
Myositis
Synovitis

Central nervous system
Stroke
Seizures
Peripheral neuropathy
Psychosis
Organic brain syndrome

Hematopoietic system
Anemia
Leukopenia
Lymphadenopathy
Splenomegaly
Thrombocytopenia

Gastrointestinal system
Abdominal pain
Diarrhea
Dysphagia
Nausea and vomiting

Reproductive system
Menstrual abnormalities

FIG. 65-9 Multisystem involvement in systemic lupus erythematosus.

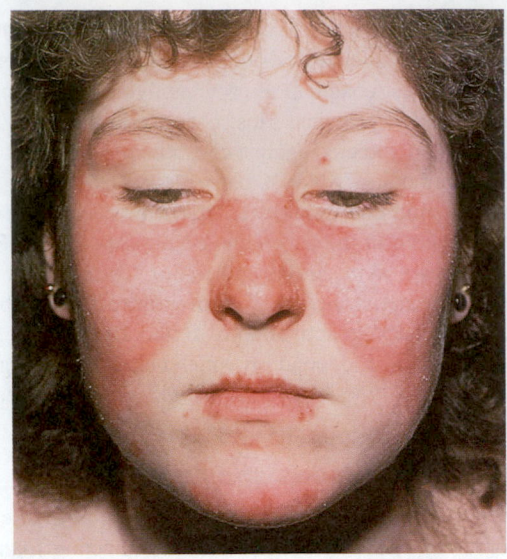

FIG. 65-10 Butterfly rash of systemic lupus erythematosus.

plaints such as fever, weight loss, arthralgia, and excessive fatigue may precede an exacerbation of disease activity.

Dermatologic Manifestations. Cutaneous vascular lesions can appear in any location but are most likely to develop in sun-exposed areas. Severe skin reactions can occur in persons who are photosensitive. The classic butterfly rash over the cheeks and bridge of the nose occurs in 50% of patients with SLE (Fig. 65-10). A small number of patients have persistent lesions, photosensitivity, and mild systemic disease in a syndrome referred to as *subacute cutaneous lupus.*

Ulcers of the oral or nasopharyngeal membranes occur in up to one third of patients with SLE. Transient diffuse or patchy hair loss *(alopecia)* is also common, with or without underlying scalp lesions. The hair may grow back during remission, but hair loss may be permanent over lesions. The scalp becomes dry, scaly, and atrophied.

Musculoskeletal Problems. Polyarthralgia with morning stiffness is often the patient's first complaint and may precede the onset of multisystem disease by many years. Arthritis occurs in more than 90% of patients with SLE. Diffuse swelling is accompanied by joint and muscle pain, and some stiffness may be experienced. Lupus-related arthritis is generally nonerosive, but it may cause deformities such as swan neck deformity of the fingers (see Fig. 65-4, *D*), ulnar deviation, and subluxation with hyperlaxity of the joints.

Cardiopulmonary Problems. Tachypnea and cough in patients with SLE are suggestive of restrictive lung disease. Pleurisy with or without pleural effusion is also possible. Cardiac involvement may include dysrhythmias resulting from fibrosis of the sinoatrial and atrioventricular nodes. This occurrence is an ominous sign of advanced disease, contributing significantly to the morbidity and mortality seen in SLE. Pericarditis can also occur. Clinical factors such as hypertension and hypercholesterolemia require aggressive therapy and careful monitoring. People with SLE are more likely to develop coronary artery disease (CAD) if they are taking corticosteroids or have renal problems.[33]

Renal Problems. Lupus nephritis (LN) occurs in 40% to 85% of patients with SLE.[34] Manifestations of renal involvement vary from mild proteinuria to rapid, progressive glomerulonephritis.

The primary goal in treating LN is to slow the progression of nephropathy and preserve renal function by managing the underlying disease. The importance of obtaining a renal biopsy is controversial, but findings can help guide treatment, which typically includes corticosteroids, cytotoxic agents (cyclophosphamide [Cytoxan]), and immunosuppressive agents (azathioprine [Imuran], cyclosporine [Sandimmune]). Cyclophosphamide is the most effective cytotoxic therapy, but azathioprine is considered to be less toxic. Oral prednisone or pulsed IV methylprednisolone may also be used as an intervention for LN, especially in the initial treatment period when cytotoxic agents have not had time to take effect.

Mycophenolate mofetil (CellCept), which is typically used to prevent organ transplant rejection, has recently been shown in a small study to be more effective and safer in the long-term treatment of LN when compared to cyclophosphamide.[35] Larger clinical studies are currently underway.

Nervous System Problems. Along with renal involvement, neuropsychiatric manifestations are prevalent in SLE. Generalized or focal seizures are the most common manifestation involving the central nervous system (CNS), and occur in as many as 15% of patients with SLE by the time of diagnosis. Seizures are generally controlled by corticosteroids or antiseizure drugs. Peripheral neuropathy can also occur, leading to sensory and motor deficits.

Cognitive dysfunction, recognized as a CNS manifestation of SLE, may result from the deposition of immune complexes within brain tissue. It is characterized by disordered thought processes, disorientation, memory deficits, and psychiatric symptoms such as severe depression and psychosis. Various psychiatric disorders are reported in SLE, including mood disorders, anxiety, and psychosis, although they may also be related to the stress of having a major illness or to associated drug therapies. Occasionally a stroke or aseptic meningitis may be attributable to SLE. Headaches are also common and can become severe during a flare (exacerbation of disease).

Hematologic Problems. The formation of antibodies against blood cells, such as erythrocytes, leukocytes, thrombocytes, and coagulation factors, is also a common feature of SLE. Anemia, mild leukopenia, and thrombocytopenia are often present in SLE. Some patients develop a tendency toward coagulopathy involving either excessive bleeding or blood clot development. A manifestation of antiphospholipid antibody syndrome is a common cause of hypercoagulability in SLE patients, many of whom benefit from high-intensity treatment with warfarin (Coumadin).

Infection. Patients with SLE appear to have increased susceptibility to infections, possibly related to defects in the ability to phagocytize invading bacteria, deficiencies in production of antibodies, and the immunosuppressive effect of many antiinflammatory drugs. Infection is a major cause of death, with pneumonia being the most common infection. Fever should be considered serious because it may indicate an underlying infectious process rather than lupus activity alone. Vaccinations are generally safe for patients with SLE. The exception is the need to avoid live virus vaccines with patients who are being treated with corticosteroids or cytotoxic agents.

Diagnostic Studies

The diagnosis of SLE is based on the presence of distinct criteria revealed through patient history, physical examination, and laboratory findings (Table 65-14). No specific test is diagnostic for SLE, but a variety of abnormalities may be present in the blood. SLE is characterized by the presence of ANA, and its identification estab-

TABLE 65-14	Criteria for Diagnosis of Systemic Lupus Erythematosus*

- Malar rash
- Discoid rash
- Photosensitivity
- Oral ulcers
- Arthritis: nonerosive, involvement of two or more joints characterized by tenderness, swelling, and effusion
- Serositis: pleuritis or pericarditis
- Renal disorder: persistent proteinuria or cellular casts in urine
- Neurologic disorder: seizures or psychosis
- Hematologic disorder: hemolytic anemia, leukopenia, lymphopenia, or thrombocytopenia
- Immunologic disorder: positive LE preparation; anti-DNA antibody or antibody to Sm nuclear antigen; or false-positive serologic tests for syphilis
- Antinuclear antibody

Data from American College of Rheumatology: Classification criteria for rheumatic diseases. Available at *www.rheumatology.org/publications/classification* (accessed April 30, 2006).

LE, Lupus erythematosus; *Sm,* Smith.

*A person is classified as having SLE if four or more of the criteria are present, serially or simultaneously, during any interval of observation. Revised criteria by a subcommittee of the American College of Rheumatology are used for the purpose of *classification* in population surveys, *not* for the diagnosis of individual patients.

TABLE 65-15	COLLABORATIVE CARE Systemic Lupus Erythematosus

Diagnostic
History and physical examination
Antibodies
- Anti-DNA antibody
- Anti-Sm antibody
- Antinuclear antibody (ANA)
Complete blood cell count
LE cell prep
Urinalysis
X-ray of affected joints
Chest x-ray
ECG to determine extraarticular involvement

Collaborative Therapy
NSAIDs for mild disease
Steroid-sparing drugs (e.g., methotrexate)
Antimalarials (e.g., hydroxychloroquine [Plaquenil])
Corticosteroids for exacerbations and severe disease
Immunosuppressive drugs
- cyclophosphamide (Cytoxan)
- azathioprine (Imuran)

ECG, Electrocardiogram; *LE,* lupus erythematosus; *NSAIDs,* nonsteroidal antiinflammatory drugs; *Sm antibody,* Smith antibody.

lishes the existence of an autoimmune disease. Other antibodies include anti-DNA, antineuronal, anticoagulant, anti-WBC, anti–red blood cell (RBC), antiplatelet, antiphospholipid, and anti–basement membrane. The tests that are most specific for SLE include the anti–double-stranded DNA and the anti-Smith (Sm). High levels of anti-DNA are rarely found in any condition other than SLE, and anti-Sm seems to be found almost exclusively in SLE. The lupus erythematosus (LE) cell prep test is a nonspecific test for SLE and is positive in other rheumatic diseases. ESR and CRP levels are not diagnostic of SLE but may be used to monitor disease activity and effectiveness of therapy.

Collaborative Care

A major challenge in treatment of SLE is to manage the active phase of the disease while preventing complications of treatments that cause long-term tissue damage. An improving prognosis of SLE may be the result of earlier diagnosis, prompt recognition of serious organ involvement, and better therapeutic regimens. Survival is influenced by several factors, including age, race, gender, socioeconomic status, accompanying morbid conditions, and severity of disease.

Drug Therapy. NSAIDs continue to be an important intervention, especially for patients with mild polyarthralgias or polyarthritis. Because prolonged therapy is likely, careful patient monitoring must include the potential for GI effects from NSAID use. Antimalarial agents such as hydroxychloroquine (Plaquenil) are often used to treat fatigue and moderate skin and joint problems. The beneficial effect may not be noticed for several months.[32] Flares may also be prevented with these drugs. Retinopathy can develop with high-dose use of these drugs, but it generally reverses when they are discontinued. If the patient cannot tolerate an antimalarial agent, an antileprosy drug such as dapsone may be used.

Corticosteroid exposure should be limited, but tapering doses of IV methylprednisolone may be useful in controlling severe exacerbations of polyarthritis. Steroid-sparing drugs such as metho-

trexate can serve as an alternate treatment and are prescribed in combination with folic acid to decrease minor side effects of corticosteroids. However, high doses of corticosteroids may be especially appropriate for the patient with very severe cutaneous SLE. Immunosuppressive drugs such as azathioprine (Imuran) and cyclophosphamide (Cytoxan) may be prescribed to reduce the need for long-term corticosteroid therapy. Azathioprine or cyclophosphamide is also appropriate for treatment of severe organ-system disease, especially LN. Close monitoring is necessary to minimize drug toxicity and side effects.

Clinical trials are currently investigating the effect of high-dose cyclophosphamide combined with autologous stem cell transplantation for patients with severe SLE who are not responsive to treatment. An earlier study showed beneficial results in a majority of patients.[36]

Disease management is most appropriately monitored by serial anti-DNA titers (Table 65-15). Simpler and less costly tests such as ESR or CRP may also help in monitoring treatment effectiveness. Patient teaching related to prescribed drugs must include their indications for use, proper administration, and possible side effects. The patient should understand that abrupt cessation may precipitate exacerbation of disease activity.

NURSING MANAGEMENT
SYSTEMIC LUPUS ERYTHEMATOSUS

■ *Nursing Assessment*

As in the majority of rheumatic diseases, the chronic and unpredictable nature of SLE presents many challenges to the patient and family. The physical, psychologic, and sociocultural problems associated with the long-term management of SLE require the varied approaches and skills of the multidisciplinary health care team.

Subjective and objective data that should be obtained from the patient with SLE are presented in Table 65-16. In particular, the

TABLE 65-16	*NURSING ASSESSMENT* Systemic Lupus Erythematosus

Subjective Data

Important Health Information

Past health history: Exposure to ultraviolet radiation, drugs, chemicals, viral infections; physical or psychologic stress; states of increased estrogen activity, including early onset of menarche, pregnancy, and postpartum period; pattern of remissions and exacerbations

Medications: Use of oral contraceptives, procainamide (Pronestyl), hydralazine (Apresoline), isoniazid (INH), antiseizure drugs, antibiotics (possibly precipitating symptoms of SLE); corticosteroids, NSAIDs

Functional Health Patterns

Health perception–health management: Family history of autoimmune disorders; frequent infections; malaise

Nutritional-metabolic: Weight loss, oral and nasal ulcers; nausea and vomiting; xerostomia (salivary gland dryness), dysphagia; photosensitivity with rash; frequent infections

Elimination: Decreased urine output; diarrhea or constipation

Activity-exercise: Morning stiffness; joint swelling and deformity; shortness of breath, dyspnea; excessive fatigue

Sleep-rest: Insomnia

Cognitive-perceptual: Visual disturbances; vertigo; headache; polyarthralgia; chest pain (pericardial, pleuritic); abdominal pain; joint pain; pain, throbbing, coldness of fingers with numbness and tingling

Sexuality-reproductive: Amenorrhea, irregular menstrual periods

Coping–stress tolerance: Depression, withdrawal

Objective Data

General

Fever, lymphadenopathy, periorbital edema

Integumentary

Alopecia; dry, scaly scalp; keratoconjunctivitis, malar "butterfly" rash, palmar or discoid erythema, urticaria, periungual erythema, purpura, or petechiae; leg ulcers

Respiratory

Pleural friction rub, decreased breath sounds

Cardiovascular

Vasculitis; pericardial friction rub; hypertension, edema, dysrhythmias, murmurs; bilateral, symmetric pallor and cyanosis of fingers (Raynaud's phenomenon)

Gastrointestinal

Oral and pharyngeal ulcers; splenomegaly

Neurologic

Facial weakness, peripheral neuropathies, papilledema, dysarthria, confusion, hallucination, disorientation, psychosis, seizures, aphasia, hemiparesis

Musculoskeletal

Myopathy, myositis, arthritis

Urinary

Proteinuria

Possible Findings

Presence of anti-DNA, anti-Sm, and antinuclear antibodies; anemia, leukopenia, thrombocytopenia; ↑ erythrocyte sedimentation rate (ESR); positive LE cell prep; ↑ serum creatinine; microscopic hematuria, cellular casts in urine; pericarditis or pleural effusion evident on chest x-ray

NSAIDs, Nonsteroidal antiinflammatory drugs; *SLE,* systemic lupus erythematosus; *Sm,* Smith.

TABLE 65-17	*PATIENT AND FAMILY TEACHING GUIDE* Systemic Lupus Erythematosus

Teaching related to the disease and appropriate management should include

1. Disease process
2. Names of drugs, actions, side effects, dosage, administration
3. Pain management strategies
4. Energy conservation and pacing techniques
5. Therapeutic exercise, use of heat therapy (for arthralgia)
6. Avoidance of physical and emotional stress
7. Avoidance of exposure to individuals with infection
8. Avoidance of drying soaps, powders, household chemicals
9. Use of sunscreen protection (at least SPF 15) and protective clothing, with minimal sun exposure from 11:00 AM to 3:00 PM
10. Regular medical and laboratory follow-up
11. Marital and pregnancy counseling as needed
12. Community resources and health care agencies

SPF, Sun protection factor.

extent to which pain and fatigue influence activities of daily living must be evaluated. A developmental approach focuses on age-appropriate education and counseling on issues such as personal relationships, family planning, occupational responsibilities, and recreational activities.

■ Nursing Diagnoses

Nursing diagnoses for the patient with SLE may include, but are not limited to, those presented in NCP 65-2.

■ Planning

As overall disease management goals, the patient with SLE will (1) have satisfactory pain relief, (2) comply with the therapeutic regimen to achieve maximum symptom management, (3) demonstrate awareness of and avoid activities that cause disease exacerbation, and (4) maintain optimal role function and a positive self-image.

■ Nursing Implementation

Health Promotion. Prevention of SLE is not possible at this time. However, education of health professionals and the community should promote a clear understanding of the disease and the need for early diagnosis and treatment.

Acute Intervention. During an exacerbation of SLE, the patient may become abruptly and dramatically ill. Nursing interventions include accurately recording the severity of symptoms and documenting the response to therapy. Fever pattern, joint inflammation, limitation of motion, location and degree of discomfort, and fatigability should be specifically assessed. The patient's weight and fluid intake and output should be monitored if corticosteroids are prescribed because of the fluid-retention effect of these drugs and the possibility of renal failure. Collection of 24-hour urine samples for protein and creatinine clearance may be ordered. The nurse should observe for signs of bleeding that result from drug therapy, such as pallor, skin bruising, petechiae, or tarry stools.

Careful assessment of neurologic status includes observation for visual disturbances, headaches, personality changes, seizures, and forgetfulness. Psychosis may indicate CNS disease or may be the effect of corticosteroid therapy. Irritation of the nerves of the extremities (peripheral neuropathy) may produce numbness, tingling, and weakness of the hands and feet.

NURSING CARE PLAN 65-2

Patient with Systemic Lupus Erythematosus

NURSING DIAGNOSIS **Fatigue** *related to* chronic inflammation and altered immunity *as evidenced by* lack of energy, inability to maintain usual routine

PATIENT GOALS
1. Uses energy conservation techniques
2. Sets and completes priority activities
3. Adapts lifestyle to energy level

OUTCOMES (NOC)

Energy Conservation
- Recognizes energy limitations _____
- Uses energy conservation techniques _____
- Balances activity and rest _____
- Organizes activities to conserve energy _____
- Adapts lifestyle to energy level _____

Measurement Scale

1 = Never demonstrated
2 = Rarely demonstrated
3 = Sometimes demonstrated
4 = Often demonstrated
5 = Consistently demonstrated

INTERVENTIONS (NIC) and *RATIONALES*

Energy Management
- Determine patient's physical limitations *to plan daily activities.*
- Assist patient in assigning priority to activities *to accommodate energy levels.*
- Assist patient to schedule rest periods *to temporarily reverse effect of fatigue.*
- Teach activity organization and time-management techniques *to prevent fatigue.*
- Encourage alternate rest and activity periods *to promote recuperation and to foster maximum participation in activities.*
- Instruct patient/significant other to recognize signs and symptoms of fatigue that require reduction in activity.
- Instruct patient/significant other to notify health care provider if signs and symptoms of fatigue persist *to increase patient's support and family's understanding of disease and related problems.*

NURSING DIAGNOSIS **Acute pain** *related to* inflammatory processes and inadequate comfort measures *as evidenced by* complaints of joint pain, lack of relief from pain-relieving measures; reduction of activity to avoid exacerbating pain

PATIENT GOAL Uses analgesics and nonpharmacologic measures appropriately to control pain at an acceptable level

OUTCOMES (NOC)

Pain Control
- Uses preventive measures _____
- Uses nonanalgesic relief measures _____
- Uses analgesics appropriately _____
- Reports uncontrolled symptoms to health care professional _____
- Reports pain controlled _____

Measurement Scale

1 = Never demonstrated
2 = Rarely demonstrated
3 = Sometimes demonstrated
4 = Often demonstrated
5 = Consistently demonstrated

INTERVENTIONS (NIC) and *RATIONALES*

Pain Management
- Perform a comprehensive assessment of pain to include location, characteristics, onset/duration, frequency, quality, intensity or severity of pain, and precipitating factors *to plan appropriate interventions.*
- Ensure that patient receives attentive analgesic care *to relieve pain.*
- Teach use of nonpharmacologic techniques (e.g., relaxation, guided imagery, distraction, and hot/cold application) before pain occurs or increases, and along with other pain-relief measures, *to replace or supplement analgesics.*

Continued

The nurse must explain the nature of the disease, modes of therapy, and all diagnostic procedures. Emotional support for the patient and family is essential.

Ambulatory and Home Care. Nursing interventions must emphasize health teaching and the importance of patient cooperation for successful home management. The patient must understand that even strong adherence to the treatment plan is not a guarantee against exacerbation, because the course of the disease is unpredictable. However, a variety of factors may increase disease activity, such as fatigue, sun exposure, emotional stress, infection, drugs, and surgery. Nursing interventions should be directed toward assisting the patient and family to eliminate or minimize exposure to precipitating factors (Table 65-17).

Lupus and Pregnancy. Because SLE is most common in women of childbearing age, treatment during pregnancy must be

considered. The women's primary health care provider (or rheumatologist) and obstetrician should thoroughly discuss with the woman her desire to become pregnant. Infertility may have already resulted from renal involvement and the use of high-dose corticosteroid and chemotherapy drugs. The SLE patient should understand that spontaneous abortion, stillbirth, and intrauterine growth retardation are common problems with pregnancy. They occur because of deposits of immune complexes in the placenta and because of inflammatory responses in the placental blood vessels. Renal, cardiovascular, pulmonary, and central nervous systems may be especially affected during pregnancy. Women who already demonstrate serious SLE involvement in these systems should be counseled against pregnancy. For the best outcome, pregnancy should be planned at a point when the disease activity is minimal. Exacerbation is common during the postpartum period. Therapeu-

NURSING CARE PLAN 65-2

Patient with Systemic Lupus Erythematosus—cont'd

NURSING DIAGNOSIS **Impaired skin integrity** *related to* photosensitivity, skin rash, and alopecia *as evidenced by* rash anywhere on body, butterfly rash on face, hair loss, areas of ulceration on fingertips, complaints of urticaria and photosensitivity

PATIENT GOALS
1. Maintains skin integrity with the use of topical treatments
2. Prevents exacerbations with the use of sunscreens and limited sun exposure

OUTCOMES (NOC)	**INTERVENTIONS (NIC) and *RATIONALES***
Tissue Integrity: Skin and Mucous Membranes	***Skin Care: Topical Treatments***
• Hair growth on skin ____	• Inspect skin of patients at risk of breakdown daily.
• Skin intactness ____	• Document degree of skin breakdown *to plan appropriate interventions.*
• Sensation ____	• Apply topical antiinflammatory agent to affected area *to control skin manifestations.*
• Texture ____	
	Teaching: Disease Process
Measurement Scale	• Discuss lifestyle changes that may be required to prevent future complications and/or control disease process (e.g., use of sunscreens and sun protective clothing when outdoors) *as sun exacerbates manifestations.*
1 = Severely compromised	
2 = Substantially compromised	
3 = Moderately compromised	
4 = Mildly compromised	
5 = Not compromised	

NURSING DIAGNOSIS **Deficient knowledge** *related to* lack of exposure to and unfamiliarity with information resources *as evidenced by* questions about SLE, misinterpretation of information, and inaccurate follow-through of instruction

PATIENT GOALS
1. Describes the disease process and the rationale for prescribed treatment
2. Expresses confidence in ability to recognize complications and use precautions to prevent their occurrence

OUTCOMES (NOC)	**INTERVENTIONS (NIC) and *RATIONALES***
Knowledge: Disease Process	***Teaching: Disease Process***
• Description of specific disease process ____	• Describe disease process.
• Description of effects of disease ____	• Discuss therapy/treatment options *to increase probability of successful long-term management.*
• Description of measures to minimize disease progression ____	• Provide family/significant other(s) with information about patient's progress *to provide support during exacerbation and increase their sense of involvement.*
• Description of signs and symptoms of complications ____	• Instruct patient on which signs and symptoms to report to health care provider (e.g., fever, edema, decreased urine output, chest pain, and dyspnea) *to ensure early intervention.*
• Description of precautions to prevent complications ____	• Refer patient to local community agencies/support groups (e.g., Lupus Foundation, Arthritis Foundation) *to provide additional sources of information and support.*
Measurement Scale	
1 = None	
2 = Limited	
3 = Moderate	
4 = Substantial	
5 = Extensive	

tic abortion offers the same risk of postdelivery exacerbation as carrying the fetus to term.

Neonatal lupus erythematosus (NLE) may rarely occur in infants born to women with SLE. The characteristic skin rash is seen in more than 30% of the cases of NLE.

Psychosocial Issues. The patient with SLE confronts many psychosocial issues. Disease onset and symptoms may be vague, and SLE may be undiagnosed for long periods. Supportive therapies may become as important as medical treatment in helping the patient cope with the disease. The nurse should counsel the patient and family that SLE has a good prognosis for the majority of persons. Families are anxious about hereditary aspects and want to know whether their children will also have SLE. Many couples require pregnancy and sexual counseling. Individuals making deci-

sions about marriage and careers worry about how SLE will interfere with their plans. The nurse may have to educate teachers, employers, and co-workers.

The obvious physical effects of skin rashes, discoid lesions, and alopecia may cause social isolation for the patient with SLE, affecting the individual's self-esteem and body image. However, pain and fatigue are cited most frequently as interfering with quality of life. Friends and relatives are confused by the patient's complaints of transient joint pain and overwhelming fatigue. Pacing techniques and relaxation therapy can help the patient remain involved in day-to-day activities. The nurse should stress the importance of planning both recreational and occupational activities. Young adults find sun restrictions and physical limitations particularly difficult to follow. Nursing interventions should assist the pa-

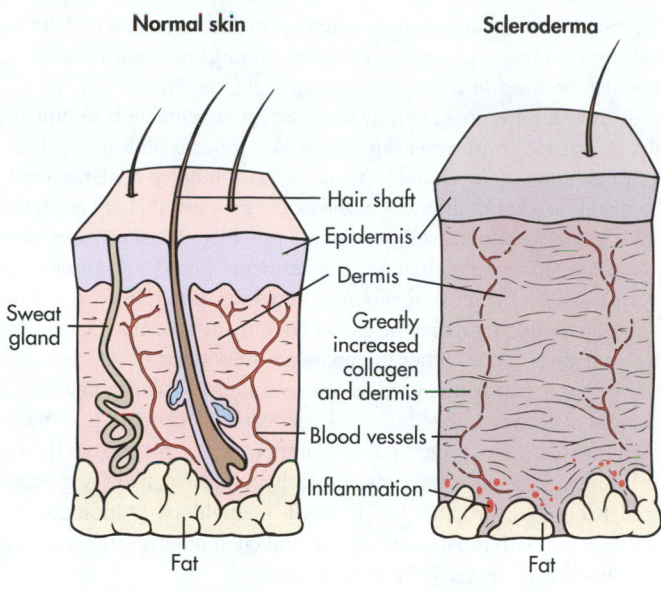

Normal skin   **Scleroderma**

Hair shaft
Epidermis
Dermis
Sweat gland
Greatly increased collagen and dermis
Blood vessels
Inflammation
Fat   Fat

FIG. 65-11 Scleroderma skin changes.

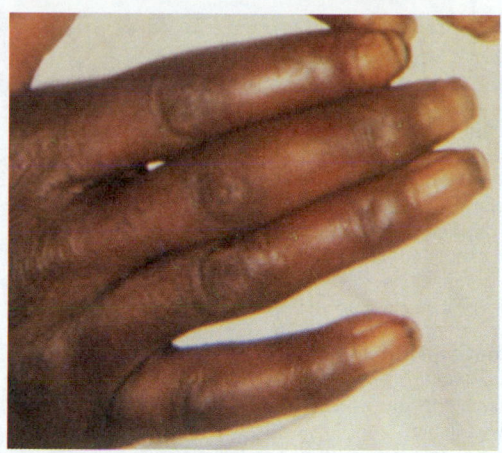

FIG. 65-12 Hand of a patient with systemic sclerosis showing sclerodactyly.

tient in developing and accomplishing reasonable goals for improving or maintaining mobility, energy levels, and self-esteem.

■ Evaluation

The expected outcomes for the patient with SLE are presented in NCP 65-2.

SYSTEMIC SCLEROSIS

Systemic sclerosis (SS), or *scleroderma,* is a disorder of connective tissue characterized by fibrotic, degenerative, and occasionally inflammatory changes in the skin, blood vessels, synovium, skeletal muscle, and internal organs. Two types of SS exist, one being the more common *limited cutaneous disease* (80%) and the second being *diffuse cutaneous disease.* The disease course of SS is variable. SS affects women four times more often than men. SS has been reported in all ethnic groups but is more common in African Americans than whites. Hispanics and Native Americans may also be at higher risk than whites. Although symptoms may begin at any time, the usual age at onset is between 30 and 50 years. Overall incidence increases with age. SS affects approximately 300,000 people in the United States.[37]

Etiology and Pathophysiology

The exact cause of SS remains unknown. Immunologic dysfunction and vascular abnormalities are believed to play a role in development of widespread systemic disease. Other risk factors associated with skin thickening include environmental occupational exposure to coal, plastics, and silica dust. In SS, collagen, the protein that gives normal skin its strength and elasticity, is overproduced (Fig. 65-11). Disruption of the cell is followed by platelet aggregation and fibrosis. Proliferation of collagen disrupts the normal functioning of internal organs, such as the lungs, kidney, heart, and GI tract.

Clinical Manifestations

Manifestations of SS range from a diffuse cutaneous thickening with rapidly progressive and widespread organ involvement to the more benign variant of limited cutaneous SS. The signs of limited

disease appear on the face and hands, while diffuse disease initially involves the trunk and extremities. Clinical manifestations can be described by the acronym **CREST.**[38]

    Calcinosis—painful deposits of calcium in the skin
    Raynaud's phenomenon—abnormal blood flow in response to cold or stress (Raynaud's phenomenon is described further in Chapter 38)
    Esophageal dysfunction—difficulty with swallowing caused by internal scarring
    Sclerodactyly—tightening of the skin on the fingers and toes
    Telangiectasia—red spots on the hands, forearms, palms, face, and lips

Raynaud's Phenomenon. Raynaud's phenomenon (paroxysmal vasospasm of the digits) is the most common initial complaint in limited disease. Patients have diminished blood flow to the fingers and toes on exposure to cold (blanching or white phase), followed by cyanosis as hemoglobin releases oxygen to the tissues (blue phase), and then erythema during rewarming (red phase). The color changes are often accompanied by numbness and tingling. Raynaud's phenomenon may precede the onset of systemic disease by months, years, or even decades.

Skin and Joint Changes. Symmetric painless swelling or thickening of the skin of the fingers and hands may progress to diffuse scleroderma of the trunk. In limited disease, skin thickening does not generally extend above the elbow or above the knee, although the face can be affected in some individuals. In more diffuse disease, the skin loses elasticity and becomes taut and shiny, producing the typical expressionless facies with tightly pursed lips. Skin changes in the face may also contribute to reduced ROM in the temporomandibular joint. The hands may be affected by *sclerodactyly* in which the fingers are in a semiflexed position, with tightened skin to the wrist (Fig. 65-12). Reduced peripheral joint function may occur as an early symptom of polyarthritis.

Internal Organ Involvement. Esophageal fibrosis causes dysphagia and frequent reflux of gastric acid. If swallowing becomes difficult, the patient often decreases food intake and loses weight. GI effects include constipation resulting from colonic hypomotility and diarrhea caused by malabsorption from bacterial overgrowth.

    Lung involvement includes pleural thickening, pulmonary fibrosis, and pulmonary function abnormalities. The patient devel-

TABLE 65-18	*COLLABORATIVE CARE* Systemic Sclerosis

Diagnostic
History and physical examination
Antinuclear antibody titers
Anticentromere antibody
Nail bed capillary microscopy
X-rays of chest and hands
Skin or visceral biopsy
Urinalysis (proteinuria, hematuria, casts)

Collaborative Therapy
Physical therapy
Occupational therapy
Vasoactive agents
Calcium channel blockers (diltiazem [Cardizem])
Nonsteroidal antiinflammatory drugs
D-penicillamine (Cuprimine)
Corticosteroids

ops a cough and dyspnea. Pulmonary artery hypertension may occur in up to 50% of patients with limited SS, and interstitial lung disease can occur additionally in another 10% of these patients.

Primary heart disease consists of pericarditis, pericardial effusion, and cardiac dysrhythmias. Myocardial fibrosis resulting in heart failure occurs most frequently in patients with diffuse SS.

Renal disease is a major cause of death in diffuse SS. Malignant hypertension associated with rapidly progressive and irreversible renal insufficiency is often present. Recent improvements in dialysis, bilateral nephrectomy in patients with uncontrollable hypertension, and kidney transplantation have offered some hope to patients with renal failure.

Diagnostic Studies

Laboratory findings are relatively normal. Blood studies may reveal a mildly elevated ESR and mild hemolytic anemia as a result of RBC damage from diseased small vessels. The scleroderma antibody SCL-70 is found in about 35% of patients with diffuse disease, and serum RF is found in 30% of affected patients. An anticentromere antibody is seen in many patients with CREST. If renal involvement is present, urinalysis may show proteinuria, microscopic hematuria, and casts. Serum levels of creatinine may be elevated. X-ray evidence of subcutaneous calcification, distal esophageal hypomotility, or bilateral pulmonary fibrosis is diagnostic of SS. Pulmonary function studies reveal decreased vital capacity and lung compliance.

Collaborative Care

The collaborative care of SS (Table 65-18) offers no specific treatment with long-term effects. Care is directed toward attempts to prevent or treat secondary complications of involved organs. Physical therapy helps maintain joint mobility and preserve muscle strength. Occupational therapy assists the patient in maintaining functional abilities.

Drug Therapy. No specific drug or combination of drugs has been proven effective for the treatment of SS. Vasoactive agents are often prescribed in early disease, and calcium channel blockers (nifedipine [Adalat, Procardia] and diltiazem [Cardizem]) are now a common treatment choice for Raynaud's phenomenon. Reserpine (Serpasil), an alpha-adrenergic blocking agent, increases blood flow to the fingers. Iloprost (Ventavis), a prostacyclin ana-

log, causes vasodilation and, when given intravenously, it helps heal digital ulcers. Losartan (Cozaar), an angiotension II blocker, may also be used in treating Raynaud's phenomenon.

Corticosteroids are generally reserved for patients with significant joint or muscle involvement or severe skin disease with ulcerations. D-penicillamine (Cuprimine) increases the solubility of dermal collagen and may cause thinning of the skin. However, it is not accepted as a treatment option by all health care providers because of its possible toxic side effects, including myasthenia gravis and blood and liver dyscrasias. Topical agents may provide some relief from joint pain. Capsaicin cream may be useful not only as a local analgesic but also as a vasodilator. Other therapies are prescribed to address specific systemic problems, such as tetracycline for diarrhea caused by bacterial overgrowth, histamine (H_2)-receptor blockers (e.g., cimetidine [Tagamet]) and proton pump inhibitors (e.g., omeprazole [Prilosec]) for esophageal symptoms, an antihypertensive agent (e.g., captopril [Capoten], propranolol [Inderal], methyldopa [Aldomet]) for hypertension with renal involvement, and chemotherapy (e.g., cyclophosphamide [Cytoxan]) for lung disease.

NURSING MANAGEMENT
SYSTEMIC SCLEROSIS

Because prevention is not possible, nursing intervention often begins during a hospitalization for diagnostic purposes. The nurse can help the patient resolve feelings of helplessness by providing information about the illness and encouraging active participation in planning care. Vital signs, weight, intake and output, respiratory and bowel function, and joint ROM should be assessed at regular intervals as indicated by specific symptoms to plan appropriate care. Emotional stress and cold ambient temperatures may aggravate Raynaud's phenomenon. Patients with SS should not have finger-stick blood testing done because of compromised circulation and poor healing of the fingers.

Health teaching is an important nursing intervention as the patient and family begin to live with this disease. Obvious changes in the face and hands often lead to poor self-image and the loss of mobility and function. The patient must actively carry out therapeutic exercises at home to prevent skin retraction and promote vascularization. Mouth excursion (yawning with an open mouth) is a good exercise to help with temporomandibular joint function. Isometric exercises are most appropriate if the patient has arthropathy because no joint movement occurs. The nurse should encourage the use of moist heat applications or paraffin baths to promote skin flexibility in the hands and feet. The patient should use assistive devices as appropriate and organize activities to preserve strength and reduce disability.

Hands and feet should be protected from cold exposure and possible burns or cuts that might heal slowly. Smoking should be avoided because of its vasoconstricting effect. Signs of infection should be promptly reported. Lotions may help alleviate skin dryness and cracking, but they must be rubbed in for an unusually long time because of the thickness of the skin.

Dysphagia may be reduced by eating small, frequent meals; chewing carefully and slowly; and drinking fluids. Heartburn may be minimized by using antacids 45 to 60 minutes after each meal and by sitting upright for at least 2 hours after eating. Using additional pillows or raising the head of the bed on blocks may help reduce nocturnal gastroesophageal reflux.

Job modifications are often necessary because stair climbing, typing, writing, and cold exposure may pose particular problems.

The patient may become socially withdrawn as skin tightening alters the appearance of the face and hands. Dining out may become a socially embarrassing event because the patient's small mouth, difficulty swallowing, and reflux make eating less enjoyable. Some individuals with SS wear gloves to protect fingertip ulcers and to provide extra warmth. Sensitive areas on fingertips resulting from ulcers or calcinosis may require padded utensils or special assistive devices to reduce discomfort. Daily oral hygiene must be emphasized, or neglect may lead to increased tooth and gingival problems. The patient needs a dentist who is familiar with SS and can deal with a small oral aperture. Psychologic support reduces stress and may positively influence peripheral motor response. Biofeedback training and relaxation techniques can reduce tension, improve sleeping habits, and raise the temperature of the fingers and toes.

Sexual dysfunction resulting from body changes, pain, muscular weakness, limited mobility, decreased self-esteem, erectile dysfunction, and decreased vaginal secretions may require sensitive counseling by the nurse. Specific suggestions based on individual patient assessment should be offered.

POLYMYOSITIS AND DERMATOMYOSITIS

Polymyositis (PM) and **dermatomyositis** (DM) are diffuse, idiopathic, inflammatory myopathies of striated muscle that produce bilateral weakness usually most severe in the proximal or limb-girdle muscles. These disorders occur twice as often in women as in men but are still relatively rare.[39] The diseases typically affect adults ages 45 to 65 years. The diseases can be similar in signs and symptoms and treatment, but they are two distinct disorders.[40] Patients with PM generally have more severe disease.

Etiology and Pathophysiology

The exact cause of PM and DM is unknown. Theories include an infectious agent, neoplasms, drugs or vaccinations, and stress. Because disease severity is not well correlated with altered immune complexes, it is unclear if the complexes occur as primary or secondary phenomena. Because T cytotoxic cells and macrophages have been found near the damaged muscle fibers of PM, this disease is believed to be caused by cell-mediated injury. In contrast, DM has been associated with B cells (humoral immunity) and destruction of the muscle microvasculature.

Clinical Manifestations and Complications

Muscular. Patients with DM and PM experience weight loss and increasing fatigue, with a gradually developing weakness of the muscles that leads to difficulty in performing routine activities. The most commonly affected muscles are those of the shoulders, legs, arms, and pelvic girdle. The patient may have difficulty rising from a chair or bathtub, climbing stairs, combing hair, or reaching into a high cupboard. Neck muscles may become so weak that the patient is unable to raise the head from the pillow. Muscle discomfort or tenderness is uncommon. Muscle examination reveals an inability to move against resistance or even gravity. Weak pharyngeal muscles may produce dysphagia and dysphonia (nasal or hoarse voice).

Dermal. Skin changes of DM include a classic violet-colored, cyanotic, or erythematous symmetric rash *(heliotrope)* with edema around the eyelids (Fig. 65-13). Violet-colored or erythematous papules and small plaques can develop over the DIP or MCP areas, and at elbow or knee joints in about 70% of patients with DM (Gottron's papules). These early skin changes usually prompt earlier recognition of DM as compared to PM, in which a rash does not appear.

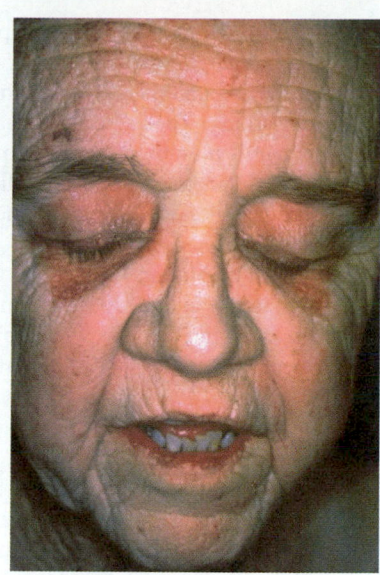

FIG. 65-13 Dermatomyositis. Periorbital edema and purplish rash around the eyelids with erythema of the face.

Reddened, smooth, or scaly patches appear with the same symmetric distribution but sparing the interphalangeal spaces (Gottron's sign); they can be confused with psoriasis or seborrheic dermatitis. On the back, buttocks, and a V-shaped area of the anterior neck and chest, an erythematous scaling rash (poikiloderma) may develop as a late finding. Hyperemia and telangiectasias are often present at the nail beds. Calcium nodules (calcinosis cutis), which can develop throughout the skin, are especially common in long-standing DM.

Other Manifestations. Joint redness, pain, and inflammation often occur and contribute to limitations in joint ROM in DM and PM. Contractures and muscle atrophy may occur with advanced disease. Weakened pharyngeal muscles can lead to a poor cough effort, difficulty swallowing, and increased risk for aspiration pneumonia in both disorders. Persons with DM have an increased risk of an occult malignancy, which may be present at time of diagnosis. Both diseases may be associated with other connective tissue disorders (e.g., systemic sclerosis).

Diagnostic Studies

A diagnosis of DM or PM is confirmed by electromyography (EMG) findings, muscle biopsy, and serum enzyme levels.[39] An EMG suggestive of PM will show bizarre high-frequency discharges and spontaneous fibrillation, with positive spikes at rest. Muscle biopsy reveals necrosis, degeneration, regeneration, and fibrosis with pathology findings distinct for DM or PM. Enzymes such as creatinine kinase and myoglobin are elevated. Elevation of the ESR is also expected with active disease. The typical skin rash seen with DM is not commonly seen with other disorders.

NURSING *and* COLLABORATIVE MANAGEMENT
POLYMYOSITIS AND DERMATOMYOSITIS

PM and DM are initially treated with high-dose corticosteroids. Improvement is generally achieved if corticosteroid therapy is promptly instituted, and the dosage can typically be reduced as improvement is noted. Long-term corticosteroid therapy may often be required as relapses are common when the drug is withdrawn. If corticosteroids prove ineffective and/or organ involvement is occurring, immunosuppressive drugs may also be administered (methotrexate, azathioprine [Imuran], cyclophosphamide [Cytoxan]) using oral or intermittent intravenous dosing. DM has been shown to improve with IV immunoglobulin when the patient does not respond to corticosteroids. Topical corticosteroids and hydroxychloroquine (Plaquenil) may be prescribed to treat the skin rash. Biologic therapy (e.g., etanercept [Enbrel], infliximab [Remicade]) is being explored for its possible role in the treatment of DM and PM.

Physical therapy can be helpful and should be tailored to the activity of the disease. Massage and passive movement are appropriate during active disease. More aggressive exercises should be reserved for periods when disease activity is minimal, as evidenced by low serum enzyme levels.

Nursing interventions should include a thorough explanation of the nature of the disease, the prescribed therapies, all diagnostic tests, and the importance of regular medical care. It is important for the patient to understand that the benefits of therapy are often delayed. For example, weakness may increase during the first few weeks of corticosteroid therapy. Special attention is paid to patient safety. Use of assistive devices should be encouraged as a fall prevention strategy. To prevent aspiration, the patient should be encouraged to rest before meals, maintain an upright position when eating, and choose a diet of easily swallowed foods.

The nurse should assist the patient to organize activities and use pacing techniques to conserve energy. Daily ROM exercises are encouraged to prevent contractures. When active inflammation is not evident, muscle-strengthening (repetitive) exercises may be started. Home care and bed rest may become necessary during the acute phase of PM because profound muscle weakness renders the patient unable to carry out activities of daily living.

MIXED (OVERLAPPING) CONNECTIVE TISSUE DISEASE

Patients having a combination of clinical features of several rheumatic diseases are described as having *mixed or overlapping connective tissue disease.* Although this combination was originally believed to be a distinct clinical disorder, follow-up revealed that for most patients this disorder is a stage in the progression to a connective tissue disorder such as SLE or SS.[41] This early undifferentiated or transitional form of connective tissue disease has a typical serologic pattern, including high titers of a speckled pattern of ANA, high levels of antibody to ribonuclease-sensitive extractable nuclear antibody, and autoantibodies to ribonucleoprotein.

SJÖGREN'S SYNDROME

Sjögren's syndrome is a relatively common autoimmune disease that targets moisture-producing glands, leading to the common symptoms of *xerostomia* (dry mouth) and *keratoconjunctivitis sicca* (dry eyes). The nose, throat, airways, and skin can also become dry. The disease can affect other glands as well, including those in the stomach, pancreas, and intestines (extraglandular involvement). The disease is usually diagnosed in women who are 40 to 60 years old.

In primary Sjögren's syndrome, symptoms can be traced to problems with the lacrimal and salivary glands. The patient with primary disease is likely to have antibodies against the cytoplasmic antigens SS-A (or RO) and SS-B (or LA), as well as ANA. The patient with secondary Sjögren's syndrome typically has had another autoimmune disease (e.g., RA, SLE) before Sjögren's develops.[42]

Sjögren's syndrome appears to be caused by genetic and environmental factors. Several genes seem to be involved. One gene predisposes whites to the disease, whereas other genes are linked to the disease in people of Japanese, Chinese, and African American heritage. The trigger may be a viral or bacterial infection that adversely stimulates the immune system. In Sjögren's syndrome, lymphocytes attack and damage the lacrimal and salivary glands.

Dry eyes cause decreased tearing which leads to a "gritty" sensation in the eyes, burning, blurred vision, and photosensitivity.[43] Dry mouth produces buccal membrane fissures, altered sense of taste, dysphagia, and increased frequency of mouth infections or dental caries. Dry skin and rashes, joint and muscle pain, and thyroid problems may also be present. Other exocrine glands can be affected. For example, vaginal dryness may lead to dyspareunia (painful intercourse). Autoimmune thyroid disorders are common with Sjögren's syndrome, including Graves' disease and Hashimoto's thyroiditis. Histologic study reveals lymphocyte infiltration of salivary and lacrimal glands. The disease may become more generalized and involve the lymph nodes, bone marrow, and visceral organs (pseudolymphoma). The risk of developing lymphoma is high in Sjögren's syndrome.

Ophthalmologic examination (Schirmer's test), measures of salivary gland function, and lower lip biopsy of minor salivary glands aid in diagnosis. The treatment is symptomatic, including (1) instillation of preservative-free artificial tears as necessary to maintain adequate hydration and lubrication, (2) surgical punctual occlusion, and (3) increased fluids with meals. Dental hygiene is important. Pilocarpine (Salagen) and cevimeline (Evoxac) can be used to treat symptoms of dry mouth. Increased humidity at home may reduce respiratory infections. Vaginal lubrication with a water-soluble product such as KY jelly may increase comfort during intercourse. Corticosteroids and immunosuppressive drugs are indicated for treatment of pseudolymphoma.

Soft Tissue Rheumatic Syndromes

Myofascial pain syndrome, fibromyalgia syndrome (FMS), and chronic fatigue syndrome (CFS) are three soft tissue disease syndromes that have many commonalities and may be related. Ongoing research continues to explore links among these three syndromes. A multidisciplinary team approach consisting of a rheumatologist, nurse, mental health professional, and physical therapist may be especially helpful for patients with these syndromes, whose disease course may be chronic.

MYOFASCIAL PAIN SYNDROME

Myofascial pain syndrome is characterized by musculoskeletal pain and tenderness in one anatomic region of the body. The pain has been shown to originate in anterior and posterior trigger points resulting from muscle trauma or chronically strained muscles (e.g., desk or computer work). Regions of pain are often within the taut bands and fascia of skeletal muscles. When activated by pressure, trigger points are thought to activate a characteristic pattern of pain that can be worse with activity or stress.[44] The incidence, and the age-groups and gender that are most affected, are not known. Patients complain of the pain as deep and aching and accompanied by a sensation of burning, stinging, and stiffness. The muscles frequently involved are located in the chest, neck, lower back, and shoulders. Referred pain from these muscle groups can also travel to the buttock, hand, and head, causing severe headaches. Additional systemic manifestations have not been reported.

Diagnosis of myofascial pain syndrome is done by palpation of trigger points, which reveals induration and frequently a muscle

TABLE 65-19	Comparison of Fibromyalgia and Myofascial Pain Syndromes	
Variable	**Fibromyalgia**	**Myofascial Pain**
Location	Generalized	Regional
Examination	Tender points	Trigger points
Response to local therapy	Not sustained	Curative
Gender	Female/male ratio: 10:1	Equal or unknown
Systemic features	Characteristic	Unknown

From McCance KL, Huether SE: *Pathophysiology: the biologic basis for disease in adults and children*, ed 5, St Louis, 2006, Mosby.

TABLE 65-20	Commonalities Between Fibromyalgia Syndrome and Chronic Fatigue Syndrome
Occurrence	Previously healthy, young, and middle-aged women
Etiology (theories)	Infectious trigger, dysfunction in HPA axis, alteration in CNS
Clinical manifestations	Malaise and fatigue, cognitive dysfunction, headaches, sleep disturbances, depression, anxiety, fever, generalized musculoskeletal pain
Course of disease	Variable intensity of symptoms, fluctuates over time
Diagnosis	No definitive laboratory tests or joint and muscle examinations, mainly a diagnosis of exclusion
Collaborative care	Treatment is symptomatic and may include antidepressant drugs such as amitriptyline (Elavil) and fluoxetine (Prozac). Other measures are heat, massage, regular stretching, biofeedback, stress management, and relaxation training. Patient and family teaching is essential.

CNS, Central nervous system; *HPA*, hypothalamic-pituitary-adrenal.

twitch in the area of a trigger point. Once a trigger point is palpated, pain will be felt locally and may also be referred to a region often at some distance away. These finding have also been noted in normal healthy persons and in persons with FMS. Similarities in myofascial pain syndrome and FMS have led to the suggestion that myofascial pain may be a form of or evolve into FMS. A comparison of the two syndromes is shown in Table 65-19.

Physical therapy is one treatment used for myofascial pain syndrome. A typical treatment is the "spray and stretch" method, in which the painful area is iced or sprayed with a coolant such as ethyl chloride and then stretched. Positive results have been seen by injecting the trigger points with a local anesthetic (e.g., 1% lidocaine). Massage, acupuncture, biofeedback, and ultrasound therapy have also shown to benefit some patients.

Patient and family teaching is an important nursing responsibility. Instruction should focus on the prevention of muscle tension in work and leisure activities. Good posture and resting and sleeping positions should also be reviewed. Most patients with myofascial pain syndrome are able to lead a normal and active lifestyle.

FIBROMYALGIA SYNDROME

Fibromyalgia syndrome (FMS) is a chronic disorder characterized by widespread, nonarticular musculoskeletal pain and fatigue with multiple tender points. People with FMS may also experience nonrestorative sleep, morning stiffness, irritable bowel syndrome, and anxiety. The former name for this disorder, fibrositis, implied inflammation of the muscles and soft tissues. However, FMS is now known to be nondegenerative, nonprogressive, and noninflammatory.

Fibromyalgia is a commonly diagnosed musculoskeletal disorder and a major cause of disability, affecting approximately 2% of the population in the United States.[45] FMS occurs 6 times more frequently in women than in men, but can affect persons of all ages and ethnic groups. FMS and CFS share many commonalities (Table 65-20).

Etiology and Pathophysiology

Research continues to focus on identifying the underlying causes and pathophysiologic mechanisms of FMS. There is general agreement that FMS is a disorder of central processing with neuroendocrine/neurotransmitter dysregulation. The pain amplification experienced by the affected patient is due to abnormal sensory processing in the central nervous system. Numerous studies now identify multiple physiologic abnormalities in the FMS patient, including increased levels of substance P in the spinal cord, low levels of blood flow to the thalamus, dysfunction of the hypothalamic-pituitary-adrenal (HPA) axis, low levels of serotonin and tryptophan, and abnormalities in cytokine function. Serotonin and substance P play a role in mood regulation, sleep, and pain perception. Changes in the HPA axis can also negatively affect a person's physical and mental health, leading to an increased incidence of depression and a decreased response to stress. There may also be a genetic susceptibility for FMS. A recent viral illness or Lyme disease may serve as an infectious trigger in susceptible persons.

Clinical Manifestations and Complications

Clinical manifestations of FMS overlap with those of CFS.[46] The patient complains of a widespread burning pain that worsens and improves through the course of a day. It is often difficult for the patient to discriminate if pain occurs in the muscles, joints, or soft tissues. Head or facial pain often results from stiff or painful neck and shoulder muscles. It can accompany temporomandibular joint dysfunction, which affects an estimated one third of FMS patients. Nonrestorative sleep and resulting fatigue are typical. Physical examination characteristically reveals point tenderness at 11 or more of 18 identified sites[47] (Fig. 65-14). Patients with FMS are sensitive to painful stimuli throughout the body and not merely at the identified tender sites. In addition, point tenderness can vary from day to day. On some occasions, the FMS patient may respond to fewer than 11 tender points; at other times, palpation of all sites may elicit pain.

Cognitive effects range from difficulty concentrating to memory lapses and a feeling of being overwhelmed when dealing with multiple tasks. Many individuals report migraine headaches. Depression and anxiety often occur and may require drug therapy. Numbness or tingling in the hands or feet (paresthesia) often accompanies FMS. Restless legs syndrome is also typical, with the patient describing an irresistible urge to move the legs when at rest or lying down.

Irritable bowel syndrome with manifestations of constipation and/or diarrhea, abdominal pain, and bloating is common. FMS patients may also experience difficulty swallowing, perhaps because of abnormalities in esophageal smooth muscle function. Increased frequency of urination and urinary urgency, in the absence of a bladder infection, are typical complaints. Women with FMS may experience more difficult menstruation, with a worsening of disease symptoms during this time.

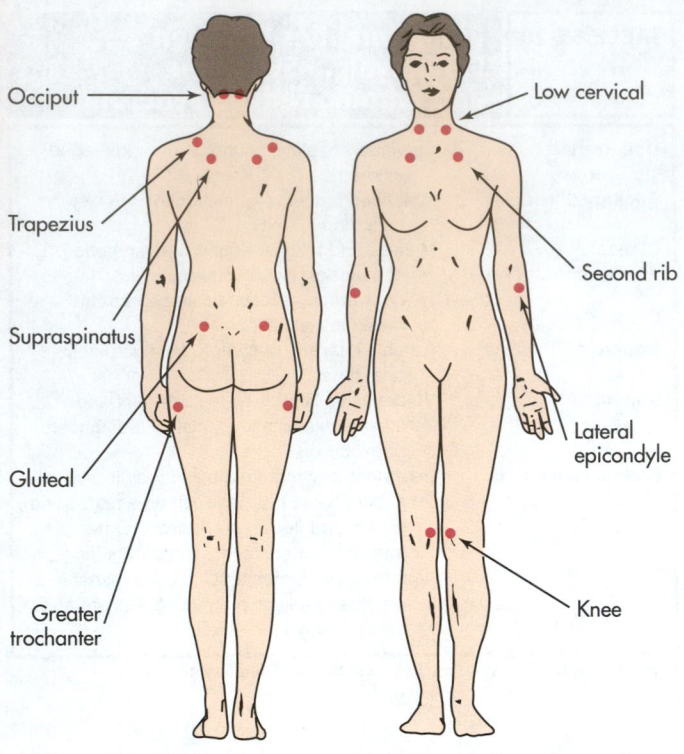

FIG. 65-14   Tender points in fibromyalgia syndrome.

Labels: Occiput, Trapezius, Supraspinatus, Gluteal, Greater trochanter, Low cervical, Second rib, Lateral epicondyle, Knee

Diagnostic Studies

A definitive diagnosis of FMS is often difficult to establish. Lack of knowledge among health care providers may also cause delays in diagnosis and treatment. Laboratory results in most cases serve to rule out other suspected disorders based on the patient's history and physical examination. Occasionally a low ANA titer is seen, but it is not considered diagnostic. Muscle biopsy may reveal a nonspecific moth-eaten appearance or fiber atrophy. The American College of Rheumatology classifies an individual as having FMS if two criteria are met: (1) pain is experienced in 11 of the 18 tender points on palpation (see Fig. 65-14) and (2) a history of widespread pain is noted for at least 3 months. Widespread pain is defined as occurring on both sides of the body and above and below the waist.

Collaborative Care

The treatment of FMS is symptomatic and requires a high level of patient motivation. The nurse can play a key role in teaching the patient to be an active participant in the therapeutic regimen. Pain, aching, and tenderness can be helped by rest. Analgesics such as acetaminophen (Tylenol) and NSAIDs (e.g., tramadol [Ultram]) are effective for some patients. Stress, fatigue, and sleep disturbances can be helped by taking a low-dose tricyclic antidepressant such as amitriptyline (Elavil).[48] If amitriptyline is not well tolerated, other similar drugs can be substituted (e.g., doxepin [Sinequan], imipramine [Tofranil], trazodone [Desyrel]). Selective serotonin reuptake inhibitor (SSRI) antidepressants (e.g., sertraline [Zoloft] or paroxetine [Paxil]) tend to be reserved for FMS patients who also have depression. SSRIs are often prescribed at low doses during the day and sometimes combined with a tricyclic antidepressant at bedtime. The skeletal muscle relaxant cyclobenzaprine (Flexeril) is also commonly used to treat sleep disturbances. Both antidepressants and muscle relax-

ants have sedative effects that can help in improving nighttime rest for the patient with FMS. Clinical trials are examining the antidepressant duloxetine (Cymbalta) for the treatment of FMS, and dextromethorphan (active ingredient in cough remedies) for reducing FMS pain.

Benzodiazepines (e.g., diazepam [Valium], alprazolam [Xanax], clonazepam [Klonopin]) are often prescribed with low doses of ibuprofen (Motrin, Advil) to treat anxiety, as well as the muscle spasms that affect many FMS patients. The drug zolpidem (Ambien) is sometimes prescribed for short-term intervention in patients with severe sleep disturbances.

NURSING MANAGEMENT
FIBROMYALGIA SYNDROME

Because of the chronic nature of FMS and the necessity of maintaining an ongoing rehabilitation program, the patient with FMS needs consistent support from the nurse and other members of the health care team. Massage is often combined with ultrasound or the application of alternating heat and cold packs to soothe tense, sore muscles and increase blood circulation. Gentle stretching can be performed by a physical therapist or practiced by the FMS patient at home to relieve muscle tension and spasm. Yoga and Tai Chi are often appropriate choices. Low-impact aerobic exercise such as walking can help prevent muscle atrophy.

Dietitians often urge FMS patients to limit their consumption of sugar, caffeine, and alcohol because these substances have been shown to be muscle irritants. Vitamin and mineral supplements may be appropriate to combat stress, correct deficiencies, and support the immune system. However, unproven "miracle diets" or supplements should be carefully investigated by the patient with FMS and discussed with the health care provider before using them. The patient should understand that some foods and supplements may cause serious or even dangerous side effects when mixed with certain drugs.

Pain and the related symptoms of FMS can cause significant stress. There is also some indication that patients simply do not process stress well. Effective relaxation strategies include biofeedback, guided imagery, and autogenic training. Patients need to receive initial training for these interventions, but they can then continue to practice in their own homes. (Stress management is discussed in Chapter 9.) Psychologic counseling (individual or group) may also prove beneficial for the FMS patient.

CHRONIC FATIGUE SYNDROME

Chronic fatigue syndrome (CFS), also called chronic fatigue and immune dysfunction syndrome, is a disorder characterized by debilitating fatigue and a variety of associated complaints. Immune abnormalities are also frequently present. The prevalence of CFS is difficult to establish because of the lack of validated diagnostic tests. It affects approximately 0.2% to 0.7% of adults in the United States, and women more often than men. It occurs in all ethnic and socioeconomic groups. CFS is a poorly understood condition that can have a devastating impact on the lives of patients and their families. CFS and FMS share some common features (see Table 65-20).

Etiology and Pathophysiology

Despite numerous attempts to determine the etiology and pathology of CFS, the precise mechanisms remain unknown. However, there are many theories about the cause of CFS. Neuroendocrine

TABLE 65-21	Diagnostic Criteria for Chronic Fatigue Syndrome*

Major Criteria
- Unexplained, persistent, or relapsing chronic fatigue is of new and definite onset (not lifelong).
- Fatigue is not due to ongoing exertion.
- Fatigue is not substantially alleviated by rest.
- Fatigue results in substantial reduction in occupational, educational, social, or personal activities.

Minor Criteria
- Substantial impairment in short-term memory or concentration
- Sore throat
- Tender cervical or axillary lymph nodes
- Muscle pain
- Multijoint pain without joint swelling or tenderness
- Headaches of a new type, pattern, or severity
- Unrefreshing sleep
- Postexertional malaise lasting more than 24 hr

Adapted from Fukuda K, Straus SE, Hickie I, et al: The chronic fatigue syndrome: a comprehensive approach to its definition and study. International Chronic Fatigue Syndrome Study Group, *Ann Intern Med* 121:953, 1994.

*For a diagnosis to be made, the patient must fulfill all the major criteria, plus four or more of the minor criteria. Each minor criterion must have persisted or recurred during 6 or more consecutive months of illness and must not have predated the fatigue. These criteria were prepared by the Centers for Disease Control and Prevention, National Institutes of Health, and International Chronic Fatigue Syndrome Study Group.

abnormalities have been implicated involving a hypofunction of the HPA axis and HPG (hypothalamic-pituitary-gonadal) axis, which together regulate the stress response and reproductive hormone levels.[49] Several microorganisms have been investigated as etiologic agents, including herpesviruses (e.g., Epstein-Barr [EBV], cytomegalovirus [CMV]), retroviruses, enteroviruses, *Candida albicans,* and mycoplasma. Because cognitive deficits (e.g., decreased memory attention, concentration) occur in many of these patients, it has also been proposed that CFS is due to changes in the CNS.

Clinical Manifestations

It is often difficult to distinguish between CFS and FMS because many clinical features are similar (see Table 65-20). In about half of the cases, CFS develops insidiously, or the patient may have intermittent episodes that gradually become chronic. Incapacitating fatigue is the most common symptom of CFS and is the problem that causes the patient to seek health care. Associated symptoms (Table 65-21) may fluctuate in intensity over time. In other situations, CFS arises suddenly in a previously active, healthy individual. An unremarkable flu-like illness or other acute stress is often identified as a triggering event.

The patient may become angry and frustrated with the inability of health care providers to diagnose a problem. The disorder may have a major impact on work and family responsibilities. Some individuals may even need help with activities of daily living.

Diagnostic Studies

Physical examination and diagnostic studies can be used to rule out other possible causes of the patient's symptoms. No laboratory test can diagnose CFS or measure its severity. The Centers for Disease Control and Prevention have developed diagnostic criteria based on the patient's symptoms (see Table 65-21). In general, it remains a diagnosis of exclusion.

NURSING *and* COLLABORATIVE MANAGEMENT
CHRONIC FATIGUE SYNDROME

Because there is no definitive treatment for CFS, supportive management is essential. The patient should be informed about what is known about the disease, and all complaints should be taken seriously. NSAIDs can be used to treat headaches, muscle and joint aches, and fever. Because many patients with CFS also have allergies and sinusitis, antihistamines and decongestants can be used to treat allergic symptoms. Tricyclic antidepressants (e.g., doxepin [Sinequan], amitriptyline [Elavil]) and SSRIs (e.g., fluoxetine [Prozac], paroxetine [Paxil]) can improve mood and sleep problems. Clonazepam (Klonopin) can also be used to treat sleep disturbances and panic disorders. The use of low-dose hydrocortisone is being studied to decrease fatigue and disability.

Total rest is not advised because it can potentiate the self-image of being an invalid, while strenuous exertion can exacerbate the exhaustion. Therefore it is important to plan a carefully graduated exercise program. A well-balanced diet including fiber and fresh dark-colored fruits and vegetables for antioxidant action is essential in treatment. Behavioral therapy may be used to promote a positive outlook, as well as improve overall disability, fatigue, and other symptoms.[50]

One of the major problems facing many CFS patients is financial instability. When the illness strikes, they cannot work or must decrease the amount of time working. Loss of a job often leads to loss of medical insurance. Obtaining disability benefits can be frustrating because of the difficulty of establishing a diagnosis of CFS.

CFS does not appear to progress. Although most patients recover or at least gradually improve over time, some do not show substantial improvement. Recovery is more common in individuals with a sudden onset of CFS. Patients with CFS may experience substantial occupational and psychosocial impairments and loss, including the social pressure and isolation from being characterized as lazy or "crazy."

CRITICAL THINKING EXERCISE

CASE STUDY

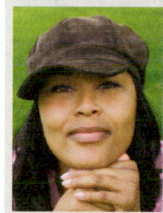

Case Study photo ©iStockphoto.com/ Jason Stitt.

Rheumatoid Arthritis

Patient Profile. Sharon Steele, a 36-year-old married African American woman, is seen at the rheumatology clinic with complaints of swelling and stiffness in the small joints of her hands.

Subjective Data
- Concert pianist
- Gave birth to her first child 2 months ago
- Complains of joint pain and stiffness in both hands for the last 6 weeks
- Experiencing fatigue, anorexia, and morning stiffness

Objective Data

Physical Examination
- Swelling and tenderness of third and fourth metacarpophalangeal joints of both hands
- Mild pain with neck motion

Diagnostic Studies
- Positive ESR and RF
- Moderate bone demineralization evidence in bilateral hand x-rays

Continued

CRITICAL THINKING EXERCISE—cont'd

Collaborative Care
- Diagnosed with RA
- Started on meloxicam (Mobic) 15 mg daily, hydroxychloroquine (Plaquenil) 400 mg daily, prednisone 10 mg daily

Critical Thinking Questions

1. How might the nurse explain the pathophysiology of RA to Sharon?
2. How might the recent childbirth have influenced the symptoms that she is currently experiencing?
3. What are some home and work modifications that the nurse can suggest to Sharon that will reduce her symptoms?
4. What suggestions can the nurse make to Sharon about coping with fatigue?
5. Based on the assessment data presented, write one or more nursing diagnoses. Are there any collaborative problems?

NXCLEX EXAMINATION REVIEW QUESTIONS

The number of the question corresponds to the same-numbered objective at the beginning of the chapter.

1. In assessing the joints of a patient with rheumatoid arthritis, the nurse understands that the joints are damaged by
   a. the development of Heberden's nodes in the joint capsule.
   b. the deterioration of cartilage by the enzyme hyaluronidase.
   c. invasion of pannus into the joint capsule and subchondral bone.
   d. bony ankylosis following inflammation of the joints in HLA-B27–positive individuals.

2. Assessment data noted by the nurse in the patient with osteoarthritis commonly include
   a. elevated ESR.
   b. evening but no morning stiffness.
   c. progressive joint pain with activity.
   d. symmetric swelling of metacarpophalangeal joints.

3. An important nursing intervention in caring for the patient with ankylosing spondylitis is to teach the patient to
   a. avoid extremes in environmental temperatures.
   b. continue with physical activity during flare-ups.
   c. apply cool compresses for relief of local symptoms.
   d. maintain proper posture and engage in back exercises.

4. When administering medications to the patient with gout, the nurse would recognize which of the following as a treatment for acute disease?
   a. Colchicine
   b. Sulfasalazine
   c. Allopurinol
   d. Cyclosporine

5. In teaching a patient with SLE about the disorder, the nurse uses the knowledge that the pathophysiology of SLE includes
   a. the production of autoantibodies directed against constituents of cellular DNA.
   b. an autoimmune reaction resulting in degeneration, necrosis, and fibrosis of muscle fibers.
   c. chronic inflammation and cytokine activity resulting in cartilage, bone, and muscle damage.
   d. a deposition in tissues of immune complexes formed from IgG autoantibodies reacting with IgG.

6. The nurse caring for a patient with Sjögren's syndrome will discuss the likelihood that the patient may also develop which of the following autoimmune disorders?
   a. Uveitis
   b. Ulcerative colitis
   c. Glomerulonephritis
   d. Hashimoto's thyroiditis

7. In teaching a patient with chronic fatigue syndrome (CFS) about this disorder, the nurse understands that
   a. more men than women are affected.
   b. tender points are a definitive diagnostic test.
   c. many symptoms are similar to fibromyalgia syndrome.
   d. CFS is characterized by a progression of worsening inflammation.

REFERENCES

1. Flynn J, Johnson T: *The Johns Hopkins white papers: arthritis,* Baltimore, 2006, Johns Hopkins Medicine.
2. National Center for Chronic Disease Prevention and Health Promotion: Arthritis. Available at *www.cdc.gov/arthritis* (accessed September 5, 2006).
3. Roberts D: Arthritis and connective tissue disorders. In Taggart HM, editor: *NAON core curriculum for orthopaedic nursing,* ed 5, Boston, 2006, Pearson Custom Publishing.
4. Centers for Disease Control and Prevention: Arthritis risk factors. Available at *www.cdc.gov/arthritis* (accessed September 5, 2006).
5. National Institute of Arthritis and Musculoskeletal and Skin Diseases: Handout on health: Arthritis. Available at *www.niams.nih.gov/hi/topics/arthritis/oahandout* (accessed September 5, 2006).
6. Bartz R, Laudicina L: Osteoarthritis after sports knee injuries, *Clin Sports Med* 24:39, 2005.
7. Dyer E, Heflin M: Osteoarthritis: its course in older patients and current treatment methods, *Clin Geriatr* 13:18, 2005.
8. American College of Rheumatology Subcommittee on Osteoarthritis guidelines: Recommendations for the medical management of osteoarthritis of the hip and knee. Available at *www.rheumatology.org/guidelines* (accessed May 8, 2006).
9. Witt C, Brinkhaus B, Jena S, et al: Acupuncture in patients with osteoarthritis of the knee: a randomized trial, *Lancet* 366:136, 2005.
10. National Institutes of Health: Glucosamine/chondroitin Arthritis Intervention Trial (GAIT). Available at *www.arthritis.org/arthritistoday* (accessed September 5, 2006).
11. U.S. Food and Drug Administration: Decision memo: analysis and recommendations for agency actions—COX-2 selective and non-selective NSAIDS. Available at *www.fda.gov/cder/drug/infopage/cox2* (accessed September 5, 2006).
12. Brandt K, Mazzuca S, Katz B, et al: Effects of doxycycline on progression of osteoarthritis: results of a randomized placebo-controlled, double-blind trial, *Arthritis Rheum* 52:2015, 2005.
13. Ling SM: Rehabilitation of older adult patients, Johns Hopkins Arthritis. Available at *www.hopkins-arthritis.org/mngmnt/rehab.html* (accessed September 5, 2006).
14. Padyukov L, Silva C, Stolt P, et al: A gene-environment interaction between smoking and shared epitope genes in HLA-DR provides a high risk of seropositive rheumatoid arthritis, *Arthritis Rheum* 50:3085, 2004.
15. Rooney J: Oh, those aching joints: what you need to know about arthritis, *Nursing* 34(11):59, 2004.
16. Olsen N, Stein M: New drugs for rheumatoid arthritis, *N Engl J Med* 350:2167, 2004.
17. Anderson D: TNF inhibitors: a new age in rheumatoid arthritis treatment, *Am J Nurs* 104(11):60, 2004.
18. U.S. Food and Drug Administration: Prosorba column, summary of safety and effectiveness data. Available at *www.fda.gov* (accessed September 5, 2006).
19. Westby M: Exercise and arthritis, American College of Rheumatology. Available at *www.rheumatology.org/public/factsheets/exercise* (accessed September 5, 2006).
20. Anandarajah AP, Ritchlin CT: Treatment update on spondyloarthropathy, *Postgrad Med* [online] 116:5, 2004. Available at *www.postgradmed.com/issues* (accessed September 5, 2006).

21. Ritchlin C: Newer therapeutic approaches: spondyloarthritis and uveitis, *Rheum Dis Clin North Am* 32:75, 2006.

22. National Psoriasis Foundation: The five types of psoriatic arthritis. Available at *www.psoriasis.org/about/psa/types.php* (accessed May 18, 2006).

23. Petersel D, Sigal L: Reactive arthritis, *Infect Dis Clin North Am* 19:863, 2005.

24. Ross J: Septic arthritis, *Infect Dis Clin North Am* 19:799, 2005.

25. Centers for Disease Control and Prevention, Division of Vector-Borne Infectious Diseases: Lyme disease. Available at *www.cdc.gov/ncidod/dvbid/lyme* (accessed March 21, 2006).

26. Postgraduate Medicine Patient Notes: Lyme disease, *Postgrad Med* 117:47, 2005.

27. Rodriguez F: Rheumatic manifestations of human immunodeficiency virus infection, *Rheum Dis Clin North Am* 29:145, 2003.

28. Monu J, Pope T: Gout: a clinical and radiologic review, *Radiol Clin North Am* 42:169, 2004.

29. Choi HK, Atkinson K, Karlson EW, et al: Obesity, weight gain, hypertension, diuretic use, and risk of gout in men: the health professionals follow-up study, *Arch Intern Med* 165:742, 2005.

30. Becker MA, Schumacher HR, Wortmann RL, et al: Febuxostat compared with allopurinol in patients with hyperuricemia and gout, *N Engl J Med* 353:2450, 2005.

31. National Institute of Arthritis and Musculoskeletal and Skin Diseases: The many shades of lupus. Available at *www.niams.nih.gov/hi/topics/lupus* (accessed September 5, 2006).

32. Rooney J: Systemic lupus: unmasking a great imitator, *Nursing* 35(11):54, 2005.

33. Lupus Foundation of America: Cardiopulmonary disease and lupus. Available at *www.lupus.org/education/brochures/cardio05.html#coronary* (accessed September 5, 2006).

34. Brady H, O'Meara Y, Brenner B: Glomerular diseases. In Kasper DL, et al, editors: *Harrison's principles of internal medicine,* ed 16, New York, 2005, McGraw-Hill.

35. Contreras G: Sequential therapies for proliferative lupus nephritis, *N Engl J Med* 350:971, 2004.

36. Burt R, Traynor A, Stratkute L, et al: Nonmyeloablative hematopoietic stem cell transplantation for systemic lupus erythromatosus, *N Engl J Med* 295:527, 2006.

37. Cassidy J: Systemic lupus erythematosus, juvenile dermatomyositis, scleroderma and vasculitis. In Harris E, et al, editors: *Kelley's textbook of rheumatology,* ed 7, St Louis, 2005, Elsevier.

38. Scleroderma Foundation: Your questions answered: CREST syndrome! Available at *www.scleroderma.org/medical/crest* (accessed September 5, 2006).

39. DiMartino S, Kagen L: Newer therapeutic approaches: inflammatory muscle disorders, *Rheum Dis Clin North Am* 32:121, 2006.

40. Younger D: The myopathies, *Med Clin North Am* 87:899, 2003.

41. Swanton J, Isenberg D: Mixed connective tissue disease: still crazy after all these years, *Rheum Dis Clin North Am* 31:421, 2005.

42. Carsons S: Sjögren's syndrome. In Harris E, Budd R, Firestein G, et al, editors: *Kelly's textbook of rheumatology,* ed 7, St Louis, 2005, Elsevier Mosby.

43. Derk C, Vivino F: A primary care approach, *Postgrad Med* 116:49, 2004.

44. The Cleveland Clinic: Myofascial pain syndrome. Available at *www.clevelandclinic.org/health* (accessed May 28, 2006).

45. American College of Rheumatology: What is fibromyalgia? Available at *www.rheumatology.org/public/factsheets/fibromya.asp* (accessed September 8, 2006).

46. Hellmann D, Stone J: Arthritis and musculoskeletal disorders. In Tierney L, et al, editors *Current medical diagnosis and treatment,* ed 44, New York, 2005, McGraw-Hill.

47. American College of Rheumatology: Criteria for classification of fibromyalgia. Available at *www.nfra.net/Diagnost.htm* (accessed May 28, 2006).

48. Gill J, Quisel A: Fibromyalgia and diffuse myalgia, *Clin Fam Pract* 7:181, 2005.

49. Gur A, Cevik R, Nas K, et al: Cortisol and hypothalamic-pituitary-gonadal axis hormones in follicular-phase women with fibromyalgia and chronic fatigue syndrome and effect of depressive symptoms on these hormones, *Arthritis Res* 6:R232, 2004.

50. Centers for Disease Control and Prevention: Treatment of patients with chronic fatigue syndrome. Available at *www.cdc.gov/ncidod/diseases/cfs/treat.htm* (accessed September 8, 2006).

RESOURCES

American Autoimmune Related Diseases Association
586-776-3900
www.aarda.org

American College of Rheumatology
404-633-3777
www.rheumatology.org

American Pain Society
847-375-4715
www.ampainsoc.org

Arthritis Foundation
800-283-7800
www.arthritis.org

The Arthritis Society of Canada
416-979-7228
www.arthritis.ca

International Association for Chronic Fatigue Syndrome
847-258-7248
www.aacfs.org

Lupus Foundation of America, Inc.
202-349-1155
www.lupus.org

National Fibromyalgia Association
714-921-0150
www.fmaware.org

National Fibromyalgia Research Association
www.nfra.net

National Institute of Arthritis and Musculoskeletal and Skin Diseases Information Clearinghouse, National Institutes of Health
877-22-NIAMS (226-4267) or 301-495-4484
www.niams.nih.gov

National Psoriasis Foundation
800-723-9166 or 503-244-7404
www.psoriasis.org

Partnership for Prescription Assistance
888-477-2669
www.pparx.org

Scleroderma Foundation
978-463-5843
Info line: 800-722-HOPE (4673)
www.scleroderma.org

Scleroderma Research Foundation
415-834-9444
www.srfcure.org

Sjögren's Syndrome Foundation
800-475-6473
www.sjogrens.org

Spondylitis Association of America
800-777-8189 or 818-981-1616
www.spondylitis.org

For additional Internet resources, see the website for this book at *http://evolve.elsevier.com/Lewis/medsurg.*

Nursing Care
in Specialized Settings

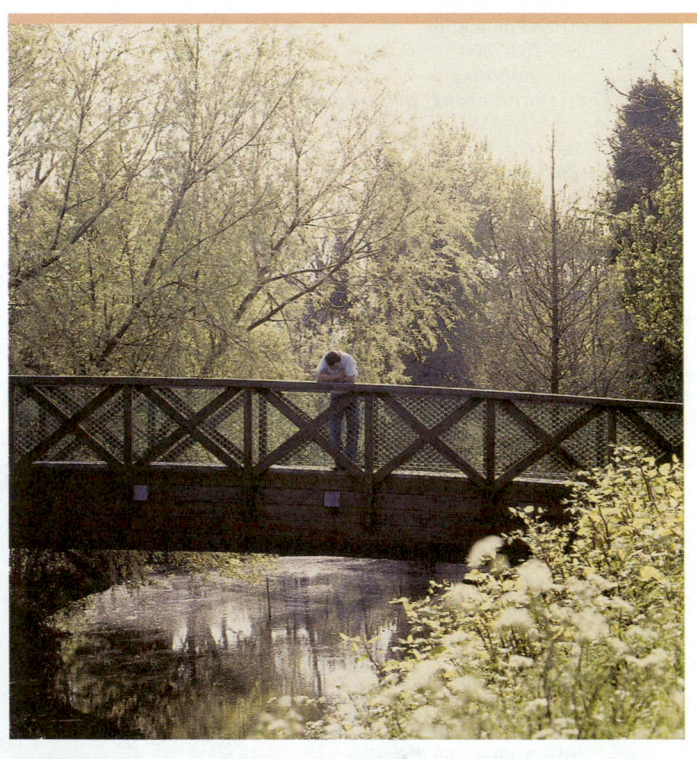

Section Outline

66 **Nursing Management**
Critical Care, p. 1733

67 **Nursing Management**
Shock, Systemic Inflammatory Response
Syndrome, and Multiple Organ Dysfunction
Syndrome, p. 1772

68 **Nursing Management**
Respiratory Failure and Acute Respiratory
Distress Syndrome, p. 1799

69 **Nursing Management**
Emergency and Disaster Nursing, p. 1821

The more serious the illness, the more important it is for you to fight back, mobilizing all your resources—spiritual, emotional, intellectual, physical.

Norman Cousins

Nursing Management
Critical Care

66

Linda Bucher and Maureen A. Seckel

LEARNING OBJECTIVES

1. Differentiate among the certification roles of critical care nurses: CCRN, PCCN, CCNS, and ACNP.
2. Select appropriate nursing interventions to manage common problems and needs of critically ill patients.
3. Develop effective strategies to manage issues related to the families of critically ill patients.
4. Discuss the principles of hemodynamic monitoring and collaborative care and nursing management of the patient receiving hemodynamic monitoring.
5. Describe the purpose, indications, and function of circulatory assist devices and related collaborative care and nursing management.
6. Describe types of artificial airways and appropriate nursing interventions to manage the care of an intubated patient.
7. Differentiate the indications for and modes of mechanical ventilation.
8. Describe the principles of mechanical ventilation and collaborative care and nursing management of a patient receiving mechanical ventilation.

KEY TERMS

circulatory assist devices, p. 1747
continuous positive airway pressure, p. 1762
endotracheal intubation, p. 1751
hemodynamic monitoring, p. 1738
high-frequency ventilation, p. 1763
intraaortic balloon pump, p. 1748
mechanical ventilation, p. 1759
negative pressure ventilation, p. 1759
phlebostatic axis, p. 1739
positive end-expiratory pressure, p. 1762
positive pressure ventilation, p. 1760
pressure ventilation, p. 1760
ventricular assist device, p. 1750
volume ventilation, p. 1760

Electronic Resources

Supplemental content related to Chapter 66 can be found . . .

Companion CD
- Stress-Busting Kit for Nursing Students
- NCLEX Examination Review Questions
- Comprehensive Glossary

Evolve Website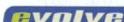
http://evolve.elsevier.com/Lewis/medsurg
- Content Updates
- Key Points (Printable and CD/MP3 Download)
- Concept Map Creator
- Expanded Audio Glossary
- Key Term Flash Cards

- Customizable Nursing Care Plan: Mechanical Ventilation
- Electronic Calculators
- WebLinks

CRITICAL CARE NURSING

Critical Care Units

Critical care units (CCUs) or intensive care units (ICUs) are designed to meet the special needs of acutely and critically ill patients. Florence Nightingale developed the concept of clustering the most acutely ill patients as far back as the 1800s.[1] During poliomyelitis and tuberculosis pandemics in the middle of the twentieth century, special units were established, equipped with technical equipment to manage the airway and ventilate the pa-tient, and staffed by specialized care providers. Finally, lessons learned from World War II and the Korean War solidified the concepts of triage and specialty nursing units, and by the late 1950s, these concepts were being incorporated into hospital systems.[2]

In the 1960s technologic developments allowed for more accessible monitoring of electrocardiogram (ECG), arterial and central venous pressures, pulmonary artery pressures, and arterial blood gases (ABGs). Coronary care units were developed for patients with acute myocardial infarction and heart failure. In these units

Reviewed by Mary Ellen Kern, RN, MSN, CCRN, APRN, Clinical Nurse Specialist, Thomas Jefferson University Hospital, Methodist Division, Philadelphia, Pa.; and Janet Riggs, RN, MSN, CCRN, CCNS, Research Project Manager, Penn Presbyterian Medical Center, Philadelphia, Pa.

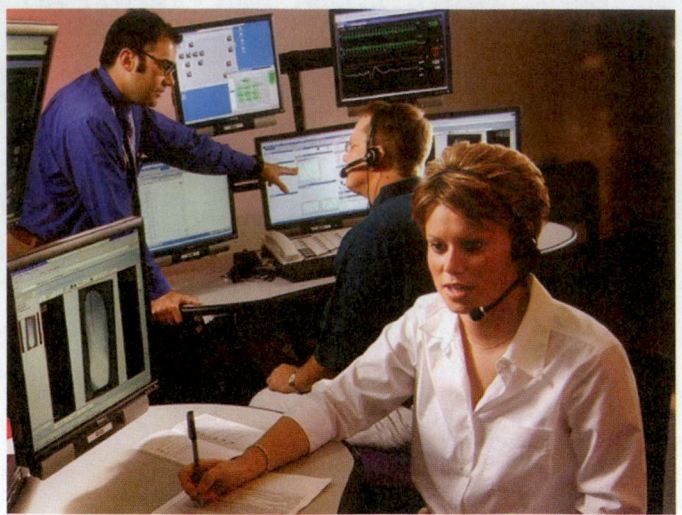

FIG. 66-1   Electronic intensive care unit (E-ICU) control room.

TABLE 66-1	Abbreviations Commonly Used in the Intensive Care Unit
Abbreviation	**Term**
CI	• Cardiac index
CO	• Cardiac output
CVP	• Central venous pressure
$ETCO_2$	• End-tidal carbon dioxide
FIO_2	• Fraction of inspired oxygen
IABP	• Intraaortic balloon pump
MAP	• Mean arterial pressure
PA	• Pulmonary artery
PAS, PAD	• Pulmonary artery systolic (pressure), pulmonary artery diastolic (pressure)
PAWP	• Pulmonary artery wedge pressure
PVR	• Pulmonary vascular resistance
$ScvO_2$	• Percent oxygen saturation of hemoglobin in venous blood (e.g., in the superior vena cava)
SpO_2	• Percent oxygen saturation of hemoglobin measured by pulse oximetry
SvO_2	• Percent oxygen saturation of hemoglobin in mixed venous blood (e.g., in the pulmonary artery)
SV, SVI	• Stroke volume, stroke volume index
SVR, SVRI	• Systemic vascular resistance, systemic vascular resistance index
VAD	• Ventricular assist device

patients were continually monitored for cardiac dysrhythmias. Nurses followed protocols to aggressively manage dysrhythmias. By the 1970s the ICU was a standard unit in most general hospitals worldwide. Since that time, technical advances have continued at a rapid pace, bringing improved monitoring capabilities and new strategies to manage life-threatening problems.

In many acute care settings, the concept of ICU care has expanded from delivering care in a standard unit to bringing ICU care to patients wherever they might be. The *electronic* or *virtual ICU* is designed to augment the bedside ICU team by monitoring the patient from a remote location (Fig. 66-1). Another development is the role of the *rapid response team* (RRT). The RRT is usually composed of a critical care nurse, a respiratory therapist, and a critical care physician or an advanced practice nurse (APN). The team goes outside the ICU to bring rapid and immediate care to unstable patients in noncritical care units. Research has shown that patients often exhibit subtle early signs of deterioration (e.g., mild confusion) 6 to 8 hours before cardiac and/or respiratory arrest, and early critical care intervention has made significant contributions to reducing mortality rates in these patients.[3]

The term *critical care nursing* is often used interchangeably with the term *intensive care nursing,* but it is not exclusively restricted to that specialty area. The critical care nurse is responsible for assessing life-threatening conditions, instituting appropriate interventions, and evaluating the outcomes of the interventions. The biotechnology available in the ICU is extensive and continually evolving. The capability exists to continuously monitor ECG, blood pressure, oxygenation saturation, mechanical ventilation, cardiac output, intracranial pressure, and temperature. More advanced monitoring devices allow for the measurement of cardiac index, stroke volume, ejection fraction, end-tidal carbon dioxide (CO_2), and tissue oxygen consumption. (See Table 66-1 for common abbreviations used in critical care nursing.) Patients may be receiving continual support from mechanical ventilators, intraaortic balloon pumps, ventricular assist devices, or dialysis machines. A typical ICU is illustrated in Fig. 66-2.

Critical Care Nurse

The critical care nurse cares for patients and the families of patients with acute and unstable physiologic problems in an environment equipped for technically advanced methods of assessing and

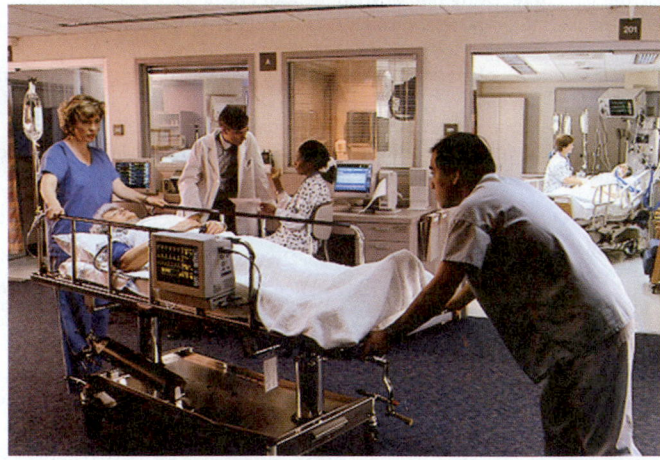

FIG. 66-2   Typical intensive care unit.

managing patient problems. The American Association of Critical Care Nurses (AACN) defines *critical care nursing* as that specialty dealing with human responses to life-threatening problems. Critical care nursing requires in-depth knowledge of anatomy, physiology, pathophysiology, pharmacology, and advanced assessment skills, as well as the ability to use advanced biotechnology. The critical care nurse provides ongoing assessment and early recognition and management of complications while fostering healing and recovery. Appropriate actions by an astute nurse can prevent many complications and contribute to good patient outcomes. The nurse must also be able to provide psychologic support to the patient and the family. To be effective, the critical care nurse must be able to communicate and collaborate effectively with all health team providers (e.g., physician, dietitian, social worker, respiratory therapist, occupational therapist). Along with rapidly evolving technology, critical care nurses are often faced with ethical dilemmas related to the care of their patients. Moral distress over perceived issues of delivering futile or nonbeneficial care can lead to emotional exhaustion or "burnout."[4] It is important that all members of the health team coexist in a healthy work environment. AACN has proposed six standards for establishing and sustaining a healthy work environment: (1) skilled communication, (2) true collaboration, (3) effective decision making, (4) appropriate staffing, (5) meaningful recognition, and (6) authentic leadership.[5]

Nursing practice in the ICU often follows a total care model with the patient cared for by a limited group of nurses who become thoroughly familiar with the patient's condition and the needs of the patient and the family. The ICU nurse spends most working hours near or at the patient's bedside. Specialization in ICU nursing usually requires formal, in-service education combined with a preceptored clinical orientation.

The AACN Certification Corporation offers critical care certification (CCRN) in adult, pediatric, and neonatal critical care nursing. The designation requires registered nurse licensure, practice experience in critical care nursing, and successful completion of a written test. Continued critical care practice and retesting or continuing education are required for recertification. CCRN certification validates basic knowledge of critical care nursing; it is not the same as advanced practice.

Advanced practice critical care nurses have a graduate (master's or doctorate) degree. These nurses are employed in a variety of roles: patient and staff educators, consultants, administrators, researchers, or expert practitioners. The advanced practice critical care nurse who is a clinical nurse specialist (CNS) typically functions in one or more of these roles. Certification for the CNS in acute and critical care (CCNS) is available through the AACN Certification Corporation. Another advanced practice role is the acute care nurse practitioner (ACNP). This advanced practice nurse provides comprehensive care to select critically ill patients and their families. The ACNP conducts comprehensive assessments, orders and interprets diagnostic tests, manages health problems and disease-related symptoms, prescribes treatments, and coordinates care during transitions in settings. The ACNP may practice independently (e.g., providing comprehensive care to the chronically critically ill) or collaboratively (e.g., providing symptom management in conjunction with physicians). Certification as an ACNP is available through the AACN Certification Corporation. Prescriptive authority regulations for advanced practice nurses vary by state.

Critical Care Patient

A patient is generally admitted to the ICU for one of three reasons. First, the patient may be physiologically unstable, requiring advanced and sophisticated clinical judgments by the nurse or physician. Second, the patient may be at risk for serious complications and require frequent and often invasive assessments. Third, the patient may require intensive and complicated nursing support related to the use of intravenous (IV) polypharmacy (e.g., neuromuscular blockade, sedation, thrombolytics, drugs requiring titration) and advanced biotechnology (e.g., ventricular assist devices, mechanical ventilation, intracranial pressure monitoring, continuous renal replacement therapy, hemodynamic monitoring).

ICU patients can be clustered by disease condition (e.g., neurology, pulmonary) or age-group (e.g., neonatal, pediatrics). ICU patients are sometimes clustered by acuity (e.g., acute and unstable versus technology dependent but stable). Patients commonly treated in the ICU include those with respiratory distress, myocardial ischemia or infarction, or acute neurologic impairment or

those receiving care after cardiac surgery or major organ transplantation. The care of the critically injured patient is provided in trauma and burn ICUs. The patient with a medical emergency (e.g., sepsis, diabetic ketoacidosis, drug overdoses, or poisonings or thyroid, adrenal, or hematologic crises) is often treated in a medical ICU. The patient with multiple comorbidities may be monitored in the ICU while receiving care for unrelated conditions. The patient who is not expected to recover from an illness is usually not admitted to an ICU. For example, the ICU should not be used to manage the patient in a persistent coma, nor should ICU care be used to prolong the natural process of death.

Despite the emphasis on caring for the patient who is expected to survive, the incidence of death is higher in ICU patients than in non-ICU patients. It is reported that 33% to 50% of Americans will spend time in an ICU during the final year of their life and 20% will die there. Another 20% may leave the ICU but will not survive to discharge. This suggests a need for caution and coordination of care when transferring patients from ICUs to general care units. In general, nonsurvivors are older, have preexisting health problems, and experience longer ICU stays.[6]

Progressive care units (PCUs), also called high-dependency units, intermediate care units, or stepdown units, have been established as transition units between the ICU and the general care unit or discharge. Generally, patients in PCUs are at risk for serious complications, but their risk is lower than that of ICU patients. Examples of patients found in PCUs include patients scheduled for interventional cardiac procedures (e.g., stent placement, pacemaker implantation), awaiting heart transplant, receiving stable doses of vasoactive IV drugs (e.g., diltiazem [Cardizem]), or being weaned from prolonged mechanical ventilation. Patients in these units can be monitored for cardiac rhythm, arterial blood pressure, oxygen saturation, and end-tidal CO_2. The use of PCUs provides specialized nursing care for an at-risk patient population in a more cost-effective environment. The AACN Certification Corporation offers certification for progressive care nurses (PCCNs) working with acutely ill adult patients.

Common Problems of Critical Care Patients. The patient admitted to the ICU is at risk for numerous complications and special problems. Critically ill patients are usually immobile and at risk for skin problems (see Chapter 24). The use of multiple, invasive devices predisposes the patient to hospital-acquired infections. Sepsis and multiple organ dysfunction syndrome (MODS) may follow (see Chapter 67). Adequate nourishment for the critically ill patient is paramount but frequently inadequate. Other special problems for ICU patients relate to anxiety, pain, impaired communication, sensory-perceptual problems, and sleep disorders.

Nutrition. Patients are often admitted to ICUs with conditions that result in either hypermetabolic states (e.g., burns, trauma, sepsis) or catabolic states (e.g., acute renal failure). Other times, patients may be admitted in severely malnourished states, such as those that occur with wasting syndrome and chronic cardiac, pulmonary, or liver disease. In general, malnutrition has been linked to increases in mortality and morbidity rates. Determining who to feed, what to feed, when to feed, and how to feed (e.g., route of administration) are crucial questions that must be asked when caring for a critically ill patient.[7] The critical care nurse must collaborate with the physician and the dietitian to determine how best to meet the nutritional needs of ICU patients. Research has demonstrated that an additional factor in underfeeding patients is the frequent interruptions in enteral feedings due to medication administration and ICU tests and procedures.[8]

The primary goal of nutritional support is to prevent or correct nutritional deficiencies. This is usually accomplished by the early provision of enteral nutrition (i.e., delivery of calories via the gastrointestinal [GI] tract) or parenteral nutrition (i.e., delivery of calories intravenously).[9] Enteral nutrition is thought to preserve the structure and function of the gut mucosa and help to possibly prevent the translocation of gut bacteria. In addition, enteral nutrition is associated with fewer complications and is less expensive than parenteral nutrition.[10] (Enteral and parenteral nutrition are discussed in Chapter 40.)

Parenteral nutrition should be considered only when the enteral route is unsuccessful in providing adequate nutrition or is contraindicated. Examples of these conditions are paralytic ileus, diffuse peritonitis, intestinal obstruction, pancreatitis, GI ischemia, intractable vomiting, and severe diarrhea.[9]

Anxiety. It has been reported that as many as 70% to 80% of ICU patients experience some degree of anxiety. The primary sources of anxiety for patients include the perceived or anticipated threat to physical health, actual loss of control of body functions, and an environment that is foreign. Many patients and families feel uncomfortable in the ICU environment with its complex equipment, high noise and light levels, isolation from family, and intense pace of activity. Pain and sleeplessness enhance anxiety, as do immobilization, loss of control, and impaired communication.[11]

In one study of over 700 critical care nurses, 71% reported that assessing patients for anxiety was very important. The nurses also identified agitation, increased blood pressure, increased heart rate, patient verbalization of anxiety, and restlessness as the five most important clinical indicators of anxiety. To help reduce anxiety, the nurse should encourage patients and families to express concerns, ask questions, and state their needs. The nurse should include the patient and family in all conversations and explain the purpose of equipment and procedures. The nurse should also structure the patient's surrounding environment in a way that may decrease anxiety. For example, family members can be encouraged to bring in photographs and personal items. Judicious use of antianxiety drugs (e.g., lorazepam [Ativan]) and complementary therapies (e.g., imagery, music, massage) may reduce the stress response that can be triggered by anxiety and should be considered.[12,13]

Pain. The control of pain in the ICU patient is paramount. It is reported that as many as 70% of ICU patients recount having moderate to severe unrelieved pain.[6,14] Inadequate pain control is often linked with agitation and anxiety and is known to contribute to the stress response. ICU patients at high risk for pain include patients (1) who have medical conditions that include ischemic, infectious, or inflammatory processes; (2) who are immobilized; (3) who have invasive monitoring devices, including endotracheal tubes; and (4) who are scheduled for any invasive or noninvasive procedures.[14]

For some critically ill patients, continuous IV sedation (e.g., propofol [Diprivan]) and an analgesic agent (e.g., fentanyl [Sublimaze]) are a practical and effective strategy for sedation and pain control. However, patients receiving deep sedation are unresponsive, and this prevents the nurse and other health care providers from properly assessing the patient's neurologic status. To address this limitation, guidelines that include a daily, scheduled interruption of sedation, or "drug holiday," have been developed. Daily sedative interruption allows the patient to awaken and the health care provider to conduct a neurologic examination and assess readiness for weaning.[13,15] In one study, patients who had interrupted sedation were extubated faster and discharged sooner from the ICU than patients who did not have their sedation interrupted.[13,16,17] (Chapter 10 has more detailed information on pain management.)

Impaired Communication. Inability to communicate can be a distressing problem for the patient who may be unable to speak because of the use of sedative and paralyzing drugs or an endotracheal tube. As part of any procedure the nurse should explain what will happen or is happening to the patient. When the patient cannot speak, the nurse should explore alternative methods of communication, including the use of devices such as picture boards, notepads, magic slates, or computer keyboards. When speaking with the patient, the nurse should look directly at the patient and use hand gestures when appropriate. For patients who do not speak English, the use of an interpreter is strongly recommended (see Chapter 3).

Nonverbal communication is important. High levels of procedure-related touch and decreased levels of affection-related or comfort-related touch characterize the ICU. Patients have different levels of tolerance for being touched, usually related to cultural background and personal history. It may be appropriate to provide comforting touch with ongoing evaluation of the patient's response. Often the ICU nurse encourages the family to touch and talk with the patient even if the patient is unresponsive or comatose.

Sensory-Perceptual Problems. Acute and reversible sensory-perceptual changes are common in ICU patients. The combination of alterations in mentation (e.g., delusions, short attention span, loss of recent memory), psychomotor behavior (e.g., restlessness, lethargy), and sleep-wake cycle (e.g., daytime sleepiness, nighttime agitation) has been inappropriately labeled *ICU psychosis*. The patient experiencing these alterations is not psychotic but is suffering from delirium. It is estimated that the prevalence of delirium in ICU patients ranges from 15% to 40%.[18] Demographic factors predisposing the patient to delirium include advanced age, preexisting cerebral illnesses (e.g., dementia), use of medications that block rapid eye movement (REM) sleep (e.g., opioids), and a history of drug or alcohol abuse. Environmental factors that can contribute to delirium include sleep deprivation, anxiety, sensory overload, and immobilization. Physical conditions such as hemodynamic instability, hypoxemia, hypercarbia, electrolyte disturbances, and severe infections can precipitate delirium. Last, certain drugs (e.g., sedatives [benzodiazepines], furosemide [Lasix], antimicrobials [aminoglycosides]) have been associated with the development of delirium.[18] (Delirium is discussed in Chapter 60.)

The task of the ICU nurse is to identify all predisposing factors that may precipitate delirium and attempt to improve the patient's mental clarity and cooperation with therapy. It is imperative that physiologic factors be addressed (e.g., correction of oxygenation, perfusion, and electrolyte problems). The use of clocks and calendars may help the patient remain oriented. If the patient demonstrates unsafe behavior, hyperactivity, insomnia, or delusions, symptoms may be managed pharmacologically with neuroleptic drugs (e.g., haloperidol [Haldol]).[18] In addition, the presence of family members may help reorient the patient and reduce agitation.

Sensory overload can also result in patient distress and anxiety. Environmental noise levels are particularly high in the ICU.[19] The nurse can limit noise and assist the patient in understanding noises that cannot be prevented. Conversation is a particularly stressful noise, especially when the discussion concerns the patient and is conducted in the presence of, but without participation from, the patient. The nurse can eliminate this source of stress by identifying suitable places for patient-related discussions and, whenever possible, by including the patient in the discussion. The nurse can also limit noise levels directly by muting phones, setting alarms appropriate to the patient's condition, and eliminating unnecessary alarms. For example, the nurse should silence the blood pressure alarms while manipulating invasive lines and then reactivate the alarms when the procedures are complete. Similarly, ventilator alarms should be transiently silenced during endotracheal suctioning. Overhead paging and other unnecessary noise should be limited in patient care areas.

Sleep Problems. Nearly all ICU patients experience sleep disturbances. Patients may have difficulty falling asleep or have disrupted sleep because of noise, anxiety, pain, frequent monitoring, or treatment procedures. Sleep disturbance is a significant stressor in the ICU, contributing to delirium and possibly affecting recovery. The ICU nurse can structure the environment to promote the patient's sleep-wake cycle. Strategies include clustering activities, scheduling rest periods, dimming lights at nighttime, opening curtains during the daytime, obtaining physiologic measurements without disrupting the patient, limiting noise, and providing comfort measures (e.g., massage, evening care). If necessary, benzodiazepines (e.g., temazepam [Restoril]) and benzodiazepine-like drugs (e.g., zolpidem [Ambien]) can be used to induce and maintain sleep.[20]

Issues Related to Families

When someone becomes critically ill, care must be extended beyond the patient to the patient's family because they are intimately connected. Family members play a valuable role in the patient's recovery and should be considered members of the health care team. They can contribute to the patient's well-being by

1. Providing a link to the patient's personal life (e.g., news of friends, family, and job)
2. Advising the patient in health care decisions or functioning as the decision maker when the patient cannot
3. Helping with activities of daily living (e.g., bathing, oral suctioning)
4. Providing positive, loving, and caring support

To be effective in caring for their loved one, family members need guidance and support from the nurse. The experience of having a friend or family member in the ICU is physically and emotionally difficult often to the point of caretaker exhaustion. Anxiety regarding the patient's condition and prognosis and concerns regarding the patient's pain and other discomforts are some of the issues families confront. They may question the quality of care that the patient is receiving. In addition, it is common for families to experience anxiety regarding the financial issues related to the provision of care during a critical illness. Consulting with the case manager or social worker is helpful in these instances.

The family will typically be experiencing disruption of their daily routines to support the patient. They may be far from their own home and supportive friends and family members. Ultimately, families of the critically ill are considered in crisis, and family-centered care is imperative. To provide family-centered care effectively, the nurse must be skilled in crisis intervention. The nurse should conduct a family assessment and intervene as necessary. Interventions can include active listening, reduction of anxiety, and

support of those who become upset or angry.[21] The family's feelings should be acknowledged and accepted and their decisions supported. Other health team members (e.g., chaplains, psychologists, patient representatives) may be helpful in assisting the family to adjust and should be consulted as necessary. The extent to which family-centered care is provided will, in turn, affect the patient's clinical course in the ICU.

The major needs of families of critically ill patients have been categorized as informational needs, reassurance needs, and convenience needs.[22] Lack of information is a major source of anxiety for the family. The nurse should assess the family's understanding of the patient's status, treatment plan, and prognosis and provide information as appropriate. The nurse should also provide information to the family when the patient's condition changes. It is recommended that a spokesperson for the family be identified so that information between the health care team and the family can be coordinated.

The family needs reassurance regarding the way in which the patient's care is managed and decisions are made. The family should have the opportunity to be involved in decision making. If the patient has an advance directive or a living will, the family will need to see that the patient's wishes are understood and respected. When patients are incapable of making their own health care decisions, they may have designated a durable power of attorney, and this person should be involved in the patient's plan of care. The family should also be invited to meet the health care team members, including physicians, dietitian, respiratory therapist, social worker, physical therapist, and chaplain. The nurse should evaluate the appropriateness of including family members in multidisciplinary care conferences. It helps family members to accept and cope with problems if they observe that health care providers are hopeful, caring, and competent; decisions are deliberate; and they have the opportunity to help shape the course of care.

Research has demonstrated that families of critically ill patients need the convenience of access to the patient and that limiting family visitation does not protect that patient from adverse physiologic consequences.[23] Rigid visitation policies in ICUs should be reviewed, and a move toward less restrictive, individualized visiting policies is strongly recommended by the AACN.[21] This can be accomplished by assessing the patient's and family members' needs and preferences and incorporating these into the plan of care. The first time that family members visit it is important for the nurse to prepare them for the experience by briefly describing the patient's appearance and the physical environment (e.g., equipment, noise). It is helpful if the nurse can accompany the family members as they enter the room. They should be invited to participate in the patient's care if they desire. The nurse should observe the responses of both the patient and family. In some ICUs, visitation has been expanded to include family pet visitation or animal-assisted therapy. The positive benefits of pet visitation (e.g., decreases in blood pressure and anxiety) far outweigh the risks (e.g., transmission of infection from pet to patient) and should be considered as part of the visitation policy.[24]

In addition to traditional family visiting, research has also demonstrated that family members of patients undergoing invasive procedures, including cardiopulmonary resuscitation (CPR), should be given the option of being present at the bedside during these events. Even when the outcomes were not favorable, being present helped family members remove doubts about the patient's condition, decreased their anxiety and fear, facilitated the need to be together and to support their loved one, and facilitated the grief process when death occurred. AACN encourages ICUs to develop policies and procedures that provide for the option of family presence during invasive procedures and cardiopulmonary resuscitation.[25]

CULTURALLY COMPETENT CARE
CRITICAL CARE PATIENTS

Providing culturally competent care to critically ill patients and families is challenging. Often, the nurse is focused on meeting the physiologic needs of the patient and may not appreciate the influence of the patient's culture on the illness experience. The cultural dimensions of the meaning of sickness and health, pain, dying and death, and grief need to be considered when caring for critically ill patients and their families. (Chapter 3 discusses cultural issues.)

Cultural perspectives on dying and death are complex. Telling some patients that they are dying as a way of letting them prepare for death may be considered an infringement on the role of the family. Others view a discussion about advance directives as a legal device to deny care. One study found that most would opt to extend life even at the expense of the quality of life.[26]

Customs surrounding dying and death vary widely, from leaving a window open to allow the spirit of the dead person to leave to providing the final bath for the deceased. The nurse caring for the dying patient must make every attempt to understand and accommodate the family's cultural traditions. The expressions of grief that follow the loss of a loved one are highly individualized and influenced by several variables. These include the relationship between the grieving person and the deceased, whether the loss is sudden or anticipated, the support systems available to the grieving person, past experiences with loss, and the person's religious and cultural beliefs. It is of utmost importance that the critical care nurse proceed cautiously when approaching patients facing death and their families. Asking patients, "What do you want to know?" and "Who do you want with you when discussing options?" is a good starting point.[26] (Chapter 11 provides additional information about end-of-life care.)

HEMODYNAMIC MONITORING

Hemodynamic monitoring refers to the measurement of pressure, flow, and oxygenation within the cardiovascular system. Both invasive (internally placed devices) and noninvasive (external devices) hemodynamic measurements are made in the ICU. Values commonly measured include systemic and pulmonary arterial pressures, central venous pressure (CVP), pulmonary artery wedge pressure (PAWP), cardiac output/index, stroke volume/index, and oxygen saturation of the hemoglobin of arterial blood (SaO_2) and mixed venous blood (SvO_2). From these measurements the clinician calculates several values, including the resistance of the systemic and pulmonary arterial vasculature and oxygen content, delivery, and consumption. When these data are integrated with clinical assessment data, the nurse can derive a picture of the patient's hemodynamic status and the effect of therapy over time. It is important that all measures be made with attention to technical accuracy. False or inaccurate data are potentially misleading and may result in unnecessary or inappropriate treatment.

Hemodynamic Terminology

Cardiac Output and Cardiac Index. *Cardiac output* (CO) is the volume of blood pumped by the heart in 1 minute. *Cardiac index* (CI) is the measurement of the CO adjusted for body size (e.g., height and weight) and is a more precise measurement of the efficiency of the pumping action of the heart. Although minor beat-to-beat changes may occur, generally the left and right ventricles pump the same volume. The volume ejected with each heartbeat is the stroke volume (SV). Like CI, stroke volume index (SVI) is the measurement of SV adjusted for body size. CO and the forces opposing blood flow determine blood pressure, the force exerted by blood on the vessel wall. The opposition to blood flow offered by the vessels is called *systemic vascular resistance* (SVR) (opposition encountered by the left ventricle) or *pulmonary vascular resistance* (PVR) (opposition encountered by the right ventricle). Preload, afterload, and contractility (see Chapter 32) determine SV (and thus CO and blood pressure). Understanding these concepts and relationships is essential for the critical care nurse. In addition, the nurse must understand the effects of manipulation of each of these variables. The formulas and normal values for common hemodynamic parameters are given in Table 66-2.

Preload. *Preload* is the volume within the ventricle at the end of diastole. Unfortunately, chamber volume measurements are difficult to obtain. Instead, various pressures are used to estimate volume. Left ventricular preload is called *left ventricular end-diastolic pressure*. PAWP, a measurement of pulmonary capillary pressure, reflects left ventricular end-diastolic pressure under normal conditions (i.e., when there is no mitral valve dysfunction, intracardiac defect, or dysrhythmia). CVP, measured in the right atrium or in the vena cava close to the heart, is the right ventricular preload or right ventricular end-diastolic pressure when there is no tricuspid valve dysfunction, intracardiac defect, or dysrhythmia.

The effects of preload are explained by *Frank-Starling's law,* which states that the more a myocardial fiber is stretched during filling, the more it shortens during systole and the greater the force of the contraction. As preload increases, force generated in the subsequent contraction increases, thus SV and CO increase. The greater the preload, the greater the myocardial (heart muscle) stretch and the greater the oxygen requirement of the myocardium. Hence, increases in CO via increased preload require increased delivery of oxygen to the myocardium. It should be remembered that the change in SV with preload comes about because of stretching and recoil of the heart muscle. However, the clinical measurement made is not a direct measurement of the muscle length; the measurement made is pressure at the time of the peak stretch (end diastole) (see Table 66-2). This pressure indirectly indicates the amount of stretch and the volume. This pressure is also important because it indicates pressure in the blood vessels of the lung or in the blood returning to the heart. Preload can be increased by fluid administration and decreased by diuresis.

Afterload. *Afterload* refers to the forces opposing ventricular ejection. These forces include systemic arterial pressure, the resistance offered by the aortic valve, and the mass and density of the blood to be moved. Clinically, although the measures fail to include all the components of afterload, SVR and arterial pressure are indices of left ventricular afterload. Similarly, PVR and pulmonary arterial pressure are indices of right ventricular afterload. Increased afterload often results in a decreased CO. CO can be restored by decreasing afterload (i.e., decreasing forces opposing contraction). When afterload is reduced, myocardial oxygen needs

TABLE 66-2	**Hemodynamic Parameters at Rest**

Indicators	Normal Range
Preload	
Right atrial pressure (RAP) or central venous pressure (CVP)	2-8 mm Hg
Pulmonary artery wedge pressure (PAWP) or left atrial pressure (LAP)	6-12 mm Hg
Pulmonary artery diastolic pressure (PADP)	4-12 mm Hg
Afterload	
Pulmonary vascular resistance (PVR) $= \dfrac{\text{(Pulmonary artery mean pressure [PAMP]} - \text{PAWP)} \times 80}{\text{Cardiac output (CO)}}$	<250 dynes/sec/cm^{-5}
Pulmonary vascular resistance index (PVRI) = (PAMP − PAWP) × 80/Cardiac index (CI)	160-380 dynes/sec/cm^{-5}/m^2
Systemic vascular resistance (SVR) = (Mean arterial pressure [MAP] − CVP) × 80/CO	800-1200 dynes/sec/cm^{-5}
Systemic vascular resistance index (SVRI) = (MAP − CVP) × 80/CI	1970-2390 dynes/sec/cm^{-5}/m^2
Mean arterial pressure (MAP) $= \dfrac{\text{Systolic blood pressure} + 2\ \text{(Diastolic blood pressure)}}{3^*}$	70-105 mm Hg
Pulmonary artery mean pressure (PAMP) $= \dfrac{\text{Pulmonary artery systolic pressure (PASP)} + 2\text{PADP}}{3^*}$	10-20 mm Hg
Other	
Stroke volume (SV) = CO/Heart rate	60-150 ml/beat
Stroke volume index (SVI) = CI/Heart rate	30-65 ml/beat/m^2
Heart rate (HR)	60-100 beats/min
CO = SV × HR	4-8 L/min
Cardiac index (CI) = CO/Body surface area (BSA)	2.2-4 L/min/m^2
Arterial hemoglobin oxygen saturation	95%-99%
Mixed venous hemoglobin oxygen saturation	60%-80%
Venous hemoglobin oxygen saturation	70%

*This formula is an approximation because it does not take into consideration the heart rate. The monitor looks at the area under the pressure curve, as well as the heart rate, to calculate MAP and PAMP.

are decreased. Thus CO is increased, and myocardial oxygen requirements are decreased. Drug therapy directed at reducing afterload (e.g., milrinone [Primacor]) is often used in the management of heart failure (see Chapter 35).

Vascular Resistance. *Systemic vascular resistance* (SVR) is the resistance of the systemic vascular bed. *Pulmonary vascular resistance* (PVR) is the resistance of the pulmonary vascular bed. Both of these measures reflect afterload as described earlier and can be adjusted for body size (see Table 66-2).

Contractility. *Contractility* describes the strength of contraction. Contractility is said to increase when preload is not changed yet the heart contracts more forcefully. Epinephrine, norepinephrine [Levophed], isoproterenol (Isuprel), dopamine (Intropin), dobutamine (Dobutrex), digitalis-like drugs, calcium, and milrinone (Primacor) increase or improve contractility. These agents are termed *positive inotropes*. Contractility is diminished by *negative inotropes,* such as certain drugs (e.g., barbiturates, alcohol, calcium channel blockers, β-adrenergic blockers) and conditions (e.g., acidosis). Increased contractility results in increased SV and increased myocardial oxygen requirements. There are no direct clinical measures of cardiac contractility. To indirectly determine contractility, the nurse measures the patient's preload (PAWP) and CO and graphs the results. If preload, heart rate, and afterload remain constant yet CO changes, contractility is altered. Contractility is diminished in the failing heart.

Principles of Invasive Pressure Monitoring

Invasive lines are commonly used in the ICU to measure systemic and pulmonary blood pressures. Components of a typical invasive arterial pressure monitoring system are illustrated in Fig. 66-3. Catheter, pressure tubing, flush system, and usually the transducer are disposable.

To accurately measure pressure, equipment must be referenced and zero balanced to the environment and dynamic response characteristics optimized. *Referencing* means positioning the transducer so that the zero reference point is at the level of the atria of the heart. The stopcock nearest the transducer is usually the zero reference for the transducer. To place this level with the atria, the nurse uses an external landmark, the phlebostatic axis. To identify the **phlebostatic axis,** two imaginary lines are drawn with the patient supine (Fig. 66-4, *A*). The first line, a horizontal line, is drawn through the midchest, halfway between the outermost anterior and posterior surfaces. The second line, a vertical line, is drawn through the fourth intercostal space at the sternum. The phlebostatic axis is the intersection of the two imaginary lines. Once the phlebostatic axis is identified, it should be marked on the patient's chest with a permanent marker. The port of the stopcock nearest the transducer must be positioned level with the phlebostatic axis. It is recommended that the transducer be taped to the patient's chest at the phlebostatic axis or mounted on a bedside pole.[27]

Zeroing confirms that when pressure within the system is zero, the monitor reads zero. This is accomplished by opening the reference stopcock to room air (off to the patient) and observing the monitor for a reading of zero. Most transducers in current use are disposable and have little zero drift. Zeroing the transducer is recommended during initial setup, immediately after insertion of the arterial line, when the transducer has been disconnected from the pressure cable or the pressure cable has been disconnected from the monitor, and when the accuracy of the measurements is questioned, and it should be done according to the manufacturer's guidelines.[27]

Optimizing dynamic response characteristics involves checking that the equipment reproduces, without distortion, a signal that changes rapidly. A *dynamic response test (square wave test)* is

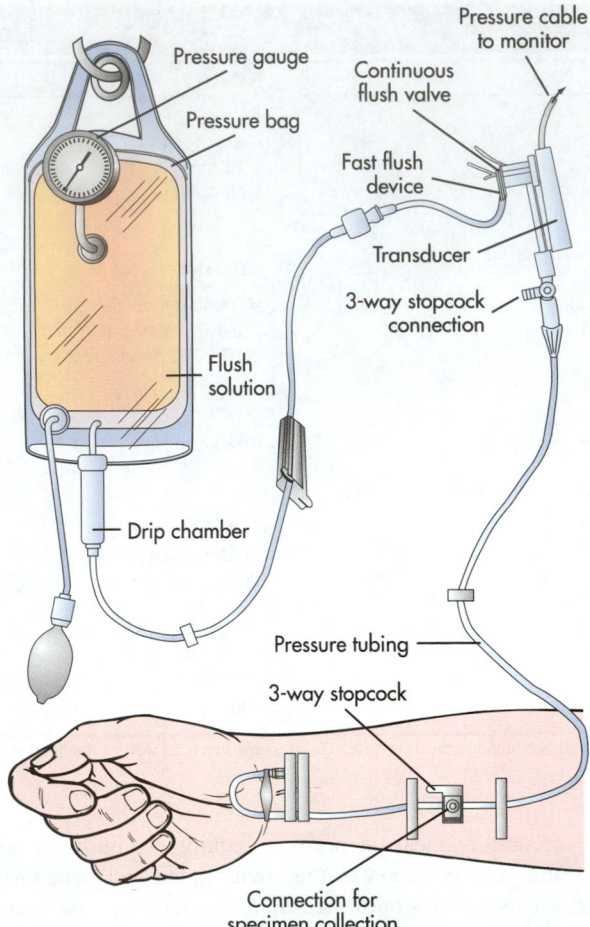

FIG. 66-3 Components of a pressure monitoring system. The cannula, shown entering the radial artery, is connected via pressure (nondistensible) tubing to the transducer. The transducer converts the pressure wave into an electronic signal. The transducer is wired to the electronic monitoring system, which amplifies, conditions, displays, and records the signal. Stopcocks are inserted into the line for specimen withdrawal and for referencing and zero-balancing procedures. A flush system, consisting of a pressurized bag of intravenous fluid, tubing, and a flush device, is inserted into the line. The flush system provides continuous slow (approximately 3 ml/hr) flushing and provides a mechanism for fast flushing of lines. All items except the electronic monitoring system are commonly disposable equipment.

performed every 8 to 12 hours and when the system is opened to air or the accuracy of the measurements is questioned. It involves activating the fast flush and checking that the equipment reproduces a distortion-free signal[28] (Fig. 66-5).

Steps in obtaining blood pressure measurements with an invasive line are given in Table 66-3. Pressure measurements can be obtained from both digital and printed analog outputs, but accurate readings are best obtained from a printed pressure tracing at the end of expiration. Initial readings are made with the patient flat (supine). Unless the patient's blood pressure is extremely sensitive to orthostatic changes, values at modest degrees of backrest elevation (up to 45 degrees) are generally equivalent to measurements with the patient supine. Most studies do not support the accuracy of readings for patients in the lateral position but do support the accuracy of readings for patients in the prone position.[27] It is not necessary to reposition the patient for each pressure reading. However, it is necessary to move the zero reference stopcock to keep it positioned at the phlebostatic axis (see Fig. 66-4, *B*).

Types of Invasive Pressure Monitoring

Arterial Blood Pressure. Continuous arterial pressure monitoring is indicated for patients in many situations, including acute hypertension and hypotension, respiratory failure, shock, neurologic injury, coronary interventional procedures, continuous infusion of vasoactive drugs (sodium nitroprusside [Nipride]), and frequent ABG sampling. A 20-gauge, 2-inch (5.1 cm) nontapered Teflon catheter is typically used to cannulate a peripheral artery (e.g., radial, femoral) using a percutaneous approach. After insertion, the catheter is sutured in place.[29] It is important that the insertion site be immobilized so that the catheter line is not dislodged and lines are not kinked.

Measurements. The nurse can use the arterial line to obtain systolic, diastolic, and mean blood pressures (see Fig. 66-5). High- and low-pressure alarms should be set based on the patient's current status and activated. Measurements are obtained at end expiration to limit the effect of the respiratory cycle on arterial pressure.[29] In heart failure, the systolic upstroke may be slower. In volume depletion, systolic pressure varies greatly with mechanical ventilation, diminishing during inspiration. In severe heart failure, systolic amplitude does not vary with ventilation. With dysrhythmias it is useful to observe simultaneous ECG and pressure tracings. Dysrhythmias that significantly diminish arterial pressure are more urgent than those that cause only a slight decrease in systolic amplitude.

Complications. Arterial lines carry the risk of hemorrhage, infection, thrombus formation, neurovascular impairment, and loss of limb. Hemorrhage is most likely to occur when the catheter becomes dislodged or the line becomes disconnected. To avoid this serious complication, the nurse uses Luer-Lok connections and always checks the arterial waveform and that the alarms are activated. If the pressure in the line falls (e.g., when the line is disconnected), the low-pressure alarm sounds immediately, allowing prompt correction of the problem. Pressure is always monitored when an arterial line is in place, even if the line was placed for ABG sampling.

Infection is a risk with any invasive line. The nurse should inspect the insertion site for local signs of inflammation and monitor the patient for signs of systemic infection. To limit the risk of contamination and catheter-related infection, the catheter site, pressure tubing, flush bag, and transducer should be changed every 96 hours.[29] When infection is suspected, the catheter should be removed and the equipment changed.

Circulatory impairment can result from formation of a thrombus around the catheter, release of an embolus, spasm, or occlusion of the circulation by the catheter. Before inserting a line into the radial artery, an *Allen test* should be performed to confirm that ulnar circulation is sufficient to sustain the hand. In this test, pressure is applied to the radial and ulnar arteries simultaneously. The patient is instructed to open and close the hand repeatedly. The hand should blanch. The nurse then releases the pressure on the ulnar artery while compressing the radial artery. If pinkness fails to return within 6 seconds, the ulnar artery is insufficient, indicating that the radial artery should not be used for line insertion.

To help maintain line patency and limit thrombus formation, the nurse should assess the continuous flush irrigation system every 1 to 4 hours to determine that the pressure bag is inflated to 300 mm Hg, the flush bag contains fluid, and the system is delivering 3 to 6 ml per hour. It is recommended that a solution of heparinized saline be used for the flush solution unless contraindicated (e.g., history of heparin-induced thrombocytopenia).[28]

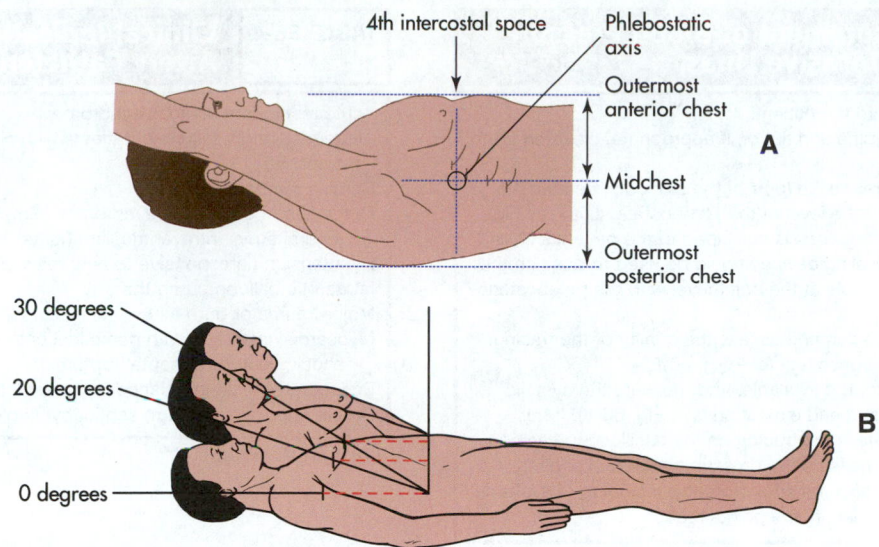

FIG. 66-4   Identification of the phlebostatic axis. **A,** Phlebostatic axis is an external landmark used to identify the level of the atria in the supine patient. The *phlebostatic axis* is defined as the intersection of two imaginary lines: one drawn vertically through the fourth intercostal space at the sternum, and another drawn horizontally through the midchest, halfway between the outermost anterior and outermost posterior points of the chest. **B,** As the backrest of the supine patient is elevated, the phlebostatic axis remains at the same anatomic location, becoming progressively elevated from the floor. The zero reference point must be repositioned with changes in backrest elevation, in order to keep it at the phlebostatic level.

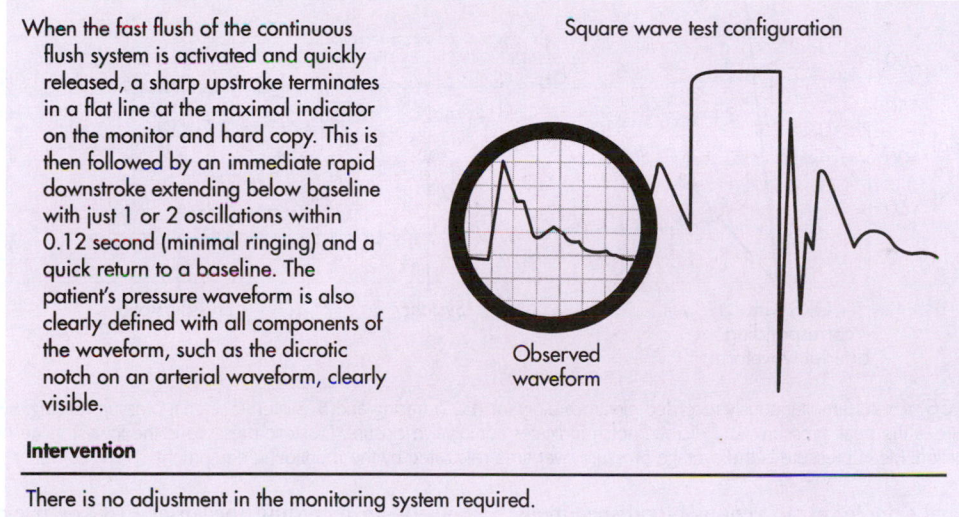

When the fast flush of the continuous flush system is activated and quickly released, a sharp upstroke terminates in a flat line at the maximal indicator on the monitor and hard copy. This is then followed by an immediate rapid downstroke extending below baseline with just 1 or 2 oscillations within 0.12 second (minimal ringing) and a quick return to a baseline. The patient's pressure waveform is also clearly defined with all components of the waveform, such as the dicrotic notch on an arterial waveform, clearly visible.

Square wave test configuration

Observed waveform

Intervention

There is no adjustment in the monitoring system required.

FIG. 66-5   Optimally damped system. Dynamic response test (square wave test) using the fast flush system: normal response.

Once the catheter is inserted, the nurse should evaluate the neurovascular status distal to the arterial insertion site hourly. The limb with compromised arterial flow will appear cool and pale, with capillary refill greater than 3 seconds. There may be symptoms of neurologic impairment, such as tingling, pain, or paresthesia. Neurovascular impairment can result in loss of a limb and is an emergency.

Pulmonary Artery Flow-Directed Catheter. Pulmonary artery (PA) pressure monitoring is used to guide acute-phase management of patients with complicated cardiac, pulmonary, and intravascular volume problems (Table 66-4). PA diastolic (PAD) pressure and PAWP are sensitive indicators of cardiac function and

fluid volume status. PAD pressure and PAWP are increased in heart failure and fluid volume overload. They are decreased with volume depletion. Fluid therapy based on PA pressure allows restoration of fluid balance while avoiding overcorrection of the problem. Monitoring PA pressures can allow precise therapeutic manipulation of preload, which allows CO to be maintained without placing the patient at risk for pulmonary edema.

A PA flow-directed catheter (e.g., Swan-Ganz) is used to measure PA pressures, including PAWP. The standard PA catheter is number 7.5-French, 43 inches (110 cm) long, with four or five lumens (Fig. 66-7). When properly positioned, the distal lumen port (catheter tip) is within the PA (Fig. 66-8). This port is used to

TABLE 66-3	**Measurement of Blood Pressure with Invasive Lines**

1. Explain the procedure to the patient.
2. Position the patient supine and flat or, if appropriate, elevated up to 45 degrees or prone.
3. Confirm that the zero reference (port of the stopcock nearest the transducer) is placed at the level of the phlebostatic axis (see Fig. 66-4). If the reference stopcock is not taped to the patient's chest, a low-intensity laser leveling device should be used to position the stopcock on a bedside pole at the point level with the phlebostatic axis.
4. Observe the monitor tracing and assess the quality of the tracing. Perform a dynamic response test (see Fig. 66-5).
5. Obtain an analog printout, if available, and measure the systolic and diastolic pressures at end expiration (see Fig. 66-6). If no printout is available, freeze the tracing on the oscilloscope screen and use the cursor to measure the pressures at end expiration.
6. Record the pressure measurements promptly, including (if available) the printout marked to identify the points read.

TABLE 66-4	**Clinical Indications for Pulmonary Artery Catheterization***

Acute respiratory distress syndrome
Acute respiratory failure in patients with chronic obstructive pulmonary disease
Cardiac tamponade
Evaluation of circulatory syndromes (e.g., heart failure, mitral valve regurgitation, intraventricular shunts)
Hypotension unresponsive to fluid resuscitation
Intraaortic balloon pump therapy
Major trauma or burn injury
Myocardial infarction with complications (e.g., heart failure, cardiogenic shock, ventricular septal rupture)
Perioperative fluid imbalance in high-risk patients (e.g., cardiac history)
Severe shock states (e.g., septic, hypovolemic)

*List is not all-inclusive.

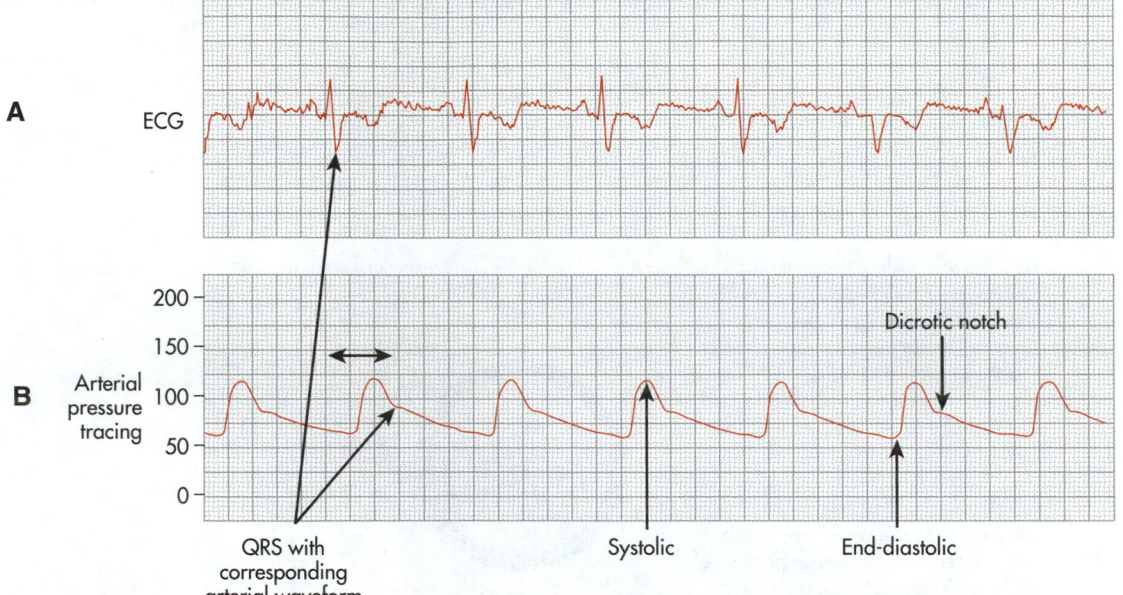

FIG. 66-6   **A,** Simultaneously recorded electrocardiogram (ECG) tracing and **B,** systemic arterial pressure tracing. Systolic pressure is the peak pressure. The dicrotic notch indicates aortic valve closure. Diastolic pressure is the lowest value before contraction. Mean pressure is the average pressure over time calculated by the monitoring equipment.

monitor PA pressures and sample mixed venous blood specimens (e.g., to evaluate oxygen saturation). A balloon connected to an external valve via the second lumen surrounds the distal lumen port. Balloon inflation has two purposes: (1) to allow moving blood to float the catheter forward and (2) to allow PAWP measurement. There will be one or two proximal lumens, with exit ports in the right atrium or right atrium and right ventricle (if two). The right atrium port is used for measurement of CVP, injection of fluid for CO determination, and withdrawal of blood specimens. If a second proximal port is available, it is used for infusion of fluids and drugs or blood sampling. A thermistor (temperature sensor) lumen port located near the distal tip is wired to an external connector. This port is used for monitoring blood or core temperature and in the thermodilution method of measuring CO.

In addition to these relatively standard and common features of the PA flow-directed catheter, catheters with other features are available. One modification is the inclusion of an atrial electrode,

useful in recording the atrial ECG or pacing the heart. Another common modification is inclusion of a fiberoptic sensor in the distal tip that detects mixed venous oxygen saturation. Another type of catheter provides continuous measurement of right ventricular volume and ejection fraction, and some catheters provide continuous CO monitoring.[30] The PA catheter sheath (introducer) usually has a side port that serves as another IV line. Most catheters also have a plastic "sleeve" connected to the sheath, which permits manipulation of the catheter while maintaining sterility.

Pulmonary Artery Catheter Insertion. Before PA catheter insertion, the nurse notes the patient's electrolyte, acid-base, oxygenation, and coagulation status. Imbalances such as hypokalemia, hypomagnesemia, hypoxemia, or acidosis can make the heart more irritable and increase the risk of ventricular dysrhythmia during catheter insertion. Coagulopathy increases the risk of hemorrhage. The nurse prepares for the procedure by arranging the monitor, cables, and infusion and pressurized flush solutions. The system is

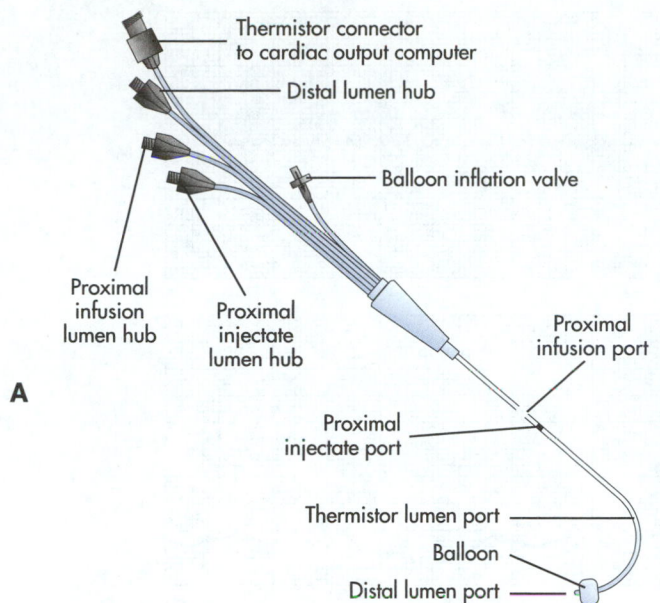

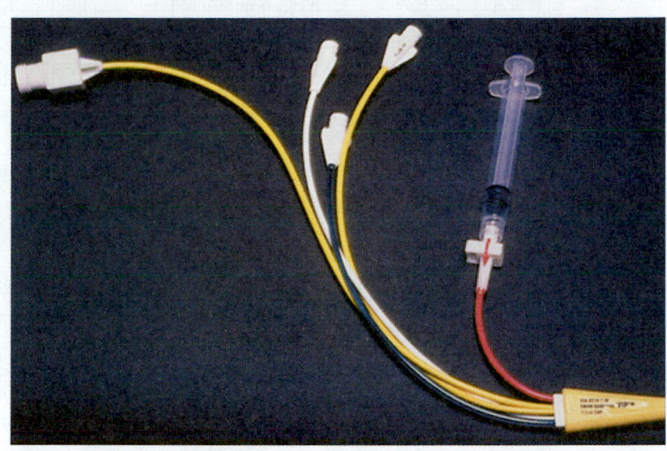

A

B

FIG. 66-7 Pulmonary artery (PA) catheter. **A,** Illustrated catheter has five lumens. When properly positioned, the distal lumen exit port is in the PA and the proximal lumen ports are in the right atrium and right ventricle. The distal and one of the proximal ports are used to measure PA and central venous pressures, respectively. A balloon surrounds the catheter near the distal end. The balloon inflation valve is used to inflate the balloon with air to allow reading of the pulmonary artery wedge pressure. A thermistor located near the distal tip senses PA temperature and is used to measure thermodilution cardiac output when solution cooler than body temperature is injected into a proximal port. **B,** Photo of an actual catheter.

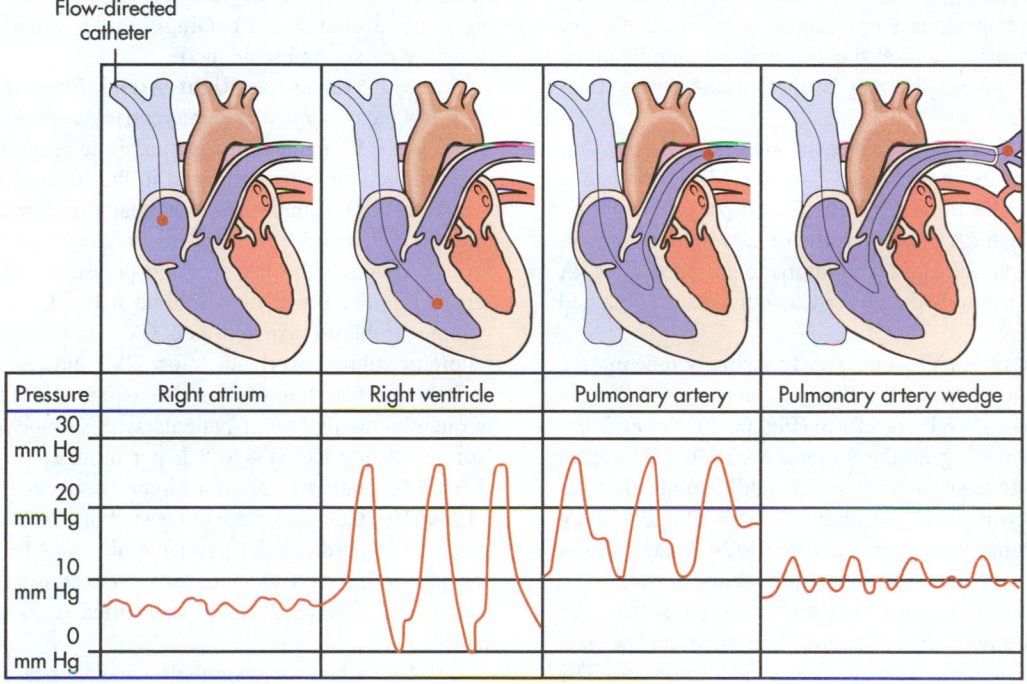

FIG. 66-8 Position of the pulmonary artery flow-directed catheter during progressive stages of insertion with corresponding pressure waveforms.

zero referenced to the phlebostatic axis. The procedure is explained to the patient, and informed consent is obtained. The patient is positioned supine with the head of the bed flat.[30] The PA catheter is inserted through a sheath percutaneously into the internal jugular, subclavian, antecubital, or femoral vein using surgical asepsis. Venous cut-down is rarely required. The line is then advanced through the venous system to the right side of the heart.

Catheter insertion is guided by continuously observing the characteristic waveforms on the monitor as the catheter is ad-

vanced through the heart to the PA (see Fig. 66-8). When the tip reaches the right atrium, the balloon is inflated.[30] Inflation of the balloon should not exceed the balloon's capacity (usually 1 to 1.5 ml of air). The catheter is then floated through the tricuspid valve into the right ventricle and then through the pulmonic valve and into the PA. It is necessary to monitor the ECG continuously during insertion because of the risk for dysrhythmias, particularly when the catheter reaches the right ventricle. Once a typical PAWP tracing is observed, the balloon is deflated, and the PA waveform

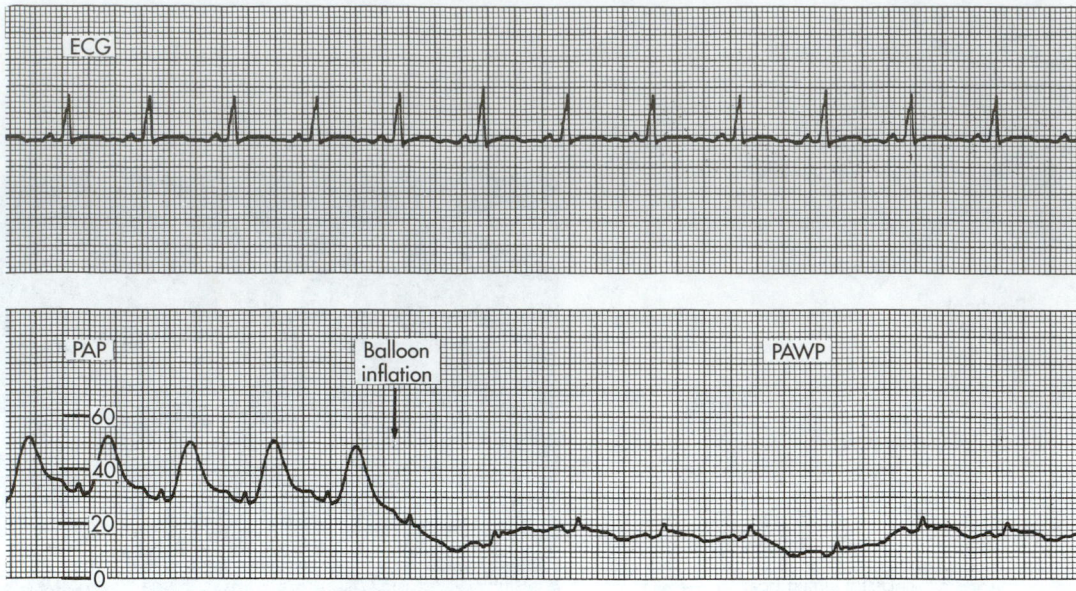

FIG. 66-9 Change in pulmonary artery pressure *(PAP)* waveform to pulmonary artery wedge pressure *(PAWP)* waveform with balloon inflation. The balloon is inflated while observing the bedside monitor for change in the waveform. Balloon inflation *(arrow)* in patient with a normal PAWP.

should return on the monitor. Following insertion, a chest x-ray is obtained to confirm the position. To maintain the catheter in its proper position, the catheter is then secured at its point of entry into the skin. The measurement at the exit point should be noted and recorded. An occlusive dressing is applied and changed according to unit protocol.

Pulmonary Artery Pressure Measurements. Systolic, diastolic, and mean pressures are routinely monitored. PA systolic is the peak pressure and PA diastolic is the lowest pressure point on the PA waveform. Mean PA pressure is the time-weighted average. Because PA ports are in the chest, intrathoracic pressures alter PA pressure. To produce accurate data, PA measurements are obtained at the end of expiration.[29]

The measurement of PAWP is obtained by slowly inflating the balloon with air (not to exceed balloon capacity) until the PA waveform changes to a PAWP waveform (Fig. 66-9). Before inflation the PA pressure tracing on the monitor looks like an arterial tracing, with a systolic peak, dicrotic notch, and then the diastolic low point. As the waveform becomes "wedged," the tracing changes shape and amplitude. Generally, the PAWP waveform is characterized by two small positive waves, the *a* and *v* waves. The *a wave* indicates atrial contraction, and it is followed by the *x descent*, indicating atrial relaxation. At times, a *c wave* may be seen following the *a* wave and indicates closure of the mitral valve. The *v wave* is seen during the interval between the T and P waves of the ECG. The *v* wave indicates inflow into the left atrium when the mitral valve is closed and the ventricle is contracting. The *v* wave is followed by the *y descent,* indicating the emptying of the left atrium when the mitral valve opens and the ventricle fills.[31]

When measuring the PAWP, the balloon should be inflated for no more than four respiratory cycles or 8 to 15 seconds.[31] There is danger of rupture of the PA if the catheter migrates distally into a smaller vessel or if the balloon is overinflated. This is suspected when less than 1 ml is needed to wedge the tracing or an "overwedge" tracing is obtained (Fig. 66-10). Readings should be ac-

quired from an analog strip pressure recording, and the strip should be placed into the patient's record. If a printout of the tracing is not available, the readings can be taken from the monitor using the cursor and scale mode.

Central Venous or Right Atrial Pressure Measurement. CVP is a measurement of right ventricular preload. It can be measured with a PA catheter using one of the proximal lumens or with a central venous catheter placed in the internal jugular or subclavian vein. CVP is measured as a mean pressure at the end of expiration. CVP waveforms (Fig. 66-11) are similar to PAWP waveforms. Although the PA diastolic pressure and PAWP are more sensitive indicators of fluid volume status, CVP also reflects fluid volume problems. An elevated CVP indicates right ventricular failure or volume overload. A low CVP indicates hypovolemia.

Invasive Cardiac Output Measurement Techniques. CO is frequently monitored in patients with hemodynamic instability. Normal resting CO is 4 to 8 L per minute and varies with body size. CI accounts for variations in body size and is normally 2.2 to 4 L/min/m². CO and CI are decreased in conditions such as shock states (e.g., cardiogenic, hypovolemic) and heart failure. Under normal conditions, CO increases with exercise. Increases in CO at rest indicate a hyperdynamic state often seen with fever or early sepsis.

The PA catheter is commonly used to measure CO via the intermittent bolus *thermodilution* CO (TDCO) method or the *continuous* CO (CCO) method. With the TDCO method, a fixed volume (5 to 10 ml) of cold (0° to 12° C [32° to 53.6° F]) or room temperature solution of 5% dextrose (or saline, only if contraindicated) is injected rapidly (≤4 seconds) and smoothly into the proximal lumen port of the PA catheter.[32] The thermistor sensor located near the distal tip of the PA catheter detects the differences in blood temperature. The CO is mathematically calculated from the area under the temperature curve by the computer. The larger the area under the curve, the lower the CO, and, conversely, the smaller the area under the curve, the higher the CO[32] (Fig. 66-12).

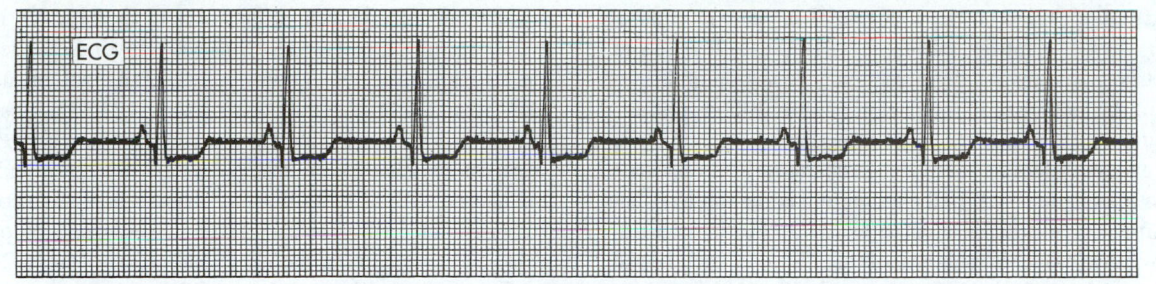

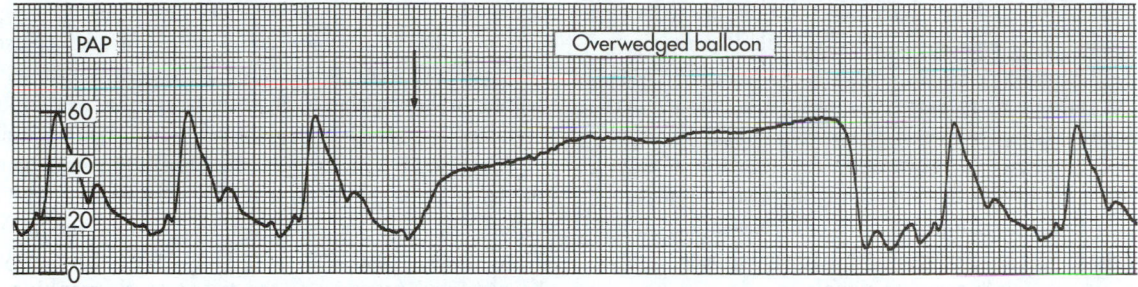

FIG. 66-10   Balloon inflation *(arrow)* in patient with elevated wedge pressure. Overwedging of balloon (balloon has been overinflated). The danger of overinflating the balloon is that the pulmonary artery (PA) vessel may rupture from the pressure of the balloon. *PAP,* Pulmonary artery pressure.

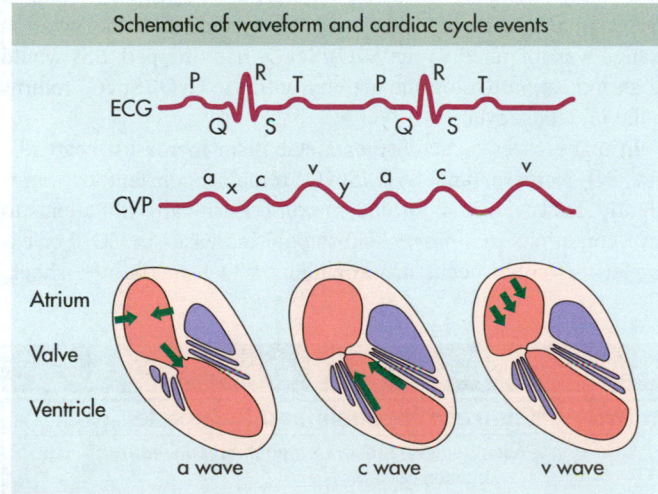

FIG. 66-11   Cardiac events that produce the central venous pressure (CVP) waveform with *a, c,* and *v* waves. The *a* wave represents atrial contraction. The *x* descent represents atrial relaxation. The *c* wave represents the bulging of the closed tricuspid valve into the right atrium during ventricular systole. The *v* wave represents atrial filling. The *y* descent represents opening of the tricuspid valve and filling of the ventricle.

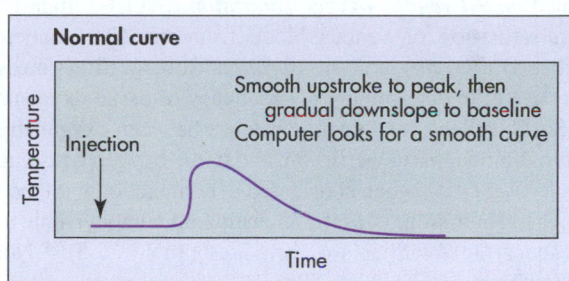

FIG. 66-12   Normal cardiac output curve. Cardiac output is calculated from the temperature change in the pulmonary artery when a fixed volume and known temperature of a solution is injected into the proximal port in the right atrium. The nurse should observe the curve during injection to make sure that it is smooth.

This procedure is repeated three or four times, with each measurement 1 to 2 minutes apart. Any CO measurement that does not have a normal curve is discarded. An average of three acceptable measurements (within 0.5 L of each other) is calculated to determine the CO.

The CCO method uses a heat-exchange CO catheter. This PA catheter contains a thermal filament that is located in the right atrium. This filament emits a pulsed signal every 30 to 60 seconds that allows for the mixing of blood with heat as it passes through the right ventricle. The thermistor sensor detects the change in temperature. A bedside computer displays digital measurements every 30 to 60 seconds that reflect the average CO for the past 3 to

6 minutes. The CCO method eliminates the need for fluid boluses, reduces the risk of contamination, and permits ongoing evaluation (or trending) of the CO. Comparisons of the TDCO method with the CCO method have shown the CCO method to be reliable.[32]

SVR, SVR index (SVRI), SV, and SV index (SVI) can be calculated each time that CO is measured. The formulas for calculating these parameters are shown in Table 66-2. Increased SVR (>1200 dynes/sec/cm^{-5}) indicates vasoconstriction from shock, hypertension, increased release or administration of epinephrine and other vasoactive inotropes, or left ventricular failure. A low SVR (<800 dynes/sec/cm^{-5}) indicates vasodilation, which may occur during shock states (e.g., septic, neurogenic) or with drugs that reduce afterload. Changes in SV are rapidly becoming more important indicators of the pumping status of the heart than other parameters. A high SV may be seen in bradycardia and exercise and with the use of positive inotropes (e.g., dobutamine). Low SV is seen with tachydysrhythmias, extreme vasodilation, and cardiac tamponade.

Noninvasive Hemodynamic Monitoring: Impedance Cardiography. Impedance cardiography (ICG) is a continuous or intermittent, noninvasive method of obtaining CO and assessing thoracic fluid status. Based on the concepts of *impedance* (the resistance to the flow of electrical current [Ω]), ICG uses four sets of external electrodes to deliver a high-frequency, low-amplitude current that is similar to that used in apnea monitors. Blood is an excellent conductor of electricity (lower impedance), and pulsatile blood flow generates electrical impedance changes. ICG measures the change in impedance ($d\Omega$) in the ascending aorta and left ventricle over time (dt) and is represented as $d\Omega$/dt. Ωo is the measurement of the average impedance of the fluid in the thorax. Impedance-based hemodynamic parameters (CO, SV, and SVR) can be calculated from Ωo, $d\Omega$/dt, mean arterial pressure (MAP), CVP, and the ECG. Major indications for ICG include early signs and symptoms of pulmonary or cardiac dysfunction, differentiation of cardiac or pulmonary cause of shortness of breath, evaluation of etiology and management of hypotension, monitoring after discontinuing a PA catheter or justification for insertion of a PA catheter, evaluation of pharmacotherapy, and diagnosis of rejection following cardiac transplantation.[33] ICG is not recommended in patients who have generalized edema or third spacing because the excess volume interferes with accurate signals.

Venous Oxygen Saturation. Both CVP and PA catheters can include sensors to measure oxygen saturation of hemoglobin in venous blood. The oxygen saturation of blood from the PA catheter is termed *mixed venous oxygen saturation* (SvO_2). Similarly, the oxygen saturation of venous blood from the CVP catheter is termed *central venous oxygen saturation* ($ScvO_2$). Either measurement is useful in determining the adequacy of tissue oxygenation. SvO_2/$ScvO_2$ reflects the dynamic balance between oxygenation of the arterial blood, tissue perfusion, and tissue oxygen consumption (VO_2). SvO_2/$ScvO_2$, when considered in conjunction with the arterial oxygen saturation, is useful in analyzing hemodynamic status and response to treatments or activities (Table 66-5).[34] Normal SvO_2/$ScvO_2$ at rest is 60% to 80%.

Sustained decreases and increases in SvO_2/$ScvO_2$ must be analyzed carefully. Decreased SvO_2/$ScvO_2$ may indicate decreased arterial oxygenation, low CO, low hemoglobin level, or increased oxygen consumption or extraction. If the SvO_2/$ScvO_2$ falls below 60%, the nurse determines which of these factors has changed. The nurse observes for changes in arterial oxygenation by monitoring pulse oximetry or ABGs. By noting any changes in level of consciousness, strength and quality of peripheral pulses, urine output, and skin color and temperature, the nurse can grossly assess CO and tissue perfusion. If arterial oxygenation, CO, and hemoglobin level are unchanged, a fall in SvO_2/$ScvO_2$ indicates increased oxygen consumption or extraction, which could represent an increased metabolic rate, pain, movement, or fever. If oxygen consumption increases without a comparable increase in oxygen delivery, more oxygen is extracted from the blood, and SvO_2/$ScvO_2$ will continue to fall.[34]

Increased SvO_2/$ScvO_2$ is also clinically significant and may indicate a clinical improvement (e.g., increased arterial oxygen saturation, improved perfusion, decreased metabolic rate) or problems (e.g., sepsis, ventricular septal defect). In sepsis, oxygen may not be extracted properly at the tissue level, resulting in increased mixed venous oxygen saturation.

Nursing interventions may be guided by changes in SvO_2/$ScvO_2$. The nurse might note that the patient's heart rate increased moderately during repositioning but that the SvO_2/$ScvO_2$ remained stable. In this case the nurse might conclude that the position change was tolerated. If the SvO_2/$ScvO_2$ had dropped, this would be an indication to stop the activity until the SvO_2/$ScvO_2$ returns to the previous level.

In many cases as activity or metabolism increases, heart rate and CO increase, and SvO_2/$ScvO_2$ remains constant or varies slightly. However, it is not uncommon for critically ill patients to have conditions that prevent substantial increases in CO. For example, this could occur in the patient with heart failure, shock,

TABLE 66-5	Clinical Interpretation of SvO_2/$ScvO_2$* Measurements	
SvO_2/$ScvO_2$ Measurement	**Physiologic Basis for Change in SvO_2**	**Clinical Diagnosis and Rationale**
High SvO_2/$ScvO_2$ (80%-95%)	Increased oxygen supply	Patient receiving more oxygen than required by clinical condition
	Decreased oxygen demand	Anesthesia, which causes sedation and decreased muscle movement
		Hypothermia, which lowers metabolic demand (e.g., with cardiopulmonary bypass)
		Sepsis caused by decreased ability of tissues to use oxygen at the cellular level
		False high positive because pulmonary artery catheter is wedged in a pulmonary capillary (SvO_2 only)
Normal SvO_2/$ScvO_2$ (60%-80%)	Normal oxygen supply and metabolic demand	Balanced oxygen supply and demand
Low SvO_2/$ScvO_2$ (<60%)	Decreased oxygen supply caused by	
	• Low hemoglobin	Anemia or bleeding with compromised cardiopulmonary system
	• Low arterial saturation (SaO_2)	Hypoxemia resulting from decreased oxygen supply or lung disease
	• Low cardiac output	Cardiogenic shock caused by left ventricular pump failure
	• Increased oxygen demand	Metabolic demand exceeds oxygen supply in conditions that increase muscle movement and metabolic rate, including physiologic states such as shivering, seizures, and hyperthermia and nursing interventions such as being weighed on a bedside scale and turning

From Urden LD, Stacy KM, Lough ME: *Thelan's critical care nursing: diagnosis and management,* ed 5, St Louis, 2006, Elsevier Mosby.
*$ScvO_2$ values are generally slightly higher than SvO_2 values.

dysrhythmias, or cardiac transplantation. In these cases, SvO_2/$ScvO_2$ can provide a useful indicator of the balance between oxygen delivery and consumption.

Complications with PA Catheters. Infection and sepsis are serious problems associated with PA catheters. Careful surgical asepsis for insertion and maintenance of the catheter and attached tubing is mandatory to prevent infection. The skin is cleansed according to unit procedure, usually with chlorhexidine or an iodine preparation. The insertion site is covered with a sterile occlusive dressing. The nurse should monitor the patient for local and systemic signs of infection (e.g., redness and exudate at the insertion site, fever, increased white blood cell count). The PA catheter must be removed if there are local or systemic signs of infection. To reduce the risk of infection, the flush bag, pressure tubing, transducer, and stopcock should be changed every 96 hours, and the PA catheter should be removed once hemodynamic monitoring is no longer needed.[27]

Air embolus is another risk associated with PA catheters. Air embolus can be caused by balloon rupture or injection of air into any of the lumens, including the lumen of a ruptured balloon. The nurse decreases the risk of air embolus by first aspirating to check for the absence or presence of blood and by injecting only the prescribed volume of air into the balloon before obtaining the PAWP. Catheters are also checked for balloon integrity before insertion; defective catheters are not used. If the nurse aspirates blood from the balloon port or observes that injected air does not passively flow back into the syringe, the catheter should be so labeled and the physician notified. Air can also be introduced into the system if connections are not tight. Luer-Lok connections should be used on all pressure lines. In addition, the low-pressure alarm is activated for all pressure lines to signal any substantial drop in the pressure. Any time the line needs to be disconnected to change the apparatus, the nurse closes the line to the patient via clamping or stopcocks.

The patient with a PA catheter is at risk for pulmonary infarction or PA rupture from the following causes: (1) the balloon may rupture, releasing air and fragments that could embolize; (2) prolonged balloon inflation may obstruct blood flow; (3) the catheter may advance into a wedge position, obstructing blood flow; and (4) a thrombus could form and embolize. To reduce the risk of pulmonary infarction and rupture, the balloon must never be inflated beyond the balloon's capacity (usually 1 to 1.5 ml of air). The balloon must not be left inflated for more than four breaths (except during insertion) or 8 to 15 seconds.[31] PA pressure waveforms are monitored continuously for evidence of catheter occlusion, dislocation, or spontaneous wedging. The pressure tracing will be blunted if the catheter starts to be occluded. The pressure tracing will appear wedged if the PA catheter advances and becomes spontaneously wedged. In each of these cases, the catheter must be immediately repositioned by the physician or a qualified nurse. To reduce the risk of thrombus and embolus formation, the PA catheter is continuously flushed with a slow infusion of heparinized (unless contraindicated) saline solution (similar to an arterial line) to prevent thrombus formation.[30]

Ventricular dysrhythmias can occur during PA catheter insertion or removal or if the tip migrates back from the PA to the right ventricle and irritates the ventricular wall. In addition, the nurse may observe that the PA catheter cannot be wedged. In these situations, the catheter may need to be repositioned by the physician or a qualified nurse.

Noninvasive Arterial Oxygenation Monitoring. *Pulse oximetry* is a noninvasive and continuous method of determining arterial oxygenation (SpO_2), and monitoring SpO_2 may reduce the frequency of ABG sampling (see Chapter 26). SpO_2 is normally 95% to 100%. A common use for pulse oximetry is to evaluate the effectiveness of oxygen therapy. Decreased SpO_2 indicates inadequate oxygenation of the blood in the pulmonary capillaries. This may be corrected by increasing the fraction of inspired oxygen (FIO_2) and evaluating the patient's response. Similarly, the nurse uses SpO_2 to monitor how the patient tolerates decreases in FIO_2 and responds to changes in position and treatments. For example, the nurse might note that SpO_2 falls when the patient is positioned in a left lateral recumbent position. The nurse could then plan position changes that pose less risk for the patient.

Accurate SpO_2 measurements may be difficult to obtain on patients who are hypothermic, receiving IV vasopressor therapy (e.g., norepinephrine), or experiencing hypoperfusion (e.g., shock). Alternate locations for placement of the pulse oximetry probe may need to be considered (e.g., forehead, earlobe).

NURSING MANAGEMENT
HEMODYNAMIC MONITORING

Assessment of hemodynamic status requires integration of data from many sources and trending of the data over time. Thorough, basic nursing observations provide important clues about the patient's hemodynamic status. The nurse should begin by obtaining baseline data regarding the patient's general appearance, level of consciousness, skin color and temperature, vital signs, peripheral pulses, and urine output. Does the patient appear tired, weak, exhausted? There may be too little cardiac reserve to sustain even minimum activity. Pallor, cool skin, and diminished pulses may indicate decreased CO. Changes in mental clarity may reflect problems with cerebral perfusion or oxygenation. Monitoring urine output reflects the adequacy of perfusion to the kidneys. The patient with diminished perfusion to the GI tract may develop hypoactive or absent bowel sounds. If the patient is bleeding and developing shock, blood pressure might initially be relatively stable, yet the patient may become increasingly pale and cool from peripheral vasoconstriction. Conversely, the patient experiencing septic shock may remain warm and pink yet develops tachycardia and blood pressure instability. Although heart rates of 100 beats per minute are common among stressed, compromised, critically ill patients, sustained tachycardia greatly increases myocardial oxygen demand and may result in diminished CO.

The astute critical care nurse correlates observational data with data obtained from biotechnology (e.g., ECG; arterial, CVP, PA, PAWP pressures; SvO_2/$ScvO_2$). Single hemodynamic values are rarely significant. The nurse must monitor trends in these values and evaluate the whole clinical picture with the goals of recognizing early clues and intervening before problems escalate.

CIRCULATORY ASSIST DEVICES

Mechanical **circulatory assist devices** (CADs), such as the intraaortic balloon pump (IABP) and left or right ventricular assist device (VAD), are used to decrease cardiac work and improve organ perfusion in patients with heart failure when conventional

TABLE 66-6	Indications and Contraindications for Intraaortic Balloon Pump Therapy*

Indications

Refractory unstable angina (when drugs have failed)
Short-term bridge to cardiac transplantation
Acute myocardial infarction with any of the following:†
- Ventricular aneurysm accompanied by ventricular dysrhythmias
- Acute ventricular septal defect
- Acute mitral valve dysfunction
- Cardiogenic shock
- Refractory chest pain with or without ventricular dysrhythmias

Preoperative, intraoperative, and postoperative cardiac surgery (e.g., prophylaxis before surgery, failure to wean from cardiopulmonary bypass, left ventricular failure after cardiopulmonary bypass)
High-risk interventional cardiology procedures

Contraindications

Irreversible brain damage
Terminal or untreatable diseases of any major organ system
Abdominal aortic and thoracic aneurysms
Moderate to severe aortic insufficiency
Generalized peripheral vascular disease‡

*List is not all-inclusive.
†Allows time for emergent angiography and corrective cardiac surgery to be performed.
‡May inhibit placement of balloon and is considered a relative contraindication; sheathless insertion may be used.

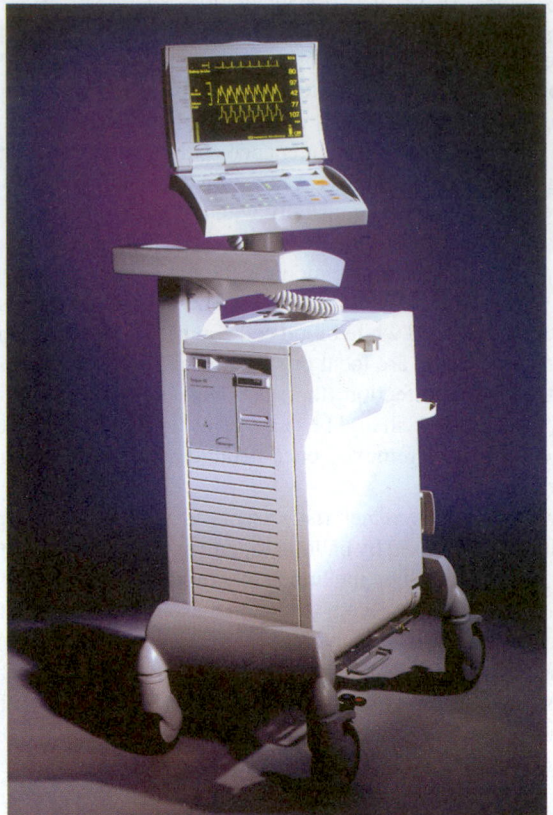

FIG. 66-13 Intraaortic balloon pump machine.

drug therapy is no longer adequate. The type of device used depends on the extent and nature of the myocardial problem and the capabilities of the institution and staff. CADs provide interim support in three types of situations: (1) the left, right, or both ventricles require support while recovering from acute injury; (2) the heart requires surgical repair (e.g., a ruptured septum), but the patient must be stabilized; and (3) the heart has failed, and the patient is awaiting cardiac transplantation. All CADs decrease ventricular workload, increase myocardial perfusion, and augment circulation. The most commonly used CAD is the IABP. Several types of VADs are available, and additional devices are under development.

Intraaortic Balloon Pump

The **intraaortic balloon pump** (IABP) provides temporary circulatory assistance to the compromised heart by reducing afterload (via reduction in systolic pressure) and augmenting the aortic diastolic pressure, resulting in improved coronary blood flow. Table 66-6 lists clinical conditions for which the IABP is used. The IABP consists of a sausage-shaped balloon, a pump that inflates and deflates the balloon, control panel for synchronizing the balloon inflation to the cardiac cycle, and fail-safe features (Fig. 66-13). The balloon is inserted percutaneously or surgically, under strict aseptic technique, into the femoral artery, advanced toward the heart, and positioned in the descending thoracic aorta just below the left subclavian artery and above the renal arteries (Fig. 66-14). Following placement, the position is confirmed by x-ray. A pneumatic device cyclically fills the balloon with helium at the start of diastole (immediately after aortic valve closure) and deflates it just before the next systole. The ECG is the primary trigger used to initiate the deflation on the upstroke of the R wave (of the QRS) and inflation on the T wave. The dicrotic notch of the arterial pressure tracing is used to refine timing (Fig. 66-15, *A*). IABP therapy is referred to as *counterpul-*

sation because the timing of balloon inflation is opposite to ventricular contraction. The IAPB assist ratio is 1:1 in the acute phase of treatment, that is, one IABP cycle of inflation and deflation for every heartbeat.[35]

Effects of Counterpulsation. In late diastole when the balloon is totally inflated, blood is forcibly displaced distally to the extremities and proximally to the coronary arteries and main branches of the aortic arch. Diastolic arterial pressure rises (diastolic augmentation), increasing coronary artery perfusion pressure and perfusion of vital organs. The rise in coronary artery perfusion pressure causes an increase in blood flow to the myocardium. The balloon is rapidly deflated just before systole. The suddenly created vacuum causes aortic pressure to drop. With aortic resistance to left ventricular ejection reduced (reduced afterload), the left ventricle empties more easily and completely. As with other types of afterload reduction, the SV increases, yet the myocardial oxygen consumption decreases.[35] Hemodynamic effects of IABP therapy are summarized in Table 66-7.

Complications with Intraaortic Balloon Pump Therapy. Complications that may occur with the IABP are listed in Table 66-8. Vascular injuries such as dislodging of plaque, aortic dissection, and compromised distal circulation are common, occurring in 3% to 65% of cases. Thrombus and embolus formation add to the risk of circulatory compromise to the extremity. Peripheral nerve damage can occur, particularly when a cut-down is performed for insertion. To reduce these risks, cardiovascular, neurovascular, and hemodynamic assessments are necessary every 15 to 60 minutes depending on the patient's status. The action of the balloon pump can cause physical destruc-

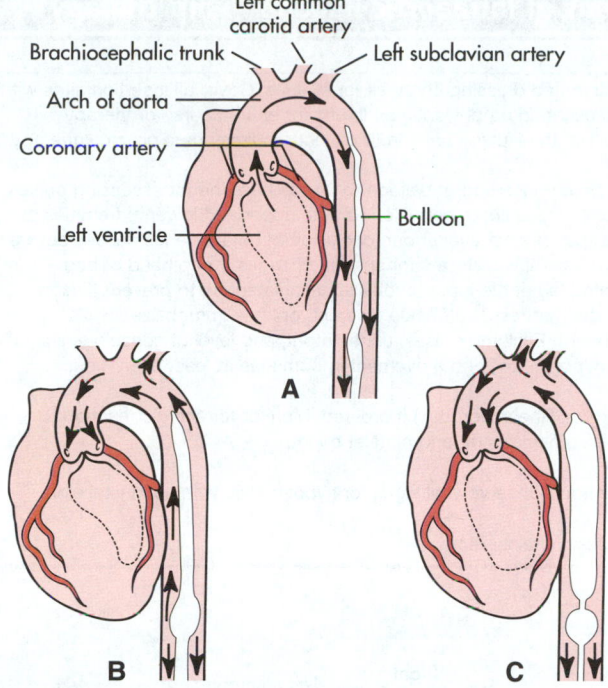

FIG. 66-14 Intraaortic balloon pump. **A,** During systole the balloon is deflated, which facilitates ejection of the blood into the periphery. **B,** In early diastole, the balloon begins to inflate. **C,** In late diastole, the balloon is totally inflated, which augments aortic pressure and increases the coronary perfusion pressure with the end result of increased coronary and cerebral blood flow.

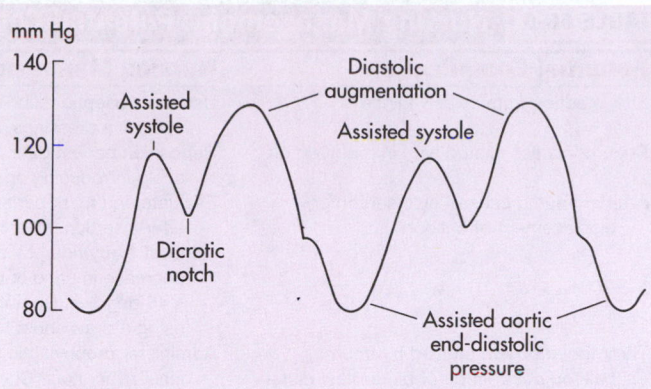

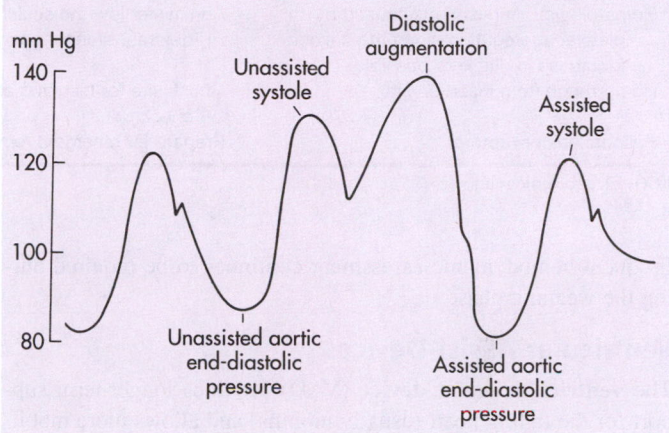

FIG. 66-15   A, Correct 1:1 intraaortic balloon pump frequency. **B,** Correct 1:2 intraaortic balloon pump frequency.

tion of platelets and thrombocytopenia. Coagulation profiles should be monitored, and the patient should be assessed for evidence of systemic bleeding. Displacement of the balloon can occlude the left subclavian, renal, or mesenteric arteries and can result in diminished or absent radial pulse, decreased urine output, and diminished or absent bowels sounds. Patients receiving IABP therapy are prone to infection, and local or systemic signs of infection necessitate catheter removal.[35]

Mechanical complications are rare but may occur. Improper timing of balloon inflation may cause increased afterload, decreased CO, myocardial ischemia, and increased myocardial oxygen demand. These must be immediately recognized by the nurse. If the balloon develops a leak, the pump will automatically stop. The catheter must be removed immediately to avoid an embolus. Signs of a leak include less effective augmentation, repeated alarms for gas loss, and blood backing up into the catheter. A malfunction of the balloon or console triggers fail-safe alarms and automatic shutdown of the unit.

The patient with an IABP is relatively immobile, limited to side-lying or supine positions with the head of the bed elevated less than 45 degrees. The leg in which the catheter is inserted must not be flexed at the hip to avoid kinking or dislodgement of the catheter. The patient may be receiving ventilatory support and will likely have multiple invasive lines that increase the challenge of comfortable positioning. The patient may experience sleeplessness and anxiety. Adequate sedation, pain relief, skin care, and comfort measures are required.

IABP therapy is weaned as the patient improves; that is, circulatory support provided by the IABP is gradually reduced. Weaning involves reducing the IABP assist ratio from 1:1 to 1:2 and as-

TABLE 66-7	**Hemodynamic Effects of Counterpulsation**

Effects of Inflation During Diastole
Increased diastolic pressure (may exceed systolic pressure)
Increased pressure in the aortic root during diastole
Increased coronary artery perfusion pressure
Improved oxygen delivery to the myocardium
- Decreased angina
- Decreased electrocardiographic evidence of ischemia
- Decreased ventricular ectopy

Effects of Deflation During Systole
Decreased afterload
Decreased peak systolic pressure
Decreased myocardial oxygen consumption
Increased stroke volume, possibly associated with
- Improved sensorium
- Warmed skin
- Increased urine output
- Decreased heart rate
Increased forward flow of blood, decreasing preload
- Decreased PA pressures, including PAWP
- Decreased crackles

PA, Pulmonary artery; *PAWP,* PA wedge pressure.

sessing the patient's response (see Fig. 66-15, *B*). If hemodynamic parameters remain stable, the ratio can be changed from 1:3 to 1:8 until the IABP catheter is removed. Even if the patient is stable without IABP, pumping is continued until the line is removed.[35] This reduces the risk of thrombus formation around the catheter.

TABLE 66-8	Nursing Management: Potential Complications of Intraaortic Balloon Pump Therapy
Potential Complication	**Nursing Management**
Site infection from invasive lines	Use strict aseptic technique for insertion and dressing changes for all lines. Cover all insertion sites with occlusive dressings. Administer prescribed prophylactic antibiotic for entire course of therapy.
Pneumonia associated with immobilization	Reposition patient q2hr, being careful not to displace balloon. If patient requires chest physical therapy, avoid introducing an ECG artifact.
Arterial trauma caused by insertion or displacement of balloon	Evaluate and mark peripheral pulses before insertion of balloon to use as baseline for assessing pulses after insertion. After insertion of balloon, evaluate perfusion to both upper and lower extremities at least every hour. Measure urine output at least every hour (occlusion of renal arteries causes severe decrease in urine output). Observe arterial waveforms for sudden changes. Keep head of bed <45 degrees. Do not flex cannulated leg at the hip. Immobilize cannulated leg to prevent flexion using a draw sheet tucked under the mattress, soft ankle restraint, or knee immobilizer.
Thromboembolism caused by trauma, balloon obstruction of blood flow distal to catheter	Administer prophylactic heparin if ordered. Evaluate pulses, urine output, and level of consciousness at least every hour. Check circulation, sensation, and movement in both legs at least every hour.
Hematologic complications caused by platelet aggregation along the balloon (decrease in platelets possible)	Administer low-molecular-weight dextran (Rheomacrodex) if ordered. Monitor for allergic reaction to dextran. Monitor coagulation profiles, hematocrit, and platelet count.
Hemorrhage from insertion site	Check site for bleeding at least every hour. Observe vital signs for hypovolemia with each vital sign check.
Balloon leak or rupture	Prepare for emergent removal and possible reinsertion.

ECG, Electrocardiogram.

Frequent hemodynamic assessment continues to be required during the weaning phase.

Ventricular Assist Devices

The **ventricular assist device** (VAD) provides longer-term support for the failing heart (usually months) and allows more mobility than the IABP. VADs are inserted into the path of flowing blood to augment or replace the action of the ventricle. Some VADs are implanted (e.g., peritoneum), and others are positioned externally. A typical VAD would shunt the blood from the left atrium or ventricle to the device and then to the aorta (Fig. 66-16). Some VADs provide biventricular support.

Failure to wean from cardiopulmonary bypass (CPB) after surgery has been the primary indicator for VAD support. Increasingly the VAD is used to support patients with ventricular failure caused by myocardial infarction and patients awaiting cardiac transplantation. A VAD is a temporary device with the capability to partially or totally support circulation until the heart recovers or a donor heart can be obtained. Cannula sites depend on the type of device used. For support of the right side of the heart, the right atrium and PA are cannulated. The left ventricular apex can be cannulated for left VADs. Direct cannulation of the atria and great vessels occurs in the operating room through a sternotomy.

Appropriate patient selection for VAD therapy is critical. Indications for VAD therapy include (1) extension of CPB for failure to wean or postcardiotomy cardiogenic shock, (2) bridge to recovery or cardiac transplantation, and (3) patients with New York Heart Association Classification IV (see Table 35-4) who have failed medical therapy. Relative contraindications for VAD therapy include (1) body surface area less than 1.5 m², (2) renal or liver failure unrelated to a cardiac incident, and (3) comorbidities that would limit life expectancy to less than 3 years.[36]

Implantable Artificial Heart

Every year in the United States approximately 2000 patients receive cardiac transplants, yet the demand for these hearts far exceeds the supply. Research on mechanical CADs has led to the development of a fully implantable artificial heart that can sustain the

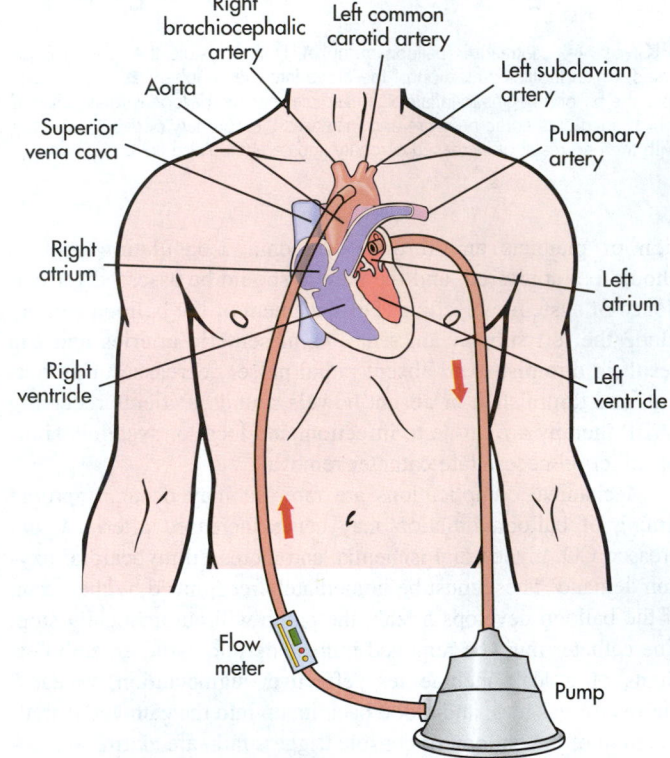

FIG. 66-16   Schematic diagram of a left ventricular assist device.

body's circulatory system. This device is designed not only to extend life but also to provide a satisfactory quality of life for the thousands of patients with irreversible heart disease who never receive a donor heart. One major anticipated advantage of the artificial heart compared with heart transplantation is decreased costs for implantation and drug therapies. Patients will not require immunosuppression therapy, nor will they experience the inevitable, long-term effects of this therapy. However, patients will require lifelong anticoagulation.[37]

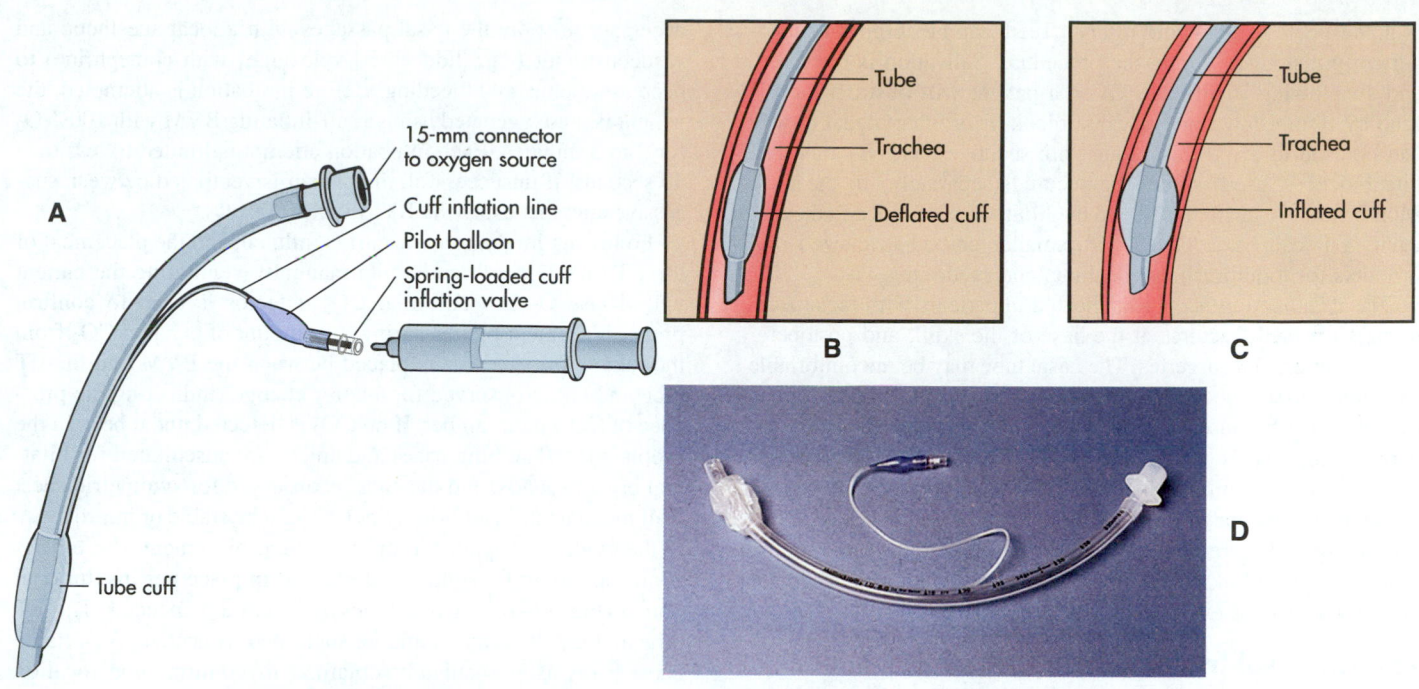

FIG. 66-17   Endotracheal tube. **A,** Parts of an endotracheal tube. **B,** Tube in place with cuff deflated. **C,** Tube in place with the cuff inflated. **D,** Photo of tube before placement.

NURSING MANAGEMENT
CIRCULATORY ASSIST DEVICES

The patient with an IABP requires highly skilled nursing care. Detailed cardiovascular assessment, including measurement of hemodynamic parameters (e.g., PA and arterial pressures, CO, CI, SVR, SV), cardiac and thoracic auscultation, and evaluation of the ECG (e.g., rate, rhythm), is performed frequently. Assessment of adequate tissue perfusion (e.g., skin color and temperature, mentation, peripheral pulses, urine output, bowel sounds) is also performed at regular intervals.[35] It is expected that with IABP therapy these parameters should improve.

Nursing care of the patient with a VAD is similar to that of the patient with an IABP. The patient is observed for bleeding, cardiac tamponade, ventricular failure, infection, dysrhythmias, renal failure, hemolysis, and thromboembolism. Unlike the patient with an IABP, who must remain in bed with limited position change, the patient with VAD may be mobile and require an activity plan.[36] In some cases, patients with VADs may go home. Preparation for discharge is complex and requires in-depth teaching about the device and ancillary equipment (e.g., battery chargers). Patients must have a competent caregiver present at all times.

Ideally, patients with CADs will recover through ventricular improvement, heart transplantation, or artificial heart implantation. However, many patients die, or the decision to terminate the device is made and death follows. Both the patient and family require psychologic support. Nursing care should include the family as much as possible. Other members of the health care team, such as social workers or clergy, should be consulted as needed.

ARTIFICIAL AIRWAYS

The patient in the ICU often requires mechanical assistance to maintain airway patency. Inserting a tube into the trachea, bypassing upper airway and laryngeal structures, creates an artificial airway. The tube is placed into the trachea via the mouth or nose past the larynx (**endotracheal [ET] intubation**) or through a stoma in the neck *(tracheostomy)*. ET intubation is more common in ICU patients. It can be performed quickly and safely at the bedside. Indications for ET intubation include (1) upper airway obstruction (e.g., secondary to burns, tumor, bleeding), (2) apnea, (3) high risk of aspiration, (4) ineffective clearance of secretions, and (5) respiratory distress. ET tubes are illustrated in Fig. 66-17.

A *tracheotomy* is a surgical procedure that is performed when the need for an artificial airway is expected to be long term. There is ongoing debate regarding the timing of a tracheotomy in the patient requiring an ET tube. Research has suggested that early tracheotomy (2 to 10 days) may have advantages over delayed tracheotomy, particularly when mechanical ventilation is predicted to be needed for longer than 10 to 14 days.[38,39] The situation varies with the patient, physician, and institution. Tracheostomy tubes and related nursing management are discussed in Chapter 27.

Endotracheal Tubes

In *oral intubation* the ET tube is passed through the mouth and vocal cords and into the trachea with the aid of a laryngoscope or bronchoscope. In *nasal ET intubation,* the ET is placed blindly (i.e., without visualizing the larynx) through the nose, nasopharynx, and vocal cords. Oral ET intubation is the procedure of choice for most emergencies because the airway can be secured rapidly. Compared with the nasal route, a larger-diameter tube can be used for oral intubation. With a larger-bore ET tube, work of breathing (WOB) is reduced because there is less airway resistance. It is easier to remove secretions and perform fiberoptic bronchoscopy if needed. Nasal ET intubation is indicated when head and neck manipulation is risky.

There are risks associated with oral ET intubation. It may be difficult to place an oral tube if head and neck mobility is limited (e.g., suspected spinal cord injury). Teeth can be chipped or inadvertently dislodged during the procedure. Salivation is increased, and swallowing is difficult. Often a patient will obstruct the ET tube by biting down on it. A bite block or oropharyngeal airway can be used to avoid this, along with sedatives. The ET tube and bite block (if used) should be secured (separately) to the face. Mouth care is a challenge due to the limitations of space in the oral cavity but can be achieved with smaller or pediatric-sized oral products for toothbrushing, cleaning, and suctioning.

Nasal intubation is contraindicated in patients with facial fractures, suspected fractures at the base of the skull, and postoperatively after cranial surgeries. The nasal tube may be uncomfortable for some patients because it presses on the septum, whereas others may prefer it because there is no need for a bite block and mouth care is more easily accomplished. However, nasal ET tubes are more subject to kinking than oral tubes; the WOB is greater because the longer, narrower tube offers more airflow resistance; and suctioning and secretion removal are more difficult. Finally, nasal tubes have been linked with an increased incidence of sinus infection and ventilator-associated pneumonia.[40-42]

Endotracheal Intubation Procedure

Unless endotracheal intubation is emergent, consent for the procedure should be obtained. The patient and family should be told the reason for ET intubation, the steps that will occur in the procedure, and the patient's role in the procedure (if indicated). It is also important to explain that while intubated, the patient will not be able to speak, but that other means of communication will be provided, and that the patient's hands may be restrained for safety purposes.[43,44]

All patients undergoing intubation and receiving mechanical ventilation need to have a self-inflating **bag-valve-mask** (BVM) (e.g., *Ambu bag*) available and attached to oxygen, suctioning equipment ready at the bedside, and IV access. The BVM should contain a reservoir to sequester oxygen so that oxygen concentrations of 90% to 95% can be delivered. The slower the bag is deflated and inflated, the higher the oxygen concentration that will be delivered. The nurse assembles and checks the equipment to be used, removes the patient's dentures and/or partial plates (for oral intubation), and administers drugs as ordered. Premedication varies, depending on the patient's level of consciousness (e.g., awake, obtunded) and the nature of the procedure (e.g., emergent, nonemergent). Rapid-sequence intubation (RSI) is the rapid, concurrent administration of a combination of both a paralytic agent and a sedative agent during emergency airway management to decrease the risks of aspiration, combativeness, and injury to the patient. RSI is not indicated in patients who are comatose or during cardiac arrest.[45,46] A sedative-hypnotic-amnesic (e.g., midazolam [Versed]) is used if the patient is agitated, disoriented, or combative. A rapid-onset narcotic such as fentanyl (Sublimaze) may be used to blunt the pain of laryngoscopy and intubation. A paralytic drug such as succinylcholine (Anectine) may be used to produce skeletal muscle paralysis. Atropine may be used to limit secretions. Pulse oximetry is used during the procedure to assess oxygenation.

For oral intubation, the patient is placed supine with the head extended and the neck flexed ("sniffing position"). This position allows for visualization of the vocal cords by aligning the axes of the mouth, pharynx, and trachea. For nasal intubation it may be necessary to spray the nasal passages with a local anesthetic and vasoconstrictor (e.g., lidocaine [Xylocaine] with epinephrine) to decrease trauma and bleeding. Before intubation is attempted, the patient is preoxygenated using a self-inflating BVM with 100% O_2 for 3 to 5 minutes. Each intubation attempt is limited to less than 30 seconds. If unsuccessful, the patient is ventilated between successive attempts using the BVM with 100% O_2.[43,47]

Following intubation, the cuff is inflated, and the placement of the ET tube is confirmed while manually ventilating the patient with 100% O_2. An end-tidal CO_2 detector is used to confirm proper placement by measuring the amount of exhaled CO_2 from the lungs. The detector is placed between the BVM and the ET tube and either observed for a color change (indicating the presence of CO_2) or a number. If no CO_2 is detected, the tube is in the esophagus.[48] The lung bases and apices are auscultated for bilateral breath sounds, and the chest is observed for symmetric chest wall movement. In addition, SpO_2 should be stable or improved.[43] If the evidence supports proper ET tube placement, the tube is connected to an O_2 source and secured in place per institutional policy (Fig. 66-18). A bite block is inserted as needed. The ET tube and the pharynx should be suctioned as needed. A portable chest x-ray is immediately obtained to confirm tube location (3 to 5 cm above the carina in the adult). This position allows the patient to move the neck without dislodging the tube or causing it to enter the right mainstem bronchus. Once proper positioning is confirmed with x-ray, the position of the tube at the lip or teeth (usually 21 cm for women and 23 cm for men) or nose ("exit mark") is recorded and marked.[43,49] Excess tubing is cut to reduce dead space.

The ET tube is connected either to humidified air, O_2, or a mechanical ventilator. ABGs should be obtained within 25 minutes after intubation to determine oxygenation and ventilation status. ABG values are reviewed and used to guide oxygenation and ventilation changes. Continuous pulse oximetry monitoring provides a valuable estimate of arterial oxygenation.

NURSING MANAGEMENT
ARTIFICIAL AIRWAY

Nursing responsibilities for the patient with an artificial airway include (1) maintaining correct tube placement, (2) maintaining proper cuff inflation, (3) monitoring oxygenation and ventilation, (4) maintaining tube patency, (5) assessing for complications, (6) providing oral care and maintaining skin integrity, and (7) fostering comfort and communication (NCP 66-1).

■ *Maintaining Correct Tube Placement*

The nurse must monitor the patient with an ET tube for proper placement at least every 2 to 4 hours.[40,43] If the tube is dislodged, it could terminate in the pharynx or enter the esophagus or the right mainstem bronchus (thus ventilating only the right lung). The nurse maintains proper tube position by confirming that the exit mark on the tube remains constant while at rest, during patient care, repositioning, and patient transport. The nurse observes for symmetric chest wall movement and auscultates to confirm bilateral breath sounds. It is an emergency if the ET tube is not positioned properly. The nurse stays with the patient, maintains the airway, supports ventilation, and secures the appropriate assistance to immediately reposition the tube. It may be necessary to ventilate

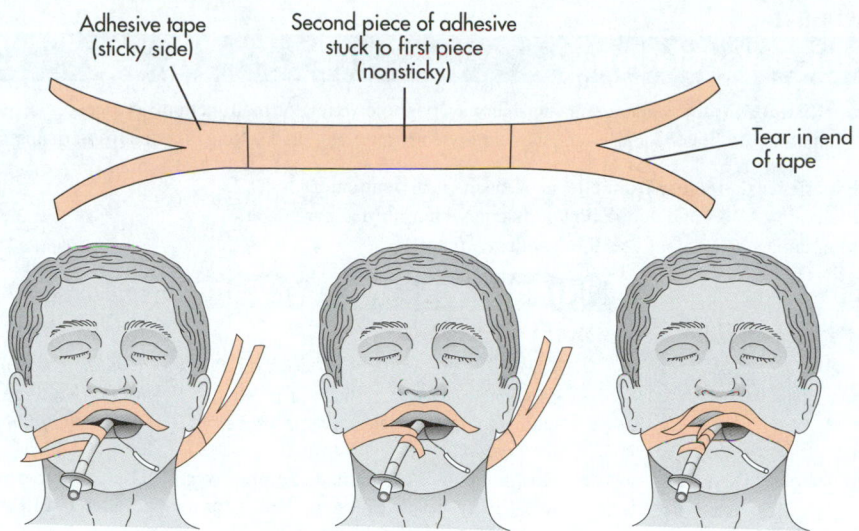

Adhesive tape
(sticky side)

Second piece of adhesive
stuck to first piece
(nonsticky)

Tear in end
of tape

FIG. 66-18   Example of protocol for securing endotracheal tube using adhesive tape:
1. Clean the patient's skin with mild soap and water.
2. Remove oil from the skin with alcohol and allow to dry.
3. Apply a skin adhesive product to enhance tape adherence. (When tape is removed, an adhesive remover will be necessary.)
4. Place a hydrocolloid membrane over the cheeks to protect friable skin.
5. Secure with adhesive tape as shown here.

the patient with a BVM. If a malpositioned tube is not repositioned, minimal or no oxygen will be delivered to the lungs or the entire tidal volume will be delivered to one lung, placing the patient at risk for pneumothorax.

■ *Maintaining Proper Cuff Inflation*

The cuff is an inflatable, pliable sleeve encircling the outer wall of the ET tube (see Fig. 66-17). The high-volume, low-pressure cuff stabilizes and seals the ET tube within the trachea and prevents escape of ventilating gases. However, the cuff can cause tracheal damage. To avoid damage, the cuff is inflated with air, and the pressure in the cuff is measured and monitored. Normal arterial tracheal perfusion is estimated at 30 mm Hg. To ensure adequate tracheal perfusion, cuff pressure should be maintained at 20 to 25 mm Hg.[49] The nurse or respiratory therapist, depending on the institution's policy, measures and records cuff pressure after intubation and on a routine basis (e.g., every 8 hours) using the *minimal occluding volume* (MOV) *technique* or the *minimal leak technique* (MLT).

The steps in the MOV technique for cuff inflation are as follows: (1) for the mechanically ventilated patient, place a stethoscope over the trachea and inflate the cuff to MOV by adding air until no air leak is heard at peak inspiratory pressure (end of ventilator inspiration); (2) for the spontaneously breathing patient, inflate until no sound is heard after a deep breath or after inhalation with a BVM; (3) use a manometer to verify that cuff pressure is between 20 and 25 mm Hg; and (4) record cuff pressure in the chart. If adequate cuff pressure cannot be maintained or larger volumes of air are needed to keep the cuff inflated, the cuff could be leaking or there could be tracheal dilation at the cuff site. In these situations the ET tube should be repositioned or changed and the physician should be notified.

The procedure for MLT is similar with one exception. A small amount of air is removed from the cuff until a slight leak is auscultated at peak inflation. Both techniques are intended to prevent the risks of tracheal trauma due to high cuff pressures.

■ *Monitoring Oxygenation and Ventilation*

The patient with an ET tube is vigilantly monitored for adequate oxygenation by assessing clinical findings, ABGs, SpO_2, and $SvO_2/ScvO_2$ The nurse must assess for clinical signs of hypoxemia such as a change in mental status (e.g., confusion), anxiety, dusky skin, and dysrhythmias. Periodic ABGs (specifically PaO_2) and continuous SpO_2 provide objective data regarding oxygenation. Lower values are expected in patients with some disease states, such as chronic obstructive pulmonary disease (COPD). PA or CVP catheters with SvO_2 or $ScvO_2$ capability also can give an indirect indication about the patient's oxygenation status (see Table 66-5).

Indicators of ventilation include assessment of clinical findings, $PaCO_2$, and continuous partial pressure of end-tidal CO_2 ($PETCO_2$). The patient's respirations should be assessed for rate and rhythm and use of accessory muscles. The patient who is hyperventilating will be breathing rapidly and deeply and may experience circumoral and peripheral numbness and tingling. The patient who is hypoventilating will be breathing shallowly or slowly and may appear dusky. $PaCO_2$ is the best indicator of alveolar hyperventilation (e.g., decreased $PaCO_2$, increased pH indicate respiratory alkalosis) or hypoventilation (e.g., increased $PaCO_2$, decreased pH indicate respiratory acidosis).

PETCO$_2$ monitoring is done by analyzing exhaled gas directly at the patient-ventilator circuit (*mainstream sampling*) or by transporting a sample of gas via a small-bore tubing to a bedside monitor (*sidestream sampling*). Continuous $PETCO_2$ monitoring can be used to assess the patency of the airway and the presence of breathing. In addition, gradual changes in $PETCO_2$ values may accompany an increase in CO_2 production (e.g., sepsis, hypoventilation, neuromuscular blockade) or a decrease in CO_2 production (e.g.,

Critical Care

NURSING CARE PLAN 66-1

Patient on Mechanical Ventilation

NURSING DIAGNOSIS   **Risk for injury** *related to* artificial airway, possible ventilator malfunction, accidental disconnection/extubation, inability to breathe unassisted, asynchrony with ventilator, and settings ineffective in maintaining adequate oxygenation

PATIENT GOALS   1. Experiences no injury from effects of mechanical ventilation
2. Maintains ABGs and ventilation/perfusion within normal parameters
3. Maintains synchronous breathing with ventilator

OUTCOMES (NOC)

Mechanical Ventilation Response: Adult

- Auscultated breath sounds ____
- Respiratory rate ____
- Lung compliance ____
- End-tidal carbon dioxide ____
- FIO$_2$ meets oxygen demand ____
- PaO$_2$ ____
- PaCO$_2$ ____
- Oxygen saturation ____
- Ventilation/perfusion balance ____

Measurement Scale

1 = Severely compromised
2 = Substantially compromised
3 = Moderately compromised
4 = Mildly compromised
5 = Not compromised

INTERVENTIONS (NIC) and *RATIONALES*

Mechanical Ventilation

- Check all ventilator connections regularly *to avoid accidental disconnections.*
- Monitor for adverse effects of mechanical ventilation: infection, barotrauma, reduced cardiac output *to determine presence of risk factors and plan for appropriate intervention.*
- Routinely monitor ventilator settings (e.g., FIO$_2$, respiratory rate, tidal volume, O$_2$ flow rate, PEEP, airway pressure, thermistor temperature, and I:E ratio) *to determine if appropriate to clinical situation.*
- Administer muscle-paralyzing agents, sedatives, and opioid analgesics as needed *to promote respirations synchronous with ventilator.*
- Ensure that ventilator alarms are on *to rapidly assess patient and intervene appropriately.*
- Silence ventilator alarms during suctioning *to decrease frequency of false alarms.*
- Empty condensed water from water traps *to prevent aspiration of accumulated fluid.*
- Monitor effects of ventilator changes on oxygenation: ABG, SaO$_2$, SvO$_2$, ScvO$_2$, end-tidal CO$_2$, patient's subjective response *to determine appropriateness of changes.*

Artificial Airway Management

- Provide an oropharyngeal airway or bite block *to prevent biting on the endotracheal tube, if needed.*
- Provide additional intubation equipment and Ambu bag in a readily available location *for use in case of an emergency.*
- Auscultate for presence of lung sounds bilaterally after insertion and after changing endotracheal/tracheostomy ties *to ensure appropriate placement of endotracheal tube.*

NURSING DIAGNOSIS   **Decreased cardiac output** *related to* impeded venous return by PPV *as evidenced by* ↓ BP, ↓ SV and PAWP, ↑ heart rate, decreased urine output, presence of dysrhythmias, mental confusion

PATIENT GOAL   Experiences cardiac output adequate to meet systemic oxygen needs

OUTCOMES (NOC)

Cardiac Pump Effectiveness

- Systolic blood pressure ____
- Diastolic blood pressure ____
- Urinary output ____
- Cognitive status ____
- Cardiac index ____

Fluid Balance

- Central venous pressure ____
- Pulmonary artery wedge pressure ____

Measurement Scale

1 = Severely compromised
2 = Substantially compromised
3 = Moderately compromised
4 = Mildly compromised
5 = Not compromised

INTERVENTIONS (NIC) and *RATIONALES*

Hemodynamic Regulation

- Monitor heart rate, rhythm, and pulses *to track trends.*
- Monitor cardiac output and/or cardiac index and left ventricular stroke work index *to identify decreased venous return to the heart, decreased left ventricular end-diastolic volume, and lowered blood pressure.*
- Monitor pulmonary artery wedge pressure and central venous/right-arterial pressure *to anticipate need for plasma expanders, vasopressors, and IV fluids as ordered because hemodynamic complications of decreased venous return induced by positive pressure ventilation are exaggerated by hypovolemia.*

PAWP, Pulmonary artery wedge pressure; *PEEP,* positive end-expiratory pressure; *PPV,* positive pressure ventilation; *SV,* stroke volume.

NURSING CARE PLAN 66-1

Patient on Mechanical Ventilation—cont'd

NURSING DIAGNOSIS   **Ineffective airway clearance** *related to* presence of artificial airway, problems with positioning, accumulation of secretions, and immobility *as evidenced by* presence of abnormal breath sounds, absent cough, presence of thick or copious secretions

PATIENT GOAL   Experiences normal breath sounds with repositioning, chest physical therapy, and appropriate suctioning

OUTCOMES (NOC)

Respiratory Status: Airway Patency

- Ease of breathing _____
- Moves sputum out of airway _____

Measurement Scale

1 = Severely compromised
2 = Substantially compromised
3 = Moderately compromised
4 = Mildly compromised
5 = Not compromised

- Adventitious breath sounds _____

Measurement Scale

1 = Severe
2 = Substantial
3 = Moderate
4 = Mild
5 = None

INTERVENTIONS (NIC) and *RATIONALES*

Ventilation Assistance

- Auscultate breath sounds, noting areas of decreased or absent ventilation and presence of adventitious breath sounds *to detect risk for inadequate ventilation.*
- Monitor the effects of position changes on oxygenation: ABG, SaO_2, SvO_2, $ScvO_2$, and end-tidal CO_2 levels *to monitor trends and effectiveness of interventions.*
- Assist with frequent position changes *to mobilize respiratory sections.*

Mechanical Ventilation

- Perform chest physical therapy *to prevent pooling of secretions in the lungs.*
- Stop NG tube feedings during suctioning and 30 to 60 minutes before chest physical therapy *to prevent aspiration.*
- Perform suctioning based on presence of adventitious breath sounds and/or increased inspiratory pressure *to remove secretions.*
- Use aseptic technique *to prevent introducing microorganisms into respiratory system.*

NURSING DIAGNOSIS   **Impaired physical mobility** *related to* imposed movement restrictions *as evidenced by* limited range of motion, difficulty turning, muscle weakness

PATIENT GOALS   1. Maintains normal range of motion
2. Experiences no physiologic consequences of immobility

OUTCOMES (NOC)

Immobility Consequences: Physiologic

- Pressure sores _____
- Contracted joints _____
- Lung congestion _____
- Hypoactive bowel _____
- Venous thrombosis _____

Measurement Scale

1 = Severe
2 = Substantial
3 = Moderate
4 = Mild
5 = None

- Muscle strength _____
- Muscle tone _____
- Joint movement _____

Measurement Scale

1 = Severely compromised
2 = Substantially compromised
3 = Moderately compromised
4 = Mildly compromised
5 = Not compromised

INTERVENTIONS (NIC) and *RATIONALES*

Exercise Therapy: Joint Mobility

- Perform passive or assisted range-of-motion (ROM) exercises *to maintain patient's joint and muscle functioning and improve circulation.*
- Encourage active ROM exercises according to regular, planned schedule *to increase muscle strength and tone.*
- Assist patient to optimal body position for passive/active joint movement *to prevent contractures and other musculoskeletal complications (e.g., external rotation of hips).*
- Encourage patient to sit in bed, on side of bed ("dangle"), or in chair *to improve circulation and oxygenation and facilitate exercises.*

Positioning

- Use appropriate devices to support limbs (e.g., hand roll, trochanter roll) *to prevent contracted joints.*
- Turn the immobilized patient at least every 2 hours, according to a specific schedule, *to maintain skin integrity, mobilize respiratory secretions, and prevent venous stasis.*

Continued

NURSING CARE PLAN 66-1

Patient on Mechanical Ventilation—cont'd

NURSING DIAGNOSIS   **Anxiety** *related to* clinical condition, pain, inability to communicate, fear of death/suffocation/choking, ICU environment *as evidenced by* anxious appearance, agitation, rigid body posture, asynchronous breathing with ventilator

PATIENT GOALS   1. Expresses relaxed facial and muscle tension
2. Reports manageable anxiety level with nonverbal communication

OUTCOMES (NOC)	INTERVENTIONS (NIC) and *RATIONALES*
Anxiety Level	**Mechanical Ventilation**

Anxiety Level

- Restlessness _____
- Distress _____
- Muscle tension _____
- Facial tension _____
- Verbalized apprehension _____

Measurement Scale

1 = Severe
2 = Substantial
3 = Moderate
4 = Mild
5 = None

Mechanical Ventilation

- Instruct the patient and family about the rationale and expected sensations associated with use of mechanical ventilators *to foster a realistic understanding of therapy and reassure patient that breathing will be maintained.*
- Provide patient with a means of communication (e.g., paper and pencil, alphabet board) *to reduce anxiety associated with inability to speak and to provide means for patient to communicate anxieties.*
- Initiate relaxation techniques *to help patient manage anxiety.*
- Administer muscle-paralyzing agents, sedatives, and opioid analgesics *to manage patient's anxiety and/or pain during a critical time.*

Coping Enhancement

- Evaluate the patient's decision-making ability *to allow for patient participation in plan of care as appropriate.*
- Arrange situations that encourage patient's autonomy *to help patient regain and maintain a sense of control.*
- Encourage family to verbalize feelings about ill family member *to lessen their anxiety and increase their cooperation.*

NURSING DIAGNOSIS   **Dysfunctional ventilatory weaning response** *related to* too-rapid pace of weaning plan, and insufficient knowledge of the weaning plan *as evidenced by* restlessness, tachypnea, dyspnea, cyanosis, pallor, fatigue, ↑/↓ BP, use of accessory muscles, tachycardia, O_2 desaturation

PATIENT GOALS   1. Meets progressive ventilatory weaning goals
2. Remains extubated following initial weaning process

OUTCOMES (NOC)	INTERVENTIONS (NIC) and *RATIONALES*

Mechanical Ventilation Weaning Response: Adult

- Drive to breathe _____
- Spontaneous respiratory rate _____
- Spontaneous respiratory rhythm _____
- PaO_2 _____
- $PaCO_2$ _____
- Oxygen saturation _____
- Vital capacity _____
- Tidal volume _____
- Response to setting changes in mechanical ventilation _____
- Chest abdominal synchrony _____

Measurement Scale

1 = Severely compromised
2 = Substantially compromised
3 = Moderately compromised
4 = Mildly compromised
5 = Not compromised

Mechanical Ventilatory Weaning

- Monitor degree of shunt, vital capacity, MVV, inspiratory force, and FEV_1 *to determine readiness to wean from mechanical ventilation based on agency protocol.*
- Instruct the patient and family about what to expect during various stages of weaning *to decrease anxiety and facilitate cooperation.*
- Provide some means of patient control during weaning *to provide patient a level of control in establishing the plan.*
- Set discrete, attainable goals with the patient for weaning *to maintain patient confidence.*
- Monitor for signs of respiratory muscle fatigue (e.g., abrupt rise in $PaCO_2$, rapid, shallow ventilation; paradoxic abdominal wall motion), hypoxemia, and tissue hypoxia while weaning is in progress *to evaluate patient's weaning progress.*
- Avoid delaying return of patient with fatigued respiratory muscles to mechanical ventilation *to ensure adequate ventilation.*
- Consider using alternative methods of weaning as determined by patient's response to the current method *to minimize frustration and disappointment and enhance cooperation.*

FEV$_1$, Forced expiratory volume in 1 second; *MVV*, maximal voluntary ventilation volume.

TABLE 66-9	Suctioning Procedures for a Patient on a Mechanical Ventilator

General Measures
1. Gather all equipment.
2. Wash hands and don personal protective equipment.
3. Explain procedure and patient's role in assisting with secretion removal by coughing.
4. Monitor patient's cardiopulmonary status (e.g., vital signs, SpO_2, SvO_2, $ScvO_2$, ECG, level of consciousness) before, during, and after the procedure.
5. Turn on suction and set vacuum to 100-120 mm Hg.
6. Pause ventilator alarms.

Open-Suction Technique
1. Open sterile catheter package using the inside of the package as a sterile field. NOTE: Suction catheter should be no wider than half the diameter of the ET tube (e.g., for a 7-mm ET tube, select a 10-French suction catheter).
2. Fill the sterile solution container with sterile normal saline or water.
3. Don sterile gloves.
4. Pick up sterile suction catheter with dominant hand. Using nondominant hand, secure the connecting tube (to suction) to the suction catheter.
5. Check equipment for proper functioning by suctioning a small volume of sterile saline solution from the container. **(Go to step 7.)**

Closed-Suction Technique
6. Connect the suction tubing to the closed suction port.
7. Hyperoxygenate the patient for 30 sec using one of the following methods:
   - Activate the suction hyperoxygenation setting on the ventilator using nondominant hand.
   - Increase FIO_2 to 100%. NOTE: FIO_2 must be returned to baseline level at the completion of the procedure.
   - Disconnect the ventilator tubing from the ET tube and manually ventilate the patient with 100% O_2 using a BVM device.* Administer 5-6 breaths over 30 sec. NOTE: Use of a second person to deliver the manual breaths will significantly increase the tidal volume delivered.
8. With suction off, gently and quickly insert the catheter using the dominant hand. When resistance is met, pull back ½ inch.
9. Apply continuous or intermittent suction using the nondominant thumb. Rotate the catheter between the dominant thumb and forefinger and withdraw the catheter over 10 sec or less.
10. Hyperoxygenate for 30 sec as described in step 7.
11. If secretions remain and the patient has tolerated the procedure, two to three suction passes may be performed as described in steps 8 and 9. NOTE: Rinse the suction catheter with sterile saline solution between suctioning passes as needed.
12. Reconnect patient to ventilator (open-suction technique).
13. At the completion of ET tube suctioning, rinse the catheter and connecting tubing with the sterile saline solution.
14. Suction nasal and/or oral pharynx. NOTE: A separate catheter must be used for this step when using the closed-suction technique.
15. Discard the suction catheter and rinse the connecting tubing with the sterile saline solution (open-suction technique).
16. Reset FIO_2 (if necessary) and ventilator alarms.
17. Reassess patient for signs of effective suctioning.

Adapted from Chulay M: Suctioning: Endotracheal or tracheostomy tube. In Wiegand DL, Carlson KK, editors: *AACN procedure manual for critical care,* ed 5, St Louis, 2005, Mosby.
BVM, Bag-valve-mask; *ECG,* electrocardiogram; *ET,* endotracheal.
*Attach a PEEP valve to the BVM for patients on >5 cm H_2O PEEP.

hypothermia, decreased CO, metabolic acidosis). In patients with normal ventilation-to-perfusion ratios (see Chapter 68), $PETCO_2$ can be used as an estimate of $PaCO_2$, with $PETCO_2$ generally 1 to 5 mm Hg lower than $PaCO_2$. However, in patients with unusually large dead space or serious mismatch between ventilation and perfusion, $PETCO_2$ is not a reliable estimate of $PaCO_2$.[48,50]

■ Maintaining Tube Patency

The patient should be assessed routinely to determine a need for suctioning, but the patient should not be suctioned routinely. Indications for suctioning include (1) visible secretions in the ET tube, (2) sudden onset of respiratory distress, (3) suspected aspiration of secretions, (4) increase in peak airway pressures, (5) auscultation of adventitious breath sounds over the trachea and/or bronchi, (6) increase in respiratory rate and/or sustained coughing, and (7) sudden or gradual decrease in PaO_2 and/or SpO_2.

Two recommended suctioning methods, the **closed-suction technique** (CST) and the **open-suction technique** (OST), are described in Table 66-9. The CST uses a suction catheter that is enclosed in a plastic sleeve connected directly to the patient-ventilator circuit (Fig. 66-19). With the CST, oxygenation and ventilation are maintained during suctioning, and exposure to the patient's secretions is reduced. The CST should be considered for patients who require high levels of positive end-expiratory pressure (PEEP) (>7 to 8 cm H_2O), who have bloody or infected

pulmonary secretions, who require frequent suctioning, and who experience clinical instability with the OST.[49,51]

Potential complications associated with suctioning include hypoxemia, bronchospasm, increased intracranial pressure, dysrhythmias, hypertension, hypotension, mucosal damage, pulmonary bleeding, and infection.[51] The nurse must closely assess the patient before, during, and after the suctioning procedure. If the patient does not tolerate suctioning (e.g., decreased SpO_2, increased or decreased blood pressure, sustained coughing, development of dysrhythmias), the procedure is halted, and the patient is manually hyperventilated with 100% oxygen or, if performing CST, hyperoxygenated until equilibration occurs and before another suction pass is attempted. Hypoxemia is prevented by hyperoxygenating the patient before and after each suctioning pass and limiting each suctioning pass to 10 seconds or less (see Table 66-9). Research has shown that there are no differences in outcomes between the use of hyperventilation or hyperoxygenation to prevent suction-induced hypoxia.[52] If $SvO_2/ScvO_2$ and/or SpO_2 is used, trends should be assessed throughout the suctioning procedure.

Causes of dysrhythmias during suctioning include hypoxemia resulting in myocardial hypoxia; vagal stimulation caused by tracheal irritation; and sympathetic nervous system stimulation caused by anxiety, discomfort, or pain. Dysrhythmias include tachydysrhythmias and bradydysrhythmias, premature beats, and

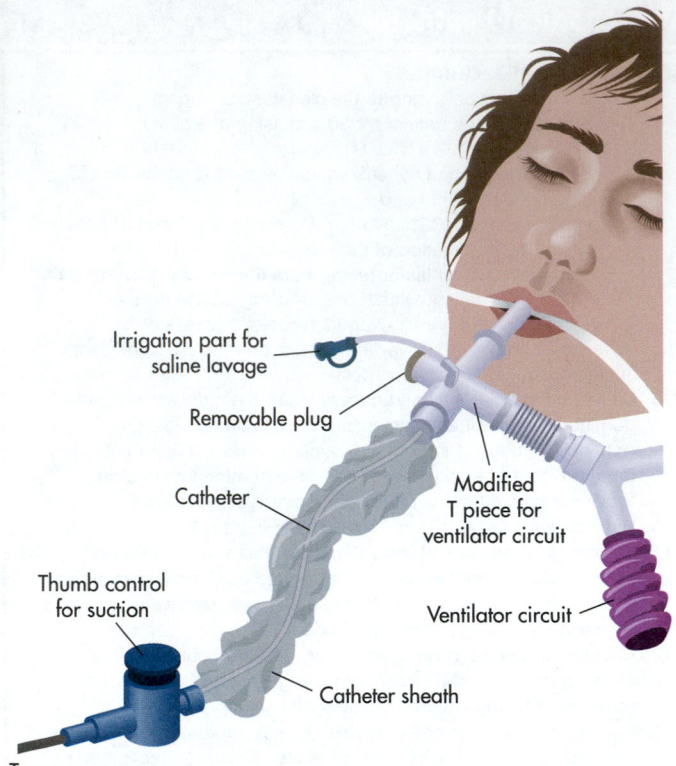

Irrigation part for
saline lavage

Removable plug

Catheter

Modified
T piece for
ventilator circuit

Thumb control
for suction

Ventilator circuit

Catheter sheath

To vacuum source

FIG. 66-19   Closed tracheal suction system.

Adapted from Scott JM, Vollman KM: Endotracheal tube and oral care. In Wiegand DL, Carlson KK, editors: *AACN procedure manual for critical care*, ed 5, St Louis, 2005, Elsevier Mosby.

TABLE 66-10	Oral Care Procedures for a Patient on a Mechanical Ventilator

General Measures

1. Gather all equipment.
2. Wash hands and don personal protective equipment.
3. Explain procedure to the patient and family, if present.
4. Perform oral care using pediatric or adult soft toothbrushes at least twice a day by gently brushing to clean and remove plaque.
5. Use oral swabs with a 1.5% hydrogen peroxide solution every 2-4 hr. NOTE: Postoperative cardiac surgery patients are the only population in which 2% chlorhexidine gluconate is recommended twice a day.
6. Apply a mouth moisturizer to oral mucosa and lips with each cleaning.
7. Suction oral cavity/pharynx frequently. See Fig. 66-20 for example of an endotracheal tube that can provide continuous subglottic suctioning.

NOTE:
- All oral suction equipment and suction tubing should be changed every 24 hr.
- Nondisposable oral suction apparatus should be rinsed with sterile normal saline after each use and placed on a dry paper towel.

asystole. Suctioning should be halted if any new dysrhythmias develop. Excessive suctioning should be avoided in patients with severe hypoxemia or bradycardia.

Tracheal mucosal damage may occur because of excessive suction pressures (>120 mm Hg), overly vigorous catheter insertion, and the characteristics of the suction catheter itself. The presence of blood streaks or tissue shreds in aspirated secretions may indicate that mucosal damage has occurred. Mucosal damage increases the risk of infection and bleeding, particularly if the patient is receiving anticoagulants.[49,51] Trauma to the mucosa can be prevented by following the steps described in Table 66-9.

Secretions may be thick and difficult to suction because of inadequate hydration, inadequate humidification, infection, or inaccessibility of the left mainstem bronchus or lower airways. Adequately hydrating the patient (e.g., oral or IV fluids) and providing supplemental humidification of inspired gases may assist in thinning secretions. Instillation of normal saline into the ET tube is discouraged. SpO$_2$ has been shown to decrease during suctioning with instillation of normal saline.[53] Normal saline is unable to liquefy or thin secretions due to lack of mucolytic properties.[49,54] If infection is the cause of thick secretions, the patient should be given appropriate antibiotics. Postural drainage, percussion, and turning the patient every 2 hours may help move secretions into larger airways.[51]

■ *Providing Oral Care and Maintaining Skin Integrity*

When an oral ET tube is in place, the patient's mouth is always open, and the lips, tongue, and mouth should be moistened with saline or water swabs to prevent mucosal drying. Oral care should include toothbrushing twice a day along with use of moistened mouth swabs

and oral/pharyngeal suctioning every 2 to 4 hours and as needed to provide comfort and to prevent injury to the gums and plaque accumulation (Table 66-10). Meticulous care is required to prevent skin breakdown on the face, lips, tongue, and/or nares as a result of pressure from the ET tube and/or bite block or from the method used to secure the ET tube to the patient's face. The ET tube should be repositioned and retaped every 24 hours and as needed.[40] Repositioning and retaping of the ET tube may be shared practice between nursing and respiratory therapy or limited to respiratory therapy.

If the patient is nasally intubated, the nurse should remove the old tape or ties and clean the skin around the ET tube with saline-soaked gauze or cotton swabs. If the patient is orally intubated, the nurse should remove the bite block (if present) and the old tape or ties. Oral hygiene should be provided, and the ET tube should be repositioned to the opposite side of the mouth. The nurse replaces the bite block (if appropriate) and reconfirms proper cuff inflation and tube placement.[40] The ET tube is resecured per institutional policy (see Fig. 66-18). If a manufactured tube holder is used, the straps can be loosened, the area under the straps massaged, and the straps reapplied. If the patient is anxious or uncooperative, it is recommended that two nurses perform the repositioning procedure to prevent accidental dislodgement. The patient should be monitored for any signs of respiratory distress throughout the procedure.

■ *Fostering Comfort and Communication*

Patients have reported that intubation is a major stressor in the ICU.[55,56] The intubated patient may experience anxiety because of the inability to communicate and not knowing what to expect. Communicating with the intubated patient can be a frustrating experience for the patient, the family, and the nurse. To communicate more effectively, the nurse should employ a variety of methods (see Common Problems of Critical Care Patients earlier in this chapter).[57,58]

The physical discomfort associated with ET intubation and mechanical ventilation often necessitates sedating the patient and administering an analgesic until the ET tube is no longer required. The patient may require morphine, lorazepam (Ativan), propofol, or other sedatives to blunt the anxiety and discomfort related to intubation. The nurse should evaluate the effectiveness of the drugs used to achieve an acceptable level of patient comfort.[13] In addition, the nurse should consider initiating alternative therapies (e.g., music therapy, guided imagery) to complement drug therapy.[12]

Complications of Endotracheal Intubation

Two major complications of ET intubation are unplanned (inadvertent) extubation and aspiration. Unplanned **extubation** (i.e., removal of the ET tube from the trachea) can be a catastrophic event and usually complicates the patient's recovery. Unplanned extubations can be due to patient removal of the ET tube or accidental (i.e., result of movement or procedural-related) removal. Usually the unplanned extubation is obvious (the patient is holding the ET tube). Other times, the tip of the ET tube is in the hypopharynx or esophagus and the extubation is not so obvious. Signs of unplanned extubation may include patient vocalization, activation of the low-pressure ventilator alarm, diminished or absent breath sounds, respiratory distress, and gastric distention.[59] The nurse is responsible for preventing unplanned extubation by ensuring adequate securement of the ET tube and observation and support of the ET tube during repositioning, procedures, patient transfer, and so on. Additionally, immobilizing the patient's hands through the use of soft wrist restraints and providing sedation and analgesia as ordered may be needed. The nurse should provide explanations to the patient and family when restraints are used for patient safety. Reassessment for continued need of restraints is done per institution policy.

Should an unplanned extubation occur, the nurse should stay with the patient and call for help. Interventions are directed at maintaining the patient's airway, supporting ventilation (usually by manually ventilating the patient with 100% oxygen), securing the appropriate assistance to immediately reintubate the patient (if necessary), and providing psychologic support to the patient.

Aspiration is a potential hazard for the patient with an ET tube. The ET tube passes through the epiglottis, splinting it in an open position. Thus the intubated patient cannot protect the airway from aspiration. The high-volume, low-pressure ET or tracheal cuff cannot totally prevent the trickle of oral or gastric secretions into the trachea. Furthermore, secretions accumulate above the cuff. When the cuff is deflated, those secretions can move into the lungs. Some ET tubes provide continuous suctioning of secretions above the cuff (Fig. 66-20).

Oral intubation increases salivation, yet swallowing is difficult, so the mouth must be suctioned frequently. This may be performed with a Yankauer (tonsil-tip) suction catheter or a sterile single-use catheter. Other contributing factors to aspiration include improper cuff inflation, patient positioning, and tracheoesophageal fistula. The patient with an ET tube is at risk for aspiration of gastric contents. Even when the cuff is properly inflated, the nurse must take precautions to avoid emesis, which can lead to aspiration. Frequently, an orogastric (OG) or nasogastric (NG) tube is inserted and connected to low, intermittent suction when a patient is intubated. Preference should be given to placement of an OG tube to reduce the risk of sinusitis. All intubated patients and patients receiving enteral feedings

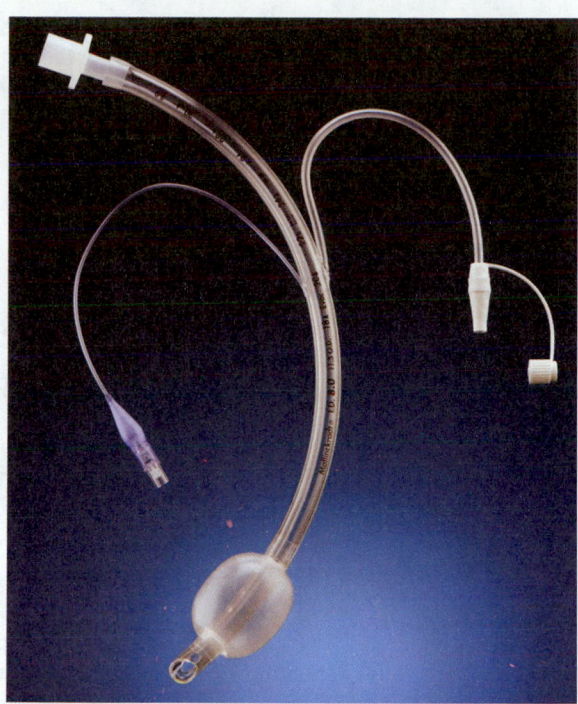

FIG. 66-20 Continuous subglottal suctioning can be provided by the Hi Lo Evac Tube. A dorsal lumen above the cuff allows for suctioning of secretions from the subglottic area.

should have the head of the bed (HOB) elevated a minimum of 30 degrees to 45 degrees unless medically contraindicated.[60]

MECHANICAL VENTILATION

Mechanical ventilation is the process by which the fraction of inspired oxygen (FIO_2) is at 21% (room air) or greater and moved into and out of the lungs by a mechanical ventilator. Mechanical ventilation is not curative. It is used as a means of supporting patients until they recover the ability to breathe independently, as a bridge to long-term mechanical ventilation, or until a decision is made to withdraw ventilatory support. Indications for mechanical ventilation include (1) apnea or impending inability to breathe, (2) acute respiratory failure (generally defined as pH ≤ 7.25 with a $PaCO_2 \geq 50$ mm Hg), (3) severe hypoxia, and (4) respiratory muscle fatigue.[59] Patients with chronic pulmonary disease and their families should be given the opportunity to decide the issue of mechanical ventilation before terminal respiratory disease develops. All patients, particularly those with grave or chronic illnesses, should also be encouraged to discuss the subject with their families and health care providers along with formalizing the results of that discussion in an advance directive. The decision to use, withhold, or withdraw mechanical ventilation must be made carefully, respecting the informed wishes of the patient and family. When there is disagreement between the health care team, the patient, and/or the family over the plan of care, the institution's ethics committee should be consulted for assistance.

Types of Mechanical Ventilation

The two major types of mechanical ventilation are negative pressure and positive pressure ventilation.

Negative Pressure Ventilation. **Negative pressure ventilation** involves the use of chambers that encase the chest or body

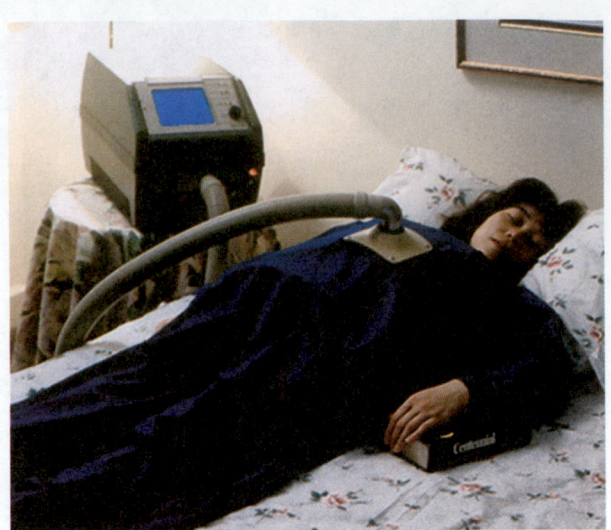

FIG. 66-21   Negative pressure ventilator.

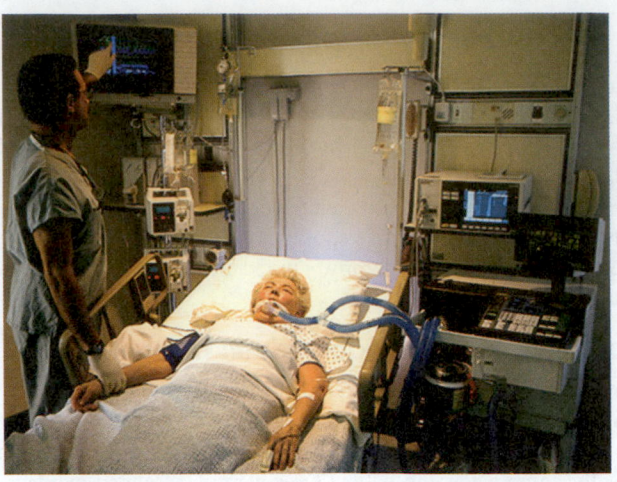

FIG. 66-22   Patient receiving mechanical ventilation.

and surround it with intermittent subatmospheric or negative pressure. The "iron lung" was the first form of negative pressure ventilation that evolved during the polio epidemic. Intermittent negative pressure around the chest wall causes the chest to be pulled outward. This reduces intrathoracic pressure. Air rushes in via the upper airway, which is outside the sealed chamber. Expiration is passive; the machine cycles off, allowing chest retraction. This type of ventilation is similar to normal ventilation in that decreased intrathoracic pressures produce inspiration and expiration is passive. Negative pressure ventilation is delivered as noninvasive ventilation and an artificial airway is not required.

There are several portable negative pressure ventilators that are used in the home for patients with neuromuscular diseases, central nervous system disorders, diseases and injuries of the spinal cord, and severe COPD (Fig. 66-21). Negative pressure ventilators are not used extensively for acutely ill patients. However, some research has demonstrated positive outcomes with the use of negative pressure ventilation in acute exacerbations of chronic respiratory failure.[61]

Positive Pressure Ventilation. Positive pressure ventilation (PPV) is the primary method used with acutely ill patients (Fig. 66-22). During inspiration the ventilator pushes air into the lungs under positive pressure. Unlike spontaneous ventilation, intrathoracic pressure is raised during lung inflation rather than lowered. Expiration occurs passively as in normal expiration. Modes of PPV are categorized into two groups: volume and pressure ventilation.

Volume Ventilation. With **volume ventilation,** a predetermined tidal volume (V_T) is delivered with each inspiration, and the amount of pressure needed to deliver the breath varies based on the compliance and resistance factors of the patient-ventilator system. Consequently, the V_T is consistent from breath to breath, but airway pressures will vary.[59,62]

Pressure Ventilation. With **pressure ventilation,** the peak inspiratory pressure is predetermined, and the V_T delivered to the patient varies based on the selected pressure and the compliance and resistance factors of the patient-ventilator system. With this understanding, careful attention must be given to the V_T to prevent unplanned hyperventilation or hypoventilation. For example, when the patient breathes out of synchrony with the ventilator, the pressure limit may be reached quickly, and the volume of gas delivered may be small. Initially, pressure ventilation was used only in stable

patients being weaned from the ventilator. Today, pressure ventilation is frequently selected to treat critically ill patients.[59,62,63]

Settings of Mechanical Ventilators

Mechanical ventilator settings regulate the rate, depth, and other characteristics of ventilation (Table 66-11). Settings are based on the patient's status (e.g., ABGs, body weight, level of consciousness, muscle strength). The ventilator is tuned as finely as possible to match the patient's ventilatory pattern. Settings are evaluated and adjusted frequently until the patient achieves optimal ventilation. Some settings serve as a fail-safe mechanism, alerting staff to problems with ventilation. It is important that the nurse ensure that all ventilator alarms are on at all times. Alarms alert the staff of potentially dangerous situations such as mechanical malfunction, apnea, or patient asynchrony with the ventilator. On many ventilators the alarms can be temporarily suspended or silenced for up to 2 minutes for suctioning or testing. After that period of time, the alarm system automatically becomes functional again.

Modes of Volume Ventilation

The variable methods by which the patient and the ventilator interact to deliver effective ventilation are called *modes.* The selected *ventilator mode* is based on how much WOB the patient ought to or can perform and is determined by the patient's ventilatory status, respiratory drive, and ABGs. WOB refers to inspiratory effort needed to overcome the elasticity and viscosity of the lungs along with the airway resistance. Generally, ventilator modes are controlled or assisted. With controlled ventilatory support, the ventilator does all of the WOB, and with assisted ventilatory support, the ventilator and the patient share the WOB. For the past 25 years, volume modes such as controlled mandatory ventilation (CMV), assist-control ventilation (ACV), and synchronized intermittent mandatory ventilation (SIMV) have been used to treat critically ill patients. Over the last decade, pressure modes such as pressure support ventilation (PSV) and pressure-controlled inverse ratio ventilation (PC-IRV) have become more widespread.[59,62,63] These modes are described in Table 66-12.

Controlled Mandatory Ventilation. With **controlled mandatory ventilation** (CMV), breaths are delivered at a set rate per minute and a set V_T, which are independent of the patient's ventilatory efforts. Although CMV is used infrequently, it is used when the patient has no drive to breathe (e.g., the anesthetized patient) or is

TABLE 66-11   Settings of Mechanical Ventilation

Parameter	Description
Respiratory rate (f)	Number of breaths the ventilator delivers per minute; usual setting is 6-20 breaths/min
Tidal volume (V_T)	Volume of gas delivered to patient during each ventilator breath; usual volume is 10-12 ml/kg; 6-8 ml/kg in acute lung injury
Oxygen concentration (FIO_2)	Fraction of inspired oxygen delivered to patient; may be set between 21% (essentially room air) and 100%; usually adjusted to maintain PaO_2 level >60 mm Hg or SpO_2 level >90%
Positive end-expiratory pressure (PEEP)	Positive pressure applied at the end of expiration of ventilator breaths; usual setting is 3-5 cm H_2O
Pressure support	Positive pressure used to augment patient's inspiratory pressure; usual setting is 5-10 cm H_2O
I:E ratio	Duration of inspiration (I) to duration of expiration (E); usual setting is 1:2 to 1:1.5 unless IRV is desired
Inspiratory flow rate and time	Speed with which the V_T is delivered; usual setting is 40-80 L/min and time is 0.8-1.2 sec
Sensitivity	Determines the amount of effort the patient must generate to initiate a ventilator breath; it may be set for pressure triggering or flow triggering; usual setting for a pressure trigger is 0.5-1.5 cm H_2O below baseline pressure and for a flow trigger is 1-3 L/min below baseline flow
High pressure limit	Regulates the maximal pressure the ventilator can generate to deliver the V_T; when the pressure limit is reached, the ventilator terminates the breath and spills the undelivered volume into the atmosphere; usual setting is 10-20 cm H_2O above peak inspiratory pressure

From Urden LD, Stacy KM, Lough ME: *Thelan's critical care nursing: diagnosis and management*, ed 5, St Louis, 2006, Elsevier Mosby.
IRV, Inverse ratio ventilation.

unable to breathe spontaneously (e.g., the paralyzed patient). Additionally, ACV can achieve similar results and not "lock out" the patient's inspiratory efforts. In the CMV mode, the patient performs no WOB and cannot adjust respirations to meet changing demands.

Assist-Control Mechanical Ventilation. With **assist-control ventilation** (ACV), the ventilator delivers a preset V_T at a preset frequency, and when the patient initiates a spontaneous breath, the preset V_T is delivered. The ventilator senses a decrease in intrathoracic pressure and then delivers the preset V_T. The patient can breathe faster than the preset rate but not slower. This mode has the advantage of allowing the patient some control over ventilation while providing some assistance. ACV is used in patients with a variety of conditions, including neuromuscular disorders (e.g., Guillain-Barré syndrome), pulmonary edema, and acute respiratory failure. In the ACV mode, the patient has the potential for hypoventilation and hyperventilation. The spontaneously breathing patient can easily be overventilated, resulting in hyperventilation. If the volume or minimum rate is set low and the patient is apneic or weak, the patient will be hypoventilated. Thus these patients require vigilant assessment and monitoring of ventilatory status, including respiratory rate, ABGs, SpO_2, and SvO_2/$ScvO_2$. It is also important that the sensitivity or amount of negative pressure required to initi-

TABLE 66-12   Modes of Mechanical Ventilation

Volume Modes
Control Ventilation (CV) or Controlled Mandatory Ventilation (CMV)
With this mode, the ventilator provides all of the patient's minute ventilation. The clinician sets the rate, V_T, inspiratory time, and positive end-expiratory pressure (PEEP). Generally, this term is used to describe those situations in which the patient is chemically relaxed or is paralyzed from a spinal cord or neuromuscular disease and is therefore unable to initiate spontaneous breaths. The ventilator mode setting may be set on CMV, assist-control (AC), or synchronized intermittent mandatory ventilation (SIMV) because all these options provide volume breaths at the clinician-selected rate.

Assist-Control (AC) or Assisted Mandatory Ventilation (AMV)
This option requires that a rate, V_T, inspiratory time, and PEEP be set for the patient. The ventilator sensitivity is also set, and when the patient initiates a spontaneous breath, a full-volume breath is delivered.

Intermittent Mandatory Ventilation (IMV) and Synchronized Intermittent Mandatory Ventilation (SIMV)
This mode requires that rate, V_T, inspiratory time, sensitivity, and PEEP are set by the clinician. In between "mandatory breaths," patients can spontaneously breathe at their own rates and V_T. With SIMV, the ventilator synchronizes the mandatory breaths with the patient's own inspirations.

Pressure Modes
Pressure Support Ventilation (PSV)
This mode provides an augmented inspiration to a spontaneously breathing patient. With PSV the clinician selects an inspiratory pressure level, PEEP, and sensitivity. When the patient initiates a breath, a high flow of gas is delivered to the preselected pressure level and pressure is maintained throughout inspiration. The patient determines the parameters of V_T, rate, and inspiratory time.

Pressure-Controlled Inverse Ratio Ventilation (PC-IRV)
This mode combines pressure-limited ventilation with an inverse ratio of inspiration to expiration. The clinician selects the pressure level, rate, inspiratory time (1:1, 2:1, 3:1, 4:1), and the PEEP level. With the prolonged inspiratory times, auto-PEEP may result. The auto-PEEP may be a desirable outcome of the inverse ratios. Some clinicians use PC without IRV. Conventional inspiratory times are used and rate, pressure level, and PEEP are selected.

Positive End-Expiratory Pressure (PEEP) and Continuous Positive Airway Pressure (CPAP)
PEEP
This ventilatory option creates positive pressure at end exhalation. PEEP restores functional residual capacity (FRC). The term *PEEP* is used when end-expiratory pressure is provided during ventilator positive pressure breaths.

CPAP
Similar to PEEP, CPAP restores FRC. This pressure is continuous during spontaneous breathing; no positive pressure breaths are present.

From Burns SM: Ventilatory management: volume and pressure modes. In Wiegand DL, Carlson KK, editors: *AACN procedure manual for critical care*, ed 5, St Louis, 2005, Elsevier Mosby.

ate a breath is appropriate to the patient's condition. For example, if it is too difficult for the patient to initiate a breath, the WOB is increased and the patient may tire and or develop ventilator asynchrony (i.e., the patient "fights" the ventilator).[59]

Synchronized Intermittent Mandatory Ventilation. With **synchronized intermittent mandatory ventilation** (SIMV), the ventilator delivers a preset V_T at a preset frequency in synchrony with the patient's spontaneous breathing. Between ventilator-delivered breaths, the patient is able to breathe spontaneously through the ventilator circuit. Thus the patient receives the preset FIO_2 concentration during the spontaneous breaths but self-regulates the rate and volume of those breaths. This mode of ventilation differs from ACV, in which all breaths are of the same preset volume. It is used during continuous ventilation and during weaning from the ventilator. SIMV may also be combined with PSV (described below). Potential benefits of SIMV include improved patient-ventilator synchrony, lower mean airway pressure, and prevention of muscle atrophy as the patient takes on more of the WOB.[59]

There are disadvantages with SIMV. If spontaneous breathing decreases when the preset rate is low, ventilation might not be adequately supported. Low-rate SIMV should be used only in patients with regular, spontaneous breathing. Weaning with SIMV demands close monitoring and may take longer because the rate of breathing is gradually reduced. Patients being weaned with SIMV may also have increased muscle fatigue associated with spontaneous breathing efforts.[64]

Modes of Pressure Ventilation

Pressure Support Ventilation. With **pressure support ventilation** (PSV), positive pressure is applied to the airway only during inspiration and is used in conjunction with the patient's spontaneous respirations. The patient must be able to initiate a breath in this modality. A preset level of positive airway pressure is selected so that the gas flow rate is greater than the patient's inspiratory flow rate. As the patient initiates a breath, the machine senses the spontaneous effort and supplies a rapid flow of gas at the initiation of the breath and variable flow throughout the breath. With PSV the patient determines inspiratory length, V_T, and respiratory rate. V_T depends on the pressure level and airway compliance. PSV is used with continuous ventilation and during weaning. PSV may also be used with SIMV during weaning. PSV is not used as a sole ventilatory support during acute respiratory failure because of the risk of hypoventilation. Advantages to PSV include increased patient comfort, decreased WOB (because inspiratory efforts are augmented), decreased oxygen consumption (because inspiratory work is reduced), and increased endurance conditioning (because the patient is exercising respiratory muscles).[59,63]

Pressure-Controlled Inverse Ratio Ventilation. *Pressure-controlled inverse ratio ventilation* (PC-IRV) combines pressure-limited ventilation with an inverse ratio of inspiration (I) to expiration (E). Some clinicians use PC without IRV. The I/E ratio is the ratio of duration of inspiration (I) to the duration of expiration (E). This value is normally a ratio of 1:2. With IRV, the I/E ratio begins at 1:1 and may progress to 4:1. With IRV, a prolonged positive pressure is applied, increasing inspiratory time. IRV progressively expands collapsed alveoli. The short expiratory time has a PEEP-like effect, preventing alveolar collapse. Because IRV imposes a nonphysiologic breathing pattern, the patient requires sedation with or without paralysis. PC-IRV is indicated for patients with acute respiratory distress syndrome (ARDS) who continue to have refractory hypoxemia despite high levels of PEEP. Not all patients with poor oxygenation respond to PC-IRV.

Other Modes. Increases in ventilator technology have led to the development of additional pressure modes. However, due to the nonstandardization of these options, the names and features are manufacturer specific. The superiority of these modes has not been established. Some examples include *volume-assured pressure ventilation* (VAPS) and *pressure release ventilation* (PRV).

Other Ventilatory Maneuvers

Positive End-Expiratory Pressure. **Positive end-expiratory pressure** (PEEP) is a ventilatory maneuver in which positive pressure is applied to the airway during exhalation. Normally during exhalation, airway pressure drops to zero, and exhalation occurs passively. With PEEP, exhalation remains passive, but pressure falls to a preset level greater than zero, often 3 to 20 cm H_2O. With PEEP, lung volume during expiration and between breaths is greater than normal. Thus PEEP increases functional residual capacity (FRC), and this often improves oxygenation with restoration of lung volume that normally remains at the end of passive exhalation. The mechanisms by which PEEP increases FRC and oxygenation include increased aeration of patent alveoli, aeration of previously collapsed alveoli, and prevention of alveolar collapse throughout the respiratory cycle.[59,63]

PEEP is titrated to the point that oxygenation improves without compromising hemodynamics.[59,63] This is termed *best* or *optimal PEEP*. Often 5 cm H_2O PEEP (referred to as *physiologic PEEP*) is used prophylactically to replace the glottic mechanism, help maintain a normal FRC, and prevent alveolar collapse. PEEP of 5 cm H_2O is also used for patients with a history of alveolar collapse during weaning. PEEP has demonstrated improvements in gas exchange, vital capacity, and inspiratory force when used during weaning.

In contrast, *auto-PEEP* is not purposely set on the ventilator but is a result of inadequate exhalation time. Auto-PEEP is additional PEEP over what is set by the clinician and can be measured at the end-expiratory hold button located on most ventilators. This additional PEEP may result in increased WOB, barotrauma, and hemodynamic instability. However, during some ventilator modes (PC-IRV), auto-PEEP may be desirable. Interventions to limit auto-PEEP include sedation and analgesia, large-diameter ET tube, bronchodilators, short inspiratory times, decreased respiratory rates, and reducing water accumulation in the ventilator circuit by frequent emptying or use of heated circuits. In patients with short exhalation times and early airway closure (e.g., COPD, asthma), setting PEEP can offset auto-PEEP by splinting the airway open during exhalation and preventing "air trapping."[65]

In general, the major purpose of PEEP is to maintain or improve oxygenation while limiting risk of oxygen toxicity. FIO_2 can often be reduced when PEEP is used. PEEP is thought to be useful in pulmonary edema, providing a counterpressure opposing fluid extravasation. PEEP is indicated in lungs with diffuse disease, severe hypoxemia unresponsive to FIO_2 greater than 50%, and loss of compliance or stiffness. The classic indication for PEEP therapy is ARDS (see Chapter 68). PEEP is generally contraindicated or used with extreme caution in patients with highly compliant lungs (e.g., COPD), unilateral or nonuniform disease, hypovolemia, and low CO. In these situations the adverse effects of PEEP may outweigh any benefits.

Continuous Positive Airway Pressure. **Continuous positive airway pressure** (CPAP) restores FRC and is similar to PEEP. However, the pressure in CPAP is delivered continuously during spontaneous breathing, thus preventing the patient's airway pressure from falling to zero. For example, if CPAP is 5 cm H_2O, airway pressure during expiration is 5 cm H_2O. During inspiration,

1 to 2 cm H_2O of negative pressure is generated, thus reducing airway pressure to 3 or 4 cm H_2O. The patient receiving SIMV with PEEP receives CPAP when breathing spontaneously. CPAP is commonly used in the treatment of obstructive sleep apnea. CPAP can be administered noninvasively by a tight-fitting mask or an ET or tracheal tube. CPAP increases WOB because the patient must forcibly exhale against the CPAP and so must be used with caution in patients with myocardial compromise.

Bilevel Positive Airway Pressure. *Bilevel positive airway pressure* (BiPAP) provides two levels of positive pressure support, higher inspiratory positive airway pressure (IPAP) and lower expiratory positive airway pressure (EPAP), along with oxygen. It is a noninvasive modality and is delivered through a tight-fitting face mask, nasal mask, or nasal pillows. Similar to PSV that is delivered through an artificial airway, the patient must be able to spontaneously breathe and cooperate with this treatment. Indications include acute respiratory failure in patients with COPD and heart failure, and sleep apnea. BiPAP may also be used after extubation to prevent reintubation. Patients with shock, altered mental status, or increased airway secretions are not candidates for BiPAP.[59,66]

High-Frequency Ventilation. **High-frequency ventilation** (HFV) involves delivery of a small tidal volume (usually 1 to 5 ml/kg of body weight) at rapid respiratory rates (100 to 300 breaths/min) in an effort to recruit and maintain lung volume and reduce intrapulmonary shunting (see Chapter 68). One benefit of HFV may be the ability to support gas exchange while minimizing the risk of volutrauma. HFV has been widely accepted in neonatal and pediatric ICUs, but its use in adults is still considered investigational and limited to patients with ARDS.[59,67]

There are three types of HFV. *High-frequency jet ventilation* (HFJV) delivers humidified gas from a high-pressure source through a small-bore cannula positioned in the airway. With HFJV, precise V_T is difficult to predict and is a function of numerous variables. *High-frequency percussive ventilation* (HFPV) attempts to combine the positive effects of both HFV and conventional mechanical ventilation. A piston mechanism positioned at the end of the ET tube is driven by a high-pressure gas supply at a rate of 200 to 900 beats/min. These high-frequency beats are superimposed on a conventional pressure-controlled ventilator mode. *High-frequency oscillatory ventilation* (HFOV) uses a diaphragm or a piston in the ventilator to generate vibrations (or oscillations) of subphysiologic volumes of gas. HFOV can produce respiratory frequencies in excess of 3000 breaths/min.[59,67] Patients receiving HFV must be paralyzed to suppress spontaneous respiration. In addition, patients must receive concurrent sedation and analgesia as necessary adjuncts when inducing paralysis (see Chapter 68).

Partial Liquid Ventilation. Currently, clinical trials are investigating the use of perflubron (LiquiVent) in **partial liquid ventilation** (PLV) for patients with ARDS. Perflubron is an inert, biocompatible, clear, odorless liquid derived from organic compounds that has an affinity for both oxygen and carbon dioxide and surfactant-like qualities.[68] Perflubron is trickled down a specially designed ET tube through a side port into the lungs of a mechanically ventilated patient. The amount used is usually equivalent to a patient's FRC. Perflubron evaporates quickly and must be replaced to maintain a constant level during the therapy (usually 3 to 5 days). Additional research is needed to assess the efficacy of this therapy.[68]

Nitric Oxide. *Nitric oxide* (NO) is a gaseous molecule that is synthesized intravascularly and participates in the regulation of pulmonary vascular tone. Inhibition of NO production results in pulmonary vasoconstriction, and administration of continuous inhaled NO results in pulmonary vasodilation. Current indications include ARDS, as a diagnostic screening tool for pulmonary hypertension during a cardiac catheterization, and during or after cardiac surgery.[69] Administration may be given invasively through an ET tube or a tracheostomy, or via a face mask. NO therapy does not appear to pose a risk to health care providers during routine delivery of up to 20 ppm.[70]

Prone Positioning. *Prone positioning* is the repositioning of a patient from a supine or lateral position to a prone (on the stomach with face down) position. This repositioning is used to improve lung recruitment through various mechanisms. The effects of fluid in the dependent parts of the lungs are reversed via gravity as the patient is changed from supine to prone. In this position, the heart rests on the sternum, away from the lungs, contributing to an overall uniformity of pleural pressures. This relatively safe (although nurse-intensive) therapy is used as supportive therapy in critically ill patients with acute lung injury or ARDS to improve oxygenation.[67,71]

Extracorporeal Membrane Oxygenation. *Extracorporeal membrane oxygenation* (ECMO) is an alternative form of pulmonary support for the patient with severe respiratory failure. It is more commonly used in the pediatric and neonatal populations with increasing use in the adult patient. ECMO is a modification of cardiac bypass and involves partially removing blood from a patient through the use of large-bore catheters, infusing oxygen, removing CO_2, and returning the blood back to the patient. This intensive therapy requires systemic anticoagulation and is a time-limited intervention. A skilled team of specialists including a perfusionist is required continuously at the bedside.[72]

Complications of Positive Pressure Ventilation

Although mechanical ventilation may be essential to maintain ventilation and oxygenation, it can cause adverse effects. It is often difficult to distinguish complications of mechanical ventilation from the underlying disease.

Cardiovascular System. PPV can affect circulation because of the transmission of increased mean airway pressure to the thoracic cavity. With increased intrathoracic pressure, thoracic vessels are compressed. This results in decreased venous return to the heart, decreased left ventricular end-diastolic volume (preload), decreased CO, and hypotension. Mean airway pressure is further increased if titrating PEEP (>5 cm H_2O) to improve oxygenation.

If the lungs are noncompliant (as in ARDS), airway pressures are not as easily transmitted to the heart and blood vessels. Thus effects of PPV on CO are reduced. Conversely, with compliant lungs (e.g., emphysema), there is increased danger of transmission of high airway pressures and negative effects on hemodynamics.

Compromise of venous return by PPV is exaggerated by hypovolemia (e.g., hemorrhage, multiple trauma) and decreased venous tone (e.g., sepsis, spinal shock). Restoration and maintenance of the circulating blood volume are important in minimizing cardiovascular complications.

Pulmonary System

Barotrauma. As lung inflation pressures increase, risk of *barotrauma* increases. Patients with compliant lungs (e.g., COPD) are at greater risk for barotrauma because the increased airway pressure readily distends the lungs and may rupture alveoli or emphysematous blebs. Patients with stiff lungs (e.g., ARDS) who are given high inspiratory pressures and high levels of PEEP (>5 cm H_2O) and patients with suppurative lung abscesses resulting from necrotizing organisms (e.g., staphylococci) are also susceptible to barotrauma.

Air can escape into the pleural space from alveoli or interstitium, accumulate, and become trapped. Pleural pressure increases and collapses the lung, causing pneumothorax. (Clinical manifestations of pneumothorax are discussed in Chapter 28.) The lung receives air during inspiration but cannot expel it during expiration. Respiratory bronchioles are larger on inspiration than expiration. They may close on expiration, and air becomes trapped. With PPV, a simple pneumothorax can become a life-threatening tension pneumothorax. With tension pneumothorax, the mediastinum and contralateral lung are compressed, compromising CO. Immediate treatment of the pneumothorax is required. For some patients, chest tubes may be placed prophylactically.

Pneumomediastinum usually begins with rupture of alveoli into the lung interstitium; progressive air movement then occurs into the mediastinum and subcutaneous neck tissue. This is commonly followed by pneumothorax. Occurrence of new, unexplained subcutaneous emphysema is an indication for immediate chest x-ray. Pneumomediastinum and subcutaneous emphysema in the neck may be too small to be detected radiographically or clinically before the development of a pneumothorax.

Volutrauma. The concept of *volutrauma* in PPV relates to the lung injury that occurs when large tidal volumes are used to ventilate noncompliant lungs (e.g., ARDS). Volutrauma results in alveolar fractures and movement of fluids and proteins into the alveolar spaces. The ARDS Network Study demonstrated a change in mortality rate of patients with ARDS by using smaller V_T of 6 ml/kg.[73] The use of low-volume ventilation rather than pressure ventilation is the suggested strategy for lung protection in ARDS patients.[67]

Alveolar Hypoventilation. *Hypoventilation* can be caused by inappropriate ventilator settings, leakage of air from the ventilator tubing or around the ET tube or tracheostomy cuff, lung secretions or obstruction, and low ventilation/perfusion ratio. Low V_T or respiratory rate decreases minute ventilation, causing hypoventilation. A leaking cuff or tubing that is not secured may cause air leakage, lowering the delivered V_T. Too low an SIMV rate in a patient who is unable to produce adequate spontaneous respirations causes hypoventilation, respiratory acidosis, and additional problems related to acidosis such as cardiac dysrhythmias. Excess lung secretions can cause hypoventilation. Turning the patient every 1 to 2 hours, providing chest physical therapy to lung areas with increased secretions, encouraging deep breathing and coughing, and suctioning as needed may alleviate this. Atelectasis may develop. Increasing the V_T, adding small increments of PEEP, and adding a preset number of sighs to the ventilator settings lessen the likelihood of atelectasis.

Alveolar Hyperventilation. Respiratory alkalosis can occur if the respiratory rate or V_T is set too high (*mechanical overventilation*) or if the patient receiving assisted ventilation is *hyperventilating*. It is easy to overventilate a patient on PPV. Particularly at risk are patients with chronic alveolar hypoventilation and CO_2 retention (e.g., patients with COPD). The patient with COPD may have a chronic $PaCO_2$ elevation (acidosis) and compensatory bicarbonate retention by the kidneys. When the patient is ventilated, the patient's "normal baseline" rather than the standard normal

values should be the therapeutic goal. If the COPD patient is returned to a standard normal $PaCO_2$, the patient will develop alkalosis because of the retained bicarbonate. Such a patient could move from compensated respiratory acidosis to serious metabolic alkalosis. The presence of alkalosis makes weaning from the ventilator difficult. Alkalosis, especially if the onset is abrupt, can have additional serious consequences, including hypokalemia, hypocalcemia, and dysrhythmias. Neuromuscular irritability, seizures, coma, and death can occur. Usually the patient with COPD who is supported on the ventilator does better with a short inspiratory and longer expiratory time.

If hyperventilation is spontaneous, it is important to determine the cause and treat it. Causes might include hypoxemia, pain, fear, anxiety, or compensation for metabolic acidosis. Patients who fight the ventilator or breathe out of synchrony may be anxious or in pain. If the patient is anxious and fearful, sitting with the patient and verbally coaching the patient to breathe with the ventilator may help. If these measures fail, manually ventilating the patient slowly with a 100% oxygen source may slow breathing enough to bring it in synchrony with the ventilator.

Ventilator-Associated Pneumonia. The risk for hospital-acquired pneumonia is highest in patients requiring mechanical ventilation because the ET or tracheostomy tube bypasses normal upper airway defenses. In addition, poor nutritional state, immobility, and the underlying disease process (e.g., immunosuppression, organ failure) make the patient more prone to infection. *Ventilator-associated pneumonia* (VAP) is defined as a pneumonia that occurs 48 hours or more after ET intubation.[74] VAP occurs in 9% to 27% of all intubated patients, with 50% of the occurrences developing within the first 4 days of mechanical ventilation. In addition, patients who develop VAP have significantly longer hospital stays and higher mortality rates than those who do not develop VAP.[42]

In patients with early VAP (within 96 hours of mechanical ventilation), sputum cultures often grow gram-negative bacteria such as *Escherichia coli, Klebsiella, Proteus, Streptococcus pneumoniae, Haemophilus influenzae,* and oxacillin-sensitive *Staphylococcus aureus.* Organisms associated with late VAP include antibiotic-resistant organisms such as *Pseudomonas aeruginosa* and oxacillin-resistant *S. aureus.* These organisms are abundant in the hospital environment and/or the patient's GI tract. Organisms can spread in a number of ways, including contaminated respiratory equipment, inadequate hand washing, adverse environmental factors such as poor room ventilation and high traffic flow, and decreased patient ability to cough and clear secretions. Colonization of the oropharynx tract by gram-negative organisms is a predisposing factor in the development of gram-negative pneumonia.

Clinical evidence suggesting VAP includes fever, elevated white blood cell count, purulent sputum, odorous sputum, crackles or rhonchi on auscultation, and pulmonary infiltrates noted on chest x-ray. The patient is treated with antibiotics after appropriate cultures are taken by tracheal suctioning or bronchoscopy and when infection is evident.

Guidelines on VAP prevention include (1) head of bed (HOB) elevation at a minimum of 30 degrees to 45 degrees unless medically contraindicated, (2) no routine changes of the patient's ventilator circuit tubing, and (3) the use of an ET tube with a dorsal lumen above the cuff to allow continuous suctioning of secretions in the subglottic area[60] (see Fig. 66-20). Research has demonstrated that continuous subglottic suctioning appears to be effective in preventing early-onset VAP.[75] Prevention also includes effective and frequent hand washing before and after suctioning, whenever ventilator equipment is touched, and after contact with any respiratory secretions (see Nursing Management: Artificial Airway earlier in this chapter).[41] The nurse should wear gloves when in contact with the patient and change gloves between activities (e.g., bathing the patient, administering an IV drug). Research continues to note that compliance with the simplest preventive measures (e.g., washing hands and changing gloves) continues to be inconsistent among health care workers.[76] Finally, condensation that collects in the ventilator tubing should be drained away from the patient as it collects.

Sodium and Water Imbalance. Progressive fluid retention often occurs after 48 to 72 hours of PPV, especially PPV with PEEP. It is associated with decreased urinary output and increased sodium retention. Fluid balance changes may be due to decreased CO, which in turn results in diminished renal perfusion. Consequently, renin release is stimulated with subsequent production of angiotensin and aldosterone (see Fig. 45-4). This results in sodium and water retention. It is also possible that pressure changes within the thorax are associated with decreased release of atrial natriuretic peptide, which also causes sodium retention. Mild water retention is also associated with PPV. There is less insensible water loss via the airway because ventilated delivered gases are humidified with body temperature water. In addition, as a part of the stress response, release of antidiuretic hormone and cortisol may be increased, contributing to sodium and water retention.

Neurologic System. In patients with head injury, PPV, especially with PEEP, can impair cerebral blood flow. This is related to increased intrathoracic positive pressure impeding venous drainage from the head as evidenced by jugular venous distention. As a result of the impaired venous return and increase in cerebral volume, the patient may exhibit increases in intracranial pressure. Elevating the head of the bed and keeping the patient's head in alignment may decrease the deleterious effects of PPV on intracranial pressure.

Gastrointestinal System. Patients receiving PPV are often stressed because of serious illness, immobility, and discomforts associated with the ventilator. Thus the ventilated patient is at risk for developing stress ulcers and GI bleeding. Patients with a preexisting ulcer or those receiving corticosteroid therapy are at an especially increased risk. Any kind of circulatory compromise, including reduction of CO caused by PPV, may contribute to ischemia of the gastric and intestinal mucosa and possibly increase the risk of translocation of GI bacteria.[77]

Peptic ulcer prophylaxis includes the administration of histamine H_2-receptor blockers (e.g., ranitidine [Zantac]), proton pump inhibitors (e.g., omeprazole [Prilosec]), and tube feedings to decrease gastric acidity and diminish the risk of stress ulcer and hemorrhage. Although the research regarding the use of H_2-receptor blockers or proton pump inhibitors is conflicting, guidelines support the use of routine peptic ulcer prophylaxis in patients who are mechanically ventilated to decrease the risk of VAP.[15]

Gastric and bowel dilation may occur as a result of gas accumulation in the GI tract from swallowed air. The irritation of an artificial airway may cause excessive air swallowing and subsequent gastric dilation. Gastric or bowel dilation may put pressure on the vena cava, decrease CO, and prohibit adequate diaphragmatic excursion during spontaneous breathing. Elevation of the diaphragm as a result of paralytic ileus or bowel dilation leads to compression of the lower lobes of the lungs, which may cause atelectasis and

compromise respiratory function. Decompression of the stomach can be accomplished by the insertion of an NG/OG tube.

Immobility, sedation, circulatory impairment, decreased oral intake, use of opioid pain medications, and stress contribute to decreased peristalsis. The patient's inability to exhale against a closed glottis may make defecation difficult. As a result, the ventilated patient could be predisposed to constipation.

Musculoskeletal System. Maintenance of muscle strength and prevention of the problems associated with immobility are important. Exercise tolerance is enhanced by adequate analgesia and adequate nutrition. Progressive ambulation of patients receiving long-term PPV can be attained without interruption of mechanical ventilation. The ventilator can be pushed around the room, or the patient can be manually ventilated with a BVM while ambulating. Passive and active exercises, consisting of movements to maintain muscle tone in the upper and lower extremities, should be done in bed. Simple maneuvers such as leg lifts, knee bends, quadriceps setting, or arm circles are appropriate. Prevention of contractures, pressure ulcers, footdrop, and external rotation of the hip and legs by proper positioning is important.

Psychosocial Needs. The patient receiving mechanical ventilation may experience physical and emotional stress. In addition to the problems related to critical care patients discussed at the beginning of this chapter, the patient supported by a mechanical ventilator is unable to speak, eat, move, or breathe normally. Tubes and machines may cause pain, fear, and anxiety. Ordinary activities of daily living such as eating, elimination, and coughing are extremely complicated.

In studying the psychosocial needs of ICU patients, one researcher discovered that feeling safe was an overpowering need of ICU patients. In addition, four related needs were the need to know (information), the need to regain control, the need to hope, and the need to trust. Patients reported that when these needs were met, they felt safe. The nurse should work to strengthen the various factors that affect feeling safe. Communication must be creative in the case of the intubated patient and information must be forthright. Patients should be involved in decision making as much as possible. The nurse should encourage hope and build trusting relationships with the patient and family.[78]

Patients receiving PPV usually require some type of sedation (e.g., propofol) and/or analgesia (e.g., fentanyl) to facilitate optimal ventilation.[13,17] Before initiating sedation and/or analgesia in the mechanically ventilated patient who is agitated or anxious, it is important to assess for the cause of distress. Common problems that can result in patient agitation or anxiety include PPV, nutritional deficits, pain, hypoxemia, hypercapnia, drugs, and environmental stressors (e.g., sleep deprivation). It is important to note that delirium is an acute change in mental status and is a marker of cerebral insufficiency with associated longer hospital stays and a higher mortality rate. ICU patients are particularly vulnerable to delirium, and every effort should be made to assess and treat it.[79,80]

At times the decision is made to paralyze the patient with a neuromuscular blocking agent (e.g., cisatracurium [Nimbex]) to provide more effective synchrony with the ventilator and increased oxygenation. If the patient is paralyzed, the nurse should remember that the patient can hear, see, think, and feel. Intravenous sedation and analgesia must always be administered concurrently when the patient is paralyzed. Assessment of the patient should include train-of-four (TOF) peripheral nerve stimulation, physiologic signs

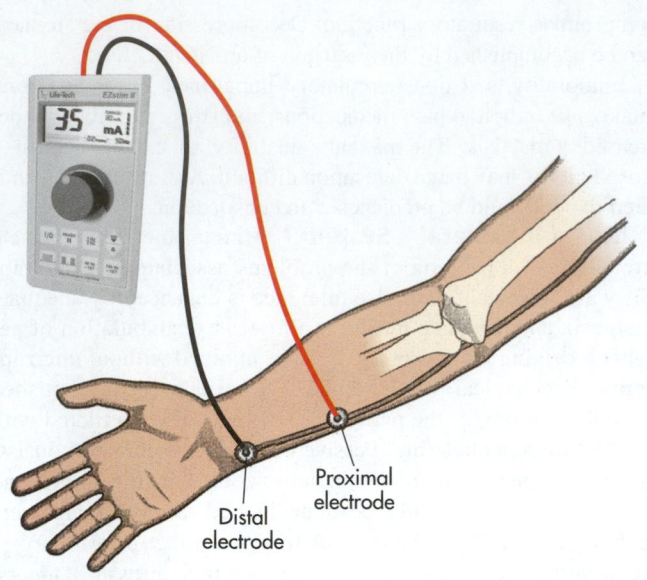

Distal electrode

Proximal electrode

FIG. 66-23 Placement of electrodes along ulnar nerve.

of pain or anxiety (changes in heart rate and blood pressure), and ventilator synchrony.[13,81] The TOF assessment involves the use of a peripheral nerve stimulator to deliver four successive stimulating currents to elicit muscle twitches (Fig. 66-23). The number of twitches will vary with the percentage of neuromuscular blockade; the usual goal is one or two twitches out of four. Excessive administration of neuromuscular blocking agents may predispose the patient to prolonged paralysis and muscle weakness even after these agents are discontinued.

Many patients have few memories of their time in the ICU, whereas others remember vivid details.[17] Although appearing to be asleep, sedated, or paralyzed, patients may be aware of their surroundings and should always be addressed as if they are awake and alert.

Machine Disconnection or Malfunction. Mechanical ventilators may become disconnected or malfunction. When turned on and operative, alarms alert the nurse to problems. Most deaths from accidental ventilator disconnection occur while the alarm is turned off, and most accidental disconnections in critical care settings are discovered by low-pressure alarm activation. The most frequent site for disconnection is between the tracheal tube and the adapter. Connections should be pushed together and then twisted to secure more tightly. The nurse should ascertain that alarms are set at all times and should chart that this is the case. Alarms can be paused (not inactivated) during suctioning or removal from the ventilator and should always be reactivated before leaving the patient's bedside.

Ventilator malfunction may also occur and may be related to several factors. Although most institutions have emergency generators in the event of a power failure and newer ventilators may have battery backup, the nurse should always consider the possibility that power may fail and have a plan for manually ventilating all the patients who are dependent on a ventilator. If, at any time, the nurse determines that the ventilator is malfunctioning (e.g., failure of oxygen supply), the patient should be disconnected from the machine and manually ventilated with 100% oxygen until the ventilator is fixed or replaced.

Nutritional Therapy: Patient Receiving Positive Pressure Ventilation

PPV and the hypermetabolism associated with critical illness can contribute to inadequate nutrition. Presence of an ET tube eliminates the normal route for eating. A patient with a tracheostomy may be able to eat normally once the stoma has healed and swallowing has been assessed via a speech therapy consultation. When eating with a tracheostomy tube in place, the patient should tilt the head slightly forward to facilitate swallowing and to prevent aspiration. Diet may be restricted to soft foods (e.g., puddings, ice cream) and thickened liquids.

Patients likely to be without food for 3 to 5 days should have a nutritional program initiated. Inadequate nutrition makes the patient receiving prolonged mechanical ventilation more prone to poor oxygen transport secondary to anemia and to poor tolerance of minimal exercise. Poor nutrition and the disuse of respiratory muscles contribute to decreased respiratory muscle strength. In addition, the hypermetabolism associated with critical illness, trauma, and surgery and the presence of anxiety, pain, and increased WOB greatly increase caloric expenditure. Serum protein levels (e.g., albumin, prealbumin, transferrin, total protein) are usually decreased. Inadequate nutrition can delay weaning, decrease resistance to infection, and decrease the speed of recovery.[7,10] Enteral feeding via a small-bore feeding tube is the preferred method to meet caloric needs of ventilated patients (see Chapter 40 for discussion of enteral feeding). There is no evidence to support gastric feedings over small bowel feedings in ventilated patients.[41,74,77]

Verification of feeding tube placement includes (1) x-ray confirmation before initial use, (2) marking and ongoing assessment of the tube's exit site, and (3) ongoing review of routine x-rays and aspirate.[82] The auscultatory method of assessment (i.e., listening for air after injection) is not a reliable method for verifying placement of feeding tubes.

A concern regarding the nutritional support of patients receiving PPV is the carbohydrate content of the diet. Metabolism of carbohydrates may contribute to an increase in serum CO_2 levels. The resulting CO_2 load results in a higher required minute ventilation. This, in turn, can cause an increase in WOB. Limiting carbohydrate content in the diet may lower CO_2 production. The dietitian should be consulted to determine the caloric and nutrient needs of these patients.

Weaning from Positive Pressure Ventilation and Extubation

The process of reducing ventilator support and resuming spontaneous ventilation is termed **weaning.** The weaning process differs for patients requiring short-term ventilation (≤3 days) versus long-term ventilation (>3 days). Patients requiring short-term ventilation (e.g., after cardiac surgery) will experience a linear weaning process. Patients likely to require prolonged PPV (e.g., patients with COPD who develop respiratory failure) will most likely experience a weaning process that consists of peaks and valleys.[83] Conceptually, preparation for weaning should begin when PPV is initiated and should involve a team approach (e.g., nurse, physician, patient, family, respiratory therapist, dietitian, physical therapist).

Weaning can be viewed as consisting of three phases: the *preweaning phase,* the *weaning process,* and the *outcome phase.* The preweaning or assessment phase determines the patient's ability to breathe spontaneously. Assessment in this phase depends on a combination of respiratory (Table 66-13) and nonrespiratory fac-

TABLE 66-13	Indicators for Weaning

Weaning Readiness

Patients receiving mechanical ventilation for respiratory failure should undergo a formal assessment of weaning potential if the following are satisfied*:

1. Reversal of the underlying cause of respiratory failure
2. Adequate oxygenation:
   - $PaO_2/FIO_2 > 150-200$
   - $PEEP \leq 5-8$ cm H_2O
   - $FIO_2 \leq 40\%-50\%$
   - $pH \geq 7.25$
3. Hemodynamic stability:
   - Absence of myocardial ischemia
   - Absence of clinically significant hypotension (no vasopressor therapy or low dose)
4. Patient ability to initiate an inspiratory effort

Weaning Assessment

Measurement	Significance	Normal Values	Indices for Weaning
Spontaneous respiratory rate (f)	Respiratory rate/frequency over 1 min	12-20 min	<38 min
Spontaneous tidal volume (V_T)	Amount of air exchanged during normal breathing at rest; measure of muscle endurance	7-9 ml/kg	≥5 ml/kg
Minute ventilation (V_E)	Tidal volume multiplied by respiratory rate over 1 min For example: 0.350 (V_T) × 28 (f) = 8.8 L/min	5-10 L/min	≤10 L/min
Negative inspiratory force or pressure (NIF, NIP)	Amount of negative pressure that a patient is able to generate to initiate spontaneous respirations. Measured by clinician: After complete occlusion of inspiratory valve, a pressure manometer is attached to airway or mouth for 10-20 sec while negative inspiratory efforts are noted.	−75 to −100 cm H_2O	>−20 cm H_2O The more negative the number, the better indication for weaning.
Positive expiratory pressure (PEP)	Measure of expiratory muscle strength and ability to cough. Measured by clinician: After complete occlusion of expiratory valve, a pressure manometer is attached to the airway or mouth for 10-20 sec while positive expiratory efforts are noted.	60-85 cm H_2O	≥30 cm H_2O
Compliance, rate, oxygenation, and pressure (CROP) index	Combined index that is complex to calculate. C_{Dyn} × NIF × (PaO_2/PAO_2)/f C_{Dyn} = Compliance PaO_2/PAO_2 = Oxygenation ratio of arterial O_2/alveolar O_2	Not applicable	>13
Rapid shallow breathing index (f/V_T)	Spontaneous respiratory rate over 1 min divided by tidal volume (in liters). Easier calculation and more widely used. For example: 30(f)/0.400(V_T) = 75/L	60-105/L	<105/L
Vital capacity (VC)	Maximum inspiration and then measurement of air during maximal forced expiration; measure of respiratory muscle endurance or reserve or both; requires patient cooperation.	65-75 ml/kg	≥10-15 ml/kg

Adapted from Collective Task Force, American College of Chest Physicians, American Association of Respiratory Care, American College of Critical Care: Evidence-based guidelines for weaning and discontinuing ventilatory support, *Chest* 120:375S, 2001; and Burns SM: Weaning process. In Wiegand DL, Carlson KK, editors: *AACN procedure manual for critical care,* ed 5, St Louis, 2005, Elsevier.

*The decision to use these criteria must be individualized to the patient.

tors. Weaning assessment parameters should include criteria to assess muscle strength (negative inspiratory force [NIF]) and endurance (spontaneous tidal volume [V_T], vital capacity [VC], minute ventilation [V_E], and rapid shallow breathing index [RSBI]).[64,83,84] In addition, the patient's lungs should be reasonably clear on auscultation and chest x-ray. Nonrespiratory factors include the assessment of the patient's neurologic status, hemodynamics, fluid and electrolytes/acid-base balance, nutrition, and hemoglobin. It is important to have an alert, well-rested, and well-informed patient relatively free from pain and anxiety who can cooperate with the weaning plan. This does not mean complete withdrawal from sedatives or analgesics. Instead, drugs should be titrated to achieve comfort without causing excessive drowsiness.[13]

Evidenced-based clinical guidelines recommend a spontaneous breathing trial (SBT) in patients who demonstrate weaning readiness. An SBT should be at least 30 minutes but no longer than 120 minutes and may be done with low levels of CPAP, low levels of PSV, or a "T" piece.[64] Tolerance of the trial may lead to extubation. Failure to tolerate an SBT should prompt a search for reversible or complicating factors and a return to a nonfatiguing ventilator modality for the patient. The SBT should be reattempted the next day.

Additionally, the use of a standard approach for weaning or weaning protocols has been shown to decrease ventilator days. The components of the protocol are not as important as the use of a protocol to prevent delays in weaning. All methods can be delivered with the patient remaining connected to the ventilator circuit. The patient receiving SIMV can have the ventilator breaths gradually reduced as the patient's ventilatory status permits. CPAP or PSV can be added to SIMV. Another method involves PSV, CPAP, or both delivered without SIMV. PSV is thought to provide gentle, slow respiratory muscle conditioning and may be especially beneficial for patients who are deconditioned or have cardiac problems. Some patients may be weaned by simply providing humidified oxygen (T-piece or flow-by method).[64,83,84]

Weaning is usually carried out during the day, with the patient ventilated at night in a rest mode. The rest mode should be a stable, nonfatiguing, and comfortable form of support for the patient. Regardless of the weaning mode selected, all team members should be familiar with the weaning plan. Additionally, regardless of the method used, it is important to permit the patient's respiratory muscles to rest between weaning trials. Once the respiratory muscles become fatigued, they may require 12 to 24 hours to recover.

The patient being weaned and the family should be provided ongoing psychologic support. The weaning process should be explained, and the patient and family informed of progress. The patient should be placed in a sitting or semirecumbent position and made comfortable. Baseline vital signs and respiratory parameters are measured. During the weaning trial, the patient must be monitored closely for noninvasive criteria that may signal intolerance and result in cessation of the trial (e.g., tachypnea, dyspnea, tachycardia, dysrhythmias, sustained desaturation [SpO_2 <91%], hypertension or hypotension, agitation, diaphoresis, anxiety, sustained V_T <5 ml/kg, changes in level of consciousness).[83,84] Documentation of the patient's tolerance throughout the weaning process is important and should include statements regarding the patient's and the family's perceptions.

The weaning outcome phase refers to the period when weaning stops and the patient is extubated or weaning is stopped because no further progress is being made. The patient who is ready for extubation should receive hyperoxygenation and suctioning (e.g., oropharynx, ET tube). The patient should be instructed to take a deep breath, and at the peak of inspiration, the cuff should be deflated and the tube removed in one motion. After removal, the patient should be encouraged to deep breathe and cough, and the pharynx should be suctioned as needed. Supplemental oxygen should be applied and naso-oral care provided. The nurse must carefully monitor the patient's vital signs, respiratory status, and oxygenation immediately following extubation, within 1 hour, and per institutional policy.[49] If the patient cannot tolerate extubation, immediate reintubation may be necessary.

Chronic Mechanical Ventilation

Mechanical ventilators are no longer limited to the ICU but are now a part of long-term and home care. In some instances, terminally ill, ventilated patients may be discharged to hospice. The emphasis on controlling hospital health care costs has increased the early discharge of patients and the need to provide highly technical care such as mechanical ventilation in home settings.[85] The success of home mechanical ventilation will depend, in part, on careful predischarge assessment and planning for both the patient and caregivers.

Both negative pressure and positive pressure ventilators can be used in the home. Negative pressure ventilators do not require an

TABLE 66-14	**Cross-References to Other Critical Care Content**
Topic	**Discussed in Chapter**
Acute heart failure	35
Acute respiratory distress syndrome	68
Acute respiratory failure	68
Basic life support and cardiopulmonary resuscitation	Appendix A
Burns	25
Cardiac dysrhythmias	36
Cardiac pacemakers	36
Cardiac surgery	34
Delirium	60
Emergencies	69
End-of-life care	11
Enteral nutrition	40
Head injury, including ICP monitoring	57
Myocardial infarction	34
Multiple organ dysfunction syndrome	67
Oxygen delivery	29
Pain management	10
Parenteral nutrition	40
Pulmonary edema	35
Renal dialysis, including renal replacement therapy	47
Shock	67
Systemic inflammatory response syndrome	67
Tracheostomy	27
Trauma	69

ICP, Intracranial pressure.

artificial airway and may be less complicated to use. Several types of small, portable (battery-powered) positive pressure ventilators are available and can be attached to a wheelchair or placed on a bedside table. Settings and alarms on these ventilators are simpler to use than the standard ICU ventilators.[85]

Home mechanical ventilation has advantages and disadvantages. Having the patient in the home eliminates the strain that the hospital setting may impose on family dynamics. The feeling of helplessness by family members when they first hear about the necessity for long-term mechanical ventilation is frequently countered by the ability of the family to participate fully in the patient's care in the home setting. At home the patient may be able to participate more in activities of daily living around a more individualized schedule and, because of the smaller size of the home ventilator, be more mobile. Another advantage of home mechanical ventilation is the reduction in the patient's risk of hospital-acquired infection.

Disadvantages of home mechanical ventilation include problems related to reimbursement, equipment, caregiver stress and fatigue, and the complex needs of these patients. Ventilated patients are usually dependent, requiring extensive nursing care, at least initially. Disposable products may not be reimbursable. Financial resources must be carefully assessed when arranging home mechanical ventilation, and a meeting with the discharge team should be scheduled before initiating a teaching plan for discharge. Another disadvantage of home mechanical ventilation is its potential impact on the family. Family members may seem enthusiastic about caring for their loved one in the home but may be motivated by numerous, complex factors. They may lack understanding of the potential sacrifices they may have to make financially and in personal time and commitment. Families should be encouraged to consider respite care to periodically relieve caregiver stress and fatigue.[85]

NURSING MANAGEMENT
MECHANICAL VENTILATION

Nursing management of the patient receiving mechanical ventilation is presented in NCP 66-1.

OTHER CRITICAL CARE CONTENT

Table 66-14 lists additional critical care content presented in other chapters of this book.

CRITICAL THINKING EXERCISE

CASE STUDY

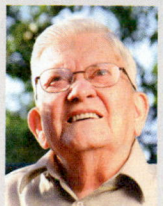

Case Study photo ©iStockphoto.com/ Shannon Dominick.

Critical Care and Mechanical Ventilation

Patient Profile. Mr. R. is a 72-year-old white man found lying on the street by the police. He was unresponsive on admission and remains unresponsive. He has an oral ET tube in place and is receiving mechanical ventilation. He weighs 198 lb (90 kg). A subclavian central line was placed to monitor CVP and administer fluids.

Subjective Data

None; patient is unresponsive to painful stimuli

Objective Data

Physical Examination

- Noninvasive blood pressure is 100/75; heart rate is 110 (uncontrolled atrial fibrillation); temperature is 102° F (38.8° C); SpO_2 is 98%
- Purulent secretions from ET tube
- Breath sounds: rhonchi bilaterally, decreased breath sounds on the right

Diagnostic Studies

- Chest x-ray reveals right lower lung consolidation
- ABGs: pH 7.48; PaO_2 94 mm Hg; $PaCO_2$ 30 mm Hg; HCO_3 34 mEq/L
- Computed tomography (CT) scan is positive for cerebrovascular accident

Collaborative Care

- Positive pressure ventilation settings: assist-control mode
- Set rate 16 breaths/min; tidal volume 900 ml; FIO_2 60%
- Enteral nutrition at 25 ml/hr via small-bore feeding tube
- Indwelling urinary catheter to bedside drainage
- Change position every 2 hours
- Perform chest physical therapy every 2 to 4 hours
- Azithromycin (Zithromax) 500 mg IV q24hr
- Cefotaxime (Claforan) 2 g IV q6hr
- D_5NS with KCl 20 mEq/L at 100 ml/hr

Critical Thinking Questions

1. Identify two reasons for intubating and providing mechanical ventilation for Mr. R.
2. What do Mr. R.'s ABGs indicate, and which ventilator setting(s) should be changed?
3. What is his PaO_2/FIO_2 ratio, and what does it signify?
4. Mr. R.'s blood pressure drops to 80 mm Hg, and he remains in uncontrolled atrial fibrillation with a ventricular rate of 158. A PA catheter is inserted for hemodynamic monitoring. What would be the purpose of hemodynamic monitoring in this patient? Identify two priority nursing considerations for a patient with a PA catheter.
5. Mr. R.'s initial PAWP is 14 mm Hg, CI is 2 L/min/m², and SVRI is 2667 dynes/sec/cm⁻⁵/m². How would you interpret these values? What medical interventions might be considered?
6. Mr. R.'s pulmonary condition deteriorates. PaO_2 drops to 70 mm Hg, and SpO_2 is 89%. PEEP at 5 cm H_2O is added to the ventilator settings. What implications does this have for Mr. R. given his hemodynamic status?
7. Based on the data presented, identify two priority nursing diagnoses. Are there any collaborative problems?
8. After 4 days, Mr. R. remains unresponsive and has developed renal failure. The physician believes the patient will not recover and wishes to discuss goals of care with the patient's family. What would be the nurse's role in this meeting?

NCLEX EXAMINATION REVIEW QUESTIONS

The number of the question corresponds to the same-numbered objective at the beginning of the chapter.

1. Certification in critical care nursing by the American Association of Critical Care Nurses indicates that a nurse
   a. is an advanced practice nurse in the care of acutely ill patients.
   b. may practice independently to provide symptom management for the critically ill.
   c. has earned a master's degree in the field of providing advanced critical care nursing.
   d. has practiced in critical care and successfully completed a test of critical care knowledge.

2. An appropriate nursing intervention for the patient with delirium in the ICU is to
   a. use tranquilizers to establish normal sleep patterns.
   b. identify the factors contributing to the patient's confusion and irritability.
   c. silence all alarms, overhead paging, and conversations around the patient.
   d. sedate the patient with psychotropic drugs to protect the patient from harmful behaviors.

3. The critical care nurse recognizes that an ideal plan for family involvement includes
   a. a family member at the bedside at all times.
   b. allowing family at the bedside at preset, brief intervals.
   c. an individually devised plan with family involved with care and comfort measures.
   d. restriction of visiting in the ICU because the environment is overwhelming to visitors.

4. To establish hemodynamic monitoring for a patient, the nurse zeros the
   a. cardiac output monitoring system to the level of the left ventricle.
   b. pressure monitoring system to the level of the catheter tip located in the patient.
   c. pressure monitoring system to the level of the atrium, identified as the phlebostatic axis.
   d. pressure monitoring system to the level of the atrium, identified as the midclavicular line.

5. The hemodynamic changes the nurse expects to find after successful initiation of intraaortic balloon pump therapy in a patient with cardiogenic shock include
   a. decreased SVR and decreased SV.
   b. decreased PAWP and increased CO.
   c. increased diastolic BP and decreased systolic BP.
   d. decreased CVP and increased right atrial pressure.

Critical Care

6. The nursing management of a patient with an artificial airway includes
   a. maintaining ET tube cuff pressure at 30 cm H_2O.
   b. routine suctioning of the tube at least every 2 hours.
   c. observing for cardiac dysrhythmias during suctioning.
   d. preventing tube dislodgement by limiting mouth care to lubrication of the lips.

7. The purpose of adding PEEP to positive pressure ventilation is to
   a. increase functional residual capacity and improve oxygenation.
   b. increase FIO_2 in an attempt to wean the patient and avoid oxygen toxicity.
   c. determine if the patient is in synchrony with the ventilator or needs to be paralyzed.
   d. determine if the patient is able to be weaned and avoid the risk of pneumomediastinum.

8. The nurse monitors the patient with positive pressure mechanical ventilation for
   a. paralytic ileus because pressure on the abdominal contents affects bowel motility.
   b. diuresis and sodium depletion because of increased release of atrial natriuretic peptide.
   c. signs of cardiovascular insufficiency because pressure in the chest impedes venous return.
   d. respiratory acidosis in a patient with COPD because of alveolar hyperventilation and increased PaO_2 levels.

REFERENCES

1. Nightingale F: *Notes on hospitals,* ed 3, London, 1863, Longman, Roberts, & Green.
2. Lynaugh JE, Fairman J: *Critical care nursing: a history,* Philadelphia, 1998, University of Pennsylvania Press.
3. Seckel MA, Johnson K: Ask the experts: RRT, *Crit Care Nurs* 25:52, 2005.
*4. Meltzer LS, Huckabay LM: Critical care nurses' perceptions of futile care and its effect on burnout, *Am J Crit Care* 13:202, 2004.
5. American Association of Critical Care Nurses: AACN standards for establishing and sustaining healthy work environments: a journey to excellence, *Am J Crit Care* 14:187, 2005.
6. Garland A: Improving the ICU, *Chest* 127:2151, 2005.
7. Heyland DK, Dhaliwal R, Drover JW, et al: The Canadian Critical Care Clinical Practice Guidelines Committee: Canadian clinical practice guidelines for nutritional support in mechanically ventilated, critically ill adult patients, *J Parenter Enteral Nutr* 27:355, 2003.
*8. O'Leary-Kelley CM, Puntillo KA, Barr J, et al: Nutritional adequacy in patients receiving mechanical ventilation who are fed enterally, *Am J Crit Care* 14:222, 2005.
9. Doig GS: Evidence-based guidelines for nutritional support of the critically ill: results of a bi-national guideline development conference, 2005. Available at *www.guideline.gov/summary/summary.aspx?doc_id=8012&nbr=004499&string=nutrition* (accessed September 12, 2006).
10. Stamps DC: Enteral nutrition. In Wiegand DL, Carlson KK, editors: *AACN procedure manual for critical care,* ed 5, St Louis, 2005, Elsevier Mosby.
*11. Frazier SK, Moser DK, Riegel B, et al: Critical care nurses' assessment of patients' anxiety: reliance on physiological and behavioral parameters, *Am J Crit Care* 11:57, 2002.
12. Keegan L: Alternative and complementary modalities for managing stress and anxiety in acute and critical care. In Chulay M, Molter NC, editors: *Protocols for practice: creating a healing environment,* Aliso Viejo, Calif, 1998, AACN.
13. Jacobi J, Fraser GL, Coursin DB, et al: Clinical practice guidelines for the sustained use of sedatives and analgesics in the critically ill adult, *Crit Care Med* 30:119, 2002.
14. Stanik-Hutt J: Pain management in the acutely ill. In Chulay M, Molter NC, editors: *Protocols for practice: creating a healing environment,* Aliso Viejo, Calif, 1998, AACN.
15. Institute for Healthcare Improvement: Getting started kit: preventing ventilator-associated pneumonia. Available at *www.ihi.org/NR/rdonlyres/A448DDB1-E2A4-4D13-8F02-16417EC52990/0/VAPHowtoGuideFINAL.pdf* (accessed August 18, 2005).

16. Kress JP, Pohlman AS, O'Connor MK, et al: Daily interruption of sedative infusions in critically ill patients undergoing mechanical ventilation, *N Engl J Med* 342:1471, 2000.
*17. Puntillo KA, White C, Morris AB, et al: Patients' perceptions and responses to procedural pain: results from Thunder II Project, *Am J Crit Care* 10:238, 2001.
18. Roberts BL: Managing delirium in adult intensive care patients, *Crit Care Nurse* 21:48, 2001.
19. Dines-Kalinowski CM: Nature's nurse: promoting sleep in the ICU, *DCCN* 21:32, 2002.
20. Lehne RA: *Pharmacology for nursing care,* ed 6, St Louis, 2007, Elsevier Saunders.
21. Titler MG: Family visitation and partnership in the critical care unit. In Chulay M, Molter NC, editors: *Protocols for practice: creating a healing environment,* Aliso Viejo, Calif, 1998, AACN.
22. Doherty MH, Plowfield L, Ware C, et al: Impact of critical illness on the patient and family. In Bucher L, Melander S, editors: *Critical care nursing,* Philadelphia, 1999, WB Saunders.
*23. Gonzalez CE, Carroll DL, Elliott JS, et al: Visiting preferences of patients in the intensive care unit and in a complex care medical unit, *Am J Crit Care* 13:194, 2004.
24. Titler MG, Drahozal R: Family pet visiting, animal-assisted activities, and animal-assisted therapy in critical care. In Chulay M, Molter NC, editors: *Protocols for practice: creating a healing environment,* Aliso Viejo, Calif, 1998, AACN.
*25. American Association of Critical-Care Nurses: AACN practice alert: family presence during CPR and invasive procedures. Available at *www.aacn.org/AACN/practiceAlert.nsf/Files/Family%20Presence%20During%20CPR%2011-2004.pdf* (accessed December 4, 2006).
26. Mitty EL: Ethnicity and end-of-life decision-making, *Reflec Nurs Leadersh* 27:28, 2001.
27. Preuss T, Wiegand DL: Single- and multiple-pressure transducer system. In Wiegand DL, Carlson KK, editors: *AACN procedure manual for critical care,* ed 5, St Louis, 2005, Elsevier Mosby.
28. Shaffer RB: Arterial catheter insertion (assist), care, and removal. In Wiegand DL, Carlson KK, editors: *AACN procedure manual for critical care,* ed 5, St Louis, 2005, Elsevier Mosby.
29. Becker DE: Arterial catheter insertion (perform). In Wiegand DL, Carlson KK, editors: *AACN procedure manual for critical care,* ed 5, St Louis, 2005, Elsevier Mosby.
30. Fleck DA: Pulmonary artery catheter insertion (perform). In Wiegand DL, Carlson KK, editors: *AACN procedure manual for critical care,* ed 5, St Louis, 2005, Elsevier Mosby.
31. Preuss T, Wiegand DL: Pulmonary artery catheter and pressure lines, troubleshooting. In Wiegand DL, Carlson KK, editors: *AACN procedure manual for critical care,* ed 5, St Louis, 2005, Elsevier Mosby.
32. Albert NM: Cardiac output measurement techniques (invasive). In Wiegand DL, Carlson KK, editors: *AACN procedure manual for critical care,* ed 5, St Louis, 2005, Elsevier Mosby.
33. Von Ruedon KT et al: Noninvasive hemodynamic monitoring: impedance cardiology. In Wiegand DL, Carlson KK, editors: *AACN procedure manual for critical care,* ed 5, St Louis, 2005, Elsevier Mosby.
34. Urden LD, Stacy KM, Lough ME: *Thelan's critical care nursing,* ed 5, St Louis, 2006, Elsevier Mosby.
35. Quaal S: Intraaortic balloon pump management. In Wiegand DL, Carlson KK, editors: *AACN procedure manual for critical care,* ed 5, St Louis, 2005, Elsevier Mosby.
36. Fleck DA, Hargraves J: Ventricular assist devices. In Wiegand DL, Carlson KK, editors: *AACN procedure manual for critical care,* ed 5, St Louis, 2005, Elsevier Mosby.
37. Abiomed: AbioCor FAQs. Available at *www.abiomed.com/products/heart_replacement/faqs.cfm* (accessed March 1, 2006).
38. Hsu C, Chen K, Chang C, et al: Timing of tracheostomy as a determinant of weaning success in critically ill patients: a retrospective study, *Crit Care* 9:R46, 2005.
39. Rumbak MJ, Newton M, Truncale T, et al: A prospective, randomized, study comparing early percutaneous dilational tracheotomy to prolonged translaryngeal intubation (delayed tracheotomy) in critically ill medical patients, *Crit Care Med* 32:1689, 2004.
40. Scott JM, Vollman KM: Endotracheal tube and oral care. In Wiegand DL, Carlson KK, editors: *AACN procedure manual for critical care,* ed 5, St Louis, 2005, Elsevier Mosby.
41. Centers for Disease Control and Prevention: Guidelines for preventing health-care-associated pneumonia, *MMWR* 53:1, 2004.
42. Kollef MH: Prevention of hospital-associated pneumonia and ventilator-associated pneumonia, *Crit Care Med* 32:1396, 2004.

*Nursing research–based reference.

43. Scott JM: Endotracheal intubation (assist). In Wiegand DL, Carlson KK, editors: *AACN procedure manual for critical care,* ed 5, St Louis, 2005, Elsevier Mosby.

44. Maccioli GA, Dorman T, Brown BR, et al: Clinical practice guidelines for the maintenance of patient physical safety in the intensive care unit: use of restraining therapies—American College of Critical Care Medicine Task Force 2001-2002, *Crit Care Med* 31:2665, 2003.

45. American Society of Anesthesiologists Task Force: Practice guidelines for management of the difficult airway, *Anesth* 98:1269, 2003.

46. Tamburri LM, Hix CD: Acute respiratory failure. In Sole ML, Klein DG, Moseley MJ, editors: *Introduction to critical care nursing,* ed 4, St Louis, 2005, Elsevier Mosby.

47. Burns SM: Manual self-inflation resuscitation bag. In Wiegand DL, Carlson KK, editors: *AACN procedure manual for critical care,* ed 5, St Louis, 2005, Elsevier Mosby.

48. Ahrens T, Sona C: Capnography application in acute and critical care, *AACN Clin Issues* 14:123, 2003.

49. St John R, Seckel MA: Airway management. In Burns S, editor: *Protocols for practice: care of the mechanically ventilated patient,* ed 2, Sudbury, Mass, 2006, Jones & Bartlett.

50. Good VS: Continuous end-tidal carbon dioxide monitoring. In Wiegand DL, Carlson KK, editors: *AACN procedure manual for critical care,* ed 5, St Louis, 2005, Elsevier Mosby.

51. Chulay M: Suctioning: endotracheal or tracheostomy tube. In Wiegand DL, Carlson KK, editors: *AACN procedure manual for critical care,* ed 5, St Louis, 2005, Elsevier Mosby.

*52. Oh H, Sco W: A meta-analysis of the effects of various interventions in preventing endotracheal suction-induced hypoxia, *J Clin Nurs* 12:912, 2003.

*53. Akgul S, Akyolcu N: Effects of normal saline on endotracheal suctioning, *J Clin Nurs* 11:826, 2002.

54. Ridling DA, Martin LD: Endotracheal suctioning with or without instillation of isotonic chloride solution in critically ill children, *Am J Crit Care* 12:212, 2003.

*55. Lusk B, Lash AA: The stress response. Psychoneuroimmunology and stress among ICU patients, *DCCN* 24:25, 2005.

*56. Thomas LA: Clinical management of stressors perceived by patients on mechanical ventilation, *AACN Clin Issues* 14:73, 2003.

*57. Happ MB: Communicating with mechanically ventilated patients: state of the science, *AACN Clin Issues* 12:247, 2001.

58. Happ MB, Tuite P, Dobbin K, et al: Communication ability, method, and content among nonspeaking nonsurviving patients treated with mechanical ventilation in the intensive care unit, *Am J Crit Care* 13:210, 2004.

59. Burns SM: Ventilatory management—volume and pressure modes. In Wiegand DL, Carlson KK, editors: *AACN procedure manual for critical care,* ed 5, St Louis, 2005, Elsevier Mosby.

60. American Association of Critical-Care Nurses: AACN practice alert: ventilator-associated pneumonia. Available at *www.aacn.org/AACN/practiceAlert.nsf/Files/VAP%20PDF/$file/Ventilator%20Associated%20Pneumonia.pdf* (accessed December 4, 2006).

61. Todisco T, Baglioni S, Eslami A, et al: Treatment of acute exacerbations of chronic respiratory failure: integrated use of negative pressure ventilation and noninvasive positive pressure ventilation, *Chest* 125:2217, 2004.

62. Pierce LN: Traditional and nontraditional modes of mechanical ventilation, *Crit Care Nurs* 22:56, 2002.

63. Fenstermacher D, Hong D: Mechanical ventilation—what have we learned? *Crit Care Nurs Q* 27:157, 2004.

64. Collective Task Force, American College of Chest Physicians, American Association of Respiratory Care, American College of Critical Care: Evidence-based guidelines for weaning and discontinuing ventilatory support, *Chest* 120:375S, 2001.

65. Burns SM: Auto-PEEP calculation. In Wiegand DL, Carlson KK, editors: *AACN procedure manual for critical care,* ed 5, St Louis, 2005, Elsevier Mosby.

66. Majid A, Hill NS: Noninvasive ventilation for acute respiratory failure, *Curr Opin Crit Care* 11:77, 2005.

67. Burns SM: Mechanical ventilation of patients with acute respiratory distress syndrome and patients requiring weaning, *Crit Care Nurse* 25:14, 2005.

68. Davies MW, Fraser JF: Partial liquid ventilation for preventing death and morbidity in adults with acute lung injury and acute respiratory distress syndrome, *Cochrane Database of Systematic Reviews* 1, 2006.

69. Hart CM: Nitric oxide in adult lung disease, *Chest* 115:1407, 1999.

70. Qureshi MA, Shah NJ, Hemmen CW, et al: Exposure of intensive care unit nurses to nitric oxide and nitrogen dioxide during therapeutic use of inhaled nitric oxide in adults with acute respiratory distress syndrome, *Am J Crit Care* 12:2, 2003.

*71. Vollman K: Prone positioning in the patient who has acute respiratory distress syndrome: the art and the science, *Crit Care Nurs Clin North Am* 16:319, 2004.

*72. Gay SE, Ankney N, Cochran JB, et al: Critical care challenges in the adult ECMO patient, *DCCN* 24:157, 2005.

73. ARDS Clinical Trial Network, National Heart, Lung, and Blood Institute, National Institutes of Health: Effects of recruitment maneuvers in patients with acute lung injury and acute respiratory distress syndrome ventilated with high positive end-expiratory pressure, *Crit Care Med* 31:2592, 2003.

74. American Thoracic Society, Infectious Diseases Society of America: Guidelines for the management of adults with hospital-acquired, ventilator-associated, and healthcare-associated pneumonia, *Am J Respir Crit Care Med* 171:388, 2005.

75. Dezfulian C, Shojania K, Collard HR, et al: Subglottic secretion drainage for preventing ventilator-associated pneumonia: a meta-analysis, *Am J Med* 118:11, 2005.

76. Kim PW, Roghmann M, Perencevich E, et al: Rates of hand disinfection associated with glove use, patient isolation, and changes between exposure to various body site, *Am J Infect Control* 31:97, 2003.

*77. Metheny NA, Schalom M, Edwards SJ: Effect of gastrointestinal motility and feeding tube site on aspiration risk in critically ill patients: a review, *Heart Lung* 33:131, 2004.

*78. Hupcey JE: Feeling safe: the psychosocial needs of ICU patients, *J Nurs Scholarsh* 32:361, 2000.

79. Ely EW, Shintani A, Truman B, et al: Delirium as a predictor of mortality in mechanically ventilated patients in the intensive care unit, *JAMA* 291:1753, 2004.

80. Ely EW, Gautam S, Margolin R, et al: The impact of delirium in the intensive care unit on hospital length of stay, *Intens Care* 27:1892, 2001.

*81. Whetstone Foster JG: Peripheral nerve stimulators. In Wiegand DL, Carlson KK, editors: *AACN procedure manual for critical care,* ed 5, St Louis, 2005, Elsevier Mosby.

82. American Association of Critical-Care Nurses: AACN practice alert: verification of feeding tube placement. Available at *www.aacn.org/AACN/practiceAlert.nsf/Files/VOTP/$file/Verification%20of%20Feeding%20Tube%20Placement%2005-2005.pdf* (accessed December 4, 2006).

83. Burns SM: Weaning process. In Wiegand DL, Carlson KK, editors: *AACN procedure manual for critical care,* ed 5, St Louis, 2005, Elsevier Mosby.

84. Burns SM: Weaning criteria—negative pressure, spontaneous tidal volume, and vital capacity measurement. In Wiegand DL, Carlson KK, editors: *AACN procedure manual for critical care,* ed 5, St Louis, 2005, Elsevier Mosby.

85. Ecklund MM: Beyond the ICU, homecare management of patients receiving mechanical ventilation. In Burns SM, editor: *Protocols for practice: care of the mechanically ventilated patient,* ed 2, Sudbury, Mass, 2006, Jones & Bartlett.

RESOURCES

American Association of Critical Care Nurses (AACN)
800-899-2226 or 949-362-2000
www.aacn.org
Australian College of Critical Care Nurses (ACCCN)
800-357-968
www.acccn.com.au
Canadian Association of Critical Care Nurses (CACCN)
866-477-9077
www.caccn.ca
Society of Critical Care Medicine (SCCM)
847-827-6869
www.sccm.org

For additional Internet resources, see the website for this book at *http://evolve.elsevier.com/Lewis/medsurg.*

*Nursing research–based reference.

67

Nursing Management

Shock, Systemic Inflammatory Response Syndrome, and Multiple Organ Dysfunction Syndrome

Kathleen M. Geib

LEARNING OBJECTIVES

1. Define *shock.*
2. Differentiate the two major classifications of shock: low blood flow and maldistribution of blood flow.
3. Describe the pathophysiology and clinical manifestations of the different types of shock.
4. Compare and contrast the effects of shock, systemic inflammatory response syndrome, and multiple organ dysfunction syndrome on the major body systems.
5. Compare the collaborative care, drug therapy, and nursing management of patients with different types of shock.
6. Describe the nursing management of a patient experiencing multiple organ dysfunction syndrome.

KEY TERMS

anaphylactic shock, p. 1777
cardiogenic shock, p. 1773
hypovolemic shock, p. 1775
multiple organ dysfunction
   syndrome, p. 1794
neurogenic shock, p. 1777
sepsis, p. 1778
septic shock, p. 1778
shock, p. 1772
systemic inflammatory response
   syndrome, p. 1794

Electronic Resources

Supplemental content related to Chapter 67 can be found . . .

Companion CD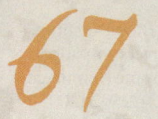
- Stress-Busting Kit for Nursing Students
- Interactive Case Study: Cardiogenic Shock
- NCLEX Examination Review Questions
- Comprehensive Glossary

Evolve Website *evolve*
http://evolve.elsevier.com/Lewis/medsurg
- Content Updates
- Key Points (Printable and CD/MP3 Download)
- Concept Map Creator
- Expanded Audio Glossary

- Key Term Flash Cards
- Customizable Nursing Care Plan:
  Shock
- Electronic Calculators
- WebLinks

Shock, systemic inflammatory response syndrome (SIRS), and multiple organ dysfunction syndrome (MODS) are serious and interrelated problems. Fig. 67-1 shows the relationship among shock, SIRS, and MODS. Shock is a complex process that often leads to the development of SIRS and MODS. This chapter provides an overview of shock, SIRS, and MODS.

SHOCK

Shock is a syndrome characterized by decreased tissue perfusion and impaired cellular metabolism. This results in an imbalance between the supply of and demand for oxygen and nutrients. The exchange of oxygen and nutrients at the cellular level is essential to life. When a cell experiences a state of hypoperfusion, the demand for oxygen and nutrients exceeds the supply.

Classification of Shock

Although the cause, initial presentation, and management strategies of the various types of shock differ, the physiologic responses of the cell to hypoperfusion are similar. For the purposes of discussion, shock will be classified as *low blood flow* (cardiogenic and

---

Reviewed by John J. Gallagher, RN, MSN, CCNS, CCRN, RRT, Clinical Nurse Specialist, Surgical Critical Care, Hospital of the University of Pennsylvania, Philadelphia, Pa.; and Anita K. Witzke, RN, CCRN, Nurse Manager/Operations Director of eCare Virtual ICU, Christiana Care Health Care System, Newark, Del.

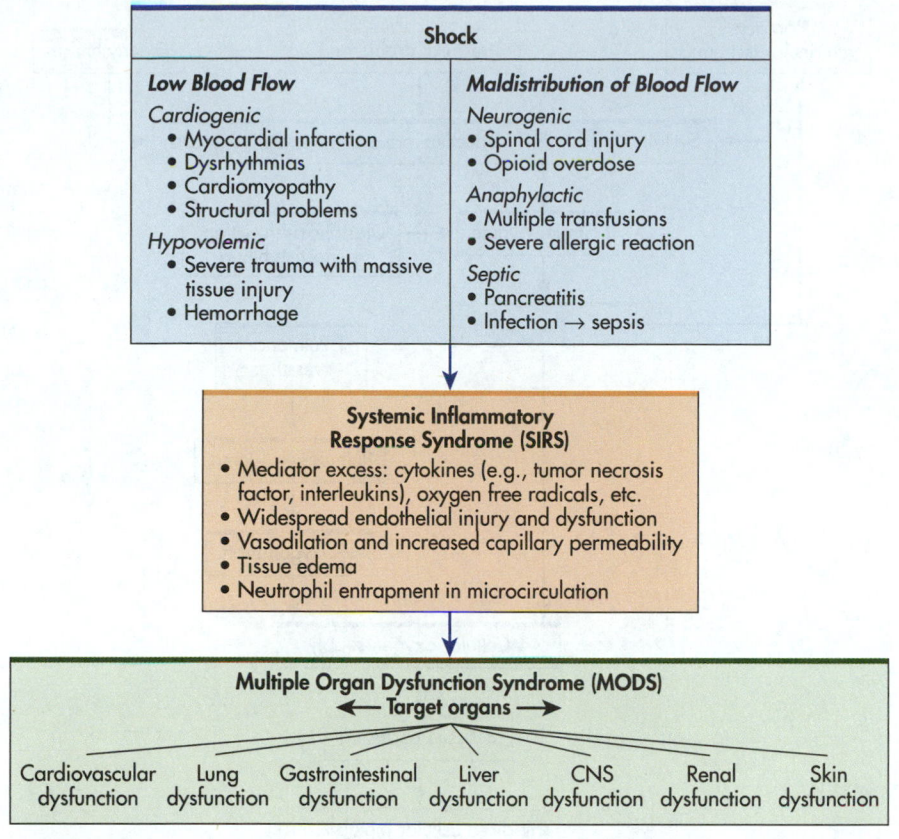

FIG. 67-1 Relationship of shock, systemic inflammatory response syndrome, and multiple organ dysfunction syndrome. *CNS,* Central nervous system.

TABLE 67-1	Classification and Precipitating Factors of Shock

Low Blood Flow	**Maldistribution of Blood Flow**
Cardiogenic Shock Systolic dysfunction: inability of the heart to pump blood forward (e.g., myocardial infarction, cardiomyopathy) Diastolic dysfunction: inability of the heart to fill during diastole (e.g., pericardial tamponade) Dysrhythmias (e.g., bradydysrhythmias, tachydysrhythmias) Structural factors: valvular abnormality (e.g., stenosis or regurgitation), ventricular septal rupture, tension pneumothorax **Hypovolemic Shock** *Absolute Hypovolemia* External loss of whole blood (e.g., hemorrhage from trauma, surgery, GI bleeding) Loss of other body fluids (e.g., vomiting, diarrhea, excessive diuresis, diabetes insipidus, diabetes mellitus) *Relative Hypovolemia* Pooling of blood or fluids (e.g., bowel obstruction) Fluid shifts (e.g., burn injuries, ascites) Internal bleeding (e.g., fracture of long bones, ruptured spleen, hemothorax, severe pancreatitis) Massive vasodilation (e.g., sepsis)	**Neurogenic Shock** Hemodynamic consequence of injury and/or disease to the spinal cord at or above T5 Spinal anesthesia Vasomotor center depression (e.g., severe pain, drugs, hypoglycemia, injury) **Anaphylactic Shock** Contrast media, blood/blood products, drugs, insect bites, anesthetic agents, food/food additives, vaccines, environmental agents, latex **Septic Shock** Infection (e.g., urinary tract, respiratory tract, invasive procedure, indwelling lines and catheters) At-risk patients: older adults, patients with chronic diseases (e.g., diabetes mellitus, chronic kidney disease, heart failure), patients receiving immunosuppressive therapy or who are malnourished or debilitated Gram-negative bacteria most common; also gram-positive bacteria, viruses, fungi, and parasites

GI, Gastrointestinal.

hypovolemic shock) or *maldistribution of blood flow* (septic, anaphylactic, and neurogenic shock)[1,2] (Table 67-1).

Low Blood Flow Shock

Cardiogenic Shock. Cardiogenic shock occurs when either systolic or diastolic dysfunction of the pumping action of the heart

results in compromised cardiac output (CO). The heart's inability to pump the blood forward is classified as *systolic dysfunction.* Systolic dysfunction primarily affects the left ventricle, because systolic pressure and tension are greater on the left side of the heart. When systolic dysfunction affects the right side of the heart,

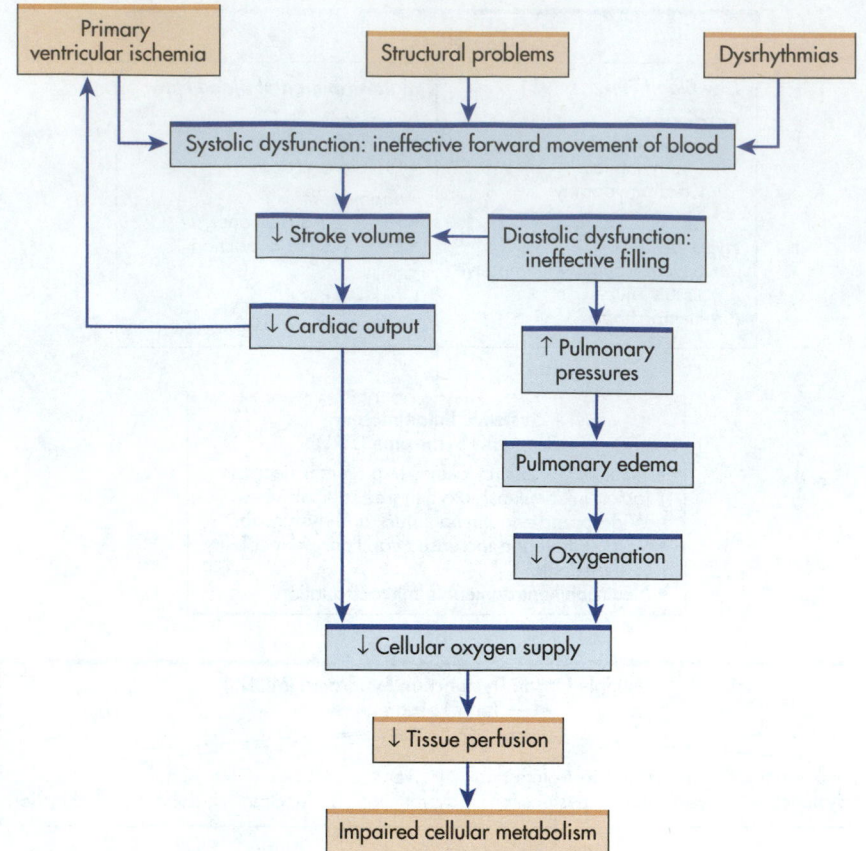

FIG. 67-2   The pathophysiology of cardiogenic shock.

TABLE 67-2	**Effects of Shock on Hemodynamic Parameters**									
Type	**HR**	**Pulse Pressure**	**BP**	**SVR**	**PVR**	**CVP**	**PAP**	**PAWP**	**CO**	**SvO₂/ScvO₂**
Low Blood Flow										
Cardiogenic shock	↑	↓	↓	↑	↑	~↑	↑	↑	↓	↓
Hypovolemic shock	↑	↓	↓	↑	↑	↓	↓	↓	↓	↓
Maldistribution of Blood Flow										
Neurogenic shock	↓	↓	↓	↓	~	↓	↓	↓	↓	↓
Anaphylactic shock	↑	↓	↓	↓	~↑	↓	↓	↓	↓	↓
Septic shock	↑	↓	↓	↓	~↑	↓	↑ ~ ↓	↓	↑ ~ ↓	↑ ~ ↓

NOTE: Hemodynamic effects in some illnesses are highly variable.

KEY: ↓, decrease; ↑, increase; ~, no change.

BP, Blood pressure; *CO,* cardiac output; *CVP,* central venous pressure; *HR,* heart rate; *PAP,* pulmonary artery pressure; *PAWP,* pulmonary artery wedge pressure; *PVR,* pulmonary vascular resistance; *SIRS,* systemic inflammatory response syndrome; *ScvO₂,* central venous oxygen saturation; *SvO₂,* mixed venous oxygen saturation; *SVR,* systemic vascular resistance.

blood flow through the pulmonary circulation is compromised. Precipitating causes of systolic dysfunction include myocardial infarction (MI), cardiomyopathies, blunt cardiac injury, severe systemic or pulmonary hypertension, and myocardial depression from metabolic problems. Despite treatment, mortality rates for patients with cardiogenic shock can range from 50% to 85%.[3] *Diastolic dysfunction* is an impaired ability of the right or left ventricle to fill during diastole. Decreased filling of the ventricle will result in decreased stroke volume. Precipitating causes of diastolic dysfunction include cardiac tamponade and cardiomyopathy (see Chapter 37).

Fig. 67-2 describes the pathophysiology of cardiogenic shock. Whether the initiating event is myocardial dysfunction, a structural problem (e.g., valvular abnormality, ventricular septal rupture, tension pneumothorax), or dysrhythmias, the physiologic responses

are similar. The patient experiences impaired tissue perfusion and impaired cellular metabolism because of cardiogenic shock.

The early clinical presentation of a patient with cardiogenic shock is similar to that of a patient with acute decompensated heart failure (see Chapter 35). The patient's response to low blood flow may include tachycardia, hypotension, and a narrowed pulse pressure. An increase in systemic vascular resistance (SVR) increases the workload of the heart, thus increasing the myocardial oxygen consumption. The heart's inability to pump blood forward will result in a low CO (less than 4 L/min) and *cardiac index* (less than 2.1 L/min/m²). On examination, the patient will be tachypneic and pulmonary congestion will be evident by the presence of crackles. The hemodynamic profile will demonstrate an increase in the pulmonary artery wedge pressure (PAWP) and pulmonary vascular resistance (Table 67-2). Signs of peripheral hypoperfusion (e.g.,

TABLE 67-3	*DIAGNOSTIC STUDIES* Laboratory Abnormalities in Shock	

Laboratory Study	Finding	Significance of Finding
Blood		
Red blood cell count, hematocrit, hemoglobin	Normal	Remains within normal limits in shock because of relative hypovolemia and pump failure and in hemorrhagic shock before fluid resuscitation
	Decreased	Decreases in hemorrhagic shock after fluid resuscitation when fluids other than blood are used
	Increased	Increases in nonhemorrhagic shock due to actual hypovolemia because fluid lost does not contain erythrocytes
DIC screen		Acute DIC can develop within hours to days after an initial assault on the body (e.g., shock)
• Fibrin split products (FSP)	Increased	
• Fibrinogen level	Decreased	
• Platelet count	Decreased	
• PTT and PT/INR	Prolonged	
• Thrombin time	Increased	
• D-dimer	Increased	
Creatine kinase	Increased	Increases in trauma, myocardial infarction in response to cellular damage and/or hypoxia
Troponin	Increased	Increases in myocardial infarction
BUN	Increased	Indicates impaired kidney function due to hypoperfusion as a result of severe vasoconstriction or occurs secondary to catabolism of cells (e.g., trauma, infection)
Creatinine	Increased	Indicates impaired kidney function due to hypoperfusion as a result of severe vasoconstriction; is more sensitive indicator of renal function than BUN
Glucose	Increased	Found in early shock because of release of liver glycogen stores in response to sympathetic nervous system stimulation and cortisol; insulin insensitivity develops
	Decreased	Occurs because of depleted glycogen stores with hepatocellular dysfunction possible as shock progresses
Serum Electrolytes		
Sodium	Increased	Found in early shock because of increased secretion of aldosterone, causing renal retention of sodium
	Decreased	May occur iatrogenically when excess hypotonic fluid is administered after fluid loss
Potassium	Increased	Results when cellular death liberates intracellular potassium; also occurs in acute renal failure and in the presence of acidosis
	Decreased	Found in early shock because of increased secretion of aldosterone, causing renal excretion of potassium
Arterial blood gases	Respiratory alkalosis	Found in early shock secondary to hyperventilation
	Metabolic acidosis	Occurs later in shock when organic acids, such as lactic acid, accumulate in blood from anaerobic metabolism
Base deficit	>−6	Indicates acid production secondary to hypoxia
Blood cultures	Growth of organisms	May grow organisms in patients who are in septic shock
Lactic acid	Increased	Usually increases once significant hypoperfusion and impaired oxygen utilization at the cellular level have occurred; by-product of anaerobic metabolism
Liver enzymes (ALT, AST, GGT)	Increased	Elevations indicate liver cell destruction in progressive stage of shock
Urine		
Specific gravity	Increased	Occurs secondary to the action of ADH
	Fixed at 1.010	Occurs in renal failure

ADH, Antidiuretic hormone; *ALT,* alanine aminotransferase; *AST,* aspartate aminotransferase; *BUN,* blood urea nitrogen; *DIC,* disseminated intravascular coagulation; *GGT,* γ-glutamyl transferase; *INR,* international normalized ratio; *PT,* prothrombin time; *PTT,* partial thromboplastin time.

cyanosis, pallor, cool and clammy skin, decreased capillary refill time) will be apparent. Decreased renal blood flow will result in sodium and water retention and decreased urine output. Anxiety, confusion, and agitation may develop as cerebral perfusion is impaired. Studies that may be helpful in diagnosing cardiogenic shock include laboratory studies (e.g., cardiac enzymes, troponin levels), electrocardiogram (ECG), chest x-ray, and echocardiogram (Table 67-3). The overall clinical presentation of a patient with cardiogenic shock is presented in Table 67-4.

Hypovolemic Shock. The second type of low blood flow shock is hypovolemic shock. **Hypovolemic shock** occurs when there is a loss of intravascular fluid volume. In hypovolemic shock, the volume is inadequate to fill the vascular space. The volume loss may be either an absolute or a relative volume loss. **Absolute hypovolemia** results when fluid is lost through hemorrhage, gastrointestinal (GI) loss (e.g., vomiting, diarrhea), fistula drainage, diabetes insipidus, hyperglycemia, or diuresis. In **relative hypovolemia,** fluid volume moves out of the vascular space into the extravascular space (e.g., interstitial or intracavitary space). This type of fluid shift is called *third spacing.* One example of relative volume loss is leakage of fluid from the vascular space to the interstitial space from increased capillary permeability, as seen in sepsis. Table 67-1 provides examples of low blood flow shock such as confinement of fluid into the colon from a bowel obstruction, ascites, loss of blood

Shock and MODS

TABLE 67-4   Clinical Presentation of the Major Types of Shock

	Low Blood Flow		Maldistribution of Blood Flow		
	Cardiogenic Shock	**Hypovolemic Shock**	**Neurogenic Shock**	**Anaphylactic Shock**	**Septic Shock**
Cardiovascular (see Table 67-2 for complete hemodynamic profile)	↓ Capillary refill time ↑ MVO₂ Chest pain may or may not be present	↓ Preload ↓ Stroke volume ↓ Capillary refill time	↓/↑ Temperature Bradycardia	Chest pain Third spacing of fluid	↓/↑ Temperature Biventricular dilation: ↓ ejection fraction
Pulmonary	Tachypnea Cyanosis Crackles Rhonchi	Tachypnea → brady-pnea (late)	Dysfunction related to level of injury	Swelling of lips and tongue Shortness of breath Edema of larynx and epiglottis Wheezing Rhinitis Stridor	Hyperventilation Respiratory alkalosis → respiratory acidosis Hypoxemia Respiratory failure ARDS Pulmonary hypertension Crackles ↓ Urine output
Renal	↑ Na⁺ and H₂O retention ↓ Renal blood flow ↓ Urine output	↓ Urine output	Bladder dysfunction		↓ Urine output
Skin	Pallor Cool, clammy	Pallor Cool, clammy	↓ Skin perfusion Cool or warm Dry	Flushing Pruritus Urticaria Angioedema	Warm and flushed → cool and mottled (late)
Neurologic	↓ Cerebral perfusion: anxiety, confusion, agitation	Anxiety Confusion Agitation	Flaccid paralysis below the level of the lesion Loss of reflex activity	Anxiety Feeling of impending doom Confusion ↓ LOC Metallic taste	Alteration in mental status (e.g., confusion) Agitation Coma (late)
Gastrointestinal	↓ Bowel sounds Nausea/vomiting	Absent bowel sounds	Bowel dysfunction	Cramping Abdominal pain Nausea Vomiting Diarrhea	GI bleeding Paralytic ileus
Diagnostic findings (also see Table 67-3)	↑ Cardiac markers ↑ Blood glucose ↑ BUN ECG (e.g., dysrhythmias) Echocardiogram (e.g., left ventricular dysfunction) Chest x-ray (e.g., pulmonary infiltrates)	↓ Hematocrit ↓ Hemoglobin ↑ Lactate ↑ Urine specific gravity Changes in electrolytes		Sudden onset History of allergies Exposure to contrast media	↑/↓ WBC ↓ Platelets ↑ Lactate ↑ Glucose ↑ Urine specific gravity ↓ Urine Na⁺ Positive blood cultures

ARDS, Acute respiratory distress syndrome; *BUN,* blood urea nitrogen; *ECG,* electrocardiogram; *GI,* gastrointestinal; *LOC,* level of consciousness; *MVO₂,* myocardial oxygen consumption; *WBC,* white blood cell.

volume into a fracture site (e.g., pelvic fracture), and burns (see Chapter 25).

In hypovolemic shock, the size of the vascular compartment remains unchanged while the volume of blood or plasma decreases. Whether the loss of intravascular volume is absolute or relative, the physiologic consequences are similar. A reduction in intravascular volume results in a decreased venous return to the heart, decreased preload, decreased stroke volume, and decreased CO (see Table 67-2). A cascade of events results in decreased tissue perfusion and impaired cellular metabolism, the hallmarks of shock (Fig. 67-3).

The patient's response to low blood flow due to acute volume loss is dependent on a number of factors, including extent of injury or insult, age, and general state of health. However, the clinical presentation of hypovolemic shock will be similar (see Table

67-4). An overall assessment of physiologic reserves may indicate the patient's ability to compensate. A patient may compensate for a loss of up to 15% of the total blood volume (approximately 750 ml). Further loss of volume (15% to 30%) will result in a sympathetic nervous system (SNS)–mediated response. This response results in an increase in heart rate, CO, and respiratory rate and depth. The stroke volume and PAWP are decreased because of the decreased circulating blood volume. The patient may appear anxious and urine output will begin to decrease. If hypovolemia is corrected by crystalloid fluid replacement at this time, tissue dysfunction is generally reversible. If volume loss is greater than 30%, compensatory mechanisms may begin to fail and immediate replacement with blood or blood products should be initiated. Loss of autoregulation in the microcirculation and irreversible tissue destruction occurs with loss of more than 40%

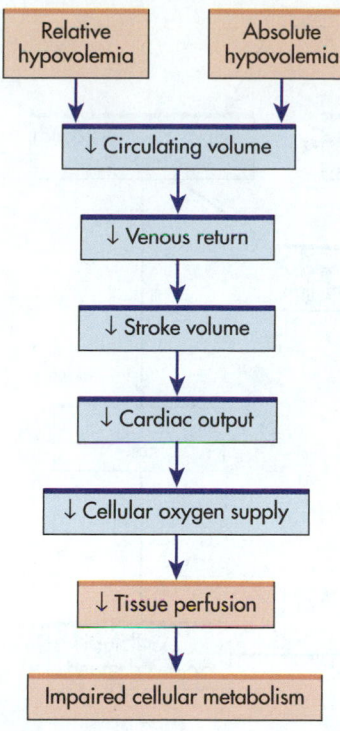

FIG. 67-3   The pathophysiology of hypovolemic shock.

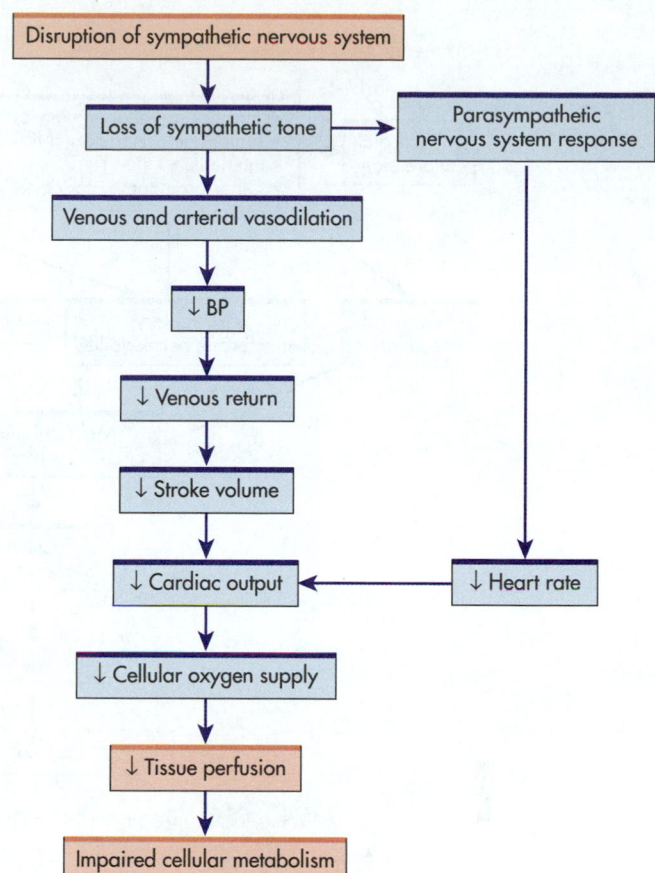

FIG. 67-4   The pathophysiology of neurogenic shock. *BP,* Blood pressure.

of the total blood volume.[4-6] Laboratory studies that may be done include measurements of serial hemoglobin and hematocrit levels, urine specific gravity, serum electrolytes, blood gases, and lactic acid (see Table 67-3).

Maldistribution of Blood Flow Shock

Neurogenic Shock. Neurogenic shock is a hemodynamic phenomenon that can occur within 30 minutes of a spinal cord injury at the fifth thoracic (T5) vertebra or above and last up to 6 weeks. The injury results in a massive vasodilation without compensation due to the loss of SNS vasoconstrictor tone. This massive vasodilation leads to a pooling of blood in the blood vessels, tissue hypoperfusion, and ultimately impaired cellular metabolism (Fig. 67-4).

In addition to spinal cord injury, spinal anesthesia can block transmission of impulses from the SNS. Depression of the vasomotor center of the medulla from drugs (e.g., benzodiazepines, opioids) also can result in decreased vasoconstrictor tone of the peripheral blood vessels, resulting in neurogenic shock (see Table 67-1).

The most important clinical manifestations in neurogenic shock are hypotension (from the massive vasodilation) and bradycardia (from unopposed parasympathetic stimulation).[7] The patient in neurogenic shock may have an inability to regulate temperature. The inability to regulate temperature, combined with massive vasodilation, promotes heat loss. Initially, the patient's skin will be warm due to the massive dilation without compensation. As the heat dissipates, the patient is at risk for hypothermia. Later, the patient's skin may be cool or warm depending on the ambient temperature (*poikilothermia*—taking on the temperature of the environment). In either case, the skin will usually be dry. Tables 67-2, 67-3, and 67-4 further describe the clinical presentation of a patient with neurogenic shock.

Although spinal shock and neurogenic shock often occur in the same patient, they are not the same disorder. *Spinal shock* is a transient condition that is present after an acute spinal cord injury

(see Chapter 61). The patient with spinal shock will experience the absence of all voluntary and reflex neurologic activity below the level of the injury.[7]

Anaphylactic Shock. Anaphylactic shock is an acute and life-threatening hypersensitivity (allergic) reaction to a sensitizing substance (e.g., drug, chemical, vaccine, food, insect venom). Usually an immediate reaction causes massive vasodilation, release of vasoactive mediators, and an increase in capillary permeability. As capillary permeability increases, fluid leaks from the vascular space into the interstitial space. Anaphylactic shock can lead to respiratory distress, because of laryngeal edema or severe bronchospasm, and circulatory failure, because of massive vasodilation.[8] The patient experiences a sudden onset of symptoms, including dizziness, chest pain, incontinence, swelling of the lips and tongue, wheezing, and stridor. Skin changes include flushing, pruritus, urticaria, and angioedema.[9] In addition, the patient may become very anxious and confused and feel an impending sense of doom.

A patient can develop a severe allergic reaction, possibly leading to anaphylactic shock, after contact, inhalation, ingestion, or injection with an antigen (allergen) to which the person has previously been sensitized (see Table 67-1). Parenteral administration of the antigen (allergen) is the route most likely to cause anaphylaxis. However, oral, topical, and inhalation routes can also cause anaphylactic reactions. Tables 67-2, 67-3, and 67-4 describe the clinical presentation of a patient in anaphylactic shock. Quick and decisive action by the nurse is critical to preventing the progression of an anaphylactic reaction to anaphylactic shock. (Anaphylaxis is discussed in Chapter 14.)

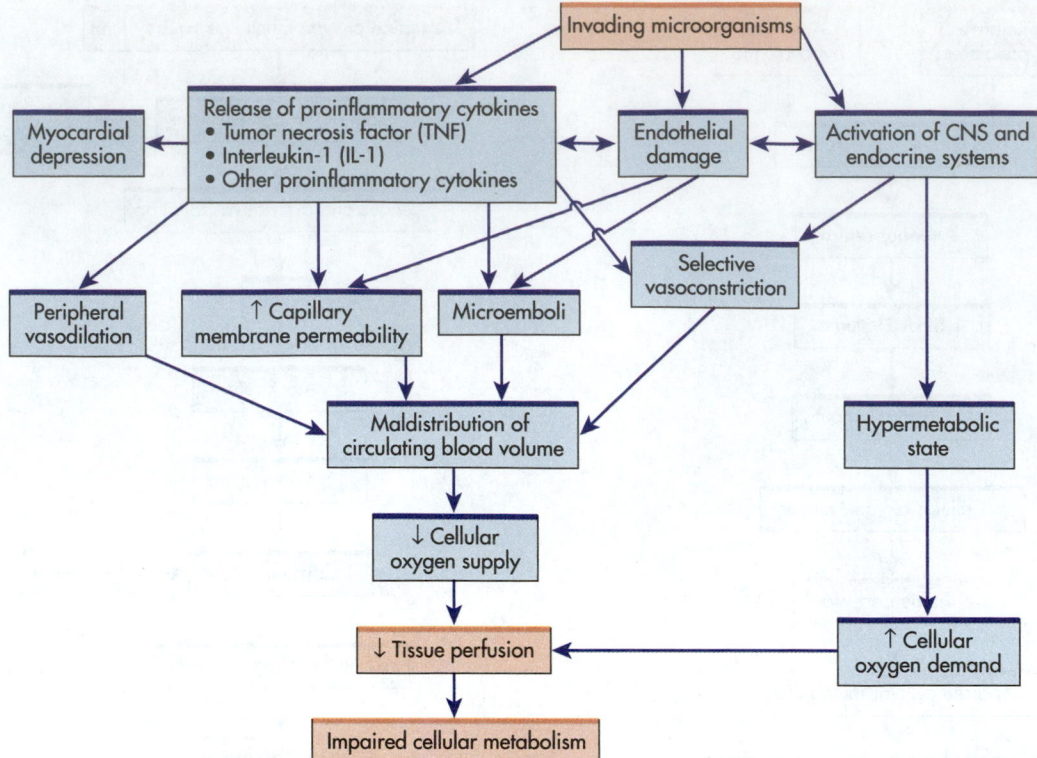

FIG. 67-5   The pathophysiology of septic shock. *CNS,* Central nervous system.

Septic Shock. Sepsis is a systemic inflammatory response to a documented or suspected infection.[10] In as many as 10% to 30% of patients with sepsis, the causative organism is not identified. *Severe sepsis,* defined as sepsis complicated by organ dysfunction, is diagnosed in more than 750,000 patients per year and has mortality rates as high as 28% to 50%.[10-12] **Septic shock** is the presence of sepsis with hypotension despite fluid resuscitation along with the presence of tissue perfusion abnormalities. Thus managing the patient with sepsis and septic shock is a challenge for the entire health care team. The primary organisms that cause sepsis are gram-negative and gram-positive bacteria. The morbidity and mortality rates from infections with gram-negative organisms are greater than those from gram-positive organisms. Parasites, fungi, and viruses can also lead to the development of sepsis and septic shock.[13,14] The pathogenesis of septic shock is complex (Fig. 67-5).

When an antigen (microorganism) enters the body the normal immune/inflammatory cascade responses are initiated and work together to destroy the antigen. However, in severe sepsis and septic shock the initiated body response to an antigen is exaggerated. There is an increase in inflammation and coagulation, and a decrease in fibrinolysis. Endotoxins from the microorganism cell wall stimulate the release of cytokines, including tumor necrosis factor (TNF), interleukin-1 (IL-1), and other proinflammatory mediators that act through secondary mediators such as platelet-activating factor, IL-6, and IL-8.[2,12-15] (See Chapter 13 for discussion of the inflammatory response.) The release of platelet activating factor results in the formation of microthrombi and obstruction of the microvasculature. The combined effects of the mediators result in damage to the endothelium, vasodilation, increased capillary permeability, and neutrophil and platelet aggregation and adhesion to the endothelium.

The clinical presentation of sepsis is complex, and no single symptom or group of symptoms is specific to the diagnosis[10] (Ta-

ble 67-5). Patients will usually experience an initial hyperdynamic state characterized by increased CO and decreased SVR.[16] Despite this, the combination of TNF and IL-1 is thought to have a role in sepsis-induced myocardial dysfunction. The ejection fraction is decreased for the first few days after the initial insult. Because of a decreased ejection fraction, the ventricles will dilate in order to maintain the stroke volume. The ejection fraction typically improves and the ventricular dilation resolves over 7 to 10 days. Persistence of a high CO and a low SVR beyond 24 hours is an ominous finding and is often associated with an increased development of hypotension and MODS. Coronary artery perfusion and myocardial oxygen metabolism are not primarily altered in septic shock.[16]

In addition to the cardiovascular dysfunction that accompanies sepsis, respiratory failure is common. The patient will initially hyperventilate as a compensatory mechanism, resulting in respiratory alkalosis. Once the patient can no longer compensate, respiratory acidosis will develop. Respiratory failure will develop in 85% of patients with sepsis, and 40% will develop acute respiratory distress syndrome (ARDS). Other clinical signs of septic shock include alteration in neurologic status, decreased urine output, and GI dysfunction, such as GI bleeding and paralytic ileus. Tables 67-2 and 67-4 further delineate the clinical presentation of a patient with septic shock.

Stages of Shock

In addition to understanding the underlying pathogenesis of the type of shock the patient is experiencing, monitoring and management are also guided by knowing where the patient is on the shock "continuum." This continuum begins with the initial stage of shock that occurs at a cellular level and is usually not clinically apparent. Metabolism changes at the cellular level from aerobic to anaerobic, causing lactic acid buildup. Lactic acid is a waste product and

TABLE 67-5 Diagnostic Criteria for Sepsis

Infection, documented or suspected, and some of the following:

General Variables
- Fever (core temperature >100.9° F [38.3° C])
- Hypothermia (core temperature <97.0° F [36° C])
- Heart rate >90 beats/min
- Tachypnea
- Altered mental status
- Significant edema or positive fluid balance (>20 ml/kg over 24 hr)
- Hyperglycemia (blood glucose >120 mg/dl) in the absence of diabetes

Inflammatory Variables
- Leukocytosis (WBC count >12,000 cells/μl)
- Leukopenia (WBC count <4000 cells/μl)
- Normal WBC count with >10% immature forms
- Elevated C-reactive protein

Hemodynamic Variables
- Arterial hypotension (SBP <90 mm Hg, MAP <70, or a decrease in SBP of >40 mm Hg)
- SvO_2 >70%
- Cardiac index >3.5 L/min/m²

Organ Dysfunction Variables
- Arterial hypoxemia (PaO_2/FIO_2 <300)
- Acute oliguria (urine output <0.5 ml/kg/hr for at least 2 hr)
- Coagulation abnormalities (INR >1.5 or PTT >60 sec)
- Paralytic ileus (absent bowel sounds)
- Hyperbilirubinemia (total bilirubin >4 mg/dl)

Tissue Perfusion Variables
- Hyperlactatemia (>1 mmol/L)
- Decreased capillary refill or mottling

Source: Levy MM et al: 2001 SCCM/ESICM/ACCP/ATS/SIS International Sepsis Definitions Conference, *Crit Care Med* 31:1250, 2003. Used with permission. *INR,* International normalized ratio; *MAP,* mean arterial pressure; *PTT,* partial thromboplastin time; *SBP,* systolic blood pressure; *SvO2,* mixed venous oxygen saturation; *WBC,* white blood cell.

must be removed by the liver. However, this process requires oxygen, which is unavailable because of the decrease in tissue perfusion. Shock can be categorized into three clinically apparent but overlapping stages: the compensatory stage, the progressive stage, and the refractory (irreversible) stage.[5,17]

Compensatory Stage. In the *compensatory stage,* the body activates neural, hormonal, and biochemical compensatory mechanisms in an attempt to overcome the increasing consequences of anaerobic metabolism and to maintain homeostasis (Fig. 67-6). The patient's clinical presentation begins to reflect the body's responses to the imbalance in oxygen supply and demand (Table 67-6).

One of the first clinical signs of shock may be a fall in blood pressure (BP), which occurs because of a decrease in CO and a narrowing of the pulse pressure. The baroreceptors in the carotid and aortic bodies immediately respond by activating the SNS. The SNS stimulates vasoconstriction and the release of the potent vasoconstrictors epinephrine and norepinephrine. Blood flow to the most essential (vital) organs, the heart and the brain, is maintained, while blood flow to the nonvital organs, such as the kidneys, GI tract, skin, and lungs, is diverted or shunted.[5,17]

Decreased blood flow to the kidneys activates the renin-angiotensin system. Renin is released, which activates angiotensinogen to produce angiotensin I, which is then converted to angiotensin II (see Chapter 45, Fig. 45-4). Angiotensin II is a potent

vasoconstrictor that causes both arterial and venous vasoconstriction. The net result is an increase in venous return to the heart and an increase in BP. Angiotensin II also stimulates the adrenal cortex to release aldosterone, which results in sodium and water reabsorption, and potassium excretion by the kidneys. The increase in sodium reabsorption raises the serum osmolality and stimulates the release of antidiuretic hormone (ADH) from the posterior pituitary gland. ADH works by increasing water reabsorption by the kidneys, thus further increasing blood volume. The increase in total circulating volume results in an increase in CO and BP.[5,17]

The shunting of blood from other organ systems also results in clinically important changes. The decrease in blood flow to the GI tract results in impaired motility and a slowing of peristalsis, thus increasing the risk for the development of a paralytic ileus. Decreased blood flow to the skin results in the patient feeling cool and clammy. The exception is the patient in early septic shock who will feel warm and flushed due to a hyperdynamic state.[16]

Shunting blood away from the lungs has an important clinical effect in the patient in shock. Decreased blood flow to the lungs increases the patient's physiologic dead space. *Physiologic dead space* is the anatomic dead space (the amount of air that will not reach gas-exchanging units) and any inspired air that cannot participate in gas exchange. The clinical result of an increase in dead space ventilation is a *ventilation-perfusion mismatch.* There will be areas of the lungs participating in ventilation that will not be perfused because of the decreased blood flow to the lungs. Arterial oxygen levels will decrease, and the patient will have a compensatory increase in the rate and depth of respirations.

The myocardium responds to the SNS stimulation and the increase in oxygen demand by increasing the heart rate and contractility.[17] However, increased contractility increases myocardial oxygen consumption (MVO_2). The coronary arteries dilate in an attempt to meet the increased oxygen demands of the myocardium.

A multisystem response to decreasing tissue perfusion is initiated in the compensatory stage of shock. At this stage, the body is able to compensate for the changes in tissue perfusion. If the perfusion deficit (the cause of the shock) is corrected, the patient will recover with little or no residual aftereffects. If the perfusion deficit is not corrected and the body is unable to compensate, the patient enters the progressive stage of shock.

Progressive Stage. The *progressive stage* of shock begins as compensatory mechanisms fail (Fig. 67-7). In this stage, aggressive interventions are necessary to prevent the development of MODS. Continued decreased cellular perfusion and resulting altered capillary permeability are the distinguishing features of this stage. Altered capillary permeability allows leakage of fluid and protein out of the vascular space into the surrounding interstitial space. In addition to the decrease in circulating volume, there is an increase in systemic interstitial edema. The patient may have *anasarca,* or diffuse profound edema. Fluid leakage from the vascular space also affects the solid organs (e.g., liver, spleen, GI tract, lungs) and peripheral tissues by further decreasing perfusion.

The pulmonary system is often the first system to display signs of critical dysfunction. During the compensatory stage, blood flow to the lungs is already reduced. In response to the decreased blood flow and the SNS stimulation, the pulmonary arterioles constrict, resulting in increased pulmonary artery (PA) pressure. As the pressure within the pulmonary vasculature increases, blood flow to the pulmonary capillaries decreases and ventilation-perfusion mismatch worsens. Another key response in the lungs is the movement of fluid from the pulmonary vasculature into the interstitial space.

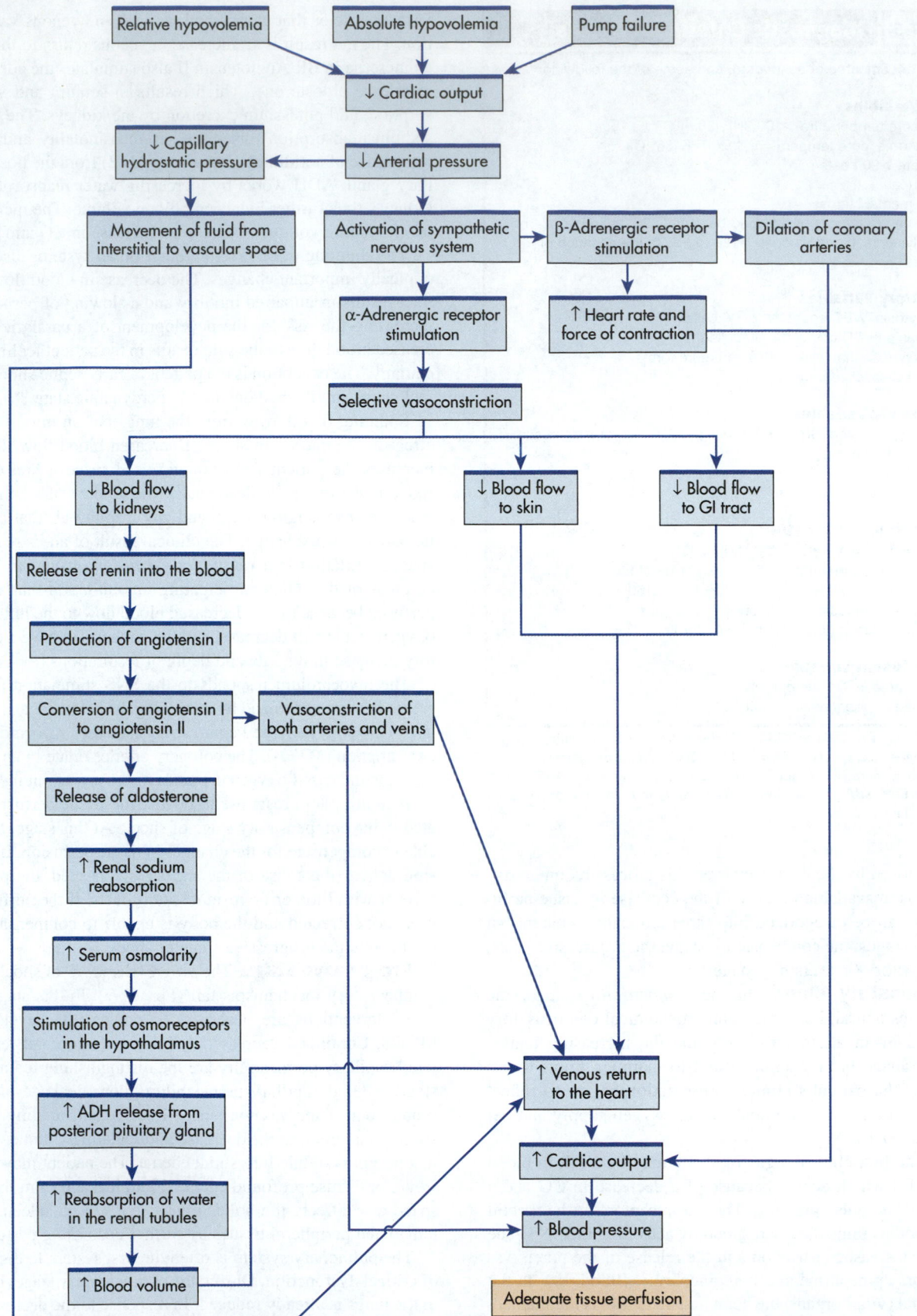

FIG. 67-6   Compensated stage: reversible stage during which compensatory mechanisms are effective and homeostasis is maintained.

TABLE 67-6	Clinical Manifestations of the Stages of Shock		
System	**Compensatory Stage**	**Progressive Stage**	**Refractory Stage**
Neurologic	Oriented to person, place, time Restless, apprehensive, confused Change in level of consciousness	↓ Cerebral perfusion pressure ↓ Cerebral blood flow Listless or agitated ↓ Responsiveness to stimuli	Unresponsive Areflexia (loss of reflexes) Pupils unreactive and dilated
Cardiovascular	Sympathetic nervous system response: Release of epinephrine/norepinephrine, which promotes vasoconstriction ↑ MVO_2 ↑ Contractility ↑ HR Coronary artery dilation Narrowed pulse pressure BP adequate to perfuse vital organs (heart, brain)	Loss of autoregulation in microcirculation ↑ Capillary permeability → systemic interstitial edema ↓ Cardiac output → ↓ BP and ↑ HR MAP <60 mm Hg (or 40 mm Hg drop in BP from baseline) ↓ Coronary perfusion → • Dysrhythmias • Myocardial ischemia • Myocardial infarction • Myocardial dysfunction → impaired cardiac output ↓ Peripheral perfusion → ischemia of distal extremities, diminished pulses, ↓ capillary refill	Profound hypotension ↓ Cardiac output Bradycardia; irregular rhythm ↓ BP inadequate to perfuse vital organs
Respiratory	↓ Blood flow to the lungs • ↑ Physiologic dead space • ↑ Ventilation-perfusion mismatch • Hyperventilation • ↑ Minute ventilation (V_E)	Acute respiratory distress syndrome (ARDS) • ↑ Capillary permeability • Pulmonary vasoconstriction • Pulmonary interstitial edema • Alveolar edema • Diffuse infiltrates • ↑ Respiratory rate • ↓ Compliance Moist crackles	Severe refractory hypoxemia Respiratory failure
Gastrointestinal	↓ Blood supply Hypoactive bowel sounds	Vasoconstriction and ↓ perfusion → ischemic gut (e.g., stomach, small and large intestines, gallbladder, pancreas) • Erosive ulcers • GI bleeding • Translocation of GI bacteria • Impaired absorption of nutrients	Ischemic gut
Renal	↓ Renal blood flow ↑ Renin resulting in release of angiotensin (vasoconstrictor) ↑ Aldosterone resulting in Na^+ and H_2O reabsorption ↑ Antidiuretic hormone resulting in H_2O reabsorption	Renal tubules become ischemic → acute tubular necrosis ↓ Urine output ↑ BUN/creatinine ratio ↑ Urine sodium ↓ Urine osmolarity and specific gravity ↓ Urine potassium Metabolic acidosis	Anuria
Hepatic		Failure to metabolize drugs and waste products Jaundice (decreased clearance of bilirubin) ↑ NH_3 and lactate	Metabolic changes from accumulation of waste products (e.g., NH_3, lactate, CO_2)
Hematologic		DIC • Thrombin clots in microcirculation • Consumption of clots in microcirculation	DIC
Temperature	Normal or abnormal	Hypothermia Sepsis: hypothermia or hyperthermia	Hypothermia
Skin	Pale and cool Warm and flushed (early onset of septic shock)	Cold and clammy	Mottled, cyanotic
Key laboratory findings	↑ Blood glucose ↑ pH ↓ PaO_2 ↓ $PaCO_2$	↑ Liver enzymes: ALT, AST, GGT ↑ Bleeding times Thrombocytopenia	↓ Blood glucose ↑ NH_3, lactate, and K^+ Metabolic acidosis

ALT, Alanine aminotransferase; *AST,* aspartate aminotransferase; *BUN,* blood urea nitrogen; *DIC,* disseminated intravascular coagulation; *GGT,* γ-glutamyl transferase; *GI,* gastrointestinal; *HR,* heart rate; *MAP,* mean arterial pressure; *MVO₂,* myocardial oxygen consumption; *Na⁺,* sodium ions.

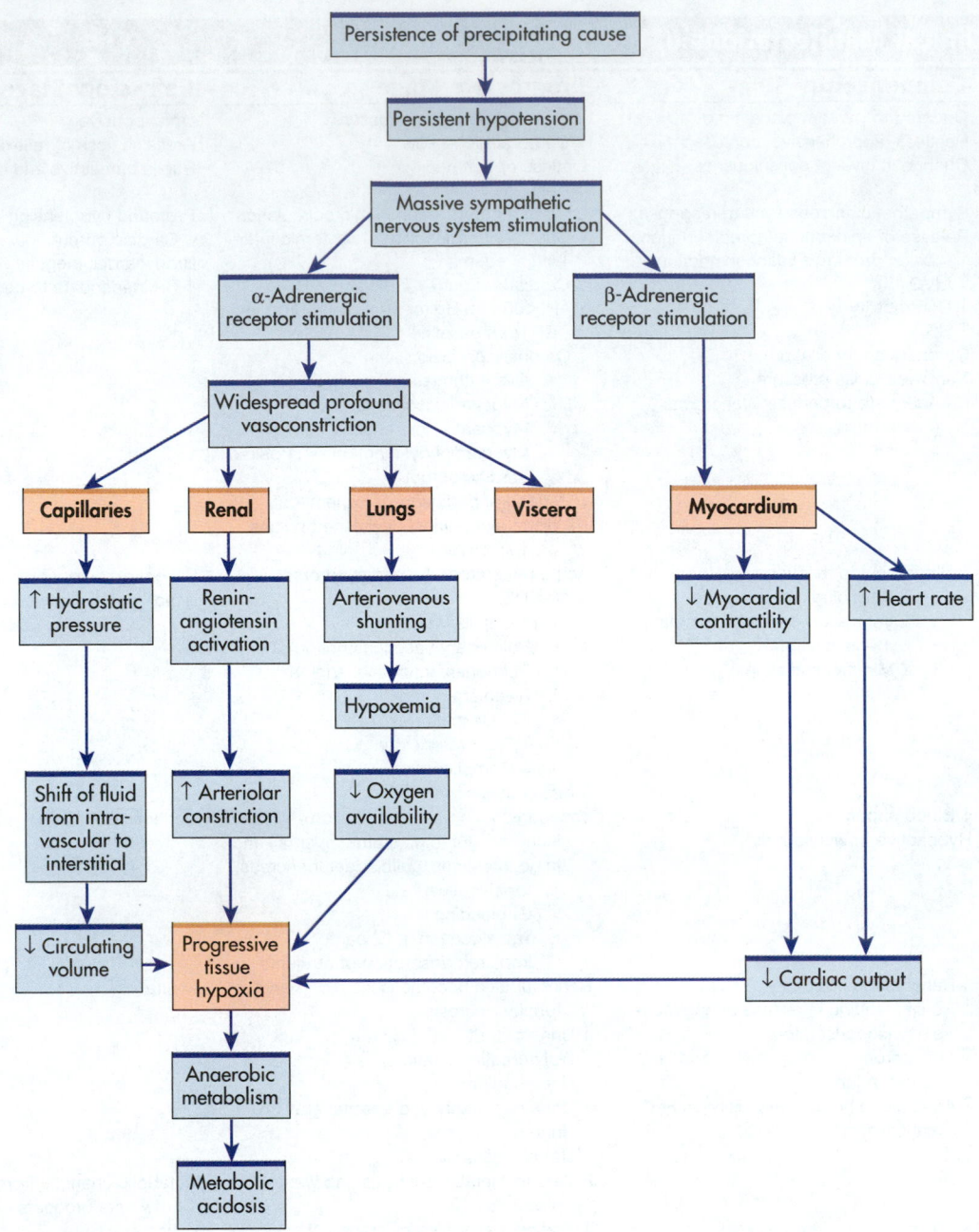

FIG. 67-7   Progressive stage: compensatory mechanisms are becoming ineffective and fail to maintain perfusion to vital organs.

As capillary permeability increases, the movement of fluid to the interstitial spaces results in interstitial edema, bronchoconstriction, and a decrease in functional residual capacity. With further increases in capillary permeability the fluid moves to the alveoli, with resultant alveolar edema and a decrease in surfactant production. The combined effects of pulmonary vasoconstriction and bronchoconstriction are impaired gas exchange, decreased compliance, and worsening ventilation-perfusion mismatch. Clinically, the patient has tachypnea, crackles, and an overall increased work of breathing.

The cardiovascular system is profoundly affected in the progressive stage of shock. CO begins to fall, with a resultant decrease in BP and coronary artery, cerebral, and peripheral perfusion. Changes in the patient's mental status are important findings in this stage. Capillary permeability continues to increase, enhancing the

movement of fluid from the vascular space into the interstitial space. Sustained hypoperfusion results in weak peripheral pulses, and ischemia of the distal extremities eventually occurs. Myocardial dysfunction from decreased perfusion results in dysrhythmias, myocardial ischemia, and potentially MI. The end result is a complete deterioration of the cardiovascular system.

The effect of prolonged hypoperfusion on the kidneys is renal tubular ischemia. The resulting acute tubular necrosis (ATN) may lead to the development of acute renal failure, which can be worsened by nephrotoxic drugs, including certain antibiotics, anesthetics, and diuretics (see Chapter 47). Renal function is markedly impaired during the progressive stage of shock. The patient will have a decreased urine output and an elevated blood urea nitrogen (BUN) and serum creatinine. Metabolic acidosis occurs from an inability to excrete acids and reabsorb bicarbonate.

The GI system is also affected by prolonged decreased tissue perfusion. As the blood supply to the GI tract is decreased, the normally protective mucosal barrier becomes ischemic. This ischemia predisposes the patient to erosive ulcers and GI bleeding and increases the potential risk of bacterial translocation from the GI tract to the blood. The decreased perfusion to the GI tract also leads to a decreased ability to absorb nutrients.[2]

Other systems are also affected by the sustained hypoperfusion in the progressive stage of shock. The loss of the functional ability of the liver leads to a failure of the liver to metabolize drugs and waste products such as ammonia (NH_3) and lactate. Jaundice results from an accumulation of bilirubin. As the liver cells die, enzymes become elevated, in particular alanine aminotransferase (ALT), aspartate aminotransferase (AST), and γ-glutamyl transferase (GGT). The liver also loses its ability to function as an immune organ. Bacteria that may translocate from the GI system are unable to be scavenged by the Kupffer cells. Instead, they are released into the bloodstream, thus increasing the possibility of the development of bacteremia.[18]

Dysfunction of the hematologic system adds to the complexity of the clinical picture. The patient is at risk for the development of disseminated intravascular coagulation (DIC). In DIC, there is a consumption of the platelets and clotting factors with secondary fibrinolysis. This results in clinically significant bleeding from many orifices, including, but not limited to, the GI tract, lungs, and puncture sites (see Chapter 31). Altered laboratory values in DIC include decreased platelets, prolonged prothrombin time, prolonged partial thromboplastin time, decreased fibrinogen, elevated D-dimer fragments, and increased fibrin split products[13] (see Tables 67-3 and 67-6).

Refractory Stage. In the final stage of shock, the *refractory stage,* decreased perfusion from peripheral vasoconstriction and decreased CO exacerbate anaerobic metabolism (Fig. 67-8). The accumulation of lactic acid contributes to an increased capillary permeability and dilation of the capillaries. Increased capillary permeability allows fluid and plasma proteins to leave the vascular space and move to the interstitial space. Blood pools in the capillary beds secondary to the constricted venules and dilated arterioles. The loss of intravascular volume worsens hypotension and tachycardia and decreases coronary blood flow. Decreased coronary blood flow leads to worsening myocardial depression and a further decline in CO. Cerebral blood flow cannot be maintained, and cerebral ischemia results.

The patient in this stage of shock will demonstrate profound hypotension and hypoxemia. The failure of the liver, lungs, and kidneys will result in an accumulation of waste products, such as lactate, urea, ammonia, and carbon dioxide. The failure of one organ system will have an effect on several other organ systems. In this final stage, recovery is unlikely. The organs are in failure and the body's compensatory mechanisms are overwhelmed (see Table 67-6).

Diagnostic Studies

There is no single diagnostic study to determine whether a patient is in shock. The process of establishing a diagnosis begins with a thorough history and physical examination. The history may be obtained from the patient, family, or friends. Obtaining the patient's medical and surgical history, and a history of recent events (e.g., upper respiratory tract infection, surgery, chest pain, trauma), will provide valuable data.

Decreased tissue perfusion in shock leads to an elevation of lactate and a base deficit (the amount needed to bring the pH back to normal). These laboratory changes may reflect an increase in anaerobic metabolism. Other laboratory findings seen in shock are summarized in Table 67-3.

Additional diagnostic studies include a 12-lead ECG, continuous cardiac monitoring, chest x-ray, continuous pulse oximetry, and hemodynamic monitoring (e.g., arterial pressure monitoring, central venous or PA pressure monitoring). (See Chapter 66 for information on hemodynamic monitoring.)

Collaborative Care: General Measures

Critical factors in the successful management of a patient experiencing shock relate to the early recognition and treatment of the shock state. Prompt intervention in the early stages of shock may prevent the decline to the progressive or refractory stage. Successful management of the patient in shock includes the following:

1. Identification of patients at risk for the development of shock
2. Integration of the patient's history, physical examination, and clinical findings to establish a diagnosis
3. Interventions to control or eliminate the cause of the decreased perfusion
4. Protection of target and distal organs from dysfunction
5. Provision of multisystem supportive care

Table 67-7 provides an overview of the initial assessment findings and interventions for the emergency care of patients in shock.[19,20] General management strategies for a patient in shock begin with ensuring that the patient has a patent airway. Once the airway is established, either with a natural airway or an endotracheal tube, oxygen delivery must be optimized. Supplemental oxygen and mechanical ventilation may be necessary to support the delivery of oxygen to maintain an arterial oxygen saturation of 90% or greater (PaO_2 >60 mm Hg) to avoid hypoxemia (see Chapter 66). The mean arterial pressure and circulating blood volume are optimized with fluid replacement and drug therapy.

Oxygen and Ventilation. Oxygen delivery is dependent on CO, available hemoglobin, and arterial oxygen saturation (SaO_2). Methods to optimize oxygen delivery are directed at increasing supply and decreasing demand. Supply can be increased by (1) optimizing the CO with drug therapy or fluid replacement, (2) increasing the hemoglobin by the transfusion of blood or packed red blood cells (RBCs), and/or (3) increasing the arterial oxygen saturation with supplemental oxygen and mechanical ventilation.

Care must be planned so as not to disrupt the balance of oxygen supply and demand. Activities that increase oxygen consumption (e.g., endotracheal suctioning, position changes) should be appropriately spaced for oxygen conservation. Continuous monitoring of central venous oxygenation ($ScvO_2$) by a central venous catheter or mixed venous oxygen saturation (SvO_2) by a PA catheter is helpful. Both reflect the dynamic balance between oxygen supply and demand. These values are considered in conjunction with the arterial oxygen saturation, CO, hemoglobin, and oxygen consumption to evaluate the patient's response to treatments or activities (see Chapter 66).

Fluid Resuscitation. Except for cardiogenic and neurogenic shock, all other classifications of shock involve decreased circulating blood volume. The cornerstone of therapy for septic, hypovolemic, and anaphylactic shock is volume expansion with the administration of the appropriate fluid. Before beginning fluid resuscitation, two large-bore (e.g., 14- to 16-gauge) intravenous (IV) catheters must be inserted, preferably into the antecubital veins. Both crystalloids (e.g., normal saline solution) and colloids (e.g., albumin) have a role in fluid resuscitation (Table 67-8) (see Chapter 17). The choice

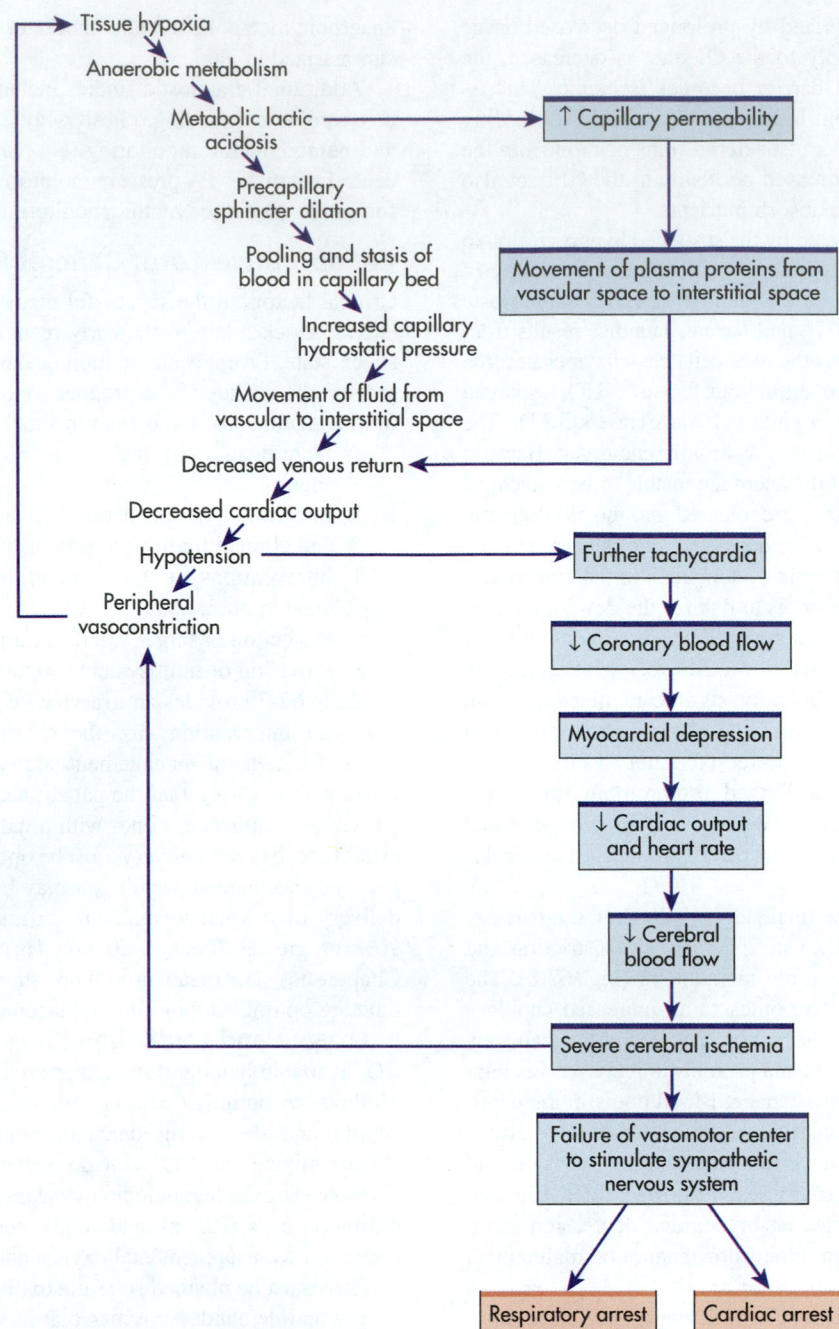

FIG. 67-8   Irreversible or refractory stage: compensatory mechanisms are not functioning or are totally ineffective, leading to multiple organ dysfunction syndrome.

of fluid for resuscitation remains controversial. Currently, it is generally accepted that isotonic crystalloids, such as normal saline, are used in the initial resuscitation of shock. Lactated Ringer's solution should be used cautiously in all shock situations because the failing liver cannot convert lactate to bicarbonate, thus increasing the serum lactate levels. In some cases, hypertonic saline may be administered to expand plasma volume.[21] Colloids are effective volume expanders because the size of their molecules keeps them in the vascular space for a longer period of time. Despite this fact, colloids are costly and no definitive studies demonstrate that using colloids for resuscitation improves patient outcomes.[4]

The choice of fluid for resuscitation must also be based on the type and volume of fluid lost and the patient's clinical status. If the patient does not respond to 2 to 3 L of crystalloids, blood adminis-

tration and central venous or PA pressure monitoring may be instituted.[4,19,20] Serial blood pressures with an automatic BP cuff or an intraarterial catheter can be used to monitor the patient's response. An indwelling bladder catheter to monitor urine output will also assist in monitoring the patient's fluid status.

When large amounts of fluids are required, the patient must be protected against complications. Two major complications are hypothermia and coagulopathy. The patient can be protected from hypothermia by warming both crystalloid and colloid solutions used during massive fluid resuscitation. If the patient is receiving large volumes of packed RBCs, it is important to remember that they do not contain clotting factors. Therefore clotting factors will need to be replaced based on the clinical situation and blood studies. If the patient has persistent hypotension after adequate fluid

TABLE 67-7	*EMERGENCY MANAGEMENT* **Shock**

Etiology*

Surgical
- Postoperative bleeding
- Ruptured organ/vessel
- Gastrointestinal bleeding
- Aortic dissection
- Vaginal bleeding
- Ruptured ectopic pregnancy or ovarian cyst

Medical
- Myocardial infarction
- Dehydration
- Addisonian crisis
- Diabetes insipidus
- Sepsis
- Diabetes mellitus
- Pulmonary embolus

Trauma
- Ruptured or lacerated vessel or organ (e.g., spleen)
- Fractures, spinal injury
- Multisystem or multiorgan injury

Assessment Findings
- Restlessness
- Confusion
- Anxiety
- Feeling of impending doom
- Decreased level of consciousness
- Weakness
- Rapid, weak, thready pulses
- Dysrhythmias
- Hypotension
- Narrowed pulse pressure
- Cool, clammy skin (warm skin in early onset of septic and neurogenic shock)
- Tachypnea, dyspnea, or shallow, irregular respirations
- Decreased O_2 saturation
- Extreme thirst
- Nausea and vomiting
- Chills
- Pallor
- Cyanosis
- Obvious hemorrhage or injury
- Temperature dysregulation

Interventions

Initial
- Establish and maintain patent airway.
- Administer high-flow oxygen (100%) by non-rebreather mask or bag-valve-mask.
- Anticipate need for intubation and mechanical ventilation.
- Stabilize cervical spine as appropriate.
- Establish IV access with two large-bore catheters (14-16 gauge) and begin fluid resuscitation with crystalloids (e.g., normal saline solution).
- Draw blood for laboratory studies (e.g., blood cultures, lactate, WBC)
- Control any external bleeding with direct pressure or pressure dressing.
- Assess for life-threatening injuries (e.g., pericardial tamponade, liver laceration, tension pneumothorax).
- Consider vasopressor therapy only after hypovolemia has been corrected.
- Insert an indwelling bladder catheter and nasogastric tube.
- Antibiotic therapy if sepsis is suspected.
- Treat dysrhythmias.

Ongoing Monitoring
- Level of consciousness
- Vital signs, including pulse oximetry, peripheral pulses, capillary refill
- Respiratory status
- Cardiac rhythm
- Urine output

WBC, White blood cell.
*See Table 67-1 for additional etiologies of shock.

resuscitation, a vasopressor (e.g., dopamine [Intropin], norepinephrine [Levophed]) or an inotrope (e.g., dobutamine [Dobutrex]) may be added. The goal for fluid resuscitation remains the restoration of tissue perfusion. Thus decisions on which agent to use should be based on the physiologic goal. Although BP helps determine whether the patient's CO is adequate, an assessment of end-organ perfusion (e.g., urine output, neurologic function, peripheral pulses) provides information that is more relevant.

Drug Therapy. The primary goal of drug therapy for shock is the correction of decreased tissue perfusion. Medications used to improve perfusion in shock are administered intravenously via an infusion pump and often via a central venous line. One of the key reasons for administration of these medications via a central line is that many of the medications that have vasoconstrictor properties may have deleterious effects if administered peripherally and the drug extravasates (Table 67-9).

Sympathomimetic Drugs. Many of the drugs used in the treatment of shock have an effect on the SNS. Drugs that mimic the action of the SNS are termed *sympathomimetic*. The effects of these drugs are mediated through their binding to α-adrenergic or β-adrenergic receptors. The various drugs differ in their relative α-adrenergic and β-adrenergic effects. (See Chapter 33, Table 33-1, for a discussion of adrenergic receptors.)

Many of the sympathomimetic drugs cause peripheral vasoconstriction and are referred to as vasopressor drugs (e.g., epinephrine [Adrenalin], norepinephrine). These drugs have the potential to cause severe peripheral vasoconstriction and an increase in SVR.

This further jeopardizes tissue perfusion, either directly or indirectly. The increased SVR increases the workload of the heart and can be detrimental to a patient in cardiogenic shock by causing further myocardial damage. Use of vasopressor drugs is generally reserved for patients who have been unresponsive to other therapies. Adequate fluid resuscitation must be achieved before the use of any vasopressor because peripheral vasoconstrictor effects in patients with low blood volume will cause further reduction in tissue perfusion.

The goals of vasopressor therapy are to achieve and maintain a mean arterial pressure (MAP) of 60 to 65 mm Hg.[17] The nurse must continuously monitor end-organ perfusion (e.g., urine output, SvO$_2$, serum lactate levels) to ensure that tissue perfusion is adequate.

Vasodilator Drugs. Some patients in shock show evidence of excessive vasoconstriction and poor tissue perfusion in spite of fluid replacement and normal or even high systemic BP. This is especially true of patients in cardiogenic shock. Although generalized sympathetic vasoconstriction is a useful compensatory mechanism for maintaining systemic pressure, excessive constriction can reduce tissue blood flow and increase the workload of the heart. The rationale for using vasodilator therapy for a patient in shock is to break the deleterious cycle in which widespread vasoconstriction causes a decrease in CO and BP, resulting in further sympathetic-induced vasoconstriction.

The goal of vasodilator therapy, as in vasopressor therapy, is to maintain a MAP of 60 to 65 mm Hg or greater. It is also important to closely monitor PA pressures along with MAP so that fluid administration can be increased or the dose of the vasodilator de-

TABLE 67-8	**Fluid Therapy in Shock**		
Fluid Type	**Mechanism of Action**	**Type of Shock**	**Nursing Implications**
Crystalloids ***Isotonic*** • 0.9% NaCl (NSS) • Lactated Ringer's (LR)	Fluid primarily remains in the intravascular space, increasing intravascular volume	Used for initial volume replacement in most types of shock	Monitor patient closely for circulatory overload. LR should not be used in patients with liver failure.
Hypertonic • 1.8%, 3%, 5% NaCl	Fluid remains in the intravascular space, rapid volume expansion	May be used for initial volume expansion in hypovolemic shock	Monitor patient closely for signs of hypernatremia (e.g., disorientation, convulsions).
Blood/Blood Products • Whole blood/packed red blood cells • Fresh frozen plasma	Replaces blood loss, increases oxygen-carrying capability Replaces coagulation factors	All types of shock if hemoglobin is <12 g/dl (120 g/L) or if the patient does not respond to crystalloids	Same precautions as any blood administration (see Chapter 31).
Colloids • Hetastarch (Hespan)	Made from starch and acts as volume expander; is at least as effective as albumin; can exert osmotic effect for up to 36 hr	All types of shock except cardiogenic and neurogenic shock	May be 50% less costly than albumin. Use cautiously in patients with heart failure, renal failure, or bleeding disorders (due to antiplatelet effect).
• Human serum albumin (5%, 25%), plasma protein fraction (5% albumin in 500 ml NSS)	Can increase plasma colloid osmotic pressure; rapid volume expansion	All types of shock except cardiogenic and neurogenic shock	Monitor for circulatory overload. Mild side effects of chills, fever, and urticaria may develop. More expensive than other colloids.

• dextran
  dextran 40
  dextran 70
	Hyperosmotic glucose polymer; has similar degrees of volume expansion with dextran 40 and dextran 70; longer duration of action with dextran 70	Limited use because of side effects including reducing platelet adhesion, diluting clotting factors	Increases risk of bleeding. Important to monitor patient for allergic reactions and acute renal failure.

NSS, Normal saline solution.

creased if a serious fall in CO or BP occurs. The vasodilator agent most often used for the patient in cardiogenic shock is nitroglycerin (Tridil). Vasodilation may be enhanced with nitroprusside (Nipride) in noncardiogenic shock.

Nutritional Therapy. Protein-calorie malnutrition is one of the primary manifestations of hypermetabolism in shock. Nutrition is vital to decreasing morbidity. Enteral nutrition should be initiated within the first 24 hours.[19,22] Generally, parenteral nutrition is used if enteral feedings are contraindicated or fail to meet at least 80% of the patient's caloric requirements.[22] (Parenteral nutrition and enteral tube feedings are discussed in Chapter 40.) The patient is started on continuous drip of very small amounts of enteral feedings. Early enteral feedings are thought to enhance perfusion of the GI tract and help maintain the integrity of the gut mucosa.

A patient in shock should be weighed daily on the same scale at the same time of day. If the patient experiences a significant weight loss, dehydration should be ruled out before additional calories are provided. Large weight gains are common because of third spacing of fluids. Therefore daily weights may function better as an indicator of fluid status than caloric needs and balance. Serum protein, nitrogen balance, BUN, serum glucose, and serum electrolytes are all used to assess nutritional status.

Collaborative Care: Specific Measures

Cardiogenic Shock. For a patient in cardiogenic shock, the overall goal is to restore blood flow to the myocardium by restoring the balance between oxygen supply and demand. Definitive measures to restore blood flow include thrombolytic therapy, angioplasty with stenting, emergency revascularization, and valve replacement (see Chapter 34). Cardiac catheterization should be performed as soon as possible after the initial insult. Coronary angioplasty with or without stenting may be performed during the cardiac catheterization. Until these interventions can be performed, the heart must be supported to optimize stroke volume and CO in an effort to facilitate optimal perfusion (Tables 67-9 and 67-10).

Hemodynamic management of a patient in cardiogenic shock is geared toward reducing the workload of the heart through drug therapy or mechanical interventions. Drug selection is based on the clinical goal and a thorough understanding of the pharmacodynamics of each drug. Drugs can be used to decrease the workload of the heart by dilating coronary arteries (e.g., nitrates), reducing preload (e.g., diuretics), reducing afterload (e.g., vasodilators), and reducing heart rate and contractility (e.g., β-adrenergic blockers).[3]

The patient may also benefit from a circulatory assist device such as an intraaortic balloon pump (IABP) or a ventricular assist device (VAD) (see Chapter 66). The IABP is a circulatory assist device that is inserted into the femoral artery and placed in the aorta just distal to the aortic arch. The goal of this intervention is to decrease the SVR and thus left ventricular workload. Another type of circulatory assist device, the VAD, may also be used as a temporary measure for the patient in cardiogenic shock and/or awaiting cardiac transplantation. Cardiac transplantation is an option for a small and select group of patients with cardiogenic shock.

TABLE 67-9	**DRUG THERAPY** **Shock**

Drug*	Mechanism of Action	Hemodynamic Effects	Type of Shock	Nursing Implications
dobutamine (Dobutrex)	↑ Myocardial contractility ↓ Ventricular filling pressures	↓ SVR/PAWP ↑ CO/stroke volume/CVP ↑/↓ HR	Used in cardiogenic shock with severe systolic dysfunction Used in septic shock with normal CO that is not meeting ↑ metabolic demands	Correct hypovolemia Do not administer in same line with NaHCO$_3$ Administration via central line recommended (infiltration leads to tissue sloughing) Monitor HR, BP (hypotension may worsen, requiring addition of a vasopressor) Monitor for tachydysrhythmias

dopamine (Intropin)	Precursor to epinephrine and norepinephrine
	Hemodynamic effects from release of norepinephrine
	Positive inotropic effects:
	  ↑ Myocardial contractility
	  ↑ Automaticity
	  ↑ Atrioventricular conduction
	Low doses: ↑ blood flow to renal, mesenteric, and cerebral circulation
	High doses: can cause progressive vasoconstriction
		↑ HR
		↑ CO
		↑ BP
			Cardiogenic shock:
			↑ Mean arterial pressure
			↑ HR
			↑ MVO$_2$
				Correct hypovolemia
				Administer via central line (infiltration leads to tissue sloughing); do not administer in same line with NaHCO$_3$
				Monitor for tachydysrhythmias
				Monitor for peripheral vasoconstriction at moderate to high doses (e.g., paresthesias, coldness in extremities)

Drotrecogin alpha (Xigris)	Anticoagulant effect by inhibiting factor Va/VIIIa Profibrinolytic and antiinflammatory properties	None	Septic shock	Monitor for signs of bleeding Monitor hemoglobin, platelets, PT, PTT
epinephrine (Adrenalin)	Low doses: β-adrenergic agonist (cardiac stimulation, bronchial dilation, peripheral vasodilation)	↑ HR/contractility/CO ↓ SVR	Cardiogenic shock combined with afterload reduction Anaphylactic shock	Correct hypovolemia if appropriate Monitor for HR >110 beats/min Monitor for dyspnea, pulmonary edema
	High doses: α-adrenergic agonist (peripheral vasoconstriction)	↑ Stroke volume ↑ SVR		Monitor for chest pain, dysrhythmias secondary to ↑ MVO$_2$
		↑ Systolic/↓ diastolic BP, widened pulse pressure ↑ CVP/PAWP	Cardiac arrest, pulseless ventricular tachycardia, ventricular fibrillation, asystole	Monitor for renal failure secondary to ischemia
hydrocortisone (Solu-Cortef)	Decreases inflammation; reverses increased capillary permeability	↑ BP, HR	Septic shock requiring vasopressor therapy, despite fluid resuscitation, to maintain adequate BP Anaphylactic shock if hypotension persists past initial therapy	Monitor for hypokalemia, hyperglycemia

BP, Blood pressure; *CO*, cardiac output; *CVP*, central venous pressure; *HR*, heart rate; *MVO$_2$*, myocardial oxygen consumption; *PAWP*, pulmonary artery wedge pressure; *PT*, prothrombin time; *PTT*, partial thromboplastin time; *SVR*, systemic vascular resistance.

*Consult individual facility's guidelines, pharmacist, pharmacology references, and drug manufacturer's administration materials for additional information and dosing recommendations.

Continued

TABLE 67-9	*DRUG THERAPY* Shock—cont'd			
Drug*	**Mechanism of Action**	**Hemodynamic Effects**	**Type of Shock**	**Nursing Implications**
norepinephrine (Levophed)	β_1-Adrenergic agonist (cardiac stimulation) α-Adrenergic agonist (peripheral vasoconstriction) Renal/splanchnic vasoconstriction	↑ BP, MAP ↑ CVP/PAWP ↑ SVR ↑/↓ CO	Cardiogenic shock after myocardial infarction Septic shock: works by increasing vascular tone	Used for hypotension unresponsive to adequate fluid resuscitation Administer via a central line (infiltration leads to tissue sloughing) Monitor for dysrhythmias secondary to ↑ MVO_2 requirements
phenylephrine (Neo-Synephrine)	α-Adrenergic agonist Vasoconstriction: renal, mesenteric, splanchnic, cutaneous, and pulmonary vessels	↑ HR ↑ BP ↑ SVR ↑/↓ CO	Neurogenic shock	Monitor for reflex bradycardia, headache, restlessness Monitor for renal failure secondary to ↓ renal blood flow Administer via central line (infiltration leads to tissue sloughing)
nitroglycerin (Tridil)	Venodilation Dilates coronary arteries ↓ Preload ↓ MVO_2	↓ SVR ↓ BP	Cardiogenic shock	Continuously monitor BP; reflex tachycardia Use glass bottles for storage
sodium nitroprusside (Nipride)	Arterial and venous vasodilation ↓ Preload/afterload	↓CVP/PAWP ↑/↓ CO ↓ BP ↓ CO	Cardiogenic shock with ↑ SVR	Continuously monitor BP Protect solution from light; wrap infusion bottle with opaque covering Administer with D_5W only Monitor for cyanide toxicity (e.g., tinnitus, hyperreflexia, confusion, seizures)
vasopressin (Pitressin [Pressyn])	Antidiuretic hormone, nonadrenergic vasoconstrictor	↑ MAP ↑ Urine output ↓ Need for other vasopressors	Shock states (most commonly septic shock) refractory to other vasopressors	Usually administer low dose Monitor hemodynamic pressures; urine output

Hypovolemic Shock. The underlying principles of managing patients with hypovolemic shock focus on stopping the loss of fluid and restoring the circulating volume. Fluid resuscitation in hypovolemic shock initially is calculated using a 3:1 rule (3 ml of isotonic crystalloid for every 1 ml of estimated blood loss). Table 67-8 delineates the different types of fluid used for volume resuscitation, the mechanisms of action, and specific nursing implications for each fluid type.

Septic Shock. Patients in septic shock require large amounts of fluid replacement, sometimes as much as 6 to 10 L of isotonic crystalloids and 2 to 4 L of colloids.[13] Predetermined end points of fluid resuscitation are suggested in Table 67-10. To optimize and evaluate large-volume fluid resuscitation, hemodynamic monitoring with a PA or central venous catheter and arterial pressure monitoring may be necessary. The overall goal of fluid resuscitation is to restore perfusion. If that cannot be accomplished with IV fluids, vasopressor drug therapy may be added. Vasodilation and low CO, or vasodilation alone, can cause low BP in spite of adequate volume resuscitation. Vasopressin (Pitressin) may be given for patients refractory to vasopressor therapy.[16,19] Exogenous vasopressin is used to replace the stores of physiologic vasopressin that are often depleted in septic shock.

Vasopressor drugs may increase BP but may also result in a decrease in stroke volume. An inotropic agent (e.g., dobutamine) is often added to offset the decrease in stroke volume (see Table 67-9). In addition, IV corticosteroids are recommended for patients who require vasopressor therapy, despite fluid resuscitation, to maintain adequate BP.[15,19] In an attempt to meet the increasing tissue demands coupled with a low SVR, the patient initially demonstrates a normal or high CO. If the patient is unable to achieve and maintain an adequate CO and has unmet tissue oxygen demands, the CO may need to be increased using drug therapy (e.g., dobutamine).[13] The adequacy of the CO can be assessed using SvO_2 monitoring. The SvO_2 (normal, 65% to 75%) is a reflection of the balance between oxygen delivery and consumption (see Chapter 66). If the balance is maintained, the tissue demands will be met.

Antibiotics are an important and early component of therapy. Before beginning definitive treatment for the infection, the cause of the infection must first be identified. Cultures (e.g., blood, wound exudate, urine, stool, sputum) are obtained before antibiotics are started. Broad-spectrum antibiotics are given initially, followed by antibiotics that are more specific once the organism has been identified.[19]

TABLE 67-10	COLLABORATIVE CARE — Specific Strategies for the Treatment of Shock

Cardiogenic Shock	Hypovolemic Shock	Septic Shock	Neurogenic Shock	Anaphylactic Shock
Oxygenation				
• Provide supplemental O_2 (e.g., nasal cannula, non-rebreather mask) • Intubation/mechanical ventilation, if necessary • Monitor SvO_2 or $ScvO_2$	• Provide supplemental O_2 • Monitor SvO_2 or $ScvO_2$	• Provide supplemental O_2 • Intubation/mechanical ventilation, if necessary • Monitor SvO_2 or $ScvO_2$	• Maintain patent airway • Provide supplemental O_2 • Intubation/mechanical ventilation, if necessary	• Maintain patent airway • Optimize oxygenation with supplemental O_2 • Intubation/mechanical ventilation, if necessary
Circulation				

• Restore blood flow with thrombolytics, angioplasty with stenting, emergent coronary revascularization
• Reduce workload of the heart with circulatory assist devices: IABP, VAD
	• Restore fluid volume (e.g., blood/blood products, crystalloids)
	• Rapid fluid replacement using two large-bore (14-16 gauge) peripheral IVs
	• Endpoints of fluid resuscitation:
	  CVP 15 mm Hg
	  PAWP 10-12 mm Hg
		• Aggressive fluid resuscitation
		• Endpoints of fluid resuscitation:
		  CVP 15 mm Hg
		  PAWP 10-12 mm Hg
			• Cautious administration of fluids	• Aggressive fluid resuscitation with colloids

Drug Therapies				
• Nitrates (e.g., nitroglycerin) • Inotropes (e.g., dobutamine) • Diuretics (e.g., furosemide) • β-Adrenergic blockers (contraindicated with ↓ ejection fraction)		• Antibiotics as ordered • Vasopressors (e.g., dopamine) • Inotropes (e.g., dobutamine) • Anticoagulation (e.g., low-molecular-weight heparin)	• Vasopressors (e.g., phenylephrine) • Atropine (for bradycardia)	• Antihistamines (e.g., diphenhydramine) • Epinephrine (subcutaneous, IV, nebulized) • Bronchodilators: nebulized (e.g., albuterol) • Corticosteroids (if hypotension persists)
Supportive Therapies				
• Correct dysrhythmias	• Correct the cause (e.g., stop bleeding, GI losses) • Use warmed fluids	• Obtain cultures (e.g., blood, wound) before beginning antibiotics • Monitor temperature • Control blood glucose • Stress ulcer prophylaxis	• Minimize spinal cord trauma with stabilization • Monitor temperature	• Identify and remove offending cause • Prevention via avoidance of known allergens • Premedication with history of prior sensitivity (e.g., contrast media)

CVP, Central venous pressure; *GI*, gastrointestinal; *IABP*, intraaortic balloon pump; *PAWP*, pulmonary artery wedge pressure; *VAD*, ventricular assist device.

Mortality rates from septic shock remain high, and until recently research efforts had not helped to improve outcomes for patients with septic shock. Drotrecogin alpha (Xigris), a recombinant form of activated protein C, has demonstrated promise in treating patients with severe sepsis. Activated protein C is a naturally occurring substance whose exact mechanism of action is unknown. It is thought to produce an antiinflammatory effect by inhibiting TNF production and limiting inflammation. Activated protein C is found in subnormal levels in patients with sepsis. Drotrecogin interrupts the body's response to severe sepsis, including bleeding and clotting abnormalities. The use of drotrecogin has resulted in a significant decrease in mortality rate when used for patients with severe sepsis and septic shock.[13,19,23,24] Bleeding is the most common serious adverse effect associated with its use.

Glucose levels should be maintained at less than 150 mg/dl (8.33 mmol/L).[15,19] Research has shown improved survival rates when continuous infusions of insulin and glucose were used to keep glucose levels between 80 and 110 mg/dl (4.44 and 6.11 mmol/L).[19] Therefore frequent monitoring of glucose levels of all patients in septic shock is necessary. Stress ulcer prophylaxis with histamine H_2-receptor blockers (e.g., famotidine [Pepcid]) and deep vein thrombosis prophylaxis with low-dose unfractionated heparin or low-molecular-weight heparin (e.g., enoxaparin [Lovenox]) are also recommended for these patients.[19]

Neurogenic Shock. The specific treatment of neurogenic shock is dependent on the cause. If the cause is spinal cord injury, general measures to promote spinal stability (e.g., spinal precautions, cervical stabilization with a collar) are initially used. Once the spine is stabilized, definitive treatment of the hypotension and bradycardia is essential to prevent further spinal cord damage. Hypotension, which occurs as a result of a loss of sympathetic tone, is associated with peripheral vasodilation and decreased venous return. Treatment involves the use of vasopressors (e.g., phenylephrine [Neo-Synephrine]) to maintain BP and organ perfusion (see Table 67-9). Bradycardia may be treated with atropine (AtroPen). Fluids are administered cautiously because the cause of the hypotension is not related to fluid loss.[25]

The patient with a spinal cord injury will also need to be monitored for hypothermia due to hypothalamic dysfunction (see Table 67-10). Although corticosteroids do not have an effect in neurogenic shock, methylprednisolone (Solu-Medrol) is used for patients with a spinal cord injury to prevent secondary spinal cord damage caused by the release of chemical mediators (see Chapter 61).

Anaphylactic Shock. The first strategy in managing patients at risk for anaphylactic shock is prevention. A thorough history is key in avoiding the risk factors for anaphylaxis (see Table 67-1). The clinical presentation of anaphylactic shock is dramatic, and immediate intervention is required. Epinephrine is the drug of choice to treat anaphylactic shock.[9] It causes peripheral vasoconstriction and bronchodilation and opposes the effect of histamine. Diphenhydramine (Benadryl) is administered to block the massive release of histamine from the allergic reaction.

Maintaining a patent airway is important because the patient can quickly develop airway compromise from laryngeal edema or bronchoconstriction. Nebulized bronchodilators are highly effective. Aerosolized epinephrine can also be used to treat laryngeal edema. Endotracheal intubation or cricothyroidotomy may be necessary to secure and maintain a patent airway.[8]

Hypotension results from leakage of fluid out of the intravascular space into the interstitial space as a result of increased vascular permeability and vasodilation. Aggressive fluid resuscitation, predominantly with colloids, is necessary. Intravenous corticosteroids may be helpful in anaphylactic shock if significant hypotension persists after 1 to 2 hours of aggressive therapy (see Tables 67-9 and 67-10).

NURSING MANAGEMENT
SHOCK

▪ Nursing Assessment

The role of the nurse is vital in caring for patients who are at risk for developing shock or are in a state of shock. The initial assessment should be geared toward the ABCs: airway, breathing, and circulation. Further assessment should focus on the assessment of tissue perfusion and includes evaluation of vital signs, level of consciousness, peripheral pulses, capillary refill, skin (e.g., temperature, color, moisture), and urine output. As shock progresses, the patient's skin will become cooler and mottled, urine output will decrease, peripheral pulses will diminish, and neurologic status will continue to deteriorate.

To understand the complexity of the patient's clinical status, the nurse must integrate all of the assessment data. As care is initiated (see Tables 67-7 and 67-10), it is essential for the nurse to obtain a brief history from the patient or other knowledgeable person. This information should include a description of the events leading to the shock condition, time of onset and duration of symptoms, and a health history (e.g., medications, allergies, date of last tetanus vaccination). In addition, details regarding any care that the patient received before hospitalization are also important.

▪ Nursing Diagnoses

Nursing diagnoses for the patient with shock may include, but are not limited to, those presented in NCP 67-1.

▪ Planning

The overall goals for a patient in shock include (1) assurance of adequate tissue perfusion, (2) restoration of normal or baseline BP, (3) return/recovery of organ function, and (4) avoidance of complications from prolonged states of hypoperfusion.

▪ Nursing Implementation

Health Promotion. It is important for nurses to become involved in the prevention of shock. To prevent shock, the nurse needs to identify patients at risk. In general, patients who are older, those with debilitating illnesses, and those who are immunocompromised are at an increased risk. Any person who sustains surgical or accidental trauma is at high risk for shock resulting from hemorrhage, spinal cord injury, and other conditions (see Table 67-1). Any patient who is at risk for decreased oxygen delivery or tissue hypoxia is also at risk for the development of shock.

Planning is essential to help prevent shock after a susceptible individual has been identified. For example, a person with an MI, especially an anterior wall MI, is at risk for cardiogenic shock. The primary goal for the patient with an MI is to limit the size of the infarction. The infarct size can be limited by restoring coronary blood flow through thrombolytic therapy, percutaneous coronary intervention, or surgical revascularization. Rest, analgesics, sedation, and judicious use of paralytic agents (if the patient is intubated) can reduce the myocardial demand for oxygen. The nurse can modify the patient's environment to provide care at intervals that will not increase the patient's oxygen demand. For example, if the patient becomes anxious with bathing, that activity can be planned at a time so as not to interfere with x-rays or other activities that may also increase oxygen demand.

A person with a severe allergy to such substances as drugs, shellfish, and insect bites is at increased risk to develop anaphylactic shock. The risk of anaphylactic shock can be decreased if the patient is carefully questioned about allergies before administering a new drug (even if the patient has received this drug in the past) or before undergoing diagnostic procedures involving the use of contrast media. Patients with severe allergies should wear a medical alert tag and report their allergies to their health care providers. These patients should also be instructed about the availability of special kits that contain equipment and medication (e.g., epinephrine [EpiPen]) for the treatment of acute hypersensitivity reactions.[26] If a patient's condition warrants receiving a medication to which he or she is at high risk for an allergic reaction (e.g., contrast media), the patient should receive a premedication such as diphenhydramine or methylprednisolone.

Careful monitoring of fluid balance can help prevent hypovolemic shock. Ongoing monitoring of intake and output and daily weights are important. In addition, monitoring of the patient's clinical status is essential because trends in clinical findings are more meaningful than any single piece of clinical information.

All patients must be carefully monitored for the development of infection. Progression from an infection to sepsis and septic shock is dependent on the patient's host defense mechanisms. Patients who are immunocompromised or immunosuppressed are at especially high risk to develop an opportunistic infection. Interventions to decrease the risk of infection for hospitalized patients include decreasing the number of indwelling catheters (e.g., central lines, urinary catheters), using aseptic technique during invasive procedures, and strict attention to hand washing. In addition, all equipment must be changed according to institutional policy, or thoroughly cleaned or discarded (if disposable) between patient use.

NURSING CARE PLAN 67-1

Patient in Shock*

NURSING DIAGNOSIS   **Ineffective tissue perfusion: renal, cerebral, cardiopulmonary, gastrointestinal, hepatic, and peripheral** *related to* low blood flow or maldistribution of blood *as evidenced by* the following possible findings:

- *Renal:* urinary output <0.5 mg/kg/hr; ↑ BUN, ↑ plasma creatinine, ↑ BUN/creatinine ratio, ↑ urine specific gravity
- *Cerebral:* anxiety, confusion, agitation, altered mentation, ↓ LOC, ↑↓ temperature
- *Cardiopulmonary:* ↓ BP, orthostatic hypotension, tachycardia; dysrhythmias, ↓ CVP and PAWP; weak, thready pulses; flat neck veins; tachypnea, ↓ SpO₂; crackles; ↑ ventilation-perfusion mismatch, refractory hypoxemia, respiratory failure
- *Gastrointestinal:* ↓ bowel sounds, paralytic ileus, hyperglycemia or hypoglycemia
- *Hepatic:* ↑ liver enzymes (e.g., ALT, AST, GGT), ↑ NH₃ and lactate
- *Peripheral:* ↓ peripheral pulses, cool and clammy skin, decreased capillary refill, pallor or cyanosis

PATIENT GOALS   1. Experiences adequate tissue perfusion with restoration of normal blood pressure
2. Recovers normal organ function with no complications from hypoperfusion

OUTCOMES (NOC)	INTERVENTIONS (NIC) and *RATIONALES*
Tissue Perfusion: Cerebral	**Shock Management**
• Restlessness ____	• Monitor vital signs, orthostatic blood pressure, mental status, and urinary output *to assess trends in patient's condition and evaluate patient's response to treatment.*
• Unexplained anxiety ____	• Monitor trends in hemodynamic parameters (e.g., CVP, PAP, PAWP) *to assess patient's status and detect fluid deficits or excesses and to evaluate patient's response to treatment.*
• Agitation ____	• Administer fluids *to maintain blood pressure and cardiac output.*
• Fever ____	• Monitor laboratory evidence of inadequate tissue perfusion (e.g., increased lactic acid levels, decreased arterial pH levels) *to assess trends in patient's status and evaluate patient's response to treatment.*
Measurement Scale	• Monitor determinants of tissue oxygen delivery (e.g., PaO₂, SpO₂, ScvO₂ SvO₂, hemoglobin levels, cardiac output) *to assess trends in patient's status and evaluate patient's response to treatment.*
1 = Severe	• Monitor for symptoms of respiratory failure (e.g., low PaO₂, elevated PaCO₂ levels, respiratory muscle fatigue) *to plan respiratory interventions.*
2 = Substantial	• Monitor fluid status, including intake and output, *to evaluate response to treatment.*
3 = Moderate	• Monitor renal function (e.g., BUN, Cr levels) *to evaluate response to treatment.*
4 = Mild	• Provide oxygen therapy and/or mechanical ventilation *to maximize oxygenation and maintain SpO₂ ≥90%.*
5 = None	• Monitor blood glucose levels, as indicated, *to maintain normal levels.*
Tissue Perfusion: Cardiac	
• Pulmonary artery wedge pressure ____	
• Cardiac index ____	
• ECG findings ____	
• Systolic blood pressure ____	
• Diastolic blood pressure ____	

ALT, Alanine aminotransferase; *AST,* aspartate aminotransferase; *BUN,* blood urea nitrogen; *Cr,* creatinine; *CVP,* central venous pressure; *GGT,* γ-glutamyl transferase; *ECG,* electrocardiogram; *PAP,* pulmonary artery pressure; *PAWP,* pulmonary artery wedge pressure; *ScvO₂,* percent oxygen saturation of hemoglobin in venous blood; *SpO₂,* percent oxygen saturation of hemoglobin measured by pulse oximetry; *SvO₂,* percent oxygen saturation of hemoglobin in mixed venous blood.

*The outcomes and related interventions are not all-inclusive and will vary based on the type of shock that the patient is experiencing.

Continued

Acute Intervention. The role of the nurse in shock involves (1) monitoring the patient's ongoing physical and emotional status to detect subtle changes in the patient's condition, (2) planning and implementing nursing interventions and therapy, (3) evaluating the patient's response to therapy, (4) providing emotional support to the patient and family, and (5) collaborating with other members of the health team to coordinate care (see NCP 67-1).

Neurologic Status. Neurologic status, including orientation and level of consciousness, should be assessed every hour or more often. The patient's neurologic status is the best indicator of cerebral blood flow. The nurse should be aware of the clinical manifestations that may indicate neurologic involvement, such as changes in behavior, restlessness, hyperalertness, blurred vision, confusion, and paresthesias. The astute nurse must also be alert to any subtle changes in the neurologic status (e.g., mild agitation).

Attempts should be made to orient the patient to time, place, person, and events. If the patient is in an ICU, orientation to the environment is particularly important. Measures such as minimizing noise and light levels should be taken to control sensory input. A day-night cycle of activity and rest should be maintained as much as possible. Sensory overload and disruption of the patient's diurnal cycle may contribute to delirium.

Cardiovascular Status. Most shock therapy is based on information about the patient's cardiovascular status. If the patient is unstable, the heart rate, BP, central venous pressure, and PA pressures including continuous cardiac output (if available) should be assessed at least every 15 minutes. PAWP should be measured every 1 to 2 hours. (Hemodynamic monitoring is discussed in Chapter 66.) Monitoring trends in hemodynamic parameters yields more important information than individual numbers. Integration of hemodynamic data with physical assessment data is essential in planning strategies to manage the patient with shock.

Patients in shock often have hypotension. There is no definitive research to support placement of patients in the Trendelenburg (head-down) position during hypotensive crisis. It has been suggested that patients placed into this position may experience compromised pulmonary function and increased intracranial pressure. Therefore the Trendelenburg position should be used judiciously or not at all.[27,28]

The patient's ECG should be continuously monitored to detect dysrhythmias that may result from the cardiovascular and meta-

NURSING CARE PLAN 67-1

Patient in Shock—cont'd

OUTCOMES (NOC)

Tissue Perfusion: Pulmonary

- Pulmonary artery pressure _____
- Respiratory rate _____
- PaO$_2$ _____
- PaCO$_2$ _____
- Arterial pH _____
- Oxygen saturation _____

Tissue Perfusion: Abdominal Organs

- Urine output _____
- Fluid balance _____
- Electrolyte and acid/base balance _____
- Urine specific gravity _____
- BUN _____
- Plasma Cr _____
- Bowel sounds _____
- Liver function test findings _____
- Blood glucose _____

Tissue Perfusion: Peripheral

- Capillary refill fingers _____
- Capillary refill toes _____
- Sensation _____
- Skin color _____
- Extremity skin temperature _____
- Peripheral pulses _____

Measurement Scale

1 = Severely compromised
2 = Substantially compromised
3 = Moderately compromised
4 = Mildly compromised
5 = Not compromised

INTERVENTIONS (NIC) and *RATIONALES*

Shock Management: Cardiac

- Monitor for symptoms of inadequate coronary artery perfusion (e.g., ST changes on ECG or angina).
- Promote optimal preload *to improve contractility while minimizing heart failure* (e.g., administer nitroglycerin and maintain PAWP within prescribed range).
- Promote coronary artery perfusion (e.g., maintain mean arterial pressure >60 mm Hg and control tachycardia) *to prevent myocardial ischemia.*

Shock Management: Vasogenic

- Remove stimuli precipitating neurogenic reaction *to control symptoms.*
- Administer antibiotics, antihistamines, epinephrine, and antiinflammatory drugs, if appropriate, *to control symptoms.*

Shock Management: Volume

- Monitor the patient closely for hemorrhage.
- Note hemoglobin/hematocrit level before and after blood loss *to evaluate response to treatment.*
- Administer blood products (e.g., platelets or fresh frozen plasma) *to replace lost volume.*

NURSING DIAGNOSIS **Fear** *related to* severity of condition *as evidenced by* verbalization of anxiety about condition and fear of death, or withdrawal with no communication; restlessness; sleeplessness; increase in heart and respiratory rate

PATIENT GOALS 1. Verbalizes fears related to severity of condition
2. Reports decreased fear and increased psychologic comfort

OUTCOMES (NOC)

Anxiety Level

- Restlessness _____
- Verbalized apprehension _____
- Increased pulse rate _____
- Increased respiratory rate _____
- Withdrawal _____
- Sleep pattern disturbance _____

Measurement Scale

1 = Severe
2 = Substantial
3 = Moderate
4 = Mild
5 = None

INTERVENTIONS (NIC) and *RATIONALES*

Anxiety Reduction

- Seek to understand the patient's perspective of a stressful situation *to validate patient's feelings.*
- Use a calm, reassuring approach.
- Listen attentively.
- Administer medications if appropriate *to reduce anxiety.*
- Stay with patient *to promote safety and reduce fear.*
- Control stimuli for patient needs *to reduce patient's anxieties and oxygen need.*
- Provide factual information concerning diagnosis, treatment, and prognosis *to reduce patient's fear of the unknown and assist patient in making informed decisions.*
- Encourage family to stay with patient *to reduce anxiety level.*

bolic derangements associated with shock. Heart sounds should be assessed for the presence of an S_3 or S_4 sound or new murmurs. The presence of an S_3 sound in an adult usually indicates heart failure. The frequency of this monitoring is decreased as the patient's condition improves.

In addition to monitoring the patient's cardiovascular status, the nurse must administer the prescribed therapy that is designed to correct the dysfunctions of the cardiovascular system. The patient's response to fluid and medication administration is assessed as often as every 10 to 15 minutes. Appropriate adjustments (e.g., medication titration) should be made as needed. Once tissue perfusion is restored and the patient is stabilized, the frequency of monitoring is decreased and the patient is slowly weaned off medications to support BP and tissue perfusion.

Respiratory Status. The respiratory status of the patient in shock must be frequently assessed to ensure adequate oxygenation, detect complications early, and provide data regarding the patient's acid-base status. The rate, depth, and rhythm of respirations are initially monitored as frequently as every 15 to 30 minutes. Increased rate and depth provide information regarding the patient's attempts to correct metabolic acidosis. Breath sounds should be assessed every 1 to 2 hours for any changes that may indicate fluid overload or accumulation of secretions.

Pulse oximetry is used to continuously monitor oxygen saturation. Pulse oximetry using a patient's finger or toe may not be accurate in an advanced shock state because of poor peripheral circulation. In this situation, the probe should be attached to the nose, ear, or forehead (according to the manufacturer's guidelines) to increase accuracy. Arterial blood gases (ABGs) provide definitive information on ventilation and oxygenation status and acid-base balance. Initial interpretation of ABGs is often the nurse's responsibility. A PaO_2 below 60 mm Hg (in the absence of chronic lung disease) indicates the presence of hypoxemia and the need for the administration of higher oxygen concentrations or for a different mode of oxygen administration. Low $PaCO_2$ in the presence of a low pH and low bicarbonate level may indicate that the patient is attempting to compensate for a metabolic acidosis. A rising $PaCO_2$ in the presence of a persistently low pH and PaO_2 may indicate the need for intubation and mechanical ventilation.

Most patients in shock will be intubated and on mechanical ventilation. Maintaining a patent airway and monitoring for ventilator-related complications are critical. (Artificial airways and mechanical ventilation are discussed in Chapter 66.)

Renal Status. Hourly measurements of urinary output are essential in assessment of the adequacy of renal perfusion. An indwelling bladder catheter is inserted to facilitate measurements. Urine output of less than 0.5 ml/kg/hr may indicate inadequate perfusion of the kidneys. BUN and serum creatinine values are additional indicators used to assess renal function. Serum creatinine is a better indicator of renal function because BUN levels can be influenced by the catabolic state of the patient.

Body Temperature and Skin Changes. In the presence of an elevated or subnormal temperature, tympanic or pulmonary arterial temperatures should be obtained hourly. If normal, the temperature should be monitored every 4 hours. The patient should be kept comfortably warm with the use of light covers and the control of environmental temperature. If the patient's temperature rises above 101.5° F (38.6° C) and the patient becomes uncomfortable or experiences cardiovascular compromise, the fever may be managed with nonsteroidal antiinflammatory drugs

(e.g., ibuprofen [Motrin]), with acetaminophen (Tylenol), or by removing some of the patient's covers.

The patient's skin should be monitored for temperature, pallor, flushing, cyanosis, diaphoresis, and piloerection. In addition, capillary refill should be assessed as an indicator of peripheral perfusion.

Gastrointestinal Status. Bowel sounds should be auscultated at least every 4 hours, and abdominal distention should be assessed. If a nasogastric tube is inserted, drainage should be measured and checked for occult blood. Similarly, stools should also be checked for occult blood.

Personal Hygiene. Hygiene is especially important to the patient in shock because impaired tissue perfusion predisposes the patient to skin breakdown and infection. However, bathing and other nursing measures must be carried out judiciously because a patient in shock is experiencing problems with oxygen delivery to tissues. The nurse must use clinical judgment in determining priorities of care in order to limit the demands for increased oxygen.

Oral care for the patient in shock is essential because mucous membranes may become dry and fragile in the volume-depleted patient. In addition, the intubated patient usually has difficulty swallowing, resulting in pooled secretions in the mouth. A water-soluble lubricant applied to the lips prevents drying and cracking. Moist swabbing of the tongue and oral mucosa with saline solution or diluted mouthwash is also beneficial. Lemon glycerin swabs should not be used because they can cause further drying of the mucosa.

Passive range of motion should be performed three to four times per day to maintain joint mobility. The patient should be turned at least every 1 to 2 hours and positioned in good body alignment to help prevent pressure ulcers. Use of a pressure-relieving mattress or a specialty bed may also be needed. If possible, oxygen consumption (e.g., SvO_2 or $ScvO_2$) should be monitored during all nursing interventions to monitor the patient's tolerance to activity.

Emotional Support and Comfort. The effects of anxiety and fear in the face of a critical, life-threatening situation on the patient and family are frequently overlooked or underestimated. Anxiety, fear, and pain may aggravate respiratory distress and increase the release of catecholamines. When implementing care, the nurse should assess and monitor the patient's anxiety and pain. Medications to decrease anxiety and pain are common modes of therapy. Continuous infusions of a benzodiazepine (e.g., lorazepam [Ativan]), an opioid or anesthetic (e.g., morphine, propofol [Diprivan]), and occasionally a neuromuscular blocking agent (e.g., cisatracurium [Nimbex]) are extremely helpful in decreasing anxiety, pain, and oxygen demand.

The nurse should talk to the patient and encourage the family to talk to the patient, even if the patient is intubated, is sedated, or appears comatose. Hearing is often the last sense to be diminished, and even if the patient cannot respond, he or she may still be able to hear. If the intubated patient is capable of writing, a "magic slate" or a pencil and paper should be provided. Alphabet boards or signboards with common requests (e.g., turn, fan, lights) are also useful. The patient should also receive simple explanations of procedures before they are carried out, as well as information regarding the current plan of care and its rationale. If the patient or family asks questions about progress and prognosis, simple and honest answers should be given.

The patient's spiritual needs should not be overlooked. Patients may desire a visit from a priest, rabbi, or minister. One way to provide support is to offer to call a member of the clergy rather than wait for the patient or family to express a wish for spiritual counseling.

Family and significant others can have a therapeutic effect on the patient. To perform this role, they need to be supportive and comforting. Family and significant others (1) link the patient to the outside world, (2) facilitate decision making and advise the patient, (3) assist with activities of daily living, (4) act as liaisons to advise the health care team of the patient's wishes for care, and (5) provide safe, caring, familiar relationships for the patient.[29] The family primarily needs to be kept informed of the patient's condition. If possible, the same nurses should continuously care for the patient to decrease anxiety, limit contradictory information, and increase trust. Should the prognosis become increasingly grave, the patient's family should be given support when making difficult decisions regarding continuation of life support. The nursing staff must support the family's decisions and facilitate realistic expectations and outcomes. It is important for the nurse to remember that compassionate understanding is as essential as scientific and technical expertise in the total care of a patient and family.

Family time with the patient should be facilitated, provided this time is perceived as comforting by the patient. The nurse should explain in simple terms the purpose of tubes and equipment surrounding the patient, and the family should be informed of what they may and may not touch. If possible, the patient's hands and arms can be kept outside the sheets to encourage therapeutic touch. If desired, the family may be encouraged to perform simple comfort measures. Privacy should be provided as much as possible, but the patient and family should be assured that assistance is readily available should it be required. The call bell should be in reach at all times.

Ambulatory and Home Care. Rehabilitation of the patient who has experienced critical illness necessitates correction of the precipitating cause and prevention or early treatment of complications. The nurse should continue to monitor the patient for indications of complications throughout the recovery period. Complications may include decreased range of motion, decreased physical endurance, renal failure following acute tubular necrosis, and the development of fibrotic lung disease as a result of ARDS (see Chapters 47 and 68). Thus patients recovering from shock may require diverse services on discharge. These can include admission to transitional care units (e.g., for mechanical ventilation weaning), rehabilitation centers (inpatient or outpatient), or home health care agencies. The nurse should begin to anticipate and facilitate a safe transition from the hospital to home on admission.

■ Evaluation

Expected outcomes for the patient with shock are addressed in NCP 67-1.

SYSTEMIC INFLAMMATORY RESPONSE SYNDROME AND MULTIPLE ORGAN DYSFUNCTION SYNDROME

Etiology and Pathophysiology

Systemic inflammatory response syndrome (SIRS) is a systemic inflammatory response to a variety of insults, including infection (referred to as sepsis), ischemia, infarction, and injury (see Table 67-5). SIRS is characterized by generalized inflammation in organs remote from the initial insult.[10] Normally, the inflammatory process is contained within a confined environment.

A systemic inflammatory response can be triggered by many mechanisms. Examples include the following:

- Mechanical tissue trauma: burns, crush injuries, surgical procedures
- Abscess formation: intraabdominal, extremities
- Ischemic or necrotic tissue: pancreatitis, vascular disease, myocardial infarction
- Microbial invasion: bacteria, viruses, fungi, parasites
- Endotoxin release: gram-negative bacteria
- Global perfusion deficits: post–cardiac resuscitation, shock states
- Regional perfusion deficits: distal perfusion deficits

Multiple organ dysfunction syndrome (MODS) is the failure of two or more organ systems in an acutely ill patient such that homeostasis cannot be maintained without intervention. MODS results from SIRS. These two syndromes represent the ends of a continuum. Transition from SIRS to MODS does not occur in a clear-cut manner[10] (see Fig. 67-1).

Organ and Metabolic Dysfunction. When the inflammatory response is not controlled, consequences occur. These include activation of inflammatory cells and release of mediators, direct damage to the endothelium, and hypermetabolism. Vasodilation becomes excessive and leads to decreased SVR and hypotension. In addition, there is also an increase in vascular permeability that allows mediators and protein to leak out of the endothelium and into the interstitial space. The white blood cells begin to phagocytize the foreign debris, and the coagulation cascade is activated (see Chapter 30). Organ perfusion may be compromised because of hypotension, decreased perfusion, microemboli, and redistributed or shunted blood flow.

The respiratory system is often the first system to show signs of dysfunction in SIRS and MODS.[30] Inflammatory mediators have a direct effect on the pulmonary vasculature. The endothelial damage from the release of inflammatory mediators results in an increase in capillary permeability and facilitates movement of proteinaceous fluid from the pulmonary vasculature into the pulmonary interstitial spaces. The fluid then moves to the alveoli, causing alveolar edema. Type I pneumocytes (alveolar cells) are destroyed. Type II pneumocytes become dysfunctional, and there is a decrease in surfactant production. The alveoli collapse, creating an increase in *shunt* (blood flow to the lungs that does not participate in gas exchange) and a worsening of the ventilation-perfusion mismatch. The end result is ARDS. Patients with ARDS require aggressive pulmonary management with mechanical ventilation. (See Chapter 68 for a complete discussion of ARDS.)

Cardiovascular changes include myocardial depression and massive vasodilation in response to increasing tissue demands. Vasodilation results in decreased SVR and BP. The baroreceptor reflex causes release of *inotropic* (increasing force of contraction) and *chronotropic* (increasing heart rate) factors that enhance CO. To compensate for hypotension, CO increases by an increase in heart rate and stroke volume. Increases in capillary permeability cause a shift of albumin and fluid out of the vascular space, further diminishing venous return and thus preload. The patient becomes warm and tachycardic with a high CO and a low SVR. Other signs include decreased capillary refill, skin mottling, increased central venous pressure and PAWP, and dysrhythmias. SvO_2 may be abnormally high because the patient is perfusing areas not consuming much oxygen (e.g., skin, nonworking muscle) while other areas may have blood shunted away from them. Eventually, either perfusion of vital organs becomes insufficient or the cells are unable to use oxygen and their function is further compromised.

Neurologic dysfunction commonly manifests as mental status changes with SIRS and MODS. Acute alteration in mental status can be an early sign of MODS. The patient may become confused and agitated, combative, disoriented, lethargic, or comatose. These changes may be due to hypoxemia, the direct effect of the inflammatory mediators, or impaired perfusion.[31]

Acute renal failure (ARF) is frequently seen in SIRS and MODS. ARF can be caused not only by hypoperfusion but also by the effects of the mediators. When there is decreased perfusion to the kidneys, the SNS and the renin-angiotensin system are activated. The stimulation of the renin-angiotensin system results in systemic vasoconstriction and aldosterone-mediated sodium and water reabsorption. Another risk factor for the development of ARF is the use of nephrotoxic drugs. Antibiotics commonly used to treat gram-negative bacteria, such as aminoglycosides, can also be nephrotoxic. Careful monitoring of drug levels is essential to avoid the nephrotoxic effects.

The GI tract also plays a key role in the development of MODS. GI motility is often decreased in critical illness, causing abdominal distention and paralytic ileus. In the early stages of SIRS and MODS, blood also is shunted away from the GI mucosa, making it highly vulnerable to ischemic injury. Decreased perfusion leads to a breakdown of this normally protective mucosal barrier, thus increasing the risk for ulceration and GI bleeding. With the breakdown of the mucosal barrier of the gut, the potential for bacterial translocation from the GI tract into circulation exists. Some research has implicated bacterial translocation in the development of MODS. However, other studies indicate the possibility that insult to the GI system may induce the production of inflammatory mediators, thus contributing to the systemic inflammation leading to MODS.[18]

Metabolic changes are pronounced in SIRS and MODS. Both syndromes trigger a hypermetabolic response. Glycogen stores are rapidly converted to glucose (glycogenolysis). Once glycogen is depleted, amino acids are converted to glucose (gluconeogenesis), reducing protein stores. Fatty acids are mobilized for fuel. Catecholamines and glucocorticoids are released and result in hyperglycemia and insulin resistance. The net result is a catabolic state, and lean body mass (muscle) is lost.

The hypermetabolism that is associated with SIRS and MODS may last for several days and results in liver dysfunction. Liver dysfunction in MODS may exist long before clinical evidence is present. Protein synthesis is impaired. The liver is unable to synthesize albumin, one of the key proteins that has an essential role in maintaining plasma oncotic pressure. Consequently, plasma oncotic pressure is altered and fluid and protein leak from the vascular spaces to the interstitial space. Administration of albumin does not normalize oncotic pressure in these patients.

As the state of hypermetabolism persists, the patient is unable to convert lactate to glucose, and lactate accumulates (lactic acidosis). Despite increases in glycogenolysis and gluconeogenesis, eventually the liver is unable to maintain a glucose level and the patient becomes hypoglycemic.

Failure of the coagulation system manifests as DIC. DIC results in simultaneous microvascular clotting and bleeding because of the depletion of clotting factors and platelets in addition to excessive fibrinolysis. (DIC is discussed in Chapter 31.)

Electrolyte imbalances, which are common, are related to hormonal and metabolic changes and fluid shifts. These changes exacerbate mental status changes, neuromuscular dysfunction, and dysrhythmias. The release of antidiuretic hormone and aldosterone results in sodium and water retention. Aldosterone increases urinary potassium loss, and catecholamines cause potassium to move into the cell, resulting in hypokalemia. Hypokalemia is associated with dysrhythmias and muscle weakness. Metabolic acidosis results from impaired tissue perfusion, hypoxia, and a shift to anaerobic metabolism with a resultant increase in hydrogen ion production. Progressive renal dysfunction also contributes to metabolic acidosis. Hypocalcemia, hypomagnesemia, and hypophosphatemia are common.

Clinical Manifestations of SIRS and MODS

The clinical manifestations of MODS are presented in Table 67-11.

NURSING and COLLABORATIVE MANAGEMENT
SIRS AND MODS

The prognosis for the patient with MODS is poor, with estimated mortality rates at 90% to 95% when three or more organ systems fail.[30] Research with immunotherapy (e.g., anticytokine and antiendotoxin therapy) may become helpful in the future care of patients with SIRS and MODS.[32] Therefore the most important goal is to prevent the progression of SIRS to MODS.

A critical component of the nursing role is vigilant assessment and ongoing monitoring to detect early signs of deterioration or organ dysfunction. Collaborative care for patients with MODS focuses on (1) prevention and treatment of infection, (2) maintenance of tissue oxygenation, (3) nutritional and metabolic support, and (4) appropriate support of individual failing organs. Table 67-11 summarizes the management for patients with MODS.

■ *Prevention and Treatment of Infection*

Aggressive infection control strategies are essential to decrease the risk for nosocomial infections. Despite aggressive strategies, host dysfunction may lead to the development of an infection. Once an infection is suspected, interventions to control the source must be instituted. Appropriate cultures should be sent, and broad-spectrum antibiotic therapy should be initiated. Early, aggressive surgery is recommended to remove necrotic tissue (e.g., early debridement of burn tissue) that may provide a culture medium for microorganisms. Once a specific organism is identified, therapy should be modified if necessary. Aggressive pulmonary management, including early ambulation, can reduce the risk of infection. Strict asepsis can decrease infections related to intraarterial lines, endotracheal tubes, urinary catheters, IV lines, and other invasive devices or procedures.

■ *Maintenance of Tissue Oxygenation*

Hypoxemia frequently occurs in patients with SIRS and MODS. These patients have greater oxygen needs and decreased oxygen supply to the tissues. Interventions that decrease oxygen demand and increase oxygen delivery are essential. Sedation, mechanical ventilation, analgesia, paralysis, and rest may decrease oxygen demand and should be considered. Oxygen delivery may be optimized by maintaining normal levels of hemoglobin (e.g., transfusion of packed RBCs) and PaO_2 (80 to 100 mm Hg), using

| TABLE 67-11 | Multiple Organ Dysfunction Syndrome: Clinical Manifestations and Management |

System	Clinical Manifestations of Organ Failure	Management
Respiratory	Development of ARDS (see Chapter 68): • Severe dyspnea • PaO_2/FIO_2 ratio <200 • Bilateral fluffy infiltrates on chest x-ray • PAWP <18 mm Hg • Ventilation-perfusion (V/Q) mismatch • Pulmonary hypertension • Increased minute ventilation • Increased respiratory rate • Decreased compliance • Refractory hypoxemia	Prevention Optimize oxygen delivery/minimize oxygen consumption Mechanical ventilation (see Chapter 66) • Positive end-expiratory pressure • Lung protective modes (e.g., pressure control/inverse ratio ventilation, low tidal volumes) • Permissive hypercapnia Positioning (e.g., continuous lateral rotation therapy, prone positioning)
Renal	Prerenal: renal hypoperfusion • BUN/creatinine ratio >20:1 • ↓ Urine Na^+ <20 mEq/L • ↑ Urine specific gravity >1.020 • ↑ Urine osmolality Intrarenal: acute tubular necrosis • BUN/creatinine ratio <10:1-15:1 • ↑ Urine Na^+ >20 mEq/L • ↓ Urine osmolality • Urine specific gravity (~1.010)	Diuretics • Loop diuretics (e.g., furosemide [Lasix]) • May need to increase dose due to ↓ glomerular filtration rate Dopamine (Intropin) • Enhances renal blood flow • Improves renal perfusion • Increases urine output (if volume resuscitated) • May work synergistically with diuretics Continuous renal replacement therapy (see Chapter 47)
Hepatic	Bilirubin >2 mg/dl (34 μmol/L) ↑ Liver enzymes (ALT, AST, GGT) ↑ Serum NH_3 ↓ Serum albumin, prealbumin, transferrin Jaundice Hepatic encephalopathy	Maintain adequate tissue perfusion Provide nutritional support (e.g., enteral feedings) Judicious use of hepatically metabolized drugs
Gastrointestinal	Mucosal ischemia • ↓ Intramucosal pH • Potential translocation of gut bacteria Hypoperfusion → ↓ peristalsis, paralytic ileus Mucosal ulceration on endoscopy GI bleeding	Stress ulcer prophylaxis • Antacids (e.g., Maalox) • Histamine H_2-receptor blockers (e.g., famotidine [Pepcid]) • Proton pump inhibitors (e.g., omeprazole [Prilosec]) • Sucralfate (Carafate) Dietary consultation Enteral feedings • Stimulate mucosal activity • Provide essential nutrients and optimal calories
Central Nervous	Acute change in neurologic status Fever Hepatic encephalopathy Seizures Confusion/disorientation Failure to wean/prolonged rehabilitation	Evaluate for hepatic/metabolic encephalopathy Optimize cerebral blood flow ↓ Cerebral oxygen requirements Prevent secondary tissue ischemia • Calcium channel blockers (reduce cerebral vasospasm) Prevent further compromise

ALT, Alanine aminotransferase; *ARDS*, acute respiratory distress syndrome; *AST*, aspartate aminotransferase; *BUN*, blood urea nitrogen; *CO*, cardiac output; *ECG*, electrocardiogram; *GGT*, γ-glutamyl transferase; *GI*, gastrointestinal; *MAP*, mean arterial pressure; *PA*, pulmonary artery; *PAWP*, pulmonary artery wedge pressure; *PT*, prothrombin time; *PTT*, partial thromboplastin time; *SvO₂*, oxygen saturation of hemoglobin in mixed venous blood; *SVR*, systemic vascular resistance.

individualized tidal volumes with positive end-expiratory pressure,[19] increasing preload or myocardial contractility to enhance CO, or reducing afterload to increase CO.

■ *Nutritional and Metabolic Needs*

Hypermetabolism in SIRS or MODS can result in profound weight loss, cachexia, and further organ failure. Protein-calorie malnutrition is one of the primary manifestations of hypermetabolism and MODS. Total energy expenditure is often increased 1.5 to 2.0 times the normal metabolic rate. Because of their relatively short half-life, plasma transferrin and prealbumin levels are monitored to assess hepatic protein synthesis.

The goal of nutritional support is to preserve organ function. Providing early and optimal nutrition decreases morbidity and mortality rates in patients with SIRS and MODS.[19] The use of the enteral route is preferable to parenteral nutrition. If the enteral route cannot be used or cannot meet the caloric needs, parenteral nutrition should be initiated or added.[22] (Enteral and parenteral nutrition are discussed in Chapter 40.) Attention to tight glycemic control (blood glucose <150 mg/dl [8.33 mmol/L]) using insulin infusions is important in these patients.[19]

■ *Support of Failing Organs*

Support of any failing organ is a primary goal of therapy. For example, the patient with ARDS requires aggressive oxygen therapy and mechanical ventilation (see Chapter 68). DIC should be treated appropriately (e.g., blood products) (see Chapter 31). Renal failure may require dialysis. Continuous renal replacement therapy is better tolerated than hemodialysis, especially in a patient with hemodynamic instability (see Chapter 47).

TABLE 67-11	Multiple Organ Dysfunction Syndrome: Clinical Manifestations and Management—cont'd	
System	**Clinical Manifestations of Organ Failure**	**Management**
Cardiovascular	Myocardial depression Biventricular failure Systolic/diastolic dysfunction ↑ HR/CO/SVR ↓ Stroke volume ↓ MAP ↓ Ejection fraction/contractility	Volume management • PA catheter for hemodynamic monitoring • ↑ Preload via volume replacement • Maximize myocardial function • Maintain CO • Arterial pressure monitoring • Maintain MAP >60 mm Hg Vasopressors Continuous SvO$_2$ monitoring; balance O$_2$ supply and demand Continuous ECG monitoring Circulatory assist devices • Intraaortic balloon pump • Ventricular assist device
Hematologic	↑ Bleeding times, ↑ PT, ↑ PTT ↓ Platelet count (thrombocytopenia) ↑ Fibrin split products ↑ D-dimer test	Observe for bleeding from obvious and/or occult sites Replace factors being lost (e.g., platelets) Minimize traumatic interventions (e.g., intramuscular injections, multiple venipunctures)
Endocrine	Hyperglycemia → hypoglycemia	Continuous infusion of insulin and glucose to maintain blood glucose <150 mg/dl

CRITICAL THINKING EXERCISE

CASE STUDY

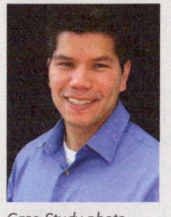

Case Study photo
©iStockphoto.com/
Yvonne Chamberlain.

Shock

Patient Profile. Kim, a 25-year-old Korean American, was not wearing his seat belt when he was the driver involved in a motor vehicle collision. The windshield was broken and Kim was found 15 feet from his car. He was face down, conscious, and moaning. His wife and daughter were found in the car with their seat belts on. They sustained no obvious injuries, but were very upset. All passengers were taken to the emergency department (ED). The following information pertains to Kim.

Subjective Data
- States, "I can't breathe."
- Cries out when abdomen is palpated.

Objective Data

Physical Examination
- Cardiovascular: BP 80/56; apical pulse 135 but no radial or brachial pulses palpable; carotid pulse present but weak
- Lungs: respiratory rate 35 breaths/min; labored breathing with severe respiratory distress; asymmetric chest wall movement; absence of breath sounds on left side
- Trachea deviated slightly to the right
- Abdomen: slightly distended and painful on palpation
- Musculoskeletal: open compound fracture of the lower left leg

Diagnostic Studies
- Chest x-ray: hemopneumothorax and rib fractures on left side
- Hematocrit: 28%

Collaborative Care
- In the ED, placement of left chest tube, which drained bright red blood

Surgical Procedure
- Splenectomy
- Repair of torn intercostal artery
- Repair of compound fracture

Critical Thinking Questions

1. What type of shock was present in Kim? What clinical manifestations did he display?
2. What were the causes of Kim's shock? What are other causes of this type of shock?
3. What are the initial nursing responsibilities for Kim?
4. What continual nursing assessment parameters are essential for this patient?
5. What are his potential complications?
6. Based on the assessment data presented, write two or more priority nursing diagnoses.

NCLEX EXAMINATION REVIEW QUESTIONS

The number of the question corresponds to the same-numbered objective at the beginning of the chapter.

1. *Shock* is best defined as
   a. cardiovascular collapse.
   b. loss of sympathetic tone.
   c. inadequate tissue perfusion.
   d. blood pressure less than 90 mm Hg systolic.
2. A patient has a spinal cord injury at T4. Vital signs include a falling blood pressure with bradycardia. The nurse recognizes that the patient is experiencing
   a. a relative hypervolemia.
   b. an absolute hypovolemia.
   c. neurogenic shock from low blood flow.
   d. neurogenic shock from a maldistribution of blood flow.
3. An early effect that shock has on the body is
   a. sympathetic nervous system activation that results in stimulation of adrenergic receptors.
   b. massive vasoconstriction in the heart and brain that causes stimulation of the renin-angiotensin system.
   c. decreased tissue perfusion that results in aerobic metabolism, leading to the development of lactic acidosis.
   d. heart rate that is usually slow and irregular in the compensatory stage because of parasympathetic nervous stimulation.

Shock and MODS

4. A 78-year-old man has confusion and temperature of 104° F (40° C). He is a diabetic with purulent drainage from his right great toe. His assessment findings are BP 84/40; heart rate 110; respiratory rate 42 and shallow; CO 8 L/min; and PAWP 4 mm Hg. This patient's symptoms are most likely indicative of
   a. sepsis.
   b. septic shock.
   c. multiple organ dysfunction syndrome.
   d. systemic inflammatory response syndrome.

5. Appropriate treatment modalities for the management of cardiogenic shock include
   a. dobutamine to increase myocardial contractility.
   b. vasopressors to increase systemic vascular resistance.
   c. corticosteroids to stabilize the cell wall in the infarcted myocardium.
   d. plasma volume expanders such as albumin to decrease an elevated preload.

6. The most accurate assessment parameters for the nurse to use to determine adequate tissue perfusion in the patient with MODS are
   a. blood pressure, pulse, and respirations.
   b. breath sounds, blood pressure, and body temperature.
   c. pulse pressure, level of consciousness, and pupillary response.
   d. level of consciousness, urine output, and skin color and temperature.

REFERENCES

1. Rice V: *Shock, a clinical syndrome,* ed 2, Aliso Viejo, Calif, 1997, AACCN.
2. Baldwin KM, Cheek DJ, Morris SE: Shock, multiple organ dysfunction syndrome, and burns in adults. In McCance KL, Huether SE, editors: *Pathophysiology: the biologic basis for disease in adults and children,* ed 5, St Louis, 2006, Mosby.
3. Bromet DS, Klein LW: Cardiogenic shock: art and science, *Crit Care Med* 32:293, 2004.
4. Kelley DM: Hypovolemic shock: an overview, *Crit Care Nurse Q* 28:2, 2005.
5. Guyton AC, Hall JE: *Textbook of medical physiology,* ed 11, Philadelphia, 2005, Saunders.
6. Muhlberg A, Ruth-Sahd L: Holistic care: treatment and interventions for hypovolemic shock secondary to hemorrhage, *DCCN* 23:55, 2004.
7. Sheerin F: Spinal cord injury: causation and pathophysiology, *Emerg Nurse* 12:29, 2005.
8. Tang A: A practical guide to anaphylaxis, *Am Fam Physician* 68:1325, 2003.
9. Brown SG: Cardiovascular aspects of anaphylaxis: implications for treatment, *Curr Opin Allergy Clin Immunol* 5:359, 2005.
10. Levy MM et al: 2001 SCCM/ESICM/ACCP/ATS/SIS International Sepsis Definitions Conference, *Crit Care Med* 31:1250, 2003.
11. Hoyert DL, Kung HC, Smith BL: National vital statistics reports for 2003, *Centers Disease Control* 53:243, 2005.
12. Ely EW, Kleinpell RM, Goyette RE: Advances in the understanding of clinical manifestations and therapy of severe sepsis: an update for critical care nurses, *Am J Crit Care* 12:120, 2003.
13. Cunneen J, Cartwright M: The puzzle of sepsis, *AACN Clin Issues* 15:18, 2004.
14. Wright BE, West MA: Pathophysiology of septic shock. In Deitch EA, Vincent JL, Windsor A, editors: *Sepsis and multiple organ dysfunction: a multidisciplinary approach,* Philadelphia, 2002, Saunders.
15. Ahrens T, Tuggle D: Surviving severe sepsis: early recognition and treatment, *Crit Care Nurse* 2 (suppl), Oct 2004.
16. Bridges EJ, Dukes S: Cardiovascular aspects of septic shock: pathophysiology, monitoring and treatment, *Crit Care Nurse* 25:14, 2005.
17. Bench S: Clinical skills: assessing and treating shock: a nursing perspective, *Br J Nurs* 13:715, 2004.
18. Deitch EA, Sambol JT: The gut-origin hypothesis of MODS. In Deitch EA, Vincent JL, Windsor A, editors: *Sepsis and multiple organ dysfunction: a multidisciplinary approach,* Philadelphia, 2002, Saunders.
19. Dellinger RP et al: Surviving sepsis campaign guidelines for management of severe sepsis and septic shock, *Crit Care Med* 32:858, 2004.
20. Robson W, Newell J, Beavis S: Severe sepsis in A&E, *Emerg Nurse* 13:24, 2005.
21. Johnson AL, Criddle LM: Pass the salt: indications for and implications of using hypertonic saline, *Crit Care Nurse* 24:36, 2004.
22. Doig GS: Evidence-based guidelines for nutritional support of the critically ill: results of a bi-national guideline development conference, 2005. Available at *www.guideline.gov/summary/summary.aspx?doc_id=8012&nbr=004499&string=nutrition* (accessed January 22, 2006).
23. Ahrens T, Vollman K: Severe sepsis management: are we doing enough? *Crit Care Nurse* 2 (suppl), Oct 2003.
24. Tazbir J: Sepsis and the role of activated protein C, *Crit Care Nurse* 24:40, 2004.
25. Carlson BA: Shock. In Urden LD, Stacy KM, Lough ME, editors: *Thelan's critical care nursing,* ed 5, St Louis, 2006, Elsevier Mosby.
26. Hathaway LR: Anaphylaxis, *Nursing* 35:46, 2005.
27. Johnson S, Henderson SO: Myth: the Trendelenburg position improves circulation in cases of shock, *Can J Emerg Med* 6:48, 2004.
28. Bridges N, Jarquin-Valdivia AA: Use of the Trendelenburg position as the resuscitation position: to T or not to T? *Am J Crit Care* 14:364, 2005.
*29. Eichorn DJ et al: Family presence during invasive procedures and resuscitation: hearing the voice of the patient, *Am J Nurs* 101:48, 2001.
30. Fry DE: MODS: an introduction. In Deitch EA, Vincent JL, Windsor A, editors: *Sepsis and multiple organ dysfunction: a multidisciplinary approach,* Philadelphia, 2002, Saunders.
31. Philips B, Bennett DE: CNS dysfunction in sepsis. In Deitch EA, Vincent JL, Windsor A, editors: *Sepsis and multiple organ dysfunction: a multidisciplinary approach,* Philadelphia, 2002, Saunders.
32. Oberholzer A, Oberholzer C, Ertel W: Immunotherapy—new concepts and agents. In Deitch EA, Vincent JL, Windsor A, editors: *Sepsis and multiple organ dysfunction: a multidisciplinary approach,* Philadelphia, 2002, Saunders.

RESOURCES

Additional resources for this chapter are listed after Chapter 66 on p. 1771 and Chapter 69 on p. 1844.

---

*Nursing research–based reference.

> *Wisdom is to the soul what health is to the body.*
>
> De Saint-Real

Nursing Management

Respiratory Failure and Acute Respiratory Distress Syndrome

68

Richard B. Arbour

LEARNING OBJECTIVES

1. Compare the pathophysiologic mechanisms that result in hypoxemic and hypercapnic respiratory failure.
2. Differentiate between early and late clinical manifestations of acute respiratory failure.
3. Describe the nursing and collaborative management of the patient with hypoxemic or hypercapnic respiratory failure.
4. Relate the pathophysiologic mechanisms that result in acute respiratory distress syndrome (ARDS) to the clinical manifestations.
5. Describe the nursing and collaborative management of the patient with ARDS.
6. Identify complications that may result from acute respiratory failure or ARDS and measures to prevent or reverse these complications.

KEY TERMS

acute respiratory distress syndrome, p. 1812
alveolar hypoventilation, p. 1802
diffusion limitation, p. 1802
hypercapnia, p. 1799
hypercapnic respiratory failure, p. 1800
hypoxemia, p. 1799
hypoxemic respiratory failure, p. 1799
hypoxia, p. 1804
refractory hypoxemia, p. 1813

Electronic Resources

Supplemental content related to Chapter 68 can be found . . .

Companion CD
- Stress-Busting Kit for Nursing Students
- Interactive Case Study: Acute Respiratory Failure
- NCLEX Examination Review Questions
- Comprehensive Glossary

Evolve Website **evolve**
http://evolve.elsevier.com/Lewis/medsurg
- Content Updates
- Key Points (Printable and CD/MP3 Download)
- Concept Map Creator
- Expanded Audio Glossary
- Key Term Flash Cards

- Customizable Nursing Care Plan: Acute Respiratory Failure
- Electronic Calculators
- WebLinks

ACUTE RESPIRATORY FAILURE

The major function of the respiratory system is gas exchange, which involves the transfer of oxygen (O_2) and carbon dioxide (CO_2) between the atmosphere and the blood[1,2] (Fig. 68-1). *Respiratory failure* results when one or both of these gas-exchanging functions are inadequate. For example, insufficient O_2 is transferred to the blood or inadequate CO_2 is removed from the lungs. Clinical states that interfere with adequate O_2 transfer result in **hypoxemia,** which is manifested by a decrease in arterial O_2 tension (PaO_2) and saturation (SaO_2). Insufficient CO_2 removal results in **hypercapnia,** which is manifested by an increase in arterial CO_2 tension ($PaCO_2$).[1-5] Arterial blood gases (ABGs) can be used to assess changes in pH, PaO_2, $PaCO_2$, bicarbonate, and SaO_2, and pulse oximetry can be used to intermittently or continuously assess arterial oxygen saturation (SpO_2). Data should be interpreted within the context of the clinical assessment findings, as well as the patient's baseline. For example, an individual with chronic lung disease may have a baseline $PaCO_2$ higher than what is considered the "normal" range.

Respiratory failure is not a disease; it is a condition that occurs as a result of one or more diseases involving the lungs or other body systems (Tables 68-1 and 68-2). Respiratory failure can be classified as hypoxemic or hypercapnic (Fig. 68-2). Hypoxemic respiratory failure is also referred to as *oxygenation failure* because the primary problem is inadequate O_2 transfer between the alveoli and the pulmonary capillary bed.[1,2] Although no universal definition exists, **hypoxemic respiratory failure** is commonly defined as a PaO_2 of 60 mm Hg or less when the patient is receiving

Reviewed by Katherine M. Crawford, RN, MSN, Cardiac Care Coordinator, Christiana Care Health System, Newark, Del.; and Eleanor R. Fitzpatrick, RN, MSN, CRNP, CCRN, Clinical Nurse Specialist, Thomas Jefferson University Hospital, Philadelphia, Pa.

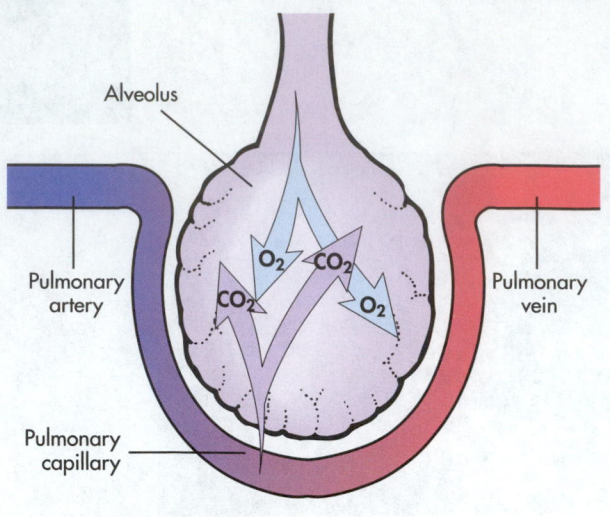

FIG. 68-1 Normal gas exchange unit in the lung.

Glossary of Abbreviations

Arterial Blood Monitoring

ABGs	Arterial blood gases
pH	Negative log of the free hydrogen ion [H+]
PaO_2	Partial pressure of oxygen in arterial blood
$PaCO_2$	Partial pressure of carbon dioxide in arterial blood
SaO_2	Oxygen saturation in arterial blood measured by ABGs
SpO_2	Oxygen saturation in arterial blood measured by pulse oximetry

Oxygen and Lung Function Monitoring

FIO_2	Fraction of inspired oxygen concentration
FRC	Functional residual capacity (volume of air in lung at end of expiration)
PEEP	Positive end-expiratory pressure (pressure in lungs at end of expiration)
PEFR	Peak expiratory flow rate (maximum airflow during a forced expiration)
V/Q	Ventilation/perfusion ratio (relationship of ventilation to perfusion in the lungs)
V_E	Minute ventilation (product of tidal volume times respiratory rate)
V_T	Tidal volume (volume of air inspired with each breath)

TABLE 68-1 Types of Respiratory Failure and Common Causes

Hypoxemic Respiratory Failure*	Hypercapnic Respiratory Failure*
Respiratory System Acute respiratory distress syndrome Pneumonia Toxic inhalation (e.g., smoke inhalation) Hepatopulmonary syndrome (e.g., low-resistance flow state, V/Q mismatch) Massive pulmonary embolism (e.g., thrombus emboli, fat emboli) Pulmonary artery laceration and hemorrhage **Cardiac System** Anatomic shunt (e.g., ventricular septal defect) Cardiogenic pulmonary edema Shock (decreasing blood flow through pulmonary vasculature)	**Respiratory System** Asthma COPD Cystic fibrosis **Central Nervous System** Brainstem injury/infarction Sedative and opioid overdose Spinal cord injury Severe head injury **Chest Wall** Thoracic trauma (e.g., flail chest) Kyphoscoliosis Pain Morbid obesity **Neuromuscular System** Myasthenia gravis Critical illness polyneuropathy Acute myopathy Toxic ingestion (e.g., tree tobacco) Amyotrophic lateral sclerosis Phrenic nerve injury Guillain-Barré syndrome Poliomyelitis Muscular dystrophy Multiple sclerosis

COPD, Chronic obstructive pulmonary disease.
*This list is not all-inclusive.

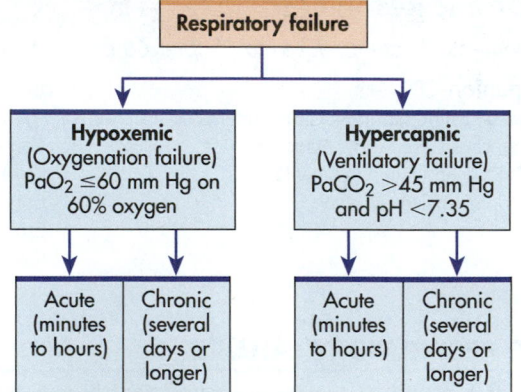

FIG. 68-2 Classification of respiratory failure.

an inspired O_2 concentration of 60% or greater. This definition incorporates two important concepts: (1) the PaO_2 is at a level that indicates inadequate O_2 saturation of hemoglobin; and (2) this PaO_2 level exists despite administration of supplemental O_2 at a percentage (60%) that is about three times that in room air (21%). Disorders that interfere with O_2 transfer into the blood include pneumonia, pulmonary edema, pulmonary emboli, and alveolar injury related to inhalation of toxic gases (e.g., smoke), as well as lung damage related to alveolar stress/ventilator-induced lung injury. In addition, low cardiac output states (e.g., heart failure, shock) can also cause hypoxemic respiratory failure.[1,2]

Hypercapnic respiratory failure is also referred to as *ventilatory failure* because the primary problem is insufficient CO_2 removal. **Hypercapnic respiratory failure** is commonly defined as a $PaCO_2$ above normal (greater than 45 mm Hg) in combination with acidemia (arterial pH less than 7.35). This definition incorporates three important concepts: (1) the $PaCO_2$ is higher than normal; (2) there is evidence of the body's inability to compensate for this increase (acidemia); and (3) the pH is at a level where a further decrease may

lead to severe acid-base imbalance. (See Chapter 17 for a discussion of acid-base balance.) Disorders that compromise lung ventilation and subsequent CO_2 removal include drug overdoses with central nervous system (CNS) depressants, neuromuscular diseases (e.g., myasthenia gravis), and trauma or diseases involving the spinal cord and its role in lung ventilation. Acute asthma is also associated with hypercapnic respiratory failure.[3-8] Many patients experience both hypoxemic and hypercapnic respiratory failure.

Etiology and Pathophysiology

Hypoxemic Respiratory Failure. Common diseases and conditions that cause hypoxemic respiratory failure are listed in Table 68-1. Four physiologic mechanisms may cause hypoxemia and

TABLE 68-2	Predisposing Factors for Acute Respiratory Failure

Predisposing Factors	Mechanisms of Respiratory Failure
Airways and Alveoli	
Acute respiratory distress syndrome • *Direct lung injury:* aspiration; severe, disseminated pulmonary infection; near-drowning; toxic gas inhalation; airway contusion • *Indirect lung injury:* sepsis/septic shock, severe nonthoracic trauma, cardiopulmonary bypass	Fluid enters the interstitial space and subsequently the alveoli, markedly impairing gas exchange. The result is an initial ↓ in PaO_2 and later an ↑ in $PaCO_2$. A low-flow state to pulmonary capillaries can result in ischemic injury to lung tissues with loss of integrity of the alveolar-capillary membrane.
Asthma	Bronchospasm escalates in severity rather than responding to therapy. Bronchospasm, edema of the bronchial mucosa, and plugging of small airways with secretions greatly reduce airflow. Work of breathing increases, causing respiratory muscle fatigue. ↓ PaO_2 and ↑ $PaCO_2$.
Chronic obstructive pulmonary disease (COPD)	Alveoli are destroyed by protease-antiprotease imbalance or respiratory infection, or an exacerbation of COPD escalates in severity rather than responding to therapy. Secretions obstruct airflow. Work of breathing increases and causes respiratory muscle fatigue. ↓ PaO_2 and ↑ $PaCO_2$.
Cystic fibrosis	Abnormal Na^+ and Cl^- transport produces secretions that are viscous, poorly cleared, and therefore foci for infection. Over time the airways become clogged with copious, purulent, often greenish colored sputum. Secretions obstruct airflow. Repeated infections destroy alveoli. Work of breathing increases, causing respiratory muscle fatigue. ↓ PaO_2 and ↑ $PaCO_2$.
Central Nervous System	
Opioid or other drug overdose with CNS depressant	Respirations slowed by drug effect. Insufficient CO_2 is excreted, resulting in ↑ $PaCO_2$.
Brainstem infarction, head injury	Medulla cannot alter respiratory rate in response to changes in $PaCO_2$. Total loss of respiratory drive secondary to severe brainstem injury.
Chest Wall	
Severe soft tissue injury, flail chest, rib fracture, pain	Prevent normal rib cage expansion resulting in inadequate gas exchange.
Kyphoscoliosis	Change in spinal configuration compresses the lungs and prevents normal expansion of the chest wall.
Morbid obesity	Weight of the chest and abdominal contents prevents normal rib cage movement.
Neuromuscular Conditions	
Cervical cord injury, phrenic nerve injury	Neural control is lost, preventing use of the diaphragm, the major muscle of respiration. As a consequence, the patient inspires a smaller tidal volume, which predisposes to an ↑ in $PaCO_2$.
Amyotrophic lateral sclerosis (ALS), Guillain-Barré, muscular dystrophy, multiple sclerosis, poliomyelitis, myasthenia gravis, myopathy, critical illness polyneuropathy, prolonged effects of neuromuscular blocking agents	Respiratory muscle weakness or paralysis occurs, preventing normal CO_2 excretion. Dysfunction may be slowly progressive (e.g., muscular dystrophy, multiple sclerosis), progressive with no potential of recovery (e.g., ALS), rapid with good expectation of recovery (e.g., Guillain-Barré), or stable for extended periods of time (e.g., poliomyelitis, myasthenia gravis).

CNS, Central nervous system.

subsequent hypoxemic respiratory failure: (1) mismatch between ventilation (V) and perfusion (Q), commonly referred to as V/Q mismatch; (2) shunt; (3) diffusion limitation; and (4) hypoventilation. The most common causes are V/Q mismatch and shunt.[1-4]

Ventilation-Perfusion (V/Q) Mismatch. In the normal lung, the volume of blood perfusing the lungs each minute (4 to 5 L) is approximately equal to the amount of fresh gas that reaches the alveoli each minute (4 to 5 L). In a perfectly matched system, each portion of the lung would receive about 1 ml of air for each 1 ml of blood flow. This match of ventilation and perfusion would result in a V/Q ratio of 1:1 (e.g., 1 ml of air per 1 ml of blood), which is expressed as V/Q = 1. Ventilation is ideally matched with perfusion.

Although this example implies that ventilation and perfusion are ideally matched in all areas of the lung, this situation does not normally exist. In reality, there is some regional mismatch. At the lung apex, V/Q ratios are greater than 1 (more ventilation than perfusion). At the lung base, V/Q ratios are less than 1 (less ventilation than

perfusion). Because changes at the lung apex balance changes at the base, the net effect is a close overall match (Fig. 68-3).

Many diseases and conditions alter overall V/Q matching and thus cause *V/Q mismatch* (Fig. 68-4). The most common are those in which increased secretions are present in the airways (e.g., chronic obstructive pulmonary disease [COPD]) or alveoli (e.g., pneumonia), and when bronchospasm is present (e.g., asthma). V/Q mismatch may also result from alveolar collapse (atelectasis) or as a result of pain. Unrelieved or inadequately relieved pain interferes with chest and abdominal wall movement, compromising lung ventilation. Additionally, pain increases muscle and motor tension, producing generalized muscle rigidity; causes systemic vasoconstriction and activation of the stress response; and increases O_2 consumption and CO_2 production.[9] In this circumstance, increased metabolic (oxygen) demand and CO_2 production increase the demand side of the equation and may increase both oxygen and ventilation demands. All of these conditions result in limited airflow

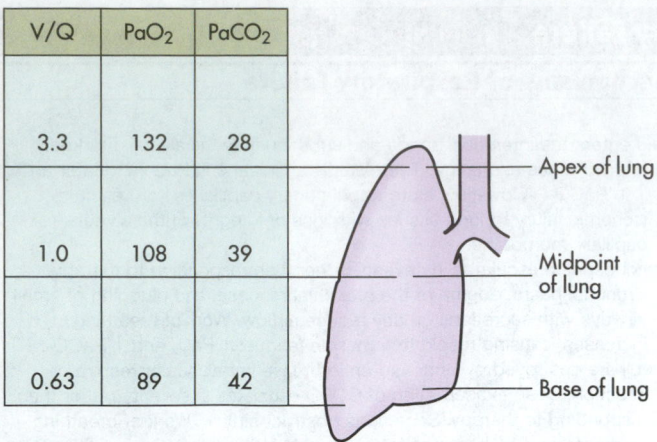

V/Q	PaO₂	PaCO₂
3.3	132	28
1.0	108	39
0.63	89	42

Apex of lung

Midpoint of lung

Base of lung

FIG. 68-3 Regional V/Q differences in the normal lung. At the lung apex, the V/Q ratio is 3.3, at the midpoint 1.0, and at the base 0.63. This difference causes the PaO_2 to be higher at the apex of the lung and lower at the base. Values for $PaCO_2$ are the opposite (i.e., lower at the apex and higher at the base). Blood that exits the lung is a mixture of these values.

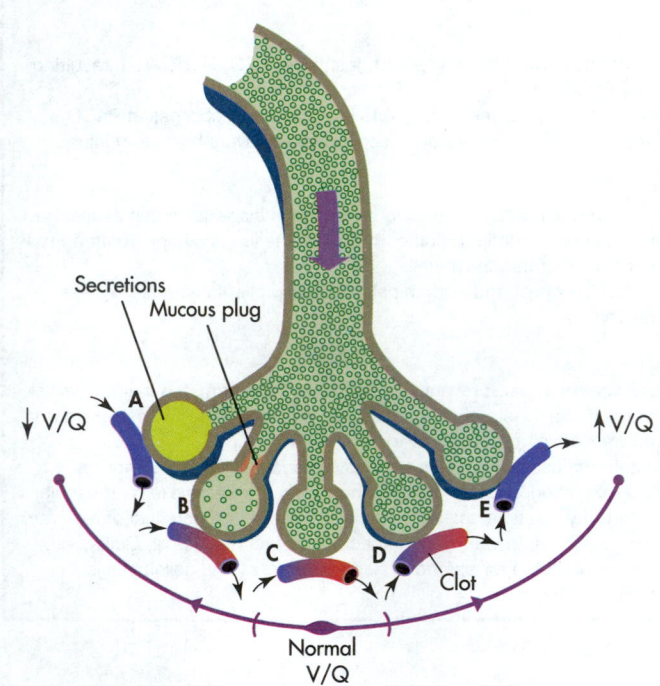

FIG. 68-4 Range of ventilation to perfusion (V/Q) relationships. **A,** Absolute shunt, no ventilation due to fluid filling the alveoli. **B,** V/Q mismatch, ventilation partially compromised by secretions in the airway. **C,** Normal lung unit. **D,** V/Q mismatch, perfusion partially compromised by emboli obstructing blood flow. **E,** Dead space, no perfusion due to obstruction of the pulmonary capillary.

(ventilation) to alveoli but have no effect on blood flow (perfusion) to the gas exchange units.[1,2] The consequence is V/Q mismatch. A pulmonary embolus affects the perfusion portion of the V/Q relationship. The embolus limits blood flow but has no effect on airflow to the alveoli, again causing V/Q mismatch (see Fig. 68-4).

O_2 therapy is an appropriate first step to reverse hypoxemia caused by V/Q mismatch because not all gas exchange units are affected. O_2 therapy increases the PaO_2 in blood leaving normal gas exchange units, thus causing a higher than normal PaO_2. The well-oxygenated blood mixes with poorly oxygenated blood, raising the overall PaO_2 of blood leaving the lungs.[2-4] Ultimately, the optimal approach to hypoxemia caused by a V/Q mismatch is mechanism based and directed at the cause.

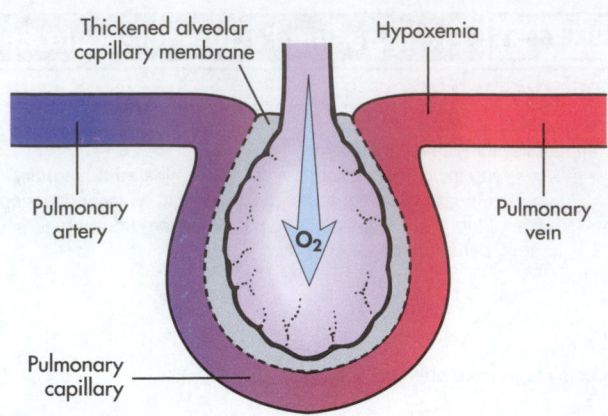

FIG. 68-5 Diffusion limitation. Exchange of CO_2 and O_2 cannot occur because of the thickened alveolar-capillary membrane.

Shunt. Shunt occurs when blood exits the heart without having participated in gas exchange. A shunt can be viewed as an extreme V/Q mismatch (see Fig. 68-4). There are two types of shunt: anatomic and intrapulmonary. An *anatomic shunt* occurs when blood passes through an anatomic channel in the heart (e.g., a ventricular septal defect) and therefore does not pass through the lungs. An *intrapulmonary shunt* occurs when blood flows through the pulmonary capillaries without participating in gas exchange. Intrapulmonary shunt is seen in conditions in which the alveoli fill with fluid (e.g., acute respiratory distress syndrome [ARDS], pneumonia, pulmonary edema).[2] O_2 therapy alone may be ineffective in increasing the PaO_2 if hypoxemia is due to shunt because (1) blood passes from the right to the left side of the heart without passing through the lungs (anatomic shunt); or (2) the alveoli are filled with fluid, which prevents gas exchange (intrapulmonary shunt). Patients with shunt are usually more hypoxemic than patients with V/Q mismatch, and they may require mechanical ventilation and a high fraction of inspired oxygen (FIO_2) to improve gas exchange.

Diffusion Limitation. Diffusion limitation occurs when gas exchange across the alveolar-capillary membrane is compromised by a process that thickens or destroys the membrane (Fig. 68-5). Diffusion limitation can also be worsened by conditions that affect the pulmonary vascular bed such as severe emphysema or recurrent pulmonary emboli. Some diseases cause the alveolar-capillary membrane to become thicker (fibrotic), which slows gas transport. These diseases include pulmonary fibrosis, interstitial lung disease, and ARDS. Diffusion limitation is more likely to cause hypoxemia during exercise than at rest. During exercise, blood moves more rapidly through the lungs. Because transit time is increased, red blood cells are in the lungs for a shorter time, decreasing the time for diffusion of O_2 across the alveolar-capillary membrane. The classic sign of diffusion limitation is hypoxemia that is present during exercise but not at rest.

Alveolar Hypoventilation. Alveolar hypoventilation is a generalized decrease in ventilation that results in an increase in the $PaCO_2$ and a consequent decrease in PaO_2. Alveolar hypoventilation may be the result of restrictive lung diseases, CNS diseases, chest wall dysfunction, acute asthma, or neuromuscular diseases. Although alveolar hypoventilation is primarily a mechanism of hypercapnic respiratory failure, it is mentioned here because it can also cause hypoxemia.

Interrelationship of Mechanisms. Frequently, hypoxemic respiratory failure is caused by a combination of two or more of the following: V/Q mismatch, shunting, diffusion limitation, and hypoventilation. The patient with acute respiratory failure secondary to pneumonia may have a combination of V/Q mismatch and shunt because the inflammation, edema, and hypersecretion of exudate within the bronchioles and terminal respiratory units obstruct the airways (V/Q mismatch) and fill the alveoli with exudate (shunt). In addition, shunt may be increased because of improper positioning (e.g., bad lung down) and endogenous vasodilator mediators as is the case with pneumococcal pneumonia.[2] The patient with cardiogenic pulmonary edema or ARDS may have a combination of shunt and V/Q mismatch because some alveoli are completely filled with fluid from edema (shunt) and others are partially filled with fluid (V/Q mismatch).

Hypercapnic Respiratory Failure. Hypercapnic respiratory failure results from an imbalance between ventilatory supply and ventilatory demand. *Ventilatory supply* is the maximum ventilation (gas flow in and out of the lungs) that the patient can sustain without developing respiratory muscle fatigue. *Ventilatory demand* is the amount of ventilation needed to keep the $PaCO_2$ within normal limits. Normally, ventilatory supply far exceeds ventilatory demand. As a consequence, individuals with normal lung function can engage in strenuous exercise, which greatly increases CO_2 production without an elevation in $PaCO_2$. Patients with preexisting lung disease such as severe COPD do not have this advantage and cannot effectively increase lung ventilation in response to exercise or metabolic demands. However, considerable dysfunction is typically present before ventilatory demand exceeds ventilatory supply.

When ventilatory demand does exceed ventilatory supply, the $PaCO_2$ can no longer be sustained within normal limits and hypercapnia occurs. Hypercapnia reflects substantial lung dysfunction. Hypercapnic respiratory failure is sometimes called *ventilatory failure* because the primary problem is the inability of the respiratory system to ventilate out sufficient CO_2 to maintain a normal $PaCO_2$. Hypercapnic respiratory failure can also be differentiated as acute or chronic respiratory failure. For example, an episode of respiratory failure may represent an acute decompensation in a patient whose underlying lung function has deteriorated to the point that some degree of decompensation is always present (chronic respiratory insufficiency).

Many different diseases can cause a limitation in ventilatory supply (see Tables 68-1 and 68-2). These diseases can be grouped into four categories: (1) abnormalities of the airways and alveoli, (2) abnormalities of the CNS, (3) abnormalities of the chest wall, and (4) neuromuscular conditions.[2]

Airways and Alveoli. Patients with asthma, COPD, and cystic fibrosis are at high risk for hypercapnic respiratory failure because the underlying pathophysiology of these conditions results in airflow obstruction and air trapping.

Central Nervous System. A variety of problems may suppress the drive to breathe. A common example is an overdose of an opioid or other respiratory depressant drug. In a dose-related manner, CNS depressants such as opioids and benzodiazepines decrease CO_2 reactivity in the brainstem, allowing arterial CO_2 levels to rise. A brainstem infarction or severe head injury may also interfere with normal function of the respiratory center in the medulla. Patients with these conditions are at risk for respiratory failure because the medulla does not alter the respiratory rate in response to a change in $PaCO_2$. Independent of direct brainstem dysfunction, metabolic or structural brain injury resulting in significant depression of consciousness or loss of consciousness may interfere with the patient's ability to manage secretions or adequately protect his

or her airway. CNS dysfunction may also include high-level spinal cord injuries that limit innervation to the respiratory muscles of the chest wall and diaphragm.

Chest Wall. A variety of conditions may prevent normal movement of the chest wall and hence limit lung expansion. In patients with flail chest, fractures prevent the rib cage from expanding normally because of pain, mechanical restriction, and muscle spasm. In patients with kyphoscoliosis, the change in spinal configuration compresses the lungs and prevents normal expansion of the chest wall. In patients with morbid obesity, the weight of the chest and abdominal contents may limit lung expansion. Patients with these conditions are at risk for respiratory failure because these dysfunctions limit lung expansion or diaphragmatic movement and consequently gas exchange.

Neuromuscular Conditions. Various types of neuromuscular diseases may result in respiratory muscle weakness or paralysis (see Table 68-1). For example, patients with Guillain-Barré syndrome, muscular dystrophy, myasthenia gravis (acute exacerbation), or multiple sclerosis are at risk for respiratory failure because the respiratory muscles are weakened or paralyzed as a consequence of the underlying neuromuscular condition. Therefore they are unable to maintain normal $PaCO_2$ levels.

In summary, respiratory failure may occur in three of these categories (CNS, chest wall, neuromuscular conditions) despite the presence of normal lungs. Respiratory failure occurs because the medulla, chest wall, peripheral nerves, or respiratory muscles are not functioning normally. The patient may have no damage to lung tissue but may be unable to inspire a tidal volume sufficient to expel CO_2 from the lungs.

Tissue Oxygen Needs. It is important to remember that even though PaO_2 and $PaCO_2$ determine the definition of respiratory failure, the major threat of respiratory failure is the inability of the lungs to meet the oxygen demands of the tissues. This inability may occur as a result of inadequate tissue O_2 delivery or because the tissues are unable to use the O_2 delivered to them. It may also occur as a result of the stress response and dramatic increases in tissue oxygen consumption.[9] Tissue O_2 delivery is determined by the amount of O_2 carried in the hemoglobin, as well as cardiac output. Therefore respiratory failure places the patient at greater risk if there are coexisting cardiac problems or anemia. Failure of O_2 utilization most commonly occurs as a result of septic shock. In this situation, adequate O_2 may be delivered to the body tissues, but due to impaired oxygen extraction, an abnormally high amount of O_2 returns in the venous blood because it is not used or off-loaded at the tissue level. (Shock is discussed in Chapter 67.) Acid-base alterations (e.g., alkalosis, acidosis) may also interfere with oxygen delivery to peripheral tissues (see Chapter 26).

Clinical Manifestations

Respiratory failure may develop suddenly (minutes or hours) or gradually (several days or longer). A sudden decrease in PaO_2 or a rapid rise in $PaCO_2$ implies a serious condition, which can rapidly become a life-threatening emergency. An example is the patient with asthma who develops severe bronchospasm and a marked decrease in airflow, resulting in respiratory arrest. A more gradual change in PaO_2 and $PaCO_2$ is better tolerated because compensation can occur. An example is the patient with COPD who develops a progressive increase in $PaCO_2$ over several days following the onset of a respiratory infection. Because the change occurred over several days, there is time for renal compensation (e.g., retention of bicarbonate), which will minimize the change in arterial pH. The patient will have compensated respiratory acidosis.[10,11] (See Chapter 17 for a discussion of renal compensation for acid-base disorders.)

Manifestations of respiratory failure are related to the extent of change in PaO_2 or $PaCO_2$, the rapidity of change (acute versus chronic), and the ability to compensate to overcome this change. When the patient's compensatory mechanisms fail, respiratory failure occurs. Because clinical manifestations are variable, it is important to monitor trends in ABGs and/or pulse oximetry to evaluate the extent of change. These measurements cannot substitute for clinical assessment and should be interpreted within the context of clinical assessment findings. Frequently, the initial indication of respiratory failure is a change in the patient's mental status. Because the cerebral cortex is so sensitive to variations in oxygenation, arterial CO_2 levels, and acid-base balance, mental status changes will occur early and frequently before ABG results are obtained. Restlessness, confusion, agitation, and combative behavior suggest inadequate delivery of O_2 to the brain and should be fully investigated.[12,13]

The nurse may detect manifestations of respiratory failure that are specific (arise from the respiratory system) or nonspecific (arise from other body systems) (Table 68-3). An understanding of the significance of these manifestations is critical to the ability to detect the onset of respiratory failure and effectiveness of treatment.

Tachycardia and mild hypertension can also be early signs of respiratory failure. Such changes may indicate an attempt by the heart to compensate for decreased O_2 delivery. A severe morning headache may suggest that hypercapnia may have occurred during the night, increasing cerebral blood flow by vasodilation and causing a morning headache. At night the respiratory rate is slower and the lungs of patients at risk for respiratory failure may remove less $PaCO_2$. Rapid, shallow breaths suggest that the tidal volume may be inadequate to remove CO_2 from the lungs. Cyanosis is an unreliable indicator of hypoxemia and is a late sign of respiratory failure because it does not occur until hypoxemia is severe ($PaO_2 \leq 45$ mm Hg).

Consequences of Hypoxemia and Hypoxia. *Hypoxemia* occurs when the amount of O_2 in arterial blood is less than the normal value (see Chapter 26 for normal values). **Hypoxia** occurs when the PaO_2 falls sufficiently to cause signs and symptoms of inadequate oxygenation (see Table 68-3). Hypoxemia can lead to hypoxia if not corrected. If hypoxia or hypoxemia is severe, the cells shift from aerobic to anaerobic metabolism. Anaerobic metabolism uses more fuel and produces less energy and is less efficient than aerobic metabolism. The waste product of anaerobic metabolism, lactic acid, is more difficult to remove from the body than CO_2 because lactic acid has to be buffered with sodium bicarbonate. When the body does not have adequate amounts of sodium bicarbonate to buffer the lactic acid produced by anaerobic metabolism, metabolic acidosis results and cell death may occur.[10]

Hypoxia and metabolic acidosis have adverse effects on the vital organs, especially the heart and CNS. The heart tries to compensate for the decreased O_2 level in the blood by increasing the heart rate and cardiac output.[12] A cardiovascular hyperdynamic state may also occur due to catecholamine release that is associated with the physiologic stress response. As the PaO_2 decreases and acidosis increases, the heart muscle may become dysfunctional and cardiac output may decrease. In addition, angina and dysrhythmias may occur. All of these consequences result in a further decrease in oxygen delivery. Permanent brain damage may occur because of O_2 deprivation. Renal function may also be impaired, and sodium retention, edema formation, acute tubular necrosis, and uremia may occur. Gastrointestinal (GI) system altera-

tions include tissue ischemia, increased permeability of the intestinal wall, and possible translocation of bacteria from the GI tract into circulation.

Specific Clinical Manifestations. The patient in respiratory failure may have several clinical findings indicating distress. The patient may have a rapid, shallow breathing pattern or a respiratory rate that is slower than normal. Both changes predispose to insufficient CO_2 removal. The patient may increase the respiratory rate in an effort to blow off accumulated CO_2. This breathing pattern requires a substantial amount of work and predisposes to respiratory muscle fatigue. A change from a rapid rate to a slower rate in a patient in acute respiratory distress such as that seen with acute asthma suggests extreme progression of respiratory muscle fatigue and increased probability of respiratory arrest.[2-6]

The position that the patient assumes is an indication of the effort associated with breathing. The patient may be able to lie down (mild distress), be able to lie down but prefer to sit (moderate distress), or be unable to breathe unless sitting upright (severe dis-

TABLE 68-3	Clinical Manifestations of Hypoxemia and Hypercapnia*
Specific	**Nonspecific**
Hypoxemia	
Respiratory	***Cerebral***
Dyspnea	Agitation
Tachypnea	Disorientation
Prolonged expiration (I:E = 1:3, 1:4)	Delirium
Intercostal muscle retraction	Restless, combative behavior
Use of accessory muscles in respiration	Confusion
↓ SpO_2 (<80%)	↓ Level of consciousness
Paradoxic chest/abdominal wall movement with respiratory cycle (late)	Coma (late)
Cyanosis (late)	***Cardiac***
	Tachycardia
	Hypertension
	Skin cool, clammy, and diaphoretic
	Dysrhythmias (late)
	Hypotension (late)
	Other
	Fatigue
	Unable to speak in complete sentences without pausing to breathe
Hypercapnia	
Respiratory	***Cerebral***
Dyspnea	Morning headache
↓ Respiratory rate or ↑ rapid rate with shallow respirations	Disorientation
↓ Tidal volume	Progressive somnolence
↓ Minute ventilation	Coma (late)
	Cardiac
	Dysrhythmias
	Hypertension
	Tachycardia
	Bounding pulse
	Neuromuscular
	Muscle weakness
	↓ Deep tendon reflexes
	Tremor, seizures (late)
	Other
	Pursed-lip breathing
	Use of tripod position

I:E, Inspiratory:expiratory ratio.
*List is not all-inclusive.

tress). A common position is to sit with the arms propped on the overbed table. This position, called the *tripod position*, helps decrease the work of breathing because propping the arms increases the anterior-posterior diameter of the chest and changes pressure in the thorax. Pursed-lip breathing may be used. This strategy causes an increase in SaO_2 because it slows respirations, allows more time for expiration, and prevents the small bronchioles from collapsing, thus facilitating air exchange. (Pursed-lip breathing is discussed in Chapter 29.) Another assessment parameter is the number of pillows the patient requires to breathe comfortably when attempting to lie flat. This is termed *orthopnea* and may be documented as one-, two-, three-, or four-pillow orthopnea.

The person who is experiencing dyspnea is working hard to breathe and may be able to speak only a few words at a time between breaths. The ability of the patient to speak without pausing to breathe is an indication of the severity of dyspnea. The patient may speak in sentences (mild or no distress), phrases (moderate distress), or words (severe distress). The number of words is also a clue (e.g., how many words can the patient say without pausing to breathe?). The patient may have "two-word" or "three-word" dyspnea, signifying that only two or three words can be said before pausing to breathe. There may also be earlier onset of fatigue with walking. An additional assessment parameter is how far the patient is able to walk without stopping to rest.

There may be a change in the *inspiratory (I) to expiratory (E) (I:E) ratio*. Normally, the I:E ratio is 1:2, which means that expiration is twice as long as inspiration. In patients in respiratory distress, the ratio may increase to 1:3 or 1:4. This change signifies airflow obstruction and that more time is required to empty the lungs.

The nurse may observe *retraction* (inward movement) of the intercostal spaces or the supraclavicular area and use of the accessory muscles (e.g., sternocleidomastoid) during inspiration or expiration. Use of the accessory muscles signifies moderate distress. Paradoxic breathing indicates severe distress. Normally, the thorax and abdomen move outward on inspiration and inward on exhalation. During *paradoxic breathing,* the abdomen and chest move in the opposite manner—outward during exhalation and inward during inspiration.[12,14] Paradoxic breathing results from maximal use of the accessory muscles of respiration. The patient may also be diaphoretic from the work associated with breathing.

Auscultation should be performed in order to assess the patient's baseline breath sounds, as well as any changes from baseline. The nurse should note the presence and location of any adventitious breath sounds. Crackles may indicate pulmonary edema and rhonchi may indicate COPD. Absent or diminished breath sounds may indicate atelectasis or pleural effusion. The presence of bronchial breath sounds over the lung periphery often results from lung consolidation that is seen with pneumonia. A pleural friction rub may also be heard in the presence of pneumonia that has involved the pleura.

A thorough nursing assessment may result in early detection of manifestations associated with respiratory insufficiency, allowing therapy to be instituted before the patient experiences respiratory failure. Patients with end-stage (severe) chronic lung disease may have low PaO_2 values or elevated $PaCO_2$ levels and crackles as their "normal" baseline. It is especially important to monitor specific and nonspecific signs of respiratory failure in patients with COPD because a small change can cause significant decompensation (see Table 68-3). Any deterioration in mental status, such as agitation, combative behavior, confusion, or decreased level of consciousness, should be reported immediately because this change may indicate the onset of rapid deterioration in clinical status and the need for mechanical ventilation.

Diagnostic Studies

After physical assessment, the most common diagnostic studies used to evaluate respiratory failure are ABG analysis and chest x-ray. ABGs are used to determine the levels of $PaCO_2$, PaO_2, bicarbonate, and pH. An indwelling catheter may be inserted into a peripheral artery for continuous monitoring of systemic blood pressure (BP) and obtaining blood for ABGs. Pulse oximetry is frequently used for monitoring oxygenation status, but reveals little about lung ventilation. In respiratory failure, ABGs are necessary to obtain both oxygenation (PaO_2) and ventilation ($PaCO_2$) status, as well as information related to acid-base balance. A chest x-ray is done to help identify possible causes of respiratory failure (e.g., atelectasis, pneumonia).

Other diagnostic studies that may be done include a complete blood cell count, serum electrolytes, urinalysis, and electrocardiogram (ECG). Cultures of the sputum and blood are obtained as necessary to determine sources of possible infection.[12,14] If pulmonary embolus is suspected, a ventilation/perfusion (V/Q) lung scan or pulmonary angiography may be done.[15] For the patient in severe respiratory failure requiring endotracheal intubation, end-tidal CO_2 ($ETCO_2$) may be used to assess tube placement within the trachea immediately following intubation. (Intubation is discussed in Chapter 66.) $ETCO_2$ may also be used during ventilator management to assess trends in lung ventilation as determined by expired CO_2. Although not commonly done in acute situations, pulmonary function tests may be performed.

In severe respiratory failure, a pulmonary artery catheter may be inserted to measure heart pressures and cardiac output, as well as mixed venous oxygen saturation (SvO_2). This information is helpful in determining the adequacy of tissue perfusion and the patient's response to treatment measures. Pulmonary artery, pulmonary artery wedge, and left atrial pressures are monitored to determine whether the accumulation of fluid in the lungs is the result of cardiac or pulmonary problems.[16] These parameters are also monitored to determine the response of the lung and heart to hypoxemia and the patient's response to therapy. Pulmonary arterial pressure monitoring can also provide feedback on the physiologic effects of mechanical ventilation on hemodynamic status. (Hemodynamic monitoring is discussed in detail in Chapter 66.)

NURSING *and* COLLABORATIVE MANAGEMENT
ACUTE RESPIRATORY FAILURE

Because many different problems cause respiratory failure, specific care of these patients varies. This section discusses general assessment and collaborative care measures that apply to patients with acute respiratory failure. In acute care settings there is often an overlap of function between nursing and other members of the health care team.

■ *Nursing Assessment*

Subjective and objective data that should be obtained from the patient with acute respiratory failure are presented in Table 68-4.

■ *Nursing Diagnoses*

Nursing diagnoses for the patient with acute respiratory failure include, but are not limited to, those presented in NCP 68-1.

TABLE 68-4	**NURSING ASSESSMENT** **Acute Respiratory Failure**

Subjective Data
Important Health Information
Past health history: Chronic lung disease; potential occupational exposures to lung toxins; tobacco use (pack-years); previous hospitalizations related to lung disease; thoracic or spinal cord trauma; morbid obesity; altered consciousness; age (physiologic and chronologic); use/abuse of alcohol, other drugs
Medications: Use of oxygen, inhalers (bronchodilators), home nebulization, over-the-counter medications; immunosuppressant (corticosteroid) therapy, CNS depressants
Surgery or other treatments: Previous intubation and mechanical ventilation; recent thoracic or abdominal surgery

Functional Health Patterns
Health perception–health management: Exercise, self-care activities; immunizations (flu, pneumonia, hepatitis)
Nutritional-metabolic: Eating habits; bloating, indigestion; weight gain or loss; decreased appetite; vitamin/herbal supplements
Activity-exercise: Fatigue, dizziness; dyspnea at rest or with activity, wheezing, cough (productive or nonproductive); sputum (volume, color, viscosity); palpitations, swollen feet
Sleep-rest: Changes in sleep pattern
Cognitive-perceptual: Headache, chest pain or tightness
Coping–stress tolerance: Anxiety, depression, hopelessness

Objective Data
General
Restlessness, agitation

Integumentary
Pale, cool, clammy skin or warm, flushed skin; peripheral and central cyanosis; peripheral dependent edema

Respiratory
Shallow, increased respiratory rate progressing to decreased rate; use of accessory muscles with evidence of retractions, altered I:E ratio; increased diaphragmatic excursion or asymmetric chest expansion; paradoxic breathing; tactile fremitus, crepitus, or deviated trachea on palpation; resonant, hyperresonant, or dull percussion note; absent, diminished, or adventitious breath sounds; bronchial or bronchovesicular sounds heard in other than normal location, inspiratory stridor, pleural friction rub

Cardiovascular
Tachycardia progressing to bradycardia, dysrhythmias, extra heart sounds (S3, S4); bounding pulse; hypertension progressing to hypotension; pulsus paradoxus; jugular vein distention; pedal edema

Gastrointestinal
Abdominal distention with tympany; ascites, epigastric tenderness, hepatojugular reflex

Neurologic
Somnolence, confusion, slurred speech, restlessness, delirium, agitation, tremors, seizures, coma; asterixis, decreased deep tendon reflexes; papilledema

Possible Findings
↑/↓ pH, ↑/↓ $PaCO_2$, ↑/↓ bicarbonate, ↓ PaO_2, ↓ SaO_2, ↓ PEFR, ↓ tidal volume, ↓ forced vital capacity, ↓ minute ventilation, ↓ negative inspiratory force; altered values of serum electrolytes, hemoglobin, hematocrit, and white blood cell count; abnormal findings on chest x-ray; abnormal pulmonary artery and pulmonary artery wedge pressures

CNS, Central nervous system; *I:E,* inspiratory:expiratory; *PEFR,* peak expiratory flow rate.

TABLE 68-5	**COLLABORATIVE CARE** **Acute Respiratory Failure**

Diagnostic
History and physical examination
Arterial blood gases
Pulse oximetry
Chest x-ray
CBC
Serum electrolytes and urinalysis
ECG
Blood and sputum cultures (if indicated)
Hemodynamic parameters: PAP, PAWP, LAP

Collaborative Therapy
Respiratory Therapy
O_2 therapy
Mobilization of secretions
- Effective coughing
- Incentive spirometry
- Hydration/humidification
- Chest physical therapy
- Airway suctioning
Positive pressure ventilation
- Noninvasive positive pressure ventilation
- Intubation with mechanical ventilation

Drug Therapy
Relief of bronchospasm (e.g., albuterol [Proventil])
Reduction of airway inflammation (corticosteroids)
Reduction of pulmonary congestion (e.g., furosemide [Lasix])
Treatment of pulmonary infections (e.g., antibiotics)
Reduction of severe anxiety, pain, and agitation (e.g., lorazepam [Ativan], fentanyl [Sublimaze])

Medical Supportive Therapy
Management of the underlying cause of respiratory failure
Maintenance of adequate cardiac output
Maintenance of adequate hemoglobin concentration

Nutritional Therapy
Enteral nutrition support
Parenteral nutrition support

CBC, Complete blood count; *ECG,* electrocardiogram; *LAP,* left atrial pressure; *PAP,* pulmonary artery pressure; *PAWP,* pulmonary artery wedge pressure.

■ *Planning*

The overall goals for the patient in acute respiratory failure include (1) ABG values within the patient's baseline, (2) breath sounds within the patient's baseline, (3) no dyspnea or breathing patterns within the patient's baseline, and (4) effective cough and ability to clear secretions.

■ *Prevention*

As part of the plan of care for any patient who may be at risk for respiratory failure, prevention and early recognition of respiratory distress are important. Prevention involves a thorough physical assessment and history to identify the patient at risk for respiratory failure and, then, the initiation of appropriate nursing interventions. For example, a patient at risk for respiratory failure should receive appropriate patient teaching regarding coughing, deep breathing, incentive spirometry, and ambulation. Prevention of atelectasis, pneumonia, and complications of immobility, as well as optimizing hydration and nutrition, can potentially decrease the risk of respiratory failure in the acutely or critically ill patient.

NURSING CARE PLAN 68-1

Patient with Acute Respiratory Failure

NURSING DIAGNOSIS   **Impaired gas exchange** *related to* alveolar hypoventilation, intrapulmonary shunting, V/Q mismatch, and diffusion impairment *as evidenced by* hypoxemia and/or hypercapnia

PATIENT GOAL   Maintains adequate tissue oxygenation as indicated by normal or baseline arterial blood gases

OUTCOMES (NOC)	INTERVENTIONS (NIC) and *RATIONALES*
Respiratory Status: Gas Exchange	**Ventilation Assistance**
• Oxygen saturation ____ • PaO$_2$ ____ • PaCO$_2$ ____ • Arterial pH ____ • Oxygen saturation ____ • Ventilation/perfusion balance ____	• Monitor respiratory and oxygenation status *to detect systemic manifestations of decreased oxygen and increased carbon dioxide.* • Initiate and maintain supplemental oxygen, as prescribed, *to increase PaO$_2$ and SaO$_2$ levels.* • Monitor the effects of position change on oxygenation: ABGs, SpO$_2$, SvO$_2$, end-tidal CO$_2$ *to assess pulmonary gas exchange.*
Measurement Scale 1 = Severely compromised 2 = Substantially compromised 3 = Moderately compromised 4 = Mildly compromised 5 = Not compromised	**Acid-Base Management: Respiratory Acidosis** • Monitor for symptoms of respiratory failure (e.g., low PaO$_2$ and elevated PaCO$_2$ levels and respiratory muscle fatigue) *to identify need for ventilatory assistance.* • Monitor determinants of tissue oxygen delivery (e.g., PaO$_2$, SaO$_2$, hemoglobin levels, cardiac output) *to plan appropriate interventions.* • Provide mechanical ventilatory support, if necessary, *to maintain adequate gas exchange.* **Cardiac Care** • Monitor for angina and/or cardiac dysrhythmias, including disturbances of both rhythm and conduction, *because hypoxemia may precipitate cardiac dysrhythmias and angina.*

NURSING DIAGNOSIS   **Ineffective airway clearance** *related to* excessive secretions, decreased level of consciousness, presence of an artificial airway, neuromuscular dysfunction, and pain *as evidenced by* difficulty in expectorating sputum, presence of rhonchi or crackles, ineffective or absent cough

PATIENT GOALS   1. Maintains effective airway with removal of excessive secretions
2. Experiences normal or baseline breath sounds

OUTCOMES (NOC)	INTERVENTIONS (NIC) and *RATIONALES*
Respiratory Status: Airway Patency	**Airway Management**
• Ease of breathing ____ • Respiratory rate ____ • Moves sputum out of airway ____	• Encourage slow, deep breathing; turning; and coughing *to promote secretion removal.* • Perform endotracheal or nasotracheal suctioning *to remove secretions and improve oxygenation.* • Position patient to maximize ventilation potential (e.g., head of bed elevated at least 45 degrees or in the tripod position) *to promote maximal chest expansion and effective cough.* • Administer humidified air or oxygen *to prevent drying of the mucosa.* • Perform chest physical therapy *to enhance removal of secretions.* • Regulate fluid intake to optimize fluid balance *to liquefy secretions.* • Administer aerosol treatments (e.g., nebulizer) as ordered *to promote better airflow and secretion removal.*
Measurement Scale 1 = Severely compromised 2 = Substantially compromised 3 = Moderately compromised 4 = Mildly compromised 5 = Not compromised • Adventitious breath sounds ____ **Measurement Scale** 1 = Severe 2 = Substantial 3 = Moderate 4 = Mild 5 = None	

CVP, Central venous pressure; *MAP,* mean arterial pressure; *PAP,* pulmonary artery pressure; *PAWP,* pulmonary artery wedge pressure.   *Continued*

■ Respiratory Therapy

The major goals of care for acute respiratory failure include maintaining adequate oxygenation and ventilation. This goal is accomplished by collaboration among the nursing, medical, and respiratory care teams. The interventions used include O$_2$ therapy, mobilization of secretions, and positive pressure ventilation (PPV) (Table 68-5).

Oxygen Therapy.   The primary goal of O$_2$ therapy is to correct hypoxemia. If hypoxemia is secondary to V/Q mismatch, supplemental O$_2$ administered at 1 to 3 L/min by nasal cannula or 24% to 32% by simple face mask or Venturi mask should improve the PaO$_2$, SaO$_2$, and SpO$_2$. Hypoxemia secondary to an intrapulmonary shunt is usually not responsive to high O$_2$ concentrations, and the patient

NURSING CARE PLAN 68-1
Patient with Acute Respiratory Failure—cont'd

NURSING DIAGNOSIS **Ineffective breathing pattern** *related to* neuromuscular impairment of respirations, pain, anxiety, decreased level of consciousness, respiratory muscle fatigue, and bronchospasm *as evidenced by* respiratory rate <12 or >24 breaths/min, altered I:E ratio, irregular breathing pattern, use of accessory muscles, asynchronous thoracoabdominal movement, wheezing, apnea

PATIENT GOAL Demonstrates normal or baseline respiratory rate, rhythm, and depth of respirations

OUTCOMES (NOC)

Respiratory Status: Ventilation

- Respiratory rhythm ____
- Respiratory rate ____
- Depth of inspiration ____
- Symmetric chest expansion ____
- Ease of breathing ____
- Auscultated breath sounds ____

Measurement Scale

1 = Severely compromised
2 = Substantially compromised
3 = Moderately compromised
4 = Mildly compromised
5 = Not compromised

INTERVENTIONS (NIC) and *RATIONALES*

Ventilation Assistance

- Auscultate breath sounds, noting areas of decreased or absent ventilation and presence of adventitious sounds *to assess for presence of inability to sustain ventilation.*
- Monitor for respiratory muscle fatigue *to provide ventilatory support as needed.*
- Position to minimize respiratory efforts (e.g., elevate the head of the bed and provide overbed table for patient to lean on) *to preserve energy for breathing.*
- Teach pursed-lip breathing techniques *to reverse altered I:E ratio.*
- Initiate resuscitation efforts *because airway support may be needed in the event of severely impaired ventilation or apnea.*

Airway Insertion and Stabilization

- Assist with insertion of an endotracheal tube by gathering necessary intubation and emergency equipment, positioning patient, administering medications as ordered, and monitoring the patient for complications during insertion *to maintain adequate oxygenation and ventilation.*

NURSING DIAGNOSIS **Risk for fluid volume imbalance** *related to* sodium and water retention

PATIENT GOALS 1. Maintains stable body weight and balanced intake and output
2. Experiences normal hemodynamic status

OUTCOMES (NOC)

Fluid Balance

- Blood pressure ____
- Mean arterial pressure ____
- Central venous pressure ____
- Pulmonary wedge pressure ____
- Stable body weight ____
- 24-hr intake and output balance ____

Measurement Scale

1 = Severely compromised
2 = Substantially compromised
3 = Moderately compromised
4 = Mildly compromised
5 = Not compromised

INTERVENTIONS (NIC) and *RATIONALES*

Fluid Management

- Monitor for indications of fluid overload/retention (e.g., crackles, edema, neck vein distention, and ascites) *to identify problem.*
- Monitor hemodynamic status, including CVP, MAP, PAP, and PAWP, *to detect changes in systemic fluid volume.*
- Weigh patient daily *to evaluate trends in fluid status.*
- Maintain accurate intake and output record daily *to evaluate trends in fluid status.*
- Administer prescribed diuretics *to prevent or reduce fluid overload.*

---

will usually require PPV.[1,2] PPV offers a means of providing O_2 therapy and humidification, decreasing the work of breathing, and reducing respiratory muscle fatigue. In addition, the positive pressure may assist in opening collapsed airways and decreasing shunt. PPV may be provided via an endotracheal tube (most frequently) or noninvasively by means of a tight-fitting mask.[17] (Mechanical ventilation is discussed in detail in Chapter 66.)

The type of O_2 delivery system chosen for the patient in acute respiratory failure should (1) be tolerated by the patient, because anxiety caused by feelings of claustrophobia related to the face mask or dyspnea may prompt the patient to remove the O_2 device, and (2) maintain PaO_2 at 55 to 60 mm Hg or more and SaO_2 at 90% or more at the lowest O_2 concentration possible. High O_2 concentrations replace the nitrogen gas normally present in the alveoli,

causing instability and atelectasis. In intubated patients, exposure to 60% or greater O_2 for longer than 48 hours poses a significant risk for O_2 toxicity. In nonintubated patients, the risk is less clear. The effects of prolonged exposure to high levels of O_2 include increased pulmonary microvascular permeability, decreased surfactant production and surfactant inactivation, and fibrotic changes in the alveoli. (O_2 delivery devices are discussed in Chapter 29.)

A possible risk of O_2 therapy is specific to the patient with chronic hypercapnia such as the patient with COPD. Chronic hypercapnia may blunt the response of chemoreceptors in the medulla. In this situation, respirations are primarily stimulated by hypoxia. Patients with chronic hypercapnia should receive O_2 through a low-flow device such as a nasal cannula at 1 to 2 L/min or a Venturi mask at 24% to 28%. They should be closely monitored for

NURSING CARE PLAN 68-1

Patient with Acute Respiratory Failure—cont'd

NURSING DIAGNOSIS   **Imbalanced nutrition: less than body requirements** *related to* poor appetite, shortness of breath, presence of artificial airway, decreased energy level, and increased caloric requirements *as evidenced by* weight loss, weakness, muscle wasting, dehydration, poor muscle tone, poor skin integrity

PATIENT GOALS
1. Maintains intake adequate to meet body's nutritional needs
2. Experiences stable weight and muscle tone

OUTCOMES (NOC)	INTERVENTIONS (NIC) and *RATIONALES*
Nutritional Status: Energy	**Nutrition Therapy**
• Stamina ____	• Determine—in collaboration with the dietitian—the number of calories and type of nutrients needed *to meet nutrition requirements.*
• Tissue healing ____	• Provide needed nourishment within limits of prescribed diet *to meet increased nutritional requirements.*
Nutritional Status: Nutrient Intake	• Select nutritional supplements *to maintain adequate caloric intake.*
• Nutrient intake ____	• Administer enteral feedings *to meet nutritional needs if patient cannot tolerate oral feedings.*
• Food intake ____	• Administer parenteral feeding *to meet nutritional needs if patient cannot tolerate oral or enteral feedings.*
• Energy ____	
• Hematocrit ____	**Oxygen Therapy**
• Muscle tone ____	• Monitor patient's ability to tolerate removal of oxygen while eating *to prevent shortness of breath and blood oxygen desaturation while eating.*
Measurement Scale	**Acid-Base Management: Respiratory Acidosis**
1 = Severe deviation from normal range	• Provide low-carbohydrate, high-fat diet (e.g., Pulmocare feedings) *to reduce CO_2 production, if indicated, for patients with respiratory acidosis.*
2 = Substantial deviation from normal range	
3 = Moderate deviation from normal range	
4 = Mild deviation from normal range	
5 = No deviation from normal range	

changes in mental status, respiratory rate, and ABG results until their PaO_2 level has reached their baseline normal value.

Mobilization of Secretions. Retained pulmonary secretions may cause or exacerbate acute respiratory failure by blocking movement of O_2 into the alveoli and pulmonary capillary blood and removal of CO_2 during the respiratory cycle. Secretions can be mobilized through effective coughing, adequate hydration and humidification, chest physical therapy (chest physiotherapy), and tracheal suctioning.

Effective Coughing and Positioning. If secretions are obstructing the airway, the patient should be encouraged to cough. The patient with a neuromuscular weakness from a disease or exhaustion may not be able to generate sufficient airway pressures to produce an effective cough. *Augmented coughing (quad coughing)* may be of benefit to these patients. Augmented coughing is performed by placing the palm of the hand (or the palms of both hands) on the abdomen below the xiphoid process (Fig. 68-6). As the patient ends a deep inspiration and begins the expiration, the hands should be moved forcefully downward, increasing abdominal pressure and facilitating the cough. This measure helps increase expiratory flow and thereby facilitates secretion clearance.

Some patients may benefit from therapeutic cough techniques. *Huff coughing* is a series of coughs performed while saying the word "huff." This technique prevents the glottis from closing during the cough. Patients with COPD generate higher flow rates with a huff cough than is possible with a normal cough. The huff cough is effective in clearing only the central airways, but it may assist in moving secretions upward. The staged cough also assists secretion mobilization. To perform the *staged cough,* the patient sits in a chair, breathes three or four times in and out through the mouth, and coughs while bending forward and pressing a pillow inward against the diaphragm.

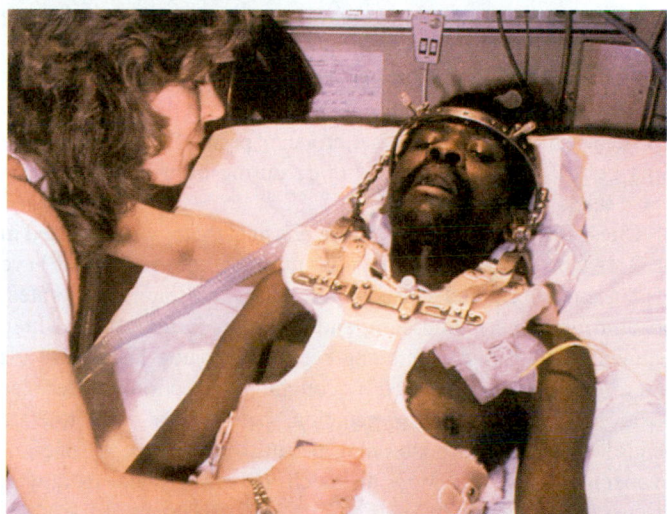

FIG. 68-6   Augmented coughing is performed by placing the palm of the hand on the abdominal musculature below the xiphoid process. As the patient ends a deep inspiration and begins the expiration, the hand should be moved forcefully downward, increasing abdominal pressure, resulting in a forceful cough.

Positioning the patient either by elevating the head of the bed at least 45 degrees or by using a reclining chair or chair bed may help maximize thoracic expansion, thereby decreasing dyspnea and improving secretion mobilization. A sitting position improves pulmonary function and assists in venous pooling in dependent body areas such as the lower extremities. When lungs are upright, ventilation and perfusion are best in the lung bases. Lateral or side-lying positioning may be used in patients with disease involving only one lung. This position, termed *good lung down,* allows for improved V/Q matching in the affected lung. Pulmonary blood flow and ventilation are optimal in dependent lung areas. This positioning also allows for secretions to drain out of the affected lung to the point where they may be removed by suctioning. For example, in patients with significant right-sided pneumonia, optimal positioning would be to place them on their left side to maximize ventilation and perfusion in the "good" lung and facilitate secretion removal from the affected lung (postural drainage). All patients should be side-lying if there is any possibility that the tongue will obstruct the airway or that aspiration may occur. An oral or nasal airway should be kept at the bedside for use if necessary.

Hydration and Humidification. Thick and viscous secretions are difficult to move and should be thinned. Adequate fluid intake (2 to 3 L/day) is necessary to keep secretions thin and easy to expel. If the patient is unable to take sufficient fluids orally, intravenous (IV) hydration will be used. Thorough assessment of the patient's cardiac and renal status is essential to determine whether he or she can tolerate the intravascular volume and avoid heart failure and pulmonary edema. Assessment for signs of fluid overload (e.g., crackles, dyspnea, increased central venous pressure) at regular intervals is also essential. These considerations would also apply to the patient with renal dysfunction.

An appropriate humidification device is an adjunct in secretion management. Aerosols of sterile normal saline, administered by a nebulizer, may be used to liquefy secretions. Oxygen may also be administered by aerosol mask to thin secretions and facilitate their removal. Aerosol therapy may induce bronchospasm and severe coughing, causing a decreased PaO_2. As such, frequent assessment of patient tolerance to therapy is critical.[12,16] Mucolytic agents such as nebulized acetylcysteine (Mucomyst) mixed with a bronchodilator may be used to thin secretions but, as a side effect, may also cause airway erythema and bronchospasm. Therefore they are used only in special situations (e.g., during bronchoscopy to remove thick, copious secretions).

Chest Physical Therapy. Chest physical therapy is indicated in patients who produce more than 30 ml of sputum per day or have evidence of severe atelectasis or pulmonary infiltrates. If tolerated, postural drainage, percussion, and vibration to the affected lung segments may assist in moving secretions to the larger airways where they may be removed by coughing or suctioning. Because positioning may affect oxygenation, patients may not tolerate head-down or lateral positioning because of extreme dyspnea or hypoxemia caused by V/Q mismatch. (Chest physical therapy is discussed in Chapter 29.)

Airway Suctioning. If the patient is unable to expectorate secretions, nasopharyngeal, oropharyngeal, or nasotracheal suctioning (blind suctioning without a tracheal tube in place) is indicated. Suctioning through an artificial airway, such as endotracheal or tracheostomy tubes, may also be performed (see Chapters 27 and 66). A mini-tracheostomy (or mini-trach) may be used to suction patients who have difficulty mobilizing secretions and when blind suctioning is difficult or ineffective. The *mini-trach* is a 4-mm indwelling plastic cuffless cannula inserted through the cricothyroid membrane. It is used to instill sterile normal saline solution to elicit a cough and to perform suctioning using a size 10 or less French catheter. Contraindications for a mini-trach include an absent gag reflex, history of aspiration, and the need for long-term mechanical ventilation. At all times, suctioning is done cautiously because it may precipitate hypoxia.

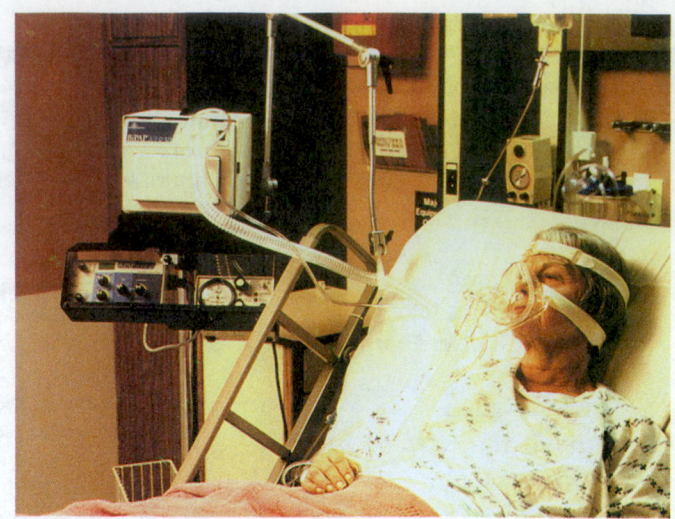

FIG. 68-7 Noninvasive bilevel positive pressure ventilation. A mask is placed over the nose or nose and mouth. Positive pressure from a mechanical ventilator assists the patient's breathing efforts, decreasing the work of breathing.

Positive Pressure Ventilation. If intensive measures fail to improve ventilation and oxygenation and the patient continues to exhibit manifestations of acute respiratory failure, ventilatory assistance may be initiated. PPV may be provided invasively through orotracheal or nasotracheal intubation or noninvasively through a nasal or face mask.[17,18] Patients who require PPV are typically cared for in a critical care unit. (See Chapter 66 for a discussion of artificial airways and mechanical ventilation.)

Noninvasive positive pressure ventilation (NIPPV) may be used as a treatment for patients with acute or chronic respiratory failure. During NIPPV a mask is placed tightly over the patient's nose or nose and mouth and the patient breathes spontaneously while PPV is delivered (Fig. 68-7). With NIPPV it is possible to decrease the work of breathing without the need for endotracheal intubation. Bilevel positive airway pressure (BiPAP) is a form of NIPPV in which different positive pressure levels are set for inspiration and expiration (Fig. 68-7). Continuous positive airway pressure (CPAP) is another form of NIPPV in which a constant positive pressure is delivered to the airway during inspiration and expiration.[17]

NIPPV is most useful in managing chronic respiratory failure in patients with chest wall and neuromuscular disease (see Table 68-1). NIPPV has been used in patients with hypoxemic respiratory failure (e.g., ARDS, cardiogenic pulmonary edema), but with less success. NIPPV may also be used for patients who refuse endotracheal intubation but still desire some palliative ventilatory support (e.g., patients with end-stage COPD).[18-20] NIPPV is not appropriate for the patient who has absent respirations, excessive secretions, decreased level of consciousness, high O_2 requirements, facial trauma, or hemodynamic instability.[17]

■ *Drug Therapy*

Goals of drug therapy for patients in acute respiratory failure include (1) relief of bronchospasm, (2) reduction of airway inflammation and pulmonary congestion, (3) treatment of pulmonary infection, and (4) reduction of severe anxiety and restlessness.

Relief of Bronchospasm. Alveolar ventilation will be increased with relief of bronchospasm. Short-acting bronchodilators, such as metaproterenol (Alupent) and albuterol (Ventolin), are frequently administered to reverse bronchospasm using either a handheld nebulizer or a metered-dose inhaler with a spacer.[3-8,13] In acute bronchospasm these drugs may be given at 15- to 30-minute intervals until it can be determined that a response is occurring. The bronchodilator effects of these medications can sometimes cause a worsening of arterial hypoxemia by redistributing the inspired gas to areas of decreased perfusion. Administering the bronchodilator with an O_2-enriched gas mixture usually alleviates this effect.[4] (See Chapter 29 for nursing management related to bronchodilators.)

Reduction of Airway Inflammation. Corticosteroids (e.g., methylprednisolone [Solu-Medrol]) may be used in conjunction with bronchodilating agents when bronchospasm and inflammation are present. When administered IV, corticosteroids have an immediate onset of action. Inhaled corticosteroids are not used for acute respiratory failure, because they require 4 to 5 days before optimum therapeutic effects are seen.[3-8,13]

Reduction of Pulmonary Congestion. Pulmonary interstitial fluid can occur as a consequence of direct or indirect injury to the alveolar capillary membrane (e.g., ARDS) or from right- or left-sided heart failure, and therefore can be either cardiac or noncardiac in origin. The result is decreased alveolar ventilation and hypoxemia. IV diuretics (e.g., furosemide [Lasix]) and nitroglycerin (e.g., Tridil) are used to decrease the pulmonary congestion caused by heart failure. If atrial fibrillation is also present, calcium channel blockers (e.g., diltiazem) and β-adrenergic blockers (e.g., metoprolol) may be used to decrease heart rate and improve cardiac output. (See Chapter 35 for discussion of heart failure.)

Treatment of Pulmonary Infections. Pulmonary infections (pneumonia, acute bronchitis) result in excessive mucus production, fever, increased oxygen consumption, and inflamed, fluid-filled, or collapsed alveoli. Alveoli that are fluid filled or collapsed cannot participate in gas exchange. Pulmonary infections can either cause or exacerbate acute respiratory failure. IV antibiotics, such as vancomycin (Vancocin) or ceftriaxone (Rocephin), are frequently administered to inhibit bacterial growth. Chest x-rays are performed to determine the location and extent of a suspected infectious process. Sputum cultures are used to determine the type of organisms causing the infection and their sensitivity to antimicrobial medications.

Reduction of Severe Anxiety, Pain, and Agitation. Anxiety, restlessness, and agitation result from cerebral hypoxia. In addition, fear caused by the inability to breathe and a sense of loss of control may exacerbate anxiety. Anxiety, pain, and agitation increase O_2 consumption, which may worsen the degree of hypoxemia. Anxiety, pain, and agitation also increase CO_2 production, affect ventilator management, and increase morbidity.[3-5] Several nursing strategies can assist the patient in reducing the level of anxiety and pain (see NCP 68-1).

Sedation and analgesia with drug therapy such as propofol (Diprivan), benzodiazepines (e.g., lorazepam [Ativan], midazolam [Versed]), and opioids (e.g., morphine, fentanyl [Sublimaze]) may be used to decrease anxiety, agitation, and pain. Continued agitation will increase the patient's work of breathing, O_2 consumption, CO_2 production, and risk of injury (e.g., accidental extubation). When receiving any sedative or analgesic agent, patients must be monitored closely for cardiovascular and respiratory depression.[4,7,9] In the critical care setting, sedation and analgesia are commonly used for severely restless, anxious, and agitated patients who may be experiencing pain and are in acute respiratory

failure. It is important to note that agitation is best characterized as a symptom and may be caused by pain, hypoxemia, electrolyte imbalance, evolution of structural or metabolic brain injury, and adverse drug reactions. As such, aggressive assessment and treatment of all potentially reversible causes should always be undertaken. Sedative and analgesic agents may have prolonged duration of action in critically ill patients. This may contribute to increased length of stay and prolonged ventilator days. Patients receiving these agents are best managed by following a research-based, protocol-driven plan of care.[21]

Patients who breathe asynchronously with mechanical ventilation may also benefit from titration of ventilator flow rates and other settings, as well as addressing treatable causes of agitation such as hypoxemia, pain, or hypercapnia. Patients who remain asynchronous with mechanical ventilation may require neuromuscular blockade with agents such as vecuronium (Norcuron) or cisatracurium (Nimbex) to produce skeletal muscle relaxation by interference with neuromuscular transmission, ultimately producing synchrony with mechanical ventilation. Neuromuscular blockade may also decrease the patient's risk of lung injury related to excessive inspiratory/intrathoracic pressures. In this way, the ventilator can then provide optimal respiratory support.

Patients receiving neuromuscular blockade should receive sedation and analgesia to the point of unconsciousness for patient comfort, to eliminate patient awareness, and to avoid the terrifying experience of being awake and in pain while paralyzed.[9,22] Monitoring levels of sedation in patients receiving neuromuscular blockade is challenging. Noninvasive electroencephalogram-based technology is available that may help guide sedative and analgesic therapy in this population.[22] Monitoring levels of pharmacologic paralysis is commonly done through the use of a peripheral nerve stimulator. Clinical assessment is essential to determine the adequacy of sedation, analgesia, and neuromuscular blockade in critically ill patients.

■ Medical Supportive Therapy

Therapeutic goals and interventions to maximize O_2 delivery and treat the underlying cause of the respiratory failure are essential to improving the patient's oxygenation and ventilation status. The primary goal is to treat the underlying cause of the respiratory failure. Other goals include maintaining an adequate cardiac output and hemoglobin concentration.

Treating the Underlying Cause. Interventions are directed toward reversing the disease process that resulted in the development of acute respiratory failure. Patients with hypoventilation can be diagnosed and treated rapidly. Patients with V/Q mismatch, shunting, or diffusion limitation are managed differently depending on the underlying cause. In all patient situations, monitoring treatment effects, including trends in ABGs and changes in respiratory status, is a continuous process.

Maintaining Adequate Cardiac Output. Cardiac output reflects the blood flow reaching the tissues. BP and mean arterial pressure (MAP) are important indicators of the adequacy of cardiac output. Interpretation of BP and MAP readings must be done within the context of the overall physical examination indicating adequacy of cardiac output and tissue perfusion. Usually a systolic BP of at least 90 mm Hg or a MAP greater than 60 mm Hg is adequate to maintain perfusion to the vital organs. If the systolic BP is at least 90 mm Hg or the MAP is at least 60 mm Hg, changes in mental status may be attributed to the level of O_2 and CO_2 rather than decreased cerebral perfusion. In a patient with chronic, uncontrolled hypertension, a systolic BP of 90 to 100 mm Hg may be inadequate to maintain systemic and cerebral perfusion. Stability of cerebral perfusion may not only tolerate but may require higher systemic arterial pressures and MAPs to prevent episodes of brain ischemia.

Decreased cardiac output is treated by administration of IV fluids, medications, or both. (See Chapter 67 for a discussion of drugs used to treat decreased cardiac output and shock.) Cardiac output may also be decreased by changes in intrathoracic or intrapulmonary pressures from PPV. Patients experiencing exacerbation of COPD or asthma and those receiving controlled ventilation are at risk of alveolar hyperinflation, increased right ventricular afterload, and excessive intrathoracic pressures. These alterations in thoracic pressure dynamics may cause increased right ventricular afterload, which limits blood flow from the right side of the heart through the pulmonary vasculature to the left side of the heart; this may potentially result in dramatic hemodynamic compromise. In addition, blood return from the systemic circulation to the right side of the heart may be impaired, decreasing preload.[3,4] Each of these physiologic consequences can potentially lead to severe hemodynamic compromise. Consequently, BP and clinical indicators of adequate cardiac output and tissue perfusion should be monitored closely with initiation or titration of mechanical ventilation by mask or endotracheal intubation.

Maintaining Adequate Hemoglobin Concentration. Hemoglobin is the primary carrier when delivering O_2 to the tissues. If the patient is anemic, tissue O_2 delivery will be compromised. A hemoglobin concentration of 9 g/dl (90 g/L) or greater typically ensures adequate O_2 saturation of the hemoglobin. The patient should be monitored for sites of blood loss and transfused with packed red blood cells if an adequate hemoglobin concentration cannot be maintained and the patient is symptomatic.

■ Nutritional Therapy

Maintenance of protein and energy stores is especially important in patients who experience acute respiratory failure because nutritional depletion causes a loss of muscle mass, including the respiratory muscles, and may prolong recovery. The nurse and dietitian work together to determine the optimal method of feeding, as well as the optimal caloric and fluid requirements. During the acute manifestations of respiratory failure, the risk of aspiration typically prevents oral nutritional intake. Therefore enteral or parenteral nutrition is usually initiated within 24 hours in malnourished patients and within 3 days in well-nourished patients. When the acute manifestations subside, the patient may resume oral intake as tolerated.

A multitude of nutritional supplements are available for this patient population. A high-carbohydrate diet may need to be avoided in the patient who retains CO_2 because carbohydrates metabolize into CO_2 and increase the CO_2 load of the patient. However, research in this area remains controversial. Additional issues affecting nutritional state include hypermetabolic state encountered in critical illness. A hypermetabolic state may potentially dramatically increase caloric requirements to maintain body weight and muscle mass.

■ Evaluation

The expected outcomes for the patient with acute respiratory failure are presented in NCP 68-1.

The elderly population is the fastest growing age-group in North America, a trend that is increasingly reflected within the patient populations in acute care and critical care settings. Multiple factors contribute to an increased risk of respiratory failure in older adults. They are at higher risk of developing respiratory failure because of the reduction in ventilatory capacity that accompanies aging, especially if other risk factors are present. Physiologic aging of the lung may produce alveolar dilation, larger air spaces, and loss of surface area. Diminished elastic recoil within the airways, decreased chest wall compliance, and decreased respiratory muscle strength also occur. In older adults, the PaO_2 falls further and the $PaCO_2$ rises to a higher level before the respiratory system is stimulated to alter the rate and depth of breathing. This delayed response can contribute to the development of respiratory failure. In addition, a history of tobacco use is a risk factor that can accelerate age-related respiratory changes. Poor nutritional status and less available physiologic reserve in the cardiovascular, respiratory, and autonomic nervous systems increase the risk of additional disease states such as pneumonia and cardiac disease that may compromise respiratory function and precipitate respiratory failure. Poor nutrition can also result in a decrease in muscle mass and related respiratory drive.[23,24]

The elderly are more vulnerable to delirium, nosocomial infections, the effects of medications, and an intensive care unit (ICU) environment that may be perceived as threatening. Delirium has been identified as an independent risk factor for increased mortality and morbidity rates in critically ill patients.[25] It can complicate ventilator management and weaning by interfering with patient cooperation. Agitated delirium increases CO_2 elimination and O_2 consumption, increases risk for unplanned extubation and device removal, and contributes to increased length of stay and ventilator days.[24,25]

Assessment parameters must also be adjusted for age. For example, heart rate and BP generally increase with age and related changes in the cardiovascular system. Therefore determination of the patient's baseline vital signs and using them as a basis for comparison of physical assessment findings is most appropriate in evaluating changes in cardiopulmonary function in the older adult.

ACUTE RESPIRATORY DISTRESS SYNDROME

Acute respiratory distress syndrome (ARDS) is a sudden and progressive form of acute respiratory failure in which the alveolar capillary membrane becomes damaged and more permeable to intravascular fluid (Fig. 68-8). The alveoli fill with fluid, resulting in severe dyspnea, hypoxemia refractory to supplemental O_2, reduced lung compliance, and diffuse pulmonary infiltrates.[14,26,27]

The incidence of ARDS in the United States is estimated at more than 150,000 cases annually. Despite supportive therapy, the mortality rate from ARDS is approximately 50%. Patients who have both gram-negative septic shock and ARDS have a mortality rate of 70% to 90%.[14,25,26]

Etiology and Pathophysiology

Table 68-6 lists conditions that predispose patients to the development of ARDS. The most common cause of ARDS is sepsis. Patients with multiple risk factors are three to four times more likely to develop ARDS.

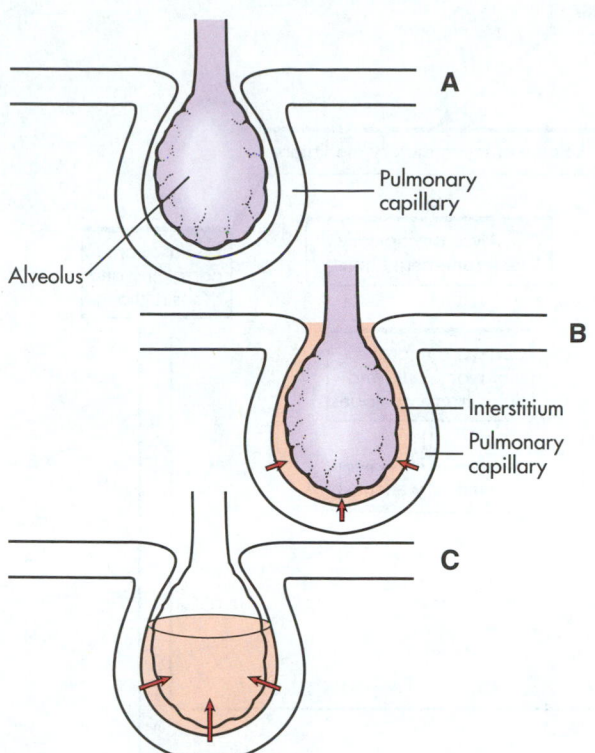

FIG. 68-8   Stages of edema formation in acute respiratory distress syndrome. **A,** Normal alveolus and pulmonary capillary. **B,** Interstitial edema occurs with increased flow of fluid into the interstitial space. **C,** Alveolar edema occurs when the fluid crosses the blood-gas barrier.

Labels: A, Pulmonary capillary, Alveolus, B, Interstitium, Pulmonary capillary, C

TABLE 68-6	Conditions Predisposing to Acute Respiratory Distress Syndrome

Direct Lung Injury
Common Causes
Aspiration of gastric contents or other substances
Viral/bacterial pneumonia

Less Common Causes
Chest trauma
Embolism: fat, air, amniotic fluid, thrombus
Inhalation of toxic substances
Near-drowning
O_2 toxicity
Radiation pneumonitis

Indirect Lung Injury
Common Causes
Sepsis (especially gram-negative infection)
Severe massive trauma

Less Common Causes
Acute pancreatitis
Anaphylaxis
Cardiopulmonary bypass
Disseminated intravascular coagulation
Multiple blood transfusions
Opioid drug overdose (e.g., heroin)
Nonpulmonary systemic diseases
Severe head injury
Shock states

Direct lung injury may cause ARDS (Fig. 68-9), or ARDS may develop as a consequence of the systemic inflammatory response syndrome (SIRS) (see Chapter 67, Fig. 67-1). SIRS may have an infectious or a noninfectious etiology and is characterized by widespread inflammation or clinical responses to inflammation following a variety of physiologic insults, including severe trauma, gut ischemia, lung injury, and sepsis.[26,27] ARDS may also develop as a consequence of multiple organ dysfunction syndrome (MODS). MODS results from organ system dysfunction that progressively increases in severity and ultimately results in multisystem organ failure. (SIRS and MODS are discussed in Chapter 67.)

An exact cause for the damage to the alveolar-capillary membrane is not known. However, the pathophysiologic changes of ARDS are thought to be due to stimulation of the inflammatory and immune systems, which causes an attraction of neutrophils to the pulmonary interstitium.[14,27] The neutrophils cause a release of biochemical, humoral, and cellular mediators (Table 68-7) that produce changes in the lung, including increased pulmonary capillary membrane permeability, destruction of elastin and collagen, formation of pulmonary microemboli, and pulmonary artery vasoconstriction[27] (see Fig. 68-9). (These mediators are discussed in Chapters 13 and 14.)

The pathophysiologic changes in ARDS are divided into three phases: (1) injury or exudative phase, (2) reparative or proliferative phase, and (3) fibrotic phase.[14,26-28]

Injury or Exudative Phase. The *injury or exudative phase* occurs approximately 1 to 7 days (usually 24 to 48 hours) after the initial direct lung injury or host insult. Neutrophils adhere to the

pulmonary microcirculation, causing damage to the vascular endothelium and increased capillary permeability. In the earliest phase of injury, there is engorgement of the peribronchial and perivascular interstitial space, which produces interstitial edema. Next, fluid from the interstitial space crosses the alveolar epithelium and enters the alveolar space. Intrapulmonary shunt develops because the alveoli fill with fluid, and blood passing through them cannot be oxygenated (see Figs. 68-4 and 68-8).

Alveolar type I and type II cells (which produce surfactant) are damaged by the changes caused by ARDS. This damage, in addition to further fluid and protein accumulation, results in surfactant dysfunction. The function of *surfactant* is to maintain alveolar stability by decreasing alveolar surface tension and preventing alveolar collapse. Decreased synthesis of surfactant and inactivation of existing surfactant cause the alveoli to become unstable and collapse (atelectasis). Widespread atelectasis further decreases lung compliance, compromises gas exchange, and contributes to hypoxemia.[14,26,27]

Also during this stage, hyaline membranes begin to line the alveoli. The hyaline membrane is composed of necrotic cells, protein, and fibrin and lies adjacent to the alveoli wall. These hyaline membranes are thought to result from the exudation of high-molecular-weight substances (particularly fibrinogen) in the edema fluid. Hyaline membranes contribute to the development of fibrosis and atelectasis, leading to a decrease in gas exchange capability and lung compliance.

The primary pathophysiologic changes that characterize the *injury or exudative phase* of ARDS are interstitial and alveolar edema (noncardiogenic pulmonary edema) and atelectasis.[14,27] Severe V/Q mismatch and shunting of pulmonary capillary blood result in hypoxemia unresponsive to increasing concentrations of O_2 (termed **refractory hypoxemia**). Diffusion limitation, caused by hyaline membrane formation, further contributes to the severity of

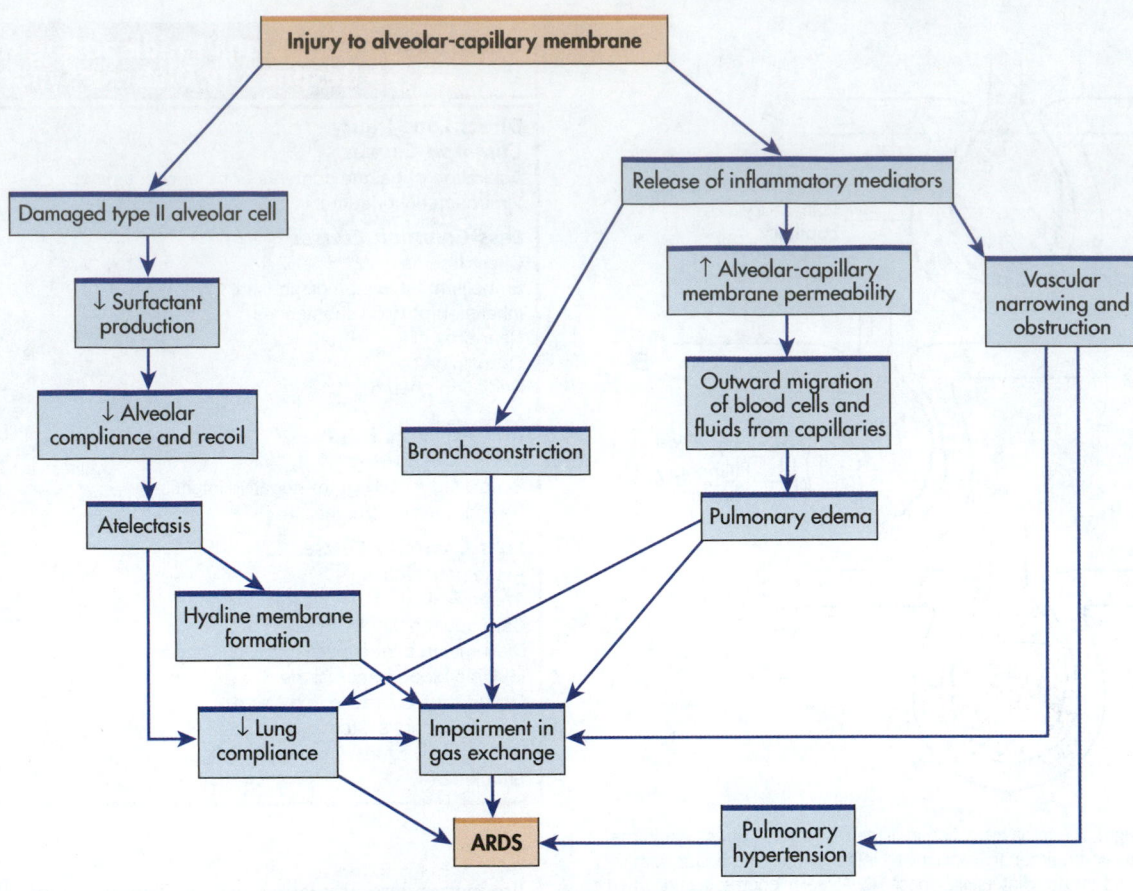

FIG. 68-9 Pathophysiology of acute respiratory distress syndrome (ARDS).

TABLE 68-7	Mediators of Acute Lung Injury

- Complement component C5a
- Neutrophil products, including proteases and O_2 radicals
- Monocyte and macrophage products, including tumor necrosis factor, interleukin-1, and colony-stimulating factor
- Arachidonic acid metabolites, including prostaglandins and leukotrienes
- Coagulation products, including kallikreins, kinins, fibrin degradation products, and plasminogen-activating factor
- Histamine
- Serotonin
- Endotoxin
- Elastase
- Collagenase

the hypoxemia. As the lungs become less compliant because of decreased surfactant, pulmonary edema, and atelectasis, the patient must generate higher airway pressures to inflate "stiff" lungs. Reduced lung compliance greatly increases the patient's work of breathing. During ventilator management at this stage, higher inspiratory and plateau pressures may be noted. Progressive increase in pressures required to deliver a controlled ventilation may occur as a result of worsening lung compliance.

Hypoxemia and the stimulation of juxtacapillary receptors in the stiff lung parenchyma (J reflex) initially cause an increase in respiratory rate and a decrease in tidal volume. This breathing pattern increases CO_2 removal, producing respiratory alkalosis. Cardiac output increases in response to hypoxemia, a compensatory

effort to increase pulmonary blood flow. However, as atelectasis, pulmonary edema, and pulmonary shunt increase, compensation fails, and hypoventilation, decreased cardiac output, and decreased tissue O_2 perfusion eventually occur.

Reparative or Proliferative Phase. The *reparative or proliferative phase* of ARDS begins 1 to 2 weeks after the initial lung injury. During this phase, there is an influx of neutrophils, monocytes, and lymphocytes and fibroblast proliferation as part of the inflammatory response. The injured lung has an immense regenerative capacity after acute lung injury. The proliferative phase is complete when the diseased lung becomes characterized by dense, fibrous tissue. Increased pulmonary vascular resistance and pulmonary hypertension may occur in this stage because fibroblasts and inflammatory cells destroy the pulmonary vasculature. Lung compliance continues to decrease as a result of interstitial fibrosis. Hypoxemia worsens because of the thickened alveolar membrane, causing diffusion limitation and shunting. If the reparative phase persists, widespread fibrosis results. If the reparative phase is arrested, the lesions resolve.[14,26]

Fibrotic Phase. The *fibrotic phase* of ARDS occurs approximately 2 to 3 weeks after the initial lung injury. This phase is also called the *chronic or late phase* of ARDS. By this time, the lung is completely remodeled by sparsely collagenous and fibrous tissues. There is diffuse scarring and fibrosis, resulting in decreased lung compliance. In addition, the surface area for gas exchange is significantly reduced because the interstitium is fibrotic, and therefore hypoxemia continues. Pulmonary hypertension results from pulmonary vascular destruction and fibrosis.[14,26]

Clinical Progression

Progression of ARDS varies among patients. Some persons survive the acute phase of lung injury; pulmonary edema resolves and complete recovery occurs in a few days. The chance for survival is poor in patients who enter the fibrotic (chronic or late) stage, which requires long-term mechanical ventilation. It is not known why injured lungs repair and recover in some patients, and in others ARDS progresses. Several factors seem to be important in determining the course of ARDS, including the nature of the initial injury, extent and severity of coexisting diseases, and pulmonary complications.[14,26,27]

Clinical Manifestations

The initial presentation of ARDS is often insidious. At the time of the initial injury, and for several hours to 1 to 2 days afterward, the patient may not experience respiratory symptoms, or the patient may exhibit only dyspnea, tachypnea, cough, and restlessness. Chest auscultation may be normal or reveal fine, scattered crackles. ABGs usually indicate mild hypoxemia and respiratory alkalosis caused by hyperventilation. Respiratory alkalosis results from hypoxemia and the stimulation of juxtacapillary receptors. The chest x-ray may be normal or exhibit evidence of minimal scattered interstitial infiltrates. Edema may not show on the x-ray until there is a 30% increase in fluid content in the lung.[14,26]

As ARDS progresses, symptoms worsen because of increased fluid accumulation and decreased lung compliance. Respiratory discomfort becomes evident as the work of breathing increases. Tachypnea and intercostal and suprasternal retractions may be present. Pulmonary function tests in ARDS reveal decreased compliance and decreased lung volumes, particularly a decreased functional residual capacity (FRC). Tachycardia, diaphoresis, changes in sensorium with decreased mentation, cyanosis, and pallor may be present. Chest auscultation usually reveals scattered to diffuse crackles and rhonchi. The chest x-ray demonstrates diffuse and extensive bilateral interstitial and alveolar infiltrates. A pulmonary artery catheter may be inserted. Pulmonary artery wedge pressure does not increase in ARDS because the cause is noncardiogenic (not related to cardiac function).

Hypoxemia and a PaO_2/FIO_2 ratio below 200 (e.g., 80/0.8 = 100) despite increased FIO_2 by mask, cannula, or endotracheal tube are hallmarks of ARDS. ABGs may initially demonstrate a normal or decreased $PaCO_2$ despite severe dyspnea and hypoxemia. Hypercapnia signifies that hypoventilation is occurring, and the patient is no longer able to maintain the level of ventilation needed to provide optimum gas exchange.

As ARDS progresses, it is associated with profound respiratory distress requiring endotracheal intubation and PPV. The chest x-ray is often termed *whiteout* or *white lung,* because consolidation and coalescing infiltrates are widespread throughout the lungs, leaving few recognizable air spaces (Fig. 68-10). Pleural effusions may also be present. Severe hypoxemia, hypercapnia, and metabolic acidosis, with symptoms of target organ or tissue hypoxia, may ensue if prompt therapy is not instituted.

In summary, no precise criteria define ARDS. ARDS is considered to be present if the patient has (1) refractory hypoxemia, (2) a chest x-ray with new bilateral interstitial or alveolar infiltrates, (3) a pulmonary artery wedge pressure of 18 mm Hg or less and no evidence of heart failure, and (4) a predisposing condition for ARDS within 48 hours of clinical manifestations (Table 68-8).

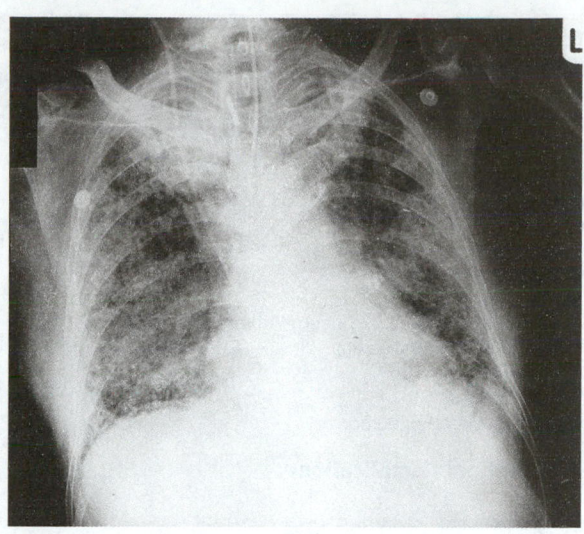

FIG. 68-10 Chest x-ray of a patient with acute respiratory distress syndrome (ARDS). The x-ray shows new, bilateral, diffuse, homogeneous pulmonary infiltrates without cardiac failure, fluid overload, chest infection, or chronic lung disease.

TABLE 68-8	Diagnostic Findings in Acute Respiratory Distress Syndrome

Refractory Hypoxemia
PaO_2 <50 mm Hg on FIO_2 >40% with PEEP >5 cm H_2O
PaO_2/FIO_2 ratio <200

Chest X-Ray
New bilateral interstitial and alveolar infiltrates

Pulmonary Artery Wedge Pressure
≤18 mm Hg and no evidence of heart failure

Predisposing Condition
Identification of a predisposing condition for ARDS within 48 hr of clinical manifestations

ARDS, Acute respiratory distress syndrome; *PEEP,* positive end-expiratory pressure.

Complications

Complications may develop as a result of ARDS itself or its treatment. (Table 68-9 lists the common complications of ARDS.) The major cause of death in ARDS is MODS, often accompanied by sepsis. The vital organs most commonly involved are the kidneys, liver, and heart. The organ systems most often involved are the CNS, hematologic system, and GI system.[28]

Hospital-Acquired Pneumonia. A frequent complication of ARDS is hospital-acquired pneumonia, occurring in as many as 68% of patients with ARDS. Risk factors include impaired host defenses, contaminated medical equipment, invasive monitoring devices, aspiration of GI contents (especially in patients receiving tube feedings), and prolonged mechanical ventilation, as well as colonization of the respiratory tract. Strategies to prevent hospital-acquired pneumonia include infection control measures (e.g., strict hand washing and sterile technique during endotracheal suctioning) and elevating the head of the bed 30 to 45 degrees to prevent aspiration.[26,29] (See Chapter 28 for discussion of pneumonia and Chapter 66 for discussion of ventilator-associated pneumonia.)

TABLE 68-9	Complications Associated with Acute Respiratory Distress Syndrome

Infection
Catheter-related infection
Hospital-acquired pneumonia
Sepsis (bacteremia)

Respiratory Complications
O_2 toxicity
Pulmonary barotrauma (e.g., pneumothorax, pneumomediastinum, subcutaneous emphysema)
Pulmonary emboli
Pulmonary fibrosis
Ventilator-associated pneumonia

Gastrointestinal Complications
Paralytic ileus
Pneumoperitoneum
Stress ulceration and hemorrhage
Hypermetabolic state, dramatically increased nutrition requirements

Renal Complications
Acute renal failure

Cardiac Complications
Dysrhythmias
Decreased cardiac output

Hematologic Complications
Anemia
Disseminated intravascular coagulation
Thrombocytopenia

Endotracheal Tube Intubation Complications
Laryngeal ulceration
Tracheal malacia
Tracheal stenosis
Tracheal ulceration

Central Nervous System/Psychologic Complications
Delirium
Sleep deprivation
Posttraumatic stress disorder

Barotrauma. *Barotrauma* may result from rupture of overdistended alveoli during mechanical ventilation. The high peak airway pressures that may be required in patients with ARDS predispose to this complication. Barotrauma results in the presence of alveolar air in locations where it is not usually found. This can lead to pulmonary interstitial emphysema, pneumothorax, subcutaneous emphysema, pneumoperitoneum, pneumomediastinum, pneumopericardium, and tension pneumothorax. (See Chapter 28 for discussion of pneumothorax.)

To avoid barotrauma and minimize risk associated with elevated plateau and peak inspiratory pressures, the patient with ARDS may be ventilated with smaller tidal volumes (e.g., 6 ml/kg) and varying amounts of positive end-expiratory pressure (PEEP) in order to minimize oxygen requirements and intrathoracic pressures. This approach, known as the Acute Respiratory Distress Syndrome Clinical Network (ARDSNet) protocol, has been shown to reduce mortality rate and number of ventilator days in these patients.[14,30] One consequence of this protocol is an elevation in $PaCO_2$. This is termed *permissive hypercapnia* because the $PaCO_2$ is allowed (permitted) to rise above normal limits.[31] It is generally well tolerated as long as

the rise in $PaCO_2$ is gradual to allow systemic and brain circulation to compensate and the pH is supported at or above 7.2 to 7.25.

Volu-Pressure Trauma. *Volu-pressure trauma* can occur in patients with ARDS when large tidal volumes (e.g., 10 to 15 ml/kg) are used to ventilate noncompliant lungs. Volu-pressure trauma results in alveolar fractures and movement of fluids and proteins into the alveolar spaces. To limit this complication, it is recommended that smaller tidal volumes or pressure ventilation be used in patients with ARDS[27,30] (see Chapter 66).

Physiologic Stress Ulcers. Critically ill patients with acute respiratory failure are at high risk for stress ulcers. Bleeding from stress ulcers occurs in 30% of patients with ARDS who require PPV, a higher incidence than other causes of acute respiratory failure. Management strategies include correction of predisposing conditions such as hypotension, shock, and acidosis. Prophylactic management includes antiulcer agents such as H_2-histamine receptor antagonists (e.g., ranitidine [Zantac]), as well as proton pump inhibitors (e.g., pantoprazole [Protonix]) and mucosal-protecting agents (e.g., sucralfate [Carafate]). Early initiation of enteral nutrition also helps prevent mucosal damage (see Chapters 40 and 66).

Renal Failure. Renal failure can occur from decreased renal tissue oxygenation as a result of hypotension, hypoxemia, or hypercapnia. Renal failure may also be caused by administration of nephrotoxic drugs (e.g., aminoglycosides), which are used to treat infections associated with ARDS.

NURSING *and* COLLABORATIVE MANAGEMENT
ACUTE RESPIRATORY DISTRESS SYNDROME

The collaborative care for acute respiratory failure (see Table 68-5) is applicable to ARDS. The following section discusses additional collaborative care measures for the patient with ARDS (Table 68-10). Patients with ARDS are commonly cared for in critical care units. The nursing care plan for acute respiratory failure (see NCP 68-1) is applicable to patients with ARDS.

▪ Nursing Assessment

Because ARDS causes acute respiratory failure, the subjective and objective data that should be obtained from a person with ARDS are the same as those for acute respiratory failure (see Table 68-4). Abnormal findings on physical examination are indications that ARDS has progressed beyond the initial stages.

▪ Nursing Diagnoses

Nursing diagnoses for the patient with ARDS may include, but are not limited to, those described for acute respiratory failure (see NCP 68-1).

▪ Planning

With appropriate therapy, the overall goals for the patient with ARDS include a PaO_2 of at least 60 mm Hg and adequate lung ventilation to maintain normal pH. The goals for a patient recovering from ARDS include (1) PaO_2 within normal limits for age or baseline values on room air (FIO_2 of 21%), (2) SaO_2 greater than 90%, (3) patent airway, and (4) clear lungs on auscultation.

▪ Respiratory Therapy

Oxygen Administration. The primary goal of O_2 therapy is to correct hypoxemia. O_2 administered via a simple face mask or nasal cannula is usually inadequate to treat refractory hypoxemia

TABLE 68-10	COLLABORATIVE CARE Acute Respiratory Distress Syndrome

Diagnostic
See Table 68-8

Collaborative Therapy
Respiratory Therapy
O$_2$ administration
Prone positioning
Lateral rotation therapy
Positive pressure ventilation with PEEP
Permissive hypercapnia
Alternative modes of mechanical ventilation: pressure support ventilation, pressure release ventilation, pressure control ventilation, inverse ratio ventilation, high-frequency ventilation*

Supportive Therapy
Identification and treatment of underlying cause
Hemodynamic monitoring
Inotropic/vasopressor medications
• dopamine (Intropin)
• dobutamine (Dobutrex)
• norepinephrine (Levophed)
Diuretics
IV fluid administration
Sedation/analgesia
Neuromuscular blockade

IV, Intravenous; *PEEP,* positive end-expiratory pressure.
*See Chapter 66.

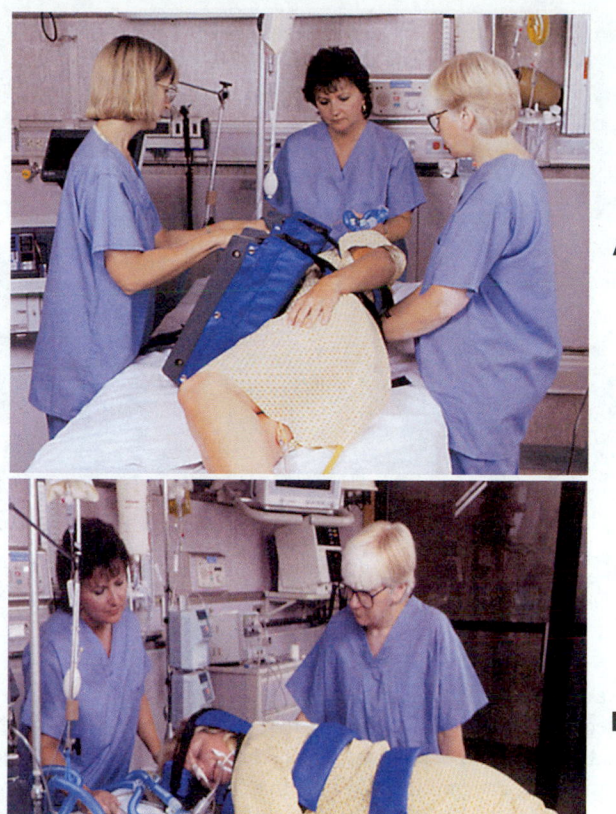

FIG. 68-11   A, Turning patient prone on Vollman Prone Positioner. **B,** Patient lying prone on Vollman Prone Positioner. *(©2001 Hill-Rom Services, Inc. Reprinted with permission. All rights reserved.)*

that is associated with ARDS. Masks with high-flow systems that deliver higher O$_2$ concentrations are initially used to maximize O$_2$ delivery. Pulse oximetry (SpO$_2$) is continuously monitored to assess the effectiveness of O$_2$ therapy. The general standard for O$_2$ administration is to give the patient the lowest concentration that results in a PaO$_2$ of 60 mm Hg or greater. When the FIO$_2$ exceeds 60% for more than 48 hours, the risk for O$_2$ toxicity increases. Patients with ARDS commonly need intubation with mechanical ventilation because the PaO$_2$ cannot otherwise be maintained at acceptable levels.

Mechanical Ventilation. Endotracheal intubation and mechanical ventilation provide additional respiratory support. However, even with these interventions it may be necessary to maintain the FIO$_2$ at 60% or greater to maintain the PaO$_2$ at 60 mm Hg or greater. During mechanical ventilation, it is common to apply PEEP at 5 cm H$_2$O to compensate for loss of glottic function caused by the presence of the endotracheal tube. In patients with ARDS, higher levels of PEEP (e.g., 10 to 20 cm H$_2$O) may be used. The mechanism of action of PEEP is related to its ability to increase FRC and recruit (open up) collapsed alveoli. PEEP is typically applied in 3 to 5 cm H$_2$O increments until oxygenation is adequate with FIO$_2$ of 60% or less. PEEP may improve V/Q in respiratory units that collapse at low airway pressures, thus allowing the FIO$_2$ to be lowered.

However, PEEP is not a benign therapy. The additional intrathoracic and intrapulmonic pressures can compromise venous return to the right side of the heart, thereby decreasing preload, cardiac output, and BP. PEEP can also cause hyperinflation of the alveoli, compression of the pulmonary capillary bed, a reduction in blood return to the left side of the heart, and a dramatic reduction in BP. In addition, high levels of PEEP or excessive inspiratory pressures can result in barotrauma and volu-pressure trauma.[14,26,27]

If hypoxemic failure persists in spite of high levels of PEEP, alternative modes and therapies may be used. These include pressure support ventilation, pressure release ventilation, pressure control ventilation, inverse ratio ventilation, high-frequency ventilation, and permissive hypercapnia (low tidal volumes that allow PaCO$_2$ to increase slowly, maintaining normal pH and low airway pressures).[14,26,27] Additional information on mechanical ventilation and PEEP is provided in Chapter 66.

Extracorporeal membrane oxygenation (ECMO) and extracorporeal CO$_2$ removal (ECCO$_2$R) pass blood across a gas-exchanging membrane outside the body and then return oxygenated blood back to the body. ECCO$_2$R with low-frequency PPV allows the lungs to heal while the lungs are not functional.[32]

Positioning Strategies. Some patients with ARDS demonstrate a marked improvement in PaO$_2$ when turned from the supine to the prone position (e.g., PaO$_2$ 70 mm Hg supine, PaO$_2$ 90 mm Hg the prone) with no change in inspired O$_2$ concentration (Fig. 68-11). The response may be sufficient to allow a reduction in inspired O$_2$ concentration or PEEP.

In the early phases of ARDS, fluid moves freely throughout the lung. Because of gravity, this fluid pools in dependent regions of the lung. As a consequence, some alveoli are fluid filled (dependent areas), whereas others are air filled (nondependent areas). In addition, when the patient is supine the heart and mediastinal contents place more pressure on the lungs than in the prone position, which changes pleural pressure and predisposes

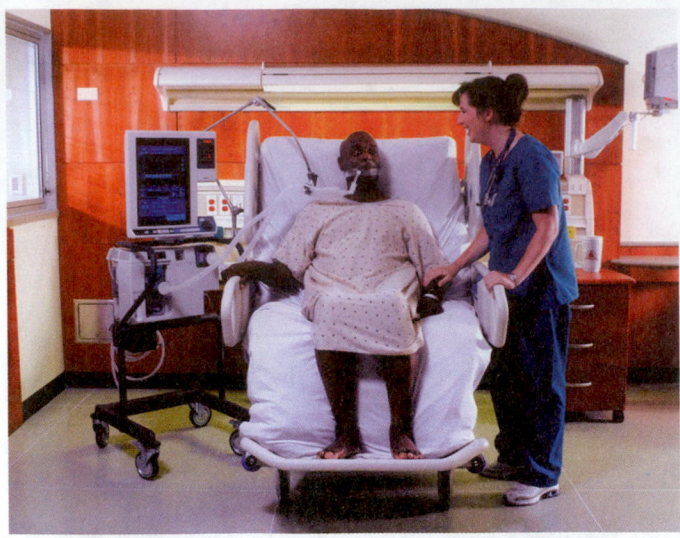

FIG. 68-12 TotalCare SpO₂RT® Bed System offers continuous lateral rotation therapy and percussion and vibration therapies. Patients can easily and quickly be repositioned.

to atelectasis. If the patient is turned from supine to prone, air-filled, nonatelectatic alveoli in the ventral (anterior) portion of the lung become dependent. Perfusion may be better matched to ventilation, causing less V/Q mismatch. Not all patients respond to prone positioning with an increase in PaO_2, and there is no reliable way of predicting who will respond. Prone positioning is typically reserved for patients with refractory hypoxemia who do not respond to other strategies to increase PaO_2.[33] When this positioning strategy is used, there must be a plan in place for immediate repositioning for cardiopulmonary resuscitation in the event of a cardiac arrest.

Other positioning strategies that can be considered for patients with ARDS include continuous lateral rotation therapy (CLRT) and kinetic therapy.[34] The purpose of CLRT is to provide continuous, slow, side-to-side turning of the patient by rotating the actual bed frame less than 40 degrees. The lateral movement of the bed is maintained for 18 of every 24 hours to simulate postural drainage and to help mobilize pulmonary secretions. In addition, the bed may also contain a vibrator pack that can provide chest physical therapy to further assist with secretion mobilization and removal (Fig. 68-12). Kinetic therapy is similar to CLRT in that patients are rotated side-to-side at least 40 degrees or more. Baseline assessment of the patient's pulmonary status (e.g., respiratory rate and rhythm, breath sounds, ABGs, SpO_2) should be obtained before initiation of the therapy and continued throughout the use of the therapy.

■ Medical Supportive Therapy

Maintenance of Cardiac Output and Tissue Perfusion. Patients on PPV and PEEP frequently experience decreased cardiac output. One cause is decreased venous return, which results from the PEEP-induced increase in intrathoracic pressure. Cardiac output may also be decreased by impaired contractility and decreased preload. Continuous hemodynamic monitoring is essential to detect changes and titrate therapy appropriately. An arterial catheter is inserted to permit continuous monitoring of BP and sampling of blood for ABGs. A pulmonary artery catheter is normally inserted to allow monitoring of pulmonary artery pressure and pulmonary artery wedge pressures (which indicate the fluid status of the left side of the heart), SvO_2

monitoring, and cardiac output. If the cardiac output falls, it may be necessary to administer crystalloid fluids or colloid solutions or to lower PEEP. Use of inotropic drugs such as dobutamine (Dobutrex) or dopamine (Intropin) may also be necessary. (See Chapter 66 for discussion of hemodynamic monitoring.)

The hemoglobin level is usually kept at levels of 9 g/dl (90 g/L) or more with an oxygen saturation of 90% or greater (when PaO_2 is more than 60 mm Hg). Packed red blood cells may be administered to increase hemoglobin and thus the O_2-carrying capacity of the blood.

Maintenance of Nutrition and Fluid Balance. Maintenance of nutrition and fluid balance is challenging in the patient with ARDS. Nutrition consultations are initiated to determine optimal caloric needs. Parenteral or enteral feedings are started to meet the high energy requirements of these patients. Early research has shown that enteral formulas enriched with omega-3 fatty acids may improve the clinical outcomes of patients with ARDS.[35]

Increasing pulmonary capillary permeability results in fluid in the lungs and causes pulmonary edema. At the same time, the patient may be volume depleted and therefore prone to hypotension and decreased cardiac output from mechanical ventilation and PEEP. Pulmonary artery wedge pressures, daily weights, and intake and output are monitored to assess the patient's fluid status. Controversy exists as to the benefits of fluid replacement with crystalloids versus colloids. Critics of colloid replacement believe that proteins in colloid fluid may leak into the pulmonary interstitium, exacerbating the movement of proteinaceous fluid into the alveoli. Advocates of colloid replacement believe that colloids help keep fluid from leaking into the alveoli. The pulmonary artery wedge pressure is kept as low as possible without impairing cardiac output in order to limit pulmonary edema. The patient is usually placed on mild fluid restriction, and diuretics are used as necessary.[14,26]

■ Evaluation

The expected outcomes for the patient with ARDS are similar to those for a patient with acute respiratory failure and are presented in NCP 68-1.

SEVERE ACUTE RESPIRATORY SYNDROME

Severe acute respiratory syndrome (SARS) is a serious, acute respiratory infection caused by a coronavirus (CoV). The virus spreads by close contact between people. SARS-CoV is most likely spread via droplets in the air. It is possible that SARS may also be spread more broadly through the air or from touching objects that have become contaminated. The vast majority of patients with SARS-CoV will have a clear history of exposure either to a SARS patient or to a setting in which SARS-CoV transmission is occurring (e.g., China, Hong Kong) and will develop pneumonia.[36]

In general, SARS begins with a fever greater than 100.4° F (>38.0° C). Other manifestations may include sore throat, rhinorrhea, chills, rigors, myalgia, headache, and diarrhea. After 2 to 7 days, SARS patients may develop a dry cough and have trouble breathing.

Because the disease is severe, treatment needs to be started based on the symptoms and before the cause of the illness is confirmed. First, people who are suspected of having SARS should be placed in isolation to protect other patients and health care workers. Although there is no definitive treatment, antiviral medications (such as ribavirin), antibiotics, and corticosteroids may be used. Although antibiotics will not help with SARS (because it is believed to be caused by a virus), they may be used in cases where the person also has a bacterial infection.

About 80% to 90% of infected people start to recover after 6 to 7 days. However, 10% to 20% go on to develop respiratory failure and may need intubation and mechanical ventilation. The risk of death is higher for this group, and appears to be linked to the person's preexisting health conditions. People over age 40 are more likely to develop severe breathing problems.[36]

CRITICAL THINKING EXERCISE

CASE STUDY

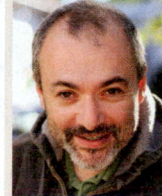

Case Study photo ©iStockphoto.com/ Galina Barskaya.

Acute Respiratory Distress Syndrome

Patient Profile. Mr. Jacobi is a 55-year-old white man who was admitted 72 hours ago to a general surgical unit after surgery for an acutely ischemic bowel. The surgical procedure involved extensive abdominal surgery to repair a perforated colon, irrigate the abdominal cavity, and provide hemostasis. During surgery his systolic BP dropped to 70 mm Hg. Seven units of packed red blood cells and 4 L of normal saline were administered IV. He is receiving 60% O_2 through an aerosol face mask. He is being monitored with a cardiac monitor and pulse oximeter. He has a central IV catheter in place and is receiving 0.9% normal saline intravenously at 125 ml/hr. A urinary catheter is in place.

His pulmonary status continues to worsen. He requires progressively higher fractions of inspired oxygen. Emergent endotracheal intubation and controlled ventilation are necessary. Sedation, analgesia, and neuromuscular blockade are initiated to achieve pain control and ventilator synchrony.

His lung function continues to worsen and his hypoxemia is refractory to 100% FIO_2 and high levels of PEEP. He experiences kidney and liver failure. There is little hope of weaning him from controlled ventilation. He has an advance directive that indicates he does not want to be kept alive by artificial means.

Subjective Data
- Patient is sedated and paralyzed. Unable to communicate. His wife and two adult children are at the bedside and voicing concerns and questions regarding his progress.

Objective Data
Physical Assessment
- General: Sedated, paralyzed, well-nourished man; head of bed elevated 45 degrees; skin cool with moderate diaphoresis
- Respiratory: No accessory muscle use, retractions, or paradoxic breathing; respiratory rate 18 breaths/min; SpO_2 85%; fine crackles at lung bases
- Cardiovascular: BP 100/60 mm Hg; cardiac monitor shows sinus tachycardia at 120 beats/min, with equal apical-radial pulse; temperature 101° F (38° C) rectally
- Gastrointestinal: Surgical dressing dry and intact; colostomy draining serosanguineous drainage
- Urologic: Urinary catheter draining concentrated urine <30 ml/hr

Diagnostic Findings
- ABGs: pH 7.15, PaO_2 59 mm Hg, $PaCO_2$ 57 mm Hg, HCO_3 16 mEq/L, O_2 saturation 86%
- PaO_2/FIO_2 ratio <200

- Chest x-ray shows new bilateral, scattered interstitial infiltrates compatible with an ARDS pattern as interpreted by the radiologist

CRITICAL THINKING QUESTIONS

1. How does the pathophysiology of ARDS predispose to the development of refractory hypoxemia?
2. What clinical manifestations does Mr. Jacobi exhibit that support a diagnosis of ARDS?
3. What are the possible causes of ARDS in Mr. Jacobi?
4. What are the possible complications that Mr. Jacobi is at risk for developing secondary to ARDS?
5. What respiratory care interventions might be implemented to improve Mr. Jacobi's hypoxemia?
6. Based on the assessment data presented, write one or more priority nursing diagnoses.
7. Given his progressive decline in cardiopulmonary function, what information should be given to the family?
8. Given the patient's advance directive, what legal/ethical issues might be encountered in this patient scenario?

NCLEX EXAMINATION REVIEW QUESTIONS

The number of the question corresponds to the same-numbered objective at the beginning of the chapter.

1. Hypercapnic respiratory failure can be caused by
   a. ARDS.
   b. asthma.
   c. pneumonia.
   d. pulmonary emboli.
2. An early sign of acute respiratory failure is
   a. coma.
   b. cyanosis.
   c. restlessness.
   d. paradoxic breathing.
3. The oxygen delivery system chosen for the patient in acute respiratory failure should
   a. always be a low-flow device, such as a nasal cannula.
   b. correct the PaO_2 to a normal level as quickly as possible.
   c. administer positive pressure ventilation to prevent CO_2 narcosis.
   d. maintain the PaO_2 at 60 mm Hg or greater at the lowest O_2 concentration possible.
4. The most common early clinical manifestations of ARDS that the nurse may observe are
   a. dyspnea and tachypnea.
   b. cyanosis and apprehension.
   c. hypotension and tachycardia.
   d. respiratory distress and frothy sputum.
5. Maintenance of fluid balance in the patient with ARDS involves
   a. hydration using colloids.
   b. administration of surfactant.
   c. mild fluid restriction and diuretics as necessary.
   d. keeping the hemoglobin at levels of 15 to 16 g/dl (150 to 160 g/L).
6. Which of the following interventions is designed to prevent or limit barotrauma in the patient with ARDS who is mechanically ventilated?
   a. Increasing PEEP
   b. Increasing the tidal volume
   c. Use of permissive hypercapnia
   d. Use of positive pressure ventilation

Respiratory Failure and ARDS

REFERENCES

1. Roussos C, Koutsoukou A: Respiratory failure, *Eur Respir J* 47(suppl):3s, 2003.
2. Markou NK, Myrianthefs PM, Baltopoulos GJ: Respiratory failure: an overview, *Crit Care Nurs Q* 27(4):353, 2004.
3. Corbridge SJ, Corbridge TC: Severe exacerbations of asthma, *Crit Care Nurs Q* 27(3):207, 2004.
4. Rodrigo GJ, Rodrigo C, Hall JB: Acute asthma in adults: a review, *Chest* 125:1081, 2004.
5. Schwartz A, Leih-Lai MW: Status asthmaticus. Available at *www.emedicine.com* (accessed September 20, 2006).
6. Saadeh C, Malacara J, Goldman M: Status asthmaticus. Available at *www.emedicine.com/med/topic2169.htm* (accessed September 20, 2006).
7. Leatherman JW, McArthur C, Shapiro RS: Effect of prolongation of expiratory time on dynamic hyperinflation in mechanically ventilated patients with severe asthma, *Crit Care Med* 32:1542, 2004.
8. McFadden ER: Acute severe asthma, *Am J Respir Crit Care Med* 168:740, 2003.
*9. Arbour R: Using bispectral index monitoring to detect potential break-through awareness and limit duration of neuromuscular blockade, *Am J Crit Care* 13(1):66, 2004.
10. *The Merck manual of diagnosis and therapy,* Chapter 12. Water, electro-lyte and acid-base metabolism. Available at *www.merck.com* (accessed September 20, 2006).
11. Martinu T, Menzies D, Dial S: Re-evaluation of acid-base prediction rules in patients with chronic respiratory acidosis, *Can Respir J* 10(6):311, 2003.
12. Priestly MA, Huh J: Respiratory failure. Available at *www.emedicine.com/ped/topic1994.htm* (accessed September 20, 2006).
13. Gronkiewicz C, Borkgren-Okonek M: Acute exacerbation of COPD: nursing application of evidence-based guidelines, *Crit Care Nurs Q* 27(4):336, 2004.
14. Kane C, Galanes S: Adult respiratory distress syndrome, *Crit Care Nurs Q* 27(4):325, 2004.
15. Cardin T, Marinelli A: Pulmonary embolism, *Crit Care Nurs Q* 27(4):310, 2004.
16. Harman E, Walia R: Acute respiratory distress syndrome. Available at *www.emedicine.com/med/topic70.htm* (accessed September 20, 2006).
17. Fenstermacher D, Hong D: Mechanical ventilation: what have we learned? *Crit Care Nurs Q* 27(3):258, 2004.
18. Phua J et al: Noninvasive ventilation in hypercapnic acute respiratory failure due to chronic obstructive pulmonary disease vs. other conditions: effectiveness and predictors of failure, *Intensive Care Med* 31(4):533, 2005.
19. Chu CM et al: Noninvasive ventilation in patients with acute hypercapnic exacerbation of chronic obstructive pulmonary disease who refused endotracheal intubation, *Crit Care Med* 32(2):372, 2004.
20. Schettino G, Altobelli N, Kacmarek RM: Noninvasive positive pressure ventilation reverses acute respiratory failure in select "do-not-intubate" patients, *Crit Care Med* 33(9):1976, 2004.
21. DeJohnge B et al: Sedation algorithm in critically ill patients without acute brain injury, *Crit Care Med* 33(1):120, 2005.
22. Arbour R: Continuous nervous system monitoring: EEG, the bispectral index and neuromuscular transmission, *AACN Clin Issues* 14(2):185, 2003.
23. *The Merck manual of geriatrics.* Respiratory failure. Available at *www.merck.com/mrkshared/mmg/sec10/ch79/ch79a.jsp#ind10-078-5153* (accessed September 19, 2006).
24. Sevransky JE, Haponik EF: Respiratory failure in elderly patients, *Clin Geriatr Med* 19(1):205, 2003.
25. Lin SM et al: The impact of delirium on the survival of mechanically ventilated patients, *Crit Care Med* 32(11):2254, 2004.
26. Conrad SA: Adult respiratory distress syndrome. Available at *www.emedicine.com/emerg/topic503.htm* (accessed September 20, 2006).
27. Rothenhaus T, Okafor N: Acute respiratory distress syndrome. Available at *www.emedicine.com/emerg/topic15.htm* (accessed September 20, 2006).
28. Sharma S, Kumar A: Septic shock, multiple organ failure and acute respiratory distress syndrome, *Curr Opin Pulm Med* 9(3):199, 2003.
29. Myrianthefs PM et al: Nosocomial pneumonia, *Crit Care Nurs Q* 27(3):241, 2004.
30. Acute Respiratory Distress Syndrome Clinical Network (ARDSNet). Available at *www.nhlbi.nih.gov/resources/deca/descriptions/ards.htm* (accessed September 20, 2006).
31. Mutlu GM et al: Severe status asthmaticus: management with permissive hypercapnia and inhalation anesthesia, *Crit Care Med* 30:477, 2002.
32. Hemmila MR et al: Extracorporeal life support for severe acute respiratory distress syndrome in adults, *Ann Surg* 240(4):595, 2004.
33. Fan E, Mehta S: High-frequency oscillatory ventilation and adjunctive therapies: inhaled nitric oxide and prone positioning, *Crit Care Med* 33(3):s182, 2005.
*34. Ahrens T, Kollef M, Stewart J: Effect of kinetic therapy on pulmonary complications, *Am J Crit Care* 13:376, 2004.
35. Hasselmann M, Reimund JM: Lipids in the nutritional support of critically ill patients, *Curr Opinion Crit Care* 10:449, 2004.
36. Clinical guidance on the identification and evaluation of possible SARS-CoV disease among persons presenting with community-acquired illness. Version 2. Available at *www.cdc.gov/ncidod/sars/clinicalguidance.htm* (accessed September 20, 2006).

*Nursing research–based references.

RESOURCES

Resources for this chapter are listed after Chapter 66 on p. 1771.

Nursing Management
Emergency and Disaster Nursing

69

Linda Bucher

LEARNING OBJECTIVES

1. Apply the sequential steps in triage, the primary survey, and the secondary survey to a patient in an emergency situation.
2. Describe the pathophysiology, assessment, and collaborative care of select environmental emergencies, including hyperthermia, hypothermia, submersion injury, and animal bites.
3. Describe the pathophysiology, assessment, and collaborative care of select toxicologic emergencies.
4. Differentiate between the various types and victims of violence.
5. Identify the agents most likely to be used in a terrorist attack.
6. Differentiate the responsibilities of health care providers, the community, and select federal agencies in emergency and mass casualty incident preparedness.

KEY TERMS

bioterrorism, p. 1838
emergency, p. 1842
heat cramps, p. 1828
heat exhaustion, p. 1829
heatstroke, p. 1829
hypothermia, p. 1831
jaw-thrust maneuver, p. 1823
mass casualty incident, p. 1842
triage, p. 1822

Electronic Resources

Supplemental content related to Chapter 69 can be found . . .

Companion CD
- Stress-Busting Kit for Nursing Students
- NCLEX Examination Review Questions
- Comprehensive Glossary

Evolve Website *evolve*
http://evolve.elsevier.com/Lewis/medsurg
- Content Updates
- Key Points (Printable and CD/MP3 Download)
- Concept Map Creator
- Expanded Audio Glossary

- Key Term Flash Cards
- Electronic Calculators
- WebLinks

Most patients with life-threatening or potentially life-threatening problems arrive at the hospital through the emergency department (ED). Many more patients report to the ED for less urgent conditions.[1] Over 80 million people visit EDs annually, and this number is increasing for a variety of reasons (e.g., the inability to see a primary care provider, the aging population, shorter hospital stays resulting in frequent readmissions, and lack of health insurance or a primary care provider).[2,3] These factors have resulted in chronic overcrowding and long wait times in many EDs.[1]

Emergency nurses care for patients of all ages and with a variety of problems. However, some EDs specialize in certain patient populations or conditions, such as pediatric ED or trauma ED. The Emergency Nurses Association (ENA) is the specialty nursing organization aimed at advancing emergency nursing practice. The ENA provides standards of care for nurses working in the ED, as well as a certification process that allows nurses to become a certified emergency nurse (CEN).[4] This certification validates the knowledge that a nurse needs to provide competent care in emergency settings.

Emergency management of patients with various medical, surgical, and traumatic emergencies is presented throughout this book. Tables that highlight emergency management of specific problems are presented in the related chapters. Table 69-1 lists each emergency management table by title, number, and page. This chapter focuses on triage, initial assessment, and management of the trauma patient and selected emergency conditions not addressed elsewhere in this book, including heat- and cold-related emergencies, submersion injuries, bites, stings, and poisonings. In addition, an overview of issues related to violence and emergency and disaster preparedness is presented.

Reviewed by Carolyn Carty, RN, MSN, CEN, Staff Nurse, Emergency Department, Virtua West Jersey Hospital Marlton, Marlton, N.J.; and Virginia Crocker, RN, MS, CEN, Clinical Nurse Specialist, Emergency Department, Winchester Hospital, Winchester, Mass.

CARE OF THE EMERGENCY PATIENT

Recognition of life-threatening illness or injury is one of the most important aspects of emergency care. Before a diagnosis can be made, recognition of dangerous clinical signs and symptoms with initiation of interventions to reverse or prevent a crisis is essential. This process begins with the first patient contact. The emergency nurse is usually confronted with multiple patients who have a variety of problems. Prompt identification of patients requiring immediate treatment and determination of appropriate treatment area are essential nurse competencies in a busy ED.

Triage

Triage, a French word meaning "to sort," refers to the process of rapidly determining patient acuity. It is one of the most important assessment skills needed by the emergency nurse.[5,6] The triage process is based on the premise that patients who have a threat to life, vision, or limb should be treated before other patients.

A *triage system* identifies and categorizes patients so that the most critical are treated first. The ENA and American College of Emergency Physicians support the use of a five-level triage system.[7] The *Emergency Severity Index* (ESI) is a five-level triage system that incorporates concepts of illness severity and resource utilization (e.g., electrocardiogram, laboratory work, radiology studies, intravenous fluids) to determine who should be treated first[5] (Table 69-2). The ESI includes a triage algorithm that the nurse uses to assign an ESI level to patients presenting to the ED (Fig. 69-1). Initially, patients are assessed for any threats to life (e.g., Is the patient apneic?). Patients who do not meet the criteria for ESI-1 or ESI-2 are next evaluated for the number of anticipated resources they may need. Patients are assigned to ESI level 3, 4, or 5 based on this determination. Vital signs are required for patients assigned to ESI level 3. Patients with abnormal vital signs may be reassigned to ESI level 2.[5] The use of triage systems such as the ESI can provide a mechanism for EDs to predict short-term hospital resource and staffing needs.[8]

After the emergency nurse completes the initial assessment to determine the presence of actual or potential threats to life, appropriate interventions are initiated for the patient's condition. A his-

| TABLE 69-1 | EMERGENCY MANAGEMENT Emergency Management Tables |

Title	Chapter	Page
Abdominal trauma	43	1048
Acute abdominal pain	43	1045
Acute soft tissue injury	63	1632
Anaphylactic shock	14	230
Chemical burns	25	489
Chest pain	34	806
Chest trauma	28	586
Cocaine and amphetamine toxicity	12	175
Depressant drugs, overdose of	12	179
Diabetic ketoacidosis	49	1280
Dysrhythmias	36	848
Electrical burns	25	490
Eye injury	22	421
Fractured extremity	63	1642
Head injury	57	1484
Hyperthermia	69	1830
Hypothermia	69	1832
Inhalation injury	25	489
Sexual assault	54	1410
Shock	67	1785
Spinal cord injury	61	1596
Stroke	58	1511
Submersion injuries	69	1833
Thermal burns	25	490
Thoracic injuries	28	586
Tonic-clonic seizures	59	1537

TABLE 69-2	Five-Level Emergency Severity Index (ESI)				
	Level				
Definition	**ESI-1**	**ESI-2**	**ESI-3**	**ESI-4**	**ESI-5**
Stability of vital functions (ABCs)	Unstable	Threatened	Stable	Stable	Stable
Life threat or organ threat	Obvious	Likely but not always obvious	Unlikely but possible	No	No
How soon patient should be seen by physician	Immediately	Minutes	Up to 1 hr	Could be delayed	Could be delayed
Expected resource intensity	High resource intensity; staff at bedside continuously; often mobilization of team response	High resource intensity; multiple, often complex diagnostic studies; frequent consultation; continuous (remote) monitoring	Medium/high resource intensity; multiple diagnostic studies or brief observation; or complex procedure	Low resource intensity; one simple diagnostic study; or a simple procedure	Low resource intensity; examination only
Examples	Cardiac arrest, intubated trauma patient, severe overdose, SIDS	Chest pain probably resulting from ischemia, multiple trauma unless responsive, child with fever and lethargy, disruptive psychiatric patient	Abdominal pain or gynecologic disorders unless in severe distress, hip fracture in elderly patient	Closed extremity trauma, simple laceration, cystitis, typical migraine	Cold symptoms, minor burn, recheck (e.g., wound)

Reprinted with permission. Copyright 1999, Richard C. Wuerz, MD, and David R. Eitel, MD.
ABCs, Airway, breathing, circulation; *SIDS*, sudden infant death syndrome.

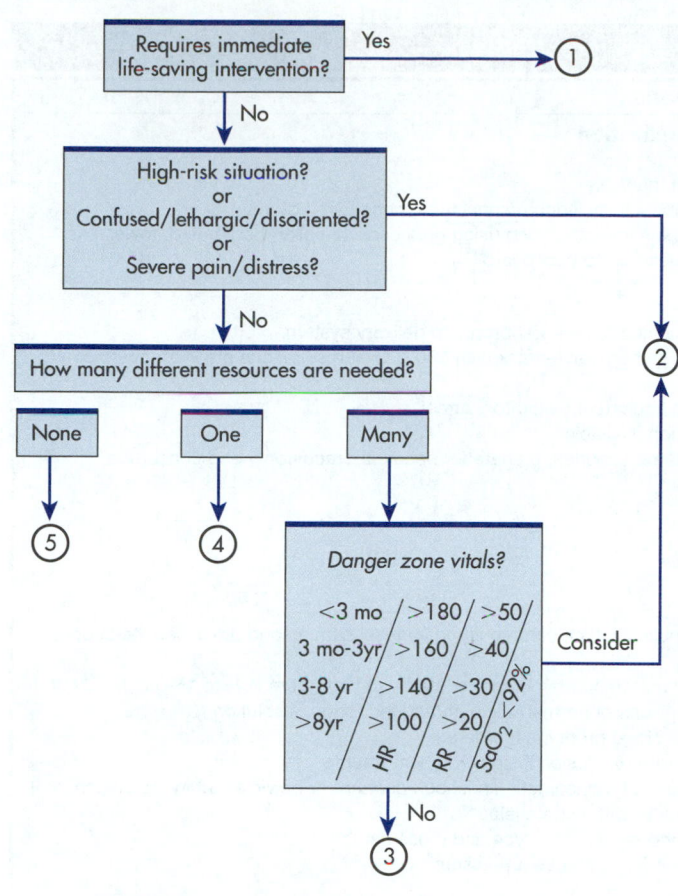

FIG. 69-1   Emergency Severity Index Triage Algorithm, version 4.

tory is obtained simultaneously with the assessment. A systematic approach to the initial patient assessment decreases the time required to identify potential threats and minimizes the risk of overlooking a life-threatening condition. Two systematic approaches, a primary survey and a secondary survey, were initially developed for use with the trauma patient, but these can be easily applied to assessment of any emergency patient.

Primary Survey

The **primary survey** (Table 69-3) focuses on airway, breathing, circulation, and disability and serves to identify life-threatening conditions so that appropriate interventions can be initiated. Life-threatening conditions related to airway, breathing, circulation, and disability (Table 69-4) may be identified at any point during the primary survey. When this occurs, interventions are started immediately and before proceeding to the next step of the survey.

A = Airway with Cervical Spine Stabilization and/or Immobilization.
Nearly all immediate trauma deaths occur because of airway obstruction. Saliva, bloody secretions, vomitus, laryngeal trauma, dentures, facial trauma, fractures, and the tongue can obstruct the airway. Patients at risk for airway compromise include those who have seizures, near-drowning, anaphylaxis, foreign body obstruction, or cardiopulmonary arrest. If an airway is not maintained, obstruction of airflow occurs and hypoxia, acidosis, and death may result.

Primary signs and symptoms in a patient with a compromised airway include dyspnea, inability to vocalize, presence of foreign

body in the airway, and trauma to the face or neck. Airway maintenance should progress rapidly from the least to the most invasive method. Treatment includes opening the airway using the **jaw-thrust maneuver** (avoiding hyperextension of the neck) (Fig. 69-2), suctioning and/or removal of foreign body, insertion of a nasopharyngeal or an oropharyngeal airway (will cause gagging if patient is conscious), and endotracheal intubation. If unable to intubate because of airway obstruction, an emergency cricothyroidotomy or tracheotomy should be performed (see Chapter 27). Patients should be ventilated with 100% oxygen using a bag-valve-mask (BVM) device before intubation or cricothyroidotomy.[9]

Rapid-sequence intubation is the preferred procedure for securing an unprotected airway in the ED. It involves the use of sedation (e.g., etomidate [Amidate]) and paralysis (e.g., succinylcholine [Anectine]) to facilitate intubation while minimizing the risk of aspiration and airway trauma.[10]

Any patient with face, head, or neck trauma and/or significant upper torso injuries should always be suspected of cervical spine trauma. The cervical spine must be stabilized (head maintained in a neutral position) and/or immobilized during assessment of the airway. At the scene of the injury, the cervical spine is immobilized with a rigid cervical collar or a *cervical immobilization device* (CID) (also known as "head blocks"). Towel rolls are taped to a backboard on either side of the head. Finally, the patient's forehead is secured to the backboard. Sandbags should not be used because the weight of the bags could move the head if the patient must be logrolled.

B = Breathing.
Adequate airflow through the upper airway does not ensure adequate ventilation. Breathing alterations are caused by many conditions, including fractured ribs, pneumothorax, penetrating injury, allergic reactions, pulmonary emboli, and asthma attacks. Patients with these conditions may experience a variety of signs and symptoms, including dyspnea (e.g., pulmonary emboli), paradoxic or asymmetric chest wall movement (e.g., flail chest), decreased or absent breath sounds on the affected side (e.g., pneumothorax), visible wound to chest wall (e.g., penetrating injury), cyanosis (e.g., asthma), tachycardia, and hypotension.

Every critically injured or ill patient has an increased metabolic and oxygen demand and should have supplemental oxygen. High-flow oxygen (100%) via a non-rebreather mask should be administered and the patient's response monitored. Life-threatening conditions, such as tension pneumothorax and flail chest, can severely compromise ventilation. Interventions in these situations include BVM ventilation with 100% oxygen, intubation, and treatment of the underlying cause.

C = Circulation.
An effective circulatory system includes the heart, intact blood vessels, and adequate blood volume. Uncontrolled internal and/or external bleeding places a person at risk for hemorrhagic shock (see Chapter 67). A central pulse (e.g., carotid) should be checked because peripheral pulses may be absent as a result of direct injury or vasoconstriction. If a pulse is palpated, the quality and rate of the pulse are assessed. Skin should be assessed for color, temperature, and moisture. Altered mental status and delayed capillary refill (longer than 3 seconds) are the most significant signs of shock. Care must be taken when evaluating capillary refill in cold environments because cold delays refill.

Intravenous (IV) lines are inserted into veins in the upper extremities unless contraindicated, such as in a massive fracture or an injury that affects limb circulation. Two large-bore (14- to

TABLE 69-3	Primary Survey of an Emergency Patient

Assessment	Interventions
Airway with Simultaneous Cervical Spine Stabilization and/or Immobilization	
• Clear and open airway • Assess for obstructed airway • Assess for respiratory distress • Check for loose teeth or foreign objects • Assess for bleeding, vomitus, or edema	• Suction • Jaw-thrust maneuver • Nasal or oral airway, endotracheal tube, cricothyroidotomy • Cervical spine immobilization using rigid cervical collar; backboard, towel rolls, forehead secured to backboard
Breathing	

• Assess ventilation
  • Look for paradoxic movement of the chest wall during inspiration and expiration
  • Note use of accessory muscles or abdominal muscles
  • Listen for air being expired through nose and mouth
  • Feel for air being expelled
• Observe and count respiratory rate
• Note color of nail beds, mucous membranes, skin
• Auscultate lungs
• Assess for jugular venous distention and position of trachea
	• Give supplemental O$_2$ via appropriate delivery system
	• Ventilate with bag-valve-mask with 100% O$_2$ if respirations are inadequate or absent
	• Prepare to intubate if respiratory arrest
	• Have suction available
	• If absent breath sounds, prepare for needle thoracostomy and chest tube insertion

Circulation	
• Check carotid or femoral pulse • Palpate pulse for quality and rate • Assess color, temperature, and moisture of skin • Check capillary refill • Assess for external bleeding • Measure blood pressure	• If absent pulse, initiate cardiopulmonary resuscitation and advanced life-support measures • If shock symptoms or hypotensive, start two large-bore (14- to 16-gauge) IVs and initiate infusions of normal saline or lactated Ringer's solution • Administer blood products if ordered • Consider autotransfusion if isolated chest trauma • Consider use of a pneumatic antishock garment or pelvic splint in the presence of pelvic fracture with hypotension • Obtain blood samples for type and crossmatch • Control bleeding with direct pressure
Disability	
Brief Neurologic Assessment • Assess level of consciousness by determining response to verbal and/or painful stimuli • Assess pupils for size, shape, equality, and response to light	• Periodically reassess level of consciousness, mental status
Identify Deformities • Inspect extremities for any obvious deformities • Determine range of movement and strength in extremities	• Immobilize (e.g., splint) any obvious deformities
Brief Pain Assessment • Assess pain (e.g., PQRST [see Table 34-8])	• Periodically reassess pain using standardized pain scale

IVs, Intravenous.

16-gauge) IV catheters should be inserted and aggressive fluid resuscitation initiated using normal saline or lactated Ringer's solution. Direct pressure with a sterile dressing should be applied to obvious bleeding sites. Blood samples are obtained for typing to determine ABO and Rh group. Type-specific packed red blood cells should be administered if needed. In an emergency (life-threatening) situation, uncrossmatched blood may be given if immediate transfusion is warranted.

The use of the *pneumatic antishock garment* (PASG) is a temporary strategy that may be considered for pelvic fracture bleeding with hypotension.[11] The PASG is a three-chambered suit that is applied to the patient's legs and abdomen and is inflated with a foot pump. Physiologically, the PASG increases peripheral vascular resistance in the patient's lower extremities, thus elevating blood pressure, and works to control pelvic fracture bleeding. Care must be taken when deflating the garment. Rapid deflation can result in a severe drop in peripheral vascular resistance and blood pressure. Alternative devices to the PASG include pelvic splints and belts.[11]

D = Disability. A brief neurologic examination completes the primary survey. The degree of disability is measured by the patient's level of consciousness. Determining the patient's response to verbal and/or painful stimuli is one approach to assessing level of consciousness. A simple mnemonic to remember is AVPU: **A** = alert, **V** = responsive to voice, **P** = responsive to pain, and **U** = unresponsive. In addition, the Glasgow Coma Scale (GCS) is used to further assess the arousal aspect of the patient's consciousness (see Chapter 57). Finally, the pupils should be also assessed for size, shape, response to light, and equality.

Secondary Survey

After each step of the primary survey is addressed and any lifesaving interventions are initiated, the secondary survey begins. The **secondary survey** is a brief, systematic process that is aimed at identifying *all* injuries (Table 69-5).

E = Exposure/Environmental Control. All trauma patients should have their clothes removed so that a thorough physical assessment can be performed. Once the patient is exposed, it is important to limit heat loss and prevent hypothermia by using warming blankets, overhead warmers, and warmed IV fluids.

F = Full Set of Vital Signs/Five Interventions/Facilitate Family Presence. A complete set of vital signs, including blood pressure, heart rate, respiratory rate, and temperature, should

TABLE 69-4	Causes of Life-Threatening Conditions Identified During the Primary Survey*

Airway
- Inhalation injury
- Obstruction (partial or complete) from foreign bodies, debris (e.g., vomitus), or tongue
- Penetrating wounds and/or blunt trauma to upper airway structures

Breathing
- Anaphylaxis
- Flail chest with pulmonary contusion
- Hemothorax
- Pneumothorax (e.g., open, tension)

Circulation
- Direct cardiac injury (e.g., myocardial infarction, trauma)
- Pericardial tamponade
- Shock (e.g., massive burns, hypovolemia)
- Uncontrolled external hemorrhage

Disability
- Head injury
- Stroke

*List is not all-inclusive.

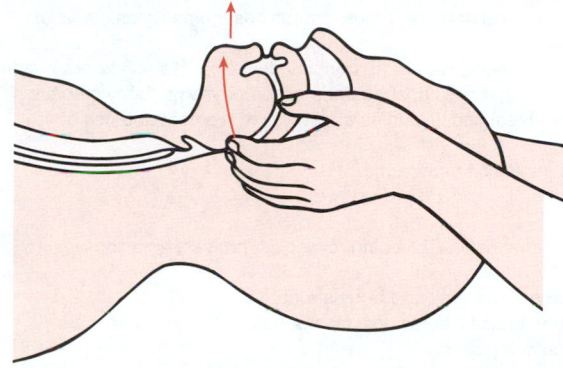

FIG. 69-2 Jaw-thrust maneuver is the recommended procedure for opening the airway of an unconscious patient with a possible neck or spinal injury. The patient should be lying supine with the rescuer kneeling at the top of the head. The rescuer places one hand on each side of the patient's head, resting his or her elbows on the surface. The rescuer grasps the angles of the patient's lower jaw and lifts the jaw forward with both hands without tilting the head.

be obtained after the patient is exposed. Blood pressure should be obtained in both arms if the patient has sustained or is suspected of having sustained chest trauma, or if the blood pressure is abnormally high or low.

At this point, it must be determined whether to proceed with the secondary survey or to perform additional interventions. The availability of other team members often influences this decision. For patients who have sustained significant trauma and/or have required lifesaving interventions during the primary survey, the following five interventions should be performed at this time:

1. The patient should be monitored by electrocardiogram (ECG) for heart rate and rhythm.
2. The pulse oximetry should be initiated and oxygen saturation (SpO$_2$) monitored.
3. An indwelling catheter should be inserted to monitor urine output and to check for hematuria. An indwelling catheter should not be inserted if a urethral tear is suspected. Patients with pelvic injuries, with blood at the meatus, or who are unable to void, and men with a high-riding prostate gland on

digital rectal examination, are at risk for a urethral tear or transection. A retrograde urethrogram should be obtained before a catheter is inserted.
4. An orogastric or a nasogastric tube should be inserted to provide gastric decompression and emptying to reduce the risk of aspiration and to test the contents for blood. A nasogastric tube should not be placed in the nares of a patient suspected of having facial fractures or a basilar skull fracture because the tube could enter the brain through the cribriform plate; rather, it should be placed orally.
5. Laboratory studies for typing and crossmatching, hematocrit, hemoglobin, blood urea nitrogen, creatinine, blood alcohol, toxicology screening, arterial blood gases, electrolytes, coagulation profile, liver enzymes, cardiac enzymes, and pregnancy should be facilitated.

Facilitating **family presence** (FP) completes this step of the secondary survey. Research supports the benefits of FP during resuscitation and invasive procedures to patients, families, and staff.[12,13] Patients reported that having family members present comforted them, served as an advocate for them, and helped to remind the health care team of their "personhood."[14] Family members who wished to be present during invasive procedures and resuscitation viewed themselves as active participants in the care process. They also believed that they provided comfort to the patient and that it was their right to be with the patient.[15] Staff nurses reported that family members who participated in FP functioned as "patient helpers" (e.g., providing support) and "staff helpers" (e.g., acting as a translator) and reinforced that FP helped to convey the sense of the patient's personhood.[15] Should a family member request FP during resuscitation or invasive procedures, it is essential that a member of the team be designated to explain care delivered and be available to answer questions.

G = Give Comfort Measures. Provision of comfort measures is of paramount importance when caring for patients in the ED. It has been reported that pain is the primary complaint of all patients who come to the ED.[16] Many EDs have developed nurse-initiated pain management protocols to treat pain early, beginning at triage.[16,17] Pain management strategies should include a combination of pharmacologic (e.g., nonsteroidal antiinflammatory drugs, IV opioids) and nonpharmacologic (e.g., imagery, distraction) measures. Emergency nurses play a pivotal role in ongoing pain management because of their frequent contact with patients. General comfort measures such as verbal reassurance, listening, reducing stimuli (e.g., dimming lights), and developing a trusting relationship with the patient and family should be provided to all patients in the ED.

H = History and Head-to-Toe Assessment. The history of the incident, injury, or illness provides clues to the cause of the crisis (e.g., Were the injuries self-inflicted?) and suggests specific assessment and intervention needs. The patient may be unable to give a history. However, family, friends, witnesses, and prehospital personnel can frequently provide important information. Prehospital information should focus on the mechanism and pattern of injury, injuries suspected, vital signs, and treatment initiated and patient responses.

Details of the incident are extremely important because the mechanism of injury and injury patterns can predict specific injuries. For example, a restrained front-seat passenger may have a head injury from hitting the steering wheel; knee, femur, or hip fractures or dislocation from striking the dashboard; and an abdominal injury from the seat belt. If there were fatalities at the scene, the patient has a high chance of significant injury.

TABLE 69-5	Secondary Survey of an Emergency Patient

Parameter	Interventions
Exposure and Environmental Control	• Remove clothing for adequate examination. Keep patient warm with blankets, warmed IV fluids, overhead lights.
Full Set of Vital Signs	• Obtain vital signs: temperature, heart rate, respiratory rate, blood pressure bilaterally.
Five Interventions	• Determine heart rhythm and initiate ECG monitoring, O_2 saturation; insert urinary catheter (if not contraindicated), insert gastric tube; obtain blood for laboratory studies.
Facilitate Family Presence	• Determine family's desire to be present during invasive procedures and/or cardiopulmonary resuscitation; assign team member to support family.
Give Comfort Measures	• Assess and treat pain, anxiety; provide emotional support to patient and family.
History and Head-to-Toe Assessment	
History	• Obtain details of the incident/illness, mechanism and pattern of injury, length of time since incident occurred, injuries suspected, treatment provided and patient's response, level of consciousness. • Use the mnemonic **AMPLE** to determine **A**llergies, **M**edication history, **P**ast health history (e.g., preexisting medical/psychiatric conditions, last menstrual period), **L**ast meal, and **E**vents/**E**nvironment preceding illness or injury.
Head, neck, and face	• Note general appearance, including skin color. • Examine face and scalp for lacerations, bone or soft tissue deformity, tenderness, bleeding, and foreign bodies. • Examine eyes, ears, nose, and mouth for bleeding, foreign bodies, drainage, pain, deformity, ecchymosis, lacerations. • Examine head for depressions of cranial or facial bones, contusions, hematomas, areas of softness, bony crepitus. • Examine neck for stiffness, pain in cervical vertebrae, tracheal deviation, distended neck veins, bleeding, edema, difficulty swallowing, bruising, subcutaneous emphysema, bony crepitus.
Chest	• Observe rate, depth, and effort of breathing, including chest wall movement and use of accessory muscles. • Palpate for bony crepitus, subcutaneous emphysema. • Auscultate breath sounds. • Obtain 12-lead ECG. • Inspect for external signs of injury: petechiae, bleeding, cyanosis, bruises, abrasions, lacerations, old scars.
Abdomen and flanks	• Evaluate symmetry of external abdominal wall and bony structures. • Inspect for external signs of injury: bruises, abrasions, lacerations, punctures, old scars. • Assess for masses, guarding, femoral pulses. • Assess type and location of pain, rigidity, or distention of abdomen. • Auscultate for bowel sounds.
Pelvis and perineum	• Gently palpate pelvis. • Assess genitalia for blood at the meatus, priapism, ecchymosis, rectal bleeding, anal sphincter tone. • Determine ability to void.
Extremities	• Inspect for signs of external injury: deformity, ecchymosis, abrasions, lacerations, swelling. • Assess for quality and location of pain, tenderness. • Evaluate movement, strength, and sensation in arms and legs. • Observe skin color and palpate skin for temperature and crepitus. • Presence, quality, and symmetry of peripheral pulses.
Inspect Posterior Surfaces	• Logroll and inspect and palpate back for deformity, bleeding, lacerations, bruises.

ECG, Electrocardiogram; *IV*, intravenous.

Patients who jump from buildings or bridges may have bilateral calcaneal (heel) fractures, bilateral wrist fractures, and lumbar spine compression fractures, and they may be at risk for aortic tears. Older patients who have climbed ladders and fallen may have had a stroke or myocardial infarction that led to the fall.

Prehospital personnel will often provide a detailed description of the patient's general condition, level of consciousness, and apparent injuries. An experienced ED team can complete a history within 5 minutes of the patient's arrival. If the patient is emergently ill, a thorough history is obtained from family or friends after the patient is taken to the treatment area. The history should include the following questions:

1. What is the chief complaint? What caused the patient to seek attention?
2. What are the patient's subjective complaints?
3. What is the patient's description of pain (e.g., location, duration, quality, character)?
4. What are witnesses' (if any) descriptions of the patient's behavior since the onset?
5. What is the patient's health history? The mnemonic *AMPLE* is a memory aid that prompts the nurse to ask about the following:

   A: Allergies
   M: Medication history

P: Past health history (e.g., preexisting medical and/or psychiatric conditions, previous hospitalizations/surgeries, smoking history, recent use of drugs/alcohol, tetanus immunization, last menstrual period, baseline mental status)

L: Last meal

E: Events/environment preceding illness or injury

Head, Neck, and Face. The patient should be assessed for general appearance, skin color, and temperature. The eyes should be evaluated for extraocular movements. A disconjugate gaze is an indication of neurologic damage. Battle's sign, or bruising directly behind the ear(s), may indicate a fracture of the base of the posterior portion of the skull. "Raccoon eyes," or periorbital ecchymosis, is usually an indication of a fracture of the base of the frontal portion of the skull. The tympanic membranes and external canal are checked for blood and cerebrospinal fluid (see Chapter 57). Clear drainage from the ear or nose should not be blocked.

The airway is assessed for foreign bodies, bleeding, edema, and loose or missing teeth. Assess for difficulty swallowing, movement of the palate, and ability to open the mouth. The neck should be examined for bruising, edema, bleeding, or distended neck veins. The trachea is palpated and visualized to determine whether it is midline. A deviated trachea may signal a life-threatening tension pneumothorax. Subcutaneous emphysema may indicate laryngotracheal disruption. A stiff or painful neck area may signify a fracture of one or more cervical vertebrae. The cervical spine must be protected using a rigid collar and supine positioning. Patients must be logrolled while maintaining cervical spine immobilization when movement is necessary.

Chest. The chest is examined for paradoxic chest movements and large sucking chest wounds. The sternum, clavicles, and ribs are palpated for deformity and point tenderness. The chest is assessed for pain on palpation, respiratory distress, decreased breath sounds, distant heart sounds, and distended neck veins. In addition to tension pneumothorax and open pneumothorax, the patient should be evaluated for rib fractures, pulmonary contusion, blunt cardiac injury, and hemothorax. A 12-lead ECG should be obtained, particularly on a patient with known or suspected heart disease. The ECG should be done to detect dysrhythmias and evidence of myocardial ischemia or infarction.

Abdomen and Flanks. The abdomen and flanks are more difficult to assess. Frequent evaluation for subtle changes in the abdominal examination is essential. Motor vehicle collisions and assaults can cause blunt trauma. Penetrating trauma tends to injure specific, solid organs (e.g., spleen). Decreased bowel sounds may indicate a temporary paralytic ileus. Bowel sounds in the chest may indicate a diaphragmatic rupture. The abdomen is percussed for distention (e.g., tympany [excessive air], dullness [excessive fluid]) and palpated for peritoneal irritation.

If intraabdominal hemorrhage is suspected, a *focused abdominal sonography for trauma* (FAST) to determine the presence of blood in the peritoneal space (hemoperitoneum) is preferred. This procedure is noninvasive and can be performed quickly at the bedside.[18] However, a FAST cannot rule out a retroperitoneal bleed. If suspected, a computed tomography (CT) scan is usually performed. An alternative, a diagnostic peritoneal lavage, may be considered. Before this procedure, a gastric tube and a bladder catheter must be inserted to decompress these organs and reduce the possibility of perforation.[18]

Pelvis and Perineum. The pelvis is gently palpated, not rocked. If pain is elicited, it may indicate a pelvic fracture. The genitalia are inspected for bleeding and obvious injuries. A rectal examination is performed to check for blood, a high-riding prostate gland, and loss of sphincter tone. Assess for bladder distention, hematuria, dysuria, or the inability to void.

Extremities. The upper and lower extremities are assessed for point tenderness, crepitus, and deformities. Injured extremities are splinted above and below the injury to decrease further soft tissue injury and pain. Grossly deformed, pulseless extremities should be realigned and splinted. Pulses are checked before and after movement or splinting of an extremity. A pulseless extremity is a time-critical vascular or orthopedic emergency.

Extremities are also assessed for *compartment syndrome*. This occurs as pressure and swelling increase inside a section of an extremity (e.g., anterior compartment of lower leg), compromising the viability of the extremity muscles, nerves, and arteries. Potential causes of compartment syndrome include crush injuries, fractures, edema (e.g., burns), and hemorrhage.

Injured extremities should be immobilized and elevated, and ice packs need to be applied. Prophylactic antibiotics are administered for open fractures. Patients with fractures should receive IV analgesia.[17]

I = Inspect the Posterior Surfaces. The trauma patient should always be logrolled (while maintaining cervical spine immobilization) to inspect the patient's posterior surfaces. The back is inspected for ecchymoses, abrasions, puncture wounds, cuts, and obvious deformities. The entire spine is palpated for misalignment, deformity, and pain.

Intervention and Evaluation

Once the secondary survey is complete, all findings are recorded. All patients should be evaluated to determine their need for tetanus prophylaxis. Information about the patient's past vaccination history and the condition of any wounds is needed in order to make an appropriate decision[19] (Table 69-6).

Regardless of the patient's chief complaint, ongoing patient monitoring and evaluation of interventions are critical in an emergency situation. The nurse is responsible for providing appropriate interventions and assessing the patient's response. The evaluation of airway patency and the effectiveness of breathing will always assume highest priority. The nurse will monitor O_2 saturation and arterial blood gases (ABGs) to help determine the patient's progress in these areas. Level of consciousness, vital signs, quality of peripheral pulses, urine output, and skin temperature, color, and moisture provide key information about circulation and perfusion and are also closely monitored.

Depending on the patient's injuries and/or illness, the patient may be (1) transported for diagnostic tests such as x-ray or CT scan; (2) admitted to a general unit, telemetry, or an intensive care unit; or (3) transferred to another facility. The emergency nurse is responsible for monitoring the critically ill patient during intrafacility and interfacility transport and notifying the team should the patient's condition change from baseline. Nurses accompanying patients on transports must be competent in advanced life-support measures.

Death in the Emergency Department

Unfortunately, there are a number of emergency patients who do not benefit from the skill, expertise, and technology available in the ED. It is important for the emergency nurse to be able to deal with feelings about sudden death so that the nurse can help families and significant others begin the grieving process.

TABLE 69-6	Prophylaxis Against Tetanus in Wound Management		
		Type of Wound	
Tetanus Vaccination History	**Clean, Minor Wound**	**All Other Wounds**	
Unknown or <3 doses	Td or Tdap* (Tdap preferred for ages 11-18)	Td or Tdap* (Tdap preferred for ages 11-18) plus TIG†	
Three or more doses and ≤5 yr since last dose	No prophylaxis needed	No prophylaxis needed	
Three or more doses and 6-10 yr since last dose	No prophylaxis needed	Td or Tdap* (Tdap preferred for ages 11-18)	
Three or more doses and >10 yr since last dose	Td or Tdap* (Tdap preferred for ages 11-18)	Td or Tdap* (Tdap preferred for ages 11-18)	

Td, Tetanus-diphtheria toxoid absorbed (for adult use); *Tdap*, tetanus toxoid, reduced diphtheria toxoid, and acellular pertussis vaccine; *TIG*, tetanus immune globulin (human).
*Tdap should be used in adults 19-64 if they have not previously received Tdap.
†When TIG and Td are administered concurrently, separate sites and syringes must be used.

The emergency nurse should recognize the importance of certain hospital rituals in preparing the bereaved to grieve, such as collecting the belongings, arranging for an autopsy, viewing the body, and making mortuary arrangements. The death must seem real so that the significant others can begin to grieve and accept the death. The emergency nurse plays a significant role in providing comfort to the surviving loved ones after a death in the ED.

Many patients who die in the ED could potentially be a candidate for *non–heart beating donation* (NHBD). Certain tissues and organs such as corneas, heart valves, skin, bone, and kidneys can be harvested from patients after death.[20] Approaching families about donation after an unexpected death is distressing to both the staff and the family. For many families, however, the act of donation may be the first positive step in the grieving process. *Organ procurement organizations* (OPOs) are available to assist in the process of screening potential donors, counseling donor families, obtaining informed consent, and harvesting organs from patients who have died in the ED.

GERONTOLOGIC CONSIDERATIONS
EMERGENCY CARE

The proportion of the population over age 65 is growing, with most leading active lives. Regardless of a patient's age, aggressive interventions are warranted for all injuries or illnesses unless the patient is known to have a preexisting terminal illness, an extremely low probability of survival, or an advance directive indicating a different course of action.

The elderly population is at high risk for injury due to many of the anatomic and physiologic changes that occur with aging (e.g., reduced visual acuity, limited neck rotation, slower gait, reduced reaction time). Of the injury-related admissions for people age 65 or older, most are for fractures, with many of these resulting from falls.[21] The three most common causes of falls in the elderly are generalized weakness, environmental hazards (e.g., loose mats, furniture), and orthostatic hypotension (e.g., side effect of medications, dehydration).[21] When assessing a patient who has experienced a fall, it is important to determine whether the physical findings may have actually caused the fall or may be due to the fall itself. For example, a patient may exhibit acute confusion. The confusion may be due to myocardial infarction or stroke that caused the patient to lose consciousness and fall, or the patient may have suffered a head injury as a result of the fall.

Knowledge of the concepts of aging will improve the care delivered to the elderly in the ED (see Chapter 6). Unfortunately, many older adults dismiss symptoms as simply "normal for their age." Any complaint by an older adult must be fully investigated. Research has shown that the use of an ED-based nurse discharge plan coordinator for elderly patients can reduce the number of returns to the ED and facilitate the transition from the ED to home.[22]

Environmental Emergencies

Increased interest in outdoor activities such as running, hiking, cycling, skiing, sailing, and swimming has increased the number of environmental emergencies seen in the ED. Illness or injury may be caused by the activity, exposure to weather, or attack from various animals or humans. Specific environmental emergencies discussed in this section include heat-related emergencies, cold-related emergencies, submersion injuries, bites, and stings.

HEAT-RELATED EMERGENCIES

Brief exposure to intense heat or prolonged exposure to less intense heat leads to heat stress when thermoregulatory mechanisms such as sweating, vasodilation, and increased respirations cannot compensate for exposure to increased ambient temperatures.[23] Ambient temperature is a product of environmental temperature and humidity. Strenuous activities in hot or humid environments, clothing that interferes with perspiration, high fevers, and preexisting illnesses predispose individuals to heat stress (Table 69-7). Effects can be mild (heat rash and heat edema) or severe (heat exhaustion and heatstroke). The management of heat-related emergencies is summarized in Table 69-8.

Heat rash (miliaria or prickly heat) is a fine, red, papular rash that occurs on the torso, neck, and skinfolds. The rash occurs when sweat ducts are obstructed and become inflamed so that sweat excretion does not occur. The rash usually occurs in warm weather, but has also been reported in cold weather as a result of clothing.

Heat syncope is associated with prolonged standing and heat exposure. Manifestations include dizziness, orthostatic hypotension, and syncope. Inadequate vasomotor tone associated with aging places the elderly at greater risk for heat syncope.

Heat edema is characterized by swelling of the hands, feet, and ankles, usually in nonacclimatized individuals as a result of prolonged standing or sitting. Swelling usually resolves in days with rest, elevation, and support hose. Diuretics are not recommended because this condition is self-limiting and requires no additional treatment.

Heat Cramps

Heat cramps are severe cramps in large muscle groups fatigued by heavy work. Cramps are brief, intense, and tend to occur during rest after exercise or heavy labor. Nausea, tachycardia, pallor, weakness, and profuse diaphoresis are often present. The condition

TABLE 69-7	**Risk Factors for Heat-Related Emergencies**

Age
- Elderly
- Infants

Environmental Conditions
- High environmental temperature
- High relative humidity
- Low wind

Preexisting Illness
- Cardiovascular disease
- Cystic fibrosis
- Diabetes
- Obesity
- Previous stroke or other central nervous system lesion
- Skin disorders (e.g., large burn scars)

Prescription Drugs
- Anticholinergics
- Antihistamines
- Antiparkinsonian drugs
- Antispasmodics
- β-Adrenergic blockers
- Butyrophenones
- Diuretics
- Phenothiazines
- Tricyclic antidepressants

Street Drugs
- Amphetamines
- Jimsonweed
- Lysergic acid diethylamide (LSD)
- Phencyclidine (PCP)
- 3,4-methylenedioxymethamphetamine (MDMA, ecstasy)

Alcohol

Adapted from Emergency Nurses Association, Newberry L, editor: *Sheehy's emergency nursing: principles and practice,* ed 6, St Louis, 2006, Mosby.

is seen most often in healthy, acclimated athletes with inadequate fluid intake. Cramps resolve rapidly with rest and oral or parenteral replacement of sodium and water. Elevation, gentle massage, and analgesia minimize pain associated with heat cramps. The patient should avoid strenuous activity for at least 12 hours after the development of heat cramps. Education should emphasize salt replacement during strenuous exercise in hot, humid environments. Commercially prepared electrolyte solutions (e.g., sports drinks) are recommended.

Heat Exhaustion

Prolonged exposure to heat over hours or days leads to **heat exhaustion,** a clinical syndrome characterized by fatigue, lightheadedness, nausea, vomiting, diarrhea, and feelings of impending doom (see Table 69-8). Tachypnea, hypotension, tachycardia, elevated body temperature, dilated pupils, mild confusion, ashen color, and profuse diaphoresis are also present. Hypotension and mild to severe temperature elevation (99.6° to 104° F [37.5° to 40° C]) are due to dehydration.[23] Heat exhaustion usually occurs in individuals engaged in strenuous activity in hot, humid weather, but it also occurs in sedentary individuals.

Treatment begins with placement of the patient in a cool area and removal of constrictive clothing. The patient is monitored for airway, breathing, and circulation (ABCs), including cardiac dysrhythmias (due to electrolyte imbalances). Oral fluid and electro-lyte replacement is initiated unless the patient is nauseated. Salt tablets are not recommended because of potential gastric irritation and hypernatremia. A 0.9% normal saline solution is initiated intravenously when oral solutions are not tolerated. An initial fluid bolus may be used to correct hypotension. However, fluid replacement should be correlated to clinical and laboratory parameters. A moist sheet placed over the patient decreases core temperature through evaporative heat loss. Hospital admission is considered for the elderly, the chronically ill, or those who do not improve within 3 to 4 hours.

Heatstroke

Heatstroke, the most serious form of heat stress, results from failure of the hypothalamic thermoregulatory processes and is considered a medical emergency. Increased sweating, vasodilation, and increased respiratory rate (the body's attempt to lower temperature) deplete fluids and electrolytes, specifically sodium. Eventually, sweat glands stop functioning, and core temperature increases rapidly, within 10 to 15 minutes. The patient has core temperature greater than 104° F (40° C), altered mentation, absence of perspiration, and circulatory collapse. The skin is hot, dry, and ashen. Because the brain is extremely sensitive to thermal injuries, a range of neurologic symptoms occur, such as hallucinations, loss of muscle coordination, and combativeness. Cerebral edema and hemorrhage may occur as a result of direct thermal injury to the brain and decreased cerebral blood flow.

The development of heatstroke is directly related to the amount of time that the patient's body temperature remains elevated.[23] Prognosis is related to age, baseline health status, and length of exposure. Older adults and individuals with diabetes mellitus, chronic kidney disease, cardiovascular disease, pulmonary disease, or other physiologic compromise are particularly vulnerable.

Collaborative Care. Treatment of heatstroke focuses on stabilizing the patient's ABCs and rapidly reducing the core temperature. Administration of 100% O_2 compensates for the patient's hypermetabolic state. Ventilation with a BVM or intubation and mechanical ventilation may be required. Fluid and electrolyte imbalances are corrected, and continuous cardiac monitoring for dysrhythmias is initiated.

Various cooling methods are available, such as removal of clothing, covering with wet sheets, and placing the patient in front of a large fan (evaporative cooling); immersion in an ice water bath (conductive cooling); and administering cool fluids or lavaging with cool fluids.[23] Whatever method is selected, the nurse is responsible for closely monitoring the patient's temperature and controlling shivering. Shivering increases core temperature (due to the associated heat generated by muscle activity) and complicates cooling efforts. Chlorpromazine (Thorazine) IV is the drug of choice to suppress shivering. Aggressive temperature reduction should continue until core temperature reaches 102° F (38.9° C).[23] Antipyretics are not effective in this situation because the elevated temperature is not related to infection.

The patient is also monitored for signs of *rhabdomyolysis* (a serious disease characterized by breakdown of skeletal muscle). The muscle breakdown leads to myoglobinuria, which places the kidneys at risk for acute failure. Therefore urine should be carefully monitored for color (e.g., tea colored), amount, pH, and myoglobin. Finally, clotting studies are performed to monitor the patient for signs of disseminated intravascular coagulation (see Chapter 31).

Patient and family teaching focuses on how to avoid future problems. Essential information regarding proper hydration during

TABLE 69-8	*EMERGENCY MANAGEMENT* Hyperthermia	

Etiology	Assessment Findings	Interventions
Environmental • Lack of acclimatization • Prolonged exposure to extreme temperatures • Physical exertion, especially during hot weather **Trauma** • Head injury • Spinal cord injury **Metabolic** • Dehydration • Thyrotoxicosis • Diabetes **Drugs** • Phenothiazines • Tricyclic antidepressants • Diuretics • Amphetamines • β-Adrenergic blockers • Antihistamines **Other** • Cardiovascular disease • CNS disorders • Alcoholism	**Heat Cramps** • Severe muscle contractions in exerted muscles • Thirst **Heat Exhaustion** • Pale, ashen • Fatigue, weakness • Profuse sweating • Altered mental status (e.g., feelings of impending doom) • Hypotension • Tachycardia • Weak, thready pulse • Temperature 99.6° F (37.5° C) to 104° F (40° C) **Heatstroke** • Hot, dry skin • Altered mental status (e.g., ranging from confusion to coma) • Hypotension • Tachycardia • Weakness • Temperature >104° F (40° C)	**Initial** • Manage and maintain ABCs. • Provide high-flow O₂ via non-rebreather mask or BVM. • Establish IV access and begin fluid replacement for significant heat injury. • Place patient in a cool environment. • For patient with heatstroke, initiate rapid cooling measures: remove patient's clothing, place wet sheets over patient, and place in front of fan; immerse in ice water bath; administer cool IV fluids or lavage with cool fluids. • Obtain ECG. • Obtain blood for electrolytes and CBC. • Insert urinary catheter. **Ongoing Monitoring** • Monitor ABCs, vital signs, level of consciousness. • Monitor cardiac rhythm, O₂ saturation, electrolytes, and urinary output. • Monitor urine for development of myoglobinuria. • Monitor clotting studies for development of disseminated intravascular coagulation.

ABCs, Airway, breathing, circulation; *BVM*, bag-valve-mask; *CBC*, complete blood count; *CNS*, central nervous system; *ECG*, electrocardiogram; *IV*, intravenous.

hot weather and physical exercise is imperative. Patients should also be instructed on the early signs of and interventions for heat-related stress.

COLD-RELATED EMERGENCIES

Cold injuries may be localized (frostbite) or systemic (hypothermia). Contributing factors include age, duration of exposure, environmental temperature, homelessness, preexisting conditions (e.g., diabetes mellitus, peripheral vascular disease), medications that suppress shivering (opioids, heroin, psychotropic agents, and antiemetics), and alcohol intoxication, which causes peripheral vasodilation, increases sensations of warmth, and depresses shivering. Smokers have an increased risk of cold-related injury as a result of the vasoconstrictive effects of nicotine.

Frostbite

Frostbite can be described as "true tissue freezing," which results in the formation of ice crystals in the tissues and cells. Peripheral vasoconstriction is the initial response to cold stress and results in a decrease in blood flow and vascular stasis. As cellular temperature decreases and ice crystals form in intracellular spaces, intracellular sodium and chloride increase, the cell membrane is destroyed, and organelles are damaged. These alterations result in edema. Depth of frostbite is the result of ambient temperature, length of exposure, type and condition (wet or dry) of clothing, and contact with metal surfaces. Other factors that affect severity include skin color (dark-skinned people are more prone to frostbite), lack of acclimatization, previous episodes, exhaustion, and poor peripheral vascular status.

Superficial frostbite involves skin and subcutaneous tissue, usually the ears, nose, fingers, and toes. The skin appearance will

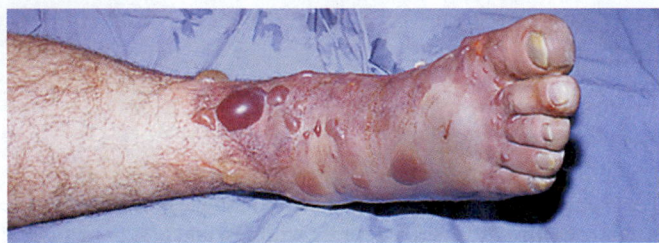

FIG. 69-3 Edema and blister formation 24 hours after frostbite injury occurring in an area covered by a tightly fitted boot.

range from waxy pale yellow to blue to mottled, and the skin will feel crunchy and frozen. The patient may complain of tingling, numbness, or a burning sensation. Injured tissue is easily damaged, so the area should be handled carefully and never squeezed, massaged, or scrubbed. Clothing and jewelry should be removed because they may constrict the extremity and decrease circulation. The affected area should be immersed in a water bath (102° to 108° F) [38.9° to 42.2° C]).[24] Warm soaks may be used for the face. The patient often experiences a warm, stinging sensation as tissue thaws. Blisters form within a few hours (Fig. 69-3). The blisters should be debrided and a sterile dressing applied. Heavy blankets and clothing should be avoided because friction and weight can lead to sloughing of damaged tissue. Rewarming is extremely painful. Residual pain may last weeks or even years. Analgesia should be administered and tetanus prophylaxis should be given as appropriate (see Table 69-6). The patient should be evaluated for systemic hypothermia.

Deep frostbite involves muscle, bone, and tendon. The skin is white, hard, and insensitive to touch. The area has the appearance

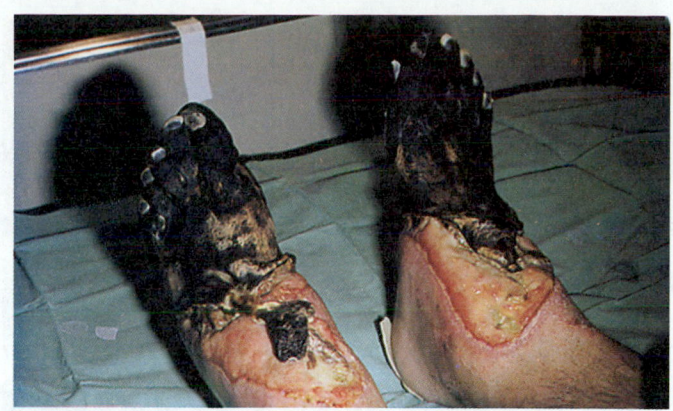

FIG. 69-4   Gangrenous necrosis 6 weeks after the frostbite injury shown in Fig. 69-3.

of deep thermal injury with mottling gradually progressing to gangrene (Fig. 69-4). The affected extremity is immersed in a circulating water bath (102° to 108° F [38.9° to 42.2° C]) until distal flush occurs. After rewarming, the extremity should be elevated to reduce edema.[24] Significant edema may begin within 3 hours, with blistering in 6 hours to days. Intravenous analgesia is always required in severe frostbite because of the pain associated with tissue thawing. Tetanus prophylaxis should be given, and the patient should be evaluated for systemic hypothermia. Amputation may be required if the injured area is untreated or treatment is unsuccessful. The patient may be admitted to the hospital for observation over 24 to 48 hours with bed rest, elevation of the injured part, and prophylactic antibiotics if the wound is at risk for infection.

Hypothermia

Hypothermia, defined as a core temperature less than 95° F (35° C), occurs when heat produced by the body cannot compensate for heat lost to the environment. From 55% to 60% of all body heat is lost as radiant energy, with the greatest loss from the head, thorax, and lungs (with each breath).[25] Wet clothing increases evaporative heat loss 5 times greater than normal; immersion in cold water increases heat loss by a factor of 25. Environmental exposure to freezing temperatures, cold winds, and wet, damp terrain in the presence of physical exhaustion, inadequate clothing, and/or inexperience predisposes individuals to hypothermia.[25,26] Near-drowning and water immersion are also associated with hypothermia.

The elderly are more prone to hypothermia due to decreased body fat, diminished energy reserves, decreased basal metabolic rate, decreased shivering response, decreased sensory perception, chronic medical conditions, and medications that alter body defenses. In addition, certain drugs, alcohol, and diabetes are considered risk factors for hypothermia.

Hypothermia mimics cerebral or metabolic disturbances causing ataxia, confusion, and withdrawal, so the patient may be misdiagnosed. Peripheral vasoconstriction is the body's first attempt to conserve heat. As cold temperatures persist, shivering and movement are the body's only mechanisms for producing heat. Coma results when core temperature falls below 82.4° F (28° C), and death usually occurs when core temperature falls below 78° F (25.6° C).[26]

Core temperature below 86° F (30° C) is severe and potentially life threatening. Assessment findings in hypothermia are variable and dependent on core temperature (Table 69-9). Patients with

mild hypothermia (93.2° to 96.8° F [34° to 36° C]) have shivering, lethargy, confusion, rational to irrational behavior, and minor heart rate changes. Shivering disappears at temperatures less than 92° F (33.3° C). Moderate hypothermia (86° to 93.2° F [30° to 34° C]) causes rigidity, bradycardia, slowed respiratory rate, blood pressure obtainable only by Doppler, metabolic and respiratory acidosis, and hypovolemia.[26]

As core temperature drops, basal metabolic rate decreases two or three times. The cold myocardium is extremely irritable, making it vulnerable to dysrhythmias (e.g., atrial and ventricular fibrillation). Decreased renal blood flow decreases glomerular filtration rate, which impairs water reabsorption and leads to dehydration. The hematocrit increases as intravascular volume decreases. Cold blood becomes thick and acts as a thrombus, placing the patient at risk for stroke, myocardial infarction, pulmonary emboli, acute tubular necrosis, and renal failure. Decreased blood flow leads to lactic acid accumulation from anaerobic metabolism and subsequent metabolic acidosis.

Profound hypothermia (less than 86° F [30° C]) makes the person appear dead. Metabolic rate, heart rate, and respirations are so slow that they may be difficult to detect. Reflexes are absent and the pupils fixed and dilated. Profound bradycardia, asystole, or ventricular fibrillation may be present. Every effort is made to warm the patient to at least 90° F (32.2° C) before the person is pronounced dead. The cause of death is usually refractory ventricular fibrillation.

Collaborative Care. Treatment of hypothermia focuses on managing and maintaining ABCs, rewarming the patient, correcting dehydration and acidosis, and treating cardiac dysrhythmias (see Table 69-9). Passive or active external rewarming is used for mild hypothermia. Passive external rewarming involves moving the patient to a warm, dry place, removing damp clothing, and placing warm blankets on the patient. Gentle handling is essential to prevent stimulation of the cold myocardium. Active external rewarming involves body-to-body contact, fluid- or air-filled warming blankets, or radiant heat lamps. The patient should be closely monitored for marked vasodilation and hypotension during rewarming.

Active core rewarming is used for moderate to profound hypothermia and refers to heat applied directly to the core. Techniques include heated (107.6° to 114.8° F [42° to 46° C]), humidified oxygen; warmed IV fluids (109.4° F [43° C]); and peritoneal, gastric, or colonic lavage with warmed fluids. Hemodialysis or cardiopulmonary bypass may also be considered in profound hypothermia.[26]

Core temperature should be carefully monitored during rewarming procedures. Warming places the patient at risk for afterdrop, a further drop in core temperature, which occurs when cold peripheral blood returns to the central circulation. Rewarming shock can produce hypotension and dysrhythmias. Thus patients with moderate to profound hypothermia should have the core warmed before the extremities. Rewarming should be discontinued once the core temperature reaches 95° F (35° C).[26]

Patient teaching should focus on how to avoid future cold-related problems. Essential information includes dressing in layers for cold weather, covering the head, carrying high-carbohydrate foods for extra calories, and developing a plan for survival should an injury occur.

SUBMERSION INJURIES

Submersion injury results when a person becomes hypoxic due to submersion in a substance, usually water. Approximately 8000 deaths occur from submersion injuries annually in the United

TABLE 69-9	EMERGENCY MANAGEMENT
	Hypothermia

Etiology	Assessment Findings	Interventions
Environmental • Prolonged exposure to cold • Prolonged submersion • Inadequate clothing for environmental temperature **Metabolic** • Hypoglycemia • Hypothyroidism **Hospital Acquired** • Cold IV fluids • Blood administration • Inadequate warming or rewarming in the ED or surgery • Administration of neuromuscular blocking agents **Other** • Phenothiazines • Barbiturates • Alcohol • Trauma • Shock	• Core body temperature: Mild hypothermia: 93.2°-96.8° F (34°-36° C) Moderate hypothermia: 86°-93.2° F (30°-34° C) Profound hypothermia: <86° F (<30° C) • Shivering, diminished or absent at core body temperature ≤92° F (33.3° C) • Hypoventilation • Hypotension • Altered mental status (ranging from confusion to coma) • Areflexia (absence of reflexes) • Pale, cyanotic skin • Blue, white, or frozen extremities • Dysrhythmias: bradycardia, atrial fibrillation, ventricular fibrillation, asystole • Fixed, dilated pupils	**Initial** • Remove patient from cold environment. • Manage and maintain ABCs. • Provide high-flow O_2 via non-rebreather mask or BVM. • Anticipate intubation for diminished or absent gag reflex. • Rewarm patient: *Passive:* Remove wet clothing, apply dry clothing and warm blankets, administer warm fluids. *Active external:* Use body-to-body contact, apply heating devices (e.g., air-filled warming blankets) or radiant lights. *Active core warming:* Administer warmed IV fluids; heated, humidified O_2; peritoneal, gastric, or colonic lavage with warmed fluids. • Anticipate the need for hemodialysis or cardiopulmonary bypass. • Warm central trunk first in patients with profound hypothermia to limit rewarming shock. • Establish IV access with two large-bore catheters for fluid resuscitation. • Assess for other injuries. • Keep patient's head covered with warm, dry towels, or stocking cap to limit loss of heat. • Treat patient gently to avoid increased cardiac irritability. **Ongoing Monitoring** • Monitor ABCs, level of consciousness, temperature, vital signs. • Monitor O_2 saturation, cardiac rhythm. • Monitor electrolytes, glucose.

ABCs, Airway, breathing, circulation; *BVM*, bag-valve-mask; *ED*, emergency department; *IV*, intravenous.

States. Forty percent of these victims are children under 5 years of age. The primary risk factors for submersion injury include inability to swim, use of alcohol or drugs, trauma, seizures, hypothermia, and stroke.

Drowning is death from suffocation after submersion in water or other fluid medium. *Near-drowning* is defined as survival from potential drowning. *Immersion syndrome* occurs with immersion in cold water, which leads to stimulation of the vagus nerve and potentially fatal dysrhythmias (e.g., bradycardia).

Death from a submersion injury is caused by hypoxia secondary to aspiration and swallowing of fluid, usually water. Swallowed water may cause vomiting and additional aspiration. A majority of drowning victims aspirate water into the pulmonary tree and develop pulmonary edema. Victims who do not aspirate fluid develop intense bronchospasm and airway obstruction, the cause of death in "dry drowning." Regardless of what fluid is aspirated into the pulmonary tree, the ultimate result is pulmonary edema. The osmotic gradient caused by aspirated fluid causes fluid imbalances in the body. Hypotonic fresh water is rapidly absorbed into the circulatory system through the alveoli. Fresh water may be contaminated with chlorine, mud, and algae, causing the breakdown of lung surfactant, fluid seepage, and pulmonary edema. Hypertonic salt water draws protein-rich fluid from the vascular space into the alveoli, impairing alveolar ventilation and resulting in hypoxia. Fig. 69-5 shows the pulmonary effects of saltwater and freshwater aspiration.

The body attempts to compensate for hypoxia by shunting blood to the lungs. This results in increased pulmonary pressures and deteriorating respiratory status. More and more blood is shunted through the alveoli. However, the blood is not adequately oxygenated, so the hypoxemia worsens. Anaerobic metabolism occurs, which leads to lactic acidosis.

The assessment findings of a patient with a submersion injury are listed in Table 69-10. Aggressive resuscitation efforts and the mammalian diving reflex improve survival of near-drowning victims even after submersion in cold water for long periods of time.[27] Cold water lowers the body's metabolic rate and oxygen demand. The mammalian diving reflex causes apnea, bradycardia, and peripheral vasoconstriction and further decreases metabolic rate. Blood flow is redistributed to the most vital organs (i.e., heart, lungs, brain).

Collaborative Care

Treatment of submersion injuries focuses on correcting hypoxia, acid-base imbalances, and fluid imbalances; supporting basic physiologic functions; and rewarming when hypothermia is present. Initial evaluation involves assessment of airway, cervical spine, breathing, and circulation. Other interventions are listed in Table 69-10.

Mechanical ventilation with positive end-expiratory pressure or continuous positive airway pressure may be used to improve gas exchange across the alveolar-capillary membrane when significant pulmonary edema is present. Ventilation and oxygenation are the primary techniques used to treat respiratory acidosis. Mannitol (Osmitrol) or furosemide (Lasix) may be given to decrease free water and treat cerebral edema.

Deterioration in neurologic status suggests cerebral edema, worsening hypoxia, or profound acidosis. Near-drowning victims may also have head and neck injuries that cause prolonged alterations in level of consciousness. All victims of near-drowning should be observed in a hospital for a minimum of 4 to 6 hours. Additional observation is needed for patients who have preexisting comorbidities (e.g., cardiovascular disease). Pneumonia and cerebral edema have been reported in patients who were essentially free of symptoms immediately after the near-drowning episode but later developed problems. *Delayed pulmonary edema* (also known as *secondary drowning*) can occur and is defined as delayed death from drowning due to pulmonary complications.

Teaching should focus on water safety and minimizing the risks for drowning. Swimming pool gates should be locked; life jackets should be used on all water craft, including inner tubes and rafts; and water survival skills (e.g., swimming lessons) should be a priority. The dangers of combining alcohol and drugs with swimming and other water sports should be emphasized.[27]

BITES AND STINGS

Animals, spiders, and insects cause injury and even death by biting or stinging. Morbidity is a result of either direct tissue damage or lethal toxins. Direct tissue damage is a product of animal size, characteristics of the animal's teeth, and strength of the jaw. Tissue may be lacerated, crushed, or chewed while toxins released

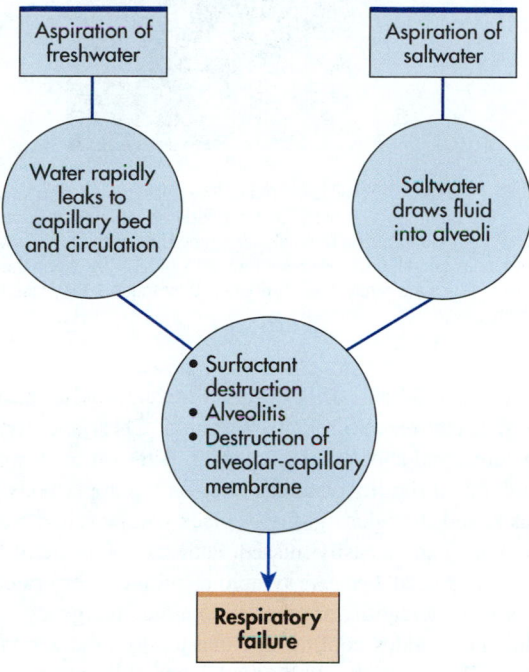

FIG. 69-5 Pulmonary effects of water aspiration.

TABLE 69-10	*EMERGENCY MANAGEMENT* **Submersion Injuries**

Etiology	Assessment Findings	Interventions
• Inability to swim or exhaustion while swimming • Entrapment or entanglement with objects in water • Loss of ability to move secondary to trauma, stroke, hypothermia, myocardial infarction • Poor judgment due to alcohol or drugs • Seizure while in water	**Pulmonary** • Ineffective breathing • Dyspnea • Respiratory distress • Respiratory arrest • Crackles, rhonchi • Cough with pink-frothy sputum • Cyanosis **Cardiac** • Tachycardia • Bradycardia • Dysrhythmia • Hypotension • Cardiac arrest **Other** • Panic • Exhaustion • Coma • Coexisting illness (e.g., MI) or injury (e.g., cervical spine injury) • Core temperature slightly elevated or below normal depending on water temperature and length of submersion	**Initial** • Manage and maintain ABCs. • Assume cervical spine injury in all drowning victims and stabilize and/or immobilize cervical spine. • Provide 100% O_2 via non-rebreather mask or BVM. • Anticipate need for intubation if gag reflex is absent. • Establish IV access with two large-bore catheters for fluid resuscitation and infuse warmed fluids if appropriate. • Assess for other injuries. • Remove wet clothing and cover with warm blankets. • Obtain temperature and begin rewarming if needed. • Obtain cervical spine and chest x-rays. • Insert gastric tube. **Ongoing Monitoring** • Monitor ABCs, vital signs, level of consciousness. • Monitor O_2 saturation, cardiac rhythm. • Monitor temperature and maintain normothermia. • Monitor for signs of acute respiratory failure.

ABCs, Airway, breathing, circulation; *BVM*, bag-valve-mask; *IV*, intravenous; *MI*, myocardial infarction.

through teeth, fangs, stingers, spines, or tentacles have local or systemic effects. Death associated with animal bites is due to blood loss, allergic reactions, or lethal toxins. Injuries caused by insects, spiders, ticks, snakes, animals (e.g., dogs, cats, rodents), and humans are described here.

Hymenopteran Stings

The *Hymenoptera* family includes bees, yellow jackets, hornets, wasps, and fire ants. Stings can cause mild discomfort or life-threatening anaphylaxis (see Chapters 14 and 67). Venom may be cytotoxic, hemolytic, allergenic, or vasoactive. Symptoms may begin immediately or be delayed up to 48 hours. Reactions are more severe with multiple stings. Most hymenopterans sting repeatedly. However, the domestic honey bee stings only once, usually leaving a barbed stinger with an attached venom sac in the skin so that release of venom continues. Africanized honey bees (killer bees) which look and sting like domestic bees have migrated into North America. If threatened, these bees aggressively swarm and repeatedly sting their victims (e.g., humans, animals). These attacks can be fatal.

If stung, the stinger should be removed with a scraping motion with a fingernail, knife, or needle. Tweezers squeeze the stinger and may cause more venom release. However, the fastest method of removing the stinger is ultimately the best, so if tweezers are available, they can be used.

Manifestations vary from stinging, burning, swelling, and itching to edema, headache, fever, syncope, malaise, nausea, vomiting, wheezing, bronchospasm, laryngeal edema, and hypotension. Treatment depends on the severity of the reaction. Mild reactions are treated with elevation, cool compresses, antipruritic lotions, and oral antihistamines. Rings, watches, and restrictive clothing are removed. More severe reactions require intramuscular or IV antihistamines (e.g., diphenhydramine [Benadryl]), subcutaneous epinephrine, and corticosteroids (e.g., dexamethasone [Decadron]). Allergic reactions and anaphylaxis are discussed in Chapter 14.

Spider Bites (Arachnid)

Although there are 20,000 species of venomous spiders in the world, only 50 species cause illness. Two venomous spiders found in the United States are the black widow spider and the brown recluse spider.[28] Their venom can cause a localized reaction or systemic anaphylaxis. Tarantulas appear more dangerous than they actually are because their bite causes only localized stinging and pain. Other types of spiders release venom when they bite and may cause allergic reactions in some individuals, but they are not considered poisonous.

Black Widow Spiders. Black widow spiders are the most feared of all spiders. The female's venom is especially poisonous to people. Both the female and male are black in color (Fig. 69-6). The female rarely leaves the web, biting defensively if disturbed. Black widow spiders are found among fallen branches, among firewood, and under objects of many kinds, including furniture, outhouse seats, and trash.

The black widow spider venom is neurotoxic. When bitten, the patient will feel a pinprick-like sensation and a tiny, red bite mark will appear. Approximately 15 to 60 minutes later, the patient will report severe pain that will increase over the next 12 to 48 hours. Systemic symptoms will develop 30 minutes after *envenomation* (the introduction of poisonous venoms into the body by a bite or a sting). These can include nausea, vomiting, abdominal cramping, hypertension, dyspnea, paresthesias, and tachycardia. Symptoms

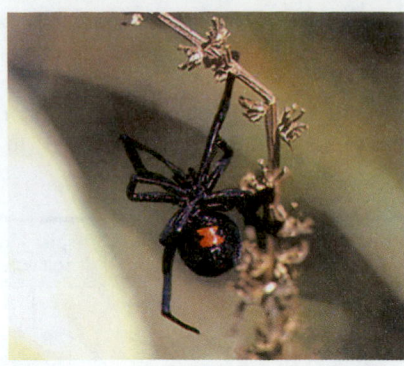

FIG. 69-6 Female black widow spider. The fully grown female is about 1.2 cm (0.5 in) long and is jet black, with an hourglass-shaped red mark on the underside of the abdomen. The female's sting is poisonous to humans. Males are only about half as long and usually have four pairs of red dots along the sides of the abdomen. Males are rarely seen and when they mature, they lose their poisonous ability.

usually peak 2 to 3 hours after onset; however, muscle spasms and hypertension can recur for 12 to 24 hours. Chest and abdominal pain, seizures, and shock can also occur. Bites on the lower body cause abdominal rigidity, whereas bites on the upper body lead to chest, back, and shoulder rigidity. A black widow spider bite is not prominent and can be easily missed. Patients not aware of the bite can be misdiagnosed, because symptoms mimic a perforated ulcer, appendicitis, pancreatitis, or other abdominal emergency.

Treatment includes cooling the area to slow the action of the neurotoxin. IV access should be established and oxygen administered as needed. The wound should be cleaned and tetanus prophylaxis given as appropriate. Muscle spasms are treated with calcium gluconate, diazepam (Valium), or methocarbamol (Robaxin). Severe pain may require opioid analgesia. Although antivenin is rarely used, it can be used for severe reactions, young children, or adults with hypertension or cardiac disease.[28]

Brown Recluse Spiders. Brown recluse spiders are usually found in dark areas such as garages, closets, and boxes. The spider, common in the southeastern, south-central, and southwestern United States, is a light brown color with a characteristic dark brown fiddle shape that extends from the eyes down the back. The venom is cytotoxic, so local tissue effects can be dramatic. Initially, the bite is insignificant, with a local reaction (e.g., itching, erythema) beginning in 6 to 12 hours. A painful, bluish-purple purpura develops in a ring around the bite and eventually may progress to a necrotic ulcerating wound by 7 to 14 days, though it may take as long as 6 months. The wound can extend deep into tissue and may persist for weeks. Occasionally, systemic manifestations of envenomation occur and can include fever, chills, joint pain, malaise, nausea, and vomiting.[29]

Treatment depends on severity of the reaction. Treatment is necessary when there is bleb or bulla formation, intense pain, and signs of rapidly progressive ischemia and necrosis. Initial interventions include cleansing the bite with mild antiseptic soap, providing cool compresses, and elevating the affected extremity. Analgesia, tetanus prophylaxis, antihistamines, corticosteroids, and antibiotics for prevention of secondary infection may also be required. Surgical debridement with grafting is necessary for some patients. Hyperbaric oxygen therapy may also be considered to enhance tissue healing. Dapsone (Avlosulfon), a polymorphonuclear leukocyte inhibitor, has been used for patients with deep crater wounds, but efficacy has not been validated. Pa-

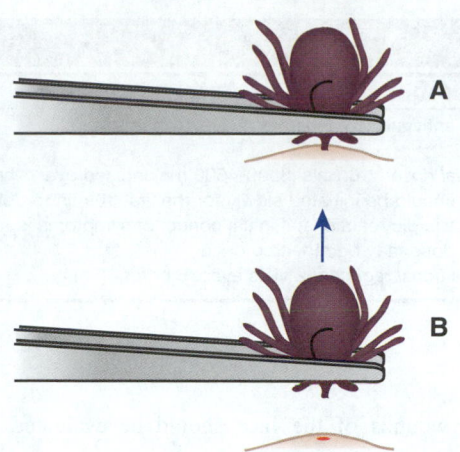

FIG. 69-7 Tick removal. **A,** Use tweezers to grasp the tick close to the skin. **B,** With a steady motion, pull the tick's body away from the skin. Do not be alarmed if the tick's mouthparts remain in the skin. Once the mouthparts are removed from the rest of the tick, it can no longer transmit disease.

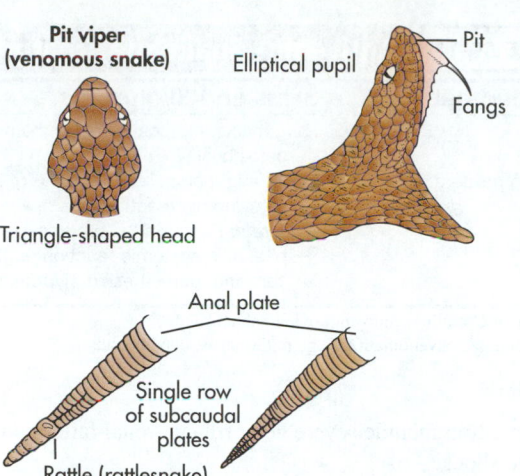

FIG. 69-8 Pit viper (a type of venomous snake).

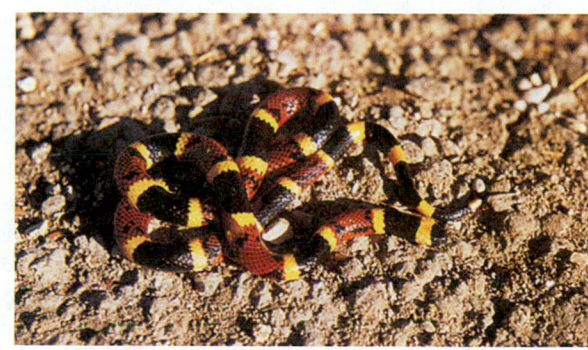

FIG. 69-9 Western coral snake. The venom from this snake is neurotoxic.

tients with systemic manifestations are hospitalized and monitored for hemolysis, disseminated intravascular coagulation, and acute renal failure.[29]

Tick Bites

Ticks are found throughout the United States, but they are most common in the northwestern, Rocky Mountain, and the northeastern regions. Emergencies associated with tick bites include Lyme disease, Rocky Mountain spotted fever, and tick paralysis. Disease is caused by an infected tick or by the release of neurotoxin. Ticks release a neurotoxic venom as long as the tick head is attached to the body. Therefore removal of the attached tick is essential for effective treatment. Forceps or tweezers may be used to safely remove the tick by grasping at the point of entry and pulling upward in a steady motion (Fig. 69-7). After the tick is removed, the skin should be cleaned with soap and water. Do not use a hot match, petroleum jelly, nail polish, or other products to remove the tick.[30]

Lyme disease is the most common arthropod-borne disease in the United States. Symptoms appear within 2 to 30 days of a bite from the *Ixodid* (hard) tick and result from exposure to the spirochete *Borrelia burgdorferi* that is found on the tick. The initial stage of this disease is characterized by nonspecific flu-like symptoms (e.g., headache, stiff neck, fatigue) and a characteristic bull's-eye rash—an expanding circular area of redness of 5 cm diameter or more. Symptoms will disappear in 2 weeks if not treated. Monoarticular arthritis, meningitis, and neuropathies occur days or weeks after the initial symptoms. Chronic arthritis and myocarditis characterize the later stage of the disease, which can develop several months to 2 years after the initial skin lesion. Treatment includes doxycycline (Vibramycin) and cefuroxime. (Lyme disease is discussed in Chapter 65.)

Rocky Mountain spotted fever is caused by *Rickettsia rickettsii*, a bacteria that is spread to humans by the *Ixodid* tick. It has an incubation period of 2 to 14 days, and a pink, macular rash appears on the palms, wrists, soles, feet, and ankles within 10 days of exposure. Other symptoms include fever, chills, malaise, myalgias, and headache. Diagnosis is often difficult in the early stages, and without treatment it can be fatal. Antibiotic therapy with doxycycline (Vibramycin) is the treatment of choice.

Tick paralysis occurs 5 to 7 days after exposure to a neurotoxin introduced by a wood tick or dog tick. Classic symptoms are flac-cid ascending paralysis, which develops over 1 to 2 days. Without tick removal, the patient dies as respiratory muscles become paralyzed. Tick removal leads to return of muscle movement, usually within 48 to 72 hours.

Snakebites

Only 375 of the 3000 species of snakes in the world are poisonous. Poisonous snakes indigenous to the United States are members of the Crotalidae and Elapidae family. Crotalidae, or pit vipers, include rattlesnakes, copperheads, and water moccasins (Fig. 69-8). Coral snakes belong to the Elapidae family. Coral snakes do not exhibit the triangular head of pit vipers but are recognized by their bright colors. Coral snakes always have a blunt black snout and red, yellow, and black rings that completely encircle the body (Fig. 69-9). Coral snakes are poisonous non–pit vipers.

Venom from the pit viper is hemolytic, whereas coral snake venom is neurotoxic. Envenomation occurs in approximately 75% to 80% of all snakebites. If swelling does not occur within 30 minutes after the bite, envenomation is unlikely. Local reaction is characterized by one or two fang marks associated with pain, bruising, and edema within 36 hours of injury, petechiae, ecchymosis, and erythema. Loss of function and necrosis of the affected limb may occur 16 to 36 hours after the bite. Systemic reactions include nausea and vomiting, dizziness, tachycardia, muscle fasciculations, gastrointestinal (GI) bleeding, and respiratory problems. The patient may experience a metallic or rubber taste. Neurologic symptoms such as constricted pupils, drowsiness, weakness, fasciculations, muscle weakness, and seizures occur with neurotoxic venom. Life-threatening problems associated with systemic

TABLE 69-11	Antivenin* Snakebite Treatment	
Envenomation	**Signs and Symptoms**	**Number of Vials of Antivenin†**
None	Fang marks, no local swelling, hemorrhage, or paresthesia	No antivenin, tetanus prophylaxis, observation
Mild to moderate	*Mild:* Fang marks, local swelling of hands or feet, pain, no systemic reactions *Moderate:* Fang marks, progressive swelling beyond bite, mild systemic reaction (e.g., nausea, vomiting, paresthesias, hypotension)	*Initial dose:* 4-6 vials (3000-4500 mg) infused over 1 hr; infusion should be initiated slowly for the first 10 min to detect any allergic reactions; if initial control of symptoms is not achieved, dose may be repeated once *Additional regimen:* 2 vials every 6 hr for 18 hr

*Polyvalent Crotalidae antivenin ovine Fab (CroFab).
†For Crotalidae envenomation (e.g., rattlesnakes, copperheads).

envenomation include severe hemorrhage, renal failure, and hypovolemic shock.

Treatment focuses on preventing the spread of venom. Rings, watches, and restrictive clothing should be removed, and then the affected limb should be immobilized at the level of the heart. Ice and tourniquets are not recommended. Incision of the wound is controversial. If done within 3 minutes of injury with the appropriate device (e.g., Sawyer extractor), 25% to 30% of the venom may be removed. Caffeine, alcohol, and smoking increase the spread of venom and should be avoided.

ED management includes vascular access with a large-bore (14- to 16-gauge) catheter and administration of crystalloids to maintain blood pressure. Diagnostic tests include complete blood count, urinalysis, coagulation studies, blood urea nitrogen, creatinine, creatine kinase, and electrolytes. Other measures include assessment of extremity swelling, usually through documentation of circumference every 30 to 60 minutes. Pain should be treated with acetaminophen (Tylenol). Aspirin and nonsteroidal antiinflammatory drugs should be avoided because they may exacerbate bleeding; opioids may cause respiratory depression. Tetanus prophylaxis should be administered as needed (see Table 69-6). Secondary infection caused by microorganisms in the snake's mouth or other contaminants may require antibiotic therapy. Debridement or fasciotomy (see Chapter 25) is necessary in some patients. Antivenin (polyvalent Crotalidae antivenin ovine Fab [CroFab]) therapy is used in mild to moderate reactions; the amount of antivenin required depends on the timing, type, and severity of envenomation (Table 69-11). Incomplete dosage is the most common cause of treatment failure.

Animal and Human Bites

Every year over 2 million animal bites are reported in the United States.[31] Children are at greatest risk. The most significant problems associated with animal bites are infection and mechanical destruction of the skin, muscle, tendons, blood vessels, and bone. The bite may cause a simple laceration or be associated with crush injury, puncture wound, or tearing or avulsion of tissue. The severity of injury depends on animal size, victim size, and anatomic location of the bite. Animal bites from dogs and cats are most common, with wild or domestic rodents (e.g., squirrels, hamsters) following dogs and cats as the third most frequent offenders in reported animal bites.[31]

Dog bites usually occur on the extremities; however, facial bites are common in small children. Most victims own the dogs that bite them. Dog bites may involve significant tissue damage with fatalities reported, usually in children. Skull fractures with intracranial injury and death may occur in children less than 2 years old. Disfiguring wounds of the face should be evaluated by a plastic surgeon.

Cat bites cause deep puncture wounds that can involve tendons and joint capsules and result in a greater incidence of infection (30% to 50%). Septic arthritis, osteomyelitis, and tenosynovitis have been reported in cat bites. The most common causative organisms of infections from cat and dog bites are from the *Pasteurella* species (e.g., *P. canis*). This organism is found in the mouths of most healthy cats and dogs.[31]

Human bites also cause puncture wounds or lacerations and carry a high risk of infection from oral bacterial flora, most commonly *Staphylococcus aureus* and streptococci, and hepatitis virus.[31] Hands, fingers, ears, nose, vagina, and penis are the most common sites of human bites and are frequently a result of violence or sexual activity. Boxer's fracture (fracture of the fourth or fifth metacarpal) is often associated with an open wound when the knuckles strike teeth. The human jaw has great crushing ability, causing laceration, puncture, crush injury, soft tissue tearing, and even amputation. More than 40 potential pathogens found in the human mouth account for an infection rate of approximately 50% in cases where victims did not seek medical intervention within 24 hours of injury.

Collaborative Care. Initial treatment for animal and human bites includes cleaning with copious irrigation, debridement, tetanus prophylaxis, and analgesics as needed. Prophylactic antibiotics are used for animal and human bites at risk for infection, such as wounds over joints, those greater than 6 to 12 hours old, puncture wounds, and bites of the hand or foot. Individuals at greatest risk of infection are infants, older adults, immunosuppressed patients, alcoholics, diabetics, and people taking corticosteroids.

Puncture wounds are left open, whereas lacerations are loosely sutured. Wounds over joints are splinted. However, initial closure is reserved only for facial wounds. The patient is admitted for IV antibiotic therapy when an infection is present. There is an increased incidence of cellulitis, osteomyelitis, and septic arthritis in these patients. Animal and human bites must be reported to the police in many states.

Consideration of rabies prophylaxis is an essential component in management of animal bites. A neurotoxic virus found in the saliva of some mammals causes rabies. If untreated, the condition is fatal in humans. Rabies exposure should be considered if an animal attack was not provoked, involved a wild animal, or involved a domestic animal not immunized against rabies. Rabies prophylaxis is always given when the animal cannot be found or a carnivorous wild animal causes the bite. An initial injection of rabies immune globulin (RIG [BayRab]) to provide passive immunity starts the prophy-

TABLE 69-12	Common Poisons

Poison	Manifestations	Treatment
Acetaminophen (Tylenol)	*Phase 1:* within 24 hr of ingestion: malaise, diaphoresis, nausea and vomiting *Phase 2:* 24-28 hr: right upper quadrant pain, decreased urine output, diminished nausea, LFTs rise *Phase 3:* 72-96 hr: nausea and vomiting, malaise, jaundice, hypoglycemia, enlarged liver, possible coagulopathies, including DIC *Phase 4:* 7-8 days after ingestion: recovery, resolution of symptoms, LFTs return to normal	Activated charcoal, *N*-acetylcysteine (oral form may cause vomiting, IV form available on experimental basis)
Acids and alkalis • *Acids:* toilet bowel cleaners, antirust compounds • *Alkalis:* drain cleaners, dishwashing detergents, ammonia	Excess salivation, dysphagia, epigastric pain, pneumonitis; burns of mouth, esophagus, and stomach	Immediate dilution (water, milk), corticosteroids (for alkali burns), induced vomiting is contraindicated
• Aspirin and aspirin-containing medications	Tachypnea, tachycardia, hyperthermia, seizures, pulmonary edema, occult bleeding/hemorrhage, metabolic acidosis	Gastric lavage, activated charcoal, urine alkalinization, hemodialysis for severe acute ingestion, intubation and mechanical ventilation, supportive care
Bleaches	Irritation of lips, mouth, and eyes, superficial injury to esophagus; chemical pneumonia and pulmonary edema	Washing of exposed skin and eyes, dilution with water and milk, gastric lavage, prevention of vomiting and aspiration
Carbon monoxide	Dyspnea, headache, tachypnea, confusion, impaired judgment, cyanosis, respiratory depression	Removal from source, administration of 100% O_2 via non-rebreather mask, BVM, or intubation and mechanical ventilation; consider hyperbaric oxygen therapy
Cyanide	Almond odor to breath, headache, dizziness, nausea, confusion, hypertension, bradycardia followed by hypotension and tachycardia, tachypnea followed by bradypnea and respiratory arrest	Amyl nitrate (nasally), IV sodium nitrate, IV sodium thiosulfate, supportive care
Ethylene glycol	Sweet aromatic odor to breath, nausea and vomiting, slurred speech, ataxia, lethargy, respiratory depression	Gastric lavage, activated charcoal, supportive care
Iron	Vomiting (often bloody), diarrhea (often bloody), fever, hyperglycemia, lethargy, hypotension, seizures, coma	Gastric lavage, chelation therapy (deferoxamine [Desferal])
Nonsteroidal antiinflammatory drugs	Gastroenteritis, abdominal pain, drowsiness, nystagmus, hepatic and renal damage	Gastric lavage, activated charcoal, supportive care
Tricyclic antidepressants (e.g., amitriptyline [Elavil])	In low doses: anticholinergic effects, agitation, hypertension, tachycardia; in high doses: central nervous system depression, dysrhythmias, hypotension, respiratory depression	Multidose activated charcoal, gastric lavage, serum alkalinization with sodium bicarbonate, intubation and mechanical ventilation, supportive care; never induce vomiting
Alcohol, barbiturates, benzodiazepines, cocaine, hallucinogens, stimulants	See Chapter 12	See Chapter 12

BVM, Bag-valve-mask; *DIC,* disseminated intravascular coagulation; *IV,* intravenous; *LFTs,* liver function tests.

laxis regimen. This is followed by a series of five injections of human diploid cell vaccine (HDCV [RabAvert]) on days 0, 3, 7, 14, and 28 to provide active immunity. Dosage is based on the patient's weight. (Rabies is discussed in Chapter 57.)

POISONINGS

A poison is any chemical that harms the body. In 2002, more than 2 million cases of human poison exposure were reported in the United States.[32] Poisonings can be accidental, occupational, recreational, or intentional. Natural or manufactured toxins can be ingested, inhaled, injected, splashed in the eye, or absorbed through the skin. Common poisons are reviewed in Table 69-12. Other poisonings related to the use of illegal drugs such as amphetamines, opioids, and hallucinogens are discussed in Chapter 12. Poisoning may also be due to toxic plants or contaminated foods. (Food poisoning is discussed in Chapter 42.)

Severity of the poisoning depends on type, concentration, and route of exposure. Toxins can affect every tissue of the body, so symptoms can be seen in any body system. Specific management of toxins involves decreasing absorption, enhancing elimination, and implementation of toxin-specific interventions. The local poison control center is available 24 hours a day and should be consulted for the most current treatment protocols for specific poisons.

Options for decreasing absorption of poisons include gastric lavage, activated charcoal, dermal cleansing, and eye irrigation. Gastric lavage involves oral insertion of a large-diameter (36- to 42-French) gastric tube for installation of copious amounts of saline. The head of the bed should be elevated or the patient placed on the side to prevent aspiration. Patients with an altered level of consciousness or diminished gag reflex must be intubated before lavage. Lavage is contraindicated in patients who ingested caustic agents, co-ingested sharp objects, or ingested nontoxic substances.

Gastric lavage must be performed within 2 hours of ingestion of most poisons to be effective.[33] Problems associated with lavage include epistaxis, esophageal perforation, and aspiration.

The most effective intervention for management of poisonings is administration of activated charcoal orally or via a gastric tube within 60 minutes of poison ingestion.[33] Many toxins adhere to charcoal and are excreted through the GI tract rather than absorbed into the circulation. Activated charcoal does not absorb ethanol, hydrocarbons, alkali, iron, boric acid, lithium, methanol, or cyanide. Adults receive 50 to 100 g of charcoal. For some toxins (e.g., phenobarbital) multiple-dose charcoal may be required.[33,34] Contraindications to charcoal administration include diminished bowel sounds, ileus, and ingestion of a substance poorly absorbed by charcoal. Charcoal can absorb and neutralize antidotes (e.g., *N*-acetylcysteine [Mucomyst] for acetaminophen toxicity) and these should not be given immediately before, with, or shortly after charcoal.[33]

Skin and ocular decontamination involves removal of toxins from eyes and skin using copious amounts of water or saline. With the exception of mustard gas, most toxins can be safely removed with water or saline.[35] Water mixes with mustard gas and releases chlorine gas. As a general rule, dry substances should be brushed from the skin and clothing before water is used. Powdered lime should not be removed with water; it should just be brushed off. Personal protective equipment (e.g., gloves, gowns, goggles, respirators) should be worn for decontamination to prevent secondary exposure. Decontamination procedures are usually done by those specially trained in hazardous material decontamination before the patient arrives at the hospital and again, at the hospital, if necessary. Decontamination takes priority over all interventions except basic life-support techniques.

Elimination of poisons is increased through administration of cathartics, whole-bowel irrigation, hemodialysis, hemoperfusion, urine alkalinization, chelating agents, and antidotes. Cathartics, such as sorbitol, are given together with the first dose of activated charcoal to stimulate intestinal motility and increase elimination.[34] Multiple doses of cathartics should be avoided because of potentially fatal electrolyte abnormalities. Whole-bowel irrigation is controversial and involves administration of a nonabsorbable bowel evacuant solution (e.g., GoLYTELY). The solution is administered every 4 to 6 hours until stools are clear. This process can be effective for swallowed objects such as cocaine-filled balloons or condoms, and heavy metals such as lead and mercury.[33,34] There is a high risk of electrolyte imbalance due to fluid and electrolyte losses with this procedure.[34]

Hemodialysis and hemoperfusion are reserved for patients who develop severe acidosis from ingestion of toxic substances (e.g., aspirin). Other interventions include alkalinization and chelation therapy. Sodium bicarbonate administration raises the pH (greater than 7.5), which is particularly effective for phenobarbital and salicylate poisoning. Vitamin C may be added to IV fluids to enhance excretion of amphetamines and quinidine. Chelation therapy may be considered for heavy metal poisoning (e.g., edetate calcium disodium [Calcium EDTA] for lead poisoning). A limited number of true antidotes are available, and many of these agents are themselves toxic.[33]

Education for toxic emergencies focuses on how the poisoning occurred. Patients who experience poisoning because of a suicide attempt or related to substance abuse should be evaluated by a mental health counselor and then referred for alcohol or drug detoxification or scheduled for follow-up with a mental health professional. The Occupational Safety and Health Administration should evaluate all poisoning related to an occupational hazard.

VIOLENCE

Violence is the acting out of the emotions of fear and/or anger to cause harm to someone or something. It may be the result of organic disease (e.g., temporal lobe epilepsy), psychosis (e.g., schizophrenia), or antisocial behavior (e.g., assault, homicide).[36] The patient cared for in the ED may be the victim of violence or the perpetrator of violence. Violence can take place in a variety of settings, including the home, community, and workplace. EDs have been identified as high-risk areas for *workplace violence*.[37] Measures to protect staff include the use of on-site security personnel and police officers, metal detectors, surveillance cameras, and locked access doors. Research has shown that ED nurses believe many of these measures are inadequate, making them vulnerable to violence at work. Comprehensive workplace violence prevention plans should be implemented and evaluated in every ED.[37]

Domestic violence is a pattern of coercive behavior in a relationship that involves fear, humiliation, intimidation, neglect, and/or intentional physical, emotional, financial, or sexual injury (see Chapter 54 for information on sexual assault). Domestic violence is found in all professions, cultures, socioeconomic groups, agegroups, and genders. Although men can be victims of domestic violence, most victims are women, children, and the elderly. It has been reported that 1.5 million women and 834,000 men treated at EDs have been *battered* (assaulted) by spouses, significant others, or individuals known to them. As many as 20% of battered females are pregnant at the time of the assault.[38]

ED nurses are well situated to conduct domestic violence screening (e.g., Do you feel safe at home? Are you being hurt by anyone?), and routine screening for this risk factor is required. Barriers to conducting effective screening include limited privacy for screening, lack of time, and lack of knowledge about how to obtain information regarding domestic violence. The development and implementation of specific policies, procedures, and staff education programs can improve the domestic violence screening practices of ED staff.[38] For any patient who is found to be a victim of abuse, appropriate interventions such as making referrals, providing emotional support, and informing victims about their options (e.g., safe house, legal rights) should be initiated.[38] See Resources at the end of this chapter for additional information on domestic violence.

AGENTS OF TERRORISM

The threat of terrorism is an ongoing concern. Terrorism involves overt actions such as the dispensing of disease pathogens (e.g., **bioterrorism**) or other agents (e.g., chemical, radiologic/nuclear, explosive devices) as weapons for the express purpose of causing harm. Prompt recognition and identification of potential health hazards are essential in the preparedness of health care professionals.

Table 69-13 summarizes general information regarding biologic agents of terrorism. The pathogens most likely to be used in a bioterrorist attack are anthrax, smallpox, botulism, plague, tularemia, and hemorrhagic fever.

Among the agents considered likely to be biologic weapons, those that cause anthrax, plague, and tularemia could be treated effectively with commercially available antibiotics if sufficient supplies were available and the organisms were not resistant. Smallpox can be prevented or ameliorated by vaccination even when first given after exposure. Botulism can be treated with antitoxin. There

TABLE 69-13	Agents of Bioterrorism

Pathogen and Description	Clinical Manifestations	Transmissibility	Treatment
Anthrax *Bacillus anthracis* ***Inhalation*** • Bacterial spores multiply in the alveoli • Toxins cause hemorrhage and destruction of lung tissue • High mortality rate	• Incubation period: 1-2 days to 6 wk • Abrupt onset • Dyspnea • Diaphoresis • Fever • Cough • Chest pain • Septicemia • Shock • Meningitis • Respiratory failure • Widened mediastinum (seen on chest x-ray) • Incubation period: up to 12 days	• No person-to-person spread • Found in nature and most commonly infects wild and domestic hoofed animals • Spread through direct contact with bacteria and its spores • Spores are dormant, encapsulated bacteria that become active when they enter a living host	• Antibiotics prevent systemic manifestations • Effective only if treated early • Ciprofloxacin (Cipro) is the treatment of choice • Penicillin • Doxycycline • Postexposure prophylaxis for 30 days (if vaccine available) or 60 days (if vaccine not available) • Vaccine has limited availability
Cutaneous • 95% of anthrax infections • Least lethal form • Spores enter skin through cuts or abrasions • Handling of contaminated animal skin products • Toxins destroy surrounding tissue	• Small papule resembles an insect bite • Advances to a depressed, black ulcer • Swollen lymph nodes in adjacent areas • Edema		
Gastrointestinal • Ingestion of contaminated, undercooked meat • Intestinal lesions in ileum or cecum • Acute inflammation of intestines	• Nausea • Vomiting • Anorexia • Hematemesis • Diarrhea • Abdominal pain • Ascites • Sepsis		
Smallpox Variola major and minor viruses • United States ended routine vaccination in 1971 • Global eradication declared in 1980	• Incubation period: 7-17 days • Sudden onset of symptoms • Fever • Headache • Myalgia • Lesions that progress from macules to papules to pustular vesicles • Malaise • Back pain	• Highly contagious • Direct person-to-person spread • Transmitted in air droplets • Transmitted by handling contaminated materials	• No known cure • Cidofovir (Vistide) under testing • Isolation for containment • Vaccine available for those exposed • Vaccinia immune globulin (VIG) available
Botulism *Clostridium botulinum* • Spore-forming anaerobe • Found in soil • Seven different toxins • Lethal bacterial neurotoxin • Can die within 24 hr	• Incubation period: 12-36 hr • Abdominal cramps • Diarrhea • Nausea • Vomiting • Cranial nerve palsies (diplopia, dysarthria, dysphonia, dysphagia) • Skeletal muscle paralysis • Respiratory failure	• Spread through air or food • No person-to-person spread • Improperly canned foods • Contaminated wound	• Induce vomiting • Enemas • Antitoxin • Mechanical ventilation • Penicillin • No vaccine available • Toxin can be inactivated by heating food or drink to 212° F (100° C) for at least 10 min

Continued

is no established treatment for viruses that cause hemorrhagic fever.[39]

Chemicals may also be used as agents of terrorism and are categorized according to their target organ or effect[40] (Table 69-14). For example, sarin is a highly toxic nerve gas that can cause death within minutes of exposure. It enters the body through the eyes and skin and acts by paralyzing the respiratory muscles. Antidotes for nerve agent poisoning include atropine (AtroPen) and pralidoxime chloride (2-PAM chloride). Multiple doses may be needed to reverse the effects of the nerve agents.

Phosgene is a colorless gas normally used in chemical manufacturing. If inhaled at high concentrations for a long enough pe-

TABLE 69-13   Agents of Bioterrorism—cont'd

Pathogen and Description	Clinical Manifestations	Transmissibility	Treatment
Plague *Yersinia pestis* • Bacteria found in rodents and fleas *Forms* • Bubonic (most common) • Pneumonic • Septicemic (most deadly)	• Incubation period: 2-4 days • Hemoptysis • Cough • High fever • Chills • Myalgia • Headache • Respiratory failure • Lymph node swelling	• Direct person-to-person spread • Transmitted through flea bites • Ingestion of contaminated meat	• Antibiotics only effective if administered immediately • Drug of choice: streptomycin or gentamicin • Vaccine under development • Hospitalization • Isolation for containment
Tularemia *Francisella tularensis* • Bacterial infectious disease of animals • Mortality rate about 35% without treatment	• Incubation period: 3-10 days • Sudden onset • Fever • Swollen lymph nodes • Fatigue • Sore throat • Weight loss • Pneumonia • Pleural effusion • Ulcerated sore from tick bite	• No person-to-person spread • Aerosol or intradermal route • Spread by rabbits and ticks • Contaminated food, air, water	• Gentamicin treatment of choice • Streptomycin, doxycycline, and ciprofloxacin are alternatives • Vaccine in development stage
Hemorrhagic Fever • Caused by several viruses, including Marburg, Lassa, Junin, and Ebola • Ebola virus is life threatening	• Fever • Conjunctivitis • Headache • Malaise • Prostration • Hemorrhage of tissues and organs • Nausea • Vomiting • Hypotension • Organ failure	• Carried by rodents and mosquitoes • Direct person-to-person spread by body fluids • Virus can be aerosolized	• No intramuscular injections • No antiplatelet drugs • Isolation for containment • Ribavirin (Virazole) effective in some cases • No known treatment available

TABLE 69-14   Chemical Agents of Terrorism by Target Organ or Effect

Nerve	Blood	Pulmonary	Blister/Vesicants
Sarin (isopropyl methylphosphanofluoridate) Tabun (ethyl *N,N*-dimethylphosphoramidocyanidate) Soman (pinacolyl methyl phosphonofluoridate) GF (cyclohexylmethylphosphonofluoridate) VX (O-ethyl S-[2-diisopropylaminoethyl] methylphosphonothiolate)	Hydrogen cyanide Cyanogen chloride	Phosgene Chlorine Vinyl chloride	Nitrogen and sulfur mustards Lewisite (an aliphatic arsenic compound, 2-chlorovinyldichloroarsine) Phosgene oxime

riod, it causes severe respiratory distress, pulmonary edema, and death. Mustard gas is yellow to brown in color and has a garlic-like odor. The gas irritates the eyes and causes skin burns and blisters. Protocols to treat casualties of chemical exposure are varied and relate to the specific agent.[40]

Radiologic/nuclear agents represent another category of agents of terrorism. *Radiologic dispersal devices* (RDDs), also known as "dirty bombs," consist of a mix of explosives and radioactive material (e.g., pellets). When the device is detonated, the blast scatters radioactive dust, smoke, and other material into the surrounding environment, resulting in radioactive contamination.[41]

The main danger from an RRD results from the explosion, which can cause serious injuries to the casualties. The radioactive materials used in an RRD (e.g., uranium, iodine-131) do not usually generate enough radiation to cause immediate serious illness, except to those casualties who are in close proximity to the explo-

sion. However, the radioactive dust and smoke can spread and cause illness if inhaled. Since radiation cannot be seen, smelled, felt, or tasted, measures to limit contamination (e.g., covering the patient's nose and mouth) and decontamination (e.g., shower) should be initiated.[41]

Ionizing radiation, such as that from a nuclear bomb or damage to a nuclear reactor, represents a serious threat to the safety of the casualties and the environment. Exposure to ionizing radiation may or may not include skin contamination with radioactive material. If external radioactive contaminants are present, decontamination procedures must be initiated immediately. Acute radiation syndrome develops after a substantial exposure to ionizing radiation and follows a predictable pattern[42] (Table 69-15).

Explosive devices (e.g., TNT, dynamite) that are used as agents of terrorism result in one or more of the following types of injuries: blast, crush, or penetrating. Blast injuries result from the super-

TABLE 69-15 Acute Radiation Syndrome

Phase of Syndrome	Feature	Whole Body Radiation from External Radiation or Internal Absorption					
		Subclinical Range		Sublethal Range		Lethal Range	
		0-100 rad	100-200 rad	200-600 rad	600-800 rad	600-3000 rad	>3000 rad
Prodromal phase	Nausea, vomiting	None	5%-50%	50%-100%	75%-100%	90%-100%	100%
	Time of onset		3-6 hr	2-4 hr	1-2 hr	<1 hr	Minutes
	Duration		<24 hr	<24 hr	<48 hr	<48 hr	N/A
	Lymphocyte count	Unaffected	Minimally decreased	<1000 at 24 hr	<500 at 24 hr	Decreases within hours	Decreases within hours
	CNS function	No impairment	No impairment	Cognitive impairment for 6-20 hr	Cognitive impairment for >24 hr	Rapid incapacitation, often after a lucid period of up to several hours	
Latent phase (subclinical)	Absence of symptoms	>2 wk	7-15 days	0-7 days	0-2 days	None	
Acute radiation illness or "manifest illness" phase	Signs and symptoms	None	Moderate leukopenia	Severe leukopenia, purpura, hemorrhage Pneumonia Hair loss after 300 rad		Diarrhea Fever Electrolyte disturbance	Convulsions, ataxia, tremor, lethargy
	Time of onset		>2 wk	2 days-2 wk		1-3 days	1-48 hr
	Critical period		None	4-6 wk—Most potential for effective medical intervention		2-14 days	
	Organ system	None		Hematopoietic and respiratory (mucosal) systems		GI tract Mucosal systems	CNS
Hospitalization	%	0%	<5%	90%	100%	100%	100%
	Duration	None	45-60 days	60-90 days	90+ days	Weeks to months	Days to weeks
Mortality rate		None	Minimal	Low with aggressive therapy	High	Very high, significant neurologic symptoms indicate lethal dose	

From Armed Forces Radiobiology Research Institute: Terrorism with ionizing radiation general guidance: pocket guide. Available at *www.afrri.usuhs.mil/www/outreach/pocketguide.htm* (accessed September 26, 2006). *CNS,* Central nervous system; *GI,* gastrointestinal.

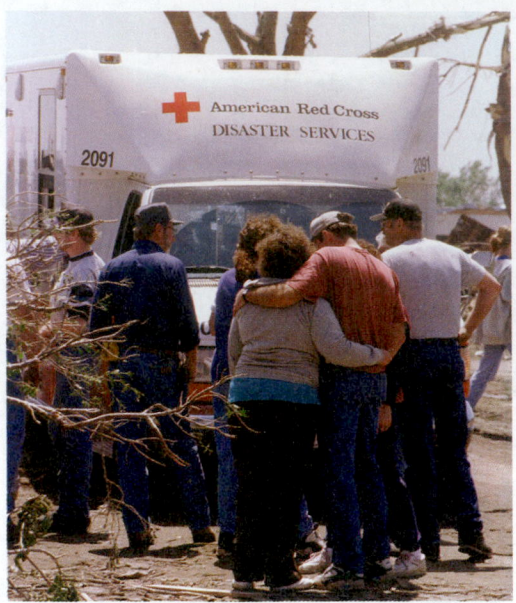

FIG. 69-10 American Red Cross.

sonic overpressurization shock wave that results from the explosion. This shock wave primarily causes damage to the lungs, GI tract, and middle ear. Crush injuries (i.e., blunt trauma) often result from explosions that occur in confined spaces and result from structural collapse (e.g., falling debris). Some explosive devices contain materials that are projected during the explosion (e.g., shrapnel) leading to penetrating injuries.

EMERGENCY AND MASS CASUALTY INCIDENT PREPAREDNESS

The term **emergency** usually refers to any extraordinary event (e.g., multicasualty train crash) that requires a rapid and skilled response and that can be managed by a community's existing resources. An emergency is differentiated from a **mass casualty incident** (MCI) in that an MCI is a manmade (e.g., biologic warfare) or natural (e.g., hurricane) event or disaster that overwhelms a community's ability to respond with existing resources. MCIs usually involve large numbers of casualties, physical and emotional suffering, and permanent changes within a community. In addition, MCIs always require assistance from people and resources outside the affected community (e.g., American Red Cross, Federal Emergency Management Agency [FEMA]) (Fig. 69-10).

When an emergency or MCI occurs, first responders (i.e., police, emergency medical personnel) are dispatched to the scene. Triage of casualties of an emergency or MCI differs from the usual triage described earlier. A system of colored tags is used to designate both the seriousness of the injury and the likelihood of survival. A green (minor injury [e.g., sprains]) or yellow (non–life-threatening injury [e.g., open fractures]) tag is used to indicate a noncritical injury. A red tag indicates a life-threatening injury requiring immediate intervention (e.g., shock). A black tag is used to identify those casualties who are deceased or who are expected to die (e.g., massive head trauma).[43]

Triage of casualties of an emergency or MCI must be rapid and conducted in less than 15 seconds. In general, two thirds of casualties will be tagged green or yellow and the remaining will

be tagged red or black. Casualties need to be treated and stabilized, and if there is known or suspected contamination, decontaminated at the scene. After this, they are transported to hospitals. Many other casualties will arrive at hospitals on their own (i.e., walking wounded). The total number of casualties a hospital can expect is estimated by doubling the number of casualties that arrive in the first hour. Generally, 30% of casualties will require admission to the hospital and one half of these will need surgery within 8 hours.

In addition to the services provided by first responders, many communities have initiated programs to develop *community emergency response teams* (CERTs). CERTs have been recognized by FEMA as important partners in emergency preparedness. The CERT training helps citizens to understand their personal responsibility in preparing for a natural or manmade disaster. In addition, they are taught what to expect following a disaster and how to safely help themselves, their family, and their neighbors. Training includes the teaching of lifesaving skills with emphasis on decision making and rescuer safety. CERTs are considered an extension of the first responder services. They are able to offer immediate help to casualties and organize untrained volunteers to assist until professional services arrive.[44]

All health care providers have a role in emergency and MCI preparedness. Knowledge of the hospital's *emergency response plan* is necessary, including individual roles and responsibilities of the members of the response team and participation in emergency/MCI preparedness drills on a regular basis. Several types of drills are used to assess a hospital's level of emergency preparedness. These drills can include hospital disaster drills, computer simulations, and tabletop exercises. It has been shown that these drills allow health care providers to become familiar with the emergency response procedures.[45]

Response to MCIs often requires the aid of a federal agency. The National Disaster Medical System (NDMS) is a section within the U.S. Department of Homeland Security that is responsible for the coordination of the federal medical response to MCIs. The NDMS works with local emergency response personnel to deliver comprehensive disaster relief to a community. One component of the NDMS is to organize and train volunteer disaster medical assistance teams (DMATs). Each DMAT is composed of members with a variety of health or medical skills, as well as those with specialized support skills (e.g., communications, logistics, maintenance, security).[46]

DMATs are categorized according to their ability to respond to an MCI. A Level-1 DMAT can be deployed within 8 hours of notification and remain self-sufficient for 72 hours with enough food, water, shelter, and medical supplies to treat about 250 patients per day. Level-2 DMATs lack enough equipment to be self-sufficient but are used to replace a Level-1 team, using and supplementing the equipment that is left on site.[46]

All disasters result in psychologic stress to the individuals involved immediately after the event. This stress can persist for an extended period of time and is influenced in part by the nature of the event, the individual's age, preexisting coping mechanisms, role in the event, and medical and psychologic history. Many hospitals and DMATs have a *critical incident stress management unit*. This unit arranges group discussions to allow participants to verbalize and validate their feelings and emotions about the experience and is important for emotional recovery.[46]

CRITICAL THINKING EXERCISE

CASE STUDY

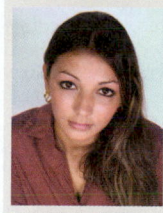

Case Study photo ©iStockphoto.com/ Lacey Gadwill.

Trauma

Patient Profile. A 20-year-old Hispanic female trauma patient is brought to the ED in an ambulance. She was the driver in a motor vehicle collision and was not wearing a seat belt. Two children in the car were pronounced dead at the scene. The paramedics stated that there was significant damage to the car on the driver's side.

Subjective Data
• Patient asks, "What happened? Where am I?"
• Complains of shortness of breath and leg pain

Objective Data
Physical Examination
• Vital signs: blood pressure 90/40, heart rate 130 beats/min, respiratory rate 36 breaths/min; O_2 saturation 85% with 100% non-rebreather mask
• Decreased breath sounds on left side of chest
• Asymmetric chest wall movement
• Glasgow Coma Score = 14; unequal pupils
• Badly deformed left lower leg with a pedal pulse by Doppler only
• 4-cm head laceration, bleeding controlled

Critical Thinking Questions

1. What life-threatening injury or injuries does this patient probably have?
2. What is the priority of care?
3. What interventions are needed immediately?
4. What other interventions should the nurse consider?
5. Several family members have arrived in the ED, including the mother of one of the children who died. The second child who died was the patient's child. How should the nurse approach the family?
6. Based on assessment data presented, write one or more priority nursing diagnoses. Are there any collaborative problems?

NCLEX EXAMINATION REVIEW QUESTIONS

The number of the question corresponds to the same-numbered objective at the beginning of the chapter.

1. An elderly man arrives in triage disoriented and tachypneic (respiratory rate = 36 breaths/min). His skin is hot and dry. His wife states that he was fine earlier today. The priority for treatment at this point is to
   a. obtain a detailed medical history from his wife.
   b. assess his vital signs, including a rectal temperature.
   c. determine the kind of insurance he has before treating him.
   d. start supplemental oxygen and have the ED physician see him.

2. A patient has a core temperature of 90° F (32.2° C). The most appropriate rewarming technique would be
   a. passive rewarming with body-to-body contact.
   b. active core rewarming using warmed IV fluids.
   c. passive rewarming using air-filled warming blankets.
   d. active external rewarming by submersing in a warm bath.

3. The most effective intervention in decreasing absorption of an ingested poison is
   a. hemodialysis.
   b. milk dilution.
   c. gastric lavage.
   d. activated charcoal.

4. An elderly woman arrives in the ED complaining of severe pain in her right shoulder. You note that her clothes are soiled with urine and feces. She tells you that she lives with her son and that she "fell." She is tearful and asks you if she can be admitted. The nurse should consider
   a. paranoia.
   b. possible cancer.
   c. domestic violence.
   d. orthostatic hypertension.

5. Which of the following biologic agents of bioterrorism has no effective treatment?
   a. Anthrax
   b. Botulism
   c. Smallpox
   d. Hemorrhagic fever

6. A chemical explosion occurs at a nearby industrial site. The first responders report that casualties are being decontaminated at the scene and approximately 125 victims will be transported to the ED. As the nurse receiving this report, you know that this will first require activation of
   a. a code red alert.
   b. a critical incident management team.
   c. the local police and fire departments.
   d. the hospital's emergency response plan.

REFERENCES

1. Mills AC, McSweeney M: Primary reasons for ED visits and procedures performed for patients who saw nurse practitioners, *J Emerg Nurs* 31:145, 2005.
2. The Advisory Board Company: Study suggests uninsured not main cause of ED overcrowding. Available at *www.Advisory.com* (accessed June 23, 2006).
3. Martin-Gill C, Reiser RC: Risk factors for 72-hour admission to the ED, *Am J Emerg Med* 22:448, 2004.
4. This is ENA. Available at *www.ena.org/about* (accessed June 23, 2006).
5. Gilboy N, Tanabe P, Travers DA, et al: *Emergency Severity Index, version 4. Implementation handbook,* AHRQ Pub No 05-0046-2, Rockville, Md, May 2005, Agency for Healthcare Research and Quality. Available at *www.ahrq.gov/research/esi* (accessed February 23, 2006).
6. Rund DA, Rausch TS: *Triage,* St Louis, 1981, Mosby.
7. Standardized ED triage scale and acuity categorization: Joint ENA/ACEP statement. Available at *www.ena.org/about/position/ACEP/Joint5-Level TriageTask.asp* (accessed June 23, 2006).
8. Toulson K, Laskowski-Jones L, McConnell L: Implementation of the five-level Emergency Severity Index in a level I trauma center emergency department with a three-tiered triage scheme, *J Emerg Nurs* 31:259, 2005.
9. Scott JM: Endotracheal intubation (assist). In Wiegand DL, Carlson KK, editors: *AACN procedure manual for critical care,* ed 5, St Louis, 2005, Elsevier.
10. Danzl DF, Vissers RJ: Tracheal intubation and mechanical ventilation. In Tintinalli JE, Kelen GD, Stapczynski SJ, editors: *Emergency medicine: a comprehensive study guide,* ed 6, New York, 2004, McGraw-Hill.
11. Steele MT, Ellison SR: Trauma to the pelvis, hip, and femur. In Tintinalli JE, Kelen GD, Stapczynski SJ, editors: *Emergency medicine: a comprehensive study guide,* ed 6, New York, 2004, McGraw-Hill.
12. Halm M: Family presence during resuscitation: a critical review of the literature, *Am J Crit Care* 14:494, 2005.
13. Emergency Nurses Association position statement family presence at the bedside during invasive procedures and resuscitation. Available at *www.ena.org/special/ps-no1226-meisje/familypresence.doc* (accessed June 23, 2006).
14. Eichhorn DJ, Meyers TA, Guzzetta CE, et al: Family presence during invasive procedures and resuscitation: hearing the voice of the patient, *Am J Nurs* 101:48, 2001.

15. Meyers TA, Eichorn DJ, Guzzetta CE, et al: Family presence during invasive procedures and resuscitation, *Am J Nurs* 100:32, 2000.

16. Campbell P, Dennie M, Dougherty K, et al: Implementation of an ED protocol for pain management at triage at a busy level I trauma center, *J Emerg Nurs* 30:431, 2004.

17. Sequin D: A nurse-initiated pain management advanced triage protocol for ED patients with an extremity injury at a level I trauma center, *J Emerg Nurs* 30:330, 2004.

18. Clontz AS, Tasota FJ: Eye on diagnostics. FAST results: using focused assessment with sonography for trauma, *Nursing* 34:21, 2004.

19. Centers for Disease Control and Prevention: Disaster information. Tetanus prevention. Available at *www.bt.cdc.gov/disasters/hurricanes/katrina/tetanus.asp* (accessed February 14, 2006).

20. Non–heart beating organ donors. Available at *www.transweb.org/news/calendar/archive/nhbd/nhbd_live_notes1.html* (accessed December 13, 2005).

21. Schwartz SW, Rosenberg DM, Wang CP, et al: Demographic differences in injuries among the elderly: an analysis of emergency department visits, *J Trauma* 58:346, 2005.

22. Guttman A, Afilalo M, Guttman R, et al: An emergency department–based nurse discharge coordinator for elder patients: does it make a difference? *Acad Emerg Med* 11:1318, 2004.

23. Walker JS, Hogan DE: Heat emergencies. In Tintinalli JE, Kelen GD, Stapczynski SJ, editors: *Emergency medicine: a comprehensive study guide,* ed 6, New York, 2004, McGraw-Hill.

24. Rabold MB: Frostbite and other localized cold-related injuries. In Tintinalli JE, Kelen GD, Stapczynski SJ, editors: *Emergency medicine: a comprehensive study guide,* ed 6, New York, 2004, McGraw-Hill.

25. Bessen HA: Hypothermia. In Tintinalli JE, Kelen GD, Stapczynski SJ, editors: *Emergency medicine: a comprehensive study guide,* ed 6, New York, 2004, McGraw-Hill.

26. Snyder ML: Learn the chilling facts about hypothermia. *Nursing* 35:32hn1, 2005.

27. Causey AL, Nichter MA: Near-drowning. In Tintinalli JE, Kelen GD, Stapczynski SJ, editors: *Emergency medicine: a comprehensive study guide,* ed 6, New York, 2004, McGraw-Hill.

28. Clark RF, Schneir AB: Arthropod bites and stings. In Tintinalli JE, Kelen GD, Stapczynski SJ, editors: *Emergency medicine: a comprehensive study guide,* ed 6, New York, 2004, McGraw-Hill.

29. Zeglin D: Brown recluse spider bites, *Am J Nurs* 105:64, 2005.

30. Centers for Disease Control and Prevention, Division of Vector-Borne Infectious Disease: Lyme disease. Available at *www.cdc.gov/ncidod/dvbid/lyme/ld_tickremoval.htm* (accessed April 17, 2006).

31. Taplitz RA: Managing bite wounds, *Postgrad Med* 116:49, 2004.

32. American Association of Poison Control Centers: 2002 poison control survey. Available at *www.aapcc.org/pccsurveyresults/2002/2002Table1.pdf* (accessed January 26, 2006).

33. Lehne RA: *Pharmacology for nursing care,* ed 6, St Louis, 2007, Elsevier.

34. Sturt PA: Toxicologic conditions. In Fultz J, Sturt PA, editors: *Mosby's emergency nursing reference,* ed 3, St Louis, 2005, Elsevier.

35. Parshall MB: Eye conditions. In Fultz J, Sturt PA, editors: *Mosby's emergency nursing reference,* ed 3, St Louis, 2005, Elsevier.

36. Fultz J, Sturt PA, editors: *Mosby's emergency nursing reference,* ed 3, St Louis, 2005, Elsevier.

37. Catlette M: A descriptive study of the perceptions of workplace violence and safety strategies of nurses working in level I trauma centers, *J Emerg Nurs* 31:519, 2005.

38. Berlinger JS: Taking an intimate look at domestic violence, *Nursing* 34:42, 2004.

39. Centers for Disease Control and Prevention: Viral hemorrhagic fevers. Available at *www.cdc.gov/ncidod/dvrd/spb/mnpages/dispages/vhf.htm* (accessed June 26, 2006).

40. Sturt PA: Exposures: chemical, radiation, and biologic. In Fultz J, Sturt PA, editors: *Mosby's emergency nursing reference,* ed 3, St Louis, 2005, Elsevier.

41. Centers for Disease Control and Prevention: Frequently asked questions about dirty bombs. Available at *www.bt.cdc.gov/radiation/dirtybombs.asp* (accessed May 31, 2006).

42. U.S. Environmental Protection Agency: Understanding radiation. Available at *www.epa.gov/radiation/understand/health_effects.htm* (accessed June 1, 2006).

43. Ganahl BH: Triage. In Fultz J, Sturt PA, editors: *Mosby's emergency nursing reference,* ed 3, St Louis, 2005, Elsevier.

44. CERT: community emergency response team. Available at *www.citizencorps.gov/cert/about.shtm* (accessed May 30, 2006).

45. Agency for Healthcare Research and Quality: Evidence report/technology assessment number 95. Training of hospital staff to respond to a mass casualty incident. Available at *www.ahcpr.gov/clinic/epcsums/hospmcisum.htm* (accessed June 1, 2006).

46. Cox E, Briggs S: Disaster nursing: new frontiers for critical care, *Crit Care Nurse* 24:16, 2004.

RESOURCES

American College of Emergency Physicians
800-798-1822 or 972-550-0911
www.acep.org

American Nurses Association
800-274-4ANA (4262)
Bioterrorism and Disaster Response website
www.nursingworld.org/news/disaster

American Red Cross
800-HELP-NOW
www.redcross.org

American Trauma Society
800-556-7890 or 301-420-4189
www.amtrauma.org

Association of Emergency Physicians (AEP)
866-772-1818
www.aep.org

CDC Public Health Awareness and Response website
404-639-3311
www.bt.cdc.gov

Center for the Prevention of Sexual and Domestic Violence
206-634-1903
www.cpsdv.org

Emergency Nurses Association (ENA)
800-900-9659
www.ena.org

Federal Emergency Management Agency
800-621-FEMA
www.fema.gov

International Association of Forensic Nurses
410-626-7805
www.forensicnurse.org

National Coalition Against Domestic Violence
303-839-1852
www.ncadv.org

National Domestic Violence Hotline
800-799-SAFE (7233)
www.ndvh.org

National Response Center
800-424-8802
www.nrc.uscg.mil/index.htm

U.S. Department of Health and Human Services, Office of Emergency Preparedness
301-443-1167 or 800-USA-NDMS
www.ndms.dhhs.gov/index.html

U.S. Department of Justice, Office on Violence Against Women
877-739-3895
www.usdoj.gov/ovw

Wilderness Medicine Institute
866-831-9001
http://wmi.nols.edu

For additional Internet resources, see the website for this book at *http://evolve.elsevier.com/Lewis/medsurg.*

Appendix A
Cardiopulmonary Resuscitation and Basic Life Support

The steps of *basic life support* (BLS) consist of a series of actions and skills performed by the rescuer(s) based on assessment findings. The first action performed by the rescuer upon finding an adult victim is to assess for responsiveness. This is accomplished by tapping or gently shaking the victim's shoulder and asking, "Are you all right?" If the victim does not respond and the rescuer is alone, the rescuer should activate emergency medical services (EMS), get an *automatic external defibrillator* (AED) (if available), return to the victim, and begin *cardiopulmonary resuscitation* (CPR) and defibrillation if necessary.[1]

The American Heart Association includes training in the use of AEDs with instruction of health care personnel and laypersons in BLS. Survival from cardiac arrest is the highest when immediate CPR is provided and defibrillation occurs within 3 to 5 minutes.[1] AEDs now can be found in many out-of-hospital, public settings (Fig. A-1).

Airway

The next step in BLS is to assess the victim's airway to confirm the absence of breathing and to establish a patent airway. Fig. A-2 demonstrates opening the airway and performing mouth-to-mouth ventilation. An adult's airway is opened by hyperextending the head. The *head tilt–chin lift maneuver* is used and involves tilting the head back with one hand and lifting the chin forward with the fingers of the other hand. If the victim is gasping occasionally or not breathing, the rescuer attempts to ventilate the victim with mouth-to-barrier (recommended) or mouth-to-mouth resuscitation.[1]

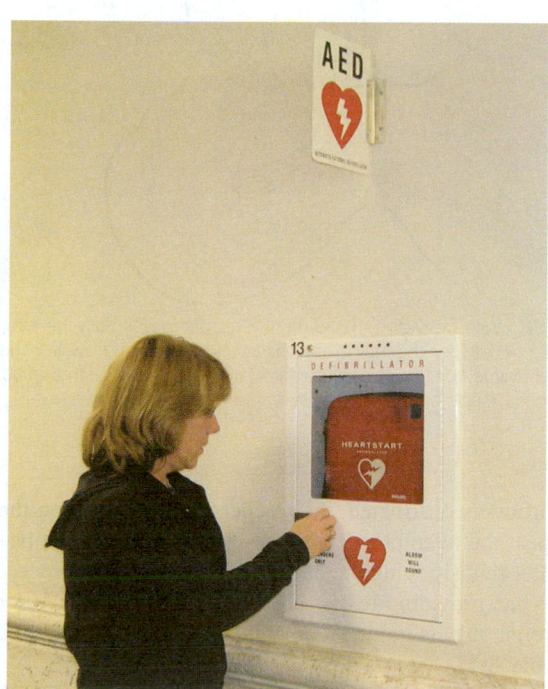

FIG. A-1   Automatic external defibrillator (AED) located in an airport.

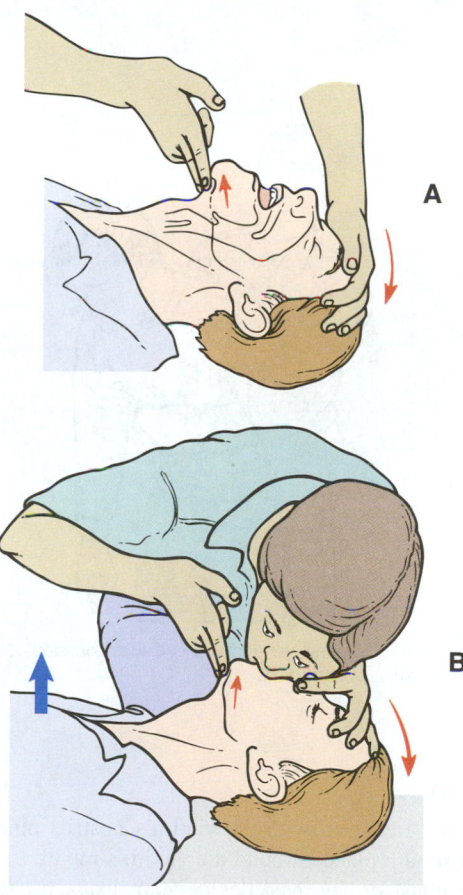

FIG. A-2   The head tilt–chin lift maneuver is used to open the victim's airway to give mouth-to-mouth resuscitation. **A,** Rescuer places one hand on the victim's forehead and applies firm, backward pressure with the palm to tilt the head back. The chin is lifted and brought forward with the fingers of the other hand. **B,** Rescuer pinches the victim's nostrils, seals mouth over victim's mouth, and delivers a regular breath. Rescuer should observe for a rise in the victim's chest *(arrow)*.

TABLE A-1	**Management of Foreign Body Airway Obstruction (FBAO)**

Conscious Adult Victim
Assess Victim for Severe Airway Obstruction

Signs of severe airway obstruction:

- Universal choking sign (victim clutches neck with hands)
- Inability to speak

Ask the victim, "Are you choking?"

- Silent cough
- High-pitched sound or no sound while inhaling
- Increased difficulty breathing
- Cyanosis

If the victim displays any of the above signs, severe or complete airway obstruction may be present and the rescuer must take action.

Heimlich Maneuver (Abdominal Thrusts) with Standing/Sitting Victim (Fig. A-3)

1. Stand behind victim and wrap arms around waist.
2. Make fist with one hand.
3. Place thumb side of fist against victim's abdomen. Position fist midline, slightly above umbilicus and well below xiphoid process.
4. Grasp fist with other hand.
5. Press fist into victim's abdomen using quick upward thrusts. Each thrust should be a separate, distinct movement. Note: If victim is in the late stages of pregnancy or obese, chest thrusts should be used. Position hands (as described) over lower portion of the sternum and apply quick backward thrusts.
6. Repeat thrusts until object is expelled or victim becomes unresponsive.

Unconscious Adult Victim
Assessment

If rescuer sees victim collapse and knows that FBAO is the cause:

1. Activate the EMS system by calling 911.
2. Be sure victim is supine.
3. Perform tongue-jaw lift; look to see if a foreign body is visible and, if seen, remove it (Fig. A-4).
4. Open airway and attempt to ventilate:
   - Give two rescue breaths.
   - If breaths are unsuccessful in making victim's chest rise:
     a. Reposition victim's head.
     b. Reopen airway.
     c. Reattempt to ventilate.
5. If efforts to ventilate are still unsuccessful, begin CPR (see Tables A-2 and A-3).

Source: 2005 American Heart Association Guidelines for Cardiopulmonary Resuscitation and Emergency Cardiovascular Care, Part 4: Adult Basic Life Support, *Circulation* 112:IV-19, 2005.

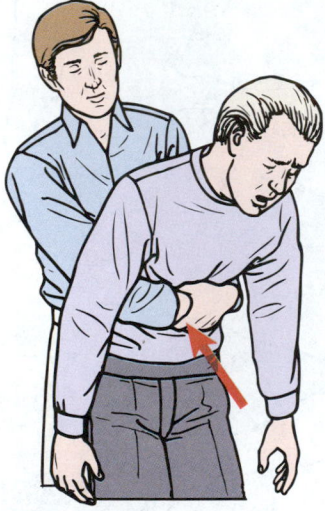

FIG. A-3 Heimlich maneuver administered to a conscious (standing) victim of foreign body airway obstruction.

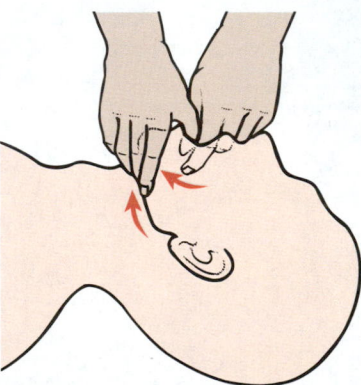

FIG. A-4 With the victim's head up, the rescuer grasps both the tongue and the lower jaw between the thumb and fingers and lifts (tongue-jaw lift). This action draws the tongue from the back of the throat and away from the foreign body. The rescuer looks to see if any foreign body is visible and, if seen, removes it.

Breathing

Ventilations are given with the victim's nostrils pinched and the rescuer's mouth placed around the victim's mouth to make a tight seal. Face mask or bag-mask devices can also be used. Two breaths are given by the rescuer (1 second per breath). The volume of air of each ventilation should be equal to a regular breath and enough to produce a visible rise in the victim's chest.[1] When the victim has a tracheostomy, ventilation should be given through the stoma.

If airflow is obstructed, the rescuer should reposition the head and repeat the attempt to ventilate. If the victim cannot be ventilated after repositioning the head, the rescuer should proceed with CPR. When providing rescue breaths, the rescuer should look for any foreign objects in the victim's mouth and remove them if visible (Table A-1).

In those rare instances when airway obstruction is not relieved, additional procedures are necessary. These include transtracheal catheter ventilation and cricothyroidotomy, which should only be attempted by health care professionals experienced in these procedures.[1]

Cardiac Compressions

Cardiac arrest is characterized by the absence of a pulse in the large arteries of an unconscious victim who is not breathing. Health care providers are instructed to perform a pulse check in victims that are unresponsive and not breathing. Lay rescuers are not taught this skill. Instead they are instructed to begin chest compressions immediately after delivering two rescue breaths.

The carotid artery is used to determine the absence of a pulse. After an airway has been established and two ventilations have been delivered, the rescuer checks the pulse of the carotid artery. While maintaining the head-tilt position with one hand on the forehead, the rescuer locates the victim's trachea with two or three fingers of the other hand. The rescuer then slides these fingers into the groove between the trachea and the muscles of the side of the neck where the carotid pulse can be felt. The technique is more easily performed on the side nearest the rescuer. If a pulse is palpated, the rescuer should provide rescue breaths at a rate of 10 to 12 breaths/minute and recheck the pulse every 2 minutes. If no pulse is palpated within 10 seconds, chest compressions should be initiated.[1]

The proper technique for administering chest compressions is shown in Fig. A-5. Chest compression technique consists of serial, rhythmic applications of pressure on the lower half of the sternum. The victim must be in the supine position when the compressions are performed. The victim must be lying on a flat, hard surface, such as a CPR board (specially designed for use in CPR), a headboard from a unit bed, or, if necessary, the floor. The rescuer should be positioned close to the side of the victim's chest.

The guidelines for proper compression technique are presented in Tables A-2 and A-3 and Fig. A-5. Rescue breathing and chest compressions are combined for an effective resuscitation effort of the victim of cardiopulmonary arrest. The compression-ventilation ratio for one- or two-person CPR is 30 compressions to 2 ventilations (see Tables A-2 and A-3). If the patient is intubated and the airway is secure, compressions should not be paused for ventilations.[1]

It is preferable to have two persons performing CPR (see Table A-3). One person, positioned at the victim's side, performs chest compressions while the other rescuer, positioned at the victim's head, maintains an open airway and performs ventilations. In order to maintain the quality and rate of compressions, rescuers should change roles approximately every 2 minutes.[1]

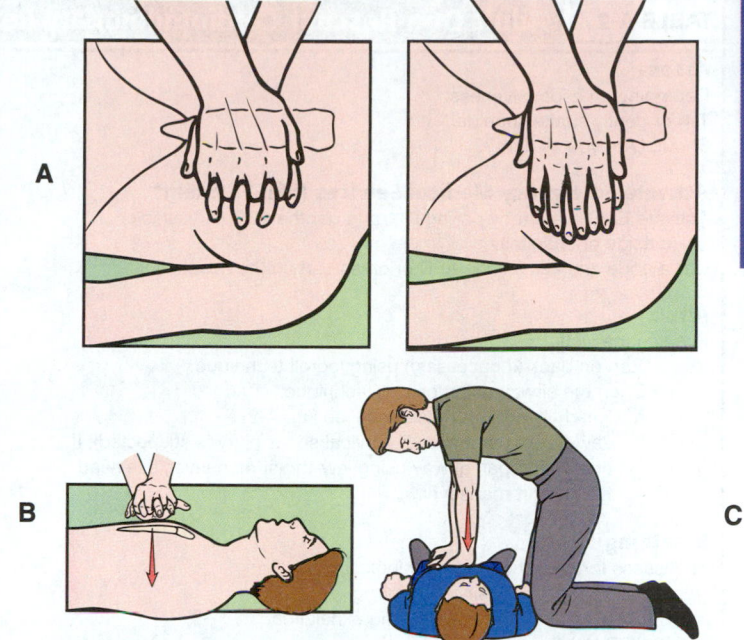

FIG. A-5 Cardiopulmonary resuscitation (CPR). **A,** Position of the hands during application of cardiac compressions. **B,** When pressure is applied, the lower portion of the sternum is displaced posteriorly with the palm of the hand. **C,** To apply maximum downward pressure, the rescuer leans forward so that both arms are at right angles to the patient's sternum and the elbows are locked.

Interruptions in CPR should be limited. When the AED or advanced cardiac life support (ACLS) team arrives, the victim's rhythm should be assessed. If the victim has a shockable rhythm (i.e., ventricular tachycardia or ventricular fibrillation), one shock should be delivered followed by five cycles of CPR before checking the rhythm. If the rhythm is not a shockable rhythm, CPR should be resumed and the rhythm rechecked every five cycles. CPR should continue between rhythm checks and shocks, and until the ACLS team arrives or the victim shows signs of movement.[1]

ACLS involves the use of detailed medical algorithms for the provision of lifesaving cardiac care in settings ranging from the pre-hospital environment to the hospital setting. Nurses are often required to obtain ACLS certification in addition to BLS depending on their area of practice.

| TABLE A-2 | Adult One-Rescuer Cardiopulmonary Resuscitation (CPR) |

Assess

Determine unresponsiveness:

Tap or gently shake shoulder.

Shout, "Are you all right?"

Activate Emergency Medical Services (EMS) System*

Activate EMS system by calling 911 and get the AED (if available) (outside of hospital).

Call a code and ask for the AED or crash cart (in the hospital).

Airway

Position the victim:

- Turn on back (if necessary) using logroll technique.
- Open the airway using proper technique:
  a. Head tilt–chin lift maneuver (see Fig. A-2)
  b. Jaw-thrust maneuver (if cervical spine injury is suspected); if unable to open airway using jaw-thrust maneuver, use head tilt–chin lift maneuver.

Breathing

1. Assess for cessation of breathing:
   - LOOK for chest rising and falling.
   - LISTEN for air escaping during exhalation.
   - FEEL for flow of air.
2. If victim is breathing adequately:
   - Continue to protect airway.
   - Place victim in recovery position.
3. If victim is unresponsive and gasping occasionally or not breathing:
   - Provide two regular breaths each over 1 second.
     a. Observe chest rise.
     b. Allow for complete exhalation between breaths.
   - If unable to give two effective breaths:
     a. Reposition victim to try to open airway.
     b. Look for foreign body and, if seen, remove.
     c. Reattempt to ventilate.
   - If ventilation is still unsuccessful, assess circulation.†
   - If adequate spontaneous breathing is restored and signs of circulation are present:
     a. Maintain open airway.
     b. Place victim in recovery position.

Circulation

Lay Rescuer

Begin chest compressions after delivering two initial breaths.

Health Care Professional

1. Assess for signs of circulation after delivery of the two initial breaths.
2. Feel for carotid pulse (10 seconds).
3. If victim has signs of circulation but is not breathing adequately, continue rescue breathing (1 breath/5 to 6 seconds) and recheck circulation every 2 minutes.
4. If there are no signs of circulation, begin chest compressions.

Compression/Ventilation

Compression-Ventilation Cycle

Compression-ventilation ratio is 30:2.

Begin Compressions

1. Get into position for compressions at victim's side (by shoulders).
2. Locate landmark notch (hands in the center of chest, right between the nipples, and two fingers above the xiphoid-sternal notch).
3. Position hands, arms, and shoulders.
   - Elbows are locked and arms are straight.
   - Rescuer's shoulders positioned directly over hands.
4. Begin compressions:
   - Compressions should depress victim's sternum approximately $1^{1}/_{2}$ to 2 inches.
   - Allow chest to rebound to normal position after each compression.
   - Perform compressions hard and fast at the rate of 100 per minute.
   - Maintain correct position at all times.

Provide Ventilation

1. Open airway using proper technique.
2. Deliver two slow regular breaths (1 second each) at the end of a cycle of 30 compressions.
3. Return hands to chest.
4. Find proper landmark and hand position.
5. Restart compressions.

Defibrillation

If witnessed arrest, use AED as soon as possible.

If unwitnessed arrest, deliver five cycles of CPR before using AED.

If rhythm is shockable, deliver one shock, then resume CPR for five cycles before rechecking rhythm.

If the rhythm is not shockable, resume CPR and recheck rhythm every five cycles.

Continuation of CPR

- CPR should be continued between rhythm checks and shocks, and until ACLS providers arrive or the victim shows signs of movement.
- Do not interrupt CPR except in special circumstances.

Source: 2005 American Heart Association Guidelines for Cardiopulmonary Resuscitation and Emergency Cardiovascular Care, Part 4: Adult Basic Life Support, *Circulation* 112:IV-19, 2005.

ACLS, Advanced cardiac life support; *AED*, automatic external defibrillator.

*Rescuers should phone 911 for unresponsive adults before beginning CPR, except in the case of drowning or a likely asphyxiation.

†Lay rescuers are no longer taught a pulse check.

TABLE A-3	**Adult Two-Rescuer Cardiopulmonary Resuscitation (CPR)**

Assess/Activate Emergency Medical Services (EMS) System*
One Rescuer
Determine unresponsiveness:
Tap or gently shake shoulder.
Shout, "Are you OK?"

Other Rescuer
Activate EMS system by calling 911 and get the AED (if available) (outside of hospital).
Call a code and ask for the AED or crash cart (in hospital).

Airway
Position the victim:
- Turn on back (if necessary) using logroll technique.
- Open the airway using proper technique:
  a. Head tilt–chin lift maneuver (see Fig. A-2).
  b. Jaw-thrust maneuver (if cervical spine injury is suspected); if unable to open airway using the jaw-thrust maneuver, use the head tilt–chin lift maneuver.

Breathing
1. Assess for cessation of breathing:
   - LOOK for chest rising and falling.
   - LISTEN for air escaping during exhalation.
   - FEEL for flow of air.
2. If victim is breathing adequately:
   - Continue to protect airway.
   - Place victim in recovery position.
3. If victim is unresponsive and gasping occasionally or not breathing:
   - Provide two regular breaths each over 1 second.
     a. Observe chest rise.
     b. Allow for complete exhalation between breaths.
   - If unable to give two effective breaths:
     a. Reposition victim to try to open airway.
     b. Look for foreign body and, if seen, remove.
     c. Reattempt to ventilate.
   - If ventilation is still unsuccessful, assess circulation.†
   - If adequate spontaneous breathing is restored and signs of circulation are present:
     a. Maintain open airway.
     b. Place victim in recovery position.

Circulation
Lay Rescuers
Begin chest compressions after delivering two initial breaths.

Health Care Professionals
1. Assess for signs of circulation after delivery of the two initial breaths.
2. Feel for carotid pulse (10 seconds).
3. If victim has signs of circulation but is not breathing adequately, continue rescue breathing (1 breath/5 to 6 seconds) and recheck circulation every 2 minutes.
4. If there are no signs of circulation, say "No pulse" and prepare for chest compressions.

Compression/Ventilation
Compression-Ventilation Cycle
Compression-ventilation ratio is 30:2.

One Rescuer/Compressor
1. Get into position for compressions at victim's side (by shoulders).
2. Locate landmark notch (hands in the center of chest, right between the nipples, and two fingers above the xiphoid-sternal notch).
3. Position hands, arms, and shoulders:
   - Elbows are locked and arms are straight.
   - Rescuer's shoulders positioned directly over hands.
4. Begin compressions:
   - Compressions should depress victim's sternum approximately $1^1/_2$ to 2 inches.
   - Allow chest to rebound to normal position after each compression.
   - Perform compressions hard and fast at the rate of 100 per minute.
   - Maintain correct position at all times.

Other Rescuer/Ventilator
1. Get into position at victim's head.
2. Maintain an open airway.
3. Deliver two slow regular breaths (1 second each) at the end of a cycle of 30 compressions.
4. Ensure that chest is rising with each ventilation.
5. Monitor carotid pulse during compressions to verify effectiveness.

Switching
Rescuers should change compressor and ventilator roles every 2 minutes to avoid compressor fatigue.
Rescuers should exchange positions simultaneously with minimal delay:
- Ventilator moves to chest.
- Compressor moves to head.

Defibrillation
If witnessed arrest, use AED as soon as possible.
If unwitnessed arrest, deliver five cycles of CPR before using AED.
If rhythm is shockable, deliver one shock, then resume CPR for five cycles before rechecking rhythm.
If the rhythm is not shockable, resume CPR and recheck rhythm every five cycles.

Continuation of CPR
- CPR should be continued between rhythm checks and shocks, and until ACLS providers arrive or the victim shows signs of movement.
- Do not interrupt CPR except in special circumstances.

Source: 2005 American Heart Association Guidelines for Cardiopulmonary Resuscitation and Emergency Cardiovascular Care, Part 4: Adult Basic Life Support, *Circulation* 112:IV-19, 2005.
ACLS, Advanced cardiac life support; *AED*, automatic external defibrillator.
*Rescuers should phone 911 for unresponsive adults before beginning CPR, except in the case of drowning or a likely asphyxiation.
†Lay rescuers are no longer taught a pulse check.

REFERENCE

1. 2005 American Heart Association Guidelines for Cardiopulmonary Resuscitation and Emergency Cardiovascular Care, Part 4: Adult Basic Life Support, *Circulation* 112:IV-19, 2005.

Appendix B
Nursing Diagnoses

ALPHABETICAL LISTING

Activity Intolerance
Activity Intolerance, Risk for
Airway Clearance, Ineffective
Allergy Response, Latex
Allergy Response, Risk for Latex
Anxiety
Anxiety, Death
Aspiration, Risk for
Attachment, Risk for Impaired Parent/Infant/Child
Autonomic Dysreflexia
Autonomic Dysreflexia, Risk for
Body Image, Disturbed
Body Temperature, Risk for Imbalanced
Bowel Incontinence
Breastfeeding, Effective
Breastfeeding, Ineffective
Breastfeeding, Interrupted
Breathing Pattern, Ineffective
Cardiac Output, Decreased
Caregiver Role Strain
Caregiver Role Strain, Risk for
Comfort, Readiness for Enhanced
Communication, Impaired Verbal
Communication, Readiness for Enhanced
Conflict, Decisional
Conflict, Parental Role
Confusion, Acute
Confusion, Chronic
Confusion, Risk for Acute
Constipation
Constipation, Perceived
Constipation, Risk for
Contamination
Contamination, Risk for
Coping, Compromised Family
Coping, Defensive
Coping, Disabled Family
Coping, Ineffective
Coping, Ineffective Community
Coping, Readiness for Enhanced
Coping, Readiness for Enhanced Community

Coping, Readiness for Enhanced Family
Decision Making, Readiness for Enhanced
Denial, Ineffective
Dentition, Impaired
Development, Risk for Delayed
Diarrhea
Disuse Syndrome, Risk for
Diversional Activity, Deficient
Energy Field, Disturbed
Environmental Interpretation Syndrome, Impaired
Failure to Thrive, Adult
Falls, Risk for
Family Processes, Dysfunctional: Alcoholism
Family Processes, Interrupted
Family Processes, Readiness for Enhanced
Fatigue
Fear
Fluid Balance, Readiness for Enhanced
Fluid Volume, Deficient
Fluid Volume, Excess
Fluid Volume, Risk for Deficient
Fluid Volume, Risk for Imbalanced
Gas Exchange, Impaired
Grieving
Grieving, Complicated
Grieving, Risk for Complicated
Growth and Development, Delayed
Growth, Risk for Disproportionate
Health Behavior, Risk Prone
Health Maintenance, Ineffective
Health-Seeking Behaviors
Home Maintenance, Impaired
Hope, Readiness for Enhanced
Hopelessness
Human Dignity, Risk for Compromised
Hyperthermia
Hypothermia
Identity, Disturbed Personal
Immunization Status, Readiness for Enhanced
Impaired Liver Function, Risk for
Incontinence, Functional Urinary
Incontinence, Overflow Urinary
Incontinence, Reflex Urinary
Incontinence, Risk for Urge Urinary
Incontinence, Stress Urinary
Incontinence, Total Urinary

Source: NANDA International. Available at *www.nanda.org; NANDA nursing diagnoses: definitions and classification 2005–2006,* Philadelphia, NANDA; and Gordon M: *Manual of nursing diagnosis,* ed 10, St Louis, 2002, Mosby.

Incontinence, Urge Urinary
Infant Behavior, Disorganized
Infant Behavior, Readiness for Enhanced Organized
Infant Behavior, Risk for Disorganized
Infant Feeding Pattern, Ineffective
Infection, Risk for
Injury, Risk for
Injury, Risk for Perioperative-Positioning
Insomnia
Intracranial Adaptive Capacity, Decreased
Knowledge, Deficient
Knowledge, Readiness for Enhanced
Lifestyle, Sedentary
Loneliness, Risk for
Memory, Impaired
Mobility, Impaired Bed
Mobility, Impaired Physical
Mobility, Impaired Wheelchair
Moral Distress
Nausea
Neglect, Unilateral
Noncompliance
Nutrition, Imbalanced: Less than Body Requirements
Nutrition, Imbalanced: More than Body Requirements
Nutrition, Readiness for Enhanced
Nutrition, Risk for Imbalanced: More than Body Requirements
Oral Mucous Membrane, Impaired
Pain, Acute
Pain, Chronic
Parenting, Impaired
Parenting, Readiness for Enhanced
Parenting, Risk for Impaired
Peripheral Neurovascular Dysfunction, Risk for
Poisoning, Risk for
Post-Trauma Syndrome
Post-Trauma Syndrome, Risk for
Power, Readiness for Enhanced
Powerlessness
Powerlessness, Risk for
Protection, Ineffective
Rape-Trauma Syndrome
Rape-Trauma Syndrome: Compound Reaction
Rape-Trauma Syndrome: Silent Reaction
Religiosity, Impaired
Religiosity, Readiness for Enhanced
Religiosity, Risk for Impaired
Relocation Stress Syndrome
Relocation Stress Syndrome, Risk for
Role Performance, Ineffective
Self-Care Deficit, Bathing/Hygiene

Self-Care Deficit, Dressing/Grooming
Self-Care Deficit, Feeding
Self-Care Deficit, Toileting
Self-Care, Readiness for Enhanced
Self-Esteem, Chronic Low
Self-Esteem, Risk for Situational Low
Self-Esteem, Situational Low
Self-Learning, Readiness for Enhanced
Self-Mutilation
Self-Mutilation, Risk for
Sensory Perception, Disturbed
Sexual Dysfunction
Sexuality Pattern, Ineffective
Skin Integrity, Impaired
Skin Integrity, Risk for Impaired
Sleep Deprivation
Sleep, Readiness for Enhanced
Social Interaction, Impaired
Social Isolation
Sorrow, Chronic
Spiritual Distress
Spiritual Distress, Risk for
Spiritual Well-Being, Readiness for Enhanced
Stress Overload
Sudden Infant Death Syndrome, Risk for
Suffocation, Risk for
Suicide, Risk for
Surgical Recovery, Delayed
Swallowing, Impaired
Therapeutic Regimen Management, Effective
Therapeutic Regimen Management, Ineffective
Therapeutic Regimen Management, Ineffective Community
Therapeutic Regimen Management, Ineffective Family
Therapeutic Regimen Management, Readiness for Enhanced
Thermoregulation, Ineffective
Thought Processes, Disturbed
Tissue Integrity, Impaired
Tissue Perfusion, Ineffective
Transfer Ability, Impaired
Trauma, Risk for
Unstable Glucose Level, Risk for
Urinary Elimination, Impaired
Urinary Elimination, Readiness for Enhanced
Urinary Retention
Ventilation, Impaired Spontaneous
Ventilatory Weaning Response, Dysfunctional
Violence, Risk for Other-Directed
Violence, Risk for Self-Directed
Walking, Impaired
Wandering

Appendix B

GROUPED BY FUNCTIONAL HEALTH PATTERNS

Health Perception–Health Management Pattern

Contamination
Contamination, Risk for
Energy Field, Disturbed
Falls, Risk for
Health Maintenance, Ineffective
Health-Seeking Behaviors
Immunization Status, Readiness for Enhanced
Infection, Risk for
Injury, Risk for
Injury, Risk for Perioperative-Positioning
Noncompliance
Poisoning, Risk for
Protection, Ineffective
Self-Care, Readiness for Enhanced
Suffocation, Risk for
Therapeutic Regimen Management, Effective
Therapeutic Regimen Management, Ineffective
Therapeutic Regimen Management, Ineffective Family
Therapeutic Regimen Management, Ineffective Community
Therapeutic Regimen Management, Readiness for Enhanced
Trauma, Risk for

Nutritional-Metabolic Pattern

Allergy Response, Latex
Allergy Response, Risk for Latex
Aspiration, Risk for
Body Temperature, Risk for Imbalanced
Breastfeeding, Effective
Breastfeeding, Ineffective
Breastfeeding, Interrupted
Dentition, Impaired
Failure to Thrive, Adult
Fluid Volume, Deficient
Fluid Volume, Excess
Fluid Volume, Readiness for Enhanced
Fluid Volume, Risk for Deficient
Fluid Volume, Risk for Imbalanced
Hyperthermia
Hypothermia
Infant Feeding Pattern, Ineffective
Liver Function, Risk for Impaired
Nausea
Nutrition, Imbalanced: Less than Body Requirements
Nutrition, Imbalanced: More than Body Requirements
Nutrition, Readiness for Enhanced
Nutrition, Risk for Imbalanced: More than Body Requirements
Oral Mucous Membrane, Impaired
Skin Integrity, Impaired
Skin Integrity, Risk for Impaired
Swallowing, Impaired
Thermoregulation, Ineffective
Tissue Integrity, Impaired
Unstable Glucose Level, Risk for

Elimination Pattern

Constipation
Constipation, Perceived
Constipation, Risk for
Diarrhea
Incontinence, Bowel
Incontinence, Functional Urinary
Incontinence, Overflow Urinary
Incontinence, Reflex Urinary
Incontinence, Risk for Urge Urinary
Incontinence, Stress Urinary
Incontinence, Total Urinary
Incontinence, Urge Urinary
Urinary Elimination, Impaired
Urinary Elimination, Readiness for Enhanced
Urinary Retention

Activity-Exercise Pattern

Activity Intolerance
Activity Intolerance, Risk for
Airway Clearance, Ineffective
Autonomic Dysreflexia
Autonomic Dysreflexia, Risk for
Breathing Pattern, Ineffective
Cardiac Output, Decreased
Development, Risk for Delayed
Disuse Syndrome, Risk for
Diversional Activity, Deficient
Fatigue
Gas Exchange, Impaired
Growth and Development, Delayed
Growth, Risk for Disproportionate
Home Maintenance, Impaired
Infant Behavior, Disorganized
Infant Behavior, Readiness for Enhanced Organized
Infant Behavior, Risk for Disorganized
Intracranial Adaptive Capacity, Decreased
Mobility, Impaired Bed
Mobility, Impaired Physical
Mobility, Impaired Wheelchair
Peripheral Neurovascular Dysfunction, Risk for
Self-Care Deficit, Bathing/Hygiene
Self-Care Deficit, Dressing/Grooming
Self-Care Deficit, Feeding
Self-Care Deficit, Toileting
Surgical Recovery, Delayed
Tissue Perfusion, Ineffective
Transfer Ability, Impaired
Ventilation, Impaired Spontaneous
Ventilatory Weaning Response, Dysfunctional
Walking, Impaired
Wandering

Sleep-Rest Pattern

Sleep Deprivation
Sleep, Readiness for Enhanced
Insomnia

Cognitive-Perceptual Pattern

Comfort, Readiness for Enhanced
Confusion, Acute
Confusion, Chronic
Confusion, Risk for Acute

Conflict, Decisional
Decision Making, Readiness for Enhanced
Environmental Interpretation Syndrome, Impaired
Knowledge, Deficient
Knowledge, Readiness for Enhanced
Memory, Impaired
Neglect, Unilateral
Pain, Acute
Pain, Chronic
Thought Processes, Disturbed

Self-Perception–Self-Concept Pattern

Anxiety
Anxiety, Death
Body Image, Disturbed
Fear
Hope, Readiness for Enhanced
Hopelessness
Human Dignity, Risk for Compromised
Identity, Disturbed Personal
Loneliness, Risk for
Power, Readiness for Enhanced
Powerlessness
Powerlessness, Risk for
Self-Esteem, Chronic Low
Self-Esteem, Risk for Situational Low
Self-Esteem, Situational Low
Violence, Risk for Self-Directed

Role-Relationship Pattern

Attachment, Risk for Impaired Parent/Infant/Child
Caregiver Role Strain
Caregiver Role Strain, Risk for
Communication, Impaired Verbal
Communication, Readiness for Enhanced
Conflict, Parental Role
Family Processes, Dysfunctional: Alcoholism
Family Processes, Interrupted
Family Processes, Readiness for Enhanced
Grieving
Grieving, Complicated
Grieving, Risk for Complicated

Parenting, Impaired
Parenting, Readiness for Enhanced
Parenting, Risk for Impaired
Relocation Stress Syndrome
Relocation Stress Syndrome, Risk for
Role Performance, Ineffective
Social Interaction, Impaired
Social Isolation
Sorrow, Chronic
Violence, Risk for Other-Directed

Sexuality-Reproductive Pattern

Rape-Trauma Syndrome
Rape-Trauma Syndrome: Compound Reaction
Rape-Trauma Syndrome: Silent Reaction
Sexual Dysfunction
Sexuality Patterns, Ineffective

Coping–Stress Tolerance Pattern

Coping, Compromised Family
Coping, Defensive
Coping, Disabled Family
Coping, Ineffective
Coping, Ineffective Community
Coping, Readiness for Enhanced
Coping, Readiness for Enhanced Community
Coping, Readiness for Enhanced Family
Denial, Ineffective
Health Behavior, Risk Prone
Post-Trauma Syndrome
Post-Trauma Syndrome, Risk for
Self-Mutilation
Self-Mutilation, Risk for
Stress Overload
Suicide, Risk for

Value-Belief Pattern

Moral Distress
Spiritual Distress
Spiritual Distress, Risk for
Spiritual Well-Being, Readiness for Enhanced

Appendix C
Laboratory Values

The tables in this appendix list some of the most common tests, their normal values, and possible etiologies of abnormal values. Laboratory values may vary with different techniques or different laboratories. Possible etiologies are presented in alphabetic order. Abbreviations appearing in the tables are defined as follows:

<	=	less than
>	=	greater than
L	=	liter
mEq	=	milliequivalent
ml	=	milliliter
dl	=	deciliter
mm Hg	=	millimeter of mercury
fl	=	femtoliter
mm	=	millimeter
g	=	gram

mg	=	milligram (10^{-3})
mcg	=	microgram (one millionth of a gram) (10^{-6})
ng	=	nanogram (one billionth of a gram) (10^{-9})
pg	=	picogram (one trillionth of a gram) (10^{-12})
μU	=	microunit
μl	=	microliter
IU	=	international unit
mOsm	=	milliosmole
U	=	unit
mmol	=	millimole
μmol	=	micromole
nmol	=	nanomole
pmol	=	picomole
kPa	=	kilopascal
μkat	=	microkatal

TABLE C-1	Serum, Plasma, and Whole Blood Chemistries			

	Normal Values		Possible Etiology	
Test	Conventional Units	SI Units	Higher	Lower
Acetone			Diabetic ketoacidosis, high-fat diet, low-carbohydrate diet, starvation	
Quantitative	0.3-2.0 mg/dl	52-344 μmol/L		
Qualitative	Negative	Negative		
Albumin	3.5-5.0 g/dl	35-50 g/L	Dehydration	Chronic liver disease, malabsorption, malnutrition, nephrotic syndrome, pregnancy
Aldolase	1.0-7.5 U/L	0.02-0.13 μkat/L	Skeletal muscle disease	Renal disease
α_1-Antitrypsin	78-200 mg/dl	0.78-2.0 g/L	Acute and chronic inflammation, arthritis, stress syndrome	Chronic lung disease (early onset), malnutrition, nephrotic syndrome
α_1-Fetoprotein	<15 ng/ml	<15 mcg/L	Cancer of testes and ovaries, carcinoma of liver	
Ammonia	30-70 mcg/dl	17.6-41.1 μmol/L	Severe liver disease	
Amylase	0-130 U/L (method dependent)	0-2.17 μkat/L	Acute and chronic pancreatitis, mumps (salivary gland disease), perforated ulcers	Acute alcoholism, cirrhosis of liver, extensive destruction of pancreas
Ascorbic acid	0.4-1.5 mg/dl	23-85 μmol/L	Excessive ingestion of vitamin C	Connective tissue disorders, hepatic disease, renal disease, rheumatic fever, vitamin C deficiency
Bicarbonate	22-26 mEq/L	22-26 mmol/L	Compensated respiratory acidosis, metabolic alkalosis	Compensated respiratory alkalosis, metabolic acidosis
Bilirubin			Biliary obstruction, hemolytic anemia, impaired liver function, pernicious anemia, prolonged fasting	
Total	0.2-1.3 mg/dl	3.4-22.0 μmol/L		
Indirect	0.1-1.0 mg/dl	1.7-17.0 μmol/L		
Direct	0.1-0.3 mg/dl	1.7-5.1 μmol/L		
Blood gases*				
Arterial pH	7.35-7.45	Same as conventional units	Alkalosis	Acidosis
Venous pH	7.35-7.45	Same as conventional units	Alkalosis	Acidosis
Arterial $PaCO_2$	35-45 mm Hg	4.67-6.00 kPa	Compensated metabolic alkalosis	Compensated metabolic acidosis
Venous $PaCO_2$	42-52 mm Hg	5.60-6.93 kPa	Respiratory acidosis	Respiratory alkalosis
Arterial PaO_2	75-100 mm Hg	10.0-13.33 kPa	Administration of high concentration of oxygen	Chronic lung disease, decreased cardiac output
Venous PaO_2	30-50 mm Hg	4.0-6.67 kPa		
b-Type natriuretic peptide (BNP)	<100 pg/ml		Heart failure	
Calcium	9-11 mg/dl (4.5-5.5 mEq/L)	2.25-2.74 mmol/L	Acute osteoporosis, hyperparathyroidism, multiple myeloma, vitamin D intoxication	Acute pancreatitis, hypoparathyroidism, liver disease, malabsorption syndrome, renal failure, vitamin D deficiency
Calcium, ionized	4.5-5.5 mg/dl (2.25-2.75 mEq/L)	1.13-1.38 mmol/L		
Carbon dioxide (CO_2 content)	20-30 mEq/L	20-30 mmol/L	Same as bicarbonate	
Carotene	10-85 mcg/dl	0.19-1.58 μmol/L	Cystic fibrosis, hypothyroidism, pancreatic insufficiency	Dietary deficiency, malabsorption disorders
Chloride	95-105 mEq/L	95-105 mmol/L	Corticosteroid therapy, metabolic acidosis, respiratory alkalosis, uremia	Addison's disease, diarrhea, metabolic alkalosis, respiratory acidosis, vomiting
Cholesterol	140-200 mg/dl (age dependent)	3.6-5.2 mmol/L	Biliary obstruction, hypothyroidism, idiopathic hypercholesterolemia, renal disease, uncontrolled diabetes	Corticosteroid therapy, extensive liver disease, hyperthyroidism, malnutrition
HDL (high-density lipoproteins)				
Male	>45 mg/dl	>1.2 mmol/L		
Female	>55 mg/dl	>1.4 mmol/L		
LDL (low-density lipoproteins)	<130 mg/dl	<3.4 mmol/L		
Cholinesterase (RBC)	0.65-1.00 pH	Same as conventional units	Exercise	Acute infections, insecticide intoxication, liver disease, muscular dystrophy
Copper	80-150 mcg/dl	12.6-23.6 μmol/L	Cirrhosis, female on contraceptives	Wilson's disease

*Because arterial blood gases are influenced by altitude, the value for PaO_2 decreases as altitude increases. The lower value is normal for an altitude of 1 mile.

Continued

TABLE C-1	Serum, Plasma, and Whole Blood Chemistries—cont'd

	Normal Values		Possible Etiology	
Test	**Conventional Units**	**SI Units**	**Higher**	**Lower**
Cortisol	8 AM: 5-25 mcg/dl 8 PM: <10 mcg/dl	0.14-0.69 μmol/L <0.28 μmol/L	Cushing syndrome, pancreatitis, stress	Adrenal insufficiency, panhypopituitary states
Creatine	0.2-1.0 mg/dl	15.3-76.3 μmol/L	Active rheumatoid arthritis, biliary obstruction, hyperthyroidism, renal disorders, severe muscle disease	Diabetes mellitus
Creatine kinase (CK)			Brain damage, exercise, musculoskeletal injury or disease, myocardial infarction, numerous intramuscular injections, severe myocarditis	
Male	15-105 U/L	0.26-1.79 μkat/L		
Female	10-80 U/L	0.17-1.36 μkat/L		
CK-MB (CK-2)	0-9 U/L	<0.1 μkat/L	Acute myocardial infarction	
Creatinine	0.5-1.5 mg/dl	44-133 μmol/L	Severe renal disease	
Ferritin (serum)			Anemia of chronic disease (infection, inflammation, liver disease), sideroblastic anemia	Iron-deficiency anemia
Male	20-300 ng/ml	20-300 mcg/L		
Female	10-120 ng/ml	10-120 mcg/L		
Folic acid (folate)	3-25 ng/ml	7-57 nmol/L	Hypothyroidism	Alcoholism, hemolytic anemia, inadequate diet, malabsorption syndrome, megaloblastic anemia
Gamma-glutamyl transpeptidase (GGT)	0-30 U/L	0-0.5 μkat/L		Liver disease, infectious mononucleosis
Glucose, fasting	70-100 mg/dl	3.89-5.55 mmol/L	Acute stress, cerebral lesions, Cushing disease, diabetes mellitus, hyperthyroidism, pancreatic insufficiency	Addison's disease, hepatic disease, hypothyroidism, insulin overdosage, pancreatic tumor, pituitary hypofunction, postgastrectomy dumping syndrome
Glucose tolerance (GTT)			Diabetes mellitus	Hyperinsulinism
Fasting	70-100 mg/dl	3.89-5.55 mmol/L		
30 min	30-60 mg/dl above fasting	1.67-3.33 mmol/L		
60 min	20-50 mg/dl above fasting	1.11-2.78 mmol/L		
120 min	5-15 mg/dl above fasting	0.28-0.83 mmol/L		
180 min	Fasting level or lower	Fasting level or lower		
Haptoglobin	26-185 mg/dl	260-1850 mg/L	Infectious and inflammatory processes, malignant neoplasms	Chronic liver disease, hemolytic anemia, mononucleosis, toxoplasmosis
Insulin	4-24 μU/ml	29-172 pmol/L	Acromegaly, adenoma of islet cells, untreated mild case of type 2 diabetes	Diabetes mellitus, obesity
Iron, total	50-150 mcg/dl	9.0-26.9 μmol/L	Excessive RBC destruction	Anemia of chronic disease, iron-deficiency anemia
Iron-binding capacity	250-410 mcg/dl	45-73 μmol/L	Iron-deficient state, oral contraceptive use, polycythemia	Cancer, chronic infections, pernicious anemia, uremia
Lactic acid	5-20 mcg/dl	0.56-2.2 mmol/L	Acidosis, heart failure, shock	
Lactic dehydrogenase (LDH)	50-150 U/L	0.83-2.5 μkat/L	Heart failure, hemolytic disorders, hepatitis, metastatic cancer of liver, myocardial infarction, pernicious anemia, pulmonary embolus, skeletal muscle damage	

RBC, Red blood cell.

| TABLE C-1 | **Serum, Plasma, and Whole Blood Chemistries—cont'd** |

Test	Normal Values Conventional Units	SI Units	Possible Etiology Higher	Lower
Lactic dehydrogenase isoenzymes				
LDH$_1$	20%-35%	0.20-0.35	Myocardial infarction, pernicious anemia	
LDH$_2$	30%-40%	0.30-0.40	Pulmonary embolus, sickle cell crisis	
LDH$_3$	15%-25%	0.15-0.25	Malignant lymphoma, pulmonary embolus	
LDH$_4$	0%-10%	0-0.10	Lupus erythematosus, pulmonary infarction	
LDH$_5$	4%-12%	0.04-0.12	Heart failure, hepatitis, pulmonary embolus and infarction, skeletal muscle damage	
Lipase	0-160 U/L	0-2.66 μkat/L	Acute pancreatitis, hepatic disorders, perforated peptic ulcer	
Magnesium	1.5-2.5 mEq/L	0.62-1.03 mmol/L	Addison's disease, hypothyroidism, renal failure	Chronic alcoholism, hyperparathyroidism, hyperthyroidism, hypoparathyroidism, severe malabsorption
Osmolality	285-295 mOsm/kg	285-295 mmol/kg	Chronic renal disease, diabetes mellitus	Addison's disease, diuretic therapy
Oxygen saturation (arterial)	95%-98%	0.95-0.98 saturated	Polycythemia	Anemia, cardiac decompensation, respiratory disorders
pH	See blood gases			
Phenylalanine	0-2 mg/dl	0-121 μmol/L	Phenylketonuria	
Phosphatase, acid	0-0.6 U/L	0-90 μkat/L	Advanced Paget's disease, cancer of prostate, hyperparathyroidism	
Phosphatase, alkaline	30-120 U/L	0.5-2.0 μkat/L	Bone diseases, marked hyperparathyroidism, obstruction of biliary system, rickets	Excessive vitamin D ingestion, hypothyroidism, milk-alkali syndrome
Phosphorus, inorganic	2.8-4.5 mg/dl	0.90-1.45 mmol/L	Healing fractures, hypoparathyroidism, renal disease, vitamin D intoxication	Diabetes mellitus, hyperparathyroidism, vitamin D deficiency
Potassium	3.5-5.0 mEq/L	3.5-5.0 mmol/L	Addison's disease, diabetic ketosis, massive tissue destruction, renal failure	Cushing syndrome, diarrhea (severe), diuretic therapy, gastrointestinal fistula, pyloric obstruction, starvation, vomiting
Progesterone				
Female			Adrenal hyperplasia, choriocarcinoma of ovary, cysts of ovary, pregnancy	Amenorrhea, hypogonadism, ovarian tumor, threatened abortion
Follicular phase	<50 ng/dl	1.6 nmol/L		
Luteal phase	200-2500 ng/dl	6.4-79.5 nmol/L		
Postmenopause	<40 ng/dl	1.28 nmol/L		
Male	10-50 ng/dl	0.32-1.6 nmol/L		
Prostate-specific antigen (PSA)	<4 ng/mL	<4 mcg/L	Prostate cancer	
Proteins			Burns, cirrhosis (globulin fraction), dehydration	Congenital agammaglobulinemia, liver disease, malabsorption
Total	6.0-8.0 g/dl	60-80 g/L		
Albumin	3.5-5.0 g/dl	35-50 g/L		
Globulin	2.0-3.5 g/dl	20-35 g/L		
Albumin/globulin ratio	1.5:1-2.5:1	Same as conventional units	Multiple myeloma (globulin fraction), shock, vomiting	Malnutrition, nephrotic syndrome, proteinuria, renal disease, severe burns
Renin			Renal hypertension, volume decrease (e.g., hemorrhage)	Increased salt intake, primary aldosteronism
Supine position	1.4-2.9 ng/ml/hr	0.39-0.81 ng/L/sec		
Upright position	0.4-4.5 ng/ml/hr	0.11-1.25 ng/L/sec		
Sodium	135-145 mEq/L	135-145 mmol/L	Corticosteroid therapy, dehydration, impaired renal function, primary aldosteronism	Addison's disease, diabetic ketoacidosis, diuretic therapy, excessive loss from gastrointestinal tract, excessive perspiration, water intoxication

Continued

TABLE C-1	Serum, Plasma, and Whole Blood Chemistries—cont'd			
	Normal Values		**Possible Etiology**	
Test	**Conventional Units**	**SI Units**	**Higher**	**Lower**
Testosterone				
Male	300-1200 ng/dl	10.4-41.6 nmol/L		Hypofunction of testes, hypogonadism
Female	25-90 ng/dl	0.87-3.1 nmol/L	Polycystic ovary, virilizing tumors	
Thyroid hormones				
T_4 (thyroxine), total	5-12 mcg/dl	64-154 nmol/L	Hyperthyroidism, thyroiditis	Cretinism, hypothyroidism, myxedema
T_4 (thyroxine), free	0.8-2.3 ng/dl	10-30 pmol/L		
T_3 uptake	25%-35%	0.25-0.35	Hyperthyroidism, metastatic neoplasms	Hypothyroidism, pregnancy
T_3 (triiodothyronine)	*Ages 20-50:* 70-204 ng/dl *Ages >50:* 40-180 ng/dl	*Ages 20-50:* 1.1-3.1 nmol/L *Ages >50:* 0.6-2.8 nmol/L	Hyperthyroidism	Hypothyroidism
Thyroid-stimulating hormone (TSH)	0.3-5.4 µU/ml	0.3-5.4 mU/L	Graves' disease, myxedema, primary hypothyroidism	Secondary hypothyroidism
Transaminases				
Aspartate aminotrans- ferase (AST)	7-40 U/L	0.12-0.67 µkat/L	Acute hepatitis, liver disease, myocardial infarction, pulmonary infarction	
Alanine aminotrans- ferase (ALT)	5-36 U/L	0.08-0.6 µkat/L	Liver disease, shock	
Triglycerides	40-150 mg/dl	0.45-1.69 mmol/L	Diabetes mellitus, hyperlipidemia, hypothyroidism, liver disease	Malnutrition
Urea nitrogen (BUN)	10-30 mg/dl	1.8-7.1 mmol/L	Increase in protein catabolism (fever, stress), renal disease, urinary tract infection	Malnutrition, severe liver damage
Uric acid			Eclampsia, gout, gross tissue destruction, high-protein weight reduction diet, leukemia, renal failure	Administration of uricosuric drugs
Male	4.5-6.5 mg/dl	268-387 µmol/L		
Female	2.5-5.5 mg/dl	149-268 µmol/L		
Vitamin A	15-60 mcg/dl	0.52-2.09 µmol/L	Excess ingestion of vitamin A	Vitamin A deficiency
Vitamin B_{12}	200-1000 pg/ml	148-738 pmol/L	Chronic myeloid leukemia	Malabsorption syndrome, pernicious anemia, strict vegetarianism, total or partial gastrectomy
Zinc	50-150 mcg/dl	7.6-22.9 µmol/L		Alcoholic cirrhosis

TABLE C-2	Hematology

Test	Normal Values — Conventional Units	Normal Values — SI Units	Possible Etiology — Higher	Possible Etiology — Lower
Bleeding time (Simplate)	3.0-9.5	180-570 sec	Aspirin ingestion, defective platelet function, thrombocytopenia, vascular disease, von Willebrand's disease	
Activated partial thromboplastin time (aPTT)	24-36 sec*	Same as conventional units	Deficiency of factors I, II, V, VIII, IX, X, XI, and XII; hemophilia; heparin therapy; liver disease	
Prothrombin time (protime, PT)	10-14 sec*	Same as conventional units	Deficiency of factors I, II, V, VII, and X; liver disease; vitamin K deficiency; warfarin therapy	
Fibrinogen	200-400 mg/dl		Burns (after first 36 hr), inflammatory disease	Burns (during first 36 hr), DIC, severe liver disease
Fibrin split (degradation) products	<10 mcg/ml	Same as conventional units	Acute DIC, massive hemorrhage, primary fibrinolysis	
D-Dimer	Negative	Negative	DIC, deep vein thrombosis, myocardial infarction, unstable angina	
Erythrocyte count† (altitude dependent)			Dehydration, high altitudes, polycythemia vera, severe diarrhea	Anemia, leukemia, posthemorrhage
Male	$4.5\text{-}6.0 \times 10^6/\mu L$	$4.5\text{-}6.0 \times 10^{12}/L$		
Female	$4.0\text{-}5.0 \times 10^6/\mu L$	$4.0\text{-}5.0 \times 10^{12}/L$		
Mean corpuscular volume (MCV)	82-98 fl	Same as conventional units	Macrocytic anemia	Microcytic anemia
Mean corpuscular hemoglobin (MCH)	27-33 pg	Same as conventional units	Macrocytic anemia	Microcytic anemia
Mean corpuscular hemoglobin concentration (MCHC)	32%-36%	0.32-0.36	Spherocytosis	Hypochromic anemia
Erythrocyte sedimentation rate (ESR), Westergren			*Moderate increase:* acute hepatitis, myocardial infarction; rheumatoid arthritis	Malaria, severe liver disease, sickle cell anemia
Male			*Marked increase:* acute and severe bacterial infections, malignancies, pelvic inflammatory disease	
≤50 yr	<15 mm/hr	Same as conventional units		
>50 yr	<20 mm/hr			
Female				
≤50 yr	<20 mm/hr	Same as conventional units		
>50 yr	<30 mm/hr			
Hematocrit (altitude dependent)†			Dehydration, high altitudes, polycythemia	Anemia, hemorrhage, overhydration
Male	40%-54%	0.40-0.54		
Female	38%-47%	0.38-0.47		
Hemoglobin (altitude dependent)†			COPD, high altitudes, polycythemia	Anemia, hemorrhage
Male	13.5-18.0 g/dl	135-180 g/L		
Female	12.0-16.0 g/dl	120-160 g/L		
Hemoglobin, glycosylated	4.0%-6.0%	Same as conventional units	Poorly controlled diabetes mellitus	Chronic kidney disease, pregnancy, sickle cell anemia
Red cell distribution width (RDW)	10.2%-14.5%	Same as conventional therapy		Anisocytosis, macrocytic anemia, microcytic anemia
Platelet count (thrombocytes)	$150\text{-}400 \times 10^3/\mu L$	$150\text{-}400 \times 10^9/L$	Acute infections, chronic granulocytic leukemia, chronic pancreatitis, cirrhosis, collagen disorders, polycythemia, postsplenectomy	Acute leukemia, DIC, thrombocytopenic purpura
Reticulocyte count (manual)	0.5%-1.5% of total RBCs	Same	Hemolytic anemia, polycythemia vera	Hypoproliferative anemia, macrocytic anemia, microcytic anemia

COPD, Chronic obstructive pulmonary disease; *DIC,* disseminated intravascular coagulation; *RBCs,* red blood cells.
*Values depend on reagent and instrumentation used.
†Components of complete blood count (CBC).

Continued

| TABLE C-2 | Hematology—cont'd | | | | |

	Normal Values		Possible Etiology	
Test	Conventional Units	SI Units	Higher	Lower
White blood cell (WBC) count†	4.0-11.0 × 10³/μL	4.0-11.0 × 10⁹/L	Inflammatory and infectious processes, leukemia	Aplastic anemia, side effect of chemotherapy and irradiation
WBC differential				
Segmented neutrophils	50%-70%	0.50-0.70	Bacterial infections, collagen diseases, Hodgkin's lymphoma	Aplastic anemia, viral infections
Band neutrophils	0%-8%	0-0.08	Acute infections	
Lymphocytes	20%-40%	0.20-0.40	Chronic infections, lymphocytic leukemia, mononucleosis, viral infections	Corticosteroid therapy, whole-body irradiation
Monocytes	4%-8%	0.04-0.08	Acute infections, chronic inflammatory disorders, Hodgkin's lymphoma, malaria, monocytic leukemia	
Eosinophils	0%-4%	0-0.04	Allergic reactions, eosinophilic and chronic granulocytic leukemia, Hodgkin's lymphoma, parasitic disorders	Corticosteroid therapy
Basophils	0%-2%	0-0.02	Hypothyroidism, myeloproliferative diseases, ulcerative colitis	Hyperthyroidism, stress
Sickle cell solubility test	Negative	Negative	Sickle cell anemia	

| TABLE C-3 | Serology-Immunology | | | | |

	Normal Values		Possible Etiology	
Test	Conventional Units	SI Units	Higher	Lower
Antibodies				
Antinuclear antibody (ANA)	Negative or titer <1:10	Same as conventional units	Chronic hepatitis, rheumatoid arthritis, scleroderma, systemic lupus erythematosus	
Anti-DNA antibody	Negative or titer <1:10 or <20% binding	Same as conventional units	Systemic lupus erythematosus	
Anti-RNP	Negative	Negative	Mixed connective tissue disease, rheumatoid arthritis, scleroderma, Sjögren syndrome, systemic lupus erythematosus	
Anti-Sm (Smith)	Negative	Negative	Systemic lupus erythematosus	
Antistreptolysin-O (ASO)	≤166 Todd units or ≤1:85	Same as conventional units	Acute glomerulonephritis, rheumatic fever, streptococcal infection	
Carcinoembryonic antigen (CEA)	≤2.5 ng/ml	≤2.5 mcg/L	Carcinoma of colon, liver, pancreas; chronic cigarette smoking; inflammatory bowel disease; other cancers	
Complement components				Acute glomerulonephritis, rheumatoid arthritis, serum sickness, subacute bacterial endocarditis, systemic lupus erythematosus
C1q	11-21 mg/dl	0.11-0.21 g/L		
C3	80-180 mg/dl	0.8-1.8 g/L		
C4	15-50 mg/dl	0.15-0.5 g/L		
C-reactive protein (CRP)	Negative or ≤1.2 mg/dl	Same as conventional units	Acute infections, any inflammatory condition, widespread malignancy	

IV, Intravenous; *RNP,* ribonuclear protein; *RPR,* rapid plasma reagin test; *VDRL,* Veneral Disease Research Laboratory (test).

TABLE C-3	Serology-Immunology—cont'd			
	Normal Values		**Possible Etiology**	
Test	**Conventional Units**	**SI Units**	**Higher**	**Lower**
Direct antihuman globulin test (DAT) or direct Coombs test	Negative	Negative	Acquired hemolytic anemia, drug reactions, hemolytic disease of the newborn, transfusion reactions	
Fluorescent treponemal antibody absorption (FTA-Abs)	Nonreactive	Negative	Syphilis	
Hepatitis A antibody	Negative	Negative	Hepatitis A	
Hepatitis B surface antigen (HBsAg)	Negative	Negative	Hepatitis B	
Hepatitis C antibody	Negative	Negative	Hepatitis C	
Immunoglobulins				
IgA	90-400 mg/dl	0.9-4.0 g/L	Autoimmune disorders, chronic infection, chronic liver disease, IgA myeloma, rheumatoid arthritis	Burns, hereditary telangiectasia, malabsorption syndromes
IgD	0.5-12.0 mg/dl	5-120 mg/L	Chronic infection, connective tissue disease	
IgE	<1.0 mg/dl	<10 mg/L	Anaphylactic shock, atopic disease (allergies), parasite infections	
IgG	650-1800 mg/dl	6.5-18.0 g/L	Hepatitis, IgG monoclonal gammopathy, infections—acute and chronic, systemic lupus erythematosus	Acquired deficiencies, burns, congenital deficiencies, immunosuppression, nephrotic syndromes
IgM	55-300 mg/dl	0.5-3.0 g/L	Acute infections, liver disease, rheumatoid arthritis	Congenital and acquired antibody deficiencies, lymphocytic leukemia, protein-losing enteropathies
Monospot or monotest	Negative	Negative	Infectious mononucleosis	
Rheumatoid factor (RA factor)	Negative or titer <1:20	Same as conventional units	Rheumatoid arthritis, Sjögren syndrome, systemic lupus erythematosus	
RPR	Nonreactive	Same as conventional units	Febrile diseases, IV drug abuse, leprosy, malaria, rheumatoid arthritis, syphilis, systemic lupus erythematosus	
Thyroid antibodies	≤1:10 titer	Same as conventional units	Early hypothyroidism, Graves' disease, Hashimoto's thyroiditis, pernicious anemia, systemic lupus erythematosus, thyroid carcinoma	
VDRL	Nonreactive	Same as conventional units	Syphilis	

TABLE C-4	**Urine Chemistry**				

Test	Specimen	Normal Values — Conventional Units	Normal Values — SI Units	Possible Etiology — Higher	Possible Etiology — Lower
Acetone	Random	Negative	Negative	Diabetes mellitus, high-fat and low-carbohydrate diets, starvation states	
Aldosterone	24 hr	1-80 mcg/day (depends on urinary sodium)	2.7-222 nmol/day	*Primary aldosteronism:* adrenocortical tumors *Secondary aldosteronism:* cardiac failure, cirrhosis, large dose of ACTH, salt depletion	ACTH deficiency, Addison's disease, corticosteroid therapy
Amylase	24 hr	1-17 U/hr	Same as conventional units	Acute pancreatitis	
Bence Jones protein	Random	Negative	Negative	Biliary duct obstruction, multiple myeloma	
Bilirubin	Random	Negative	Negative	Hepatitis	
Calcium	24 hr	100-250 mg/day	2.5-6.3 mmol/day	Bone tumor, hyperparathyroidism, milk-alkali syndrome	Hypoparathyroidism, malabsorption of calcium and vitamin D
Catecholamines	24 hr			Heart failure, pheochromocytoma, progressive muscular dystrophy	
Epinephrine		<20 mcg/day	<118 nmol/day		
Norepinephrine		<100 mcg/day	<591 nmol/day		
Chloride	24 hr	110-250 mEq/day	110-250 mmol/day	Addison's disease	Burns, diarrhea, excessive perspiration, menstruation, vomiting
Copper	24 hr	<30 mcg/day	<0.5 μmol/day	Cirrhosis, Wilson's disease	
Coproporphyrin	24 hr	50-200 mcg/day	76-305 nmol/day	Lead poisoning, oral contraceptive use, poliomyelitis	
Creatine	24 hr	<100 mg/day	<763 μmol/day	Addison's disease, burns, carcinoma of liver, diabetes, hyperthyroidism, infections, muscular dystrophy, skeletal muscle atrophy	Hypothyroidism
Creatinine	24 hr	0.8-2.0 g/day	7.1-17.7 mmol/day	Anemia, leukemia, muscular atrophy, salmonellae	Renal disease
Creatinine clearance	24 hr	85-135 ml/min	1.42-2.25 ml/sec		Renal disease
Estrogens	24 hr				
Female				Gonadal or adrenal tumor	Agenesis of ovaries, endocrine disturbance, menopause, ovarian dysfunction
Ovulation peak		28-100 mcg/day	104-370 nmol/day		
Luteal peak		22-80 mcg/day	81-296 nmol/day		
Pregnancy		Up to 45,000 mcg/day	Up to 166,455 nmol/day		
Menopause		1.4-19.6 mcg/day	5.2-72.5 nmol/day		
Male		5-18 mcg/day	18-67 nmol/day		
Glucose	Random	Negative	Negative	Diabetes mellitus, low renal threshold for glucose resorption, physiologic stress, pituitary disorders	
Hemoglobin	Random	Negative	Negative	Extensive burns, glomerulonephritis, hemolytic anemias, hemolytic transfusion reaction	
5-Hydroxyindole-acetic acid (5-HIAA)	24 hr	2-9 mg/day	10.5-47.1 μmol/day	Malignant carcinoid syndrome	
Ketone bodies	24 hr	20-50 mg/day	0.34-0.86 mmol/day	Marked ketonuria	
Lead	24 hr	<100 mcg/day	<0.48 μmol/day	Lead poisoning	
Metanephrine	24 hr	<1.3 mg/day	<7.1 μmol/day	Pheochromocytoma	
Myoglobin	Random	Negative	Negative	Crushing injuries, electrical injuries, extreme physical exertion	

ACTH, Adrenocorticotropic hormone.

TABLE C-4	Urine Chemistry—cont'd				

		Normal Values		Possible Etiology	
Test	**Specimen**	**Conventional Units**	**SI Units**	**Higher**	**Lower**
pH	Random	4.0-8.0	Same as conventional units	Chronic renal failure, compensatory phase of alkalosis, salicylate intoxication, vegetarian diet	Compensatory phase of acidosis, dehydration, emphysema
Phenylpyruvic acid	Random	Negative	Negative	Phenylketonuria	
Phosphorus, inorganic	24 hr	0.9-1.3 g/day	29-42 mmol/day	Fever, hypoparathyroidism, nervous exhaustion, rickets, tuberculosis	Acute infections, nephritis
Porphobilinogen	Random	Negative	Negative	Acute intermittent porphyria, liver disorders	
	24 hr	<2.0 mg/day	<9 μmol/day		
Protein (dipstick)	Random	Negative	Negative	Heart failure, nephritis, nephrosis, physiologic stress	
Protein (quantitative)	24 hr	<150 mg/day	<0.15 g/day	Cardiac failure, inflammatory processes of urinary tract, nephritis, nephrosis, toxemia of pregnancy	
Sodium	24 hr	40-250 mEq/day	40-250 mmol/day	Acute tubular necrosis	Hyponatremia
Specific gravity	Random	1.003-1.030	Same as conventional units	Albuminuria, dehydration, glycosuria	Diabetes insipidus
Titratable acidity	24 hr	20-50 mEq/day	Same as conventional units	Metabolic acidosis	Metabolic alkalosis
Uric acid	24 hr	250-750 mg/day	1.5-4.5 mmol/day	Gout, leukemia	Nephritis
Urobilinogen	24 hr	0.5-4.0 mg/day	0.8-6.8 μmol/day	Hemolytic disease, hepatic parenchymal cell damage, liver disease	Complete obstruction of bile duct
	Random	<1.0 mg	1.7 μmol		
Uroporphyrins	Random	Random	Same as conventional units	Porphyria	
Vanillylmandelic acid	24 hr	1-8 mg/day 1.5-7.0 mcg/mg creatine	5-40 μmol/day	Pheochromocytoma	

TABLE C-5	Gastric Analysis				

	Normal Values		Possible Etiology	
Test	**Conventional Units**	**SI Units**	**Higher**	**Lower**
Basal				
Free hydrochloric acid	0.30 mEq/L	Same as conventional units	Hypermotility of stomach	Pernicious anemia
Total acidity	15-45 mEq/L	Same as conventional units	Gastric and duodenal ulcers, Zollinger-Ellison syndrome	Gastric carcinoma, severe gastritis
Poststimulation				
Free hydrochloric acid	10-130 mEq/L	Same as conventional units		
Total acidity	20-150 mEq/L	Same as conventional units		

TABLE C-6	**Fecal Analysis**			
	Normal Values		**Possible Etiology**	
Test	**Conventional Units**	**SI Units**	**Higher**	**Lower**
Blood*	Negative	Negative	Anal fissures, hemorrhoids, inflammatory bowel disease, malignant tumor, peptic ulcer	
Fecal fat	<6 g/24 hr	Same as conventional units	Chronic pancreatic disease, malabsorption syndrome, obstruction of common bile duct	
Mucus	Negative	Negative	Mucous colitis, spastic constipation	
Pus	Negative	Negative	Chronic bacillary dysentery, chronic ulcerative colitis, localized abscesses	
Urobilinogen	30-220 mg/100 g of stool	51-372 μmol/100 g of stool	Hemolytic anemias	Complete biliary obstruction
Color				
Brown			Various shades depending on diet	
Clay			Biliary obstruction or presence of barium sulfate	
Tarry			More than 100 ml of blood in gastrointestinal tract	
Red			Blood in large intestine	
Black			Blood in upper gastrointestinal tract or iron medication	

*Ingestion of meat may produce false-positive results. Patient may be placed on a meat-free diet for 3 days before the test.

TABLE C-7	**Cerebrospinal Fluid Analysis**			
	Normal Values		**Possible Etiology**	
Test	**Conventional Units**	**SI Units**	**Higher**	**Lower**
Pressure	60-150 mm H_2O	Same as conventional units	Hemorrhage, intracranial tumor, meningitis	Head injury, spinal tumor, subdural hematoma
Blood	Negative	Negative	Intracranial hemorrhage	
Cell count (age dependent)			Inflammation or infections of CNS	
WBC	0-5 cells/μl	0.5×10^6/L		
RBC	0 cells/μl	0×10^6/L		
Chloride	100-130 mEq/L	100-130 mmol/L	Uremia	Bacterial infections of CNS (meningitis, encephalitis)
Glucose	40-75 mg/dl	2.5-4.2 mmol/L	Diabetes mellitus, viral infections of CNS	Bacterial infections and tuberculosis of CNS
Protein				
Lumbar	15-45 mg/dl	0.15-0.45 g/L	Guillain-Barré syndrome, poliomyelitis, traumatic tap	
Cisternal	15-25 mg/dl	0.15-0.25 g/L	Syphilis of CNS	
Ventricular	5-15 mg/dl	0.05-0.15 g/L	Acute meningitis, brain tumor, chronic CNS infections, multiple sclerosis	

CNS, Central nervous system; *RBC,* red blood cells; *WBC,* white blood cells.

Chapter 1
1. b
2. c
3. c
4. c
5. a
6. c
7. c
8. c
9. b
10. a
11. c
12. b
13. d

Chapter 2
1. a
2. b
3. b
4. c
5. d

Chapter 3
1. d
2. d
3. a
4. b
5. d
6. b
7. b

Chapter 4
1. d
2. a
3. a
4. c
5. a

Chapter 5
1. d
2. c
3. a
4. a
5. b
6. a
7. b
8. d
9. b
10. a

Chapter 6
1. c
2. a
3. d

4. c
5. d
6. a
7. a
8. c
9. c

Chapter 7
1. d
2. c
3. a
4. c

Chapter 8
1. b
2. d
3. c
4. b
5. d
6. c
7. c
8. c

Chapter 9
1. b
2. a
3. c
4. b
5. b
6. c
7. d

Chapter 10
1. b
2. d
3. d
4. c
5. c
6. b
7. b
8. c
9. c
10. d

Chapter 11
1. b
2. a
3. d
4. c
5. c
6. d
7. d
8. a
9. c

Chapter 12
1. d
2. c
3. a
4. b
5. d
6. b
7. b
8. d
9. b
10. b

Chapter 13
1. b
2. b
3. d
4. d
5. a
6. c
7. b
8. a
9. c

Chapter 14
1. d
2. c
3. d
4. c
5. a
6. d
7. a
8. d
9. d
10. c
11. a
12. d
13. b

Chapter 15
1. a
2. a
3. a
4. c
5. d
6. a
7. c
8. b
9. c
10. a
11. a
12. d

Chapter 16
1. d
2. d
3. d
4. a
5. d
6. b
7. c
8. d
9. b
10. d
11. a
12. c
13. a
14. d
15. a

Chapter 17
1. d
2. a
3a. a
3b. a
3c. c
3d. c
3e. c
3f. a
4. a
5. d
6. b

Chapter 18
1. d
2. c
3. c
4. a
5. b
6. c
7. a
8. d

Chapter 19
1. b
2. c
3. c
4. c
5. a
6. d
7. b
8. b
9. c
10. b

Chapter 20
1. b
2. b
3. d
4. a
5. c
6. a

Chapter 21
1. b
2. d
3. c
4. a
5. b
6. d
7. a

Chapter 22
1. b
2. d
3. c
4. b
5. d
6. b
7. a
8. a
9. b
10. a
11. d

Chapter 23
1. b
2. b
3. d
4. c
5. a
6. a
7. a
8. a
9. b

Chapter 24
1. c
2. b
3. d
4. a
5. b
6. a
7. c
8. b
9. a
10. a

Chapter 25
1. c
2. a
3. c
4. d
5. c
6. c
7. b
8. b
9. a
10. b
11. b

Chapter 26
1. c
2. d

3. c
4. a
5. c
6. b
7. c
8. a
9. b
10. d
11. a

Chapter 27
1. d
2. d
3. a
4. c
5. b
6. d
7. d
8. d

Chapter 28
1. a
2. d
3. a
4. a
5. b
6. a
7. b
8. c
9. a
10. c
11. d
12. c
13. b

Chapter 29
1. a
2. a
3. a
4. d
5. c
6. d
7. d
8. c

Chapter 30
1. b
2. d
3. b
4. a
5. a
6. c
7. b
8. b

Chapter 31
1. a
2. b
3. d
4. c
5. a
6. a
7. d
8. c
9. d
10. d
11. c
12. c
13. b

14. c
15. d
16. d

Chapter 32
1. c
2. d
3. c
4. b
5. a
6. b
7. d
8. b
9. a
10. c
11. a

Chapter 33
1. d
2. b
3. d
4. b
5. d
6. d
7. a
8. d

Chapter 34
1. c
2. a
3. b
4. d
5. c
6. c
7. b
8. d

Chapter 35
1. b
2. c
3. d
4. a
5. c

Chapter 36
1. d
2. c
3. d
4. d
5. a
6. b
7. a

Chapter 37
1. b
2. c
3. a
4. b
5. c
6. b
7. a
8. c
9. c
10. b
11. a
12. c

Chapter 38
1. a
2. c
3. b
4. d
5. c
6. b
7. a
8. d
9. d
10. c
11. b
12. d
13. c

Chapter 39
1. d
2. b
3. b
4. a
5. b
6. c
7. b
8. a
9. b

Chapter 40
1. c
2. d
3. a
4. c
5. a
6. b
7. c

Chapter 41
1. c
2. d
3. d
4. d
5. c
6. d
7. c

Chapter 42
1. b
2. a
3. d
4. c
5. d
6. c
7. c
8. d
9. d
10. b

Chapter 43
1. a
2. d
3. b
4. c
5. a
6. c
7. a
8. b
9. d
10. a
11. d

Chapter 44
1. a
2. b
3. b
4. b
5. b
6. a
7. d
8. c
9. c
10. a
11. b

Chapter 45
1. d
2. b
3. d
4. c
5. b
6. a
7. c
8. d

Chapter 46
1. d
2. b
3. b
4. a
5. d
6. a
7. d
8. d
9. b
10. a
11. b
12. d

Chapter 47
1. a
2. b
3. b
4. c
5. d
6. c
7. d
8. c
9. a
10. d
11. b

Chapter 48
1. b
2. c
3. a
4. d
5. a
6. c
7. a
8. b
9. a

Chapter 49
1. b
2. d
3. d
4. d
5. d
6. c
7. c
8. a

Chapter 50
1. a
2. b
3. c
4. d
5. d
6. d
7. a
8. c

Chapter 51
1. c
2. c
3. d
4. c
5. c
6. a
7. a
8. d

Chapter 52
1. d
2. d
3. c
4. a
5. c
6. c
7. d
8. a

Chapter 53
1. b
2. a
3. c
4. d
5. d
6. c
7. b

Chapter 54
1. b
2. d
3. d
4. c
5. c
6. b
7. c
8. d
9. b
10. a
11. c
12. d
13. a

Chapter 55
1. b
2. d
3. c
4. a
5. c
6. c
7. c

Chapter 56
1. d
2. d
3. d
4. c

5. b
6. b
7. d
8. a
9. c
10. a
11. b

Chapter 57
1. b
2. d
3. b
4. c
5. a
6. a
7. c
8. d
9. b
10. b

Chapter 58
1. d
2. c
3. d
4. c
5. c
6. c
7. b
8. c
9. b

Chapter 59
1. a
2. b
3. c
4. c
5. d

Chapter 60
1. d
2. c
3. d
4. b
5. b
6. a
7. b
8. d

Chapter 61
1. d
2. d
3. d
4. c
5. b
6. c
7. a
8. b
9. c

Chapter 62
1. d
2. b
3. d
4. d
5. c
6. d
7. c
8. d
9. a

Chapter 63
1. d
2. a
3. d
4. c
5. d
6. b
7. a
8. d
9. b

Chapter 64
1. d
2. d
3. a
4. d
5. c
6. a
7. b

Chapter 65
1. c
2. c
3. d
4. a
5. a
6. d
7. c

Chapter 66
1. d
2. b
3. c
4. c
5. b
6. c
7. a
8. c

Chapter 67
1. c
2. d
3. a
4. b
5. a
6. d

Chapter 68
1. b
2. c
3. d
4. a
5. c
6. c

Chapter 69
1. d
2. b
3. d
4. c
5. d
6. d

Glossary

α_1**-antitrypsin:** a serum protein produced by the liver normally found in the lungs that inhibits proteolytic enzymes of white blood cells from lysing lung tissue; genetic deficiency of this protein can cause emphysema

absence (petit mal) seizure: seizure characterized by a brief staring spell and a very brief loss of consciousness that usually occurs only in children and rarely continues beyond adolescence

acoustic neuroma: a benign tumor that occurs where the acoustic nerve (CN VIII) enters the internal auditory canal or the temporal bone from the brain

acquired immunodeficiency syndrome (AIDS): end stage of chronic HIV infection; a syndrome involving a defect in cell-mediated immunity that has a long incubation period and is manifested by various opportunistic infections and cancers

acromegaly: a condition caused by excessive secretion of growth hormone characterized by an overgrowth of the bones and soft tissues

actinic keratosis: a slowly developing, localized thickening and scaling of the outer layers of the skin consisting of hyperkeratotic papules and plaques as a result of chronic, prolonged exposure to the sun, also known as solar keratosis

acute bronchitis: an inflammation of the lower respiratory tract that is usually due to infection

acute coronary syndrome: develops when the oxygen supply to the myocardium is diminished and not immediately reversible

acute pancreatitis: an acute inflammatory process of the pancreas caused by autodigestion and marked by symptoms of acute abdomen and escape of pancreatic enzymes into the pancreatic tissues

acute renal failure: clinical syndrome characterized by a rapid decline in renal function with progressive azotemia and increasing levels of serum creatinine

acute respiratory distress syndrome (ARDS): a sudden and progressive form of acute respiratory failure in which the alveolar-capillary membrane becomes damaged and more permeable to intravascular fluid

acute tubular necrosis: a type of intrarenal acute renal failure affecting the renal tubules caused by renal ischemia and nephrotoxic injury

adhesion: a band of scar tissue between or around organs

adventitious sounds: extra breath sounds that are not normally heard, such as crackles, rhonchi, wheezes, and pleural friction rubs

afterload: the peripheral resistance against which the left ventricle must pump

allergic rhinitis: the reaction of the nasal mucosa to a specific allergen

alopecia: partial or complete lack of hair resulting from normal aging, endocrine disorder, drug reaction, anticancer medication, or skin disease

Alzheimer's disease (AD): a chronic, progressive, degenerative disease of the brain

amyotrophic lateral sclerosis (ALS): a rare progressive neurologic disorder characterized by loss of motor neurons and by weakness and atrophy of the muscles of the hands, forearms, and legs, spreading to involve most of the body and face

anaphylactic shock: an acute and life-threatening hypersensitivity (allergic) reaction to a sensitizing substance, such as a drug, chemical, vaccine, food, or insect venom

andropause: a decline in androgen secretion that occurs in most males due to aging

aneurysm: congenital or acquired weakness of the arterial wall resulting in dilation and ballooning of the vessel

angina: chest pain that is the clinical manifestation of reversible myocardial ischemia

angiopathy: blood vessel disease

ankylosing spondylitis: a chronic inflammatory disease that primarily affects the axial skeleton, including the sacroiliac joints, intervertebral disk spaces, and costovertebral articulations

ankylosis: stiffness or fixation of a joint usually resulting from destruction of articular cartilage and subchondral bone

aortic dissection: the result of a tear in the intimal (innermost) lining of the arterial wall that allows blood to enter between the intima and media, thus, creating a false lumen

aortic stenosis: a narrowing or stricture of the aortic valve resulting in obstruction of the flow from the left ventricle to the aorta during systole

aortic valve regurgitation: backward flow of blood into the left ventricle when the valve should be closed

aphasia: an abnormal neurologic condition in which language function is disordered or absent because of an injury to certain areas of the cerebral cortex

aplastic anemia: a disease with a deficiency of all of the formed elements of blood (specifically red blood cells, white blood cells, and platelets), representing a failure of the cell-generating capacity of bone marrow

apnea: an absence of spontaneous respirations

appendicitis: an inflammation of the appendix that if undiagnosed, leads rapidly to perforation and peritonitis

arterial blood pressure: a measure of the pressure exerted by blood against the walls of the arterial system

arthritis: inflammation of a joint; most prevalent types are osteoarthritis, rheumatoid arthritis, and gout

arthrocentesis: incision or puncture of joint capsule to obtain samples of synovial fluid from within joint cavity or to remove excess fluid

arthrodesis: the surgical fusion of a joint

arthroplasty: surgical reconstruction or replacement of a joint

arthroscopy: insertion of an arthroscope into a joint for visualization or surgery

Aschoff's bodies: tiny rounded or spindle-shaped nodules formed by a reaction to myocardial inflammation with accompanying swelling and fragmentation of collagen fibers

ascites: an abnormal intraperitoneal accumulation of a fluid containing large amounts of protein and electrolytes as a result of portal hypertension

asterixis: flapping tremor (liver flap) commonly affecting the arms and hands that is a manifestation of hepatic encephalopathy

asthma: a chronic inflammatory lung disease that results in airflow obstruction

asystole: represents the total absence of ventricular electrical activity

atelectasis: an abnormal condition characterized by the collapse of alveoli

atherosclerosis: formation of focal deposits of cholesterol and lipids known as atheromas or plaque, primarily within the intimal wall of arteries, that obstruct circulation

atrial fibrillation: a cardiac dysrhythmia characterized by a total disorganization of atrial electrical activity without effective atrial contraction

atrial flutter: an atrial tachydysrhythmia identified by recurring, regular, sawtooth-shaped flutter waves

atrophy: wasting of muscle, characterized by decreased circumference and flabby appearance leading to decreased function and tone

atypical absence seizures: a type of seizure characterized by a staring spell accompanied by other signs and symptoms, including brief warnings, peculiar behavior during the seizure, or confusion afterward

aura: a sensation of light or warmth or other perception that may be a warning of an attack of a migraine or an epileptic seizure

auscultation: the act of listening for sounds within the body to evaluate the condition of the heart, blood vessels, lungs, pleura, intestines, or other organs

autoimmunity: an inappropriate immune reaction to self-proteins

automaticity: a property of specialized cells of the heart found in the sinoatrial (SA) node, parts of the atria, the atrioventricular (AV) node, and the His-Purkinje system, that are able to discharge spontaneously

azotemia: an accumulation of nitrogenous waste products such as blood urea nitrogen (BUN) and creatinine

bariatric surgery: a surgical procedure that is used to treat morbid obesity

Barrett's esophagus: a precancerous esophageal disorder characterized by metaplastic cell changes

basal cell carcinoma: a malignant epithelial cell tumor arising from epidermal basal cells that begins as a papule and enlarges peripherally, developing a central crater that erodes, crusts, and bleeds

Bell's palsy: a disorder characterized by a disruption of the motor branches of the facial nerve (CN VII) on one side of the face in the absence of any other disease, such as a stroke

benign neoplasm: a localized tumor that has a fibrous capsule, limited potential for growth, a regular shape, and cells that are well differentiated

benign prostatic hyperplasia (BPH): a nonmalignant, noninflammatory enlargement of the prostate gland caused by an increase in the number of epithelial cells and stromal tissue

biologic therapy: treatment using biologic agents such as interferons, interleukins, monoclonal antibodies, and growth factors to modify the relationship between the host and the tumor

blepharitis: a chronic inflammatory condition of the lash follicles and meibomian glands of the eyelids, characterized by swelling, redness, and crusts of dried mucus on the lids

bone marrow transplant: the transplantation of bone marrow from healthy donors to stimulate production of normal blood cells

borborygmi: audible abdominal sounds produced by hyperactive intestinal peristalsis

botulism: a serious food poisoning caused by GI absorption of the neurotoxin produced by *Clostridium botulinum* that results in disturbed muscle innervation

brachytherapy: radiation delivery system that means "closed" treatment and consists of the implantation or insertion of radioactive materials directly into the tumor or in close proximity to the tumor

brain abscess: an accumulation of pus within the brain tissue that can result from a local or a systemic infection from another source, such as the skull, sinuses, or other structures in the head

brain attack: term used to describe a stroke

brain death: an irreversible form of unconsciousness characterized by a complete loss of brain function while the heart continues to beat

bronchospasm: narrowing and obstruction of the lumen of the bronchi caused by spasm of the peribronchial smooth muscle

Brown-Séquard syndrome: damage to one half of the spinal cord characterized by spastic paralysis on the body's injured side, loss of postural sense (proprioception), and loss of the senses of pain and heat on the other side of the body

bursitis: inflammation of the bursa

calculus: an abnormal stone formed in body tissues by an accumulation of mineral salts

carcinogens: agents capable of producing cellular alterations leading to the development or increasing the incidence of neoplastic growth

carcinoma in situ: a lesion with all the histologic features of cancer except invasion

carcinomas: malignant tumors that originate from embryonal ectoderm and endoderm

cardiac index: a measure of the cardiac output of a patient per square meter of body surface area

cardiac output: the amount of blood pumped by each ventricle in 1 minute

cardiac pacemaker: an electronic device used to increase the heart rate in severe bradycardia by electrically stimulating the heart muscle

cardiac reserve: the ability to respond to demands (exercise, stress, hypovolemia) by altering cardiac output threefold or fourfold

cardiac tamponade: compression of the heart produced by fluid accumulation in the pericardial sac

cardiogenic shock: shock occurring when either systolic or diastolic dysfunction of the myocardium results in compromised cardiac output

cardiomyopathy: a group of diseases that directly affect the structural or functional ability of the myocardium

carpal tunnel syndrome: a condition caused by compression of the median nerve beneath the transverse carpal ligament within the narrow confines of the carpal tunnel located in the wrist

cataract: an abnormal progressive condition of the lens of the eye, characterized by an opacity within the lens

celiac disease: an inborn error of metabolism characterized by the inability to hydrolyze peptides contained in gluten

cell-mediated immunity: immunity that is initiated through specific antigen recognition by T lymphocytes, macrophages, and natural killer cells

central cord syndrome: damage to the central spinal cord characterized by microscopic hemorrhage, edema of the central spinal cord, and compression on anterior horn cells

cerebral edema: increased accumulation of fluid in the extravascular spaces of brain tissue that can lead to increased intracranial pressure

chancre: painless indurated lesions found on the penis, vulva, lips, mouth, vagina, and rectum characteristic of syphilis

cheilosis: a disorder of the lips and mouth characterized by bilateral scales and fissures, resulting from a deficiency of riboflavin in the diet

chemotherapy: the treatment of disease with chemical agents

chest physiotherapy: a series of maneuvers including percussion, vibration, and postural drainage designed to promote clearance of excessive respiratory secretions

Cheyne-Stokes respiration: an abnormal pattern of breathing characterized by alternating periods of apnea and deep, rapid breathing

chlamydial infections: superficial mucosal infections caused by *Chlamydia trachomatis*

cholecystitis: inflammation of the gallbladder

cholelithiasis: stones in the gallbladder

cholesteatoma: a cystic mass composed of epithelial cells and cholesterol that is found in the middle ear and occurs as a congenital defect or as a serious complication of chronic otitis media

chronic bronchitis: obstructive pulmonary disease characterized by excessive production of mucus and chronic inflammatory changes in the bronchi

chronic fatigue syndrome: a disorder characterized by debilitating fatigue and a variety of associated complaints

chronic kidney disease: the presence of kidney damage or decreased glomerular filtration rate for at least 3 months with functional or structural abnormalities, with or without decreased glomerular filtration rate

chronic obstructive pulmonary disease (COPD): pulmonary disease state characterized by the presence of airflow obstruction caused by chronic bronchitis or emphysema

chronic pancreatitis: progressive destruction of the pancreas with fibrotic replacement of pancreatic tissue

chronic stable angina: chest pain that occurs intermittently over a long period with the same pattern of onset, duration, and intensity of symptoms

cirrhosis: chronic progressive disease of the liver characterized by extensive degeneration and destruction of the liver parenchymal cells

cluster headache: repeated headaches that can occur for weeks to months at a time, followed by periods of remission

collateral circulation: development of arterial branching that occurs within the coronary circulation when occlusion of the coronary arteries occurs slowly over a long period

coma: profound state of unconsciousness

community-acquired pneumonia: a lower respiratory tract infection of the lung parenchyma with onset in the community or during the first 2 days of hospitalization

compartment syndrome: a condition in which elevated intracompartmental pressure within a confined myofascial compartment compromises the neurovascular function of tissues within that space

complete heart block: third-degree atrioventricular heart block in which no impulses from the atria are conducted to the ventricles

concussion: a sudden transient mechanical head injury, such as a blow or explosion, with disruption of neural activity and a change in the level of consciousness

conjunctivitis: an infection or inflammation of the conjunctiva, caused by bacterial or viral infection, allergy, or environmental factors

conscious sedation: a minimally depressed level of consciousness with maintenance of the patient's protective airway reflexes

continuous renal replacement therapy: provides a means by which solutes and fluids can be removed slowly and continuously in the hemodynamically unstable patient

contracture: an abnormal, usually permanent condition of a joint, characterized by flexion and fixation

contusion: the bruising of the brain tissue within a focal area without altering the integrity of the pia mater and arachnoid layers

coronary artery disease: an abnormal condition that may affect the heart's arteries and produce various pathologic effects, especially the reduced flow of oxygen and nutrients to the myocardium

cor pulmonale: hypertrophy of the right side of the heart, with or without heart failure, resulting from pulmonary hypertension

crackles: short, low-pitched sounds consisting of discontinuous bubbling caused by air passing through airway intermittently occluded by mucus, unstable bronchial wall, or fold of mucosa

crepitation: crackling sound or grating sensation as a result of friction between bones

cretinism: hypothyroidism that develops in infancy

Crohn's disease: a chronic inflammatory bowel disorder that can affect any part of the GI tract from the mouth to the anus

cryosurgery: the use of subfreezing temperatures to perform surgery

cultured epithelial autograft: skin grafts grown from biopsy specimens obtained from the patient's own skin

curettage: scraping of material from the wall of a cavity or other surface, performed to remove tumors or other abnormal tissue or to obtain tissue

Cushing syndrome: a metabolic disorder resulting from the chronic and excessive production of cortisol by the adrenal cortex or by the administration of glucocorticoids in large doses for several weeks or longer

cystic fibrosis: an autosomal recessive, multisystem disease characterized by altered function of the exocrine glands involving primarily the lungs, pancreas, and sweat glands

cystitis: an inflammatory condition of the urinary bladder, characterized by pain, urgency and frequency of urination, and hematuria

cystocele: herniation or protrusion of the urinary bladder through the wall of the vagina, resulting from weakened connective tissue support between the vagina and bladder

death rattle: a sound produced by air moving through mucus that has accumulated in the throat of a dying person who has lost the cough reflex

debridement: removal of dirt, foreign objects, damaged tissue, and cellular debris from a wound or a burn to prevent infection and promote healing

deep vein thrombosis: a disorder involving a thrombus in a deep vein; most commonly the iliac and femoral veins

degenerative disk disease: progressive degeneration that is a normal process of aging; results in the intervertebral disks losing their elasticity, flexibility, and shock-absorbing capabilities

dehiscence: the separation and disruption of previously joined wound edges, typically an abdominal incision

delirium: a state of temporary but acute mental confusion

dementia: a syndrome caused by brain disease, evidenced by chronic personality disintegration, confusion, memory impairment, deterioration of intellectual capacity and function

dermatome: the area of skin innervated by the sensory fibers of a single dorsal root of a spinal nerve

dermatomyositis: a disease of the connective tissues, characterized by pruritic or eczematous inflammation of the skin and tenderness of the muscles

diabetes insipidus: a group of conditions associated with deficient production or secretion of antidiuretic hormone (ADH), or a decreased renal response to ADH caused by injury of the neurohypophyseal system

diabetes mellitus: a multisystem disease related to abnormal insulin production, impaired insulin utilization, or both

diabetic ketoacidosis (DKA): an acute metabolic complication of diabetes occurring when fats are metabolized in the absence of insulin resulting in formation of acid by-products, such as ketones

diabetic nephropathy: a microvascular complication of diabetes mellitus associated with damage to the small blood vessels that supply the glomeruli of the kidney

diabetic neuropathy: nerve damage that occurs because of the metabolic derangements associated with diabetes mellitus and characterized by sensory and/or motor disturbances in the peripheral nervous system

diabetic retinopathy: the process of microvascular damage to the retina in patients with diabetes

dialysis: technique in which substances move from the blood through a semipermeable membrane and into a dialysis solution

diastolic blood pressure: the residual pressure of the arterial system during ventricular relaxation

dislocation: a severe injury of the ligamentous structures that surround a joint resulting in the complete displacement or separation of the articular surfaces of the joint

disseminated intravascular coagulation (DIC): a grave coagulopathy resulting from the overstimulation of clotting and anticlotting processes in response to disease or injury

diverticulum: a saccular dilation or outpouching of the mucosa through the circular smooth muscle of the intestinal wall

dysarthria: a disturbance in the muscular control of speech, resulting from interference in the control and execution over the muscles of speech

dysmenorrhea: abdominal cramping pain or discomfort associated with menstrual flow

dyspareunia: abnormal pain during sexual intercourse

dysphagia: difficulty swallowing

dysphasia: difficulty related to the comprehension or use of language

dysplastic nevi: nevi that are larger than usual with irregular borders and various shades of color; also known as atypical moles

dyspnea: shortness of breath; difficulty breathing that may be caused by certain heart or lung conditions, strenuous exercise, or anxiety

ecchymosis: bruising

ectopic pregnancy: the implantation of the fertilized ovum anywhere outside the uterine cavity

ejection fraction: percentage of end-diastolic blood volume that is ejected during systole

electrocardiogram: a graphic tracing of the electrical impulses produced in the heart

embolic stroke: a stroke that occurs when an embolus lodges in and occludes a cerebral artery, resulting in infarction and edema of the area supplied by the involved vessel

emergence delirium: a neurologic alteration in recovery from anesthesia that can include behaviors such as restlessness, agitation, disorientation, thrashing, and shouting

emerging infection: an infectious disease whose incidence has increased in the past 20 years or threatens to increase in the immediate future

emphysema: an abnormal condition of the pulmonary system, characterized by overinflation and destructive changes in alveolar walls

empyema: an accumulation of purulent exudates in a body cavity, especially the pleural space, as a result of bacterial infection, such as pleurisy or tuberculosis

encephalitis: an acute inflammation of the brain usually caused by a virus

endometriosis: the presence of normal endometrial tissue in sites outside the endometrial cavity

endoscopy: the direct visualization of a body structure through a lighted instrument (scope)

endotracheal intubation: artificial airway created by inserting a tube into the trachea through the mouth or nose past the larynx, bypassing upper airway and laryngeal structures

end-stage renal disease (ESRD): last stage of kidney disease occurring when the GFR is less than 5% to 10% of normal or when creatinine clearances are less than 15 ml/min

enteral nutrition: the administration of a nutritionally balanced liquefied food or formula through a tube inserted into the stomach, duodenum, or jejunum

enucleation: removal of the eye

epididymitis: acute or chronic inflammation of the epididymis, usually secondary to an infectious process, trauma, or urinary reflux down the vas deferens

epidural analgesia: the infusion of pain-relieving medications through a catheter placed into the epidural space surrounding the spinal cord

epidural block: injection of a local anesthetic into the epidural (extradural) space by either a thoracic or lumbar approach

epidural hematoma: collection of blood between the dura and the inner surface of the skull, producing compression of the dura matter and thus of the brain

epilepsy: a condition in which a person has spontaneously recurring seizures caused by a chronic underlying condition

epistaxis: nosebleed

erectile dysfunction: the inability to attain or maintain an erect penis that allows satisfactory sexual performance

escharotomy: incisions into necrotic tissue from a severe burn performed when eschar formation compromises circulation

esophageal diverticulum: saclike outpouching of one or more layers of the esophagus

esophageal speech: a method of swallowing air, trapping it in the esophagus, and releasing it to create sound

esophageal varices: distended, tortuous, fragile veins at the lower end of the esophagus that result from portal hypertension

esophagitis: inflammation of the mucosal lining of the esophagus, caused by infection, irritation from a nasogastric tube, or, most commonly, backflow of gastric juice from the stomach

evisceration: the separation and disruption of previously joined wound edges to the extent that an internal organ, typically intestinal contents, protrudes through the wound

excision and grafting: procedure during which eschar is removed down to the subcutaneous tissue or fascia, depending on the degree of injury; a graft is then placed on clean, viable tissue to achieve good adherence

exophthalmos: protrusion of the eyeballs from the orbits caused by increased fat deposits and fluid in the retroorbital tissues

external otitis: inflammation or infection of the epithelium of the auricle and ear canal

fat embolism syndrome: embolization of fat globules that occurs in a small percentage of patients with fractures

fibrinolysis: a continual process resulting in the dissolution of fibrin to maintain blood in its fluid form

fibroadenoma: a small, painless, round, well-delineated, mobile benign breast tumor commonly found in young women

fibrocystic changes: a benign condition of the breasts characterized by development of excess fibrous tissue, hyperplasia of the epithelial lining of the mammary ducts, proliferation of mammary ducts, and cyst formation

fibromyalgia syndrome: a chronic disorder characterized by widespread, nonarticular musculoskeletal pain and fatigue with multiple tender points

flail chest: instability of the chest wall resulting from multiple rib fractures

fracture: a disruption or break in the continuity of the structure of bone

fremitus: vibration of the chest wall produced by vocalization

frontotemporal dementia: dementia of the temporal and/or frontal lobes

frostbite: freezing that results in the formation of ice crystals in the tissues and cells

full-thickness burn: destruction of all skin elements and subcutaneous tissues, with possible involvement of muscles, tendons, and bones

galactorrhea: a milky secretion from the nipple caused by inappropriate lactation

gastritis: inflammation of the gastric mucosa

gastroenteritis: an inflammation of the mucosa of the stomach and small intestine

gastroesophageal reflux disease (GERD): any clinically significant symptomatic condition or histopathologic alteration presumed to be secondary to reflux of gastric contents into the lower esophagus

generalized seizures: seizures characterized by bilateral synchronous epileptic discharge in the brain with loss of consciousness for a few seconds to several minutes

genital herpes: a sexually transmitted disease caused by the herpes simplex virus, type 2 (HSV-2) resulting in painful genital or anal vesicular lesions

Glasgow Coma Scale: assessment tool for altered states of consciousness that evaluates motor responses, verbal responses, and eye opening

glaucoma: a group of disorders characterized by (1) increased intraocular pressure and the consequences of elevated pressure, (2) optic nerve atrophy, and (3) peripheral visual field loss

glomerular filtration rate: the amount of blood filtered by the glomeruli in a given time

glomerulonephritis: an immune-related inflammation of the glomeruli characterized by proteinuria, hematuria, decreased urine production, and edema

glycemic index: term used to describe the rise in blood glucose levels after a person has consumed a carbohydrate-containing food

goiter: enlargement of the thyroid gland that may be associated with hyperthyroidism, hypothyroidism, or normal thyroid function

gonorrhea: infection of the genitalia, the rectum, and/or the oropharynx by *Neisseria gonorrhoeae*, which, if left untreated, leads to the formation of fibrous tissue and adhesions

Goodpasture syndrome: an example of cytotoxic autoimmune disease, characterized by the presence of circulating antibodies against the glomerular basement membrane and alveolar basement membrane

gout: recurrent attacks of acute arthritis associated with increased levels of serum uric acid

Graves' disease: an autoimmune disease of unknown etiology marked by diffuse thyroid enlargement and excessive thyroid hormone secretion

Guillain-Barré syndrome: an acute, rapidly progressing, and potentially fatal form of polyneuritis believed to be caused by a cell-mediated immunologic reaction directed at the peripheral nerves

gynecomastia: a transient enlargement of one or both breasts in men

heart failure: an abnormal clinical condition involving impaired cardiac pumping that results in pathophysiologic changes in vasoconstriction and fluid retention

heat cramps: severe cramps in large muscle groups caused by depletion of both water and salt; usually follow vigorous exertion in an extremely hot environment

heat exhaustion: a clinical syndrome characterized by fatigue, light-headedness, nausea, vomiting, diarrhea, and feelings of impending doom precipitated by prolonged exposure to heat over hours or days

heatstroke: the most serious form of heat stress; results from failure of the central thermoregulatory mechanisms and is considered a medical emergency

heaves: sustained lifts of the chest wall in the precordial area that can be seen or palpated

hematemesis: vomiting of blood that indicates bleeding in the upper GI tract

hematopoietic stem cell transplant: transplantation of peripheral stem cells

hemochromatosis: an autosomal recessive disease characterized by increased intestinal iron absorption and, as a result, increased tissue iron deposition

hemodialysis: dialysis that uses an artificial membrane as the semipermeable membrane through which the patient's blood circulates

hemolytic anemia: an anemia caused by destruction of RBCs at a rate that exceeds production

hemophilia: hereditary bleeding disorders caused by defective or deficient clotting factors

hemorrhagic stroke: a stroke that results from bleeding into the brain tissue itself or into the subarachnoid space or ventricles

hemorrhoids: varicosities in the lower rectum or anus caused by congestion in the veins of the hemorrhoidal plexus

hemostasis: a homeostatic process of blood clotting and blood lysing

hemothorax: accumulation of blood in the pleural space

hepatic encephalopathy: changes in neurologic and mental function resulting from high levels of ammonia in the blood that a damaged liver cannot detoxify

hepatitis: inflammation of the liver

hepatorenal syndrome: a serious complication of cirrhosis characterized by functional renal failure with advancing azotemia, oliguria, and intractable ascites

hernia: a protrusion of a viscus through an abnormal opening or a weakened area in the wall of the cavity in which it is normally contained

herniated intervertebral disk: herniation of nuclear material from the intervertebral disk that may compress or place tension on a cervical, lumbar, or sacral spinal nerve root

hiatal hernia: herniation of a portion of the stomach into the esophagus through an opening, or hiatus, in the diaphragm

Hodgkin's lymphoma: a malignant condition characterized by proliferation of abnormal giant, multinucleated cells, called *Reed-Sternberg cells,* which are located in lymph nodes

hordeolum: an infection of the sebaceous glands in the lid margin

hospice: a system of family-centered care designed to assist the terminally ill person to be comfortable and to maintain a satisfactory lifestyle through the phases of dying

hospital-acquired pneumonia: pneumonia occurring 48 hours or longer after hospital admission and not incubating at the time of hospitalization

human immunodeficiency virus: a retrovirus that causes HIV infection and acquired immunodeficiency syndrome

human leukocyte antigens: system that consists of a series of linked genes that occur together on the sixth chromosome in humans and is used to assess tissue compatibility

humoral immunity: antibody-mediated immunity

Huntington's disease: a genetically transmitted, autosomal dominant disorder that affects both men and women of all races characterized by chronic, devastating loss of all neurologic function resulting in dementia

hydrocele: a nontender, fluid-filled mass that results from interference with lymphatic drainage of the scrotum and swelling of the tunica vaginalis that surrounds the testis

hydronephrosis: dilation or enlargement of the renal pelvis and calyces resulting from obstruction in the lower urinary tract with backflow of urine to the kidney

hydrostatic pressure: the force that fluid exerts within a compartment

hydroureter: dilation of the renal pelvis due to backflow of urine

hyperaldosteronism: excessive aldosterone secretion caused by an adenoma of the adrenal zona glomerulosa or bilateral adrenal hyperplasia

hypercapnia: greater than normal amounts of carbon dioxide in the blood; also called hypercarbia

hypercapnic respiratory failure: a condition in which the $PaCO_2$ is above normal in combination with acidemia

hyperopia: inability of the eye to focus on nearby objects

hyperosmolar hyperglycemic ketotic syndrome: a life-threatening syndrome that can occur in the patient with diabetes who is able to produce enough insulin to prevent diabetic ketoacidosis but not enough to prevent severe hyperglycemia, osmotic diuresis, and extracellular fluid depletion

hyperparathyroidism: a condition involving increased secretion of parathyroid hormone resulting in increased serum calcium levels

hypertension: a common disorder characterized by sustained elevation of BP

hypertensive crisis: a severe and abrupt elevation in blood pressure

hyperthyroidism: a clinical syndrome where there is a sustained increase in synthesis and release of thyroid hormones by the thyroid gland

hypertonic: a solution that increases the degree of osmotic pressure on a semipermeable membrane

hypertrophic scar: an inappropriately large, red, raised, and hard scar that occurs when the body produces excess collagen tissue

hypocapnia: low arterial carbon dioxide pressure; also called hypocarbia

hypoparathyroidism: a condition of insufficient secretion of the parathyroid glands

hypopituitarism: a rare disorder that involves a decrease in one or more of the pituitary hormones and marked by excessive deposits of fat and persistence or acquisition of adolescent characteristics

hypothermia: a core temperature <95° F (35° C) that occurs when heat produced by the body cannot compensate for heat lost to the environment

hypothyroidism: insufficient circulation of thyroid hormones resulting in a hypometabolic state

hypotonic: a solution that has a lower concentration of solute than another solution, thus exerting less osmotic pressure on a semipermeable membrane

hypovolemic shock: shock that is caused by a loss of intravascular fluid volume

hypoxemia: low oxygen tension in the blood characterized by a variety of nonspecific clinical signs and symptoms

hypoxemic respiratory failure: a condition in which the PaO_2 is 60 mm Hg or less when the patient is receiving an inspired oxygen concentration of 60% or greater

hypoxia: the state in which the PaO_2 has fallen sufficiently to cause signs and symptoms of inadequate oxygenation

hysterectomy: surgical removal of the uterus

ileal conduit: urinary diversion procedure in which ureters are implanted into part of ileum or colon that has been resected from intestinal tract and abdominal stoma is created

impaired fasting glucose: an intermediate stage between normal glucose homeostasis and diabetes

infective endocarditis: an infection of the endocardial surface of the heart

inflammatory bowel disease (IBD): chronic, recurrent inflammatory diseases of the intestinal tract that include ulcerative colitis and Crohn's disease

insulin pump: a small battery-operated device that is programmed to deliver a continuous infusion of short-acting insulin 24 hr/day through a catheter inserted into the subcutaneous tissue in the abdominal wall

insulin resistance: a condition in which body tissues do not respond to the action of insulin

intensive insulin therapy: multiple daily insulin injections together with frequent self-monitoring of blood glucose

intermittent claudication: ischemic muscle ache or pain that is precipitated by a consistent level of exercise, resolves within 10 minutes or less with rest, and is reproducible

interstitial cystitis: chronic, painful inflammatory disease of the bladder, believed to be associated with an autoimmune or allergic response

intraaortic balloon pump: a temporary circulatory assist device that is used to enhance the function of a compromised heart by reducing afterload and augmenting the aortic diastolic pressure

intracerebral hematoma: collection of blood within the parenchyma of the brain possibly from the rupture of an intracerebral vessel at the time of a head injury

intracerebral hemorrhage: a type of hemorrhagic stroke in which bleeding within the brain caused by a rupture of a blood vessel occurs

intracranial pressure: the hydrostatic force measured in the brain cerebrospinal fluid compartment

intravenous pyelogram (IVP): diagnostic study using an IV contrast medium that is excreted through the urinary system used to examine the structure and function of the urinary system

iron-deficiency anemia: a microcytic hypochromic anemia caused by inadequate supplies of iron needed to synthesize hemoglobin; characterized by pallor, fatigue, and weakness

irritable bowel syndrome (IBS): a symptom complex characterized by intermittent and recurrent abdominal pain associated with an alteration in bowel function (diarrhea or constipation)

ischemic stroke: stroke that results from inadequate blood flow to the brain due to partial or complete occlusion of an artery

isometric contractions: muscular contraction that increases tension but does not produce movement

isotonic contractions: muscular contraction with shortening that produces movement

Janeway's lesions: flat, painless, small, red spots that may be found on the palms and soles in patients with infective endocarditis

jaundice: symptom of yellowish discoloration of body tissues that results from an increased concentration of bilirubin in the blood

jaw-thrust maneuver: a technique used to maintain an open airway that should be used in emergency situations when neck trauma is suspected

keloid: an overgrowth of collagenous scar tissue at the site of a skin injury, particularly a wound or a surgical incision; the new tissue is elevated, rounded, and firm

keratinocytes: cells synthesized from epidermal cells in the basal layer; they produce a specialized protein, keratin, that is vital to the protective barrier function of the skin

keratitis: an inflammation or infection of the cornea that can be caused by a variety of microorganisms or by other factors

keratoconus: a noninflammatory, usually bilateral disease of the cornea that is familial but has no exclusive inheritance pattern; the cause of the condition is unknown

Korotkoff sounds: sounds heard during the taking of a blood pressure reading using a sphygmomanometer and stethoscope

Korsakoff's psychosis: a form of amnesia often seen in people with chronic alcoholism; characterized by loss of short-term memory and an inability to learn

Kupffer cells: a type of macrophage found in the liver that removes bacteria and toxins from the blood

kwashiorkor: a type of protein-calorie malnutrition caused by a deficiency of protein intake that is superimposed on a catabolic stress event

kyphosis: anterior-posterior or forward bending of spine with convexity of curve in posterior direction

lactase deficiency: an inherited abnormality in which the amount of the digestive enzyme lactase is inadequate for the normal digestion of milk products, resulting in the inability to digest lactose

lacunar stroke: a stroke resulting from occlusion of a small penetrating artery with development of a cavity in the place of the infarcted brain tissue

leiomyoma: a benign smooth muscle tumor that occurs most commonly within the uterus, stomach, esophagus, or small intestine; uterine fibroid

leukemia: a broad term given to a group of malignant diseases characterized by diffuse replacement of bone marrow with proliferating leukocyte precursors

leukopenia: an abnormal decrease in the number of total white blood cells to $<4000/\mu l$

leukoplakia: a whitish precancerous lesion on the oral mucosa or tongue that results from chronic irritations

Lewy body disease: a condition characterized by the presence of Lewy bodies (intraneural cytoplasmic inclusions) in the brainstem and cortex

lichenification: the thickening of the skin as a result of proliferation of keratinocytes with accentuation of the normal markings of the skin often caused by repeated scratching of a pruritic lesion

lipectomy: adipectomy; performed to remove unsightly flabby folds of adipose tissue for cosmetic reasons

lipodystrophy: hypertrophy or atrophy of subcutaneous tissue

lithotripsy: the use of sound waves to break renal stones into small particles that can be eliminated from the urinary tract

lordosis: lumbar spinal deformity resulting in anterior-posterior curvature with concavity in posterior direction

lumpectomy: breast conservation surgery that involves the removal of the entire tumor along with a margin of normal tissue

lung abscess: a pus-containing lesion of the lung parenchyma that results in a cavity formed by necrosis of lung tissue

Lyme disease: a spirochetal infection caused by *Borrelia burgdorferi* and transmitted by the bite of an infected deer tick; characterized by fever, chills, headache, stiff neck, and migratory joint and muscle pain

lymphedema: accumulation of lymph in soft tissue with swelling resulting from inflammation, obstruction, or removal of lymph channels and nodes

lymphogranuloma venereum: chronic sexually transmitted infection caused by strains of *Chlamydia trachomatis* that spreads by way of the regional lymphatics and may spread to the central nervous system through the blood

lymphomas: malignant neoplasms originating in the bone marrow and lymphatic structures resulting in the proliferation of lymphocytes

malabsorption syndrome: a complex of symptoms resulting from disorders in the intestinal absorption of nutrients, characterized by anorexia, weight loss, abdominal bloating, muscle cramps, bone pain, and steatorrhea

malignant hyperthermia: a rare genetic metabolic disease characterized by hyperthermia with rigidity of skeletal muscles that can result in death

malignant melanoma: a tumor arising in cells producing melanin, usually the melanocytes of the skin

malignant neoplasm: a tumor that tends to grow, invade, and metastasize; usually has an irregular shape and is composed of poorly differentiated cells

Mallory-Weiss tear: tear that occurs in the esophageal mucosa at the junction of the esophagus and stomach caused by severe retching and vomiting and results in severe bleeding

mammoplasty: a change in the size or shape of the breast due to surgery

marasmus: a type of protein-calorie malnutrition resulting from a concomitant deficiency of both caloric and protein intake leading to generalized loss of body fat and muscle

mass casualty incident: a human-caused (e.g., biologic warfare) or natural (e.g., hurricane) event or disaster that overwhelms a community's ability to respond with existing resources

mastalgia: breast pain, can be caused by congestion or "caking" during lactation, an infection, or fibrocystic disease, especially during or before menstruation, or in advanced cancer

mastectomy: surgical removal of the breast

mastitis: an inflammatory condition of the breast that occurs most frequently in lactating women caused by streptococcal or staphylococcal infection

mean arterial pressure (MAP): a calculated average of systolic and diastolic blood pressures; calculated by adding the diastolic pressure to one third of the pulse pressure.

megaloblastic anemias: a group of disorders caused by impaired DNA synthesis and characterized by the presence of large red blood cells

melena: black, tarry stools that indicate slow bleeding from an upper GI source

menarche: the first episode of menstrual bleeding, indicating a female has reached puberty

Ménière's disease: a disease characterized by symptoms caused by inner ear disease including episodic vertigo, tinnitus, fluctuating sensorineural hearing loss, and aural fullness

meningitis: an acute inflammation of the pia mater and the arachnoid membrane surrounding the brain and the spinal cord

menopause: the physiologic cessation of menses associated with declining ovarian function

menorrhagia: increased duration or amount of menstrual bleeding at the time of a normal period

metabolic equivalent (MET): a unit of measurement of heat production by the body; used to determine the energy costs of various exercises

metabolic syndrome: a collection of risk factors that increase an individual's chance of developing cardiovascular disease and diabetes mellitus

metastasis: the spread of the cancer from the initial or primary site to a distant site

metered-dose inhaler: aerosolized drug delivered in a specific amount by activating the inhaler or by inhaling

metrorrhagia: uterine bleeding other than that caused by menstruation

migraine headache: a recurring headache characterized by unilateral or bilateral throbbing pain and a triggering event or factor; can occur with and without an aura

mild cognitive impairment: a state of cognition and functional ability between normal aging and early Alzheimer's disease

mitral valve prolapse (MVP): a structural abnormality of the mitral valve leaflets and the papillary muscles or chordae that allows the leaflets to prolapse, or buckle, back into the left atrium during ventricular systole

morbidly obese: classification describing individuals with a body mass index of >40 kg/m^2

multiple myeloma: a condition in which malignant neoplastic plasma cells infiltrate the bone marrow and destroy bone

multiple organ dysfunction syndrome (MODS): the failure of more than one organ system in an acutely ill patient such that homeostasis cannot be maintained without intervention

multiple sclerosis (MS): a chronic, progressive, degenerative disorder of the central nervous system characterized by disseminated demyelination of nerve fibers of the brain and spinal cord

murmur: a gentle blowing, fluttering, or humming sound, heard on auscultation and produced by turbulent blood flow through the heart or the walls of large arteries

muscular dystrophy (MD): a group of genetically transmitted diseases characterized by progressive symmetric wasting of skeletal muscle without evidence of neurologic involvement

myasthenia gravis (MG): an autoimmune disease of the neuromuscular junction characterized by the fluctuating weakness of certain skeletal muscle groups

myasthenic crisis: an acute exacerbation of myasthenia gravis triggered by infection, surgery, emotional distress, or overdose or inadequate medication

myelodysplastic syndrome: a group of related hematologic disorders characterized by a change in the quantity and quality of bone marrow elements

myocardial infarction (MI): irreversible cardiac cellular death caused by sustained myocardial ischemia

myocarditis: a focal or diffuse inflammation of the myocardium

myofascial pain syndrome: musculoskeletal pain and tenderness in one anatomic region of the body originating in anterior and posterior trigger points that have resulted from muscle trauma and/or chronically strained muscles

myopia: inability of the eye to focus on objects far away

myxedema: the progression of the mental sluggishness, drowsiness, and lethargy of hypothyroidism to a notable impairment of consciousness or coma that is a medical emergency

nadir: the lowest point, such as the blood count after it has been depressed by chemotherapy

nasal polyps: benign mucous membrane masses that form slowly in response to repeated inflammation of the sinus or nasal mucosa and project into the nasal cavity

nephrolithiasis: the formation of stones in the urinary tract

nephrosclerosis: a vascular disease of the kidney characterized by sclerosis of the small arteries and arterioles of the kidney resulting in renal tissue necrosis

nephrotic syndrome: an abnormal condition of the kidney characterized by peripheral edema, massive proteinuria, hyperlipidemia, and hypoalbuminemia

neurofibrillary tangles: tangled bundles of fibers seen in the cytoplasm of abnormal neurons in those areas of the brain most affected by Alzheimer's disease

neurogenic bladder: any type of bladder dysfunction related to abnormal or absent bladder innervation caused by a lesion of the nervous system

neurogenic bowel: condition that results from less voluntary neurologic control over the bowel

neurogenic shock: neurologic syndrome caused by the loss of vasomotor tone caused by spinal cord injury at the fifth thoracic (T5) vertebra or above and characterized by hypotension, bradycardia, and warm, dry extremities

neuroglia: cells in the central nervous system that provide support, nourishment, and protection to neurons; they perform the less specialized function of the nerve network

neuropathic pain: pain caused by damage to nerve cells or changes in spinal cord processing

neurosyphilis: an infection of any part of the nervous system by the organism *Treponema pallidum*

neutropenia: an abnormal reduction of the neutrophil count to <1000/μl

nociception: activation of the primary afferent nerves with peripheral terminals that respond to noxious stimuli

nociceptive pain: pain that is caused by damage to somatic or visceral tissue and occurs abruptly after an injury or disease, persists until healing occurs, and often is intensified by anxiety or fear

nonalcoholic fatty liver disease: a group of disorders that is characterized by hepatic *steatosis* (accumulation of fat in the liver) that is not associated with other causes such as hepatitis, autoimmune disease, or alcohol

non-Hodgkin's lymphoma: a heterogeneous group of malignant neoplasms involving lymphoid tissue

normal pressure hydrocephalus: an uncommon disorder characterized by an obstruction in the flow of cerebrospinal fluid, which causes a buildup of this fluid in the brain

nuchal rigidity: resistance to flexion of the neck

nulliparous: never having given birth

nystagmus: an abnormal involuntary repetitive movement of the eyes

O$_2$ toxicity: a condition of oxygen overdosage caused by prolonged exposure to a high level of oxygen

obese: classification used to describe individuals with body mass index values of 30 kg/m^2 or more

obstructive sleep apnea: a condition characterized by partial or complete upper airway obstruction during sleep

oligomenorrhea: long intervals between menses, generally >35 days

oliguria: <400 ml of urine in 24 hr

oncogenes: potentially cancer-inducing genes

oncotic pressure: the osmotic pressure of a colloid in solution, such as when there is a higher concentration of a protein in the plasma on one side of a cell membrane than in the neighboring interstitial fluid

opioids: category including opiates in addition to the many semisynthetic and synthetic narcotic agents used as analgesics

oral hairy leukoplakia: an Epstein-Barr virus infection that causes painless, white, raised lesions on the lateral aspect of the tongue

orchitis: an acute inflammation of the testis

orthostatic hypotension: abnormally low blood pressure occurring when an individual suddenly assumes a standing position

Osler's nodes: painful, tender, red or purple, peasize lesions that may be found on the fingertips or toes in patients with infective endocarditis and usually last only 1 or 2 days

osteoarthritis: a slowly progressive noninflammatory disorder of the diarthrodial (synovial) joints

osteochondroma: primary benign bone tumor that is characterized by an overgrowth of cartilage and bone near the end of the bone at the growth plate

osteogenic sarcoma: a primary neoplasm of bone that is extremely malignant and is characterized by rapid growth and metastasis

osteomalacia: a rare condition of adult bone associated with vitamin D deficiency, resulting in decalcification and softening of bone

osteomyelitis: a severe infection of the bone, bone marrow, and surrounding soft tissue

osteoporosis: a metabolic bone disease characterized by low bone mass and structural deterioration of bone tissue leading to increased bone fragility and pathologic fractures

osteotomy: removing or adding a wedge or slice of bone to change its alignment and shift weight bearing, thereby correcting deformity and relieving pain

ostomy: a surgical procedure in which an opening is made to allow the passage of urine from the bladder or intestinal contents from the bowel to an incision or stoma surgically created in the wall of the abdomen

otosclerosis: a hereditary condition in which irregular ossification occurring on the footplate of the stapes in the oval window results in decreased hearing acuity

Paget's disease of the bone: a skeletal bone disorder in which there is excessive bone resorption followed by replacement of normal marrow by vascular, fibrous connective tissue and new bone that is larger, disorganized, and weaker

Paget's disease of the breast: a breast malignancy characterized by a persistent lesion of the nipple and areola with or without a palpable mass

palliative care: health care aimed at symptom management rather than curative treatment for diseases that no longer respond to treatment

palpation: a technique used in physical examination in which the examiner feels the texture, size, consistency, and location of certain body parts with the hands

pancytopenia: marked decrease in the number of red blood cells, white blood cells, and platelets

paracentesis: a procedure in which fluid is withdrawn from a cavity of the body

paralytic ileus: lack of intestinal peristalsis

paraplegia: paralysis characterized by motor and/or sensory loss in the lower limbs and trunk

parenteral nutrition: the administration of nutrients by a route (e.g., bloodstream) other than the GI tract

Parkinson's disease: a disease of the basal ganglia characterized by a slowing down in the initiation and execution of movement, increased muscle tone tremor at rest, and impaired postural reflexes

paroxysmal nocturnal dyspnea: a disorder characterized by sudden attacks of respiratory distress that awakens the person, usually after several hours of sleep in a reclining position

partial seizures: seizures that begin in a specific region of the cortex and may be confined to one side of the brain and remain partial or focal in nature, or they may spread to involve the entire brain

partial-thickness burn: varying degrees of epidermal and dermal skin injury in which some skin elements remain viable for regeneration

pelvic inflammatory disease (PID): an infectious condition of the pelvic cavity that may involve infection of the fallopian tubes, ovaries, and pelvic peritoneum

peptic ulcer disease: a condition characterized by erosion of the GI mucosa resulting from the digestive action of HCl acid and pepsin

percussion: a technique in physical examination of tapping the body with the fingertips or fist

percutaneous coronary intervention: a common elective intervention for coronary artery disease in which a catheter equipped with an inflatable balloon tip is inserted into a narrowed coronary artery and the balloon is inflated

pericardial effusion: an accumulation of excess fluid in the pericardial sac

pericardial friction rub: a scratching, grating, high-pitched sound believed to arise from friction between the roughened pericardial and epicardial surfaces

pericardiocentesis: procedure in which a 16- to 18-gauge needle is inserted into the pericardial space to remove fluid for analysis and to relieve cardiac pressure

pericarditis: a condition caused by inflammation of the pericardial sac

perimenopause: a normal life transition that begins with the first signs of change in menstrual cycles and ends after cessation of menses

perineal prostatectomy: surgical removal of the prostate gland through a perineal approach

peripheral arterial disease: progressive narrowing and degeneration of the arteries of the neck, abdomen, and extremities

peritoneal dialysis: dialysis using the peritoneal membrane as the semipermeable membrane

peritonitis: the inflammation of the peritoneum

pernicious anemia: a progressive megaloblastic macrocytic anemia resulting from inadequate gastric secretion of intrinsic factor necessary for absorption of cobalamin

petechiae: small purplish lesions

phantom limb sensation: perception of sensations or pain in an amputated limb

pheochromocytoma: a rare condition characterized by a tumor of the adrenal medulla that produces excessive catecholamines causing persistent or intermittent hypertension

phimosis: a constriction of the uncircumcised foreskin around the head of the penis making retraction difficult

Pick's disease: a rare brain disorder characterized by disturbances in behavior, sleep, personality, and eventually memory

pleural effusion: an abnormal accumulation of fluid in the intrapleural spaces of the lungs

pleural friction rub: creaking or grating sound from roughened, inflamed surfaces of the pleura rubbing together, evident during inspiration, expiration, or both and no change with coughing

pleurisy (pleuritis): inflammation of the pleura

pneumoconiosis: a general term for lung diseases caused by inhalation and retention of dust particles

pneumonia: an acute inflammation of the lungs, often caused by inhaled pneumococci of the species *Streptococcus pneumoniae*

pneumothorax: a collection of air or gas in the pleural space causing the lung to collapse

point of maximal impulse: the site on the chest wall where the thrust or pulsation of the left ventricle is most prominent

polycystic kidney disease: a genetic kidney disorder in which the cortex and the medulla are filled with thin-walled cysts that enlarge and destroy surrounding tissue

polycythemia: an abnormal condition with excessive levels of red blood cells

polymyositis: diffuse, idiopathic, inflammatory myopathies of striated muscle, producing bilateral weakness usually most severe in the proximal or limb-girdle muscles; some forms of polymyositis are associated with malignancy

portal hypertension: increased venous pressure in the portal circulation caused by compression and destruction of the portal and hepatic veins and sinusoids

positive end-expiratory pressure (PEEP): a ventilatory maneuver in which positive pressure is applied to the airway during exhalation

postpolio syndrome: recurrence of neuromuscular symptoms experienced by polio survivors who previously had the disease

postural drainage: the use of various positions to promote gravity drainage of bronchial secretions

prediabetes: impaired glucose tolerance; occurs when a 2-hr plasma glucose level is higher than normal but lower than that considered diagnostic for diabetes

prehypertension: disorder characterized by a systolic blood pressure of 120-139 mm Hg and a diastolic blood pressure of 80-90 mm Hg

preload: the volume of blood in the ventricles at the end of diastole before the next contraction

premature atrial contraction: contraction originating from an ectopic focus in the atrium in a location other than the sinus node

premature ventricular contraction: a contraction originating in an ectopic focus in the ventricles

premenstrual syndrome (PMS): a common disorder in women in which a group of physical and psychologic symptoms occur during the last few days of the menstrual cycle and prior to the onset of menstruation

presbycusis: hearing loss associated with aging

presbyopia: a hyperopic shift to farsightedness resulting from a loss of elasticity of the lens of the eye

pressure ulcer: a localized area of tissue necrosis caused by unrelieved pressure that occludes blood flow to the tissues

primary (essential) hypertension: an elevated systemic arterial pressure for which no cause can be found and which is often the only significant clinical finding

Prinzmetal's angina: variant angina; occurs at rest, usually in response to reversible, severe spasm of a major coronary artery

prostate specific antigen (PSA): a glycoprotein found only in the epithelial cells of the prostate that, when elevated, indicates a pathologic condition of the prostate, but not necessarily cancer of the prostate

prostatitis: acute or chronic inflammation of the prostate gland, usually as a result of infection

protein-calorie malnutrition: the most common form of undernutrition

pruritus: itching

pulmonary edema: an acute, life-threatening situation in which the lung alveoli become filled with serous or serosanguineous fluid caused most commonly by heart failure

pulmonary embolism: a thromboembolic occlusion of the pulmonary vasculature resulting from thrombi in the venous circulation or right side of the heart that travel as emboli until lodging in the pulmonary vessels

pulmonary hypertension: elevated pulmonary pressure resulting from an increase in pulmonary vascular resistance to blood flow through small arteries and arterioles

pulse pressure: the difference between the systolic and diastolic pressures

pursed-lip breathing: a technique of exhaling against pursed lips to prolong exhalation, preventing bronchiolar collapse and air trapping

pyelonephritis: a diffuse pyogenic infection of the renal parenchyma and collecting system

pyrosis: burning in epigastric or substernal area; heartburn

radical prostatectomy: surgical removal of the entire prostate gland, seminal vesicles, and part of the bladder neck (ampulla)

Raynaud's phenomenon: an episodic vasospastic disorder of small cutaneous arteries, most frequently involving the fingers and toes

rectocele: herniation or protrusion of the rectum through the wall of the vagina resulting from weakened connective tissue support between the vagina and rectum

refractive error: a defect in the ability of the lens of the eye to focus an image accurately, as occurs in nearsightedness and farsightedness

Reiter syndrome: a symptom complex more commonly found in young men that includes urethritis, conjunctivitis, and mucocutaneous lesions

renal artery stenosis: a partial occlusion of one or both renal arteries and their major branches and is a major cause of abrupt onset hypertension

renal osteodystrophy: syndrome of skeletal changes found in chronic kidney disease as a result of alterations in calcium and phosphate metabolism

repetitive strain injury: a cumulative trauma disorder resulting from prolonged, forceful, or awkward movements resulting in strain of tendons, ligaments, and muscles, causing tiny tears that become inflamed

restless legs syndrome: unpleasant sensory and motor abnormalities of one or both legs; characterized by an irritating sensation of uneasiness, tiredness, and itching deep within the muscles of the leg

retinal detachment: a separation of the retina from the retinal pigment epithelium in the back of the eye, allowing the vitreous humor to leak between the two layers

retinopathy: the process of microvascular damage of the retina; may develop slowly or rapidly

retrograde pyelogram: radiologic technique for examining the structures of the collecting system of the kidneys that is especially useful in locating a urinary tract obstruction

retropubic prostatectomy: removal of the prostate gland through a low abdominal incision without entry into the bladder

rheumatic fever: an inflammatory disease of the heart potentially involving all layers

rheumatic heart disease: the resulting damage to the heart muscle and heart valves from rheumatic fever, a chronic condition characterized by scarring and deformity of the heart valves

rheumatoid arthritis: a chronic, systemic autoimmune disease characterized by inflammation of connective tissue in the diarthrodial (synovial) joints, typically with periods of remission and exacerbation

rhinoplasty: the surgical reconstruction of the nose

rhonchi: continuous rumbling, snoring, or rattling sounds from obstruction of large airways with secretions

sarcoma: a malignant tumor that originates from embryonal mesoderm that becomes connective tissue, muscle, bone, and fat

scoliosis: a lateral S-shaped curvature of the thoracic and lumbar spine

secondary hypertension: elevated blood pressure associated with any of several primary diseases, such as renal, pulmonary, endocrine, and vascular diseases

seizure: a paroxysmal, uncontrolled electrical discharge of neurons in the brain that interrupts normal function leading to a sudden, violent involuntary series of contractions of a group of muscles

sepsis: a systemic inflammatory response to infection

septic arthritis: infectious or bacterial arthritis caused by invasion of the joint cavity with microorganisms; characterized by bacterial inflammation of a joint caused by the spread of bacteria through the bloodstream from an infection elsewhere in the body or by contamination of a joint during trauma or surgery

septic shock: the presence of sepsis with hypotension despite adequate fluid resuscitation along with the presence of tissue perfusion abnormalities

sexually transmitted diseases: infectious diseases transmitted most commonly through sexual intercourse or genital contact

shock: a syndrome characterized by decreased tissue perfusion and impaired cellular metabolism resulting in an imbalance between the supply of and demand for oxygen and nutrients

sickle cell disease: a group of inherited, autosomal recessive disorders characterized by the presence of an abnormal form of hemoglobin in the erythrocyte

silent ischemia: asymptomatic ischemia that may damage the heart

Sjögren's syndrome: an autoimmune disease that targets moisture-producing glands, leading to the common symptoms of xerostomia (dry mouth) and keratoconjunctivitis sicca (dry eyes)

Somogyi effect: a condition in which an excessive insulin dose causes a decline in blood glucose levels during sleep, causing the release of counterregulatory hormones that increase the blood glucose levels, resulting in high blood glucose levels at morning testing; indicates a need for reduced insulin dose

spermatogenesis: formation of sperm

spider angiomas: small, dilated blood vessels with a bright red center point the size of a pinhead from which small blood vessels radiate

spinal shock: immediate failure of all spinal cord function at the time of injury below the level of cord damage resulting in flaccid paralysis, loss of reflexes, and loss of sympathetic innervation

spondyloarthropathies: a group of interrelated multisystem inflammatory disorders that affect the spine, peripheral joints, and periarticular structures

squamous cell carcinoma: a slow-growing malignant tumor of squamous epithelium; found in the lungs and skin and occurring also in the anus, cervix, larynx, nose, and bladder

status asthmaticus: a severe, life-threatening asthma attack that is refractory to usual treatment and places the patient at risk for developing respiratory failure

status epilepticus: a state of continuous seizure activity or a condition in which seizures recur in rapid succession without return to consciousness between seizures

steatorrhea: greater than normal amounts of fat in the feces

stenosis: constriction or narrowing

stent: expandable mesh-like structure designed to maintain vessel patency by compressing the arterial walls and resisting vasoconstriction

stricture: an abnormal temporary or permanent narrowing of the lumen of a hollow organ

stroke: death of brain cells that occurs when there is ischemia to a part of the brain or hemorrhage into the brain

subarachnoid hemorrhage: a stroke resulting from intracranial bleeding into the cerebrospinal fluid–filled space between the arachnoid and pia mater membranes on the surface of the brain

subdural hematoma: collection of blood between the dura mater and the arachnoid layer of the meninges of the brain that is usually of venous origin, usually caused by injury

subluxation: a partial or incomplete displacement of the joint surface

submersion injury: hypoxia resulting from submersion in a substance, usually water

sudden cardiac death: unexpected death from cardiac causes

sundowning: condition in which the patient becomes more confused and agitated in the late afternoon or evening

superficial thrombophlebitis: inflammation of a superficial vein; occurs in about 65% of all patients receiving IV therapy

surfactant: a lipoprotein that lowers the surface tension in the alveoli, reduces the amount of pressure needed to inflate the alveoli and decreases the tendency of the alveoli to collapse

syncope: fainting that may occur with decreased cardiac output, fluid deficits, or defects in cerebral perfusion

synovectomy: surgical removal of synovial membrane

syphilis: infection of organs and tissues of the body by *Treponema pallidum*

systemic inflammatory response syndrome (SIRS): a systemic inflammatory response to a variety of insults, including infection, ischemia, infarct, and injury

systemic lupus erythematosus (SLE): a chronic multisystem inflammatory disease associated with abnormalities of the immune system

systemic sclerosis: a disorder of connective tissue characterized by fibrotic, degenerative, and occasionally inflammatory changes in the skin, blood vessels, synovium, skeletal muscle, and internal organs

systolic blood pressure: the peak pressure exerted against the arteries when the heart contracts

systolic failure: a type of ventricular failure caused by impaired contractile function, increased afterload, or mechanical abnormalities

teletherapy: radiation therapy administered by a machine that is positioned at some distance from the patient; the most common form of radiation therapy treatment

tenesmus: spasmodic contraction of the anal sphincter with pain and persistent desire to empty the bowel

tension pneumothorax: rapid accumulation of air in the pleural space causing severely high intrapleural pressures with resultant tension on the heart and great vessels

tension-type headache: headache that is characterized by a bilateral feeling of pressure around the head

tetanus: lockjaw; an extremely severe polyradiculitis and polyneuritis affecting spinal and cranial nerves that results from the effects of a potent neurotoxin released by the anaerobic bacillus *Clostridium tetani*

tetany: increased nerve excitability and sustained muscle contraction that results from low calcium levels that allow sodium to move into excitable cells, increasing depolarization

tetraplegia (quadriplegia): paralysis of the arms, legs, and trunk occurring with spinal cord damage at C8 or above

thalassemia: an autosomal recessive genetic disorder of inadequate production of normal hemoglobin

thoracentesis: a surgical procedure done to remove fluid from the pleural space

thoracotomy: surgical opening into the thoracic cavity

thromboangiitis obliterans: a somewhat rare nonatherosclerotic, segmental inflammatory disorder of the medium-size arteries, veins, and nerves of the upper and lower extremities

thrombocytopenia: a reduction of the platelet count $<100,000/\mu l$

thrombocytosis: a condition marked by excessive platelets; a disorder that occurs with inflammation and some malignant disorders

thrombotic stroke: a stroke resulting from thrombosis or narrowing of the blood vessel

thyroiditis: an inflammation of the thyroid gland that may cause hyperthyroid or hypothyroid manifestations

thyrotoxic crisis: an acute, rare condition in which all hyperthyroid manifestations are heightened

thyrotoxicosis: a hypermetabolic state caused by excessive circulating levels of T_4, T_3, or both

tinnitus: a subjective noise sensation, often described as ringing, heard in one or both ears

tonic-clonic seizure: seizure characterized by loss of consciousness and falling to the ground, followed by stiffening of the body for 10 to 20 seconds and subsequent jerking of the extremities for another 30 to 40 seconds

tracheostomy: surgical opening into the trachea through which an indwelling tube may be inserted

tracheotomy: a surgical incision into the trachea for the purpose of establishing an airway; performed below a blockage by a foreign body, tumor, or edema of the glottis

traction: the application of a pulling force to an injured or diseased part of the body or an extremity while countertraction pulls in the opposite direction

transient ischemic attack (TIA): a temporary focal loss of neurologic function caused by ischemia of the brain, lasting less than 24 hours, and often lasting less than 15 minutes

transurethral incision of the prostate: a surgical procedure in which transurethral incisions or slits are made into prostatic tissue to relieve obstruction

transurethral resection of the prostate (TURP): a surgical procedure involving the removal of prostate tissue with the use of a resectoscope inserted through the urethra

triage: system that identifies and categorizes patients so the most critical are treated first

trigeminal neuralgia: a neurologic condition of the trigeminal facial nerve, characterized by paroxysms of flashing, stablike pain radiating along the course of a branch of the nerve from the angle of the jaw

trigger point: a circumscribed hypersensitive area within a tight band of muscle that is caused by acute or chronic muscle strain

tuberculosis: an infectious disease caused by *Mycobacterium tuberculosis;* usually involves the lungs, but also occurs in the larynx, kidneys, bones, adrenal glands, lymph nodes, and meninges and can be disseminated throughout the body

tumor angiogenesis: the process of the formation of blood vessels within the tumor itself

tumor suppressor genes: genes that suppress neoplastic growth

ulcerative colitis: chronic inflammatory bowel disease that causes ulceration of the colon and rectum

unstable angina: angina that is new in onset, occurs at rest, or has a worsening pattern

uremia: the presence of excessive amounts of urea and other nitrogenous waste products in the blood; renal function declines to the point that symptoms develop in multiple body systems

urethritis: inflammation of the urethra

urinalysis: analysis of urine for color, pH, specific gravity, osmolality, and normal and abnormal constituents

urinary incontinence: an uncontrolled leakage of urine as a result of cerebral clouding and/or physical factors that make it difficult to get to the bathroom facilities on time

urinary retention: the inability to empty the bladder despite micturition or the accumulation of urine in the bladder because of an inability to urinate

urosepsis: urinary tract infection that has spread into the systemic circulation; life-threatening condition requiring emergency treatment

uterine prolapse: the downward displacement of the uterus into the vaginal canal as a result of impaired pelvic support

Valsalva maneuver: a maneuver that involves contraction of the chest muscles on a closed glottis with simultaneous contraction of the abdominal muscles

varicocele: a dilation of the veins that drain the testes

varicose veins: dilated, tortuous subcutaneous veins most frequently found in the saphenous system

vascular dementia: the loss of cognitive function resulting from ischemic, ischemic-hypoxic, or hemorrhagic brain lesions caused by cardiovascular disease

vasectomy: bilateral surgical ligation or resection of the vas deferens performed for the purpose of sterilization

venous thrombosis: the formation of a thrombus in association with inflammation of the vein

ventricular assist device: device that is applied externally or internally into the path of flowing blood to augment or replace the action of the ventricle of the heart

ventricular fibrillation: a severe derangement of the heart rhythm characterized on ECG by irregular undulations of varying contour and amplitude

ventricular tachycardia: a condition that occurs when an ectopic focus or foci fire repetitively and the ventricle takes control as the pacemaker

vertigo: a sensation that a person or objects around the person are moving or spinning; usually stimulated by movement of the head

vesicants: agents that when accidentally infiltrated into the skin cause severe local tissue breakdown and necrosis

vibration: pressing on the chest with the flat of the hands while repeatedly tensing the hand and arm muscles to facilitate movement of secretions to larger airways

viral load: quantity of viral particles in a biologic sample

Virchow's triad: three important factors in the etiology of venous thrombosis: (1) venous stasis, (2) damage of the endothelium (inner lining of the vein), and (3) hypercoagulability of the blood

viremia: large amounts of virus in the blood, resulting from initial infection with a virus

Wernicke's encephalopathy: an inflammatory, hemorrhagic, degenerative condition of the brain resulting from a deficiency of thiamine; is seen in association with chronic alcoholism

wheezes: a form of rhonchus characterized by continuous high-pitched squeaking sound caused by rapid vibration of bronchial walls

window period: time period of 2 months after infection during which an infected individual will not test HIV-antibody positive

wound dehiscence: separation and disruption of previously joined wound edges

Illustration Credits

Chapter 1
1-4, 1-5, from Rick Brady, Riva, Md; **1-6,** Courtesy Elizabeth Burkhart, RN, MPH, PhD, Chicago, Ill.

Chapter 2
2-1, From McGinnis JM, Williams-Russo P, Knickman JR: The case for more active policy attention to health promotion, *Health Affairs* 21:78, 2002; **2-2,** from Health Quality Survey, Diverse Communities, Common Concerns: Assessing Health Care Quality for Minority Americans, Collins KS, Hughes DL, Doty MM et al, *The Commonwealth Fund,* March 2002; **2-3,** from Rick Brady, Riva, Md; **2-4,** from Giger JN, Davidhizar RE: *Transcultural nursing,* ed 4, St Louis, 2004, Mosby; **Case study photo,** © 2007 JupiterImages Corporation.

Chapter 3
3-1, 3-3, 3-4, 3-6, © 2007 JupiterImages Corporation; **3-5,** from Rick Brady, Riva, Md; **Case study photo,** ©iStockphoto.com/ Joseph Jean Rolland Dubé.

Chapter 4
4-1, From Wilson SF, Giddens JF: *Health assessment for nursing practice,* ed 3, St Louis, 2005, Mosby.

Chapter 5
5-1, © 2007 JupiterImages Corporation; **5-3, 5-5,** from Rick Brady, Riva, Md; **5-6,** from Wilson SF, Giddens JF: *Health assessment for nursing practice,* ed 3, St Louis, 2005, Mosby.

Chapter 6
6-1, From Centers for Disease Control and Prevention, National Center for Health Statistics. *Health,* United States, 2004; **6-3, 6-4, 6-5, 6-6, 6-7, 6-9, 6-10,** from Rick Brady, Riva, Md; **6-8,** from Fulmer SPICES: an overall assessment tool of older adults. Developed by Meredith Wallace and Terry Fulmer, Hartford Institute for Geriatric Nursing, New York University, New York. In Ebersole P et al: *Gerontological nursing and healthy aging,* ed 2, St Louis, 2005, Mosby; **6-11,** redrawn from Benzon J: Approaching drug regiments with a therapeutic dose of suspicion, *Geriatr Nurs* 12(4):1813, 1991.

Chapter 7
7-1, 7-3, From Potter PA, Perry AG: *Fundamentals of nursing: concepts, process, and practice,* ed 4, St. Louis, 1997, Mosby; **7-2,** from Potter PA, Perry AG: *Basic nursing, a critical thinking approach,* ed 4, St. Louis, 1999, Mosby **7-4,** from Rick Brady, Riva, Md.

Chapter 8
8-1, 8-2, From National Center for Complementary and Alternative Medicine: *The use of complementary and alternative medicine in the United States,* Bethesda, Md.; **8-4, 8-5,** courtesy Cory Shaw, San Antonio, Tex.; **8-6,** from Blake S: *Alternative remedies CD-ROM,* St Louis, 1999, Mosby; **8-7,** courtesy Effie Wood, San Antonio, Tex.; **8-8, 8-9** courtesy Lori Karhu, RMT, RN, San Antonio, Tex.; **Case study photos,** courtesy Scripps Center for Integrative Medicine, La Jolla, Calif.

Chapter 9
9-1, 9-2, 9-7, 9-8, 9-9, © 2007 JupiterImages Corporation; **Case study photo,** ©iStockphoto.com/Rosemarie Colombraro.

Chapter 10
10-1, Developed by McCaffery M, Pasero C, Paice JA. From McCaffery M, Pasero C: *Pain: clinical manual,* ed 2, St Louis, 1999, Mosby; **10-5,** from McCaffery M, Pasero C: *Pain: clinical manual,* ed 2, St Louis, 1999, Mosby; **10-6,** from Acute Pain Management Guideline Panel, 1992; **10-8,** from Salerno E, Willins J: *Pain management handbook,* St Louis, 1996, Mosby; **10-10,** from Rick Brady, Riva, Md; **Case study photo,** © 2007 JupiterImages Corporation.

Chapter 11
11-1, 11-4, 11-5, Courtesy Kathleen A. Pollard, RN, MSN, CHPN, Phoenix, Ariz.; **11-2,** from Potter PA, Perry AG: *Fundamentals of nursing: concepts, process, and practice,* ed 4, St. Louis, 1997, Mosby; **11-3, 11-6,** from Rick Brady, Riva, Md.

Chapter 12
12-1, 12-4, from Rick Brady, Riva, Md; **12-2,** From Department of Health and Human Services: *Clinical practice guideline: treating tobacco use and dependence,* Washington, DC, 2000, U.S. Public Health Service; **12-3,** © iStockphoto.com/Rebecca Ellis; **12-5,** © 2007 JupiterImages Corporation; **Case study photo,** ©iStockphoto.com/Lisa Kyle Young.

Chapter 13
13-8, Courtesy Scott Health Care—A Molnlyche Company, Philadelphia. In Potter PA, Perry AG: *Fundamentals of nursing,* ed 6, St Louis, 2005, Mosby; **13-9A,** from Habif TP: *Clinical dermatology: a color guide to diagnosis and therapy,* ed 2, St Louis, 1992, Mosby; **13-9B,** from Lemmi FO, Lemmi CAE: *Physical assessment findings CD-ROM,* Philadelphia, 2000, Saunders; **13-10,** from Morison MJ: *Prevention and treatment of pressure ulcers,*

London, 2001, Mosby; **13-11,** courtesy Robert B. Babiak, RN, BSN, CWOCN, San Antonio, Tex.; **13-12,** from Potter PA, Perry AG: *Fundamentals of nursing,* ed 6, St Louis, 2005, Mosby; **Case study photo,** ©iStockphoto.com/Gisele Gaze.

Chapter 14
14-1, From Thibodeau GA, Patton KT: *The human body in health and disease,* ed 3, St Louis, 2002, Mosby; **14-12, 14-13,** from Morison MJ: *Nursing management of chronic wounds,* Edinburgh, 2001, Mosby; **14-16,** from the U.S. Department of Health and Human Services, Washington DC; **14-18,** from McKenry L, Tessier E, Hogan M: *Mosby's pharmacology in nursing,* St Louis, 2006, Mosby.

Chapter 15
15-5, 15-6, Set of slides published in 1992 by Jon Fuller, MD and Howard Libman, MD at Boston University School of Medicine, Boston, Mass.; **15-7, 15-8,** from Grimes DE, Grimes RM: *AIDS and HIV infection,* St Louis, 1994, Mosby; **15-9,** from the Centers for Disease Control and Prevention. Courtesy Jonathan WM Gold, MD, New York, N.Y.; **Case study photo 1,** ©iStockphoto.com/Roberta Osborne; **Case study photo 2,** ©iStockphoto.com/Mike Manzano.

Chapter 16
16-1, Adapted from Kumar V, Abbas AK, and Fausto N: *Robbins and Cotran pathologic basis of disease,* ed 7, Philadelphia, 2005, Saunders; **16-4,** from Stevens A, Lowe J: *Pathology: an illustrated review in color,* ed 2, London, 2000, Mosby; **16-5,** adapted from DeVita VT, Helman S, Rosenberg SA, eds: *Cancer: principles and practice of oncology,* Philadelphia, 1997, Lippincott-Raven; **16-12,** Sauerland C, Engelking C, Wickham R, Corbi D: Vesicant extravasation part I: Mechanisms, pathogenesis, and nursing care to reduce risk, *Oncology Nursing Forum* 33(6): 1134-41, 2006.; **16-15A,** courtesy Pharmaceia Deltec, Inc, St. Paul, Minn.; **16-16B,** courtesy Strato/Infusaid, Inc, Norwood, Mass; **16-17, 16-18,** courtesy of Jormain Cady, Virginia Mason Medical Center, Seattle, Wash.; **16-23,** from Forbes CD, Jackson WF: *Color atlas and text of clinical medicine,* ed 3, London, 2003, Mosby.

Chapter 17
17-14, Redrawn from McCance KL, Huether SE: *Pathophysiology: the biologic basis for disease in adults and children,* ed 5, St Louis, 2006, Mosby; **Case study photo,** ©iStockphoto.com/ Jessica Jones Photography.

Chapter 18
18-1, © 2007 JupiterImages Corporation; **Case study photo,** ©iStockphoto.com/bbear.

Chapter 19
19-1, Courtesy Greg McVicar; **19-2,** © 2007 JupiterImages Corporation; **19-4,** courtesy The Methodist Hospital, Houston, Tex. Photograph by Donna Dahms, RN, CNOR; **19-5,** from Rothrock JC: *Alexander's Care of the Patient in Surgery,* ed 13, St Louis, 2007, Mosby.

Chapter 20
Case study photo, ©iStockphoto.com/Malcolm Romain.

Chapter 21
21-1, From Thibodeau GA, Patton KT: *Anatomy and physiology,* ed 6, St Louis, 2007, Mosby; **21-5,** Adapted from Kanski J:

Clinical ophthalmology: a synopsis, New York, 2004, Butterworth-Heinemann; **21-6,** courtesy Eye Institute, Department of Ophthalmology and Visual Services, University of Iowa Health Care, Iowa City, Iowa; **21-7,** from Thibodeau GA, Patton KT: *The human body in health and disease,* ed 4, St Louis, 2005, Mosby; **21-8,** from Seidel HM et al: *Mosby's guide to physical examination,* ed 5, St Louis, 2003, Mosby.

Chapter 22
22-2, 22-3, From Kanski J: *Clinical ophthalmology: a synopsis,* New York, 2004, Butterworth-Heinemann; **22-9,** courtesy of Siemens Hearing Solutions, Piscataway, N.J.; **22-10,** courtesy Advanced Vionics, Valencia, Calif.; **Case study photo,** © 2007 JupiterImages Corporation.

Chapter 23
23-1, From Jarvis C: *Physical examination and health assessment,* ed 4, Philadelphia, 2004, Saunders; **23-3, 23-5,** from Habif TP: *Clinical dermatology: a color guide to diagnosis and therapy,* ed 4, St Louis, 2004, Mosby; **23-4,** from Habif TP: *Clinical dermatology: a color guide to diagnosis and therapy,* ed 3, St Louis, 1996, Mosby.

Chapter 24
24-1, From Hooper BJ, Goldman NP: *Primary dermatologic care,* St Louis, 1999, Mosby; **24-2,** from Goldstein BG, Goldstein AO: *Practical dermatology,* ed 2, St Louis, 1997, Mosby. Courtesy Department of Dermatology, Medical College of Georgia, Augusta, Ga.; **24-3,** from The Skin Cancer Foundation, New York, N.Y.; **24-4, 24-5,** from Habif TP: *Clinical dermatology: a color guide to diagnosis and therapy,* ed 4, St Louis, 2004, Mosby; **24-6,** from Habif TP: *Clinical dermatology: a color guide to diagnosis and therapy,* ed 3, St Louis, 1996, Mosby; **24-7, 24-11,** from Lemmi FO, Lemmi CAE: *Physical assessment findings CD-ROM,* Philadelphia, 2000, Saunders; **24-8, 24-9, 24-10, 24-13,** from Gawkrodger D: *Dermatology: an illustrated colour text,* ed 3, Edinburgh, 2003, Churchill Livingstone; **24-14, 24-15,** from Fortunato N, McCullough SM: *Plastic and reconstructive surgery,* St Louis, 1998, Mosby; **Case study photo,** © 2007 JupiterImages Corporation.

Chapter 25
25-8, 25-10, 25-11D, Courtesy Judy A. Knighton, RegN, MScN, Toronto, Ontario, Canada; **Case study photo,** © 2007 JupiterImages Corporation.

Chapter 26
26-1, Redrawn from Price SA, Wilson LM: *Pathophysiology: clinical concepts of disease processes,* ed 6, St Louis, 2003, Mosby; **26-2, 26-3, 26-11, 26-12,** from Thompson JM et al: *Mosby's clinical nursing,* ed 5, St Louis, 2002, Mosby; **26-4A,** from Bone RC et al, editors: *Pulmonary and critical care medicine,* Vol. 1, St Louis, 1993, Mosby; **26-4B,** from Albertine KH, Williams MC, Hyde DM: Anatomy of the lungs. In Mason RJ et al (editors): *Murray and Nadel's textbook of respiratory medicine,* ed 4, Philadelphia, 2005, Saunders; **26-7A,** courtesy Nonin Medical, Inc, Plymouth, Minn.; **26-7B,** used with permission of Respironics, Inc, Murrysville, Pa.; **26-9,** modified from Wilkins RL, Stoller JK, Scanlan CL: *Egan's fundamentals of respiratory care,* ed 8, St Louis, 2003, Mosby; **26-13,** from Beare PG, Myers JL: *Adult*

health nursing, ed 3, St Louis, 1998, Mosby; **26-14A,** courtesy Olympus America Inc, Melville, N.Y.; **26-14B,** from Meduri GU et al: Protected bronchoalveolar lavage, *Am Rev Respir Dis* 143:855, 1991; **26-15,** redrawn from Du Bois RM, Clarke SW: *Fiberoptic bronchoscopy in diagnosis and management,* Orlando, 1987, Grune & Stratton.

Chapter 27

27-4, Courtesy Robert Margulies, Miami, Fla. From Smolley LA: How to help patients with obstructive sleep apnea, *J Respir Dis* 11: 723-732, 1990; **27-8D,** Dale Medical Products, Inc, Plainville, Mass.; **27-11,** courtesy Passy-Muir, Inc, Irvine, Calif.; **27-13,** from the American Cancer Society; **27-16,** courtesy CLG Photographics, St Louis.

Chapter 28

28-2, From Damjanov I, Linder J: *Anderson's pathology,* ed 10, St Louis, 1996, Mosby; **28-8, 28-9,** from Atrium Medical Corporation, Hudson, N.H.; **28-10,** from the teaching collection of the Department of Pathology, University of Texas Southwestern Medical School, Dallas, Tex. In Kumar V, Abbas AK, and Fausto N: *Robbins and Cotran pathologic basis of disease,* ed 7, Philadelphia, 2005, Saunders; **Case Study Photo,** ©iStockphoto.com/ Peeter Viisimaa.

Chapter 29

29-1, Adapted from McCance KL, Huether SE, editors: *Pathophysiology: the biologic basis for disease in adults and children,* ed 5, St Louis, 2005, Mosby; **29-3,** redrawn from Price SA, Wilson LM: *Pathophysiology: clinical concepts of disease processes,* ed 6, St Louis, 2003, Mosby; **29-5,** trom Togger DA, Brenner PS: Metered dose inhalers, *Am J Nurs* 101(10):26-32, 2001; **29-11A, 29-11B,** from Potter PA, Perry AG: *Fundamentals of nursing,* ed 5, St. Louis, 2001, Mosby; **29-14, 29-15,** courtesy Nellcor Puritan Bennett, Inc, Pleasanton, Calif; **29-18,** courtesy Axcan Scandipharm, Inc, Birmingham, Ala.; **29-19C,** from Kumar V, Abbas AK, and Fausto N: *Robbins and Cotran pathologic basis of disease,* ed 7, Philadelphia, 2005, Saunders; **Case Study Photo,** ©iStockphoto.com/Sandy Jones.

Chapter 30

30-2, From Thibodeau GA, Patton KT: *Anatomy and physiology,* ed 6, St Louis, 2007, Mosby; **30-3,** copyright Dennis Kunkel Microscopy, Inc, Kailua, Hawaii; **30-7,** from Seidel HM et al: *Mosby's guide to physical examination,* ed 6, St Louis, 2006, Mosby; **30-9,** from Herlihy B, Maebius N: *The human body in health and illness,* ed 3, Philadelphia, 2007, Saunders.

Chapter 31

31-3, Redrawn from Raven PH, Johnson GB: *Biology,* ed 2, St Louis, 1991, Mosby; **31-4,** modified from McCance KL, Huether SE: *Pathophysiology: the biologic basis for disease in adults and children,* ed 5, St Louis, 2006, Mosby; **31-6, 31-9, 31-11,** from Forbes CD, Jackson WF: *Color atlas and text of clinical medicine,* ed 3, London, 2003, Mosby; **31-8,** from Bingham BJG, Hawke M, Kwok P: *Clinical atlas of otolaryngology,* St Louis, 1992, Mosby; **31-13, 31-14, 31-17,** from Skarin AT: *Atlas of diagnostic oncology,* ed 2, London, 1996, Mosby-Wolfe; **31-16,** from Cotran RS, Kumar V, Collins T: *Robbins pathologic basis of disease,* ed 6, Philadelphia, 1999, Saunders; **Case Study Photo,** ©iStockphoto.com/ Beata Pastuszek.

Chapter 32

32-1, 32-3, modified from Price SA, Wilson LM: *Pathophysiology: clinical concepts of disease processes,* ed 6, St Louis, 2003, Mosby; **32-5, 32-9,** modified from Kinney MR: *Andreoli's comprehensive cardiac care,* ed 8, St Louis, 1996, Mosby; **32-12, 32-15,** from Drake RL, Vogl W, Mitchell AWM: *Gray's anatomy for students,* Edinburgh, 2005, Churchill Livingstone; **32-13,** modified from Kinney MR: *Andreoli's comprehensive cardiac care,* ed 7, St Louis, 1991, Mosby; **32-14,** from Zipes DB et al: *Braunwald's heart disease: a textbook of cardiovascular medicine,* ed 7, St Louis, 2005, Saunders.

Chapter 33

33-1, Redrawn from West JB: *Physiological basis of medical practice,* ed 12, Baltimore, 1991, Williams & Wilkins; **33-3,** from Kissane JM: *Anderson's pathology,* ed 9, St Louis, 1990, Mosby; **33-4, 33-5,** from U.S. Department of Health and Human Services: *Seventh report of the Joint National Committee on Prevention, Detection, Evaluation, and Treatment of High Blood Pressure (JNC 7),* Washington, DC, 2003, National Institutes of Health; **Case Study Photo,** ©iStockphoto.com/Matthew Gough.

Chapter 34

34-1, 34-4, From *2005 Heart and Stroke Statistics,* American Heart Association, Dallas, Tex.; **34-2,** from Huether SE, McCance KL: *Understanding pathophysiology,* ed 3, St Louis, 2003, Mosby, **34-10,** from Zipes DB et al: *Braunwald's heart disease: a textbook of cardiovascular medicine,* ed 7, St Louis, 2005, Saunders; **34-12, 34-14,** courtesy Mayo Clinic, Rochester, Minn.; **34-13,** from Kumar V, Abbas AK, Fausto N: *Robbins and Cotran pathologic basis of disease,* ed 7, Philadelphia, 2005, Saunders; **34-16,** from Bucher L, Melander S: *Critical care nursing,* Philadelphia, 1999, Saunders; **Case Study Photo,** ©iStockphoto.com/ Floyd Anderson.

Chapter 35

35-1, Modified from Huether SE, McCance KL: *Understanding pathophysiology,* ed 3, St Louis, 2004, Mosby; **35-2,** modified from Urden LD, Stacy KM, Lough ME: *Thelan's critical care nursing: diagnosis and management,* ed 5, St Louis, 2006, Mosby; **35-3,** from ABIOMED, Inc, Danvers, Mass.; **Case Study Photo,** ©iStockphoto.com/Andres Rodriguez.

Chapter 36

36-1, 36-5, 36-7, 36-8, 36-9, 36-11, 36-14B, 36-15, 36-16C, 36-16D, 36-17, 36-19, From Huszar RJ: *Basic dysrhythmias: interpretation and management,* ed 3, St Louis, 2002, Mosby; **36-2,** modified from Goldberger AL: *Clinical electrocardiography: a simplified approach,* ed 7, St Louis, 2006, Mosby; **36-4, 36-10,** modified from Urden LD, Stacy KM, Lough ME: *Thelan's critical care nursing: diagnosis and management,* ed 5, St Louis, 2006, Mosby; **36-6, 36-12, 36-13, 36-14A, 36-16A, 36-16B, 36-18, 36-23, 36-29, 36-30,** from Bucher L, Melander S: *Critical care nursing,* Philadelphia, 1999, Saunders; **36-21,** courtesy Medtronic Physio-Control, Redmond, Wash.; **36-22A, 36-24A, 36-25,** courtesy Medtronic, Inc, Minneapolis, Minn.; **36-27A, 36-27B,** from Craig, K: How to provide transcutaneous pacing, *Nursing 2005,* 35:10, 2005; **36-27C,** from Woods, et al: *Cardiac nursing,* ed 5, Philadelphia, 2005, Lippincott; **Case Study Photo,** ©iStockphoto.com/Joseph Jean Rolland Dubé.

Chapter 37

37-1, Modified from Thibodeau GA, Patton KT: *The human body in health and disease,* ed 4, St Louis, 2005, Mosby; **37-2, 37-4,** from Damjanov I, Linder J: *Pathology: a color atlas,* St Louis, 1999, Mosby; **37-5,** from Guzzetta CE, Dossey BM: *Cardiovascular nursing: holistic practice,* St Louis, 1992, Mosby; **37-6,** redrawn from Braunwald E: *Heart disease: a textbook of cardiovascular medicine,* ed 3, Philadelphia, 1988, Saunders; **37-7, 37-9,** from Stevens A, Lowe J: *Pathology: illustrated review in color,* ed 2, St Louis, 2000, Mosby; **37-8,** from McCance KL, Huether SE: *Pathophysiology: the biologic basis for disease in adults and children,* ed 5, St Louis, 2006, Mosby; **37-10, 37-12, 37-14,** from Kumar V, Abbas AK, and Fausto N: *Robbins and Cotran pathologic basis of disease,* ed 7, Philadelphia, 2005, Saunders; **37-11,** from Zipes DB et al: *Braunwald's heart disease: a textbook of cardiovascular medicine,* ed 7, St Louis, 2005, Saunders; **37-13,** modified from Urden LD, Stacy KM, Lough ME: *Thelan's critical care nursing: diagnosis and management,* ed 5, St Louis, 2006, Mosby; **Case Study Photo,** ©iStockphoto.com/Kati Neudert.

Chapter 38

38-2, Courtesy Jo Menzoian, Boston, MA; **38-5,** from Medtronic, Minneapolis, Minn.; **38-6,** from Damjanov I, Linder J, eds: *Anderson's pathology,* ed 10, St Louis, 1996, Mosby; **38-7,** courtesy FW LoGerfo, Boston; **38-8, 38-13,** from Kamal A, Brockelhurst JC: *Color atlas of geriatric medicine,* ed 2, 1991, Mosby-Year Book-Europe; **38-9,** from Greig JD, Garden OJ: *Color atlas of surgical diagnosis,* London, 1996, Times Mirror International Publishers; **38-11,** from Lofgren KA: Varicose veins. In Haimovici H, editor: *Vascular surgery: principles and techniques,* New York, 1976, McGraw-Hill; **Case Study Photo,** ©iStockphoto.com/Kevin Russ.

Chapter 39

39-1, 39-3, From Thibodeau GA, Patton KT: *The human body in health and disease,* ed 4, St Louis, 2005, Mosby; **39-9,** from Doughty DB, Jackson DB: *Mosby's clinical nursing series: gastrointestinal disorders,* St Louis, 1993, Mosby; **39-10, 39-11, 39-12,** from Drake RL, Vogl W, Mitchell AWM: *Gray's anatomy for students,* Edinburgh, 2005, Churchill Livingstone; **39-13,** from Given Imaging, Inc, Norcross, Ga.

Chapter 40

40-1, Modified from U.S. Department of Agriculture, Center for Nutrition Policy and Promotion, *http://www.MyPyramid.gov;* **40-2,** from Morgan SL, Weinsier RL: *Fundamentals of clinical nutrition,* ed 2, St Louis, 1998, Mosby; **40-3,** adapted with permission of the American Society for Parenteral and Enteral Nutrition [ASPEN]. ASPEN Board of Directors: Guidelines for the use of parenteral and enteral nutrition in adult and pediatric patients, *J Parenter Enteral Nutr* 26:8SA, 2002; **40-4,** modified from Mahan LK, Escott-Stump S: *Krause's food, nutrition, and diet therapy,* ed 11, Philadelphia, 2004, Saunders; **40-5, 40-6, 40-7,** redrawn from Mahan LK, Arlin M: *Krause's food, nutrition, and diet therapy,* ed 8, Philadelphia, 1992, Saunders; **Case Study Photo,** ©iStockphoto.com/Stan Rohrer.

Chapter 41

41-1, From Forbes CD, Jackson WF: *Color atlas and text of clinical medicine,* ed 3, London, 2003, Mosby.

Chapter 42

42-1, From McKenry L, Tessier E, Hogan M: *Mosby's pharmacology in nursing,* ed 22, St Louis, 2006, Mosby; **42-2,** from Kumar V, Abbas AK, and Fausto N: *Robbins and Cotran pathologic basis of disease,* ed 7, Philadelphia, 2005, Saunders; **42-3,** courtesy University of Washington, Division of Gastroenterology, St Louis; **42-4,** from Doughty DB, Jackson DB: *Mosby's clinical nursing series: gastrointestinal disorders,* St Louis, 1993, Mosby; **42-6,** courtesy Curon Medical, Inc, Sunnyvale, Calif.; **42-7, 42-9, 42-11, 42-15,** redrawn from Price SA, Wilson LM: *Pathophysiology: clinical concepts of disease processes,* ed 6, St Louis, 2003, Mosby; **42-12, 42-17,** from Kumar V, Abbas AK, and Fausto N: *Robbins and Cotran pathologic basis of disease,* ed 7, Philadelphia, 2005, Saunders; **Case Study Photo,** ©iStockphoto.com/Joseph Jean Rolland Dubé.

Chapter 43

43-2, 43-15, From Stevens A, Lowe J: *Pathology,* ed 2, London, 2000, Mosby; **43-3,** from Damjanov I, Linder J, editors: *Anderson's pathology,* ed 10, St Louis, 1996, Mosby; **43-7, 43-10,** from McCance KL, Huether SE: *Pathophysiology: the biologic basis for disease in adults and children,* ed 5, St Louis, 2006, Mosby. Courtesy David Bjorkman, MD, University of Utah School of Medicine, Department of Gastroenterology; **43-9,** from Kumar V, Abbas AK, and Fausto N: *Robbins and Cotran pathologic basis of disease,* ed 7, Philadelphia, 2005, Saunders; **43-12,** redrawn from Hampton BG, Bryant RA: *Ostomies and continent diversions,* St Louis, 1992, Mosby; **43-13,** redrawn from Meeker MH, Rothrock JC: *Alexander's care of the patient in surgery,* ed 9, St Louis, 1991; **43-17B,** from Swartz MH: *Textbook of physical diagnosis: history and examination,* ed 5, Philadelphia, 2006, Saunders; **43-19,** from Townsend CM, Beauchamp RD, Evers BM et al: *Sabiston textbook of surgery: the biological basis of modern surgical practice,* ed 17, Saunders, 2004, Philadelphia.

Chapter 44

44-1, From Kamal A, Brockelhurst JC: *Color atlas of geriatric medicine,* ed 2, St Louis, 1991, Mosby-Year Book–Europe; **44-2, 44-3, 44-5,** from McCance KL, Huether SE: *Pathophysiology: the biologic basis for disease in adults and children,* ed 5, St Louis, 2006, Mosby; **44-4, 44-13, 44-17,** from Kumar V, Abbas AK, and Fausto N: *Robbins and Cotran pathologic basis of disease,* ed 7, Philadelphia, 2005, Saunders; **44-7,** adapted from McCance KL, Huether SE: *Pathophysiology: the biologic basis for disease in adults and children,* ed 5, St Louis, 2006, Mosby; **44-11,** from LaBerge JM et al: Transjugular intrahepatic portosystemic shunts: preliminary results in 25 patients, *J Vasc Surg* 16:258, 1992; **44-15,** from Stevens A, Lowe J: *Pathology: illustrated review in color,* ed 2, London, 2000, Mosby.

Chapter 45

45-1A, 45-2, 45-5, Modified from Thibodeau GA, Patton KT: *Anatomy and physiology,* ed 6, St Louis, 2007, Mosby; **45-3,** modified from Thibodeau GA, Patton KT: *The human body in health and disease,* ed 4, St Louis, 2005, Mosby; **45-4,** adapted from Herlihy B, Maebius N: *The human body in health and disease,* ed 3, Philadelphia, 2007, Saunders; **45-6,** from Brundage DJ: *Renal disorders,* St Louis, 1992, Mosby; **45-7,** from Price SA, Wilson LM: *Pathophysiology: clinical concepts of disease processes,* ed 6, St Louis, 2003, Mosby; **45-9,** courtesy Circon Corporation, Santa Barbara, Calif.

Chapter 46

46-2, 46-4, 46-7B, 46-9, 46-10B, From Kumar V, Abbas AK, and Fausto N: *Robbins and Cotran pathologic basis of disease,* ed 7, Philadelphia, 2005, Saunders; **46-5, 46-10A,** from Stevens A, Lowe J: *Pathology: illustrated review in color,* ed 2, London, 2000, Mosby; **46-7A,** from Brundage DJ: *Renal disorders,* St Louis, 1992, Mosby. B, From Kumar V, Abbas AK, and Fausto N: *Robbins and Cotran pathologic basis of disease,* ed 7, Philadelphia, 2005, Saunders; **46-8,** from Lemmi FO, Lemmi CAE: *Physical assessment findings CD-ROM,* Philadelphia, 2000, Saunders; **46-13, 46-15, 46-16,** courtesy Lynda Brubacher, Virginia Mason Hospital, Seattle, Wash.; **Case study photo,** © 2007 JupiterImages Corporation.

Chapter 47

47-2, From Stevens A, Lowe J: *Pathology,* ed 2, Mosby, 2000, London; **47-4,** from United States Renal Data System, Minneapolis, Minn.; **47-9, 47-12,** ©1994 Baxter Healthcare Corp., Deerfield, Ill.; **47-10, 47-11,** courtesy Mary Jo Holechek, Baltimore, Md.; **47-13D, 47-17,** courtesy Vascular Access Services, LLC, St Louis; **47-14A,** courtesy Quinton Instrument Co., Seattle, Wash.; **Case Study Photo,** ©iStockphoto.com/Michael Blackburn.

Chapter 48

48-2, 48-10, Modified from Thibodeau GA, Patton KT: *Anatomy and physiology,* ed 6, St Louis, 2007, Mosby; **48-3, 48-4,** from Herlihy B, Maebius N: *The human body in health and disease,* ed 3, Philadelphia, 2007, Saunders; **48-6,** redrawn from McCance KL, Huether SE: *Pathophysiology: the biologic basis for disease in adults and children,* ed 5, St Louis, 2006, Mosby; **48-8, 48-10, 48-11,** from Thibodeau GA, Patton KT: *The human body in health and disease,* ed 4, St Louis, 2005, Mosby; **48-12,** from Thompson JM, Wilson SF: *Health assessment for nursing practice,* St Louis, 1996, Mosby.

Chapter 49

49-8A, 49-16, 49-17, From Chew SL, Leslie D: *Clinical endocrinology and diabetes: an illustrated colour text,* Edinburgh, 2006, Churchill Livingstone; **49-8B,** courtesy Medtronic MiniMed, Northridge, Calif.; **49-9,** from Medtronic Diabetes, Minneapolis, Minn.; **49-10,** from Home Diagnostics, Ft. Lauderdale, Fla.; **49-12, 49-14,** from Kumar V, Abbas AK, and Fausto N: *Robbins and Cotran pathologic basis of disease,* ed 7, Philadelphia, 2005, Saunders; **49-13,** from Urden LD, Stacy KM, Lough ME: *Thelan's critical care nursing: diagnosis and management,* ed 5, St Louis, 2006, Mosby; **Case study photo,** © 2007 JupiterImages Corporation.

Chapter 50

50-1, Courtesy Linda Haas, Seattle, Wash.; **50-3, 50-4,** redrawn from Urden LD, Stacy KM, Lough ME: *Thelan's critical care nursing: diagnosis and management,* ed 5, St Louis, 2006, Mosby; **50-6, 50-7,** from Forbes CD, Jackson WF: *Color atlas and text of clinical medicine,* ed 3, London, 2003, Mosby; **50-8, 50-12, 50-13,** from Chew SL, Leslie D: *Clinical endocrinology and diabetes: an illustrated colour text,* Edinburgh, 2006, Churchill Livingstone; **50-9,** courtesy Paul W. Ladenson, MD, The Johns Hopkins University and Hospital, Baltimore, Md. From Seidel HM et al: *Mosby's guide to physical examination,* ed 6, St Louis, 2006, Mosby; **50-10,** from Seidel HM et al: *Mosby's guide to physical examination,* ed 6, St Louis, 2006, Mosby; **Case Study Photo,** ©iStockphoto.com/Lanica Klein.

Chapter 51

51-1, From Thibodeau GA, Patton KT: *The human body in health and disease,* ed 4, St Louis, 2005, Mosby; **51-2, 51-5, 51-6, 51-9,** modified from Thibodeau GA, Patton KT: *Anatomy and physiology,* ed 6, St Louis, 2007, Mosby; **51-3, 51-4,** from Seidel HM et al: *Mosby's guide to physical examination,* ed 6, St Louis, 2006, Mosby.

Chapter 52

52-2, From Powell DE, Stilling CB: *Diagnosis and detection of breast diseases,* St Louis, 1993, Mosby; **52-4,** from Evans A et al: *Atlas of breast disease management,* Philadelphia, 1998, Saunders; **52-6,** from Swartz MH: *Textbook of physical diagnosis: history and examination,* ed 5, Philadelphia, 2006, Saunders; **52-7,** courtesy of Cytyc Corporation and affliates, Marlborough, Mass.; **52-9, 52-10B,** courtesy Brian Davies, MD. From Fortunato N, McCullough S: *Plastic and reconstructive surgery,* St Louis, 1998, Mosby; **52-10A,** from Cameron J: *Current surgical therapy,* ed 5, St Louis, 1995, Mosby; **52-11,** modified from Beare PG, Myers JL: *Adult health nursing,* ed 3, St Louis, 1998, Mosby; and Fortunato N, McCullough S: *Plastic and reconstructive surgery,* St Louis, 1998, Mosby; **Case Study Photo,** ©iStockphoto.com/Jessica Jones.

Chapter 53

53-1, 53-2, 53-3, 53-6, 53-7B, From Morse S, Moreland A, Holmes K, editors: *Atlas of sexually transmitted diseases and AIDS,* London, 1996, Mosby-Wolfe; **53-4,** courtesy USPHS, Washington DC; **53-5,** from Habif T: *Clinical dermatology: a color guide to diagnosis and therapy,* ed 4, St Louis, 2004, Mosby; **53-7A, C, 53-9C,** from the Center for Disease Control and Prevention. Courtesy of Susan Lindsley. **53-8, 53-10,** Reproduced with permission of GlaxoSmithKline, Research Triangle Park, N.C.; **53-9A,** from the Center for Disease Control and Prevention. Courtesy Joe Millar. **53-9B,** from the Center for Disease Control and Prevention. Courtesy of Dr. Wiesner. **Case Study Photo,** ©iStockphoto.com/Roberta Osborne.

Chapter 54

54-2, Courtesy Ethicon, Inc, Cornelia, Ga.; **54-3,** from Seidel HM et al: *Mosby's guide to physical examination,* ed 6, St Louis, 2006, Mosby; **54-4,** from Lowdermilk DL, Perry SE: *Maternity and women's health care,* ed 8, St Louis, 2004, Mosby; **54-6,** modified from Stenchever MA et al: *Comprehensive gynecology,* ed 4, St Louis, 2001, Mosby; **54-7,** from McCance KL, Huether SE: *Pathophysiology: the biologic basis for disease in adults and children,* ed 5, St Louis, 2006, Mosby; **54-8, 54-13B,** from Symonds EM, McPherson MBA: *Color atlas of obstetrics and gynecology,* London, 1994, Mosby; **54-9,** from Drake RL, Vogl W, Mitchell AWM: *Gray's anatomy for students,* Edinburgh, 2005, Churchill Livingstone; **54-10,** from Phipps WJ, Sands JK, and Marek JF: *Medical-surgical: nursing concepts and clinical practice,* ed 6, St Louis, 1999, Mosby; **54-12,** modified from Seidel HM et al: *Mosby's guide to physical examination,* ed 6, St Louis, 2006, Mosby; **54-14B,** from Huffman JW: *Gynecology and obstetrics,* Philadelphia, 1962, Saunders; **Case Study Photo,** ©iStockphoto.com/Brandon Clark.

Chapter 55

55-5, Modified from Iwamoto RR, Maher KE: Radiation therapy for prostate cancer, *Semin Oncol Nurs* 17(2):90-100, 2001; **55-6A,**

Inc, Allendale, Pa.; **63-15,** from Ryan DW, Park GR: *Color atlas of critical and intensive care: diagnosis and investigation,* London, 1995, Mosby-Wolfe; **63-18,** from Thompson JM et al: *Mosby's clinical nursing,* ed 4, St Louis, 1997, Mosby; **63-19,** courtesy R.A. Weinstein, Denver, Colo.; **63-21,** from Macklin EJ et al: *Hunter, Macklin, and Callahan's rehabilitation of the hand and upper extremity,* vol. 2, ed 5, St Louis, 2002, Mosby; **63-23,** from Thibodeau GA, Patton KT: *Anatomy and physiology,* ed 6, St Louis, 2007, Mosby; **63-25,** courtesy Zimmer, Inc, Warsaw, Ind.; **Case Study Photo,** ©iStockphoto.com.

Chapter 64

64-1, Redrawn from Mourad L: *Orthopedic disorders,* St Louis, 1992, Mosby; **64-2, 64-5,** from Thibodeau GA, Patton KT: *Human body in health and disease,* ed 4, St Louis, 2005, Mosby; **64-3, 64-4,** from Damjanov I, Linder J: *Anderson's pathology,* ed 10, St Louis, 1996, Mosby; **64-6,** from Eidelson SG, Spinasanta SA: *Advanced technologies to treat neck and back pain: a patient's guide,* Wheaton, Ill., 2005, SYA Press and Research; **64-7,** from DePuy Spine, Inc. Raynham, Mass.; **64-8,** from Mercier LR: *Practical orthopedics,* ed 5, St Louis, 2000, Mosby; **64-9,** from Mercier LR: *Practical orthopedics,* ed 4, St Louis, 1996, Mosby; **64-10,** from Maher A et al: *Orthopaedic nursing,* ed 3, Philadelphia, 2002, Saunders; **Case Study Photo,** ©iStockphoto.com/Roberta Osborne.

Chapter 65

65-1, 65-3, From Stevens A, Lowe J: *Pathology: an illustrated review in color,* ed 2, London, 2000, Mosby; **65-6,** from Forbes CD, Jackson WF: *Color atlas of clinical medicine,* ed 3, London, 2003, Mosby; **65-7,** from Habif TP: *Clinical dermatology: a color guide to diagnosis and therapy,* ed 4, St Louis, 2004, Mosby; **65-8,** reprinted from the Clinical Slide Collection on the Rheumatic Diseases, copyright 1991, 1995, 1997. Used by permission of the American College of Rheumatology; **65-10,** from Habif TP: *Clinical dermatology: a color guide to diagnosis and therapy,* ed 3, St Louis, 1996, Mosby; **65-12,** from Zitelli BJ, Davis HW: *Atlas of pediatric physical diagnosis,* ed 4, St Louis, 2002, Mosby; **65-13,** from Kumar V, Abbas AK, and Fausto N: *Robbins and Cotran pathologic basis of disease,* ed 7, Philadelphia, 2005, Saunders; **65-14,** redrawn from Freundlich B, Leventhal L: The fibromyalgia syndrome. In Schumacher HR Jr, Klippel JH, Koopman WJ, editors: *Primer on the rheumatic diseases,* ed 11, Atlanta, 1997, Arthritis Foundation. Reprinted with permission from The Arthritis Foundation, 1330 W. Peachtree St., Atlanta, Ga. 30309; **Case Study Photo,** ©iStockphoto.com/Jason Stitt.

Chapter 66

66-1, From Avera Health, Sioux Falls, S.Dak.; **66-2, 66-22,** courtesy Spacelabs Medical, Redmond, Wash.; **66-3,** redrawn from Gardner PE: *Hemodynamic pressure monitoring,* Redmond, Wash., 1994, Spacelabs Medical; **66-4,** redrawn from Flynn JBM, Bruce NP: *Introduction to critical care skills,* St Louis, 1993, Mosby; **66-5,** from Darovic GO, Vanriper S, Vanriper J: *Fluid-filled monitoring systems.* In Darovic GO: *Hemodynamic monitoring,* ed 2, Phila-

delphia, 1995, Saunders; **66-6, 66-8, 66-11,** modified from Urden LD, Stacy KM, Lough ME: *Thelan's critical care nursing: diagnosis and management,* ed 5, St Louis, 2006, Mosby; **66-7,** courtesy Edwards Critical Care Division, Baxter Healthcare Corporation, Santa Ana, Calif.; **66-9, 66-10,** from Lynn-McHale DJ, Carlson KK (editors): *AACN procedure manual for critical care,* ed 5, Philadelphia, 2005, Saunders; **66-13,** courtesy Datascope Corp., Fairfield, N.J.; **66-15,** from Datascope Corp., Montvale, N.J.; **66-16,** redrawn from Urden LD, Stacy KM, Lough ME: *Thelan's critical care nursing: diagnosis and management,* ed 4, St Louis, 2002, Mosby; **66-17A,** from Beare PG, Myers JL: *Adult health nursing,* ed 3, St Louis, 1998, Mosby; **66-18,** from Henneman E, Ellstrom K, St. John RE: *AACN protocols for practice: care of the mechanically ventilated patient series,* Aliso Viejo, Calif., 1999, American Association of Critical-Care Nurses; **66-19,** from Sills JR: *Respiratory care certification guide: the complete review resource for the entry level exam,* ed 2, St Louis, 1991, Mosby. In Urden LD, Stacy KM, Lough ME: *Thelan's critical care nursing: diagnosis and management,* ed 5, St Louis, 2006, Mosby; **66-20,** reprinted by permission of Nellcor Puritan Bennett Inc, Pleasanton, California; **66-21,** courtesy Lifecare, Westminster, Colo.; **66-23,** from Wiegand DL, Carlson K (editors): *AACN procedure manual for critical care,* ed 5, 2005, Saunders; **Case Study Photo,** ©iStockphoto.com/Sharon Dominick.

Chapter 67

67-2, 67-3, 67-4, 67-5, Modified from Urden LD, Stacy KM, Lough ME: *Thelan's critical care nursing: diagnosis and management,* ed 5, St Louis, 2006, Mosby; **Case Study Photo,** ©iStockphoto.com/Yvonne Chamberlain.

Chapter 68

68-6, From Richmond TS: The patient with a cervical spinal cord injury, *Focus on Critical Care* 12:27, 1985; **68-7,** courtesy Respironics, Inc, Pittsburgh, Pa.; **68-10,** from Cohen J, Powderly WG: *Infectious diseases,* ed 2, St Louis, 2004, Mosby; **68-11, 68-12,** © 2006 Hill-Rom Services, Inc. Reprinted with permission. All rights reserved; **Case Study Photo,** ©iStockphoto.com/Galina Barskaya.

Chapter 69

69-1, ©ESI Triage Research Team, 2004. Reproduced with permission; **69-3, 69-4,** courtesy Cameron Bangs, MD. From Auerbach PS, Donner HJ, Weiss EA: *Field guide to wilderness medicine,* ed, 2, St Louis, 2003, Mosby; **69-6,** from Auerbach PS, Donner HJ, Weiss EA: *Field guide to wilderness medicine,* St Louis, 1999, Mosby; **69-7,** courtesy of Centers for Disease Control, Division of Viral and Rickettsial Diseases. Available at *www.cdc.gov/ncidod/dvbid/lyme/ld_tickremoval.htm*; **69-8,** modified from Marx JA et al: *Rosen's emergency medicine: concepts and clinical practice,* vol 1, ed 6, St Louis, 2006, Mosby; **69-9,** courtesy Sherman Minton, MD. From Auerbach PS, Donner HJ, Weiss EA: *Field guide to wilderness medicine,* St Louis, 1999, Mosby; **69-10,** photo used with the permission of the American Red Cross; **Case Study Photo,** ©iStockphoto.com/Lacey Gadwill.

A

AAA. *See* Abdominal aortic aneurysms
AAT. *See* Animal-assisted therapy
AAT deficiency. *See* α₁-Antitrypsin deficiency
AB5000™ Circulatory Support System, 839
Abacavir (Ziagen)
 adverse effects of, 258*t*
 lamivudine, zidovudine, and abacavir (Trizivir), 258*t*
 lamivudine and abacavir (Epizicom), 258*t*
Abandonment, fear of, 159
Abarelix (Plenaxis), 1426, 1426*t*
Abatacept (Orencia)
 for arthritis and connective tissue disorders, 1700*t*
 for rheumatoid arthritis, 1706
ABC codes, 8*t*
ABCDs of melanoma, 465, 466*f*
Abciximab (ReoPro), 800*t*
ABD Combine Pads, 205*t*
Abdomen
 assessment abnormalities, 676*t*, 940*t*
 auscultation of, 937
 distention of, 676*t*, 940*t*
  postoperative, 1188
 inspection of, 937
 palpation of, 937-938
  deep, 937, 938*t*
  light, 937, 938*f*
 percussion of, 937
 physical examination of, 936-938, 1246
  adaptations, 50*t*
  normal, 939*t*
  outline for, 49*t*
  recording, 51*t*
 quadrants of, 936, 936*f*
 rebound tenderness of, 940*t*
 regions of, 936, 936*f*, 937*t*
 secondary survey head-to-toe assessment, 1826*t*, 1827
Abdominal aorta atherosclerosis, 893, 893*f*
Abdominal aortic aneurysms, 894, 894*f*
 fusiform, 894, 894*f*
 surgical repair of, 895, 896*f*
Abdominal (diaphragmatic) breathing, 117, 646
Abdominal hysterectomy
 nursing care plan for patient with, 1398*b*
 total, 1405*f*
  and bilateral salpingo-oophorectomy, 1404*t*
  case study, 1411
Abdominal incision, 381, 382*f*
Abdominal pain
 acute, **1043-1046**
  acute intervention for, 1045-1046
  causes of, 1043-1044, 1044*t*
  clinical manifestations of, 1043
  collaborative management of, 1043-1044
  diagnostic studies, 1043-1044
  emergency management of, 1044, 1045*t*
  etiology and pathophysiology of, 1043

Abdominal pain (*Continued*)
 nursing assessment of, 1044
 nursing diagnoses, 1044
 nursing evaluation of, 1046
 nursing implementation for, 1045-1046
 nursing management of, **1044-1046**
 nursing planning for, 1044
 postoperative care of, 1045-1046
 preoperative care of, 1045
 assessment of, 1335*t*
 chronic, **1046-1048**
 in peritoneal dialysis, 1219
Abdominal paradox, 524*t*
Abdominal tenderness, 1335*t*
Abdominal trauma, 1047-1048
 clinical manifestations of, 1047
 diagnostic studies, 1048
 emergency management of, 1048, 1048*t*
 etiology and pathophysiology of, 1047
 nursing and collaborative management of, **1048**
Abdominal ultrasound, 682*t*, 940, 941*t*
Abdominal wall, 932, 933*t*
Abducens nerve (cranial nerve VI), 1450*t*
Abducens nerve (cranial nerve VI) testing, 1457
Abduction, 1622, 1622*t*
 after total hip replacement, 1663, 1663*f*
ABGs. *See* Arterial blood gases
ABI. *See* Ankle-brachial index
AbioCor Heart Replacement System, 839, 840*f*
Ablation
 radiofrequency catheter ablation therapy, 861
 surgical, 1551
ABO blood groups and compatibilities, 679, 680*t*
Abortion, 1383-1385
 as ethical dilemma, 1385*b*
 habitual recurrent, 1383
 induced, 1383, **1384-1385**
 methods for inducing, 1384, 1384*t*
 spontaneous, **1383-1384**
Above-the-knee amputation, residual limb bandaging, 1660, 1661*f*
Abraxane (paclitaxel)
 for breast cancer, 1355
 for cervical cancer, 1402
 classification of, 287*t*
ABRs. *See* Auditory brainstem responses
Abscesses
 anorectal, **1083-1084,** 1084*f*
 brain, 1494*t*, **1499,** 1870
 lactational breast, 1346
 lung, **576-577,** 1873
 peritonsillar, **542**
Absence (petit mal) seizures, 1534-1535
 atypical, 1535
Absent grief, 154
Absorbent products, 1183*t*
Absorption, 926, 928-930, 930
 problems of, **925-1134**
 resources for, 970
 by small intestine, 929
Absorption atelectasis, 644
Absorptive dressings, 205*t*
Abstinence, 166*t*

Abuse
 alcohol abuse, 176, 176*f*
  chronic, 177, 177*t*
  complications of, 168*t*, 177
  contributing factors, 166-167, 167*f*
 drug abuse (*See also* Substance abuse)
  contributing factors, 166-167, 167*f*
  health problems related to, 168*t*
 elder mistreatment/abuse, 73-74
  resources for, 84
 financial, 73*t*
 of medications, 80
 physical, 73*t*
 psychologic, 73*t*
 sexual, 73*t*
Ac globulin, 670*t*
Acamprosate (Campral), 178
Acanthamoeba keratitis, 423, 423*f*
Acanthosis nigricans, 462, 1287
Acapella, 649
Acarbose (Precose), 1265, 1266*t*
Accelerated fractionation, 292
Accelerated idioventricular rhythm, 849*t*, 855
Access to health care, 20*b*, 33-34
Accessory muscle use, 524*t*
Accessory nerve (cranial nerve XI), 1450*t*
Accessory pathways, 851
Accolate (zafirlukast), 620
 for allergic rhinitis and sinusitis, 537*t*
 for asthma and COPD, 619*t*
 food/nutrient interactions, 954*t*
Accommodation, 399, 1457
Acculturation, 27
Accupril (quinapril), 776*t*
Accuretic (quinapril/hydrochlorothiazide), 777*t*
Accutane (isotretinoin)
 for acne, 472*t*
 drug alert, 470
ACE inhibitors. *See* Angiotensin-converting enzyme inhibitors
Acebutolol (Sectral)
 classification of, 856*t*
 for hypertension, 774*t*
Aceon (perindopril), 776*t*
Acetaminophen (Tylenol, Phenaphen, Midrin)
 blood glucose level effects, 1267*t*
 codeine plus acetaminophen (Tylenol #3), 137*t*, 138
 ethnic differences in response to, 35*t*
 for headache, 1530
 hepatotoxicity, 933, 934*t*
 for hyperthermia, 1512
 mechanism of action, 202*t*
 for osteoarthritis, 1697*b*
 for pain, 135, 136*t*, 141
 poisoning, 1837*t*
 toxicology, 1865*t*
 Vicodin (hydrocodone plus acetaminophen), 138
Acetazolamide (Diamox)
 for acute pancreatitis, 1121*t*
 blood glucose level effects, 1267*t*
 for glaucoma, 435*t*
Acetic acid, 1117
Acetone, 1855*t*, 1862*t*
Acetylcholine, 1445*t*
Acetylsalicylic acid (aspirin), 1512

Achalasia, 1012-1013
 esophageal, 1012-1013, 1012*f*
 treatment of, 1012, 1012*f*
Achilles tendon reflex testing, 1459
Achilles tendonitis, 1623*t*
Acid, 333*t*
Acid poisoning, 1837*t*
Acid-base imbalances, 333-337, 335*t*, 336*f*
 alterations, 334-336
 assessment of, **337-338**
 blood gas values in, 336-337
 in chronic kidney disease, 1207
 clinical manifestations of, 336-337
 diagnosis of, 336-337
 mixed disorders, 335-336
 terminology related to, 333*t*
Acid-base regulation, 333-334
Acidemia, 333*t*
Acid-fast smear and culture, 527*t*
Acidity. *See* pH
Acidosis, 333, 333*f*
 clinical manifestations of, 336, 336*t*
 definition of, 333*t*
 diabetic ketoacidosis, 1255, **1278-1280**
 metabolic, 335, 335*t*
  in acute renal failure, 1200
  in chronic kidney disease, 1207
  clinical manifestations of, 336*t*
 respiratory, 334-335, 335*t*, 336*t*
Aciphex (rabeprazole)
 for gastroesophageal reflux disease, 1006, 1006*t*
 for gastrointestinal bleeding, 998*t*
 for peptic ulcer disease, 1019*t*, 1020
Acne, 472*t*
Acne lesions, 457*t*
ACNP. *See* Acute care nurse practitioner
Acoustic nerve testing, 1457
Acoustic neuroma, 442, 1488*t*
Acova (argatroban), 914
ACP. *See* Anesthesia care provider
Acquired immunodeficiency syndrome (AIDS), 252-253
 diagnostic criteria for, 252, 253*t*
 ocular manifestations of, 437*t*
 renal disease in, **1168**
 resources for, 270
Acrochordons, 462, 472*t*
Acromegaly, 1291
 dermatologic manifestations of, 473*t*
 drug therapy for, 1292
 facial changes associated with, 1291, 1291*f*
Acropachy, 1299, 1300*f*
ACT. *See* Assist-control ventilation; Automated coagulation time
Acticoat, 205*t*, 499
Actinic keratosis, 452, **463,** 464*t*
Actinomyces israelii, 576*t*
Actinomycosis, 576*t*
Action potential, 741, 1443
 phases of, 843, 843*f*
Actiq (fentanyl), 137*t*, 141
Activase (alteplase), 800*t*
Activated charcoal, 1037*t*, 1838
Activated clotting time, 911*t*, 913*t*
Activated partial thromboplastin time, 679*t*, 913*t*
 in deep vein thrombosis, 911*t*
 laboratory values, 1859*t*
Active core rewarming, 1831
Active transport, 317

Note: Disorder names are in **bold face.** Page numbers in **bold face** indicate main discussions. Page numbers followed by *f, t, b,* or *n* indicate figures, tables, boxed material, or notes, respectively.

I-1

Activity considerations. *See also* Physical activity
  for COPD, 652-655
Activity-exercise pattern
  in assessment of auditory system, 410*t*, 411, 746
  in assessment of cardiovascular system, 746*t*
  in assessment of endocrine system, 1244
  in assessment of fluid, electrolyte, and acid-base imbalances, 337-338
  in assessment of gastrointestinal system, 934, 935*t*
  in assessment of hematologic system, 673, 673*t*
  in assessment of integumentary system, 453*t*, 454
  in assessment of musculoskeletal system, 1621
  in assessment of nervous system, 1454-1455
  in assessment of preoperative patient, 350*t*
  in assessment of reproductive system, 1333, 1333*t*
  in assessment of respiratory system, 518*t*, 520
  in assessment of urinary system, 1143*t*, 1144
  in assessment of visual system, 403, 403*t*
  and asthma, 624*t*
  comparison with NANDA International Taxonomy II, 42*t*
  concerns of patients requiring home health care, 90*t*
  nursing diagnoses, **1852**
  nursing history, 45, 45*t*
Actonel (risedronate), 1689
Actos (pioglitazone), 1265, 1266*t*
Actron (ketoprofen), 1698*t*
Acupressure, 98, 98*t*
Acupressure points, 98, 100*f*
Acupuncture, 96, 99*f*, 1682*b*
  clinical applications of, 98
  conditions that may benefit from, 99*t*
  for pain, 144
Acute abdominal pain, 1043-1046
  acute intervention for, 1045-1046
  causes of, 1043-1044, 1044*t*
  clinical manifestations of, 1043
  collaborative management of, 1043-1044
  diagnostic studies, 1043-1044
  emergency management of, 1044, 1045*t*
  etiology and pathophysiology of, 1043
  nursing assessment of, 1044
  nursing diagnoses, 1044
  nursing evaluation of, 1046
  nursing implementation for, 1045-1046
  nursing management of, **1044-1046**
  nursing planning for, 1044
  postoperative care of, 1045-1046
  preoperative care of, 1045
Acute alcohol toxicity, 177

Acute arterial ischemic disorders, 907-908
  clinical manifestations of, 907
  collaborative care for, 908
  etiology and pathophysiology of, 907
Acute blood loss, 694-695
  clinical manifestations of, 694, 695*t*
  collaborative care for, 695
  diagnostic studies, 694
  laboratory study findings in, 690*t*
  nursing management of, **695**
Acute bronchitis, 561
Acute care
  for older adults, 79
  for stroke, 1511-1513
Acute care nurse practitioner (ACNP), 1735
Acute chest syndrome, 697
Acute cholecystitis, 1127, 1127*t*
Acute cocaine toxicity, 174-175
Acute coronary syndrome, 784-785, 802, 802*f*
  acute intervention for, 813-814
  ambulatory and home care for, 815-817
  collaborative care for, 799*f*, **806-817**
  diagnostic studies, **805-806**
  drug therapy of, 800*t*, 808
  ECG changes associated with, **861-862, 861*f*, 861*t***
  emotional and behavioral reactions to, 814, 814*t*
  etiology and pathophysiology of, 802
  fibrinolytic therapy of, 807-808
  FITT physical activity guidelines for, 816*t*
  gender differences in, 802*t*
  manifestations of, **802-818**
  monitoring, 813
  monitoring guidelines for, 862
  nursing assessment of, 810, 810*t*
  nursing care plan for patient with, 811*b*-812*b*
  nursing diagnoses, 810
  nursing evaluation of, 817
  nursing implementation for, 813-817
  nursing management of, **810-817**
  nursing planning for, 810
  nutritional therapy of, 808
  patient and family teaching guide for, 815*t*
  patient and family teaching guide for sexual activity after, 817*t*
  rehabilitation after, 813*t*
  resources, 820
Acute coryza. *See* Viral rhinitis, acute
Acute decompensated heart failure
  clinical manifestations of, 824-825
  collaborative care for, 827*t*
  nursing and collaborative management of, **827-829**
Acute disseminated intravascular coagulation
  laboratory abnormalities in, 712*t*
  predisposing conditions to, 710*t*
Acute glaucoma, 434*t*-435*t*
Acute glomerulonephritis, 1166*t*
Acute hemodialysis, 1221, 1221*f*
Acute hemolytic reactions, 732, 733*t*
Acute hepatitis, 1092, 1093*t*
Acute HIV infection, 252
Acute illness, 1272-1274
Acute infectious diarrhea
  causes of, 1036, 1037*t*
  nursing assessment of, 1037-1038
  nursing care plan for, 1039*b*
  nursing diagnoses, 1038

Acute infectious diarrhea *(Continued)*
  nursing implementation for, 1038
  nursing management of, **1037-1038**
  nursing planning for, 1038
Acute inflammation, 197
Acute intracranial problems, 1467-1501
Acute leukemia, 718*f*
Acute liver failure, 1115
Acute low back pain, 1676-1680
  acute intervention for, 1676-1677
  ambulatory and home care for, 1677-1680
  collaborative care for, 1676
  health promotion in, 1676
  nursing assessment of, 1676, 1676*t*
  nursing diagnoses, 1676
  nursing evaluation of, 1680
  nursing implementation for, 1676-1680
  nursing management of, **1676-1680**
  nursing planning for, 1676
  physical activity and, 1681*b*
Acute lung injury
  mediators of, 1813, 1814*t*
  transfusion-related, 732, 733*t*
Acute lymphocytic leukemia, 718, 718*t*, 721*t*
Acute marginal gingivitis, 939*t*
Acute myelogenous leukemia, 718, 718*t*, 721*t*
Acute myocardial infarction, 803, 803*f*
Acute necrotizing ulcerative gingivitis, 1000*t*
Acute osteomyelitis, 1669
Acute otitis media, 439
Acute pain, 130*t*, 131
Acute pancreatitis, 1118-1124
  acute intervention for, 1122-1124
  ambulatory and home care for, 1124
  clinical manifestations of, 1119
  collaborative care for, 1120-1121, 1120*t*
  complications of, 1119-1120
  conservative therapy of, 1120-1121
  diagnostic studies, 1120, 1120*t*
  drug therapy of, 1121, 1121*t*
  etiology and pathophysiology of, 1118-1119, 1119*f*
  health promotion in, 1122
  nursing assessment of, 1121, 1121*t*
  nursing care plan for patient with, 1122*b*-1123*b*
  nursing diagnoses, 1121
  nursing evaluation of, 1124
  nursing implementation for, 1122-1124
  nursing management of, **1121-1124**
  nursing planning for, 1122
  nutritional therapy of, 1121
  surgical therapy of, 1121
Acute pericarditis, 871-874, 872*f*
  clinical manifestations of, 872
  collaborative care for, 873-874, 874*t*
  complications of, 872
  diagnostic studies, 872-873, 873*f*
  etiology of, 871-872, 872*t*
  nursing management of, **874**
Acute pharyngitis, 541-542
  clinical manifestations of, 541
  nursing and collaborative management of, **541-542**
Acute poststreptococcal glomerulonephritis, 1165-1166
  clinical manifestations of, 1165
  complications of, 1165

Acute poststreptococcal glomerulonephritis, *(Continued)*
  diagnostic studies, 1165-1166
  nursing and collaborative management of, **1166**
Acute pulmonary embolism, 599*t*
Acute pyelonephritis, 1161-1162, 1161*f*
  acute intervention and home care for, 1162
  acute intervention for, 1162
  clinical manifestations of, 1161
  collaborative care for, 1161-1162, 1162*f*
  diagnostic studies, 1161
  drug therapy of, 1161-1162
  etiology and pathophysiology of, 1161
  health promotion in, 1162
  nursing assessment of, 1162
  nursing diagnoses, 1162
  nursing evaluation of, 1162
  nursing implementation for, 1162
  nursing management of, **1162**
  nursing planning for, 1162
Acute radiation syndrome, 1840, 1841*t*
Acute rehabilitation, 87*t*
Acute rejection, 238
Acute renal failure, 1197-1204
  in acquired immunodeficiency syndrome, 1168
  acute intervention for, 1203-1204
  clinical course, 1199-1201
  collaborative care for, 1201-1203, 1202*t*
  diagnostic studies, 1201
  diuretic phase, 1200-1201
  etiology and pathophysiology of, 1198-1199, 1198*f*, 1198*t*
  gerontologic considerations for, **1204**
  health promotion in, 1203
  indications for dialysis in, 1202
  initiating phase, 1199
  intrarenal causes, 1198, 1198*f*, 1198*t*
  manifestations of, 1201*t*
  nursing assessment of, 1203
  nursing diagnoses, 1203
  nursing evaluation of, 1204
  nursing implementation for, 1203
  nursing management of, **1203-1204**
  nursing planning for, 1203
  nutritional therapy of, 1202-1203
  oliguria of, 1199-1200, 1200*t*
  oliguric phase, 1199-1200
  postrenal causes, 1198*f*, 1198*t*, 1199
  prerenal causes, 1198, 1198*f*, 1198*t*
  recovery phase, 1201
  resources for, 1232
Acute renal lithiasis, 1173*b*-1174*b*
Acute respiratory distress syndrome (ARDS), 1812-1818
  case study, 1819
  chest x-ray findings in, 1815, 1815*f*, 1815*t*
  chronic or late phase, 1814
  clinical manifestations of, 1815
  clinical progression of, 1815
  collaborative care for, 1817*t*
  complications of, 1815-1816, 1816*t*
  conditions predisposing to, 1812, 1813*t*
  diagnostic criteria for, 1815
  diagnostic findings in, 1815, 1815*t*
  etiology of, 1812-1814, 1814*f*
  fibrotic phase, 1814
  fluid therapy in, 1818
  injury or exudative phase, 1813-1814

Note: Disorder names are in **bold face.** Page numbers in **bold face** indicate main discussions. Page numbers followed by *f*, *t*, *b*, or *n* indicate figures, tables, boxed material, or notes, respectively.

Acute respiratory distress syndrome (ARDS), *(Continued)*
medical supportive therapy for, 1818
nursing and collaborative management of, **1816-1818**
nursing assessment of, 1816
nursing diagnoses, 1816
nursing evaluation of, 1818
nursing planning for, 1816
oxygen therapy for, 1816-1817
positioning strategies for, 1817-1818
reparative or proliferative phase, 1814
respiratory therapy for, 1816-1818
and restrictive lung disease, 596*t*
stages of edema formation in, 1812, 1813*f*
Acute respiratory failure, 1799-1812
chest physical therapy in, 1810
clinical manifestations of, 1803-1805
collaborative care for, 1806*t*
in COPD, 636-637
diagnostic studies, 1805
drug therapy for, 1810-1811
etiology and pathophysiology of, 1800-1803
medical supportive therapy for, 1811-1812
nursing and collaborative management of, **1805-1812**
nursing assessment of, 1805, 1806*t*
nursing care plan for patient with, 1807*b*-1809*b*
nursing diagnoses, 1805
nursing evaluation of, 1812
nursing planning for, 1806
nutritional therapy for, 1812
oxygen therapy for, 1807-1809
predisposing factors, 1801*t*
prevention of, 1806
respiratory therapy for, 1807-1810
treatment of underlying cause of, 1811
Acute rheumatic fever, 875-876
cardiac lesions, 876
complications of, 876-877
diagnosis of, 876
diagnostic criteria for
major, 876
minor, 876, 876*t*
modified Jones criteria, 876, 876*t*
valvular deformities, 876
Acute sinusitis, 540, 541*t*
Acute soft tissue injuries, 1631, 1632*t*
Acute thyrotoxicosis, 1302-1304
Acute toxicity of chemotherapy, 291
Acute transfusion reactions, 732-734, 733*t*
Acute tubular necrosis, 1198-1199, 1199*f*
pathophysiology of, 1199
Acute ulcerative colitis, 1052, 1052*f*
Acute urinary retention, 1180
Acute viral hepatitis, 1097*b*-1098*b*
Acute viral rhinitis, 536-538
ACV. *See* Assist-control ventilation
Acyclovir (Zovirax)
for Bell's palsy, 1585
for encephalitis, 1498
for genital herpes, 1375
for keratitis, 423
AD. *See* Alzheimer's disease
ADA deficiency. *See* Adenosine deaminase deficiency
Adalat (nifedipine)
for Raynaud's phenomenon, 1724
for voiding dysfunction, 1185*t*

Adalat CC (nifedipine long acting), 776*t*
Adalimumab (Humira)
for arthritis and connective tissue disorders, 1700*t*
for rheumatoid arthritis, 1705-1706
Adaptic, 205*t*
Adaptive grief, 154
ADC programs. *See* Adult day care programs
Addiction, 145-146, 165
ambulatory and home care for, 189
contributing factors to, 166-167
definition of, 166, 166*t*
fear of, 146*t*
health complications of, 167
neurobiology of, 166
treatment of, 167
Addictive behaviors, 165-191
definition of, 166*t*
gender differences, 167*b*
gerontologic considerations, **189**
health promotion in, 184-185
motivational interviewing for, 188-189
nursing assessment of, 181-183
nursing diagnoses, 183-184
nursing implementation for, 184-189
nursing management of, **181-189**
nursing planning for, 184
overview of, **166-167**
Addictive substances, 169*t*-170*t*
Addisonian crisis, 1316-1317
Addison's disease, 1316
acute intervention for, 1317
ambulatory and home care for, 1317
clinical manifestations of, 1313*t*, 1316, 1316*f*
collaborative care for, 1316-1317, 1317*t*
dermatologic manifestations of, 473*t*
diagnostic studies, 1316
nursing implementation for, 1317
nursing management of, **1317**
patient and family teaching guide for, 1317*t*
Adduction, 1622, 1622*t*
Adefovir (Hepsera)
for chronic hepatitis B, 1094-1095
drug alert, 1095
Adenocard (adenosine)
classification of, 856*t*
drug alert, 850
for sinus tachycardia, 850
Adenohypophysis. *See* Anterior pituitary gland
Adenoma, pituitary, 1488*t*
Adenosine (Adenocard)
classification of, 856*t*
drug alert, 850
for paroxysmal supraventricular tachycardia, 851
for sinus tachycardia, 850
Adenosine deaminase deficiency, 217, 217*f*
Adenosine diphosphate receptor antagonists, 800*t*
Adenoviruses, 244*t*
Adherence, patient, 575*b*
Adhesions, 201-202
Adipectomy, 984
Adiphex-P (phentermine), 169*t*, 981
Adipokines, 972-973

Adiponectin, 972-973
Adjustable gastric banding, 982*t*, 983, 983*f*
Administration on Aging (AoA), 74, 84
Admission, same-day, 344
Admitting procedure, 364
Adnexa, 1326
Adrenal androgens, 1241
Adrenal cortex, 1241
disorders of, **1312-1320**
effects of aging on, 1242*t*
regulation of water balance by, 320
Adrenal cortex hormones, 1236*t*
Adrenal gland, 1241, 1241*f*
hypothalamic-pituitary-adrenal axis, 113, 113*f*
radiology, 1251*t*
serum studies, 1250*t*-1251*t*
urine studies, 1251*t*
Adrenal medulla, 1241
disorders of, **1320**
effects of aging on, 1242*t*
Adrenal medulla hormones, 1236*t*
Adrenal studies, 1250, 1250*t*-1251*t*
Adrenalectomy, medical, 1312
Adrenaline (epinephrine)
for allergic disorders, 231
for asthma and COPD, 619*t*
for shock, 1787*t*
target tissue and functions, 1236*t*
α-Adrenergic receptor agonists
effects on lower urinary tract function, 1180*t*
for glaucoma, 434*t*-435*t*
for voiding dysfunction, 1185*t*
α₂-Adrenergic receptor agonists, 139, 139*t*
β-Adrenergic receptor agonists, 833
β₂-Adrenergic receptor agonists, 620-621
for asthma and COPD, 619*t*
drug alert, 621
long-acting, 615
Adrenergic receptor antagonists
combined α- and β-, 775*t*
for hypertension, 773*t*-775*t*
α-Adrenergic receptor antagonists
for benign prostatic hyperplasia, 1417
effects on lower urinary tract function, 1180*t*
for hypertension, 773*t*-774*t*
for voiding dysfunction, 1185*t*
α₁-Adrenergic receptor antagonists, 774*t*
β-Adrenergic receptor antagonists (β-Adrenergic blockers)
for acute coronary syndrome, 800*t*, 808
and asthma attacks, 610
blood glucose level effects, 1267*t*
for chronic HF, 832
for chronic stable angina, 799-801, 800*t*
classification of, 856*t*
effects on lower urinary tract function, 1180*t*
ethnic differences in response to, 35*t*
food/nutrient interactions, 954*t*
for glaucoma, 434*t*
for hypertension, 774*t*, 777*t*, 1210
for hyperthyroidism, 1301
Adrenocortical insufficiency, 1316-1317
clinical manifestations of, 1316
collaborative care for, 1316-1317
complications of, 1316
diagnostic studies, 1316
etiology and pathophysiology of, 1316

Adrenocorticotropic hormone
cysyntropin stimulation test, 1250*t*
for multiple sclerosis, 1544, 1544*t*
serum levels, 1250*t*
suppression test, 1250*t*
target tissue and functions, 1236*t*
Adriamycin (doxorubicin)
adverse cardiovascular effects of, 745*t*
for bladder cancer, 1179
for breast cancer, 1355
for cervical cancer, 1402
classification of, 287*t*
drug alert, 1355
for leukemia, 720*t*
method of administration, 288*t*
for multiple myeloma, 729
for non-Hodgkin's lymphoma, 727*t*
Adrucil (fluorouracil), 287*t*
Adult day care programs, 76
Adult learners, 54-55
characteristics of, 55*t*
motivation of, 55
Adult learning principles, 54
Adult stem cells, 218
Advair (fluticasone/salmeterol)
for asthma and COPD, 620*t*
for exercise-induced asthma, 608
Advair Diskus, 621
Advance care planning, 155
Advance directives, 155, 156*t*, 637*b*
Advanced practice nurses, 3-4, 4*t*
Advancing HIV Prevention (AHP) initiative (CDC), 260, 270
Adventitious sounds, 524
Advil (ibuprofen)
analgesic effects of, 128
for arthritis and connective tissue disorders, 1698*t*
for fever, 203
and gastritis, 1013
mechanism of action, 202*t*
for pain, 136, 136*t*
for premenstrual syndrome, 1386
AEDs. *See* Antiepileptic drugs; Automatic external defibrillators
AEPs. *See* Auditory evoked potentials
AeroBid (flunisolide), 618*t*
AeroBid-M (flunisolide), 618*t*
AeroChamber spacers, 617, 620*f*, 621
Aerosol nebulization therapy, 649
Aerosol propellants, 170*t*
Affect
assessment of, 1456
after stroke, 1508, 1523
African Americans
caregivers of, 72
cultural values, 27*t*
culture-bound syndromes, 35*t*
diabetes mellitus in, 1255
end-of-life care, 155
ethnic differences in response to drugs, 34, 35*t*
folk healers, 30
health disparities, 20, 21, 21*t*, 33-34
medications for, 34
nurses, 26
older adults, 66
Afterdrop, 1831
Afterload, 742, 828, 1738-1739
decreasing, 828-829
normal range at rest, 1739*t*
AGB. *See* Adjustable gastric banding
Age
and coronary artery disease, 787-788
and health disparities, 22
and wound healing, 201*t*

Ageism, 67
Agency for Healthcare Research and
  Quality (AHRQ)
  *Clinical Practice Guideline: Treating
    Tobacco Use and Dependence,*
    172, 172*f,* 172*t*
  PORT (Pneumonia Patient Outcomes
    Research Team) Severity Index
    (PSI), 562, 562*t*
Agenerase (amprenavir), 258*t*
Agent Orange, 674
Agents of bioterrorism, 1838, 1839*t*-
  1840*t*
Agents of terrorism, **1838-1842**
  chemical, 1839, 1840*t*
Age-related macular degeneration,
  431-432
  clinical manifestations of, 432
  collaborative care for, 432
  diagnostic studies, 432
  etiology and pathophysiology of,
    431-432
Age-related physiologic changes, 69
  nursing diagnoses associated with,
    78, 78*t*
  and nutritional status, 959
Agglutination, 227, 669, 1339*t*
Aggrastat (tirofiban), 800*t*
Aggregation, 669
Aggrenox (dipyridamole and aspirin)
  for long-term therapy after TIAs,
    1505
  to prevent stroke, 1510
Aging
  attitudes toward, **67**
  biologic theories, **67-69,** 68*f,* 68*t*
  and COPD, 632
  cross-link theory of, 68*t,* 69
  definition of, 67
  demographics of, **66-67,** 67*f*
  effects on adult mental functioning,
    70, 70*t*
  effects on auditory system, **409**
  effects on cardiovascular system,
    744
  effects on drug metabolism, 80, 81*f*
  effects on endocrine system, **1242,**
    1242*t*
  effects on gastrointestinal system,
    932-933
  effects on hematologic studies, 672*t*
  effects on hematologic system, **671**
  effects on immune system, **224,** 224*t*
  effects on integumentary system,
    451-452
  effects on musculoskeletal system,
    1618-1619
  effects on nervous system, 1452-1453
  effects on reproductive system, **1330-**
    1331
  effects on respiratory system, **516-**
    517
  effects on sexual function, 1330,
    1331*t*
  effects on sexual response, **1330-**
    1331
  effects on urinary system, **1141**
  effects on visual system, **402**
  immunologic theory of, 68*t,* 69
  neuroendocrine theory of, 68*t,* 69
  nonstochastic theories of, 68, 68*t,* 69
  process of, 67, 68*f*

Aging *(Continued)*
  resources, 84
  stochastic theories of, 68-69
  strategies for slowing or reversing,
    67-68, 68*t*
  telomere-telomerase hypothesis of,
    68*t,* 69
Aging male syndrome, 1437
Agitation, 1811
Agnosia, 1508
Agranulocytes, 667, 668*t*
AIDS. *See* Acquired immunodeficiency
  syndrome
Air conduction, 408
Air filtration, 516
Air pollutants, 609
Air pollution, 631
Airborne infection isolation, 574
Airborne precautions, 249
Airway management
  artificial airways, **1751-1759**
  basic life support, 1845-1846
  in burns, 488, 493
  head tilt–chin lift maneuver for,
    1845-1846, 1845*f*
  in hypercapnic respiratory failure,
    1803
  initial postanesthesia care unit assess-
    ment, 377-378, 377*t*
  primary survey of, 1825*t*
  primary survey of airway with cervi-
    cal spine stabilization and/or
    immobilization, 1823, 1824*t*
  reduction of inflammation, 1811
  stenting for lung cancer, 583
  suctioning
    in acute respiratory failure, 1810
    closed tracheal suction system,
      1757, 1758*f*
    closed-suction technique, 1757,
      1757*t*
    indications for, 1757
    open-suction technique, 1757,
      1757*t*
    procedures for patients on me-
      chanical ventilators, 1757*t*
    subglottal, continuous, 1759, 1759*f*
    tracheostomy, 545*t,* 546, 546*f*
Airway obstruction, 543
  foreign body, 1846, 1846*f,* 1846*t*
  postoperative, 378, 379*t,* 380*f*
AIVR. *See* Accelerated idioventricular
  rhythm
Akarpine (pilocarpine), 435*t*
AK-Homatropine (homatropine hydro-
  bromide), 427*t*
Akinesia, 1507
Akineton (biperiden), 1552*t*
AK-Pentolate (cyclopentolate HCl),
  427*t*
Alanine aminotransferase, 1858*t*
Alarm reaction, 112, 112*t*
Alaska Natives. *See also* Native
  Alaskans
  diabetes mellitus in, 1255
  nurses, 26
Albinism, 437*t*
Albumin
  laboratory values, 1855*t*
  preoperative levels, 351
  protein levels, 1857*t*
  serum levels, 956*t*
  for shock, 1783-1784, 1786*t*
Albumin products, 731*t*
Albumin/globulin ratio, 1857*t*
Albustix (dipstick) test, 1146*t*

Albuterol (Proventil, Ventolin), 620
  for asthma, 619*t*
  for COPD, 619*t,* 640
  ipratropium and albuterol (Combi-
    vent, DuoNeb), 620*t,* 621, 640
Alcohol, **176-178**
  blood alcohol concentration, 177,
    177*t*
  characteristics of, 176
  complications of, 177-178
  in diabetic meal plan, 1268
  effects on lower urinary tract func-
    tion, 1180*t*
  ethnic differences in response to, 35*t*
  moderation of consumption of, 770
  toxicology, 1865*t*
Alcohol abuse, 176, 176*f*
  chronic, 177, 177*t*
  collaborative care, 178
  complications of, 168*t,* 177
  contributing factors, 167, 167*f*
  effects of, 169*t,* 176-177
Alcohol poisoning, 1837*t*
  acute intervention for, 185-186
Alcohol toxicity, acute, 177
Alcohol Use Disorders Identification
  Test (AUDIT), 182, 182*t*
Alcohol withdrawal
  acute intervention for, 186
  clinical manifestations and suggested
    drug treatment of, 178, 178*t*
  nursing care plan for patient in, 183*b*-
    184*b*
  onset of, 185*t*
Alcohol withdrawal delirium, 177
Alcoholic cirrhosis, 1102
Aldactazide (spironolactone/hydrochlo-
  rothiazide), 777*t*
Aldactone (spironolactone)
  for chronic HF, 831
  for cirrhosis, 1110*t*
  drug alert, 831
  for hyperaldosteronism, 1319
  for hypertension, 773*t*
Aldara (imiquimod), 1376
Aldesleukin (Proleukin), 223*t,* 303*t*
Aldolase, 1627*t,* 1855*t*
Aldomet (methyldopa)
  autoreactivity to, 234
  for hypertension, 774*t*
Aldoril (methyldopa/hydrochlorothia-
  zide), 777*t*
Aldosterone, 1138, 1241
  factors affecting secretion of, 320,
    320*f*
  mechanism of action of, 764, 764*f*
  renin-angiotensin-aldosterone system,
    1139, 1139*f*
  serum levels, 1250*t*
  target tissue and functions, 1236*t*
  urine levels, 1251*t,* 1862*t*
Aldosterone receptor blockers, 773*t*
Aldosteronism, primary, 325
Alefacept (Amevive), 472*t*
Alemtuzumab (Campath), 303*t,* 720*t,*
  721, 721*t*
Alendronate (Fosamax)
  for hyperparathyroidism, 1310
  for osteoporosis, 1689
  for Paget's disease, 1690
Aleve (naproxen)
  analgesic effects of, 128
  for arthritis and connective tissue dis-
    orders, 1698*t*
  and gastritis, 1013
Alfentanil (Alfenta), 370*t*

Alfuzosin (UroXatral)
  for benign prostatic hyperplasia, 1417
  for voiding dysfunction, 1185*t*
AlgiCELL, 205*t*
Alginates, 205*t*
AlgiSite, 205*t*
Alimta (pemetrexed), 287*t*
Alka-2, 1020*t*
Alkalemia, 333*t*
Alkali poisoning, 1837*t*
Alkaline phosphatase, 947*t,* 1626*t*
Alkalosis, 333, 333*f*
  clinical manifestations of, 336, 336*t*
  definition of, 333*t*
  metabolic, 335, 335*t,* 336*t*
  respiratory, 335, 335*t,* 336*t*
Alka-Seltzer, 1020*t*
Alkeran (melphalan)
  classification of, 287*t*
  for multiple myeloma, 729
Alkets, 1020*t*
Alkylamines, 537*t*
Alkylating agents
  classification of, 287*t*
  for leukemia, 720*t*
  methods of administration, 288*t*
ALL. *See* Acute lymphocytic leukemia
Allegra (fexofenadine)
  for allergic rhinitis and sinusitis, 538*t*
  for dermatologic problems, 475
Alleles, 214
  definition of, 214*t*
  dominant, 214, 214*t*
  recessive, 214, 214*t*
Allergens, 462
  and asthma attacks, 608
  recognition and control of, 230-231
  that cause anaphylactic shock, 227*t*
Allergic conjunctivitis, 423
Allergic contact dermatitis, 228, 462,
  471*t*
Allergic dermatologic problems, 470-
  471, 471*t*
Allergic disorders, 228-232
  assessment, 228-229
  collaborative care, 230-232
  diagnostic studies, 229-230
  drug therapy of, 231
  immunotherapy of, 231-232
Allergic reactions
  acute transfusion reactions, 732
    mild, 733*t*
    severe, 733*t*
  in eyelids, 406*t*
  to insulin therapy, 1263
  to latex, 232*t*
  mediators of, 225, 226*t*
  type I, 225-227, 225*f,* 225*t*
Allergic rhinitis, 226-227, **535-536**
  clinical manifestations of, 535
  drug therapy of, 535-536, 537*t*-538*t*
  how to reduce symptoms of, 536*t*
  intermittent, 535
  nursing and collaborative manage-
    ment of, **535-536**
  persistent, 535
Allergies
  chronic, 230-231
  latex, **232**
    guidelines for preventing reactions,
      232*t*
    nursing and collaborative manage-
      ment of, **232**
    screening for, 347
    types of, 232
  nursing assessment of, 229*t*
  and preoperative care, 347

Allergy shots, 536
Allevyn, 205t
Allocation of resources for transplantation, 1226b
AlloDerm, 498t
Allodynia, 129
Allogeneic transplantation, 304-305
Allografts, 498, 498t
Allopurinol (Zyloprim), 598, 1764, 1802
    blood glucose level effects, 1267t
    for gout, 1716
    hematologic effects of, 674t
    for multiple myeloma, 729
Allow natural death, 156
Almotriptan (Axert), 1530
Aloe, 102t
Alopecia, 452, 457t
    chemotherapy-induced, 295t, 300
Alosetron (Lotronex)
    drug alert, 1047
    for irritable bowel syndrome, 1047
Aloxi (palonosetron), 297, 992t
ALP. See Alkaline phosphatase
Alpha hydroxy acids, 479t
Alphagan (brimonidine), 434t
Alport syndrome, 1177
Alprazolam (Xanax)
    effects of use, 169t
    ethnic differences in response to, 35t
    withdrawal from, 179
Alprostadil (Caverject)
    for erectile dysfunction, 1435
    intraurethral insertion of pellets with MUSE device, 1435, 1436f
ALS. See Amyotrophic lateral sclerosis
ALT. See Argon laser trabeculoplasty
Altace (ramipril), 776t
Alteplase (Activase), 800t, 915
Altered consciousness, 1460t
Altered sensory input problems, 397-507
AlternaGEL, 1210
Alternative healers, 1309b
Alternative medical systems, 96-98, 96t, 97t
Alternative therapy, 94. See also Complementary and alternative therapies
Altretamine (Hexalen), 1403
Alu-Cap, 1020t, 1210
Aludrox, 1020t
Aluminum carbonate, 1020t
Aluminum chloride (Drysol), 476
Aluminum hydroxide, 1020t
Aluminum phosphate, 1020t
Aluminum preparations, 1210
Aluminum salts (Vurow's solution), 1375
Alupent (metaproterenol), 620
    for asthma and COPD, 619t
    food/nutrient interactions, 954t
Alveolar edema, 598
Alveolar hyperventilation, 1764
Alveolar hypoventilation, 1764, 1802
Alveolar macrophages, 516
Alveoli, 511, 511f
    in hypercapnic respiratory failure, 1803
Alzheimer's Association, 1575
Alzheimer's disease (AD), 1564-1575
    acute intervention for, 1570
    ambulatory and home care for, 1570-1575
    brain tissue effects of, 1565, 1566f
    case study, 1578
    cellular and other factors, 1566

Alzheimer's disease (AD),
    (Continued)
    characteristic findings, 1565
    clinical manifestations of, 1567-1568
    collaborative care for, 1568-1570, 1568t
    diagnostic studies, 1568
    drug therapy for, 1568-1570, 1569t
    early warning signs of, 1567t
    early-onset, 1565
    eating difficulties in, 1573-1574
    elimination problems in, 1574
    epidemiologic factors, 1567
    etiology and pathophysiology of, 1564-1569, 1566f
    familial, 1565
    family and caregiver teaching guide for, 1574t
    gender differences in, 1565b
    genetic factors, 1565, 1565b
    health promotion in, 1570
    infection prevention in, 1574
    late-onset, 1565
    nursing assessment of, 1570, 1570t
    nursing care plan for patient with, 1571b-1572b
    nursing diagnoses, 1570
    nursing evaluation of, 1575
    nursing implementation for, 1570-1575
    nursing management of, 1570-1575
    nursing planning for, 1570
    oral care in, 1574
    pain management in, 1573
    skin care in, 1574
    swallowing difficulties in, 1573-1574
Amanita phalloides, 1115
Amantadine (Nemedia, Symmetrel)
    for influenza, 540
    for multiple sclerosis, 1544-1545, 1545t
    for pain, 140
    for Parkinson's disease, 1551, 1552t
    for pneumonia, 566
Amaryl (glimepiride), 1265, 1266t
Amaurosis fugax, 1505
Ambien (zolpidem)
    for Alzheimer's disease, 1569t
    for fibromyalgia syndrome, 1728
Amblyopia, 417
Ambu bag, 1752
Ambulation
    assistive devices for, 1648-1649
    with fractures, 1648
    weight-bearing, 1648
Ambulatory care, 88. See also specific disorders
    blood pressure monitoring, 768
    characteristics of settings, 87t
    continuous ambulatory peritoneal dialysis, 1219, 1219f
    ECG monitoring, 753t, 757
Ambulatory surgery, 344
    discharge, 394
    discharge criteria, 393t
    postoperative care, 394
    preoperative teaching information, 352
Amcort (diacetate), 1437
AMD. See Age-related macular degeneration
Amenorrhea, 1330, 1334, 1387, 1390
    causes of, 1387t
    primary, 1387
    secondary, 1387, 1387-1388
Amerge (naratriptan), 1530
American Academy of Dermatology, 478

American Association of Colleges of Nursing (AACN), 3
American Association of Critical Care Nurses (AACN)
    definition of critical care nursing, 1734
    standards for healthy work environments, 1735
American Burn Association (ABA), Burn Unit referral criteria, 486t
American Cancer Society, 281
    Reach to Recovery program, 1360
American College of Allergy, Asthma, and Immunology (ACAAI), recommendations for screening for latex allergies, 347
American College of Cardiology, stages of heart failure, 826t, 827
American College of Chest Physicians (ACCP), recommendations for screening for lung cancer, 581
American Heart Association
    AED training, 1845
    Council on Cardiovascular Nursing, 840
    stages of heart failure, 826t, 827
American Indians. See also Native Americans
    nurses, 26
    older adults, 66
American Nurses Association (ANA)
    Code of Ethics, 106
    definition of nursing, 3
    nursing terminologies recognized by, 8, 8t
American Red Cross, 1842f, 1844
American Rheumatism Association, 1705t
American Society of Anesthesiologists, 350t
American Society of Clinical Oncology (ASCO), 284
American Spinal Injury Association (ASIA)
    Impairment Scale, 1592, 1592f
    standard neurologic classification of spinal cord injury, 1592, 1593f
American Stroke Association, 1524
American Urological Association (AUA)
    Bladder Health Council, 1196
    Symptom Index for BPH, 1415, 1416t
Amevive (alefacept), 472t
Amicar (epsilon aminocaproic acid), 709
Amidate (etomidate), 369t
Amikacin (Amikin)
    nephrotoxicity, 1142t
    for tuberculosis, 573t
Amiloride (Midamor)
    for bilateral adrenal hyperplasia, 1319
    for cirrhosis, 1110t
    for hypertension, 773t
Amiloride/hydrochlorothiazide (Moduretic), 777t
Amines, 1445t
Amino acids, 1445t
γ-Aminobutyric acid (GABA), 1445t
γ-Aminobutyric acid (GABA) receptor agonists, 140
Aminoglutethimide (Cytadren)
    for bilateral adrenal hyperplasia, 1319
    for Cushing syndrome, 1312-1314
Aminoglycosides, 674t
Aminophylline, 619t

Aminosalicylates, 1053
5-Aminosalicylates (5-ASA), 1054, 1055t
Amiodarone (Cordarone)
    for atrial fibrillation, 852
    for atrial flutter, 851
    classification of, 856t
    hepatotoxicity, 934t
    for paroxysmal supraventricular tachycardia, 851
    photosensitivity, 461t
    for ventricular tachycardia, 855
Amitiza (lubiprostone), 1042t
Amitriptyline (Elavil)
    adverse cardiovascular effects of, 745t
    for Alzheimer's disease, 1569t
    for depression, 1551
    effects of, 130
    ethnic differences in response to, 35t
    food/nutrient interactions, 954t
    for interstitial cystitis/painful bladder syndrome, 1164
    local, 139t
    photosensitivity, 461t
    for premenstrual dysphoric disorder, 1386
    for voiding dysfunction, 1185t
AML. See Acute myelogenous leukemia
Amlodipine (Norvasc)
    for chronic stable angina and acute coronary syndrome, 800t
    for hypertension, 776t
    and reproductive system, 1332
Amlodipine/benazepril (Lotrel), 777t
Ammonia
    blood levels, 946t
    laboratory values, 1855t
Ammonia salt encrustations, 1193f
Amobarbital (Amytal), 169t
Amoxicillin
    for Lyme disease, 1714
    for peptic ulcer disease, 1019t
Amphetamines, 175
    adverse cardiovascular effects of, 745t
    and angina, 797t
    characteristics of, 175
    collaborative care, 175
    complications of, 168t, 175
    effects of use, 169t, 175
    onset, peak, duration, and withdrawal, 185t
    toxicity, 175, 175t
Amphojel
    preparation, 1020t
    for renal osteodystrophy, 1210
Amphotericin B (Fungizone)
    hematologic effects of, 674t
    for infective endocarditis, 869t
    nephrotoxicity, 1142t
Ampicillin (Omnipen)
    for bacterial meningitis, 1495
    for infective endocarditis, 869t
AMPLE mnemonic, 1826-1827
Amprenavir (Agenerase), 258t
Amputation, 1658-1662
    above-the-knee bandaging, 1660, 1661f
    acute intervention for, 1659-1661
    ambulatory and home care for, 1661
    clinical indications for, 1658
    collaborative care for, 1658-1659, 1658t
    diagnostic studies, 1658
    gerontologic considerations for, 1662

Amputation *(Continued)*
  health promotion in, 1659
  lower extremity sites, 1658-1659, 1659*f*
  nursing assessment of, 1659
  nursing diagnoses, 1659
  nursing evaluation of, 1662
  nursing implementation for, 1659-1662
  nursing management of, **1659-1662**
  nursing planning for, 1659
  patient and family teaching guide for, 1661*t*
  postoperative management of, 1660-1661
  preoperative management of, 1659-1660
  resources for, 1667
  sites of, 1658-1659, 1659*f*
  Syme's, 1659
  upper limb
    sites of, 1658-1659, 1659*f*
    special considerations for, 1661-1662
Amsler grid test, 408*t*
AMV. *See* Assisted mandatory ventilation
Amyl nitrite, 170*t*
Amylase
  laboratory values, 1855*t*
  serum levels, 944*t*
  urine levels, 1862*t*
Amylin analog, 1265, 1266t
β-Amyloid, 1565
Amyloidosis, 1177
Amyotrophic lateral sclerosis (ALS), 1558
  nursing interventions for, 1558
  pathogenesis of, 1558, 1558*f*
  and restrictive lung disease, 595*t*
Amytal (amobarbital), 169*t*
ANA. *See* American Nurses Association; Antinuclear antibody
Anabolic steroids, 1267*t*
Anafranil (clomipramine), 461*t*
Anakinra (Kineret)
  for arthritis and connective tissue disorders, 1700*t*
  clinical uses of, 223*t*
  for rheumatoid arthritis, 1705-1706
Anal fissures, 1083
Anal fistula, 1084, 1084*f*
Analgesia, 367, 1460*t*
  adjuvant therapy, 138-140
  for burns, 498-499, 499*t*
  deep, 367
  epidural
    for postoperative pain, 389
  patient-controlled, 142, 389
  postoperative, 389, 389*b*
  surgical, 99*t*
Analgesics
  adjuvant drugs, 138-140, 139*t*
  administration of, 140-142
  administration routes, 140-142
  buccal, 140-141
  for burns, 498-499
  ceiling effect, 135
  epidural delivery of, 141
  equianalgesic dosing, 140
  ethnic differences in response to, 35*t*

Analgesics *(Continued)*
  fear of hastening death by administering, 147
  intranasal, 141
  intraspinal delivery of, 141-142
  intrathecal delivery of, 141
  nonopioid, 135-137, 136*t*
  opioid, 137-138, 137*t*, 800*t*
  oral administration of, 140
  parenteral routes, 141
  rectal, 141
  scheduling, 140
  sublingual, 140-141
  titration of, 140
  topical, 1698*t*
  transdermal, 141
Anaphylactic reactions, 225
  acute transfusion reaction, 733*t*
  in operating room, 373
  systemic, 226, 226*f*
Anaphylactic shock, 1773*f*, **1777**
  allergens causing, 227*t*
  classification of, 1773*t*
  clinical presentation of, 1776*t*
  collaborative care for, 1789*t*, 1790
  emergency management of, 230*t*
  precipitating factors, 1773*t*
  treatment of, 1789*t*
Anaphylatoxins, 195, 226*t*
Anaphylaxis, 226, 226*f*
  collaborative care, 230
  slow-reacting substance of (SRS-A), 195, 197*f*
  therapeutic management of, 230
Anaprox (naproxen), 1698*t*
Anasarca, 1779
Anastrozole (Arimidex)
  for breast cancer, 1355
  classification of, 288*t*
Anatomic dead space (V_D), 511
Anatomic shunts, 1802
Ancef (cefazolin), 1670
Ancobon (flucytosine), 674*t*
AND. *See* Allow natural death
Androgen receptor blockers, 1426, 1426*t*
Androgens
  adrenal, 1241
  deficiency of, 473*t*
  excess of, 473*t*
  target tissues and functions, 1236*t*
Androgogy (adult learning), 54, 54*t*
Android obesity, 974, 975*t*
Andropause, 1437
  clinical manifestations of, 1437*t*
Androsterone, 1236*t*
Anectine (succinylcholine), 370, 370*t*
Anemia, 297, **685-687**
  aplastic, **693-694**
    laboratory study findings in, 690*t*
  cardiopulmonary manifestations of, 686
  caused by blood loss, **694-695**
  caused by decreased erythrocyte production, **687-694**
  caused by increased erythrocyte destruction, **695-701**
  causes of, 685, 685*f*
  in chemotherapy and radiation therapy, 295*t*
  of chronic disease, 690*t*, **693**
  in chronic kidney disease, 1207
  classification of, 685-686, 685*t*, 686*t*
  clinical manifestations of, 686, 686*t*
  definition of, 685-686
  dermatologic manifestations of, 473*t*
  drug therapy of, 1210-1211

Anemia, 297, *(Continued)*
  effects on wound healing, 201*t*
  etiologic classification of, 685*t*, 686*t*
  gerontologic considerations for, 687
  hemolytic, 695
    acquired, **699**
  iron deficiency, **687-691**
    collaborative care for, 690-691, 690*t*
    nursing management of, **691**
    laboratory study findings in, 690*t*
  megaloblastic, **691-693**
    classification of, 692*t*
    nursing management of, **693**
  morphologic, 685
  morphologic classification of, 686*t*
  nursing assessment of, 686, 687*t*
  nursing care plan for patient with, 688*b*-689*b*
  nursing diagnoses, 686
  nursing implementation for, 686-687
  nursing management of, **686-687**
  nursing planning, 686
  pernicious, 692
  sickle cell, 690*t*
Anergy, 224
Anesthesia, **366-367**, 367
  additional considerations, 372
  classification of, **367-372**
  cryoanesthesia, 372
  description of, 1460*t*
  dissociative, 369*t*, 371
  effects of use, 170*t*
  epidural, 371-372, 372*f*
  etiology and significance of, 1460*t*
  fear of, 345
  general, **367-371**
    adjuncts to, 370*t*
    patient positioning for recovery from, 381, 381*f*
  levels of, 367
  local, 367, **371-372**
    adjuvant drugs for, 139*t*
    for pain, 139-140, 139*t*
    methods of administration of, 371-372, 371*t*
  postanesthesia care
    phase I, 377, 377*t*
    phase II, 377, 377*t*
    phase III, 377, 377*t*
  postanesthesia discharge criteria, 393*t*
  regional, 142-143, 367
  spinal, 371-372, 372*f*
  total IV anesthesia, 367
Anesthesia care provider (ACP), 362-363
  assisting, 365
  role in general anesthesia, 368*t*
Anesthesiology, 362-363
Aneuploidy, 1351
Aneurysms
  aortic, **894-898**
    classification of, 894-895, 894*f*
    clipping and wrapping, 1512-1513, 1512*f*
    dissecting, 898
    endovascular stent grafting of, 896, 896*f*
    false, 894*f*, 895
    fusiform, 894, 894*f*
    pseudoaneurysms, 895
    saccular, 894-895, 894*f*
    and stroke, 1507
    surgical therapy for, 1512-1513

Aneurysms *(Continued)*
    true, 894, 894*f*
    ventricular, 805
Anger
  in acute coronary syndrome, 814*t*
  in burn patients, 505*t*
Angina, 796
  acute intervention for, 810
  chronic stable, **796-797**, 798*t*, 802*f*
    collaborative care for, 799*f*
    collaborative management of, **797-802**
    in coronary artery disease, **796-802**
    drug therapy of, 798-801, 800*t*
    nursing management of, **810-817**
    treatment elements, 798*t*
  nocturnal, 797
  pain during, 796, 797*f*
  PQRST assessment of, 796*t*
  precipitating factors, 797*t*
  Prinzmetal's, 797, 798*t*
  types of, 798*t*
  unstable, 798*t*, **802-803**
    diagnostic studies, 805-806
Angina decubitus, 797
Angioedema, 227, 832
Angiogenesis, 786, 1067
Angiogenesis inhibitors, 303*t*
Angiography, 895
  cerebral, 1461-1464, 1463*t*, 1464*f*
  coronary, 755*t*, **759**, 759*f*
    in unstable angina and myocardial infarction, 806
  fluorescein, 408*t*
  magnetic resonance, 755*t*
    of nervous system, 1463*t*
    of urinary system, 1148*t*
  pulmonary, 526, 528*t*
  renal, 1148*t*
Angioma, 454, 457*t*, 675*t*
  spider, with cirrhosis, 1102
Angiomax (bivalirudin), 914
Angiopathy, 1282
Angioplasty
  balloon, 801
  patch graft, 904
  percutaneous transluminal balloon, 903-904
Angiotensin II receptor blockers
  for chronic HF, 833
  combination drug therapy of hypertension, 777*t*
  for hypertension, 776*t*, 1210
Angiotensin inhibitors
  for hypertension, 776*t*
  types of, 771
Angiotensin-converting enzyme inhibitors
  for acute coronary syndrome, 800*t*, 808
  and asthma attacks, 610
  for chronic HF, 832
  for chronic stable angina, 800*t*, 801
  ethnic differences in response to, 35*t*
  for hypertension, 776*t*, 777*t*, 1210
Angle of Louis, 511, 748, 748*f*
Angle-closure glaucoma
  acute, 434
  acute care, 434*t*
  primary, 432-433
Anglo Americans
  cultural values, 27*t*
  ethnic differences in response to drugs, 34, 35*t*
  health disparities, 21*t*
  medications for, 34

Angulation, fracture, 1638*t*
Anicteric hepatitis, 1092
Animal bites, 1836
    collaborative care for, 1836-1837
Animal sera that cause anaphylactic
        shock, 227*t*
Animal-assisted therapy, 97*t*
Animalcules, 244
Anion gap, 333*t*
Anions, 315, 316*t*
Anismus, 1041
Anisocoria, 406*t,* 1460*t*
Ankle arthroplasty, 1664
Ankle-brachial index, 901
Ankylosing spondylitis, 1711-1713
    advanced, 1712, 1712*f*
    clinical manifestations of, 1711-1712
    collaborative care for, 1712
    complications of, 1711-1712
    diagnostic studies, 1712
    etiology and pathophysiology of,
        1711
    genetics of, 1712*b*
    nursing management of, **1712-1713**
    postural abnormalities and deformity
        in, 1712, 1712*f*
Ankylosis, 1623*t*
Annuloplasty, 882
Annulus, 412
Anorectal abscess, 1083-1084, 1084*f*
Anorectal problems, 1082-1084
Anorexia
    in chemotherapy and radiation
        therapy, 295*t,* 299
    cultural and ethnic health disparities
        in, 969*b*
    at end of life, 161*t*
Anorexia nervosa, 968-969
Anosognosia, 1460*t*
ANP. *See* Atrial natriuretic peptide
ANS. *See* Autonomic nervous system
Antabuse (disulfiram), 178
Antacids, 997
    for acute pancreatitis, 1121*t*
    for gastroesophageal reflux disease,
        1006*t*
    for gastrointestinal bleeding, 997,
        998*t*
    magnesium-containing, 1210
    for peptic ulcer disease, 1019*t,* 1020-
        1021
    preparations, 1020*t*
    for renal osteodystrophy, 1210
    side effects of, 1020*t*
Antagon (ganirelix), 1383*t*
Antalgic gait, 1623*t*
Antegrade pyelogram, 1147*t*
Anterior cerebral artery, 1507*t*
Anterior cord syndrome, 1591, 1592*f*
Anterior pituitary gland disorders,
    1291-1294
Anterior pituitary gland hormones,
    1236*t,* 1239
Anterior thorax examination, 49*t*
Anthracyclines, 720*t*
Anthrax, 1839*t*
Anthropometric measurements, 955
Antiaging strategies, 67-68, 68*t*
Antibiotics
    antitumor, 287*t*
    for arthritis and connective tissue dis-
        orders, 1698*t*
    for dermatologic problems, 475
    for *H. pylori,* 1019*t,* 1020
    for infective endocarditis, 868, 869*t*
    for leukemia, 720*t,* 721*t*
    nephrotoxicity, 1142, 1142*t*

Antibiotics *(Continued)*
    for osteoarthritis, 1697
    patient and family teaching guide to
        decrease risk for resistant infec-
        tion, 247*t*
    prophylaxis for infective endocardi-
        tis, 868
        conditions requiring, 869*t*
        procedures requiring, 866, 867*t*
    for recurrent UTIs, 1158, 1158*b*
    resistant organisms, 246, 246*t*
    for rheumatoid arthritis, 1706
    for UTIs, 1158
Antibodies
    HIV-antibody test, 253, 256*t*
        pretest and posttest counseling as-
            sociated with, 263, 264*t*
    laboratory values, 1860*t*
    monoclonal, 240, 240*f,* 303*t*
        hybridoma technology of, 240-241
        immunosuppressive therapy, 239*t*
    polyclonal, 239*t,* 240
    thyroid, 1861*t*
Antibody-mediated rejection, 238
Anticancer drugs
    adverse cardiovascular effects of,
        745*t*
    photosensitivity, 461*t*
Anticholinergics, 621
    for allergic rhinitis and sinusitis, 537*t*
    antidiarrheal, 1037*t*
    for asthma and COPD, 618*t*
    drug alert, 426
    for multiple sclerosis, 1544*t,* 1545
    for nausea and vomiting, 992, 992*t*
    for Parkinson's disease, 1551, 1552*t*
    for peptic ulcer disease, 1019*t,* 1021
    preoperative, 355*t*
Anticoagulant therapy, 670, 913*t*
    for deep vein thrombosis, 912
    drug alert, 908
    drugs, vitamins, and minerals that in-
        teract with, 914*t*
    for DVT prophylaxis, 914
    for DVT treatment, 914-915
    food/nutrient interactions, 954*t*
    nursing interventions to prevent
        bleeding complications in, 916,
        916*t*
    patient and family teaching guide for,
        917*b*
Antidepressants
    food/nutrient interactions, 954*t*
    for pain, 138-139, 139*t*
    that may cause photosensitivity, 461*t*
    tricyclic
        blood glucose level effects, 1267*t*
        effects on lower urinary tract func-
            tion, 1180*t*
        food/nutrient interactions, 954*t*
        hematologic effects of, 674*t*
        for peptic ulcer disease, 1019*t*
        poisoning, 1837*t*
        for voiding dysfunction, 1185*t*
Antidiabetic agents, 954*t*
Antidiarrheals, 1036, 1037*t*
    for inflammatory bowel disease,
        1054, 1055*t*
Antidiuretic hormone, 1239-1240
    disorders associated with secretion
        of, **1294-1297**
    factors affecting release of, 1240,
        1240*t*
    plasma osmolality and, 1240, 1240*f*
    syndrome of inappropriate antidi-
        uretic hormone, **1294-1296**
    target tissue and functions, 1236*t*

Anti-DNA antibody, 1626*t,* 1860*t*
Antidysrhythmics, 856
    for acute coronary syndrome, 808
    hematologic effects of, 674*t*
    major classifications of, 856*t*
    that may cause photosensitivity, 461*t*
Antiemetics
    adjuncts to general anesthesia, 370*t,*
        371
    preoperative, 355*t*
Antiepileptic drugs, 139
Antiestrogens, 288*t*
Antifibrinolytic therapy, 709
Antifungals, 461*t*
Antigens, 219
    CD antigens, 220
    human leukocyte antigen system, **233**
    oncofetal, 279
    tumor-associated, 277, 278*f*
Antihemophilic factor, 670*t*
Antihemophilic factor B, 670*t*
Antihemophilic factor C, 670*t*
Antihemophilic globulin, 670*t*
Antihistamines
    for allergic disorders, 231
    for allergic rhinitis, 535
    for allergic rhinitis and sinusitis,
        537*t*-538*t*
    for dermatologic problems, 475
    drug alert, 541
    for nausea and vomiting, 992, 992*t*
    for opioid-induced pruritus, 138
    for Parkinson's disease, 1551, 1552*t*
    that may cause photosensitivity, 461*t*
Antihypertensive drugs
    ethnic differences in response to, 35*t*
    hematologic effects of, 674*t*
    site and method of action, 771, 772*f*
Anti-incontinence devices, 1183*t*
Antiinflammatory drugs
    for asthma, 617-620, 617*t*
    for asthma and COPD, 618*t*
    corticosteroid action, 1318
    mechanisms of action, 202*t*
Antimalarials, 1700*t*
Antimetabolites
    classification of, 287*t*
    for leukemia, 720*t*
Antimicrobials, 205*t*
    for burns, 499
    hematologic effects of, 674*t*
    for inflammatory bowel disease,
        1053, 1054, 1055*t*
    that may cause photosensitivity, 461*t*
Antineoplastics, 674*t*
Antinuclear antibody, 1626*t,* 1860*t*
Antiparkinsonian agents
    effects on lower urinary tract func-
        tion, 1180*t*
    for multiple sclerosis, 1545*t*
Antiplatelet therapy
    for chronic stable angina and acute
        coronary syndrome, 800*t*
    for coronary artery disease, 794-795
Antipruritic drugs, 231
Antipsychotics
    adverse cardiovascular effects of,
        745*t*
    for Alzheimer's disease, 1569*t*
    ethnic differences in response to, 35*t*
    that may cause photosensitivity, 461*t*
Antipyretic drugs, 202*t*
Antireflux procedures, 1006
Antiretroviral therapy
    adherence to, 264-265
    adverse effects of, 258*t*
    hematologic effects of, 674*t*
    for HIV infection, 256-257, 264

Antiretroviral therapy *(Continued)*
    indications for initiation of, 257*t*
    nursing interventions for, 264
    patient and family teaching guide, 265*t*
    strategies to improve adherence to,
        265*t*
    when to start, 264
Anti-RNP, 1860*t*
Antisecretory drugs
    antidiarrheal, 1037*t*
    for peptic ulcer disease, 1019*t*
Antiseizure drugs
    adjuvants for pain management, 139*t*
    analgesic effects of, 128
    drug alert, 1535
    food/nutrient interactions, 954*t*
    gerontologic considerations for,
        1537-1538
    hematologic effects of, 674*t*
    for pain, 139
    side effects of, 1537
Anti-Sm (Smith), 1860*t*
Antispasmodics, 1121*t*
Antistreptolysin-O, 1860*t*
Antithrombin III, 679*t*
Antithyroid drugs, 1301
α₁-Antitrypsin
    laboratory values, 1855*t*
α₁-Antitrypsin deficiency, 632,
        632*b*
Antitumor antibiotics
    classification of, 287*t*
    for leukemia, 720*t,* 721*t*
Antivenin snakebite treatment, 1836,
        1836*t*
Antivert (meclizine), 992*t*
Antiviral drug therapy, 1545*t*
Antiviral protein, 223
Antrectomy, 934*t*
Anuria, 1145*t*
Anus
    age-related changes in, 932, 933*t*
    assessment abnormalities, 940*t*
    physical examination of, 938-939,
        939*t,* 1335, 1335*t*
Anxiety
    in acute coronary syndrome, 813-
        814, 814*t*
    in acute respiratory failure, 1811
    in burn patients, 505*t*
    in COPD, 637
    in critical care patients, 1736
    at end of life, 158
    preoperative, 345
    reduction of, 829, 1811
Anzemet (dolasetron)
    as adjunct to general anesthesia, 370*t*
    for nausea and vomiting, 297, 992,
        992*t*
AORN. *See* Association of periOpera-
        tive Registered Nurses
Aorta, disorders of, **894-900**
Aortic aneurysms, 894-898
    acute intervention for, 897-898
    ambulatory and home care for, 898
    classification of, 894-895
    clinical manifestations of, 895
    collaborative care for, 895-897
    complications of, 895
    diagnostic studies, 895
    etiology and pathophysiology of, 894
    health promotion in, 897
    nursing assessment of, 897
    nursing evaluation of, 898
    nursing implementation for, 897-898
    nursing management of, **897-898**
    nursing planning for, 897
    surgical therapy of, 895-897

Aortic dissection, **898-900**
  clinical manifestations of, 899
  collaborative care for, 899-900, 900t
  complications of, 899
  conservative therapy of, 900
  diagnostic studies, 899
  etiology and pathophysiology of, 899
  nursing management of, **900**
  surgical therapy of, 900
  of thoracic aorta, 898, 899f
Aortic valve regurgitation, **880-881**
  clinical manifestations of, 879t, 881
  etiology and pathophysiology of, 880-881
Aortic valve stenosis, **880**
  clinical manifestations of, 879t, 880
  etiology and pathophysiology of, 880
Aortoiliac disease
  acute intervention for, 897-898
  ambulatory and home care for, 898
  health promotion in, 897
  nursing assessment of, 897
  nursing evaluation of, 898
  nursing implementation for, 897-898
  nursing management of, **897-898**
  nursing planning for, 897
Apathetic hyperthyroidism, 1299
APD. *See* Automated peritoneal dialysis
Aphakia, **417**
Aphasia, 1460t
  communication with patient with, 1520t
  expressive, 1508
  global, 1508
  receptive, 1508
  after stroke, 1508
Apheresis, 234-235, 1706
Aphthous stomatitis, 1000t
Apical pulse, 750
Apidra (insulin glulisine), 1260t
Aplastic anemia, **693-694**
  acquired, 693
  clinical manifestations of, 693-694
  congenital, 693
  diagnostic studies, 694
  etiology of, 693, 694t
  nursing and collaborative management of, **694**
Apnea, 542
  sleep apnea, 542f
    management of, 543, 543f
    nursing and collaborative management of, **542-543**
  obstructive, **542-543**
Apo-Chlorthalidone (chlorthalidone), 773t
Apocrine sweat glands, 451
Apo-Diclo SR (diclofenac), 1698t
Apo-Hydro (hydrochlorothiazide), 773t
Apomorphine (Apokyn), 1551, 1552t
Apoptosis, 1590
Apo-Sulin (sulindac), 1698t
Appendectomy, 934t
Appendicitis, **1048-1049**
  clinical manifestations of, 1048-1049
  collaborative care for, 1049

Appendicitis, *(Continued)*
  diagnostic studies, 1049
  etiology and pathophysiology of, 1048, 1049f
  nursing management of, **1049**
Appetite-suppressing drugs, 981
Approach magnification, 421
Apraclonidine (Lopidine), 434t
Apraxia, 1460t
Aprepitant (Emend), 297, 992t
Apresoline (hydralazine), 775t
APSGN. *See* Acute poststreptococcal glomerulonephritis
Aptivus (tipranavir), 258t
Aquacel Ag, 499
AquaMEPHYTON (vitamin K), 1108
AquaSite, 205t
Aquatag (benzthiazide), 773t
Aqueous humor, 399, 399f
Ara-C (cytarabine)
  classification of, 287t
  for leukemia, 720t
  for non-Hodgkin's lymphoma, 727t
Arachidonic acid, 135-136, 136f, 195, 197f
Arachnid bites, **1834-1835**
Arachnoid layer, 1452
Arachnoid villi, 1448
Arava (leflunomide)
  for arthritis and connective tissue disorders, 1699t
  for rheumatoid arthritis, 1705
Arbovirus, 244t
ARDS. *See* Acute respiratory distress syndrome
Arduan (pipecuronium), 370t
Area Agencies on Aging, 74
Aredia (pamidronate)
  for hypercalcemia, 330
  for osteoporosis, 1689
Areflexia, **1586**
Areola, 1327
Arfonad (trimethaphan), 775t
Argatroban (Acova), 914
Arginine, 1267t
Argon laser trabeculoplasty, 433
Aricept (donepezil)
  for Alzheimer's disease, 1569t
  for Parkinson's dementia, 1551
Arimidex (anastrozole)
  for breast cancer, 1355
  classification of, 288t
Aristospan (triamcinolone), 1698t, 1699t
Arixtra (fondaparinux), 914
Aromasin (exemestane)
  for breast cancer, 1355
  classification of, 288t
Aromatase inhibitors, 288t
Aromatherapy, 97t
Arranon (nelarabine), 720t
Arrow injury, 1484t
Arsenic, 934t
Arsenic trioxide (Trisenox)
  classification of, 288t
  for leukemia, 720t, 721t
Art therapy, 97t, 116t
Artane (trihexyphenidyl), 1552t
Arterial access therapies, 1224, 1224t
Arterial blood gases, 337, 513, 527t
  abbreviations, 1800t
  in acute asthmatic attack, 614t
  normal values, 337t, 514t
  preoperative analysis, 351
  in shock, 1775t

Arterial blood pressure, 743, 1740-1741
  measurement of, 743, 1740, 1742f
  complications of, 1740-1741
Arterial bruit, 750t
Arterial bruits, 748
Arterial hemoglobin oxygen saturation, 1739t
Arterial ischemia, acute, 907
Arterial ischemic disorders, acute, **907-908**
Arterial leg ulcers, 901t, 903
Arterial oxygen saturation (SaO₂), 1857t
Arterial oxygen tension (PaO₂), 515, 515t
Arterial oxygenation monitoring, noninvasive, 1747
Arteries, 742, 742f
  at base of brain, 1452f
  cerebral, 1504, 1504f
  of head and neck, 1451f
Arteriography
  peripheral, 755t
  renal, 1148t, 1151f
Arterioles, 742, 742f
Arteriovenous fistulas, **1220-1221**, 1220f
Arteriovenous grafts, 1220-1221, 1220f, 1221
Arteriovenous hemodialysis, continuous, 1224t
Arteriovenous hemofiltration, continuous, 1224t
Arteriovenous malformations, **1507**
Arthralgia, 673-674, 676t, 869
Arthritis, **1693-1711**
  drug therapy for, 1696, 1698t-1700t
  gerontologic considerations for, **1711**
  infectious or bacterial, 1713-1714
  osteoarthritis, **1693-1702**
  prevention of, 1701b
  psoriatic, **1713**
  reactive, **1713**
  resources for, 1731
  rheumatoid, **1702-1711**
    case study, 1729-1730
  septic, **1713-1714**, 1876
Arthritis Foundation Self-Help Course, 1701
Arthrocentesis, 1627-1628, 1627t
Arthrodesis, 1664
Arthropan (choline salicylate), 1698t
Arthroplasty, **1662-1664**
  ankle, 1664
  elbow and shoulder, 1664
  finger joint, 1664
  hip, 1663-1664, 1663f
  knee, 1664
Arthroscopy, 1624-1627, 1625t, 1628f
Artificial airways, **1751-1759**
  nursing management of, **1752-1759**
Artificial disks, 1683, 1683f
Artificial heart, 839, 840f
  implantable, 1750
Artificial larynx, 557, 557f
Artificial skin, 501-502
AS. *See* Ankylosing spondylitis
5-ASA. *See* 5-Aminosalicylates
Asacol (mesalamine), 1055t
Asaphen (salsalate), 1698t
Asbestosis, 578t
Aschoff's bodies, 876
Ascites, 940t
  bilirubin metabolism abnormalities in, 1106, 1107t
  with cirrhosis, 1104, 1105f

Ascites *(Continued)*
  collaborative care for, 1106-1107
  development of
    factors involved in, 1104, 1105f
    mechanisms for, 1104, 1105f
Ascorbic acid, 1855t
Aseptic technique, basic, 365, 365b, 366t
ASH. *See* Asymmetric septal hypertrophy
Ash Split catheter, 1222
ASIA. *See* American Spinal Injury Association
Asian Americans
  caregivers of, 72
  diabetes mellitus in, 1255
  ethnic differences in response to drugs, 34, 35t
  folk healers, 30
  health disparities, 20, 21, 23f
  nurses, 26
  older adults, 66
  and touch, 33
Asian Indians, 34, 35t
Asmanex Twisthaler (mometasone), 618t
L-Asparaginase (Elspar)
  blood glucose level effects, 1267t
  classification of, 288t
  for leukemia, 720t, 721t
Aspartate, 1445t
Aspartate aminotransferase, 947t, 1858t
Aspercreme (trolamine salicylate), 141
Aspergillosis, 576t
Aspergillus fumigatus, 245t, 576t
Aspergillus niger, 576t
Aspiration
  with ET tube, 1759
  in postanesthesia care unit (PACU), 378
  postoperative, 379t
Aspiration pneumonia, 561, 564
  case study, 604
Aspirin (acetylsalicylic acid)
  for arthritis and connective tissue disorders, 1698t
  for chronic stable angina and acute coronary syndrome, 800t
  complications of, 1512
  dipyridamole and aspirin (Aggrenox)
    for long-term therapy after TIAs, 1505
    to prevent stroke, 1510
  for hyperthermia, 1512
  for long-term therapy after TIAs, 1505
  mechanism of action, 202t
  for osteoarthritis, 1697
  for pain, 135, 136t
  poisoning, 1837t
  to prevent stroke, 1510
  for stroke, 1512
  for tension-type headache, 1530
Aspirin-containing medications, 1837t
Assault, 1484t
Assessment
  breathing assessment, 117, 117t
  of characteristics that affect patient teaching, 57-58, 58t
  cultural, 29t-30t
  culturally competent, **43**
  episodic or problem-centered, 40
  general survey, 46, 48t
  gerontologic differences in, 50t, 69t, 224t
  head-to-toe secondary survey, 1825-1827, 1826t

Assessment (Continued)
home health care activities, 90t
individual patient evaluation for hypertension, 777-778
nursing phase, 9, **10**
pain assessment, **131-134**
in cancer, 309, 309t
patient education process, 57-59
physical, 57-58
postanesthesia care unit, 377, 377t
preoperative, 351
psychologic, 58
sociocultural, 58-59
wound measurements, 203, 204f
Assimilation, 27
Assist-control ventilation, 1760, 1761t
Assisted listening devices, 445
Assisted mandatory ventilation, 1761t
Assisted suicide, 147
Assisted-living facilities, 75
Assistive devices. See also Prostheses
for ambulation, 1648-1649
for eating, 1522, 1522f
gait patterns with, 1648-1649
for hearing loss and deafness, 444-445
for older adults, 80
Association of periOperative Registered Nurses (AORN), 396
AST. See Aspartate aminotransferase; Association of Surgical Technologists
Astelin (azelastine), 538t
Astereognosis, 1460t
Asterixis, 1106, 1208
Asthma, 227, 608, **608-629**
action plan for, 626, 627-628, 627t
acupuncture for, 99t
acute attacks, 609t
acute episode, 615-616
acute intervention for, 626
allergic, 611, 611f
ambulatory and home care for, 626-629
case study, 661
chest examination findings in, 526t
classification of, 612, 613t
clinical manifestations of, 612, 635t
collaborative care for, 614t, 615-617
comparison with COPD, 634, 635t
complications of, 612-613
cough variant, 612
diagnostic studies, 613-615, 635t
drug therapy of, 617-624, 617t, 618t-620t
nonprescription combination drugs, 623-624, 624t
patient teaching related to, 621-623
early-phase response in, 611, 611f
exercise-induced, 608
factors causing obstruction in, 611, 611f
gender differences in, 608b
health disparities and, 21t
health promotion in, 625-626
late-phase response in, 611
mild intermittent and persistent, 615
nursing assessment of, 624, 624t
important health information for, 624t
objective data in, 624t
subjective data in, 624t
nursing care plan for patient with, 625b-626b

Asthma (Continued)
nursing diagnoses, 624
nursing implementation for, 625-629
nursing management of, **624-629**
nursing planning for, 624-625
occupational factors, 609
pathophysiology of, 609, 610f, 611-612
patient and family teaching guide for, 630t
physical training and respiratory and general health in persons with, 609b
possible findings in, 624t
psychologic factors, 610-611
stepwise approach for managing, 616t
triggers of attacks, **608-611**, 609t
Asthma triad, 610
Astigmatism, 400, **417**
Astrocytes, 1442
Asymmetric septal hypertrophy, 888
Asystole, 855-856
clinical associations, 856
clinical significance of, 856
treatment of, 856
Atacand (candesartan), 776t
Atacand HCT (candesartan/hydrochlorothiazide), 777t
Atarax (hydroxyzine), 475
Atazanavir (Reyataz), 258t
Ataxia, 676t, 1460t
Ataxic gait, 1623t
Atelectasis, 511-512, **597**
absorption, 644
chest examination findings in, 526t
effects of, 511, 511f
in pneumonia, 565
postoperative, 378, 379t, 381f
and restrictive lung disease, 596t
Atenolol (Tenormin)
for acute coronary syndrome, 800t
for chronic stable angina, 799, 800t
classification of, 856t
effects on lower urinary tract function, 1180t
for hypertension, 774t
for hyperthyroidism, 1301
Atenolol/chlorthalidone (Tenoretic), 777t
Atgam (lymphocyte immune globulin), 239t
Atheromas, 785
Atherosclerosis, 785, 1504
complicated lesions, 785-786, 786f
developmental stages of, 785, 786f
in extracranial and intracranial arteries, 1504, 1505f
homocysteine and, 791
locations of lesions, 893, 893f
in peripheral arterial disease, 893
progression of, 785, 786f
Athetosis, 1458, 1578
Ativan (lorazepam)
as adjunct to general anesthesia, 370t
for alcohol withdrawal, 178, 186
for Alzheimer's disease, 1569t
for burns, 499t
preoperative, 355t
Atkins diet, 979t
Atonic (drop attack) seizures, 1535
Atopic dermatitis, 227, 471t
Atopic reactions, 226-227
Atorvastatin (Lipitor), 793, 795t
Atracurium (Tracrium), 370t

Atrial contractions, premature, 850, 850f
characteristics of, 849t
Atrial fibrillation, 851f, 852
characteristics of, 849t
clinical associations, 852
clinical significance of, 852
ECG characteristics, 852
treatment of, 852
Atrial flutter, 851-852, 851f
characteristics of, 849t
clinical associations, 851
clinical significance of, 851
ECG characteristics, 851
treatment of, 851-852
Atrial gallop, 751
Atrial natriuretic peptide, 1138
Atrioventricular block
first-degree, 853, 853f
characteristics of, 849t
clinical associations, 853
clinical significance of, 853
ECG characteristics, 853
treatment of, 853
second-degree, type I, 853, 853f
characteristics of, 849t
clinical associations, 853
clinical significance of, 853
ECG characteristics, 853
treatment of, 853
second-degree, type II, 853-854, 853f
characteristics of, 849t
clinical associations, 853
clinical significance of, 854
ECG characteristics, 853
treatment of, 854
third-degree, 853f, 854
characteristics of, 849t
clinical associations, 854
clinical significance of, 854
ECG characteristics, 854
treatment of, 854
Atripla (tenovir, emtricitabine, and efavirenz), 258t
Atrium Chest Drainage Unit, 589f, 590
Atrium Dry System, 591t
Atromid-S (clofibrate), 1267t
Atrophy, 455t
Atropine (Atropisol, Atropair, Bufopto, Atropine, Isopto Atropine, Ocu-Tropine, Atro-Pen), 427t
diphenoxylate with atropine (Lomotil, Colonaid), 1037t, 1055t
for neurogenic shock, 1790
preoperative, 355t
Atrovent (ipratropium bromide), 621
for allergic rhinitis and sinusitis, 537t
for asthma, 618t
for COPD, 618t, 640
Attitudes toward aging, **67**
Atypical absence seizures, 1535
Audiometry, 414-415
impedance, 414t
pure-tone, 414t, 415
screening, 415
Audiovisual materials, 62
Auditory brainstem responses, 414t
Auditory evoked potentials, 414t
Auditory problems
cultural and ethnic health disparities in, 417b
of external ear and canal, **438-439**
resources, 448

Auditory system
age-related changes in, 410t
assessment abnormalities, 413t
assessment of, **409-412**
health history questions to ask, 410t
important health information, 409-411
objective data, 412
subjective data, 409-412
diagnostic studies, **412-415**, 414t
effects of aging on, **409**
physical examination of, 412, 412t
specialized tests of, 415
structures and functions of, **407-409**, 408f
Augmented coughing (quad coughing), 1809, 1809f
Aura, 1528
migraine with, 1529
migraine without, 1529
Auranofin (Ridaura)
for arthritis and connective tissue disorders, 1699t
for rheumatoid arthritis, 1706
Aurothioglucose (Solganal), 1699t
Auscultation, 48, 48f
of abdomen, 937
cardiac areas, 748, 758f
of chest, 522-523
assessment abnormalities, 524t-525t
findings in pulmonary problems, 526t
normal sounds, 522-523, 523f
of peripheral vascular system, 748
of thorax, 750-751
assessment abnormalities, 750t
normal, 751t
of urinary system, 1145
Auscultation sounds, 522-523, 523f
Auscultatory gap, 781
Austin-Flint murmur, 881
Autografts, 498t, 501
cultured epithelial autografts, 498t, 501, 502f
skin grafts, 481
Autoimmune diseases, 224, 234
examples, 234t
of liver, **1100-1101**
theories of causation of, 234
Autoimmune gastritis, 1013
Autoimmune hepatitis, 1100
Autoimmune reactions, 699
Autoimmune thyroiditis, chronic (Hashimoto's), 1298
Autoimmunity, 234-235
development of, 234
theory for rheumatoid arthritis, 1702
Autologous donation, 734
Autologous stem cell transplantation, 305, 305f
Autologous transplantation, 305
Autolytic debridement, 205
Automated coagulation time (ACT), 679t
Automated peritoneal dialysis, 1218-1219, 1218f
Automatic external defibrillators, 856, 1845, 1845f
Automaticity, 842, 843t, 846, 1869
Automatisms, 1535
Autonomic dysreflexia
patient and family teaching guide for, 1604t
in spinal cord injury, 1603-1604
Autonomic hyperreflexia, 1603-1604

Autonomic nervous system, 743, 1449-1450
  age-related changes in, 1454*t*
  control of heart by, 843
  effects on blood vessels, 743
  effects on heart, 743
  gerontologic differences in assessment findings, 1454*t*
Autonomic neuropathy, 1285-1286
Auto-PEEP, 1762
Autoreactivity, 234
Autoregulation, cerebral, 1468-1469, 1504
Autosomal disorders, 215
Autosomal dominant disorders, 215, 216*t*
Autosomal recessive disorders, 215, 216*f,* 216*t*
Autosomes, 214, 214*t*
Autosplenectomy, 697
Autotransfusion, 734
AV node, 846, 847*t*
Avalide (irbesartan/hydrochlorothiazide), 777*t*
Avandamet (rosiglitazone and metformin), 1266*t*
Avandia (rosiglitazone), 1265, 1266*t*
Avapro (irbesartan), 776*t*
Avastin (bevacizumab), 302, 303*t*
  for colorectal cancer, 1067
  FOLFOX treatment regimen, 291, 291*t*
Avaxim (hepatitis A virus vaccine), 1095-1096
Aveeno (colloidal oatmeal), 1375
Avelox (moxifloxacin), 573*t*
Aventyl (nortriptyline)
  for Alzheimer's disease, 1569*t*
  for interstitial cystitis/painful bladder syndrome, 1164
  for smoking cessation, 171*t*
AVGs. *See* Arteriovenous grafts
Avinza (morphine), 137*t,* 140
AVMs. *See* Arteriovenous malformations
Avodart (dutasteride)
  for benign prostatic hyperplasia, 1417
  for voiding dysfunction, 1185*t*
Avonex (β-Interferon)
  clinical uses of, 223*t*
  drug alert, 1544
  for multiple sclerosis, 1544, 1544*t*
Avulsion fracture, 1631
Axert (almotriptan), 1530
Axid (nizatidine)
  for gastroesophageal reflux disease, 1005-1006, 1006*t*
  for gastrointestinal bleeding, 998*t*
  for peptic ulcer disease, 1019*t*
Axilla
  contracture of, 504, 504*f*
  physical examination of, 51*t*
Axillary lymph node dissection, 1352
  exercise after mastectomy or lumpectomy with, 1359, 1360*f*
Axonal injury, diffuse, 1483
Axons, 1442
Aygestin (norethindrone), 1392
Ayurveda, 97*t*
Azacitidine (Vidaza), 717
Azatadine (Optimine), 537*t*

Azathioprine (Imuran), 238, 239*t*
  for arthritis and connective tissue disorders, 1700*t*
  hepatotoxicity, 934*t*
  for inflammatory bowel disease, 1054, 1055*t*
  for lupus nephritis, 1718
  for myasthenia gravis, 1556
  for polymyositis and dermatomyositis, 1726
  for rheumatoid arthritis, 1706
  for systemic lupus erythematosus, 1719
Azelastine (Astelin), 538*t*
Azilect (rasagiline), 1551, 1552*t*
Azithromycin (Zithromax)
  for cervicitis, 1394*t*
  for chlamydial infections, 1373
  for gonorrhea, 1368
  photosensitivity, 461*t*
  for rheumatic fever, 878
Azmacort (triamcinolone), 618*t*
Azopt (brinzolamide), 435*t*
Azotemia, 1197-1198
AZT (zidovudine), 258*t*
Azulfidine (sulfasalazine)
  for arthritis and connective tissue disorders, 1699*t*
  drug alert, 1054
  for inflammatory bowel disease, 1054, 1055*t*
  for rheumatoid arthritis, 1705

B
B lymphocytes, 220, 221*f*
Babinski's sign, 1460*t*
BAC. *See* Blood alcohol concentration
Bacitracin, 1142*t*
Back exercises, 1677*t*
Back pain, 1675-1686
Back School, 1676
Baclofen (Lioresal)
  local, 139*t*
  for multiple sclerosis, 1545, 1545*t*
  for pain, 140
  for spasms, 1603
Bacteremia, 565
Bacteria, 243-244
  antibiotic-resistant organisms, 246, 246*t*
  culture for, 458*t*
  disease-causing, 244, 244*t*
  emerging infections, 245*t*
  organisms associated with infective endocarditis, 866, 866*t*
  reemerging infections, 246*t*
Bacterial arthritis, 1713-1714
Bacterial conjunctivitis, acute, 422
Bacterial endocarditis, 865. *See also* Infective endocarditis
Bacterial food poisoning, 1031, 1032*t*
Bacterial infections
  conjunctivitis, 422
  keratitis, 423
  sexually transmitted diseases, **1367-1373**
  of skin, 466, 467*t*
Bacterial meningitis, 1493-1497
  acute intervention for, 1495-1497
  clinical manifestations of, 1494
  collaborative care for, 1495, 1495*t*
  complications of, 1494
  diagnostic studies, 1494-1495
  etiology and pathophysiology of, 1493-1494
  health promotion in, 1495
  nursing assessment of, 1495

Bacterial meningitis *(Continued)*
  nursing care plan for patient with, 1496*b*-1497*b*
  nursing diagnoses, 1495
  nursing evaluation of, 1497
  nursing implementation for, 1495-1497
  nursing management of, **1495-1497**
  nursing planning for, 1495
Bacterial persistence, 1155
Bacterial vaginosis, 1394*t*
Bacteriuria
  asymptomatic, 1155
  unresolved, 1155
Bactrim (trimethoprim/sulfamethoxazole)
  hematologic effects of, 674*t*
  for *P. jiroveci* pneumonia, 564
Bag-valve-mask ventilation, 1752
BAL. *See* Bronchoalveolar lavage
Balance assessment, 410*t*
Balanced Budget Act of 1997 (P.L. 105-33), 89
Balloon angioplasty, 801
  percutaneous transluminal, 903-904
Balloon pumps, intraaortic, 1748-1750, 1748*f,* 1749*f*
  for cardiogenic shock, 1786
  complications of, 1748-1750
  contraindications to, 1748*t*
  indications for, 1748*t*
Balloon thermotherapy, 1388, 1388*f*
Balloon valvuloplasty, percutaneous transluminal, 881-882
Bamboo spine, 1712
Band, 668
Band neutrophils, 1860*t*
Bandaging, for above-the-knee amputation residual limb, 1660, 1661*f*
Baraclude (entecavir), 1094, 1095
Barbiturates
  blood glucose level effects, 1267*t*
  effects of use, 169*t*
  food/nutrient interactions, 954*t*
  for general anesthesia, 369*t*
  poisoning, 1837*t*
  and restrictive lung disease, 595*t*
  toxicology, 1865*t*
Bard catheter, 1221
Bariatric surgery
  procedures, 982, 983*f*
  special considerations for ambulatory and home care, 986
  special considerations for postoperative care, 986
  special considerations for preoperative care, 985
Barium enema x-ray, 941*f,* 941*t*
Barium swallow, 941*t*
Baroreceptors, 763
  regulation of blood pressure by, 764
  regulation of cardiovascular system by, 743
Barotrauma
  in acute respiratory distress syndrome, 1816
  in positive pressure ventilation, 1763-1764
"Barrel chest," 634
Barrett's esophagus, 1004-1005
Basal body temperature assessment, 1341*t*
Basal body temperature record, 1382, 1382*f*
Basal cell carcinoma, 463, 464*t,* 465*f*
  therapy of, 465*b*
Basal ganglia, 1447*t*

Basaljel
  preparation, 1020*t*
  for renal osteodystrophy, 1210
Base, 333*t*
Base deficit, 1775*t*
Basic life support, 1845
  airway management, 1845-1846
  breathing, 1846
  cardiac compressions, 1846-1849, 1849*f*
Basilar artery, 1450, 1451*f*
Basiliximab (Simulect), 239*t,* 240
Basophils, 668
  function of, 668*t*
  laboratory values, 1860*t*
  response to injury, 195
Baths, 477
Battle's sign, 1481, 1482*f*
BayRab (rabies immune globulin), 1836-1837
BCG vaccine (TheraCys), 303*t*
BCNU (carmustine), 720*t*
Becker muscular dystrophy, 1675*t*
Beclomethasone (Vanceril, Beclovent, Vanceril DS, Qvar, Qvar HFA, Vancenase)
  for allergic rhinitis and sinusitis, 537*t*
  for asthma and COPD, 618*t*
Bedbugs, 470*t*
Bee stings, 470*t,* 1834
Beepen-VK (penicillin V potassium), 878
Behavior(s)
  addictive, **165-191,** 166*t*
    nursing management of, **181-189**
    overview of, **166-167**
  in Alzheimer's disease, 1569, 1569*t*
    acute intervention for, 1573
    assessment of, 1456
  in chronic HF, 826
  in fluid and electrolyte imbalances, 338*t*
  reactions to acute coronary syndrome, 814, 814*t*
  stages of, 55, 55*t*
Behavioral management
  for obesity, 980
  for older adults, 82
Beliefs. *See also* Values-belief pattern
  affecting health and health care, 31*t*
  health-related, of religious groups, 32*t*
  and pain, 134
Bell's palsy, 1584-1585
  clinical manifestations of, 1584
  collaborative care for, 1584-1585
  diagnostic studies, 1584
  drug therapy for, 1584-1585
  etiology and pathophysiology of, 1584
  facial characteristics of, 1584, 1584*f*
  nursing assessment of, 1585
  nursing diagnoses, 1585
  nursing evaluation of, 1585
  nursing implementation for, 1585
  nursing management of, **1585**
  nursing planning for, 1585
Benadryl (diphenhydramine)
  for allergic rhinitis and sinusitis, 537*t*
  for anaphylactic shock, 1790
  for dermatologic problems, 475
  for opioid-induced pruritus, 138
  for Parkinson's disease, 1552*t*
  photosensitivity, 461*t*
Benazepril (Lotensin)
  amlodipine/benazepril (Lotrel), 777*t*
  for chronic HF, 832
  for hypertension, 776*t*

Note: Disorder names are in **bold face.**
Page numbers in **bold face** indicate main discussions. Page numbers followed by
f, t, b, or *n* indicate figures, tables, boxed material, or notes, respectively.

Benazepril/hydrochlorothiazide (Lotensin HCT), 777*t*

Bence Jones protein, 78, 682*t*, 1862*t*

Bendroflumethiazide (Naturetin)
  for hypertension, 773*t*
  nadolol/bendroflumethiazide (Corzide), 777*t*

Benemid (probenecid), 1371*t*

Benicar (olmesartan), 776*t*

Benicar HCT (olmesartan medoxomil/hydrochlorothiazide), 777*t*

Benign dermatologic problems, 471, 472*t*

Benign neoplasms, 274, 275*t*

Benign nephrosclerosis, 1175

Benign prostatic hyperplasia (BPH), 1414-1422, 1415*f*
  acute intervention for, 1421-1422
  ambulatory and home care for, 1422
  case study, 1438
  clinical manifestations of, 1415
  collaborative care for, 1416-1419, 1417*t*
  complications of, 1415
  diagnostic studies, 1415-1416
  drug therapy for, 1416-1417
  etiology and pathophysiology of, 1414-1415
  health promotion in, 1421
  herbal therapy for, 1417
  invasive therapy for, 1417-1418, 1418*t*
  irritative symptoms of, 1415
  minimally invasive therapy for, 1418-1419, 1418*t*
  nursing assessment of, 1419, 1419*t*
  nursing diagnoses, 1419
  nursing evaluation of, 1422
  nursing implementation for, 1421-1422
  nursing management of, **1419-1422**
  nursing planning for, 1419
  obstructive symptoms of, 1415
  postoperative care of, 1421-1422
  preoperative care of, 1421
  Symptom Index for BPH (AUA), 1415, 1416*t*
  transurethral microwave thermotherapy for, 1418-1419

Benign tumors
  of female reproductive system, **1398-1400**
  ovarian, **1399-1400**

Bentyl (dicyclomine)
  for acute pancreatitis, 1121*t*
  for voiding dysfunction, 1185*t*

Benzodiazepines
  adjuncts to general anesthesia, 369, 370*t*
  for Alzheimer's disease, 1569*t*
  effects of use, 169*t*
  ethnic differences in response to, 35*t*
  poisoning, 1837*t*
  preoperative, 355*t*

Benzphetamine (Didrex), 981

Benzquinamide (Emete-Con), 992*t*

Benzthiazide (Aquatag, Exna), 773*t*

Benztropine (Cogentin), 1552*t*

Bereavement, 153

Berylliosis, 577, 578*t*

β-blockers. *See* β-Adrenergic receptor antagonists (β-Adrenergic blockers)

Betagan (levobunolol), 434*t*

Betapace (sotalol)
  classification of, 856*t*
  food/nutrient interactions, 954*t*
  for ventricular tachycardia, 855

Betaseron (β-Interferon)
  clinical uses of, 223*t*
  drug alert, 1544
  for multiple sclerosis, 1544, 1544*t*

Betaxolol (Betoptic)
  for glaucoma, 434*t*
  for hypertension, 774*t*

Bethanechol (Urecholine)
  for gastroesophageal reflux disease, 1006, 1006*t*
  for multiple sclerosis, 1544*t*

Betoptic (betaxolol)
  for glaucoma, 434*t*
  for hypertension, 774*t*

Bevacizumab (Avastin), 302, 303*t*
  for colorectal cancer, 1067
  FOLFOX treatment regimen, 291*t*

Bexarotene (Targretin), 727

Bextra (valdecoxib), 136, 136*t*, 1697

Bexxar (tositumomab/tositumomab-^{131}I), 303*t*, 727

Bias, 23

Biaxin (clarithromycin)
  for inflammatory bowel disease, 1054, 1055*t*
  for peptic ulcer disease, 1019*t*

Bicalutamide (Casodex), 1426, 1426*t*

Bicarbonate (HCO_3^-), 1147*t*
  laboratory values, 1855*t*
  normal values, 321*t*

Biceps reflex test, 1459*f*

Bicillin (penicillin G benzathine), 1371, 1371*t*

Bicillin LA (penicillin G benzathine), 878

BiCNU (carmustine), 287*t*

BiDil (isosorbide dinitrate and hydralazine), 833

Bier block, 371

Biguanides
  blood glucose level effects, 1267*t*
  for diabetes mellitus, 1265, 1266*t*

Bilberry, 102*t*, 425*b*

Bile, 932*t*, 946*t*

Bile duct system, 931*f*

Bile flow obstruction, 1128, 1128*t*

Bile reflux gastritis, 1026

Bile-acid sequestrants, 793, 795*t*

Bi-leaflet valve, 883*t*

Bilevel positive airway pressure, 1763, 1810, 1810*f*

Biliary catheters, transhepatic, 1129

Biliary cirrhosis, primary, **1101**

Biliary colic, 1127

Biliary necrosis, 1102

Biliary tract, **931-932,** 931*f*
  disorders of, **1126-1132**
  obstruction of, 473*t*
  problems of, **1087-1134**

Biliopancreatic diversion, 982*t*, 983*f*, 984

Bilirubin, 680*t*
  in anemias, 690*t*
  laboratory values, 1855*t*
  metabolism, 931-932
  metabolism abnormalities in ascites, 1106, 1107*t*
  serum, 946*t*
  urinary, 946*t*, 1862*t*

Bilis, 35*t*

Billroth I operation, 1025, 1026*f*

Billroth II operation, 1025, 1026*b*

BioBrane, 498*t*

Biochemical problems, 296*t*

Biochemical theory for fat embolism syndrome, 1651

Bioclusive, 205*t*

Bioethics Resources on the Web, 38

Biofeedback, 97*t*
  for headache, 1530
  for seizures, 1538
  for urinary incontinence, 1182*b*, 1183*t*

Biologic response modifier therapy, 302

Biologic theories of aging, **67-69,** 68*t*

Biologic therapy, 303*t*
  for arthritis and connective tissue disorders, 1700*t*
  for breast cancer, 1356
  for cancer, **302-304**
  for colorectal cancer, 1067
  drug alert, 1705-1706
  host-tumor response effects, 302
  for inflammatory bowel disease, 1053, 1054, 1055*t*
  for leukemia, 720*t*
  for lung cancer, 582
  nursing management of, **304**
  side effects of, 302-304

Biologic valves, 882, 883*t*

Biologic-based therapies, 96*t*, 97*t*, **100-101**

BIOPATCH, 205*t*

Biopsy
  breast, 1340*t*
  cancer, 283
  closed (needle), 681, 682*t*
  endometrial, 1341*t*
  endomyocardial, 875
  excisional, 283, 458*t*
  hematologic, 681, 682*t*
  incisional, 283, 458*t*
  liver, 944*t*, 946
  lung, 528*t*, 529-530
  lymph node, 681, 682*t*
  needle
    for cancer diagnosis, 283
    lymph node, 681, 682*t*
    transbronchial, 529-530, 530*f*
  punch, 458*t*, 476
  renal, 1149*t*
  shave, 458*t*

Bioterrorism, 1838
  agents of, 1838, 1839*t*-1840*t*

BiPAP. *See* Bilevel positive airway pressure

Biperiden (Akineton), 1552*t*

Bird fancier's, breeder's, or handler's lung, 578*t*

Bisacodyl (Dulcolax)
  for constipation, 1042*t*
  for opioid-induced constipation, 138

Bismuth subsalicylate (Pepto-Bismol), 1019*t*, 1037*t*

Bisoprolol (Zebeta), 774*t*

Bisoprolol/hydrochlorothiazide (Ziac), 777*t*

Bisphosphonates
  drug alert, 1689
  for osteoporosis, 1689
  for Paget's disease, 1690

Bites and stings, 1833-1837

Bitolterol (Tornalate), 619*t*, 620

Bivalirudin (Angiomax), 914

Biventricular failure, 823, 824

Bivona Fome-Cuf tracheostomy tube, 544*t*

Black cohosh, 102*t*, 1393*b*

Black lung, 578*t*

Black widow spiders, 1834, 1834*f*

Black wounds, 200, 200*t*, 204-205

Bladder, **1140,** 1140*f*
  age-related changes in, 1141*t*
  assessment of, 1461*t*
  comparison of functional health patterns and NANDA International Taxonomy II, 42*t*

Bladder (*Continued*)
  neurogenic
    collaborative care for, 1604, 1605*t*
    after spinal cord injury, 1604-1605
    types of, 1604, 1605*t*
  orthotopic reconstruction of, 1190
  pain related to, 1145*v*
  painful bladder syndrome, **1163-1164**
  spastic (uninhibited), 1543

Bladder cancer, 1178-1180
  chemotherapy of, 291, 1179
  clinical manifestations of, 1178-1179, 1179*f*
  collaborative care for, 1179*t*
  diagnostic studies, 1178-1179
  intravesical therapy of, 291, 1180
  nursing and collaborative management of, **1179-1180**
  radiation therapy of, 1179
  surgical therapy of, 1179

Bladder management
  retraining, 1183*t*, 1519
  after spinal cord injury, 1602-1603, 1605-1606
  after stroke, 1523

Bladder neck support prostheses, 1183*t*

Bladder outlet obstruction, 1168

Blast wounds, 1642*t*

Blastomyces dermatitidis, 245*t*, 576*t*

Blastomycosis, 576*t*

Bleaches, 1837*t*

Blebs, 501, 633, 634*f*

Bleeding. *See also* Hemorrhage
  with anticoagulant therapy, 916, 916*t*
  in chronic kidney disease, 1207
  duodenal, 996
  epistaxis, 534-535, 675*t*, 1871
  gastrointestinal
    drug therapy of, 997, 998*t*
    scintigraphy of, 942*t*
  in peritoneal dialysis, 1219
  postcoital, 1334
  stomach, 996
  upper gastrointestinal, **995-1000**
  uterine, 1387
  vaginal
    abnormal, **1387-1389**
    breakthrough, 1388

Bleeding time, 679*t*
  in deep vein thrombosis, 911*t*
  in hemophilia, 709*t*
  laboratory values, 1859*t*

Bleeding varices
  acute intervention for, 1114
  collaborative care for, 1106-1110

Blenoxane (bleomycin)
  classification of, 287*t*
  for esophageal cancer, 1010
  method of administration, 288*t*
  for oral cancer, 1002
  for testicular cancer, 1432

Bleomycin (Blenoxane)
  classification of, 287*t*
  for esophageal cancer, 1010
  method of administration, 288*t*
  for non-Hodgkin's lymphoma, 727*t*
  for oral cancer, 1002
  for testicular cancer, 1432

Blepharitis, 406*t*, **422**

Blepharoplasty, 480

Blindness
  functional, 419
  legal, 405, 419, 419*t*
  total, 419

BlisterFilm, 205*t*

Blocadren (timolol), 774*t*

Blom-Singer voice prosthesis, 557, 557*f*

Blood, 666-668
  cerebrospinal fluid analysis, 1864t
  fecal analysis, 1864t
  functions of, 666, 666t
  hypercoagulability of, 909-910, 910t
  protective role, 666
  regenerative ability of, 198, 198t
  thin blood, 35t
  transmission of HIV by contact with, 250
Blood alcohol concentration, 177, 177t
Blood ammonia levels, 946t
Blood cells
  development of, 666, 666f
  types of, 667
Blood chemistries
  of gastrointestinal system, 944t
  urinary, 1147t
Blood cholesterol, high, 789, 790t
Blood coagulation tests, 913t
Blood component therapy, **730-734**
  administration procedure, 730-732
Blood components, 667, 667f
Blood culture, 1775t
Blood flow
  low blood flow shock, 1772-1773, **1773-1777,** 1773f
    classification of, 1773t
    clinical presentation of, 1776t
    effects on hemodynamic parameters, 1774-1775, 1774t
    precipitating factors, 1773t
  maldistribution of blood flow shock, 1773, 1773f, 1777-1778
    classification of, 1773t
    clinical presentation of, 1776t
    effects on hemodynamic parameters, 1774-1775, 1774t
    precipitating factors, 1773t
  measurement of, 759-760
  peripheral vessel, 759-760
Blood gases
  in acid-base imbalances, 336-337
  arterial, 337, 513, 527t
    abbreviations, 1800t
    in acute asthmatic attack, 614t
    normal values, 337t, 514t
    preoperative analysis, 351
    in shock, 1775t
  laboratory values, 1855t
  mixed venous, 513-514, 514t
Blood glucose
  drugs affecting, 1266, 1267t
  fasting, 1251t
  feedback between insulin and, 1237, 1237f
  low, 1278. See also Hypoglycemia
  monitoring, 1269-1271
    patient and family teaching guide for monitoring, 1277t
    patient and family teaching guide for self-monitoring, 1270t
    preoperative, 351
    self-monitoring of, 1269
    tight control, 1283
Blood glucose monitors, 1269, 1270f
Blood loss
  acute, **694-695**
    anemia caused by, 685t
    laboratory study findings in, 690t
  anemia caused by, 694-695
  chronic, **695**

Blood loss (Continued)
  anemia caused by, 685t
  laboratory study findings in, 690t
  in hemodialysis, 1223
Blood pressure, 743, 762
  altered, 676t
  arterial, 743, 1740-1741
    measurement of, 743, 1742f
  central venous
    measurement of, 1744, 1745f
    normal range at rest, 1739t
    in shock, 1774t
  classification of, 769t
  in compartment syndrome, 1650
  diagnostic criteria for metabolic syndrome, 987t
  diastolic, 743, 1871
  factors influencing, 762-763, 763f
  in fluid and electrolyte imbalances, 338t
  left atrial pressure, 1739t
  left ventricular end-diastolic pressure, 1738
  management of, 769t
  mean arterial pressure (MAP), 744
    calculation of, 744, 781
    normal range at rest, 1739t
  measurement of, 759-760, 778
    with invasive lines, 1742f, 1742t
    manual, 779t
  normal, 789
  pulmonary artery, 1741-1747, 1744f
    measurement of, 1744, 1744f
    normal range at rest, 1739t
    in shock, 1774t
  pulmonary artery diastolic pressure, 1739t
  pulmonary artery wedge pressure
    in acute respiratory distress syndrome, 1815t
    elevated, 1744, 1745f
    measurement of, 1744, 1744f
    normal range at rest, 1739t
    in shock, 1774t
  pulse pressure, 743-744
    in shock, 1774t
  reduction of dietary salt and, 780b
  regulation of, 762-764
    by corticosteroids, 1318
  right atrial pressure
    measurement of, 1744
    normal range at rest, 1739t
  segmental, 901
  in shock, 1774t
  sympathetic nervous system receptors affecting, 763, 763t
  systolic, 743, 1876
Blood pressure monitoring
  ambulatory, 768
  home monitoring, 780
  invasive, 1742f, 1742t
    principles of, 1739-1740
    types of, 1740-1747
  system components, 1739, 1740f
Blood products, 731t
  for shock, 1786t
  transmission of HIV by contact with, 250
Blood studies
  cardiovascular, 751-756, 752t
  in deep vein thrombosis, 911t
  laboratory studies, 680t
  preoperative, 351
  reproductive, 1336-1341
  respiratory, 525, 527t
Blood transfusion, 730
Blood transfusion reactions, 732-734
Blood typing, 351, 679

Blood urea nitrogen, 1147t
  BUN/creatinine ratio, 1147t
  in shock, 1775t
Blood vessels
  age-related changes in, 744t
  autonomic nervous system and, 743
  regenerative ability of linings, 198, 198t
Blood-borne metastasis, 276, 277f
Blood-borne pathogens, 247, 248t
Blood-brain barrier, 1452
BLS. See Basic life support
Blunt trauma
  to chest, 585, 585t
  to eye, 421t
  fractured extremity, 1642, 1642t
  head injury, 1484t
  spinal cord injury, 1596t
  steering-wheel injury, 585t
Blurred vision, 406t, 675t
BMT. See Bone marrow transplantation
BNP. See b-Type natriuretic peptide
Body fluid chemistry terminology, 316t
Body fluid compartments, 315, 315f
  electrolyte composition of, 316, 316f
Body image concerns, 345, 345t
Body jacket cast, 1640, 1640f
Body mass index, 956-957
  calculation of, 956
  classification of overweight and obesity by, 974, 975t
Body mass index chart, 974, 974f
Body position. See also Patient positioning
  in increased ICP, 1480
Body shape, 974, 975t
Body surface area, total, 487
Body temperature
  basal body temperature assessment, 1341t
  in shock, 1793
Body water content, 315
  age-related changes in, 315, 315f
  functions of, 315
Body weight
  classification of, 974-975
  Hamwi "rule of thumb" for, 956, 957t
Bone, **1615-1616**
  age-related changes in, 1618-1619, 1619t
  cancellous, 1615
  cortical, 1615, 1615f
  enlargement of, 1247t
  function of, 1615
  gross structure of, 1615-1616
  microscopic structure of, 1615
  regenerative ability of, 198, 198t
  self-healing stages, 1636-1638
  structure of, 1615, 1615f
  types of, 1616
Bone cancer
  acute intervention for, 1674
  ambulatory and home care for, 1674-1675
  health promotion in, 1674
  metastatic, **1674-1675**
  nursing assessment of, 1674
  nursing diagnoses, 1674
  nursing evaluation of, 1675
  nursing implementation for, 1674-1675
  nursing management of, **1674-1675**
  nursing planning for, 1674
Bone conduction studies, 414t
Bone diseases, metabolic, **1686-1690**
  gerontologic considerations for, **1690**
Bone healing, 1636-1638, 1637f

Bone marrow, 665-666
Bone marrow aspiration, 681, 681f
Bone marrow examination, 681, 681f, 682t
Bone marrow failure, 719
Bone marrow suppression, 294-297
Bone marrow transplantation, 304
Bone mineral density measurements, 1625t
Bone remodeling, 1615
  fracture healing, 1637-1638, 1637f
  in osteoporosis, 1687
Bone scans, 682t, 1625t
Bone tumors, 1672-1675, 1673t
Bonefos (clodronate), 1689
Bonine (meclizine), 992t
Boniva (ibandronate), 1689
Bontril (phendimetrazine), 981
Borborygmi, 937, 940t
  in intestinal obstruction, 1061
  postoperative, 1026
Borg category-ratio scale, 520, 520f
Borrelia burgdorferi, 245t
Bortezomib (Velcade), 303t, 729
Bosentan (Tracleer), 602
Botox (BoNT-A), 1531
Botulinum toxin (Botox)
  for botulism, 1587-1588
  injection procedures, 479t
Botulism, 1031, 1032t, **1587-1588,** 1839t
  clinical manifestations of, 1587
  collaborative care for, 1587-1588
  diagnostic studies, 1587
  drug therapy for, 1587-1588
  etiology and pathophysiology of, 1587
  nursing management of, **1588**
  ocular manifestations of, 437t
Bouchard's nodes, 1695
Bounding, 749t
Boutonnière deformity, 1623t
Bowlegs, 1624t
Bowel
  comparison of functional health patterns and NANDA International Taxonomy II, 42t
  neurogenic, with spinal cord injury, 1605-1606
  patterns at end of life, 161t
Bowel management
  after spinal cord injury, 1602-1603, 1605, 1606t
  after stroke, 1522-1523
Bowel obstructions, 1060, 1060f
  pseudo-obstruction, 1061
Bowel sounds, 937
  absent, 940t
BP. See Arterial blood pressure
BPD. See Biliopancreatic diversion
BPH. See Benign prostatic hyperplasia
Braces
  halo vest (Ace), 1601, 1601f
  sternal-occipital-mandibular immobilizer brace, 1601, 1601f
Brachioradialis reflex, 1459
Brachiocephalic artery, 1451f
Brachytherapy, 293-294
  afterloading, 1405
  for breast cancer, 1354, 1354f
  for cancers of female reproductive system, **1404-1405**
  high-dose, 1354, 1354f

Note: Disorder names are in **bold face.** Page numbers in **bold face** indicate main discussions. Page numbers followed by f, t, b, or n indicate figures, tables, boxed material, or notes, respectively.

Brachytherapy *(Continued)*
 preloading, 1405
 for prostate cancer, 1425-1426, 1426*f*
Braden Risk Assessment Scale, 207-
 209, 208*t*, 212
Bradycardia
 absolute, 849
 relative, 849
 sinus bradycardia, 849-850
Bradykinesia, 1549, 1550
Bradykinin, 195*t*
Brain, 1445-1448
 age-related changes in, 1454*t*
 arteries at base of, 1452*f*
 components of, 1467, 1468*f*
 functional areas of, 1488,
  1488*f*
 inflammatory conditions of, **1493-
  1499**
Brain abscess, 1494*t*, **1499**
"Brain attack," 1502
Brain death, 153
 ethical dilemma, 1485*b*
Brain fag, 35*t*
Brain reward system, 166
Brain stents, 1510, 1510*f*
Brain tumors, 1487-1491
 chemotherapy for, 1490
 clinical manifestations of, 1488,
  1489*t*
 collaborative care for, 1489-
  1490
 complications of, 1489
 cultural and ethnic health disparities
  in, 1487*b*
 diagnostic studies, 1489
 metastatic, 1488, 1488*t*, 1489*t*
 nursing assessment of, 1490
 nursing diagnoses, 1490
 nursing evaluation of, 1491
 nursing implementation for, 1490-
  1491
 nursing management of, **1490-
  1491**
 nursing planning for, 1490
 radiation therapy for, 1489-
  1490
 radiosurgery for, 1489-1490
 surgical therapy for, 1489
 types of, 1487-1488, 1488*t*
Brainstem, 1447
Brainstem auditory evoked potentials,
 1463*t*
Brainstem tumors, 1488, 1489*t*
Bravelle (urofollitropin), 1383*t*
BRCA-1 mutation, 216
BRCA-2 mutation, 216
Breakthrough pain, 132
Breast(s)
 age-related changes in, 1331*t*, **1348**
 assessment abnormalities, 1335*t*
 cysts, 1345*t*
 dimpling of, 1335*t*
 female, 1327, 1327*f*
  age-related changes in, 1331*t*
  lymphatic drainage of, 1327, 1327*f*
  normal physical assessment of,
   1335*t*
  physical examination of, 1335
 fibrocystic changes, 1345*t*, **1346-
  1347,** 1346*f*
 physical examination of, 51*t*
Breast abscess, lactational, 1346
Breast augmentation, **1361**
 nursing management of, **1362**
Breast biopsy, 1340*t*

Breast cancer, 1348-1361
 acute intervention for, 1359-1360
 adjuvant therapy for, 1353-1356
 ambulatory and home care for, 1360-
  1361
 biologic therapy for, 1356
 brachytherapy for, high-dose, 1354,
  1354*f*
 case study, 1363-1364
 chemotherapy for, 1354-1355
 clinical manifestations of, 1350
 collaborative care for, 1351-1356,
  1351*t*
 complications of, 1350
 cultural and ethnic health disparities
  in, 1348*b*
 culturally competent care for, **1356**
 diagnostic studies, 1350-1351
 diploid, 1351
 distribution of, 1350, 1350*f*
 etiology and pathophysiology of,
  1348-1349
 genetics of, 1349*b*
 gerontologic considerations for, **1361**
 hormonal therapy for, 1355
 inflammatory, 1350
 noninvasive, 1350
 nursing assessment of, 1356, 1356*t*
 nursing diagnoses, 1356
 nursing evaluation of, 1361
 nursing implementation for, 1359-
  1361
 nursing management of, **1356-1361**
 nursing planning for, 1359
 palliative radiation therapy for, 1354
 psychologic care in, 1360
 radiation therapy for, 1353-1354
 receptor-negative tumors, 1351
 receptor-positive tumors, 1351
 risk factors for, 1348-1349, 1349*t*
 screening for
  guidelines for early detection,
   282*t*, 1343-1344
  increasing participation in, 1359*b*
 sites of recurrence and metastasis,
  1350, 1351*t*
 staging of, 1352, 1352*t*
 surgical therapy for, 1352-1353
  follow-up care, 1353
  procedures, 1353*t*
 systemic therapy for, 1354-1356
 targeted therapy for, 1356
 types of, 1349, 1350*t*
Breast conservation surgery, 1352-1353,
 1353*t*
Breast disorders, 1343-1365
 assessment of, **1343-1345**
 benign, **1345-1348,** 1345*t*
 diagnostic studies, 1344-1345
 resources, 1365
Breast implants, 1353*t*, 1362, 1363*f*
Breast infections, 1345-1346
Breast nodules, masses, lumps, 1335*t*
Breast pain, 1345
Breast reconstruction, **1362-1363,** 1362*f*
 indications for, 1362
 musculocutaneous flap procedure,
  1362-1363
 types of, 1362-1363
Breast reduction, **1361**
 nursing management of, **1362**
Breast self-examination, 1344, 1344*f*
Breath sounds
 abnormal, 524
 absent, 525*t*
Breathing
 abdominal, 117, 646
 basic life support, 1846

Breathing *(Continued)*
 diaphragmatic, 117, 646
 paradoxic, 1805
 primary survey of, 1823, 1824*t*, 1825*t*
 pursed-lip, 524*t*, 646
 rapid shallow breathing index (f/V$_T$),
  1767*t*
 shortness of breath, 518, 519*t*
  fear of, 159
 spontaneous breathing trial, 1767
Breathing assessment, 117, 117*t*
 in burns, 488
 initial postanesthesia care unit assessment, 377-378, 377*t*
Breathing exercises, 646
Breathing retraining, 646
Breslow measurement, 466
Brethine (terbutaline), 619*t*
Bretylium (Bretylol), 856*t*
Brevibloc (esmolol)
 for aortic dissection, 899
 for chronic stable angina and acute
  coronary syndrome, 800*t*
 classification of, 856*t*
 for hypertension, 774*t*
Brevital (methohexital), 369*t*
Bricanyl (terbutaline), 619*t*
Brief Pain Inventory, 134
Brimonidine (Alphagan), 434*t*
Brinzolamide (Azopt), 435*t*
Broad ligament, 1326
Broca's area, 1445
Bromocriptine (Parlodel)
 drug alert, 1551
 for Parkinson's disease, 1551, 1552*t*
 for prolactinoma, 1293
 for restless legs syndrome, 1558
Brompheniramine (Dimetane), 537*t*
Bronchial carcinoma, 307, 307*f*
Bronchial sounds, 523
Bronchiectasis, 659-661
 clinical manifestations of, 660
 collaborative care for, 660
 diagnostic studies, 660
 etiology and pathophysiology of,
  659-660
 nursing management of, **660-661**
 pathologic changes in, 656, 657*f*
Bronchiolitis obliterans, 577, 603
Bronchitis
 acute, **561**
 chronic, 608, 629
Bronchoalveolar lavage, 529, 529*f*
Bronchoconstriction, 511
Bronchodilation, 511
Bronchodilators, 620-621
 for asthma, 617*t*
 for COPD, 618*t*
 for drug therapy, 639-640
 food/nutrient interactions, 954*t*
Bronchophony, 525*t*
Bronchoscopic laser therapy, 582
Bronchoscopy, 528-529, 528*t*
 fiberoptic, 529, 529*f*
Bronchospasm
 postoperative, 378-380, 379*t*
 relief of, 1810-1811
Bronchovesicular sounds, 523
Brooke (modified) formula, 496, 497*t*
Brown recluse spiders, 1834-1835
Brown-Séquard syndrome, 1591-
 1592, 1592*f*
Brudzinski's sign, 1460*t*, 1461*f*, 1494
Bruising, 676*t*, 677
Bruits, 748, 750*t*, 940*t*, 1145, 1221
b-Type natriuretic peptide, 752*t*
 for chronic HF, 832
 human, 832

b-Type natriuretic peptide *(Continued)*
 laboratory values, 1855*t*
 levels, 827, 827*t*
Buboes, 1373
Buck's traction, 1639, 1639*f*
Buclizine (Bucladin-S), 992*t*
Budesonide (Pulmicort Turbuhaler,
  Pulmicort Respules, Entocort,
  Rhinocort)
 for allergic rhinitis and sinusitis, 537*t*
 for asthma and COPD, 618*t*
 for inflammatory bowel disease,
  1055*t*
Budesonide/formoterol (Symbicort), 620*t*
Buerger's disease, 473*t*, 908
Buffers, 333*t*, 334
Bufopto (atropine), 427*t*
Bulbourethral gland, 1324
Bulimia, 969*b*
Bulimia nervosa, 969
Bullae, 633, 634*f*
Bullectomy, 646
Bumetanide (Bumex)
 for heart failure, 828
 for hypertension, 773*t*
BUN/creatinine ratio, 1147*t*
Bundle of His, 846, 847*t*
Bunion, 1685*t*, 1686*f*
Bupivacaine (Sensorcaine), 128
Buprenorphine (Buprenex)
 for pain, 137*t*, 138
 for pain management, 187
Buprenorphine plus naloxone
  (Suboxone)
 for opioid withdrawal, 180
 for pain, 137*t*
Bupropion (Zyban)
 for smoking cessation, 171*t*
 for tobacco cessation, 170
Burn shock, 488, 491, 491*f*
Burn Unit referral criteria, 486*t*
"Burning" on urination, 1145*t*
Burns, 483-507
 acute phase, **499-503**
  clinical manifestations of,
   500
  collaborative care for, 493*t*
  complications of, 500-501
  excision of, 501
  grafting of, 501
  laboratory values, 500
  nursing and collaborative management of, **501-503**
  pathophysiology of, 499
 care measures for, 498
 case study, 506
 causes of, 484*t*
 chemical, 484, 489*t*
 classification of injury, **486-488**
  by depth, 486, 487*t*
 collaborative care for, 493*t*
 common places of, 484*t*
 depth of, 486, 487*f*
 drug therapy for, 498-499, 499*t*
 electrical, 485-486, 485*f*, 490*t*
 emergent (resuscitative) phase, **488-
  499**
  clinical manifestations of, 491
  collaborative care for, 493*t*
  complications of, 491-492
  nursing and collaborative management of, **492-499**
  pathophysiology of, 488-491
 emotional needs of patient and
  family, 505

Burns (*Continued*)
emotional responses of patients with, 505*t*
extent of, 487, 487*f*
to eye, 421*t*
full-thickness, 486, 487*t*
emergency management of, 490*t*
gerontologic considerations for, **504-505**
healing, 491
location of, 487-488
management phases, **488-506**
nursing care plan for patient with, 494*b*-496*b*
open wound care, 497
operative debridement of, 496, 497*f*
partial-thickness, 486, 487*t*
emergency management of, 490*t*
prehospital care of, **488**
rehabilitation phase, **503-505**
clinical manifestations of, 503-504
collaborative care for, 493*t*
complications of, 504
nursing and collaborative management of, **504**
pathophysiologic changes, 503-504
resources for, 507
risk factors for, 488
risk reduction strategies for, 484*t*
rule of nines for, 487, 487*f*
severity of, 486
special needs of nursing staff in, **505-506**
thermal, 484, 490*t*
types of injury, **484-486**, 484*t*, 485*f*
types of pain in, 502-503
upper respiratory tract injury, 492, 492*t*
wound care, 496-498
Burr holes, 1491*t*
Bursae, 1618
Bursitis, 1635
Burst suppression, 1475
Buserelin (Suprefact), 1426*t*
Buspirone (BuSpar), 1386
Busulfan (Myleran)
classification of, 287*t*
for leukemia, 720*t*
Butalbital, 1530
Butorphanol (Stadol), 137*t*, 138, 141, 187
Butterfly rash, 1718, 1718*f*
Butyl nitrite, 170*t*
Butyrophenones, 992, 992*t*
BVM ventilation. *See* Bag-valve-mask ventilation
BVS® 5000 Biventricular Support System, 839
Byetta (exenatide), 1265-1266, 1266*t*
Bypass graft surgery
coronary artery
for acute coronary syndrome, 808-809
off-pump, 809-810
peripheral artery, 907*t*
Byssinosis, 578*t*

C

Cabergoline (Dostinex)
for acromegaly, 1292
for prolactinoma, 1293

CABG. *See* Coronary artery bypass graft
Cadaver valve, 883*t*
CADs. *See* Circulatory assist devices
Caffeine, **176**
blood glucose level effects, 1267*t*
characteristics of, 176
collaborative care, 176
complications of, 168*t*, 176
effects of use, 169*t*, 176
effects on lower urinary tract function, 1180*t*
onset, peak, duration, and withdrawal, 185*t*
for opioid-induced sedation, 138
CAGE questionnaire adapted to include drugs (CAGEAID), 182, 183*t*
Caged ball valve, 883*t*
Calan (verapamil)
for acute coronary syndrome, 800*t*
for chronic stable angina, 800*t*, 801
classification of, 856*t*
effects on lower urinary tract function, 1180*t*
for hypertension, 776*t*
for voiding dysfunction, 1185*t*
Calciferol (ergocalciferol), 1311
Calcifying pancreatitis, chronic, 1124
Calcijex (calcitriol), 1210
Calcimar (calcitonin), 1689
Calcimimetic agents, 1210
Calcineurin inhibitors, 238, 239*t*
Calcitonin (Calcimar), 1240*f*
blood glucose level effects, 1267*t*
for osteoporosis, 1689
for Paget's disease, 1690
target tissue and functions, 1236*t*
Calcitriol (Rocaltrol, Calcijex)
for hypocalcemia, 1210
for hypoparathyroidism, 1311
Calcium (Ca^{2+}), 670*t*, 1147*t*, 1626*t*
daily requirements in chronic kidney disease, 1211-1212, 1212*t*
feedback between parathyroid hormone and, 1237, 1237*f*
foods moderate or high in, 1171*t*
ionized, 1250*t*
laboratory values, 1855*t*
normal values, 321*t*
laboratory values, 1855*t*
as positive inotrope, 1739
preparations, 1689*t*
for prevention and treatment of osteoporosis, 1688
sources of, 1688, 1689*t*
total, 321*t*
total serum, 1250*t*
urine levels, 1862*t*
Calcium carbonate (Tums)
antacid preparations, 1020*t*
antacid side effects, 1020*t*
elemental calcium content, 1689*t*
Calcium carbonate + 5 mcg vitamin D_2 (Os-Cal 250), 1689*t*
Calcium channel blockers
for acute coronary syndrome, 800*t*
blood glucose level effects, 1267*t*
for chronic stable angina, 800*t*, 801
classification of, 856*t*
effects of, 801
for hypertension, 776*t*, 777*t*, 1210
for Raynaud's phenomenon, 1724
for voiding dysfunction, 1185*t*
Calcium citrate, 1689*t*
Calcium gluconate
elemental calcium content, 1689*t*
for elevated potassium levels, 1202*t*

Calcium glycerophosphate (Prelief), 1164
Calcium imbalances, 329-331
in acute renal failure, 1200
causes and clinical manifestations of, 330*t*
in chronic kidney disease, 1207
Calcium lactate, 1689*t*
Calcium oxalate stones, 1169, 1170*t*
Calcium phosphate stones, 1169, 1170*t*
Calcium polycarbophil (Mitrolan-OTC), 1037*t*
Calcium sensitizers, 833
Calculus(i)
acute renal lithiasis, 1173*b*-1174*b*
calcium oxalate stones, 1169, 1170*t*
calcium phosphate stones, 1169, 1170*t*
choledocholelithiasis, 1127
cholelithiasis, **1126-1132**
cystine stones, 1169, 1170*t*
gallstones, 941*f*, 1126-1132, 1127*f*
kidney stones, 1169, 1170*f*
nephrolithiasis, 1169
staghorn, 1169, 1170*f*
struvite stones, 1169, 1170*t*
uric acid stones, 1169, 1170*t*
urinary tract, **1169-1173**
Calluses
foot, 1685*t*
formation of, 1637, 1637*f*
Caloric restriction
1200-calorie-restricted weight-reduction diet, 978*t*
as antiaging strategy, 67-68, 68*t*
Caloric test stimulus, 414*t*
Calories
activities that affect expenditure of, 1269, 1269*t*
daily requirements in chronic kidney disease, 1211-1212, 1212*t*
high-calorie, high-protein diet, 958*t*
high-calorie foods, 306, 307*t*
in parenteral nutrition, 965
Camalox, 1020*t*
Campath (alemtuzumab), 303*t*, 720*t*, 721
Campral (acamprosate), 178
Camptosar (irinotecan)
classification of, 287*t*
for colorectal cancer, 1067
for esophageal cancer, 1010
for lung cancer, 582
Campylobacter infection, 1037*t*
Campylobacter jejuni **infection,** 245*t*
Canadian Infectious Disease Society/ Canadian Thoracic Society (CIDS/ CTS) guidelines for community-acquired pneumonia, 562
Canaliculi, 1615
Canasa (mesalamine suppositories), 1055*t*
Cancer, 271-313. *See also* Carcinoma
anatomic classification of, 279
association with obesity, 976
biologic therapy of, **302-304**
biology of, **272-279**
bladder cancer, **1178-1180**
bone cancer
metastatic, **1674-1675**
nursing management of, **1674-1675**
breast cancer, **1348-1361**
screening guidelines for early detection of, 1343-1344
cervical, **1400-1401**

Cancer (*Continued*)
chemotherapy of, **285-291**
in chronic kidney disease, 1207
classification of, **279-280**
clinical staging of, 280
collaborative care for, **283-284**, 283*f*
colorectal, **1063-1069**
combined modality therapy of, 284
complications of, **306-308**
control of, 284
cultural and ethnic health disparities, 273*b*
cure and control of, 284-285
deaths from, 272, 272*t*
detection of, **281-283**
development of, 274-279, 275*f*
diagnosis of, 281-283
coping with, 310
studies or procedures, 283
early detection of, 282*b*
endometrial, **1401-1402**
escape mechanisms from immunologic surveillance, 279, 279*f*
esophageal, **1009-1011**
extent of disease classification of, 280
of female reproductive system, **1400-1407**
cultural and ethnic health disparities in, 1400*b*
nursing management of, **1405-1407**
radiation therapy for, **1404-1407**
gallbladder cancer, **1132**
gastric, **1028-1031**
gender differences in, 272, 272*t*
gene therapy of, **306**
gerontologic considerations, **310**
guidelines for cancer-related check-ups, 282*t*
head and neck, **551-558**
nursing assessment of, 553*t*
nursing management of, **553-558**
health disparities and, 21*t*
hereditary nonpolyposis colorectal cancer, 1064*b*
histologic classification of, 279
immune system role in, 277-279
incidence of, 272, 272*t*
initiation of, 275-276
kidney cancer, **1177-1178**
laryngeal
case study, 558
excision of, 551, 551*f*
latent period, 276
lung cancer, **578-584**, 579*b*
of male reproductive system, 1423*b*
multimodality therapy of, 284
nonmelanoma skin cancers, **463-464**
nutritional problems in, 306-307
nutritional therapy of, 306, 306*t*, 307*t*
oral cancer, **1001-1003**
ovarian, **1402-1404**
pain assessment in, 309, 309*t*
pain management in, **309**
palliation of, 284, 285
pancreatic, **1125-1126**
of penis, **1430**
prevention of, **281-283**, 282*b*, 284
progression of, 276-277
promotion of, 276
prostate, **1422-1428**
psychologic support for, **309-310**
radiation therapy of, **292-301**
rehabilitative care of, 285
resources, 313
resources for survivors, 311, 311*t*
response to chemotherapy, 286

Note: Disorder names are in **bold face**. Page numbers in **bold face** indicate main discussions. Page numbers followed by *f*, *t*, *b*, or *n* indicate figures, tables, boxed material, or notes, respectively.

Cancer (*Continued*)
screening guidelines for early detection of, 281, 282*t*
staging, 280
stress associated with diagnosis and treatment of (case study), 122
supportive care of, 285
surgical therapy of, **284-285**
targeted therapy of, **302-304**
testicular, **1432**
TNM classification system, 280, 280*t*
treatment of
evidence-based guidelines for, 284
goals of, 283-284, 283*f*
hematopoietic growth factors used in, 304*t*
vaginal, **1404**
vulvar, **1404**
warning signs of, 281, 282*t*
Cancer biopsy, 283
Cancer survivorship, **310-311**
Candesartan (Atacand), 776*t*
Candesartan/hydrochlorothiazide (Atacand HCT), 777*t*
Candida, 252
Candida albicans, 245*t*, 254*t*, 576*t*, 1155*t*, 1394*t*
Candidiasis, 469*f*, 469*t*, 576*t*, 939*t*
oral, 1000*t*
vulvovaginal, 1394*t*
Canker sores, 1000*t*
Cannabis, 180-181
acute intervention for intoxication, 186
characteristics of, 180-181
collaborative care, 181
complications of, 168*t*
effects of use, 169*t*, 181
Capastat (capreomycin), 573*t*
CAPD. *See* Continuous ambulatory peritoneal dialysis
Capecitabine (Xeloda)
for breast cancer, 1355
classification of, 287*t*
for colorectal cancer, 1067
drug alert, 1067
method of administration, 288*t*
for pancreatic cancer, 1126
Capillaries, 743
fluid movement in, **318-319,** 319*f*
Capillary filling time, abnormal, 749*t*
Capillary fragility test, 679*t*
Capillary glucose monitoring, 1251*t*
Capillary refill, 748
Capoten (captopril)
for acute coronary syndrome, 808
for chronic HF, 832
for chronic stable angina, 801
for chronic stable angina and acute coronary syndrome, 800*t*
drug alert, 832
effects on lower urinary tract function, 1180*t*
for hypertension, 776*t*, 1210
nephrotoxicity, 1142*t*
Capozide (captopril/hydrochlorothiazide), 777*t*
Capreomycin (Capastat), 573*t*
Capsaicin (Icy-Hot, Zostrix, Capzasin)
for arthritis and connective tissue disorders, 1698*t*
local, 139*t*
for osteoarthritis, 1696
for pain, 141
Capsule endoscopy, 943*t*, 945*f*, 946
Captopril (Capoten)
for acute coronary syndrome, 800*t*, 808
for chronic HF, 832

Captopril (Capoten) (*Continued*)
for chronic stable angina, 800*t*, 801
drug alert, 832
effects on lower urinary tract function, 1180*t*
for hypertension, 776*t*, 1210
nephrotoxicity, 1142*t*
Captopril/hydrochlorothiazide (Capozide), 777*t*
Carafate (sucralfate)
for gastroesophageal reflux disease, 1006, 1006*t*
for peptic ulcer disease, 1019*t*
Carbachol (Isopto Carbachol), 435*t*
Carbamazepine (Tegretol)
for Alzheimer's disease, 1569
analgesic effects of, 128
for diabetes insipidus, 1297
drug alert, 1536
gerontologic considerations for, 1538
hepatotoxicity, 934*t*
local, 139*t*
for seizures, 1536, 1538*t*
for trigeminal neuralgia, 1581-1582
Carbex (selegiline), 1552*t*
Carbidopa/levodopa (Sinemet, Paracopa)
drug alert, 1551
for Parkinson's disease, 1551, 1552*t*
Carbohydrates, 949
in diabetic meal plan, 1267
metabolism of, 932*t*
in chronic kidney disease, 1206
by corticosteroids, 1318
in peritoneal dialysis, 1220
CarboMedic valve, 883*t*
Carbon dioxide
laboratory values, 1855*t*
partial pressure of end-tidal CO_2 (PETCO$_2$), 1753-1754
Carbon dioxide narcosis, 643
Carbon monoxide poisoning, 484-485, 1837*t*, 1865*t*
Carbonic acid excess, 334-335
Carbonic anhydrase inhibitors
for acute pancreatitis, 1121*t*
for glaucoma, 435*t*
Carboplatin (Paraplatin)
for cervical cancer, 1402
classification of, 287*t*
for lung cancer, 582
for oral cancer, 1002
for ovarian cancer, 1403
Carboprost (Hemabate), 1384*t*
Carboxyhemoglobin, 1865*t*
Carbuncles, 467*t*
Carcinoembryonic antigen, 1860*t*
Carcinogens, 275
chemical, 275
viral, 276
Carcinoma. *See also* Cancer
classification of, 279
Carcinoma in situ, 280
ductal, 1350
lobular, 1350
Cardene (nicardipine)
for acute coronary syndrome, 800*t*
for chronic stable angina, 800*t*, 801
for hypertension, 776*t*
Cardiac assessment, 747*t*
Cardiac auscultatory areas, 748, 758*f*
Cardiac borders, abnormal, 749*t*
Cardiac catheterization, 755*t*, **759**
in chronic stable angina, 801-802
Cardiac cells, 842, 843*t*
Cardiac compensation, 824
Cardiac compressions, 1846-1849, 1849*f*

Cardiac cycle
absolute refractory period, 741
relative refractory period, 741
Cardiac death, sudden, **817-818,** 856, 1876
Cardiac decompensation, 824
Cardiac index, 742, 1738, 1774
normal range at rest, 1739*t*
Cardiac lesions, 876
Cardiac markers, 751
serum, 805-806, 805*f*
Cardiac murmurs, 750*t*
Cardiac muscle, 1617
regenerative ability of, 198, 198*t*
Cardiac natriuretic peptide markers, 756
Cardiac output, 742, 1738
factors affecting, 742
formula for, 742
maintenance of
in acute respiratory distress syndrome, 1818
in acute respiratory failure, 1811-1812
measurement of
continuous, 1744-1745
invasive techniques, 1744-1745
thermodilution method, 1744
normal curve, 1744-1745, 1745*f*
normal range at rest, 1739*t*
in shock, 1774*t*
Cardiac pacemakers, 858-861
Cardiac regulation, 320-321
Cardiac rehabilitation, 794*b*, 815
Cardiac reserve, 742
Cardiac resynchronization therapy, 830, 859
Cardiac rhythm
absolute refractory phase or period, 847, 847*f*
assessment of, 846, 848*t*
dysrhythmias, **842-864**
in heart failure, 826
in myocardial infarction, 804
postoperative, 382
identification and treatment of, **842-861**
refractory phase or period, 847
relative refractory period, 847, 847*f*
Cardiac tamponade
in acute pericarditis, 872
in cancer, 308
emergency management of, 586*t*
Cardiac transplantation, **837-840**
bridge devices, 839
indications for, 839*t*
research, 839-840
Cardiac valves, 740, 740*f*
Cardiac-specific troponins, 752*t*
Cardiogenic shock, 1773-1775, 1773*f*
classification of, 1773*t*
clinical presentation of, 1776*t*
collaborative care for, 1786
in myocardial infarction, 804
pathophysiology of, 1774, 1774*f*
precipitating factors, 1773*t*
treatment of, 1789*t*
Cardiography, impedance, 1745-1746
Cardiology, nuclear, **758**
Cardiomegaly
in dilated cardiomyopathy, 886
in infective endocarditis, 868
Cardiomyopathy, 885-889
collaborative care for, 886*t*
comparisons, 886*t*
dilated, **886-888,** 886*t*, 887*f*
hypertrophic, 886*t*, **888,** 888*f*
hypertrophic obstructive, 888

Cardiomyopathy (*Continued*)
idiopathic, 885
patient and family teaching guide for, 889*t*
primary, 885
restrictive, 886*t*, **889**
secondary, 885, 886*t*
types of, 887*f*
Cardiopulmonary bypass, 808-809
Cardiopulmonary resuscitation, **1845-1849,** 1849*f*
adult one-rescuer, 1847*t*
adult two-rescuer, 1848*t*
Cardiopulmonary system, 1718
Cardiotoxicity, 296*t*
Cardiovascular disease, 784-785, 785*f*
in diabetes mellitus, 1284*t*
health disparities and, 21*t*
in kidney transplantation, 1229
mortality trends, 788, 788*f*
Cardiovascular system, **739-760**
in acute renal failure, 1201*t*
age-related changes in, 744*t*
nursing diagnoses associated with, 78*t*
in anemia, 686*t*
after aortic surgery, 897
assessment abnormalities, 749*t*-750*t*, 1246*t*
assessment of, **744-751**
gender differences in, 747*t*
gerontologic differences in, 744*t*
key questions to ask, 746*t*
objective data, 747-751
preoperative, 349, 351*t*
subjective data, 744-747
and asthma, 624*t*
burn injury complications, 491-492, 500
changes at end of life, 152*t*
in chronic kidney disease, 1207-1208
and COPD, 650*t*
diagnostic studies, **751-760,** 752*t*-755*t*
effects of aging on, **744**
effects of chronic alcohol abuse on, 177*t*
in extracellular fluid volume imbalances, 322-323
functions of, **740-744**
gerontologic considerations, **744**
in HIV infection, 259*t*
and lung cancer, 583*t*
in multiple organ dysfunction syndrome, 1797*t*
physical examination of, 747-748, 751*t*
in pneumonia, 567*t*
positive pressure ventilation effects on, 1763
preoperative review, 347-348
problems of
associated with obesity, 975
in chemotherapy and radiation therapy, 296*t*, 300-301
in clinical unit, 382-386
cues to, 745*t*
with dermatologic manifestations, 473*t*
nursing assessment of, 386
nursing diagnoses, 386
nursing implementation for, 386-387
nursing management of, 386-387
in postanesthesia care unit (PACU), 382
postoperative, **382-386**
regulation of, 743-744

Cardiovascular system *(Continued)*
  in shock, 1781*t*, 1782
    acute intervention for, 1791-1793
  in spinal cord injury, 1594-1595, 1602
  after stroke, 1515-1518
  structures of, **740-744**
Cardioversion, synchronized, 857
CardioWest Total Artificial Heart, 839
Carditis, 876
  chronic rheumatic, 876-877
Cardizem (diltiazem)
  for acute coronary syndrome, 800*t*
  for chronic stable angina, 800*t*, 801
  classification of, 856*t*
  effects on lower urinary tract function, 1180*t*
  for hypertension, 776*t*
  for Raynaud's phenomenon, 1724
  for voiding dysfunction, 1185*t*
Cardura (doxazosin)
  for benign prostatic hyperplasia, 1417
  drug alert, 772
  effects on lower urinary tract function, 1180*t*
  for hypertension, 774*t*
  for voiding dysfunction, 1185*t*
Caregiver support
  in Alzheimer's disease, 1574-1575
  family and caregiver teaching guide for Alzheimer's disease, 1574*t*
  special needs for, in end-of-life care, **161-162**
  support groups, 1575, 1575*f*
Caregivers, 72-73, 73*t*
Caregiving
  positive aspects of, 73
  tasks of, 72
Carina, 511
Carmustine (BiCNU, Gliadel)
  classification of, 287*t*
  for leukemia, 720*t*, 721*t*
  nephrotoxicity, 1142*t*
Carnitine, 902
Carotene, 1855*t*
Carotenemia, 457*t*
Carotenosis, 457*t*
Carotid artery disease, **893-894**
Carotid artery rupture, 308
Carotid duplex studies, 1463*t*
Carotid endarterectomy, 1510, 1510*f*
Carpal tunnel syndrome, 1633-1634, 1633*f*
  nursing and collaborative management of, **1633-1634**
Carpentier-Edwards valve, 883*t*
CarraFilm, 205*t*
CarraSorb, 205*t*
Carrasyn Gel, 205*t*
Carrier, 214*t*, 215
Carteolol (Ocupress)
  food/nutrient interactions, 954*t*
  for glaucoma, 434*t*
  for hypertension, 774*t*
Cartilage, **1616-1617**
  elastic, 1617
  enlargement of, 1247*t*
  fibrous, 1617
  hyaline, 1617
  regenerative ability of, 198, 198*f*

Carvedilol (Coreg)
  for acute coronary syndrome, 800*t*
  for chronic HF, 832
  for chronic stable angina, 799, 800*t*
  drug alert, 832
  for hypertension, 775*t*
Cascade disease pattern, 71
Cascara sagrada, 1042*t*
Case management, 4, 87
  for older adults, 76-77
Case studies
  acute respiratory distress syndrome, 1819
  Alzheimer's disease, 1578
  aspiration pneumonia, 604
  asthma, 661
  benign prostatic hyperplasia, 1438
  breast cancer, 1363-1364
  burn and inhalation injury, 506
  chlamydia and gonorrhea, 1379
  chronic kidney disease, 1231
  cirrhosis, 1132
  colorectal cancer, 1084
  complementary and alternative therapies, 108
  critical care, 1769
  culturally competent care, 37
  diabetic ketoacidosis, 1288
  dysrhythmias, 863
  fluid and electrolyte imbalance, 340
  glaucoma and diabetic retinopathy, 446-447
  Graves' disease, 1320-1321
  head injury, 1499
  health disparities, 24*b*
  heart failure, 840
  hiatal hernia, 1033
  hip fracture, 1665
  inflammation and infection, 211
  laryngeal cancer, 558
  leukemia, 734-735
  malignant melanoma and dysplastic nevi, 481
  mechanical ventilation, 1769
  myocardial infarction, 818
  obesity, 988
  osteoporosis, 1690-1691
  pain, 148-149
  Parkinson's disease, 1559
  peripheral arterial disease, 920
  postoperative patients, 395
  preoperative patients, 356-357
  primary hypertension, 782
  rheumatoid arthritis, 1729-1730
  at risk for HIV disease, 268
  shock, 1797
  spinal cord injury, 1611
  stress, 122
  stroke, 1524
  substance misuse and abuse, 190
  symptomatic HIV disease, 268
  trauma, 1843
  undernutrition, 969
  urinary tract infection, 1194
  valvular heart disease, 890
Casodex (bicalutamide), 1426, 1426*t*
Cast care, 1646-1647, 1646*t*
Cast syndrome, 1640
Casts, 1639-1641
  body jacket, 1640, 1640*f*
  hip spica, 1640
  for injuries to lower extremities, 1640-1641
  long arm, 1640, 1640*f*
  petaling edges with waterproof adhesive strips, 1639, 1639*f*
  short arm, 1640, 1640*f*
  types of, 1639-1640, 1640*f*

Cat bites, 1836
Cataflam (diclofenac K), 135, 136*t*
Catapres (clonidine)
  blood glucose level effects, 1267*t*
  drug alert, 782
  for hypertension, 773*t*
  for migraine prevention, 1531
  for opioid withdrawal, 180
  for pain, 139
  and reproductive system, 1332
  for restless legs syndrome, 1558
  for smoking cessation, 171*t*
Cataracts, 406*t*, 425-429
  acute care for, 426*t*
  acute intervention for, 428-429
  ambulatory and home care for, 429
  clinical manifestations of, 425
  collaborative care for, 425-427, 426*t*
  diagnostic studies, 425
  etiology and pathophysiology of, 425
  gerontologic considerations, **429**
  health promotion in, 428
  nonsurgical therapy of, 425-426
  nursing assessment of, 427
  nursing diagnoses, 427
  nursing implementation for, 428-429
  nursing management of, **427-429**
  nursing planning for, 428
  phacoemulsification of, 426, 427*f*
  surgical therapy of, 426-427, 426*t*
    intraoperative phase, 426
    postoperative phase, 427
    preoperative phase, 426
    surgical location for, 428*b*
Catarrhal exudate, 197*t*
Catastrophic events, 372-373
Catecholamines, 1241, 1862*t*
Catechol-*O*-methyl transferase inhibitors, 1551, 1552*t*
Catheter ablation therapy, 861
Catheterization
  cardiac, 755*t*, **759**
  intermittent, 1187-1188
  urethral, **1186-1187**
  urinary, 1185, 1186*t*
Catheters
  drainage from, 392, 393*t*
  peritoneal
    exit site, 1218, 1218*f*
    for peritoneal dialysis, 1217, 1218*f*
  placement for parenteral nutrition, 966, 966*f*
  placement for peritoneal dialysis, 1217-1218, 1217*f*
  pulmonary artery, 513-514, 1741-1747, 1743*f*
    complications of, 1747
    insertion of, 1742-1743
  semipermanent, 1222, 1222*f*
  Silastic catheter, 290
  suprapubic, 1187
  temporary double-lumen vascular access, 1221, 1221*f*
  Tenckhoff, 290, 1217, 1217*f*
  transhepatic biliary, 1129
  transtracheal, 641*t*, 643*f*
  tunneled, 289-290
  types of, 1186, 1186*f*
  ureteral, 1187
Cations, 315
  definition of, 316*t*
  normal values, 321*t*
Cauda equina, 1681
Cauda equina syndrome, 1592
Caverject (alprostadil), 1435

CAVH. *See* Continuous arteriovenous hemofiltration
CAVHD. *See* Continuous arteriovenous hemodialysis
CBF. *See* Cerebral blood flow
CCC. *See* Clinical Care Classification
CCRN. *See* Critical care certification
CCUs. *See* Critical care units
CD antigens, 220
CD20, 303*t*
CDSR. *See* Cochrane Database of Systematic Reviews
CEA. *See* Cultured epithelial autografts
Cecostomy, 934*t*
CeeNu (lomustine), 287*t*
Cefazolin (Ancef), 1670
Cefixime (Suprax), 1368
Cefizox (ceftizoxime), 1495
Cefotaxime (Claforan), 1495
Cefoxitin (Mefoxin), 1670
Ceftazidime (Ceptaz), 1495
Ceftin (cefuroxime)
  for bacterial meningitis, 1495
  for Lyme disease, 1714
Ceftizoxime (Cefizox), 1495
Ceftriaxone (Rocephin)
  for bacterial meningitis, 1495
  for gonorrhea, 1368
  for infective endocarditis, 869*t*
Cefuroxime (Ceftin)
  for bacterial meningitis, 1495
  for Lyme disease, 1714
Celecoxib (Celebrex)
  for arthritis and connective tissue disorders, 1698*t*
  and gastritis, 1013
  for osteoarthritis, 1697
  for pain, 136, 136*t*
  for rheumatoid arthritis, 1706
Celexa (citalopram), 1569, 1569*t*
Celiac disease, 1079-1081
  clinical manifestations of, 1080
  collaborative care for, 1080-1081
  diagnostic studies, 1080-1081
  etiology and pathophysiology of, 1080
  nutritional therapy of, 1080*t*
Cell(s)
  effects of water status on, 318, 318*f*
  generation time of, 273
  life cycle and metabolic activity, 273, 273*f*
  response in inflammation, 194-195, 194*f*
Cell death, programmed, 68*t*, 69
Cell injury
  inflammatory response, **193-197**
  vascular response, 193-194
Cell-based therapies, antiaging, 67-68, 68*t*
CellCept (mycophenolate mofetil), 238, 239*t*, 1718
Cell-mediated immune response, 228
Cell-mediated immunity, 224
  comparison with humoral immunity, 223-224, 223*t*
Cellular differentiation
  defect in, 274
  normal, 274, 274*f*
Cellular proliferation
  defect in, 273-274
  rapid rate of, 291, 291*t*
Cellular tissue, 227
Cellules, 1168
Cellulitis, 467*t*, 468*f*

Note: Disorder names are in **bold face.** Page numbers in **bold face** indicate main discussions. Page numbers followed by *f*, *t*, *b*, or *n* indicate figures, tables, boxed material, or notes, respectively.

Centers for Disease Control and Prevention (CDC), 65, 606
Advancing HIV Prevention (AHP) initiative, 260
Division of Healthcare Quality Promotion, 396
Public Health Awareness and Response website, 1844
recommendations for isolation precautions in health care facilities, 247, 248*t*-249*t*
Centers for Medicare and Medicaid Services, 84
Centigray (cGy), 292
Central cord syndrome, 1591, 1592*f*, 1870
Central hearing loss, 408
Central lymphoid organs, 219
Central nervous system, **1444-1448**
in acute respiratory distress syndrome, 1816*t*
age-related changes in, 1454*t*
autoimmune diseases of, 234*t*
effects of chronic alcohol abuse on, 177*t*
in hypercapnic respiratory failure, 1803
in multiple organ dysfunction syndrome, 1796*t*
protective structures, 1452
and restrictive lung disease, 595*t*
structure of, 1442, 1448*f*
Central nervous system depressants, 186-187
Central nervous system lymphoma
associated with HIV infection, 254*t*
primary, 1488*t*
Central nervous system stimulants, 1545*t*
Central parenteral nutrition, 965
Central vascular access devices, 288
Central venous oxygen saturation (ScvO₂), 1746
SvO₂/ScvO₂ measurements
clinical interpretation of, 1746-1747, 1746*t*
in shock, 1774*t*
Central venous pressure
measurement of, 1744, 1745*f*
normal range at rest, 1739*t*
in shock, 1774*t*
Central visual field defect, 406*t*
Cephalexin (Keflex), 1670
Cephalic secretion, 929, 930*t*
Cephalosporins, 1142*t*
Cephulac (lactulose)
for cirrhosis, 1110*t*
for variceal bleeding, 1108
Ceptaz (ceftazidime), 1495
Cerebellar tumors, 1488, 1489*t*
Cerebellopontine tumors, 1488, 1489*t*
Cerebellum, 1447
Cerebral angiography, 1461-1464, 1463*t*, 1464*f*
Cerebral arteries, 1504, 1504*f*
Cerebral blood flow, 1468-1469
autoregulation of, 1468-1469, 1504
brain stents to treat blockages in, 1510, 1510*f*
factors affecting, 1469
regulation of, 1504
Cerebral circulation, 1450-1452
anatomy of, 1504, 1504*f*
Cerebral cortex, 113, 114*f*

Cerebral edema, 1469-1470
causes of, 1469, 1470*t*
cytotoxic, 1469-1470
interstitial, 1470
vasogenic, 1469
Cerebral inflammatory conditions, 1493, 1494*t*
Cerebral perfusion pressure, 1468, 1468*t*
Cerebrospinal fluid, 1448
analysis of, 1461, 1462*t*, 1864*t*
drainage of, 1473-1474
flow of, 1448, 1449*f*
normal values, 1464*t*
Cerebrovascular disease, hypertensive, 766*t*, 767
Cerebrum, 1445-1447, 1447*f*, 1447*t*
Certified registered nurse anesthetist (CRNA), 363
CERTs. *See* Community emergency response teams
Cerubidine (daunorubicin)
adverse cardiovascular effects of, 745*t*
classification of, 287*t*
drug alert, 720
for leukemia, 720*t*
Cerumen
in external ear canal, **438-439**
impacted, 413*t*, 439*t*
Cervical cancer, 1400-1401
clinical manifestations of, 1400, 1400*f*
collaborative care for, 1401
diagnostic studies, 1400-1401
etiology and pathophysiology of, 1400
health disparities and, 21*t*
staging and treatment of, 1401, 1401*t*
Cervical cord injury, 1597*t*
Cervical immobilization devices, 1823
Cervical polyps, 1399
Cervical spine stabilization and/or immobilization, 1823, 1824*t*
Cervical traction, 1601, 1601*f*
Cervicitis, 1394*t*
Cervidil (dinoprostone), 1384*t*
Cervix, conditions of, **1393-1395**
clinical manifestations of, 1393-1394
collaborative care for, 1394
etiology and pathophysiology of, 1393
nursing management of, **1394-1395**
Cesamet (nabilone), 992*t*
Cetirizine (Zyrtec)
for allergic rhinitis and sinusitis, 538*t*
for dermatologic problems, 475
Cetrorelix (Cetrotide), 1383*t*
Cetuximab (Erbitux), 303*t*, 1067
Cevimeline (Evoxac), 1726
CFS. *See* Chronic fatigue syndrome
Chalazion, 422
Chamomile, 102*t*, 103*f*
Chancres, 1369, 1370*f*
Change, transtheoretical model of, 55, 55*t*, 188
Chantix (varenicline), 170-171, 171*t*
Charcoal, activated, 1037*t*, 1838
Charcot's joints, 1589
Charité disk, 1683, 1683*f*
Chart review, 363-364
Cheilitis, 689, 939*t*
Cheilosis, 939*t*

Chemical burns, 484
emergency management of, 489*t*
to eye, 421*t*
risk reduction strategies, 484*t*
Chemical peels, 479*t*
Chemical (noninfectious) pneumonitis, 564, 577
Chemical sensitivities, multiple, 233
Chemicals
agents of terrorism, 1839, 1840*t*
carcinogens, 275
hepatotoxicity of, 933-934, 934*t*
occupational, 631
Chemistry, body fluid, 316*t*
Chemoembolization, 1117
Chemoreceptors
regulation of cardiovascular system by, 743
regulation of respiratory system by, 515-516
Chemotaxis, 194, 194*f*
Chemotherapy, **285-291**
acute toxicity, 291
administration of, 286
anemia caused by, 685*t*
for bladder cancer, 1179
for brain tumors, 1490
for breast cancer, 1354-1355
cardiovascular effects of, 300-301
cell cycle phase–nonspecific drugs, 286, 287*t*, 288*t*
cell cycle phase–specific drugs, 286, 287*t*
chronic toxicities, 291
classification of drugs, 286, 287*t*-288*t*
for colorectal cancer, 1067
coping with, 301
delayed effects of, 291
effects on cells, 286
effects on normal tissues, 291
example drug schedule, 291, 291*t*
FOLFOX treatment regimen, 291, 291*t*
gastrointestinal effects of, 297-299
goals of, 285-286, 286*f*
guidelines for safe handling, 286
intraarterial, 290
intraperitoneal, 290-291
intrathecal or intraventricular, 291
intravesical bladder, 291
late effects of, **301-302**
for lung cancer, 582
methods of administration, 286-289, 288*t*
myeloablative, 305
nadir, 297
nursing implementation for, 294-301
nursing management of patients undergoing, **294-301**
nursing management of problems caused by, 295*t*-296*t*
preparation of, 286
for prostate cancer, 1427
BEP combination therapy, 1432
pulmonary effects of, 300
regional administration of, 290-291
reproductive effects of, 301
response of cancer cells to, 286
skin reactions to, 299-300
for testicular cancer, 1432
treatment plan, 291
VIP, 1432
Chemotherapy-induced nausea, 99*t*
Chest
assessment abnormalities, 676*t*
auscultation of, 522-523
assessment abnormalities, 524*t*-525*t*

Chest (*Continued*)
findings in pulmonary problems, 526*t*
normal sounds, 522-523, 523*f*
flail chest, **588,** 588*f*
inspection of, 521
assessment abnormalities, 524*t*
findings in pulmonary problems, 526*t*
palpation of, 521-522
assessment abnormalities, 524*t*
findings in pulmonary problems, 526*t*
percussion of, 522
assessment abnormalities, 524*t*
findings in pulmonary problems, 526*t*
physical examination of, 521, 522, 522*f*, 525*t*
findings in pulmonary problems, 526*t*
secondary survey head-to-toe assessment, 1826*t*, 1827
Chest compression, high-frequency, 649
Chest drainage, 591*t*
clinical guidelines for care of patient with, 591*t*
dry systems, 591*t*
nursing management of, **590-592**
wet systems, 591*t*
Chest drainage units, 589, 589*f*
portable, 590, 590*f*
Chest movement, altered, 524*t*
Chest pain, 1246*t*
in chronic HF, 826
emergency management of, 806*t*
pleuritic, 519*t*
Chest physiotherapy, 646-647
in acute respiratory failure, 1810
indications for, 646
steps in, 647*t*
Chest surgery, **592-593,** 593*t*
postoperative care, 593
preoperative care for, 592
surgical therapy, 592-593
Chest trauma, 585-593, 585*t*
blunt, 585, 585*t*
contrecoup, 585
emergency management of, 586*t*
penetrating, 585, 585*t*
Chest tube dressings, 592*t*
Chest tubes, **588-592**
clinical guidelines for care of patient with, 591*t*-592*t*
complications of, 590-592
insertion of, 588
nursing management of, **590-592**
obtaining samples from, 592*t*
placement of, 588, 589*f*
removal of, 592
small, 590
Chest wall, 512
age-related changes in, 744*t*
in hypercapnic respiratory failure, 1803
landmarks and structures of, 510, 510*f*
and restrictive lung disease, 595*t*
Chest x-ray, 526, 527*t*, 571, 753*t*, **756,** 756*f*
in acute pericarditis, 873, 873*f*
in acute respiratory distress syndrome, 1815, 1815*f*, 1815*t*
preoperative, 351
Cheyne-Stokes respiration, 152
Chinese Americans
culture-bound syndromes, 35*t*
ethnic differences in response to drugs, 34, 35*t*

Chinese herbs, 96-98
Chinese medicine, traditional, 96-98, 97t
Chiropractic therapy, 95, 96f, 98t
Chlamydia, 562
Chlamydia pneumoniae, 562t, 565
Chlamydia trachomatis, 1367t, 1394t
Chlamydial infections, 1371-1373
　case study, 1379
　clinical manifestations of, 1372
　collaborative care for, 1372-1373, 1372t
　complications of, 1372
　conjunctivitis, 422-423
　diagnostic studies, 1372-1373
　drug therapy for, 1373
　epididymitis, 1372, 1372f
　etiology and pathophysiology of, 1372
　risk factors for, 1372, 1372t
Chloral hydrate (Somnote), 169t
Chlorambucil (Leukeran)
　classification of, 287t
　for leukemia, 720t, 721t
Chloramphenicol (Chloromycetin)
　blood glucose level effects, 1267t
　hematologic effects of, 674t
Chlordiazepoxide (Librium)
　effects of use, 169t
　toxicology, 1865t
　withdrawal from, 179
Chlorhexidine (Hibiclens), 205
Chloride
　cerebrospinal fluid analysis, 1864t
　laboratory values, 1855t
　normal values, 321t
　urine levels, 1862t
Chloroform
　effects of use, 170t
　hepatotoxicity, 934t
Chloroma, 675t
Chloromycetin (chloramphenicol), 674t
Chlorothiazide (Diuril)
　for cirrhosis, 1110t
　for diabetes insipidus, 1297
　for hypertension, 773t
Chlorpheniramine (Chlor-Trimeton)
　for allergic rhinitis and sinusitis, 537t
　drug alert, 541
　photosensitivity, 461t
Chlorpromazine (Thorazine)
　adverse cardiovascular effects of, 745t
　effects on lower urinary tract function, 1180t
　for heatstroke, 1829
　for nausea and vomiting, 992, 992t
　photosensitivity, 461t
　toxicology, 1865t
Chlorpropamide (Diabinese)
　for diabetes insipidus, 1297
　photosensitivity, 461t
Chlorthalidone (Hygroton, Apo-Chlorthalidone)
　atenolol/chlorthalidone (Tenoretic), 777t
　clonidine/chlorthalidone (Combipres), 777t
　for hypertension, 773t
　reserpine/chlorthalidone (Demi-Regroton), 777t

Chlor-Trimeton (chlorpheniramine)
　for allergic rhinitis and sinusitis, 537t
　drug alert, 541
Cholangiography, 942t
　percutaneous transhepatic, 942t
　surgical, 942t
Cholangiopancreatography
　endoscopic retrograde, 943f, 944, 944t
　magnetic resonance, 942t
Cholangitis, 1127
　primary sclerosing, 1102
Cholecystectomy, 934t
　incisional
　　ambulatory and home care for, 1131-1132
　　postoperative care of, 1131
　laparoscopic
　　ambulatory and home care for, 1131
　　postoperative care of, 1131
　　postoperative patient and family teaching guide for, 1132b
　open, 1129, 1130t
Cholecystitis, 1126-1132
　acute, 1127, 1127t
　clinical manifestations of, 1127
　complications of, 1128
　conservative therapy of, 1128
　etiology and pathophysiology of, 1126-1127
　nursing assessment of, 1130t
　nutritional therapy of, 1130
Cholecystokinin, 929, 930t
　in obesity, 972, 973f, 973t
Cholecystostomy, 934t
Choledochojejunostomy, 934t
Choledocholelithiasis, 1127
Choledocholithotomy, 934t
Choledyl (oxtriphylline), 954t
Cholelithiasis, 1126-1132, 1127f
　clinical manifestations of, 1127, 1127t
　collaborative care for, 1127t
　complications of, 1128
　conservative therapy of, 1128-1129
　diagnostic studies, 1127, 1128
　etiology and pathophysiology of, 1127
　gender differences in, 1127b
　nursing assessment of, 1130t
　nutritional therapy of, 1130
　silent, 1127
　surgical therapy of, 1129, 1129t
Cholestasis, 1101
Cholesteatoma, 439
Cholesterol, 752t
　blood levels, high, 789, 790t
　high-density lipoprotein, 987t
　laboratory values, 1855t
　low-density lipoprotein, 789
Cholesterol absorption inhibitors, 794, 795t
Cholesterol-lowering drugs, 793-794, 808
Cholestyramine (Questran), 794, 795t
　for bile reflux gastritis, 1026
　blood glucose level effects, 1267t
　food/nutrient interactions, 954t
　for pruritus, 1129
Choline magnesium trisalicylate (Trilisate)
　for arthritis and connective tissue disorders, 1698t
　for pain, 135, 136t
Choline salicylate (Arthropan), 1698t

Cholinergic agents
　for gastroesophageal reflux disease, 1006, 1006t
　for glaucoma, 435t
　for multiple sclerosis, 1544t, 1545
Cholinergic crisis, 1557t
Cholinesterase, 1855t
Cholinesterase inhibitors
　for Alzheimer's disease, 1568, 1569t
　mechanism of action, 1568, 1569f
Chondroitin sulfate, 103t
Chondromas, 585
Chondrosarcoma, 1673f, 1673t
Chordae tendineae, 740, 740f
Chordee, 1429
Chordoma, 1673t
Chorea, 876, 1458
Choroid, 399f, 401
Christmas disease. *See* Hemophilia B
Chromosomes, 214, 214t
Chronic abdominal pain, 1046-1048
Chronic alcohol abuse, 177, 177t
Chronic allergies, 230-231
Chronic autoimmune thyroiditis (Hashimoto's), 1298
Chronic blood loss, 690t, **695**
Chronic bronchitis, 608, 629
Chronic calcifying pancreatitis, 1124
Chronic constrictive pericarditis, 874
　clinical manifestations of, 874
　diagnostic studies, 874
　etiology and pathophysiology of, 874
　nursing and collaborative management of, **874**
Chronic dermatologic problems
　physiologic effects of, 478
　psychologic effects of, 478
Chronic disease. See also specific diseases
　anemia of, 690t, **693**
　older adults with, 71
　prevention and management of, 86
　tasks required for daily living with, 71, 72t
Chronic disseminated intravascular coagulation, 710t
Chronic fatigue syndrome, 1727t, **1728-1729**
　clinical manifestations of, 1729
　diagnostic criteria for, 1729t
　diagnostic studies, 1729
　etiology and pathophysiology of, 1728-1729
　nursing and collaborative management of, **1729**
Chronic glaucoma, 434t-435t
Chronic glomerulonephritis, 1167
Chronic headache, 1531b
Chronic heart failure. *See* Heart Failure
Chronic hepatitis B, 1094-1095
Chronic hepatitis C, 1095
Chronic hereditary nephritis, 1177
Chronic HIV infection, 252-253
　antiretroviral therapy of, 257t
　early, 252
　intermediate, 252
　late, 252-253
Chronic inflammation, 197
Chronic kidney disease, 1197, **1204-1216**
　acute intervention for, 1213-1216
　case study, 1231

Chronic kidney disease (*Continued*)
　causes of, 1204, 1205f
　clinical manifestations of, 1205-1209
　clinical practice guidelines for bone metabolism and disease in, 1210
　conservative therapy of, 1209-1213, **1213-1216**
　cultural and ethnic health disparities in, 1204b
　daily requirements for patient with, 1211-1212, 1212t
　dermatologic manifestations of, 473t
　diagnostic studies, 1209
　drug therapy of, 1210-1211
　gerontologic considerations for, **1230-1231**
　health promotion in, 1213
　nursing assessment of, 1213
　nursing care plan for patient with, 1214b-1215b
　nursing diagnoses, 1213
　nursing evaluation of, 1216
　nursing implementation for, 1213-1216
　nursing management of, **1213-1216**
　nursing planning for, 1213
　nutritional therapy of, 1211-1213
　patient and family teaching guide for, 1216r
　prevention and detection of, 1205b
　resources for, 1232
　stages of, 1205f
Chronic low back pain, 1680
Chronic lymphocytic leukemia, 718t, 719, 721t
Chronic mechanical ventilation, 1768
Chronic myelogenous leukemia, 718-719, 718t, 721t
Chronic neurologic disorders, 1532-1559
Chronic neurologic problems, 1527-1560
Chronic obstructive pancreatitis, 1124
Chronic obstructive pulmonary disease (COPD), 629-655
　activity considerations for, 652-655
　acute intervention for, 650
　aerosol nebulization therapy of, 649
　ambulatory and home care for, 650-655
　chest examination findings in, 526t
　classification of, 634-635
　classification of severity of, 634-635, 635t
　clinical manifestations of, 634-635, 635t
　collaborative care for, 638-649, 638t
　comparison with asthma, 634, 635t
　complications of, 635-637
　diagnostic studies, 635t, 637-638, 638t
　drug therapy of, 618t-620t, 639-640
　etiology and pathophysiology of, 631-632, 633f
　exacerbations of, 636
　gender differences in, 629b
　health promotion in, 650
　management of, 639b

Chronic obstructive pulmonary disease (COPD) (Continued)
morphologic types, 632, 633f
nursing assessment of, 650, 650t
nursing care plan for patient with, 651b-653b
nursing diagnoses, 650
nursing implementation for, 650-655
nursing management of, **650-655**
nursing planning, 650
nutritional therapy of, 649
oxygen therapy of, 640-644
patient and family teaching guide for, 654t
physical therapy of, 646-649
psychosocial considerations for, 655
reducing risk factors for, 640b
respiratory therapy of, 646-649
surgical therapy of, 644-646
therapy at each stage for, 638, 639t
typical findings in, 638
Chronic open-angle glaucoma, 433-434
Chronic osteomyelitis, 1669, 1669f
Chronic otitis media, 439-440
clinical manifestations of, 439
collaborative care for, 439-440, 440t
complications of, 439
diagnostic studies, 439
etiology and pathophysiology of, 439
nursing management of, **440**
surgical therapy of, 439-440
Chronic oxygen therapy, 644
Chronic pain, 130t, 131
Chronic pancreatitis, 1124-1125
clinical manifestations of, 1124
collaborative care for, 1125
diagnostic studies, 1124
drug therapy of, 1121t
etiology and pathophysiology of, 1124
nursing management of, **1125**
Chronic pelvic pain syndrome, 1428
Chronic peritoneal dialysis
adaptation to, 1220
effectiveness of, 1220
Chronic prostatitis, 1428
Chronic pyelonephritis, 1161, **1162**
Chronic rejection, 238
Chronic rheumatic carditis, 876-877
Chronic sensory polyneuropathy, 473t
Chronic sinusitis, 540, 541t
Chronic stable angina, 796-797, 798t, 802f
acute intervention for, 810
ambulatory and home care for, 810-813
collaborative care for, 799f
collaborative management of, **797-802**
in coronary artery disease, 796-802
diagnostic studies, 801-802
drug therapy of, 798-801, 800t
etiology and pathophysiology of, 796
health promotion in, 810
nursing implementation for, 810-813
nursing management of, **810-817**
treatment elements, 798t
Chronic stress, 115, 115f
Chronic toxicities, 291
Chronic uremia, 1206, 1206f
Chronic urinary retention, 1180-1182
Chronic venous insufficiency, 911, **919-920**
clinical manifestations of, 919
collaborative care for, 919-920

Chronic venous insufficiency (Continued)
complications of, 919
etiology and pathophysiology of, 919
nursing management of, **920**
Chvostek sign, 331, 331f
Chylomicrons, 756
Chylothorax, 587
CI. See Cardiac index
Cialis (tadalafil), 1435
Cigarette smoking. See Smoking
Ciliary body, 401
Cilostazol (Pletal), 902
Cimetidine (Tagamet)
for acute gastritis, 1014
for gastroesophageal reflux disease, 1005-1006, 1006t
for gastrointestinal bleeding, 998t
nephrotoxicity, 1142t
for peptic ulcer disease, 1019t
preoperative, 355t
for upper gastrointestinal bleeding, 997
for variceal bleeding, 1108
CIMT. See Constraint-induced movement therapy
Cinacalcet (Sensipar)
for hyperparathyroidism, 1310-1311
for secondary hyperparathyroidism, 1210
Cingulate herniation, 1472
Ciprofloxacin (Cipro)
for gonorrhea, 1368
for inflammatory bowel disease, 1054, 1055t
for osteomyelitis, 1670
photosensitivity, 461t
for UTIs, 1157
Circadian rhythms, 1238, 1238f
and angina, 797t
Circ-Aid, 919
Circle of Willis, 1450-1452, 1452f, 1504, 1504f
Circulation
cerebral, 1450-1452
anatomy of, 1504, 1504f
changes at end of life, 152
collateral, 786-787, 787f, 1870
coronary, 740-741, 741f
function of, 361
initial postanesthesia care unit assessment, 377-378, 377t
primary survey of, 1823-1824, 1824t, 1825t
Circulation management, in burns, 488
Circulatory assist devices, **1747-1751**
nursing management of, **1751**
Circulatory overload, 732, 733t
Circumduction, 1622t
Cirrhosis, 1101-1115, 1102f
acute intervention for, 1111-1114
alcoholic, 1102
ambulatory and home care for, 1114-1115
case study, 1132
clinical manifestations of, 1102-1103, 1104f
collaborative care for, 1106-1107, 1107t
complications of, 1103-1106
diagnostic studies, 1106
drug therapy of, 1110, 1110t
early manifestations of, 1102

Cirrhosis (Continued)
etiology and pathophysiology of, 1102, 1103f
health promotion in, 1111
later manifestations of, 1102, 1103f
nursing assessment of, 1110, 1111t
nursing care plan for patient with, 1112b-1113b
nursing diagnoses, 1111
nursing evaluation of, 1115
nursing implementation for, 1111-1115
nursing management of, **1110-1115**
nursing planning for, 1111
nutritional therapy of, 1110
patient and family teaching guide for, 1115b
portal or nutritional, 1102
postnecrotic, 1102
systemic manifestations of, 1102, 1104f
types of, 1102
Cisplatin (Platinol)
for bladder cancer, 1179
for cervical cancer, 1402
classification of, 287t
for lung cancer, 582
method of administration, 288t
nephrotoxicity, 1142t
for non-Hodgkin's lymphoma, 727t
for oral cancer, 1002
for testicular cancer, 1432
Citalopram (Celexa), 1569, 1569t
Citrucel (methylcellulose), 1042t
CK. See Conductive keratoplasty
CK-MB, 752t, 1856t
Cladribine (Leustatin), 287t
Claforan (cefotaxime), 1495
Clarinex (desloratadine), 538t
Clarithromycin (Biaxin)
for inflammatory bowel disease, 1054, 1055t
for peptic ulcer disease, 1019t
Claritin (loratadine)
for allergic rhinitis and sinusitis, 538t
for dermatologic problems, 475
Clark level, 466
Claw-toe deformity, 1686f
Clemastine (Tavist)
for allergic rhinitis and sinusitis, 537t
photosensitivity, 461t
Clindamycin (Cleocin, Clindesse), 1394t
Clinical Care Classification (CCC), 8t
Clinical manifestations, 40
Clinical nurse leader (CNL), 3-4
Clinical nurse specialist (CNS), 1735
Clinical (critical) pathways, 16
Clinical Practice Guideline: Treating Tobacco Use and Dependence (AHRQ), 172, 172f, 172t
Clinical questions
examples, 6, 7t
PICO format for, 6, 6t
Clinical unit
cardiovascular problems in, 382-386
discharge to, 393
neurologic/psychologic problems in, 387-388
nursing assessment and care of patient on admission to, 393t
respiratory problems in, 380-381
Clinoril (sulindac)
for arthritis and connective tissue disorders, 1698t
and gastritis, 1013
photosensitivity, 461t

Clitoris, 1327
CLL. See Chronic lymphocytic leukemia
Clodronate (Bonefos), 1689
Clofibrate (Atromid-S), 1267t
Clomiphene (Clomid, Serophene)
drug alert, 1400
for infertility, 1383t
Clomipramine (Anafranil)
ethnic differences in response to, 35t
photosensitivity, 461t
Clonal disorders, 716-717
Clonazepam (Klonopin), 1536, 1538t
Clonic seizures, 1535
Clonidine (Catapres, Duraclon)
blood glucose level effects, 1267t
drug alert, 782
for hypertension, 773t
local, 139t
for migraine prevention, 1531
for opioid withdrawal, 180, 186
for pain, 139
and reproductive system, 1332
for restless legs syndrome, 1558
for smoking cessation, 171t
Clonidine/chlorthalidone (Combipres), 777t
Clopidogrel (Plavix)
for chronic stable angina and acute coronary syndrome, 800t
drug alert, 1505
for long-term therapy after TIAs, 1505
for peripheral arterial disease of lower extremities, 902
to prevent stroke, 1510
for stroke, 1512
Closed (needle) biopsy, 681, 682t
Closed book fractures, 1652
Closed pneumothorax, 585
Closed-suction technique, 1757, 1757t, 1758f
Clostridia, 244t
Clostridial food poisoning, 1031, 1032t
Clostridium difficile **infection,** 1036-1037, 1037t, 1038
Clostridium perfringens **infection,** 1037t
Clotrimazole (Mycelex), 1163
Clotting
activated clotting time, 911t, 913t
extrinsic pathway, 670
herbs that may affect, 903b
intrinsic pathway, 670
lysis of, 670
mechanism of, 669f
normal mechanisms, 668-670
retraction of, 679t
Clotting disorders, 473t
Clotting factors, 669-670, 672t
Clotting studies, 672t, 678, 679t, 913t
Clozapine (Clozaril), 35t
Clubbing
of fingers, 524t
of nail beds, 749t
Cluster headache, 1528t, **1529**
clinical manifestations of, 1529
diagnostic studies, 1529
drug therapy for, 1531
etiology and pathophysiology of, 1529
Clustering, 1581
Clusters of differentiation, 220
CML. See Chronic myelogenous leukemia
CMV. See Controlled mandatory ventilation; Cytomegalovirus

CNL. *See* Clinical nurse leader
CNS. *See* Clinical nurse specialist
CO. *See* Cardiac output
Coagulation. *See also* Clotting
  mechanism of, 669*f*
  tests of, 913*t*
Coagulation factors, 670*t*
Coalworker's pneumoconiosis (black lung), 578*t*
Co-analgesics, 138
Cobalamin (vitamin B$_{12}$), 680*t*
  for inflammatory bowel disease, 1055*t*
  laboratory values, 680*t*, 1858*t*
  recommended dietary reference intakes, 953*t*
Cobalamin (vitamin B$_{12}$) deficiency, 691-692
  classification of, 692*t*
  clinical manifestations of, 692
  collaborative care for, 692
  diagnostic studies, 692
  etiology of, 692
  laboratory study findings in, 690*t*
Cobalamin (vitamin B$_{12}$) overdose, 953*t*
Coblation nucleoplasty, 1682
Cocaine, **174-175**
  adverse cardiovascular effects of, 745*t*
  and angina, 797*t*
  characteristics of use, 174, 174*f*
  collaborative care, 175
  complications of, 168*t*, 174-175
  "crack," 174
  effects of use, 169*t*, 174
  "freebase," 174
  nephrotoxicity, 1142*t*
  onset, peak, duration, and withdrawal onset of, 185*t*
  poisoning, 1837*t*
  "poor man's cocaine," 175
Cocaine toxicity
  acute, 174-175
  emergency management of, 175, 175*t*
Coccidioides immitis, 245*t*, 254*t*, 576*t*
Coccidioidomycosis, 576*t*
Cochlea, 409
Cochlear implants, 445, 446*f*
Cochrane, Archie, 5
Cochrane Database of Systematic Reviews (CDSR), 7*t*
Codeine
  effects of use, 169*t*
  ethnic differences in response to, 35*t*
  for pain, 138
Codeine plus acetaminophen (Tylenol #3), 137*t*, 138
Codominance, 214*t*
Coenzyme Q$_{10}$, 103*t*
Cogentin (benztropine), 1552*t*
Cognitive impairment
  mild, **1564,** 1564*t*
  older adults with, 70
  pain in, 148
Cognitive therapy, 143*t*, 144
Cognitive-perceptual pattern
  in assessment
    of auditory system, 410*t*, 411
    of cardiovascular system, 746*t*, 747
    of endocrine system, 1244

Cognitive-perceptual pattern (*Continued*)
  of fluid, electrolyte, and acid-base imbalances, 338
  of gastrointestinal system, 935, 935*t*
  of hematologic system, 673-674, 673*t*
  of integumentary system, 453*t*, 454
  of musculoskeletal system, 1621
  of nervous system, 1455
  of preoperative patient, 350*t*
  of reproductive system, 1333*t*, 1334
  of respiratory system, 518*t*, 520
  of urinary system, 1143*t*, 1144
  of visual system, 403-404, 403*t*
  comparison with NANDA International Taxonomy II, 42*t*
  concerns of patients requiring home health care, 90*t*
  nursing diagnoses, **1852**
  nursing history, 45*t*, 46
Cogwheel rigidity, 1550
Coiling, 1512
Colace (docusate), 138, 1042*t*
Colchicine, 1716
Cold, common. *See* Viral rhinitis, acute
Cold sores, 1000*t*
Cold therapy
  for osteoarthritis, 1696
  for pain, 144
  patient and family teaching guide, 144*t*
  for rheumatoid arthritis, 1710-1711
  for soft tissue injuries, 203
Cold-related emergencies, 1830-1831
Colectomy, 934*t*
  total, with ileoanal reservoir, 1055
Colera, 35*t*
Colesevelam (WelChol), 794, 795*t*
Colestipol (Colestid), 794, 795*t*, 1167
Colic, biliary, 1127
Colitis, ulcerative, 1051, 1051*t*
  acute, 1052, 1052*f*
  dermatologic manifestations of, 473*t*
  surgical therapy of, 1055
Collaborative management. *See specific disorders*
Collaborative problems, 12
Collagen (Zyplast, CosmoDerm), 479*t*
Collateral circulation, 786-787, 787*f*
Collecting duct, 1138*t*
Collection devices
  types of urinary diversion surgery requiring, 1188, 1189*t*
  for urinary incontinence, 1183*t*
Colles' fracture, 1651-1652
Colloid solutions, 1783-1784, 1786*t*
Colloidal oatmeal (Aveeno), 1375
Colloidal osmotic pressure, 318
Colloquial prayer, 100
Cologel (methylcellulose), 1042*t*
Colon cancer. *See also* Colorectal cancer
  classification systems used to stage, 1066, 1067*t*
  FOLFOX treatment regimen, 291, 291*t*
Colon disorders, 1051*b*
Colonic polyps, 1062, 1063*f*
Colonoscopy, 943*t*
  virtual, 940-943, 942*t*
Colony-stimulating factors
  clinical uses of, 223*t*
  types and functions of, 222*t*
Color vision testing, 405*t*, 407

Colorectal cancer, 1063-1069, 1065*f*
  acute intervention for, 1068
  ambulatory and home care for, 1068-1069
  biologic therapy of, 1067
  case study, 1084
  chemotherapy of, 1067
  clinical manifestations of, 1064-1065
  collaborative care for, 1065*t*, 1066
  diagnostic studies, 1065-1066
  etiology and pathophysiology of, 1064
  health disparities and, 21*t*
  health promotion in, 1068
  hereditary nonpolyposis, 1064*b*
  incidence of, 1063-1064, 1064*b*
  nursing assessment of, 1067, 1067*t*
  nursing diagnoses, 1067-1068
  nursing evaluation of, 1069
  nursing implementation for, 1068-1069
  nursing management of, **1067-1069**
  nursing planning for, 1068
  postoperative care, 1068
  preoperative care, 1068
  radiation therapy of, 1067
  risk factors for, 1064*t*
  screening guidelines for early detection of, 282*t*
  signs and symptoms, 1064-1065, 1065*f*
  surgical therapy of, 1066-1067
  targeted therapy of, 1067
  TNM classification of, 1066, 1066*t*
Colostomy, 934*t*, 1070*t*
  care of, 1072
  irrigations of, 1072
  loop, 1069, 1070*f*
  nursing care plan for patient with, 1073*b*-1075*b*
  patient and family teaching guide for irrigation, 1075*t*
  sigmoid, 1069, 1070*f*
  transverse, 1069, 1069*f*
Colporrhaphy, 1408
Colposcopy, 1340*t*
Coma
  definition of, 1476
  diabetic, 1278-1279, 1279*f*
  Glasgow Coma Scale, 1476, 1477*t*
Combipres (clonidine/chlorthalidone), 777*t*
Combistix (dipstick) test, 1146*t*
Combivent (ipratropium and albuterol)
  for asthma, 620*t*, 621
  for COPD, 620*t*, 640
Combivir (lamivudine and zidovudine), 258*t*
Combunox (oxycodone), 137*t*
Comedo, 457*t*
Comfeel, 205*t*
Comfort
  comparison of functional health patterns and NANDA International Taxonomy II, 43*t*
  with ET tube, 1758-1759
  secondary survey measures, 1825, 1826*t*
  in shock, 1793-1794
Commissurotomy, 882
Common cold. *See* Viral rhinitis, acute
Commonwealth Fund, 25
Communication
  with aphasia patient, 1520*t*
  with critical care patients, 1736

Communication (*Continued*)
  cross-cultural, 31-32, 32*f*
  cultural assessment of, 29*t*
  cultural factors, 31*t*
  culturally competent, 36
  at end of life, 159-160, 159*f*
  during ET intubation, 1758-1759
  guidelines for, 37*t*
  with hearing-impaired patients, 445*t*
  nursing interventions that support, 1524
  for pain management, 145
  skills required for teaching, 55-56
  after stroke, 1508, 1520, 1524
Community emergency response teams (CERTs), 1842
Community-acquired pneumonia, 562-563
  drug therapy of, 562-563, 563*t*
  management of
    guidelines for, 562
    three-step approach, 562
  organisms associated with, 562*t*
Community-based care, **87-88**
Community-based nurses, 87-88
Community-based nursing, **85-93**
  prevention and management of chronic illness in, 86
  resources, 93
Community-based older adults with special needs, 76
Community-oriented nursing, 85
Comparative genomic hybridization, 682*t*
Compartment syndrome, 1650-1651
  clinical manifestations of, 1650
  collaborative care for, 1650-1651
  types of, 1650
Compazine (prochlorperazine)
  as adjunct to general anesthesia, 370*t*
  for nausea and vomiting, 138, 992, 992*t*
Competence, 830*b*
Complement, 1626*t*
Complement components, 1860*t*
Complement system, 195
  activation of, 195, 196*f*
  biologic effects of, 195, 196*f*
  component mediators of inflammation, 195*t*
Complementary and alternative therapies, 94-109, 103*b*. *See also specific therapies*
  case study, 108
  definition of, 94
  gerontologic considerations for, **105-106**
  herbs that may affect clotting, 903*b*
  natural lipid-lowering agents, 796*b*
  NCCAM categories, 96, 96*t*
  nurses as providers of, 107
  nurses as resources for, 106
  nursing management of, **106-108**
  for osteoarthritis, 1696
  for peripheral arterial disease, 903
  rates of use of, 95, 95*f*, 96*f*
  resources, 109
  at Scripps Center for Integrative Medicine, 108
  that can be integrated into nursing practice, 107*t*

Complete blood count studies, 677-678, 678*t*
  effects of aging on, 672*t*
Complete heart block
  characteristics of, 849*t*
Compliance, 512, 1469
Compliance, rate, oxygenation, and pressure index, 1767*t*
Composite urine collection, 1146*t*
Comprehensive database, 40
Compression therapy
  for preventing deep vein thrombosis, 912*b*
  for soft tissue injuries, 203
Computed tomography
  adrenal, 1251*t*
  of cardiovascular system, 758
  of chest, 526, 527*t*
  electron-beam, 755*t*, 758, 759*f*
  of gastrointestinal system, 942*t*
  hematologic, 682*t*
  of kidneys, 1148*t*
  of musculoskeletal system, 1625*t*
  myelography with, 1625*t*
  of nervous system, 1463*t*
  pancreatic, 1252*t*
  pelvic, 1340*t*, 1341
  single-photon emission, 1463*t*
  spiral (or helical), 599
Comtan (entacapone), 1551, 1552*t*
Concentration test, 1146*t*
Concept maps, 15-16, 16*f*
Concussion, 1482
  postconcussion syndrome, 1482
Condoms
  female, 262
    patient teaching guide for proper use of, 263*t*
    placement of, 263*f*
  male, 262
    patient teaching guide for proper use of, 262*t*
    placement of, 262, 262*f*
Conductive hearing loss, 408, 443
Conductive keratoplasty, 419
Conductivity, 842, 843*t*, 1442
Condylox, 1376
Confidentiality, 1378*b*
Conflicted grief, 154
Confrontation visual field test, 405*t*
Confusion, in surgical patients, 1577*b*
Congenital (term), 214*t*
Congenital problems
  of penis, **1429**
  of scrotum and testes, **1430-1431**
Congenital rubella, 437*t*
Congestion
  in pneumonia, 564
  pulmonary, 1811
Conization, 1340*t*
Conjunctiva, 400
  assessing, 407
  assessment abnormalities, 406*t*
  gerontologic differences in assessment, 401*t*
Conjunctival pallor, 675*t*
Conjunctivitis, 406*t*, **422-423**
  allergic, 423
  bacterial, 422
  chlamydial, 422-423
  keratoconjunctivitis, 423
  viral, 422
Connective tissue, 198, 198*t*

Connective tissue diseases
  with dermatologic manifestations, 473*t*
  drug therapy for, 1696, 1698*t*-1700*t*
  mixed (overlapping), **1726**
  in older adults, 1711
  renal involvement in, **1177**
  resources for, 1731
Conscious sedation, 367
Consciousness
  altered, 1460*t*
  change in level of, 1470-1471
  state of, 1456
Consent
  informed, 352-353, 353*b*
  for surgery, 352-354
Consolidation therapy, 720*t*
Constipation, 1040-1043, 1247*t*
  causes of, 1040, 1041*t*
  in chemotherapy, 295*t*
  clinical manifestations of, 1041
  collaborative care for, 1041-1042
  diagnostic studies, 1041-1042
  dietary management of, 1523
  drug therapy of, 1041, 1042*t*
  etiology and pathophysiology of, 1040-1041
  nursing assessment of, 1042, 1043*t*
  nursing diagnoses, 1042
  nursing implementation for, 1042-1043
  nursing management of, 295*t*, **1042-1043**
  nursing planning for, 1042
  nutritional therapy of, 1041-1042, 1043*t*
  opioid-induced, 138
  patient and family teaching guide for, 1044*t*
  in radiation therapy, 295*t*
  with tube feedings, 964*t*
Constraint-induced movement therapy, 1522
Constrictive pericarditis, chronic, 874
Constulose (lactulose), 138, 1042*t*
Contact dermatitis, 228, 228*f*
  allergic, 228, 462, 471*t*
  irritant, 462
Contact inhibition, 273
Contact lenses, 417, 418*t*
Contact precautions, 249
Containment devices for urinary incontinence, 1183*t*
Contemplation stage of change, 188
Continence, 1141
Continuing care retirement communities (CCRCs), 75, 88*t*
Continuous ambulatory peritoneal dialysis, 1219, 1219*f*
Continuous arteriovenous hemodialysis, 1224*t*, 1225
Continuous arteriovenous hemofiltration, 1224*t*, 1225
Continuous positive airway pressure, 1761*t*, 1762-1763
Continuous renal replacement therapy, **1224-1225,** 1224*f*
  features of, 1225
  types of, 1224, 1224*t*
Continuous ultrafiltration, slow, 1224*t*, 1225
Continuous venovenous hemodialysis, 1224-1225, 1224*f*, 1224*t*, 1225
Continuous venovenous hemofiltration, 1224-1225, 1224*f*, 1224*t*, 1225
Continuous venovenous ultrafiltration, 1224*t*, 1225

Contractility, 842, 843*t*, 1739
Contractions, 1618
  isometric, 1618
  isotonic, 1618
Contracture, 1623*t*
  with burns, 504, 504*f*
  with musculoskeletal injury, 1649*t*
  Volkmann's ischemic, 1650
  wound, 201
Contrast echocardiography, 758
Contrast medium, 1142*t*
Contrecoup trauma, 585
Control
  external locus of, 111
  internal locus of, 111
Control ventilation, 1761*t*
Controlled mandatory ventilation, 1760-1761, 1761*t*
Contusion, 1482
  with fractures, 1637*t*
Conus medullaris syndrome, 1592
Convergence, 1457
Coombs test, 680*t*
Cooper-Rand artificial larynx, 557
Coordination, 49*t*
Coordination problems, 1440-1731
Copaxone (glatiramer acetate), 1544*t*
COPD. *See* Chronic obstructive pulmonary disease
Coping, **116**
  with cancer diagnosis, 310
  compromised family coping, 121
  emotion-focused, 116, 116*t*
  example strategies, 116*t*
  ineffective, 121
  problem-focused, 116, 116*t*
  resources for, 116
  after stroke, 1520-1521, 1523
  with therapy, 301
Coping–stress tolerance pattern
  in assessment
    of auditory system, 410*t*, 412
    of cardiovascular system, 746*t*, 747
    of endocrine system, 1244
    of gastrointestinal system, 935*t*, 936
    of hematologic system, 673*t*, 674
    of integumentary system, 453*t*, 454
    of musculoskeletal system, 1621
    of nervous system, 1456
    of preoperative patient, 350*t*
    of reproductive system, 1333*t*, 1334
    of respiratory system, 518*t*, 520-521
    of urinary system, 1143*t*
    of visual system, 403*t*, 404
  comparison with NANDA International Taxonomy II, 43*t*
  concerns of patients requiring home health care, 90*t*
  nursing diagnoses, **1853**
  nursing diagnoses in, 121*t*
  nursing history, 45*t*, 46
Copper
  laboratory values, 1855*t*
  urine levels, 1862*t*
Coproporphyrin, 1862*t*
Cor pulmonale, 601, **602-603,** 824
  clinical manifestations of, 602
  collaborative care for, 602-603, 603*t*
  secondary to COPD, 635-636, 636*f*
Coral snakes, 1835, 1835*f*
Cordarone (amiodarone)
  classification of, 856*t*
  photosensitivity, 461*t*

Cordectomy, 551
Cordotomies, 143
Core rewarming, active, 1831
Coreg (carvedilol)
  for acute coronary syndrome, 800*t*
  for chronic HF, 832
  for chronic stable angina, 799, 800*t*
  drug alert, 832
  for hypertension, 775*t*
Corgard (nadolol)
  for acute coronary syndrome, 800*t*
  for chronic stable angina, 799, 800*t*
  for hypertension, 774*t*
Corlopam (fenoldopam), 775*t*
Corn, 1685*t*
Cornea, 399*f*, 400
  age-related changes in, 401*t*
  assessment abnormalities, 406*t*
  assessment of, 407
Corneal abrasion, 406*t*
Corneal disorders, 424-425
Corneal molding, 417
Corneal scars and opacities, 424-425
Corneal ulcers, 423-424
Coronary angiography, 755*t*, **759,** 759*f*
  in unstable angina and myocardial infarction, 806
Coronary arteries, 740-741, 741*f*
Coronary artery bypass graft surgery
  for acute coronary syndrome, 808-809
  minimally invasive direct, 809-810
  off-pump, 809-810
Coronary artery disease, 784-785, **785-796,** 802*f*
  chronic stable angina in, **796-802**
  cultural and ethnic health disparities in, 787*b*
  developmental stages, 785-786
  etiology and pathophysiology of, 785-787
  fibrous plaque stage, 785
  gender differences in, 785*t*
  gerontologic considerations for, **795**
  health promotion in, 791-792
  high-risk persons
    identification of, 791
    management of, 791-792
  in hypertension, 767
  nursing and collaborative management of, **791-794**
  nutritional therapy of, 792-793
  resources, 820
  risk factors for, 787-791, 787*t*
    modifiable, 787, 788-790, 790-791
    nonmodifiable, 787-788
  patient and family teaching guide for decreasing, 791-792, 792*t*
Coronary artery stents, 801-802, 801*f*, 802*f*
Coronary circulation, 740-741, 741*f*
Coronary revascularization
  for acute coronary syndrome, 808-810, 814-815
  for coronary artery disease, 801
  recommendations for, 808
Coronary veins, 740-741, 741*f*
Coronavirus, 244*t*
Correctol (phenolphthalein), 1042*t*
Cortef (hydrocortisone), 287*t*
Cortenema (hydrocortisone enema), 1055*t*
Cortex, 129
Cortical areas, 1447*t*
Cortical sensory function testing, 1459
Corticosteroid therapy, 1241, 1312, **1317-1319**
  adverse cardiovascular effects of, 745*t*
  for allergic disorders, 231

Corticosteroid therapy (Continued)
for allergic rhinitis and sinusitis, 535-536, 537t
analgesic effects of, 128
antiinflammatory action, 1318
for arthritis and connective tissue disorders, 1698t-1699t
for asthma and COPD, 617, 618t
blood glucose level effects, 1267t
classification of, 287t
complications associated with, 1318, 1475
in kidney transplantation, 1230
for dermatologic problems, 475
diseases and disorders treated with, 1318t
drug alert, 1318
effects of, 1318
effects on wound healing, 201t
food/nutrient interactions, 954t
hematologic effects of, 674t
immunosuppressive therapy, 239t
for increased ICP, 1475
for inflammatory bowel disease, 1053, 1054, 1055t
intraarticular injections, 1698t
for leukemia, 720t
major immunosuppressive agents, 238
mechanism of action, 202t
for multiple sclerosis, 1544, 1544t
nursing and collaborative management of, **1319**
for pain, 139, 139t
patient and family teaching guide for, 1319t
for Raynaud's phenomenon, 1724
for rheumatoid arthritis, 1706
side effects of, 1318t
systemic, 1699t
target tissues and functions, 1236t
Corticotropin, 1250t
Cortifoam (hydrocortisone suppository or foam), 1055t
Cortisol, 1241
circadian rhythm of secretion of, 1238, 1238f
free, 1251t
laboratory values, 1856t
serum levels, 1250t
target tissue and functions, 1236t
Cortisone (Cortone)
adverse cardiovascular effects of, 745t
classification of, 287t
Corvert (ibutilide)
for atrial flutter, 851
classification of, 856t
Corynebacterium diphtheriae, 244t
Corynebacterium vaginale, 1394t
Coryza, acute. *See* Viral rhinitis, acute
Corzide (nadolol/bendroflumethiazide), 777t
Cosmegen (dactinomycin), 287t
Cosmetic procedures, **478-480**
elective surgery, 343, 479-480
injections, 479t
laser surgery, 479
to reduce fatty tissue and skinfolds, 984
topical, 479t

Cosmetic surgery, 343
elective surgery, 479-480
laser surgery, 479
nursing management of, **480**
postoperative management of, 480
preoperative management of, 480
to reduce fatty tissue and skinfolds, 984
CosmoDerm (collagen), 479t
Cosopt (timolol maleate and dorzolamide), 435t
Costovertebral angle, 1144
Cotazym (pancrelipase), 1121t
Cough, 518, 519t
augmented, 1809, 1809f
effective coughing, 646, 646t, 1809-1810
"huff" coughing, 646, 1809
quad coughing, 1809
staged cough, 1809
techniques for wound splinting with, 381, 382f
Cough reflex, 516
Cough variant asthma, 612
Coumadin (warfarin)
and gastritis, 1013
for pulmonary embolism, 600
for stroke, 1512
Counseling
HIV, 263
pretest and posttest, with HIV-antibody testing, 263, 264t
rehabilitative, 1649
sexual, for erectile dysfunction, 1436
Counterpulsation, 1748, 1749t
Counterregulatory hormones, 1254
Coup-contrecoup injury, 1482
Couplets, 854, 854f
Covaderm, 205t
Covera-HS (verapamil long acting), 776t
Cowper's gland, 1324
COX-2 inhibitors. *See* Cyclooxygenase-2 inhibitors
Coxsackievirus A, 244t
Coxsackievirus B, 244t
Cozaar (losartan)
for chronic HF, 833
for diabetes mellitus, 1285
for gout, 1716
for hypertension, 776t, 1210
for Raynaud's phenomenon, 1724
CPAP. *See* Continuous positive airway pressure
CPB. *See* Cardiopulmonary bypass
CPP. *See* Cerebral perfusion pressure
CPR. *See* Cardiopulmonary resuscitation
"Crack" cocaine, 174
Crackles, 524
coarse, 524t
fine, 524t
Cramps
heat cramps, 1828-1829, 1830t
muscle cramps, 1223
Cranial nerve disorders, 1581-1585
Cranial nerve I. *See* Olfactory nerve
Cranial nerve II. *See* Optic nerve
Cranial nerve III. *See* Oculomotor nerve
Cranial nerve IV. *See* Trochlear nerve
Cranial nerve testing, 1456-1458
Cranial nerve V. *See* Trigeminal nerve
Cranial nerve VI. *See* Abducens nerve

Cranial nerve VII. *See* Facial nerve
Cranial nerve VIII. *See* Vestibulocochlear nerve
Cranial nerve IX. *See* Glossopharyngeal nerve
Cranial nerve X. *See* Vagus nerve
Cranial nerve XI. *See* Accessory nerve
Cranial nerve XII. *See* Hypoglossal nerve
Cranial nerves, 1448-1449, 1450f, 1450t
age-related changes in, 1454t
assessment abnormalities, 1460t
normal assessment of, 1459t
Cranial radiation, prophylactic, 582
Cranial surgery, **1491-1493**
acute intervention for, 1492-1493
ambulatory and home care for, 1493
indications for, 1491t
nursing assessment of, 1492
nursing diagnoses, 1492
nursing evaluation of, 1493
nursing implementation for, 1492-1493
nursing management of, **1492-1493**
nursing planning for, 1492
types of, 1491-1492, 1491t
Craniectomy, 1491t
Cranioplasty, 1491t
Craniotomy, 1491t, 1492
suboccipital, 1582t
Craving, 166
cue-induced, 166
definition of, 166t
C-reactive protein, 752t, 756, 1626t, 1860t
Creatine
laboratory values, 1856t
urine levels, 1862t
Creatine kinase, 1627t
laboratory values, 1856t
in shock, 1775t
Creatinine, 1147t, 1151
laboratory values, 1856t
in shock, 1775t
urine levels, 1862t
Creatinine clearance, 1146t, 1151-1152
calculation of, 1151
urine levels, 1862t
Credé's method, 1144
Crepitation, 1623t
with fractures, 1637t
in osteoarthritis, 1694
Crestor (rosuvastatin), 793, 795t
Cretinism, 1305
Creutzfeldt-Jakob disease, 1575-1576
Critical care, **1733-1771**
case study, 1769
common problems in, 1735-1736
culturally competent care, **1738**
issues related to families, 1737-1738
Critical care certification, 1735
Critical care nurse, 1734-1735
Critical care nursing, **1733-1738**
CCRN certification, 1735
definition of, 1734
Critical care patients, 1735-1737
Critical care units, 1733-1734
Critical incident stress management units, 1842
Critical limb ischemia, 903
Critical pathways, 16
Critical thinking, 5
Crixivan (indinavir), 258t
CRNA. *See* Certified registered nurse anesthetist

Crohn's disease, 1051, 1051t, 1052, 1052f
clinical manifestations of, 1052
dermatologic manifestations of, 473t
stress management strategies for, 1054b
Cromolyn (Intal), 620
for asthma, 617t, 618t
for COPD, 618t
for exercise-induced asthma, 608
Cromolyn spray (NasalCrom), 535, 537t
CROP index. *See* Compliance, rate, oxygenation, and pressure index
Cross Cultural Health Care Program, 38
Cross-cultural communication, 31-32, 32f
Crossing over, 215
Cross-link theory, 68t, 69
Crossmatch, 237, 351
Cross-tolerance, 178
CRP. *See* C-reactive protein
CRRT. *See* Continuous renal replacement therapy
CRT. *See* Cardiac resynchronization therapy
Crush injury, 585t, 1631, 1632t
emergency management of fractured extremity in, 1642, 1642t
Cryoablation, 1117
Cryoanesthesia, 372
Cryopexy, 430
Cryoprecipitates, 731t
Cryosurgery
for dermatologic problems, 476
description of, 1332t
prostatic, 1425
Cryotherapy
for cervical cancer, 1401
for diabetic retinopathy, 1284
for lung cancer, 583
for sprains and strains, 1631
Cryptococcosis, 576t
Cryptococcus neoformans, 254t, 576t
Cryptorchidism, 1430-1431
Cryptosporidium infection, 1037t
Cryptosporidium muris, 254t
Cryptosporidium parvum, 245t
Crystalloid solutions
composition and use of, 339t,
for shock, 1783-1784, 1786t
CSFs. *See* Colony-stimulating factors
CST. *See* Closed-suction technique
CT. *See* Computed tomography
CTS. *See* Carpal tunnel syndrome
Cue-induced craving, 166
Culdocentesis, 1340t
Culdoscopy, 1340t
Culdotomy, 1340t
Cullen's sign
in abdominal trauma, 1047
in acute pancreatitis, 1119
Cultural and ethnic health disparities, 20-21, 21f
in anorexia and bulimia, 969b
in brain tumors, 1487b
in breast cancer, 1348b
in cancer, 273b
in cancers of female reproductive system, 1400b
in cancers of male reproductive system, 1423b
in chronic kidney disease, 1204b
in colon disorders, 1051b
in coronary artery disease, 787b

Cultural and ethnic health disparities (Continued)
in diabetes mellitus, 1254b
in gallbladder disorders, 1089b
in heart failure, 822b
in hematologic problems, 685b
in hypertension, 762b
in integumentary problems, 461b
in liver disorders, 1089b
in lung cancer, 579b
in obesity, 971, 972b, 972f
in obstructive pulmonary diseases, 608b
in oral, pharyngeal, and esophageal problems, 1001t
in osteoporosis, 1687b
in pancreas disorders, 1089b
reducing, 23, 24t
in rheumatoid arthritis, 1702b
in stroke, 1503b
in tuberculosis, 570b
in urologic disorders, 1155b
in visual and auditory problems, 417b
Cultural assessment, 29t-30t
nurse self-assessment, 36
patient assessment, 36
Cultural awareness, 28, 28t
Cultural competence, 28-29, 28t
Cultural diversity, 30, 30f
Cultural encounters, 28t, 29
Cultural groups, 28
Cultural imposition, 28
Cultural knowledge, 28-29, 28t
Cultural skill, 28t, 29
Cultural stereotyping, 951
Cultural values, 27, 27t
Culturally competent care, 26-38
assessment, 43
for breast cancer, 1356
case study, 37
for critical care patients, 1738
for diabetes mellitus, 1271
at end of life, 154-155
for menopause, 1392
nurse self-assessment, 36
nursing implementation, 36
nursing management, 36
nutrition, 951
of older adults, 72
patient assessment, 36
patient education, 59
of preoperative patients, 356
for prostate cancer, 1427
resources, 38
transcultural nursing, 28
Culture, 20-21, 27-28, 27f
basic characteristics of, 27t
factors affecting health and health care, 30-36, 31t
Culture-bound syndromes, 35, 35t
Cultured epithelial autografts, 498t, 501, 502f
Cultures
reproductive, 1339t, 1341
skin culture, 458t
sputum culture, 527t
Cupped-hand position for percussion, 647, 647f
Cuprimine (penicillamine)
for arthritis and connective tissue disorders, 1699t
for rheumatoid arthritis, 1706
Curafoam, 205t
Curanderos (or curanderas), 30
Curasol Gel, 205t
Curettage, 476, 476f
Curie (Ci), 292t

Curity Abdominal Pads, 205t
Curity AMD, 205t
Cushing syndrome, 1312-1316
acute intervention for, 1314-1315
ambulatory and home care for, 1315-1316
causes of, 1312, 1312t
clinical manifestations of, 1312, 1313f, 1313t, 1314f
clinical presentation of, 1312
collaborative care for, 1312-1314, 1314f
dermatologic manifestations of, 473t
diagnostic studies, 1312
etiology and pathophysiology of, 1312
health promotion in, 1314
nursing assessment of, 1314, 1315t
nursing diagnoses, 1314
nursing evaluation of, 1316
nursing implementation for, 1314-1316
nursing management of, 1314-1316
nursing planning for, 1314
postoperative care in, 1315
preoperative care in, 1315
Cushing's triad, 1469
Cutaneous disease
diffuse, 1723
limited, 1723
Cutaneous lupus, subacute, 1718
Cutaneous melanoma, 465
Cutaneous T-cell lymphoma, 464t
Cutaneous ureterostomy, 1189t
CV. See Control ventilation
CVA. See Costovertebral angle
CVADs. See Central vascular access devices
CVI. See Chronic venous insufficiency
CVP. See Central venous pressure
CVVH. See Continuous venovenous hemofiltration
CVVHD. See Continuous venovenous hemodialysis
CVVU. See Continuous venovenous ultrafiltration
Cyanide poisoning, 1837t
Cyanosis, 457t, 524t, 675t
central, 749t
peripheral, 749t
variations in light- and dark-skinned individuals, 456t
Cyclizine (Marezine), 992t
Cyclobenzaprine (Flexeril), 1728
Cyclogyl (cyclopentolate HCl), 427t
Cyclohexylmethylphosphonofluoridate (GF), 1840t
Cyclooxygenase metabolic pathway, 195-196
Cyclooxygenase-2 inhibitors, 135-136, 136f, 136t
Cyclopentolate HCl (AK-Pentolate, Cyclogyl, Ocu-Pentolate, Pentolair), 427t
Cyclophosphamide (Cytoxan, Neosar), 238, 239t, 308
for arthritis and connective tissue disorders, 1700t
for breast cancer, 1355
classification of, 287t
for Goodpasture syndrome, 228
for leukemia, 720t, 721t
for lung cancer, 582
for lupus nephritis, 1718
method of administration, 288t
for multiple myeloma, 729
for myasthenia gravis, 1556
for non-Hodgkin's lymphoma, 727, 727t

Cyclophosphamide (Continued)
for polymyositis and dermatomyositis, 1726
for prostate cancer, 1427
for systemic lupus erythematosus, 1719
Cycloplegics, 426
drug alert, 426
for pupil dilation, 427t
Cycloserine (Seromycin), 573t
Cyclosporine (Sandimmune, Neoral, Gengraf), 238, 239t
blood glucose level effects, 1267t
drug alert, 238
for inflammatory bowel disease, 1055t
for lupus nephritis, 1718
nephrotoxicity, 1142t
Cyclotron, 293
Cyklokapron (transexamic acid), 709
Cylert (pemoline), 1544-1545, 1545t
Cymbalta (duloxetine), 130
Cystectomy
partial, 1179
radical, 1179
Cystic disease
medullary, 1177
polycystic kidney disease, 1176-1177
Cystic fibrosis, 608, 655-659
clinical manifestations of, 657
collaborative care for, 658
complications of, 657-658
dermatologic manifestations of, 473t
diagnostic studies, 658
etiology and pathophysiology of, 656-657, 657f
genetics of, 656b
nursing assessment of, 658, 659t
nursing diagnoses, 659
nursing implementation for, 659
nursing management of, 658-659
nursing planning for, 659
Cystic mastalgia, 1345
Cystine stones, 1169, 1170t
Cystitis, 1155
chemical, 1145t
hemorrhagic, 296t
interstitial, 1163-1164
Cystocele, 1408, 1408f
repair of, 1332t
Cystogram, 1148t
Cystolitholapaxy, 1171
Cystometrogram, 1150t
Cystoscopic lithotripsy, 1171
Cystoscopy, 1149t, 1151f
Cystotomy, 1172
Cysts, 457t
breast, 1345t
ovarian, 1399, 1399f
pilonidal, 940t
polycystic kidney disease, 1176-1177
polycystic ovary syndrome, 1399-1400
pseudocysts, 1119
sebaceous, 413t
Cysyntropin, 1250t
Cytadren (aminoglutethimide)
for bilateral adrenal hyperplasia, 1319
for Cushing syndrome, 1312-1314
Cytapheresis, 234
Cytarabine (Ara-C, Cytosar-U, Depo-Cyt)
classification of, 287t
for leukemia, 720t, 721t
methods of administration, 288t
for non-Hodgkin's lymphoma, 727t

Cytogenetics, molecular, 682t, 683
Cytokines, 115, 195t, 223
clinical uses, 223, 223t
types and functions of, 222t
Cytology, 527t
reproductive studies, 1339t, 1341
urine, 1146t
Cytolytic reactions, 227-228
Cytomegalovirus
associated with HIV infection, 254t
diseases caused by, 244t
Cytomegalovirus infection, 437t, 1367t
Cytomegalovirus pneumonia, 564
Cytomegalovirus retinitis, 436
Cytoprotective agents
for gastroesophageal reflux disease, 1006t
for peptic ulcer disease, 1019t, 1021
Cytoreductive procedures, 285
Cytosar (cytarabine), 720t
Cytosar-U (cytarabine), 287t
Cytosine arabinoside, 721t
Cytotec (misoprostol)
for inducing abortrion, 1384t
for osteoarthritis, 1697
for peptic ulcer disease, 1019t
Cytotoxic cerebral edema, 1469-1470
Cytotoxic drugs, 239t
Cytotoxic reactions, 225t, 227-228
Cytovene (ganciclovir), 564
Cytoxan (cyclophosphamide), 238, 239t, 308
for arthritis and connective tissue disorders, 1700t
for breast cancer, 1355
classification of, 287t
for Goodpasture syndrome, 228
for leukemia, 720t
for lupus nephritis, 1718
method of administration, 288t
for multiple myeloma, 729
for non-Hodgkin's lymphoma, 727t
for polymyositis and dermatomyositis, 1726
for prostate cancer, 1427

D

d4T. See Stavudine
Dacarbazine (DTIC-Dome), 287t
Daclizumab (Zenapax), 239t, 240
Dactinomycin (Cosmegen), 287t
DAI. See Diffuse axonal injury
Dalteparin (Fragmin), 800t
Danazol (Danocrine), 1345
Dantrolene (Dantrium)
for multiple sclerosis, 1545t
for spasms, 1603
Daranide (dichlorphenamide), 435t
Darbepoetin alfa (Aranesp)
for cancer treatment, 304t
clinical uses of, 223t
DARE. See Database of Abstracts of Reviews of Effects
Darifenacin (Enablex)
for urinary incontinence, 1182
for voiding dysfunction, 1185t
Dark skin color
assessment of, 209, 209t, 456-457
assessment variations, 456t
Dark-field microscopy, 1339t
Darvon (propoxyphene), 138
Dasatinib (Sprycel), 720t, 721t
DASH (Dietary Approaches to Stop Hypertension) diet, 770, 770t, 833

Data
  objective, 40
  subjective, 40
  types of, 40
Data analysis, 10
Data collection, 10, **39-43**
Data organization, 43
Database of Abstracts of Reviews of
    Effects (DARE), 7t
Databases, 39, 40
Daunorubicin (Cerubidine, Dauno-
    Xome)
  adverse cardiovascular effects of, 745t
  classification of, 287t
  drug alert, 720
  for leukemia, 720t, 721t
Davol catheter, 1221
Dawn phenomenon, 1263-1265
Daypro (oxaprozin), 1698t
D&C. *See* Dilation and curettage
DCIS. *See* Ductal carcinoma in situ
DDAVP (desmopressin acetate), 1479
DDD. *See* Degenerative disk disease
ddI. *See* Didanosine
D-dimer, 599, 679t
  in deep vein thrombosis, 911t
  laboratory values, 1859t
  in shock, 1775t
DDP-4 inhibitor. *See* Dipeptidyl pepti-
    dase-4 inhibitor
D&E. *See* Dilation and evacuation
de Quervain's thyroiditis, 1298
Deafferentation pain, 131
Deafness, 442-445
  assistive devices and techniques for,
      444-445
  clinical manifestations of, 443
  nursing and collaborative manage-
      ment of, **443-444**
Death, 152
  brain death, 153
  from cancer, 272, 272t
  in emergency department, 1827-1828
  fear of hastening by administering
      analgesics, 147
  leading causes, 784-785, 785f
  physical manifestations of approach
      of, 152, 152t
  preoperative fear of, 345
  psychosocial manifestations of ap-
      proach of, 153, 153t
"Death cap," 1115
Death rattle, 152
Debridement, 199, 1650
  approaches to, 204-205
  autolytic, 205
  of burns, 496
  enzymatic, 205, 501
  mechanical, 204
  operative, 496, 497f
  surgical, 204, **1662**
Debulking, 285
Decadron (dexamethasone)
  for arthritis and connective tissue dis-
      orders, 1699t
  classification of, 287t
  for increased ICP, 1475
  for leukemia, 720t
  for multiple myeloma, 729
  for nausea and vomiting, 297, 992,
      992t
  for pain, 139

Decannulation, 551
Deceased donors, 1227
Decerebrate posturing, 1472, 1472f
Decongestants
  for allergic disorders, 231
  for allergic rhinitis and sinusitis, 538t
Decorticate posturing, 1472, 1472f
Decortication, 593t
Dedifferentiation, 274
Deep brain stimulation, 1551-1552
Deep breathing, 95, 96f
Deep tendon reflexes, increased, 1247t
Deep vein thrombosis, 909, 910t, **911-
    915**
  anticoagulant prophylaxis of, 914
  anticoagulant treatment of, 912, 913t,
      914-915
  clinical manifestations of, 911
  collaborative care for, 911-915
  complications of, 911
  diagnostic studies, 911, 911t
  drug therapy of, 912
  nonpharmacologic therapy of, 912
  nursing assessment of, 915t
  prevention and prophylaxis of, 911-
      912, 912b
  risk factors for, 909, 910t
  surgical therapy of, 915
Defecation, 930. *See also* Elimination
Defense mechanisms
  normal, 561
  respiratory, 516
Defibrillation, 856-858, 857f
Defibrillators, 856, 857f
Defining characteristics, 11
Deformity
  in ankylosing spondylitis, 1712,
      1712f
  with fractures, 1637t
  identification of, 1824t
  with osteoarthritis, 1695
  of rheumatoid arthritis, 1703-1704,
      1704f
Degenerative disk disease, 1680,
    1681f
Degenerative joint disease, 1694
Deglutition, 928
Dehiscence, 201
Dehydration, 322
  at end of life, 160t
  with tube feedings, 964t
Dehydroepiandrosterone, 103t
Delavirdine (Rescriptor), 258t
Delayed emergence, 387
Delayed hemolytic reactions, 734t
Delayed hypersensitivity reactions,
    225t, 228
Delayed transfusion reactions, 734,
    734t
Delcid, 1020t
Delegation, 14
Delirium, 1455, **1576-1578**
  alcohol withdrawal delirium, 177
  clinical features of, 1561, 1562f
  clinical manifestations of, 1576-1577
  diagnostic studies, 1577
  drug therapy for, 1578
  emergence delirium, 387
  at end of life, 160t
  etiology and pathophysiology of,
      1576
  factors that can precipitate, 1576,
      1576t
  music and, 1577b
  nursing and collaborative manage-
      ment of, **1577-1578**
  in surgical patients, 1577b

Delta virus, 1090
Demadex (torsemide), 773t
Dementia, 1561-1564
  causes of, 1562, 1563t
  clinical features of, 1561, 1562f
  clinical manifestations of, 1562,
      1563t
  diagnostic studies, 1562-1564
  etiology and pathophysiology of,
      1562
  frontotemporal, 1576
  gender differences in, 1565b
  guidelines for dealing with patients
      with, 1575t
  Lewy body, 1575
  nursing and collaborative manage-
      ment of, **1564**
  vascular, 1562
Dementia paralytica, 1589
Demerol (meperidine), 138
  as adjunct to general anesthesia,
      370t
  contraindications to, 698
  effects of use, 169t
  nephrotoxicity, 1211
  preoperative, 355t
Demi-Regroton (reserpine/chlorthali-
    done), 777t
Demographics
  of aging, **66-67,** 67f
  and health care system, 86
Demonstration/return demonstration,
    61-62, 62f
Demulcents, 1037t
Dendrites, 1442
Dendritic cells, 222
Dengue fever, 246t
Denileukin diftitox (Ontak), 727
Deoxyribonucleic acid (DNA), 214
Depakene (valproic acid)
  for Alzheimer's disease, 1569
  for seizures, 1538t
  for trigeminal neuralgia, 1581
Depakote (divalproex), 1536, 1538t
Department of Health and Human Ser-
    vices (U.S.), 74
Department of National Health and
    Welfare (Canada), 74
Depen (penicillamine), 1699t
Dependence
  definition of, 166, 166t
  health complications of, 167, 168t
  maladjusted independence, 1523
  nicotine, **167-174,** 168t
  physical
    definition of, 166t
    and pain, 145
  physiologic, 168
  psychologic, 166t, 168
  symptoms and behaviors that may
      suggest, 181-182, 181t
Dependent rubor, 901
DepoCyt (cytarabine), 287t
Depolarization, 742, 843, 1443, 1443f
Depo-Medrol (methylprednisolone ace-
    tate), 1698t
Depo-Provera (medroxyprogesterone)
  drug alert, 1392
  for perimenopause and postmeno-
      pause, 1392
Depot (octreotide), 1292
Depressant overdose, 179, 179t
Depressants, **176-180**
  acute intervention for withdrawal
      from, 186-187
  effects of use, 169t

Depression
  in acute coronary syndrome, 814t
  in Alzheimer's disease, 1569, 1569t
  in burn patients, 505t
  clinical features of, 1561, 1562f
  in COPD, 637
  at end of life, 158
  in older adults, 80-81
  after radical neck dissection, 557
  after spinal cord injury, 1608-1609
Dermatitis
  allergic contact, 462, 471t
  atopic, 227, 471t
  contact, 228, 228f
  irritant contact, 462
Dermatologic problems
  allergic, **470-471,** 471t
  ambulatory and home care for, 477-
      478
  benign, **471,** 472t
  chronic
    physiologic effects of, 478
    psychologic effects of, 478
  collaborative care for, **471-478**
  collaborative therapy of, 471-476
  diagnostic studies, 471
  diseases with manifestations of, **471,**
      473t
  drug therapy of, 475-476
  nursing management of, **477-478**
  radiation therapy of, 474
  resources, 482
  surgical therapy of, 476-477
Dermatomes, 128, 129f, 1448
Dermatomyositis, 1725-1726
  clinical manifestations of, 1725
  complications of, 1725
  dermatologic manifestations of, 473t
  diagnostic studies, 1725
  etiology and pathophysiology of,
      1725
  nursing and collaborative manage-
      ment of, **1725-1726**
  skin changes of, 1725, 1725f
Dermis, 450, 486
DES. *See* Diethylstilbestrol
Descartes, Rene, 94
Desflurane (Suprane), 369t
Desipramine, 35t
Desirudin (Iprivask), 914
Desloratadine (Clarinex), 538t
Desmopressin acetate (DDAVP), 1479
Desoxyn (methamphetamine), 169t
Desquamation
  dry, 299, 299f
  wet, 299, 299f
Destination therapy, 831
Desyrel (trazodone)
  for Alzheimer's disease, 1569, 1569t
  food/nutrient interactions, 954t
DET. *See* Diethyltryptamine
Detoxification, 166t, 178, 932t, 946t
Detrol (tolterodine)
  drug alert, 1183
  for urinary incontinence, 1182
  for voiding dysfunction, 1185t
Detrusor muscle, 1140
Detrusor muscle hypertrophy, 1168
Deviated septum, 533
DEXA. *See* Dual-energy x-ray absorpti-
    ometry
Dexamethasone (Decadron)
  for arthritis and connective tissue dis-
      orders, 1699t
  for bilateral adrenal hyperplasia,
      1319
  classification of, 287t
  for increased ICP, 1475

Note: Disorder names are in **bold face.**
Page numbers in **bold face** indicate main
discussions. Page numbers followed by
f, t, b, or *n* indicate figures, tables, boxed
material, or notes, respectively.

Dexamethasone (Decadron)
(Continued)
for leukemia, 720t, 721t
for multiple myeloma, 729
for nausea and vomiting, 297, 992, 992t
for non-Hodgkin's lymphoma, 727t
for pain, 139
Dexchlorpheniramine (Polaramine), 537t
Dexcom, 1269, 1270
Dexedrine (dextroamphetamine)
effects of use, 169t
for opioid-induced sedation, 138
Dexfenfluramine (Redux), 981
Dextran
hematologic effects of, 674t
for shock, 1786t
Dextroamphetamine (Dexedrine)
effects of use, 169t
for opioid-induced sedation, 138
Dextrose in saline, 339t
Dextrose in water, 339t
Dextrostix, 1481
DHA. See Docosahexaenoic acid
DHEA. See Dehydroepiandrosterone
DI. See Diabetes insipidus
DiaBeta (glyburide)
for diabetes mellitus, 1265, 1266t
food/nutrient interactions, 954t
Diabetes insipidus, 1294, **1296-1297**
acute intervention for, 1479
central, 1296, 1296t
clinical manifestations of, 1296-1297
collaborative care for, 1297
diagnostic studies, 1297
etiology and pathophysiology of, 1296, 1296f, 1296t
nephrogenic, 1296, 1296t
neurogenic, 1296
nursing management of, **1297**
psychogenic, 1296, 1296t
types of, 1296t
Diabetes mellitus, 1253-1278
acute complications of, **1278-1282**
acute intervention for, 1272-1274
ambulatory and home care for, 1274-1278
association with obesity, 975
chronic complications of, **1282-1288**
collaborative care for, 1258-1259, 1259t
complications of, 1258
complications of feet and lower extremities, **1286-1287**
and coronary artery disease, 790
criteria for testing for, 1272t
cultural and ethnic health disparities in, 1254b
culturally competent care for, **1271**
dermatologic manifestations of, 473t
diagnosis of, 1258
diagnostic criteria for, 1258
diagnostic studies, 1258
diet instructions for patients, 1277t
drug therapy for, 1259-1265, 1265-1266, 1266t
early detection of, 1275b
effects on wound healing, 201t
etiology and pathophysiology of, 1254-1258, 1255
exercise therapy for, 1277t
food composition for, 1267-1268
gerontologic considerations for, **1287-1288**

Diabetes mellitus (Continued)
group-based educational programs and health of patients with, 1259b
guidelines for patients, 1277t
health disparities and, 21t
health promotion in, 1271-1272
health-promoting behaviors for, 792t
instructions for patients with, 1277t
insulin therapy for, 1259-1265, 1275
integumentary complications of, **1287**
long-term complications of, 1282, 1283, 1283f, 1284t
macrovascular complications of, 1282, **1283-1284**
management of
general guidelines for, 1277t
patient and family teaching guides for, 1277t
medical identification and travel with, 1276
microvascular complications of, 1282, **1284**
nursing assessment of, 1271, 1272t
nursing care plan for patient with, 1273b-1274b
nursing diagnoses, 1271
nursing evaluation of, 1278
nursing implementation for, 1271-1278
nursing management of, **1271-1278**
nursing planning for, 1271
nutritional therapy for, 1266-1269, 1268t
ocular manifestations of, 437t
oral agents for, 1265, 1275
pancreas transplantation for, 1271
prevention of, 1275b
resources, 1289
secondary, 1258
type 1, **1255**
characteristics of, 1254t
clinical manifestations of, 1258
etiology and pathophysiology of, 1255, 1256f
genetics of, 1256b
nutritional therapy for, 1267
onset of disease, 1255
type 2, **1255-1257**
characteristics of, 1254t
clinical manifestations of, 1258
etiology and pathophysiology of, 1255-1257, 1256f
genetics of, 1256b
nutritional therapy for, 1267
onset of disease, 1257
Diabetes risk test, 1272
Diabetic coma, 1278-1279, 1279f
Diabetic foot complications, 1286, 1286f
Diabetic ketoacidosis (DKA), 1255, **1278-1280**
case study, 1288
clinical manifestations of, 1279
collaborative care for, 1280, 1280t
emergency management of, 1280t
etiology and pathophysiology of, 1278-1279, 1279f
nursing management of, **1281**
Diabetic nephropathy, 1285
prevention, detection, and monitoring of, 1284t
renal involvement in, 1177
Diabetic neuropathy, 1285-1286, 1286f
classification of, 1285-1286

Diabetic neuropathy (Continued)
etiology and pathophysiology of, 1285
prevention, detection, and monitoring of, 1284t
Diabetic retinopathy, 429, **1284-1285**
case study, 446-447
collaborative care for, 1284-1285
etiology and pathophysiology of, 1284
prevention, detection, and monitoring of, 1284t
Diabinese (chlorpropamide)
for diabetes insipidus, 1297
photosensitivity, 461t
Diacetate (Amcort), 1437
Diagnosis
nursing phase, **10-12**
patient education, 59-60
Diagnostic statements, 11-12
Diagnostic studies. See also specific tests
auditory, **412-415**, 414t
cardiovascular, **751-760**, 752t-755t
endocrine, **1246-1250**
gastrointestinal, **939-946**, 941t-945t
hematologic, **677-683**, 682t
nervous system, **1459-1465**
of nervous system, 1462t-1463t
preoperative, 349-350, 351t
reproductive, **1336-1341**, 1338t-1341t
respiratory, **525-531**, 527t-528t
urinary, **1145-1152**, 1146t-1149t
vestibular function tests, 414t, 415
visual, **407**, 408t
Dialcor XR (diltiazem extended release), 776t
Dialysate, 1222
Dialysis, **1216-1225**
in acute renal failure, 1202
for elevated potassium levels, 1202t
general principles of, 1216
hemodialysis, 1216, 1217t, **1220-1224**
complications of, 1229t
methods of, 1216
peritoneal, 1216, **1216-1220**, 1217t
complications of, 1229t
withdrawing treatment, 1230b
Dialyzers, 1222
Diamox (acetazolamide)
for acute pancreatitis, 1121t
blood glucose level effects, 1267t
for glaucoma, 435t
Diapedesis, 194, 194f
Diaphragmatic (abdominal) breathing, 117, 646
Diaphysis, 1615
Diapid (lysine vasopressin), 1297
Dia-Quel Liquid (tincture of opium, homatropine, methylbromide, and pectin), 1037t
Diarrhea, 1036-1038
acute infectious
causes of, 1036, 1037t
nursing care plan for, 1039b
nursing management of, **1037-1038**
causes of, 1036, 1036t
in chemotherapy, 295t
clinical manifestations of, 1036
collaborative care for, 1036-1037
diagnostic studies, 1036
drug therapy of, 1036, 1037t
etiology and pathophysiology of, 1036

Diarrhea (Continued)
nursing assessment of, 1037-1038, 1038t
radiation treatment-induced, 295t, 298
with tube feedings, 964t
Diarthrodial (synovial) joints, 1616, 1616f, 1617f
Diastole, 742
Diastolic blood pressure, 743
Diastolic dysfunction, 1774
Diastolic failure, 822-823
Diazepam (Valium)
as adjunct to general anesthesia, 370t
effects of use, 169t
ethnic differences in response to, 35t
for multiple sclerosis, 1545t
for panic attacks, 181
preoperative, 355t
for status epilepticus, 1537
for tetanus, 1588
toxicology, 1865t
withdrawal from, 179
Dibenzyline (phenoxybenzamine), 1320
DIC. See Disseminated intravascular coagulation
Dichlorphenamide (Daranide), 435t
Diclofenac (Voltaren, Apo-Diclo SR)
for arthritis and connective tissue disorders, 1698t
and gastritis, 1013
photosensitivity, 461t
Diclofenac K (Cataflam), 135, 136t
Dicyclomine (Bentyl)
for acute pancreatitis, 1121t
for voiding dysfunction, 1185t
Didanosine (ddI, Videx, Videx-EC), 258t
Didrex (benzphetamine), 981
Didronel (etidronate)
food/nutrient interactions, 954t
for osteoporosis, 1689
Diencephalon, 1448f
Diet(s), 95, 96f
1200-calorie-restricted weight-reduction diet, 978t
DASH (Dietary Approaches to Stop Hypertension) diet, 770, 770t, 833
fad diets, 979, 979t
health impact of, 958b
high-calorie, high-protein, 958t
incomplete, 953
low-sodium diets, 833, 834t
special diets, 950-951
for urinary tract calculi, 1172
Dietary fiber, 1044t
Dietary guidelines, 949
Dietary Guidelines for Americans 2005, 958t
Dietary management
of constipation, 1523
of diabetes mellitus, 1277t
restriction for elevated potassium levels, 1202t
therapeutic lifestyle changes, 792, 793t
Dietary Reference Intakes (DRIs), 953, 953t
Dietary Supplement Health and Education Act of 1994 (DSHEA), 101
Dietary supplements, 44b, 103t
Diethylpropion (Tenuate, Tepanil), 981

Diethylstilbestrol (DES, Stilphostrol)
  for breast cancer, 1355
  classification of, 288*t*
  DES sons, 1431
  for prostate cancer, 1426, 1426*t*
Diethyltryptamine (DET), 170*t*
Dietitian services, 91*t*
Diffuse axonal injury, 1483
Diffuse parenchymal lung diseases, 597
Diffusion, 316-317, 317*f*, 513, 1216, 1217*f*
  facilitated, 317
  limitation of, 1802, 1802*f*
Diflucan (fluconazole)
  for pulmonary infections, 576
  for urethritis, 1163
  for vulvovaginal candidiasis, 1394*t*
Digestion, 928-930
  gastrointestinal secretions related to, 929, 929*t*
  physiology of, 929-930
  problems of, **925-1134**
  resources for, 970
Digestive system. *See* Gastrointestinal system
Digitalis glycosides, 832-833
Digitalis toxicity, 832-833, 833*t*, 1865*t*
Digitoxin, 1865*t*
Digoxin (Lanoxin)
  for atrial fibrillation, 887
  for chronic HF, 832
  classification of, 856*t*
  dose and frequency adjustments, 1211
  toxicology, 1865*t*
Dihydrotachysterol (Hytakerol), 1311
Dihydroxyaluminum aminoacetate, 1020*t*
Dihydroxyaluminum sodium carbonate, 1020*t*
Dilantin (phenytoin)
  blood glucose level effects, 1267*t*
  classification of, 856*t*
  food/nutrient interactions, 954*t*
  for seizures, 1536, 1538*t*
  toxicology, 1865*t*
  for trigeminal neuralgia, 1581
Dilated cardiomyopathy, 886-888, 886*t*, 887*f*
  clinical manifestations of, 886
  diagnostic studies, 886-887
  etiology and pathophysiology of, 886
  nursing and collaborative management of, **887-888**
Dilation, ventricular, 823
Dilation and curettage, 1340*t*
  for abnormal vaginal bleeding, 1388
  description of, 1332*t*
Dilation and evacuation, 1384*t*
Dilaudid (hydromorphone)
  for burns, 499*t*
  effects of use, 169*t*
  for pain, 137*t*, 138, 141
Diltiazem (Cardizem)
  for acute coronary syndrome, 800*t*
  for chronic stable angina, 800*t*, 801

Diltiazem (Cardizem) *(Continued)*
  classification of, 856*t*
  effects on lower urinary tract function, 1180*t*
  enalapril/diltiazem (Teczem), 777*t*
  extended release (Cardizem CD, Cardizem LA, Dialcor XR, Tiazac), 776*t*
  for hypertension, 776*t*
  for Raynaud's phenomenon, 1724
  for voiding dysfunction, 1185*t*
Dimenhydrinate (Dramamine), 992*t*
Dimetane (brompheniramine), 537*t*
Dimethyl sulfoxide (DMSO), 1164
Dimethyltryptamine (DMT), 170*t*
Dinoprostone (Prostin E₂, Cervidil), 1384*t*
Diovan (valsartan)
  for chronic HF, 833
  for hypertension, 776*t*
Diovan HCT (valsartan/hydrochlorothiazide), 777*t*
Dipentum (olsalazine), 1055*t*
Dipeptidyl peptidase-4 inhibitor, 1265, 1266*t*
Diphenhydramine (Benadryl)
  for allergic rhinitis and sinusitis, 537*t*
  for anaphylactic shock, 1790
  for burns, 504
  for dermatologic problems, 475
  for opioid-induced pruritus, 138
  for Parkinson's disease, 1552*t*
  photosensitivity, 461*t*
Diphenidol (Vontrol), 992*t*
Diphenoxylate with atropine (Lomotil, Colonaid)
  for diarrhea, 1037*t*
  for inflammatory bowel disease, 1055*t*
Diphtheria, 246*t*
Dipivefrin (Propine), 434*t*
Diplopia, 406*t*, 675*t*, 1460*t*, 1520
Diprivan (propofol), 369*t*
Dipstick (Albustix, Combistix) test, 1146*t*, 1157, 1863*t*
Dipyridamole (Persantine)
  for long-term therapy after TIAs, 1505
  to prevent stroke, 1510
  for stroke, 1512
Dipyridamole and aspirin (Aggrenox)
  for long-term therapy after TIAs, 1505
  to prevent stroke, 1510
Direct antihuman globulin test, 1861*t*
Direct Coombs test, 1861*t*
Direct thrombin inhibitors, 914
Directives to physicians (DTPs), 155, 156*t*
"Dirty bombs," 1840
Disability survey, 1824, 1824*t*, 1825*t*
Disaccharides, 949
Disalcid (salsalate), 1698*t*
Disaster medical assistance teams (DMATs), 1842
Disaster nursing, **1821-1844**
Discharge planning, 394
  for ambulatory surgery, 393*t*, 394
  for older adults, 79
  from PACU, **393**
  patient education and clinical outcomes in chronic HF, 830*b*
  postanesthesia, 393*t*
  after prostate surgery, 1422
Discomfort
  fear of, 345
  postoperative, **388-389**

Disconjugate gaze, 1457
Disease. *See also specific diseases*
  with dermatologic manifestations, **471,** 473*t*
  HLA associations, 233
  occurrence of, 33-34
  pathophysiologic mechanisms of, **192-341**
  susceptibility to, 33-34
Disease-modifying antirheumatic drugs
  for arthritis and connective tissue disorders, 1699*t*
  for rheumatoid arthritis, 1705
Disequilibrium syndrome, 1223-1224
Disk disease, degenerative, 1680, 1681*f*
Disk herniation, 1680-1681, 1682*t*
Diskectomy, 1682
Diskogram, 1625*t*
Dislocation, 1623*t*, **1632-1633**
  nursing and collaborative management of, **1632-1633**
Disopyramide (Norpace), 856*t*
Dissecting aneurysm, 898
Disseminated intravascular coagulation (DIC), 703, **710-713**
  acute
    laboratory abnormalities in, 712*t*
    predisposing conditions to, 710*t*
  in cancer, 308
  chronic, 710*t*
  clinical manifestations of, 711, 711*f*
  collaborative care for, 712, 713*f*
  diagnostic studies, 711-712
  etiology and pathophysiology of, 710-711, 711*f*
  nursing diagnoses, 712
  nursing implementation for, 712-713
  nursing management of, **712-713**
  predisposing conditions to, 710*t*
  subacute, 710*t*
Dissociative anesthesia, 369*t*, 371
Distention
  abdominal, 676*t*, 940*t*
    postoperative, 1188
  jugular venous, 748
Distention
  abdominal, 676*t*, 940*t*
Disulfiram (Antabuse), 178
Ditropan (oxybutynin)
  for multiple sclerosis, 1544*t*
  for urinary incontinence, 1182
  for voiding dysfunction, 1185*t*
Diuretic (methyclothiazide), 773*t*
Diuretics
  for chronic HF, 831
  for cirrhosis, 1110*t*
  combination drug therapy of hypertension, 777*t*
  hematologic effects of, 674*t*
  for hypertension, 773*t*, 1210
  photosensitivity, 461*t*
  thiazide, 1267*t*
Diuril (chlorothiazide)
  for cirrhosis, 1110*t*
  for diabetes insipidus, 1297
  for hypertension, 773*t*
Divalproex (Depakote), 1536, 1538*t*
Diversity, cultural, **30,** 30*f*
Diverticular disease, 1076*f*
Diverticulitis, 1076-1077, 1076*f*
  clinical manifestations of, 1076-1077
  collaborative care for, 1077*t*
  complications of, 1076, 1077*f*
  diagnostic studies, 1077

Diverticulitis *(Continued)*
  etiology and pathophysiology of, 1076
  nursing and collaborative management of, **1077**
Diverticulosis, 1076-1077
  clinical manifestations of, 1076-1077
  collaborative care for, 1077*t*
  diagnostic studies, 1077
  etiology and pathophysiology of, 1076
  nursing and collaborative management of, **1077**
Diverticulum(a), 1076, 1168
  esophageal, **1011-1012**
  urethral, **1163**
Diving injury, 1596*t*
DKA. *See* Diabetic ketoacidosis
DM. *See* Diabetes mellitus; Dermatomyositis
DMARDs. *See* Disease-modifying antirheumatic drugs
DMATs. *See* Disaster medical assistance teams
DMT. *See* Dimethyltryptamine
DNA, 214, 215*f*
  anemia caused by defective synthesis of, 685*t*
  drug-induced suppression of synthesis of, 692*t*
  recombinant DNA technology, 241, 241*f*
DNR orders. *See* Do-not-resuscitate orders
Dobutamine (Dobutrex)
  as positive inotrope, 1739
  for shock, 1787*t*
Docetaxel (Taxotere)
  for breast cancer, 1355, 1356
  classification of, 287*t*
  for esophageal cancer, 1010
  for lung cancer, 582
  for oral cancer, 1002
  for prostate cancer, 1427
Docosahexaenoic acid, 792
Documentation, **15-16**
  asthma action plan, 626, 627*t*
  chart review, 363-364
  end-of-life care, 155, 156*t*
  of normal findings on screening physical examination, 51*t*
  postanesthesia admission report, 377, 377*t*
Docusate (Colace, Surfak, Peri-Colace, Doxidan), 138, 1042*t*
Dofetilide (Tikosyn), 856*t*
Dog bites, 1836
Dolasetron (Anzemet)
  as adjunct to general anesthesia, 370*t*
  for nausea and vomiting, 297, 992, 992*t*
Doll's-eye reflex, 1477
Dolophine (methadone)
  as adjunct to general anesthesia, 370*t*
  effects of use, 169*t*
  for opioid withdrawal, 180
  for pain, 137*t*
Domeboro powder, 477
Domestic violence, 1838
Domperidone (Motilium), 992*t*
Donation
  non–heart beating, 1828
  organ and tissue, 155
Donepezil (Aricept)
  for Alzheimer's disease, 1568, 1569*t*
  for Parkinson's dementia, 1551

Donnagel, Donnagel-PG, 1037*t*
Donor sources
    deceased donors, 1227
    for kidney transplantation, 1226-1227
Do-not-resuscitate (DNR) orders, 155, 156*t*, 882*b*
    out-of-hospital, 156
Dopamine (Intropin), 1445*t*
    drug alert, 829
    as positive inotrope, 1739
    for shock, 1787*t*
    for spinal cord injury, 1596
Dopaminergics, 1551, 1552*t*
Doppler ultrasound
    duplex venous, 1627*t*
    transcranial, 1463*t*
Dorsal horn processing, 128-129
Dorsiflexion, 1622*t*
Dorzolamide (Trusopt), 435*t*
Dosing, equianalgesic, 140
Dostinex (cabergoline)
    for acromegaly, 1292
    for prolactinoma, 1293
Double voiding, 1184-1185
Double-lumen catheters
    semipermanent, 1222, 1222*f*
    temporary vascular access, 1221, 1221*f*
Doubling time, 274
Dowager's hump, 1623*t*, 1687
Down syndrome, 437*t*
Doxacurium (Nuromax), 370*t*
Doxazosin (Cardura)
    for benign prostatic hyperplasia, 1417
    drug alert, 772
    effects on lower urinary tract function, 1180*t*
    for hypertension, 774*t*
    for voiding dysfunction, 1185*t*
Doxepin (Sinequan)
    adverse cardiovascular effects of, 745*t*
    for Alzheimer's disease, 1569*t*
    local, 139*t*
    for peptic ulcer disease, 1019*t*, 1021
    photosensitivity, 461*t*
Doxercalciferol (Hectorol), 1210
Doxidan (docusate), 1042*t*
Doxorubicin (Adriamycin, Rubex, Doxil)
    adverse cardiovascular effects of, 745*t*
    for bladder cancer, 1179
    for breast cancer, 1355
    for cervical cancer, 1402
    classification of, 287*t*
    drug alert, 1355
    for leukemia, 720*t*, 721*t*
    method of administration, 288*t*
    for multiple myeloma, 729
    for non-Hodgkin's lymphoma, 727*t*
Doxycycline (Vibramycin)
    for arthritis and connective tissue disorders, 1698*t*
    for chlamydial infections, 1373
    drug alert, 1368
    for gonorrhea, 1368
    for Lyme disease, 1714
    for osteoarthritis, 1697
    for Rocky Mountain spotted fever, 1835
    for syphilis, 1371*t*
DPAHC. *See* Durable power of attorney for health care

D-penicillamine (Duprimine), 1724
DPIs. *See* Dry powder inhalers
Drainage
    chest, 591*t*
        clinical guidelines for care of patient with, 591*t*
        dry systems, 591*t*
        nursing management of, **590-592**
        portable units, 590, 590*f*
        wet systems, 591*t*
    chest units, 589, 589*f*
    lymphatic, 671, 671*f*
    pleural, **588-592,** 589*f*
    postural, 647
        positions for, 647, 648*f*
    from tubes and catheters, 392, 393*t*
    water-seal, 591*t*-592*t*
Dramamine (dimenhydrinate), 992*t*
Dressings
    absorptive, 205*t*
    chest tube, 592*t*
    multiple dressing change method, 497, 498*f*
    nonadherent, 205*t*
    occlusive, 205
    semiocclusive, 205
    silver-impregnated, 499
    transparent film dressings, 204, 204*f*
    types of, 205*t*
    wet, 477
Dressler syndrome, 805, 872
DRIs. *See* Dietary Reference Intakes
Dristan (oxymetazoliine), 538*t*
Dronabinol (Marinol), 992, 992*t*
Drop arm test, 1634
Drop attack (atonic) seizures, 1535
Droperidol (Inapsine)
    as adjunct to general anesthesia, 370*t*
    for nausea and vomiting, 992, 992*t*
    preoperative, 355*t*
Droplet precautions, 249
Drotrecogin alpha (Xigris), 1787*t*, 1789
Drowning, 1832
    "dry drowning," 1832
    near-drowning, 1832
    secondary, 1833
Droxia (hydroxyurea), 287*t*
Drug abuse. *See also* Substance abuse
    contributing factors, 167, 167*f*
    health problems related to, 168*t*
Drug Enforcement Administration, 989
Drug reactions, 471*t*
Drug therapy. *See also* Medications; *specific drugs*
    for acute and chronic pancreatitis, 1121*t*
    for acute coronary syndrome, 800*t*, 808
    for acute pancreatitis, 1121
    for acute pyelonephritis, 1161-1162
    for acute respiratory failure, 1810-1811
    adjuvant drugs for pain management, 138-140, 139*t*
    adverse cardiovascular effects of, 745*t*
    aging and, 80, 81*f*
    for allergic disorders, 231
    for allergic rhinitis and sinusitis, 535-536, 537*t*-538*t*
    for Alzheimer's disease, 1568-1570, 1569*t*
    analgesics, 135, 136*t*
    anticoagulant therapy, 912, 913*t*
    antidysrhythmia drugs, 856
    antipruritic, 231

Drug therapy *(Continued)*
    antiretroviral agents used in HIV infection, 258*t*
    antiseizure, 1537-1538
        drug alert, 1535
        side effects of, 1537
    appetite-suppressing drugs, 981
    for arthritis and connective tissue disorders, 1696, 1698*t*-1700*t*
    for asthma, 617-624, 617*t*, 618*t*-620*t*
    and asthma attacks, 610
    for benign prostatic hyperplasia, 1416-1417
    for botulism, 1587-1588
    for burns, 498-499, 499*t*
    CAGE questionnaire adapted to include drugs (CAGEAID), 182, 183*t*
    chemotherapeutic
        cell cycle phase–nonspecific, 286
        cell cycle phase–specific, 286
        classification of, 286, 287*t*-288*t*
    for chlamydial infections, 1373
    cholesterol-lowering, 793-794
    for chronic HF, 831-833
    for chronic kidney disease, 1210-1211
    for chronic stable angina, 798-801, 800*t*
    for cirrhosis, 1110, 1110*t*
    combination therapy
        for asthma, 623-624, 624*t*
        for hypertension, 777*t*
    for community-acquired pneumonia, 562-563, 563*t*
    for connective tissue disorders, 1696, 1698*t*-1700*t*
    for constipation, 1041, 1042*t*
    for COPD, 618*t*-620*t*, 639-640
    corticosteroid, 1312
    decongestant, 231
    decreasing risks related to, 262
    for deep vein thrombosis, 912
    for delirium, 1578
    for dermatologic problems, 475-476
    for diabetes mellitus, 1259-1265, 1265-1266, 1266, 1266*t*
    for diarrhea, 1036, 1037*t*
    for endometriosis, 1397
    for epilepsy, 1536-1537
    for erectile dysfunction, 1435
    errors by older adults, 80, 81*t*
    ethnic differences in response to, 34, 35*t*
    food-drug interactions, 953, 954*t*
    for fractures, 1641
    for gallbladder disease, 1129-1130
    for gastroesophageal reflux disease, 1005-1006, 1006*t*
    for gastrointestinal bleeding, 997, 998*t*
    for genital herpes, 1375
    goitrogens, 1298, 1298*t*
    for gonorrhea, 1368-1369
    for gout, 1716
    for growth hormone excess, 1292
    for headache, 1530-1531
    for healing, 202*t*
    for heart failure, 831*t*
    for hepatitis, 1093-1095
    hepatotoxicity of, 933-934, 934*t*
    for HIV infection, 256-257, 257*t*
    for hyperlipidemia, 793, 795*t*
    for hypertension, 771-776, 773*t*-776*t*
    for hyperthyroidism, 1301
    immunosuppressive, 239*t*
    for increased ICP, 1474-1475
    for infective endocarditis, 868, 869*t*
    for infertility, 1383, 1383*t*
    for inflammation, 202, 202*t*

Drug therapy *(Continued)*
    for inflammatory bowel disease, 1053-1054, 1055*t*
    injecting, 168*t*
    for intermittent claudication, 902
    for interstitial cystitis/painful bladder syndrome, 1163-1164
    for iron-deficiency anemia, 690-691
    for leukemia, 720-721, 720*t*, 721*t*
    mast cell–stabilizing, 231
    for multiple sclerosis, 1544-1545, 1544*t*-1545*t*
    for myasthenia gravis, 1556
    for nausea and vomiting, 992
    nephrotoxic agents, 1142, 1142*t*
    nutrient absorption–blocking drugs, 981-982
    for obesity, 981-982
    for opportunistic diseases, 257
    oral anticoagulants interactions, 914*t*
    for osteoarthritis, 1696-1697
    for osteoporosis, 1689-1690
    for pain, 135-142
        side effects of, 135, 135*t*
    for Parkinson's disease, 1552*t*
    patient and family teaching guide for proper use of equipment, 263*t*
    patient teaching related to, 772-776
    for peptic ulcer disease, 1019-1021, 1019*t*
    for perimenopause and postmenopause, 1391-1392
    for peripheral arterial disease of lower extremities, 902
    photosensitivity, 461-462
    platinum drugs, 287*t*
    for pneumonia, 566-567
    for premenstrual syndrome, 1386
    to prevent stroke, 1510
    for prostate cancer, 1426-1427
    for rheumatoid arthritis, 1705-1706
    risk reduction rules for, 262
    for seizure disorders and epilepsy, 1536-1537, 1538*t*
    for shock, 1785-1786, 1787*t*-1788*t*
    side effects of, 266-267
    snorting, 168*t*
    for spinal cord injury, 1596-1597
    for stroke, 1512
    for syphilis, 1371, 1371*t*
    for systemic lupus erythematosus, 1719
    for systemic sclerosis, 1724
    targeted therapy, **302-304,** 303*t*
    for tetanus, 1588-1589
    that cause anaphylactic shock, 227*t*
    that may cause photosensitivity, 461*t*
    for tuberculosis, 571-572, 573*t*
    for upper gastrointestinal bleeding, 997
    for urinary incontinence, 1182
    for urinary retention, 1185
    for UTIs, 1157-1158
    for voiding dysfunction, 1185*t*
Drug-eluting stents, 802
Drug-induced hepatitis, 1099-1100
Dry chest drainage systems, 591*t*
Dry desquamation, 299, 299*f*
Dry drowning, 1832
Dry excretion tests, 946*t*
Dry eyes, 406*t*, 424, 1726
Dry mouth, 1726
Dry powder inhalers, 617, 620*f*, 623, 623*f*, 623*t*
    advantages over MDIs, 623
    patient and family teaching guide for, 623*t*

Dry suction system, 591*t*
Drysol (aluminum chloride), 476
DSHEA. *See* Dietary Supplement
    Health and Education Act of 1994
DTIC, 288*t*
DTIC-Dome (dacarbazine), 287*t*
DTIs. *See* Direct thrombin inhibitors
DTPs. *See* Directives to physicians
Dual-energy x-ray absorptiometry,
    1625*t*
Duchenne muscular dystrophy,
    1675*b*, 1675*t*
Ducon, 1020*t*
Ductal carcinoma in situ, 1350
Ductal ectasia, 1345*t*, 1347
Ducts, 1324
Ductus deferens, 1324, 1325*f*
Duetact (pioglitazone and glimepiride),
    1266*t*
Dulcolax (bisacodyl)
    for constipation, 1042*t*
    for opioid-induced constipation, 138
Dullness, 524*t*, 937
Duloxetine (Cymbalta), 130
Dumping syndrome
    postgastrectomy, 1027*t*
    postoperative, 1026
Duodenal bleeding, 996
Duodenal switch, 982*t*, 983*f*, 984
Duodenal ulcers, 1015, 1015*t*
    complications of, 1017-1018, 1017*f*
    etiology and pathophysiology of,
        1017
Duodenum, 1015, 1015*f*
DuoDerm, 204, 205*t*
DuoNeb (ipratropium and albuterol)
    for asthma and COPD, 620*t*
    for COPD, 640
Duplex scanning
    in deep vein thrombosis, 911*t*
    venous Doppler, 1627*t*
Duprimine (D-penicillamine), 1724
Dura mater, 1452
Durable power of attorney for health
    care, 155, 156*t*, 655*b*
Duraclon (clonidine), 139*t*
Duragesic (fentanyl)
    drug alert, 141
    for pain, 137*t*, 141
Duramorph (morphine), 800*t*
Dutasteride (Avodart)
    for benign prostatic hyperplasia,
        1417
    for voiding dysfunction, 1185*t*
DVT. *See* Deep vein thrombosis
Dyazide (triamterene/hydrochlorothia-
    zide), 777*t*
DynaCirc CR (isradipine), 776*t*
Dynamic response test (square wave
    test), 1739-1740, 1741*f*
Dyphylline (Lufyllin), 954*t*
Dyrenium (triamterene)
    for cirrhosis, 1110*t*
    for hypertension, 773*t*
Dysarthria, 1460*t*
    after stroke, 1508
Dysfunctional grief, 154
Dyskinesia, 1460*t*
Dyslipidemia, 1211
Dysmenorrhea, 1386-1387
    clinical manifestations of, 1386
    collaborative care for, 1387

Dysmenorrhea *(Continued)*
    etiology and pathophysiology of,
        1386
    nursing management of, **1387**
    primary, 1386
    secondary, 1386
Dyspareunia, 1334
    in perimenopause and postmeno-
        pause, 1391
Dyspepsia, 939*t*
    in gastroesophageal reflux disease,
        1004
    in stomach cancer, 1028
Dysphagia, 939*t*, 1460*t*
    at end of life, 160*t*
    in oral cancer, 1001
Dysphasia, 1460*t*
    fluent, 1508
    nonfluent, 1508
    after stroke, 1508
Dysphoria, premenstrual, 1385
Dysplastic nevus, 464*t*, **466**
    case study, 481
Dyspnea, 512, 519*t*, 745*t*
    assessment of, 520, 520*f*
    in chronic HF, 825
    at end of life, 160*t*
    paroxysmal nocturnal, 746, 825
Dysreflexia, autonomic, 1603-1604
Dysrhythmias, 842-864, 1246*t*
    case study, 863
    causes of, 847*t*
    characteristics of, 849*t*
    electrophysiologic mechanisms of,
        846-847
    emergency management of, 848*t*
    evaluation of, 847-849
    in heart failure, 826
    identification and treatment of, **842-
        861**
    junctional, 849*t*, 852-853
    in myocardial infarction, 804
    postoperative, 382
    types of, 849-856
Dyssynergia, 1604
Dystonia, 1458
Dysuria, 1145*t*

E
EACA (epsilon aminocaproic acid),
    709
Ear(s)
    in allergies, 229*t*
    external, 408*f*
        age-related changes in, 410*t*
        assessment abnormalities, 413*t*
        malignancy of, **439**
        physical examination of, 412
        problems of, **438-439**
        trauma to, **438**
    inner, 408*f*, 409
        age-related changes in, 410*t*
        problems of, **441-445**
    middle, 408*f*, 409
        age-related changes in, 410*t*
        problems of, **439-441**
    physical examination of, 49*t*, 51*t*
    protection for, 444*b*
    sebaceous cysts behind, 413*t*
Ear surgery, 440*t*
Eardrum, retracted, 413*t*
Early Lung Cancer Action Project, 581-
    582
Eating difficulties
    in Alzheimer's disease, 1573-1574
    assistive devices for, 1522, 1522*f*
Eating disorders, 968-969
    resources for, 970

EBCT. *See* Electron-beam computed to-
    mography
Ebola virus, 245*t*
EBP. *See* Evidence-based practice
Ecchymosis, 457*t*, 675*t*, 677, 702
    with fractures, 1637*t*
    in hemophilia, 707, 708*f*
    postauricular, 1481, 1482*f*
    variations in light- and dark-skinned
        individuals, 456*t*
Eccrine sweat glands, 451
ECF. *See* Extracellular fluid
ECG. *See* Electrocardiography
Echinacea, 102*t*, 103*f*, 536*b*
Echocardiography, 753*t*-754*t*, **757-758,**
    757*f*
    contrast, 758
    M-mode, 757
    pharmacologic, 754*t*
    transesophageal, 754*t*, 758
    two-dimensional (2-D), 757
    types, 757
Echoviruses, 244*t*
ECMO. *See* Extracorporeal membrane
    oxygenation
Economic factors, cultural, 31*t*
"Ecstasy," 170*t*, 181
Ectocervix, 1326
Ectoderm, 279
Ectopic focus, 846
Ectopic pregnancy, 1389-1390
    clinical manifestations of,
        1389
    diagnostic studies, 1389-1390
    etiology and pathophysiology of,
        1389
    nursing and collaborative manage-
        ment of, **1390**
    sites of implantation, 1389,
        1389*f*
Ectropion, 406*t*
Eczema, 227, 227*f*
ED. *See* Erectile dysfunction
Edecrin (ethacrynic acid), 1267*t*
Edema, 318, 1246*t*
    in acute decompensated heart failure,
        825
    in acute respiratory distress syn-
        drome, 1812, 1813*f*
    alveolar, 598
    assessment of, 323
    cerebral, **1469-1470**
    in chronic HF, 826
    formation of, 1812, 1813*f*
    with fractures, 1637*t*
    after frostbite, 1830, 1830*f*
    heat edema, 1828
    interstitial, 598, 825
    laryngeal, 379*t*
    lymphedema, 1352, 1352*f*
    myxedema, 1246*t*, 1305, 1305*f*
    peripheral, with cirrhosis, 1104
    pitting, 749*t*, 826
    pulmonary, **597-598**
        in acute decompensated heart fail-
            ure, 824, 825*f*
        chest examination findings in,
            526*t*
        collaborative care for, 827*t*
        delayed, 1833
        nursing and collaborative manage-
            ment of, **827-829**
        in postanesthesia care unit, 378
        postoperative, 379*t*
Edematous pancreatitis, 1119
Edrophonium (Tensilon), 370, 1556

Education, 22. *See also* Patient
    education
    group-based programs, 1259*b*
    pain, **147**
    patient and family teaching, **53-66**
    about STDs, 1378
Educational assessment, 30*t*, 57*t*
EEG. *See* Electroencephalography
Efavirenz (Sustiva)
    adverse effects of, 258*t*
    drug alert, 257
    tenovir, emtricitabine, and efavirenz
        (Atripla), 258*t*
Effexor (venlafaxine), 130
Effleurage, 104, 104*f*
Effusion
    exudative, 595
    otitis media with, **440**
    pericardial, 872, 873*f*
    pleural, 512, 588, **595-596**
        chest examination findings in,
            526*t*
        in heart failure, 826
        in pneumonia, 565
        in restrictive lung disease, 596*t*
        in tuberculosis, 571
EGD. *See* Esophagogastro-
    duodenoscopy
Egophony, 525*t*
EHRs. *See* Electronic health records
EIA. *See* Exercise-induced asthma
Eicosapentaenoic aicd, 792
E-ICUs. *See* Electronic intensive care
    units
Ejaculation, 1324, 1330
    retrograde, 1422
Ejection fraction, 757, 822
Elastic recoil, 512
Elavil (amitriptyline)
    adverse cardiovascular effects of,
        745*t*
    for Alzheimer's disease, 1569*t*
    for depression, 1551
    effects of, 130
    food/nutrient interactions, 954*t*
    for interstitial cystitis/painful bladder
        syndrome, 1164
    local, 139*t*
    photosensitivity, 461*t*
    for premenstrual dysphoric disorder,
        1386
    for voiding dysfunction, 1185*t*
Elbow and shoulder arthroplasty,
    1664
Eldepryl (selegiline)
    food/nutrient interactions, 954*t*
    for Parkinson's disease, 1551,
        1552*t*
Elder mistreatment/abuse, 73-74
    institutional, 74
    nursing management of, 74, 74*t*
    resources for, 84
    risk factors for, 74
    types of, 73, 73*t*
Elder neglect, 73
Elderly. *See also* Older adults
    frail elderly, 67, 71
Elective surgery
    cosmetic procedures, 479-480
    phlebotomy, 734
    withholding fluids before, 353*b*
Electrical burns, 485-486, 485*f*
    emergency management of, 490*t*
    risk reduction strategies, 484*t*
Electrical stimulation for urinary
    incontinence, 1183*t*

Note: Disorder names are in **bold face.**
Page numbers in **bold face** indicate main
discussions. Page numbers followed by
f, t, b, or *n* indicate figures, tables, boxed
material, or notes, respectively.

Electrocardiography, 741-742, 753t, **756-757**, 843-846
in acute coronary syndrome, **861-862**, 861f, 861t
ambulatory monitoring, 753t, 757
in anterolateral wall myocardial infarction, 862, 862f
artifacts, 844-846, 846f
heart rate determination from, 843-844, 845f
in injury and infarction, 862, 862f
intervals, 846, 847t
in ischemia, 861, 862f
lead placement, 843, 845f
leads, 843, 845f
monitoring guidelines for acute coronary syndrome, 862
normal pattern, 741, 742f
normal sinus rhythm, 843, 844f, 846, 846f
in potassium imbalances, 327-328, 328f
preoperative, 351
recording leads, 843, 844f
signal-averaged, 848-849
time and voltage on, 843, 845f
12-lead, 843, 844f
in unstable angina and myocardial infarction, 805
waveforms, 846, 847t
Electrocautery, 1179
Electrocoagulation, 476
Electrodessication, 476
Electroencephalography, 1463t, 1464, 1465f
Electrographic nervous system studies, 1463t, 1464-1465
Electrohydraulic lithotripsy, 1172
Electrolyte balance
effects of stress on, 320, 320f
in increased ICP, 1478-1479
preoperative review, 349
Electrolyte imbalances, 321-340
assessment abnormalities in, 338t
assessment of, **337-338**
case study, 340
in chronic kidney disease, 1207
Electrolyte replacement
intravenous, **338-340**
oral, **338**
Electrolyte shifts, in burns, 488
Electrolyte solutions, 339t
Electrolytes, **315-316**
composition of fluid compartments, 316, 316f
daily requirements, 965
definition of, 316t
gerontologic considerations for, **321**
measurement of, 315-316
mechanisms controlling movement of, **316-318**
in parenteral nutrition, 965
preoperative, 351
serum levels
normal values, 321t
in shock, 1775t
Electromyography, 1463t, 1464, 1627t
sphincter, 1150t
Electron-beam computed tomography, 755t, 758, 759f
Electronic health records, 8-9
Electronic intensive care units, 1734, 1734f
Electronystagmography, 414t
Electrophysiology studies
of dysrhythmia, 848
of heart, 755t, 759f
Electrosurgery, loop excision, 1340t

Electrovaporization, transurethral, of prostate, 1418t
Eletriptan (Relpax), 1530
Elevation, for soft tissue injuries, 203
Elevation pallor, 901
Eligard (leuprolide), 1426, 1426t
Elimination, 926, 930
home health care activities, 90t
after stroke, 1508
Elimination pattern
in assessment
of auditory system, 410t, 411, 746
of endocrine system, 1244
of fluid, electrolyte, and acid-base imbalances, 337
of gastrointestinal system, 934, 935t
of hematologic system, 673, 673t
of integumentary system, 453t, 454
of musculoskeletal system, 1621
of nervous system, 1454
of preoperative patient, 350t
of reproductive system, 1333, 1333t
of respiratory system, 518t, 519
of urinary system, 1142-1144, 1143t
of visual system, 403, 403t
comparison with NANDA International Taxonomy II, 42t
concerns of patients requiring home health care, 90t
and COPD, 650t
nursing diagnoses, **1852**
nursing history, 44-45, 45t
Elimination problems, 925-1134
in Alzheimer's disease, 1574
resources for, 970
Elixophyllin, 619t
Ellence (epirubicin)
for breast cancer, 1355
classification of, 287t
for prostate cancer, 1427
Elmiron (pentosan), 1164
Eloxatin (oxaliplatin)
classification of, 287t
for colorectal cancer, 1067
FOLFOX treatment regimen, 291, 291f
Elspar (L-asparaginase)
blood glucose level effects, 1267t
classification of, 288t
for leukemia, 720t
EM. *See* Elder mistreatment/abuse
EMB. *See* Endomyocardial biopsy
Embolic stroke, 1505f, 1506, 1506t
Embolism
fat embolism syndrome, 1651
in infective endocarditis, 866
pulmonary, **598-600**
nursing management of, **600**
pathophysiology of, 598, 598f
postoperative, 379t
Embryonic stem cells, 218
Emcyt (estramustine)
classification of, 288t
for prostate cancer, 1427
Emend (aprepitant), 297, 992t
Emergence, delayed, 387
Emergence delirium, 387
Emergency and disaster nursing, **1821-1844**
Emergency and mass casualty incident preparedness, **1842**

Emergency care, **1822-1828**
gerontologic considerations for, **1828**
intervention and evaluation, 1827
primary survey, 1823-1824, 1824t, 1825t
secondary survey, 1824-1827, 1826t
Emergency department
death in, 1827-1828
layout of, 360
Emergency management
of abdominal trauma, 1048, 1048t
of acute abdominal pain, 1044, 1045t
of acute soft tissue injury, 1632t
agents of terrorism, **1838-1842**
of amphetamine toxicity, 175, 175t
of anaphylactic shock, 230t
bites and stings, **1833-1837**
of chemical burns, 489t
of chest pain, 806t
of chest trauma, 586t
of cocaine toxicity, 175, 175t
cold-related emergencies, **1830-1831**
of depressant overdose, 179, 179t
of diabetic ketoacidosis, 1280t
of dysrhythmias, 848t
of electrical burns, 490t
environmental emergencies, **1828-1842**
of eye injury, 421t
of fractured extremity, 1642, 1642t
of head injury, 1484-1485, 1484t
heat-related emergencies, **1828-1830**
of hyperthermia, 1830t
of hypothermia, 1832t
of inhalation injury, 489t
oncologic emergencies, 307-308
preparedness, **1842**
of sexual assault, 1410t
of shock, 1783, 1785t
of spinal cord injury, 1596t
of stroke, 1511, 1511t
of submersion injuries, 1833t
of thermal burns, 490t
of thoracic injuries, 586t
of tonic-clonic seizures, 1536, 1537t
of upper gastrointestinal bleeding, 996
violence, **1838**
Emergency response plan, 1842
Emergency Severity Index (ESI), 1822, 1822t, 1823f
Emergency surgery, 343
Emergent percutaneous coronary intervention, 807
Emerging infection, 245
Emesis, **990**
Emete-Con (benzquinamide), 992t
EMG. *See* Electromyography
EMLA (eutectic mixture of local anesthetics), 139t, 141
Emmetropia, 399
Emotional reactions
in acute coronary syndrome, 814, 814t
and angina, 797t
atypical emotional responses, 1523
of burn patients, 505t
patient and family needs in burns, 505
Emotional stress. *See* Stress
Emotional support, in shock, 1793-1794
Emotion-focused coping, 116
Empacho, 35
Empathy, 56, 159

Emphysema, 608, 629
centrilobular, 632, 633f
panlobular, 632, 633f
Empyema, 512, 588, 596
in pneumonia, 565
in tuberculosis, 571
Emtricitabine (FTC, Emtriva)
adverse effects of, 258t
tenofovir and emtricitabine (Truvada), 258t
tenovir, emtricitabine, and efavirenz (Atripla), 258t
E-Mycin (erythromycin), 878
Enablex (darifenacin)
for urinary incontinence, 1182
for voiding dysfunction, 1185t
Enalapril (Vasotec)
for chronic HF, 832
for chronic stable angina and acute coronary syndrome, 800t
effects on lower urinary tract function, 1180t
for hypertension, 776t, 1210
Enalaprilat (Vasotec I.V.), 776t
Enalapril/diltiazem (Teczem), 777t
Enalapril/felodipine (Lexxel), 777t
Enalapril/hydrochlorothiazide (Vaseretic), 777t
Enbrel (etanercept)
for arthritis and connective tissue disorders, 1700t
clinical uses of, 223t
drug alert, 1706
for rheumatoid arthritis, 1706
Encapsulating sclerosing peritonitis, 1220
Encephalitis, 1494t, **1497-1498**
clinical manifestations of, 1498
diagnostic studies, 1498
etiology and pathophysiology of, 1497-1498
nursing and collaborative management of, **1498**
Encephalopathy
hepatic
acute intervention for, 1114
with cirrhosis, 1104-1106
collaborative care for, 1108-1109
factors precipitating, 1105, 1106t
grading scale for, 1106t
hypertensive, 781
Wernicke's, 177-178
End of life
definition of, 151
nursing assessment of, 157-158
nursing diagnoses, 158t
nursing implementation for, 158-162
nursing management of, **157-162**
physical manifestations at, **152-153**, 158t
psychosocial manifestations of, **153**, 158t
End stoma, 1069
Endarterectomy, 904
Endocarditis
bacterial, 865
infective, **865-871**
ocular manifestations of, 437t
in pneumonia, 565
rheumatic, 876, 876f
Endocardium, 740, 865
Endocervical gonorrhea, 1367-1368, 1368f
Endocervix, 1326
Endocet (oxycodone), 137t
Endochroma, 1673t

Endocrine glands, 1234, **1235**, 1235f
Endocrine hormones, **1235-1238**
  classification of, 1235
  functions of, 1235
  target tissues and functions, 1236t
Endocrine problems, 1290-1322
  with cirrhosis, 1103
  with dermatologic manifestations, 473t
  gender differences, 1299b
  resources, 1322
Endocrine system, **1234-1252**
  assessment abnormalities, 1246t-1247t
  assessment of, **1242-1246**
    gerontologic considerations for, **1242**
    gerontologic differences in, 1242t
    important health information for, 1243-1244
    key questions to ask, 1243t
    objective data, 1245-1246
    subjective data, 1243-1245
  autoimmune diseases of, 234t
  burn injury complications, 500-501
  in chronic kidney disease, 1209
  diagnostic studies, **1246-1250**
  effects of aging on, **1242**, 1242t
  effects of chronic alcohol abuse on, 177t
  functions of, **1235-1242**
  laboratory studies, **1246-1250**
  in multiple organ dysfunction syndrome, 1797t
  physical examination of, 1245-1246
  preoperative review, 348-349
  regulation of blood pressure by, 764
  response to stress, 113-114
  structures of, **1235-1242**
Endoderm, 279
End-of-life care, **151-164**, 159f
  culturally competent, **154-155**
  definition of, **151**
  documents in, 156t
  ethical dilemmas, 159b
  goals for, 151-152, 152f
  legal and ethical issues affecting, **155-156**
  legal documents used in, 155
  nursing diagnoses associated with, 158, 158t
  physical care, 160-162, 161t-162t
  planning for, 158
  psychosocial care, 160t
  resources, 164
  special needs of caregivers in, **161-162**
  variables affecting, **154**
Endolymphatic hydrops, 441-442
Endometrial biopsy, 1341t
Endometrial cancer, 1401-1402
  clinical manifestations of, 1401
  collaborative care for, 1402
  etiology and pathophysiology of, 1401
Endometrial cycle, 1329
Endometriosis, 1396-1398
  clinical manifestations of, 1396-1397
  collaborative care for, 1397, 1397t
  drug therapy for, 1397
  etiology and pathophysiology of, 1396

Endometriosis *(Continued)*
  nursing management of, **1397-1398**
  sites of, 1396, 1397f
  surgical therapy for, 1397
Endomyocardial biopsy, 875
Endomysium, 1617
Endophthalmitis, 436
Endorphins, 1445t
Endoscopic gastrostomy, percutaneous, 961, 962f
Endoscopic hemostasis, 997
Endoscopic retrograde cholangiopan-creatography, 943f, 944, 944t
Endoscopic sclerotherapy, 1108
Endoscopic sphincterotomy, 1128, 1129f
Endoscopic therapy
  for gastroesophageal reflux disease, 1006
  for upper gastrointestinal bleeding, 997
Endoscopic ultrasound, 941t, 944t
Endoscopy
  capsule, 943t, 945f, 946
  for esophageal cancer, 1010
  gastrointestinal studies, 943t-944t, 944-946
  musculoskeletal studies, 1625t
  respiratory studies, 528-529, 528t
  urinary studies, 1149t
Endothelial cell dysfunction, 766
Endothelial damage, 909, 910t
Endothelin, 764, 823
Endotracheal intubation, 1751
  in acute respiratory distress syndrome, 1816t
  complications of, 1759, 1816t
  fostering comfort and communication with, 1758-1759
  indications for, 1751
  maintaining cuff inflation, 1753
    minimal leak technique, 1753
    minimal occluding volume technique, 1753
  maintaining skin integrity, 1758
  maintaining tube patency, 1757-1758
  monitoring oxygenation and ventilation with, 1753-1757
  nasal, 1751
  oral, 1751
  oral care during, 1758
  procedure, 1752
  protocol for securing adhesive tape, 1753f
  tube placement, 1752-1753
Endotracheal tubes, 1751-1752, 1751f
Endoureterotomy, 1174
Endourologic procedures, 1171
Endovascular graft procedure, 896-897
Endovascular stent grafting, 896, 896f
End-stage heart failure, 837, 839t
End-stage renal disease (ESRD), 1204
  causes of, 1205, 1205f
End-tidal CO_2 partial pressure monitoring (PETCO$_2$), 1753-1754
Enduron (methyclothiazide), 773t
Enemas
  barium enema x-ray, 941f, 941t
  for constipation, 1042t
  for inflammatory bowel disease, 1055t
"Energy" beverages, 176
Energy conservation, 1701b
Energy expenditure, 816t
Energy field disturbance, 105
Energy therapies, 96t, 98t, **105**
Enflurane (Ethrane), 369t

Enfuvirtide (Fuzeon)
  adverse effects of, 258t
  drug alert, 257
Engerix-B (hepatitis B virus vaccine), 1096
Enhancing Motivation for Change in Substance Abuse Treatment, 188
Enkephalins, 1445t
Enoxaparin (Lovenox)
  for chronic stable angina and acute coronary syndrome, 800t
  for pulmonary embolism, 600
Entacapone (Comtan), 1551, 1552t
***Entamoeba histolytica* infection,** 1037t
Entecavir (Baraclude), 1094
  for chronic hepatitis B, 1095
Enteral nutrition
  gerontologic considerations for, **965**
  nursing care plan for patient receiving, 963b-964b
  placement locations for feeding tubes, 961, 961f
Enterobacter, 244t, 562t, 1155t
Enterococcus, 1155t
Enterococcus faecalis, 246, 246t
Enterococcus faecium, 246, 246t
Enterohemorrhagic *Escherichia coli* infection, 1037t
Entitlement to treatment, 1652b
Entocort (budesonide), 1055t
Entropion, 406t
Entry inhibitors
  adverse effects of, 258t
  mechanism of action, 257t
Enucleation, 437
Enuresis, 1145t
Environmental control
  noise control, 443-444
  secondary survey, 1824, 1826t
Environmental emergencies, 1828-1842
Environmental hazards, 460-462
Environmental lung diseases, 577-578, 578t
  clinical manifestations of, 577
  collaborative care for, 577-578
Environmental tobacco smoke, 185b, 631
Enzymatic debridement, 205, 501
EOL care. *See* End-of-life care
Eosinophils, 668
  function of, 668t
  laboratory values, 1860t
  response to injury, 195
EPA. *See* Eicosapentaenoic aicd
Ependymal cells, 1442
Ephedra (ma huang), 745t
Ephedrine
  dangers of, 624
  effects on lower urinary tract function, 1180t
Epicardial pacing, 859
Epidermis, 449-450, 486
Epidermophyton, 245t
Epididymis, 1324, 1325f
Epididymitis, 1430
  chlamydial, 1372, 1372f
Epidural analgesia
  for postoperative pain, 389
Epidural anesthesia, 371-372, 372f
Epidural hematoma, 1483, 1483f, 1871
Epifrin (epinephrine), 434t
Epilepsy, 1532-1542
  acute intervention for, 1539
  ambulatory and home care for, 1539-1541

Epilepsy *(Continued)*
  collaborative care for, 1536t
  complications of, 1535-1536
  diagnostic studies, 1536
  drug therapy for, 1538t
  etiology and pathophysiology of, 1533-1534
  health promotion in, 1538-1539
  nursing assessment of, 1538, 1539t
  nursing care plan for patient with, 1540b-1541b
  nursing diagnoses, 1538
  nursing implementation for, 1538-1541
  nursing management of, **1538-1542**
  nursing planning for, 1538
  patient and family teaching guide for, 1541f
  surgical procedures for, 1538t
  surgical therapy for, 1538
EpiMorph (morphine), 137t
Epimysium, 1617
Epinephrine (Adrenalin), 1445t
  for allergic disorders, 231
  for asthma and COPD, 619t
  blood glucose level effects, 1267t
  dangers of, 624
  for gastrointestinal bleeding, 997, 998t
  for glaucoma, 434t
  as positive inotrope, 1739
  for shock, 1787t
  target tissue and functions, 1236t
  urine levels, 1862t
Epiphyseal plate, 1616
Epiphysis, 1615
Epirubicin (Ellence)
  for breast cancer, 1355
  classification of, 287t
  for prostate cancer, 1427
Epispadias, 1429
Epistaxis, 534-535, 675t
  nursing and collaborative management of, **534-535**
Epithelial autografts, cultured, 498t, 501, 502f
Epithelial tissue, 198, 198t
Epitrate (epinephrine), 434t
Epivir (lamivudine)
  adverse effects of, 258t
  for chronic hepatitis B, 1094
  drug alert, 1094
Epizicom (lamivudine and abacavir), 258t
Eplerenone (Inspra)
  for hyperaldosteronism, 1319
  for hypertension, 773t
Epoetin alfa (Epogen, Procrit)
  for anemia, 1211
  for cancer treatment, 304t
  clinical uses of, 223t
Epoprostenol (Flolan), 601-602, 601f
Eprosartan (Teveten), 776t
Eprosartan/hydrochlorothiazide (Teveten HCT), 777t
EPS. *See* Electrophysiology studies
Epsilon aminocaproic acid (EACA, Amicar), 709
Epstein-Barr virus, 244t
Eptifibatide (Integrelin), 800t
Equipment. *See also specific instruments*
  for physical examination, 48
  for screening physical examination, 48t

Note: Disorder names are in **bold face.** Page numbers in **bold face** indicate main discussions. Page numbers followed by *f, t, b,* or *n* indicate figures, tables, boxed material, or notes, respectively.

Erb muscular dystrophy, 1675*t*
Erbitux (cetuximab), 303*t*, 1067
Erb's point, 748, 748*f*
ERCP. *See* Endoscopic retrograde cholangiopancreatography
Erectile dysfunction, 1434-1437
clinical manifestations of, 1435
collaborative care for, 1435-1436,
1435*t*
complications of, 1435
diagnostic studies, 1435
etiology and pathophysiology of,
1434
medicated urethral system for, 1435,
1436*f*
nursing management of, **1437**
oral drug therapy for, 1435
physiologic, 1434
psychologic, 1434
risk factors for, 1434*t*
self-injection therapy for, 1435, 1436*f*
sexual counseling for, 1436
treatments for, 1607
Ergamisol (levamisole), 303*t*, 1067
Ergocalciferol (Calciferol), 1311
Erlotinib (Tarceva), 303*t*, 1126
Erosions, 1336*t*
Eructation, 939*t*
ERV. *See* Expiratory reserve volume
Erwinia asparaginase, 288*t*
Erysipelas, 467*t*
Erythema, 457*t*
penile or scrotal, 1336*t*
radiation-induced, 299, 299*f*
variations in light- and dark-skinned
individuals, 456*t*
vulvar, 1335*t*
Erythema marginatum, 876
Erythema migrans, 1714, 1714*f*
Erythrocyte sedimentation rate, 678-
679, 680*t*, 1626*t*
effects of aging on, 672*t*
laboratory values, 1859*t*
Erythrocytes, 666*f*, 667, 667*f*
anemia caused by decreased number
of precursors of, 685*t*
anemia caused by decreased production of, 685*t*, **687-694**
anemia caused by increased destruction of, 685*t*, **695-701**
laboratory values, 1859*t*
Erythroleukemia, 691, 692*t*
Erythromelalgia, 700
Erythromycin (E-Mycin)
for chlamydial infections, 1373
for rheumatic fever, 878
Erythroplakia, 551
Erythroplasia, 1001
Erythropoiesis, 667, 688, 689*t*
Erythropoietin, 667, 680*t*
for anemia, 1211
for cancer treatment, 304*t*
clinical uses of, 223*t*
effects of aging on, 672*t*
function of, 222*t*
Eschar, 204, 487-488
Escharotomy, 491, 492*f*
Escherichia coli, O157:H7, 245*t*, 246*t*,
562*t*, 1155*t*
diseases caused by, 244*t*
food poisoning, 1031, 1032*t*,
1037*t*
in UTIs, 1156
Esidrix (hydrochlorothiazide), 773*t*
Esimil (guanethine/hydrochlorothia-
zide), 777*t*

Esmolol (Brevibloc)
for aortic dissection, 899
for chronic stable angina and acute
coronary syndrome, 800*t*
classification of, 856*t*
for hypertension, 774*t*
Esomeprazole (Nexium)
for gastroesophageal reflux disease,
1006, 1006*t*
for gastrointestinal bleeding, 998*t*
for peptic ulcer disease, 1019*t*, 1020
Esophageal achalasia, 1012-1013, 1012*f*
Esophageal cancer, 1009-1011
acute intervention for, 1011
ambulatory and home care for, 1011
clinical manifestations of, 1009
collaborative care for, 1010, 1010*t*
complications of, 1009
diagnostic studies, 1009-1010
etiology and pathophysiology of,
1009
health promotion in, 1011
nursing assessment of, 1010
nursing diagnoses, 1010-1011
nursing evaluation of, 1011
nursing implementation for, 1011
nursing management of, **1010-1011**
nursing planning for, 1011
nutritional therapy of, 1010
postoperative care, 1011
preoperative care, 1011
Esophageal disorders, 1011-1013
Esophageal diverticulum(a), 1011-1012
sites for, 1011, 1012*f*
Esophageal endoscopic ultrasound, 941*t*
Esophageal speech, 557
Esophageal strictures, 1012
in gastroesophageal reflux disease,
1004
sites for, 1012
Esophageal tamponade, 1108, 1109*f*
Esophageal ulcerations, 1004, 1004*f*
Esophageal varices, 1013
with cirrhosis, 1103-1104
collaborative care for, 1107-1110
long-term management of, 1108
Esophagectomy, 1010
Esophagitis
associated with HIV infection, 254*t*
in chemotherapy and radiation therapy, 295*t*
with esophageal ulcerations, 1004,
1004*f*
Esophagoenterostomy, 934*t*, 1010
Esophagogastro-duodenoscopy, 943*t*
Esophagogastrostomy, 1010
Esophagus
age-related changes in, 932, 933*t*
assessment abnormalities, 939*t*
bleeding from, 995
cultural and ethnic health disparities
in problems of, 1001*t*
ingestion propulsion of food by, 928
Esotropia, 424
ESR. *See* Erythrocyte sedimentation
rate
ESRD. *See* End-stage renal disease
Essential fatty acids, deficiency of, 473*t*
Essential Nursing Competencies and
Curricula Guidelines for Genetics
and Genomics, 242
Estradiol (Estrace)
classification of, 288*t*
serum levels, 1338*t*
for voiding dysfunction, 1185*t*
Estramustine (Emcyt)
classification of, 288*t*
for prostate cancer, 1427

Estring (estrogen vaginal ring), 1185*t*
Estrogen (Premarin)
classification of, 288*t*
for perimenopause and postmenopause, 1391
for prostate cancer, 1426-1427, 1426*t*
target tissue and functions, 1236*t*
unopposed, 1388
urine levels, 1862*t*
for vaginal atrophy, 1391*b*
for voiding dysfunction, 1185*t*
Estrogen + progestin (Ortho-Novum,
Prempro), 745*t*
Estrogen deficiency, 1390*t*
Estrogen replacement therapy, 1689
ESWL. *See* Extracorporeal shock-wave
lithotripsy
ET intubation. *See* Endotracheal intubation
Etanercept (Enbrel)
for arthritis and connective tissue disorders, 1700*t*
clinical uses of, 223*t*
drug alert, 1706
for rheumatoid arthritis, 1706
Ethacrynic acid (Edecrin)
blood glucose level effects, 1267*t*
for hypertension, 773*t*
Ethambutol (Myambutol), 573*t*, 574*t*
Ethanol
percutaneous injection for liver cancer, 1117
toxicology, 1865*t*
Ethanolamines, 537*t*
Ethical dilemmas
abortion, 1385*b*
advance directives, 637*b*
allocation of resources, 1226*b*
alternative healers, 1309*b*
brain death, 1485*b*
competence, 830*b*
confidentiality, 1378*b*
do not resuscitate, 882*b*
durable power of attorney for health
care, 655*b*
end-of-life care, 159*b*
entitlement to treatment, 1652*b*
genetic testing, 218*b*
guardianship, 1009*b*
health disparities, 22*b*
impaired health care providers, 174*b*
individual vs. public health protection, 256*b*
informed consent, 353*b*
justice, 809*b*
medical futility, 309*b*
pain management, 698*b*
patient adherence, 575*b*
payment for organs, 1225*b*
rationing, 1115*b*
religious interest, 730*b*
sterilization, 1433*b*
withdrawing treatment, 1230*b*
withholding treatment, 1492*b*
Ethical issues
affecting end-of-life care, **155-156**
for older adults, **77**
in pain management, **147**
Ethionamide (Trecator), 573*t*
Ethmozine (moricizine), 856*t*
Ethnic differences. *See also* Cultural
and ethnic health disparities
and coronary artery disease, 787-788
in response to drugs, 34, 35*t*
and treatment outcome in hepatitis C,
1095*b*
Ethnic identity, 72
Ethnic older adults, 72, 72*f*, 72*t*

Ethnicity, 28, 28*f*
Ethnocentrism, 28
Ethno-geriatrics, 72
Ethosuximide (Zarontin), 1536, 1538*t*
Ethrane (enflurane), 369*t*
Ethylene glycol poisoning, 1142*t*,
1837*t*
Ethylenediamines, 537*t*
Etidronate (Didronel)
food/nutrient interactions, 954*t*
for osteoporosis, 1689
for Paget's disease, 1690
Etomidate (Amidate), 369*t*
Etoposide (VePesid)
classification of, 287*t*
for leukemia, 720*t*, 721*t*
for lung cancer, 582
for non-Hodgkin's lymphoma, 727*t*
for testicular cancer, 1432
ETS. *See* Environmental tobacco smoke
Eulexin (flutamide)
for hyperandrogenism, 1399
for prostate cancer, 1426, 1426*t*
Eutectic mixture of local anesthetics
(EMLA), 139*t*, 141, 371
Evaluation of nursing care
for older adults, 82, 82*t*
phase of, 9, **15**
Evaluation of patient education, 63-64
short-term techniques, 63-64
written measurement tools, 64
Evening primrose, 102*t*
Event monitors, 848
Eversion, 1622*t*
Evidence-based practice, 5-7
acetaminophen or NSAIDs for osteoarthritis, 1697*b*
acute low back pain and physical activity, 1681*b*
cardiac rehabilitation programs, 794*b*
dietary salt reduction and blood pressure, 780*b*
ethnicity and treatment outcome in
hepatitis C, 1095*b*
exercise effects on quality of life in
multiple sclerosis, 1547*b*
exercise programs for stroke patients,
1514*b*
group-based educational programs
and health of diabetic patients,
1259*b*
implementation of, 7
increasing participation in breast cancer screenings, 1359*b*
invasive screening for ovarian cancer,
1403*b*
localized estrogen preparations and
vaginal atrophy, 1391*b*
male condom breakage during intercourse, 1373*b*
managing stable COPD, 639*b*
music effects on confusion and delirium in surgical patients, 1577*b*
nicotine replacement therapy to assist
with smoking cessation, 172*b*
noninvasive interventions and quality
of life in lung cancer, 583*b*
noninvasive physical treatments for
chronic headache, 1531*b*
patient discharge education and clinical outcomes in chronic HF,
830*b*
physical training and respiratory and
general health in persons with
asthma, 609*b*
PICO format for questions, 6, 6*t*

Evidence-based practice (Continued)
  postoperative analgesia, 389b
  preventing deep vein thrombosis, 912b
  process of, 6-7, 6f, 6t, 7t
  prophylactic antibiotics for recurrent UTIs, 1158b
  psychologic interventions for helping overweight individuals lose weight, 981b
  reducing risk factors for COPD, 640b
  Retin-A effectiveness for sun-damaged skin, 463b
  self-management program for irritable bowel syndrome, 1047b
  sexuality after spinal cord injury, 1607b
  stress management strategies for Crohn's disease, 1054b
  therapy for urinary incontinence after radical prostatectomy, 1425b
  therapy of basal cell carcinoma, 465b
  weight loss interventions and prediabetes, 1257b
  weight-bearing exercise for hip fracture patients, 1655b
  when to start nutritional support for head injury, 1475b
  withholding fluids before elective surgery, 353b
Evista (raloxifene)
  for breast cancer, 1355
  classification of, 288t
  for osteoporosis, 1689-1690
  for perimenopause and postmenopause, 1392
Evoked potentials, 1463t, 1464-1465
Evoxac (cevimeline), 1726
Ewing's sarcoma, 1673t
ExAblate 2000 system, 1399
Excision
  of burns, 493t, 501
  for dermatologic problems, 476-477
Excisional biopsy, 283, 458t
Excitability, 842, 843t, 846-847, 1442
Excoriations, 455t, 675t
Exelon (rivastigmine)
  for Alzheimer's disease, 1551, 1569t
  for Parkinson's dementia, 1551
Exemestane (Aromasin)
  for breast cancer, 1355
  classification of, 288t
Exenatide (Byetta)
  for diabetes mellitus, 1265-1266, 1266t
  mechanisms of action, 1266
Exercise. See also Activity-exercise pattern
  activities that affect caloric expenditure, 1269, 1269t
  and asthma attacks, 608
  back exercises, 1677t
  breathing exercises, 646
  for constipation, 1044t
  for diabetes mellitus, 1269, 1269t, 1277t
  after mastectomy or lumpectomy with axillary lymph node dissection, 1359, 1360f
  neck exercises, 1684t
  for obesity, 980
  for osteoarthritis, 1696

Exercise (Continued)
  for pain, 143-144
  pelvic floor muscle (Kegel) exercises, 1183t, 1184f
  for peripheral arterial disease, 902-903
  postoperative leg exercises, 387, 387f
  and quality of life in multiple sclerosis, 1547b
  for rheumatoid arthritis, 1710-1711
  and skin, 462
  as stress management, 116t
  for stroke patients, 1514b
  for urinary incontinence, 1183t
  weight-bearing, for hip fracture patients, 1655b
Exercise nuclear imaging, 754t
Exercise testing, 530-531, 757
  stress test, 801
  treadmill test, 753t, 849
Exercise-induced asthma, 608
Exhaustion
  heat exhaustion, 1829, 1830t
  stage of, 112, 112f, 112t
Exit site infection, 1219
Ex-Lax (phenolphthalein), 1042t
Exna (benzthiazide), 773t
Exocrine glands, 1235
Exophthalmos, 404, 406t, 1246t
  of Graves' disease, 1298f, 1299
Exostosis, 413t
Exotropia, 424
Expiration, 512
Expiratory reserve volume (ERV), 531t
Exploratory surgery, 343
Exploratory thoracotomy, 593t
Explosive devices, 1840-1842
Exposure/environmental control, 1824, 1826t
Expressive aphasia, 1508
Extension, 1622, 1622t
Extensor plantar response, 1460t
External beam radiation, 293, 1425
External ear and canal, 408-409, 408f
  age-related changes in, 410t
  assessment abnormalities, 413t
  cerumen in, 438-439
  foreign bodies in, 438-439
  malignancy of, 439
  physical examination of, 412
  problems, 438-439
  trauma to, 438
External fixators, 1641, 1641f
External genitalia
  female, 1326-1327, 1326f
    normal physical assessment of, 1335t
    physical examination of, 49t, 51t, 1335
  male, 1324
    normal physical assessment of, 1335t
    physical examination of, 49t, 51t
External otitis, 438
  clinical manifestations of, 438
  collaborative care for, 438t
  complications of, 438
  etiology of, 438
  malignant, 438
  nursing management of, 438
External rewarming
  active, 1831
  passive, 1831
External rotation, 1622t
Extracellular fluid, 315
  differential assessment of, 324, 324f
  movement between intracellular fluid and, 319

Extracellular fluid volume imbalances, 321-324
  causes and clinical manifestations of, 322t
  deficit, 322
    causes and clinical manifestations of, 322t
    hypernatremia with, 325t
    hyponatremia with, 325t
    nursing diagnoses, 322
  excess, 322
    causes and clinical manifestations of, 322t
    hypernatremia with, 325t
    hyponatremia with, 325t
    nursing diagnoses, 322
  nursing diagnoses, 322
  nursing implementation for, 322-324
  nursing management of, 322-324
  nursing measures for, 324
  sodium imbalances associated with, 324, 325f
Extracorporeal membrane oxygenation, 1763
Extracorporeal shock-wave lithotripsy, 1172
Extracranial artery atherosclerosis, 1504, 1505f
Extraocular disorders, 422-425
Extraocular inflammation and infection, 422-424
  acute intervention for, 424
  ambulatory and home care for, 424
  health promotion in, 424
  nursing assessment of, 424
  nursing diagnoses, 424
  nursing evaluation of, 424
  nursing implementation for, 424
  nursing management of, 424
  nursing planning for, 424
Extraocular muscles, 400
  assessment abnormalities, 406t
  function testing, 405
Extravasation injury, 286, 288f
Extremities
  assessment abnormalities, 749t
  color changes with postural change, 749t
  fractured, 1642, 1642t
  lower
    atherosclerotic lesions of, 893, 893f
    bandaging for above-the-knee amputation residual limb, 1660, 1661f
    casts for injuries to, 1640-1641
    complications in diabetes mellitus, 1286-1287
    eczema of, 227, 227f
    peripheral arterial disease of, 900-907
    pitting edema of, 749t
    sites of amputation, 1658-1659, 1659f
  physical examination of, 1246
    adaptations, 50t
    completion of, 49t
    outline for, 49t
  secondary survey head-to-toe assessment, 1826t, 1827
  upper limb amputation
    sites of, 1658-1659, 1659f
    special considerations for, 1661-1662
Extubation, 1759, 1766-1768
Exudate
  formation of, 196
  types of, 196, 197t

Exudative effusion, 595
Exuderm, 205t
Eye(s), 398-399, 399f
  in allergies, 229t
  in anemia, 686t
  assessment abnormalities, 675t, 1460t
  autoimmune diseases of, 234t
  external, 400, 400f
  herpes simplex virus infection of, 1374
  HIV infection of, 259t
  infections in newborns, 1368
  internal structures and functions, 400-402
  patient and family teaching guide for after surgery, 428t
  physical examination of, 49t, 51t
  recommendations for isolation precautions, 248t
Eye care, 420b
Eye trauma, 421-422
  emergency management of, 421t
Eyeball, 398-399, 399f
Eyebrows, 400
  age-related changes in, 401t
  assessment of, 407
Eyelashes, 400
  age-related changes in, 401t
  assessment of, 407
Eyelid-lifts, 480
Eyelids, 400
  age-related changes in, 401t
  assessment abnormalities, 406t
  assessment of, 407
Ezetimibe (Zetia), 794, 795t
Ezetimibe/simvastatin (Vytorin), 794

F
Face masks, simple, 641t, 642f
Face shields, 248t
Face tents, 641t, 642f
Face-lift, 479-480, 480f
Facial fractures, 1656-1658, 1657t
Facial nerve (cranial nerve VII), 1450t
Facial nerve (cranial nerve VII) testing, 1457
Facilitated diffusion, 317
Facilitators, 61, 61f
Factor assays, 709t
Factor I. See Fibrinogen
Factor II. See Prothrombin
Factor III. See Thromboplastin
Factor IV. See Calcium
Factor V, 670t, 672t
Factor VI, 670t
Factor VII, 670t, 672t
Factor VIII, 670t, 672t, 709t
Factor IX, 670t, 672t, 709t
Factor X, 670t
Factor Xa inhibitors, 913t, 914
Factor XI, 670t
Factor XII, 670t
Factor XIII, 670t
FAD. See Familial Alzheimer's disease
Fad diets, 979, 979t
Fallopian tubes, 1325
Falls
  acute soft tissue injury, 1631, 1632t
  fractured extremity, 1642, 1642t
  head injury, 1484t
  spinal cord injury, 1596t
Falx cerebri, 1452, 1472
Famciclovir (Famvir)
  for Bell's palsy, 1585
  for genital herpes, 1375
Familial adenomatous polyposis, 1063b

Note: Disorder names are in **bold face**. Page numbers in **bold face** indicate main discussions. Page numbers followed by f, t, b, or n indicate figures, tables, boxed material, or notes, respectively.

Familial Alzheimer's disease, 1565
Familial hypercholesterolemia, 788b
Families
facilitating presence of, 1825, 1826t
roles and relationships of, 32-33, 33f
Family coping
with burn patients, 505
compromised, 121
critical care issues, 1737-1738
in end-of-life care, 161-162
patient and family teaching, **53-66**
with shock patient, 1794
after stroke, 1523
support groups for, 1575, 1575f
teaching guide for Alzheimer's disease, 1574t
Family history, 788
Family support, 57
facilitating, 1824-1825
Famotidine (Pepcid)
for gastroesophageal reflux disease, 1005-1006, 1006t
for gastrointestinal bleeding, 998t
for peptic ulcer disease, 1019t
preoperative, 355t
Famvir (famciclovir), 1375
Fareston (toremifene)
for breast cancer, 1355
classification of, 288t
Farmer's lung, 578t
Farsightedness, 416, 417. See also Hyperopia
Fascia, 1618
Fasciculations, 338, 1245
Fasciculi, 1617
Faslodex (fulvestrant)
for breast cancer, 1355
classification of, 288t
FAST. See Focused abdominal sonography for trauma
Fastin (phentermine), 981
Fasting, 1258
preoperative, 352t
Fasting blood glucose, 1251t
diagnostic criteria for metabolic syndrome, 987t
impaired, 1255, 1873
Fast-tracking, 377
Fat(s)
daily requirements for, 1211-1212, 1212t
in diabetic meal plan, 1268
dietary guidelines, 949
fecal analysis, 1864t
metabolism of, 932t
Fat embolism syndrome, 1651
biochemical theory for, 1651
clinical manifestations of, 1651
collaborative care for, 1651
mechanical theory for, 1651
Fat necrosis, 1345t
Fatigue, 519t, 745t
in chemotherapy, 296t
chronic fatigue syndrome, **1728-1729,** 1870
in chronic HF, 825
at end of life, 160t
in radiation therapy, 296t, 297
Fatty liver disease, nonalcoholic, 1101
Fatty streaks, 785, 786f
Fatty tissue and skinfolds, 984
FDA. See Food and Drug Administration
Fear
in acute coronary syndrome, 814t
of addiction, 146t
of alteration in body image, 345

Fear (Continued)
of anesthesia, 345
in burn patients, 505t
of death, 345
of disruption of life functioning or patterns, 346
at end of life, 158-159
of hastening death by administering analgesics, 147
of injections, 146t
of loneliness and abandonment, 159
of meaninglessness, 159
of mutilation, 345
of pain, 158-159
of pain and discomfort, 345
preoperative, 345-346
of shortness of breath, 159
of tolerance, 146t
Febrile reactions, 732, 733t
Fecal analysis, 945t, 1864t
Fecal impaction, 1038
Fecal incontinence, 1038-1040
causes of, 1038, 1040t
collaborative care for, 1038-1039
diagnostic studies, 1038-1039
nursing assessment of, 1039-1040
nursing diagnoses, 1040
nursing implementation for, 1040
nursing management of, **1039-1040**
nursing planning for, 1040
Fecal urobilinogen, 946t
Fecalith, 1048, 1076
Federal Emergency Management Agency, 1844
Feeding
administration of, 962-963
assistive devices for eating, 1522, 1522f
oral, **960**
tube, **960-965**
Feeding tubes
complications of, 963-965
enteral, 961, 961f
nasogastric, 961
nasointestinal, 961
nursing management of, 962t
patency of, 962
position of, 962
verification of placement of, 1766
Feen-a-Mint (phenolphthalein), 1042t
FEF₂₅%-₇₅%. See Forced midexpiratory flow rate
Felbamate (Felbatol), 1537, 1538t
Feldene (piroxicam)
for arthritis and connective tissue disorders, 1698t
and gastritis, 1013
mechanism of action, 202t
photosensitivity, 461t
Felodipine (Plendil)
for chronic stable angina and acute coronary syndrome, 800t
enalapril/felodipine (Lexxel), 777t
for hypertension, 776t
Felty syndrome, 1704
Female breasts, 1327, 1327f
age-related changes in, 1331t
lymphatic drainage of, 1327, 1327f
normal physical assessment of, 1335t
physical examination of, 1335
Female condoms, 262
patient teaching guide for proper use of, 263t
placement of, 263f

Female external genitalia, 1326-1327, 1326f
physical examination of, 1335
normal, 1335t
outline for, 49t
recording, 51t
Female infertility, 1382-1383
Female pelvis, 1326
Female reproductive system, 1325f, 1326f
acupuncture benefits, 99t
age-related changes in, 1330, 1331t
assessment abnormalities, 1335t
assessment of, **1331-1335**
benign tumors of, **1398-1400**
cancers of, **1400-1407**
acute intervention related to surgery for, 1406-1407
acute intervention with radiation therapy for, 1407
cultural and ethnic health disparities in, 1400b
nursing assessment of, 1405
nursing diagnoses, 1405
nursing evaluation of, 1407
nursing implementation for, 1405-1407
nursing management of, **1405-1407**
nursing planning for, 1405
radiation therapy for, **1404-1407**
diagnostic studies, **1337-1341,** 1338t-1341t
functions of, **1325-1327**
physical examination of, 1335, 1335t
problems of, **1381-1413**
roles of, 1325
structures of, **1325-1327,** 1325f
surgeries of, 1332, 1332t
surgical procedures, **1404,** 1404t
Female sexual response, 1330
Femara (letrozole)
for breast cancer, 1355
classification of, 288t
Femoral head prosthesis, 1654, 1654t
Femoral osteomyelitis, chronic, 1669, 1669f
Femoral shaft fracture, **1655-1656**
Femoral vessel cannulation, 1221
Fenestrated tracheostomy tubes, 544t, 545f
Fenestration, 441
Fenfluramine (Pondimin), 981
Fenofibrate (TriCor), 795t
Fenoldopam (Corlopam), 775t
Fentanyl (Sublimaze, Duragesic, Actiq), 179
as adjunct to general anesthesia, 370t
for burns, 499t
drug alert, 141
effects of use, 169t
for pain, 137t, 141
preoperative, 355t
Ferric subsulfate (Monsel's solution), 476
Ferritin, 680t, 681
in anemias, 690t
effects of aging on, 672t
serum values, 1856t
Ferrous gluconate, 1055t
Ferrous sulfate
for burns, 499t
for inflammatory bowel disease, 1055t
Fertility studies, 1341t
Fertinex (urofollitropin), 1383t

FES. See Fat embolism syndrome
Festinating gait, 1623t
α-Fetoprotein, 946t
α₁-Fetoprotein, 1855t
Fetor hepaticus, 1106
FEV₁. See Forced expiratory volume in first second of expiration
Fever, 196-197
acute intervention for, 203
hemorrhagic, 1840t
in myocardial infarction, 804
production of, 196, 198f
rheumatic, **875-878**
Fever blisters, 1000t
Feverfew, 102t
Fexofenadine (Allegra)
for allergic rhinitis and sinusitis, 538t
for dermatologic problems, 475
Fiber
dietary, 1044t
high-fiber foods, 1041, 1043t
Fiberall (psyllium), 1042t
Fiberoptic bronchoscopy, 529, 529f
Fibric acid derivatives, 793, 795t
Fibrin degradation products, 670, 711
Fibrin split products, 670, 679t, 711
laboratory values, 1859t
in shock, 1775t
Fibrinogen, 670t, 679t
effects of aging on, 672t
laboratory values, 1859t
in shock, 1775t
Fibrinolysis, 670
Fibrinolytic system, 670, 670f
Fibrinolytic therapy
for acute coronary syndrome, 800t, 807-808
for chronic stable angina, 800t
contraindications to, 807, 807t
indications for, 807
procedure, 807-808
Fibrinous exudate, 197t
Fibrin-stabilizing factor, 670t
Fibroadenoma, 1345t, **1347**
nursing and collaborative management of, **1347**
Fibroblasts, 198, 450
Fibrocystic changes, 1346-1347, 1346f
of the breast, 1346
nursing and collaborative management of, **1346-1347**
Fibroids, uterine, **1398-1399**
Fibromyalgia syndrome, 1727-1728
clinical manifestations of, 1727
collaborative care for, 1728
commonalities with chronic fatigue syndrome, 1727t
comparison with myofascial pain syndrome, 1727t
complications of, 1727
diagnostic studies, 1728
etiology and pathophysiology of, 1727
nursing management of, **1728**
tender points in, 1728, 1728f
Fibrothorax, 587f, 596
Fibrous plaque, 785, 786f
Fibrous tissue, 198
"Fight-or-flight" response, 112, 113, 114f, 1450
Filgrastim (Neupogen)
for cancer treatment, 304t
clinical uses of, 223t
Filipino Americans, 155
Film dressings, transparent, 204, 204f
Fimbriae, 1325

Financial abuse, 73t
Finasteride (Proscar)
    for benign prostatic hyperplasia,
        1416-1417
    drug alert, 1417
    for voiding dysfunction, 1185t
Fine needle aspiration, 681
Finger joint arthroplasty, 1664
Fingers
    clubbing of, 524t
    physical examination of, 49t
Fiorinal, 1530
First spacing, 319
FISH. *See* Fluorescent in situ hybridization
Fish oil/omega-3 fatty acids, 103t, 771b
Fissures, 455t
    anal, 940t
Fistulas
    internal arteriovenous, 1220-1221,
        1220f
    vaginal, **1409,** 1409f
FITT physical activity guidelines, 792,
    816t
Fitz-Hugh–Curtis syndrome, 1395
Five As for smoking cessation, 172,
    172t, 584
Five Rs for smoking cessation, 172,
    172t, 584
5-FU. *See* Fluorouracil
Fixation
    external fixators, 1641, 1641f
    intermaxillary, 1657, 1657f
    internal
        devices for, 1641
        for hip fracture, 1653, 1653f
        open reduction with, 1638
FK506 (tacrolimus), 238, 239t
Flagyl (metronidazole)
    for bacterial vaginosis, 1394t
    for inflammatory bowel disease,
        1054, 1055t
    for peptic ulcer disease, 1019t
    for trichomonas vaginitis, 1394t
    for urethritis, 1163
Flail chest, 588, 588f
    emergency management of, 586t
    and restrictive lung disease, 595t
Flank pain, 1145t
Flanks, secondary survey of, 1826t,
    1827
Flatfoot, 1685t
Flavoxate (Urispas), 1185t
Flecainide (Tambocor)
    for atrial fibrillation, 852
    for atrial flutter, 851
    classification of, 856t
Fleet enema (sodium phosphates),
    1042t
Fleets Oil retention enema (mineral
    oil), 1042t
Flexeril (cyclobenzaprine), 1728
Flexion, 1622, 1622t
Flexzan, 205t
Flocculation, 1338t
Flolan (epoprostenol), 601-602
    for primary pulmonary hypertension,
        601f
Flomax (tamsulosin)
    for benign prostatic hyperplasia, 1417
    for voiding dysfunction, 1185t
Flonase (fluticasone), 537t

Florinef (fludrocortisone acetate), 1316
Flovent Diskus (fluticasone), 618t
Flovent HFA (fluticasone), 618t
Floxin (ofloxacin)
    for chlamydial infections, 1373
    for gonorrhea, 1368
    for UTIs, 1157
Floxuridine (FUDR), 287t
Flu vaccines, 539
Fluconazole (Diflucan)
    for pulmonary infections, 576
    for urethritis, 1163
    for vulvovaginal candidiasis, 1394t
Flucytosine (Ancobon), 674t
Fludarabine (Fludara)
    classification of, 287t
    for leukemia, 721t
    for non-Hodgkin's lymphoma, 727t
Fludrocortisone acetate (Florinef), 1316
Fluid balance
    daily requirements in chronic kidney
        disease, 1211-1212, 1212t
    effects of stress on, 320, 320f
    gerontologic considerations for, **321**
    in increased ICP, 1478-1479
    normal, 321, 321t
    preoperative review, 349
    in spinal cord injury, 1602
Fluid imbalances, 321-340
    assessment abnormalities in, 338t
    assessment of, **337-338**
    case study, 340
Fluid movement
    calculation of gain or loss, 315
    in capillaries, **318-319,** 319f
    between extracellular fluid and intra-
        cellular fluid, **319**
    mechanisms controlling, **316-318**
    shifts, 318-319
    shifts in burns, 488, 491f
Fluid replacement therapy
    in acute respiratory distress syn-
        drome, 1818
    assessment of, 496
    for burns, 493-496, 493t
    for constipation, 1044t
    formulas for estimating, 497t
    hypertonic, 318
    hypotonic, 318
    intravenous, **338-340**
    isotonic, 318
    oral, **338**
    osmotive movement of, 318
    in shock, 1783-1785, 1786t
    withholding before elective surgery,
        353b
Fluid resuscitation
    in hypovolemic shock, 1788
    with Parkland (Baxter) formula, 496,
        497t
    in shock, 1783-1785
Fluid retention, 745t
Fluid spacing, 319
Fluid volume deficit, 322
    causes and clinical manifestations of,
        322t
    collaborative care, 322
    nursing diagnoses, 322
Fluid volume excess, 322
    in acute renal failure, 1200
    causes and clinical manifestations of,
        322t
    collaborative care, 322
    nursing diagnoses, 322
Flumadine (rimantadine)
    for influenza, 540
    for pneumonia, 566

Flumazenil (Romazicon), 369
Flumazine (silver sulfadiazine), 499
Flunisolide (AeroBid)
    for allergic rhinitis and sinusitis,
        537t
    for asthma and COPD, 618t
Fluorescein angiography, 408t
Fluorescent in situ hybridization, 682t
Fluorescent treponemal antibody ab-
    sorption test, 1339t, 1371, 1861t
Fluorinated hydrocarbons, 170t
Fluoroquinolones
    for osteomyelitis, 1670
    for tuberculosis, 573t
    for UTIs, 1157
5-Fluorouracil (5-FU) (Adrucil)
    for breast cancer, 1355
    cardiotoxicity, 301
    for cervical cancer, 1402
    classification of, 287t
    for colorectal cancer, 1067
    FOLFOX treatment regimen, 291,
        291t
    leucovorin-modulated (Orzel), 1067
    methods of administration, 288t
    for oral cancer, 1002
    topical, 475-476
Fluothane (halothane), 369t
Fluoxetine (Prozac, Sarafem)
    for Alzheimer's disease, 1569, 1569t
    for pain, 139
    for premenstrual dysphoric disorder,
        1386
Fluoxymesterone (Halotestin), 1355
Flutamide (Eulexin)
    for hyperandrogenism, 1399
    for prostate cancer, 1426, 1426t
Fluticasone (Flonase)
    for allergic rhinitis and sinusitis, 537t
    for asthma and COPD, 618t
Fluticasone/salmeterol (Advair), 621
    for asthma and COPD, 620t
    for exercise-induced asthma, 608
Flutter mucus clearance device, 648,
    648f
Fluvastatin (Lescol), 793, 795t
Fluvoxamine (Luvox), 1569, 1569t
Foams, 205t
Focused abdominal sonography for
    trauma, 1827
Folate (folic acid), 680t
    for inflammatory bowel disease,
        1055t
    manifestations of imbalance, 953t
    recommended dietary reference in-
        takes, 953t
Folex (methotrexate)
    for bladder cancer, 1179
    for esophageal cancer, 1010
    for leukemia, 720t
FOLFOX treatment regimen, 291, 291t
Folic acid (folate), 680t, 1856t
Folic acid (folate) deficiency, 692-693
    causes of, 692
    classification of, 692t
    laboratory study findings in, 690t
Folinic acid (leucovorin), 291, 291t
Folk healers, 30-31
Follicle-stimulating hormone
    assay, 1338t
    serum levels, 1248t, 1338t
    target tissue and functions, 1236t
Follicle-stimulating hormone agonists,
    1383, 1383t
Folliculitis, 467t
Follitropin (Gonal-f, Follistim), 1383t

Fondaparinux (Arixtra), for DVT pro-
    phylaxis, and treatment, 914-915
Food(s)
    for diabetes mellitus, 1267-1268
    drug interactions, 953, 954t
    effects on stoma output, 1075t
    high-calorie, 306, 307t
    high-fiber, 1041, 1043t
    high-potassium, 1213, 1213t
    ingestion of, 928
    moderate or high in purine, calcium,
        or oxalate, 1171t
    propulsion of, 928
    protein foods with high biologic
        value, 306, 306t
    that cause anaphylactic shock, 227t
Food additives, 610
Food and Drug Administration (FDA),
    101, 989
Food groups
    MyPyramid, 949, 949f
    recommended number of servings,
        949, 950t
    sodium content in, 834t
Food poisoning, 1031-1033
    bacterial, 1031, 1032t
    patient and family teaching guide for
        preventing, 1031, 1032t
    types of, 1031
Foot care, 1287t
Foot disorders, 1684, 1685t
    acute intervention for, 1685-1686
    ambulatory and home care for, 1686
    complications in diabetes mellitus,
        1286-1287
    gerontologic considerations for, 1686
    health promotion in, 1684-1685
    nursing implementation for, 1684-
        1686
    nursing management of, **1684-1686**
    paresthesias, 676t
Footdrop, 1649t
Foradil (formoterol)
    for asthma, 619t
    for COPD, 619t, 640
Forane (isoflurane), 369t
Forced expiratory volume in first sec-
    ond of expiration (FEV_1)
    correlation with probable clinical
        manifestations, 638, 638t
    FEV_1/FVC ratio, 531t, 594b
    normal values, 531t
    and ventilatory disorders, 594b
Forced midexpiratory flow rate
    ($FEF_{25\%-75\%}$), 531t
Forced vital capacity (FVC)
    FEV_1/FVC ratio, 531t, 594b
    normal values, 531t
Foreign bodies
    airway obstruction due, 1846, 1846f,
        1846t
    in external ear canal, **438-439**
    in eye, 421f
    in upper respiratory tract, **541**
Formoterol (Foradil), 621
    for asthma, 619t
    budesonide/formoterol (Symbicort),
        620t
    for COPD, 619t, 640
Formula, 962
Fortamet (metformin), 1266t
Fortovase (saquinavir), 258t
Fosamax (alendronate)
    for hyperparathyroidism, 1310
    for osteoporosis, 1689
Fosamprenavir (Lexiva), 258t

Note: Disorder names are in **bold face.**
Page numbers in **bold face** indicate main
discussions. Page numbers followed by
f, t, b, or *n* indicate figures, tables, boxed
material, or notes, respectively.

Fosinopril (Monopril), 776t
Fosinopril/hydrochlorothiazide (Monopril-HCT), 777t
Four-point gait, 1648
Fourth heart sound (S$_4$), 750t
Fourth ventricle tumors, 1488, 1489t
Fracture hematoma, 1636
Fractures, 1635-1651
  acute intervention for, 1643-1646
  ambulatory and home care for, 1646-1649
  avulsion, 1631
  classification of, 1635-1636, 1636f
  clinical manifestations of, 1636, 1637t
  clinical union of, 1637
  closed book, 1652
  closed reduction of, 1638
  collaborative care for, 1638-1642, 1638t
  Colles' fracture, **1651-1652**
  complications of, **1649-1651**
  delayed union of, 1638, 1638t
  drug therapy for, 1641
  emergency management of, 1642, 1642t
  external fixation of, 1641
  facial, **1656-1658**
  femoral shaft, **1655-1656**
  of frontal bone, 1657t
  healing, 1636-1638, 1637f
  healing complications, 1638, 1638t
  health promotion in, 1643
  of hip, **1653-1654,** 1653f, 1665
  of humerus, **1652,** 1652f
  immobilization of, 1639-1642
  internal fixation of, 1641
  intracapsular, 1653
  malunion of, 1638t
  mandibular
    clinical manifestations of, 1657t
    nursing management of, **1657-1658**
  maxillary, 1657t
  nasal, **533-534,** 1657t
  neurovascular assessment of, 1642-1643
  nonunion of, 1638, 1638t
  nursing assessment of, 1642-1643, 1643t
  nursing care plan for patient with, 1644b-1645b
  nursing diagnoses, 1643
  nursing evaluation of, 1649
  nursing implementation for, 1643-1649
  nursing management of, **1642-1643**
  nursing planning for, 1643
  nutritional therapy for, 1641-1642
  open, 1636
  open book, 1652
  open reduction of, 1638
  of pelvis, **1652-1653**
  of periorbital bone, 1657t
  postoperative management of, 1643-1645
  preoperative management of, 1643
  reduction of, 1638-1639
  refracture, 1638t
  rib, 587-588, 595t
  skull, 1481-1482, 1481t
  stable, 1635-1636
  of tibia, **1656**
  treatment goals, 1638
  types of, 1636f, **1651-1658**
  union of, 1636
  unstable, 1636

Fractures (Continued)
  vertebral, stable, **1656**
  of zygomatic arch, 1657t
Fragmin (dalteparin), 800t
Frailty, 67, 71
Frank-Starling law, 823, 1738
FRC. See Functional residual capacity
Free radical theory, 68t, 69
"Freebase" cocaine, 174
Fremitus, 522
  altered tactile, 524t
Fresh frozen plasma, 731t, 1786t
Friction, 206
"Fright sickness" or **"soul loss,"** 35
Frontal bone fracture, 1657t
Frontotemporal dementia, 1576
Frostbite, 1830-1831
  deep, 1830-1831, 1831f
  superficial, 1830, 1830f
Frovatriptan (Frova), 1530
Frozen red blood cells, 731t
FSH. See Follicle-stimulating hormone
FSPs. See Fibrin split products
FTA-Abs test. See Fluorescent treponemal antibody absorption test
FTC (emtricitabine), 258t
5-FU. See 5-Fluorouracil
FUDR. See Floxuridine
Fulguration
  open loop resection with, 1179
  transurethral resection with, 1179
Full code, 156
Fulminant hepatic failure, 1115-1116
  clinical manifestations of, 1115-1116
  collaborative care for, 1116
  diagnostic studies, 1115-1116
  nursing management of, **1116**
Fulminant viral hepatitis, 1092
Fulvestrant (Faslodex)
  for breast cancer, 1355
  classification of, 288t
Functional health patterns, 43, 44-46
  in assessment
    of auditory system, 411-412
    of cardiovascular system, 745-746
    of endocrine system, 1244-1245
    of fluid, electrolyte, and acid-base imbalances, 337-338
    of gastrointestinal system, 934-936
    of hematologic system, 672-674
    of integumentary system, 453-454
    of musculoskeletal system, 1620-1621
    of nervous system, 1453-1456
    of preoperative patient, 349
    of reproductive system, 1332-1334
    of respiratory system, 517-521
    of urinary system, 1142-1144
    of visual system, 402-404
  and asthma, 624t
  comparison with NANDA International Taxonomy II, 42t-43t
  and COPD, 650t
  in HIV infection, 259t
  nursing diagnoses, **1851-1853**
  nursing history format, 45t
Functional incontinence, 1181t
Functional residual capacity (FRC), 531t
Funduscopy, 1457
Fungal infections
  culture for, 458t
  of lung, 575, 576t
  organisms associated with infective endocarditis, 866, 866t
  pneumonia, 564
  pulmonary, **575-576**
  of skin, 469-470, 469t

Fungi, 244, 245t
Fungizone (amphotericin B)
  hematologic effects of, 674t
  for infective endocarditis, 869t
Furosemide (Lasix)
  blood glucose level effects, 1267t
  for cirrhosis, 1110t
  effects on lower urinary tract function, 1180t
  for heart failure, 828
  for hypercalcemia, 330
  for hypertension, 773t, 1210
  for multiple myeloma, 729
  photosensitivity, 461t
Furuncles, 467t
Furunculosis, 467t
Fusiform abdominal aortic aneurysms, 894, 894f
Fusion, 251, 251f
Fusion inhibitors, 257
Futility, medical, 309b
Fuzeon (enfuvirtide)
  adverse effects of, 258t
  drug alert, 257
FVC. See Forced vital capacity
f/V$_T$. See Rapid shallow breathing index

G
G2 Biographer (device), 1270
GABA. See γ-Aminobutyric acid
Gabapentin (Neurontin)
  for alcohol treatment, 178
  for burns, 499t
  local, 139t
  for seizures, 1536, 1538t
  for trigeminal neuralgia, 1582
Gabitril (tiagabine), 1536, 1538t
Gait
  antalgic, 1623t
  with assistive devices, 1648-1649
  ataxic, 1623t
  festinating, 1623t
  four-point, 1648
  short-leg, 1624t
  spastic, 1624t
  steppage, 1624t
  swing-through, 1648-1649
  swing-to, 1648
  two-point, 1648
Galactorrhea, 1335t, 1347
Galantamine (Razadyne), 1551, 1569t
Gallbladder
  secretions related to digestion, 929, 929t
  structure of, 931f
  surgery procedures, 1128, 1128t
  ultrasound of, 941f, 941t
Gallbladder cancer, 1132
Gallbladder disease
  acute intervention for, 1130-1131
  ambulatory and home care for, 1131-1132
  cultural and ethnic health disparities in, 1089b
  drug therapy of, 1129-1130
  health promotion in, 1130
  nursing assessment of, 1130
  nursing diagnoses, 1130
  nursing evaluation of, 1132
  nursing implementation for, 1130-1132
  nursing management of, **1130-1132**
  nursing planning for, 1130
Gallstones, 941f, 1126-1132, 1127f
  diagnosis of, 1128
  drug therapy of, 1129-1130
  surgical therapy of, 1128, 1129f

Galvus (vildagliptin), 1265
  for diabetes mellitus, 1266t
Gamma knife radiosurgery, 1582-1583
  for trigeminal neuralgia, 1582t
Gamma-glutamy transpeptidase, 1856t
Ganciclovir (Cytovene), 564
Ganglion cyst, 1623t
Ganglionic blockers, 775t
Ganirelix (Antagon), 1383t
Garamycin (gentamicin)
  dose and frequency adjustments, 1211
  drug alert, 1670
  for infective endocarditis, 869t
  for osteomyelitis, 1670
  toxicology, 1865t
Gardnerella vaginalis, 1394t
Garlic, 102t, 796b
GAS. See General adaptation syndrome
Gas exchange
  improving, 829
  normal, 1799, 1800f
Gaseous anesthetic agents, 369t
Gastrectomy, 934t
  postgastrectomy dumping syndrome, 1027t
  total, 1029, 1029f
Gastric analysis, 945t, 1863t
Gastric banding, adjustable, 982t, 983, 983f
Gastric bypass, Roux-en-Y, 982t, 983f, 984
Gastric cancer, 1028-1031
Gastric emptying studies, 942t
Gastric fundus, 1005
Gastric inhibitory peptide, 929, 930t
Gastric lavage, 1837-1838
Gastric outlet obstruction, 1018
  nursing implementation for, 1024-1025
  therapy of, 1022
Gastric secretion, 929, 930t
Gastric ulcers, 1015, 1015t
  etiology and pathophysiology of, 1016
Gastric varices
  with cirrhosis, 1103-1104
  collaborative care for, 1107-1110
  long-term management of, 1108
Gastrin, 929, 930t
Gastritis, 1013-1014
  acute, 1014
  autoimmune, 1013
  bile reflux, 1026
  causes of, 1013, 1013t
  chronic, 1014
  clinical manifestations of, 1014
  diagnostic studies, 1014
  drug-related, 1013
  etiology and pathophysiology of, 1013
  nursing and collaborative management of, **1014**
  risk factors for, 1013
  types of, 1013
Gastroduodenostomy, 1025, 1026f
Gastroenteritis, 1050-1051
  nursing management of, **1050-1051**
Gastroesophageal reflux disease (GERD), 1003-1007
  and asthma attacks, 610
  clinical manifestations of, 1004
  collaborative care for, 1005-1006, 1005t
  complications of, 1004-1005
  in COPD, 637
  diagnostic studies, 1005
  drug therapy of, 1005-1006, 1006t

Gastroesophageal reflux disease (GERD) *(Continued)*
endoscopic therapy of, 1006
etiology and pathophysiology of, 1003-1004
gerontologic considerations for, **1008-1009**
nursing management of, **1006-1007**
nutritional therapy of, 1005
pathogenesis of, 1003, 1004*f*
patient and family teaching guide for prevention of, 1007*t*
surgical therapy of, 1006
Gastrografin (meglumine diatrizoate), 940
Gastrointestinal bleeding
drug therapy of, 997, 998*t*
scintigraphy of, 942*t*
Gastrointestinal stromal tumors, 1082
Gastrointestinal system, **926-947**
acupuncture benefits, 99*t*
in acute renal failure, 1201*t*
in acute respiratory distress syndrome, 1816*t*
age-related changes in, 932, 933*t*
nursing diagnoses associated with, 78*t*
in anemia, 686*t*
after aortic surgery, 897-898
assessment abnormalities, 939*t*-940*t*, 1247*t*
assessment of, 926-927, **933-939**
important health information, 933-934
key questions to ask, 935*t*
objective data, 936-939
preoperative, 349, 351*t*
subjective data, 933-936
autoimmune diseases of, 234*t*
burn injury complications, 500
chemotherapy effects on, 297-299
in chronic kidney disease, 1208
and COPD, 650*t*
diagnostic studies, **939-946**, 941*t*-945*t*
effects of aging on, **932-933**
effects of chronic alcohol abuse on, 177*t*
at end of life, 152*t*
functions of, **927-933**, 928
in HIV infection, 259*t*
hormones controlling secretion and motility, 929, 930*t*
layers of, 927
location of organs of, 926, 927*f*
lower gastrointestinal problems, **1035-1086**
in multiple organ dysfunction syndrome, 1796*t*
physical examination of, 936-939, 939*t*
positive pressure ventilation effects on, 1765
postoperative problems, **390-391**
etiology of, 390-391
nursing assessment of, 391
nursing diagnoses, 391
nursing implementation for, 391
nursing management of, **391**
problems associated with obesity, 975-976

Gastrointestinal system *(Continued)*
problems in chemotherapy and radiation therapy, 295*t*
problems with dermatologic manifestations, 473*t*
procedures requiring antibiotic prophylaxis to prevent endocarditis, 866, 867*t*
regulation of, 321
in shock, 1781*t*, 1783
acute intervention for, 1793
in spinal cord injury, 1595
after stroke, 1519
structures of, **927-933**
support for burns, 499*t*
surgery of, 934, 934*t*
upper gastrointestinal bleeding, **995-1000**
upper gastrointestinal problems, **990-1034**
Gastrointestinal tract. *See* Gastrointestinal system
Gastrojejunostomy, 1025, 1026*b*
Gastroparesis, 1285
Gastropexy, 1007
Gastroplasty, vertical banded, 983, 983*f*
Gastrostomy, 934*t*, 961
feedings problems, 964
percutaneous endoscopic, 961, 962*f*
Gastrostomy tubes
ambulatory and home care, 558
placement of, 961, 961*f*
sexuality and, 557-558
Gatifloxacin (Tequin)
for tuberculosis, 573*t*
for UTIs, 1157
Gaucon (epinephrine), 434*t*
Gauzes, 205*t*
Gaviscon
for gastroesophageal reflux disease, 1006*t*
preparation, 1020*t*
Gaze
cardinal positions of, 407*f*
disconjugate, 1457
GCS. *See* Glasgow Coma Scale
G-CSF. See Granulocyte colony-stimulating factor
GDC coil, 1512-1513, 1513*f*
Gefitinib (Iressa), 303*t*
Geliperm, 205*t*
Gelusil
for gastroesophageal reflux disease, 1006*t*
preparation, 1020*t*
Gelusil M, 1020*t*
Gemcitabine (Gemzar)
classification of, 287*t*
for lung cancer, 582
for ovarian cancer, 1403
for pancreatic cancer, 1126
Gemfibrozil (Lopid), 794, 795*t*
Gemtuzumab ozogamicin (Mylotarg), 303*t*, 720*t*, 721, 721*t*
Gender differences
in acute coronary syndrome, 802*t*
in addictive behaviors, 167*b*
in Alzheimer's disease, 1565*b*
in asthma, 608*b*
in cancer, 272, 272*b*
in cardiac assessment, 747*b*
in cholelithiasis, 1127*b*
in COPD, 629*b*
and coronary artery disease, 787-788
in coronary artery disease, 785*b*
in dementia, 1565*b*
in endocrine problems, 1299*b*
in gout, 1715*b*

Gender differences *(Continued)*
in headache, 1528*b*
and health disparities, 22
in heart failure, 823*b*
in hip fracture, 1653*b*
in hypertension, 762*b*
in irritable bowel syndrome, 1046*b*
in lung cancer, 579*b*
in malabsorption syndrome, 1079*b*
in older adults, 70*b*
in osteoarthritis, 1694*b*
in osteoporosis, 1687, 1687*b*
in pain, 127*b*
in stroke, 1503*b*
in urinary incontinence, 1180*b*
in urinary tract calculi, 1169*b*
in vascular disorders, 893*b*
Gene therapy, 217, 217*f*
for cancer, **306**
delivery methods, 217
for hemophilia, 709
General adaptation syndrome, **112-113**, 112*t*
General anesthesia, **367-371**, 369*t*
adjuncts to, 368-371, 370*t*
indications for, 367
patient positioning for recovery from, 381, 381*f*
phases of, 368*t*
General survey, 46, 48*t*
General survey statement, 46
Generalized lymphadenopathy, persistent, 252
Generalized seizures, 1534-1535
Genes, 214
definition of, 214*t*
oncogenes, 214*t*, 274
protooncogenes, 214*t*, 274
sex-linked genes, 214*t*
tumor suppressor genes, 274
GeneTests website, 217
Genetic diagnosis, preimplantation, 217
Genetic disorders, 216*t*
autosomal, 215
autosomal dominant, 215, 216*t*
autosomal recessive, 215, 216*t*
of liver, **1100-1101**
X-linked, 215
X-linked recessive, 215, 216*t*
Genetic manipulation, antiaging, 67-68, 68*t*
Genetic susceptibility, 234*t*, 276
Genetic testing, 215-217, 682*t*, 683
ethical dilemma, 218*b*
resources for, 241
Genetics, **213-217**
basic principles of, 213-215
and coronary artery disease, 788
definition of, 214*t*
Essential Nursing Competencies and Curricula Guidelines for Genetics and Genomics, 242
glossary of terms, 214*t*
nursing management, **217-218**
of obesity, 972-973
resources, 242
Genetics in clinical practice, 216*b*
Alzheimer's disease, 1565*b*
ankylosing spondylitis, 1712*b*
α_1-antitrypsin deficiency, 632*b*
breast cancer, 1349*b*
cystic fibrosis, 656*b*
diabetes mellitus, 1256*b*
Duchenne muscular dystrophy, 1675*b*
familial adenomatous polyposis, 1063*b*
familial hypercholesterolemia, 788*b*

Genetics in clinical practice *(Continued)*
hemochromatosis, 699*b*
hemophilia A and B, 707*b*
hereditary nonpolyposis colorectal cancer, 1064*b*
Human Genome Project (HGP), 214*b*
Huntington's disease, 1559*b*
ovarian cancer, 1402*b*
polycystic kidney disease, 1176*b*
sickle cell disease, 696*b*
Gengraf (cyclosporine), 238, 239*t*
Genital herpes, 1373-1375
clinical manifestations of, 1373-1374, 1374*f*
collaborative care for, 1375, 1375*t*
complications of, 1374
diagnostic studies, 1374-1375
drug therapy for, 1375
etiology and pathophysiology of, 1373
primary (initial) episode, 1373-1374
recurrent, 1374
symptomatic care of, 1375
Genital warts, 1375-1379, 1376*f*
clinical manifestations of, 1375
collaborative care for, 1375-1376
complications of, 1375
diagnostic studies, 1375-1376
Genitalia
external female, 1326-1327, 1326*f*
normal physical assessment of, 1335*t*
physical examination of, 49*t*, 51*t*, 1335
external male, 1324
normal physical assessment of, 1335*t*
physical examination of, 49*t*, 51*t*
physical examination of, 1246
adaptations, 50*t*
outline for, 49*t*
recording, 51*t*
Genitourinary tract
initial postanesthesia care unit assessment of, 377-378, 377*t*
problems in chemotherapy and radiation therapy, 296*t*
procedures requiring antibiotic prophylaxis to prevent endocarditis, 866, 867*t*
Genome, 214, 214*t*
Genomics, 242
Gentamicin (Garamycin)
dose and frequency adjustments, 1211
drug alert, 1670
for infective endocarditis, 869*t*
nephrotoxicity, 1142*t*
for osteomyelitis, 1670
toxicology, 1865*t*
Geographic location as a factor in health disparities, 21-22
Geographic tongue, 939*t*
GERD. *See* Gastroesophageal reflux disease
Geriatric rehabilitation, 79-80, 79*f*
Gerontologic considerations
in acute renal failure, **1204**
in addictive behaviors, **189**
age-related breast changes, **1348**
in amputation, **1662**
in anemia, **687**
in arthritis, **1711**
in breast cancer, **1361**
in burns, **504-505**
in cancer, **310**
in cataracts, **429**
in chronic kidney disease, **1230-1231**

Gerontologic considerations (Continued)
in complementary and alternative therapies, **105-106**
in coronary artery disease, **795**
in diabetes mellitus, **1287-1288**
in emergency care, **1828**
in enteral nutrition, **965**
in fluids and electrolytes, **321**
in foot problems, **1686**
in glaucoma, **436**
in hearing loss, **446**
in hiatal hernia and GERD, **1008-1009**
in hip fracture, **1655**
in hypertension, **780-781**
in immune system, **224**, 224t
in infection, **247**
in inflammatory bowel disease, **1060**
in liver disease, **1118**
in malnutrition, **959-960**
in metabolic bone diseases, **1690**
in nausea and vomiting, **995**
in neutropenia, **716**
in pain, 147-148
in peptic ulcer disease, **1027-1028**
in postoperative patient, **394-395**
in preoperative patient, **356**
in respiratory failure, **1812**
in spinal cord injury, **1609**
in stroke, **1524**
in surgery, **372**
in thrombocytopenia, **716**
in visual impairment, **421**
Gerontologic differences
in assessment, 50t, 69t, 224t
adaptations in physical assessment techniques, 20t
of adult mental functioning, 70t
of auditory system, 410t
of cardiovascular system, 744t
of endocrine system, **1242**, 1242t
of gastrointestinal system, 932, 933t
of hematologic studies, 672t
of immune system, 224t
of integumentary system, 451-452, 452t
of musculoskeletal system, 1618-1619, 1619t
of nervous system, 1452-1453, 1454t
of reproductive system, 1330, 1331t
of respiratory system, 517t
of urinary system, 1411t
of visual system, 401t
factors affecting nutritional intake in older adults, 959, 959t
Gerontologic nursing, 66
Gestational diabetes, 1257-1258
GF (cyclohexylmethylphosphonofluoridate), 1840t
GFR. See Glomerular filtration rate
GGT. See γ-Glutamyl transpeptidase
GH. See Growth hormone
Ghost sickness, 35t
Ghrelin, 928, 972, 973f, 973t
Giant cells, multinucleated, 195
Giardia lamblia **infection,** 1037t
Giardiasis, 246t
Ginger, 102t, 993b
Gingival changes, 675t
Gingivitis, 1000t
acute marginal, 939t
acute necrotizing ulcerative, 1000t
Ginkgo biloba, 102t, 1569b
for Alzheimer's disease, 1569
for peripheral arterial disease, 903
Ginseng, 102t, 103f, 120b

GISTs. See Gastrointestinal stromal tumors
Glasgow Coma Scale, 1476, 1477t
Glasses, corrective, 417
Glatiramer acetate (Copaxone), 1544t
Glaucoma, 432-436, 433f
acute, 434t-435t
acute intervention for, 436
ambulatory and home care for, 436
angle-closure
acute, 434
acute care, 434t
primary, 432-433
case study, 446-447
chronic, 434t-435t
chronic open-angle, 433-434
clinical manifestations of, 433
collaborative care for, 433-434, 434t
diagnostic studies, 433
etiology and pathophysiology of, 432-433
gerontologic considerations for, **436**
health promotion in, 436
nursing assessment of, 435
nursing diagnoses, 436
nursing evaluation of, 436
nursing implementation for, 436
nursing management of, **435-436**
nursing planning for, 436
open-angle
ambulatory/home care for, 434t
chronic, 433-434
primary, 432
primary angle-closure, 432-433
primary open-angle, 432
secondary, 433, 434
Gleason scale, 1424
Gleevec (imatinib), 303t, 720, 720t
Gliadel (carmustine), 287t
Glial nerve cells, 198, 198t
Glimepiride (Amaryl)
for diabetes mellitus, 1265, 1266t
pioglitazone and glimepiride (Duetact), 1266t
Glioblastoma, 1488f
Glioma, 1488t
Gliosis, 1534
Glipizide (Glucotrol, Glucotrol XL)
for diabetes mellitus, 1265, 1266t
photosensitivity, 461t
Global Initiative for Asthma (GINA), 615, 663
Global Initiative for Chronic Obstructive Lung Disease (GOLD), 638, 663
Globe, eye, abnormalities in assessment, 406t
Globulin levels, 1857t
Globus sensation
in esophageal cancer, 1009
in gastroesophageal reflux disease, 1004
Glomerular filtration rate, 1138
Glomerulonephritis, 1165
acute, 1166t
acute poststreptococcal, **1165-1166**
chronic, **1167**
classification of, 1165
clinical manifestations of, 1165
etiology and pathophysiology of, 1165
rapidly progressive, **1166-1167**
Glomerulus, 1137-1138, 1138t
Glossectomy, 934t, 1002
Glossitis, 689, 939t
Glossopharyngeal nerve (cranial nerve IX), 1450t
Glossopharyngeal nerve (cranial nerve IX) testing, 1457-1458

Gloves
recommendations for isolation precautions, 248t
before surgery, 364-365
Glucagon, 1241
blood glucose level effects, 1267t
target tissue and functions, 1236t
Glucocorticoid excess, 473t
Glucophage (metformin)
for diabetes mellitus, 1265, 1266t
for hyperandrogenism, 1399-1400
Glucophage XR (metformin), 1266t
Glucosamine, 103t, 1697b
Glucose, 1257f
blood levels
altered, 1247t
drugs affecting, 1266, 1267t
fasting, 987t, 1251t, 1255, 1856t
feedback between insulin and, 1237, 1237f
low, 1278
monitoring, 1269-1271, 1277t
preoperative, 351
self-monitoring of, 1269, 1270t
urine levels, 1251t
capillary blood, monitoring, 1251t
cerebrospinal fluid analysis, 1864t
herbs that may affect, 1276b
in shock, 1775t
urine levels, 1862t
Glucose tolerance
impaired, 1255
laboratory values, 1856t
oral, 1251t
Glucose-lowering agents, 1264t
α-Glucosidase inhibitors
blood glucose level effects, 1267t
for diabetes mellitus, 1265, 1266t
Glucotrol (glipizide)
for diabetes mellitus, 1265, 1266t
photosensitivity, 461t
Glucotrol XL (glipizide), 1265, 1266t
Glucovance (metformin and glyburide), 1266t
Glutamate, 1445t
γ-Glutamyl transpeptidase, 947t
Glyburide (Micronase, DiaBeta, Glynase)
for diabetes mellitus, 1265, 1266t
for diabetes mellitus in older adults, 1288
food/nutrient interactions, 954t
metformin and glyburide (Glucovance), 1266t
Glycemic index, 979t, 1267-1268, 1872
Glycerin, 1267t
Glycerin liquid (Ophthalgan, Osmoglyn Oral), 435t
Glycerol, 1267t
Glycerol rhizotomy, 1582, 1582t, 1583f
Glycine, 1445t
Glycolic acid, 479t
Glycoprotein IIb/IIIa inhibitors, 800t
Glycopyrrolate (Robinul), 355t
Glycosylated hemoglobin (Hb A1C), 1251t, 1258
Glynase (glyburide), 1265
for diabetes mellitus, 1266t
Glyset (miglitol), 1265, 1266t
GM-CSF. See Macrophage colony-stimulating factor
GnRH agonists, 1383, 1383t
GnRH antagonists, 1383, 1383t
Goiter, 1246t
of Graves' disease, 1298, 1298f
toxic nodular, 1299
Goitrogens, 1298, 1298t

Gold
nephrotoxicity, 1142t
for rheumatoid arthritis, 1706
Gold compounds
for arthritis and connective tissue disorders, 1699t
hepatotoxicity, 934t
for rheumatoid arthritis, 1706
Gold sodium thiomalate (Myochrysine)
for arthritis and connective tissue disorders, 1699t
for rheumatoid arthritis, 1706
Goldenseal, 102t, 536b
GoLYTELY (polyethylene glycol), 1042t
Gonadal hormones, 1328, 1328t
Gonadotropic hormones, 1236t
Gonadotropin, 1248t
Gonads, 1324
effects of aging on, 1242t
hormones and target tissues of, 1236t
Gonal-f (follitropin), 1383t
Goniometry, 1622, 1622f
Gonorrhea, 1367-1369
case study, 1379
clinical manifestations of, 1367-1368
collaborative care for, 1368-1369, 1369t
complications of, 1368
diagnostic studies, 1368
drug therapy for, 1368-1369
endocervical, 1367-1368, 1368f
etiology and pathophysiology of, 1367
"Good lung down" position, 1809-1810
Goodpasture syndrome, 228, **1166**
nursing and collaborative management of, **1166**
Goserelin (Zoladex), 1426, 1426t
Gout, 1715-1716
clinical manifestations of, 1715
collaborative care for, 1716, 1716t
complications of, 1715
diagnostic studies, 1715-1716
drug therapy for, 1716
etiology and pathophysiology of, 1715
gender differences in, 1715b
nursing management of, **1716**
nutritional therapy for, 1716
pseudogout, 1716
renal involvement in, 1177
secondary, 1715
tophaceous, 1715, 1715f
Gowns
recommendations for isolation precautions, 249t
before surgery, 364-365
Grafts
arteriovenous, 1221
for burns, 493t, 501, 502f
coronary artery bypass
for acute coronary syndrome, 808-809
off-pump, 809-810
endovascular stent, 896, 896f
internal arteriovenous, 1220-1221, 1220f
patch graft angioplasty, 904
patency of, 897
pericardial heterografts, 883t
perigraft leaks, 896
peripheral artery bypass, 907t
skin grafts, **480-481**
sources of, 498t
Graft-versus-host disease, 236
Gram stain, 527t, 1339t
Granisetron (Kytril), 297, 992, 992t

Granulation (fibroblastic, proliferative, reconstructive) phase, 198, 199*t*
Granulation tissue, 1637
  excess, 201, 202*f*
Granulocyte colony–stimulating factor
  for cancer treatment, 304*t*
  clinical uses of, 223*t*
  function of, 222*t*
Granulocyte-macrophage colony–stimulating factor
  for cancer treatment, 304*t*
  clinical uses of, 223*t*
  function of, 222*t*
Granulocytes, 667-668, 668*t*
Granulocytopenia, 713
Granuloma, 570
Granulomatous thyroiditis, subacute (de Quervain's), 1298
Graphesthesia, 1459
Graves' disease, 1299
  case study, 1320-1321
  exophthalmos and goiter of, 1298, 1298*f*
Gray (Gy), 292, 292*t*
Gray hepatization, 565
Green tea, 103*t*
Greenfield filter, 915, 915*f*
Grey Turner's spots or sign, 895
  in abdominal trauma, 1047
  in acute pancreatitis, 1119
Grief, 153, **153-154**
  absent, 154
  adaptive, 154
  clusters of, 153-154
  conflicted, 154
  dysfunctional, 154
  at end of life, 160
  maladaptive, 154
  manifestations of, 153
  pathologic, 154
  after spinal cord injury, 1608-1609
  stages of, 153, 153*t*
Griseofulvin, 461*t*
Groshong catheter, 290
Group teaching, 61, 61*f,* 1259*b*
Growth and development, 43*t*
Growth hormone, 1239
  serum levels, 1248*t*
  stimulation test, 1248*t*
  target tissue and functions, 1236*t*
Growth hormone excess, 1291-1293
  acute intervention for, 1292-1293
  ambulatory and home care for, 1293
  clinical manifestations of, 1291
  collaborative care for, 1291-1292
  diagnostic studies, 1291
  drug therapy for, 1292
  etiology and pathophysiology of, 1291
  nursing assessment of, 1292
  nursing diagnoses, 1292
  nursing evaluation of, 1293
  nursing implementation for, 1292-1293
  nursing management of, **1292-1293**
  nursing planning for, 1292
  radiation therapy for, 1292
  surgical therapy for, 1291-1292
Guanabenz (Wytensin), 773*t*
Guanadrel sulfate (Hylorel), 774*t*
Guanethidine (Ismelin), 774*t*

Guanethine/hydrochlorothiazide (Esimil), 777*t*
Guanfacine (Tenex), 774*t*
Guardianship, 1009*b*
Guided imagery, 118
Guided meditation, 117
Guillain-Barré syndrome, 1585-1587
  clinical manifestations of, 1586
  collaborative care for, 1586
  complications of, 1586
  diagnostic studies, 1586
  etiology and pathophysiology of, 1585-1586
  nursing assessment of, 1586
  nursing diagnoses, 1586-1587
  nursing evaluation of, 1587
  nursing implementation for, 1587
  nursing management of, **1586-1587**
  nursing planning for, 1587
  nutritional therapy for, 1586
  and restrictive lung disease, 595*t*
Guilt, 505*t*
Gummas, 1370
Gunshot wounds
  to chest, 585*t*
  fractured extremity, 1642, 1642*t*
  to head, 1484*t*
  spinal cord injury, 1596*t*
GVH disease. *See* Graft-versus-host disease
Gynecomastia
  with cirrhosis, 1104, 1105*f*
  in men, **1347-1348,** 1347*f*
  pubertal, 1348
  senescent, 1348
Gynoid obesity, 974, 975*t*

H
Habit retraining, 1183*t*
Haemophilus, 244*t*
Haemophilus influenzae, 562, 562*t,* 565
Hageman factor, 670*t*
Hair
  age-related changes in, 451-452, 452*t*
  distribution changes, 1246*t*
  physical examination of, 51*t*
Hairy cell leukemia, 719
Hairy leukoplakia, oral, 252, 253*f*
Haldol (haloperidol)
  adverse cardiovascular effects of, 745*t*
  for burns, 499*t*
  for delirium, 1578
  photosensitivity, 461*t*
Halitosis, 1012
Hallucinogen intoxication, 186
Hallucinogens
  effects of use, 170*t*
  poisoning, 1837*t*
Hallux rigidus, 1685*t*
Hallux valgus, 1684, 1685*t,* 1686*f*
Halo or ring sign, 1481, 1482*f*
Halo vest (Ace), 1601, 1601*f,* 1606*t*
Haloperidol (Haldol)
  adverse cardiovascular effects of, 745*t*
  for Alzheimer's disease, 1569*t*
  for burns, 499*t*
  for delirium, 1578
  ethnic differences in response to, 35*t*
  photosensitivity, 461*t*
Halotestin (fluoxymesterone), 1355
Halothane (Fluothane), 369*t,* 934*t*
Hamartomas, 585
Hammer toe, 1685*t,* 1686*f*
Hamwi "rule of thumb" for body weight, 956, 957*t*
Hancock valve, 883*t*

Hand(s)
  paresthesias of, 676*t*
  rheumatoid arthritis of, 1703-1704, 1703*f,* 1704*f*
  thrombophlebitis of, 910, 911*f*
Hand massage, 104, 105*f*
Handwashing recommendations, 248*t*
Hantavirus, 245*t*
Hantavirus pulmonary syndrome, 578*t*
HAP. *See* Hospital-acquired pneumonia
Haplotype, 233
Haptoglobin, 1856*t*
Hardiness, 111
Hartmann's solution, 339*t*
Hashimoto's thyroiditis, 1298
Hashish, 169*t*
Haustral churning, 930
Haversian systems, 1615, 1615*f*
Hawthorn, 102*t,* 831*b*
Hay fever, 226-227
HCAP. *See* Health care–associated pneumonia
HCM. *See* Hypertrophic cardiomyopathy
HCO_3^-. *See* Bicarbonate
Hcy. *See* Homocysteine
HD. *See* Hemodialysis
HDCV. *See* Human diploid cell vaccine
HDLs. *See* High-density lipoproteins
Head and neck
  arteries of, 1451*f*
  assessment abnormalities, 1246*t*
  cutaneous innervation of, 1581*f*
  physical examination of, 1245
    adaptations, 50*t*
    outline for, 48*t-49t*
    recording, 51*t*
  secondary survey assessment of, 1826*t,* 1827
Head and neck cancer, 551-558
  acute intervention for, 553-558
  clinical manifestations of, 551
  collaborative care for, 551-553
  diagnostic studies, 551
  health promotion in, 553
  nursing assessment of, 553, 553*t*
  nursing diagnoses, 553
  nursing evaluation of, 558
  nursing implementation for, 553-558
  nursing management of, **553-558**
  nursing planning, 553
  radiation therapy of, 555-556
  surgical therapy of, 556
Head blocks, 1823
Head injury, 1481-1487
  acute intervention for, 1485-1487
  ambulatory and home care for, 1487
  case study, 1499
  collaborative care for, 1484-1485
  complications of, 1483-1484
  diagnostic studies, 1484-1485
  emergency management of, 1484-1485, 1484*t*
  health promotion in, 1485
  major trauma, 1482-1483
  minor trauma, 1482
  nursing assessment of, 1485, 1486*t*
  nursing diagnoses, 1485
  nursing evaluation of, 1487
  nursing implementation for, 1485-1487
  nursing management of, **1485-1487**
  nursing planning for, 1485
  nutritional support for, 1475*b*

Head injury *(Continued)*
  pathophysiology of, 1483
  patient and family teaching guide for, 1486*t*
  and restrictive lung disease, 595*t*
  types of, **1481-1483**
Head tilt–chin lift maneuver, 1845-1846, 1845*f*
Head trauma, 1481. *See also* Head injury
  major, 1482-1483
  minor, 1482
Headache, 676*t,* **1527-1532**
  chronic, 1531*b*
  cluster, 1528*t,* **1529**
  collaborative care for, 1529-1531, 1530*t*
  diagnostic studies, 1529
  drug therapy for, 1530-1531
  gender differences in, 1528*b*
  in increased ICP, 1472
  medication overuse, 1531
  migraine, **1528-1529,** 1528*t*
  nursing assessment of, 1531-1532, 1532*t*
  nursing care plan for patient with, 1533*b*
  nursing diagnoses, 1532
  nursing evaluation of, 1532
  nursing implementation for, 1532
  nursing management of, **1531-1532**
  nursing planning for, 1532
  patient and family teaching guide for, 1533*t*
  tension-type, **1527-1528,** 1528*t*
  types of, **1529-1532**
Head-to-toe secondary survey assessment, 1825-1827, 1826*t*
Head-upright tilt-table testing, 863
Healers, folk (traditional), 30
Healing
  bone, 1636-1638, 1637*f*
  of burns, 491
  complications of, 200-202
  delay of, 200, 201*t*
  drug therapy of, 202, 202*t*
  granulation (fibroblastic, proliferative, reconstructive) phase, 198, 199*t*
  initial phase, 198, 199*t*
  maturation phase, 198-199
  primary intention, 198-199, 199*t*
  process of, **197-202,** 804
  secondary intention, 199
  tertiary intention, 199
  wound
    factors delaying, 200, 201*t*
    nursing and collaborative management of, **203-206**
    process of, **197-202**
    resources, 212
    types of, 198, 199*f*
Healing touch, 98*t*
Health
  chronic stress and, 115, 115*f*
  cultural factors, **30-36,** 31*t*
  determinants of, **19-20,** 20*f*
  individual vs. public health protection, 256*b*
  stress and, **115**
Health care
  cultural factors, **30-36,** 31*t*
  disparities in, 20
  integrative model, 94-95, 95*t*
Health care facilities, 247, 248*t-249t*
Health care informatics, 8-9

Health care personnel
control of hepatitis in, 1099
measures to prevent transmission of hepatitis viruses from patients to, 1100t
Health care providers
attitudes of, 22-23
impaired, 174b
Health care system
changing, **86-87**
cultural factors affecting, 31t
factors influencing change, 86
Health care workplace, **30,** 30f
Health care–associated pneumonia, 563-564
Health disparities, 20-24
case study, 24b
definitions of, 20
ethical dilemmas, 22b
factors and conditions that lead to, 20-23
factors that contribute to, 20t
impact on health, 21, 21t, 23
nursing interventions to eliminate, 23, 23t
nursing management reducing, **23-24,** 24f
reducing, for ethnic adults, 23, 24t
resources, 25
risk for, 23, 23f
Health history, 39-52
AMPLE mnemonic for, 1826-1827
in assessment of allergic disorders, 228-229
secondary survey, 1826-1827
Health information, important, 43, 45t
in assessment
of allergies, 229t
of auditory system, 409-411
of cardiovascular system, 745
of endocrine system, 1243-1244
of fluid, electrolyte, and acid-base imbalances, 337-338
of gastrointestinal system, 933-934
of HIV infection, 259t
of musculoskeletal system, 1619-1620
of nervous system, 1454
of pressure ulcers, 209t
of reproductive system, 1331-1332
of urinary system, 1141-1144
of visual system, 402-404
Health Information Technology Institute (HITI) criteria for website evaluation, 63
Health Insurance Portability and Accountability Act (HIPAA), 40-41
Health literacy, 22, 58
Health literacy assessment, 58-59
Health maintenance organizations (HMOs), 86, 86b
Health management. *See* Health perception–health management pattern
Health perception–health management pattern
in assessment
of auditory system, 410t, 411
of cardiovascular system, 745, 746t
of endocrine system, 1244
of fluid, electrolyte, and acid-base imbalances, 337
of gastrointestinal system, 934, 935t
of hematologic system, 672, 673t
of integumentary system, 453, 453t
of lung cancer, 583t
of musculoskeletal system, 1620-1621
of nervous system, 1453-1455

Health perception–health management pattern (Continued)
of pneumonia, 567t
of preoperative patient, 350t
of reproductive system, 1332, 1333t
of respiratory system, 517-519, 518t
of urinary system, 1142, 1143t
of visual system, 402-403, 403t
and asthma, 624t
comparison with NANDA International Taxonomy II, 42t
concerns of patients requiring home health care, 90t
and COPD, 650t
nursing diagnoses, **1851-1852**
nursing history, 44, 45t
Health promotion
in acute low back pain, 1676
in acute pancreatitis, 1122
in acute pyelonephritis, 1162
in acute renal failure, 1203
in Alzheimer's disease, 1570
in amputation, 1659
in aortic aneurysms and aortoiliac disease, 897
in asthma, 625-626
in bacterial meningitis, 1495
in benign prostatic hyperplasia, 1421
in bone cancer, 1674
in cancers of female reproductive system, 1405-1406
in cataracts, 428
in chronic HF, 835
in chronic kidney disease, 1213
in chronic stable angina, 810
in cirrhosis, 1111
in colorectal cancer, 1068
comparison of functional health patterns and NANDA International Taxonomy II, 42t
in COPD, 650
in coronary artery disease, 791-792
in Cushing syndrome, 1314
in diabetes mellitus, 1271-1272
in esophageal cancer, 1011
in extraocular inflammation and infection, 424
in foot disorders, 1684-1685
in fracture, 1643
in gallbladder disease, 1130
in glaucoma, 436
in head and neck cancer, 553
in head injury, 1485
in hearing loss and deafness, 443-444
in hemophilia, 709
in HIV infection, 260-263, 261t, 265
in hypertension, 777-779
in hypothyroidism, 1306
in infective endocarditis, 870
in inflammation, 202-203
in lower extremity peripheral arterial disease, 904-906
in lung cancer, 584
in malnutrition, 957
for older adults, 78-79, 78f
in oral cancer, 1003
in osteoarthritis, 1701
in osteomyelitis, 1670
in peptic ulcer disease, 1022
in pneumonia, 567-569
in pressure ulcers, 209
in prostate cancer, 1428
in pulmonary embolism, 600
in rheumatic fever and heart disease, 877-878
in rheumatoid arthritis, 1707
in seizure disorders and epilepsy, 1538-1539

Health promotion (Continued)
in sexually transmitted diseases, 1376-1378
in shock, 1790
for skin health, **460-463**
in spinal cord injury, 1597-1609
in sprains and strains, 1631
in stomach cancer, 1030
in stroke, 1515
for stroke prevention, 1509
in substance abuse problems and addictive behaviors, 184-185
in systemic lupus erythematosus, 1720
in thrombocytopenia, 705
in trigeminal neuralgia, 1583
in tuberculosis, 574
in upper gastrointestinal bleeding, 998-999
in urinary tract infection, 1158-1159
in valvular disorders, 883-885
in visual impairment, 420
Health-related beliefs and practices
cultural assessment, 29t
of religious groups, 32t
Healthy People 2010, 20, 971
initiatives, 5, 5t
online resource, 18
Hearing acuity tests, 413-415
Hearing aids, 444-445, 445f
Hearing loss, 442-445
assistive devices and techniques for, 444-445
causes of, 443f
central, 408, 443
classification of, 443
clinical manifestations of, 443
communication with hearing-impaired patients, 445t
conductive, 408, 443
at end of life, 152t
functional, 443
gerontologic considerations for, **446**
hazardous zone for, 444t
health history questions to ask, 410t
health promotion in, 443-444
mixed, 443
nursing and collaborative management of, **443-444**
sensorineural, 408, 443
types of, 443
Heart, **740-742.** *See also under* Cardiac
age-related changes in, 744t
artificial, 839
assessment abnormalities, 676t
autonomic nervous system and, 743
blood flow through, 740, 740f
conduction system of, 741, 741f, 842-843
intrinsic rates, 846, 847t
layers of, 865, 866f
mechanical system of, 742
nervous control of, 843
orientation in thorax, 740, 740f
physical examination of, 51t
structure of, 740
Heart block, 853f. *See also* Atrioventricular block
complete
characteristics of, 849t
Mobitz I or Wenckebach, 849t, 853
Mobitz II, 849t, 853-854
Heart disease
autoimmune, 234t
health promotion in, 877-878
hypertensive, 766t, 767

Heart disease (Continued)
inflammatory disorders, **865-878**
NYHA functional classification of, 826t, 827
prevention of, 791b
resources, 891
rheumatic, **875-878,** 1876
valvular, **878-885**
case study, 890
collaborative care for, **881-885**
diagnostic studies, **881**
Heart failure, 821-841
ACC/AHA stages of, 826t, 827
acute decompensated
clinical manifestations of, 824-825
collaborative care for, 827t
nursing and collaborative management of, **827-829**
biventricular, 824
case study, 840
causes of, 822, 822t
chronic
acute intervention for, 835
ambulatory and home care for, 835-837
clinical manifestations of, 825-826
collaborative care for, 827t, 829-831
drug therapy of, 831-833
health promotion in, 835
nursing assessment of, 834
nursing diagnoses, 834
nursing evaluation of, 837
nursing implementation for, 835-837
nursing management of, **834-837**
nursing planning for, 835
nutritional therapy of, 833-834
patient discharge education and clinical outcomes in, 830b
classification of, 827
clinical manifestations of, 825, 825t
compensatory mechanisms, 823-824
complications of, 826-827
core measures for, 827-828, 828t
counterregulatory mechanisms, 824
cultural and ethnic health disparities in, 822b
diagnostic studies, 827
drug therapy of, 831t
end-stage, 837, 839t
etiology and pathophysiology of, 822-824
gender differences in, 823b
in hypertension, 767
left-sided, 824, 824f, 825, 825t
in myocardial infarction, 804
neurohormonal response to, 823
nursing assessment of, 835t
nursing care plan for patient with, 12, 836b-838b
patient and family teaching guide for, 838t
precipitating causes of, 822, 822t
resources, 840
right-sided, 824, 825, 825t
types of, 824
Heart rate
determination of, 843-844, 845f
normal range at rest, 1739t
in shock, 1774t
Heart rhythm, **842-861**
Heart sounds, 750f
fourth (S₄), 750t
third (S₃), 750t
Heart valves, 740, 740f
deformities of, 876
disease of, **878-885**
prosthetic, 882, 883f, 883t

Heartbeat
  irregular, 745*t*
  triggered beats, 846
Heartsbreath test, 839
Heat cramps, 1828-1829, 1830*t*
Heat edema, 1828
Heat exhaustion, 1829
  emergency management of, 1830*t*
Heat rash, 1828
Heat stroke, 1829-1830, 1830*t*
  collaborative care for, 1829-1830
Heat syncope, 1828
Heat therapy
  for osteoarthritis, 1696
  for pain, 144
  patient and family teaching guide, 144*t*
  for rheumatoid arthritis, 1710-1711
  for soft tissue injuries, 203
Heat-related emergencies, **1828-1830**
  risk factors for, 1828, 1829*t*
Heaves, 750
Heavy metals, 1142*t*
Heberden's nodes, 1695, 1695*f*
Hectorol (doxercalciferol), 1210
Heels, painful, 1685*t*
Heel-to-shin test, 1458
Hegu point (LI4), 98, 100*f*
Height assessment, 1245
Heimlich maneuver, 1846*f*, 1846*t*
Heimlich valves, 590
Helicobacter pylori **infection**
  diseases caused by, 244*t*
  drug therapy of, 1014, 1014*t*
  and gastritis, 1013
  related diseases, 245*t*
Helios liquid portable oxygen system, 643*f*
Heliotrope skin changes in dermatomyositis, 1725
Hemabate (carboprost), 1384*t*
Hemangioblastoma, 1488*t*
Hemarthrosis, 674, 1631
  acute, 708, 708*f*
Hematemesis, 519, 672, 939*t*, 995*t*, 1872
Hematinics, 1054, 1055*t*
Hematocrit (Hct), 527*t*, 677, 678*t*
  in anemias, 690*t*
  in deep vein thrombosis, 911*t*
  laboratory values, 1859*t*
  in shock, 1775*t*
Hematogenous spread, 561
Hematologic system, **665-683**
  in acute renal failure, 1200, 1201*t*
  in acute respiratory distress syndrome, 1816*t*
  assessment abnormalities, 675*t*-676*t*
  assessment of, **671-677**
    gerontologic differences in, 672*t*
    important health information in, 671-672
    key questions to ask, 673*t*
    objective data, 674-677
    subjective data, 671-674
  in chronic kidney disease, 1207
  in cirrhosis, 1102-1103
  diagnostic studies, **677-683**, 682*t*
  drugs affecting, 672, 674*t*
  effects of aging on, **671**, 672*t*
  effects of chronic alcohol abuse on, 177*t*
  laboratory studies, 677-681, 1859*t*-1860*t*

Hematologic system (*Continued*)
  in multiple organ dysfunction syndrome, 1797*t*
  physical examination of, 674-676
  problems of, **684-737**
    in chemotherapy and radiation therapy, 295*t*
    cultural and ethnic health disparities, 685*b*
    dermatologic manifestations of, 473*t*
    resources, 737
    in shock, 1781*t*, 1783
    in systemic lupus erythematosus, 1718
Hematoma, 457*t*, 675*t*
  epidural, 1483, 1483*f*
  fracture, 1636
  in hemophilia, 707, 708*f*
  intracerebral, 1484
  subdural, 1483-1484, 1483*f*
Hematopoiesis, 665
Hematopoietic growth factors, **304,** 304*t*
Hematopoietic stem cell transplantation, **304-306**
  complications of, 306
  harvest procedures, 305
  indications for, 305*t*
  for leukemia, 721
  preparative regimens, 305-306
  procedures, 305-306
  types of, 304-305
Hematuria, 1145*t*
Hemianopsia, homonymous, 1508
  after stroke, 1520, 1520*f*
Hemiglossectomy, 934*t*, 1002
Hemilaryngectomy, 551
Hemiplegia, 1460*t*
Hemochromatosis, 699-700, 1100-1101
  genetics of, 699*b*
Hemodialysis, 1216, 1217*t*, **1220-1224,** 1225
  acute, temporary double-lumen vascular access catheters for, 1221, 1221*f*
  adaptation to, 1224
  complications of, 1223-1224, 1229*t*
  continuous arteriovenous, 1224*t*
  continuous venovenous, 1224-1225, 1224*f*, 1224*t*, 1225
  dialyzers, 1222
  effectiveness of, 1224
  in-center, 1223, 1223*f*
  procedure, 1222-1223
  settings for, 1223
  system components, 1222, 1222*f*
  temporary vascular access for, 1221-1222, 1222*f*
  vascular access for, 1220, 1220*f*
  vascular access sites, 1220-1222
Hemodynamic monitoring, 755*t*, 760, **1738-1747**
  effects of shock on, 1774-1775, 1774*t*
  invasive
    principles of, 1739-1740
    types of, 1740-1747
  noninvasive, 1745-1746
  nursing management of, **1747**
  terminology, 1738-1739
Hemofiltration, 1225
  continuous arteriovenous, 1224*t*
  continuous venovenous, 1224-1225, 1224*f*, 1224*t*, 1225
Hemoglobin, 527*t*, 667, 677, 678*t*
  in anemias, 690*t*
  in deep vein thrombosis, 911*t*
  effects of aging on, 672*t*

Hemoglobin (*Continued*)
  glycosylated, 1251*t*, 1258, 1859*t*
  laboratory values, 1859*t*
  maintaining, 1812
  in shock, 1775*t*
  sickle cell, 696, 696*f*
  urine levels, 1862*t*
Hemoglobin electrophoresis, 680*t*
Hemoglobin S, 696
Hemolysis, 667
  extravascular, 695, 695*f*
  extrinsic causes of, 699
  intravascular, 695
Hemolytic anemia, 695
  acquired, **699**
  intrinsic, 695
  laboratory study findings in, 690*t*
Hemolytic (prehepatic) jaundice, 1088
Hemolytic transfusion reactions, 227-228
  acute, 732, 733*t*
  delayed, 734*t*
Hemophilia, 707-710
  acute intervention for, 709-710
  ambulatory and home care for, 710
  clinical manifestations of, 707-708, 708*f*
  collaborative care for, 708
  complications of, 707-708
  diagnostic studies, 708
  gene therapy of, 709
  health promotion in, 709
  laboratory results in, 709*t*
  nursing evaluation of, 710
  nursing implementation for, 709-710
  nursing management of, **709-710**
  replacement factor treatment of, 709*t*
  types of, 708*t*
Hemophilia A, 707*t*, 708*t*
Hemophilia B, 707*t*, 708*t*
Hemoptysis, 519, 519*t*
Hemorrhage. *See also* Bleeding
  intracerebral, 1506, 1506*t*, 1507*f*
  in peptic ulcer disease, 1017, 1023
  splinter, 749*t*, 867
  subarachnoid, 1506-1507, 1506*t*
  subconjunctival, 406*t*
  surgical therapy for, 1512-1513
Hemorrhagic cystitis, 296*t*
Hemorrhagic exudate, 197*t*
Hemorrhagic fever, 1840*t*
Hemorrhagic stroke, 1505*f*, 1506-1507, 1506*t*
Hemorrhoids, 940*t*, **1082-1083,** 1082*f*
  clinical manifestations of, 1082
  collaborative care for, 1082-1083
  diagnostic studies, 1082-1083
  etiology and pathophysiology of, 1082
  nursing management of, **1083**
Hemostasis, 668
  endoscopic, 997
  problems of, **701-723**
Hemostatic function tests, 946*t*
Hemothorax, 587
  emergency management of, 586*t*
Heparin
  low-molecular-weight, 913*t*
    for chronic stable angina and acute coronary syndrome, 800*t*
    for DVT prevention, 912*b*
    for DVT treatment, 914
  unfractionated (Hepalean), 800*t*, 913*t*
Heparin-induced thrombocytopenia and thrombosis syndrome
  collaborative care for, 704, 704*t*
  etiology and pathophysiology of, 702

Hepatic encephalopathy
  acute intervention for, 1114
  with cirrhosis, 1104-1106
  collaborative care for, 1108-1109
  factors precipitating, 1105, 1106*t*
  grading scale for, 1106*t*
Hepatic failure
  acute, 1115
  fulminant, **1115-1116**
Hepatic system. *See also* Liver
  effects of chronic alcohol abuse on, 177*t*
  in multiple organ dysfunction syndrome, 1796*t*
  preoperative assessment of, 349, 351*t*
  preoperative review, 348
  in shock, 1781*t*
Hepatitis, 1088-1099
  acute, 1092, 1093*t*
  acute intervention for, 1099
  acute viral, 1097*b*-1098*b*
  ambulatory and home care for, 1099
  anicteric, 1092
  autoimmune, **1100**
  characteristics of viruses, 1089, 1090*t*
  clinical manifestations of, 1091-1092, 1092*t*
  collaborative care for, 1093-1096
  complications of, 1092
  control in health care personnel, 1099
  diagnostic studies, 1092-1093
  drug therapy of, 1093-1095
  drug-induced, **1099-1100**
  etiology of, 1089-1092
  fulminant, 1092
  general considerations for, 1092
  in hemodialysis, 1223
  liver changes in, 1091
  measures to prevent transmission to health care personnel, 1100*t*
  nonalcoholic steatohepatitis, **1101**
  nursing assessment of, 1096, 1096*t*
  nursing diagnoses, 1097
  nursing evaluation of, 1099
  nursing implementation for, 1097-1099
  nursing management of, **1096-1097**
  nursing planning for, 1097
  nutritional therapy of, 1096
  pathophysiology of, 1091
  systemic effects of, 1091
  toxic, **1099-1100**
  viral
    acute, 1097*b*-1098*b*
    collaborative care for, 1094*b*
    preventive measures for, 1097, 1098*t*
    tests for, 1092, 1093*t*
Hepatitis A
  control in health care personnel, 1099
  prevention of, 1095-1096, 1099*t*
Hepatitis A antibody, 1861*t*
Hepatitis A virus, 1089
  characteristics of, 1089, 1090*t*
  course of infection with, 1089, 1090*f*
  diseases caused by, 244*t*
  measures to prevent transmission to health care personnel, 1100*t*
  nursing implementation for, 1097-1098
  tests for, 1093*t*
Hepatitis A virus vaccine (Havrix), 1095-1096

Note: Disorder names are in **bold face.**
Page numbers in **bold face** indicate main
discussions. Page numbers followed by
f, *t*, *b*, or *n* indicate figures, tables, boxed
material, or notes, respectively.

Hepatitis B
  associated with HIV infection, 254t
  chronic, 1094-1095
  control in health care personnel, 1099
  delayed transfusion reaction, 734, 734t
  nursing implementation for, 1098
  prevention of, 1096, 1099t
Hepatitis B surface antigen, 1861t
Hepatitis B virus, 1089, 1367t
  characteristics of, 1089, 1090t
  course of infection with, 1089, 1091f
  diseases caused by, 244t
  measures to prevent transmission to health care personnel, 1100t
  tests for, 1093t
Hepatitis B virus vaccine (Recombivax HB, Engerix-B), 1096
Hepatitis C
  associated with HIV infection, 254t
  chronic, 1095
  control in health care personnel, 1099
  delayed transfusion reaction, 734, 734t
  ethnicity and treatment outcome in, 1095b
  nursing implementation for, 1098-1099
  prevention of, 1096, 1099t
Hepatitis C antibody, 1861t
Hepatitis C virus, 1090
  characteristics of, 1089, 1090t
  diseases caused by, 244t
  measures to prevent transmission to health care personnel, 1100t
  related diseases, 245t
  tests for, 1093t
Hepatitis D virus, 1090
  characteristics of, 1089, 1090t
  tests for, 1093t
Hepatitis E virus, 1090
  characteristics of, 1089, 1090t
  related diseases, 245t
Hepatitis G virus, 1091
Hepatobiliary scintigraphy, 942t
Hepatobiliary ultrasound, 941t
Hepatocellular (hepatic) jaundice, 1088
Hepatocytes, 930
Hepatomegaly, 676t, 940t
  in heart failure, 826
Hepatorenal syndrome, 1106
Hepatotoxicity
  of chemicals and drugs, 933-934, 934t
  in chemotherapy and radiation therapy, 295t
Hepsera (adefovir)
  for chronic hepatitis B, 1094-1095
  drug alert, 1095
HER-2. *See* Human epidermal growth factor receptor 2
Herbal therapy, 100-101, 103f
  adverse cardiovascular effects of, 745t
  assessment of use of, 44b
  for benign prostatic hyperplasia, 1417
  Chinese herbs, 96-98
  clinical applications of, 101
  common herbs, 103f
  commonly used herbs, 102t
  description of, 97t
  effects during perioperative period, 347b
  for menopause, 1393b
  patient and family teaching guide, 101t
  supplements, 100-101

Herbal therapy (Continued)
  that may affect clotting, 903b
  that may affect glucose, 1276b
Herceptin (trastuzumab), 302, 303t
  for breast cancer, 1356
  cardiotoxicity, 301
  drug alert, 1356
Hereditary (term), 214t
Hereditary nephritis, chronic, 1177
Hereditary nonpolyposis colorectal cancer, 1064b
Hereditary renal diseases, 1175-1177
Heredity
  and COPD, 632
  and hypertension, 765
Hering-Breuer reflex, 516
Hernias, 940t, **1077-1078**
  cingulate, 1472
  clinical manifestations of, 1078
  direct, 1078, 1078f
  hiatal, 1007-1009
    case study, 1033
    collaborative care for, 1005t
  indirect, 1078, 1078f
  intracranial, 1469, 1471f
  nursing and collaborative management of, **1078**
  in peritoneal dialysis, 1219
  tentorial, 1472
  types of, 1078, 1078f
  uncal, 1472
Herniated intervertebral disk, 1680-1681
Hernioplasty, 1078
Herniorrhaphy, 934t, 1008, 1078, 1332t
Herniotomy, 1008
Heroin
  effects of use, 169t
  injecting or "mainlining," 180, 180f
  nephrotoxicity, 1142t
Herpes simplex, 468f, 469, 939t, 1000t
  in eye, 1374
  genital, **1373-1375**
  ocular manifestations of, 437t
  in pregnancy, 1374
Herpes simplex virus, 1367t
  autoinoculation of, 1374, 1374f
  type 1, 468t
    associated with HIV infection, 254t
    diseases caused by, 244t
  type 2, 468f, 468t, 1374f
    associated with HIV infection, 254t
    diseases caused by, 244t
Herpes simplex virus keratitis, 1374
Herpes zoster (shingles), 468t, 469, 469f
Herpesviruses, 244t
Herpetic whitlow, 1374, 1374f
Hertz (Hz), 414
Hespan (hetastarch), 1786t
Hetastarch (Hespan), 1786t
Heterografts, 498t
Heterozygous (term), 214t
Hexalen (altretamine), 1403
HFJV. *See* High-frequency jet ventilation
HFOV. *See* High-frequency oscillatory ventilation
HFPV. *See* High-frequency percussive ventilation
HFV. *See* High-frequency ventilation
HHS. *See* Hyperosmolar hyperglycemic syndrome
HHV. *See* Human herpesvirus

Hi Lo Evac Tube, 1759, 1759f
Hiatal hernia, 1007-1009
  case study, 1033
  clinical manifestations of, 1008
  collaborative care for, 1005t
  complications of, 1008
  conservative therapy of, 1008
  diagnostic studies, 1008
  etiology and pathophysiology of, 1007-1008
  gerontologic considerations for, **1008-1009**
  nursing and collaborative management of, **1008**
  paraesophageal or rolling, 1007, 1008f
  sliding, 1007, 1008f
  surgical therapy of, 1008
  types of, 1007
Hibiclens (chlorhexidine), 205
Hiccups, postoperative, 391
Hickman catheter, 290
HIDA. *See* Hepatobiliary scintigraphy
High-calorie foods, 306, 307t
High-density lipoprotein cholesterol, 987t
High-density lipoproteins, 756, 788
High-fiber foods, 1041, 1043t
High-frequency chest compression, 649
High-frequency jet ventilation, 1763
High-frequency oscillatory ventilation, 1763
High-frequency percussive ventilation, 1763
High-frequency ventilation, 1763
Hilus, 511, 1137
Hip arthroplasty, 1663-1664, 1663f
Hip fracture, 1653-1654
  case study, 1665
  clinical manifestations of, 1653
  collaborative care for, 1653
  gender differences in, 1653b
  gerontologic considerations for, **1655**
  internal fixation for, 1653, 1653f
  neurovascular assessment of, 1654
  nursing evaluation of, 1654
  nursing implementation for, 1653-1654
  nursing management of, **1653-1654**
  postoperative management of, 1654
  preoperative management of, 1653-1654
  types of, 1653, 1653f
  weight-bearing exercise for, 1655b
Hip injury, 1632, 1632f
Hip replacement, total, 1663, 1663f
Hip spica cast, 1640
Hirsutism, 457t
Hirudin, 914
Hispanic Americans
  culture-bound syndromes, 35, 35t
  diabetes mellitus in, 1255
  end-of-life care, 155
  ethnic differences in response to drugs, 34, 35t
  health disparities, 20, 21, 33-34
  nurses, 26
  older adults, 66
  personal space, 33
  and touch, 33
Hispanic health care, 97t
Histamine, 195t, 226t
Histamine H$_2$-receptor antagonists
  for acute pancreatitis, 1121t
  for cirrhosis, 1110t

Histamine H$_2$-receptor antagonists (Continued)
  for gastroesophageal reflux disease, 1006t
  for gastrointestinal bleeding, 997, 998t
  hematologic effects of, 674t
  for peptic ulcer disease, 1019-1020, 1019t
  preoperative, 355t
  for upper gastrointestinal bleeding, 997
Histocompatibility studies, 237, 1226
Histoplasma capsulatum, 254t, 576t
Histoplasmosis, 437t, 576t
History. *See specific types*
HITTS. *See* Heparin-induced thrombocytopenia and thrombosis syndrome
HIV. *See* Human immunodeficiency virus
HIV-associated nephropathy, 1168
HIV-associated renal syndromes, 1168
Hives, 227
HLA system. *See* Human leukocyte antigen system
HMG-CoA reductase inhibitors, 793, 795t
HMOs. *See* Health maintenance organizations
HOCM. *See* Hypertrophic obstructive cardiomyopathy
Hodgkin's lymphoma, 723-724, 723t
  clinical manifestations of, 723, 723f
  dermatologic manifestations of, 473t
  diagnostic studies, 724
  etiology and pathophysiology of, 723
  nursing and collaborative management of, **724**
  staging studies, 724
  staging system for, 725f
Holding area, 360, 364
Holistic nursing, 107
Holistic nursing practice, 106-107
Holistic self-care, 106-107
Holistic therapy, 94
Holter monitoring, 753t, 848
Homans' sign, positive, 749t
Homatropine hydrobromide (AK-Homatropine), 427t
Home BP monitoring, 780
Home care nursing, 92t
Home health aides, 91t
Home health care, **89-92,** 92f. *See also specific disorders; specific disorders*
  chronic oxygen therapy, 644
  definition of, 89
  example nursing activities, 90t
  funding mechanisms for, 89t
  nursing diagnoses for patients requiring, 91t
  for older adults, 76
  oxygen delivery systems, 644, 645t
  parenteral nutrition, 968
  patient and family teaching guide for home oxygen therapy, 645t
  patient care, 89-91, 89f
  patient concerns, 90t
  after prostate surgery, 1422
  resources, 93
  for spinal cord injury, 1604
Home Health Care Classification, 8, 8t
Home health care team, 91-92, 91t
"Homebound status," 91
Homelessness
  key factors, 71
  in older adults, 70-71

Homeopathy, 97t
Homeostasis, **314-315**
Homocysteine, 680t, 752t, 756
  and atherosclerosis, 791
  and coronary artery disease, 791
Homograft skin, 498, 498t
Homografts, 883t
Homologous immunity, 1089
Homonymous hemianopsia, 1460t,
  1508
  after stroke, 1520, 1520f
Homozygous (term), 214t
Hordeolum, 406t, **422,** 422f
Hormone replacement therapy
  adverse cardiovascular effects of,
    745t
  for osteoporosis, 1689
  for perimenopause and postmeno-
    pause, 1391-1392
  for voiding dysfunction, 1185t
Hormone therapy
  antiaging, 67-68, 68t
  for breast cancer, 1355
  classification of, 288t
  hematologic effects of, 674t
  for prostate cancer, 1426-1427, 1426t
Hormones, **1235-1238**
  blood studies, 1336
  classification of, 1235
  complex feedback, 1238
  controlling gastrointestinal secretion
    and motility, 929, 930t
  endocrine, **1235-1242,** 1236t
  functions of, 1235
  of hypothalamus, 1238, 1238t
  lipid-soluble, 1235
  negative feedback, 1237, 1238f
  in obesity, 972, 973f, 973t
  of pituitary, 1239-1240
  positive feedback, 1237-1238
  receptors, 1235-1237
  regulation of, 1237-1238, 1237f
  rhythms of secretions, 1238
  simple feedback, 1237
  target cells, 1235, 1235f
  target tissue, 1235
  targets, 1235-1237
  transport of, 1235
  urine studies, 1336
  water-soluble, 1235
Hospice, 92, **156-157,** 156f
  inpatient settings, 157, 157f
  resources, 164
Hospital-acquired pneumonia, 563-
  564
  in acute respiratory distress syn-
    drome, 1815
  organisms associated with, 562t
Hospitalization
  "23-hour" stay, 344
  older adult care, 79, 79t
  same-day admission, 344
  same-day surgery, 344
Housing
  assessment of, 59
  congregate, 75
  for older adults, 75-76, 75f
HPS. *See* Hantavirus pulmonary syndrome
HR. *See* Heart rate

HSCT. *See* Hematopoietic stem cell
  transplantation
Huber-point needles, 289, 290
Huff coughing, 646, 1809
Huhner test, 1341t
Humalog (lispro) insulin, 1260t
Human bites, 1836-1837
Human chorionic gonadotropin
  for infertility, 1383, 1383t
  preoperative, 351
  serum assay, 1338t
  urine test, 1338t
Human diploid cell vaccine (HDCV)
  (RabAvert), 1837
Human epidermal growth factor receptor 2, 302, 1349
Human Genome Project (HGP), 214,
  214b
Human herpesvirus 6, 245t
Human herpesvirus 8, 245t
Human immunodeficiency virus, 250-
  251, 251f, 1367t
  diseases caused by, 244t
  related diseases, 245t
  testing for, 263
  transmission of, 250
    by contact with blood and blood
      products, 250
    perinatal, 250, 262-263
    sexual, 250
  vaccination against, 257-259
Human immunodeficiency virus counseling, 263, 264t
**Human immunodeficiency virus in-
  fection, 249-267**
  acute, 252
  acute exacerbations of, 265
  acute intervention for, 261t, 264-265
  ambulatory and home care for, 261t,
    265-267
  antiretroviral therapy of, 256-257,
    264
  asymptomatic disease, 252
  chronic, 252-253
    early, 252
    intermediate, 252
    late, 252-253
  clinical manifestations of, 252-253
  collaborative care, 255-259
  complications of, 252-253
  course of, 252, 252f
  diagnosis of, 253
  drug therapy of, 256-257, 257t
  early detection of, 260b
  early intervention for, 264
  health promotion in, 260-263, 261t,
    265
  health promotion interventions for,
    265
  individual vs. public health protection
    against, 256b
  initial response to diagnosis of, 264
  laboratory studies, 253-255
  nursing assessment of, 259, 259t
  nursing diagnoses, 260, 260t
  nursing evaluation of, 267
  nursing implementation for, 260-267
  nursing interventions in, 261t
  nursing management of, **259-267**
  nursing planning for, 260
  opportunistic diseases associated with
    drug therapy of, 257
    manifestations and treatment of,
      253, 254t-255t
  pathophysiology of, 250-252
  postexposure prophylaxis of, 263

Human immunodeficiency virus infection *(Continued)*
  prevention of, 260-263, 260b
  resources, 270
  risk assessment, 259
  risk for, 268
  risk-reducing activities, 260
  risks at work, 263
  risks related to drug use, 262
  risks related to sexual intercourse,
    261-262
  safe activities, 260
  side effects of, 266-267
  significance of problem, 249-250
  signs and symptoms that HIV-in-
    fected patients need to report,
    266t
  symptomatic, case study, 268
  terminal care for, 267
  timeline for, 252, 252f
  treatment guidelines, 256
  viral load, 249, 250f
  window period, 253
Human immunodeficiency virus–
  antibody testing, 253, 256t, 263,
  264t
**Human immunodeficiency virus–
  associated rheumatic disease,
  1714-1715**
Human leukocyte antigen (HLA)-B27,
  1626t, 1711
Human leukocyte antigen system, **233**
  disease associations, 233
  matching, 237
  patterns of inheritance, 233, 233f
Human leukocyte antigens, 1872
Human papillomavirus, 1367t
Humegon, 1383t
Humerus
  chondrosarcoma of, 1673f
  fractures of, **1652,** 1652f
Humira (adalimumab)
  for arthritis and connective tissue dis-
    orders, 1700t
  for rheumatoid arthritis, 1705-1706
Humor, 116t
Humoral immunity, 223-224
  comparison with cell-mediated im-
    munity, 223-224, 223t
Humoral rejection, 238
Humulin N (NPH insulin), 1260t
Humulin R (regular insulin), 1260t
Huntington's disease, 1558-1559
  genetics of, 1559b
Hyaline cartilage, 1617
Hyaluronic acid (Orthovisc)
  injection procedures, 479t
  for osteoarthritis, 1697-1701
Hybridoma technology, 240-241
Hycamtin (topotecan)
  classification of, 287t
  for lung cancer, 582
  for ovarian cancer, 1403
Hydralazine (Apresoline), 775t
Hydrasorb, 205t
Hydrea (hydroxyurea)
  classification of, 287t
  for leukemia, 720t
  for sickle cell disease, 698
Hydrocele, 1431, 1431f
Hydrocephalus, normal pressure, 1576
Hydrochlorothiazide (HydroDIURIL)
  combination drug therapy of hyper-
    tension, 777t
  for diabetes insipidus, 1297
  for hypertension, 773t, 777t
  photosensitivity, 461t

Hydrocil (psyllium), 1042t
Hydrocodone (Lortab, Vicodin,
  Zydone), 137t, 138
Hydrocol, 205t
Hydrocolloids, 205t
Hydrocortisone (Cortef, Solu-Cortef)
  for asthma and COPD, 618t
  classification of, 287t
  for inflammatory bowel disease,
    1055t
  for shock, 1787t
  target tissue and functions, 1236t
Hydrocortisone enema (Cortenema),
  1055t
Hydrocortisone sodium succinate (Solu-
  Cortef), 1699t
Hydrocortisone suppository or foam
  (Cortifoam), 1055t
HydroDiuril (hydrochlorothiazide)
  for diabetes insipidus, 1297
  for hypertension, 773t, 777t
  photosensitivity, 461t
Hydrogel, 205t
Hydrogen ion concentration (H$^+$), 333
Hydromorphone (Dilaudid)
  for burns, 499t
  effects of use, 169t
  for pain, 137t, 138, 141
Hydronephrosis, 1168, 1169f
Hydropres (reserpine/hydrochlorothia-
  zide), 777t
Hydrostatic pressure, 318
  venous, 319
Hydrotherapy cart shower, 496, 497f
Hydrothoraces, 595
Hydroureter, 1168
Hydroxychloroquine (Plaquenil)
  for arthritis and connective tissue dis-
    orders, 1700t
  drug alert, 1705
  for polymyositis and dermatomyosi-
    ties, 1726
  for rheumatoid arthritis, 1705
  for systemic lupus erythematosus,
    1719
5-Hydroxyindole-acetic acid, 1862t
Hydroxyurea (Hydrea, Droxia)
  classification of, 287t
  for leukemia, 720t, 721t
  for sickle cell disease, 698
Hydroxyzine (Atarax, Vistaril)
  for dermatologic problems, 475
  for nausea and vomiting, 138,
    992t
Hygiene, 1379
  oral, 1003b
  personal, 1275-1276, 1793
  in shock, 1793
  and skin, 462
Hygroton (chlorthalidone), 773t
Hylorel (guanadrel sulfate), 774t
Hymen, 1327
Hymenopteran stings, 1834
Hyoscine HBr (Donnagel), 1037t
Hyoscyamine (Levsin, Levbid), 1185t
Hyperacute rejection, 238
Hyperaldosteronism, 1319-1320
  and ascites, 1105t
  clinical manifestations of, 1319
  diagnostic studies, 1319
  etiology and pathophysiology of,
    1319
  nursing and collaborative manage-
    ment of, **1319-1320**
  primary, 1319
  secondary, 1319
Hyperalgesia, 129
Hyperbaric oxygen therapy, 205-206

Note: Disorder names are in **bold face.**
Page numbers in **bold face** indicate main
discussions. Page numbers followed by
f, t, b, or *n* indicate figures, tables, boxed
material, or notes, respectively.

Hypercalcemia, 329-330
in cancer, 308
causes and clinical manifestations of, 330t
nursing and collaborative management of, **330**
nursing diagnoses, 330
nursing implementation for, 330
Hypercapnia, 1799
clinical manifestations of, 1804, 1804t
in obstructive sleep apnea, 542
Hypercapnic respiratory failure
causes of, 1800, 1800t
definition of, 1800
etiology and pathophysiology of, 1803
Hyperemia, reactive, 901
Hyperesthesia, 1460t
Hyperextension, 1622t
Hyperfractionated radiation therapy, 292
Hypergel, 205t
Hyperglycemia, 1278t
chronic, 1282-1283
hyperosmolar hyperglycemic syndrome, **1280-1281**
collaborative care for, 1280t
nursing management of, **1281**
pathophysiology of, 1280-1281, 1281f
treatment based on LDL levels, 789, 790t
Hyperinsulinemia, 766
Hyperkalemia, 327-328
in burn patients, 500
causes and clinical manifestations of, 327t
clinical manifestations of, 327-328, 328f
drug therapy of, 1210
nursing and collaborative management of, **328**
nursing diagnoses, 328
nursing implementation for, 328
therapies to treat, 1202t
treatment of, 328
Hyperlipidemia
drug therapy of, 793, 795t
treatment of, 1167
Hypermagnesemia, 332-333, 332t
Hypermetabolic state, 499
Hypernatremia, 324-326
in burn patients, 500
causes and clinical manifestations of, 325t
clinical manifestations of, 325-326
with decreased ECF volume, 325t
with normal/increased ECF volume, 325t
nursing and collaborative management of, **326**
nursing diagnoses, 326
nursing implementation for, 326
Hyperopia, 400, 416, **417**
Hyperosmolar agents, 435t
Hyperosmolar hyperglycemic syndrome, 1280-1281
collaborative care for, 1280t, 1281
nursing management of, **1281**
pathophysiology of, 1280-1281, 1281f
Hyperparathyroidism, 1308-1311
clinical manifestations of, 1309, 1310t
collaborative care for, 1309-1311
complications of, 1309
diagnostic studies, 1309

Hyperparathyroidism (Continued)
etiology and pathophysiology of, 1308-1309
nonsurgical therapy for, 1310-1311
nursing management of, **1311**
primary, 1309
secondary, 1210, 1309
surgical therapy for, 1309-1310
tertiary, 1309
Hyperphosphatemia, 331, 332t
Hyperpigmentation, 1246t
Hyperpituitarism, 473t
Hyperresonance, 523t, 524t, 940t
Hypersensitivity pneumonitis, 577
Hypersensitivity reactions, 224-228
atopic, 226-227
cytolytic, 227-228
cytotoxic, 225t, 227-228
delayed, 225t, 228
IgE-mediated, 225-227, 225f, 225t
microbial, 228
type I, 225-227, 225f
type II, 227-228
type III, 228
type IV, 228
types of, 225, 225t
Hypersplenism, 729
Hypertension, 764-781, 1246t
age-related changes and, 780-781
ambulatory and home care for, 779-780
cardiovascular risk factor modification for, 779
classification of, 764, 765t
clinical manifestations of, 766
collaborative care for, 768-776, 768t
collaborative problems, 778t
combination drug therapy of, 777t
complications of, 766
control of, 768b
and coronary artery disease, 789
cultural and ethnic health disparities in, 762b
DASH diet for, 770, 770t
definition of, 761
diagnostic studies, 767-768, 768t
drug therapy of, 771-776, 773t-776t, 1210
etiology of, 765
gender differences in, 762t
gerontologic considerations for, **780-781**
health disparities and, 21t
health promotion in, 777-779
health-promoting behaviors for, 792t
individual patient evaluation for, 777-778
nursing assessment of, 778t
nursing diagnoses, 778t
nursing evaluation of, 780
ocular manifestations of, 437t
patient and family teaching guide for, 779t
portal
with cirrhosis, 1103-1104, 1104
postoperative, 382
primary (essential)
case study, 782
etiology and pathophysiology of, 765
nursing assessment of, 777
nursing diagnoses, 777
nursing implementation for, 777-780
nursing management of, **777-780**
nursing planning for, 777
risk factors for, 766t

Hypertension (Continued)
pseudohypertension, 765
pulmonary, 599, **600-604,** 1875
resistant, 776, 777t
resources for, 783
screening programs, 779
secondary, 765
causes of, 765
stage 1, 769t
stage 2, 769t
subtypes, 765
systolic, isolated, 765
target organ diseases, 766-767, 766t
treatment algorithm for, 769f
treatment of, 1210
"white coat," 768
Hypertensive crisis, 781-782
causes of, 781, 781t
clinical manifestations of, 781
nursing and collaborative management of, **781-782**
Hypertensive emergency, 781
Hypertensive encephalopathy, 781
Hypertensive retinopathy, 429
Hyperthermia
emergency management of, 1830t
malignant, 373
Hyperthyroidism, 1299-1305
acute intervention for, 1302-1304
ambulatory and home care for, 1304-1305
apathetic, 1299
clinical manifestations of, 1299, 1300t
collaborative care for, 1301-1302, 1301t
complications of, 1299-1300
definition of, 1872
dermatologic manifestations of, 473t
diagnostic studies, 1300-1301
drug therapy for, 1301
etiology and pathophysiology of, 1299
nursing assessment of, 1302, 1302t
nursing care plan for patient with, 1303b
nursing diagnoses, 1302
nursing evaluation of, 1305
nursing implementation for, 1302-1304
nursing management of, **1302-1305**
nursing planning for, 1302
nutritional therapy for, 1302
postoperative care of, 1304
radioactive iodine therapy for, 1304
radioiodine therapy for, 1301
surgical therapy for, 1301
thyroid surgery for, 1304
in younger and older adults, 1301t
Hypertonia, 1458
Hypertonic fluids, 318, 1786t
Hypertonic solutions, 340
Hypertrophic cardiomyopathy, 886t, 888, 888f
characteristics of, 888
clinical manifestations of, 888
diagnostic studies, 888
etiology and pathophysiology of, 888
nursing and collaborative management of, **888-889**
Hypertrophic obstructive cardiomyopathy, 888
Hypertrophic scars, 201
Hypertrophy, 1618
detrusor muscle, 1168
ventricular, 742, 823-824
Hypertropia, 424

Hyperuricemia
in chemotherapy and radiation therapy, 296t
conditions that can cause, 1715, 1715t
Hyperventilation, alveolar, 1764
Hyperventilation therapy, 1475
Hyperviscosity, 700
Hypervolemia, 700
Hypnosis
description of, 97t
for pain, 144
Hypnotics
nonbarbiturate, 369t
sedative-hypnotics, 178-179
Hypocalcemia
causes and clinical manifestations of, 330t
drug therapy of, 1210
nursing and collaborative management of, **330-331, 331**
nursing diagnoses, 331
nursing implementation for, 331
tests for, 331, 331f
Hypochromia, 691
Hypoesthesia, 1460t
Hypofractionated radiation therapy, 292
Hypoglossal nerve (cranial nerve XII), 1450t
Hypoglossal nerve (cranial nerve XII) testing, 1458
Hypoglycemia, 1278t, 1278t, **1281-1282**
collaborative care for, 1282t
postprandial, 1026
Hypoglycemic unawareness, 1281-1282
nursing and collaborative management of, **1282**
Hypoglycemics, 461t
Hypogonadism, late-onset, 1437
Hypokalemia, 328-329
in burn patients, 500
causes and clinical manifestations of, 327t
clinical manifestations of, 328-329, 328f
nursing and collaborative management of, **329**
nursing diagnoses, 329
nursing implementation for, 329
prevention of, 329t
Hypomagnesemia, 332, 332t, **333**
Hyponatremia, 326
in burn patients, 500
causes and clinical manifestations of, 325t
clinical manifestations of, 326
with decreased ECF volume, 325t
with normal/increased ECF volume, 325t
nursing and collaborative management of, **326**
nursing diagnoses, 326
nursing implementation for, 326
Hypoparathyroidism, 1311
clinical manifestations of, 1310t, 1311
dermatologic manifestations of, 473t
etiology and pathophysiology of, 1311
nursing and collaborative management of, 1311
Hypophosphatemia, 332, 332t
Hypophysectomy, 1291-1292, 1292f
Hypophysis. See Pituitary gland
Hypopigmentation, 457t

Hypopituitarism, 1293
  panhypopituitarism, 1293
  selective, 1293
Hypopnea, 542
Hypospadias, 1429
Hypotension
  controlled, 372
  in hemodialysis, 1223
  orthostatic, 778, 1874
  postoperative, 382
Hypothalamic regulation, 319
Hypothalamic-pituitary-adrenal axis,
  113, 113*f*
Hypothalamic-pituitary-gonadal axis,
  1328, 1328*f*
Hypothalamus, 1448*f*
  hormones of, 1238, 1238*t*
  location and function of, 1447*t*
  response to stress, 113
Hypothalamus-hypophyseal portal system, 1239, 1239*f*
Hypothermia, 1831
  anesthetic considerations, 372
  collaborative care for, 1831
  emergency management of, 1832*t*
  mild, 1831
  moderate, 1831
  postoperative, 389-390
  profound, 1831
Hypothyroidism, 1305-1308
  acute intervention for, 1306-1307
  ambulatory and home care for, 1307-
    1308
  clinical manifestations of, 1300*t,*
    1305-1306
  collaborative care for, 1306, 1306*t*
  complications of, 1306
  dermatologic manifestations of,
    473*t*
  diagnostic studies, 1306
  etiology and pathophysiology of,
    1305
  health promotion in, 1306
  nursing care plan for patient with,
    1307*b*-1308*b*
  nursing diagnoses, 1306
  nursing implementation for, 1306-
    1308
  nursing management of, **1306-**
    1308
  nursing planning for, 1306
  patient and family teaching guide for,
    1309*f*
Hypotonia, 1458, 1586
Hypotonic fluids, 318
Hypotonic solutions, 339
Hypotropia, 424
Hypoventilation
  alveolar, 1764, 1802
  with nasal packs, 535
  postoperative, 379*t,* 380
Hypovolemia
  absolute, 1773*t,* 1775
  relative, 1773*t,* 1775
Hypovolemic shock, 1773*f,* **1775-**
  1777
  classification of, 1773*t*
  clinical presentation of, 1776*t*
  collaborative care for, 1788
  pathophysiology of, 1776, 1777*f*
  precipitating factors, 1773*t*
  treatment of, 1789*t*

Hypoxemia, 1799
  clinical manifestations of, 1804,
    1804*t*
  consequences of, 1804
  with nasal packs, 535
  in obstructive sleep apnea, 542
  oxygen therapy of, 640
  postoperative, 378, 379*t*
  refractory, 1813, 1815*t*
Hypoxemic respiratory failure, 1799-
  1800
  causes of, 1799-1800, 1800*t*
  definition of, 1799-1800
  etiology and pathophysiology of,
    1800-1803
Hypoxia
  consequences of, 1804
Hysterectomy, 1398, 1404
  abdominal
    and bilateral salpingo-oophorec-
      tomy, 1404*t*
    case study, 1411
    nursing care plan for patient with,
      1398*b*
  acute intervention related to, 1406
  description of, 1332*t,* 1404*t*
  subtotal, 1404*t,* 1405*f*
  total, 1405*f*
    and bilateral salpingo-oophorec-
      tomy, 1404*t*
    case study, 1411
  vaginal, 1405*f*
Hysterosalpingogram, 1340*t,* 1341*t*
Hysterotomy, 1384*t*
Hytakerol (dihydrotachysterol), 1311
Hytrin (terazosin)
  for benign prostatic hyperplasia,
    1417
  effects on lower urinary tract func-
    tion, 1180*t*
  for hypertension, 774*t*
  for voiding dysfunction, 1185*t*
Hyzaar (losartan/hydrochlorothiazide),
  777*t*

I

IABPs. *See* Intraaortic balloon pumps
Ibandronate (Boniva)
  for osteoporosis, 1689
  for Paget's disease, 1690
IBD. *See* Inflammatory bowel disease
Ibritumomab tiuxetan/yttrium-90
  (Zevalin), 303*t,* 727
IBS. *See* Irritable bowel syndrome
Ibuprofen (Advil, Motrin, Novoprofen,
  Nuprin, Vicoprofen)
  analgesic effects of, 128
  for arthritis and connective tissue dis-
    orders, 1698*t*
  for fever, 203
  and gastritis, 1013
  mechanism of action, 202*t*
  nephrotoxicity, 1142*t*
  for pain, 136, 136*t,* 138
  for premenstrual syndrome, 1386
Ibutilide (Corvert)
  for atrial fibrillation, 852
  for atrial flutter, 851
  classification of, 856*t*
IC. *See* Inspiratory capacity; Interstitial
  cystitis
ICDs. *See* Implantable cardioverter-
  defibrillators; Intermittent compression devices
Iceberg effect, 486
ICF. *See* Intracellular fluid
ICG. *See* Impedance cardiography
ICP. *See* Intracranial pressure

ICRs. *See* Intracorneal ring segments
ICUS. *See* Intracoronary ultrasound
ICUs. *See* Intensive care units
Icy-Hot (capsaicin), 141
Idarubicin (Idamycin)
  classification of, 287*t*
  for leukemia, 720*t,* 721*t*
  for prostate cancer, 1427
IDET. *See* Intradiscal electrothermo-
  plasty
Idiopathic cardiomyopathy, 885
Idiopathic myocarditis, 875
Idiopathic pulmonary fibrosis, 597
Idiopathic seizure disorders, 1533
**Idiopathic thrombocytopenic pur-
  pura,** 701
  acute, 702, 703*f*
IE. *See* Infective endocarditis
Ifex (ifosfamide)
  classification of, 287*t*
  for testicular cancer, 1432
IFN. *See* Interferon
Ifosfamide (Ifex)
  classification of, 287*t*
  for lung cancer, 582
  for non-Hodgkin's lymphoma, 727*t*
  for testicular cancer, 1432
IGF-1. *See* Insulin-like growth factor-1
IL. *See* Interleukin
ILDS. *See* Interstitial lung diseases
Ileal conduit, 1189, 1189*t*
  definition of, 1873
  nursing care plan for patient with,
    1191*b*-1192*b*
  patient and family teaching guide for
    changing appliances, 1193*t*
  postoperative management of, 1192,
    1193*t*
  skin problems with, 1193, 1193*f*
Ileal loop, 1189*t*
Ileoanal reservoir, 1055, 1056*f,* 1070
Ileocecal junction, 943*f*
Ileostomy, 934*t,* 1069, 1069*f,* 1070*t*
  continent
    surgical formation of, 1055, 1056*f*
    total proctocolectomy with, 1055-
      1056
  nursing care plan for patient with co-
    lostomy/ileostomy, 1073*b*-1075*b*
  permanent, 1055
Ileostomy care, 1072-1073
Ileus, paralytic (adynamic), 1060-1061,
  1875
Illness. *See also specific illnesses*
  and health care system, 86
  malnutrition in, 952-953
Iloprost (Ventavis), 1724
Imagery, 1361*b*
  description of, 97*t*
  examples, 119*t*
  guided, 118
  as relaxation strategy, 118-119, 118*f,*
    118*t*
Imatinib (Gleevec), 303*t,* 720, 720*t,*
  721*t*
Imdur (isosorbide mononitrate), 798
Imferon (iron dextran injection), 1055*t*
Imipramine (Tofranil)
  for Alzheimer's disease, 1569*t*
  ethnic differences in response to, 35*t*
  local, 139*t*
  for peptic ulcer disease, 1019*t,* 1021
  for voiding dysfunction, 1185*t*
Imiquimod (Aldara), 476, 1376
Imitrex (sumatriptan)
  drug alert, 1531*b*
  for migraine headache, 1530
Immersion syndrome, 1832

Immigrants, 34, 34*f*
Immigration, 34
Immobilization
  for radiation therapy, 293, 293*f*
  for soft tissue injuries, 203
  after spinal cord injury, 1598-1601
Immune responses
  altered, **224-228**
  cell-mediated, 228
  cells involved, 220-222, 221*f*
  functions of, 219
  normal, **219-224**
  primary, 224, 224*f*
  resources, 241
  secondary, 224, 224*f*
  to viruses, 220, 221*f*
Immune system
  age-related changes in, 78*t*
  effects of aging on, **224,** 224*t*
  effects of chronic alcohol abuse on,
    177*t*
  gerontologic considerations for, **224**
  organs of, 219, 220*f*
  preoperative assessment of, 349, 351*t*
  preoperative review, 349
  problems with dermatologic manifes-
    tations, 473*t*
  response to stress, 114-115
  role in cancer, 277-279
Immune thrombocytopenic purpura
  collaborative care for, 703-704, 704*t*
  etiology and pathophysiology of, 701
Immune-complex reactions, 225*t,* 228
Immunity, 219
  acquired, 219
    active, 219
      artificial, 219*t*
      natural, 219*t*
    passive, 219
    types of, 219*t*
  autoimmunity, **234-235**
  cell-mediated, 223-224, 223*t*
  homologous, 1089
  humoral, 223-224
    comparison with cell-mediated im-
      munity, 223-224, 223*t*
    definition of, 1872
  innate, 219
  passive
    artificial, 219*t*
    natural, 219*t*
  types of, 219
Immunization
  and deafness, 444
  influenza, 538, 539*t*
  tetanus, 499
Immunocompetence, 224
Immunodeficiency, 235
  acquired immunodeficiency syn-
    drome (AIDS), **252-253**
    diagnostic criteria for, 252, 253*t*
    ocular manifestations of, 437*t*
    renal disease in, **1168**
    resources for, 270
  drug-induced, 235*t*
  human immunodeficiency virus in-
    fection, **249-267**
  human immunodeficiency virus–asso-
    ciated rheumatic disease, **1714-**
    1715
  secondary, 235, 235*t*
Immunodeficiency disorders, 235-236
  primary, 235, 235*t*
  resources, 270
  secondary, 235-236
Immunofluorescent studies, 458*t*
Immunoglobulin (Sandoglobulin), 1586
Immunoglobulin A, 220*t,* 1861*t*

Immunoglobulin D, 220*t*, 1861*t*
Immunoglobulin E
　characteristics of, 220*t*
　laboratory values, 1861*t*
　-mediated reactions, 225-227, 225*f*, 225*t*
Immunoglobulin E antagonists, 618*t*, 620
Immunoglobulin G, 220*t*, 1861*t*
Immunoglobulin M, 220*t*, 1861*t*
Immunoglobulins, 220
　characteristics of, 220*t*
　laboratory values, 1861*t*
Immunologic disorders, of kidney, **1165-1168**
Immunologic escape, 279, 279*f*
Immunologic surveillance, 277
Immunologic theory of aging, 68*t*, 69
Immunology
　with burns, 491
　laboratory values, 1860*t*-1861*t*
　technologies in, **240-241**
Immunomodulators
　for dermatologic problems, 476
　for inflammatory bowel disease, 1054, 1055*t*
　for multiple sclerosis, 1544, 1544*t*
Immunosenescence, 224
Immunosuppressive therapy, 238-239, 239*t*
　for arthritis and connective tissue disorders, 1700*t*
　corticosteroid, 1318
　hematologic effects of, 674*t*
　for inflammatory bowel disease, 1053, 1054, 1055*t*
　for kidney transplantation, 1229
　major agents, 238
　for multiple sclerosis, 1544, 1544*t*
　for rheumatoid arthritis, 1706
　side effects of, 238
　sites of action, 239*f*
Immunotherapy
　for allergic disorders, 231-232
　for allergic rhinitis, 536
　mechanism of action, 231
　method of administration, 231-232
　nursing management of, **232**
Imodium (loperamide), 1037*t*, 1055*t*
Impaired fasting glucose, 1255, 1258, 1873
Impaired glucose tolerance, 1255, 1258
Impaired health care providers, 174*b*
Impedance, 1746
Impedance audiometry, 414*t*
Impedance cardiography, 1745-1746
Impetigo, 466, 466*f*, 467*t*
Impingement syndrome, 1630*t*
Implantable cardioverter-defibrillators, 857-858, 858*f*, 858*t*
Implantable pumps, 142
Implanted infusion ports, 289, 290*f*
Implanted infusion pumps, 290, 290*f*
Implants
　artificial heart, 839, 840*f*, 1750
　breast, 1353*t*
　cochlear, 445
　penile, 1436, 1436*f*
　for refractive errors, 419
IMRT. *See* Intensity-modulated radiotherapy
Imuran (azathioprine), 238, 239*t*
　for arthritis and connective tissue disorders, 1700*t*
　for inflammatory bowel disease, 1054, 1055*t*
　for lupus nephritis, 1718

Imuran (azathioprine) *(Continued)*
　for polymyositis and dermatomyositis, 1726
　for rheumatoid arthritis, 1706
　for systemic lupus erythematosus, 1719
IMV. *See* Intermittent mandatory ventilation
Inamrinone (Inocor), 829
Inapsine (droperidol)
　as adjunct to general anesthesia, 370*t*
　for nausea and vomiting, 992, 992*t*
　preoperative, 355*t*
Inborn errors of metabolism, 692*t*
In-center hemodialysis, 1223, 1223*f*
Incisional biopsy, 283, 458*t*
Incontinence, 1145*t*
　fecal, **1038-1040**
　stress, 1145*t*
　urinary, **1180-1188**
Incontinent urinary diversion, 1189
Incretin mimetic, 1265-1266, 1266*t*
Incus, 409
Inderal (propranolol)
　for chronic stable angina, 799
　for cirrhosis, 1110*t*
　effects on lower urinary tract function, 1180*t*
　for hypertension, 774*t*
　for hyperthyroidism, 1301
　for pheochromocytoma, 1320
　and reproductive system, 1332
　for restless legs syndrome, 1558
　toxicology, 1865*t*
Inderide (propranolol/hydrochlorothiazide), 777*t*
Indinavir (Crixivan), 258*t*
Indocin (indomethacin)
　for diabetes insipidus, 1297
　and gastritis, 1013
　for pain, 135, 136*t*
Indocyanine green, 946*t*
Indomethacin (Indocin, Indocid)
　for arthritis and connective tissue disorders, 1698*t*
　for diabetes insipidus, 1297
　and gastritis, 1013
　nephrotoxicity, 1142*t*
　for pain, 135, 136*t*
Induction therapy, 720
Infant mortality, 21*t*
Infection, 193, **243-249**
　in acute respiratory distress syndrome, 1816*t*
　antibiotic-resistant, 247*t*
　bacterial
　　sexually transmitted diseases, **1367-1373**
　　of skin, 466
　of breast, **1345-1346**
　in burns, 500
　in cancer, 307
　case study, 211
　causes of, **243-245**
　chlamydial, **1371-1373**
　in chronic kidney disease, 1207
　control of, 206, **247-249**
　and COPD, 631-632
　delayed transfusion reactions, 734
　in diabetes mellitus, **1287**
　ear (*See* Otitis media)
　effects on wound healing, 201*t*
　emerging, **245-246,** 245*t*
　evidence of, 876
　exit site, 1219

Infection *(Continued)*
　extraocular, **422-424**
　　acute intervention for, 424
　　ambulatory and home care for, 424
　　nursing assessment of, 424
　　nursing diagnoses, 424
　　nursing evaluation of, 424
　　nursing implementation for, 424
　　nursing management of, **424**
　　nursing planning for, 424
　eye, in newborns, 1368
　with fractures, 1649-1650
　fungal
　　of lung, 575, 576*t*
　　pulmonary, **575-576**
　herpes simplex virus
　　of eye, 1374
　　in pregnancy, 1374
　human immunodeficiency virus, **249-267**
　intraocular, **436-437**
　in kidney transplantation, 1229
　of lower genital tract, 1394*t*
　of mouth, 1000-1001, 1000*t*
　of nose and paranasal sinuses, **535-541**
　nosocomial, **246-247**
　ocular manifestations of, 437*t*
　in older adults, **247**
　oral, **1000-1001**
　with oxygen therapy, 644
　postinfectious polyneuropathy (*See* Guillain-Barré syndrome)
　prevention of, 206, **247-249,** 1795
　　in Alzheimer's disease, 1574
　prosthetic vascular graft, 897
　pulmonary, 1811
　reemerging, 245-246, 246*t*
　respiratory, 609
　sexually transmitted diseases, 1377-1378
　skin, **466-470**
　surgical wound, 392
　in systemic lupus erythematosus, 1718
　treatment of, 1795
　urinary tract, **1155-1159**
　viral
　　sexually transmitted diseases, **1373-1379**
　　of skin, 468*t*
Infection precautions, 247-249
　airborne precautions, 249
　contact precautions, 249
　droplet precautions, 249
　standard, 247, 248*t*-249*t*
　transmission-based, 247-248, 248*t*-249*t*
Infectious arthritis, 1713-1714
Infectious diarrhea, acute
　causes of, 1036, 1037*t*
　nursing care plan for, 1039*b*
　nursing management of, **1037-1038**
Infectious Disease Society of America (IDSA)
　drug therapy of community-acquired pneumonia, 562-563, 563*t*
　guidelines for community-acquired pneumonia, 562
Infectious keratitis, 423-424
Infective endocarditis, 865-871
　acute form, 866
　ambulatory and home care for, 870-871
　antibiotic prophylaxis of, 868
　classification of, 866
　clinical manifestations of, 867

Infective endocarditis *(Continued)*
　collaborative care for, 868
　conditions associated with risk for, 869*t*
　conditions requiring antibiotic prophylaxis to prevent, 869*t*
　diagnostic studies, 867-868
　drug therapy of, 868, 869*t*
　embolization, 866
　etiology and pathophysiology of, 866-867, 866*t*
　health promotion in, 870
　of mitral valve, 866, 867*f*
　nursing assessment of, 869, 869*t*
　nursing care plan for patient with, 870*b*-871*b*
　nursing diagnoses, 869
　nursing evaluation of, 871
　nursing implementation for, 870-871
　nursing management of, **869-871**
　nursing planning for, 869
　predisposing conditions for, 866, 866*t*
　procedures requiring antibiotic prophylaxis to prevent, 866, 867*t*
　prophylactic treatment of, 868
　sequence of events in, 868*f*
　subacute form, 866
　vegetations, 866
Inferior vena cava, 743
Inferior vena caval interruption, 915, 915*f*
Infertility
　female, **1382-1383**
　　collaborative care for, 1382*t*
　　diagnostic studies, 1382-1383
　　drug therapy for, 1383*t*
　　etiology and pathophysiology of, 1382
　　nursing and collaborative management of, **1383**
　male, **1437-1438**
Infestations, 470, 470*f*, 470*t*
Infiltrative emergencies, oncologic, 308
Inflammation, 193-197
　acute, 197
　acute intervention for, 203
　airway, 1811
　of brain, **1493-1499**
　of burns, 491
　case study, 211
　cellular response, 194-195, 194*f*
　cerebral, 1493, 1494*t*
　chemical mediators of, 195-196, 195*t*
　chronic, 197
　clinical manifestations of, 196-197
　collaborative care, 202
　drug therapy of, 202, 202*t*
　extraocular, **422-424**
　　acute intervention for, 424
　　ambulatory and home care for, 424
　　nursing assessment of, 424
　　nursing diagnoses, 424
　　nursing evaluation of, 424
　　nursing implementation for, 424
　　nursing management of, **424**
　　nursing planning for, 424
　health promotion in, 202-203
　of heart, **865-878**
　intraocular, **436-437**
　local manifestations of, 196, 197*t*
　lower gastrointestinal, **1048-1051**
　mediators of, 195-196, 195*t*
　of mouth, 1000-1001, 1000*t*
　of nose and paranasal sinuses, **535-541**
　nursing implementation for, 202-203

Inflammation (Continued)
nursing management of, **202-203**
nutritional therapy of, 202
observation of, 203
oral, **1000-1001**
of parotid gland, 1000*t*
resources, 212
of scrotum and testes, **1430**
subacute, 197
systemic inflammatory response syndrome, 1772, **1794-1796**
types of, 197
of urinary system, **1155-1165**
vascular response, 193-194, 194*f*
Inflammatory bowel disease (IBD), 1051-1060
clinical manifestations of, 1052
collaborative care for, 1053-1057
complications of, 1052-1053
diagnostic studies, 1053
drug therapy of, 1053-1054, 1055*t*
etiology and pathophysiology of, 1051-1052
extraintestinal complications of, 1053, 1053*t*
gerontologic considerations for, **1060**
nursing assessment of, 1057, 1057*t*
nursing care plan for patient with, 1058*b*-1059*b*
nursing diagnoses, 1057
nursing evaluation of, 1060
nursing implementation for, 1057-1060
nursing management of, **1057-1060**
nursing planning for, 1057
nutritional therapy of, 1056-1057
postoperative care of, 1056
surgical therapy of, 1054-1055, 1055*t*
treatment goals, 1053
Inflammatory breast cancer, 1350
Inflammatory prostatitis, asymptomatic, 1428
Infliximab (Remicade)
for arthritis and connective tissue disorders, 1700*t*
drug alert, 1706
for inflammatory bowel disease, 1054, 1055*t*
for rheumatoid arthritis, 1705-1706
Influenza, 538-540
associated with HIV infection, 254*t*
clinical manifestations of, 538-540
immunization, 538
nursing and collaborative management of, **539-540**
target groups for immunization, 539*t*
Influenza A virus, 244*t*
Influenza B virus, 244*t*
Influenza vaccine, 519
Informatics
health care, 8-9
nursing, 9
Informed consent, 352-353, 353*b*
Infusion Nurses Society, 341
Infusion ports, implanted, 289, 290*f*
Infusion pumps, 289-290
implanted, 290, 290*f*
Infusions, stem cell, 305-306
Ingestion, 926
problems of, **925-1134**
resources for, 970
Inguinal masses, 1336*t*
Inguinal region examination, 1335

INH. *See* Isoniazid
Inhalants, **181**
effects of use, 170*t*
for general anesthesia, 367-368, 369*t*
onset, peak, duration, and withdrawal onset of, 185*t*
Inhalation injury, 484-485, 492
above glottis, 485
below glottis, 485
case study, 506
emergency management of, 489*t*
manifestations of, 492*t*
types of, 484-485
Inhalation pneumonia, 561
Inhaled insulin, 1263
Inheritance patterns, 215
HLA system, 233, 233*f*
Punnett squares, 217, 218*f*
Inherited conditions, multifactorial, 215
Injecting drugs, 168*t*
Injection
fear of, 146*t*
patient and family teaching guide for proper use of equipment, 263*t*
Injury. *See also* Trauma
burn
classification of, **486-488**
types of, **484-486**
cellular response to, 194-195, 194*f*
coup-contrecoup, 1482
crush injury, 585*t*
extravasation injury from infiltration of chemotherapy, 286, 288*f*
to head, **1481-1487**
case study, 1499
and restrictive lung disease, 595*t*
types of, **1481-1483**
when to start nutritional support for, 1475*b*
immediate care for, 1631
in increased ICP, 1480-1481
inflammatory response, **193-197**
inhalation, 484-485, 489*t*
ligament, 1630*t*
to lower extremities, 1640-1641
meniscal, 1630*t*, **1634-1635**
muscle injury, 1627*t*
musculoskeletal, 1647-1648, 1649*t*
repetitive strain, **1633**
rotator cuff, **1634**
smoke and inhalation, 484-485
soft tissue, **1630-1635**
acute, 1631, 1632*t*
of hip, 1632, 1632*f*
RICE for, 203
spinal cord, **1589-1609**
and restrictive lung disease, 595*t*
sports-related, 1630, 1630*t*
submersion, **1831-1833**
thoracic, **585-593**
Inner ear, 408*f*, 409
age-related changes in, 410*t*
problems of, **441-445**
Inocor (inamrinone), 829
Inpatient hospice settings, 157, 157*f*
INR. *See* International normalized ratio
Insect bites, 470, 470*t*
venoms that cause anaphylactic shock, 227*t*
Insensible water loss, 321
Insertive sex, 261-262
Inspection, 47
of abdomen, 937
of chest, 521
assessment abnormalities, 524*t*
findings in pulmonary problems, 526*t*

Inspection (Continued)
of mouth, 936
of musculoskeletal system, 1621
of peripheral vascular system, 748
of posterior surfaces, 1826*t*, 1827
of skin, 48*t*, 454-456
of thorax, 748-750
assessment abnormalities, 749*t*
normal, 751*t*
of urinary system, 1144
Inspiration, 512
Inspiratory capacity (IC), 531*t*
Inspiratory reserve volume (IRV), 531*t*
Inspiratory to expiratory (I:E) ratio, 1805
InspirEase, 621
Inspra (eplerenone)
for hyperaldosteronism, 1319
for hypertension, 773*t*
Institute of Medicine
definition of end of life, 151
definition of health disparities, 20
Food and Nutrition Board, 970
Institutional elder mistreatment, 74
Instrumentation, urinary, **1185-1188**
Insulin, 1241-1242
alteration in obesity, 972, 973*f*, 973*t*
blood glucose level effects, 1267*t*
exogenous, 1255
factors influencing secretion of, 1242*t*
feedback between blood glucose and, 1237, 1237*f*
laboratory values, 1856*t*
normal metabolism of, 1254-1255, 1255*f*
target tissue and functions, 1236*t*
Insulin aspart (NovoLog), 1260*t*
Insulin detemir (Levemir), 1260*t*, 1261*t*
Insulin glargine (Lantus), 1260*t*, 1261*t*
Insulin glulisine (Apidra), 1260*t*
Insulin lispro (Humalog), 1260*t*
Insulin pen, 1263, 1263*f*
Insulin pumps, 1263, 1264*f*
Minimed Paradigm insulin pump (Medtronic), 1269, 1270*f*
Insulin reaction, 1278
Insulin resistance, 1256-1257
and hypertension, 766
Insulin resistance syndrome, 1284
Insulin sensitizers, 1265
Insulin therapy
administration of, 1262-1263
allergic reactions to, 1263
alternative delivery methods for, 1263
for chronic pancreatitis, 1121*t*
combination therapy, 1260-1261
commercially available preparations, 1259, 1260*f*
for diabetes mellitus, 1259-1265, 1275
for elevated potassium levels, 1202*t*
inhaled, 1263
by injection, 1262-1263
sites for, 1262, 1262*f*
intensive, 1263, 1873
long-acting (basal) background insulin, 1260
mealtime insulin (bolus), 1260
mixing insulins, 1262, 1262*f*
NPH insulin (Humulin N, Novolin N, ReliOn N), 1260*t*, 1261*t*
patient and family teaching guide for, 1262*t*
problems with, 1263-1264

Insulin therapy (Continued)
regimens, 1259-1260, 1261*t*
regular insulin (Humulin R, Novolin R, ReliOn R), 1260*t*
storage of, 1261-1262
types of, 1259, 1260*t*
Insulin-like growth factor-1, 1248*t*
Intake and output records, 322
Intal (cromolyn), 620
for asthma, 617*t*, 618*t*
for COPD, 618*t*
for exercise-induced asthma, 608
Integra, 498*t*
Integrase, 251
Integrative health care model, 94-95, 95*t*
Integrative nursing practice, **108**
Integrative therapy, 94
Integrelin (eptifibatide), 800*t*
Integumentary system, **449-459**
age-related changes in, 451-452, 452*t*
nursing diagnoses associated with, 78*t*
in allergies, 229*t*
in anemia, 686, 686*t*
assessment abnormalities, 457*t*, 1246*t*
assessment of, **452-457**
gerontologic differences in, 451-452, 452*t*
health history questions to ask, 453*t*
important health information in, 453
objective data, 454-456
physical, 452-453, 453*t*
preoperative, 349, 351*t*
subjective data, 453-454
and asthma, 624*t*
in chronic kidney disease, 1209
complications of diabetes mellitus, **1287**
and COPD, 650*t*
diagnostic studies, **458-459**, 458*t*
effects of aging on, **451-452**
effects of chronic alcohol abuse on, 177*t*
at end of life, 152*t*
functions of, 451
health promotion for, **460-463**
in HIV infection, 259*t*
and lung cancer, 583*t*
physical examination of, 48*t*, 454-456, 1245
postoperative problems, **392-393**
preoperative review, 348
in pressure ulcers, 209*t*
problems of, **460-482**
in chemotherapy and radiation therapy, 295*t*-296*t*
cultural and ethnic health disparities in, 461*b*
in spinal cord injury, 1595
after stroke, 1519
Intellectual capacity assessment, 1456
Intellectual function, after stroke, 1508
Intensification therapy, 720
Intensity-modulated radiotherapy, 292
Intensive care nursing, 1734
Intensive care units, 1734, 1734*f*
abbreviations commonly used in, 1734*t*
electronic or virtual ICUs, 1734, 1734*f*
Intercostal retractions, 524*t*

Note: Disorder names are in **bold face.** Page numbers in **bold face** indicate main discussions. Page numbers followed by *f, t, b,* or *n* indicate figures, tables, boxed material, or notes, respectively.

Interferon
  mass production by recombinant DNA technology, 241, 241f
  mechanism of action, 223, 223f
  types and functions of, 222t
α-Interferon (Roferon-A, Intron-A), 303t
  for chronic hepatitis B, 1094
  clinical uses of, 223t
  function of, 222t
  pegylated (PEG-Intron, Pegasys), 1095
  side effects of, 1094t
β-Interferon (Avonex, Betaseron, Rebif)
  clinical uses of, 223t
  drug alert, 1544
  function of, 222t
  for multiple sclerosis, 1544, 1544t
γ-Interferon, 222t
Interleukin, 222t
Interleukin-1, 222t
Interleukin-1 receptor antagonist, 223t
Interleukin-2, 303t
  clinical uses of, 223t
  function of, 222t
Interleukin-3, 222t
Interleukin-4, 222t
Interleukin-5, 222t
Interleukin-6, 222t
Interleukin-7, 222t
Interleukin-8, 222t
Interleukin-9, 222t
Interleukin-10, 222t
Interleukin-11
  for cancer treatment, 304t
  clinical uses of, 223t
  function of, 222t
Interleukin-12, 222t
Interleukin-13, 222t
Interleukin-14, 222t
Interleukin-15, 222t
Interleukin-16, 222t
Interleukin-17, 222t
Interleukin-18, 222t
Interleukin-19, 222t
Interleukin-20, 222t
Interleukin-21, 222t
Interleukin-22, 222t
Interleukin-23, 222t
Interleukin-24, 222t
Interleukin-25, 222t
Interleukin-26, 222t
Interleukin-27, 222t
Intermaxillary fixation, 1657, 1657f
Intermediate care facilities, 88, 88f, 88t
Intermittent catheterization, 1187-1188
Intermittent claudication, 767, 900
  drug therapy of, 902
Intermittent compression devices, 912
Intermittent mandatory ventilation, 1761t
Internal arteriovenous fistulas and grafts, 1220-1221, 1220f
Internal carotid artery, 1450, 1451f
Internal fixation
  for hip fracture, 1653, 1653f
  open reduction with, 1638
Internal fixation devices, 1641
Internal mammary artery graft, 809, 809f
Internal pelvic examination, 1335
Internal rotation, 1622t
International Association for the Study of Pain (IASP), definition of pain, 126
International normalized ratio, 679t, 913t
  in deep vein thrombosis, 911t
  preoperative, 351

Internet, 63
  criteria for website evaluation, 63
  resources for older adults, 84
Interspinous process decompression system, 1682
Interstitial cerebral edema, 1470
Interstitial cystitis, 1163-1164
  collaborative care for, 1163-1164
  diagnostic criteria for, 1164t
  drug therapy of, 1163-1164
  nursing management of, 1164
Interstitial edema, 598, 825
Interstitial fluid, 315
  shifts of plasma to, 318-319
  shifts to plasma, 319
Interstitial lung diseases, 596t, 597
Interstitial nephritis, 1162
Interstitial oncotic pressure, 319
Intertriginous areas, 454
Intertrigo, 457t, 462, 1348
Intervertebral disk herniation, 1680-1681
Intervertebral lumbar disk damage, 1680-1684
  collaborative care for, 1682t
  etiology and pathophysiology of, 1680-1681
Interviewing
  considerations for, 40-41
  motivational, 188
    for addictive behaviors, 188-189
    key aspects of, 188, 188t
  preoperative patient interview, 344
Intestinal obstruction, 1060-1062
  clinical manifestations of, 1061, 1061t
  collaborative care for, 1062
  diagnostic studies, 1061-1062
  etiology and pathophysiology of, 1061
  mechanical, 1060, 1060f
  nonmechanical, 1060-1061
  nursing assessment of, 1062
  nursing diagnoses, 1062
  nursing implementation for, 1062
  nursing management of, 1062
  nursing planning for, 1062
  pseudo-obstruction, 1061
  types of, 1060-1061
Intestinal secretion, 929, 930t
Intimate distance, 33
Intoxication. See also Poisoning
  hallucinogen, 186
  paradoxic, 1551
  water, 500
Intraaortic balloon pumps, 1748-1750, 1748f, 1749f
  for cardiogenic shock, 1786
  complications of, 1748-1750, 1750t
  contraindications to, 1748t
  indications for, 1748t
Intraarterial chemotherapy, 290
Intraarticular corticosteroid injections, 1698t
Intracapsular fractures, 1653
Intracellular fluid, 315
  fluid movement between extracellular fluid and, 319
Intracerebral hematoma, 1484
Intracerebral hemorrhage, 1506, 1506t, 1507f
Intracorneal ring segments, 419
Intracoronary ultrasound, 759
Intracranial arteriosclerosis, 1504, 1505f
Intracranial hernias, 1469, 1471f

Intracranial pressure, 1467-1469
  changes in, 1469
  factors that influence, 1467
  increased, 1469-1481
    acute intervention for, 1478-1481
    in chemotherapy, 296t
    clinical manifestations of, 1470-1472, 1471t
    collaborative care for, 1472t, 1474-1476
    complications of, 1472
    diagnostic studies, 1472
    drug therapy for, 1474-1475
    hyperventilation therapy for, 1475
    mechanisms of, 1470
    neurologic assessment of, 1476-1478
    nursing assessment of, 1476, 1476f
    nursing care plan for patient with, 1479b-1480b
    nursing diagnoses, 1478
    nursing evaluation of, 1481
    nursing implementation for, 1478-1481
    nursing management of, 296t, 1476-1481
    nursing planning for, 1478
    nutritional therapy for, 1475-1476
    ocular signs of, 1471
    progression of, 1470, 1470f
    protection from injury in, 1480-1481
    psychologic considerations for, 1481
    in radiation therapy, 296t
  maintenance of, 1468
  measurement of, 1468, 1473-1474
  monitoring, 1479-1480
    indications for, 1473
    sites for placement of devices, 1473f
  normal, 1468
  normal waveforms, 1473, 1474f, 1474t
  regulation of, 1468
Intracranial pressure-volume curve, 1469, 1469f
Intracranial problems, acute, 1467-1501
Intradiscal electrothermoplasty, 1681-1682
Intraductal papilloma, 1345t, 1347
Intrahepatic portosystemic shunts, transjugular, 1108, 1109f
Intranasal inhalers, 539f
Intraocular disorders, 425-437
Intraocular inflammation and infection, 436-437
Intraocular lenses
  phakic, 419
  refractive, 419
Intraocular procedures
  postoperative considerations, 431
  for retinal detachment, 431
Intraoperative care, 359-375
  new and future considerations, 373
  postanesthesia care
    phase I, 377, 377t
    phase II, 377, 377t
    phase III, 377, 377t
Intraperitoneal chemotherapy, 290-291
Intrapleural space, 512
Intraprostatic urethral stents, 1419
Intrapulmonary shunt, 1802
IntraSite, 205t
Intrathecal or intraventricular chemotherapy, 291
Intraurethral devices, 1435-1436, 1436f
  for urinary incontinence, 1183t

Intravaginal support devices, 1183t
Intravascular volume, decreasing, 828
Intravenous agents, 367
  for general anesthesia, 369t
Intravenous pyelogram (IVP), 1147t
Intravenous therapy
  additives, 340
  fluid and electrolyte replacement, 338-340
  home health care activities, 90t
  solutions, 339-340
  total IV anesthesia, 367
Intraventricular catheter, 1473, 1474f
Intraventricular chemotherapy, 291
Intravesical therapy, 291, 1180
Intrinsic factor, 691, 1014
Intrinsic mutagenesis theory, 68, 68t
Introacular pressure, 405-407
Intron A (α-Interferon), 223t, 303t
Intropin (dopamine)
  drug alert, 829
  as positive inotrope, 1739
  for shock, 1787t
  for spinal cord injury, 1596
Intubation. See Endotracheal intubation
Inversion, 1622t
Invirase (saquinavir), 258t
Involucrum, 1669, 1669f
Iodine
  for hyperthyroidism, 1301
  radioactive
    for hyperthyroidism, 1304
    uptake test, 1249t
Ionamin (phentermine), 981
Ionescu-Shiley valve, 883t
Ionizing radiation, 1840
  acute radiation syndrome, 1840, 1841t
Ions, 315
IPF. See Idiopathic pulmonary fibrosis
Ipratropium (Atrovent)
  for allergic rhinitis and sinusitis, 537t
  for asthma, 618t, 621
  for COPD, 618t, 640
Ipratropium and albuterol (Combivent, DuoNeb), 620t, 621, 640
Iprivask (desirudin), 914
Ipstyl (lanreotide SR), 1292
Irbesartan (Avapro), 776t
Irbesartan/hydrochlorothiazide (Avalide), 777t
Iressa (gefitinib), 303t
Irinotecan (Camptosar)
  classification of, 287t
  for colorectal cancer, 1067
  for esophageal cancer, 1010
  for lung cancer, 582
Iris, 400-401
  assessing, 407
  gerontologic differences in assessment, 401t
Irish Americans, 72
Iron
  daily requirements in chronic kidney disease, 1211-1212, 1212t
  foods high in, 951t
  normal metabolism of, 668, 668f
  serum levels, 679-680, 680t
    in anemias, 690t
    effects of aging on, 672t
  total, 1856t
Iron (ferrous sulfate), 499t
Iron dextran injection (Imferon), 1055t
Iron metabolism tests, 679-680
Iron overload, 734t
Iron poisoning, 1837t

Iron therapy
    administration of, 690
    drug alert, 690
Iron-binding capacity, 1856t
Iron-deficiency anemia, 687-691
    clinical manifestations of, 689
    collaborative care for, 690-691, 690t
    diagnostic studies, 689
    drug therapy of, 690-691
    etiology of, 688-689
    laboratory study findings in, 690t
    nursing management of, **691**
**Irritable bowel syndrome (IBS),
    1046-1047**
    gender differences in, 1046b
    self-management program for, 1047b
Irritant contact dermatitis, 462
IRV. See Inspiratory reserve volume
Ischemia
    acute arterial disorders, **907-908**
    in coronary artery disease, 786
    ECG changes associated with, 861,
        862f
    silent, 797, 1876
Ischemic cascade, 1504
Ischemic contracture, Volkmann's,
    1650
Ischemic stroke, 1505-1506, 1506t
    surgical therapy for, 1513, 1513f
Islam, 32t
Island Wound Dressing with Microban,
    205t
Islets of Langerhans, 1241
    hormones of, 1236t
Ismelin (guanethidine), 774t
Ismotic (isosorbide solution), 435t
Isoflurane (Forane), 369t
Isografts, 481
Isoimmune reactions, 699
Isolation
    airborne infection isolation for tuber-
        culosis, 574
    CDC recommendations for precau-
        tions, 247, 248t-249t
Isometric contractions, 1618
Isoniazid (INH)
    drug alert, 572
    food/nutrient interactions, 954t
    hematologic effects of, 674t
    hepatotoxicity, 934t
    for tuberculosis, 573t, 574t
Isoproterenol (Isuprel), 1739
Isoptin (verapamil)
    for chronic stable angina and acute
        coronary syndrome, 800t
    for hypertension, 776t
    for voiding dysfunction, 1185t
Isopto Atropine (atropine), 427t
Isopto Carbachol (carbachol), 435t
Isopto Carpine (pilocarpine), 435t
Isopto Homatropine (homatropine hy-
    drobromide), 427t
Isopto Hyoscine (scopolamine), 427t
Isosorbide dinitrate (Isordil, Sorbitrate)
    for acute coronary syndrome, 800t
    for chronic stable angina, 798, 800t
Isosorbide dinitrate and hydralazine
    (BiDil), 833
Isosorbide mononitrate (Imdur), 798

Isosorbide solution (Ismotic), 435t
Isotonic contractions, 1618
Isotonic fluids, 318, 1786t
Isotonic solutions, 340
Isotretinoin (Accutane)
    for acne, 472t
    drug alert, 470
Isradipine (DynaCirc CR), 776t
Istalol (timolol maleate), 434t
Isuprel (isoproterenol), 1739
Italian Americans, 72
ITP. See Immune thrombocytopenic
    purpura
Itraconazole (Sporanox), 576
IVP. See Intravenous pyelogram

J
J reflex, 1814
Jacksonian seizures, 1535
Janeway's lesions, 867
Januvia (sitagliptin), 1265, 1266t
Japanese Americans, 33
Jaundice, 457t, 675t, **1088,** 1088f
    acute intervention for, 1099
    in cirrhosis, 1102
    diagnostic findings in, 1088t
    hemolytic (prehepatic), 1088
    hepatocellular (hepatic), 1088
    obstructive (posthepatic), 1088, 1128
    variations in light- and dark-skinned
        individuals, 456t
Jaundiced sclera, 675t
Jaw thrust maneuver, 1823, 1825f
JC papovavirus, 255t
JCAHO. See Joint Commission on Ac-
    creditation of Healthcare Organi-
    zations
Jejunostomy, 961
Jejunostomy feedings, 964
Jewish Americans, 155
Job Stress Help, 124
Joint Commission on Accreditation of
    Healthcare Organizations (JCAHO)
    core measures for HF, 827-828, 828t
    National Patient Safety Goals, 366
Joint motion
    evaluation of, 1622
    limited range of, 1623t
    measurement of, 1622, 1622f
Joint protection
    in osteoarthritis, 1696
    patient and family teaching guide for,
        1701b, 1710t
    protection of small joints, 1710t
    in rheumatoid arthritis, 1709-1710,
        1710t
Joint surgery
    collaborative care for, 1664-1665
    complications of, 1664
    indications for, 1662
    nursing management of, **1665**
    postoperative management of, 1665
    preoperative management of, 1664-
        1665
    procedures, **1662-1665**
    types of, **1662-1665**
Joints, 1616. See also specific joints
    age-related changes in, 1618-1619,
        1619t
    classification of, 1616, 1616f
    diarthrodial (synovial), 1616,
        1616f
        movement at, 1622, 1622t
        types of, 1616, 1617f
    osteoarthritis of, 1694-1695, 1696f
    rheumatoid arthritis of, 1702-1704,
        1703f

Joints (Continued)
    structure of, 1616, 1616f
    swelling of, 676t
    in systemic sclerosis, 1723, 1723f
Jones criteria, modified, 876, 876t
Journaling, 97t, 116t
Judaism, 32t
Jugular venous bulb catheter, 1473
Jugular venous distention, 748
Junctional dysrhythmias, 852-853,
    852f
    characteristics of, 849t
    clinical associations, 852
    clinical significance of, 852-853
    ECG characteristics, 852
Junctional escape rhythm, 852, 852f
Justice, 809b

K
Kadian (morphine), 137t, 140
Kaletra (lopinavir and ritonavir), 258t
Kalginate, 205t
Kanamycin (Kantrex), 573t, 1142t
Kaolin, pectin, hyoscyamine sulfate,
    and hyoscine hydrobromide (Don-
    nagel), 1037t
Kaolin, pectin, hyoscyamine sulfate,
    and hyoscine hydrobromide, and
    opium (Donnagel-PG), 1037t
Kaposi sarcoma, 252, 253f, 255t
Karnofsky Functional Performance
    Scale, 280, 281t
Karyotyping, 216, 682t
Kava, 102t, 121b
Kayexalate (sodium polystyrene sulfo-
    nate), 1202t, 1210
Keflex (cephalexin), 1670
Kegel exercises, 1184f
    for cystocele and rectocele, 1408
    for prostate cancer, 1428
    for urinary incontinence, 1183t
    for uterine prolapse, 1408
Keloid, 457, 457t, 458f
    formation of, 201, 201f
Kenalog (triamcinolone acetonide)
    for andropause, 1437
    for dermatologic problems, 475
Kepivance (palifermin), 298
Keppra (levetiracetam), 1536
Keratinization, 1001
Keratinocytes, 450
Keratitis, 422, **423-424**
    Acanthamoeba, 423, 423f
    bacterial, 423
    causes of, 423
    herpes simplex virus, 1374
    infectious, 423-424
    viral, 423
Keratoconjunctivitis, 423
Keratoconjunctivitis sicca, 424,
    1726
Keratoconus, 425
Keratometry, 405t
Keratoplasty
    conductive, 419
    laser thermal, 419
Keratosis
    actinic, 452, **463,** 464t
    seborrheic, 472t
Kernig's sign, 1460t, 1461f, 1494
Ketamine (Ketalar), 369t
    for dissociative anesthesia, 371
    for pain, 140
Ketoacidosis, diabetic, 1255, **1278-
    1280**

Ketoconazole (Nizoral)
    for Cushing syndrome, 1312-1314
    hepatotoxicity, 934t
    photosensitivity, 461t
    for pulmonary infections, 576
Ketone bodies, 1862t
Ketones, 1252t
Ketoprofen (Orudis, Actron)
    for arthritis and connective tissue dis-
        orders, 1698t
    for burns, 499t
Ketorolac (Toradol), 135, 136t
17-Ketosteroids, 1251t
Kidney(s), **1136-1139.** See also under
    Renal
    age-related changes in, 1141t
    blood supply, 1137
    CT scan of, 1148t
    functions of, 1139
    hydronephrosis of, 1168, 1169f
    immunologic disorders of, **1165-1168**
    macrostructure of, 1136-1137, 1137f
    magnetic resonance imaging of,
        1148t
    in metabolic and connective tissue
        diseases, **1177**
    microstructure of, 1137
    palpation of, 1144, 1145f
    physiology of urine formation, 1137-
        1139
Kidney, ureters, bladder (KUB) film,
    1147t
Kidney cancer, 1177-1178
    clinical manifestations of, 1177-1178,
        1178f
    diagnostic studies, 1177-1178
    nursing and collaborative manage-
        ment of, **1178**
Kidney disease
    autoimmune, 234t
    chronic, 1197, **1204-1216**
        case study, 1231
        dermatologic manifestations, 473t
        gerontologic considerations for,
            1230-1231
        prevention and detection of, 1205b
        resources for, 1232
    polycystic, **1176-1177,** 1176f
Kidney stones, 1169, 1170f
    nursing care plan for patient with
        acute renal lithiasis, 1173b-
        1174b
Kidney transplantation, **1225-1230**
    complications of, 1229-1230, 1229t
    with deceased donors, 1227
    donor sources, 1226-1227
    histocompatibility studies, 1226
    immunosuppressive therapy for, 1229
    live donors for, 1226-1227
        postoperative care of, 1228
        surgical procedure, 1227
    recipient
        nursing management of, **1227-
            1229**
        postoperative care of, 1228-1229
        preoperative care of, 1228
        selection of, 1226
        surgical procedure, 1227, 1228f
    rejection, 1229
    surgical procedure, 1227
Kineret (anakinra)
    for arthritis and connective tissue dis-
        orders, 1700t
    clinical uses of, 223t
    for rheumatoid arthritis, 1705-1706

Note: Disorder names are in **bold face.**
Page numbers in **bold face** indicate main
discussions. Page numbers followed by
f, t, b, or n indicate figures, tables, boxed
material, or notes, respectively.

Kininogen, 226t
Kinins, 195t, 226t
Klebsiella, 562t, 1155t
   diagnostic studies, 565
   diseases caused by, 244t
Klebsiella pneumoniae, 246, 246t
Klonopin (clonazepam), 1536, 1538t
Knee arthroplasty, 1664
Knee immobilizer, 1641, 1641f
"Knee jerk" reflex arc, 1446f
Knee joint, 1634, 1635f
Kock pouch, 1055-1056, 1070
   creation of, 1190, 1190f
   surgical formation of, 1055, 1056f
KOH. *See* Potassium hydroxide
Kondremul Plain (mineral oil),
   1042t
Konsyl (psyllium), 1042t
Korotkoff sounds, 743
Korsakoff's psychosis, 178
KUB film. *See* Kidney, ureters, bladder
   film
Kübler-Ross, Elisabeth, 155
Kupffer cells, 931, 932t
Kussmaul respirations, 335, 524t
Kwashiorkor, 952
Kyphoplasty, 1656
Kyphoscoliosis, 595t
Kyphosis, 744t, 1623t, 1687
Kytril (granisetron), 297, 992, 992t

L
Labetalol (Normodyne, Trandate)
   drug alert, 782
   food/nutrient interactions, 954t
   for hypertension, 775t
Labyrinthitis, 442
Lacerations
   of brain, 1482-1483
   of scalp, 1481
Lacrimal apparatus, 400, 400f, 401t
Lactase deficiency, 1081
Lactated Ringer's solution
   composition and use of, 339t
   for shock, 1784, 1786t
Lactational breast abscess, 1346
Lactational mastitis, 1345-1346,
   1345t
Lactic acid, 479t
   laboratory values, 1856t
   in shock, 1775t
Lactic dehydrogenase
   isoenzymes, 1857t
   laboratory values, 1856t
Lactinex, 499
Lactobacillus, 1156
Lacto-ovo-vegetarians, 950
Lactulose (Cephulac, Constulose)
   for cirrhosis, 1110t
   for constipation, 138, 1042t
   for variceal bleeding, 1108
Lacunar stroke, 1505-1506
Laënnec's cirrhosis, 1102
Lamellae, 1615
Lamictal (lamotrigine)
   analgesic effects of, 128
   for seizures, 1536, 1538t
Laminectomy, 1682
Lamivudine (3TC, Epivir, Trizivir)
   adverse effects of, 258t
   for chronic hepatitis B, 1094
   drug alert, 1094
Lamivudine and abacavir (Epizicom),
   258t
Lamivudine and zidovudine (Combivir), 258t

Lamotrigine (Lamictal)
   analgesic effects of, 128
   for seizures, 1536, 1538t
   for trigeminal neuralgia, 1582
**Landouzy–Déjérine muscular dystro-
   phy,** 1675t
**Landry–Guillain-Barré–Stahl
   syndrome.** *See* Guillain-Barré
   syndrome
Lanoxin (digoxin)
   for chronic HF, 832
   classification of, 856t
   dose and frequency adjustments,
      1211
Lanreotide SR (Ipstyl), 1292
Lansoprazole (Prevacid)
   for acute gastritis, 1014
   for gastroesophageal reflux disease,
      1006, 1006f
   for gastrointestinal bleeding, 998t
   for peptic ulcer disease, 1019t,
      1020
Lantus (insulin glargine), 1260t,
   1261t
Lanugo, 969
LAP. *See* Left atrial pressure
Laparoscopic cholecystectomy
   ambulatory and home care for,
      1131
   postoperative care of, 1131
   postoperative patient and family
      teaching guide for, 1132b
Laparoscopic nephrectomy, 1188
Laparoscopic-assisted vaginal hysterectomy, 1404t
Laparoscopy, 944t
   of pelvic organs, 1340t
LapBand (Inamed), 983
**Large cell (undifferentiated) carci-
   noma,** of lung, 581t
Large intestine. *See also* Colon
   age-related changes in, 932, 933t
   anatomic locations of, 930, 931f
   barium enema x-ray of, 941f, 941t
   elimination by, 930
   obstruction of, 1061, 1061t
   parts of, 930
   polyps of, **1062-1063,** 1063t
Laryngeal cancer
   case study, 558
   excision of, 551, 551f
Laryngeal edema, postoperative,
   379t
Laryngeal polyps, 551
Laryngeal stridor, 1304
Laryngectomy
   hemilaryngectomy, 551
   supraglottic, 551
   total
      airflow in and out of lungs after,
         552, 552f
      nursing care plan for patient hav-
         ing, 554b-556b
Laryngospasm, postoperative, 379t
Larynx
   artificial, 557, 557f
   problems related to, **543-558**
LASEK. *See* Laser-assisted epithelial
   keratomileusis
Laser diskectomy, percutaneous,
   1682
Laser lithotripsy probes, 1172
Laser photocoagulation
   for bladder cancer, 1179
   for retinal detachment, 430
Laser prostatectomy, 1418t, 1419

Laser revascularization, transmyocardial, 810
Laser therapy
   bronchoscopic, 582
   cosmetic surgery procedures, 479
   for refractive errors, 418-419
   for skin conditions, 474-475,
      475t
Laser thermal keratoplasty, 419
Laser-assisted epithelial keratomileusis
   (LASEK), 418
Laser-assisted in-situ keratomileusis
   (LASIK), 418
LASIK. *See* Laser-assisted in-situ keratomileusis
Lasix (furosemide)
   blood glucose level effects, 1267t
   for cirrhosis, 1110t
   effects on lower urinary tract func-
      tion, 1180t
   for heart failure, 828
   for hypercalcemia, 330
   for hypertension, 773t, 1210
   for multiple myeloma, 729
   photosensitivity, 461t
Latanoprost (Xalatan), 435t
Lateral epicondylitis, 1623t
Latex allergies, 232
   guidelines for preventing reactions,
      232t
   nursing and collaborative manage-
      ment of, **232**
   screening for, 347
   types of, 232
Latino Americans, 20
   caregivers of, 72
   personal space, 33
LAVH. *See* Laparoscopic-assisted vaginal hysterectomy
Laxatives, 1041, 1042t
LBD. *See* Lewy body dementia
LCIS. *See* Lobular carcinoma in situ
LDLs. *See* Low-density lipoproteins
L-dopa. *See* Levodopa
Lead, 1862t
Lead poisoning, 1837t, 1838
Leading health indicators, 5
Learning, 54
   adult learning principles, 54
   principles of androgogy (adult learn-
      ing), 54, 54t
   teaching-learning process, **54-57**
   techniques to enhance, 63t
Learning needs assessment, 59
Learning objectives, 60
   elements of, 60
   examples of, 60
   writing, 60
Learning style, 59
Lecture-discussion, 61
LEEP. *See* Loop electrosurgical exci-
   sion procedure
LEETZ. *See* Loop electrosurgical exci-
   sion of transformation zone
Leflunomide (Arava)
   for arthritis and connective tissue dis-
      orders, 1699t
   for rheumatoid arthritis, 1705
Left atrial pressure, 1739t
Left ventricular assist devices, 1750,
   1750f
Left ventricular end-diastolic pressure,
   1738
Left ventricular hypertrophy, 767,
   767f

Left ventricular thrombus, 826
Left-brain stroke, 1508f
Left-sided heart failure, 824, 824f,
   825, 825t
Leg exercises, postoperative, 387, 387f
Leg pain, 745t
Leg ulcers, 675t
   arterial, 901, 901t
   venous, 901, 901t, **919-920,** 919f
Legal aid for older adults, 77, 77f
Legal blindness, 405, 419, 419t
Legal issues
   affecting end-of-life care, **155-156**
   documents for end-of-life care, 155
   for older adults, **77**
   preparation for surgery, 352-354
Legionella, 562, 565
Legionella pneumophila, 562t
   clinical manifestations of, 565
   diseases caused by, 244t
   related diseases, 245t
Legs, physical examination of, 49t
Leiomyomas, 585, **1398-1399,**
   1398f
   clinical manifestations of, 1398-
      1399
   collaborative care for, 1399
   etiology and pathophysiology of,
      1398
   uterine, 1388
Lenalidomide (Revimid), 717
Lens, 401
   age-related changes in, 401t
   assessment abnormalities, 406t
Lentigines, 465
Lentigo, 472t
Lepirudin (Refludan), 914
Leprosy, 437t
Leptin, 928
   in obesity, 972, 973f, 973t
Lescol (fluvastatin), 793, 795t
Lesions
   cardiac, 876
   configuration terminology, 456t
   distribution terminology, 456t
   on external ear, 413t
   Janeway's, 867
Letrozole (Femara)
   for breast cancer, 1355
   classification of, 288t
Leucovorin (folinic acid, Wellcovorin)
   for colorectal cancer, 1067
   FOLFOX treatment regimen, 291,
      291t
   for non-Hodgkin's lymphoma, 727t
Leucovorin-modulated 5-FU (Orzel),
   1067
Leukemia, 717-723
   acute, 717, 718f
   acute intervention for, 721-722
   acute lymphocytic, 718, 718t, 721t
   acute myelogenous, 718, 718t, 721t
   ambulatory and home care for, 722-
      723
   blastic phase, 719
   case study, 734-735
   chemotherapy of
      consolidation therapy, 720
      induction therapy, 720
      intensification therapy, 720
      maintenance therapy, 720
   chronic, 717
   chronic lymphocytic, 718t, 719, 721t
   chronic myelogenous, 718-719, 718t,
      721t

Leukemia *(Continued)*
classification of, 717-719
clinical manifestations of, 718t, 719
collaborative care for, 719-721
diagnostic studies, 719
drug therapy of, 720t, 721t
drug therapy regimens, 720-721
etiology and pathophysiology of, 717
hairy cell, 719
nursing assessment of, 721, 722t
nursing diagnoses, 721
nursing evaluation of, 723
nursing implementation for, 721-723
nursing management of, **721-723**
nursing planning for, 721
remission
complete, 719
minimal residual, 719
molecular, 719
partial, 719
types of, 718t
unclassified, 719
Leukeran (chlorambucil)
classification of, 287t
for leukemia, 720t
Leukine (sargramostim)
for cancer treatment, 304t
clinical uses of, 223t
Leukocytapheresis, 234
Leukocytes, 667, 668t
Leukopenia, 678, 713
in chemotherapy and radiation therapy, 295t
Leukoplakia, 551, 939t, 1001
oral hairy, 252, 253f
Leukotriene inhibitors, 619t
Leukotriene modifiers, 619t, 620
Leukotriene receptor antagonists
for allergic disorders, 231
for allergic rhinitis and sinusitis, 535, 537t
for asthma and COPD, 619t
Leukotrienes, 195-196, 195t, 197f, 226t
Leuprolide (Lupron)
drug alert, 1397
for infertility, 1383t
for prostate cancer, 1426, 1426t
Leustatin (cladribine), 287t
Levalbuterol (Xopenex, Xopenex HFA), 619t
Levamisole (Ergamisol), 303t, 1067
Levaquin (levofloxacin)
for chlamydial infections, 1373
for gonorrhea, 1368
for tuberculosis, 573t
for UTIs, 1157
Levatol (penbutolol), 774t
Levbid (hyoscyamine), 1185t
Levemir (insulin detemir), 1260t, 1261t
Levetiracetam (Keppra), 1536
Levitra (vardenafil), 1435
Levobunolol (Betagan), 434t
Levodopa (L-dopa)
blood glucose level effects, 1267t
for Parkinson's disease, 1551, 1552t
Levodopa/carbidopa (Sinemet)
drug alert, 1551
for Parkinson's disease, 1551, 1552t
Levo-Dromoran (levorphanol), 137t, 138

Levofloxacin (Levaquin)
for chlamydial infections, 1373
for gonorrhea, 1368
for tuberculosis, 573t
for UTIs, 1157
Levophed (norepinephrine)
as positive inotrope, 1739
for shock, 1788t
Levorphanol (Levo-Dromoran), 137t, 138
Levothyroxine (Synthroid)
combined with liothyronine (Liotrix), 1306
drug alert, 1306
for hypothyroidism, 1306
Levsin (hyoscyamine), 1185t
Lewy body dementia, 1575
Lexiva (fosamprenavir), 258t
Lexxel (enalapril/felodipine), 777t
LGV. *See* Lymphogranuloma venereum
LH. *See* Luteinizing hormone
Lhermitte's sign, 1543
Librium (chlordiazepoxide)
effects of use, 169t
toxicology, 1865t
withdrawal from, 179
Licensed practical nurse (LPN), 14-15, 362
Licensed vocational nurse (LVN), 14-15
Lichen sclerosis, 1394
Lichenification, 457t, 477-478
LICOX brain tissue oxygenation catheter, 1473
Lidocaine (Lidoderm, Xylocaine)
classification of, 856t
eutectic mixture of local anesthetics (EMLA), 139t, 371
for genital herpes, 1375
for pain, 140, 141
for ventricular tachycardia, 855
Life expectancy, 67
Life review, 159
Life support, basic, 1845
LifePak defibrillator, 857f
LifeSite system, 1222
Lifestyle modifications
for gastroesophageal reflux disease, 1005
for hypertension, 768-771
therapeutic lifestyle changes, 792
therapeutic lifestyle changes diet, 792, 793t
for urinary incontinence, 1183t
Ligament injury, 1630t
Ligaments, **1618**
regenerative ability of, 198, 198t
Light response, abnormal, 406t
Light skin, 456t
Light touch test, 1458
Lillehei-Kaster valve, 883t
Limb circumference, 749t
Limbic system
location and function of, 1447t
response to stress, 113
structures of, 1447, 1448f
Linear accelerator, 293, 294f
Lioresal (baclofen)
local, 139t
for multiple sclerosis, 1545, 1545t
for pain, 140
Liotrix (levothyroxine and liothyronine), 1306
Lip cancer, 1001, 1001t
Lip reading, 445
Lipase
laboratory values, 1857t
serum levels, 944t

Lipectomy, 984
Lipid-lowering agents, natural, 796b
Lipids
in peritoneal dialysis, 1220
serum, 751-756, 752t
and coronary artery disease, 788-789
health-promoting behaviors for, 792t
Lipid-soluble hormones, 1235
Lipitor (atorvastatin), 793, 795t
Lipodystrophy, 1263
manifestations of, 266, 267f
Lipoma, 472t
Lipoprotein-associated phospholipase A$_2$, 752t, 756
Lipoproteins, 751, 752t, 756, 788
drugs that increase removal of, 794
drugs that restrict production of, 793-794
high-density, 756
low-density, 756
treatment for high blood cholesterol based on, 789, 790t
very-low-density, 756
Liposuction, 480, 480f, 984
Lipoxygenase pathway, 195
Liquid oxygen, 645t
Liquid portable oxygen systems, 643f, 644, 645f
Liquids, volatile, 369t
LiquiVent (perflubron), 1763
Lisinopril (Prinivil, Zestril)
for diabetes mellitus, 1285
for hypertension, 776t
and lower urinary tract function, 1180t
and reproductive system, 1332
Lisinopril/hydrochlorothiazide (Prinzide, Zestoretic), 777t
Literacy, 58
assessment of, 58
health literacy, 22
Lithiasis
choledocholithiasis, 1127
cholelithiasis, **1126-1132**
nephrolithiasis, 1169
renal, acute, 1173b-1174b
Lithium
blood glucose level effects, 1267t
nephrotoxicity, 1142t
Lithotripsy, 1172
cystoscopic, 1171
electrohydraulic, 1172
extracorporeal shock-wave, 1172
indications for, 1171
laser probes, 1172
percutaneous ultrasonic, 1172
Live donors
for kidney transplantation, 1226-1227
postoperative care, 1228
Liver, 671, **930-931.** *See also under* Hepatic
absence of dullness of, 940t
age-related changes in, 932, 933t
disorders of, **1088-1118**
autoimmune, 234t, **1100-1101**
cultural and ethnic health disparities in, 1089b
with dermatologic manifestations, 473t
genetic, **1100-1101**
metabolic, **1100-1101**
in older adults, **1118**
resources, 1134
functions of, 931, 932t
in hepatitis, 1091

Liver *(Continued)*
microscopic structure of, 930-931, 932f
nodular, 940t
nonalcoholic fatty, **1101**
palpation of, 677, 937-938, 938f
physical examination of, 51t
problems associated with obesity, 975-976
secretions related to digestion, 929, 929t
structure of, 930, 931f
ultrasound of, 682t
Liver biopsy, 944t, 946
closed or needle biopsy, 946
open method, 946
Liver cancer, 1116-1117, 1116f
clinical manifestations of, 1116-1117
diagnostic studies, 1116-1117
nursing and collaborative management of, **1117**
Liver enzymes, 1775t
Liver failure, acute, 1115
Liver function tests, **946,** 946t-947t
preoperative, 351
Liver spots, 472t
Liver transplantation, **1117-1118**
Liver/spleen scan, 682t
Living will, 155, 156t
LN. *See* Lupus nephritis
Lobectomy, 593t
Lobular carcinoma in situ, 1350
Local anesthesia, 367, **371-372**
methods of administration, 371-372, 371t
for pain, 139-140, 139t
Logical Observation Identifiers Names and Codes (LOINC®), 8t
Logrolling, 1656
Lomotil (diphenoxylate with atropine), 1037t, 1055t
Lomustine (CeeNu), 287t
Long arm cast, 1640, 1640f
Long-term acute care, 87t
Long-term care, 88, 88t
Long-term care facilities, 76, 76f
caregiver concerns, 76
factors that precipitate placement in, 76
Long-term home health care programs (LTHHCPs), 88t
Loniten (minoxidil), 775t
Loop colostomy, 1069, 1070f
Loop diuretics
for chronic HF, 831
effects on lower urinary tract function, 1180t
for hypertension, 773t
Loop electrosurgical excision of transformation zone, 1340t
Loop electrosurgical excision procedure, 1340t, 1401
Loop of Henle, 1138t
Loop stoma, 1069
Loopogram, 1149t
Looser's transformation zones, 1686
Loperamide (Imodium), 1037t, 1055t
Lopid (gemfibrozil), 794, 795t
Lopidine (apraclonidine), 434t
Lopinavir and ritonavir (Kaletra), 258t
Lopressor (metoprolol)
for acute coronary syndrome, 800t
for chronic stable angina, 799, 800t
classification of, 856t

Lopressor (metoprolol) *(Continued)*
 effects on lower urinary tract function, 1180*t*
 for hypertension, 774*t*, 1210
Lopressor HCT (metoprolol/hydrochlo-
  rothiazide), 777*t*
Loratidine (Claritin)
 for allergic rhinitis and sinusitis, 538*t*
 for dermatologic problems, 475
Lorazepam (Ativan)
 as adjunct to general anesthesia, 370*t*
 for alcohol withdrawal, 178, 186
 for Alzheimer's disease, 1569*t*
 for burns, 499*t*
 preoperative, 355*t*
 for status epilepticus, 1537
Lordosis, 1623*t*
Lortab (hydrocodone), 137*t*
Losartan (Cozaar)
 for chronic HF, 833
 for diabetes mellitus, 1285
 for gout, 1716
 for hypertension, 776*t*, 1210
 for Raynaud's phenomenon, 1724
Losartan/hydrochlorothiazide (Hyzaar),
  777*t*
Lotensin (benazepril)
 for chronic HF, 832
 for hypertension, 776*t*
Lotensin HCT (benazepril/hydrochloro-
  thiazide), 777*t*
Lotrel (amlodipine/benazepril), 777*t*
Lotronex (alosetron)
 drug alert, 1047
 for irritable bowel syndrome, 1047
Lovastatin (Mevacor), 793, 795*t*, 1167
Lovenox (enoxaparin)
 for chronic stable angina and acute
  coronary syndrome, 800*t*
 for pulmonary embolism, 600
Low back pain, 1675-1686
 acute, **1676-1680**
  nursing assessment of, 1676, 1676*t*
  nursing management of, **1676-
   1680**
  physical activity and, 1681*b*
 chronic, **1680**
 etiology and pathophysiology of,
  1675-1676
 nursing care plan for patient with,
  1678*b*-1680*b*
 prevention of, 1677*b*
Low back problems, 1677*t*
 in peritoneal dialysis, 1219
Low blood flow shock, 1772-1773,
  1773-1777, 1773*f*
 classification of, 1773*t*
 clinical presentation of, 1776*t*
 effects on hemodynamic parameters,
  1774-1775, 1774*t*
 precipitating factors, 1773*t*
Low blood glucose, 1278. *See also* Hypoglycemia
Low-density lipoprotein cholesterol,
  789
Low-density lipoproteins, 756
 treatment for high blood cholesterol
  based on, 789, 790*t*
Lower airways, 511, 511*f*
Lower esophageal sphincter pressure,
  1004, 1004*t*
Lower extremities
 atherosclerotic lesions of, 893, 893*f*
 casts for injuries to, 1640-1641
 complications in diabetes mellitus,
  1286-1287
 eczema of, 227, 227*f*
 pitting edema of, 749*t*

Lower extremity amputation
 bandaging for above-the-knee amputation residual limb, 1660, 1661*f*
 sites of, 1658-1659, 1659*f*
**Lower extremity peripheral arterial
  disease, 900-907**
 acute intervention for, 906
 ambulatory and home care for, 906-
  907
 health promotion in, 904-906
 nursing assessment of, 904
 nursing care plan for patient with,
  905*b*-906*b*
 nursing diagnoses, 904
 nursing evaluation of, 907
 nursing implementation for, 904-907
 nursing management of, **904-907**
 nursing planning for, 904
**Lower gastrointestinal problems,
  1035-1086**
 inflammatory disorders, **1048-1051**
Lower gastrointestinal series, 940, 941*t*
Lower genital tract infections, 1394*t*
Lower motor neurons, 1445
Lower respiratory tract
 blood supply to, 512
 problems of, **560-606**
 structures and functions of, 511-512,
  511*f*
Lower urinary tract, 1180*t*
Lower urinary tract symptoms, 1156,
  1157*t*
Low-sodium diets, 833, 834*t*
Loxapine (Loxitane), 1569*t*
LPN. *See* Licensed practical nurse
Lp-PLA₂. *See* Lipoprotein-associated
  phospholipase A₂
LSD. *See* Lysergic acid diethylamide
LTHHCP. *See* Long-term home health
  care programs
LTK. *See* Laser thermal keratoplasty
LTRAs. *See* Leukotriene receptor an-
  tagonists
Lubiprostone (Amitiza), 1042*t*
Lubricants, 1041, 1042*t*
Lucentis (ranibizumab), 432
Lufyllin (dyphylline), 954*t*
LUMA Cervical Imaging System, 1401
Lumbar disk damage
 clinical manifestations of, 1681
 collaborative care for, 1681-1683
 diagnostic studies, 1681
 intervertebral, **1680-1684**
 surgical therapy for, 1681-1683
Lumbar disk herniation, 681, 1680-
  1681, 1682*t*
Lumbar puncture, 1461, 1462*t*
Luminal (phenobarbital)
 effects of use, 169*t*
 food/nutrient interactions, 954*t*
 withdrawal from, 179
Lumpectomy, 1352
 with axillary lymph node dissection,
  1359, 1360*f*
 nursing care plan for patient after
  mastectomy or, 1357*b*-1358*b*
 with radiation therapy, 1353*t*
Lumps, breast, 1335*t*
Lund-Browder chart, 487, 487*f*
Lung(s). *See also under* Pulmonary
 abbreviations, 1800*t*
 airflow in and out of, 552, 552*f*
 blood supply to, 512
 fungal infections of, 575, 576*t*
 normal gas exchange in, 1799,
  1800*f*
 percussion of, 522
 physical examination of, 51*t*, 521

Lung abscess, 576-577
 clinical manifestations of, 576-577
 complications of, 576-577
 diagnostic studies, 577
 etiology and pathophysiology of, 576
 nursing and collaborative management of, **577**
 in pneumonia, 565
Lung biopsy, 528*t*, 529-530, 530*f*
Lung cancer, 578-584
 acute intervention for, 584
 ambulatory and home care for, 584-
  585
 biologic and targeted therapy of, 582
 bronchoscopic laser therapy of, 582
 chemotherapy of, 582
 clinical manifestations of, 580
 collaborative care for, 581*t*, 582-583
 cryotherapy of, 583
 cultural and ethnic health disparities,
  579*b*
 diagnostic studies, 580-582
 etiology of, 579
 gender differences in, 579*b*
 health disparities and, 21*t*
 health promotion in, 584
 noninvasive interventions and quality
  of life in, 583*b*
 nursing assessment of, 583, 583*t*
  important health information, 583*t*
  objective data, 583*t*
  subjective data, 583*t*
 nursing diagnoses, 583-584
 nursing evaluation of, 584
 nursing implementation for, 584
 nursing management of, **583-584**
 nursing planning for, 584
 pathophysiology of, 579-580,
  580*f*
 photodynamic therapy of, 582-583
 radiation therapy of, 582
 screening for, 581-582
 staging, 580-581
 surgical therapy of, 582
 types of, 579, 580*f*, 581*t*
Lung disease
 diffuse parenchymal, 597
 environmental, **577-578,** 578*t*
 interstitial, **597**
 restrictive, 594, 595*t*, 596*t*
 vascular disorders, **597-600**
Lung injury, acute
 mediators of, 1813, 1814*t*
 transfusion-related, 732, 733*t*
Lung parenchyma, 511, 511*f*
Lung resection
 segmental, 593*t*
 wedge, 593*t*
Lung transplantation, 603-604
 for COPD, 646
 indications for, 603, 603*t*
Lung tumors, 585
Lung volume reduction surgery, 593*t*,
  644-646
Lung volumes, 531*f*, 531*t*, 594*b*
Lunula, 450
Lupron (leuprolide)
 for infertility, 1383*t*
 for prostate cancer, 1426, 1426*t*
Lupus nephritis, 1718
Luteinizing hormone
 serum levels, 1248*t*
 target tissue and functions, 1236*t*
Luteinizing hormone–releasing hormone agonists, 1426
 for prostate cancer, 1426*t*
Luteinizing hormone–releasing hormone antagonists, 1426, 1426*t*

LUTS. *See* Lower urinary tract
  symptoms
Luvox (fluvoxamine), 1569, 1569*t*
LVN. *See* Licensed vocational nurse
LVRS. *See* Lung volume reduction
  surgery
Lyme disease, 1714, 1835
 ocular manifestations of, 437*t*
 prevention of, 1714, 1714*t*
Lymph node biopsy, 681, 682*t*
 closed (needle), 681, 682*t*
 open procedure, 681, 682*t*
Lymph nodes
 assessment abnormalities, 675*t*
 assessment of, 676-677
 axillary node dissection, 1352
 functions of, 220
 sentinel lymph node dissection,
  1351
 shotty nodes, 521
 superficial, palpable, 676-677,
  677*f*
Lymph system, 670
Lymphadenopathy, 675*t*
Lymphatic drainage, 671, 671*f*
Lymphatic mapping, 1351
Lymphedema, 1352, 1352*f*, 1873
Lymphocytapheresis, 234
Lymphocyte immune globulin (Atgam),
  239*t*
Lymphocytes, 220-222, 668
 B lymphocytes, 220, 221*f*
 function of, 668*t*
 laboratory values, 1860*t*
 response to injury, 195
 T lymphocytes, 220, 221*f*
Lymphogranuloma venereum,
  1373
Lymphoid organs, 219-220
 central, 219
 peripheral, 219
Lymphoma, 723-734
 central nervous system
  associated with HIV infection,
   254*t*
  primary, 1488*t*
 dermatologic manifestations of, 473*t*
 Hodgkin's, **723-724,** 723*t*
  clinical manifestations of, 723*f*
  staging system for, 725*f*
 non-Hodgkin's, 723*t*, **724-728**
  classification of, 726*t*
  guidelines for treatment of, 727*t*
  nursing and collaborative management of, **726-728**
  staging system for, 725*f*
 T-cell, cutaneous, 464*t*
Lyofoam, 205*t*
Lysergic acid diethylamide (LSD),
  170*t*
Lysine vasopressin (Diapid), 1297
Lysodren (mitotane), 1312-1314

M
M protein, 728
Ma huang (Ephedra), 745*t*
Maalox
 for burns, 499*t*
 for gastroesophageal reflux disease,
  1006*t*
 preparation, 1020*t*
 for renal osteodystrophy, 1210
Macrodantin (nitrofurantoin)
 drug alert, 1158
 nephrotoxicity of, 1142
 for UTIs, 1157
Macrophage colony-stimulating factor,
  222*t*

Macrophages, 221f
alveolar, 516
response to malignant target cells, 278, 279f
Macugen (pegaptanib), 432
Macular degeneration, age-related, 431-432
Macules, 455t
Mad cow disease (bovine spongiform encephalitis), 1576
Mafenide acetate (Sulfamylon), 499
Magaldrate, 1020t
Magnesium
antacid side effects, 1020t
classification of, 856t
laboratory values, 1857t
normal values, 321t
Magnesium carbonate, 1020t
Magnesium citrate, 1042t
Magnesium hydroxide, 1020t
Magnesium imbalances, 332-333
causes of, 332t
in chronic kidney disease, 1207
Magnesium oxide, 1020t
Magnesium salts
antacid preparations, 1020t
for constipation, 1042t
Magnesium sulfate, 1110t
Magnesium-containing antacids (Maalox, Mylanta), 1210
Magnet therapy, 98t
Magnetic resonance angiography
of cardiovascular system, 755t
of nervous system, 1463t
of urinary system, 1148t
Magnetic resonance cholangiopancrea-tography, 942t
Magnetic resonance imaging
of brain, 1463t, 1464f
of cardiovascular system, 758
of chest, 526, 528t
clinical setting for, 1464f
functional, 1463t
of gastrointestinal system, 942t
of heart, 755t
hematologic, 682t
of kidneys, 1148t
of musculoskeletal system, 1625t
of nervous system, 1463t
pituitary, 1249t
of reproductive system, 1340t, 1341
Magnetic resonance spectroscopy, 1463t
Magnetoencephalography, 1463t
Magovern-Cromie valve, 883t
Mag-Ox, 1020t
"Mainlining," 180, 180f
Mainstream sampling, 1753-1754
Maintenance therapy, 720
Major histocompatibility complex, 233
Malabsorption syndrome, 953, **1078-1082**
causes of, 1078, 1079t
classification of, 1078
clinical manifestations of, 1079, 1079t
definition of, 1873
dermatologic manifestations of, 473t
gender differences in, 1079b
screening tests for, 1079
Malabsorptive surgery, 982-983, 982t, 983-984

Maladaptive grief, 154
Maldistribution of blood flow shock, 1773, 1773f, **1777-1778**
classification of, 1773t
clinical presentation of, 1776t
effects on hemodynamic parameters, 1774-1775, 1774t
precipitating factors, 1773t
Male condoms, 262
breakage during intercourse, 1373b
patient teaching guide for proper use of, 262t
placement of, 262, 262f
Male external genitalia, 1324
physical examination of
normal, 1335t
outline for, 49t
recording, 51t
Male infertility, 1437-1438
Male menopause, 1437
Male reproductive system
accessory glands of, 1324
age-related changes in, 1330, 1331t
assessment abnormalities, 1336t
assessment of, **1331-1335**
cancers of, 1423b
diagnostic studies, **1337-1341,** 1338t-1341t
functions of, **1324**
physical examination of, 1334-1335, 1335t
problems of, **1414-1439**
areas of, 1414, 1415f
resources, 1439
problems of sexual functioning, **1433-1438**
roles of, **1324**
structures of, **1324**
surgeries of, 1332, 1332t
Male sex organs, 1324, 1324f
Male sexual response, 1330
Malignancy. *See also* Cancer
of external ear, **439**
in kidney transplantation, 1230
macrophage response to, 278, 279f
skin conditions, 464t
Malignant external otitis, 438
Malignant hyperthermia, 373
Malignant melanoma, 464t, **465-466**
case study, 481
clinical manifestations of, 465
definition of, 1873
Malignant neoplasms, 274, 275t
Malignant nephrosclerosis, 1175
Malignant skin neoplasms, 462-463
Malleus, 409
Mallory-Weiss tears, 995
Malnutrition, 951-960, 951f
acute intervention for, 957-958
ambulatory and home care for, 958-959
anthropometric measurements in, 955
in cancer, 306-307
causes of, 952-953
clinical manifestations of, 953-954
conditions that increase risk for, 952, 952t
diagnostic studies, 954-955
etiology and pathophysiology of, 952-955
gerontologic considerations for, **959-960**
health promotion in, 957
history and physical examination in, 954
laboratory studies, 954-955
nursing assessment of, 955-957, 956t

Malnutrition (Continued)
nursing diagnoses, 957
nursing evaluation of, 959
nursing implementation for, 957-959
nursing management of, **955-959**
nursing planning for, 957
protein-calorie, 951-952
manifestations of, 953, 955t
types of, 951-952
Mammography, 1339t, 1341, 1344, 1344f
diagnostic, 1339t
screening, 1339t
Mammoplasty, **1361-1363**
MammoSite technique, 1354, 1354f
Managed care, 4
Mandibular fracture, 1657
clinical manifestations of, 1657t
nursing implementation for, 1657-1658
nursing management of, **1657-1658**
postoperative management of, 1657-1658
preoperative management of, 1657
Mandibulectomy, 934t, 1002
Manipulative and body-based methods, 96t, 98t, **101-104**
Mannitol (Osmitrol)
for glaucoma, 435t
for increased ICP, 1474
Mantoux test, 571
Mantra, 117
Manubrium, 412
MAP. *See* Mean arterial pressure
Marasmus, 952
Marezine (cyclizine), 992t
Marfan syndrome, 437t, 899
Margination, 194, 194f
Marijuana, 180-181. *See also* Cannabis
blood glucose level effects, 1267t
collaborative care, 181
effects of use, 169t, 181
onset, peak, duration, and withdrawal onset of, 185t
Marinol (dronabinol), 992
for nausea and vomiting, 992t
Mass casualty incidents, 1842
preparedness in, **1842**
Massage therapy, 95, 96f, 103-104
clinical applications of, 103-104
description of, 98t
hand massage, 104, 105f
for pain management, 143
for stress management, 120
techniques for, 104, 104f
Masses
abdominal, 940t
anal, 940t
breast, 1335t
inguinal, 1336t
penile, 1336t
rectal, 940t
scrotal, 1336t, 1430, 1431f
Massive blood transfusion reactions, 732-734
Mast cell stabilizers, 620
for allergic rhinitis and sinusitis, 537t
for asthma and COPD, 618t
Mast cells, 226t
Mast cell–stabilizing drugs, 231
Mastalgia, 1345
cystic, 1345
noncystic, 1345

Mastectomy, 1351
with axillary lymph node dissection, 1359, 1360f
description of, 1332t
nursing care plan for patient after, 1357b-1358b
postmastectomy pain syndrome, 1353
radical, modified, 1353, 1353t
Mastitis, 1345-1346
lactation, 1345t
lactational, 1345-1346
nonlactation, 1345t
Mastoid, **439-441**
Mastoidectomy, 440
Mastoiditis, 439-440
Materials
audiovisual, 62
printed, 62
Matulane (procarbazine)
for brain tumors, 1490
classification of, 288t
food/nutrient interactions, 954t
Mavik (trandolapril), 776t
Maxair (pirbuterol), 619t, 620
Maxalt (rizatriptan), 1530
Maxillary fracture, 1657t
Maximal voluntary ventilation (MVV), 531t
Maxorb, 205t
Maxzide (triamterene/hydrochlorothia-zide), 777t
Maze procedure, 852
MCI. *See* Mild cognitive impairment
MCIs. *See* Mass casualty incidents
MCS. *See* Multiple chemical sensitivi-ties
M-CSF. *See* Macrophage colony-stimu-lating factor
MD. *See* Muscular dystrophy
MDIs. *See* Metered-dose inhalers
MDMA. *See* 3,4-Methylenedioxyam-phetamine
MDS. *See* Minimum Data Set
Mean arterial pressure (MAP), 744
calculation of, 744, 781
normal range at rest, 1739t
Mean corpuscular hemoglobin, 1859t
Mean corpuscular hemoglobin concen-tration
effects of aging on, 672t
laboratory values, 1859t
Mean corpuscular volume
in anemias, 690t
effects of aging on, 672t
laboratory values, 1859t
Meaninglessness, fear of, 159
Measles, 437t
Measurement tools, written, 64
Mebaral (mephobarbital), 954t
Mechanical embolus retrieval in cere-bral ischemia (Merci) retriever, 1513, 1513f
Mechanical overventilation, 1764
Mechanical receptors, 515-516
Mechanical theory for fat embolism syndrome, 1651
Mechanical valves, 882, 883t
Mechanical ventilation, **1759-1769,** 1760f
in acute respiratory distress syn-drome, 1817
assist-control ventilation, 1760, 1761f
assisted mandatory ventilation, 1761f
case study, 1769
chronic, 1768
control ventilation, 1761f
controlled mandatory ventilation, 1760-1761, 1761t

Mechanical ventilation *(Continued)*
high-frequency ventilation, 1763
indications for, 1759
intermittent mandatory ventilation, 1761*t*
machine dislocation or malfunction, 1766
modes, 1760, 1761*t*
negative pressure ventilation, 1759-1760, 1760*f*
nursing care plan for patient on, 1754*b*-1756*b*
nursing management of, **1769**
nutritional therapy for patients receiving positive pressure ventilation, 1766
oral care procedures for patient on, 1758*t*
partial liquid ventilation, 1763
positive pressure ventilation, 1760, 1760*f*
in acute respiratory failure, 1810
complications of, 1763-1766
pressure modes, 1761*t*, 1762
pressure release ventilation, 1762
pressure support ventilation, 1761*t*, 1762
pressure ventilation, 1760, 1762
pressure-controlled inverse ratio ventilation, 1761*t*, 1762
settings, 1760, 1761*t*
suctioning procedures for patient on, 1757*t*
synchronized intermittent mandatory ventilation, 1761-1762, 1761*t*
types of, 1759-1762
volume modes, 1760-1762, 1761*t*
volume ventilation, 1760
volume-assured pressure ventilation, 1762
weaning from positive pressure ventilation, 1766-1768
Mechlorethamine (Mustargen), 287*t*
Meclizine (Antivert, Bonine), 992*t*
Meclofenamate (Meclomen), 1698*t*
Median nerve
decompression of, 1633*f*, 1634
distribution of, 1633, 1634*f*
Mediastinoscopy, 528*t*, 529, 894
Medic Alert bracelet, 1317
Medical adrenalectomy, 1312
Medical alerts, 1276, 1276*f*
Medical focus, 39-40
Medical futility, 309*b*
Medical history, 39, 40*t*
Medical interpreters, 36, 36*b*
choosing, 36*b*
strategies for working with, 36*b*
Medical power of attorney (MPOA), 155, 156*t*
Medicare, **75**
Part A, 75
Part B, 75
Part D, 75
Medicare Prescription Drug Benefit Program, 75
Medicated urethral system for erection (MUSE) device, 1435, 1436*f*
Medication errors, 80, 81*t*
Medication overuse headache, 1531
Medications. *See also* Drug therapy; *specific medications*
abuse of, 80
aspirin-containing, 1837*t*
and auditory system, 411
and cardiovascular system, 745
cultural factors, 34-35

Medications *(Continued)*
and endocrine system, 1243
ethnic differences in response to, 34, 35*t*
and fluid, electrolyte, and acid-base imbalances, 337
and gastrointestinal system, 933-934
and hematologic system, 672, 674*t*
home health care activities, 90*t*
important information, 43
and integumentary system, 453
and musculoskeletal system, 1619-1620
and nervous system, 1454
ototoxic, 411
preoperative, 346-347, 354, 355*t*
and reproductive system, 1332
and respiratory system, 517
topical, 474*t*, 477
and urinary system, 1142
use by older adults, 80, 81*t*
vasoactive, 1435
and visual system, 402
Medicine, primary goals of, 9, 9*t*
Meditation, 95, 96*f*, 117-118, 118*f*
basic guide to, 117*t*
basic ways to practice, 117
description of, 97*t*
guided, 117
Medrol (methylprednisolone)
for asthma and COPD, 618*t*
classification of, 287*t*
for pain, 139
Medroxyprogesterone (Depo-Provera, Provera)
drug alert, 1392
for perimenopause and postmenopause, 1392
Medtronic, Inc.
ICD, 858*f*
MiniMed insulin pump, 1264*f*, 1269, 1270*f*
pacemaker, 859*f*
Paradigm REAL-Time System, 1270
valve, 883*t*
Medtronic-Hall valve, 883*t*
Medullary cystic disease, 1177
autosomal dominant form, 1177
autosomal recessive form, 1177
Mefoxin (cefoxitin), 1670
MEG. *See* Magnetoencephalography
Megace (megestrol acetate), 1355
Megakaryocytes, 703
Megaloblastic anemia, 691-693
classification of, 692*t*
nursing management of, **693**
Megaloblasts, 691
Megestrol acetate (Megace), 1355
Meglitinides, 1265, 1266*t*
Meglumine diatrizoate (Gastrografin), 940
Meiosis, 215
Melanocytes, 449-450
Melanocyte-stimulating hormone, 1236*t*
Melanoma
ABCDs of, 465, 466*f*
collaborative care for, 466
cutaneous, 465
malignant, 464*t*, **465-466**
case study, 481
types of, 465
Melanonychea striata, 451, 451*f*
Melasma, 478
Melatonin, 103*t*
Melena, 688, 940*t*, 995, 995*t*
Mellaril (thioridazine), 1180*t*

Meloxicam (Mobic), 1698*t*
Melphalan (Alkeran)
classification of, 287*t*
for multiple myeloma, 729
Memantine (Namenda), 1551, 1569*t*
Memorial Pain Assessment Card, 134
Men
gonorrhea in, 1367, 1367*f*
gynecomastia in, **1347-1348**
The Mended Hearts, 820
contact info, 840, 891
Menest (estrogen), 288*t*
Ménière's disease, 441-442
collaborative care for, 442*t*
nursing and collaborative management of, **441-442**
Meningeal tumors, 1488, 1489*t*
Meninges, 1452
Meningioma, 1488*f*, 1488*t*
Meningismus, 1373
Meningitis, 1493, 1494*t*
bacterial, **1493-1497**
with HIV infection, 254*t*
in pneumonia, 565
viral, **1497**
Meniscus injury, 1630*t*, **1634-1635,** 1635*f*
Menometrorrhagia, 1388
Menopause, 1330, 1390
culturally competent care for, **1392**
herbs and supplements for, 1393*b*
male, 1437
pseudomenopause, 1397
Menorrhagia, 1334, 1387, **1388**
balloon thermotherapy for, 1388, 1388*f*
Menotropin, 1383, 1383*t*
Menstrual cycle, 1329-1330, 1329*f*
Menstruation
characteristics of, 1329*t*
problems related to, **1385-1389**
Mental functioning, adult, 70, 70*t*
Mental status
assessment abnormalities, 1460*t*
assessment of, 1456
in fluid and electrolyte imbalances, 338*t*
Mental status examination
components of, 1456
Mini-Mental State Examination, 1563, 1564*t*
normal, 1459*t*
Mental-emotional status assessment, 1245
Meperidine (Demerol, Pethidine), 138
as adjunct to general anesthesia, 370*t*
contraindications to, 698
effects of use, 169*t*
nephrotoxicity, 1211
preoperative, 355*t*
Mephobarbital (Mebaral), 954*t*
Mepilex, 205*t*
6-Mercaptopurine (6-MP) (Purinethol)
classification of, 287*t*
hepatotoxicity, 934*t*
for inflammatory bowel disease, 1054, 1055*t*
for leukemia, 720*t*, 721*t*
Merci retriever, 1513, 1513*f*
Mercury, 934*t*
Meridia (sibutramine), 981
Mesalamine (Asacol, Pentasa), 1055*t*
Mesalamine suppositories (Canasa), 1055*t*
Mescaline (peyote), 170*t*
Mesoderm, 279

Mesotheliomas, 585
Mestinon (pyridostigmine), 370
MET units. *See* Metabolic equivalent units
Metabolic acidosis, 335, 335*t*
in acute renal failure, 1200
in chronic kidney disease, 1207
clinical manifestations of, 336*t*
Metabolic alkalosis, 335, 335*t*, 336*t*
Metabolic diseases
of bone, **1686-1690**
gerontologic considerations for, **1690**
in chronic kidney disease, 1206-1207
with dermatologic manifestations, 473*t*
of liver, **1100-1101**
renal involvement in, **1177**
Metabolic emergencies, oncologic, 308
Metabolic equivalent (MET) units, 815
energy expenditure in, 816*t*
Metabolic imbalances, 334
Metabolic needs in spinal cord injury, 1595
Metabolic syndrome, 987, 1257
and coronary artery disease, 791
diagnostic criteria for, 987*t*
etiology and pathophysiology of, 987
nursing and collaborative management of, 987
Metabolic system. *See also* Nutritional-metabolic pattern
in acute renal failure, 1201*t*
Metaglip (metformin and glipizide), 1266*t*
Metahydrin (trichlormethiazide), 773*t*
Metamorphopsia, 432
Metamucil (psyllium), 1042*t*, 1519
Metanephrine, 1862*t*
Metaphysis, 1616
Metaproterenol (Alupent, Metaprel), 620
for asthma and COPD, 619*t*
food/nutrient interactions, 954*t*
Metastasis, 276
blood-borne, 276, 277*f*
breast cancer sites, 1350, 1351*t*
hematogenous, 276
pathogenesis of, 276, 278*f*
Metastatic bone cancer, 1674-1675
Metastatic brain tumors, 1488, 1488*t*, 1489*t*
Metered-dose inhalers, 617, 620*f*, 623*t*
how to use correctly, 621-622, 622*f*
problems encountered with, 622-623, 622*f*
Metformin (Glucophage, Glucophage XR, Riomet, Fortamet)
for diabetes mellitus, 1265, 1266*t*
for hyperandrogenism, 1399-1400
Metformin and glipizide (Metaglip), 1266*t*
Metformin and glyburide (Glucovance), 1266*t*
Metformin and rosiglitazone (Avandamet), 1266*t*
Methadone (Dolophine)
as adjunct to general anesthesia, 370*t*
for burns, 499*t*
effects of use, 169*t*
for opioid withdrawal, 180
for pain, 137*t*, 138
Methamphetamine (Desoxyn), 169*t*
Methaqualone (Quaalude), 169*t*

Methazolamide (Neptazane), 435t
Methicillin-resistant *Staphylococcus aureus*, 246, 246t
Methimazole (Tapazole), 1301
Methohexital (Brevital), 369t
Methotrexate (Folex, Rheumatrex, Trexall)
  for arthritis and connective tissue disorders, 1699t
  for bladder cancer, 1179
  for breast cancer, 1355
  classification of, 287t
  for esophageal cancer, 1010
  hepatotoxicity, 934t
  for inducing abortion, 1385
  for inflammatory bowel disease, 1054
  for leukemia, 720t, 721t
  methods of administration, 288t
  nephrotoxicity, 1142t
  for non-Hodgkin's lymphoma, 727t
  for oral cancer, 1002
  photosensitivity, 461t
  for polymyositis and dermatomyositis, 1726
  for rheumatoid arthritis, 1705
Methotrexate with misporostol, 1384t
Methyclothiazide (Enduron, Diuretic), 773t
Methylcellulose (Citrucel, Cologel), 1042t
Methyldopa (Aldomet)
  autoreactivity to, 234
  for hypertension, 774t
Methyldopa/hydrochlorothiazide (Aldoril), 777t
3,4-Methylenedioxyamphetamine (MDMA, Ecstasy), 170t, 181
Methylmalonic acid, 680t
Methylphenidate (Ritalin)
  effects of use, 169t
  for multiple sclerosis, 1544-1545, 1545t
  for opioid-induced sedation, 138
Methylprednisolone (MP) (Medrol, Depo-Medrol, Solu-Medrol), 238, 239t
  for arthritis and connective tissue disorders, 1698t, 1699t
  for asthma and COPD, 618t
  classification of, 287t
  for inflammatory bowel disease, 1055t
  for multiple sclerosis, 1544, 1544t
  for neurogenic shock, 1790
  for pain, 139
  for spinal cord injury, 1596
Methylxanthines, 619t, 621
Methysergide (Sansert), 1531
Metipranolol (OptiPranolol), 434t
Metoclopramide (Reglan)
  as adjunct to general anesthesia, 370t
  for gastroesophageal reflux disease, 1006, 1006t
  for nausea and vomiting, 138, 297, 992, 992t
  preoperative, 355t
Metolazone (Zaroxolyn), 773t
Metoprolol (Lopressor, Toprol)
  for acute coronary syndrome, 800t
  for chronic HF, 832
  for chronic stable angina, 799, 800t
  classification of, 856t

Metoprolol (Lopressor, Toprol)
  (Continued)
  for hypertension, 774t, 1210
  and lower urinary tract function, 1180t
Metoprolol/hydrochlorothiazide (Lopressor HCT), 777t
Metronidazole (Flagyl)
  for bacterial vaginosis, 1394t
  for inflammatory bowel disease, 1054, 1055t
  for peptic ulcer disease, 1019t
  for trichomonas vaginitis, 1394t
  for urethritis, 1163
Metrorrhagia, 1334, 1387, **1388**
METs. See Metabolic equivalent units
Metyrapone, 1312
Mevacor (lovastatin), 793, 795t, 1167
Mexican Americans
  case study, 37
  cultural values, 27t
  diabetes mellitus in, 1255
  end-of-life care, 155
  health disparities, 21t
  medications used, 34
Mexiletine (Mexitil)
  classification of, 856t
  local, 139t
MG. See Myasthenia gravis
MH. See Malignant hyperthermia
MI. See Myocardial infarction
Micardis (telmisartan), 776t
Micardis HCT (telmisartan/hydrochlorothiazide), 777t
Microbial hypersensitivity reactions, 228
Microcytosis, 691
Microdermabrasion, 479t
Microglia, 1442
Micronase (glyburide)
  for diabetes mellitus, 1265, 1266t
  for diabetes mellitus in older adults, 1288
  food/nutrient interactions, 954t
Microscopy, dark-field, 1339t
Microsporum, 245t
Microsurgery, reconstructive, 481
Microvascular decompression, 1582, 1582t
Microwave thermotherapy, transurethral, 1418-1419, 1418t
Microzide (hydrochlorothiazide), 773t
Micturition, 1140
Midamor (amiloride)
  for bilateral adrenal hyperplasia, 1319
  for cirrhosis, 1110t
  for hypertension, 773t
Midazolam (Versed)
  as adjunct to general anesthesia, 369, 370t
  for burns, 499t
  preoperative, 355t
Middle cerebral artery, 1507t
Middle ear, 408f, 409
  age-related changes in, 410t
  problems of, **439-441**
Midrin (acetaminophen), 1530
Mifepristone (Mifeprex) (RU-486), 1384t, 1385
Miglitol (Glyset), 1265, 1266t
Migraine headache, 1528-1529, 1528t
  with aura, 1529
  clinical manifestations of, 1529
  diagnostic studies, 1529
  drug therapy for, 1530-1531
  etiology and pathophysiology of, 1528-1529
  without aura, 1529

Mild cognitive impairment, 1564, 1564t
Miliary tuberculosis, 570
Milk of Magnesia
  for constipation, 1042t
  for opioid-induced constipation, 138
Milk thistle (silymarin), 102t, 1131b
Miller Fisher syndrome, 1586
Milliequivalents, 316
Millimoles, 316
Milrinone (Primacor)
  for acute decompensated HF, 829
  as positive inotrope, 1739
Mind-body interventions, 96t, 97t, **100**
Mindfulness practices, 117
Mineral metabolism studies, 1626t
Mineral oil (Fleets Oil retention enema, Kondremul Plain), 1042t
Mineral oil slides, 458t
Mineralocorticoids, 1236t
Minerals
  for burns, 499t
  major, 950, 950t
  oral anticoagulants interactions, 914t
Minimal leak technique, 547, 1753
Minimal occluding volume technique, 1753
Minimally invasive direct coronary artery bypass graft, 809-810
MiniMed insulin pump (Medtronic), 1264f, 1269, 1270f
Mini-Mental State Examination, 1563, 1564t
Minimum Data Set (MDS), 957
Minipress (prazosin)
  effects on lower urinary tract function, 1180t
  for hypertension, 774t
  for pheochromocytoma, 1320
Mini-trach, 1810
Minitran (transdermal nitroglycerin), 800t
Minizide (prazosin/polythiazide), 777t
Minnesota tube, 1108, 1109f
Minocycline (Minocin)
  for arthritis and connective tissue disorders, 1698t
  for rheumatoid arthritis, 1706
Minority Health, 38
Minoxidil (Loniten), 775t
Minute ventilation (V_E), 1767t
Miotics
  drug alert, 434
  for glaucoma, 435t
MiraLax (polyethylene glycol), 138, 1042t
Mirapex (pramipexole)
  for Parkinson's disease, 1551, 1552t
  for restless legs syndrome, 1558
Miscarriage, 1383
Misoprostol (Cytotec)
  for inducing abortrion, 1384t
  for osteoarthritis, 1697
  for peptic ulcer disease, 1019t
Misoprostol and diclofenac (Voltaren), 1697
Mithracin (plicamycin)
  classification of, 287t
  for hypercalcemia, 330
Mitomycin (Mutamycin)
  classification of, 287t
  for esophageal cancer, 1010
Mitosis, 215
Mitotane (Lysodren), 1312-1314
Mitotic inhibitors
  classification of, 287t
  for leukemia, 720t

Mitoxantrone (Novantrone)
  classification of, 287t
  for leukemia, 720t, 721t
  for multiple sclerosis, 1544, 1544t
  for non-Hodgkin's lymphoma, 727t
  for prostate cancer, 1427
Mitral valve, bacterial endocarditis of, 866, 867f
Mitral valve prolapse (MVP), 879-880, 880f
  clinical manifestations of, 879t, 880
  etiology and pathophysiology of, 879-880
  patient and family teaching guide for, 880t
Mitral valve regurgitation, 879
  clinical manifestations of, 879, 879t
  etiology and pathophysiology of, 879
Mitral valve stenosis, 878-879, 879f
  clinical manifestations of, 879, 879t
  etiology and pathophysiology of, 878-879
Mitrolan-OTC (calcium polycarbophil), 1037t
Mivacurium (Mivacron), 370t
Mixed (overlapping) connective tissue diseases, 1726
Mixed venous blood gases, 513-514, 514t
Mixed venous hemoglobin oxygen saturation, 1739t
Mixed venous oxygen saturation (SvO_2), 1746
  $SvO_2/ScvO_2$ measurements
    clinical interpretation of, 1746-1747, 1746t
    in shock, 1774t
Mobic (meloxicam), 1698t
Mobitz I heart block, 849t, 853
Mobitz II heart block, 849t, 853-854
Modafinil (Provigil)
  for multiple sclerosis, 1545, 1545t
  for opioid-induced sedation, 138
MODS. See Multiple organ dysfunction syndrome
Moduretic (amiloride/hydrochlorothiazide), 777t
Moexipril (Univasc), 776t
Moexipril/hydrochlorothiazide (Uniretic), 777t
MOH. See Medication overuse headache
Mohs' surgery, 476-477
Molecular cytogenetics, 682t, 683
Moles (nevi), 457t, 472t
Mometasone (Nasonex)
  for allergic rhinitis and sinusitis, 537t
  for asthma and COPD, 618t
Mongolian spots, 457
Monilial vaginitis, 1394t
Moniliasis, 1000t
Monoamine oxidase inhibitors
  blood glucose level effects, 1267t
  for Parkinson's disease, 1551, 1552t
Monoarthritis, 876
Monoclonal antibodies, 240, 240f, 303t
  to CD20, 303t
  hybridoma technology of, 240-241
  to IgE, 620
  immunosuppressive therapy, 239t
Monocytes, 668
  function of, 668t
  laboratory values, 1860t
  response to injury, 194
Monofilament testing, 1286

Mononuclear phagocytes, 220-222, 932t
Monopril (fosinopril), 776t
Monopril-HCT (fosinopril/hydrochlorothiazide), 777t
Monosaccharides, 949
Monospot or monotest, 1861t
Mons pubis, 1327
Monsel's solution (ferric subsulfate), 476
Montelukast (Singulair), 620
   for allergic rhinitis and sinusitis, 537t
   for asthma and COPD, 619t
Mood assessment, 1456
Moon face, 1246t
Moraxella catarrhalis, 562t
Morbid obesity
   classification of, 974, 974f, 975t
   definition of, 1874
   surgical interventions for, 982-983, 982t
Moricizine (Ethmozine), 856t
Morphine (Duramorph)
   for acute coronary syndrome, 800t
   for acute pancreatitis, 1121t
   blood glucose level effects, 1267t
   for burns, 499t
   for chronic stable angina, 800t
   drug alert, 138
   effects of use, 169t
   intrathecal, 141
   for pain, 137t, 138, 140, 141
   preoperative, 355t
Morphine sulfate
   for acute coronary syndrome, 808
   as adjunct to general anesthesia, 370t
Morrhuate (Scleromate), 1108
Mortality, infant, 21t
Morton's neuroma (Morton's toe), 1685t
Motilium (domperidone), 992t
Motion
   active range of, 1622
   limited range of, 1623t
   measurement of, 1622, 1622f
   passive range of, 1622
Motivational interviewing, 188
   for addictive behaviors, 188-189
   key aspects of, 188, 188t
Motor deficits, 1507-1508
Motor endplate, 1618
Motor function
   age-related changes in, 1454t
   in increased ICP, 1471-1472
   in stroke, 1507-1508
Motor status observations, 49t
Motor strength testing, 1477-1478
Motor system
   assessment abnormalities, 1460t
   examination of, 1458
   normal assessment of, 1459t
Motor vehicle collision
   acute soft tissue injury in, 1631, 1632t
   fractured extremity in, 1642, 1642t
   head injury in, 1484t
   spinal cord injury in, 1596t
Motrin (ibuprofen)
   analgesic effects of, 128
   for arthritis and connective tissue disorders, 1698t
   for fever, 203
   mechanism of action, 202t
   for pain, 136, 136t
   for premenstrual syndrome, 1386
Mourning process, 1608-1609, 1608t
Mouth
   age-related changes in, 932, 933t
   in anemia, 686t

Mouth *(Continued)*
   assessment abnormalities, 675t, 939t
   digestion and absorption by, 928
   infections and inflammations of, 1000-1001, 1000t
   inflammation of, 1000t
   ingestion propulsion of food by, 928
   inspection of, 936
   palpation of, 936
   physical examination of, 521, 936
      normal, 939t
      outline for, 49t
      recording, 51t
Mouth-to-mouth resuscitation, 1845-1846, 1845f
Movement problems, 1440-1731
Moxifloxacin (Avelox, Vigamox), 573t
MP. *See* Methylprednisolone
6-MP. *See* Mercaptopurine
MPOA. *See* Medical power of attorney
MRA. *See* Magnetic resonance angiography
MRCP. *See* Magnetic resonance cholangiopancreatography
MRI. *See* Magnetic resonance imaging
MRS. *See* Magnetic resonance spectroscopy
MRSA. *See* Methicillin-resistant *Staphylococcus aureus*
MS. *See* Multiple sclerosis
MSContin (morphine), 137t, 140
MSIR (morphine), 137t
Mucociliary clearance system, 516
Mucociliary escalator, 516
Mucosal disease, stress-related, 996
   etiology and pathophysiology of, 1017
Mucositis, 295t, 298-299
Mucous membranes
   changes in, 675t
   regenerative ability of, 198, 198t
Mucus
   fecal analysis, 1864t
   flutter mucus clearance device, 648, 648f
MUGA scan. *See* Multigated acquisition scan
Multicolony colony-stimulating factor, 222t
Multicultural health care environment, **30,** 30f
Multifactorial inherited conditions, 215
Multigated acquisition scan, 754t
Multimodality therapy, 284
Multinucleated giant cell, 195
Multiple chemical sensitivities, 233
Multiple dressing changes, 497, 498f
Multiple electrolyte solutions, 339t
Multiple myeloma, 728-729
   clinical manifestations of, 728
   collaborative care for, 728-729
   definition of, 1874
   diagnostic studies, 728
   etiology and pathophysiology of, 728
   nursing management of, **729**
Multiple organ dysfunction syndrome (MODS), 1772, 1773f, **1794-1796**
   clinical manifestations of, 1796t-1797t
   collaborative care for, 1795
   etiology of, 1794
   nursing and collaborative management of, **1795-1796**
   nutritional and metabolic needs in, 1796t
   organ and metabolic dysfunction in, 1794-1795
   pathophysiology of, 1794-1795

Multiple sclerosis (MS), 1542-1549
   chronic, 1542, 1542f
   clinical course of, 1542-1543, 1543t
   clinical manifestations of, 1542-1543
   collaborative care for, 1543t, 1544-1546
   diagnostic studies, 1543
   drug therapy for, 1544-1545, 1544t-1545t
   etiology and pathophysiology of, 1542
   exercise and quality of life in, 1547b
   nursing assessment of, 1546, 1546t
   nursing care plan for patient with, 1547b-1548b
   nursing diagnoses, 1546
   nursing evaluation of, 1549
   nursing implementation for, 1546-1549
   nursing management of, **1546-1549**
   nursing planning for, 1546
   nutritional therapy for, 1546
   pathogenesis of, 1542, 1542f
   signs and symptoms of, 1543
   water therapy for, 1545, 1546f
Multivitamins, 499t
Mumps, surgical, 1000t
Mumps virus, 244t
Murmurs, 744, 751
Muromonab-CD3 (Orthoclone OKT3), 239t, 240
Muscarinic receptor antagonists, 1185t
Muscle(s), **1617-1618**
   age-related changes in, 1618-1619, 1619t
   autoimmune diseases of, 234t
   cardiac, 1617
   contractions of, 1618
   energy source for, 1618
   extraocular, 400
   regenerative ability of, 198, 198t
   skeletal, 1617
   smooth, 1617
   spasticity of, 1623t
   structure of, 1617-1618
   types of, 1617
Muscle atrophy, 1649t
Muscle cramps, 1223
Muscle injury, 1627t
Muscle mass changes, 1247t
Muscle relaxants
   adjuvant drugs for pain management, 139t
   for multiple sclerosis, 1545t
Muscle relaxation, 119-120
   passive, 120
   progressive, 119, 119t
Muscle spasms, 1635
   with fractures, 1637t
   with musculoskeletal injury, 1649t
Muscle strength changes, 1247t
Muscle strength scale, 1622t
Muscle tone loss, 152-153
Muscle-strength testing, 1622
Muscular dystrophy, 1675
   Becker muscular dystrophy, 1675t
   Duchenne muscular dystrophy, 1675b, 1675t
   Erb muscular dystrophy, 1675t
   Landouzy-Déjérine muscular dystrophy, 1675t
   and restrictive lung disease, 595t
   types of, 1675, 1675t
Musculocutaneous flap procedures, 1353t, 1362-1363

Musculoskeletal system, **1614-1628**
   age-related changes in, 1618-1619, 1619t
      nursing diagnoses associated with, 78t
   in anemia, 686t
   assessment abnormalities, 676t, 1247t, 1623t-1624t
   assessment of, **1619-1624**
      gerontologic differences in, 1618-1619, 1619t
      important health information, 1619-1620
      objective data, 1621-1624
      preoperative, 349, 351t
      questions to ask, 1620t
      subjective data, 1619-1621
   burn injury complications, 500
   in chronic kidney disease, 1208-1209
   and COPD, 650t
   diagnostic studies, 1624-1628, 1625t-1628t
   effects of aging on, **1618-1619**
   effects of chronic alcohol abuse on, 177t
   at end of life, 152t
   functions of, **1615-1619**
   in HIV infection, 259t
   inspection of, 1621
   and lung cancer, 583t
   measurement of, 1622-1623
   nursing interventions to optimize, 1519
   palpation of, 1621-1622
   physical examination of, 1621-1624
      normal, 1623t
      recording, 51t
   positive pressure ventilation effects on, 1765
   preoperative review, 348
   problems associated with injury of, 1647-1648, 1649t
   problems of, **1668-1692**
      associated with obesity, 975
      with dermatologic manifestations, 473t
      prevention of, in older adults, 1630t
      resources for, 1692
      in systemic lupus erythematosus, 1718
   after stroke
      acute intervention for, 1519
      ambulatory and home care for, 1521-1522
   structures of, **1615-1619**
   trauma to, 1629-1630, 1667
MUSE device. *See* Medicated urethral system for erection device
Mushrooms (psilocybin), 170t
Music therapy, 124, 364b
   description of, 97t
   effects on confusion and delirium in surgical patients, 1577b
   for relaxation, 119
Mustard gas, 1840
Mustargen (mechlorethamine), 287t
Mutamycin (mitomycin)
   classification of, 287t
   for esophageal cancer, 1010
Mutations, 214, 214t
Mutilation, fear of, 345
MVP. *See* Mitral valve prolapse
MVV. *See* Maximal voluntary ventilation
Myalgia, 1623t
Myambutol (ethambutol), 573t

Myasthenia gravis (MG), 1555-1557
clinical manifestations of, 1555-1556
collaborative care for, 1556, 1556t
complications of, 1555-1556
diagnostic studies, 1556
drug therapy for, 1556
etiology of, 1555
nursing assessment of, 1556
nursing diagnoses, 1556
nursing evaluation of, 1557
nursing implementation for, 1556-1557
nursing management of, **1556-1557**
nursing planning for, 1556
and restrictive lung disease, 595t
surgical therapy for, 1556
Myasthenic crisis, 1556, 1557t
Mycelex (clotrimazole), 1163
Mycobacteria
atypical, **575**
diseases caused by, 244t
Mycobacterium avium complex, 255t, 575
Mycobacterium intracellulare, 575
Mycobacterium kansasii, 575
Mycobacterium scrofulaceum, 575
Mycobacterium tuberculosis, 255t, 562t, 569, 570
Mycobacterium xenopi, 575
Mycobutin (rifabutin), 573t
Mycophenolate mofetil (CellCept), 238, 239t, 240, 1718
Mycoplasma, 562
Mycoplasma pneumoniae, 561, 562t, 565
Mycosis fungoides, 464t
Mycostatin (nystatin)
for burns, 499, 499t
for urethritis, 1163
Mydfrin (phenylephrine HCl), 427t
Mydriacyl (tropicamide), 427t
Mydriatics, 426
drug alert, 426
for pupil dilation, 427t
Myectomy, 889
Myeloablative chemotherapy, 305
Myelodysplastic syndrome, 716-717
clinical manifestations of, 717
diagnostic studies, 717
etiology and pathophysiology of, 716-717
nursing and collaborative management of, **717**
Myelography, 1463t, 1625t
Myeloma protein, 728
Mylanta
for burns, 499t
for gastroesophageal reflux disease, 1006t
preparation, 1020t
for renal osteodystrophy, 1210
Myleran (busulfan)
classification of, 287t
for leukemia, 720t
Mylotarg (gemtuzumab ozogamicin), 303t, 720t, 721
Myocardial infarction (MI), 803-805, 803f
acute, 803, 803f
anterolateral wall, 862, 862f
cardiovascular manifestations of, 804
case study, 818

Myocardial infarction (MI)
(Continued)
clinical manifestations of, 803-804
complications of, 804-805
diagnostic studies, 805-806
ECG changes in, 862, 862f
healing process, 804
non–ST-segment-elevation, 802
pain during, 796, 797f
serum cardiac markers in, 805-806, 805f
ST-segment-elevation, 802
Myocardial ischemia, 796
ECG changes in, 861, 862f
Myocarditis, 874-875
in chemotherapy and radiation therapy, 296t
clinical manifestations of, 875
collaborative care for, 875
diagnostic studies, 875
etiology and pathophysiology of, 874-875
idiopathic, 875
nursing management of, **875**
Myocardium, 740
blood supply to, 740-741
factors determining oxygen needs of, 796, 796t
Myochrysine (gold sodium thiomalate)
for arthritis and connective tissue disorders, 1699t
for rheumatoid arthritis, 1706
Myoclonic seizures, 1535
Myoclonus, 161t, 1458
Myofascial pain syndrome, 1726-1727, 1727t
Myoflex cream (trolamine salicylate), 141
Myoglobin, 752t, 1862t
Myoneural or neuromuscular junction, 1618, 1618f
Myopia, 399-400, 416, **417**
Myositis ossificans, 1638t
Myotomes, 1448
MyPyramid, 949, 949f, 950t
Myringotomy, 439
Mysoline (primidone)
gerontologic considerations for, 1538
for seizures, 1538t
Myxedema, 1246t, 1305, 1305f

N
Nabilone (Cesamet), 992t
Nabumetone (Relafen), 1698t
Nadolol (Corgard)
for acute coronary syndrome, 800t
for chronic stable angina, 799, 800t
for hypertension, 774t
Nadolol/bendroflumethiazide (Corzide), 777t
Nafarelin (Synarel), 1383t
Nafcillin (Nafcil)
for infective endocarditis, 869t
for osteomyelitis, 1670
NAFLD. *See* Nonalcoholic fatty liver disease
Nail beds
pallor of, 675t
pigmented, 451, 451f
Nails, 450-451
age-related changes in, 451-452, 452t
physical examination of, 51t
structure of, 450-451, 451f

Naloxone (Narcan)
buprenorphine plus naloxone (Suboxone), 137t, 180
for opioid-induced respiratory depression, 138
Naltrexone (ReVia, Trexan, Vivitrol)
for alcohol abuse, 178
for opioid withdrawal, 180
Namenda (memantine), 1551, 1569t
NANDA. *See* North American Nursing Diagnosis Association
NANDA International, 11
NANDA-NOC-NIC linkages, 14, 14f, 14t
Nursing Diagnoses, Definitions, and Classification, 8, 10-11
purposes of, 10
Taxonomy I, 11
Taxonomy II, 11, 42t-43t, 43
Naproxen (Naprosyn, Anaprox, Aleve)
analgesic effects of, 128
for arthritis and connective tissue disorders, 1698t
for dysmenorrhea, 1387
and gastritis, 1013
Naqua (trichlormethiazide), 773t
Naratriptan (Amerge), 1530
Narcan (naloxone), 138
Narcosis, carbon dioxide, 643
Narcotics Anonymous, 191
Nasacort (triamcinolone) for allergic rhinitis and sinusitis, 537t
Nasal bone fracture, 1657t
Nasal cannulas, 641t, 642f, 644
Nasal endotracheal intubation, 1751
Nasal fracture, 533-534
Nasal masks, 543, 543f
Nasal packs, posterior, 534-535, 535f
Nasal sprays
for allergic rhinitis and sinusitis, 535-536, 537t, 538t
method for using, 539f
Nasal surgery, **534**
NasalCrom (cromolyn spray), 537t
Nasalide (flunisolide), 537t
NASH. *See* Nonalcoholic steatohepatitis
Nasogastric tubes, 961
ambulatory and home care, 558
care of, 1062
Nasointestinal tubes, 961
Nasonex (mometasone), 537t
Nateglinide (Starlix), 1265, 1266t
National Association for Home Care and Hospice (NAHC), 93, 164
definition of home care, 89
National Association of Area Agencies on Aging, *A National Eldercare Directory of Information and Referral,* 76-77
National Asthma Education and Prevention Program (NAEPP), 615
National Center for Complementary and Alternative Medicine (NCCAM), 94
complementary and alternative therapy categories, 96, 96t
National Comprehensive Cancer Network (NCCN) evidence-based cancer treatment guidelines, 284
A National Eldercare Directory of Information and Referral (National Association of Area Agencies on Aging), 76-77
National Guideline Clearinghouse, 7t

National Heart, Lung, and Blood Institute (NHLBI), 615, 663, 737, 820, 840, 891, 924
Clinical Guidelines, 663
dietary guidelines, 833
National Institute for Occupational Safety and Health (NIOSH), 578
guidelines for preventing allergic latex reactions, 232, 232t
National Institutes of Health (NIH)
definition of health disparities, 20
National Center for Complementary and Alternative Medicine (NCCAM), 95
National Osteoporosis Foundation, recommendations for treatment for osteoporosis, 1688
National Patient Safety Goals (JCAHO), 366
Native Alaskans
health disparities, 20
older adults, 66
Native Americans
communication, 36
cultural values, 27t
culture-bound syndromes, 35t
diabetes mellitus in, 1255
ethnic differences in response to drugs, 34, 35t
folk healers, 30
health care, 97t
health disparities, 20, 21, 21t, 24f, 33-34
nurses, 26
Natrecor (nesiritide), 829
Natulan (procarbazine), 288t
Natural death acts, 155
Natural killer cells, 222
Natural lipid-lowering agents, 796b
Natural products, 95, 96f
Natural Standard, 109
Naturetin (bendroflumethiazide), 773t
Naturopathy, 97t
Nausea and vomiting, 939t, **990-995**
acute intervention for, 993
ambulatory and home care for, 993-995
anticipatory, 298
chemotherapy-induced, 99t, 295t, 297-298
clinical manifestations of, 991
collaborative care for, 991-992
delayed, 298
drug therapy of, 992, 992t
at end of life, 161t
etiology and pathophysiology of, 991
gerontologic considerations for, **995**
in myocardial infarction, 804
nondrug therapy of, 992
nursing assessment of, 992-993, 993t
nursing care plan for patient with, 994b
nursing diagnoses, 993
nursing evaluation of, 995
nursing implementation for, 993-995
nursing management of, **992-995**
nursing planning for, 993
nutritional therapy of, 992
opioid-related, 138
in radiation therapy, 295t, 297-298
Navelbine (vinorelbine)
for breast cancer, 1355
classification of, 287t
for esophageal cancer, 1010
for lung cancer, 582
photosensitivity, 461t

Near syncope, 745*t*
Near-drowning, 1832
Nearsightedness, 416, 417
Nebcin (tobramycin)
  nephrotoxicity, 1142*t*
  for osteomyelitis, 1670
Nebulizers, 640-641
Neck. *See also* Head and neck
  assessment abnormalities, 1246*t*
  inspection of, 48*t*-49*t*
  palpation of, 48*t*-49*t*
  physical assessment of, 525*t*
  physical examination of, 521, 1245-
    1246
    outline for, 48*t*-49*t*
    recording, 51*t*
Neck exercises, 1684*t*
Neck pain, 1684, 1684*t*
Neck surgery
  modified dissection, 552
  radical dissection, 552, 552*f*
    nursing care plan for patient hav-
      ing total laryngectomy and/or,
      554*b*-556*b*
Neck veins, distended, 749*t*
Necrobiosis lipoidica diabeticorum,
    1287, 1287*f*
Necrosis
  acute tubular, 1198-1199, 1199*f*
  biliary, 1102
  cardiac, 1102
  diabetic foot complications, 1286,
    1286*f*
  fat, 1345*t*
  gangrenous, 1830-1831, 1831*f*
  postnecrotic cirrhosis, 1102
Necrotizing pancreatitis, 1119
Necrotizing ulcerative gingivitis,
  acute, 1000*t*
Nedocromil (Tilade), 620
  for asthma, 617*t*, 618*t*
  for COPD, 618*t*
  for exercise-induced asthma, 608
Needle ablation, transurethral, 1418*t*,
  1419
Needle biopsy
  for cancer diagnosis, 283
  liver biopsy, 946
  lymph node biopsy, 681, 682*t*
  transbronchial, 529-530, 530*f*
Needles, Huber-point, 289
Negative inotropes, 1739
Negative inspiratory force or pressure,
  1767*t*
Negative pressure ventilation, 1759-
  1760, 1760*f*
Negative-pressure wound therapy, 205
Negatives, pertinent, 47
Neglect
  elder neglect, 73, 73*t*
  personal neglect, 168*t*
Neiguan point (PC6), 98, 100*f*
Neisseria gonorrhoeae, 1367, 1367*t*
Neisseriae, 244*t*
Nelarabine (Arranon), 720*t*, 721*t*
Nelfinavir (Viracept), 258*t*
Nembutal (pentobarbital)
  effects of use, 169*t*
  withdrawal from, 179
Nemedia (amantadine), 140
Neomycin
  for cirrhosis, 1110*t*
  nephrotoxicity, 1142*t*
  for osteomyelitis, 1670
Neoplasms. *See also* Tumors
  benign, 274, 275*t*
  malignant, 274, 275*t*
Neoral (cyclosporine), 238, 239*t*

Neosar (cyclophosphamide), 239*t*, 287*t*
Neostigmine (Prostigmin), 370
  for multiple sclerosis, 1544*t*
  for myasthenia gravis, 1556
Neo-Synephrine (phenylephrine), 427*t*
  for allergic rhinitis and sinusitis, 538*t*
  for shock, 1788*t*
Neovascularization, 1284
Nephrectomy, laparoscopic, 1188
Nephritis
  chronic hereditary, 1177
  interstitial, 1162
Nephrolithiasis, 1169, 1170*f*
  nursing care plan for patient with
    acute renal lithiasis, 1173*b*-
    1174*b*
Nephrolithotomy, 1172
  percutaneous, 1171
Nephrons, 1137, 1138*f*
  destruction in acute renal failure,
    1199, 1199*f*
  functions of segments of, 1138, 1138*t*
Nephropathy
  diabetic, **1285**
    prevention, detection, and monitor-
      ing of, 1284*t*
  renal involvement in, 1177
  HIV-associated, 1168
Nephrosclerosis, 1175
  accelerated, 1175
  benign, 1175
  in hypertension, 767
  malignant, 1175
Nephrostomy, 1189*t*
Nephrostomy tubes, 1187
Nephrotic syndrome, 1167-1168
  causes of, 1167, 1167*t*
  clinical manifestations of, 1167
  collaborative care for, 1167
  etiology of, 1167
  with HIV infection, 1168
  nursing management of, **1167-1168**
Nephrotomogram, 1148*t*
Nephrotoxicity
  in chemotherapy and radiation ther-
    apy, 296*t*
  of drugs, 1142, 1142*t*
Neptazane (methazolamide), 435*t*
Nerve blocks
  epidural, 372, 372*f*
  therapeutic, 142-143
Nerve conduction studies, 1463*t*, 1464
Nerve conduction velocity, 1464
Nerve impulse, 1443-1444
Nerve regeneration, 1442
Nerve tissue, 198, 198*t*
Nervios, 35*t*
Nervous system, **1441-1466**
  acupuncture benefits, 99*t*
  in acute renal failure, 1200, 1201*t*
  age-related changes in, 1454*t*
    nursing diagnoses associated with,
      78*t*
  in anemia, 686*t*
  after aortic surgery, 898
  assessment abnormalities, 676*t*,
    1460*t*-1461*t*
  assessment of, **1453-1459**
    gerontologic differences in, 1454*t*
    key questions to ask, 1455*t*
    objective data, 1456-1459
    subjective data, 1454-1456
  burn injury complications, 500
  cells of, 1442
  chronic disorders of, **1532-1559**
  in chronic kidney disease, 1208
  chronic problems of, **1527-1560**

Nervous system *(Continued)*
  control of hormones by, 1238
  diagnostic studies, **1459-1465,** 1462*t*-
    1463*t*
  effects of aging on, 1452-1453
  in extracellular fluid volume imbal-
    ances, 323
  functions of, **1442-1453**
  in HIV infection, 254*t*, 259*t*
  and lung cancer, 583*t*
  physical examination of, 1456-1459,
    1459*t*
  in pneumonia, 567*t*
  positive pressure ventilation effects
    on, 1765
  preoperative review, 348
  problems of
    in chemotherapy and radiation
      therapy, 296*t*
    chronic, **1527-1560**
      with dermatologic manifestations,
        473*t*
    nursing assessment of, 388
    nursing diagnoses, 388
    nursing implementation for, 388
    nursing management of, **388**
    postoperative, **387-388**
    in systemic lupus erythematosus,
      1718
  response to stress, 113, 113*f*
  in shock, 1781*t*
    acute intervention for, 1791
  after stroke, 1515
  structures of, **1442-1453**
Nesiritide (Natrecor)
  for chronic HF, 832
  for heart failure, 829
Neulasta (pegfilgrastim)
  for cancer treatment, 304*t*
  clinical uses of, 223*t*
Neumega (oprelvekin), 705
  for cancer treatment, 304*t*
  clinical uses of, 223*t*
Neupogen (filgrastim)
  for cancer treatment, 304*t*
  clinical uses of, 223*t*
Neurectomies, 143
Neuroablative interventions, 143
Neuroaugmentation, 143
**Neurodegenerative diseases, 1575-
  1576**
Neuroendocrine theory of aging, 68*t*, 69
Neurofibrillary tangles, 1565
Neurogenic bladder
  areflexic, 1604, 1605*t*
  collaborative care for, 1604, 1605*t*
  reflexic, 1604, 1605*t*
  sensory, 1604, 1605*t*
  after spinal cord injury, 1604-1605
  types of, 1604, 1605*t*
Neurogenic bowel
  with spinal cord injury, 1605-1606
Neurogenic shock, 1590, 1773*f*, **1777**
  classification of, 1773*t*
  clinical presentation of, 1776*t*
  collaborative care for, 1789-1790
  pathophysiology of, 1777, 1777*f*
  precipitating factors, 1773*t*
  treatment of, 1789*t*
Neurogenic skin, 1606
Neuroglia, 1442
Neurohypophysis. *See* Posterior pituitary gland
Neurologic assessment
  abnormalities, 1247*t*
  brief, 1824*t*
  initial postanesthesia care unit assess-
    ment, 377-378, 377*t*

Neurologic assessment *(Continued)*
  outline for, 49*t*
  preoperative, 349, 351*t*
  recording, 51*t*
Neuromuscular blocking agents, 370-
  371, 370*t*
Neuromuscular junction, 1618, 1618*f*
Neurons, 1442
  characteristics of, 1442
  lower motor neurons, 1445
  regenerative ability of, 198, 198*t*
  structure of, 1442, 1442*f*
  third-order, 129
  upper motor neurons, 1445
Neurontin (gabapentin)
  for alcohol treatment, 178
  local, 139*t*
  for seizures, 1536, 1538*t*
Neuropathic pain, 128, 130-131, 130*t*
Neuropathic Pain Scale, 134
Neuropathy
  autonomic, 1285-1286
  chronic sensory polyneuropathy, 473*t*
  diabetic, 1284*t*, **1285-1286,** 1286*f*
    prevention, detection, and monitor-
      ing of, 1284*t*
  peripheral
    in chemotherapy and radiation
      therapy, 296*t*
    with cirrhosis, 1103
  sensory, in diabetes mellitus, 1285
  stocking-glove, 1285
Neuropathy Association, 1289
Neuropeptides, 1445*t*
Neurosurgical procedures for pain relief, 143, 143*f*
Neurosyphilis, 1370, 1370*t*, **1589**
Neurotoxins, 479*t*
Neurotransmitters, 1444, 1445*t*
Neurotrophic ulceration, 1285, 1286*f*
Neurovascular assessment
  of fracture, 1642-1643
  of hip fracture, 1654
Neutralizing agents, 1019*t*
Neutropenia, 297, 678, 713, **713-716**
  causes of, 713, 714*t*
  clinical manifestations of, 713-714
  collaborative care for, 715*t*
  definition of, 713
  diagnostic studies, 714
  gerontologic considerations for,
    716
  nursing and collaborative manage-
    ment of, **714-716**
  nursing care plan for patient with,
    716*b*
  patient and family teaching guide for,
    715*t*
Neutrophils, 668
  band, 1860*t*
  function of, 668*t*
  response to injury, 194
  segmented, 668, 1860*t*
  shift to the left, 194
Nevirapine (Viramune)
  adverse effects of, 258*t*
  hepatotoxicity, 934*t*
Nevus(i), 457*t*
  dysplastic, **466**
    case study, 481
  melanocytic (moles), 457*t*, 472*t*
  spider, 675*t*, 677, 1102
New York Heart Association functional
  classification of heart disease,
    826*t*, 827
Newborns, eye infections in, 1368
Nexavar (sorafenib), 303*t*

Nexium (esomeprazole)
  for gastroesophageal reflux disease, 1006, 1006t
  for gastrointestinal bleeding, 998t
  for peptic ulcer disease, 1019t, 1020
NHLBI. See National Heart, Lung, and Blood Institute
Niacin (nicotinic acid) (Nicobid, Nicotinex), 794, 795t
  blood glucose level effects, 1267t
  drug alert, 794
  hepatotoxicity, 934t
  uses, 796b
Niacin deficiency, 473t
NIC. See Nursing Interventions Classification
Nicardipine (Cardene)
  for acute coronary syndrome, 800t
  for chronic stable angina, 800t, 801
  for hypertension, 776t
Nicobid (niacin), 794, 795t
NicoDerm CQ, 171t
Nicotine, **167-174**
  blood glucose level effects, 1267t
  effects of use, 167, 169t
  onset, peak, duration, and withdrawal onset of, 185t
Nicotine dependence, 167-174
  characteristics of, 167
  collaborative care, 170-174
  complications of, 168-170, 168t
Nicotine gum, inhaler, lozenge, nasal spray, patch, 171t
Nicotine replacement therapy, 172b
Nicotine transdermal system, 171t
Nicotinex (niacin), 795t
Nicotinic acid (Slo-Niacin), 795t, 796b
Nicotinic acid deficiency, 473t
Nicotrol, 171t
NIDDK. See National Institute of Diabetes and Digestive and Kidney Diseases
NIF. See Negative inspiratory force or pressure
Nifedipine (Adalat, Procardia)
  for acute coronary syndrome, 800t
  blood glucose level effects, 1267t
  for chronic stable angina, 800t, 801
  effects on lower urinary tract function, 1180t
  for hypertension, 776t, 1210
  for Raynaud's phenomenon, 1724
  for voiding dysfunction, 1185t
Nightingale, Florence, 39, 94, 122, 1733
Nigrostriatal disorders, 1549, 1549f
NIH. See National Institutes of Health
Nilutamide (Nilandron), 1426, 1426t
Nimodipine (Nimotop)
  drug alert, 1512
  for subarachnoid hemorrhage, 1512
NIOSH. See National Institute for Occupational Safety and Health
NIP. See Negative inspiratory force or pressure
Nipent (pentostatin)
  classification of, 287t
  for leukemia, 720t

Nipple(s)
  inversion or retraction of, 1335t
  scaling or irritation of, 1335t
  secretions from, 1335t
Nipple discharge, 1347
Nipple discharge test, 1339t
Nipple-areolar reconstruction, 1363
Nipride (nitroprusside)
  drug alert, 828
  for heart failure, 828
  for shock, 1786, 1788t
Nisoldipine (Sular), 776t
Nissen fundoplication, 1006, 1006f
Nitrates
  for acute coronary syndrome, 800t
  for chronic HF, 832
  for chronic stable angina, 798-799, 800t
  extended-release buccal (Nitrogard), 800t
  long-acting, 798-799
  short-acting, 798
  transdermal controlled-release, 799
Nitric oxide, 1763
Nitrites, 170t
Nitro-Bid (nitroglycerin ointment), 800t
Nitrofurantoin (Macrodantin)
  drug alert, 1158
  nephrotoxicity of, 1142
  for urethritis, 1163
  for UTIs, 1157, 1158
Nitrogard (extended-release buccal nitrate tablets), 800t
Nitrogen mustards, 287t
Nitroglycerin (Nitro-Bid)
  for acute coronary syndrome, 800t, 808
  for acute pancreatitis, 1121t
  for chronic stable angina, 798-799, 800t
  drug alert, 798
  for heart failure, 828
  for hypertension, 775t
  for shock, 1786, 1788t
  sublingual (Nitrostat, Nitrolingual, NitroQuick), 798, 800t
  transdermal (Transderm-Nitro), 800t
Nitroprusside (Nipride)
  drug alert, 828
  for heart failure, 828
  for shock, 1786
Nitrosoureas
  classification of, 287t
  for leukemia, 720t
  nephrotoxicity, 1142t
Nitrous oxide, 170t, 369t
Nizatidine (Axid)
  for gastroesophageal reflux disease, 1005-1006, 1006t
  for gastrointestinal bleeding, 998t
  for peptic ulcer disease, 1019t
Nizoral (ketoconazole)
  for Cushing syndrome, 1312-1314
  photosensitivity, 461t
  for pulmonary infections, 576
N-methyl-D-aspartate receptor antagonists (NMDA)
  for Alzheimer's disease, 1569t
  for pain, 140
NNRTIs. See Nonnucleoside reverse transcriptase inhibitors
"No code," 156
NOC. See Nursing Outcomes Classification
Nocardia, 562t

Nocardia asteroides, 576t
Nocardiosis, 576t
Nociception, 127
  processes of, 127
  signal transmission, 128
Nociceptive pain, 128, 128f, 130, 130t
Nocturia, 826, 1145t
Nocturnal angina, 797
Nocturnal dyspnea, paroxysmal, 746, 825
Nodes of Ranvier, 1443
Nodular goiters, toxic, 1299
Nodules, breast, 1335t
Noise control, environmental, 443-444
Nolvadex (tamoxifen)
  for breast cancer, 1355
  for cervical cancer, 1402
  classification of, 288t
  drug alert, 1355
Nomenclatures, 8
Nonalcoholic fatty liver disease, 1101
  clinical manifestations of, 1101
  collaborative care for, 1101
  diagnostic studies, 1101
Nonalcoholic steatohepatitis, 1101
  clinical manifestations of, 1101
  collaborative care for, 1101
  diagnostic studies, 1101
Nondisjunction, 215
Non–heart beating donation, 1828
Non-Hodgkin's lymphoma, 723t, **724-728**
  classification of, 726t
  clinical manifestations of, 726, 726f
  diagnostic studies, 726
  etiology and pathophysiology of, 726
  guidelines for treatment of, 727t
  nursing and collaborative management of, **726-728**
  staging studies, 726
  staging system for, 725f
Noninvasive positive pressure ventilation, 1810, 1810f
Nonnucleoside reverse transcriptase inhibitors
  adverse effects of, 258t
  mechanism of action, 257, 257t
Nonopioids, 135-137, 136t
Non-rebreathing masks, 641t
Non–small cell lung cancer, 581t, 582t
Nonsteroidal anti-inflammatory drugs
  analgesic effects of, 128
  for arthritis and connective tissue disorders, 1698t
  for burns, 499t
  drug alert, 135
  for gout, 1716
  hematologic effects of, 674t
  hepatotoxicity, 933
  mechanism of action, 202t
  nephrotoxicity, 1142t, 1211
  for osteoarthritis, 1697, 1697b
  for pain, 135-137, 136f, 136t
  poisoning, 1837t
  for rheumatoid arthritis, 1706
  that may cause photosensitivity, 461t
Nonstochastic theories of aging, 68, 68t
Non–ST-segment-elevation myocardial infarction, 802
Nonverbal cues, 64
Norcuron (vecuronium), 370t
Norepinephrine (Levophed), 1445t
  as positive inotrope, 1739
  for shock, 1788t

Norepinephrine (Levophed) (Continued)
  target tissue and functions, 1236t
  urine levels, 1862t
Norethindrone (Aygestin), 1392
Norfloxacin (Noroxin), 1157
Normal pressure hydrocephalus, 1576
Normodyne (labetalol)
  drug alert, 782
  food/nutrient interactions, 954t
  for hypertension, 775t
Noroxin (norfloxacin), 1157
Norpace (disopyramide), 856t
North American Nursing Diagnosis Association (NANDA), 18
  NANDA-NOC-NIC linkages, 14, 14f, 14t
  Nursing Diagnoses, Definitions, and Classifications 2005-2006, 8t
Nortriptyline (Aventyl, Pamelor)
  for Alzheimer's disease, 1569t
  ethnic differences in response to, 35t
  for interstitial cystitis/painful bladder syndrome, 1164
  local, 139t
  for smoking cessation, 171t
Norvasc (amlodipine)
  for chronic stable angina and acute coronary syndrome, 800t
  for hypertension, 776t
  and reproductive system, 1332
Norvir (ritonavir), 258t
Norwalk virus infection, 1037t
Nose
  in allergies, 229t
  assessment abnormalities, 675t
  inflammation and infection of, **535-541**
  obstruction of, **541**
  physical examination of, 49t, 51t, 521, 525t
  problems of, and asthma attacks, 609
  structural and traumatic disorders of, **533-534**
Nosocomial infections, 246-247
  UTIs, 1156
Novantrone (mitoxantrone)
  classification of, 287t
  for leukemia, 720t
  for multiple sclerosis, 1544, 1544t
  for prostate cancer, 1427
Novarel, 1383t
Novo-Hydrazide (hydrochlorothiazide), 773t
Novolin N (NPH insulin), 1260t
Novolin R (regular insulin), 1260t
NovoLog (insulin aspart), 1260t
Novo-Niacin (nicotinic acid), 795t
Novopirocam (piroxicam), 1698t
Novoprofen (ibuprofen), 1698t
NovoSundac (sulindac), 1698t
NPPV. See Noninvasive positive pressure ventilation
NRTIs. See Nucleoside reverse transcriptase inhibitors
NSAIDs. See Nonsteroidal anti-inflammatory drugs
NSTEMI. See Non–ST-segment-elevation myocardial infarction
NtRTI. See Nucleotide reverse transcriptase inhibitors
Nuchal rigidity, 676t, 1461
  in bacterial meningitis, 1494
Nuclear cardiology, 754t, 758
Nuclear imaging
  exercise, 754t
  of gastrointestinal system, 942t
  pharmacologic, 754t

Nucleoside analogs, 1094-1095
Nucleoside reverse transcriptase inhibitors
    adverse effects of, 258t
    mechanism of action, 257, 257t
Nucleotide reverse transcriptase inhibitors
    adverse effects of, 258t
    mechanism of action, 257, 257t
NU-DERM, 205t
Nuflexxa (hyaluronic acid), 1697
Nuprin (ibuprofen), 136, 136t
Nuromax (doxacurium), 370t
Nurse anesthetist, 363
Nurses, 2, 3f
    advanced practice, 3-4
    clinical nurse leader (CNL), 3-4
    community-based, 87-88
    as facilitators, 61, 61f
    intraoperative activities of, 361t
    perioperative, 361
    as providers, 107
    registered, 361
    in research, 107-108
    as resources, 106
    role with respect to complementary
        and alternative therapies, 106
    special needs in end-of-life care, 162
    as teachers, 55-56, 56f
    as team leaders, 4
Nursing
    activities surrounding surgical experi-
        ence, 361, 362t
    collaborative functions, 10
    community-based, 85-93
    community-oriented, 85
    current practice, 2-4
    definitions of, 3
    delivery of care, 4
    dependent functions, 10
    emergency and disaster nursing,
        1821-1844
    gerontologic, 66
    holistic, 107
    independent functions, 10
    primary, 4
    primary goals of, 9, 9t
    public health, 85, 86
    resources, 18
    role during day-of-surgery prepara-
        tion, 354, 354f
    roles, 3-4
    specialty certifications, 3, 4t
    standardized terminologies, 7-8
    team nursing, 4
    transcultural, 28
    view of humanity, 3
Nursing assessment. See also specific
        disorders
    of characteristics that affect patient
        teaching, 57-58, 58t
    of complementary and alternative
        therapies, 106
    of end of life, 157-158
    of older adults, 77
    of pain, 134, 134t
    phase of, 9, 10
    of psychologic function, 58
    of psychologic status, 51t
    of stress, 120, 120f
Nursing care evaluation
    for older adults, 82, 82t
    phase of, 9, 15
Nursing care plans, 15
    electronic resources, 15
    for patient after mastectomy or
        lumpectomy, 1357b-1358b
    for patient after thoracotomy, 594b

Nursing care plans (Continued)
    for patient having orthopedic surgery,
        1647b-1648b
    for patient having prostate surgery,
        1420b
    for patient having total laryngectomy
        and/or radical neck surgery,
        554b-555b
    for patient in alcohol withdrawal,
        183b-184b
    for patient in shock, 1791b-1792b
    for patient on mechanical ventilation,
        1754b-1756b
    for patient receiving enteral nutrition,
        963b-964b
    for patient receiving parenteral nutri-
        tion, 968b
    for patient with a pressure ulcer,
        210b
    for patient with abdominal hysterec-
        tomy, 1398b
    for patient with acute coronary syn-
        drome, 811b-812b
    for patient with acute infectious diar-
        rhea, 1039b
    for patient with acute pancreatitis,
        1122b-1123b
    for patient with acute renal lithiasis,
        1173b-1174b
    for patient with acute respiratory fail-
        ure, 1807b-1809b
    for patient with acute viral hepatitis,
        1097b-1098b
    for patient with Alzheimer's disease,
        1571b-1572b
    for patient with anemia, 688b-
        689b
    for patient with asthma, 625b-626b
    for patient with bacterial meningitis,
        1496b-1497b
    for patient with burns, 494b-496b
    for patient with chronic kidney dis-
        ease, 1214b-1215b
    for patient with cirrhosis, 1112b-
        1113b
    for patient with colostomy/ileostomy,
        1073b-1075b
    for patient with COPD, 651b-653b
    for patient with diabetes mellitus,
        1273b-1274b
    for patient with fracture, 1644b-
        1645b
    for patient with headache, 1533b
    for patient with heart failure, 12,
        836b-838b
    for patient with hyperthyroidism,
        1303b
    for patient with hypothyroidism,
        1307b-1308b
    for patient with ileal conduit, 1191b-
        1192b
    for patient with increased ICP,
        1479b-1480b
    for patient with infective endocardi-
        tis, 870b-871b
    for patient with inflammatory bowel
        disease, 1058b-1059b
    for patient with low back pain,
        1678b-1680b
    for patient with multiple sclerosis,
        1547b-1548b
    for patient with neutropenia, 716b
    for patient with osteomyelitis, 1671b-
        1672b
    for patient with Parkinson's disease,
        1554b-1555b
    for patient with peptic ulcer disease,
        1023b-1024b

Nursing care plans (Continued)
    for patient with peripheral arterial
        disease of lower extremities,
        905b-906b
    for patient with pneumonia, 568b
    for patient with rheumatoid arthritis,
        1708b-1710b
    for patient with seizure disorder or
        epilepsy, 1540b-1541b
    for patient with spinal cord injury,
        1598b-1600b
    for patient with stroke, 1516b-1518b
    for patient with systemic lupus ery-
        thematosus, 1721b-1722b
    for patient with thrombocytopenia,
        706b
    for patient with tracheostomy, 548b-
        549b
    for patient with urinary tract infec-
        tion, 1160b
    for patient with valvular heart dis-
        ease, 884b-885b
Nursing diagnoses, 10-11, 50, 1850-
    1853
    associated with age-related physio-
        logic changes, 78, 78t
    associated with end-of-life care, 158,
        158t
    in coping–stress tolerance pattern,
        121t
    dealing with physical care at end of
        life, 158t
    dealing with physical manifestations
        of end of life, 158t
    dealing with psychosocial manifesta-
        tions of end of life, 158t
    definition of, 10
    etiology of, 11
    NANDA diagnoses, 10-11
    nursing phase, 9
    for older adults, 77-78
    for pain, 145t
    for patients requiring home care, 91t
    problem–etiology–signs and symp-
        toms (PES) format, 11
    related to stress, 120-121
    signs and symptoms of, 11-12
Nursing diagnostic statements, 11-12
Nursing focus, 40
Nursing history, 40
    functional health pattern format, 45t
    objective data, 46-50
    subjective data, 43-46
Nursing implementation. See also spe-
        cific disorders
    for end of life, 158-162
    for older adults, 78-82
    for patient education, 63
    phase of, 9, 14-15
Nursing informatics, 9
Nursing interventions, 13. See also spe-
        cific disorders
    considerations for, 13
    determining, 13-14
    examples, 13t
Nursing Interventions Classification
        (NIC), 8, 8t, 14
    NANDA-NOC-NIC linkages, 14, 14f,
        14t
Nursing Outcomes Classification
        (NOC), 8, 8t, 13
    NANDA-NOC-NIC linkages, 14, 14f,
        14t
Nursing practice, 1-18. See also
    Evidence-based practice
    community-oriented, population-
        focused, 85
    concepts in, 1-191

Nursing practice (Continued)
    current, 2-4
    domain of, 2-3
    future, 5-10
    holistic, 106-107
    integrative, 108
    nursing process in, 9
    population-focused, 85
Nursing process, 9, 9f
    assessment phase, 10
    diagnosis phase, 10-12
    documentation, 15-16
    evaluation phase, 15
    implementation phase, 14-15
    phases of, 9, 9f
    planning phase, 12-14
Nursing-sensitive patient outcomes, 12
Nutraceuticals, 97t
Nutrition, 33
    admission screening tool, 957t
    age-related changes of particular in-
        terest, 959
    assessment abnormalities, 1247t
    cultural assessment of, 29t
    effects of chronic alcohol abuse on,
        177t
    gerontologic differences in assess-
        ment of intake, 959, 959t
    normal, 948-950
    patient and family teaching guide for,
        958t
    preoperative review, 349
Nutritional cirrhosis, 1102
Nutritional deficiency, 201t
Nutritional problems, 948-970
    in cancer, 306-307
Nutritional support
    in acute respiratory distress syn-
        drome, 1818
    for burns, 499, 499t
    for critical care patients, 1735-1736
    culturally competent care, 951
    decision-making algorithm for, 960f
    enteral nutrition
        gerontologic considerations for,
            965
        nursing care plan for patient re-
            ceiving, 963b-964b
        placement locations for feeding
            tubes, 961, 961f
    for head injury, 1475b
    home health care activities, 90t
    parenteral nutrition, 965-967
        catheter placement for, 966, 966f
        central, 965
        complications of, 967t
        indications for, 965, 965t
        nursing care plan for patient re-
            ceiving, 968b
        nursing management of, 967-968
        peripheral, 966
    in SIRS or MODS, 1796t
    skin support, 462
    in spinal cord injury, 1602
    after stroke, 1519-1520
    types of, 960-968
Nutritional therapy
    for acute coronary syndrome, 808
    for acute pancreatitis, 1121
    for acute renal failure, 1202-1203
    for acute respiratory failure, 1812
    for burns, 493t, 499, 503
    for cancer, 306, 306t, 307t
    for celiac disease, 1080t
    for cholecystitis, 1130
    for cholelithiasis, 1130
    for chronic HF, 833-834

Nutritional therapy (Continued)
  for chronic kidney disease, 1211-
    1213
  for cirrhosis, 1110
  for constipation, 1041-1042, 1043t
  for COPD, 649
  for coronary artery disease, 792-793
  daily requirements for patient with
    chronic kidney disease, 1211-
    1212, 1212t
  DASH (Dietary Approaches to Stop
    Hypertension) diet, 770, 770t,
    833
  description of, 97t
  for diabetes mellitus, 1266-1269,
    1268t
  for erythropoiesis, 688, 689t
  for esophageal cancer, 1010
  for fractures, 1641-1642
  for gastroesophageal reflux disease,
    1005
  for gout, 1716
  for Guillain-Barré syndrome, 1586
  for hepatitis, 1096
  high-calorie, high-protein diet, 958t
  for hyperthyroidism, 1302
  for increased ICP, 1475-1476
  for inflammation, 202
  for inflammatory bowel disease,
    1056-1057
  low-sodium diets, 833, 834t
  for multiple sclerosis, 1546
  for nausea and vomiting, 992
  for obesity, 978-980
  for oral cancer, 1002
  for osteoarthritis, 1696
  for Parkinson's disease, 1552
  for peptic ulcer disease, 1021, 1026-
    1027
  for perimenopause and postmeno-
    pause, 1392
  for peripheral arterial disease, 903
  for pneumonia, 567
  for positive pressure ventilation pa-
    tients, 1766
  after radical neck surgery, 552-553
  for rheumatoid arthritis, 1706-1707
  for shock, 1786
  after stroke, 1522
  therapeutic lifestyle changes diet,
    792, 793t
  therapeutic lifestyle changes diet
    menu, 792, 793t
  for urinary tract calculi, 1171, 1171t,
    1172
Nutritional-metabolic pattern
  in assessment
    of auditory system, 410t, 411
    of cardiovascular system, 745-746,
      746t
    of endocrine system, 1244
    of fluid, electrolyte, and acid-base
      imbalances, 337
    of gastrointestinal system, 934,
      935t
    of hematologic system, 672-673,
      673t
    of integumentary system, 453t,
      454
    of musculoskeletal system, 1621
    of nervous system, 1454
    of preoperative patient, 350t

Nutritional-metabolic pattern
    (Continued)
    of reproductive system, 1332,
      1333t
    of respiratory system, 518t, 519
    of urinary system, 1142, 1143t
    of visual system, 403, 403t
  comparison with NANDA Interna-
    tional Taxonomy II, 42t
  concerns of patients requiring home
    health care, 90t
  and COPD, 650t
  nursing diagnoses, 1852
  nursing history, 44, 45t
Nystagmus, 409, 1457, 1460t
Nystatin (Mycostatin)
  for burns, 499, 499t
  for urethritis, 1163

O
OA. See Osteoarthritis
OASIS. See Outcome and Assessment
    Information Status
Oatmeal, colloidal (Aveeno), 1375
Obesity, 971-982, 972f
  android, 974, 975t
  case study, 988
  classification of, 974-975, 975t
  collaborative care for, 978t
  collaborative surgical therapy of,
    982-986
  and coronary artery disease, 790
  cultural and ethnic health disparities
    in, 971, 972b, 972f
  definition of, 790
  drug therapy of, 981-982
  effects on wound healing, 201t
  environmental factors, 973-974
  etiology of, 972-974
  genetic/biologic basis for, 972-973
  gynoid, 974, 975t
  health disparities and, 21t
  health risks associated with, 975-976,
    976f
  health-promoting behaviors for,
    792t
  hormones and peptides in, 972, 973f,
    973t
  morbid
    classification of, 974, 974f, 975t
    surgical interventions for, 982-983,
      982t
  nursing and collaborative manage-
    ment of, 976-982
  nursing assessment of, 976-977,
    977t
  nursing diagnoses, 977
  nursing evaluation of obese patient
    undergoing surgery, 986
  nursing implementation for, 977-981
  nursing management of obese patient
    undergoing surgery, 984-986
  nursing planning for, 977
  nutritional therapy of, 978-980
  in older adults, 987
  pathophysiology of, 972-974
  perioperative care, 984-986
  plan of care for, 978
  postoperative care, 985-986
  preoperative care, 984-985
  primary, 974
  psychosocial factors, 974
  resources, 989
  secondary, 974
Obesity-hypoventilation syndrome,
    595t

Objective data, 40
Obstructive cardiomyopathy, hyper-
    trophic, 888
Obstructive emergencies, oncologic,
    307-308
Obstructive (posthepatic) jaundice,
    1088, 1128
Obstructive pancreatitis, chronic,
    1124
Obstructive pulmonary disease, 607-
    663
  chronic, 629-655
    chest examination findings in, 526t
    drug therapy of, 618t-620t
    gender differences in, 629b
    cultural and ethnic health disparities
      in, 608b
    lung volumes and, 594b
    resources, 663
Obstructive sleep apnea, 542-543
  clinical manifestations of, 542
  diagnostic studies, 542
Obstructive uropathy, 1168-1175
Occlusive dressings, 205
Occupational assessment, 58
Occupational chemicals and dusts, 631
Occupational Safety and Health Admin-
    istration (OSHA)
  guidelines for infection prevention
    and control, 247
  guidelines for safe handling of che-
    motherapeutic agents, 286
  requirements for personal protective
    equipment to minimize exposure
    to blood-borne pathogens, 247,
    248t
Occupational therapists, 91t
Occupational therapy, 1604, 1604f
  for burns, 493t, 503
Octreotide (Sandostatin, Depot, Sand-
    ostatin LAR)
  for acromegaly, 1292
  for diarrhea, 1037t
  for gastrointestinal bleeding, 998t
Ocular varicella-zoster virus, 255t
Oculomotor nerve (cranial nerve III),
    1450t
Oculomotor nerve (cranial nerve III)
    testing, 1457
Oculus dexter, 405
Oculus sinister, 405
Oculus uterque, 405
Ocu-Pentolate (cyclopentolate HCl),
    427t
Ocupress (carteolol)
  food/nutrient interactions, 954t
  for glaucoma, 434t
  for hypertension, 774t
Ocu-Tropine (atropine), 427t
Odynophagia, 939t
O-ethyl S-[2-diisopropylaminoethyl]
    methylphosphonothiolate (VX),
    1840t
Office of Dietary Supplements, 109
Office of Disease Prevention and Health
    Promotion, 65
Off-pump coronary artery bypass, 809-
    810
Ofloxacin (Floxin)
  for chlamydial infections, 1373
  for gonorrhea, 1368
  for UTIs, 1157
OHS. See Obesity-hypoventilation syn-
    drome
Olanzapine (Zyprexa)
  for Alzheimer's disease, 1551-1552,
    1569t
  for delirium, 1578

Older adults, 66-84. See also Aging;
    Gerontologic considerations
  acute care for, 79
  assistive devices for, 80
  behavioral management for, 82
  care alternatives for, 75-77
  chronically ill, 71
  cognitively impaired, 70
  community-based, with special
    needs, 76
  connective tissue diseases in, 1711
  culturally competent care of, 72
  ethnic, 72, 72f, 72t
  frail, 67, 71
  gender differences in, 70b
  health promotion for, 78-79, 78f
  homeless, 70-71
  hospital discharge for, 79
  hospitalized, 79, 79t
  housing for, 75-76, 75f
  hyperthyroidism in, 1301t
  infections in, 247
  legal aid for, 77, 77f
  legal and ethical issues, 77
  liver disease in, 1118
  medication abuse by, 80
  medication errors by, 80, 81t
  medication use by, 80, 81t
  nursing assessment of, 77, 78f
  nursing care for, 82, 82t
  nursing diagnoses, 77-78
  nursing implementation for, 78-82
  nursing management of, 77-82
  nutritional assessment of, 71, 71t
  nutritional intake in, 959, 959t
  obesity in, 987
  old-old adults, 67
  patient and family teaching, 79, 79t
  physical activity programs for, 795
  planning with, 78
  prevention of musculoskeletal prob-
    lems in, 1630t
  resources, 84
  rural, 70, 70f
  safety of, 80
  sleep of, 81-82
  social services for, 74
  social support and, 72-73
  special populations, 69-72
  teaching, 79, 79t
  women, 69
  young-old adults, 67
Older Americans Act
  Title III, 74
  Title IV, 74
Old-old adults, 67
Olfactory nerve (cranial nerve I), 1450t
Olfactory nerve (cranial nerve I) test-
    ing, 1456
Oligemia, 1528
Oligodendrocytes, 1442
Oligomenorrhea, 1387, 1387-1388
Oliguria, 1145t, 1198
  of acute renal failure, 1199-1200,
    1200t
  prerenal, 1199-1200, 1200t
Olmesartan (Benicar), 776t
Olmesartan medoxomil/hydrochlorothi-
    azide (Benicar HCT), 777t
Olsalazine (Dipentum), 1055t
Omaha System, 8, 8t
Omalizumab (Xolair), 620
  for asthma, 617t
  for asthma and COPD, 618t
Omega-3 fatty acids, 771b
  for coronary artery disease, 792
  uses, 796b

Note: Disorder names are in bold face.
Page numbers in bold face indicate main
discussions. Page numbers followed by
f, t, b, or n indicate figures, tables, boxed
material, or notes, respectively.

Omeprazole (Prilosec, Zegerid)
  for acute gastritis, 1014
  for acute pancreatitis, 1121*t*
  for gastroesophageal reflux disease, 1006, 1006*t*
  for gastrointestinal bleeding, 998*t*
  for peptic ulcer disease, 1019*t*, 1020
Ommaya reservoir, 291
Omniderm, 205*t*
Omnipen (ampicillin), 869*t*
Omnitrope (somatropin), 1292
Oncaspar (pegaspargase), 720*t*
Oncofetal antigens, 279
Oncogenes, 214*t*, 274
Oncogenic viruses, 276
OncoLink (cancer information site), 313, 1365
Oncologic emergencies, 307-308
  infiltrative, 308
  metabolic, 308
  obstructive, 307-308
Oncology Nursing Society (ONS), guidelines for safe handling of chemotherapeutic agents, 286
Oncotic pressure, 318
  interstitial, 319
  plasma, 319
Oncovin (vincristine)
  classification of, 287*t*
  for leukemia, 720*t*
  method of administration, 288*t*
  for multiple myeloma, 729
  for non-Hodgkin's lymphoma, 727*t*
Ondansetron (Zofran)
  as adjunct to general anesthesia, 370*t*
  for alcohol treatment, 178
  for nausea and vomiting, 297, 992, 992*t*
  preoperative, 355*t*
Ontak (denileukin diftitox), 727
On-X valve, 883*t*
Onychomycosis, 469*f*, 469*t*
Oophorectomy, 1405*f*
  acute intervention related to, 1406
  description of, 1332*t*
Opacities, corneal, **424-425**
OPCAB. *See* Off-pump coronary artery bypass
Open book fractures, 1652
Open loop resection with fulguration, 1179
Open pneumothorax, 585-586, 587*f*
Open reduction with internal fixation, 1638
Open-angle glaucoma
  ambulatory/home care for, 434*t*
  chronic, 433-434
  primary, 432
Open-suction technique, 1757, 1757*t*
Operating room (OR), 360, 360*f*, 361*f*
  admitting patient to, 364
  catastrophic events in, **372-373**
  physical environment of, **360**
  preparation of, 364
  transferring patient to, 364
  transportation to, 354-356
Operative debridement, 496, 497*f*
Ophthalgan (glycerin liquid), 435*t*
Ophthalmopathy, 1299
Ophthalmoplegia, 1460*t*, 1586
Ophthalmoscopy, 405*t*
Opiates, 179
Opioid agonist-antagonists, 137*t*, 138
Opioid agonists, 137-138, 137*t*

Opioids, **179-180**
  adjuncts to general anesthesia, 368-369, 370*t*
  administration routes, 140-142
  analgesics for chronic stable angina and acute coronary syndrome, 800*t*
  antidiarrheal drugs, 1037*t*
  to avoid, 138
  characteristics of, 179-180
  collaborative care, 180
  complications of, 168*t*, 180
  effects of, 137
  effects of use, 169*t*, 180
  onset, peak, duration, and withdrawal onset of, 185*t*
  for pain, 137-138, 137*t*
  preoperative, 355*t*
  and restrictive lung disease, 595*t*
  side effects of, 138
  types of, 137-138
  withdrawal from, 145, 146*t*
Opisthotonus, 1460*t*, 1588
Opium
  camphorated tincture of (paregoric), 1037*t*
  effects of use, 169*t*
  tincture of, 1037*t*
Opportunistic diseases, 252
  associated with HIV infection, 253, 254*t*-255*t*
  drug therapy of, 257
Opportunistic pneumonia, 564
Opposition movement, synovial joints, 1622*t*
Oprelvekin (Neumega), 705
  for cancer treatment, 304*t*
  clinical uses of, 223*t*
OpSite, 204, 205*t*
Opsonization, 195
Optic disc cupping, 433, 433*f*
Optic nerve (cranial nerve II), 1450*t*
Optic nerve testing, 407, 1456-1457
Optical devices for vision enhancement, 420-421
Optimine (azatadine), 537*t*
OR. *See* Operating room
Oral anesthetics, 139*t*
Oral anticoagulant therapy, 914*t*
Oral cancer, 1001-1003
  acute intervention for, 1003
  characteristics of, 1001, 1001*t*
  clinical manifestations of, 1001-1002
  collaborative care for, 1002, 1002*t*
  diagnostic studies, 1002
  etiology and pathophysiology of, 1001
  health promotion in, 1003
  nonsurgical therapy, 1002
  nursing assessment of, 1002, 1003*t*
  nursing diagnoses, 1002
  nursing evaluation of, 1003
  nursing implementation for, 1003
  nursing management of, **1002-1003**
  nursing planning for, 1003
  nutritional therapy for, 1002
  surgical therapy, 1002
  types and characteristics of, 1001, 1001*t*
Oral candidiasis, 1000*t*
Oral care
  in Alzheimer's disease, 1574
  during ET intubation, 1758
  procedures for patients on mechanical ventilators, 1758*t*
Oral contraceptives, 1267*t*

Oral feeding, **960**
Oral fluid and electrolyte replacement, **338**
Oral glucose tolerance, 1251*t*
Oral hairy leukoplakia, 252, 253*f*
Oral hygiene, 1003*b*
Oral inflammations and infections, 1000-1001
Oral intubation, 1751
Oral mucosa, 525*t*
Oral problems, 1001*b*
Oramorph (morphine), 137*t*
Orasone (prednisone), 745*t*
Orchiectomy
  description of, 1332*t*
  for prostate cancer, 1426*t*, 1427
Orchitis, 1430
Orencia (abatacept)
  for arthritis and connective tissue disorders, 1700*t*
  for rheumatoid arthritis, 1705-1706
Oretic (hydrochlorothiazide), 773*t*
Organ donation, 155
Organ donor cards, 237, 237*f*
Organ donors
  deceased, 1227
  non–heart beating, 1828
Organ of Corti, 409
Organ procurement organizations, 1828
Organ transplantation, 236-240, 236*f*
  allocation of resources for, 1226*b*
  kidney transplantation, **1225-1230**
  liver transplantation, **1117-1118**
  payment for organs, 1225*b*
ORIF. *See* Open reduction with internal fixation
Orinase (tolbutamide), 461*t*
Orlistat (Xenical), 981
Oropharyngeal procedures requiring antibiotic prophylaxis to prevent endocarditis, 866, 867*t*
Orthoclone OKT3 (muromonab-CD3), 239*t*
Ortho-Novum (estrogen + progestin), 745*t*
Orthopedic surgery
  nursing care plan for patient having, 1647*b*-1648*b*
  resources for, 1667
Orthopnea, 825, 1805
Orthostatic hypotension, 778
Orthotopic bladder reconstruction, 1190
Orthovisc (hyaluronic acid), 1697
Orudis (ketoprofen)
  for arthritis and connective tissue disorders, 1698*t*
  for burns, 499*t*
Orzel (leucovorin-modulated 5-FU), 1067
OSA. *See* Obstructive sleep apnea
OSAHS. *See* Obstructive sleep apnea-hypopnea syndrome
Os-Cal 250 (calcium carbonate + 5 mcg vitamin D$_2$), 1689*t*
Oseltamivir (Tamiflu)
  for influenza, 540
  for pneumonia, 566
OSHA. *See* Occupational Safety and Health Administration
Osler's nodes, 867
Osler's sign, 765
Osmitrol (mannitol solution)
  for glaucoma, 435*t*
  for increased ICP, 1474
Osmoglyn Oral (glycerin liquid), 435*t*
Osmolality, 317
  definition of, 316*t*
  effective, 318

Osmolality (*Continued*)
  laboratory values, 1857*t*
  measurement of, 318
Osmolarity, 316*t*, 317
Osmosis, 317-318, 317*f*, 1216, 1217*f*
Osmotic pressure, 317
  colloidal, 318
Ossification, 1615
  callus, 1637
OST. *See* Open-suction technique
Osteitis deformans, 1690
Osteitis fibrosa cystica, 1208
Osteoarthritis, 1693-1702
  acute intervention for, 1701
  ambulatory and home care for, 1701-1702
  clinical manifestations of, 1694-1695, 1704*t*
  collaborative care for, 1695-1701, 1696*t*
  complementary and alternative therapies for, 1696
  deformity associated with, 1695
  diagnostic studies, 1695
  drug therapy for, 1696-1697
  etiology of, 1694, 1695*f*
  gender differences in, 1694*b*
  health promotion in, 1701
  of joints, 1694-1695, 1696*f*
  nursing assessment of, 1701
  nursing diagnoses, 1701
  nursing evaluation of, 1702
  nursing implementation for, 1701-1702
  nursing management of, **1701-1702**
  nursing planning for, 1701
  nutritional therapy for, 1696
  secondary, 1694, 1694*t*
  systemic, 1694
Osteoblasts, 1615
Osteochondroma, 1673-1674
  description of, 1673*t*
Osteoclastoma, 1673*f*, 1673*t*
Osteoclasts, 1615
Osteocysts, 1615
Osteodystrophy, renal, 1208
  drug therapy of, 1210
Osteogenic sarcoma, 1673*f*, **1674**
  description of, 1673*t*
Osteomalacia, 1208, **1686**
Osteomyelitis, 1668-1672
  acute, 1669
  acute intervention for, 1671-1672
  ambulatory and home care for, 1672
  causative organisms, 1668, 1669*t*
  chronic, 1669, 1669*f*
  clinical manifestations of, 1669
  collaborative care for, 1670
  development of, 1669, 1669*f*
  diagnostic studies, 1669-1670
  direct entry, 1669
  etiology and pathophysiology of, 1668-1669
  health promotion in, 1670
  indirect entry (hematogenous), 1668
  nursing assessment of, 1670, 1670*t*
  nursing care plan for patient with, 1671*b*-1672*b*
  nursing diagnoses, 1670
  nursing evaluation of, 1672
  nursing implementation for, 1670-1672
  nursing management of, **1670-1672**
  nursing planning for, 1670
Osteoporosis, 1686-1690, 1687*f*
  case study, 1690-1691
  clinical manifestations of, 1688
  collaborative care for, 1688, 1688*t*

Osteoporosis (Continued)
cultural and ethnic health disparities in, 1687*b*
diagnostic studies, 1688
drug therapy for, 1689-1690
etiology and pathophysiology of, 1687-1688
gender differences in, 1687, 1687*b*
nursing and collaborative management of, **1688-1690**
recommendations for treatment of, 1688
resources for, 1692
risk factors for, 1687*t*
Osteosarcoma, 1674
Osteotomy, 1662
Ostomy
adaptation to, 1073-1074
Ostomy self-care, 1072*b*
Ostomy surgery, 1069-1076
nursing management of, **1070-1076**
postoperative care, 1071-1072
preoperative care, **1070-1071**
sexual dysfunction after, 1074-1076
types of, 1069-1070, 1069*f*
OT. *See* Occupational therapy
Otalgia, 438
Otitis, external, 438
Otitis media
acute, **439**
chronic, **439-440**
collaborative care for, 439-440, 440*t*
nursing management of, **440**
with effusion, **440**
secretory, 440
serous, 440
Otorrhea, 1481, 1482*f*
Otosclerosis, 440-441
collaborative care for, 441, 441*t*
nursing management of, **441**
Otoscopic examination, 412, 413*f*
Ototoxic medications, 411
Ototoxic substances, 444
Outcome and Assessment Information Status (OASIS), 957
Outcomes
developing, 13
identifying, 12-13, 13*f*
Outflow problems, 1219
Out-of-hospital do-not-resuscitate (DNR) order, 156
Outpatient surgery, 344
Ovarian cancer, 1402-1404
clinical manifestations of, 1402-1403
collaborative care for, 1403-1404, 1403*t*
diagnostic studies, 1403
etiology and pathophysiology of, 1402
genetics of, 1402*b*
screening for, 1403*b*
Ovarian cysts, 1399, 1399*f*
Ovarian tumors, benign, **1399-1400**
Ovaries, 1325, 1325*f*
age-related changes in, 1331*t*
hormones and target tissues of, 1236*t*
"Overamping," 175
Overdose
acute intervention for, 186
manifestations of, 953*t*

Overflow urinary incontinence, 1180, 1181*t*
Overlapping connective tissue diseases, 1726
Overnutrition, 951
Overweight
classification of, 974, 974*f*, 975*t*
psychologic interventions for, 981*b*
Ovulatory studies, 1382
Oxalate, 1171*t*
Oxaliplatin (Eloxatin)
classification of, 287*t*
for colorectal cancer, 1067
FOLFOX treatment regimen, 291, 291*t*
Oxandrin (oxandrolone), 499*t*
Oxandrolone (Oxandrin), 499*t*
Oxaprozin (Daypro), 1698*t*
Oxazepam (Serax), 1569*t*
Oxcarbazepine (Trileptal)
analgesic effects of, 128
gerontologic considerations for, 1538
for seizures, 1538*t*
for trigeminal neuralgia, 1582
Oxidative stress, 68*t*, 69
Oximetry, 514, 525, 527*t*
preoperative, 351
pulse oximetry, 514, 514*f*
Oxtriphylline (Choledyl), 954*t*
Oxybutynin (Ditropan)
for multiple sclerosis, 1544*t*
for urinary incontinence, 1182
for voiding dysfunction, 1185*t*
Oxycodone (Percocet), 179
for burns, 499*t*
effects of use, 169*t*
for pain, 137*t*, 138, 140
Oxygen masks
non-rebreathing masks, 641*t*
partial rebreathing masks, 641*t*
simple face masks, 641*t*, 642*f*
Venturi masks, 642*f*, 642*t*
Oxygen saturation
arterial (SaO₂), 1857*t*
by pulse oximetry (SpO₂), 514, 514*f*
central venous (ScvO₂), 1746
critical values, 515, 515*t*
low, 676*t*
mixed venous (SvO₂), 1746
normal values, 514, 515*t*
SvO₂/ScvO₂ measurements
clinical interpretation of, 1746-1747, 1746*t*
in shock, 1774*t*
Oxygen systems, 644
Oxygen therapy
for acute respiratory distress syndrome, 1816-1817
for acute respiratory failure, 1807-1809
chronic, at home, 644
for cluster headache, 1531
complications of, 643-644
for COPD, 640-644
high-flow devices, 642*t*
home oxygen use, 645*t*
hyperbaric, 205-206
for hypoxemia, 640
indications for, 640
liquid oxygen, 645*t*
long-term, 644
low-flow devices, 641*t*
methods of administration, 640, 641*t*-642*t*, 642*f*
in shock, 1783

Oxygen toxicity, 643-644, 1808
Oxygenation
assessment of, 514-515
ET tube, 1753-1757
improving, 829
inadequate
clinical manifestations of, 377, 378*t*
signs and symptoms of, 515, 515*t*
lung function monitoring, 1800*t*
myocardial needs, 796, 796*t*
noninvasive arterial monitoring, 1747
perfusion problems, **738-924**
tissue needs, 1803
transport problems, **664-737**
ventilation problems, **508-663**
Oxygenation failure, 1799
Oxygen-conserving cannula, 641*t*, 643*f*
Oxygen-hemoglobin dissociation curve, 513, 513*f*
Oxyhemoglobin, 667
Oxymetazoliine (Dristan), 538*t*
Oxymorphone, 141
Oxypurinol, 1716
Oxytocin, 1236*t*, 1240
Oxytrol transdermal system (oxybutynin)
for urinary incontinence, 1182
for voiding dysfunction, 1185*t*

P

P wave, 846, 847*t*
PA. *See* Pulmonary artery
Pacemakers, 858-861, 858*f*, 859*f*
failure to capture, 860
failure to sense, 860
patient and family teaching guide for, 861*t*
patient monitoring, 860-861
permanent, 859
indications for, 859*t*
temporary, 859*f*
indications for, 859*t*
insertion of, 859, 860*f*
transcutaneous, 859-860, 860*f*
transvenous, 859-860
Pacific Islanders
health disparities, 20, 33-34
nurses, 26
older adults, 66
Pacing, overdrive, 857
Packed red blood cells, 731-732, 731*t*
Paclitaxel (Abraxane, Taxol)
for breast cancer, 1355
for cervical cancer, 1402
classification of, 287*t*
for esophageal cancer, 1010
for lung cancer, 582
method of administration, 288*t*
for oral cancer, 1002
for ovarian cancer, 1403
PACs. *See* Premature atrial contractions
PACU. *See* Postanesthesia care unit
PADP. *See* Pulmonary artery diastolic pressure
Paget's disease, 1350, **1690**
dermatologic manifestations of, 473*t*
PAI. *See* Percutaneous acetic acid injection
Pain, 125-150, 745*t*
abdominal
acute, **1043-1046**
assessment of, 1335*t*
chronic, **1046-1048**
in peritoneal dialysis, 1219

Pain (Continued)
acute, 130*t*, 131
in acute coronary syndrome, 813
affective component of, 127, 134
during angina or myocardial infarction, 796, 797*f*
area of, 132
associated symptoms, 132
behavioral component of, 127, 134
behavioral indicators of, 148
bladder-related, 1145*t*
bone, 676*t*
breakthrough, 132
breast, **1345**
in burn patients, 502-503
cancer pain, **309**
case study, 148-149
centrally generated, 130*t*
characteristics of, 132-134
chest pain, 1246*t*
in chronic HF, 826
emergency management of, 806*t*
pleuritic, 519*t*
chronic, 130*t*, 131
classification of, **130-131**
cognitive component of, 127, 134
in compartment syndrome, 1650
deafferentation, 131
definition of, 125, 126
dimensions of, **126-130**
dorsal horn processing, 128-129
duration of, 132
at end of life, 158-159, 160*t*
external ear, 413*t*
fear of, 158-159, 345
flank pain, 1145*t*
with fractures, 1637*t*
gender differences in, 127*b*
gerontologic considerations in, 147-148
harmful effects of unrelieved pain, 126, 126*t*
ICU patients at high risk for, 1736
impact of, 134
of inflammation, 196, 197*t*
intensity of, 132
leg pain, 745*t*
location of, 132
low back pain, **1675-1686**
magnitude of problem, **125-126**
mechanisms of, 127-130
musculoskeletal, 1649*t*
in myocardial infarction, 803-804
myofascial pain syndrome, **1726-1727**
neck pain, **1684,** 1684*t*
neuropathic, 128, 130-131, 130*t*
nociceptive, 128, 128*f*, 130, 130*t*
nursing diagnoses, 145*t*
onset of, 132
pattern of, 132
pelvic
chronic, 1395
chronic pelvic pain syndrome, 1428
perception of, 128*f*, 129
peripherally generated, 130*t*
persistent, 129
physiologic dimension of, 127
postmastectomy pain syndrome, 1353
postoperative, 379*t*, **388-389**
etiology of, 388
nursing diagnoses, 389
quality of, 132-134
referred, 129, 129*f*
resources for, 150-151

Pain *(Continued)*
sociocultural component of, 134
sociocultural dimension of, 127
somatic, 130, 130*t*
in special populations, **148**
with substance abuse problems, 148
sympathetically maintained, 131
transduction of, 127-128, 128*f*
transmission of, 128-129, 128*f*
urethral, 1145*t*
visceral, 130, 130*t*
visual system, 406*t*
Pain assessment, **131-134**
in abdominal pain, 1335*t*
brief, 1824*t*
in burns, 493*t*
in cancer, 309, 309*t*
core principles of, 131, 131*t*
elements of, 131-134
goals of, 131
initial, 133*f*
initial postanesthesia care unit assessment, 377-378, 377*t*
nursing assessment, 134, 134*t*
placebos in, 147
postoperative nursing assessment, 388-389
simple descriptive intensity scale, 132, 134*f*
testing pain sensation, 1458
tracking over time, 132, 132*f*
visual analog scale (VAS), 132, 134*f*
Pain education, institutionalizing, **147**
Pain management
acupuncture, 99*t*
in acute respiratory failure, 1811
adjuvant drugs for, 138-140, 139*t*
in Alzheimer's disease, 1573
barriers to, 145-146, 146*t*
basic principles of treatment, **134-135**
in burns, 493*t*
acute phase, 502-503
in critical care patients, 1736
drug therapy, 135-142
ethical dilemma, 698*b*
ethical issues in, **147**
home health care activities, 90*t*
institutionalizing, **147**
interventional therapy, 142-143
modulation, 128*f*, 129-130
neuroablative techniques for, 143
neurosurgical procedures for, 143, 143*f*
nondrug therapies, 143-144, 143*t*
nursing and collaborative management, **145-146**
nursing role in, 125
patient and family teaching guide, 145*t*
physical strategies for, 143-144
placebos in, 147
postburn, 498
postoperative
nursing implementation, 389
nursing management, **388-389**
strategies for, 132-134
in substance abuse, 187-188
treatment, **134-144**
undertreatment, 126
Painful bladder syndrome, 1163-1164
Painful heels, 1685*t*
PainLink, 150
Palifermin (Kepivance), 298
Palliative care, **156-157**
definition of, 156, 1875
resources, 164
surgery, 343

Pallidotomy, 1551
Pallor
in compartment syndrome, 1650
conjunctival, 675*t*
elevation pallor, 901
of nail beds, 675*t*
of skin, 675*t*
variations in light- and dark-skinned individuals, 456*t*
Palmar erythema, 1102
Palonosetron (Aloxi), 297, 992*t*
Palpation, 47, 47*f*
of abdomen, 937-938
deep, 937, 938*f*
light, 937, 938*f*
of chest, 521-522
assessment abnormalities, 524*t*
findings in pulmonary problems, 526*t*
of kidney, 1144, 1145*f*
of liver, 937-938, 938*f*
of liver or spleen, 677
of mouth, 936
of musculoskeletal system, 1621-1622
of peripheral vascular system, 748, 748*f*
of skin, 48*t*, 456
of thorax, 748-750
assessment abnormalities, 749*t*
normal, 751*t*
of thyroid gland, 1245-1246, 1245*f*
of urinary system, 1144
Palpitations, 676*t*
Pamelor (nortriptyline)
for Alzheimer's disease, 1569*t*
local, 139*t*
Pamidronate (Aredia)
for hypercalcemia, 330
for osteoporosis, 1689
for Paget's disease, 1690
Pancarditis, rheumatic, 876
Pancreas, 931*f*, **932,** 1241-1242
age-related changes in, 932, 933*t*
diagnostic studies, 1250, 1251*t*-1252*t*
disorders of, **1118-1126**
cultural and ethnic health disparities in, 1089*b*
resources for, 1134
effects of aging on, 1242*t*
hormones, 1236*t*
problems of, **1087-1134**
radiology, 1252*t*
secretions related to digestion, 929, 929*t*
serum studies, 1251*t*
structure of, 931*f*
urine studies, 1251*t*-1252*t*
Pancreas transplantation
for diabetes mellitus, 1271
indications for, 1271
Pancrease (pancrelipase), 1121*t*
Pancreatic cancer, 1125-1126
clinical manifestations of, 1125
collaborative care for, 1126
diagnostic studies, 1125-1126
etiology and pathophysiology of, 1125
nursing management of, **1126**
Pancreaticoduodenectomy, radical, 1126, 1126*f*
Pancreatin (Viokase), 1121*t*
Pancreatitis
acute, **1118-1124**
collaborative care for, 1120-1121, 1120*t*
diagnostic studies, 1120, 1120*t*

Pancreatitis *(Continued)*
drug therapy of, 1121, 1121*t*
nursing assessment of, 1121, 1121*t*
nursing care plan for patient with, 1122*b*-1123*b*
nursing management of, **1121-1124**
pathophysiology of, 1118-1119, 1119*f*
chronic, **1124-1125**
drug therapy of, 1121*t*
nursing management of, **1125**
chronic calcifying, 1124
chronic obstructive, 1124
edematous, 1119
necrotizing, 1119
severe, 1119
Pancrelipase (Cotazym, Pancrease), 1121*t*
Pancrezyme (pancreatin), 1121*t*
Pancytopenia, 693
Panhypopituitarism, 1293
Panitumumab (Vectibix), 1067
Panophthalmitis, 437
Pantoprazole (Protonix)
for cirrhosis, 1110*t*
for gastroesophageal reflux disease, 1006, 1006*t*
for gastrointestinal bleeding, 998*t*
for peptic ulcer disease, 1019*t*, 1020
for upper gastrointestinal bleeding, 997
for variceal bleeding, 1108
PaO₂. *See* Partial pressure of oxygen in arterial blood
Papanicolaou (Pap) test, 1339*t*
Papaverine, 1121*t*, 1435
Papillary muscle dysunction, 805
Papilledema, 1460*t*, 1471
Papilloma, intraductal, 1345*t*, 1347
Papovavirus, 244*t*
Papules, 455*t*
Para-aminosalicylic acid (PAS), 573*t*
Paracentesis
for ascites, 1107
Paracopa (levodopa-carbidopa), 1552*t*
Paradigm REAL-Time System (Medtronic), 1269, 1270, 1270*f*
Paradoxic breathing, 1805
Paradoxic intoxication, 1551
Paradoxic respiration, 588, 588*f*
Paraesophageal or rolling hiatal hernia, 1007, 1008*f*
Parainfluenza 1-4 virus, 244*t*
Paralysis
ascending polyneuropathic (*See* Guillain-Barré syndrome)
in compartment syndrome, 1650
Todd's paralysis, 1535
Paralytic (adynamic) ileus, 1060-1061
Paralyzed Veterans of America, 1613
Paranasal sinuses
inflammation and infection of, **535-541**
obstruction of, **541**
Paraneoplastic syndrome, 580
Paraphimosis, 1430, 1430*f*
Paraplatin (carboplatin)
for cervical cancer, 1402
classification of, 287*t*
for lung cancer, 582
for oral cancer, 1002
for ovarian cancer, 1403
Paraplegia, 1461*t*
functional level of spinal cord injury and rehabilitation potential, 1594*t*
in spinal cord injury, 1590

Parasites
emerging infections, 245*t*
reemerging infections, 246*t*
Parasympathetic nervous system, 1450
age-related changes in, 1454*t*
effects of, 1451*t*
gerontologic differences in assessment findings, 1454*t*
Parathormone, 1236*t*, 1240-1241
Parathyroid glands, 1240-1241, 1240*f*
disorders of, **1308-1311**
effects of aging on, 1242*t*
serum studies, 1250*t*
Parathyroid hormone, 1240-1241
feedback between calcium and, 1237, 1237*f*
serum levels, 1250*t*
target tissue and functions, 1236*t*
Parathyroid studies, 1247-1250, 1250*t*
Paregoric, pectin, and kaolin (Parepectolin), 1037*t*
Parenchymal lung diseases, diffuse, 597
Parenteral nutrition, **965-967**
administration of solution, 966-967
catheter placement for, 966, 966*f*
central, 965
complications of, 967*t*
composition of, 965-966
home support, 968
indications for, 965, 965*t*
methods of administration, 966
nursing care plan for patient receiving, 968*b*
nursing management of, **967-968**
peripheral, 966
Parepectolin (paregoric, pectin, and kaolin), 1037*t*
Paresthesia, 1623*t*
in compartment syndrome, 1650
of feet and hands, 676*t*
in Guillain-Barré syndrome, 1586
Paricalcitol (Zemplar), 1210
Parietal layer, 928
Parietal pleura, 512
Parkinsonism, 1549, 1549*f*
Parkinson's disease, 1549-1553
case study, 1559
clinical manifestations of, 1549-1550, 1550*f*
collaborative care for, 1550-1552, 1551*t*
complications of, 1550
diagnostic studies, 1550
drug therapy for, 1550-1551, 1552*t*
etiology and pathophysiology of, 1549, 1549*f*, 1550*f*
nursing assessment of, 1553, 1553*t*
nursing care plan for patient with, 1554*b*-1555*b*
nursing diagnoses, 1553
nursing evaluation of, 1553
nursing implementation for, 1553
nursing management of, **1553**
nursing planning for, 1553
nutritional therapy for, 1552
surgical therapy for, 1551-1552
Parkland (Baxter) formula, 496, 497*t*
Parlodel (bromocriptine)
drug alert, 1551
for Parkinson's disease, 1551, 1552*t*
for prolactinoma, 1293
for restless legs syndrome, 1558
Parotid gland inflammation, 1000*t*
Parotitis, 1000*t*
Paroxetine (Paxil), 139

Paroxysmal nocturnal dyspnea, 746, 825

Paroxysmal supraventricular tachycardia, 851, 851*f*
  characteristics of, 849*t*
  clinical associations, 851
  clinical significance of, 851
  ECG characteristics, 851
  treatment of, 851
Pars flaccida, 412
Pars tensa, 412
Partial cystectomy, 1179
Partial liquid ventilation, 1763
Partial pressure of end-tidal CO₂ (PETCO₂), 1753-1754
Partial pressure of oxygen in arterial blood (PaO₂)
  critical values, 515, 515*t*
  normal values, 514, 515*t*
Partial rebreathing masks, 641*t*
Partial seizures, 1535
  complex, 1535
  simple, 1535
Partial thromboplastin time
  activated, 679*t*, 913*t*
    in deep vein thrombosis, 911*t*
    laboratory values, 1859*t*
  effects of aging on, 672*t*
  in hemophilia, 709*t*
  preoperative, 351
  in shock, 1775*t*
Partially sighted, 419
Partial-thickness burns, 486, 487*t*
  emergency management of, 490*t*
Parvovirus, 244*t*
PAS. *See Para*-aminosalicylic acid
Passive muscle relaxation, 120
Passy-Muir speaking tracheostomy valve, 550, 550*f*
Past health history
  and auditory system, 409
  and cardiovascular system, 745
  and endocrine system, 1243
  and fluid, electrolyte, and acid-base imbalances, 337
  and gastrointestinal system, 933
  and hematologic system, 671-672
  important information, 43
  and integumentary system, 453
  and musculoskeletal system, 1619
  and nervous system, 1454
  and preoperative patient, 346, 350*t*
  and reproductive system, 1331-1332
  and respiratory system, 517
  and urinary system, 1141-1142
  and visual system, 402, 403*t*
Patch graft angioplasty, 904
Patch test, 458*t*
Patellar "knee jerk" reflex arc, 1446*f*
Patellar "knee jerk" reflex testing, 1459, 1459*f*
Pathologic grief, 154
Patient adherence, 575*b*
Patient and family teaching, 53-66
  for diabetes mellitus, 1276-1278
  with older adults, 79, 79*t*
  resources, 65
  role of, 53-54
Patient and family teaching guides
  for acute coronary syndrome, 815*t*
  acute or chronic sinusitis, 541*t*

Patient and family teaching guides (*Continued*)
  for Addison's disease, 1317*t*
  after amputation, 1661*t*
  for anticoagulant therapy, 917*b*
  for antiretroviral drugs, 265*t*
  for asthma, 630*t*
  for autonomic dysreflexia, 1604*t*
  back exercises, 1677*t*
  for bowel management after spinal cord injury, 1606*t*
  for cardiomyopathy, 889*t*
  cast care, 1646*t*
  for changing ileal conduit appliances, 1193*t*
  characteristics of menstruation, 1329*t*
  for chronic kidney disease, 1216*t*
  chronic obstructive pulmonary disease, 654*t*
  for cirrhosis, 1115*b*
  for colostomy irrigation, 1075*t*
  for constipation, 1044*t*
  for corticosteroid therapy, 1319*t*
  to decrease risk for antibiotic-resistant infection, 247*t*
  decreasing risk factors for coronary artery disease, 791-792, 792*t*
  for diabetes mellitus management, 1277*t*
  for drug-using equipment, 263*t*
  for ear surgery, 440*t*
  early warning signs of Alzheimer's disease, 1567*t*
  for exercise for diabetes mellitus, 1269*t*
  after eye surgery, 428*t*
  femoral head prosthesis, 1654*t*
  FITT physical activity guidelines, 816*t*
  for foot care, 1287*t*
  guidelines for effective coughing, 646*t*
  for halo vest care, 1606*t*
  for head injury, 1486*t*
  headaches, 1533*t*
  for heart failure, 838*t*
  for heat and cold therapy, 144*t*
  for herbal therapies, 101*t*
  home oxygen use, 645*t*
  how to reduce symptoms of allergic rhinitis, 536*t*
  how to use dry powder inhalers, 623*t*
  how to use peak flow meters, 628*t*
  for hypertension, 779*t*
  for hypothyroidism, 1309*t*
  for implantable cardioverter-defibrillators, 858*t*
  for insulin therapy, 1262*t*
  joint protection and energy conservation, 1701*b*
  low back problems, 1677*t*
  for mitral valve prolapse, 880*t*
  neck exercises, 1684*t*
  for neutropenia, 715*t*
  for nutrition, 958*t*
  for ostomy self-care, 1072*b*
  for pacemakers, 861*t*
  for pain management, 145*t*
  for peptic ulcer disease, 1025*b*
  for peripheral artery bypass surgery, 907*t*
  for postoperative laparoscopic cholecystectomy, 1132*b*
  for preoperative preparation, 352*t*
  for pressure ulcers, 210*t*
  for preventing food poisoning, 1031, 1032*t*
  for prevention of gastroesophageal reflux disease, 1007*t*

Patient and family teaching guides (*Continued*)
  prevention of hypokalemia, 329*t*
  prevention of Lyme disease, 1714, 1714*t*
  prevention of musculoskeletal problems in older adults, 1630*t*
  protection of small joints, 1710*t*
  for radiation skin reactions, 300*t*
  reducing barriers to pain management, 146*t*
  for seizure disorders and epilepsy, 1541*t*
  for self-monitoring of blood glucose, 1270*t*
  for sexual activity after acute coronary syndrome, 817*t*
  for sexual assault prevention, 1411*t*
  signs and symptoms that HIV-infected patients need to report, 266*t*
  for skin care after spinal cord injury, 1606*t*
  for smoking and tobacco use cessation, 173*t*
  steps for supraglottic swallow, 553*t*
  systemic lupus erythematosus, 1720*t*
  for thrombocytopenia, 707*t*
  for urinary tract infection, 1161*t*
  warning signs of stroke, 1515*t*
Patient care continuum, 87
Patient Care Data Set (PCDS), 8*t*
Patient education
  in acute coronary syndrome, 815
  assessment of characteristics that affect, 57-58, 57*t*
  assessment process, 57-59
  and clinical outcomes in chronic HF, 830*b*
  cultural considerations, 59
  for diabetic patients, 1259*b*
  diagnosis, 60
  discharge education, 830*b*
  evaluation, 64
  group-based programs, 1259*b*
  implementation, 63
  for inflammatory bowel disease, 1059
  for nausea and vomiting, 993
  for nutritional therapy for diabetes mellitus, 1268-1269
  planning, 60-63
  preoperative teaching, 350-352
  principles of adult education, 54, 54*t*
  process of, **57-64**
  readiness to learn, 60
  related to drug therapy, 772-776
  related to drug therapy of asthma, 621-623
  techniques to enhance learning, 63*t*
  about wound healing, 206
Patient goals, 12
Patient interviews
  considerations for, 40-41
  motivational, 188
    for addictive behaviors, 188-189
    key aspects of, 188, 188*t*
  preoperative, **344**
Patient outcomes, 12
  developing, 13
  identifying, 12-13, 13*f*
  nursing-sensitive, 12
Patient positioning
  for acute respiratory distress syndrome, 1817-1818
  effective, 1809-1810
  good lung down position, 1809-1810
  in increased ICP, 1480
  for postural drainage, 647, 648*f*

Patient positioning (*Continued*)
  prone positioning, 1763
  during recovery from general anesthesia, 381, 381*f*
  for surgery, 366
  tripod position, 524*t*, 634, 1805
  for tube feedings, 962
Patient teaching. *See* Patient education
Patient teaching guides
  for proper use of female condom, 263*t*
  for proper use of male condom, 262*t*
  for sexually transmitted diseases, 1377*t*
  for testicular self-examination, 1433*t*
Patient transport
  to operating room, 354-356
  recommendations for isolation precautions, 249*t*
Patient-controlled analgesia, 142
  for postoperative pain, 389
Pavulon (pencuronium), 370*t*
PAWP. *See* Pulmonary artery wedge pressure
Paxil (paroxetine), 139
Payment for organs, 1225*b*
PBC. *See* Primary biliary cirrhosis
PBS. *See* Painful bladder syndrome
PBZ (tripelennamine), 537*t*
PCA. *See* Patient-controlled analgesia
PC-IRV. *See* Pressure-controlled inverse ratio ventilation
PCM. *See* Protein-calorie malnutrition
PCOS. *See* Polycystic ovary syndrome
PCP. *See* Phencyclidine
PCUs. *See* Progressive care units
PEA. *See* Pulseless electrical activity
Peak expiratory flow rate, 531*t*
Peak flow meters
  how to use, 628*t*
  patient and family teaching guide for, 628*t*
Pectoriloquy, whispered, 525*t*
Pedestrian incidents
  fractured extremity in, 1642, 1642*t*
  head injury in, 1484*t*
  spinal cord injury in, 1596*t*
Pedicle, 481
Pediculosis, **470***t*
Pedigree
  definition of, 214*t*
  example, 216*f*
PEEP. *See* Positive end-expiratory pressure
Peer influence, 167, 167*f*
Peer teaching, 61-62
PEFR. *See* Peak expiratory flow rate
Pegaptanib (Macugen), 432
Pegaspargase (Oncaspar), 720*t*, 721*t*
Pegasys (α-Interferon), 1095
Pegfilgrastim (Neulasta)
  for cancer treatment, 304*t*
  clinical uses of, 223*t*
PEG-Intron (α-Interferon), 1095
Pegvisomant (Somavert), 1292
Pegylation, 1094
PEI. *See* Percutaneous ethanol injection
Pelvic computed tomography, 1340*t*, 1341
Pelvic examination, internal, 1335
Pelvic exenteration
  acute intervention related to, 1407
  anterior, 1404*t*
  description of, 1404*t*
  posterior, 1404*t*
  total, 1407, 1407*f*

Note: Disorder names are in **bold face.** Page numbers in **bold face** indicate main discussions. Page numbers followed by *f, t, b,* or *n* indicate figures, tables, boxed material, or notes, respectively.

Pelvic floor muscle (Kegel) exercises, 1183*t*, 1184*f*
Pelvic floor muscle rehabilitation, 1183*t*
Pelvic inflammatory disease (PID), 1395-1396
  clinical manifestations of, 1395
  collaborative care for, 1395-1396
  complications of, 1395
  etiology and pathophysiology of, 1395
  nursing assessment of, 1396*t*
  nursing management of, **1396**
  routes of spread of, 1395, 1395*f*
Pelvic organs, 1325-1326, 1325*f*
Pelvic pain
  chronic, 1395
  chronic pelvic pain syndrome, 1428
Pelvic support problems, 1407-1409
  nursing management of, 1408-1409
Pelvis
  female, 1326
  fractures of, 1652-1653
  secondary survey head-to-toe assessment, 1826*t*, 1827
Pemetrexed (Alimta), 287*t*
Pemoline (Cylert), 1544-1545, 1545*t*
Penbutolol (Levatol), 774*t*
Pencuronium (Pavulon), 370*t*
Penetrating injury
  chest trauma, 585, 585*t*
  to eye, 421*t*
  fractured extremity, 1642, 1642*t*
  head injury, 1484*t*
  spinal cord injury, 1596*t*
Penicillamine (Cuprimine, Depen)
  for arthritis and connective tissue disorders, 1699*t*
  for rheumatoid arthritis, 1706
Penicillin
  for bacterial meningitis, 1495
  for osteomyelitis, 1670
Penicillin G (Pfizerpen)
  for infective endocarditis, 869*t*
  for syphilis, 1371*t*
Penicillin G benzathine (Bicillin)
  for rheumatic fever, 878
  for syphilis, 1371, 1371*t*
Penicillin V potassium (Beepen-VK), 878
Penile compression devices, 1183*t*
Penile discharge, 1337*t*
Penile erythema, 1337*t*
Penile growths or masses, 1337*t*
Penile implants, 1436, 1436*f*
Penis
  age-related changes in, 1331*t*
  cancer of, 1430
  erectile mechanism problems, **1430**
  physical examination of, **1335**
  problems of, **1429-1430**
Pentazocine (Talwin)
  effects of use, 169*t*
  for pain, 137*t*, 138
Pentobarbital (Nembutal)
  effects of use, 169*t*
  withdrawal from, 179
Pentolair (cyclopentolate HCl), 427*t*
Pentosan (Elmiron), 1164
Pentostatin (Nipent)
  classification of, 287*t*
  for leukemia, 720*t*, 721*t*
Penthotal (thiopental), 369*t*
Pentoxifylline (Trental), 902
Penumbra, 1504
PEP. *See* Positive expiratory pressure; Postexposure prophylaxis

Pepcid (famotidine)
  for gastroesophageal reflux disease, 1005-1006, 1006*t*
  for gastrointestinal bleeding, 998*t*
  for peptic ulcer disease, 1019*t*
  preoperative, 355*t*
Pepcid Complete, 1005-1006
Peppermint, 102*t*
Peptic ulcer disease, 1014-1028
  acute, 1015, 1015*f*
  acute exacerbation of, 1021
  acute intervention for, 1022-1025
  ambulatory and home care for, 1025
  antibiotic therapy of, 1020
  chronic, 1015, 1015*f*
  clinical manifestations of, 1017
  collaborative care for, 1018-1022, 1019*t*, 1025-1027
  complications of, 1017-1018
    therapy related to, 1021-1022
  conservative therapy of, 1018-1022
  in COPD, 637
  cytoprotective drug therapy of, 1021
  diagnostic studies, 1018
  drug therapy of, 1019-1021, 1019*t*
  of duodenum, 1015, 1015*f*
  etiology and pathophysiology of, 1015-1017, 1016*f*
  gerontologic considerations for, **1027-1028**
  health promotion in, 1022
  nursing assessment of, 1022, 1022*t*
  nursing care plan for patient with, 1023*b*-1024*b*
  nursing diagnoses, 1022
  nursing evaluation of, 1025
  nursing implementation for, 1022-1025
  nursing management of, **1022-1027**
  nursing planning for, 1022
  nutritional therapy of, 1021
  patient and family teaching guide for, 1025*b*
  perforation of, 1017-1018, 1021-1022
    nursing implementation for, 1023-1024
  postoperative care of, 1027
  postoperative complications of, 1026
    nutritional therapy of, 1026-1027
  preoperative care of, 1027
  surgical therapy of, 1025-1027
    nursing management of, **1027**
  types of, 1015, 1015*f*
Peptide YY, 972, 973*f*, 973*t*
Peptides, 972, 973*f*, 973*t*
Pepto-Bismol (bismuth subsalicylate), 1019*t*, 1037*t*
Perception. *See also* Cognitive-perceptual pattern
  of pain, 128*f*, 129
Percocet (oxycodone)
  for burns, 499*t*
  for pain, 137*t*
Percodan (oxycodone)
  effects of use, 169*t*
  for pain, 137*t*
Percussion, 47-48, 47*f*
  of abdomen, 937
  of chest, 522, 523*f*, 647, 647*f*
    assessment abnormalities, 524*t*
    in pulmonary problems, 526*t*
  cupped-hand position for, 647, 647*f*
  of thorax, 750
    assessment abnormalities, 749*t*
    normal, 751*t*
  of urinary system, 1144-1145
Percussion sounds, 523*f*, 523*t*
Percutaneous acetic acid injection, 1117

Percutaneous coronary intervention
  advantages of, 807
  for coronary artery disease, 801
  emergent, 807
Percutaneous electrical nerve stimulation, 144
Percutaneous endoscopic gastrostomy, 961, 962*f*
Percutaneous ethanol injection, 1117
Percutaneous laser diskectomy, 1682
Percutaneous nephrolithotomy, 1171
Percutaneous radiofrequency rhizotomy, 1582, 1582*t*
Percutaneous tracheostomy, 543
Percutaneous transhepatic cholangiography, 942*t*
Percutaneous transluminal balloon angioplasty, 903-904
Percutaneous transluminal balloon valvuloplasty, 881-882
Percutaneous ultrasonic lithotripsy, 1172
Perdiem (psyllium), 1042*t*
Perflubron (LiquiVent), 1763
Perforation
  peptic ulcer, 1017-1018, 1021-1022
    nursing implementation for, 1023-1024
  tympanic membrane, 439, 440*f*
Perfusion imaging, 758
Perfusion problems, 738-924
  in acute respiratory distress syndrome, 1818
  after aortic surgery, 898
  peripheral, 898
  renal, 898
  ventilation-perfusion mismatch, 1779, 1801-1802
Pergolide (Permax)
  for Parkinson's disease, 1551, 1552*t*
  for prolactinoma, 1293
  for restless legs syndrome, 1558
Pergonal, 1383*t*
Pericardial effusion, 872, 873*f*
Pericardial friction rub, 750*t*, 751, 872
Pericardial heterografts, 883*t*
Pericardial knock, 874
Pericardial space, 740
Pericardiectomy, 874
Pericardiocentesis, 873-874, 873*f*
Pericarditis, 871
  acute, **871-874,** 872*f*
  in chemotherapy and radiation therapy, 296*t*
  chronic constrictive, 874
  etiology of, 872*t*
  late, 872
  in myocardial infarction, 805
  in pneumonia, 565
Pericardium, 740
  layers of, 865, 866*f*
Pericles, 162
Peri-Colace (docusate), 1042*t*
Perigraft leaks, 896
Perimenopause, 1390-1393
  clinical manifestations of, 1390-1391, 1390*t*
  collaborative care for, 1391-1392
  drug therapy for, 1391-1392
  nonhormonal therapy for, 1392
  nursing management of, **1393**
  nutritional therapy for, 1392
Perimysium, 1617
Perinatal transmission of HIV, 250
Perindopril (Aceon), 776*t*
Perineal prostatectomy
  approach, 1424, 1424*f*

Perineum, 1826*t*, 1827
Perioperative care, **342-396**
  herb and supplement effects during, 347*b*
  of obese patient, 984-986
Perioperative nurse, 361
  intraoperative activities of, 361*t*
  role related to anesthesia, 368*t*
Perioperative Nursing Data Set (PNDS), 8, 8*t*, 366
Periorbital bone fracture, 1657*t*
Periosteum, 1616
Peripheral adenocarcinoma, 580*f*
Peripheral arterial disease, 892, **893-894**
  case study, 920
  collaborative care for, 902*t*
  complementary and alternative therapies for, 903
  etiology and pathophysiology of, 893
  exercise therapy of, 902-903
  of lower extremities, **900-907**
    acute intervention for, 906
    clinical manifestations of, 900-901
    collaborative care for, 901-904
    complications of, 901
    diagnostic studies, 901
    drug therapy of, 902
    nursing care plan for patient with, 905*b*-906*b*
    nursing management of, **904-907**
    risk factor modification, 901
    surgical therapy of, 904, 904*f*
  nursing assessment of, 904*t*
  nutritional therapy of, 903
Peripheral arteriography and venography, 755*t*
Peripheral artery bypass surgery, 907*t*
Peripheral cyanosis, 749*t*
Peripheral edema, 1104
Peripheral lymphoid organs, 219
Peripheral nerve problems, 1580-1613
Peripheral nervous system, **1448-1450**
  age-related changes in, 1454*t*
  effects of chronic alcohol abuse on, 177*t*
  gerontologic differences in assessment findings, 1454*t*
  structure of, 1442
Peripheral neuropathy
  in chemotherapy and radiation therapy, 296*t*
  with cirrhosis, 1103
  postinfectious polyneuropathy (*See* Guillain-Barré syndrome)
Peripheral parenteral nutrition, 966
Peripheral perfusion, 898
Peripheral stem cell transplantation, 304
Peripheral vascular disease
  dermatologic manifestations of, 473*t*
  in hypertension, 766*t*, 767
Peripheral vascular system
  auscultation of, 748
  inspection of, 748
  palpation of, 748, 748*f*
  physical examination of, 748
  in spinal cord injury, 1595
Peripheral vessel blood flow, 759-760
Peripheral visual field defect, 406*t*
Peripherally inserted central venous catheters, 289, 289*f*
Peritoneal catheters
  exit site, 1218, 1218*f*
  for peritoneal dialysis, 1217, 1218*f*

Peritoneal dialysis, 1216, **1216-1220,** 1217*t*
  automated, 1218-1219, 1218*f*
  catheter exit site, 1218, 1218*f*
  catheter placement for, 1217-1218, 1217*f*
  chronic
    adaptation to, 1220
    effectiveness of, 1220
  complications of, 1219-1220, 1229*t*
  continuous ambulatory, 1219, 1219*f*
  contraindications to, 1219
  drain, 1218
  dwell, 1218
  exchange, 1218
  exit site infection, 1219
  inflow, 1218
  outflow problems, 1219
  peritoneal catheters for, 1217, 1218*f*
  phases of, 1218
  pulmonary complications of, 1219
  solutions and cycles, 1218
  systems, 1218-1219
  types of, 1218
Peritoneoscopy, 944*t*, 1340*t*
Peritoneovenous shunt, 1107, 1108*f*
Peritonitis, 1049-1050
  causes of, 1049, 1049*t*
  clinical manifestations of, 1049
  collaborative care for, 1050, 1050*t*
  diagnostic studies, 1049-1050
  encapsulating sclerosing, 1220
  etiology and pathophysiology of, 1049
  nursing assessment of, 1050
  nursing diagnoses, 1050
  nursing implementation for, 1050
  nursing management of, **1050**
  nursing planning for, 1050
  in peritoneal dialysis, 1219
Peritonsillar abscess, 542
Permax (pergolide)
  for Parkinson's disease, 1551, 1552*t*
  for prolactinoma, 1293
  for restless legs syndrome, 1558
PermCath catheter, 1221
Pernicious anemia, 692
Perphenazine (Trilafon), 992*t*
Persantine (dipyridamole)
  for long-term therapy after TIAs, 1505
  to prevent stroke, 1510
  for stroke, 1512
Persistent generalized lymphadenop-athy, 252
Persistent pain, 129
Personal distance, 33
Personal hygiene, 1275-1276, 1379
  oral hygiene, 1003*b*
  in shock, 1793
  and skin, 462
Personal neglect, 168*t*
Personal protective equipment, 247, 248*t*
Personal space, 33
Perspiration, sensible, 321
Pertussis, 246*t*
Pes cavus, 1685*t*
Pes planus, 1623*t*, 1685*t*
Pessaries
  for urinary incontinence, 1183*t*
  for uterine prolapse, 1408

PET. *See* Positron emission tomography
PETCO$_2$. *See* Partial pressure of end-tidal CO$_2$
Petechiae, 454, 457*t*, 675*t*, 677, 702
  in light- and dark-skinned individu-als, 456*t*
Pethidine (meperidine), 138
Petit mal (absence) seizures, 1534-1535
Petrissage, 104, 104*f*
Peyote (mescaline), 170*t*
Peyronie's disease, 1430
Pfizerpen (penicillin G), 869*t*
PGL. *See* Persistent generalized lymph-adenopathy
pH, 333
  definition of, 333*t*
  laboratory values, 1857*t*
  normal range, 333, 333*f*
  urine levels, 1863*t*
Phacoemulsification, 426, 427*f*
Phagocytes, mononuclear, 220-222
  functions of, 932*t*
Phagocytosis, 667-668
Phakic intraocular lenses, 419
Phalen's test, 1633
Phantom limb sensation, 1660
Pharmacologic echocardiography, 754*t*
Pharmacologic nuclear imaging, 754*t*
Pharyngitis, acute, 541-542
Pharynx
  ingestion propulsion of food by, 928
  physical examination of, 521, 525*t*
  problems related to, **541-543**
    cultural and ethnic health dispari-ties in, 1001*t*
Phenacetin, 1142*t*
Phenaphen (acetaminophen), 1530
Phenazopyridine (Pyridium)
  nephrotoxicity of, 1142
  for UTIs, 1158
Phencyclidine (PCP), 170*t*
Phendimetrazine (Bontril, Plegine), 981
Phenergan (promethazine)
  as adjunct to general anesthesia, 370*t*
  for nausea and vomiting, 992, 992*t*
Phenobarbital (Luminal)
  blood glucose level effects, 1267*t*
  effects of use, 169*t*
  food/nutrient interactions, 954*t*
  gerontologic considerations for, 1538
  for seizures, 1536, 1538*t*
  for status epilepticus, 1537
  withdrawal from, 179
Phenolphthalein (Ex-Lax, Correctol, Feen-a-Mint), 1042*t*
Phenothiazines
  blood glucose level effects, 1267*t*
  food/nutrient interactions, 954*t*
  hematologic effects of, 674*t*
  for nausea and vomiting, 138, 992, 992*t*
Phenotype, 214, 214*t*
Phenoxybenzamine (Dibenzyline), 1320
Phentermine (Adiphex-P, Fastin, Ion-amin), 169*t*, 981
Phentolamine (Regitine, Vasomax)
  for erectile dysfunction, 1435
  for hypertension, 774*t*
Phenylalanine, 1857*t*
Phenylbutazone, 1267*t*
Phenylephrine (Neo-Synephrine)
  for allergic rhinitis and sinusitis, 538*t*
  for pupil dilation, 427*t*
  for shock, 1788*t*
Phenylpropanolamine, 1185*t*

Phenylpyruvic acid, 1863*t*
Phenytoin (Dilantin)
  blood glucose level effects, 1267*t*
  classification of, 856*t*
  food/nutrient interactions, 954*t*
  for seizures, 1536, 1538*t*
  for status epilepticus, 1537
  toxicology, 1865*t*
  for trigeminal neuralgia, 1581
Pheochromocytoma, 1320
  clinical manifestations of, 1320
  diagnostic studies, 1320
  etiology and pathophysiology of, 1320
  nursing and collaborative manage-ment of, 1320
Philadelphia chromosome, 718
Phimosis, 1429, 1430*f*
Phlebography, 911*t*
Phlebostatic axis, 1739, 1741*f*
Phlebotomy, elective, 734
Phlegmasia cerulea dolens, 911
Phonophobia, 1528
Phosgene, 1839-1840
PhosLo, 1210
Phosphajel, 1020*t*
Phosphatase
  acid, 1857*t*
  alkaline, 1857*t*
  inorganic, 1857*t*
Phosphate
  normal values, 321*t*
  serum levels, 1250*t*
Phosphate binders, 1210
Phosphate imbalances, 331-332
  in acute renal failure, 1200
  causes and clinical manifestations of, 332*t*
  in chronic kidney disease, 1207
Phosphate restriction, 1213
Phospholipase A$_2$, 752*t*, 756
Phosphorus, 1147*t*, 1626*t*
  daily requirements in chronic kidney disease, 1211-1212, 1212*t*
  inorganic, 1863*t*
Phospho-Soda (sodium phosphates), 1042*t*
Photoaging, 452, 452*f*
Photodynamic therapy
  for age-related macular degeneration, 432
  for lung cancer, 582-583
Photophobia, 406*t*, 1528
Photopsia, 430
Photorefractive keratectomy, 418
Photosensitivity, 461-462, 461*t*
Phototherapy, 474, 474*f*
Physical abuse, 73*t*
Physical activity. *See also* Exercise; Sexual activity
  for acute coronary syndrome, 815-817
  and acute low back pain, 1681*b*
  for coronary artery disease, 790, 792
  FITT formula for, 792, 816*t*
  health impact of regular activity, 1631*b*
  health-promoting behaviors for, 792*t*
  for hypertension, 770-771, 779-780
  isotonic, 816
  for older adults, 795
  static, 816
Physical assessment, 57-58, 57*t*
  before surgery, 363
  of visual system, 404, 404*t*
Physical dependence
  definition of, 166*t*
  and pain, 145

Physical examination, **46-50**
  of abdomen, 936-938, 939*t*, 1246
  adaptations, 50*t*
  of anus, 938-939, 939*t*, 1335, 1335*t*
  in assessment of allergic disorders, 229
  of auditory system, 412, 412*t*
  of cardiovascular system, 747-748, 751*t*
  of chest, 521, 522, 522*f*, 525*t*
  of ears, 412
  of endocrine system, 1245-1246
  equipment for, 48
  of extremities, 1246
  of female reproductive system, 1335
  in fluid, electrolyte, and acid-base imbalances, 338
  focused, 47
  of gastrointestinal system, 936-939, 939*t*
  of genitalia, 1246
  of head and neck, 1245
  of hematologic system, 674-676
  of integumentary system, 454-456, 1245
  of lungs, 521
  of male reproductive system, 1334-1335, 1335*t*
  in malnutrition, 954
  of mouth, 521, 936
  of musculoskeletal system, 1621-1624
  of neck, 521, 1245-1246
  of nervous system, 1456-1459, 1459*t*
  of nose, 521, 525*t*
  organization of, 48-50
  of peripheral vascular system, 748
  pertinent negatives, 47
  of pharynx, 521, 525*t*
  positive findings, 47
  preoperative, 349
  of rectum, 938-939
  of respiratory system, 521-525
  screening, 47
    documentation of normal findings, 51*t*
    equipment for, 48, 48*t*
    outline for, 48*t*-49*t*
    recording, 50, 51*t*
  techniques for, 47-48
  of thorax, 748-751, 1246
  of tympanum, 412
  types of, 47
  of urinary system, 1144-1145, 1145*t*
  of visual system, 404-407
Physical therapy
  for burns, 493*t*, 503
  chest physiotherapy, 646-647
    in acute respiratory failure, 1810
    steps in, 647*t*
  for COPD, 646-649
  water exercise for multiple sclerosis, 1545, 1546*f*
Physiologic dead space, 1779
Physiologic dependence, 168
Physiologic stress ulcers, 996, 1816
Phytosterols, 796*b*
Phytotherapy, 101
PICCs. *See* Peripherally inserted central venous catheters
Pick's disease, 1576
Pickwickian syndrome, 595*t*
PICO format for evidence-based prac-tice questions, 6, 6*t*

PID. *See* Pelvic inflammatory disease
Pigmented nail beds, 451, 451*f*
Pilocarpine (Pilocar, Pilopine)
  for glaucoma, 435*t*
  for Sjögren syndrome, 1726
Pilonidal cyst, 940*t*
Pilonidal sinus, 1084
Pimicromilus (Elidel), 476
Pindolol (Visken), 774*t*
Pink-eye, 422
Pinna, swelling of, 413*t*
Pioglitazone (Actos), 1265, 1266*t*
Pioglitazone and glimepiride (Duetact), 1266*t*
Pipecuronium (Arduan), 370*t*
Piperidine, 537*t*
Pirbuterol (Maxair), 619*t*, 620
Piroxicam (Feldene, Novopirocam)
  for arthritis and connective tissue disorders, 1698*t*
  and gastritis, 1013
  mechanism of action, 202*t*
  photosensitivity, 461*t*
PIs. *See* Protease inhibitors
Pit vipers, 1835, 1835*f*
Pitressin (vasopressin)
  for cirrhosis, 1110*t*
  for diabetes insipidus, 1297, 1479
  for gastrointestinal bleeding, 998*t*
  for septic shock, 1788
  for shock, 1788*t*
Pitting edema, 749*t*, 826
Pituitary adenoma, 1488*t*
Pituitary gland
  diagnostic studies, 1247, 1248*t*-1249*t*
  hormones of, 1239-1240, 1239*f*
  hypofunction of, **1293-1294**
    clinical manifestations of, 1294
    collaborative care for, 1294
    diagnostic studies, 1294
    etiology and pathophysiology of, 1293-1294
    nursing management of, **1294**
  hypothalamic-pituitary-adrenal axis, 113, 113*f*
  radiology, 1249*t*
  regulation of water by, 319-320
  serum studies, 1248*t*
  surgery on, 1291-1292, 1292*f*
PKD. *See* Polycystic kidney disease
Placebos, 147
Plague, in bioterrorism, 1840*t*
Planning
  advance care planning, 155
  for discharge, 394
  for end-of-life care, 158
  nursing phase, 9, **12-14**
  with older adults, 78
  patient education, 60-63
Plantar fasciitis, 1623*t*
Plantar flexion, 1622*t*
Plantar neuroma, 1685*t*
Plantar warts, 468*t*, 1685*t*
Plaque
  on lips or in mouth, 939*t*
  primary, 455*t*
Plaquenil (hydroxychloroquine)
  for arthritis and connective tissue disorders, 1700*t*
  drug alert, 1705
  for polymyositis and dermatomyosities, 1726
  for rheumatoid arthritis, 1705
  for systemic lupus erythematosus, 1719
Plasma, 666-667
  shifts of interstitial fluid to, 319
  shifts to interstitial fluid, 318-319

Plasma cell myeloma, 728
Plasma cells, 220
Plasma chemistries, 1855*t*-1858*t*
Plasma clotting factors, 669-670, 670*t*
Plasma expanders, 340
Plasma oncotic pressure, 319
Plasma osmolality, 1240, 1240*f*
Plasma thromboplastin antecedent, 670*t*
Plasma thromboplastin component, 670*t*
Plasmacytoma, 675*t*
Plasmapheresis, 234-235, 1556
Plasminogen activator, recombinant, 800*t*
Plasmodium malariae, 245
Platelet count, 678, 678*t*, 679*t*
  in deep vein thrombosis, 911*t*
  in hemophilia, 709*t*
  laboratory values, 1859*t*
  preoperative, 351
  in shock, 1775*t*
Platelet growth factor
  for cancer treatment, 304*t*
  clinical uses of, 223*t*
Platelet-activating factor, 226*t*
Plateletpheresis, 234
Platelets, 226*t*, 666*f*, 668, 731*t*
  effects of aging on, 672*t*
  formation of, 669
Platinol (cisplatin)
  for bladder cancer, 1179
  for cervical cancer, 1402
  for lung cancer, 582
  nephrotoxicity, 1142*t*
  for oral cancer, 1002
  for testicular cancer, 1432
Platinol-AQ (cisplatin)
  classification of, 287*t*
  method of administration, 288*t*
Platinum drugs, 287*t*
Plavix (clopidogrel)
  for chronic stable angina and acute coronary syndrome, 800*t*
  drug alert, 1505
  for long-term therapy after TIAs, 1505
  for peripheral arterial disease of lower extremities, 902
  to prevent stroke, 1510
  for stroke, 1512
Plegine (phendimetrazine), 981
Plenaxis (abarelix), 1426, 1426*t*
Plendil (felodipine)
  for chronic stable angina and acute coronary syndrome, 800*t*
  for hypertension, 776*t*
Pletal (cilostazol), 902
Plethora, 700
Plethysmography, 1627*t*
Pleural disorders, 587*f*, 596*t*
Pleural drainage, **588-592**
  clinical guidelines for care of patient with, 591*t*
  systems, 589*f*
    first compartment, 589
    second compartment, 589
    third compartment, 589
Pleural effusion, 512, 588, **595-596**
  chest examination findings in, 526*t*
  clinical manifestations of, 596
  collaborative care for, 596
  exudative, 595
  in heart failure, 826
  in pneumonia, 565
  and restrictive lung disease, 596*t*
  in tuberculosis, 571
  types of, 595-596
Pleural friction rub, 524, 525*t*, 1875

Pleurisy, 597
  in pneumonia, 565
  and restrictive lung disease, 596*t*
Pleuritic chest pain, 519*t*
Pleuritis, 597
  and restrictive lung disease, 596*t*
Pleurodesis, 587
Plicamycin (Mithracin)
  classification of, 287*t*
  for hypercalcemia, 330
PLV. *See* Partial liquid ventilation
PM. *See* Polymyositis
PMD-D. *See* Premenstrual dysphoric disorder
PMR. *See* Progressive muscle relaxation
PMS. *See* Premenstrual syndrome
PN. *See* Parenteral nutrition
Pneumatic antishock garment, 1824
Pneumatic retinopexy, 431
Pneumaturia, 1145*t*
Pneumoccocal vaccine, 566
Pneumococcal pneumonia, 564-565, 565*f*
Pneumoconiosis, 577
  coalworker's (black lung), 578*t*
Pneumocystis pneumonia, 576*t*
Pneumocystis jiroveci, 245*t*, 576*t*
Pneumocystis jiroveci pneumonia, 255*t*, 265, 266*f*, 564
Pneumomediastinum, 1764
Pneumonectomy, 593*t*
Pneumonia, 561-569
  acquisition of organisms that cause, 561
  acute intervention for, 569
  ambulatory and home care for, 569
  aspiration, 564, 604
  associated with HIV infection, 254*t*
  chest examination findings in, 526*t*
  clinical manifestations of, 565
  collaborative care for, 566-567, 566*t*
  community-acquired, 562-563
    drug therapy of, 562-563, 563*t*
    guidelines for management of, 562
    organisms associated with, 562*t*
  complications of, 565
  cytomegalovirus, 564
  diagnostic studies, 565-566, 566*t*
  drug therapy of, 566-567
  etiology of, 561
  factors predisposing to, 561, 561*t*
  findings in, 567*t*
  fungal, 564
  health care–associated, 563-564
  health promotion in, 567-569
  hospital-acquired, 563-564
    in acute respiratory distress syndrome, 1815
    organisms associated with, 562*t*
  nursing assessment of, 567, 567*t*
    important health information, 567*t*
    objective data, 567*t*
    subjective data, 567*t*
  nursing care plan for patient with, 568*b*
  nursing diagnoses, 567
  nursing evaluation of, 569
  nursing implementation for, 567-569
  nursing management of, **567-569**
  nursing planning, 567
  nutritional therapy of, 567
  opportunistic, 564
  organisms associated with, 562*t*
  P. jiroveci, 255*t*, 265, 266*f*, 564
  pathophysiology of, 564-565
  pneumococcal, 564

Pneumonia *(Continued)*
  PORT (Pneumonia Patient Outcomes Research Team) Severity Index (PSI), 562, 562*t*
  and restrictive lung disease, 596*t*
  stages of, 564-565
  tuberculosis, 571
  types of, 562-564
  ventilator-associated, 563-564, 1764-1765
Pneumonitis
  chemical (noninfectious), 564, 577
  in chemotherapy and radiation therapy, 296*t*
  in HIV infection, 254*t*
  hypersensitivity, 577
Pneumothorax, 585-587
  clinical manifestations of, 587
  closed, 585
  collaborative care for, 587
  emergency management of, 586*t*
  open, 585-586, 587*f*
  and restrictive lung disease, 596*t*
  tension pneumothorax, 586-587, 587*f*
  types of, 585-587
Pneumovax, 519
PNI. *See* Psychoneuroimmunology
Podofilox, 1376
Podophyllotoxin, 720*t*
Poikilothermia, 1777
Poikilothermism, 1595
Point of maximal impulse, 750
Poisoning, 1837-1838, 1837*t*
  E. coli O157:H7, 1031-1033, 1037*t*
  food poisoning, **1031-1033**
Polaramine (dexchlorpheniramine), 537*t*
Poliomyelitis, 1610
  postpolio syndrome, **1610-1611**
Poliovirus, 244*t*
Polish Americans, 72
Polyarthritis, 876
Polyclonal antibodies, 239*t*, 240
Polycystic kidney disease, 1176-1177, 1176*f*
  clinical manifestations of, 1176
  collaborative care for, 1176-1177
  genetics of, 1176*b*
Polycystic ovary syndrome, 1399-1400
Polycythemia, 673, **700-701**
  clinical manifestations of, 700
  collaborative care for, 701
  complications of, 700
  diagnostic studies, 700-701
  etiology and pathophysiology of, 700
  secondary, 700, 700*f*
Polycythemia vera, 700, 700*f*
  collaborative care for, 701
  laboratory manifestations of, 700-701
  nursing management of, **701**
Polyderm, 205*t*
Polydipsia, 320, 1247*t*
Polyendocrine deficiency syndrome, 1316
Polyethylene glycol (GoLYTELY), 138, 1042*t*
Polymerase chain reaction, 241
Polymyositis, 1725-1726
  clinical manifestations of, 1725
  complications of, 1725
  diagnostic studies, 1725
  etiology and pathophysiology of, 1725
  nursing and collaborative management of, **1725-1726**

Polymyxin B, 1142*t*
Polyneuropathies, 1585-1589
   postinfectious (*See* Guillain-Barré syndrome)
Polypharmacy, 80
Polyps
   cervical, **1399**
   collaborative care for, 1063
   colonic, 1062, 1063*f*
   diagnostic studies, 1063
   of large intestine, **1062-1063**
   laryngeal, **551**
   nasal, **541**
   types of, 1063, 1063*t*
Polyskin, 205*t*
Polysomnography, 542
Polyuria, 1145*t,* 1247*t*
Pondimin (fenfluramine), 981
Porcine heterografts, 883*t*
Porphobilinogen, 1863*t*
PORT (Pneumonia Patient Outcomes Research Team) Severity Index (PSI), 562, 562*t*
Portable chest drainage units, 590, 590*f*
Portable liquid oxygen units, 643*f,* 644, 645*f*
Portal cirrhosis, 1102
Portal hypertension
   and ascites, 1105*t*
   in cirrhosis, 1103-1104
Portex fenestrated tracheostomy tube, 544*t*
Portex speaking tracheostomy tube, 544*t*
Portion sizes, 979, 980*f*
Portosystemic shunts, 1108, 1109*f,* 1110*f*
Position sense, 1458-1459
Positioning. *See* Patient positioning
Positive end-expiratory pressure (PEEP), 1761*t,* 1762-1763
   auto-PEEP, 1762
   best or optimal, 1762
   physiologic, 1762
Positive expiratory pressure therapy, 1767*t*
   flutter mucus clearance device for, 648, 648*f*
Positive findings, 47
Positive inotropes, 832-833, 1739
Positive pressure ventilation, 1760, 1760*f*
   in acute respiratory failure, 1810
   complications of, 1763-1766
   extubation, 1766-1768
   noninvasive bilevel, 1810, 1810*f*
   nutritional therapy for patients receiving, 1766
   outcome phase, 1766
   preweaning or assessment phase, 1766-1767
   psychosocial needs during, 1765-1766
   weaning from, 1766-1768
      indications for, 1767*t*
Positron emission tomography, 754*t,* 758
   hematologic, 682*t*
   of nervous system, 1463*t*
   of respiratory system, 526-528, 528*t*

Postanesthesia care
   phase I, 377, 377*t*
   phase II, 377, 377*t*
   phase III, 377, 377*t*
Postanesthesia care unit (PACU), 376
   admission report, 377, 377*t*
   admission to, 377-378
   cardiovascular problems in, 382, 386-387
   discharge from, **393**
   initial assessment in, 377, 377*t*
   neurologic/psychologic problems in, 387-388
   progression through, 377
   rapid progression through, 377
   respiratory problems in, 378-380
Postcoital bleeding, 1334
Postcoital studies, 1382
Postconcussion syndrome, 1482
Posterior cerebral artery, 1507*t*
Posterior cord syndrome, 1592
Posterior fourchette, 1327
Posterior pituitary gland hormones, 1236*t,* 1239-1240
Posterior surface inspection, 1826*t,* 1827
Posterior thorax examination, 49*t*
Postexposure prophylaxis of HIV infection, 263
Postmenopause, 1390-1393
   clinical manifestations of, 1390-1391, 1390*t*
   collaborative care for, 1391-1392
   drug therapy for, 1391-1392
   nonhormonal therapy for, 1392
   nursing management of, **1393**
   nutritional therapy for, 1392
Postmortem care, 161
Postoperative care, **376-378**
   of acute abdominal pain, 1045-1046
   ambulatory surgery, **394**
   of amputation, 1660-1661
   analgesia, 389*b*
   of benign prostatic hyperplasia, 1421-1422
   cardiovascular problems, **382-386**
   case study, 395
   for chest surgery, 593
   of colorectal cancer, 1068
   for cosmetic surgery, 480
   in Cushing syndrome, 1315
   for esophageal cancer, 1011
   of fractures, 1643-1645
   gastrointestinal problems, **390-391**
   gerontologic considerations, **394-395**
   of hip fracture, 1654
   of hyperthyroidism, 1304
   for incisional cholecystectomy, 1131
   of inflammatory bowel disease, 1056
   of joint surgery, 1665
   of kidney transplant recipient, 1228-1229
   for laparoscopic cholecystectomy, 1131
   leg exercises, 387, 387*f*
   of live donor, 1228
   of mandibular fracture, 1657-1658
   nursing care plan for postoperative patient, 383*b*-386*b*
   of obese patient, 984-985
   after ostomy surgery, 1071-1072
   of peptic ulcer disease, 1027
   potential problems in, 378, 380*f*
   for renal surgery, 1188
   respiratory problems, **378-381**
   of stomach cancer, 1030-1031
   for ureteral surgery, 1188
   of urinary diversion, 1190-1193

Postpolio syndrome, 1610-1611
   etiology and pathophysiology of, 1610-1611
   nursing and collaborative management of, **1611**
Postural abnormalities, 1712, 1712*f*
Postural drainage, 647
   positions for, 647, 648*f*
Postural stability loss, 1521-1522, 1521*f*
Posturing
   decerebrate, 1472, 1472*f*
   decorticate, 1472, 1472*f*
Posturography, 414*t*
Potassium (K+), 1147*t*
   in burn patients, 500
   daily requirements in chronic kidney disease, 1211-1212, 1212*t*
   high-potassium foods, 1213, 1213*t*
   laboratory values, 1857*t*
   normal values, 321*t*
   restriction for chronic kidney disease, 1212-1213
   serum levels, 1627*t*
   in shock, 1775*t*
Potassium channel blockers, 856*t*
Potassium hydroxide (KOH), 458*t*
Potassium imbalances, 326-329
   in acute renal failure, 1200
   causes and clinical manifestations of, 327*t*
   in chronic kidney disease, 1207
   factors causing, 327
Potassium salts, 1267*t*
Potassium-sparing diuretics, 773*t*
Potentiation, 178
Pouchogram, 1193
Power of attorney for health care, durable, 655*b*
Pox viruses, 244*t,* 1367*t*
PPH. *See* Primary pulmonary hypertension
PPIs. *See* Proton pump inhibitors
PPN. *See* Peripheral parenteral nutrition
PPO. *See* Preferred provider organizations
PQRST assessment of angina, 796*t*
PR interval, 846, 847*t*
Pramipexole (Mirapex)
   for Parkinson's disease, 1551, 1552*t*
   for restless legs syndrome, 1558
Pramlintide (Symlin)
   for diabetes mellitus, 1265, 1266*t*
   drug alert, 1265
   mechanism of action, 1265
Prandin (repaglinide), 1265, 1266*t*
Pravastatin (Pravachol), 793, 795*t*
Prayer, 95, 96*f,* 100
   clinical applications of, 100
   colloquial, 100
   description of, 97*t*
   forms of, 100
   intercessory, 100
   meditative, 100
   ritualistic, 100
Prayer groups, 95, 96*f*
Prazosin (Minipress)
   for hypertension, 774*t*
   and lower urinary tract function, 1180*t*
   for pheochromocytoma, 1320
Prazosin/polythiazide (Minizide), 777*t*
Prealbumin, 956*t*
Precontemplation stage of change, 188
Precose (acarbose), 1265, 1266*t*
Prediabetes, 1255
   weight loss interventions and, 1257*b*

Prednisone (Orasone), 238, 239*t*
   adverse cardiovascular effects of, 745*t*
   for arthritis and connective tissue disorders, 1699*t*
   for asthma and COPD, 618*t*
   for Bell's palsy, 1585
   classification of, 287*t*
   for inflammatory bowel disease, 1055*t*
   for leukemia, 720*t,* 721*t*
   for multiple myeloma, 729
   for multiple sclerosis, 1544, 1544*t*
   for myasthenia gravis, 1556
   for non-Hodgkin's lymphoma, 727*t*
   for pain, 139
   for prostate cancer, 1427
Preferred provider organizations (PPOs), 86, 86*n*
Pregnancy
   ectopic, **1389-1390**
   herpes simplex virus infection in, 1374
   lupus and, 1721-1722
   pseudopregnancy, 1397
Pregnancy testing, 1336
Pregnyl, 1383*t*
Prehypertension, 761
   definition of, 761
   management of, 769*t*
Preimplantation genetic diagnosis, 217
Prelief (calcium glycerophosphate), 1164
Preload, 742, 828, 1738
   normal range at rest, 1739*t*
Premalignant skin conditions, 464*t*
Premarin (estrogen)
   for perimenopause and postmenopause, 1391
   for voiding dysfunction, 1185*t*
Premature atrial contractions, 850, 850*f*
   characteristics of, 849*t*
   clinical associations, 850
   clinical significance of, 850
   ECG characteristics, 850
   treatment of, 850
Premature ventricular contractions, 854, 854*f*
   characteristics of, 849*t*
   clinical associations, 854
   clinical significance of, 854
   ECG characteristis, 854
   multifocal, 854, 854*f*
   treatment of, 854
   unifocal, 854
Premenstrual dysphoric disorder, 1385
Premenstrual syndrome (PMS), 1385-1386
   clinical manifestations of, 1385
   collaborative care for, 1385-1386, 1386*t*
   diagnostic studies, 1385-1386
   drug therapy for, 1386
   etiology and pathophysiology of, 1385
Prempro (estrogen + progestin), 745*t*
Preoperative care, **343-358**
   of acute abdominal pain, 1045
   of amputation, 1659-1660
   of benign prostatic hyperplasia, 1421
   case study, 356-357
   checklist for, 355*t*
   before chest surgery, 592
   of colorectal cancer, 1068
   for cosmetic surgery, 480
   culturally competent care, **356**

Preoperative care *(Continued)*
  in Cushing syndrome, 1315
  day-of-surgery preparation, 354, 354*f*
  diagnostic studies, 349-350, 351*t*
  for esophageal cancer, 1011
  fasting recommendations, 352*t*
  of fractures, 1643
  gerontologic considerations for, **356**
  of hip fracture, 1653-1654
  of joint surgery, 1664-1665
  of kidney transplant recipient, 1228
  of mandibular fracture, 1657
  medications, 354
  nursing assessment, **344-356**
    goals, 344
    objective data, 349-350
    subjective data, 344-349
  nursing management, **350-356, 364-366**
  nursing management before surgery, **363-364**
  of obese patient, 984-985
  for ostomy surgery, 1070-1071
  of peptic ulcer disease, 1027
  physiologic assessment, 349, 351*t*
  psychosocial assessment, 344-346, 345*t*
  for renal surgery, 1188
  of stomach cancer, 1030
  systems review, 347-349
  teaching, 350-352
  for ureteral surgery, 1188
  of urinary diversion, 1190
Preparation for change, 188
Prepping, 366
Prepuce problems, 1429-1430
Presbycusis, 409, 446
  classification of, 446*t*
Presbyopia, 400, 416, 417
Pressure release ventilation, 1762
Pressure support ventilation, 1761*t*, 1762
Pressure ulcers, 206-211
  acute intervention for, 209-211
  ambulatory and home care, 211
  Braden scale for predicting risk of, 207-209, 208*t*
  clinical manifestations of, 206
  collaborative management of, **206-211**
  etiology and pathophysiology of, 206
  evaluation of, 211
  health promotion in, 209
  nursing assessment of, 207-209, 209*t*
  nursing care plan for patient with, 210*b*
  nursing implementation for, 209-211
  nursing management of, **206-211**
  nursing planning for, 209
  patient and family teaching guide, 210*t*
  risk factors for, 206, 206*t*
  staging of, 206, 207*t*
Pressure ventilation, 1760, 1762
Pressure-controlled inverse ratio ventilation, 1761*t*, 1762
Pressyn (vasopressin), 1788*t*
Prevacid (lansoprazole)
  for acute gastritis, 1014
  for gastroesophageal reflux disease, 1006, 1006*t*
  for gastrointestinal bleeding, 998*t*
  for peptic ulcer disease, 1019*t*, 1020
Prevention
  collaborative preventive care for stroke, 1509-1511
  sexual assault, 1411*t*
  of stroke, 1510*b*
  surgery for, 343

Prialt (ziconotide), 141-142
Priapism, 698, 1430, 1607
Priftin (rifapentine), 573*t*
Prilocaine, 139*t*, 371
Prilosec (omeprazole)
  for acute gastritis, 1014
  for acute pancreatitis, 1121*t*
  for gastroesophageal reflux disease, 1006, 1006*t*
  for gastrointestinal bleeding, 998*t*
  for peptic ulcer disease, 1019*t*, 1020
Primacor (milrinone)
  for acute decompensated HF, 829
  as positive inotrope, 1739
Primary biliary cirrhosis, 1101
Primary pulmonary hypertension
  clinical manifestations of, 601
  collaborative care for, 601-602, 601*f*
  etiology and pathophysiology of, 600-601, 601*f*
Primary sclerosing cholangitis, 1102
Primary survey, 1823-1824, 1824*t*, 1825*t*
Primatene spray, 624
Primidone (Mysoline)
  gerontologic considerations for, 1538
  for seizures, 1538*t*
Prinivil (lisinopril)
  for diabetes mellitus, 1285
  for hypertension, 776*t*
  and reproductive system, 1332
Prinzide (lisinopril/hydrochlorothiazide), 777*t*
Prinzmetal's angina, 797, 798*t*
PRK. *See* Photorefractive keratectomy
Proaccelerin, 670*t*
Pro-Banthine (propantheline)
  for acute pancreatitis, 1121*t*
  for multiple sclerosis, 1544*t*
  for voiding dysfunction, 1185*t*
Probenecid (Benemid)
  blood glucose level effects, 1267*t*
  for syphilis, 1371*t*
Problem identification, 10, 11, **50**, 50*f*
Problem-centered assessment, 40
Problem–etiology–signs and symptoms (PES) format for nursing diagnoses, 11
Problem-focused coping, 116, 116*t*
Procainamide (Pronestyl)
  for atrial fibrillation, 852
  for atrial flutter, 851
  autoreactivity to, 234
  classification of, 856*t*
  for ventricular tachycardia, 855
Procaine penicillin G, 1371*t*
Procarbazine (Matulane, Natulan)
  for brain tumors, 1490
  classification of, 288*t*
  food/nutrient interactions, 954*t*
Procardia (nifedipine)
  for acute coronary syndrome, 800*t*
  blood glucose level effects, 1267*t*
  for chronic stable angina, 800*t*, 801
  effects on lower urinary tract function, 1180*t*
  for hypertension, 776*t*, 1210
Procedural information, 352*t*
Process information, 351, 352*t*
Prochlorperazine (Compazine)
  as adjunct to general anesthesia, 370*t*
  for nausea and vomiting, 138, 992, 992*t*
Procoagulants, 670

Procrit (epoetin alfa)
  for anemia, 1211
  for cancer treatment, 304*t*
  clinical uses of, 223*t*
Proctocolectomy, total
  with continent ileostomy, 1055-1056
  with permanent ileostomy, 1055
Prodrome, 1528
Prodysrhythmia, 856
Profasi, 1383*t*
Progesterone
  laboratory values, 1857*t*
  serum levels, 1338*t*, 1341*t*
  target tissue and functions, 1236*t*
Progestin + estrogen (Ortho-Novum, Prempro), 745*t*
Prograf (tacrolimus), 238, 239*t*, 1267*t*
Programmed theory of cell death, 68*t*, 69
Progressive care units (PCUs), 1735
Progressive muscle relaxation, 119, 119*t*
Prokinetics
  for gastroesophageal reflux disease, 1006, 1006*t*
  for nausea and vomiting, 992, 992*t*
Prolactin, 1239
  assay, 1338*t*
  serum levels, 1249*t*
  target tissue and functions, 1236*t*
Prolactinoma, 1293
Prolapse of mitral valve, 879
Proleukin (aldesleukin), 223*t*, 303*t*
Proliferative vitreoretinopathy, 431
Promazine (Sparine), 992*t*
Promethazine (Phenergan)
  as adjunct to general anesthesia, 370*t*
  for nausea and vomiting, 992, 992*t*
Prompted voiding, 1183*t*
Pronation, 1622*t*
Pronator drift, 1458
Prone positioning, 1763
Pronestyl (procainamide)
  for atrial flutter, 851
  autoreactivity to, 234
  classification of, 856*t*
Propafenone (Rythmol)
  for atrial fibrillation, 852
  for atrial flutter, 851
  classification of, 856*t*
Propantheline (Pro-Banthine)
  for acute pancreatitis, 1121*t*
  for multiple sclerosis, 1544*t*
  for voiding dysfunction, 1185*t*
Propine (dipivefrin), 434*t*
Propofol (Diprivan), 369*t*
Propoxyphene (Darvon), 138
Propranolol (Inderal)
  for acute coronary syndrome, 800*t*
  for chronic stable angina, 799, 800*t*
  for cirrhosis, 1110*t*
  ethnic differences in response to, 35*t*
  for hypertension, 774*t*
  for hyperthyroidism, 1301
  and lower urinary tract function, 1180*t*
  for pheochromocytoma, 1320
  and reproductive system, 1332
  for restless legs syndrome, 1558
  toxicology, 1865*t*
Propranolol/hydrochlorothiazide (Inderide), 777*t*
Propylthiouracil (PTU), 1301
Proscar (finasteride)
  for benign prostatic hyperplasia, 1416-1417
  drug alert, 1417
  for voiding dysfunction, 1185*t*

Prostaglandins, 195-196, 195*t*, 197*f*, 226*t*
Prostate brachytherapy, 1425-1426, 1426*f*
Prostate cancer, 1422-1428
  acute intervention for, 1428
  ambulatory and home care for, 1428
  brachytherapy for, 1425-1426
  chemotherapy for, 1427
  clinical manifestations of, 1422-1423
  collaborative care for, 1423-1427, 1424*t*
  complications of, 1422-1423
  conservative therapy of, 1424
  culturally competent care for, **1427**
  diagnostic studies, 1423
  drug therapy for, 1426-1427
  etiology and pathophysiology of, 1422
  health disparities and, 21*t*
  health promotion in, 1428
  hormonal therapy for, 1426-1427, 1426*t*
  hormone refractory, 1426, 1427
  nursing assessment of, 1427, 1427*t*
  nursing diagnoses, 1427-1428
  nursing evaluation of, 1428
  nursing implementation for, 1428
  nursing management of, **1427-1428**
  nursing planning for, 1428
  radiation therapy for, 1425-1426
  screening guidelines for early detection of, 282*t*
  surgical therapy of, 1424-1425
  Whitmore-Jewett staging classification of, 1423, 1423*t*
Prostate gland, 1324
  age-related changes in, 1331*t*
  physical examination of, 1335
  problems of, **1414-1429**
  transurethral electrovaporization of, 1418*t*
  transurethral incision of, 1418, 1418*t*
  transurethral resection of, 1417-1418, 1418*f*, 1418*t*
Prostate surgery
  discharge planning and home care issues after, 1422
  nursing care plan for patient having, 1420*b*
Prostatectomy
  approaches to, 1424-1425, 1424*f*
  description of, 1332*t*
  laser, 1418*t*, 1419
  nerve-sparing procedure, 1425
  open, 1418*t*
  perineal
    approach, 1424, 1424*f*
  radical
    urinary incontinence after, 1425*b*
  retropubic
    approach, 1424, 1424*f*
Prostate-specific antigen (PSA), 1423
  blood levels, 1338*t*
  laboratory values, 1857*t*
Prostatitis, 1428-1429
  asymptomatic inflammatory, 1428
  categories of, 1428
  chronic, 1428
  clinical manifestations of, 1428-1429
  complications of, 1428-1429
  diagnostic studies, 1429
  etiology and pathophysiology of, 1428
  nursing and collaborative management of, **1429**

Prostheses
  Blom-Singer voice prosthesis, 557, 557*f*
  femoral head, 1654, 1654*t*
  heart valves, 882, 883*f*, 883*t*
  types of, 1660, 1660*f*
Prosthetic vascular graft infection, 897
Prostigmin (neostigmine), 370, 1544*t*
Prostin E₂ (dinoprostone), 1384*t*
Protamine sulfate tests, 679*t*
Protease, 251
Protease inhibitors
  adverse effects of, 258*t*
  mechanism of action, 257, 257*t*
Proteasome inhibitors, 303*t*
Proteasomes, 302
Protein(s)
  cerebrospinal fluid analysis, 1864*t*
  complete, 949
  corticosteroid metabolism of, 1318
  daily requirements in chronic kidney disease, 1211-1212, 1212*t*
  in diabetic meal plan, 1268
  dietary guidelines, 949
  high-calorie, high-protein diet, 958*t*
  incomplete, 949
  laboratory values, 1857*t*
  loss in peritoneal dialysis, 1219-1220
  metabolism of, 932*t*
  metabolism tests, 946*t*
  in parenteral nutrition, 965
  quantitative test for, 1146*t*, 1863*t*
  sources of, 950*t*
  synthesis of, 214, 215*f*
  urinary, 1146*t*, 1863*t*
Protein deficiency, 201*t*
Protein foods with high biologic value, 306, 306*t*
Protein hormone receptors, 1236-1237, 1237*f*
Protein restriction, 1211-1212
Protein-calorie malnutrition, 951-952
  manifestations of, 953, 955*t*
Proteinuria, 1168
Proteus, 244*t*, 562*t*, 1155*t*
Prothrombin, 670*t*, 946*t*
Prothrombin conversion accelerator, 670*t*
Prothrombin time, 679*t*
  in hemophilia, 709*t*
  laboratory values, 1859*t*
  preoperative, 351
  in shock, 1775*t*
Proton pump inhibitors
  for acute pancreatitis, 1121*t*
  for cirrhosis, 1110*t*
  for gastroesophageal reflux disease, 1006*t*
  for gastrointestinal bleeding, 997, 998*t*
  for peptic ulcer disease, 1019*t*, 1020
  for upper gastrointestinal bleeding, 997
Protonix (pantoprazole)
  for cirrhosis, 1110*t*
  for gastroesophageal reflux disease, 1006, 1006*t*
  for gastrointestinal bleeding, 998*t*
  for peptic ulcer disease, 1019*t*, 1020
  for upper gastrointestinal bleeding, 997
  for variceal bleeding, 1108

Protooncogenes, 214*t*, 274
Protozoa, 245
"Proud flesh," 201, 202*f*
Proventil (albuterol), 619*t*, 620
Provera (medroxyprogesterone)
  drug alert, 1392
  for perimenopause and postmenopause, 1392
Provigil (modafinil)
  for multiple sclerosis, 1545, 1545*t*
  for opioid-induced sedation, 138
Prozac (fluoxetine)
  for Alzheimer's disease, 1569, 1569*t*
  for pain, 139
Pruritus, 454, 675*t*
  acute intervention for, 1131
  control of, 477-478
PRV. *See* Pressure release ventilation
PSA. *See* Prostate-specific antigen
PSCT. *See* Peripheral stem cell transplantation
Pseudoaneurysms, 895
Pseudoarthrosis, 1638*t*
Pseudocysts, pancreatic, 1119
Pseudoephedrine (Sudafed)
  for allergic rhinitis and sinusitis, 538*t*
  drug alert, 540
  effects on lower urinary tract function, 1180*t*
Pseudofolliculitis, 457
Pseudogout, 1716
Pseudohypertension, 765
Pseudomenopause, 1397
Pseudomonas, 1155*t*
Pseudomonas aeruginosa, 244*t*, 562*t*
Pseudopregnancy, 1397
PSI. *See* PORT (Pneumonia Patient Outcomes Research Team) Severity Index
Psilocybin (mushrooms), 170*t*
PSNS. *See* Parasympathetic nervous system
Psoriasis, 471, 471*f*, 472*t*
Psoriatic arthritis, 1713
PSV. *See* Pressure support ventilation
PSVT. *See* Paroxysmal supraventricular tachycardia
Psychedelic agents, 181
Psychoemotional problems, 296*t*
Psychologic abuse, 73*t*
Psychologic dependence, 166*t*, 168
Psychologic factors, cultural, 35
Psychologic problems
  in acute respiratory distress syndrome, 1816*t*
  in chronic kidney disease, 1209
  elder mistreatment, 73*t*
  nursing assessment of, 388
  nursing diagnoses, 388
  nursing implementation for, 388
  nursing management of, **388**
  postoperative, **387-388**
Psychologic status
  assessment of, 57*t*, 58
  and coronary artery disease, 791
  physical examination of, 51*t*
Psychologic support
  in breast cancer, 1360
  interventions for helping overweight individuals lose weight, 981*b*
  for rheumatoid arthritis patients, 1711
  for STD patients, 1378-1379
Psychomotor seizures, 1535
Psychoneuroimmunology, 114
Psychosis
  Korsakoff's psychosis, 178
  stimulant psychosis, 174

Psychosocial assessment
  preoperative, 344-346
  before surgery, 363
Psychosocial care
  for burns, 493*t*, 503
  for COPD, 655
  end-of-life care, 158-160, 160*t*
    approaching death, 153, 153*t*
    manifestations at, **153**
    nursing diagnoses related to, 158*t*
  with fractures, 1647-1648
  in positive pressure ventilation, 1765-1766
  in systemic lupus erythematosus, 1722-1723
Psychostimulants, 745*t*
Psyllium (Metamucil)
  for constipation, 1042*t*, 1519
  uses, 796*b*
PT. *See* Physical therapy
PTC. *See* Percutaneous transhepatic cholangiography
Ptosis, 406*t*, 1520
PTT. *See* Partial thromboplastin time
PTU (propylthiouracil), 1301
Pubertal gynecomastia, 1348
Pubis, 1335
Public education. *See also* Patient education
  for prevention and detection of cancer, 281
Public health nursing, 85, 86
PUD. *See* Peptic ulcer disease
Pulmicort Respules (budesonide), 618*t*
Pulmicort Turbuhaler (budesonide), 618*t*
Pulmonary angiography, 526, 528*t*, 599
Pulmonary artery catheter, 513-514
Pulmonary artery catheterization, 1742*t*
Pulmonary artery diastolic pressure, 1739*t*
Pulmonary artery flow-directed catheter, 1741-1747, 1743*f*
  complications of, 1747
  insertion of, 1742-1743
Pulmonary artery pressure, 1741-1747
  measurement of, 1744, 1744*f*
  normal range at rest, 1739*t*
  in shock, 1774*t*
Pulmonary artery wedge pressure
  in acute respiratory distress syndrome, 1815*t*
  elevated, 1744, 1745*f*
  measurement of, 1744, 1744*f*
  normal range at rest, 1739*t*
  in shock, 1774*t*
Pulmonary blebs and bullae, 633, 634*f*
Pulmonary congestion, 1811
Pulmonary disease, obstructive, 607-663
  chronic, **629-655**
    chest examination findings in, 526*t*
    drug therapy for, 618*t*-620*t*
    gender differences in, 629*b*
  cultural and ethnic health disparities in, 608*b*
Pulmonary edema, 597-598
  acute decompensated heart failure and collaborative care for, 827*t*
  nursing and collaborative management of, **827-829**
  in acute decompensated HF, 824, 825*f*
  causes of, 597, 597*t*
  chest examination findings in, 526*t*
  delayed, 1833

Pulmonary edema *(Continued)*
  in postanesthesia care unit (PACU), 378
  postoperative, 379*t*
Pulmonary embolism, 598-600
  acute, 599*t*
  acute intervention for, 600
  ambulatory and home care for, 600
  clinical manifestations of, 598
  collaborative care for, 599-600
  complications of, 598-599
  conservative therapy of, 599
  diagnostic studies, 599
  drug therapy of, 600
  etiology and pathophysiology of, 598, 598*f*
  expected outcomes, 600
  health promotion in, 600
  nursing evaluation of, 600
  nursing implementation for, 600
  nursing management of, **600**
  postoperative, 379*t*
  surgical therapy of, 600
  treatment objectives for, 599
Pulmonary fibrosis, 577
  chest examination findings in, 526*t*
  idiopathic, **597**
Pulmonary function tests, 528*t*, 530
  airflow measures, 531*t*
  normal values, 531*f*, 531*t*
  preoperative, 351
  typical findings in COPD, 638
Pulmonary hypertension, 599, **600-604**
  primary, **600-602**
  secondary, **602**
Pulmonary infarction, 598
Pulmonary infection
  fungal, **575-576**
  treatment of, 1811
Pulmonary rehabilitation, 650-652
Pulmonary stenosis, 881
Pulmonary system
  in anemia, 686*t*
  effects of water aspiration on, 1832, 1833*f*
  positive pressure ventilation effects on, 1763
  in shock, 1779-1782
Pulmonary tuberculosis, 572*t*
Pulmonary vascular resistance, 1738, 1739
  normal range at rest, 1739*t*
  in shock, 1774*t*
Pulmonary vascular resistance index, 1739*t*
Pulmonic stenosis, 879*t*
Pulmonic valve disease, 881
  etiology and pathophysiology of, 881
Pulse
  assessment abnormalities, 749*t*
  in fluid and electrolyte imbalances, 338*t*
Pulse deficit, 750*t*, 751
Pulse oximetry, 514, 514*f*, 1747
Pulse pressure, 743-744
  in shock, 1774*t*
Pulseless electrical activity, 856
Pulselessness, 1650
Pulsus alternans, 749*t*
Pulsus paradoxus, 612, 872, 873*t*
Punch biopsy, 458*t*, 476
Punnett squares, 217, 218*f*
Pupil
  assessment abnormalities, 406*t*
  function testing, 405, 405*t*
  topical medications for dilation of, 426, 427*t*

Index

Pupillary check, 1476-1477, 1477t
Pure-tone audiometry, 414t, 415
Purine, 1171t
Purinethol (6-mercaptopurine), 287t, 720t
Purkinje fibers, 741, 846, 847t
Purpura, 454, 675t, 702
Pursed-lip breathing, 524t, 646
techniques to teach, 646
Purulent exudate, 197t
Pus, 197t, 1864t
Pustules, 455t
PVCs. *See* Premature ventricular contractions
PVR. *See* Proliferative vitreoretinopathy; Pulmonary vascular resistance
PVRI. *See* Pulmonary vascular resistance index
Pyelography
antegrade, 1147t
intravenous, 1147t
retrograde, 1148t
Pyelolithotomy, 1172
Pyelonephritis, 1155, 1161
acute, **1161-1162,** 1161f
chronic, 1161, **1162**
Pyloroplasty, 934t, 1026
Pyorrhea, 939t
Pyramid effect, 274
Pyramidal tracts, 1444-1445
Pyrazinamide (PZA), 573t, 574t
Pyridium (phenazopyridine)
nephrotoxicity of, 1142
for UTIs, 1158
Pyridostigmine (Mestinon), 370, 1556
Pyrosis, 939t, 1004, 1875
PZA (pyrazinamide), 573t, 574t

Q

QFT. *See* QuantiFERON-TB
Qi, 96, 97t
Qi gong, 97t, 98
QRS interval, 846, 847t
QT interval, 846, 847t
Quaalude (methaqualone), 169t
Quad coughing (augmented coughing), 1809
Quadriplegia, 1461t
Quality of life
exercise and, in multiple sclerosis, 1547b
noninvasive interventions and, in lung cancer, 583b
QuantiFERON-TB (QFT), 571
Questran (cholestyramine), 794, 795t
for bile reflux gastritis, 1026
blood glucose level effects, 1267t
food/nutrient interactions, 954t
for pruritus, 1129
Quetiapine (Seroquel)
for Alzheimer's disease, 1569, 1569t
for delirium, 1578
Quibron, 619
Quinapril (Accupril), 776t
Quinapril/hydrochlorothiazide (Accuretic), 777t
Quinidine
classification of, 856t
photosensitivity, 461t
Quinine, 1142t
Qvar, Qvar HFA, (beclomethasone), 618t

R

RA. *See* Rheumatoid arthritis
RabAvert (human diploid cell vaccine), 1837

Rabeprazole (Aciphex)
for gastroesophageal reflux disease, 1006, 1006t
for gastrointestinal bleeding, 998t
for peptic ulcer disease, 1019t, 1020
Rabies, 1498-1499
clinical manifestations of, 1498
diagnostic studies, 1498
etiology and pathophysiology of, 1498
nursing and collaborative management of, **1498-1499**
Rabies immune globulin (RIG) (BayRab), 1499, 1836-1837
Raccoon eyes
in head injury, 1481, 1482f
in nasal fracture, 534
Race, 20-21, 28
Rad, 292t
Radiation, 292, 462
acute radiation syndrome, 1840, 1841t
as carcinogenic agent, 275-276
effects of, 292-293
high-energy beams, 292
ionizing, 1840
low-energy beams, 292
malignancies correlated with, 275-276
measurement of, 292, 292t
Radiation therapy, **292-301**
accelerated fractionation, 292
adjuvant, 293
ALARA (as low as reasonably achievable), 294
for bladder cancer, 1179
for brain tumors, 1489-1490
for breast cancer, 1353-1354
breast conservation surgery with, 1353t
for cancers of female reproductive system, **1404-1407**
cardiovascular effects of, 300-301
for colorectal cancer, 1067
coping with, 301
definitive or primary, 293
for dermatologic problems, 474
for disease control, 293
distance from patient on, 294
external, 293
for cancers of female reproductive system, **1404**
for prostate cancer, 1425
for growth hormone excess, 1292
for head and neck cancer, 555-556
hyperfractionated, 292
hypofractionated, 292
immobilization device for, 293, 293f
intensity-modulated, 292
internal, 293-294
late effects of, **301-302**
for lung cancer, 582
maximal tolerated dose, 292
nadir, 297
neoadjuvant, 293
nursing implementation for, 294-301
nursing management for patients undergoing, **294-301**
nursing management of problems caused by, 295t-296t
for palliation, 293
palliative, 1354
prophylactic cranial radiation, 582
as prophylaxis, 293
prostate brachytherapy, 1425-1426, 1426f
for prostate cancer, 1425-1426
pulmonary effects of, 300

Radiation therapy *(Continued)*
reproductive effects of, 301
shielding, 294
simulation of, 293
skin reactions, 300t
nursing management of, 295t
skin reactions to, 299
time with patient on, 294
treatment, 293-294
Radical cystectomy, 1179
Radical neck dissection, 552, 552f
Radical neck surgery, 554b-556b
Radical pancreaticoduodenectomy, 1126, 1126f
Radical prostatectomy, 1425b
Radiculopathy, 1681
Radioactive iodine therapy, 1301, 1304
Radioactive iodine uptake, 1249t
Radiobiology, 292-293
Radiofrequency catheter ablation therapy, 861, 1117
Radiofrequency discal nucleoplasty, 1682
Radioisotopes
hematologic studies, 682t
method of administration, 288t
musculoskeletal studies, 1625t
Radiologic dispersal devices, 1840
Radiologic studies
gastrointestinal, 940-943, 941t-942t
hematologic, 681, 682t
lower gastrointestinal, 940
of musculoskeletal system, 1625t
of nervous system, 1461-1465, 1462t-1463t
pituitary, 1249t
reproductive, 1339t-1340t, 1341
respiratory, 526-528, 527t-528t
upper gastrointestinal, 940
urinary, 1147t-1149t
Radiology
adrenal, 1251t
interventional procedures
indications for, 903
for peripheral arterial disease of lower extremities, 903
pancreatic, 1252t
thyroid, 1249t
Radionuclide cystography, 1150t
Radionuclide imaging, renal, 1149t
Radiosensitivity, tumor, 292-293, 293t
Radiosurgery
for brain tumors, 1489-1490
gamma knife, 1582-1583, 1582t
stereotactic, 1492
Raloxifene (Evista)
for breast cancer, 1355
classification of, 288t
for osteoporosis, 1689-1690
for perimenopause and postmenopause, 1392
Raltitrexed (Tomudex), 1067
Ramipril (Altace), 776t
Randomized controlled trials, 107
Ranexa (ranolazine), 801
Range of motion
active, 1622
assessment of, 1622
limited, 1623t
passive, 1622
Ranibizumab (Lucentis), 432
Ranitidine (Zantac)
for acute gastritis, 1014
for acute pancreatitis, 1121t
for burns, 499t
for cirrhosis, 1110t
for gastroesophageal reflux disease, 1005-1006, 1006t

Ranitidine (Zantac) *(Continued)*
for gastrointestinal bleeding, 998t
for peptic ulcer disease, 1019t
preoperative, 355t
for variceal bleeding, 1108
Ranitidine bismuth citrate (Tritec), 1014
Ranolazine (Ranexa), 801
Ranvier, nodes of, 1443
RAP. *See* Right atrial pressure
Rapamune (sirolimus), 238, 239t
Rapid plasma reagin
blood test, 1339t
laboratory values, 1861t
Rapid postanesthesia care unit progression (RPP), 377
Rapid response team, 1734
Rapid shallow breathing index (f/V_T), 1767t
Rapidly progressive glomerulonephritis, 1166-1167
Rapid-sequence intubation, 1823
Rasagiline (Azilect), 1551, 1552t
Rash
heat rash, 1828
variations in light- and dark-skinned individuals, 456t
Rationing, 1115b
Raynaud's phenomenon, 908-909, 909f
primary, 908
secondary, 908
in systemic sclerosis, 1723
treatment of, 1724
Razadyne (galantamine), 1551, 1569t
RCTs. *See* Randomized controlled trials
RDDs. *See* Radiologic dispersal devices
Reactive arthritis, 1713
Reactive hyperemia, 901
Readiness to learn, 59
Real-time three-dimensional (3-D) ultrasound, 758
Rebetol (ribavirin)
for chronic hepatitis C, 1095
drug alert, 1095
Rebif (β-Interferon)
clinical uses of, 223t
drug alert, 1544
for multiple sclerosis, 1544, 1544t
Receptive aphasia, 1508
Recombinant DNA technology, 241, 241f
Recombivax HB (hepatitis B virus vaccine), 1096
Reconstructive microsurgery, 481
Rectal suppositories, 141
Rectocele, 1408, 1408f
repair of, 1332t
Rectum
age-related changes in, 932, 933t
assessment abnormalities, 940t
physical examination of, 938-939
Red blood cell count
cerebrospinal fluid analysis, 1864t
in shock, 1775t
Red blood cell morphology, 678t
Red blood cell tests, 677-678, 678t
Red blood cells, 666, 666f. *See also* Erythrocytes
frozen, 731t
packed, 731-732, 731t
Red cell distribution width, 1859t
Red hepatization, 564
Red wounds, 200, 200t, 204
Red yeast rice, 796b
Redness of inflammation, 196, 197t

5α-Reductase inhibitors
  for benign prostatic hyperplasia, 1416-1417
  for voiding dysfunction, 1185*t*
Redux (dexfenfluramine), 981
Red-yellow-black concept of wound care, 200, 200*t*
Reed-Sternberg cells, 723
Refeeding syndrome, 967
Referred pain, 129, 129*f*
Reflex arc, 1445, 1446*f*
Reflex bronchoconstriction, 516
Reflex incontinence, 1181*t*
Reflexes, 1445
  age-related changes in, 1454*t*
  assessment abnormalities, 1460*t*
  cough reflex, 516
  J reflex, 1814
  normal, 1459*t*
  after spinal cord injury, 1603
  testing, 1459, 1459*f*
Reflexic neurogenic bladder, 1604, 1605*t*
Reflux
  antireflux procedures, 1006
  bile reflux gastritis, 1026
  gastroesophageal reflux disease, **1003-1007**
    and asthma attacks, 610
    in COPD, 637
  urinary, 1140, 1168
Refraction, 399
Refractive errors, 399-400, 416
  correctable, **416-419**
  nonsurgical corrections, 417
  surgical therapy of, 418-419
Refractive intraocular lenses, 419
Refractive media, 399
Refractometry, 408*t*
Refractory hypoxemia, 1813, 1815*t*
Refracture, 1638*t*
Regional anesthesia, 142-143, 367
Registered nurse, 361
Registered nurse first assistant (RNFA), 362
Regitine (phentolamine), 774*t*
Reglan (metoclopramide)
  as adjunct to general anesthesia, 370*t*
  for gastroesophageal reflux disease, 1006, 1006*t*
  for nausea and vomiting, 138, 297, 992, 992*t*
  preoperative, 355*t*
Regulatory problems, 1233-1439
Regurgitation
  in gastroesophageal reflux disease, 1004
  valvular, 878, 878*f*
Rehabilitation
  acute, 87*t*
  after acute coronary syndrome, 813*t*
  of cancer, 285
  cardiac, 815
  cardiac programs, 794*b*
  counseling and referrals, 1649
  definition of, 815
  geriatric, 79-80, 79*f*
  home health care activities, 90*t*

Rehabilitation (Continued)
  pulmonary, 650-652
  respiratory, 1604
  after spinal cord injury, 1592, 1594*t*, 1604
  after stroke, 1521
    collaborative care, 1513-1514
    goals for, 1521
  voice, 556-557
Reiki, 98*t*
Reiter syndrome, 1713
Rejection
  acute, 238
  chronic, 238
  hyperacute (antibody-mediated, humoral), 238
  kidney transplantation, 1229
  transplant, 237-238
Relafen (nabumetone), 1698*t*
Relapse, 166, 166*t*
Relationships. See Role-relationship pattern
Relaxation
  muscle relaxation, 119-120
    passive, 120
    progressive, 119
  music for, 119
  strategies for, **116-120,** 116*t*, 143*t*, 144
Relaxation (abdominal) breathing, 117
  description of, 97*t*
  techniques for, 117, 117*t*
Relaxation response, 116
Relaxing sigh, 117, 117*t*
Relenza (zanamivir)
  for influenza, 540
  for pneumonia, 566
Religion, 31
Religious affiliation, 30*t*
Religious groups, 32*t*
Religious interest, 730*b*
ReliOn N (NPH insulin), 1260*t*
ReliOn R (regular insulin), 1260*t*
Relpax (eletriptan), 1530
Rem, 292*t*
Remicade (infliximab)
  for arthritis and connective tissue disorders, 1700*t*
  drug alert, 1706
  for inflammatory bowel disease, 1054, 1055*t*
  for rheumatoid arthritis, 1705-1706
Remifentanil (Ultiva), 370*t*
Remodulin (treprostinil), 602
Renagel (sevelamer hydrochloride), 1210
Renal arteriogram, 1148*t*, 1151*f*
Renal artery stenosis, 1175
Renal biopsy, 1149*t*
Renal calculi
  acute, 1173*b*-1174*b*
  nursing assessment of, 1172
  nursing diagnoses, 1172
  nursing evaluation of, 1173
  nursing implementation for, 1172-1173
  nursing management of, **1172-1173**
  nursing planning for, 1172
  staghorn, 1169, 1170*f*
Renal capsule, 1137
Renal cell carcinoma, 1177-1178, 1178*f*, 1178*t*
Renal colic, 1140
Renal cortex, 1137
Renal dialysis. See Dialysis

Renal disease
  in acquired immunodeficiency syndrome, **1168**
  autoimmune, 234*t*
  chronic kidney disease, 1197, **1204-1216**
    case study, 1231
    dermatologic manifestations, 473*t*
    prevention and detection of, 1205*b*
    resources for, 1232
  end-stage, 1204
    causes of, 1205, 1205*f*
  hereditary, **1175-1177**
  HIV-associated syndromes, 1168
  in hypertension, 766*t*
  polycystic kidney disease, **1176-1177,** 1176*f*
  recurrence after kidney transplantation, 1230
Renal failure, 1197
  acute, **1197-1204**
    in acquired immunodeficiency syndrome, 1168
    gerontologic considerations for, **1204**
    nursing management of, **1203-1204**
    resources for, 1232
  in acute respiratory distress syndrome, 1816
  in heart failure, 827
Renal medulla, 1137
Renal osteodystrophy, 1208
  drug therapy of, 1210
  mechanisms of, 1208, 1208*f*
  types associated with ESRD, 1208
Renal papillae, 1137
Renal pelvis, 1137
Renal perfusion, 898
Renal radionuclide imaging, 1149*t*
Renal replacement therapy
  complications of, 1229*t*
  continuous, **1224-1225,** 1224*f*
Renal scan, 1149*t*
Renal surgery, 1188
Renal system. See also Kidney(s)
  acid-base regulation by, 334
  in acute respiratory distress syndrome, 1816*t*
  in multiple organ dysfunction syndrome, 1796*t*
  problems of, **1154-1196**
  problems with dermatologic manifestations, 473*t*
  regulation of blood pressure by, 764
  regulation of water balance by, 320
  in shock, 1781*t*, 1782
    acute intervention for, 1793
  in systemic lupus erythematosus, 1718
  vascular problems, **1175**
Renal trauma, 1175
Renal tuberculosis, 1164-1165
Renal tubules
  distal, 1138*t*
  function of, 1138-1139
  proximal, 1138*t*
Renal ultrasound, 1148*t*
Renal vein thrombosis, 1175
RenalWEB Patient Education, 1232
Renin, 1857*t*
Renin-angiotensin mechanism, 765-766
Renin-angiotensin-aldosterone system, 1139, 1139*f*
Renova (tretinoin), 479*t*
ReoPro (abciximab), 800*t*
Reoviruses, 244*t*
Repaglinide (Prandin), 1265, 1266t

Repetitive strain injury, 1633
Replacement factors, 709*t*
RepliCare, 205*t*
Repolarization, 843, 1443, 1443*f*
Reproductive system, 1323-1342. See also Sexuality-reproductive pattern
  age-related changes in, 78*t*, 1330, 1331*t*
  assessment abnormalities, 1247*t*, 1335*t*
  assessment of
    key questions to ask, 1333*t*
    normal, 1335, 1335*t*
    objective data, 1334-1335
    subjective data, 1331-1334
  in chronic kidney disease, 1209
  diagnostic studies, **1336-1341,** 1338*t*-1341*t*
  dysfunction in radiation and chemotherapy, 296*t*, 301
  effects of aging on, **1330-1331**
  effects of chronic alcohol abuse on, 177*t*
  female
    assessment of, **1331-1335**
    benign tumors of, **1398-1400**
    cancers of, **1400-1407**
    diagnostic studies, **1337-1341**
    problems of, **1381-1413**
    structures and functions of, **1325-1327**
  functional changes in, 1247*t*
  gerontologic considerations for, 1330-1331
  in HIV infection, 259*t*
  male
    assessment of, **1331-1335**
    diagnostic studies, **1337-1341**
    problems of, **1414-1439**
    structures and functions of, **1324**
  neuroendocrine regulation of, 1328-1329
  problems of, **1233-1439**
  problems with dermatologic manifestations, 473*t*
  surgeries of, 1332, 1332*t*
Repronex, 1383*t*
Requip (ropinirole)
  for Parkinson's disease, 1551, 1552*t*
  for restless legs syndrome, 1558
Rescriptor (delavirdine), 258*t*
Research, 107
Reserpine (Serpasil)
  for hypertension, 774*t*
  for systemic sclerosis, 1724
Reserpine/chlorthalidone (Demi-Regroton), 777*t*
Reserpine/hydrochlorothiazide (Hydropres), 777*t*
Residential care facilities, 88, 88*t*
Residual urine test, 1146*t*
Residual volume, 531*t*, 594*b*
Resilience, 112
Resistance, 112, 112*t*, 246
Resistin, 973
Resonance, 523*t*
Resorption, 1615
Respiration
  abnormal patterns associated with coma, 1478, 1478*f*
  control of, 515
  in fluid and electrolyte imbalances, 338*t*
  Kussmaul respirations, 335, 524*t*
  paradoxic, 588, 588*f*
  physiology of, 512-515
  spontaneous respiratory rate, 1767*t*

Note: Disorder names are in **bold face.** Page numbers in **bold face** indicate main discussions. Page numbers followed by *f, t, b,* or *n* indicate figures, tables, boxed material, or notes, respectively.

Respiratory acidosis, 334-335, 335*t*, 336*t*
Respiratory alkalosis, 335, 335*t*, 336*t*
Respiratory disorders
dermatologic manifestations of, 473*t*
inadequate oxygenation secondary to, 473*t*
obstructive, 594*b*
prevention of, 569*b*
restrictive, 593-597, 594*b*
Respiratory failure, 1799
acute, **1799-1812**
in COPD, 636-637
acute respiratory distress syndrome (ARDS), **1812-1818**
and restrictive lung disease, 596*t*
classification of, 1799, 1800*f*
gerontologic considerations for, **1812**
hypercapnic
causes of, 1800, 1800*t*
definition of, 1800
etiology and pathophysiology of, 1803
hypoxemic, 1799-1800
causes of, 1799-1800, 1800*t*
definition of, 1799-1800
etiology and pathophysiology of, 1800-1803
types of, 1799-1800, 1800*t*
Respiratory imbalances, 334
Respiratory infections
and asthma attacks, 609
at-risk for, 564
Respiratory membrane, 511, 512*f*
Respiratory rate, 1767*t*
Respiratory rehabilitation, 1604
Respiratory syncytial virus, 244*t*
Respiratory system, **509-532**
acid-base regulation, 334
in acute renal failure, 1201*t*
age-related changes in, 78*t*, 516-517, 517*t*
in allergies, 229*t*
assessment abnormalities, 524*t*-525*t*
assessment of, **517-525**
health history questions to ask, 518*t*
important health information for, 517
objective data, 521-525
physical, 525*t*
preoperative, 349, 351*t*
subjective data, 517-521
and asthma, 624*t*
burn injury, 492, 492*t*
burn injury complications, 500
in chronic kidney disease, 1208
cigarette smoke and, 631, 631*t*
and COPD, 650*t*
cues to problems, 517-518, 519*t*
defense mechanisms, 516
diagnostic studies, **525-531**, 527*t*-528*t*
effects of aging on, **516-517**
at end of life, 152, 152*t*
in extracellular fluid volume imbalances, 323
functions of, **510-517**
in HIV infection, 259*t*
in increased ICP, 1478
and lung cancer, 583*t*
in multiple organ dysfunction syndrome, 1796*t*
opioid-induced depression, 138
physical examination of, 521-525
in pneumonia, 567*t*
postoperative management of, 1188
preoperative review, 348

Respiratory system (*Continued*)
problems of
associated with obesity, 975
in chemotherapy and radiation therapy, 296*t*, 300
in clinical unit, 380-381
nursing assessment of, 381
nursing diagnoses, 381
nursing implementation for, 381-382
nursing management of, **381-382**
in postanesthesia care unit (PACU), 378-380
postoperative, **378-381**, 379*t*
procedures requiring antibiotic prophylaxis to prevent endocarditis, 866, 867*t*
radiologic studies, 526-528
in shock, 1781*t*, 1793
in spinal cord injury, 1592-1594, 1602
after stroke, 1515
structures of, 510, 510*f*
tobacco smoke and, 631*t*
Respiratory therapy, 1807-1810
for acute respiratory distress syndrome, 1816-1818
for COPD, 646-649
home health care activities, 90*t*
Rest. *See also* Sleep-rest pattern
for acute coronary syndrome, 813
for hepatitis, 1099
for osteoarthritis, 1696
for rheumatoid arthritis, 1708-1709
and skin, 462
for soft tissue injuries, 203
Rest pain, 901
Resting membrane potential, 1443, 1443*f*
Restless legs syndrome, 1557-1558
clinical manifestations of, 1557
diagnostic criteria for, 1557
diagnostic studies, 1557
etiology and pathophysiology of, 1557
nursing and collaborative management of, **1557-1558**
Restoril (temazepam), 1569*t*
Restraints, 82
Restrictive cardiomyopathy, 886*t*, **889**
clinical manifestations of, 889
diagnostic studies, 889
etiology and pathophysiology of, 889
nursing and collaborative management of, **889**
Restrictive lung disease
extrapulmonary causes of, 594, 595*t*
intrapulmonary causes of, 596*t*
Restrictive respiratory disorders, 593-597, 594*b*
Restylane (hyaluronic acid), 479*t*
Resuscitation, 155-156
cardiopulmonary, **1845-1849**, 1849*f*
adult one-rescuer, 1847*t*
adult two-rescuer, 1848*t*
fluid
in hypovolemic shock, 1788
with Parkland (Baxter) formula, 496, 497*t*
in shock, 1783-1785
mouth-to-mouth, 1845-1846, 1845*f*
Retavase (reteplase), 800*t*
Retention, 1145*t*
Reteplase (Retavase), 800*t*

Reticular activating system, 113
age-related changes in, 1454*t*
gerontologic differences in assessment findings, 1454*t*
Reticular formation, 1447
age-related changes in, 1454*t*
gerontologic differences in assessment findings, 1454*t*
response to stress, 113
Reticulocyte count, 680*t*, 1859*t*
Reticulocytes, 666*f*, 667, 690*t*
Retina, 399*f*, 401
age-related changes in, 401*t*
assessment of, 407
damage in hypertension, 767
Retin-A (tretinoin), 463*b*, 479*t*
Retinal breaks, 429, 430*t*, 431*f*
Retinal detachment, 429-431, 431*f*
clinical manifestations of, 430
collaborative care for, 430, 430*t*
diagnostic studies, 430
etiology and pathophysiology of, 429-430
exudative, 429
risk factors for, 430*t*
secondary, 429
surgical therapy of, 430-431
tractional, 429
Retinal holes, 429
Retinal tears, 429
Retinitis
associated with HIV infection, 254*t*
cytomegalovirus, 436
Retinoid, 720*t*
Retinopathy, 429
definition of, 1876
diabetic, 429, **1284-1285**
case study, 446-447
prevention, detection, and monitoring of, 1284*t*
hypertensive, 429, 767
manifestations of, 766*t*
nonproliferative, 429, 1284
proliferative, 429, 1284
Retraction, intercostal, 1805
Retrogasserian rhizotomy, 1582*t*
Retrograde pyelogram, 1148*t*
Retropubic prostatectomy
approach, 1424, 1424*f*
Retrovir (zidovudine), 258*t*
Retroviruses, 250
Return demonstration, 61-62, 62*f*
Revascularization
coronary
for acute coronary syndrome, 808-810, 814-815
for coronary artery disease, 801
recommendations for, 808
surgical, 808-810
transmyocardial laser, 810
Reverse transcriptase, 251
ReVia (naltrexone)
for alcohol abuse, 178
for opioid withdrawal, 180
Revimid (lenalidomide), 717
Rewarming
active, 390
active core, 1831
active external, 1831
passive, 390
passive external, 1831
Reyataz (atazanavir), 258*t*
Rh factor, 679
Rhabdomyolysis, 1829
Rhabdovirus, 244*t*
Rheumatic carditis, chronic, 876-877

Rheumatic disease, 1693
HIV-associated, **1714-1715**
soft tissue syndromes, **1726-1729**
Rheumatic endocarditis, 876, 876*f*
Rheumatic fever, 875-878
acute intervention for, 878
ambulatory and home care for, 878
collaborative care for, 877, 877*t*
diagnostic studies, 877
etiology and pathophysiology of, 875-876
extracardiac lesions of, 876
health promotion in, 877-878
nursing assessment of, 877, 877*t*
nursing diagnoses, 877
nursing evaluation of, 878
nursing implementation for, 877-878
nursing management of, **877-878**
nursing planning for, 877
Rheumatic heart disease, 875-878
acute intervention for, 878
ambulatory and home care for, 878
dermatologic manifestations of, 473*t*
etiology and pathophysiology of, 875-876
nursing assessment of, 877, 877*t*
nursing diagnoses, 877
nursing evaluation of, 878
nursing implementation for, 877-878
nursing management of, **877-878**
nursing planning for, 877
Rheumatic pancarditis, 876
Rheumatoid arthritis, 1702-1711, 1703*f*
acute intervention for, 1707-1708
ambulatory and home care for, 1708-1711
autoimmunity and, 1702
case study, 1729-1730
clinical manifestations of, 1702-1704, 1704*t*
cold therapy for, 1710-1711
collaborative care for, 1705-1707, 1706*t*
complications of, 1704
cultural and ethnic health disparities in, 1702*b*
definition of, 1876
deformity of, 1703-1704, 1704*f*
diagnostic criteria for, 1705, 1705*t*
diagnostic studies, 1704-1705
drug therapy for, 1705-1706
etiology and pathophysiology of, 1702
extraarticular manifestations of, 1704, 1705*f*
genetic factors, 1702
health promotion in, 1707
heat therapy for, 1710-1711
of joints, 1702-1704, 1703*f*
nursing assessment of, 1707, 1707*t*
nursing care plan for patient with, 1708*b*-1710*b*
nursing diagnoses, 1707
nursing implementation for, 1707-1711
nursing management of, **1707-1711**
nursing planning for, 1707
nutritional therapy for, 1706-1707
ocular manifestations of, 437*t*
stages of, 1702, 1703*t*
Rheumatoid factor, 1626*t*, 1861*t*
Rheumatoid nodules, 1704
Rheumatrex (methotrexate)
for arthritis and connective tissue disorders, 1699*t*
classification of, 287*t*
for rheumatoid arthritis, 1705

Rhinitis
acute viral, **536-538**
allergic, 226-227, **535-536**
drug therapy of, 537t-538t
Rhinocort (budesonide), 537t
Rhinoplasty, 534
collaborative care for, 534
Rhinorrhea, 1481, 1482f
Rhinovirus, 244t
Rhizotomies, 143
glycerol rhizotomy, 1582, 1582t, 1583f
percutaneous radiofrequency rhizotomy, 1582, 1582t
retrogasserian rhizotomy, 1582t
Rhonchi, 524, 525t
Rhythm identification and treatment, **842-861**
Rhytidectomy, 479
Rib fracture, 587-588, 595t
Ribavirin (Rebetol, Copegus)
for chronic hepatitis C, 1095
drug alert, 1095
side effects of, 1094t
Riboflavin deficiency, 473t
Ribonucleic acid (RNA), 214
RICE (rest, ice, compression, elevation), 203
Rickets, 951
Ridaura (auranofin)
for arthritis and connective tissue disorders, 1699t
for rheumatoid arthritis, 1706
Rifabutin (Mycobutin), 573t
Rifampin (Rifadin)
blood glucose level effects, 1267t
nephrotoxicity, 1142t
for tuberculosis, 573t, 574t
Rifapentine (Priftin), 573t
RIG. See Rabies immune globulin
Right atrial pressure
measurement of, 1744
normal range at rest, 1739t
Right common carotid artery, 1451f
Right subclavian artery, 1451f
Right-brain stroke, 1508, 1508f
Right-sided heart failure, 824, 825, 825t
Rigidity
cogwheel, 1550
in Parkinson's disease, 1549, 1550
Rimantadine (Flumadine)
for influenza, 540
for pneumonia, 566
Ring sign, 1481, 1482f
Ringer's solution
composition and use of, 339t
lactated
composition and use of, 339t
for shock, 1784, 1786t
Riomet (metformin), 1266t
Riopan, 1020t
Risedronate (Actonel)
for osteoporosis, 1689
for Paget's disease, 1690
Risky sexual behavior, 168t
Risperidone (Risperdal)
for Alzheimer's disease, 1551-1552, 1569t
for delirium, 1578

Ritalin (methylphenidate)
effects of use, 169t
for multiple sclerosis, 1544-1545, 1545t
for opioid-induced sedation, 138
Ritonavir (Norvir)
adverse effects of, 258t
lopinavir and ritonavir (Kaletra), 258t
Rituximab (Rituxan), 303t
for arthritis and connective tissue disorders, 1700t
drug alert, 704
for leukemia, 720t, 721t
for non-Hodgkin's lymphoma, 727, 727t
for rheumatoid arthritis, 1706
Rivastigmine (Exelon)
for Alzheimer's disease, 1551, 1569t
for Parkinson's dementia, 1551
Rizatriptan (Maxalt), 1530
RLS. See Restless legs syndrome
RNA, 214
RNC. See Radionuclide cystography
RNFA. See Registered nurse first assistant
Robalate, 1020t
Robinul (glycopyrrolate), 355t
Robson's system of staging renal carcinoma, 1178t
Rocaltrol (calcitriol)
for hypocalcemia, 1210
for hypoparathyroidism, 1311
Rocephin (ceftriaxone)
for bacterial meningitis, 1495
for gonorrhea, 1368
for infective endocarditis, 869t
Rocky Mountain spotted fever, 1835
Rocuronium (Zemuron), 370t
Roentgen (R), 292t
Rofecoxib (Vioxx), 136, 1697
Roferon-A (α-Interferon), 223t, 303t
Rolaids, 1020t
Role-relationship pattern
in assessment
of auditory system, 410t, 412
of cardiovascular system, 746t, 747
of endocrine system, 1244
of gastrointestinal system, 935t, 936
of hematologic system, 673t, 674
of integumentary system, 453t, 454
of musculoskeletal system, 1621
of nervous system, 1455-1456
of preoperative patient, 350t
of reproductive system, 1333t, 1334
of respiratory system, 518t, 520
of urinary system, 1143t, 1144
of visual system, 403t, 404
comparison with NANDA International Taxonomy II, 42t
concerns of patients requiring home health care, 90t
nursing diagnoses, **1853**
nursing history, 45t, 46
Rolling hiatal hernia, 1007, 1008f
Romazicon (flumazenil), 369
R-on-T phenomenon, 854
Ropinirole (Requip)
for Parkinson's disease, 1551, 1552t
for restless legs syndrome, 1558
Rosiglitazone (Avandia), 1265, 1266t
Rosiglitazone and metformin (Avandamet), 1266t

Rosuvastatin (Crestor), 793, 795t
Rotary chair testing, 414t
Rotation
external, 1622t
internal, 1622t
Rotator cuff injury, 1634
Rotator cuff tear, 1630t
Rotavirus infection, 1037t
Rotaviruses, 244t
Roux-en-Y gastric bypass, 982t, 983f, 984
Rowasa (5-ASA enema), 1055t
Roxanol (morphine), 137t
Roxicodone (oxycodone), 137t
RPGN. See Rapidly progressive glomerulonephritis
RPP. See Rapid postanesthesia care unit progression
RRT. See Rapid response team
RSI. See Repetitive strain injury
RU-486 (mifepristone), 1384t
Rubella, congenital, 437t
Rubella virus, 244t
Rubeola virus, 244t
Rubex (doxorubicin), 287t
Rubor, dependent, 901
Rule of nines, 487, 487t
Rumpel-Leede test, 679t
Rural older adults, 70, 70f
RYGB. See Roux-en-Y gastric bypass
Rythmol (propafenone)
for atrial flutter, 851
classification of, 856t

S
SA node, 846, 847t
Sabril (vigabatrin), 1536, 1538t
Sacral area, pitting edema of, 749t
Safety
in Alzheimer's disease, 1573
comparison of functional health patterns and NANDA International Taxonomy II, 43t
of older adults, 80
promoting, 106
surgical considerations, 365-366
Saf-Gel, 205t
Salagen (pilocarpine), 1726
Salazopyrin (sulfasalazine), 1699t
Salbutamol (albuterol), 619t
Salicylates
for arthritis and connective tissue disorders, 1698t
blood glucose level effects, 1267t
hematologic effects of, 674t
mechanism of action, 202t
nephrotoxicity, 1142t
for pain, 135, 136t
toxicology, 1865t
Salivary gland secretions, 929, 929t
Salmeterol (Serevent), 621
for asthma and COPD, 619t
for COPD, 640
fluticasone/salmeterol (Advair), 621
for asthma and COPD, 620t
for exercise-induced asthma, 608
Salmonella
diseases caused by, 244t
food poisoning, 1031, 1032t
Salpingectomy, 1405f
acute intervention related to, 1406
description of, 1332t
Salpingo-oophorectomy, bilateral, 1404t
Salsalate (Disalcid, Asaphen), 1698t
Saltatory conduction, 1443, 1443f
Same-day admission, 344
Same-day surgery, 344

Sanctura (trospium chloride)
for urinary incontinence, 1182
for voiding dysfunction, 1185t
Sandimmune (cyclosporine), 238, 239t, 1718
Sandoglobulin (immunoglobulin), 1586
Sandostatin (octreotide)
for acromegaly, 1292
for diarrhea, 1037t
for gastrointestinal bleeding, 998t
Sansert (methysergide), 1531
Saquinavir (Fortovase, Invirase), 258t
Sarafem (fluoxetine), 1386
Sarcoidosis, 597
Sarcoma, 1672
chondrosarcoma, 1673f, 1673t
classification of, 279
Ewing's, 1673t
Kaposi, 252, 253f, 255t
osteogenic, 1673f, **1674**
description of, 1673t
osteosarcoma, 1674
Sarcomeres, 1617
Sargramostim (Leukine)
for cancer treatment, 304t
clinical uses of, 223t
Sarin (isopropyl methylphosphanofluoridate), 1839, 1840t
SARS. See Severe acute respiratory syndrome
Saw palmetto (*Serenoa repens*), 102t, 1417, 1417b
SBS. See Short bowel syndrome
SBT. See Spontaneous breathing trial
Scabies, 470f, 470t
Scale, 413t, 455t
SCALES assessment, 71, 71t
Scalp lacerations, 1481
Scar tissue, 198
Scars, 455t
contraction of, 198-199, 199t
corneal, **424-425**
hypertrophic, 201
variations in light- and dark-skinned individuals, 456t
SCD. See Sudden cardiac death
Scheduled voiding regimens, 1183, 1183t
Schwann cells, 1442
Schwannoma, 1488t
Schwartz's sign, 440
Scintigraphy, 942t
of GI bleeding, 942t
hepatobiliary, 942t
Sclera, 400
assessing, 407
gerontologic differences in assessment, 401t
jaundiced, 675t
Scleral buckling, 430, 431, 431f
Sclerodactyly, 1723, 1723f
Scleroderma, 1723
dermatologic manifestations of, 473t
renal involvement in, 1177
skin changes in, 1723, 1723f
Scleromate (morrhuate), 1108
Sclerosing cholangitis, primary, 1102
Sclerosing peritonitis, encapsulating, 1220
Sclerotherapy
endoscopic, 1108
for esophageal and gastric varices, 1108
for varicose veins, 918, 918f
Scoliosis, 1623-1624, 1624f, 1624t

Note: Disorder names are in **bold face.** Page numbers in **bold face** indicate main discussions. Page numbers followed by *f, t, b,* or *n* indicate figures, tables, boxed material, or notes, respectively.

Scopolamine (Isopto Hyoscine)
for nausea and vomiting, 138, 992, 992*t*
preoperative, 355*t*
for pupil dilation, 427*t*
transdermal (Transderm-Scop), 138, 992*t*
Scotomas
in age-related macular degeneration, 432
in multiple sclerosis, 1543
Screening
for breast cancer
guidelines for early detection, 282*t*, 1343-1344
increasing participation in, 1359*b*
for latex allergies, 347
nutrition, 957*t*
for ovarian cancer, 1403*b*
Screening audiometry, 415
Screening physical examination, 47
documentation of normal findings, 51*t*
equipment for, 48, 48*t*
outline for, 48*t*-49*t*
recording, 50, 51*t*
Scripps Center for Integrative Medicine, 108
Scrotal erythema, 1337*t*
Scrotal masses, 1337*t*, 1430, 1431*f*
Scrotum
physical examination of, 1335
problems of, **1430-1432**
acquired, **1431-1432**
congenital, **1430-1431**
inflammatory, **1430**
of skin, **1430**
Scrubbing
function of, 361
before surgery, 364-365
SCUF. *See* Slow continuous ultrafiltration
Scurvy, 951
ScvO₂. *See* Central venous oxygen saturation
SeaSorb, 205*t*
Sebaceous cysts, 413*t*
Sebaceous glands, 451
Seborrheic keratoses, 472*t*
Sebum, 451
Secobarbital (Seconal)
effects of use, 169*t*
withdrawal from, 179
Second spacing, 319, 488
Secondary survey, 1824-1827, 1826*t*
Secretin, 929, 930*t*
Secretions
gastric, 929, 930*t*
hormone rhythms of, 1238
mobilization of, 1809-1810
from nipples, 1335*t*
related to digestion, 929, 929*t*
Secretory otitis media, 440
Sectral (acebutolol)
classification of, 856*t*
for hypertension, 774*t*
Sedation
for burns, 498-499, 499*t*
conscious, 367, 1870
deep, 367
levels of, 367
minimal, 367
moderate, 367
opioid-induced, 138
Sedative-hypnotics, **178-179**
for burns, 498-499
characteristics of, 178-179

Sedative-hypnotics *(Continued)*
collaborative care, 179
complications of, 168*t*, 179
effects of use, 169*t*, 179
onset, peak, duration, and withdrawal onset of, 185*t*
Seizure disorders, 1532-1542
acute intervention for, 1539
ambulatory and home care for, 1539-1541
collaborative care for, 1536-1537, 1536*t*
diagnostic studies, 1536
drug therapy for, 1536-1537, 1538*t*
etiology and pathophysiology of, 1533-1534
health promotion in, 1538-1539
idiopathic, 1533
International Classification System for, 1534, 1534*t*
nursing assessment of, 1538, 1539*t*
nursing care plan for patient with, 1540*b*-1541*b*
nursing diagnoses, 1538
nursing implementation for, 1538-1541
nursing management of, **1538-1542**
nursing planning for, 1538
patient and family teaching guide for, 1541*t*
psychosocial complications of, 1535-1536
surgical procedures for, 1538*t*
surgical therapy for, 1538
Seizure focus, 1533
Seizures, 1247*t*, 1532-1533
absence
atypical, 1535
typical, 1534-1535
atonic (drop attack), 1535
aural phase, 1534
classification of
algorithm for, 1534*f*
International Classification System, 1534, 1534*t*
clinical manifestations of, 1534-1535
clonic, 1535
collaborative care for, 1536-1537
complications of, 1535-1536
focal motor, 1535
focal sensory, 1535
generalized, 1534-1535
ictal phase, 1534
jacksonian, 1535
myoclonic, 1535
nursing evaluation of, 1542
partial, 1534, 1535
complex, 1535
simple, 1535
phases of, 1534
postictal phase, 1534
prodromal phase, 1534
psychomotor, 1535
temporal lobe, 1535
tonic, 1535
tonic-clonic, 1534
definition of, 1877
emergency management of, 1536, 1537*t*
Selective estrogen receptor modulators
for infertility, 1383, 1383*t*
for osteoporosis, 1689-1690
Selective serotonin reuptake inhibitors
for Alzheimer's disease, 1569*t*
for pain, 139

Selegiline (Eldepryl, Carbex)
food/nutrient interactions, 954*t*
for Parkinson's disease, 1551, 1552*t*
Self-concept. *See* Self-perception–self-concept pattern
Self-efficacy, 58, 188
Self-examination
breast, 1344, 1344*f*
testicular, 1432, 1433*f*, 1433*t*
Self-injection therapy, 1435, 1436*f*
Self-monitoring of blood glucose, 1269, 1270*t*
Self-perception–self-concept pattern
in assessment
of auditory system, 410*t*, 411
of cardiovascular system, 746*t*, 747
of endocrine system, 1244
of gastrointestinal system, 935-936, 935*t*
of hematologic system, 673*t*, 674
of integumentary system, 453*t*, 454
of musculoskeletal system, 1621
of nervous system, 1455
of preoperative patient, 350*t*
of reproductive system, 1333*t*, 1334
of respiratory system, 518*t*, 520
of urinary system, 1143*t*, 1144
of visual system, 403*t*, 404
comparison with NANDA International Taxonomy II, 42*t*
concerns of patients requiring home health care, 90*t*
nursing diagnoses, **1852-1853**
nursing history, 45*t*, 46
Sellar tumors, 1489*t*
Semen analysis, 1341*t*
Semilunar valves, 740, 740*f*
Seminal vesicles, 1324
Seminiferous tubules, 1325*f*
Semiocclusive dressings, 205
Semipermanent catheters, 1222, 1222*f*
Senescent gynecomastia, 1348
Sengstaken-Blakemore tube, 1108, 1109*f*
Senna (Senokot), 1042*t*
Sense of coherence, 111-112
Sensible perspiration, 321
Sensipar (cinacalcet)
for hyperparathyroidism, 1310-1311
for secondary hyperparathyroidism, 1210
Sensitivity
delayed hypersensitivity reactions, 225*t*, 228
hypersensitivity pneumonitis, 577
hypersensitivity reactions, 224-228
multiple chemical sensitivities, 233
photosensitivity, 460-462, 461*t*
tumor radiosensitivity, 292-293, 293*t*
Sensitivity testing, 1157
Sensitization
central, 128
peripheral, 127-128
Sensorcaine (bupivacaine), 128
Sensorineural hearing loss, 408, 443
Sensory deprivation, 1603
Sensory neurogenic bladder, 1604, 1605*t*
Sensory neuropathy
chronic sensory polyneuropathy, 473*t*
in diabetes mellitus, 1285, 1286

Sensory system
age-related changes in, 78*t*, 1454*t*
assessment abnormalities, 1460*t*
changes at end of life, 152, 152*t*
examination of, 1458-1459, 1459*t*
problems related to altered input, **397-507**
Sensory-perceptual alterations
in ICU patients, 1736-1737
after stroke, 1520, 1523
Sentinel lymph node dissection, 1351
Sentinel node, 1351
Sepsis
acute transfusion reaction, 732, 733*t*
diagnostic criteria for, 1779*t*
in hemodialysis, 1223
Septal hypertrophy, asymmetric, 888
Septic arthritis, 1713-1714
Septic shock, 1773*f*, **1778**
in cancer, 308
classification of, 1773*t*
clinical presentation of, 1776*t*
collaborative care for, 1788-1789
pathophysiology of, 1778, 1778*f*
precipitating factors, 1773*t*
treatment of, 1789*t*
Septra (trimethoprim-sulfamethoxazole), 674*t*
Sequestrum, 1669, 1669*f*
Serax (oxazepam), 1569*t*
Serenoa repens. See Saw palmetto
Serevent (salmeterol), 621
for asthma, 619*t*
for COPD, 619*t*, 640
Seroconversion, 252, 1094
Serologic studies
laboratory values, 1860*t*-1861*t*
musculoskeletal, 1626*t*
tests for syphilis, 1336-1341
Seromycin (cycloserine), 573*t*
Serophene (clomiphene), 1383*t*
Seroquel (quetiapine)
for Alzheimer's disease, 1569, 1569*t*
for delirium, 1578
Serotonin, 195*t*, 226*t*, 1445*t*
Serotonin antagonists, 992, 992*t*
Serotonin type 4 (5-HT₄) receptor partial agonists, 1041, 1042*t*
Serous exudate, 197*t*
Serpasil (reserpine)
for hypertension, 774*t*
for systemic sclerosis, 1724
Serratia, 1155*t*
Sertraline (Zoloft)
for Alzheimer's disease, 1569*t*
for depression, 1569
for pain, 139
for premenstrual syndrome, 1386
Serum albumin, 351, 956*t*
Serum amylase, 944*t*
Serum bilirubin, 946*t*
Serum calcium, total, 1250*t*
Serum cardiac markers, 805-806, 805*f*
Serum chemistries, 1855*t*-1858*t*
Serum electrolytes
normal values, 321*t*
in shock, 1775*t*
Serum enzyme tests, 947*t*
Serum estradiol, 1338*t*
Serum follicle-stimulating hormone, 1248*t*, 1338*t*
Serum hCG assay, 1338*t*
Serum iron, 672*t*, 679-680, 680*t*
in anemias, 690*t*
effects of aging on, 672*t*
Serum lipase, 944*t*

Serum lipids, 751-756, 752*t*, 788, 789*f*
  elevated
    and coronary artery disease, 788-789
    health-promoting behaviors for, 792*t*
  types of, 788*f*
Serum phosphate, 1250*t*
Serum potassium, 1627*t*
Serum prealbumin, 956*t*
Serum progesterone, 1338*t*, 1341*t*
Serum protein electrophoresis, 680*t*
Serum sodium, in shock, 1775*t*
Serum studies
  adrenal, 1250*t*-1251*t*
  parathyroid, 1250*t*
  pituitary, 1248*t*
  thyroid, 1249*t*
Sevelamer hydrochloride (Renagel), 1210
Severe acute respiratory syndrome, 1818-1819
Sevoflurane (Ultane), 369*t*
Sex organs, male, 1324, 1324*f*
Sex-linked gene, 214*t*
Sexual abuse, 73*t*
Sexual activity
  after acute coronary syndrome, 817*t*
  and COPD, 655
  decreasing risks related to intercourse, 261-262
  health impact of responsible behavior, 1377*b*
  health problems related to risky sexual behavior, 168*t*
  insertive sex, 261-262
  male condom breakage during, 1373*b*
  resumption of, 817
  risk-reducing activities, 262
  and STDs, 1379
Sexual assault, 1409-1411
  clinical manifestations of, 1409
  collaborative care for, 1409-1410
  definition of, 1409
  emergency management of, 1410*t*
  evaluation of alleged assault, 1411*t*
  nursing management of, **1410-1411**
  patient and family teaching guide for prevention of, 1411*t*
  physical manifestations of, 1409
  psychologic manifestations of, 1409
Sexual function
  effects of aging on, 1330, **1330-1331,** 1331*t*
  female response, 1330
  male problems of, **1433-1438**
  male response, 1330
  in men with spinal cord injury, 1607, 1607*t*
  nursing interventions for, 1524
  after ostomy surgery, 1074-1076
  phases of response, 1330
  after stroke, 1524
Sexual history, 1334, 1334*t*
Sexual transmission of HIV, 250
Sexuality
  after spinal cord injury, 1607-1608, 1607*b*
  and tracheostomy and gastrostomy tubes, 557-558

Sexuality Information and Education Council of the United States (SIECUS), 1380, 1413, 1439
Sexuality-reproductive pattern
  in assessment
    of auditory system, 410*t*, 412
    of cardiovascular system, 746*t*, 747
    of endocrine system, 1244
    of gastrointestinal system, 935*t*, 936
    of hematologic system, 673*t*, 674
    of integumentary system, 453*t*, 454
    of musculoskeletal system, 1621
    of nervous system, 1456
    of preoperative patient, 350*t*
    of reproductive system, 1333*t*, 1334
    of respiratory system, 518*t*, 520
    of urinary system, 1143*t*, 1144
    of visual system, 403*t*, 404
  comparison with NANDA International Taxonomy II, 42*t*
  concerns of patients requiring home health care, 90*t*
  nursing diagnoses, **1853**
  nursing history, 45*t*, 46
Sexually transmitted diseases, 1366-1367
  ambulatory and home care for, 1379
  bacterial infections, **1367-1373**
  case finding, 1378
  compliance, 1379
  educational and research programs, 1378
  factors affecting incidence of, 1367
  follow-up, 1379
  health promotion in, 1376-1378
  hygiene measures, 1379
  measures to prevent infection, 1377-1378
  microorganisms responsible for, 1367*t*
  nursing assessment of, 1376, 1377*t*
  nursing diagnoses, 1376
  nursing evaluation of, 1379
  nursing implementation for, 1376-1379
  nursing management of, **1376-1379**
  nursing planning for, 1376
  patient teaching guide for, 1377*t*
  psychologic support for, 1378-1379
  resources, 1380
  screening programs, 1378
  viral infections, **1373-1379**
Shallow breathing, 1767*t*
Shamans, 30
Shave biopsy, 458*t*
Shearing force, 206*t*
Sheehan syndrome, 1293
Shenjing shuairuo, 35*t*
Shielding, 294
Shigella, 244*t*, 1037*t*
Shiley fenestrated tracheostomy tube, 544*t*
Shin splints, 1630*t*
Shingles (herpes zoster), 255*t*, 468*t*, 469*f*
Shock, 1772-1794, 1773*f*
  acute intervention for, 1791-1794
  ambulatory and home care for, 1794
  anaphylactic, 1773*f*, **1777**
    allergens causing, 227*t*
    classification of, 1773*t*
    clinical presentation of, 1776*t*
    collaborative care for, 1790
    emergency management of, 230*t*

Shock *(Continued)*
    precipitating factors, 1773*t*
    treatment of, 1789*t*
  burn shock, 488, 491, 491*f*
  cardiogenic, **1773-1775,** 1773*f*
    classification of, 1773*t*
    clinical presentation of, 1776*t*
    collaborative care for, 1786
    in myocardial infarction, 804
    pathophysiology of, 1774, 1774*f*
    precipitating factors, 1773*t*
    treatment of, 1789*t*
  case study, 1797
  classification of, 1772-1778, 1773*t*
  clinical presentation of, 1776*t*
  collaborative care for, 1783-1786, 1786-1790
  compensatory stage, 1779, 1780*f*, 1781*t*
  diagnostic studies, 1783
  drug therapy for, 1785-1786, 1787*t*-1788*t*
  emergency management of, 1783, 1785*t*
  fluid therapy in, 1783-1785, 1786*t*
  general measures for, 1783-1786
  health promotion in, 1790
  hemodynamic effects of, 1774-1775, 1774*t*
  hypovolemic, 1773*f*, **1775-1777**
    classification of, 1773*t*
    clinical presentation of, 1776*t*
    collaborative care for, 1788
    pathophysiology of, 1776, 1777*f*
    precipitating factors, 1773*t*
    treatment of, 1789*t*
  irreversible or refractory stage, 1784*f*
  laboratory abnormalities in, 1775, 1775*t*
  laboratory findings in, 1781*t*
  low blood flow, 1772-1773, **1773-1777,** 1773*f*
    classification of, 1773*t*
    clinical presentation of, 1776*t*
    effects on hemodynamic parameters, 1774-1775, 1774*t*
    precipitating factors, 1773*t*
  maldistribution of blood flow, 1773, 1773*f*, **1777-1778**
    classification of, 1773*t*
    clinical presentation of, 1776*t*
    effects on hemodynamic parameters, 1774-1775, 1774*t*
    precipitating factors, 1773*t*
  neurogenic, 1590, 1773*f*, **1777**
    classification of, 1773*t*
    clinical presentation of, 1776*t*
    collaborative care for, 1789-1790
    pathophysiology of, 1777, 1777*f*
    precipitating factors, 1773*t*
    treatment of, 1789*t*
  nursing assessment of, 1790
  nursing care plan for patient in, 1791*b*-1792*b*
  nursing diagnoses, 1790
  nursing evaluation of, 1794
  nursing implementation for, 1790-1794
  nursing management of, **1790-1794**
  nursing planning for, 1790
  nutritional therapy for, 1786
  precipitating factors, 1773*t*
  progressive stage, 1779-1780, 1781*t*, 1782*f*
  refractory stage, 1781*t*, 1783, 1784*f*
  septic, 1773*f*, **1778**
    in cancer, 308
    classification of, 1773*t*

Shock *(Continued)*
    clinical presentation of, 1776*t*
    collaborative care for, 1788-1789
    pathophysiology of, 1778, 1778*f*
    precipitating factors, 1773*t*
    treatment of, 1789*t*
  spinal, 1590
  stages of, 1778-1783, 1781*t*
  treatment of, 1789*t*
Short arm cast, 1640, 1640*f*
Short bowel syndrome, 1081
  clinical manifestations of, 1081
  collaborative care for, 1081
Short-leg gait, 1624*t*
Shortness of breath, 518, 519*t*
  fear of, 159
Shotty nodes, 521
Shoulder arthroplasty, 1664
Shoulder-harness seat belt injury, 585*t*
Shoulders, 49*t*
Shunts
  anatomic, 1802
  cranial procedures, 1491*t*
  for esophageal and gastric varices, 1108
  for hemodialysis, 1220, 1220*f*
  intrapulmonary, 1802
  peritoneovenous, 1107, 1108*f*
  portosystemic, 1108, 1110*f*
  procedures, 1491*t*
  transjugular intrahepatic portosystemic, 1108
SIADH. *See* Syndrome of inappropriate antidiuretic hormone
Sibutramine (Meridia), 981
Sickle cell anemia, 690*t*
Sickle cell crisis, 696
Sickle cell disease, 696-699
  clinical manifestations of, 697, 697*f*
  complications of, 697-698, 697*f*
  diagnostic studies, 698
  etiology and pathophysiology of, 696
  genetics of, 696*b*
  nursing and collaborative management of, **698-699**
  types of, 696
Sickle cell hemoglobin, 696, 696*f*
Sickle cell solubility test, 1860*t*
Sickling episodes, 696
Sigh, 511
Sighted-guide technique, 420, 420*f*
Sigmoid colostomy, 1069, 1070*f*
Sigmoidoscopy, 944*t*
Sign language, 445
Silastic catheters, 290
Sildenafil (Viagra)
  drug alert, 1435
  for erectile dysfunction, 1435, 1607
Silent cholelithiasis, 1127
Silent ischemia, 797
Silent painless thyroiditis, 1298
Silicosis, 578*t*
Silo filler's disease, 578*t*
Silver sulfadiazine (Silvadene, Flumazine), 497, 498*f*, 499
SilverDerm, 205*t*
Silver-impregnated dressing, 499
Silverlon, 205*t*, 499
Simple Descriptive Pain Intensity Scale, 132, 134*f*
Sims-Huhner test, 1341*t*
Simulect (basiliximab), 239*t*, 240
SIMV. *See* Synchronized intermittent mandatory ventilation

Note: Disorder names are in **bold face.** Page numbers in **bold face** indicate main discussions. Page numbers followed by *f, t, b,* or *n* indicate figures, tables, boxed material, or notes, respectively.

Simvastatin (Zocor), 793, 795*t*
  drug alert, 794
  ezetimibe/simvastatin (Vytorin), 794
Sinemet (carbidopa/levodopa)
  drug alert, 1551
  for Parkinson's disease, 1551, 1552*t*
Sinequan (doxepin)
  adverse cardiovascular effects of, 745*t*
  for Alzheimer's disease, 1569*t*
  local, 139*t*
  for peptic ulcer disease, 1019*t*, 1021
  photosensitivity, 461*t*
Single-photon emission computed to-mography, 758, 1463*t*
Singulair (montelukast), 620
  for allergic rhinitis and sinusitis, 537*t*
  for asthma and COPD, 619*t*
Singultus, postoperative, 391
Sinus bradycardia, 849-850, 850*f*
  characteristics of, 849*t*
  clinical associations, 849
  clinical significance of, 850
  ECG characteristics, 850
  treatment of, 850
Sinus rhythm, normal, 843, 844*f*, 846, 846*f*
Sinus tachycardia, 850, 850*f*
  characteristics of, 849*t*
  clinical associations, 850
  clinical significance of, 850
  ECG characteristics, 850
  treatment of, 850
Sinuses
  location of, 540*f*
  paranasal
    inflammation and infection of, **535-541**
    obstruction of, **541**
  physical examination of, 49*t*
  problems of, 609
Sinusitis, 540-541
  acute, 540, 541*t*
  chronic, 540, 541*t*
  clinical manifestations of, 540
  nursing and collaborative manage-ment of, **540-541**
Sirolimus (Rapamune), 238, 239*t*
SIRS. *See* Systemic inflammatory re-sponse syndrome
Sitagliptin (Januvia), 1265, 1266*t*
6-minute walk test, 753*t*, 757
Sjögren syndrome, 1704, **1726**
  treatment of, 1726
Skeletal muscle, 1617
  contractions of, 1618
  in fluid and electrolyte imbalances, 338*t*
  regenerative ability of, 198, 198*t*
Skeletal traction, 1639
Skeletal x-ray, 682*t*
Skelid (tiludronate), 1689
Skilled nursing facilities, 88, 88*f*, 88*t*
Skin. *See also* Integumentary system
  age-related changes in, 451-452, 452*t*
  allergic conditions of, **470-471,** 471*t*
  artificial, 501-502
  assessment abnormalities, 675*t*
  assessment of, 677
    in extracellular fluid volume im-balances, 323
    general principles for, 454
    variations in light- and dark-skinned individuals, 456*t*
  assessment of turgor of, 323, 323*f*
  benign conditions of, 472*t*
  breakdown at end of life, 161*t*
  changes in texture, 1246*t*

Skin (*Continued*)
  chemotherapy-induced changes, 296*t*, 299-300
  in chronic HF, 826
  in dermatomyositis, 1725, 1725*f*
  in fluid and electrolyte imbalances, 338*t*
  health promotion for, **460-463**
  homograft, 498
  with ileal conduit, 1193, 1193*f*
  inspection of, 48*t*, 454-456
  integrity during ET intubation, 1758
  malignant conditions, 464*t*
  neurogenic, 1606
  nursing plan for prevention of break-down, 1519
  pallor of, 675*t*
  palpation of, 48*t*, 456
  physical examination of
    adaptations, 50*t*
    outline for, 48*t*
    recording, 51*t*
  premalignant conditions, 464*t*
  preparation of, 366
  prevention of spread of problems, 478
  radiation-induced changes, 295*t*, 299, 300*t*
  regenerative ability of, 198, 198*t*
  in scleroderma, 1723, 1723*f*
  of scrotum and testes, **1430**
  in shock, 1781*t*, 1793
  structures of, **449-451,** 450*f*
  sun effects on, 460-461, 461*t*
Skin appendages, 450-451
Skin cancers, nonmelanoma, **463-464**
Skin care, 478
  in Alzheimer's disease, 1574
  in extracellular fluid volume imbal-ances, 323
  after spinal cord injury, 1606, 1606*t*
Skin grafts, **480-481**
  autografts, 481
  for burns, 501, 502*f*
  cultured epithelial autografts, 498*t*, 501, 502*f*, 1870
  isografts, 481
  types of, 481
  uses of, 480-481
Skin infections, 466-470
  bacterial, 466, 467*t*
  fungal, 469-470, 469*t*
  secondary, 478
  viral, 468*t*, 469
Skin lesions
  with cirrhosis, 1102
  primary, 454, 455*t*
  secondary, 454, 455*t*
Skin neoplasms, malignant, **462-463**
Skin scraping, 476
Skin tags, 472*t*
Skin tests, 229-230
  methods for, 229
  precautions for, 230
  procedure, 229
  respiratory, 525-526
  results, 229-230
  tuberculin, 525-526, 529*t*
Skin traction, 1639
Skin ulceration, 1246*t*
Skip lesions, 1052
Skip metastasis, 277
Skull, 1452
Skull fractures, 1481-1482
  clinical manifestations of, 1481, 1482*t*
  types of, 1481, 1481*t*
  ways to describe, 1481

Skull x-rays, 1463*t*
SKY. *See* Spectral karyotyping
SLE. *See* Systemic lupus erythematosus
Sleep
  age-related changes in, 1454*t*
  with Alzheimer's disease, 1569, 1569*f*
  and COPD, 655
  of ICU patients, 1737
  with nasal mask, 543, 543*f*
  of older adults, 81-82
  and skin, 462
Sleep apnea, 542*f*
  management of, 543, 543*f*
  nursing and collaborative manage-ment of, **542-543**
  obstructive, **542-543,** 1874
  obstructive sleep apnea-hypopnea syndrome, 542
Sleep-rest pattern
  in assessment
    of auditory system, 410*t*, 411, 746-747
    of cardiovascular system, 746*t*
    of endocrine system, 1244
    of gastrointestinal system, 935, 935*t*
    of hematologic system, 673, 673*t*
    of integumentary system, 453*t*, 454
    of musculoskeletal system, 1621
    of nervous system, 1455
    of preoperative patient, 350*t*
    of reproductive system, 1333, 1333*t*
    of respiratory system, 518*t*, 520
    of urinary system, 1143*t*, 1144
    of visual system, 403, 403*t*
  and asthma, 624*t*
  comparison with NANDA Interna-tional Taxonomy II, 42*t*
  concerns of patients requiring home health care, 90*t*
  and COPD, 650*t*
  nursing diagnoses, **1852**
  nursing history, 45*t*, 46
Sliding hiatal hernia, 1007, 1008*f*
Slipped disk, 1680-1681
SLND. *See* Sentinel lymph node dissec-tion
Slo-bid, 619*t*
Slo-Niacin (nicotinic acid), 795*t*
Slo-Phyllin, 619*t*
Slow continuous ultrafiltration, 1224*t*, 1225
Slow-reacting substance of anaphylaxis (SRS-A), 195, 197*f*
Sludging, 492
Small bowel series, 941*t*
Small cell lung cancer, 581*t*
  extensive, 581
  limited, 581
Small intestine
  absorption by, 929
  age-related changes in, 932, 933*t*
  digestion and absorption by, 929
  obstruction of, 1061, 1061*t*
  secretions related to digestion, 929, 929*t*
  upper, disorders of, **1013-1033**
Small joints, protection of, 1710*t*
Smallpox, 1839*t*
SMBG. *See* Self-monitoring of blood glucose
Smears, reproductive, 1339*t*, 1341
Smell, 152
SMOG formula for written materials, 62

Smoke and inhalation injury, 484-485
"Smoker's patch," 1001
Smoking, 167-174
  complications of, 168-170, 168*t*
  and COPD, 631
  effects on respiratory system, 631, 631*f*
  effects on wound healing, 201*t*
  health impact of avoiding, 185*b*
  passive, 631
Smoking cessation
  agents used for, 171*t*
  for COPD, 639
  five As for, 584
  five Rs for, 584
  nicotine replacement therapy to assist with, 172*b*
Smooth muscle, 198, 198*t*, 1617
Snakebites, 1835-1836, 1836*t*
SNOMED CT®. *See* Systematized No-menclature of Medicine Clinical Terminology
Snorting drugs, 168*t*
SNS. *See* Sympathetic nervous system
Snuff dipping, 553
SOC. *See* Sense of coherence
Social services for older adults, **74**
Social support, 57
  and older adults, **72-73**
  as stress management, 116*t*
Social workers, 91*t*
Sociocultural assessment, 57*t*, 58-59
Socioeconomic considerations
  cultural assessment, 29*t*-30*t*
  and health care system, 86
Sodium (Na⁺), 1147*t*
  antacid side effects, 1020*t*
  in burn patients, 500
  content in food groups, 834*t*
  daily requirements in chronic kidney disease, 1211-1212, 1212*t*
  dietary reduction, 770
  label language, 834*t*
  low-sodium diet, 833, 834*t*
  laboratory values, 1857*t*
  normal values, 321*t*
  restriction for chronic kidney disease, 1212-1213
  serum levels, in shock, 1775*t*
  urine levels, 1863*t*
Sodium bicarbonate
  antacid preparations, 1020*t*
  for elevated potassium levels, 1202*t*
Sodium channel blockers, 856*t*
Sodium imbalances, 324-326
  in acute renal failure, 1200
  association with ECF volume imbal-ances, 324, 325*f*
  causes and clinical manifestations of, 325*t*
  in chronic kidney disease, 1207
  differential assessment of, 324, 324*f*
  in positive pressure ventilation, 1765
Sodium nitroprusside (Nipride)
  complications of, 828
  for heart failure, 828
  for hypertension, 775*t*
  for shock, 1788*t*
Sodium phosphates (Fleet enema, Phospho-Soda), 1042*t*
Sodium polystyrene sulfonate (Kayexa-late)
  for elevated potassium levels, 1202*t*
  for hyperkalemia, 1210
Sodium retention, 765
Sodium-potassium pump, 317*f*
Soft corn, 1685*t*

Soft tissue injuries, 1630-1635
acute, 1631, 1632*t*
of hip, 1632, 1632*f*
RICE for, 203
Soft tissue rheumatic syndromes, 1726-1729
Solganal (aurothioglucose), 1699*t*
Solifenacin (VESIcare)
for urinary incontinence, 1182
for voiding dysfunction, 1185*t*
SoloSite, 205*t*
Solu-Cortef (hydrocortisone)
for arthritis and connective tissue disorders, 1699*t*
for asthma and COPD, 618*t*
for shock, 1787*t*
Solu-Medrol (methylprednisolone), 238, 239*t*
for arthritis and connective tissue disorders, 1699*t*
for asthma and COPD, 618*t*
for neurogenic shock, 1790
for spinal cord injury, 1596
Solutes, 316*t*
Solutions
definition of, 316*t*
intravenous, 339-340
Solvents
definition of, 316*t*
effects of use, 170*t*
Soman (pinacolyl methyl phosphonofluoridate), 1840*t*
Somatic mutation theory, 68, 68*t*
Somatic pain, 130, 130*t*
Somatomedin C, 1248*t*
Somatosensory evoked potentials, 1463*t*, 1627*t*
Somatostatin, 1236*t*
Somatotropin
serum levels, 1248*t*
target tissue and functions, 1236*t*
Somatropin (Omnitrope), 1292
Somavert (pegvisomant), 1292
SOMI brace. *See* Sternal-occipital-mandibular immobilizer brace
Somogyi effect, 1263-1265, 1876
Sorafenib (Nexavar), 303*t*
Sorbalgon, 205*t*
Sorbitrate (isosorbide dinitrate), 800*t*
Sotalol (Betapace)
classification of, 856*t*
food/nutrient interactions, 954*t*
for ventricular tachycardia, 855
Sound(s)
range audible to human ear, 444*t*
transmission of, 409
South Beach diet, 979*t*
Soy
for menopause, 1393*b*
uses, 796*b*
Sparine (promazine), 992*t*
Spasms, muscle, **1635,** 1637*t*, 1649*t*
Spastic (uninhibited) bladder, 1543
Spastic gait, 1624*t*
Spatial summation, 1444
Spatial-perceptual alterations, 1508
Speaking tracheostomy tubes, 544*t*, 550, 550*f*
Speaking tracheostomy valves, 550, 550*f*

SPECT. *See* Single-photon emission computed tomography
Spectral karyotyping, 682*t*
Speech
assessment abnormalities, 1460*t*
esophageal, 557
normal, 415
with tracheostomy tube, 550-551
Speech reading, 445
Speech therapists, 91*t*
Spence procedure, 1163
SPEP. *See* Serum protein electrophoresis
Spermatic cord, 1335
Spermatocele, 1431, 1431*f*
Spermatogenesis, 1324
SPF. *See* Sun protection factor
Spherocytes, 703
Sphincter electromyography, 1150*t*
Sphincterotomy, endoscopic, 1128, 1129*f*
SPICES assessment, 77, 78*f*
Spider angiomas
with cirrhosis, 1102
Spider bites, 1834-1835
Spider nevus, 675*t*, 677, 1102
Spinal accessory nerve testing, 1458
Spinal anatomy, 141, 142*f*
Spinal anesthesia, 371-372, 372*f*
Spinal cord, 1444-1445, 1446*f*
ascending tracts of, 1444
assessment abnormalities, 1461*t*
cervical, 1823, 1824*t*
compression of, 307
descending tracts of, 1444-1445
stimulation of, 143
transmission of pain to, 128
Spinal cord injury, 1589-1609
acute intervention for, 1598-1604
American Spinal Injury Association (ASIA) Impairment Scale, 1592, 1592*f*
bladder management in, 1602-1603
blunt injury, 1596*t*
bowel management after, 1602-1603, 1605, 1606*t*
case study, 1611
cervical cord injury, 1597*t*
classification of, 1590-1592, 1593*f*
clinical manifestations of, 1592-1595
collaborative care for, 1595-1597
with complete cord involvement, 1590
degree of injury, 1590-1591
dermatologic manifestations of, 473*t*
diagnostic studies, 1595
drug therapy for, 1596-1597
early surgery for, 1596
emergency management of, 1596*t*
etiology and pathophysiology of, 1589-1592
gerontologic considerations for, **1609**
health promotion in, 1597-1609
immobilization after, 1598-1601
with incomplete cord involvement, 1590, 1592*f*
initial injury, 1590
level of injury, 1590, 1592*f*
and rehabilitation potential, 1592, 1594*t*
mechanisms of, 1590, 1591*f*
metabolic needs in, 1595
mourning process in, 1608-1609, 1608*t*
neurologic level of injury, 1590
nonoperative stabilization of, 1596
nursing assessment of, 1597, 1597*t*
nursing care plan for patient with, 1598*b*-1600*b*

Spinal cord injury *(Continued)*
nursing diagnoses, 1597
nursing evaluation of, 1609
nursing implementation for, 1597-1609
nursing management of, **1597-1609**
nursing planning for, 1597
penetrating injury, 1596*t*
potential for sexual function in men with, 1607, 1607*t*
primary injury, 1590
rehabilitation and home care for, 1604
and restrictive lung disease, 595*t*
secondary injury, 1590, 1590*f*
sexuality after, 1607*b*
skeletal level of injury, 1590
skin care after, 1606, 1606*t*
surgical therapy for, 1596
temperature control in, 1603
Spinal cord problems, 1589-1611
resources for, 1613
Spinal cord tumors, 1609-1610
classification of, 1609, 1610*t*
clinical manifestations of, 1610
etiology and pathophysiology of, 1609-1610
extradural, 1609, 1610*t*
intradural extramedullary, 1609, 1610*t*
intradural intramedullary, 1609, 1610*t*
nursing and collaborative management of, 1610
types of, 1609, 1609*f*
Spinal fusion, 1683
Spinal nerves, 1448, 1449*f*, 1454*t*
Spinal shock, 1590, 1876
Spinal stenosis, 1680
Spinal surgery, **1683-1684**
Spine x-rays, 1463*t*
Spinnbarkeit, 1326
Spinocerebellar tracts, 1444
Spinothalamic tracts, 1444
Spiritual care, 154
Spiritual healing, 100
Spirituality, 31
cultural assessment, 30*t*
end-of-life care needs, 154, 154*f*
Spiriva (tiotropium)
for asthma, 618*t*
for COPD, 618*t*, 640
Spironolactone (Aldactone)
for chronic HF, 831
for cirrhosis, 1110*t*
drug alert, 831
for hyperaldosteronism, 1319
for hypertension, 773*t*
Spironolactone/hydrochlorothiazide (Aldactazide), 777*t*
Spleen, 670
disorders of, **729-730**
filtration function of, 670
hematopoietic function of, 670
immunologic function of, 670
palpation of, 677, 938
physical examination of, 51*t*
storage function of, 670
Spleen scan, 682*t*
Spleen ultrasound, 682*t*
Splenomegaly, 676*t*, 729, 730*t*, 940*t*
Splinter hemorrhages, 749*t*, 867
Splinting, 524*t*
techniques for, 381, 382*f*
SpO$_2$. *See* Oxygen saturation
Spondyloarthropathies, 1711-1726
diagnosis of, 1711
Spontaneous abortion, 1383-1384

Spontaneous breathing trial, 1767
Spontaneous respiratory rate (f), 1767*t*
Spontaneous tidal volume, 1767*t*
Sporanox (itraconazole), 576
Sporothrix schenckii, 245*t*
Sports-related injuries, 1630, 1630*t*
acute soft tissue injury, 1631, 1632*t*
head injury, 1484*t*
Spotting, 1388
Sprains and strains, 1630-1632
acute intervention for, 1631
ambulatory and home care for, 1631-1632
first-degree (mild) sprain, 1630
health promotion in, 1631
nursing implementation for, 1631-1632
nursing management of, **1631-1632**
second-degree (moderate) sprain, 1630
third-degree (severe) sprain, 1630
Sprycel (dasatinib), 720*t*
Sputum production, 518-519, 519*t*
Sputum studies, 525, 527*t*
Squamous cell carcinoma, 464, 464*t*, 465*f*
of lung, 581*t*
Square wave test (dynamic response test), 1739-1740, 1741*f*
SRMD. *See* Stress-related mucosal disease
SRS-A. *See* Slow-reacting substance of anaphylaxis
SS. *See* Systemic sclerosis
St. John's wort, 34, 102*t*, 103*f*, 121*b*
St. Jude valve, 883*t*
ST segment, 846, 847*t*
Stab wounds
to chest, 585*t*
spinal cord injury, 1596*t*
Stadol (butorphanol), 137*t*, 138, 141, 187
Staged cough, 1809
Staghorn calculi, 1169, 1170*f*
Standardized nursing terminologies, 7-8
Stapedectomy, 441
Stapes, 409
Staphylococcal food poisoning, 1032*t*
Staphylococcal infection, 1037*t*
Staphylococcus, 1155*t*
Staphylococcus aureus, 245, 562*t*
diseases caused by, 244*t*
hematogenous spread of, 561
methicillin-resistant, 246, 246*t*
Staphylococcus epidermidis, 246, 246*t*
Staphylococcus saprophyticus, 1156
Starch blockers, 1265
Starlix (nateglinide), 1265, 1266*t*
Starr-Edwards valve, 883*t*
Starvation, 952
Statins, 793, 795*t*, 934*t*
Status asthmaticus, 612-613
collaborative care for, 615-617
Status epilepticus, 1535
Stavudine (d4T, Zerit), 258*t*
STDs. *See* Sexually transmitted diseases
Steal syndrome, 1221
Steatohepatitis, nonalcoholic, **1101**
Steatorrhea, 940*t*, 955, 1079
Stelazine (trifluoperazine), 992*t*
Stem cells, **218-219,** 666
adult, 218-219
autologous stem cell transplantation, 305, 305*f*
embryonic, 218

Stem cells (*Continued*)
hematopoietic stem cell transplantation, **304-306**
for leukemia, 721
infusions, 305-306
mutation of, 274
peripheral stem cell transplantation, 304
predetermined, 273-274
STEMI. *See* ST-segment-elevation myocardial infarction
Stenosis
aortic valve, 879*t*, **880**
mitral valve, **878-879**
pulmonary, 881
pulmonic, 879*t*
renal artery, **1175**
spinal, **1680**
tricuspid valve, 879*t*, 881
valvular, 878, 878*f*
Stents
airway, 583
coronary artery, 801-802, 801*f*, 802*f*
drug-eluting, 802
endovascular, 896, 896*f*
for peripheral arterial disease of lower extremities, 903-904
to treat blockages in cerebral blood flow, 1510, 1510*f*
urethral, 1418*t*, 1419
Stereognosis, 1459
Stereopsis, 407
Stereoscopic vision, 407
Stereotactic surgery, 1491-1492, 1491*t*, 1492*f*
Stereotyping, 28
cultural, 951
Sterilization, 1433*b*
Sternal tenderness, 676*t*
Sternal-occipital-mandibular immobilizer brace, 1601, 1601*f*
Sternotomy, 808
Steroid hormone receptors, 1235-1236, 1237*f*
Steroids. *See also* Corticosteroid therapy
anabolic, 1267*t*
metabolism of, 932*t*
Stilphostrol (diethylstilbestrol), 288*t*
Stimulant psychosis, 174
Stimulant withdrawal, 187
Stimulants, **167-175**
and angina, 797*t*
poisoning, 1837*t*
Stings, 1833-1835
Stochastic theories of aging, 68-69
Stocking-glove neuropathy, 1285
Stoma, 1069
characteristics of, 1071, 1071*t*
double-barreled, 1069*f*, 1070
effects of food on output from, 1075*t*
urinary, 1189, 1190*f*
Stoma care, 557
Stomach
age-related changes in, 932, 933*t*
assessment abnormalities, 939*t*
bleeding from, 996
digestion and absorption by, 928-929
disorders of, **1013-1033**
parts of, 927*f*, 928
secretions related to digestion, 929, 929*t*
Stomach cancer, 1028-1031, 1028*f*
acute intervention for, 1030-1031
adjuvant therapy of, 1029-1030
ambulatory and home care for, 1031
clinical manifestations of, 1028

Stomach cancer (*Continued*)
collaborative care for, 1029-1030, 1029*t*
diagnostic studies, 1028-1029
etiology and pathophysiology of, 1028
health promotion in, 1030
nursing assessment of, 1030
nursing diagnoses, 1030
nursing evaluation of, 1031
nursing implementation for, 1030-1031
nursing management of, **1030-1031**
nursing planning for, 1030
postoperative care of, 1030-1031
preoperative care of, 1030
surgical therapy of, 1029
Stomatitis, 1000*t*
aphthous, 1000*t*
associated with HIV infection, 254*t*
in chemotherapy and radiation therapy, 295*t*
Stool culture, 945*t*
Stool softeners, 808, 1041, 1042*t*
Strabismus, 406*t*, **424**
Straight-leg-raising test, 1624
Strains, 1630-1632
nursing management of, **1631-1632**
repetitive strain injury, **1633**
Strength testing, 1622
Streptococci
acute poststreptococcal glomerulonephritis, **1165-1166**
diseases caused by, 244*t*
Streptococcus pneumoniae, 562, 562*t*, 564
antibiotic resistance, 246, 246*t*
clinical manifestations of, 565
diagnostic studies, 565
Streptokinase, 915
Streptomycin
nephrotoxicity, 1142*t*
for tuberculosis, 573*t*
Streptozocin (Zanosar), 287*t*
Stress, 110-124
of acute illness and surgery, 1272-1274
case study, 122
chronic, 115, 115*f*
definition of, **110-111,** 111*f*
disorders and diseases with stress component, 115, 115*f*
effects on fluid and electrolyte balance, 320, 320*f*
effects on health, **115**
examples, 111
factors affecting response to, 111-112, 111*t*
and hypertension, 766
nursing assessment of, 120, 120*f*
nursing diagnoses related to, 120-121
nursing implementation for, 121-122
nursing management of, **120-122**
oxidative, 68*t*, 69
physiologic response to, **113-115,** 113*f*
resources for, 124
as response, 114
tips for handling, 122*t*
Stress at Work (NIOSH), 124
Stress echocardiography, 753*t*
Stress incontinence, 1145*t*, 1181*t*
Stress management, **110-124**. *See also* Coping–stress tolerance pattern
critical incident stress management units, 1842

Stress management (*Continued*)
for Crohn's disease, 1054*b*
health-promoting behaviors, 792*t*
how to implement in clinical practice, 122*t*
for hypertension, 771
principles underlying, 116*t*
resources for, 124
Stress perfusion imaging, 758
Stress testing, **757**
Stress ulcers, 996, 996*f*
in acute respiratory distress syndrome, 1816
with spinal cord injury, 1603
Stressors, 111, 111*t*
Stress-related mucosal disease, 996
etiology and pathophysiology of, 1017
Stretch reflex test, 1459*f*
Stretta procedure, 1006, 1006*f*
Striae, 1246*t*
Strictures, 1173-1175
ureteral, **1173-1174**
urethral, **1174-1175**
Stridor, 525*t*
Stroke, 1502-1526
acute intervention for, 1515-1521
ambulatory and home care after, 1521-1524
case study, 1524
clinical manifestations of, 1507-1508, 1507*t*, 1508*f*
collaborative acute care for, 1511-1513
collaborative care for, 1510*t*
collaborative preventive care for, 1509-1511
collaborative rehabilitation care after, 1513-1514
cultural and ethnic health disparities in, 1503*b*
diagnostic studies, 1509, 1509*t*
drug therapy for, 1512
drug therapy to prevent, 1510
embolic, 1505*f*, 1506, 1506*t*
emergency management of, 1511, 1511*t*
etiology and pathophysiology of, **1503-1505**
exercise programs for, 1514*b*
gender differences in, 1503*b*
gerontologic considerations for, **1524**
health disparities and, 21*t*
health promotion in, 1509, 1515
hemorrhagic, 1505*f*, 1506-1507, 1506*t*
intracerebral, 1506*t*
ischemic, 1505-1506, 1506*t*
surgical therapy for, 1513, 1513*f*
lacunar, 1505-1506
left-brain, 1508*f*
nursing assessment of, 1514-1515, 1514*t*
nursing care plan for patient with, 1516*b*-1518*b*
nursing diagnoses, 1515
nursing implementation for, 1515-1524
nursing management of, **1514-1524**
nursing planning for, 1515
nutritional therapy after, 1522
prevention of, 1509, 1510*b*
resources for, 1526
right-brain, 1508, 1508*f*
risk factors for, 1503-1504
modifiable, 1503
nonmodifiable, 1503
secondary assessment of, 1514-1515

Stroke (*Continued*)
surgery to prevent, 1510-1511
surgical therapy for, 1512-1513
thrombotic, 1505-1506, 1505*f*, 1506*t*
types of, **1505-1524,** 1505*f*, 1506*t*
warning signs of, 1515*t*
Stroke volume, 742
calculation of, 1745
normal range at rest, 1739*t*
Stroke volume index
calculation of, 1745
normal range at rest, 1739*t*
Stromal tumors, 1082
Struvite stones, 1169, 1170*t*
STS System (Dexcom), 1269, 1270
ST-segment-elevation myocardial infarction, 802
Stuart factor, 670*t*
Sty (hordeolum), 406*t*, 422, 422*f*
Subacute care, 87*t*
Subacute granulomatous thyroiditis (de Quervain's), 1298
Subacute inflammation, 197
Subarachnoid hemorrhage, 1506-1507, 1506*t*
Subarachnoid space, 1452
Subconjunctival hemorrhage, 406*t*
Subcultures, 27
Subcutaneous tissue, 450, 486
Subdural hematoma, 1483-1484, 1483*f*
acute, 1483, 1484*t*
chronic, 1483-1484, 1484*t*
subacute, 1483, 1484*t*
types of, 1483, 1484*t*
Subjective data, 40
Sublimaze (fentanyl)
as adjunct to general anesthesia, 370*t*
for burns, 499*t*
effects of use, 169*t*
for pain, 137*t*
preoperative, 355*t*
Sublingual nitroglycerin (Nitrostat, NitroQuick), 800*t*
Subluxation, 1624*t*, **1632-1633**
Submersion injuries, 1831-1833
collaborative care for, 1832-1833
emergency management of, 1833*t*
Suboccipital craniotomy, 1582*t*
Suboxone (buprenorphine plus naloxone)
for opioid withdrawal, 180
for pain, 137*t*
Substance abuse, 165-166
acupuncture for, 99*t*
acute intervention for, 185-189
case study, 190
considerations for substance-abusing patients undergoing surgery, 187, 187*t*
definition of, 166*t*
health complications of, 167, 168*t*
health impact of avoiding, 185*b*
health promotion in, 184-185
nursing diagnoses for individual with, 184
onset, peak, duration, and withdrawal onset, 185*t*
pain in patients with problems of, 148
pain management in, 187-188
perioperative care for, 187
terminology of, 166*t*
Substance dependence
definition of, 166, 166*t*
health complications of, 167, 168*t*
symptoms and behaviors that may suggest dependence on, 181-182, 181*t*

Substance misuse
  case study, 190
  definition of, 166*t*
Substance P, 1445*t*
Subthalamic nucleotomy, 1551
Succinylcholine (Anectine)
  as adjunct to general anesthesia, 370,
    370*t*
  and myasthenia gravis, 1555
Sucralfate (Carafate)
  for gastroesophageal reflux disease,
    1006, 1006*t*
  for peptic ulcer disease, 1019*t*
Suction control chambers, 589-590, 589*f*
  in dry suction system, 591*t*
  in wet suction system, 591*t*
Suctioning
  in acute respiratory failure, 1810
  closed tracheal suction system, 1757,
    1758*f*
  closed-suction technique, 1757, 1757*t*
  dry systems, 591*t*
  indications for, 1757
  open-suction technique, 1757, 1757*t*
  procedures for patients on mechani-
    cal ventilators, 1757*t*
  subglottal, continuous, 1759, 1759*f*
  tracheostomy, 545*t*, 546, 546*f*
  wet systems, 591*t*
Sudafed (pseudoephedrine)
  for allergic rhinitis and sinusitis, 538*t*
  drug alert, 540
  effects on lower urinary tract func-
    tion, 1180*t*
Sudden cardiac death, 817-818, 856
  etiology and pathophysiology of,
    817-818
  nursing and collaborative manage-
    ment of, **818**
Sufentanil (Sufenta)
  as adjunct to general anesthesia, 370*t*
  for pain, 141
Suffering, 127
Sugar Busters diet, 979*t*
Suicide, assisted, 147
Sular (nisoldipine), 776*t*
Sulfamethoxazole, 461*t*
Sulfamylon (mafenide acetate), 499
Sulfasalazine (Azulfidine, Salazopyrin)
  for arthritis and connective tissue dis-
    orders, 1699*t*
  drug alert, 1054
  for inflammatory bowel disease,
    1054, 1055*t*
  for rheumatoid arthritis, 1705
Sulfonamides, 934*t*, 1142*t*
Sulfonylureas
  blood glucose level effects, 1267*t*
  for diabetes mellitus, 1265, 1266*t*
Sulindac (Clinoril, Apo-Sulin, Novo-
    Sundac)
  for arthritis and connective tissue dis-
    orders, 1698*t*
  and gastritis, 1013
  photosensitivity, 461*t*
Sumatriptan (Imitrex)
  drug alert, 1531*b*
  for migraine headache, 1530
Sun exposure, 460-462
  effects on skin, 460-461, 461*t*
  Retin-A effectiveness for damage,
    463*b*

Sun protection factor, 461
Sundowning
  in Alzheimer's disease, 1573
  nursing interventions for, 1573
Sunitinib (Sutent), 1178
Sunscreens, 461
Supartz (hyaluronic acid), 1697
Superficial thrombophlebitis, 909,
    909*t*, **910-911**
  clinical manifestations of, 910
  collaborative care for, 911
Superior vena cava, 743
Superior vena cava syndrome, 307,
    307*f*
Superoptic nuclei cells, 1138
Supination, 1622*t*
Supplements
  effects of during perioperative period,
    347*b*
  for menopause, 1393*b*
Support devices, intravaginal, 1183*t*
Support groups
  for caregivers and family members,
    1575, 1575*f*
  for ICD patients, 858
  for obesity, 980-981
Suppurative labyrinthitis, 442
Supraglottic laryngectomy, 551
Supraglottic swallow, 553, 553*t*
Suprane (desflurane), 369*t*
Suprapubic catheters, 1187
  insertion methods, 1187
  nursing interventions for, 1187
Suprax (cefixime), 1368
Suprefact (buserelin), 1426*t*
Suresite, 205*t*
Surfactant, 511-512
Surfak (docusate), 1042*t*
*Surgeon General's Report on Smoking
    and Health—2005,* 606
Surgeons, 362
Surgeon's assistants, 362
Surgery. *See also* Postoperative care;
    Preoperative care; *specific proce-
    dures*
  ablation, 1551
  for abnormal vaginal bleeding, 1388
  for acute pancreatitis, 1121
  ambulatory, 344
    discharge criteria, 393*t*
    postoperative care, **394**
  antireflux procedures, 1006
  for aortic aneurysms, 895-897
  for aortic dissection, 900
  and auditory system, 411
  bariatric
    special considerations for ambula-
      tory and home care, 986
    special considerations for postop-
      erative care, 986
    special considerations for preoper-
      ative care, 985
  for bladder cancer, 1179
  for brain tumors, 1489
  for breast cancer, 1352-1353
    follow-up care, 1353
    procedures, 1353*t*
  breast conservation, 1352-1353,
    1353*t*
  for cancer, **284-285,** 285*f*
  for cancer of female reproductive
    system, 1406-1407
  and cardiovascular system, 745
  for cataracts, 426-427, 426*t*
  chest, **592-593,** 593*t*
  for cholelithiasis, 1129, 1129*t*
  for chronic otitis media, 439-440
  for colorectal cancer, 1066-1067

Surgery (*Continued*)
  consent for, 352-354
  considerations for substance-abusing
    patients, 187, 187*t*
  for COPD, 644-646
  coronary artery bypass graft
    for acute coronary syndrome, 808-
      809
    minimally invasive direct, 809-810
  coronary revascularization, 808-810
  cosmetic, 984
  cranial, **1491-1493**
    indications for, 1491*t*
    nursing management of, **1492-
      1493**
  for deep vein thrombosis, 915
  definition of, 343
  for dermatologic problems, 476-477
  ear, 440*t*
  elective, 343
    cosmetic procedures, 479-480
    withholding fluids before, 353*b*
  emergency, 343
  and endocrine system, 1243-1244
  for endometriosis, 1397
  for esophageal cancer, 1010
  eye, 428*t*
  female reproductive system proce-
    dures, **1404,** 1404*t*
  and fluid, electrolyte, and acid-base
    imbalances, 337
  gallbladder procedures, 1128, 1128*t*
  gamma knife radiosurgery, 1582-
    1583, 1582*t*
  for gastroesophageal reflux disease,
    1006
  of gastrointestinal system, 934, 934*t*
  gerontologic considerations, **372**
  for growth hormone excess, 1291-
    1292
  for head and neck cancer, 556
  and hematologic system, 672
  for hyperparathyroidism, 1309-1310
  for hyperthyroidism, 1301
  important information, 43
  incontinence after, 1181*t*
  for inflammatory bowel disease,
    1054-1055
  and integumentary system, 453
  intraocular procedures
    postoperative considerations, 431
    for retinal detachment, 431
  joint, **1662-1665**
  kidney transplant recipient procedure,
    1227, 1228*f*
  kidney transplantation procedure,
    1227
  legal preparation for, 352-354
  live donor kidney transplantation pro-
    cedure, 1227
  for lumbar disk damage, 1681-1683
  for lung cancer, 582
  lung volume reduction, 644-646
  malabsorptive, 982-983, 982*t*, 983-
    984
  for morbid obesity, 982-983, 982*t*
  and musculoskeletal system, 1620
  music effects on confusion and delir-
    ium in surgical patients, 1577*b*
  for myasthenia gravis, 1556
  nasal, **534**
  neck, radical, 554*b*-556*b*
  and nervous system, 1454
  neurosurgical procedures for pain re-
    lief, 143, 143*f*
  nursing evaluation of obese patient
    undergoing, 986
  nursing management before, **363-364**

Surgery (*Continued*)
  nursing management of obese patient
    undergoing, **984-986**
  for obesity, **982-986**
  for oral cancer, 1002
  orthopedic
    nursing care plan for patient hav-
      ing, 1647*b*-1648*b*
    resources for, 1667
  ostomy, 1069-1076
  outpatient, 344
  for palliative care of cancer, 285
  for Parkinson's disease, 1551-1552
  patient positioning for, 366
  for peptic ulcer disease, 1025-1027
  perioperative care, **342-396**
  for peripheral arterial disease of
    lower extremities, 904, 904*f*
  peripheral artery bypass, 907*t*
  and pneumonia, 567*t*
  postoperative care, **376-378**
  preoperative care, **343-358**
  preoperative teaching information,
    352
  and pressure ulcers, 209*t*
  to prevent stroke, 1510-1511
  for prevention of cancer, 284
  procedures for seizure disorders and
    epilepsy, 1538*t*
  procedures requiring antibiotic pro-
    phylaxis to prevent endocarditis,
    866, 867*t*
  prostate
    discharge planning and home care
      issues after, 1422
    nursing care plan for patient hav-
      ing, 1420*b*
  for prostate cancer, 1424-1425
  for pulmonary embolism, 600
  purposes of, 343
  radiosurgery for brain tumors, 1489-
    1490
  for refractive errors, 418-419
  renal, **1188**
  of reproductive system, 1332, 1332*t*
  and respiratory system, 517
  restrictive, 982-983, 982*t*, 983
  same-day, 344
  for seizure disorders and epilepsy,
    1538
  settings, **343-344**
  site assessment, 377-378, 377*t*
  site preparation, 366
  spinal, **1683-1684**
  for spinal cord injury, 1596
  stereotactic, 1491-1492, 1492*f*
  for stomach cancer, 1029
  stone removal, 1171
  stress of, 1272-1274
  for stroke, 1512-1513
  telesurgery, 373
  terminology for, 343, 343*t*
  thyroid, 1304
  for trigeminal neuralgia, 1582-1583,
    1582*t*
  for upper gastrointestinal bleeding,
    997
  ureteral, **1188**
  for urinary incontinence, 1183
  for urinary retention, 1185
  of urinary tract, 1142, **1188-1193**
  for urinary tract calculi, 1172
  for valvular heart disease, 882
  and visual system, 402
Surgical analgesia, 99*t*
Surgical attire, 364, 365*b*
Surgical cholangiography, 942*t*
Surgical debridement, 204, **1662**

Note: Disorder names are in **bold face.**
Page numbers in **bold face** indicate main
discussions. Page numbers followed by
f, t, b, or *n* indicate figures, tables, boxed
material, or notes, respectively.

Surgical mumps, 1000*t*
Surgical suite, 360
  restricted area, 360
  semirestricted area, 360
  unrestricted area, 360
Surgical team, **361-363**
Surgical technologist, 362
Surgical wounds
  infection in, 392
  nursing assessment of, 392
  nursing diagnoses, 392
  nursing implementation for, 392-393
  nursing management of, **392-393**
Sustiva (efavirenz)
  adverse effects of, 258*t*
  drug alert, 257
Susto ("fright sickness" or "soul loss"),
  35
Sutter valve, 883*t*
SV. *See* Stroke volume
SVI. *See* Stroke volume index
SvO₂. *See* Mixed venous oxygen satura-
  tion
SVR. *See* Systemic vascular resistance
SVRI. *See* Systemic vascular resistance
  index
Swallowing
  in Alzheimer's disease, 1573-1574
  supraglottic swallow, 553, 553*t*
  with tracheostomy, 547-550
Swan neck deformity, 1624*t*
Sweat glands
  apocrine, 451
  eccrine, 451
Swelling, 1624*t*
  with fractures, 1637*t*
  of inflammation, 196, 197*t*
Swimmer's ear, 438
Swing-to gait, 1648
Sydenham's chorea, 876
Symbicort (budesonide/formoterol),
  620*t*
Syme's amputation, 1659
Symlin (pramlintide)
  for diabetes mellitus, 1265, 1266t
  drug alert, 1265
Symmetrel (amantadine)
  for influenza, 540
  for multiple sclerosis, 1544-1545,
    1545*t*
  for Parkinson's disease, 1551,
    1552*t*
  for pneumonia, 566
Sympathectomies, 143
Sympathetic nervous system, 1449-
  1450
  activation of, 823
    and hypertension, 766
    in myocardial infarction, 804
  age-related changes in, 1454*t*
  effects of, 1451*t*
  receptors affecting blood pressure,
    763, 763*t*
  regulation of blood pressure by, 763-
    764
Sympathetic ophthalmia, 437
Sympathetically maintained pain, 131
Sympathoadrenal response, 113
Sympathomimetics
  for allergic disorders, 231
  hematologic effects of, 674*t*
  for shock, 1785
Symptom investigation, 41, 41*t*
Symptoms, 40
Synapse, 1443-1444, 1444*f*
Synarel (nafarelin), 1383*t*
Synchronized intermittent mandatory
  ventilation, 1761-1762, 1761*t*

Syncope, 745*t*, **862-863**
  causes of, 862
  heat syncope, 1828
  postoperative, 386
Syndesmophytes, 1712
Syndrome of inappropriate antidi-
    uretic hormone, 319, **1294-1296**
  in cancer, 308
  clinical manifestations of, 1295
  collaborative care for, 1295
  diagnostic studies, 1295
  etiology and pathophysiology of,
    1294-1295, 1295*f*, 1295*t*
  nursing assessment of, 1296*t*
  nursing management of, **1295-1296,**
    1296*t*
Synergy, 1522
Syngeneic transplantation, 305
Synovectomy, 1662
Synovial joints, 1616, 1616*f*
  movement at, 1622, 1622*t*
  types of, 1616, 1617*f*
Synthroid (levothyroxine)
  drug alert, 1306
  for hypothyroidism, 1306
Synvisc (hyaluronic acid), 1697
Syphilis, **1369-1371**
  clinical manifestations of, 1369-1370
  collaborative care for, 1371, 1371*t*
  complications of, 1370
  dermatologic manifestations of, 473*t*
  diagnostic studies, 1370-1371
  drug therapy for, 1371, 1371*t*
  etiology and pathophysiology of,
    1369
  late or tertiary, 1369-1370, 1370*t*
  latent or hidden stage, 1369, 1370*t*
  neurosyphilis, 1370, 1370*t*, **1589**
  ocular manifestations of, 437*t*
  primary stage, 1369, 1370*f*, 1370*t*
  secondary stage, 1369, 1370*f*, 1370*t*
  serology tests for, 1336-1341
  stages of, 1369-1370, 1370*t*
  tertiary, 1369-1370, 1589
  third stage (late or tertiary), 1369-
    1370
Systematized Nomenclature of Medicine Clinical Terminology
  (SNOMED CT®), 8-9, 8*t*
Systemic anaphylactic reactions, 226,
  226*f*
Systemic diseases
  autoimmune, 234*t*
  ocular manifestations of, **437,** 437*t*
Systemic inflammatory response syn-
    drome (SIRS), 1772, 1773*f*, **1794-**
    1796
  etiology and pathophysiology of,
    1794-1795
  nursing and collaborative manage-
    ment of, **1795-1796**
  nutritional and metabolic needs in,
    1796*t*
  organ and metabolic dysfunction in,
    1794-1795
Systemic lupus erythematosus (SLE),
    1716-1723
  acute intervention for, 1720-1721
  ambulatory and home care for, 1721-
    1723
  butterfly rash of, 1718, 1718*f*
  clinical manifestations of, 1717-1718
  collaborative care for, 1719, 1719*t*
  complications of, 1717-1718
  dermatologic manifestations of, 473*t*,
    1718, 1718*f*
  diagnostic criteria for, 1719*t*
  diagnostic studies, 1718-1719

Systemic lupus erythematosus (SLE)
    (*Continued*)
  drug therapy for, 1719
  etiology and pathophysiology of, 1717
  health promotion in, 1720
  multisystem involvement in, 1717,
    1717*f*
  nursing assessment of, 1719-1720,
    1720*t*
  nursing care plan for patient with,
    1721*b*-1722*b*
  nursing diagnoses, 1720
  nursing evaluation of, 1723
  nursing implementation for, 1720-1723
  nursing management of, **1719-1723**
  nursing planning for, 1720
  ocular manifestations of, 437*t*
  patient and family teaching guide for,
    1720*t*
  and pregnancy, 1721-1722
  psychosocial issues in, 1722-1723
  renal involvement in, 1177
Systemic sclerosis, **1723-1725**
  clinical manifestations of, 1723-1724
  collaborative care for, 1724, 1724*t*
  diagnostic studies, 1724
  diffuse cutaneous disease, 1723
  drug therapy for, 1724
  etiology and pathophysiology of,
    1723
  internal organ involvement, 1723-
    1724
  joint changes in, 1723, 1723*f*
  limited cutaneous disease, 1723
  nursing management of, **1724-1725**
  renal involvement in, 1177
  skin changes in, 1723, 1723*f*
Systemic vascular resistance, 762,
  1738, 1739
  calculation of, 1745
  formula for, 743
  normal range at rest, 1739*t*
  in shock, 1774*t*
Systemic vascular resistance index
  calculation of, 1745
  normal range at rest, 1739*t*
Systems review, preoperative, 347-349
Systolic blood pressure, 743, 1876
Systolic dysfunction, 1773-1774
Systolic failure, 822
  mixed systolic and diastolic failure,
    823
Systolic hypertension, isolated, 765

T
T₃. *See* Triiodothyronine
T₄. *See* Thyroxine
T lymphocytes, 220, 221*f*
  cytotoxic cells, 220, 238, 238*f*
  helper cells, 220
T tube placement, 1129, 1130*f*
T wave, 846, 847*t*
TAAs. *See* Tumor-associated antigens
Tabes dorsalis, 1370, 1589
Tabun (ethyl *N,N*-dimethylphosphor-
  amidocyanidate), 1840*t*
Tachycardia, 676*t*, 825-826
Tachypnea, 524*t*
Tacrolimus (Prograf, FK506, Protopic),
  238, 239*t*
  blood glucose level effects, 1267*t*
  for dermatologic problems, 476
Tactile fremitus, altered, 524*t*
Tadalafil (Cialis), 1435
Tagamet (cimetidine)
  for acute gastritis, 1014
  for gastroesophageal reflux disease,
    1005-1006, 1006*t*

Tagamet (cimetidine) (*Continued*)
  for gastrointestinal bleeding,
    998*t*
  nephrotoxicity, 1142*t*
  for peptic ulcer disease, 1019*t*
  preoperative, 355*t*
  for upper gastrointestinal bleeding,
    997
  for variceal bleeding, 1108
TAH-BSO. *See* Total abdominal hysterectomy and bilateral salpingo-
  oophorectomy
Tai Chi, 97*t*, 98, 1701
Talwin (pentazocine)
  effects of use, 169*t*
  for pain, 137*t*, 138
Tambocor (flecainide)
  for atrial flutter, 851
  classification of, 856*t*
Tamiflu (oseltamivir)
  for influenza, 540
  for pneumonia, 566
Tamoxifen (Nolvadex)
  for breast cancer, 1355
  for cervical cancer, 1402
  classification of, 288*t*
  drug alert, 1355
Tamsulosin (Flomax)
  for benign prostatic hyperplasia,
    1417
  for voiding dysfunction, 1185*t*
Tapazole (methimazole), 1301
Tarceva (erlotinib), 303*t*, 1126
Tardive dyskinesia, 1578
Targeted therapy, **302-304,** 303*t*
  for arthritis and connective tissue
    disorders, 1700*t*
  for breast cancer, 1356
  for colorectal cancer, 1067
  drug alert, 1705-1706
  for leukemia, 720*t*
  nursing management of, **304**
  side effects of, 302-304
  sites of action of, 302, 302*f*
Targretin (bexarotene), 727
Tarka (trandolapril/verapamil), 777*t*
Tasmar (tolcapone), 1551, 1552*t*
Tasosartan (Verdia), 776*t*
Taste sensation
  in cancer, 307
  at end of life, 152*t*
tau protein, 1565
Tavist (clemastine), 461*t*, 537*t*
Taxol (paclitaxel)
  for breast cancer, 1355
  classification of, 287*t*
  for esophageal cancer, 1010
  for lung cancer, 582
  method of administration, 288*t*
  for oral cancer, 1002
  for ovarian cancer, 1403
Taxonomies, 8, 10
Taxonomy I (NANDA International),
  11
Taxonomy II (NANDA International),
  11, 42*t*-43*t*, 43
Taxotere (docetaxel)
  for breast cancer, 1355, 1356
  classification of, 287*t*
  for esophageal cancer, 1010
  for oral cancer, 1002
  for prostate cancer, 1427
TB. *See* Tuberculosis
T-cell lymphoma, cutaneous, 464*t*
TCM. *See* Traditional Chinese medicine
TCPs. *See* Transcutaneous pacemakers

Teaching, 54. *See also* Patient education
    barriers to nurse-teacher effectiveness, 56
    group teaching, 61, 61f
    nurses as teachers, 55-56, 56f
    older adults, 79, 79t
    peer teaching, 61-62
    preoperative, 350-352
    process of, 57
    required skills for, 55-56
    strategies for, 60-63, 60f, 61f
    strategies to overcome barriers to nurse-teacher effectiveness, 56t
    techniques to enhance patient learning, 63t
Teaching materials. *See also* Patient and family teaching guides
    audiovisual materials, 62
    printed materials, 62
    writing, 62
    written materials, 62
Teaching plans, 54
Teaching-learning process, **54-57**
Team leaders, 4
Team nursing, 4
Technology, 5
    and health care system, 86
    hybridoma technology of monoclonal antibodies, 240-241
    in immunology, **240-241**
    recombinant DNA, 241, 241f
Teczem (enalapril/diltiazem), 777t
TEE. *See* Transesophageal echocardiography
Tegaderm, 204, 205t
Tegagel, 205t
Tegaserod (Zelnorm)
    for chronic constipation, 1041
    for constipation, 1042t
    for irritable bowel syndrome, 1047
Tegretol (carbamazepine)
    for Alzheimer's disease, 1569
    analgesic effects of, 128
    for diabetes insipidus, 1297
    drug alert, 1536
    gerontologic considerations for, 1538
    local, 139t
    for seizures, 1536, 1538t
    for trigeminal neuralgia, 1581-1582
Telangiectasia, 457t, 476, 675t, 677, 917, 1102
Telbivudine (Tyzeka), 1094
    for chronic hepatitis B, 1095
Telemetry monitoring, 846
Telesurgery, 373
Teletherapy, 293
Telmisartan (Micardis), 776t
Telmisartan/hydrochlorothiazide (Micardis HCT), 777t
Telomere-telomerase hypothesis of aging, 68t, 69
Temazepam (Restoril), 1569t
Temozolomide (Temodar)
    for brain tumors, 1490
    classification of, 287t
    drug alert, 1490
    method of administration, 288t
Temperature
    and angina, 797t
    postoperative alterations in, **389-390**
        etiology of, 389-390

Temperature *(Continued)*
    nursing assessment of, 390
    nursing diagnoses, 390
    nursing implementation for, 390
    nursing management of, **390**
    significance of, 390, 390t
    regulation of, 1247t, 1595
    in shock, 1781t
    in spinal cord injury, 1595, 1603
    testing, 1458
Temporal arteritis, 437t
Temporal lobe absence, 1535
Temporal lobe seizures, 1535
Temporal summation, 1444
Temporary double-lumen vascular access catheters, 1221, 1221f
Temporary pacemakers
    indications for, 859t
    insertion of, 859, 860f
Temporary vascular access, 1221-1222, 1222f
Tenckhoff catheter, 290, 1217, 1217f
Tender points, 1727, 1728f
Tenderness
    abdominal, 1335t
    with fractures, 1637t
Tendinitis, 1630t
Tendons, 198, 198t, 1618
Tenesmus, 940t
Tenex (guanfacine), 774t
Teniposide (Vumon), 287t
Tenofovir and emtricitabine (Truvada), 258t
Tenofovir DF (Viread), 258t
Tenoretic (atenolol/chlorthalidone), 777t
Tenormin (atenolol)
    for acute coronary syndrome, 800t
    for chronic stable angina, 799, 800t
    classification of, 856t
    effects on lower urinary tract function, 1180t
    for hypertension, 774t
    for hyperthyroidism, 1301
Tenosynovitis, 1624t
Tenovir, emtricitabine, and efavirenz (Atripla), 258t
TENS. *See* Transcutaneous electrical nerve stimulation
Tensilon (edrophonium), 370
Tensilon test, 1556
Tension pneumothorax, 586-587, 587f
    emergency management of, 586t
Tension-type headache, **1527-1528**, 1528t
    diagnostic studies, 1528
    drug therapy for, 1530
    etiology and pathophysiology of, 1528
Tenting, 323, 457t
Tentorial herniation, 1452, 1472
Tentorium cerebelli, 1452, 1472
Tenuate (diethylpropion), 981
Tepanil (diethylpropion), 981
Tequin (gatifloxacin)
    for tuberculosis, 573t
    for UTIs, 1157
Terazosin (Hytrin)
    for benign prostatic hyperplasia, 1417
    effects on lower urinary tract function, 1180t
    for hypertension, 774t
    for voiding dysfunction, 1185t
Terbutaline (Bricanyl, Brethine), 619t
Teriparatide (Forteo), 1690
Terminal care, 267

Terminology
    abbreviations commonly used in ICUs, 1734t
    acid-base physiology, 333t
    body fluid chemistry, 316t
    genetic terms, 214t
    glossary of abbreviations, 1800t
    hemodynamic, 1738-1739
    lesion configuration, 456t
    lesion distribution, 456t
    sodium label language, 834t
    standardized nursing terminologies, 7-8
    sunscreens, 461
    surgical procedures, 343, 343t
Terrorism
    agents of, **1838-1842**
    bioterrorism, 1838
Test of Functional Health Literacy in Adults (TOFHLA), 59
Tes-Tape, 1481
Testes, 1324, 1325f
    acquired problems of, **1431-1432**
    age-related canges in, 1331t
    congenital problems of, **1430-1431**
    hormones and target tissues of, 1236t
    inflammatory problems of, **1430**
    physical examination of, 1335
    problems of, **1430-1432**
    skin problems of, **1430**
Testicular cancer, 1432
    clinical manifestations of, 1432
    collaborative care for, 1432
    complications of, 1432
    diagnostic studies, 1432
    etiology and pathophysiology of, 1432
    nursing and collaborative management of, **1432**
Testicular self-examination, 1432, 1433f, 1433t
Testicular torsion, **1431-1432**
    repair of, 1332t
Testosterone, 1236t
    laboratory values, 1858t
    serum levels, 1338t
    target tissue and functions, 1236t
    urine levels, 1338t
Testosterone replacement therapy, 1437
Tetanus, **1588-1589**
    clinical manifestations of, 1588
    collaborative care for, 1588-1589
    drug therapy for, 1588-1589
    etiology and pathophysiology of, 1588
    immunization against, 499
    nursing management of, **1589**
    prophylaxis against, 1828t
Tetanus and diphtheria toxoid (Td) booster, 1588
Tetanus immune globulin, 1588
Tetany, 331, 1247t
Tetracycline
    for peptic ulcer disease, 1019t
    photosensitivity, 461t
    for syphilis, 1371t
Tetrahydrocannabinol, 181
Tetraplegia, 1461t
    in spinal cord injury, 1589, 1594t
Teveten (eprosartan), 776t
Teveten HCT (eprosartan/hydrochlorothiazide), 777t
ThAIRaphy Vest, 649
Thalamotomy, 1551
Thalamus, 1447, 1448f
    location and function of, 1447t
    transmission of pain to, 129
Thalamus tumors, 1489t

Thalassemia, 691
    clinical manifestations of, 691
    collaborative care for, 691
    etiology of, 691
Thalassemia major, 690t, 691
Thalassemia minor, 691
Thalidomide (Thalomid), 729
THC. *See* Tetrahydrocannabinol
Theo-24, 619t
Theochron, 619t
Theolair, 619t
Theophylline, 621
    drug alert, 621
    effects on lower urinary tract function, 1180t
    food/nutrient interactions, 954t
Theosomatic medicine, 100
TheraCys (BCG vaccine), 303t
Therapeutic touch, 105, 109
    clinical applications of, 105
    description of, 98t
Thermal burns, 484. *See also* Burns
    emergency management of, 490t
    eye injury, 421t
    risk reduction strategies, 484t
Thermal procedures for refractive errors, 419
Thermoregulation, 1247t, 1595
Thermotherapy, transurethral microwave, 1418-1419, 1418t
Thiamine deficiency, 473t
Thiazide diuretics
    blood glucose level effects, 1267t
    for diabetes insipidus, 1297
    hepatotoxicity, 934t
    for hypertension, 771, 773t
Thiazolidinediones
    blood glucose level effects, 1267t
    for diabetes mellitus, 1265, 1266t
    drug alert, 1265
    hepatotoxicity, 934t
Thickening agents, 1520
Thiethylperazine (Torecan), 992t
Thioguanine, 287t, 721t
6-Thioguanine, 721t
Thiopental (Pentothal), 369t
Thioplex (thiotepa), 287t
Thioridazine (Mellaril), 1180t
Thiotepa (Thioplex), 287t
Third heart sound (S₃), 750t
Third space syndrome, 308
Third spacing, 319, 488, 1775
Third-order neurons, 129
Thoracentesis, 528t, 530, 530f, 595-596
Thoracic aorta, dissection of, 898, 899f
Thoracic cage, 512
Thoracic expansion, estimation of, 521-522, 522f
Thoracic injuries, **585-593**, 586t
Thoracic surgery, video-assisted, 593t
Thoracotomy, 592
    exploratory, 593t
    not involving lungs, 593t
    nursing care plan for patient after, 594b
Thoratec Ventricular Assist Device, 839
Thorax
    auscultation of, 750-751
        assessment abnormalities, 750t
        normal, 751t
    inspection of, 748-750
        assessment abnormalities, 749t
        normal, 751t

Note: Disorder names are in **bold face.**
Page numbers in **bold face** indicate main discussions. Page numbers followed by *f, t, b,* or *n* indicate figures, tables, boxed material, or notes, respectively.

Thorax (Continued)
palpation of, 748-750
assessment abnormalities, 749t
normal, 751t
percussion of, 750
assessment abnormalities, 749t
normal, 751t
physical examination of, 748-751, 1246
adaptations, 50t
recording, 51t
Thorazine (chlorpromazine)
adverse cardiovascular effects of, 745t
effects on lower urinary tract function, 1180t
for heatstroke, 1829
for nausea and vomiting, 992, 992t
photosensitivity, 461t
toxicology, 1865t
3TC (lamivudine), 258t
Three-dimensional (3-D) ultrasound, real-time, 758
Thrills, 748, 749t, 1221
Throat
in allergies, 229t
physical examination of, 51t
Thrombin inhibitors
direct, 913t, 914
indirect, 913-914
Thrombin time, 679t, 709t, 1775t
Thromboangiitis obliterans, 908
dermatologic manifestations of, 473t
Thrombocytes, 667, 668
Thrombocytopenia, 297, 678, **701-707**
acquired from decreased platelet production, 704-705, 704t
acute intervention for, 705-707
ambulatory and home care for, 707
causes of, 702t
in chemotherapy and radiation therapy, 295t
clinical manifestations of, 702-703, 703f
collaborative care for, 703-705, 704t
diagnostic studies, 703
etiology and pathophysiology of, 701
food, drug, and herbal causes of, 702t
gerontologic considerations for, **716**
health promotion in, 705
heparin-induced thrombocytopenia and thrombosis syndrome, 702, 704, 704t
nursing assessment of, 705, 705t
nursing care plan for patient with, 706b
nursing diagnoses, 705
nursing evaluation of, 707
nursing implementation for, 705-707
nursing management of, **705-707**
nursing planning for, 705
patient and family teaching guide for, 707t
Thrombocytosis, 678
Thrombokinase, 670t
Thrombophlebitis
of hand, 910, 911f
superficial, 909, **910-911,** 910t
Thromboplastin, 670t
Thromboplastin generation test, 679t
Thrombosis
deep vein, 909, 910t, **911-915**
risk factors for, 909, 910t
heparin-induced thrombocytopenia and thrombosis syndrome, 702, 704, 704t
venous, **909-917**

Thrombotic stroke, 1505-1506, 1505f, 1506t
Thrombotic thrombocytopenic purpura, 702, 704, 704t
Thrush, 1000t
Thyroid acropachy, 1299, 1300f
Thyroid antibodies, 1861t
Thyroid gland, 1240, 1240f
disorders of, **1297-1308,** 1297f
ocular manifestations of, 437t
effects of aging on, 1242t
enlargement of, **1297-1298**
posterior palpation of, 1245-1246, 1245f
radiology, 1249t
serum studies, 1249t
Thyroid hormone dysfunction, 1299, 1300t
Thyroid hormones
laboratory values, 1858t
regulation of, 1238, 1238f
target tissues and functions, 1236t
Thyroid nodule(s), 1246t, **1298,** 1298f
Thyroid scan, 1249t
Thyroid storm, 1299-1300
Thyroid studies, 1247, 1249t
Thyroid surgery, 1304
Thyroidectomy
for hyperthyroidism, 1301-1302
subtotal, 1302
Thyroiditis, 1298-1299
acute, 1298
chronic autoimmune (Hashimoto's), 1298
silent painless, 1298
subacute granulomatous (de Quervain's), 1298
Thyroid-stimulating hormone
laboratory values, 1858t
serum levels, 1249t
target tissue and functions, 1236t
Thyrotoxic crisis, 1299-1300
Thyrotoxicosis, 1299-1305
acute, 1302-1304
Thyroxine (T₄), 1240
free, 1249t
laboratory values, 1858t
target tissue and functions, 1236t
total serum level, 1249t
TIA. See Transient ischemic attack
Tiagabine (Gabitril), 1536, 1538t
Tiazac (diltiazem extended release), 776t
TIBC. See Total iron-binding capacity
Tibial fracture, 1656
Tic douloureux, 1581
Tick bites, 1835
Ticks, 470t
removal of, 1835, 1835f
Ticlopidine (Ticlid)
drug alert, 1505
food/nutrient interactions, 954t
for long-term therapy after TIAs, 1505
for peripheral arterial disease of lower extremities, 902
to prevent stroke, 1510
Tidal volume (V_T), 511, 531t, 1767t
TIG. See Tetanus immune globulin
Tigan (trimethobenzamide), 992t
Tikosyn (dofetilide), 856t
Tilade (nedocromil), 620
for asthma, 617t, 618t
for COPD, 618t
for exercise-induced asthma, 608
Tilting-disk valve, 883t
Tilt-table testing, head-upright, 863

Tiludronate (Skelid)
for osteoporosis, 1689
for Paget's disease, 1690
Timed voiding, 1183t
Timolide (timolol/hydrochlorothiazide), 777t
Timolol (Blocadren), 774t
Timolol maleate (Timoptic, Istalol), 434t
Timolol maleate and dorzolamide (Cosopt), 435t
Timolol/hydrochlorothiazide (Timolide), 777t
Tincture of opium, homatropine, methylbromide, and pectin (Dia-Quel Liquid), 1037t
Tinea corporis, 469t
Tinea cruris, 469t
Tinea pedis, 469t
Tinea unguium, 469f, 469t
Tinel's sign, 1633
Tinnitus, 409
assessment of, 410t
Tiotropium (Spiriva)
for asthma, 618t
for COPD, 618t, 640
Tipranavir (Aptivus), 258t
Tirofiban (Aggrastat), 800t
Tissue
oxygen needs of, 1803
oxygenation of, 1795-1796
regenerative ability of, 198, 198t
Tissue donation, 155
Tissue expansion, 1353t, 1362, 1363f
Tissue factor, 670t
Tissue freezing, true, 1830
Tissue perfusion, 1818
Tissue plasminogen activator
for chronic stable angina and acute coronary syndrome, 800t
recombinant (Alteplase), 915
for stroke, 1512
TIVA. See Total IV anesthesia
Tizanidine (Zanaflex)
for multiple sclerosis, 1545t
for pain, 139
for spasms, 1603
TLC. See Total lung capacity
TLS. See Tumor lysis syndrome
TNF. See Tumor necrosis factor
TNKase (tenecteplase), 800t
TNK-tPA, 800t
TNM classification system, 280, 280t
Tobacco cessation, 170-174
agents used for, 171t
Clinical Practice Guideline: Treating Tobacco Use and Dependence (AHRQ), 172, 172f, 172t
five As for, 172, 172t
five Rs for, 172, 172t
Tobacco smoke
effects on respiratory system, 631t
environmental, 631
Tobacco use, 167-174
and angina, 797t
and coronary artery disease, 789-790
health-promoting behaviors for, 792t
prevention of, 170
Tobramycin (Nebcin)
nephrotoxicity, 1142t
for osteomyelitis, 1670
Tocainide (Tonocard), 856t
Todd's paralysis, 1535
TOF peripheral nerve stimulation. See Train-of-four peripheral nerve stimulation

Tofranil (imipramine)
for Alzheimer's disease, 1569t
for peptic ulcer disease, 1019t, 1021
for voiding dysfunction, 1185t
Tofranil-PM (imipramine), 139t
Tolbutamide (Orinase), 461t
Tolcapone (Tasmar), 1551, 1552t
Tolerance, 166
definition of, 166t
fear of, 146t
and pain, 145
Tolmetin (Tolectin), 1698t
Tolterodine (Detrol, Detrol LA)
drug alert, 1183
for urinary incontinence, 1182
for voiding dysfunction, 1185t
Tomudex (raltitrexed), 1067
Tongue
geographic, 939t
physical examination of, 51t
smooth, 675t, 939t
Tongue cancer, 1001, 1001t
Tonic seizures, 1535
Tonic-clonic seizures
emergency management of, 1536, 1537t
Tonocard (tocainide), 856t
Tono-pen tonometry, 405-407, 405t, 407f
Tonsils
peritonsillar abscess, **542**
physical assessment of, 525t
Topamax (topiramate), 1536, 1538t
Tophaceous gout, 1715, 1715f
Tophi, 413t, 1715, 1715f
Topical medications, 477
analgesics, 1698t
for pupil dilation, 426, 427t
Topiramate, 1538
Topiramate (Topamax)
for alcohol treatment, 178
drug alert, 1531
for migraine prevention, 1531
for seizures, 1536, 1538t
for trigeminal neuralgia, 1582
Topoisomerase inhibitors, 287t
Topotecan (Hycamtin)
classification of, 287t
for lung cancer, 582
for ovarian cancer, 1403
Toprol (metoprolol), 1180t
Toprol-XL (metoprolol), 832
Toradol (ketorolac), 135, 136t
Torecan (thiethylperazine), 992t
Toremifene (Fareston)
for breast cancer, 1355
classification of, 288t
Tornalate (bitolterol), 619t, 620
Torsades de pointes, 855
Torsemide (Demadex), 773t
Torticollis, 1624t
Tositumomab/tositumomab-¹³¹I (Bexxar), 303t, 727
Total abdominal hysterectomy, 1405f, 1411
Total abdominal hysterectomy and bilateral salpingo-oophorectomy, 1404t
Total body surface area, 487
Total Care SpO₂RT® Bed System, 1818
Total colectomy, 1055
Total hip arthroplasty, 1663, 1663f
Total hip replacement, 1663, 1663f
Total iron-binding capacity, 680, 680t
in anemias, 690t
effects of aging on, 672t

Total IV anesthesia, 367
Total laryngectomy
  airflow in and out of lungs after, 552, 552f
  nursing care plan for patient having, 554b-556b
Total lung capacity (TLC), 531t, 594b
Total proctocolectomy
  with continent ileostomy, 1055-1056
  with permanent ileostomy, 1055
Tourniquet test, 679t
Toxic hepatitis, 1099-1100
Toxic megacolon, 1052
Toxic nodular goiters, 1299
Toxic shock syndrome, 1389
Toxicity
  acute, 291
  acute alcohol, 177
  acute cocaine, 174-175
  amphetamine, 175, 175t
  cardiotoxicity, 296t
  chronic, 291
  cocaine, 175, 175t
  digitalis, 832-833, 833t, 1865t
  hepatotoxicity
    of chemicals and drugs, 933-934, 934t
    in chemotherapy and radiation therapy, 295t
  nephrotoxicity
    in chemotherapy and radiation therapy, 296t
    of drugs, 1142, 1142t
  oxygen, 643-644, 1808
Toxoplasma gondii, 255t
Toxoplasmosis, 437t
Trabeculation, 1168
Trace elements, 950, 950t, 966
Tracheal deviation, 524t
Tracheal problems, 543-558
Tracheal suction, closed, 1757, 1758f
Tracheostoma valve, 557, 557f
Tracheostomy, 543-551, 1751
  indications for, 543
  nursing care plan for patient with, 548b-549b
  nursing management of, **543-551,** 544t
  percutaneous, 543
  speaking tracheostomy tubes, 544t
  suctioning, 546, 546f
  swallowing dysfunction with, 547-550
Tracheostomy care, 543-551, 546t
  changing ties, 546, 546f
  minimal leak technique, 547
Tracheostomy collars, 641t
Tracheostomy masks, 642f
Tracheostomy T bar, 642t
Tracheostomy tubes, 544t
  ambulatory and home care, 558
  changing, 547, 547f
  fenestrated, 544t, 545f
  precautions, 547
  sexuality and, 557-558
  speaking, 544t, 550, 550f
  speech with, 550-551
  suctioning procedure for, 545t
  types of, 543, 545f
Tracheostomy valves, speaking, 550, 550f

Tracheotomy, 543, 1751
Tracleer (bosentan), 602
Tracrium (atracurium), 370t
Traction, 1638-1639
  acute intervention for, 1646
  Buck's, 1639, 1639f
  cervical, 1601, 1601f
  indications for, 1638-1639
  purpose of, 1638
  skeletal, 1639
  skin, 1639
Tractotomies, 143
Traditional Chinese medicine, 96-98, 97t
Traditional healers, 30
Train-of-four peripheral nerve stimulation, 1765-1766, 1766f
Trait, 214t
TRALI. *See* Transfusion-related acute lung injury
TRAM flap. *See* Transverse rectus abdominis musculocutaneous flap
Tramadol (Ultram), 140
Trandate (labetalol), 775t
Trandolapril (Mavik), 776t
Trandolapril/verapamil (Tarka), 777t
Transabdominal ultrasound, 1339t
Transaminases, 1858t
Transbronchial needle biopsy, 529-530, 530f
Transcellular fluid, 315
Transcranial Doppler, 1463t
Transcription, 214, 215f
Transcultural C.A.R.E. Associates, 38
Transcultural nursing, 28
Transcultural Nursing Society, 38
Transcutaneous electrical nerve stimulation, 144, 144f
Transcutaneous pacemakers, 859-860, 860f
TransCyte, 498t
Transderm Scop (scopolamine transdermal), 992t
Transdermal controlled-release nitrates, 799
Transdermal nitroglycerin (Transderm-Nitro, Minitran), 800t
Transdermal scopolamine (Transderm-Scop), 138
Transderm-Nitro (transdermal nitroglycerin), 800t
Transduction, 127-128, 128f
Transeal, 205t
Transesophageal echocardiography, 754t, 758
Transexamic acid (Cyklokapron), 709
Transferrin, 680t, 690t
Transferrin saturation, 680-681, 680t
Transfusion reactions
  acute, 732-734, 733t
  delayed, 734t
Transfusion-related acute lung injury, 732, 733t
Transhepatic biliary catheter, 1129
Transhepatic cholangiography, percutaneous, 942t
Transient ischemic attack (TIA), 1504-1505
Transitional care, 87t, 88
Transjugular intrahepatic portosystemic shunt, 1108, 1109f
Translation, 214, 215f
Translingual spray nitroglycerin (Nitrolingual), 800t
Transluminal balloon angioplasty, percutaneous, 903-904
Transluminal balloon valvuloplasty, percutaneous, 881-882

Transmyocardial laser revascularization, 810
Transparent film dressings, 204, 204f, 205t
Transplant rejection, 237-238
Transplantation
  allocation of resources for, 1226b
  allogeneic, 304-305
  autologous, 305
  autologous stem cell, 305, 305f
  bone marrow, 304
  cardiac, **837-840**
  hematopoietic stem cell, **304-306**
    for leukemia, 721
  kidney, **1225-1230**
  liver, **1117-1118**
  lung, **603-604**
    for COPD, 646
    indications for, 603, 603t
  non–heart beating donation, 1828
  organ procurement organizations for, 1828
  organ transplantation, **236-240,** 236f
  pancreas, 1271
  for Parkinson's disease, 1552
  payment for organs, 1225b
  peripheral stem cell, 304
  syngeneic, 305
Transportation
  to operating room, 354-356
  recommendations for isolation precautions, 249t
Transrectal ultrasound, 1416
Transsphenoidal surgery, 1291-1292, 1292f
Transtelephonic event recorders, 753t, 757
Transtheoretical model of change, 55, 55t, 188
Transtracheal catheters, 641t, 643f
Transudate, 595
Transurethral electrovaporization of prostate, 1418t
Transurethral incision of the prostate, 1418, 1418t
Transurethral microwave thermotherapy, 1418-1419, 1418t
Transurethral needle ablation, 1418t, 1419
Transurethral resection of the prostate (TURP), 1417-1418, 1418f, 1418t
Transurethral resection with fulguration, 1179
Transvaginal ultrasound, 1339t
Transvenous pacemakers, 859-860
Transverse colostomy, 1069, 1069f
Transverse rectus abdominis musculocutaneous flap, 1362-1363, 1363f
TrapEase filter, 915
Trastuzumab (Herceptin), 302, 303t
  for breast cancer, 1356
  cardiotoxicity, 301
  drug alert, 1356
Trauma. *See also* Injury
  abdominal, **1047-1048**
  barotrauma
    in acute respiratory distress syndrome, 1816
    in positive pressure ventilation, 1763-1764
  case study, 1843
  to chest, **585-593,** 585t
  chest wall, 595
  to external ear and canal, **438**
  to eye, **421-422,** 421t

Trauma (Continued)
  focused abdominal sonography for, 1827
  to head, 1481
    major, 1482-1483
    minor, 1482
  incontinence after, 1181t
  musculoskeletal, 1629-1630
  renal, **1175**
  volu-pressure
    in acute respiratory distress syndrome, 1816
    in positive pressure ventilation, 1764
Trazodone (Desyrel)
  for Alzheimer's disease, 1569, 1569t
  food/nutrient interactions, 954t
Trecator (ethionamide), 573t
Trelstar (triptorelin), 1426, 1426t
Tremor, 1550
Trench mouth, 1000t
Trental (pentoxifylline), 902
Treponema pallidum, 244t, 1367t
Treprostinil (Remodulin), 602
Tretinoin (Retin-A, Renova, Vesanoid), 479t, 720t, 721t
Trexall (methotrexate), 287t, 1699t
Trexan (naltrexone)
  for alcohol abuse, 178
  for opioid withdrawal, 180
Triage, 1822-1823
  Emergency Severity Index algorithm for, 1823f
  system, 1822
Triamcinolone (Aristospan, Azmacort, Nasacort)
  for allergic rhinitis and sinusitis, 537t
  for arthritis and connective tissue disorders, 1698t, 1699t
  for asthma and COPD, 618t
Triamcinolone acetonide (Kenalog)
  for andropause, 1437
  for dermatologic problems, 475
Triamterene (Dyrenium), 773t, 1110t
Triamterene/hydrochlorothiazide (Dyazide, Maxzide), 777t
Triceps reflex, 1459
Trichlormethiazide (Metahydrin, Naqua, Trichlorex), 773t
Trichomonas vaginalis, 1394t
Trichomonas vaginitis, 1394t
Trichophyton, 245t
TriCor (fenofibrate), 795t
Tricuspid valve disease, 881
  etiology and pathophysiology of, 881
  stenosis, 879t, 881
Tricyclic antidepressants
  adverse cardiovascular effects of, 745t
  blood glucose level effects, 1267t
  effects on lower urinary tract function, 1180t
  ethnic differences in response to, 35t
  food/nutrient interactions, 954t
  hematologic effects of, 674t
  for peptic ulcer disease, 1019t, 1021
  poisoning, 1837t
  for voiding dysfunction, 1185t
Tridil (nitroglycerin)
  for hypertension, 775t
  for shock, 1786, 1788t
Trifluoperazine (Stelazine), 992t
Triflupromazine (Vesprin), 992t
Trifluridine (Viroptic), 423
Trigeminal nerve (cranial nerve V), 1450t, 1581, 1581f
Trigeminal nerve (cranial nerve V) testing, 1457

Trigeminal neuralgia, 1581-1584
acute intervention for, 1583-1584
ambulatory and home care for, 1584
clinical manifestations of, 1581
collaborative care for, 1581-1583, 1582t
conservative therapy for, 1582
diagnostic studies, 1581
drug therapy for, 1581-1582
etiology and pathophysiology of, 1581
health promotion in, 1583
long-term management after surgical therapy, 1584
nursing assessment of, 1583
nursing diagnoses, 1583
nursing evaluation of, 1584
nursing implementation for, 1583-1584
nursing management of, 1583-1584
nursing planning for, 1583
surgical therapy for, 1582-1583, 1582t
Trigger points, 143
Triggered beats, 846
Triglycerides, 752t
in chronic kidney disease, 1207
diagnostic criteria for metabolic syndrome, 987t
laboratory values, 1858t
Trigone, 1140
Trihexyphenidyl (Artane), 1552t
Triiodothyronine (T₃), 1240
laboratory values, 1858t
resin uptake, 1249t
serum levels, 1249t
target tissue and functions, 1236t
Trilafon (perphenazine), 992t
Trileptal (oxcarbazepine)
analgesic effects of, 128
gerontologic considerations for, 1538
for seizures, 1538t
Trilisate (choline magnesium trisalicylate)
for arthritis and connective tissue disorders, 1698t
for pain, 135, 136t
Trimethaphan (Arfonad), 775t
Trimethobenzamide (Tigan), 992t
Trimethoprim/sulfamethoxazole (TMP/SMX) (Bactrim, Septra)
hematologic effects of, 674t
for P. jiroveci pneumonia, 564
for urethritis, 1163
for UTIs, 1157, 1158
Tripelennamine (PBZ), 537t
Tripod position, 524t, 634, 1805
Triptans, 1530
Triptorelin (Trelstar), 1426, 1426t
Trisenox (arsenic trioxide), 288t, 720t
Trismus, 1588
Tritec (ranitidine bismuth citrate), 1014
Trizivir (lamivudine, zidovudine, and abacavir), 258t
Trochlear nerve (cranial nerve IV), 1450t
Trochlear nerve testing, 1457
Trolamine salicylate (Aspercreme, Myoflex cream), 141
Tropic hormones, 1239
excess of, 1293
Tropicacyl (tropicamide), 427t
Tropicamide (Mydriacyl, Tropicacyl), 427t
Troponins
cardiac-specific, 752t
in shock, 1775t

Trospium chloride (Sanctura)
for urinary incontinence, 1182
for voiding dysfunction, 1185t
Trousseau's sign, 331, 331f
TRT. See Testosterone replacement therapy
TRUS. See Transrectal ultrasound
Trusopt (dorzolamide), 435t
Truvada (tenofovir and emtricitabine), 258t
TSS. See Toxic shock syndrome
TT. See Therapeutic touch
TTP. See Thrombotic thrombocytopenic purpura
Tubal patency studies, 1382
Tubal sterilization, 1332t
Tubarine (tubocurarine), 370t
Tube feedings, 960-965
complications of, 963-965, 964t
general nursing considerations for, 963
procedures for, 961-962
Tuberculin skin testing, 525-526, 529t, 571
Tuberculosis, 569-575
active disease, 571-572
acute intervention for, 574
ambulatory and home care for, 574-575
classification of, 570, 571t
clinical manifestations of, 570
collaborative care for, 571-572
complications of, 570-571
cultural and ethnic health disparities in, 570b
description of, 246t
diagnostic studies, 571
disease, 570
drug regimen options for initial treatment, 574t
drug therapy of, 571-572, 573t
etiology and pathophysiology of, 570
health promotion in, 574
infection, 570
latent infection, 570
drug therapy of, 572
indications for treatment of, 574t
miliary, 570
nursing assessment of, 572
nursing diagnoses, 572-574
nursing evaluation of, 575
nursing implementation for, 574-575
nursing management of, 572-575
nursing planning for, 574
ocular manifestations of, 437t
organ involvement, 571
pulmonary, 572t
renal, 1164-1165
resurgence of, 569
Tuberculosis pneumonia, 571
Tubes
chest tubes, 588-592
drainage from, expected, 392, 393t
endotracheal tubes, 1751-1752, 1751f
feeding tubes (See Feeding tubes)
gastrostomy tubes
ambulatory and home care, 558
placement of, 961, 961f
sexuality and, 557-558
nasogastric tubes, 961
ambulatory and home care, 558
care of, 1062
nasointestinal tubes, 961
nephrostomy tubes, 1187
tracheostomy tubes (See Tracheostomy tubes)
Tubocurarine (Tubarine), 370t

TUIP. See Transurethral incision of the prostate
Tularemia, 1840t
Tumor angiogenesis, 276
Tumor lysis syndrome, 308
Tumor markers, 1336
Tumor necrosis factor, 222t
Tumor necrosis factor receptor, soluble, 223t
Tumor suppressor genes, 274
Tumor-associated antigens, 277, 278f
Tumors
anatomic classification of, 279, 280t
benign, of female reproductive system, 1398-1400
bone tumors, 1672-1675
brain tumors, 1487-1491, 1487b
classification of, 279
histologic grading of, 279
lung tumors, 585
radiosensitivity of, 292-293, 293t
spinal cord tumors, 1609-1610
urinary tract tumors, 1177-1180
Tums
elemental calcium content, 1689t
preparation, 1020t
for renal osteodystrophy, 1210
TUMT. See Transurethral microwave thermotherapy
TUNA. See Transurethral needle ablation
Tuning-fork tests, 413-414
Tunneled catheters, 289-290, 289f
Turbinates, 510
Turmeric, 102t
TURP. See Transurethral resection of the prostate
Tuskegee effect, 21
TUVP. See Transurethral electrovaporization of prostate
Twinrix (hepatitis A virus vaccine), 1096
Two-dimensional (2-D) echocardiography, 757
Two-point gait, 1648
Tylenol (acetaminophen), 1530
blood glucose level effects, 1267t
for hyperthermia, 1512
mechanism of action, 202t
for pain, 135, 136t
poisoning, 1837t
toxicology, 1865t
Tylenol #3 (codeine), 137t, 138
Tylox (oxycodone), 137t
Tympanic membrane, 409
examination of, 412, 413f
perforation of, 439, 440f
Tympanometry, 414t
Tympanoplasty, 440
Tympanum
assessment abnormalities, 413t
physical examination of, 412
Tympany, 523t, 937
Tyrosine kinase inhibitors, 303t
Tyzeka (telbivudine), 1094, 1095
Tzanck test, 458t

U
UAP. See Unlicensed assistive personnel
UI. See Urinary incontinence
Ulcerative colitis, 1051, 1051t
acute, 1052, 1052f
dermatologic manifestations of, 473t
surgical therapy of, 1055
Ulcerative gingivitis, acute necrotizing, 1000t

Ulcers, 455t, 1336t
arterial, 749t
arterial leg ulcers, 901, 901t
corneal, 423-424
duodenal, 1015, 1015t
complications of, 1017-1018, 1017f
etiology and pathophysiology of, 1017
esophageal, 1004, 1004f
gastric, 1015, 1015t
etiology and pathophysiology of, 1016
leg, 675t
arterial, 901, 901t
venous, 919-920, 919f
in mouth, 939t
neurotrophic, 1285, 1286f
peptic, 1014-1028
in COPD, 637
pressure ulcers, 206-211, 1875
stress ulcers, 996, 996f
in acute respiratory distress syndrome, 1816
with spinal cord injury, 1603
venous, 749t
venous leg ulcers, 901, 901t
Ulnar deviation, 1624t
Ultane (sevoflurane), 369t
Ultec, 205t
Ultiva (remifentanil), 370t
Ultradian rhythms, 1238
Ultrafiltrate, 1224
Ultrafiltration, 1216, 1225
continuous venovenous, 1224t, 1225
loss of, 1220
slow continuous, 1224t, 1225
Ultram (tramadol), 140
Ultrasonic lithotripsy, percutaneous, 1172
Ultrasound
abdominal, 940, 941t
endoscopic, 944t
esophageal endoscopic, 941t
gallbladder, 941f, 941t
gastrointestinal, 941t
hepatobiliary, 941t
intracoronary, 755t, 759
liver, spleen, or abdominal, 682t
of nervous system, 1463t
quantitative, 1625t
real-time three-dimensional (3-D), 758
renal, 1148t
of reproductive system, 1339t, 1341
thyroid, 1249t
transabdominal, 1339t
transrectal, 1416
transvaginal, 1339t
of visual system, 408t
Ultraviolet A, 460-461, 461t
Ultraviolet B, 460-461, 461t
Ultraviolet C, 460-461, 461t
Umbo, 412
Uncal herniation, 1472
Unconsciousness, 1471
nursing assessment of, 1476, 1476f
Undernutrition, 951, 969
Understanding Gene Testing, 241
Underweight, 975t
Uniform Anatomical Gift Act, 237
Uniphyl, 619t
Uniretic (moexipril/hydrochlorothiazide), 777t
Univasc (moexipril), 776t
Universal Protocol, 366
Unlicensed assistive personnel (UAP), 15

Unna boot, 919
Upper endoscopy, 943*t*
Upper gastrointestinal bleeding, 995-1000
acute intervention for, 999-1000
ambulatory and home care for, 1000
causes of, 995, 995*t*
collaborative care for, 997
diagnostic studies, 997
drug therapy of, 997
emergency assessment and management of, 996
endoscopic therapy of, 997
of esophageal origin, 995
etiology and pathophysiology of, 995-996
health promotion in, 998-999
nursing assessment of, 997-998, 999*t*
nursing diagnoses, 998
nursing evaluation of, 1000
nursing implementation for, 998-1000
nursing management of, **997-1000**
nursing planning for, 998
of stomach and duodenal origin, 996
surgical therapy of, 997
types of, 995, 995*t*
Upper gastrointestinal problems, 990-1034
resources for, 1034
Upper gastrointestinal series, 940, 941*t*
Upper limb amputation
sites of, 1658-1659, 1659*f*
special considerations for, 1661-1662
Upper motor neurons, 1445
Upper respiratory tract
burn injury to, 492
foreign bodies in, **541**
injury to, 492*t*
problems, **533-559**
resources, 559
structures and functions of, 510-511
Upper small intestine disorders, 1013-1033
Urachus, 1140
Urea nitrogen, 1858*t*
Urease, 1016
Urecholine (bethanechol)
for gastroesophageal reflux disease, 1006, 1006*t*
for multiple sclerosis, 1544*t*
Uremia, 1198, 1206, 1206*f*
chronic, 1206, 1206*f*
Uremic fetor, 1208
Uremic red eye, 1208
Ureteral catheters, 1187
Ureteral strictures, 1173-1174
Ureteral surgery, **1188**
Ureteroileosigmoidostomy, 1189*t*
Ureterolithotomy, 1172
Ureteroneocystostomy, 1174
Ureteroscopy, 1171
Ureterostomy, 1189*t*
Ureteroureterostomy, 1174
Ureterovesical junction, 1139-1140
Ureters, **1139-1140,** 1141*t*
Urethra, **1140-1141,** 1141*t*, 1331*t*
Urethral catheterization, **1186-1187**
Urethral diverticula, 1163
Urethral pain, 1145*t*
Urethral plug, 1183*t*

Urethral stents, intraprostatic, 1418*t*, 1419
Urethral strictures, 1174-1175
Urethritis, 1155, **1162-1163**
gonococcal, 1367, 1367*f*
Urethrogram, 1148*t*
Urethroplasty, 1175
Urethrovesical unit, **1141**
Urge incontinence, 1181*t*
Urge-suppression strategies, 1183*t*
Uric acid, 1147*t*, 1626*t*
laboratory values, 1858*t*
urine levels, 1863*t*
Uric acid stones, 1169, 1170*t*
Urinalysis, 1146*t*, 1150-1151
findings, 1152*t*
Urinary acidifers, 1267*t*
Urinary alkalizing agents, 1267*t*
Urinary bilirubin, 946*t*
Urinary catheterization, 1185, 1186*t*
Urinary diversion, 1188-1193
continent, 1190
incontinent, 1189
methods of, 1188, 1189*f*
nursing management of, **1190-1193**
postoperative management of, 1190-1193
preoperative management of, 1190
types of surgery requiring collection devices, 1188, 1189*t*
Urinary incontinence, 1180-1188
collaborative care for, 1182-1183
diagnostic studies, 1182
drug therapy of, 1182
at end of life, 161*t*
functional, 1181*t*
gender differences, 1180*b*
interventions for, 1182, 1183*t*
nursing interventions for, 1523
nursing management of, **1183-1185**
overflow, 1180
after radical prostatectomy, 1425*b*
surgical therapy of, 1183
after trauma or surgery, 1181*t*
types of, 1181*t*
Urinary protein determination, 1146*t*
Urinary retention, 1180-1188
acute, 1180
chronic, 1180-1182
collaborative care for, 1184-1185
diagnostic studies, 1182
drug therapy of, 1185
nursing management of, **1185**
surgical therapy of, 1185
Urinary stoma, 1189, 1190*f*, 1193*f*
Urinary system, **1136-1153**
in acute renal failure, 1200, 1201*t*
age-related changes in, 78*t*, 1141*t*
assessment abnormalities, 1145*t*
assessment of, **1141-1145**
important health information, 1141-1144
key questions to ask, 1143*t*
objective data, 1144-1145
preoperative, 349, 351*t*
subjective data, 1141-1144
auscultation of, 1145
burn injury complications, 492
in chronic kidney disease, 1206
clinical manifestations of disorders of, 1142, 1143*t*
diagnostic studies, **1145-1152,** 1146*t*-1149*t*
effects of aging on, **1141**
effects of chronic alcohol abuse on, 177*t*
at end of life, 152*t*
functional problems of, **1135-1232**

Urinary system (Continued)
functions of, **1136-1141**
infectious disorders of, **1155-1165**
inflammatory disorders of, **1155-1165**
inspection of, 1144
organs of, 1136, 1137*f*
palpation of, 1144
percussion of, 1144-1145
physical examination of, 1144-1145, 1145*t*
postoperative problems, **391-392**
etiology of, 391
nursing assessment of, 391-392
nursing diagnoses, 392
nursing implementation for, 392
nursing management of, **391-392**
preoperative review, 348
in spinal cord injury, 1595
after stroke, 1519
structures of, **1136-1141**
surgery of, **1188-1193**
Urinary tract calculi, 1169-1173
clinical manifestations of, 1169-1170
collaborative care for, 1171-1172
diagnostic studies, 1170-1171
dietary interventions for, 1172
endourologic procedures for, 1171
etiology and pathophysiology of, 1169
gender differences in, 1169*b*
location of, 1169, 1171*f*
nursing assessment of, 1174*t*
nutritional therapy of, 1171, 1171*t*, 1172
risk factors for development of, 1169, 1169*t*
surgical therapy of, 1172
types of, 1169, 1170*t*
Urinary tract infection, 1155-1159
acute intervention for, 1159
ambulatory and home care for, 1159
case study, 1194
classification of, 1155, 1156*f*
clinical manifestations of, 1156-1157
collaborative care for, 1157-1158, 1158*t*
complicated, 1155
diagnostic studies, 1157
drug therapy of, 1157-1158
etiology and pathophysiology of, 1156
health promotion in, 1158-1159
initial, 1155
microorganisms causing, 1155, 1155*t*
nosocomial, 1156
nursing assessment of, 1158, 1159*t*
nursing care plan for patient with, 1160*b*
nursing diagnoses, 1158
nursing evaluation of, 1159
nursing implementation for, 1158
nursing management of, **1158-1159**
nursing planning for, 1158
patient and family teaching guide for, 1161*b*
predisposing factors, 1156, 1156*t*
prophylactic antibiotics for, 1158, 1158*b*
recurrent, 1155
sites of, 1155, 1156*f*
uncomplicated, 1155
Urinary tract obstruction, 1168, 1168*f*
Urinary tract tumors, 1177-1180
Urinary urobilinogen, 946*t*
Urination, 1140
burning on, 1145*t*

Urine
formation of, 1137-1139
residual, 1146*t*
in shock, 1775*t*
Urine chemistry, 1862*t*-1863*t*
Urine collection, composite, 1146*t*
Urine culture, 1146*t*, 1157
Urine cytology, 1146*t*
Urine flow study, 1150*t*
Urine output
decreased, 1247*t*
postoperative management of, 1188
Urine specific gravity, 1775*t*, 1863*t*
Urine studies, 1146*t*, 1150-1158
adrenal, 1251*t*
hematologic, 682*t*
pancreatic, 1251*t*-1252*t*
reproductive, 1336
Urispas (flavoxate), 1185*t*
Urobilinogen
fecal, 946*t*
fecal analysis, 1864*t*
urinary, 946*t*
urine levels, 1863*t*
Urodynamics, 1150*t*, 1152
Uroflow, 1150*t*
Uroflowmetry, 1416
Urofollitropin (Fertinex, Bravelle), 1383*t*
Urokinase, 915
Urologic disorders, 1155*b*
Urologic problems, 1154-1196
Uropathy, obstructive, **1168-1175**
Uroporphyrins, 1863*t*
Urosepsis, 1155, 1161
Urothelium, 1140
UroXatral (alfuzosin), 1185*t*, 1417
Urozide (hydrochlorothiazide), 773*t*
Urticaria, 227, 471*t*
USDA Food Guide, 949, 950*t*
Uterine bleeding, dysfunctional, 1387
Uterine fibroids, 1398-1399
Uterine prolapse, 1407-1408, 1408*f*, 1877
Uterus, 1325-1326, 1326*f*
age-related changes in, 1331*t*
cancer of, 282*t*
UTI. *See* Urinary tract infection
Uveitis, 436
UVJ. *See* Ureterovesical junction

V
Vaccines
flu vaccines, 539
HIV, 257-259
pneumoccocal, 566
for tuberculosis, 572
Vacuum constriction devices, 1435-1436, 1436*f*
Vacuum-assisted wound closure, 205
VADs. *See* Ventricular assist devices
Vagal nerve stimulation, 1538
Vagifem (estrogen vaginal tablets), 1185*t*
Vagina
age-related changes in, 1331*t*
conditions of, **1393-1395**
clinical manifestations of, 1393-1394
collaborative care for, 1394
etiology and pathophysiology of, 1393
nursing management of, **1394-1395**
fistulas involving, **1409,** 1409*f*
Vaginal atrophy, 1391*b*
Vaginal bleeding
abnormal, **1387-1389**
collaborative care for, 1388
diagnostic studies, 1388

Vaginal bleeding (*Continued*)
nursing management of, **1388-1389**
surgical therapy for, 1388
types of, 1387-1389
breakthrough, 1388
Vaginal cancer, 1404
Vaginal hysterectomy, 1404t, 1405f
Vaginal weight training, 1183t, 1326
Vaginectomy, 1404t
Vaginitis
monilial, 1394t
severe recurrent, 1394t
trichomonas, 1394t
Vaginosis, bacterial, 1394t
Vagotomy, 934t, 1026
Vagus nerve (cranial nerve X), 1450t
Vagus nerve (cranial nerve X) testing, 1457-1458
Valacyclovir (Valtrex)
for Bell's palsy, 1585
for genital herpes, 1375
Valdecoxib (Bextra), 136, 136t, 1697
Valence, 316t
Valerian, 102t, 1393b
Valgum deformity, 1624t
Valium (diazepam)
as adjunct to general anesthesia, 370t
effects of use, 169t
for multiple sclerosis, 1545t
for panic attacks, 181
toxicology, 1865t
withdrawal from, 179
Valproic acid (Depakene)
for Alzheimer's disease, 1569
for seizures, 1538t
for trigeminal neuralgia, 1581
Valrubicin (Valstar), 287t
Valsalva maneuver, 930, 1144, 1605, 1877
Valsartan (Diovan)
for chronic HF, 833
for hypertension, 776t
Valsartan/hydrochlorothiazide (Diovan HCT), 777t
Valstar (valrubicin), 287t
Valtrex (valacyclovir), 1375
Values-belief pattern
in assessment
of auditory system, 410t, 412
of cardiovascular system, 746t, 747
of endocrine system, 1244-1245
of gastrointestinal system, 935t, 936
of hematologic system, 673t, 674
of integumentary system, 453t, 454
of musculoskeletal system, 1621
of nervous system, 1456
of preoperative patient, 350t
of reproductive system, 1333t, 1334
of respiratory system, 518t, 521
of urinary system, 1143t
of visual system, 403t, 404
comparison with NANDA International Taxonomy II, 43t
concerns of patients requiring home health care, 90t
nursing diagnoses, **1853**
nursing history, 45t, 46
Valves, prosthetic, 882
Valvular deformities, 876
Valvular heart disease, 878-885
acute intervention for, 885
ambulatory and home care for, 885

Valvular heart disease (*Continued*)
case study, 890
clinical manifestations of, 879t
collaborative care for, **881-885**, 881t
conservative therapy of, 881-882
diagnostic studies, **881**
health promotion in, 883-885
nursing assessment of, 883, 883t
nursing care plan for patient with, 884b-885b
nursing diagnoses, 883
nursing evaluation of, 885
nursing implementation for, 883-885
nursing management of, **883-885**
nursing planning for, 883
surgical therapy of, 882
types of, 878, 878f
Valvular incompetence, 878
Valvular insufficiency, 878
Valvular regurgitation, 878, 878f
Valvular stenosis, 878, 878f
Valvuloplasty, percutaneous transluminal balloon, 881-882
Vancenase (beclomethasone), 537t
Vanceril (beclomethasone), 618t
Vanceril DS (beclomethasone), 618t
Vancomycin (Vancocin)
for bacterial meningitis, 1495
dose and frequency adjustments, 1211
for infective endocarditis, 869t
nephrotoxicity, 1142t
for osteomyelitis, 1670
Vanillylmandelic acid, 1251t, 1863t
VAP. *See* Ventilator-associated pneumonia
VAPS. *See* Volume-assured pressure ventilation
Vaqta (hepatitis A virus vaccine), 1095-1096
Vardenafil (Levitra), 1435
Varenicline (Chantix)
for smoking cessation, 171t
for tobacco cessation, 170-171
Variable expression, 215
Varicella-zoster virus
associated with HIV infection, 255t
diseases caused by, 244t
Varicocele, 1431, 1431f
Varicocelectomy, 1332t
Varicose ulcers, 919
Varicose veins, 749t, **917-919**
clinical manifestations of, 917
collaborative care for, 917-918
complications of, 917
diagnostic studies, 917-918
etiology and pathophysiology of, 917
nursing management of, **918-919**
primary, 917
sclerotherapy of, 918, 918f
secondary, 917
Varicosity, 457t, 917, 918f
Varum deformity, 1624t
VAS. *See* Visual Analog Scale
Vas deferens, 1325, 1325f
Vascular access
for hemodialysis, 1220, 1220f
temporary, 1221-1222, 1222f
Vascular access catheters, double-lumen, 1221, 1221f
Vascular dementia, 1562
Vascular disorders, 892-924
gender differences, 893t
of lungs, **597-600**
renal problems, **1175**
resources, 924

Vascular endothelium, 764
Vascular resistance, 1739
Vascular system, 742-743
in inflammation, 193-194, 194f
response, 668-669
Vasectomy, 1433-1434
description of, 1332t
procedure, 1433, 1433f
Vaseline gauze, 205t
Vaseretic (enalapril/hydrochlorothiazide), 777t
Vasoactive medications, 1435
Vasodilator drugs
for chronic HF, 831-832
for hypertension, 775t
for shock, 1785-1786
Vasogenic cerebral edema, 1469
Vasomotor instability, 1391
Vasopressin (Pitressin, Pressyn)
for cirrhosis, 1110t
for diabetes insipidus, 1297, 1479
for gastrointestinal bleeding, 998t
lysine (Diapid), 1297
for septic shock, 1788
for shock, 1788t
target tissue and functions, 1236t
Vasotec (enalapril)
for chronic HF, 832
for chronic stable angina and acute coronary syndrome, 800t
effects on lower urinary tract function, 1180t
for hypertension, 776t, 1210
Vasotec I.V. (enalaprilat), 776t
VATS. *See* Video-assisted thoracic surgery
Vaxomax (phentolamine), 1435
VBG. *See* Vertical banded gastroplasty
VC. *See* Vital capacity
VCUG. *See* Voiding cystourethrogram
VDRL test. *See* Venereal Disease Research Laboratory test
V$_E$. *See* Minute ventilation
Vectibix (panitumumab), 1067
Vecuronium (Norcuron), 370t
Vegans, 950
Vegetarian diet, 950-951
Veins, 743
coronary, 740-741, 741f
deep vein thrombosis, 909, 910t, **911-915**
disorders of, **909-920**
distended neck veins, 749t
renal vein thrombosis, **1175**
varicose veins, 749t, **917-919**
Velban (vinblastine)
for bladder cancer, 1179
classification of, 287t
for leukemia, 720t
Velcade (bortezomib), 303t, 729
Vena cava interruption devices, 915, 915f
Vena Tech filter, 915
Venereal Disease Research Laboratory (VDRL) test, 1336-1341, 1338t, 1371, 1861t
Venereal diseases, 1366
Venlafaxine (Effexor), 130
Venography
in deep vein thrombosis, 911t
peripheral, 755t
Venous access therapies, 1224, 1224t
Venous blood gases
mixed, 513-514
normal values, 514t
Venous Doppler evaluation, 911t
Venous hemoglobin oxygen saturation, 1739t

Venous hydrostatic pressure elevation, 319
Venous insufficiency, chronic, 911, **919-920**
nursing management of, **920**
Venous leg ulcers, 901, 901t, **919-920**, 919f
nursing management of, **920**
Venous oxygen saturation, 1746-1747
central, 1746
mixed, 1746
Venous return, decreasing, 828
Venous stasis, 909, 910t
Venous stasis ulcers, 919
Venous studies, noninvasive, 911t
Venous thrombosis, 909-917
acute intervention for, 916
ambulatory and home care for, 916-917
etiology of, 909-910
after fracture, 1651
nursing assessment of, 915
nursing diagnoses, 915
nursing implementation for, 916-917
nursing management of, **915-917**
nursing planning for, 916
pathophysiology of, 910
Venous ulcers, 473t, 749t
Venovenous hemodialysis, continuous, 1224-1225, 1224f, 1224t, 1225
Venovenous hemofiltration, continuous, 1224-1225, 1224f, 1224t, 1225
Venovenous ultrafiltration, continuous, 1224t, 1225
Ventavis (iloprost), 1724
Ventilation, 512
bag-valve-mask, 1752
basic life support, 1846
ET tube, 1753-1757
maximal voluntary ventilation (MVV), 531t
mechanical ventilation, **1759-1769**
problems of, **508-663**
in shock, 1783
Ventilation-perfusion lung scan, 526, 528t, 599
Ventilation-perfusion mismatch, 1779, 1801-1802
normal regional differences, 1801, 1802f
range of, 1801-1802, 1802f
Ventilator-associated pneumonia, 563-564, 1764-1765
Ventilatory demand, 1803
Ventilatory disorders, 594b
Ventilatory failure, 1800, 1803
Ventilatory supply, 1803
Ventolin (albuterol), 619t, 620
Ventricles, 1448
Ventricular aneurysm, 805
Ventricular assist devices, 831, 1750, 1750f
contraindications to, 1750
definition of, 1877
Thoratec Ventricular Assist Device, 839
Ventricular bigeminy, 854, 854f
Ventricular contractions, premature, 854, 854f
characteristics of, 849t
Ventricular failure, 822-823
Ventricular fibrillation, 855, 855f
characteristics of, 849t
clinical associations, 855
clinical significance of, 855
ECG characteristics, 855
treatment of, 855
Ventricular gallop, 751

Index

Ventricular hypertrophy, 742, 823-824
Ventricular remodeling, 804, 823
Ventricular tachycardia, 854-855, 855*f*
  characteristics of, 849*t*
  clinical associations, 855
  clinical significance of, 855
  ECG characteristics, 855
  treatment of, 855
Ventricular trigeminy, 854, 854*f*
Ventriculomyotomy and myectomy, 889
Venturi masks, 642*f*, 642*t*
Venules, 743
VePesid (etoposide)
  classification of, 287*t*
  for leukemia, 720*t*
  for lung cancer, 582
  for testicular cancer, 1432
Verapamil (Calan, Isoptin)
  for acute coronary syndrome, 800*t*
  for chronic stable angina, 800*t*, 801
  classification of, 856*t*
  effects on lower urinary tract function, 1180*t*
  for hypertension, 776*t*
  long acting (Isoptin SR, Covera-HS, Calan SR), 776*t*
  timed release (Verelan PM), 776*t*
  trandolapril/verapamil (Tarka), 777*t*
  for voiding dysfunction, 1185*t*
Verdia (tasosartan), 776*t*
Verelan PM (verapamil timed release), 776*t*
Verruca vulgaris, 468*t*
Versed (midazolam)
  as adjunct to general anesthesia, 369, 370*t*
  for burns, 499*t*
  preoperative, 355*t*
Vertebral artery, 1451*f*
Vertebral column, 1452, 1454*f*
Vertebral fractures, stable, **1656**
Vertebrobasilar artery, 1507*f*
Vertebroplasty, 1656
Verteporfin (Visudyne), 432
Vertical banded gastroplasty, 982*t*, 983, 983*f*
Vertigo, 409
Very-low-density lipoproteins, 756
Vesanoid (tretinoin), 720*t*, 721*t*
Vesicants, 286
VESIcare (solifenacin), 1182, 1185*t*
Vesicles, 455*t*, 1336*t*
Vesicular sounds, 523
Vesprin (triflupromazine), 992*t*
Vestibular function tests, 414*t*, 415
Vestibular schwannoma, 442
Vestibular (balance) system assessment, 409
Vestibule, 1327
Vestibulocochlear nerve (cranial nerve VIII), 1450*t*
Vfend (voriconazole), 576
Viadur (leuprolide), 1426, 1426*t*
Viagra (sildenafil), 1435
Vibramycin (doxycycline)
  for arthritis and connective tissue disorders, 1698*t*

Vibramycin (doxycycline) *(Continued)*
  for chlamydial infections, 1373
  drug alert, 1368
  for gonorrhea, 1368
  for Lyme disease, 1714
  for osteoarthritis, 1697
  for Rocky Mountain spotted fever, 1835
  for syphilis, 1371*t*
Vibration
  of chest, 647
Vibration sense assessment, 1458
Vibrio cholerae 0139, 245*t*
Vicodin (hydrocodone), 137*t*, 138
Vicoprofen (ibuprofen), 138
Vidarabine (Vira-A)
  for encephalitis, 1498
  for keratitis, 423
Vidaza (azacitidine), 717
Video-assisted thoracic surgery, 592-593, 593*t*
Videourodynamics, 1150*t*
Videx (didanosine), 258*t*
Videx-EC (didanosine), 258*t*
Vigabatrin (Sabril), 1536, 1538*t*
Vigamox (moxifloxacin), 573*t*
Villi, 929
Vinblastine (Velban)
  for bladder cancer, 1179
  classification of, 287*t*
  for leukemia, 720*t*
Vinca alkaloids, 720*t*
Vincent's infection, 1000*t*
Vincristine (Oncovin)
  classification of, 287*t*
  for leukemia, 720*t*, 721*t*
  method of administration, 288*t*
  for multiple myeloma, 729
  for non-Hodgkin's lymphoma, 727*t*
Vindesine, 727*t*
Vinorelbine (Navelbine)
  for breast cancer, 1355
  classification of, 287*t*
  for esophageal cancer, 1010
  for lung cancer, 582
  photosensitivity, 461*t*
Viokase (pancreatin), 1121*t*
Violation of personal rights, 73*t*
Violence, 1838
Vioxx (rofecoxib), 136, 1697
Vira-A (vidarabine)
  for encephalitis, 1498
  for keratitis, 423
Viracept (nelfinavir), 258*t*
Viral carcinogens, 276
Viral conjunctivitis, 422
Viral hepatitis. *See also* Hepatitis
  acute, 1097*b*-1098*b*
  collaborative care for, 1094*b*
  fulminant, 1092
  preventive measures for, 1097, 1098*t*
  tests for, 1092, 1093*t*
Viral infections
  sexually transmitted diseases, **1373-1379**
  of skin, 468*t*, 469
Viral keratitis, 423
Viral load, 249
Viral meningitis, 1497
Viral rhinitis, acute, **536-538**
Viramune (nevirapine), 258*t*
Virchow's triad, 909
Viread (tenofovir DF), 258*t*
Viremia, 251
Viroptic (trifluridine), 423
Virtual colonoscopy, 940-943, 942*t*
Virtual intensive care units, 1734, 1734*f*

Viruses, 244. *See also* specific viruses
  culture for, 458*t*
  disease-causing, 244, 244*t*
  emerging infections, 245*t*
  immune response to, 220, 221*f*
  oncogenic, 276
  organisms associated with infective endocarditis, 866, 866*t*
  reemerging infections, 246*t*
Visceral layer, 928
Visceral pain, 130, 130*t*
Visceral pleura, 512
Vision
  blurred, 406*t*, 675*t*
  changes at end of life, 152*t*
  distortion of, 432
  stereoscopic, 407
  structures and functions of, 398-400
Vision enhancement
  nonoptical methods for, 421
  optical devices for, 420-421
Visken (pindolol), 774*t*
Vistaril (hydroxyzine), 138, 992*t*
Visual acuity testing, 404-405, 405*t*, 1457
Visual Analog Scale (VAS), 132, 134*f*
Visual evoked potentials, 1463*t*
Visual field assessment, 1456, 1457*f*
Visual field cuts, 675*t*
Visual field defects, 406*t*
Visual impairment
  acute intervention for, 420
  ambulatory and home care for, 420-421
  gerontologic considerations, **421**
  health promotion in, 420
  levels of, 419
  nursing assessment of, 419
  nursing diagnoses, 419
  nursing evaluation of, 421
  nursing implementation for, 420-421
  nursing management of, **419-421**
  nursing planning for, 419
  severe, 419
  sighted-guide technique for, 420, 420*f*
  uncorrectable, **419-421**
Visual pathway, 400, 400*f*
Visual problems, 416-422
  cultural and ethnic health disparities in, 417*b*
  nonsurgical corrections, 417
  resources, 448
  surgical therapy of, 418-419
Visual system
  age-related changes in, 401*t*
  assessment abnormalities, 406*t*
  assessment of, **402-407**
    functional, 404-407
    health history questions to ask, 403*t*
    physical, 404, 404*t*
    techniques for, 405*t*, 407
  diagnostic studies of, **407,** 408*t*
  effects of aging on, **402**
  initial observation of, 404
  physical examination of, 404-407
  structures and functions of, **398-402**
    assessing, 407
    external, 400
    internal, 400-402
Visudyne (verteporfin), 432
Vital capacity (VC), 531*t*, 594*b*, 1767*t*
Vital signs
  assessment of, 747-748, 1245
  home health care activities, 90*t*
  in increased ICP, 1471
  in inflammation, 203
  outline for recording, 48*t*
  secondary survey of, 1824-1825, 1826*t*

Vitamin A
  for burns, 499*t*
  daily requirements in chronic kidney disease, 1211-1212, 1212*t*
  laboratory values, 1858*t*
  mechanism of action, 202*t*
  overdose, 953*t*
  recommended dietary reference intakes, 953*t*
Vitamin A deficiency, 437*t*
Vitamin B complex, 202*t*
Vitamin B deficiency, 437*t*
Vitamin B$_1$
  overdose, 953*t*
  recommended dietary reference intakes, 953*t*
Vitamin B$_1$ deficiency, 473*t*
Vitamin B$_2$ deficiency, 473*t*
Vitamin B$_6$
  overdose, 953*t*
  recommended dietary reference intakes, 953*t*
  supplementation for premenstrual syndrome, 1386
Vitamin B$_{12}$. *See* Cobalamin
Vitamin C
  for burns, 499*t*
  daily requirements in chronic kidney disease, 1211-1212, 1212*t*
  mechanism of action, 202*t*
  overdose, 953*t*
  recommended dietary reference intakes, 953*t*
Vitamin C deficiency
  dermatologic manifestations of, 473*t*
  effects on wound healing, 201*t*
  ocular manifestations of, 437*t*
Vitamin D
  for hypocalcemia, 1210
  for hypoparathyroidism, 1311
  mechanism of action, 202*t*
  overdose, 953*t*
  recommendations for older adults, 1688
  recommended dietary reference intakes, 953*t*
Vitamin D deficiency, 437*t*
Vitamin E
  for burns, 499*t*
  overdose, 953*t*
  recommended dietary reference intakes, 953*t*
Vitamin K (AquaMEPHYTON)
  for cirrhosis, 1110*t*
  overdose, 953*t*
  production test, 946*t*
  recommended dietary reference intakes, 953*t*
  for variceal bleeding, 1108
Vitamin K antagonists, 912-913, 913*t*
Vitamins
  for inflammation and healing, 202*t*
  for inflammatory bowel disease, 1054, 1055*t*
  oral anticoagulants interactions, 914*t*
  in parenteral nutrition, 966
  recommended dietary reference intakes, 953*t*
Vitiligo, 472*t*, *478*
Vitrectomy, 431, 1285
Vitreous cavity, 399, 399*f*
Vitreous humor, 399, 401*t*
Vivitrol (naltrexone), 178
VLDLs. See Very-low-density lipoproteins
Voice change, 519*t*
Voice prostheses, 557, 557*f*

Voice rehabilitation, 556-557
Voiding, 1140
    double voiding, 1184-1185
    prompted, 1183t
    scheduled regimens, 1183, 1183t
    timed, 1183t
Voiding cystourethrogram, 1149t
Voiding dysfunction, 1185t
Voiding pressure flow study, 1150t
Volatile liquids, 369t
Volkmann's ischemic contracture, 1650
Vollman Prone Positioner, 1817f
Volmax (albuterol), 619t
Voltaren (diclofenac)
    for arthritis and connective tissue disorders, 1698t
    and gastritis, 1013
    for osteoarthritis, 1697
    photosensitivity, 461t
Volume ventilation, 1760
Volume-assured pressure ventilation, 1762
Volu-pressure trauma
    in acute respiratory distress syndrome, 1816
    in positive pressure ventilation, 1764
Volutrauma, 1764
Vomiting, 990-991. See also Nausea and vomiting
    in increased ICP, 1472
    stimuli involved in, 991, 991f
    with tube feedings, 964t
von Willebrand disease, 707-710, 708t
    clinical manifestations of, 707-708
    collaborative care for, 708-709
    complications of, 707-708
    diagnostic studies, 708
Vontrol (diphenidol), 992t
Voriconazole (Vfend), 576
V_t. See Tidal volume
Vulva
    age-related changes in, 1331t
    conditions of, **1393-1395**
        clinical manifestations of, 1393-1394
        collaborative care for, 1394
        etiology and pathophysiology of, 1393
        nursing management of, **1394-1395**
Vulvar cancer, 1404
Vulvar discharge, 1335t
Vulvar erythema, 1335t
Vulvar growths, 1335t
Vulvectomy
    acute intervention related to, 1406-1407
    description of, 1404t
    radical, 1404t
    simple, 1404t
Vulvovaginal candidiasis, 1394t
Vumon (teniposide), 287t
Vurow's solution (aluminum salts), 1375
VVC. See Vulvovaginal candidiasis
VX (O-ethyl S-[2-diisopropylaminoethyl] methylphosphonothiolate), 1840t
Vytorin (ezetimibe/simvastatin), 794

W
Waist circumference, 974, 975t
    classification of overweight and obesity by, 974, 975t
    diagnostic criteria for metabolic syndrome, 987t

Waist-to-hip ratio, 974
Walking. See also Ambulation
    postoperative, 387
    6-minute walk test, 753t
Warfarin (Coumadin)
    for DVT prophylaxis, 914
    for DVT treatment, 914-915
    and gastritis, 1013
    for pulmonary embolism, 600
    for stroke, 1512
Warts, 469
    genital, **1375-1379,** 1376f
    plantar, 468t
Wasps, 470t
Waste product accumulation
    in acute renal failure, 1200
    in chronic kidney disease, 1206
Wasting, 253t
Watchful waiting, 1424
Water aspiration, 1832, 1833f
Water balance
    effects on cell size, 318, 318f
    regulation of, **319-321**
        adrenal cortical, 320
        cardiac, 320-321
        gastrointestinal, 321
        hypothalamic, 319
        pituitary, 319
        renal, 320
Water content, 315, 315f
Water deprivation test, 1248t
Water imbalances
    deficit, 318, 319
    excess, 319
    insensible loss, 321
    in positive pressure ventilation, 1765
Water intoxication, 500
Water restriction, 1212
Water retention, 765
Water therapy, 1545, 1546f
Water-hammer pulse, 881
Waterhouse-Friderichsen syndrome, 1494
Water-seal drainage, 591t-592t
Water-soluble hormones, 1235
Weakness, 676t
Website evaluation criteria, 63
Wedge resection, 593t
Weight
    assessment of, 1245, 1247t
    changes in chronic HF, 826
    daily, 323
    health impact of maintaining, 973b
Weight reduction
    1200-calorie-restricted diet, 978t
    for hypertension, 768-770
    interventions for, 1257b
    for obesity, 977-978
    psychologic interventions for, 981b
    strategies for, 977
Weight training, vaginal, 1183t
Weight-bearing ambulation, 1648
Weight-bearing exercise, 1655b
WelChol (colesevelam), 794, 795t
Wellcovorin (leucovorin), 1067
Wenckebach heart block, 849t, 853
Wernicke's area, 1445
Wernicke's encephalopathy, 177-178
West Nile virus, 245
    diseases caused by, 244t
    related diseases, 245t
Western coral snakes, 1835, 1835f
Wet chest drainage systems, 591t
Wet desquamation, 299, 299f
Wet dressings, 477
Wet mounts, 1339t, 1394

Wet suction system, 591t
Wheal-and-flare reaction, 225-226
Wheals, 455t
Wheezing, 519, 519t, 524, 525t, 1877
Whipple procedure, 1126, 1126f
Whispered pectoriloquy, 525t
Whitaker study, 1150t
White blood cell count, 678, 678t
    cerebrospinal fluid analysis, 1864t
    effects of aging on, 672t
    laboratory values, 1860t
White blood cell differential, 678, 678t, 1860t
White blood cell studies, 678
White blood cells, 666, 666f. See also Leukocytes
    margination, diapedesis, and chemotaxis of, 194, 194f
White clot syndrome, 702
"White coat" hypertension, 768
"White patch," 1001
Whiteout or white lung, 1815, 1815f
Whitmore-Jewett staging classification of prostate cancer, 1423, 1423t
Whole blood chemistries, 1855t-1858t
Willis, circle of, 1452f, 1504, 1504f
Wilson's disease, 1100
WinGel, 1020t
Withdrawal
    acute intervention for, 186-187
    alcohol
        acute intervention for, 186
        clinical manifestations and suggested drug treatment of, 178, 178t
        nursing care plan for patient in, 183b-184b
        onset of, 185t
    alcohol withdrawal delirium, 177
    definition of, 166t
    from depressants, 186-187
    from opioids, 145, 146t, 185t
    from stimulants, 187
Withdrawing treatment, 1230b
Withholding treatment, 1492b
Women
    battered, 1838
    gonorrhea in, 1367-1368, 1368f
    older adult, 69
Wood's lamp, 458t
Workplace violence, 1838
Wound care
    for burns, 493t
        acute phase, 501-502
        emergent phase, 496-498
    goals of, 501
    home health care, 89, 89f, 90t
    negative-pressure therapy, 205
    open method, 497
    prophylaxis against tetanus, 1828t
    red-yellow-black concept of, 200, 200t
    types of dressings, 205t
    vacuum-assisted closure, 205
Wound dehiscence, 392
Wound healing
    factors delaying, 200, 201t
    nursing and collaborative management of, **203-206**
    nursing assessment of, 203
    nursing implementation for, 203-206
    patient teaching about, 206
    by primary intention, 198-199
    process of, **197-202**
    resources, 212
    risk factors, 202

Wound healing (Continued)
    by secondary intention, 199
    by tertiary intention, 199
    types of, 198, 199f
Wound VAC, 1670
Woun'Dres, 205t
Wounds
    black, 200, 200t, 204-205
    classification of, 199-200, 200f
    contraction of, 201
    measurement of, 203, 204f
    postoperative infection in, 392
    psychologic implications of, 206
    red, 200, 200t, 204
    surgical, **392-393**
    yellow, 200, 200t, 204
Wright's and Giemsa's stain, 458t
Wrists
    carpal tunnel syndrome, 1633, 1633f
    physical examination of, 49t
Writing specific learning objectives, 60
Writing teaching materials, 62
Written materials, 62
Written measurement tools, 64
Wytensin (guanabenz), 773t

X
X Stop, 1682
Xalatan (latanoprost), 435t
Xanax (alprazolam)
    effects of use, 169t
    withdrawal from, 179
Xeloda (capecitabine)
    for breast cancer, 1355
    classification of, 287t
    for colorectal cancer, 1067
    drug alert, 1067
    method of administration, 288t
    for pancreatic cancer, 1126
Xenical (orlistat), 981
Xenografts, 498t
Xeroform, 205t
Xerostomia, 932
    in radiation therapy of, 555
    in Sjögren syndrome, 1726
Xigris (drotrecogin alpha), 1787t, 1789
X-linked disorders, 215
X-linked recessive disorders, 215, 216t
Xolair (omalizumab), 620
    for asthma, 617t, 618t
    for COPD, 618t
Xopenex (levalbuterol), 619t
X-rays, **1624**
    barium enema, 941f, 941t
    barium swallow, 941t
    chest x-ray, 753t, 756, 756f
    dual-energy absorptiometry, 1625t
    standard, 1625t
    upper gastrointestinal series, 940, 941t
Xylocaine (lidocaine)
    classification of, 856t
    for genital herpes, 1375
    in thoracentesis, 530

Y
Yankauer (tonsil-tip) suction catheter, 1759
Yellow wounds, 200, 200t, 204
Yin/yang, 96, 98f
Yoga, 95, 96f, 98t, 104f, 121b
Young-old adults, 67

Z

Zafirlukast (Accolate)
  for allergic rhinitis and sinusitis, 537t
  for asthma and COPD, 619t, 620
  food/nutrient interactions, 954t
Zanaflex (tizanidine)
  for multiple sclerosis, 1545t
  for pain, 139
Zanamivir (Relenza)
  for influenza, 540
  for pneumonia, 566
Zanosar (streptozocin), 287t
Zantac (ranitidine)
  for acute gastritis, 1014
  for acute pancreatitis, 1121t
  for burns, 499t
  for cirrhosis, 1110t
  for gastroesophageal reflux disease, 1005-1006, 1006t
  for gastrointestinal bleeding, 998t
  for peptic ulcer disease, 1019t
  preoperative, 355t
  for variceal bleeding, 1108
Zarontin (ethosuximide), 1536, 1538t
Zaroxolyn (metolazone), 773t
ZDV (zidovudine), 258t
Zebeta (bisoprolol), 774t
Zegerid (omeprazole), 1006

Zelnorm (tegaserod)
  for chronic constipation, 1041
  for constipation, 1042t
  for irritable bowel syndrome, 1047
Zemplar (paricalcitol), 1210
Zemuron (rocuronium), 370t
Zenapax (daclizumab), 239t, 240
Zenker's diverticulum, 1011, 1012f
Zerit (stavudine), 258t
Zeroing, 1739
Zestoretic (lisinopril/hydrochlorothiazide), 777t
Zestril (lisinopril)
  for diabetes mellitus, 1285
  effects on lower urinary tract function, 1180t
  for hypertension, 776t
Zetia (ezetimibe), 794, 795t
Zevalin (ibritumomab tiuxetan/yttrium-90), 303t, 727
Ziac (bisoprolol/hydrochlorothiazide), 777t
Ziagen (abacavir), 258t
Ziconotide (Prialt), 141-142
Zidovudine (AZT, ZDV, Retrovir)
  adverse effects of, 258t
  lamivudine, zidovudine, and abacavir (Trizivir), 258t
  lamivudine and zidovudine (Combivir), 258t
Zileuton (Zyflo), 620
  for allergic rhinitis and sinusitis, 537t
  for asthma and COPD, 619t

Zinc, 539b
  for burns, 499t
  for inflammatory bowel disease, 1055t
  laboratory values, 1858t
Zinc deficiency, 201t
Zinc supplements, 954t
Zithromax (azithromycin)
  for cervicitis, 1394t
  for chlamydial infections, 1373
  for gonorrhea, 1368
  photosensitivity, 461t
  for rheumatic fever, 878
Zocor (simvastatin), 793, 794, 795t
Zofran (ondansetron)
  as adjunct to general anesthesia, 370t
  for alcohol treatment, 178
  for nausea and vomiting, 297, 992, 992t
  preoperative, 355t
Zoladex (goserelin), 1426, 1426t
Zoledronic acid (Zometa), 728
Zollinger-Ellison syndrome, 1017
Zolmitriptan (Zomig), 1530
Zoloft (sertraline)
  for Alzheimer's disease, 1569, 1569t
  for pain, 139
  for premenstrual syndrome, 1386
Zolpidem (Ambien)
  for Alzheimer's disease, 1569t
  for fibromyalgia syndrome, 1728
Zometa (zoledronic acid), 728
Zomig (zolmitriptan), 1530

Zone diet, 979t
Zonisamide (Zonegran)
  gerontologic considerations for, 1538
  for seizures, 1536, 1538t
Zostrix (capsaicin)
  for arthritis and connective tissue disorders, 1698t
  local, 139t
  for osteoarthritis, 1696
  for pain, 141
Zovirax (acyclovir)
  for encephalitis, 1498
  for genital herpes, 1375
  for keratitis, 423
Zyban (bupropion)
  for smoking cessation, 171t
  for tobacco cessation, 170
Zydone (hydrocodone), 137t
Zyflo (zileuton), 620
  for allergic rhinitis and sinusitis, 537t
  for asthma and COPD, 619t
Zygomatic arch fracture, 1657t
Zyloprim (allopurinol)
  blood glucose level effects, 1267t
  for multiple myeloma, 729
Zyplast (collagen), 479t
Zyprexa (olanzapine)
  for Alzheimer's disease, 1551-1552, 1569t
  for delirium, 1578
Zyrtec (cetirizine)
  for allergic rhinitis and sinusitis, 538t
  for dermatologic problems, 475

Note: Disorder names are in **bold face.** Page numbers in **bold face** indicate main discussions. Page numbers followed by *f, t, b,* or *n* indicate figures, tables, boxed material, or notes, respectively.

Electronic Resources
Companion CD and Evolve

The following electronic resources are available to supplement and reinforce the content discussed in the textbook.

- Animations
- Audio and Video Clips
- Comprehensive and Chapter Glossaries with Audio Pronunciations
- Concept Map Creator
- Content Updates
- Customizable Nursing Care Plans
- Electronic Calculators
- Interactive Case Studies with Animations and Exercises
- Key Points (Printable and CD/MP3 Download)
- Key Term Flash Cards
- Patient and Family Instruction Guides in English and Spanish
- Physical Examination Videos
- Stress-Busting Kit for Nursing Students
- Additional Supplemental Information

Following is a complete listing of the specific resources available for each section and chapter in the book.

◉ = available on Companion CD
↪ = available on Evolve website

Section 1: Concepts in Nursing Practice (Chapters 1-12)
◉ NCLEX Examination Review Questions (Section 1)

Chapter 1
Nursing Practice Today
◉ Chapter Glossary with Audio Pronunciations
↪ Key Points (Printable and CD/MP3 Download)
↪ Key Term Flash Cards
↪ Nursing Interventions Classification (NIC): Complete Listing
↪ Nursing Outcomes Classification (NOC): Complete Listing
↪ WebLinks

Chapter 2
Health Disparities
◉ Chapter Glossary with Audio Pronunciations
↪ Key Points (Printable and CD/MP3 Download)
↪ Key Term Flash Cards
↪ WebLinks

Chapter 3
Culturally Competent Care
◉ Chapter Glossary with Audio Pronunciations
↪ Key Points (Printable and CD/MP3 Download)
↪ Key Term Flash Cards
↪ WebLinks

Chapter 4
Health History and Physical Examination
◉ Chapter Glossary with Audio Pronunciations
↪ Key Points (Printable and CD/MP3 Download)
↪ Key Term Flash Cards
↪ Physical Examination Video
↪ WebLinks

Chapter 5
Patient and Family Teaching
◉ Chapter Glossary with Audio Pronunciations
↪ Key Points (Printable and CD/MP3 Download)
↪ Key Term Flash Cards
↪ WebLinks

Chapter 6
Older Adults
◉ Chapter Glossary with Audio Pronunciations
↪ Key Points (Printable and CD/MP3 Download)
↪ Key Term Flash Cards
↪ WebLinks

Chapter 7
Community-Based Nursing and Home Care
◉ Chapter Glossary with Audio Pronunciations
↪ Key Points (Printable and CD/MP3 Download)
↪ Key Term Flash Cards
↪ WebLinks

Chapter 8
Complementary and Alternative Therapies
◉ Chapter Glossary with Audio Pronunciations
↪ Key Points (Printable and CD/MP3 Download)
↪ Key Term Flash Cards
◉ Stress-Busting Kit for Nursing Students: Take a Yoga Break
↪ WebLinks

Chapter 9
Stress and Stress Management
↪ Audio Lecture: *Stress*
◉ Chapter Glossary with Audio Pronunciations
↪ Key Points (Printable and CD/MP3 Download)
↪ Key Term Flash Cards
◉ Stress-Busting Kit for Nursing Students: Take a Yoga Break
↪ WebLinks

Chapter 10
Pain
◉ Chapter Glossary with Audio Pronunciations
◉ Interactive Case Study: *Pain*
↪ Key Points (Printable and CD/MP3 Download)
↪ Key Term Flash Cards
↪ WebLinks

Chapter 11
End-of-Life and Palliative Care
◉ Chapter Glossary with Audio Pronunciations
↪ Key Points (Printable and CD/MP3 Download)
↪ Key Term Flash Cards
↪ WebLinks

Chapter 12
Addictive Behaviors
◉ Chapter Glossary with Audio Pronunciations
↪ Customizable Nursing Care Plan: *Alcohol Withdrawal*
↪ Key Points (Printable and CD/MP3 Download)
↪ Key Term Flash Cards
↪ Patient and Family Instruction Guide: *Smoking and Tobacco Use Cessation*
↪ WebLinks

Section 2: Pathophysiologic Mechanisms of Disease (Chapters 13-17)
- NCLEX Examination Review Questions (Section 2)

Chapter 13
Inflammation and Wound Healing
- Chapter Glossary with Audio Pronunciations
- Customizable Nursing Care Plan: *Fever*
- Customizable Nursing Care Plan: *Pressure Ulcer*
- Interactive Case Study: *Pressure Ulcers*
- Key Points (Printable and CD/MP3 Download)
- Key Term Flash Cards
- WebLinks

Chapter 14
Genetics, Altered Immune Responses, and Transplantation
- Animation: *Function of B Cells*
- Animation: *Function of T Cytotoxic Cells*
- Chapter Glossary with Audio Pronunciations
- Key Points (Printable and CD/MP3 Download)
- Key Term Flash Cards
- WebLinks

Chapter 15
Infection and Human Immunodeficiency Virus Infection
- Chapter Glossary with Audio Pronunciations
- Interactive Case Study: *Human Immunodeficiency Syndrome and Acquired Immunodeficiency Syndrome (AIDS)*
- Key Points (Printable and CD/MP3 Download)
- Key Term Flash Cards
- Patient and Family Instruction Guide: *The Right Way to Use Antibiotics*
- Patient and Family Instruction Guide: *The Proper Use of Drug-Using Equipment*
- Patient and Family Instruction Guide: *Use of Antiretroviral Drugs*
- Patient and Family Instruction Guide: *Signs and Symptoms that HIV-Infected Patients Need to Report*
- WebLinks

Chapter 16
Cancer
- Chapter Glossary with Audio Pronunciations
- Key Points (Printable and CD/MP3 Download)
- Key Term Flash Cards
- Table: *Precautions to Minimize Risks from Neutropenia*
- Table: *Neutropenic Diet*
- WebLinks

Chapter 17
Fluid, Electrolyte, and Acid-Base Imbalances
- Chapter Glossary with Audio Pronunciations
- Fluid and Electrolyte Tutorial
- Interactive Case Study: *Hyponatremia/Fluid Volume Imbalance*
- Key Points (Printable and CD/MP3 Download)
- Key Term Flash Cards
- WebLinks

Section 3: Perioperative Care (Chapters 18-20)
- NCLEX Examination Review Questions (Section 3)

Chapter 18
Nursing Management: Preoperative Care
- Chapter Glossary with Audio Pronunciations
- Key Points (Printable and CD/MP3 Download)
- Key Term Flash Cards
- WebLinks

Chapter 19
Nursing Management: Intraoperative Care
- Chapter Glossary with Audio Pronunciations
- Key Points (Printable and CD/MP3 Download)
- Key Term Flash Cards
- WebLinks

Chapter 20
Nursing Management: Postoperative Care
- Chapter Glossary with Audio Pronunciations
- Customizable Nursing Care Plan: *Postoperative Patient*
- Interactive Case Study: *Surgery*
- Key Points (Printable and CD/MP3 Download)
- Key Term Flash Cards
- WebLinks

Section 4: Problems Related to Altered Sensory Input (Chapters 21-25)
- NCLEX Examination Review Questions (Secction 4)

Chapter 21
Nursing Assessment: Visual and Auditory Systems
- Animation: *Ears: Weber Test*
- Chapter Glossary with Audio Pronunciations
- Key Points (Printable and CD/MP3 Download)
- Key Term Flash Cards
- Physical Examination Video Clips: *Eyes*
- Physical Examination Video Clips: *Ears*
- Video Clip: *Evaluation: Central Vision and Visual Acuity*
- Video Clip: *Evaluation: Pupil Responses, Direct and Consensual*
- Video Clip: *Inspection and Palpation: External Ear*
- Video Clip: *Inspection and Palpation: External Eye*
- Video Clip: *Inspection: Ear Canal*
- WebLinks

Chapter 22
Nursing Management: Visual and Auditory Problems
- Case Study Animation: *Visual Pathway*
- Chapter Glossary with Audio Pronunciations
- Customizable Nursing Care Plan: *Patient After Eye Surgery*
- Interactive Case Study: *Cataract Surgery*
- Figure: *Refractive Errors*
- Key Points (Printable and CD/MP3 Download)
- Key Term Flash Cards
- WebLinks

Chapter 23
Nursing Assessment: Integumentary System
- Chapter Glossary with Audio Pronunciations
- Key Points (Printable and CD/MP3 Download)
- Key Term Flash Cards
- Physical Examination Video Clips: *Head and Face*
- Physical Examination Video Clips: *Back and Posterior Chest*
- Physical Examination Video Clips: *Feet, Legs, and Hips*
- WebLinks

Chapter 24
Nursing Management: Integumentary Problems
- Chapter Glossary with Audio Pronunciations
- Customizable Nursing Care Plan: *Chronic Skin Lesions*
- Key Points (Printable and CD/MP3 Download)
- Key Term Flash Cards
- WebLinks

Chapter 25
Nursing Management: Burns
- Chapter Glossary with Audio Pronunciations
- Customizable Nursing Care Plan: *Burn Patient*
- Interactive Case Study: *Burns*
- Key Points (Printable and CD/MP3 Download)
- Key Term Flash Cards
- WebLinks

Section 5: Problems of Oxygenation: Ventilation (Chapters 26-29)
- NCLEX Examination Review Questions (Section 5)

Chapter 26
Nursing Assessment: Respiratory System
- Animation: *Patterns of Respiration*
- Animation: *Percussion Tones throughout the Chest*
- Animation: *Pulmonary Circulation*
- Audio Clip: *Bronchial Breath Sounds*
- Audio Clip: *Bronchovesicular Breath Sounds*
- Audio Clip: *High Pitched Crackles*
- Audio Clip: *High Pitched Wheeze*
- Audio Clip: *Low Pitched Crackles*
- Audio Clip: *Low Pitched Wheeze*
- Audio Clip: *Pleural Friction Rub*
- Audio Clip: *Stridor*
- Audio Clip: *Vesicular Breath Sounds*
- Chapter Glossary with Audio Pronunciations
- Key Points (Printable and CD/MP3 Download)
- Key Term Flash Cards
- Physical Examination Video Clips: *Anterior Chest, Lungs, and Heart*
- Physical Examination Video Clips: *Lungs*
- Video Clip: *Inspection and Palpation: Breathing and Respiratory Excursion, Anterior Chest*
- Video Clip: *Inspection and Palpation: Respirations, Respiratory Excursion, and Tactile Fremitus, Posterior Chest*
- Video Clip: *Inspection and Percussion: Diaphragmatic Excursion*
- Video Clip: *Inspection: Nose*
- Video Clip: *Palpation: Tactile Fremitus, Posterior Chest*
- Video Clip: *Percussion: Anterior Thorax*
- WebLinks

Chapter 27
Nursing Management: Upper Respiratory Problems
- Animation: *Anatomic Location of Sinuses*
- Chapter Glossary with Audio Pronunciations
- Customizable Nursing Care Plan: *Total Laryngectomy and/or Radical Neck Surgery*
- Customizable Nursing Care Plan: *Tracheostomy*
- Interactive Case Study: *Head and Neck Cancer/Laryngectomy with Tracheostomy*
- Key Points (Printable and CD/MP3 Download)
- Key Term Flash Cards
- Patient and Family Instruction Guide: *Acute or Chronic Sinusitis*
- Patient and Family Instruction Guide: *How to Reduce Symptoms of Allergic Rhinitis*
- WebLinks

Chapter 28
Nursing Management: Lower Respiratory Problems
- Case Study Animation: *Pulmonary Embolus*
- Chapter Glossary with Audio Pronunciations
- Customizable Nursing Care Plan: *Pneumonia*
- Customizable Nursing Care Plan: *Thoracotomy*
- Interactive Case Study: *Lung Cancer*
- Interactive Case Study: *Pulmonary Embolism*
- Key Points (Printable and CD/MP3 Download)
- Key Term Flash Cards
- WebLinks

Chapter 29
Nursing Management: Obstructive Pulmonary Diseases
- Asthma Action Plan (Spanish)
- Audio Lecture: *Asthma*
- Case Study Animation: *Asthma*
- Case Study Animation: *Simple Pneumothorax and Tension Pneumothorax*
- Chapter Glossary with Audio Pronunciations
- Customizable Nursing Care Plan: *Asthma*
- Customizable Nursing Care Plan: *Chronic Obstructive Pulmonary Disease*
- Interactive Case Study: *Asthma*
- Interactive Case Study: *Chronic Obstructive Pulmonary Disease*
- Interactive Case Study: *Cystic Fibrosis*
- Key Points (Printable and CD/MP3 Download)
- Key Term Flash Cards
- Patient and Family Instruction Guide: *Home Oxygen Use*
- Patient and Family Instruction Guide: *How to Use a Dry Powder Inhaler*
- Patient and Family Instruction Guide: *How to Use Your Peak Flow Meter*
- WebLinks

Section 6: Problems of Oxygenation: Transport (Chapters 30-31)
- NCLEX Examination Review Questions (Section 6)

Chapter 30
Nursing Assessment: Hematologic System
- Chapter Glossary with Audio Pronunciations
- Key Points (Printable and CD/MP3 Download)
- Key Term Flash Cards
- Physical Examination Video Clips: *Precordium and Jugular Veins*
- Physical Examination Video Clips: *Neck*
- Physical Examination Video Clips: *Upper Extremities*
- Physical Examination Video Clips: *Anterior Chest*
- Physical Examination Video Clips: *Abdominal Reflexes, Abdominal Muscles, and Inguinal Area*
- WebLinks

Chapter 31
Nursing Management: Hematologic Problems
- Case Study Animation: *Differentiation of Blood Cells*
- Case Study Animation: *Sickle Cell Anemia*
- Chapter Glossary with Audio Pronunciations
- Customizable Nursing Care Plan: *Anemia*
- Customizable Nursing Care Plan: *Neutropenia*
- Customizable Nursing Care Plan: *Thrombocytopenia*
- Interactive Case Study: *Chronic Myelogenous Leukemia*
- Interactive Case Study: *Sickle Cell Anemia*
- Key Points (Printable and CD/MP3 Download)
- Key Term Flash Cards
- WebLinks

Section 7: Problems of Oxygenation: Perfusion (Chapters 32-38)
- NCLEX Examination Review Questions (Section 7)

Chapter 32
Nursing Assessment: Cardiovascular System
- Animation: *Auscultation of Heart Valves*
- Animation: *Blood Flow: Circulatory System*
- Animation: *Cardiac Cycle During Systole and Diastole*
- Animation: *Pulse Variations*
- Audio Clip: *Diastolic Murmur*
- Audio Clip: *Fourth Heart Sound (S_4)*
- Audio Clip: *Murmurs: Blowing, Harsh or Rough, and Rumble*
- Audio Clip: *Murmurs: High, Medium, and Low*
- Audio Clip: *S_1 at Various Locations*
- Audio Clip: *S_2 at Various Locations*
- Audio Clip: *Single S_1*
- Audio Clip: *Single S_2*
- Audio Clip: *Systolic Murmur*
- Audio Clip: *Third Heart Sound (S_3)*
- Chapter Glossary with Audio Pronunciations
- Key Points (Printable and CD/MP3 Download)
- Key Term Flash Cards
- Physical Examination Video Clips: *Neck*
- Physical Examination Video Clips: *Upper Extremities*
- Physical Examination Video Clips: *Anterior Chest, Lungs, and Heart*
- Physical Examination Video Clips: *Precordium and Jugular Veins*
- Physical Examination Video Clips: *Breasts and Heart*
- Video Clip: *Auscultation: Cardiac, with Bell*
- Video Clip: *Auscultation: Cardiac, with Diaphragm*
- Video Clip: *Auscultation: Cardiac, with Diaphragm and Bell*

- Video Clip: *Auscultation: Carotid Artery*
- Video Clip: *Inspection and Palpation: Cardiac Ausculatory Landmarks*
- Video Clip: *Inspection and Palpation: Cardiac, Anterior Chest*
- Video Clip: *Inspection and Palpation: Pulses, Lower Extremities*
- WebLinks

Chapter 33
Nursing Management: Hypertension
- Case Study Animation: *Pulmonary Hypertension*
- Chapter Glossary with Audio Pronunciations
- Interactive Case Study: *Hypertension*
- Key Points (Printable and CD/MP3 Download)
- Key Term Flash Cards
- WebLinks

Chapter 34
Nursing Management: Coronary Artery Disease and Acute Coronary Syndrome
- Audio Lecture: *Risk Factors for Coronary Artery Disease*
- Case Study Animation: *Coronary Artery Bypass Grafting*
- Case Study Animation: *Acute Myocardial Infarction*
- Chapter Glossary with Audio Pronunciations
- Customizable Nursing Care Plan: *Acute Coronary Syndrome*
- Interactive Case Study: *Myocardial Infarction*
- Key Points (Printable and CD/MP3 Download)
- Key Term Flash Cards
- Patient and Family Instruction Guide: *Decreasing Risk Factors for Coronary Artery Disease*
- Patient and Family Instruction Guide: *FITT Physical Activity Guidelines After Acute Coronary Syndrome*
- WebLinks

Chapter 35
Nursing Management: Heart Failure
- Chapter Glossary with Audio Pronunciations
- Customizable Nursing Care Plan: *Heart Failure*
- Interactive Case Study: *Heart Failure*
- Key Points (Printable and CD/MP3 Download)
- Key Term Flash Cards
- Patient and Family Instruction Guide: *Heart Failure*
- WebLinks

Chapter 36
Nursing Management: Dysrhythmias
- Algorithms for Treatment of Dysrhythmias
- Case Study Animation: *Atrial Fibrillation*
- Chapter Glossary with Audio Pronunciations
- Interactive Case Study: *Atrial Fibrillation*
- Key Points (Printable and CD/MP3 Download)
- Key Term Flash Cards
- WebLinks

Chapter 37
Nursing Management: Inflammatory and Structural Heart Disorders
- Audio Clip: *Pericardial Friction Rub*
- Chapter Glossary with Audio Pronunciations
- Customizable Nursing Care Plan: *Infective Endocarditis*
- Customizable Nursing Care Plan: *Valvular Heart Disease*
- Interactive Case Study: *Rheumatic Fever and Heart Disease*
- Key Points (Printable and CD/MP3 Download)
- Key Term Flash Cards
- WebLinks

Chapter 38
Nursing Management: Vascular Disorders
- Case Study Animation: *Abdominal Aortic Aneurysm*
- Chapter Glossary with Audio Pronunciations
- Customizable Nursing Care Plan: Peripheral Arterial Disease of the Lower Extremities
- Customizable Nursing Care Plan: Surgical Repair of the Aorta
- Interactive Case Study: *Abdominal Aortic Aneurysm*

- Interactive Case Study: *Chronic Peripheral Arterial Disease*
- Key Points (Printable and CD/MP3 Download)
- Key Term Flash Cards
- Patient and Family Instruction Guide: *Anticoagulation Therapy*
- WebLinks

Section 8: Problems of Ingestion, Digestion, Absorption, and Elimination (Chapters 39-44)
- **NCLEX Examination Review Questions (Section 8)**

Chapter 39
Nursing Assessment: Gastrointestinal System
- Animation: *Rectal Examination*
- Chapter Glossary with Audio Pronunciations
- Key Points (Printable and CD/MP3 Download)
- Key Term Flash Cards
- Physical Examination Video Clips: *Abdomen: Inspection, Auscultation, and Percussion*
- Physical Examination Video Clips: *Abdomen: Palpation*
- Video Clip: *Auscultation: Abdomen, Bowel Sounds*
- Video Clip: *Palpation: Abdomen, Superficial and Deep*
- Video Clip: *Percussion: Abdomen*
- Video Clip: *Percussion: Liver*
- Video Clip: *Percussion: Spleen*
- WebLinks

Chapter 40
Nursing Management: Nutritional Problems
- Chapter Glossary with Audio Pronunciations
- Customizable Nursing Care Plan: *Enteral Nutrition*
- Customizable Nursing Care Plan: *Parenteral Nutrition*
- Key Points (Printable and CD/MP3 Download)
- Key Term Flash Cards
- Table: Nutritional Therapy: *High-Calorie, High-Protein Diet*
- WebLinks

Chapter 41
Nursing Management: Obesity
- Chapter Glossary with Audio Pronunciations
- Interactive Case Study: *Obese Patient*
- Key Points (Printable and CD/MP3 Download)
- Key Term Flash Cards
- Table: *Nutritional therapy: 1200-Calorie-Restricted Weight-Reducion Diet*
- WebLinks

Chapter 42
Nursing Management: Upper Gastrointestinal Problems
- Case Study Animation: *Duodenal Ulcer: Pathophysiology and Symptoms*
- Chapter Glossary with Audio Pronunciations
- Customizable Nursing Care Plan: *Nausea and Vomiting*
- Customizable Nursing Care Plan: *Peptic Ulcer Disease*
- Interactive Case Study: *Oral Cancer*
- Interactive Case Study: *Peptic Ulcer Disease*
- Key Points (Printable and CD/MP3 Download)
- Key Term Flash Cards
- WebLinks

Chapter 43
Nursing Management: Lower Gastrointestinal Problems
- Audio Lecture: *Inflammatory Bowel Disease*
- Audio Lecture: *Irritable Bowel Syndrome*
- Chapter Glossary with Audio Pronunciations
- Customizable Nursing Care Plan: *Acute Infectious Diarrhea*
- Customizable Nursing Care Plan: *Colostomy/Ileostomy*
- Customizable Nursing Care Plan: *Inflammatory Bowel Disease*
- Customizable Nursing Care Plan: *Laparotomy*
- Interactive Case Study: *Ulcerative Colitis*
- Key Points (Printable and CD/MP3 Download)
- Key Term Flash Cards
- Patient and Family Instruction Guide: *Colostomy Irrigation*

- Patient and Family Instruction Guide: *Managing Constipation*
- Figure: *Intestinal Tubes*
- WebLinks

Chapter 44
Nursing Management: Liver, Pancreas, and Biliary Tract Problems
- Case Study Animation: *Laparoscopic Cholecystectomy*
- Case Study Animation: *Cholecystitis: Pathophysiology and Symptoms*
- Chapter Glossary with Audio Pronunciations
- Customizable Nursing Care Plan: *Acute Viral Hepatitis*
- Customizable Nursing Care Plan: *Cirrhosis*
- Customizable Nursing Care Plan: *Acute Pancreatitis*
- Interactive Case Study: *Acute Pancreatitis*
- Interactive Case Study: *Cholelithiasis/Cholecystitis*
- Interactive Case Study: *Hepatitis*
- Interactive Case Study: *Postnecrotic Cirrhosis*
- Key Points (Printable and CD/MP3 Download)
- Key Term Flash Cards
- WebLinks

Section 9: Problems of Urinary Function (Chapters 45-47)
- NCLEX Examination Review Questions (Section 9)

Chapter 45
Nursing Assessment: Urinary System
- Chapter Glossary with Audio Pronunciations
- Key Points (Printable and CD/MP3 Download)
- Key Term Flash Cards
- Physical Examination Video Clips: *Abdomen: Inspection, Auscultation, and Percussion*
- Physical Examination Video Clips: *Abdomen: Palpation*
- WebLinks

Chapter 46
Nursing Management: Renal and Urologic Problems
- Case Study Animation: *Nephrostomy*
- Chapter Glossary with Audio Pronunciations
- Customizable Nursing Care Plan: *Acute Renal Lithiasis*
- Customizable Nursing Care Plan: *Ileal Conduit*
- Customizable Nursing Care Plan: *Urinary Tract Infection*
- Interactive Case Study: *Bladder Cancer with Urinary Diversion*
- Interactive Case Study: *Glomerulonephritis*
- Key Points (Printable and CD/MP3 Download)
- Key Term Flash Cards
- Patient and Family Instruction Guide: *Changing Your Ileal Conduit Appliances*
- Patient and Family Instruction Guide: *Urinary Tract Infection*
- WebLinks

Chapter 47
Nursing Management: Acute Renal Failure and Chronic Kidney Disease
- Chapter Glossary with Audio Pronunciations
- Customizable Nursing Care Plan: *Chronic Kidney Disease*
- Interactive Case Study: *Kidney Transplant*
- Key Points (Printable and CD/MP3 Download)
- Key Term Flash Cards
- WebLinks

Section 10: Problems Related to Regulatory and Reproductive Mechanisms (Chapters 48-55)
- NCLEX Examination Review Questions (Section 10)

Chapter 48
Nursing Assessment: Endocrine System
- Chapter Glossary with Audio Pronunciations
- Key Points (Printable and CD/MP3 Download)
- Key Term Flash Cards
- Physical Examination Video Clips: *Abdomen: Inspection, Auscultation, and Percussion*
- Physical Examination Video Clips: *Abdomen: Palpation*
- WebLinks

Chapter 49
Nursing Management: Diabetes Mellitus
- Case Study Animation: *Insulin Function*
- Chapter Glossary with Audio Pronunciations
- Customizable Nursing Care Plan: *Diabetes Mellitus*
- Interactive Case Study: *Diabetes Ketoacidosis*
- Interactive Case Study: *Type 2 Diabetes Mellitus*
- Key Points (Printable and CD/MP3 Download)
- Key Term Flash Cards
- Patient and Family Instruction Guide: *Exercise Guidelines for Patients with Diabetes Mellitus*
- Patient and Family Instruction Guide: *Foot Care for Patients with Diabetes or Peripheral Vascular Problems*
- Patient and Family Instruction Guide: *Insulin Administration*
- Patient and Family Instruction Guide: *Management of Diabetes Mellitus*
- Patient and Family Instruction Guide: *Self-Monitoring of Blood Glucose (SMGB)*
- WebLinks

Chapter 50
Nursing Management: Endocrine Problems
- Case Study Animation: *Adrenal Function*
- Case Study Animation: *Thyroid Gland, Hormone Release*
- Chapter Glossary with Audio Pronunciations
- Customizable Nursing Care Plan: *Cushing Syndrome*
- Customizable Nursing Care Plan: *Hyperthyroidism*
- Customizable Nursing Care Plan: *Hypothyroidism*
- Interactive Case Study: *Addison's Disease*
- Interactive Case Study: *Cushing Syndrome*
- Interactive Case Study: *Hyperthyroidism*
- Key Points (Printable and CD/MP3 Download)
- Key Term Flash Cards
- Patient and Family Instruction Guide: *Corticosteroid Therapy*
- WebLinks

Chapter 51
Nursing Assessment: Reproductive System
- Animation: *Lymphatic Drainage of Breast*
- Animation: *The Menstrual Cycle*
- Chapter Glossary with Audio Pronunciations
- Key Points (Printable and CD/MP3 Download)
- Key Term Flash Cards
- Physical Examination Video Clips: *Abdominal Reflexes, Abdominal Muscles, and Inguinal Area*
- Physical Examination Video Clips: *Breasts*
- Physical Examination Video Clips: *Breasts and Heart*
- Physical Examination Video Clips: *Genitalia and Rectum (female)*
- Physical Examination Video Clips: *Rectum and Prostate Gland (male)*
- Video Clip: *Inspection and Palpation—Standing Position (Male)—1*
- Video Clip: *Inspection and Palpation—Standing Position Male)—2*
- Video Clip: *Inspection: External Genitalia (Female)*
- Video Clip: *Inspection: Female Breasts—Sitting Position*
- Video Clip: *Inspection: Speculum Examination (Female)*
- Video Clip: *Palpation: Bimanual Examination (Female)*
- Video Clip: *Palpation: Female Breasts—Supine Position*
- Video Clip: *Palpation: Inguinal Hernia Evaluation (Male)*
- WebLinks

Chapter 52
Nursing Management: Breast Disorders
- Case Study Animation: *Breast Cancer Spread*
- Chapter Glossary with Audio Pronunciations
- Customizable Nursing Care Plan: *Mastectomy or Lumpectomy*
- Interactive Case Study: *Breast Cancer*
- Key Points (Printable and CD/MP3 Download)
- Key Term Flash Cards
- WebLinks

Chapter 53
Nursing Management: Sexually Transmitted Diseases
- Chapter Glossary with Audio Pronunciations
- Key Points (Printable and CD/MP3 Download)
- Key Term Flash Cards
- WebLinks

Chapter 54
Nursing Management: Female Reproductive Problems
- Chapter Glossary with Audio Pronunciations
- Customizable Nursing Care Plan: *Abdominal Hysterectomy*
- Interactive Case Study: *Endometrial Cancer*
- Key Points (Printable and CD/MP3 Download)
- Key Term Flash Cards
- WebLinks

Chapter 55
Nursing Management: Male Reproductive Problems
- Chapter Glossary with Audio Pronunciations
- Customizable Nursing Care Plan: *Prostate Surgery*
- Interactive Case Study: *Benign Prostatic Hyperplasia (BPH)*
- Key Points (Printable and CD/MP3 Download)
- Key Term Flash Cards
- Patient and Family Instruction Guide: *Testicular Self-Examination*
- WebLinks

Section 11: Problems Related to Movement and Coordination (Chapters 56-65)
NCLEX Examination Review Questions (Section 11)

Chapter 56
Nursing Assessment: Nervous System
- Animation: *Motor Pathways and Clinical Evaluation of the Central Nervous System*
- Animation: *Reflex Arc*
- Animation: *Sensory Pathways and Clinical Evaluation of the Central Nervous System*
- Chapter Glossary with Audio Pronunciations
- Key Points (Printable and CD/MP3 Download)
- Key Term Flash Cards
- Physical Examination Video Clips: *Abdominal Reflexes, Abdominal Muscles, and Inguinal Area*
- Physical Examination Video Clips: *Ears*
- Physical Examination Video Clips: *Eyes*
- Physical Examination Video Clips: *Head and Face*
- Physical Examination Video Clips: *Neck*
- Physical Examination Video Clips: *Neurologic System: Gait and Balance*
- Physical Examination Video Clips: *Neurologic System: Motor Function and Coordination*
- Physical Examination Video Clips: *Neurologic System: Sensory Function*
- Physical Examination Video Clips: *Nose, Mouth, and Pharynx*
- Video Clip: *Evaluation: Central Vision and Visual Acuity, Cranial Nerve II—Optic Nerve*
- Video Clip: *Evaluation: Deep Tendon Reflex, Patellar Tendon*
- Video Clip: *Evaluation: Pupil Responses, Direct and Accommodation, Cranial Nerves III, IV, and VI—Oculomotor, Trochlear, and Abducens Nerves*
- Video Clip: *Evaluation: Sensory, Face, and Upper Extremities*
- Video Clip: *Evaluation: Sensory, Light Touch; Face, Upper, and Lower Extremities, Cranial Nerve V—Trigeminal Nerve*
- Video Clip: *Evaluation: Smell, Cranial Nerve I—Olfactory Nerve*
- Video Clip: *Inspection: Fine Motor Coordination, Lower Extremities*
- Video Clip: *Inspection: Fine Motor Coordination, Upper Extremities*
- WebLinks

Chapter 57
Nursing Management: Acute Intracranial Problems
- Animation: *Functional Areas of the Brain*
- Case Study Animation: *Subdural Hematoma*
- Case Study Animation: *Meningitis*
- Chapter Glossary with Audio Pronunciations
- Customizable Nursing Care Plan: *Bacterial Meningitis*
- Customizable Nursing Care Plan: *Increased Intracranial Pressure*
- Interactive Case Study: *Head Injury*
- Interactive Case Study: *Meningitis*
- Key Points (Printable and CD/MP3 Download)
- Key Term Flash Cards
- Patient and Family Instruction Guide: *Head Injury*
- WebLinks

Chapter 58
Nursing Management: Stroke
- Case Study Animation: *Blood Clot Leading to Stroke*
- Chapter Glossary with Audio Pronunciations
- Customizable Nursing Care Plan: *Stroke*
- Interactive Case Study: *Stroke*
- Key Points (Printable and CD/MP3 Download)
- Key Term Flash Cards
- Patient and Family Instruction Guide: *Warning Signs of Stroke*
- WebLinks

Chapter 59
Nursing Management: Chronic Neurologic Problems
- Case Study Animation: *Closed Reduction/Pinning of Hip Fracture*
- Case Study Animation: *Parkinson's Disease*
- Chapter Glossary with Audio Pronunciations
- Customizable Nursing Care Plan: *Headache*
- Customizable Nursing Care Plan: *Multiple Sclerosis*
- Customizable Nursing Care Plan: *Parkinson's Disease*
- Customizable Nursing Care Plan: *Seizure Disorder or Epilepsy*
- Interactive Case Study: *Parkinson's Disease and Hip Fracture*
- Interactive Case Study: *Seizures*
- Key Points (Printable and CD/MP3 Download)
- Key Term Flash Cards
- Patient and Family Instruction Guide: *Headache Management*
- WebLinks

Chapter 60
Nursing Management: Alzheimer's Disease and Dementia
- Audio Lecture: *Alzheimer's Disease*
- Case Study Animation: *Alzheimer's Disease*
- Chapter Glossary with Audio Pronunciations
- Customizable Nursing Care Plan: *Alzheimer's Disease*
- Customizable Nursing Care Plan: *Caregiver of the Patient with Alzheimer's Disease*
- Interactive Case Study: *Alzheimer's Disease*
- Key Points (Printable and CD/MP3 Download)
- Key Term Flash Cards
- Patient and Family Instruction Guide: *Early Warning Signs of Alzheimer's Disease*
- Patient and Family Instruction Guide: *Managing Alzheimer's Disease*
- WebLinks

Chapter 61
Nursing Management: Peripheral Nerve and Spinal Cord Problems
- Case Study Animation: *Spine Structure*
- Chapter Glossary with Audio Pronunciations
- Customizable Nursing Care Plan: *Spinal Cord Injury*
- Interactive Case Study: *Spinal Cord Injury*
- Key Points (Printable and CD/MP3 Download)
- Key Term Flash Cards
- Patient and Family Instruction Guide: *Autonomic Dysreflexia*
- Patient and Family Instruction Guide: *Bowel Management After Spinal Cord Injury*
- Patient and Family Instruction Guide: *Skin Care for Patient with Spinal Cord Injury*
- WebLinks